EDITION 8

Medical-Surgical Nursing

Adrianne Dill Linton, MN, PhD, RN, FAAN
Professor Emeritus and Former Chair, Department of Family and Community Health Systems
The University of Texas Health at San Antonio School of Nursing
San Antonio, Texas

Mary Ann Matteson, MSN, PhD
Professor Emeritus and Former Chair, Department of Family Nursing
The University of Texas Health at San Antonio School of Nursing
San Antonio, Texas

ELSEVIER

Elsevier
3251 Riverport Lane
St. Louis, Missouri 63043

MEDICAL-SURGICAL NURSING, EIGHTH EDITION
ISBN: 978-0-323-82671-6

Senior Content Strategist: Brandi Graham
Senior Content Development Manager: Lisa Newton
Content Development Specialist: Andrew Schubert
Publishing Services Manager: Deepthi Unni
Senior Project Manager: Umarani Natarajan
Design Direction: Renee Duenow

Printed in India

Last digit is the print number: 9 8 7 6 5 4 3 2

Dedicated to the nurses who demonstrated incredible courage and commitment to provide care during the COVID-19 pandemic.

Adrianne Dill Linton and Mary Ann Matteson

Acknowledgments

The eighth edition of *Medical-Surgical Nursing* is the product of multiple teams of amazing people. Before revisions began, chapters from the previous edition were reviewed by experienced LVN/LPN educators and content experts. The input of these individuals ensured readability, accuracy, appropriateness for the LVN/LPN student, and timeliness. Using the reviews and extensive literature searches, chapter authors crafted new manuscripts that reflect the best practices known to us as of the publication date. Once again, reviewers were invited to provide feedback on the new manuscripts.

The incredible Elsevier staff managed this entire process and then pulled all the pieces together to create this fine edition. I particularly wish to acknowledge the following individuals who each brought unique knowledge and skills to the production process and have worked to develop and carry this edition to publication with great skill and creativity. The Elsevier team included Brandi Graham, Senior Content Strategist; Lisa Newton, Senior Content Development Manager; Andrew Schubert, Content Development Specialist; Renee Duenow, Book Designer; Deepthi Unni, Production Services Manager; and Umarani Natarajan, Senior Project Manager. We also want to recognize Nancy O'Brien, Senior Content Editor (retired) who launched the initial efforts on this edition. Behind the scenes are many other individuals involved in the development of the ancillary materials.

The authors are grateful to our families for their support, encouragement, and patience as we immersed ourselves in this labor of love once again.

Contributors and Reviewers

CONTRIBUTORS

Nicole Dill, RN, MSN, FNP
Family Nurse Practitioner
Richardson, Texas Health Physicians Group
Endocrine System Introduction

Amanda Flagg, PhD, RN, MSN, EdM, ACNS, CNE
Associate Professor
School of Nursing
Middle Tennessee State University
Murfreesboro, Tennessee
Upper Digestive Tract Disorders, Lower Digestive Tract Disorders

Carl Flagg, ADN, RN
Lead Educator
PICC Infusion Care Company
Murfreesboro, Tennessee

Virginia A. Ford, RN, CRNP, MSN
Nurse Practitioner
University of Pennsylvania
Philadelphia, Pennsylvania
Hypertension, Vascular Disorders

Margit B. Gerardi
PhD, APRN, WHNP, PMHNP-BC
Director, Mental Health Nurse Practitioner Residency Program
Veterans Administration
San Antonio, Texas
Adjunct Assistant Professor, University of TX Health San Antonio School of Nursing
San Antonio Texas
Recurring Faculty
Texas Tech University School of Nursing
Lubbock, Texas

Lisa Hooter, MSN, RN, NPD-BC
Nurse Educator
Nursing Education
South Texas Veterans Health Care System
San Antonio, Texas
Diabetes and Hypoglycemia

Sherri Stevens, PhD, RN
Associate Professor
Nursing
Middle Tennessee State University
Murfreesboro, Tennessee
First Aid, Emergency, and Disaster Management

REVIEWERS

Anna Alcott, BSN, RN
Registered Nurse
Stony Brook University Nursing School
Stony Brook, New York

Kendricka Brown, RN, MSN
University of Michigan—Flint
Flint, Michigan

Argentina Fretwell
Palomar College
San Marcos, California

Samantha Hughes, BSN, RN
Student
Watts College of Nursing
Durham, North Carolina

Sarah Lalman, RN
Registered Nurse, AGNP Student
Florida International University
Miami, Florida

Almira Rezini Munda, RN
Registered Nurse
UT Southwestern Medical Center
Dallas, Texas

Desiree A. Rosario
Nursing Student
Long Island University
Brooklyn, New York

Briana VanDenHeuvel
Registered Medical Assistant
St. Mary's Medical Center
Grand Junction, Colorado

LPN Advisory Board

Nancy Bohnarczyk, MA
Adjunct Instructor
College of Mount St. Vincent
New York, New York

Nicola Contreras, BN, RN
Faculty
Galen College
San Antonio, Texas

Dolores Cotton, MSN, RN
Practical Nursing Coordinator
Meridian Technology Center
Stillwater, Oklahoma

Patricia Donovan, MSN, RN
Director of Practical Nursing and Curriculum Chair
Porter and Chester Institute
Rocky Hill, Connecticut

Nancy Haughton, MSN, RN
Practical Nursing Program Faculty
Chester County Intermediate Unit
Downingtown, Pennsylvania

Dawn Johnson, DNP, RN, Ed
Practical Nurse Educator
Reno, Nevada

Mary E. Johnson, RN, MSN
Director of Nursing
Dorsey Schools
Roseville, Michigan

Bonnie Kehm, PhD, RN
Faculty Program Director
Excelsior College
Albany, New York

Tawnya S. Lawson, MS, RN
Dean, Practical Nursing Program
Hondros College
Westerville, Ohio

Kristin Madigan, MS, RN
Nursing Faculty
Pine Technical and Community College
Pine City, Minnesota

Hana Malik, DNP, FNP-BC
Academic Director
Illinois College of Nursing
Lombard, Illinois

Mary Lee Pollard, PhD, RN, CNE
Dean, School of Nursing
Excelsior College
Albany, New York

Barbara Ratliff, MSN, RN
Program Director, Practical Nursing
Cincinnati State
Cincinnati, Ohio

Mary Ruiz-Nuve, RN, MSN
Director of Practical Nursing Program
St. Louis College of Health Careers
St. Louis, Missouri

Renee Sheehan, RN, MSN Ed
Director of Nursing, Vocational Nursing
Nursing Assistant Programs
Summit College
Colton, California

Fleur de Liza S. Tobias-Cuyco, BSc, CPhT
Dean, Director of Student Affairs, and Instructor
Preferred College of Nursing
Los Angeles, California

To the Instructor

The first seven editions of this text were designed to provide practical and vocational nursing students with accessible, comprehensive coverage of the nursing care of adults with disorders that require medical, surgical, and psychiatric management. The needs of older adults and residents of nonacute care settings received special attention.

Since the first edition of this textbook, the LVN profession has continued to evolve. Increased complexity of patient care has created a need for additional resources for LVN education.

ORGANIZATION

Unit I defines medical-surgical nursing and describes the role of the LVN/LPN in medical-surgical care. Essential knowledge and skills are explained. Ethical and legal concepts and principles of leadership and management are applied to medical-surgical care. The settings of care where medical-surgical patients are seen are described with emphasis on the role of the LVN/LPN. Attention is given to community health and community-based settings, home health, long-term care and rehabilitation facilities. **Unit II** focuses on the application of concepts from sociology and psychology that are vital in the care of medical-surgical patients. The patient's needs and the care provided must consider cultural influences and developmental stages in the context of the patient's social network (i.e., family). Major health issues at each stage of life are identified. Family stages of development and coping strategies are explored. The in-depth coverage of topics in **Unit III** provides both a foundation for understanding many disorders and a scientific basis for many aspects of nursing care. Pathological processes are described and the adaptive responses to deviations are explored. Included are concepts of health and illness; stress and coping; immunity, inflammation, and infection; fluid and electrolyte imbalances; cancer; pain; and shock. This approach avoids repetition of content such as common electrolyte imbalances that are encountered in numerous conditions.

Because LVN/LPNs are the backbone of nursing care in settings that serve older adults, **Unit IV** provides a detailed overview of the aging process and needs of the older patient as well as comprehensive coverage of four major clinical problems (falls, immobility, delirium and dementia, and incontinence). The last of the introductory units, **Unit V**, focuses on therapeutic interventions including nutrition, intravenous therapy, surgery, ostomies, complementary and alternative therapies, and palliative and hospice care. This unit creates a foundation on which the student can build when studying a variety of systems and disorders. Care of patients with specific types of cancer is addressed in later chapters. **Units VI** through **XVI** follow a systems approach to medical-surgical disorders. An introductory chapter for each system provides a thorough nursing assessment, age-related considerations, diagnostic tests and procedures, drug therapy, and other common therapeutic measures. The specific role of the LVN/LPN in data collection for focused assessments is emphasized. Common therapeutic measures are intended not to replace a fundamentals text but, instead, to provide a limited summary or review of key aspects of nursing care. The introductory systems chapters eliminate much duplication of content in each of the subsequent chapters. Introductory chapters are followed by one or more chapters that cover specific disorders requiring medical-surgical treatment. Aspects covered are pathophysiology, signs and symptoms, complications, diagnosis, and medical treatment. Nursing care is organized in the traditional nursing process format with patient problem statements, goals, and outcome criteria. Sample nursing care plans illustrate the application of the nursing process in realistic patient scenarios. **Unit XVII** consists of two chapters that address psychobiologic disorders and substance use disorders and addiction. The content on psychosocial responses to illness has been combined with earlier content in Units II and III. **Unit XIX** presents first aid, emergency care, and disaster management. This chapter has been moved to end of the text because it draws on content covered throughout the book.

KEY FEATURES

We anticipate that faculty will find *Medical-Surgical Nursing,* 8th edition to be more streamlined with less duplication of nursing fundamentals and nonnursing content. We have emphasized the application of previously learned material rather than repeating the basics.

ACCESSIBLE LANGUAGE

The text is straightforward and direct, avoiding the cumbersome third person. What's more, we have continued to improve consistency and to standardize the reading level throughout.

KEY TERMS WITH PHONETIC PRONUNCIATIONS

Complex medical, nursing, and scientific words can be tricky to understand and pronounce. A Key Terms list at the beginning of each chapter shows students how to pronounce important terms they may encounter as nurses. All phonetic pronunciations have been reviewed by a specialist in English as a Second Language (ESL). Key terms appear in color in the text and are defined.

PATIENT PROBLEMS, GOALS, AND OUTCOME CRITERIA

Nursing care is the heart of this text, which is organized according to the steps of the nursing process. For each major disorder covered, patient problems, goals, outcome criteria, and relevant interventions are presented. Faculty familiar with our textbook will note that we continue using *patient problem*, rather than NANDA nursing diagnoses. Because LVNs/LPNs do not formulate NANDA diagnoses, patient problems define issues that are more amenable to LVN/LPN identification and management. We believe this new terminology will be better understood by our student readers. A complete list of patient problem terms used in this text is provided on the inside back cover.

KEY POINTS

To succeed in the fast-paced world of health care, the nurse must be able to put it all together. Each chapter brings students a few steps closer by summarizing the most important points in a succinct and memorable way.

BOXED FEATURES CONTENT

Features described in the Student Introduction highlight important points such as pharmacology alerts ("capsules"), cultural considerations, and complementary and alternative therapies. These features emphasize and reinforce chapter content.

OTHER FEATURES

UPDATED CONTENT THROUGHOUT

Medical-Surgical Nursing, 8th edition continues the tradition of presenting innovative, accurate, and up-to-date content. Every chapter has been updated and reviewed by content and clinical experts.

REVIEW QUESTIONS

Multiple-choice, multiple-response, and short answer review questions are provided at the end of each chapter for immediate reinforcement of chapter content. Answers and rationales for these questions are located on Evolve Student Resources. Like traditional NCLEX® items, some of these questions are in multiple-choice format with single and multiple correct answers as well as in short answer format. Items with more than one correct answer direct the student to "Select all that apply." Although short-answer items are not in NCLEX format, we believe they are useful for students. We have also incorporated the Next-Generation NCLEX (NGN) item types. These items use case studies and require students to employ clinical decision making, cognitive skills, and critical thinking to make appropriate decisions. The cognitive skills are: recognize cues, analyze cues, prioritize hypotheses, generate solutions, take action, and evaluate outcomes.

See page viii for additional key features within the text.

ANCILLARIES

FOR THE INSTRUCTOR

Evolve Resources

- ExamView Test Bank with NGN and NCLEX®–style questions and answers and separate test bank in Word for alternate format questions; more than 600 review questions, including 100 Next-Generation NCLEX (NGN)® Examination-style questions. Each NGN question in the test bank includes topic, clinical judgment or nursing process step, objective, cognitive level, correct answer and rationale
- Suggestions for working with English as a Second Language (ESL) students
- Image collection
- TEACH Instructor Resources
  - Lesson Plans based on textbook chapter learning objectives, which provide a roadmap to link and integrate all parts of the educational package
  - PowerPoint Presentation including Audience Response Questions (more than 1000 slides)
- Study Guide Answer Key

FOR STUDENTS

Study Guide

Practical and student-friendly, this useful study guide, based on the textbook chapter objectives, is designed to help students master the content presented in the text. It includes learning activities (including listing, matching, and labeling exercises) and multiple-choice questions.

Evolve Resources

- Answer Keys—In-text NGN and NCLEX Review Questions, Put on Your Thinking Cap Questions, and Nursing Care Plan Critical Thinking Questions.
- Appendix—Laboratory Reference Values
- Spanish/English Glossary
- Review Questions—NCLEX-PN® Examination
- Fluid & Electrolyte Tutorial
- Bibliography and Reader References

To the Student

KEY FEATURES

Designed with the student in mind, *Medical-Surgical Nursing*, 8th edition, has a visually appealing and easy-to-use format that will help you to master medical-surgical nursing.

Following are some of the numerous special features and aids that will help you as you study.

READING AND REVIEW TOOLS

Objectives introduce the chapter topics and **Key Terms** are listed, with difficult medical, nursing, or scientific terms accompanied by simple phonetic pronunciations. Key terms are presented in color the first time they appear in the narrative and are briefly defined in the text, with complete definitions in the Glossary.

Each chapter ends with a section called **Get Ready for the NCLEX Examination! Key Points** follow the chapter objectives and serve as a useful chapter review. An extensive set of **Review Questions for the NCLEX Examination** provides an immediate opportunity to test your understanding of the chapter content. NGN style questions are included as well to stimulate clinical reasoning and the use of various cognitive skills. Most are in the same format you will see on the NCLEX-PN examination. **Answers** are located on Evolve Student Resources.

ADDITIONAL LEARNING RESOURCES

The online **Evolve Student Resources** at http://evolve.elsevier.com/Linton/medsurg gives you access to even more review questions for the NCLEX Examination, animations, and much more.

CHAPTER FEATURES

Nursing Care Plans, with critical thinking questions at the end of each care plan, encourage students to synthesize key concepts. Answer guidelines are given on the Evolve Student Resources site.

Patient Problems, Goals, and Outcome Criteria are screened and set apart in the text in a clear, easy-to-understand format to help you learn to participate in the development of a nursing care plan.

Introductory Systems Chapters prepare you for the following chapters that address specific disorders. They provide succinct reviews of system anatomy and physiology, the complete nursing assessment, related diagnostic procedures, drug classifications, and common therapeutic measures.

Drug Therapy tables developed for specific system disorders provide quick access to action, dosage, side effects, and nursing considerations for commonly used drug classes.

Diagnostic Tests and Procedures tables in the systems chapters provide quick references to relevant drugs and tests. Patient preparation and postprocedure care are included.

Health Promotion boxes highlight timely wellness and disease prevention topics.

Patient Teaching boxes appear frequently in the text to help develop awareness of the vital role of patient and family teaching in health care today.

Coordinated Care boxes help nurses to prioritize tasks and assign them safely and efficiently.

Complementary and Alternative Therapies boxes provide a breakdown of specific nontraditional therapies, along with precautions and possible side effects.

Cultural Considerations boxes explore the range of cultural preferences and how to address the needs of a culturally diverse patient and resident population when planning nursing care.

Nutrition Considerations boxes emphasize the role that nutrition plays in disease and nursing care.

Pharmacology Capsule boxes alert students to important precautions, interactions, and adverse effects of medications.

Put on Your Thinking Cap! boxes encourage analysis of content for application to clinical situations.

Contents

Aspects of Medical-Surgical Nursing

1

http://evolve.elsevier.com/Linton/medsurg

Objectives

1. Identify the most appropriate source of information about the roles of the licensed vocational nurse/licensed practical nurse (LVN/LPN) in medical-surgical nursing settings.
2. Describe the essential knowledge and skills needed by the medical-surgical nurse.
3. Describe principles of ethics that may apply when caring for medical-surgical patients.
4. Provide examples of nurse behaviors that violate laws governing the profession.
5. Describe the characteristics of effective leaders and managers.
6. Describe essential elements of delegation.
7. Describe the following in relation to LVN/LPN as a manager: making assignments, accountability, conflict resolution, and safety.
8. Describe the six cognitive skills that are essential for appropriate clinical judgment.
9. Describe the testing formats used for assessing cognitive skills.

Key Terms

bioethics
ethnocentrism
leadership
malpractice
management
tort

DESCRIPTION

Medical-surgical nursing is a specialty that employs an array of knowledge and skills to provide care for adult patients with a variety of conditions requiring medical and/or surgical management. Medical-surgical nurses are prepared to provide care from adolescence through the end of life. Depending on the setting of care, the nurse may work with families and groups as well as with individuals.

PROFESSIONAL ORGANIZATIONS

The Academy of Medical-Surgical Nurses (AMSN) is the professional organization for nurses practicing in medical-surgical settings. It delineates the scope of practice and sets the standards for nursing practice. The AMSN welcomes licensed vocational nurses/licensed practical nurses (LVNs/LPNs) as associate members. LVNs/LPNs are eligible for full membership in the National Gerontological Nursing Association, which is dedicated to the clinical care of older adults across diverse settings.

ROLES

Depending on nursing preparation, education, practice settings, and specialized education, the medical-surgical nurse may function as a caregiver, care coordinator, patient-educator, case manager, counselor, patient advocate, consultant, researcher, administrator/manager, staff educator, and expert witness. The roles that LVNs/LPNs may assume are specified in their state Nurse Practice Act. Some roles require collaboration with a registered nurse (RN), others require specialized training or certification. Because the risk of harm is inherent in the provision of nursing care, each state has a Nursing Practice Act and a set of Rules and Regulations that are enacted to protect the public. State boards of nursing specify the scope of practice and standards for practice for nurses in their respective states. The standards for practice for LVNs/LPNs in Texas is presented as an example in the Coordinated Care box. You need to know the standards for the state in which you practice.

Coordinated Care

Texas Administrative Code

RULE 217.11 STANDARDS OF NURSING PRACTICE

The Texas Board of Nursing is responsible for regulating the practice of nursing within the State of Texas for Vocational Nurses, Registered Nurses, and Registered Nurses with advanced practice authorization. The standards of practice establish a minimum acceptable level of nursing practice in any setting for each level of nursing licensure or advanced practice authorization. Failure to meet these standards may result in action against the nurse's license even if no actual patient injury resulted.

1. Standards Applicable to All Nurses. All vocational nurses, registered nurses and registered nurses with advanced practice authorization shall:
   - A. Know and conform to the Texas Nursing Practice Act and the board's rules and regulations as well as all federal, state, or local laws, rules or regulations affecting the nurse's current area of nursing practice.
   - B. Implement measures to promote a safe environment for clients and others.
   - C. Know the rationale for the effects of medications and treatments, and shall correctly administer the same.
   - D. Accurately and completely report and document:
     - i. The client's status including signs and symptoms;
     - ii. Nursing care rendered;
     - iii. Physician, dentist, or podiatrist orders;
     - iv. Administration of medications and treatments;
     - v. Client response(s); and
     - vi. Contacts with other health care team members concerning significant events regarding client's status.
   - E. Respect the client's right to privacy by protecting confidential information unless required or allowed by law to disclose the information.
   - F. Promote and participate in education and counseling to a client(s) and, where applicable, the family/significant other(s) based on health needs.
   - G. Obtain instruction and supervision as necessary when implementing nursing procedures or practices.
   - H. Make a reasonable effort to obtain orientation/training for competency when encountering new equipment and technology or unfamiliar care situations.
   - I. Notify the appropriate supervisor when leaving a nursing assignment.
   - J. Know, recognize, and maintain professional boundaries of the nurse-client relationship.
   - K. Comply with mandatory reporting requirements of Texas Occupations Code Chapter 301 (Nursing Practice Act), Subchapter 1, which include reporting a nurse:
     - i. Who violates the Nursing Practice Act or a board rule and contributed to the death or serious injury of a patient;
     - ii. Whose conduct causes a person to suspect that the nurse's practice is impaired by chemical dependency or drug or alcohol abuse;
     - iii. Whose actions constitute abuse, exploitation, fraud, or a violation of professional boundaries; or
     - iv. Whose actions indicate the nurse lacks knowledge, skill, judgment, or conscientiousness to such an extent that the nurse's continued practice of nursing could reasonably be expected to pose a risk of harm to a patient or other person, regardless of whether the conduct consists of a single incident or a pattern or behavior;
     - v. Except for minor incidents (Texas Occupations Code 301.401(2), 301.419, 22 TAC 217.16), peer review (Texas Occupations Code 301.403, 303.007, 22 TAC 217.19), or peer assistance if no practice violation (Texas Occupations Code 301.410) as stated in the Nursing Practice Act and Board rules (22 TAC Chapter 217).
   - L. Provide, without discrimination, nursing services regardless of the age, disability, economic status, gender, national origin, race, religion, health problems, or sexual orientation of the client served.
   - M. Institute appropriate nursing interventions that might be required to stabilize a client's condition and/or prevent complications.
   - N. Clarify any order or treatment regimen that the nurse has reason to believe is inaccurate, nonefficacious or contraindicated by consulting with the appropriate licensed practitioner and notifying the ordering practitioner when the nurse makes the decision not to administer the medication or treatment.
   - O. Implement measures to prevent exposure to infectious pathogens and communicable conditions.
   - P. Collaborate with the client, members of the health care team and, when appropriate, the client's significant other(s) in the interest of the client's health care.
   - Q. Consult with, utilize, and make referrals to appropriate community agencies and health care resources to provide continuity of care.
   - R. Be responsible for one's own continuing competence in nursing practice and individual professional growth.
   - S. Make assignments to others that take into consideration client safety and that are commensurate with the educational preparation, experience, knowledge, and physical and emotional ability of the person to whom the assignments are made.
   - T. Accept only those nursing assignments that take into consideration client safety and that are commensurate with the nurse's educational preparation, experience, knowledge, and physical and emotional ability.
   - U. Supervise nursing care provided by others for whom the nurse is professionally responsible.
   - V. Ensure the verification of current Texas licensure or other Compact State licensure privilege and credentials of personnel for whom the nurse is administratively responsible, when acting in the role of nurse administrator.
2. Standards Specific to Vocational Nurses. The licensed vocational nurse (LVN) practice is a directed scope of nursing practice under the supervision of a registered nurse, advanced practice registered nurse, physician's assistant, physician, podiatrist, or dentist. Supervision is the process of directing, guiding, and influencing

Coordinated Care—cont'd

Texas Administrative Code

the outcome of an individual's performance of an activity. The licensed vocational nurse shall assist in the determination of predictable health care needs of clients within health care settings and:

A. Shall utilize a systematic approach to provide individualized, goal-directed nursing care by:
   i. collecting data and performing focused nursing assessments;
   ii. participating in the planning of nursing care needs for clients;
   iii. participating in the development and modification of the comprehensive nursing care plan for assigned clients;
   iv. implementing appropriate aspects of care within the LVN's scope of practice, and
   v. assisting in the evaluation of the client's responses to nursing interventions and the identification of client needs;

B. Shall assign specific tasks, activities, and functions to unlicensed personnel commensurate with the educational preparation, experience, knowledge, and physical and emotional ability of the person to whom the assignments are made and shall maintain appropriate supervision of unlicensed personnel.

C. May perform other acts that require education and training as prescribed by board rules and policies, commensurate with the licensed vocational nurse's experience, continuing education, and demonstrated licensed vocational nurse competencies.

From Texas Board of Nursing. Standards of Nursing Practice. Last amended November 15, 2007. https://www.bon.texas.gov/rr_current/217-11.asp.

Put On Your Thinking Cap!

Use the internet to access the Nursing Practice Act and Rules and Regulations in the state where you plan to work. Read and be prepared to discuss the information about licensed vocational nurse/licensed practical nurse practice.

PRACTICE SETTINGS

Medical-surgical nurses are prepared to function in a variety of settings. Examples include acute and subacute care facilities, home health care, ambulatory care clinics, outpatient services, residential facilities, skilled nursing facilities, medical offices, adult day care, primary care, schools, correctional facilities, and private businesses. Regardless of the setting, LVNs/LPNs must practice within the scope of their state Nurse Practice Act. Chapter 2 provides additional information about the settings of care that most commonly employ LVNs/LPNs.

ESSENTIAL KNOWLEDGE AND SKILLS

Medical-surgical practice requires knowledge of an array of medical-surgical conditions including the related pathophysiology, manifestations, complications, treatments, nursing interventions, and expected patient responses. This knowledge guides the nursing assessment, planning, intervention, and evaluation. The LVN/LPN performs these functions in collaboration with or under the supervision of the RN. Other essential skills for medical-surgical nursing are communication, organization, teamwork, technical skills, and the ability to multitask. Because patients with medical-surgical conditions are commonly treated with medications, the LVN/LPN must have basic knowledge of pharmacology, access to detailed information about any medications they administer, and skill in medication administration.

ETHICAL CONSIDERATIONS

Ethics deals with values relevant to human conduct that are specific to a group. For example, nurses have professional codes of ethics. Ethics is concerned with defining what actions are right and wrong and whether the motives and outcomes of those actions are good or bad. If choices were simply two opposite actions, with one clearly good and the other clearly bad, ethical decision making would be simple, but all choices are not simple. The choices are often shades of gray rather than black and white. Sometimes a choice must be made between two good or two bad options. Ethical dilemmas are perplexing situations because ethics does not prescribe one right answer. Rather, ethics defines formal processes to explore what is proper conduct. **Bioethics** is concerned with the ethical questions that arise in the context of health care.

The concept of morality is closely related to ethics because moral beliefs provide a personal foundation for rules of action. Whereas ethics is prescribed by a given group, morals are the views of right and wrong held by an individual. For example, a patient might choose to discontinue renal dialysis knowing that they will die from renal failure. As a professional, you know that the patient has a right to make that decision. However, your personal moral beliefs might include the view that life should be preserved at all costs. In this situation, a conflict exists between the ethics of the profession and your morals. You

Box 1.1 Key Steps in the Resolution of an Ethical Dilemma

Step 1: Ask the question, "is this issue an ethical dilemma?" If a review of scientific data does not resolve the question, if the question is perplexing, and if the answer will have relevance for areas of human concern, an ethical dilemma probably exists.
Step 2: Gather information relevant to the case. Patient, family, institutional, and social perspectives are important sources of relevant information.
Step 3: Clarify values. Distinguish among fact, opinion, and values.
Step 4: Verbalize the problem. A clear, simple statement of the dilemma is not always easy, but it helps to ensure effectiveness in the final plan and facilitates discussion.
Step 5: Identify possible courses of action.
Step 6: Negotiate a plan. Negotiation requires a confidence in one's own point of view and a deep respect for the opinions of others.
Step 7: Evaluate the plan over time.

From Ecker M: Ethics and values. In Potter PA, Perry AG, Stockert PA, Hall AM, editors: *Fundamentals of nursing*, ed 9, St. Louis, 2017, Elsevier.

may feel powerless when personal moral beliefs cannot be followed as a result of institutional or other barriers. Experiences like this are thought to be one reason some nurses leave nursing. The key steps to resolve an ethical dilemma are summarized in Box 1.1.

Principles of ethics and values can guide you when faced with situations that do not have simple solutions. Principles include autonomy (respect individual rights), beneficence (act in the patient's best interests), justice (consider fairness, equity, appropriateness), nonmaleficence (do no harm), confidentiality (protect patient privacy), and veracity (be truthful, honest).

Values are specific beliefs and attitudes that are important to a person and that influence the choices a person makes on a daily basis. For example, one person may value kindness and honesty whereas another may value financial success and material possessions. A person's values affect their choice of friends, mates, and professions. Values that have been identified as essential for professional nurses include altruism, equality, esthetics, freedom, human dignity, justice, and truth. Nursing faculty often encourage students to become aware of their personal values and how those values affect their behavior through the process of values clarification. Values clarification enables people not only to understand themselves better, but also to understand their patients and to help patients explore what is important to them. Nurses need to be aware of the tendency toward **ethnocentrism**—the belief that one's own culture and its values are superior to others.

Cultural Considerations

What Does Culture Have to Do With Values?

Ethnocentric beliefs about issues such as drug use and sexual orientation can influence a nurse's attitude toward patients so subtly that they might not even be aware of it. Values clarification helps nurses to be aware of their own values and to respect the values of others so that the patient receives optimal care regardless of a nurse's personal convictions.

To reveal your own cultural bias tests, you may want to take a quiz available at https://implicit.harvard.edu/implicit/takeatest.html.

The term *values conflict* is used when the values of individuals or institutions, or both, are different. In this situation, a risk exists that the patient's values may not be recognized or respected. A positive response to values conflicts is to try to understand the other person's views and to find common ground. Nurses sometimes experience values conflicts with employers. For example, an agency may institute cost-saving measures that nurses believe negatively affect the quality of care.

LEGAL CONSIDERATIONS

The law defines the boundaries of nursing practice. Nurses are obliged to know their legal functions and limitations to protect both their patients and themselves. A nursing license is granted only to persons who have met specific educational standards and demonstrated the minimum required level of knowledge as assessed by an examination. The state board of nursing can revoke or suspend the license of a nurse who violates the provisions on the licensing statutes.

Nurses in all specialties are at risk for committing a **tort**, which is a civil wrong against a person or property. Examples of torts are: threatening contact without the patient's consent, restraining or medicating a patient against their wishes, invasion of privacy by sharing or publishing personal patient information, giving false information that can damage the patient's reputation, and acting in a negligent manner.

Professional negligence is called ***malpractice***. To be found liable for malpractice, the following conditions must be met: The nurse owed a duty to the patient, the nurse did not carry out that duty, the patient was injured, and the injury was caused by the nurse's failure to carry out that duty. Dupler (2017) provides the following examples of negligent acts that have resulted in lawsuits against hospitals and nurses:

- Failure to monitor a patient
- Failure to document findings
- Failure to notify other staff of changes in patient status
- Failure to maintain or correctly use equipment
- Failure to respond to or correctly carry out orders

- Failure to follow the six rights of medication administration
- Failure to convey discharge instructions appropriately
- Failure to ensure patient safety, especially those who are at risk for injury
- Failure to follow policies and procedures
- Failure to properly delegate and supervise.

Medical-surgical nurses often work with acutely ill patients in various functional states. They administer medications and perform procedures that carry risk, are responsible for communicating with other team members, and prepare patients for self-care after discharge. These are examples of duties that could result in patient injury if not done properly. The nurse's best protection against negligence and malpractice is to adhere to standards of care. Nursing students are held to the same standard of care as are licensed nurses. Students should never perform care for which they have not been prepared. Health care institutions commonly provide malpractice insurance for nurses they employ. This coverage generally covers legal fees and awards if a nurse is sued for professional negligence or malpractice. The agency insurance covers the nurses only when working within the employing institution. As an LVN/LPN, you are wise to seek legal advice whether to carry personal liability insurance as well as the institutional insurance.

Additional information about legal roles and responsibilities can be found at the website of the National Council of State Boards of Nursing (www.ncsbn.org) and from individual state licensing bodies.

LEADERSHIP AND MANAGEMENT IN MEDICAL-SURGICAL SETTINGS

In the evolving system of health care, nurses at all levels are being called upon to add new skills and functions. Cost control measures seek to maximize the contribution of each member of the health care team. LVNs/LPNs bring valuable knowledge and skills to many practice arenas and are positioned to be both leaders and strong collaborative followers in managing and providing care. The increase in long-term residential care required by the growing older adult population and the movement of care increasingly into the community is shifting the focus and increasing the demand for LVNs/LPNs.

LVNs/LPNs manage the care of medical-surgical patients in many health care settings. Long-term care facilities are commonly staffed by LVNs/LPNs and nursing assistants, who often provide the bulk of "hands-on" care. LVNs/LPNs have traditionally filled leadership or management positions in long-term care, often as team leaders and charge nurses. These roles require the LVN/LPN to have a working knowledge of leadership, management, and safe health care delivery. We are seeing a shift to LVNs/LPNs who not only must manage their assigned patients but also must plan, organize, direct, coordinate, and control care provided by others. As changes evolve, LVNs/LPNs must stay informed of the laws that define their practice. State Nurse Practice Acts vary and respond over time to changes in their citizens' health needs.

The terms ***leadership*** and ***management*** are sometimes used interchangeably but, in fact, have different meanings. Leadership is a broader and more future-oriented role whereas management is more local and task focused. A leader creates a vision that, when combined with unifying values, creates a mission for the group to work toward. The role of the manager is to focus on the day-to-day work of the organization. In the work setting, leadership is often considered the inspiration and management the perspiration. Ideally, leadership and management complement each other. Leaders and managers must have certain characteristics to be effective (see the Coordinated Care box).

Coordinated Care

Characteristics of an Effective Leader

- Is an effective communicator
- Is consistent in managing conflict
- Is knowledgeable and competent in all aspects of delivery of care
- Is a role model for staff
- Uses participatory approach in decision making
- Shows appreciation for a job well done
- Delegates work appropriately
- Sets objectives and guides staff
- Displays caring, understanding, and empathy for others
- Motivates and empowers others
- Is proactive and flexible
- Focuses on team development

Modified from Dunham-Taylor J: Quantum leadership: love one another. In Dunham-Taylor J, Pinczak JZ, editors: *Financial management for nurse managers,* ed 2, Boston, 2010, Jones & Bartlett; Huber DL: *Leadership & nursing care management,* ed 5, St. Louis, 2014, Elsevier.

ISSUES RELATED TO LEADERSHIP AND MANAGEMENT

MAKING ASSIGNMENTS AND DELEGATION

In management positions, such as team leader, the LVN/LPN must be able to assign tasks to others who are hired to perform them and make certain that those tasks are carried out. Delegation allows nurses to accomplish nursing care for more patients than one individual could provide alone. Activities that require clinical reasoning, nursing judgment, or critical decision making cannot be delegated.

The National Guidelines for Nursing Delegation were detailed in a joint statement by the NCSBN and the American Nurses Association (May 29, 2019). Note that the state laws related to delegation differ and the licensed nurse is responsible for knowing what is permitted in terms of delegation and making assignments.

The five rights of delegation are described in the Coordinated Care box.

Coordinated Care: Five Rights of Delegation

Right Task: The activity falls within the job description of the person being given the task (the delegatee) or is specified in the agency written policies or procedures.

Right Circumstance: The patient's condition is stable. If the condition changes, the delegatee must inform the licensed nurse who will reassess the patient.

Right Person: The licensed nurse and the employer must ensure that the delegatee has the skills and knowledge to perform the delegated activity.

Right Directions and Communication: The licensed nurse should communicate specific instructions and the delegatee should clarify any questions and agree to accept the delegated activity. The licensed nurse must confirm that the delegatee cannot make any decisions and cannot modify the activity unless approved by the licensed nurse.

Right Supervision and Evaluation: The licensed nurse must monitor the activity, follow up with the delegatee once the activity has been completed, and evaluate the outcome of the activity. The licensed nurse should be available to intervene if necessary and should ensure appropriate documentation of the activity.

From National Council of State Boards of Nursing, 1995, 1996. Retrieved October 13, 2020. www.ncsbn.org.

LVNs/LPNs can assist RNs in the management process. Following delegation by an RN to unlicensed personnel, the LVN/LPN may assist in the supervision of unlicensed personnel, may assist in training unlicensed assistive personnel, and may verify competencies of those personnel.

The NCSBN (April 29, 2019, p. 2) defines an assignment as "the routine care, activities, and procedures that are within the authorized scope of practice of the RN or LPN/VN or part of the routine functions of the AP (assistive personnel)." Making assignments requires that you know the care required by each patient and the strengths and weaknesses of each staff member. In many states the delegating RN remains accountable for the tasks delegated to unlicensed assistive personnel. See the Coordinated Care box.

Coordinated Care

Essential Elements of Effective Delegation by the LVN/LPN

- Compliance with State Nurse Practice Act statement on delegation
- Compliance with institutional policies and procedures related to delegation by LVNs/LPNs
- Knowledge of specific condition and needs of each patient
- Knowledge of training and background of individuals to whom tasks are delegated
- Determination of tasks that can be safely delegated
- Monitoring of staff performance
- Documentation of outcomes

ACCOUNTABILITY

Accountability means that persons are answerable for their actions and may be called on to explain or justify them. An LVN/LPN who makes assignments or delegates tasks to other providers is accountable not only for their own actions, but for the actions of the staff they are directing. A team leader is legally responsible for all nursing care and documentation. The LVN/LPN must ensure that proper and accurate charting is done. The RN team leader is responsible for ensuring that proper and accurate documentation is done for all nursing assessments, interventions, and evaluations.

One aspect of accountability involves communicating patient needs to others. A common form of communication is the handoff (report or handover) at the end (or beginning) of every shift. The LVN/LPN is usually responsible for reporting to the RN in charge but may also be indirectly responsible for the handoff. Guidelines for a clear and complete handoff are as follows:

- Organize information before beginning
- State the patient's name, room number, age, diagnosis, and physician
- Provide a brief, objective account of the patient's condition, including new or changed orders
- Report relevant clinical information: deviations from the patient's or expected norm (vital signs, orientation, intake and output, etc.); identify pain medications including dosage, frequency, and patient response
- For surgical patients, review preoperative checklist items. For postoperative patients, report time of return to the nursing unit, general condition, vital signs, intravenous fluids ordered (type, flow rate), dressing status, voiding, diet, tubes (type, location, patency)
- Convey any specific requests or concerns expressed by the patient or family

One systematic communication tool for the handoff is called *SBAR* (situation, background, assessment, recommendation). SBAR facilitates the exchange of important information between professionals. It may be used to alert physicians, RNs, and other care providers to changes in a patient's condition, to seek new care orders, and for shift handoffs or transfers within and across systems.

CONFLICT RESOLUTION

LVNs/LPNs in leadership or management positions must be able to facilitate conflict resolution. Conflicts arise from differences in many factors such as beliefs, knowledge, values, personalities, culture, and age. If may also be caused by unclear roles; multiple, shifting, or conflicting priorities; and competition for scarce resources. Current issues may be exacerbated by prior unresolved conflicts. When a conflict occurs, it creates stress and negative feelings that can adversely affect the work situation. A conflict may be within an individual (intrapersonal conflict), between two or more people (interpersonal conflict), or between individuals and organizations (organizational conflict).

Conflict is a process with four stages:

1. Frustration: People believe that their goals are being blocked; they feel frustrated. Individuals may become angry or resigned to the situation.
2. Conceptualization: Each party formulates a view of the basis for the conflict. Conflicts typically center on perceived differences in facts, goals, how to achieve goals, and the values on which goals are based.
3. Action: The conflict leads to various behaviors that may or may not help resolve the conflict.
4. Outcomes: Outcome follows the action; goals may be reformulated so that they are acceptable to all parties; one party may "win," the other "lose"; emotions may be positive or negative.

Identifying the root cause of the conflict and related prior history before beginning the resolution process is beneficial.

There are multiple approaches to conflict resolution, each with various advantages and disadvantages. The positive and negative consequences of each are summarized in Table 1.1. The leader must select the best approach in each situation. To understand how each of these approaches works in a "real" situation, consider the following scenario: You are the charge nurse on a 30-bed unit in a long-term care facility. Certified nursing assistants (CNAs) are assigned to equal numbers of residents in adjacent rooms. During report, Alice, a CNA, states that her assignment is unfair because all but two of her patients require almost total care. She says that all of the other CNAs have easier assignments. Using various strategies, possible solutions are:

- *Accommodation*: You shift the care of two residents to other CNAs.
- *Collaboration*: You reassess the needs of each group of assigned residents. Recognizing that Alice is correct, you work with the CNAs to identify more equitable distribution of assignments to ensure good patient care.
- *Compromise*: You tell Alice that you will alternate CNAs assigned to that group of residents.
- *Competition*: You tell Alice that everyone has some residents who require a lot of care and the assignment will stand.

Table 1.1 Modes of Conflict Resolution

MODE	POSITIVE OUTCOMES	NEGATIVE OUTCOMES	WHEN TO USE
Accommodation	Agreement is reached	Differences are suppressed; resentment	You are wrong The other person really has a better idea The issue is more important to the other party than to you You are outnumbered or outranked
Collaboration	Generates commitment to work together; focuses on shared higher goals such as good patient care, not on individual immediate needs Builds understanding and empathy	Wastes time if used for resolution of trivial issues or when the outcome has already been decided	To build understanding To find creative solutions that accommodate higher common goals To address difficult issues that affect productivity
Compromise	Can produce mutually acceptable solutions Both parties have achieved something they wanted	The compromised solution may not be the best even though it "keeps the peace"	When time pressures require quick solution When each party is firmly committed to different views A compromise can produce acceptable outcomes
Avoidance	Temporarily defuses highly charged, emotional disagreement Allows both parties to "cool off" until a reasonable approach can be considered	The conflict is not resolved Neither party is satisfied	To deal with trivial issues when more important issues are waiting To delay a decision until parties are calmer, more information has been obtained, etc. When one party's demands cannot possibly be met When others could resolve the issue more readily
Competition	Reflects a strong stance to defend important principles and protect vulnerable parties Person in power takes responsibility for a decision	Can generate bad feelings Creates a winner and a loser May generate behaviors that block the actions of the "winner"	When a quick decision is essential To implement unpopular nonnegotiable actions To defend important principles, individual rights, and group welfare

- *Avoidance*: You tell Alice that you have more important things to deal with right now and go to your office.

For each of these "solutions," think about the positive and negative outcomes. Again, realize that the best solution will vary with the situation. The art of management is to select the best approach for the situation.

SAFETY

Multiple levels of regulation are concerned with the safety of health care recipients. The mission of the state boards of nursing is to protect and promote the welfare of the people of the state by ensuring that each person holding a license as a nurse in that state is competent to practice safely. The boards fulfill their mission through the regulation of the practice of nursing and the approval of nursing education programs. Furthermore, every health care facility must meet minimum safety regulations established by law in addition to those adopted by the agency to meet its unique needs. All staff members, particularly team leaders, should learn these regulations during orientation to the job. The team leader should know the regulations and be sure that staff members are aware of them. Everyone must understand the procedures to follow in case of disasters such as fires, floods, tornadoes, or hurricanes. In addition, everyday safety related to handling equipment, using proper procedures, and working with potentially dangerous drugs must constantly be addressed to ensure that knowledge and skills are up to date. Organizations are responsible for providing timely information as changes in standards occur and new procedures are developed. Each nurse is accountable for knowing them, and leaders are accountable for ensuring adherence. Medication safety and infection control measures are increasingly complex challenges of primary focus on the national health care agenda.

CLINICAL JUDGMENT IN NURSING

The nursing process has long been used to guide nursing practice. It is defined as "a scientific, clinical reasoning approach to client care that includes assessment, analysis, planning, implementation, and evaluation" (NCSBN, 2018b, p. 5). NCLEX exams are currently based on the nursing process and intend to measure basic knowledge that a nurse needs for safe practice. However, a large study of recently graduated nurses found that they lacked basic clinical reasoning and judgment. Despite having nursing knowledge, the graduates had difficulty knowing what actions to take and why.

The NCSBN conducted a thorough review of the literature to determine the measurable skills required for clinical reasoning/judgment. In 2019, the NCSBN issued the NCSBN Clinical Judgment Measurement and Action Model (NCJMM) that identified six cognitive (thinking) skills or processes that are essential for appropriate clinical judgment. These skills are: Recognize Cues, Analyze Cues, Prioritize Hypotheses, Generate Solutions, Take Action, and Evaluate Outcomes. Rather than replacing the nursing process, the NCJMM builds on and expands it by describing the skills needed to accomplish each step.

- Recognize Cues: "Cues are elements of assessment data that provide important information for the nurse as a basis for making client decisions" (Ignatavicius & Silvestri, n.d., p. 3). Recognizing cues requires the nurse to separate relevant data from irrelevant data in a clinical situation.
- Analyze Cues: When analyzing cues, "the nurse considers the context of the client's history and situation, and interprets how the identified relevant cues relate to the client's condition" (Ignatavicius & Silvestri, n.d., p. 3). The nurse determines whether additional data support or contradict a particular cue in this situation. Potential complications related to the data are identified.
- Prioritize Hypotheses: To prioritize hypotheses, the nurse considers all possible explanations for the client's situation and determines which are most likely and which are most serious.
- Generate Solutions: Expected outcomes must be identified to generate solutions for the identified problems. Specific evidence-based actions are selected to achieve the outcomes. The nurse identifies actions that should be taken as well as actions that should be ruled out.
- Take Action: The nurse uses this skill to address the highest care priorities using the most appropriate sequence of nursing actions. "Actions include, but are not limited to, additional assessment, health teaching, documentation, requested primary healthcare provider orders, performance of nursing skills, and consultation with health care team members" (Ignatavicius & Silvestri, n.d., p. 4).
- Evaluate Outcomes: Once evidence-based actions have been taken, the nurse compares the client outcomes to the expected outcomes and determines whether the actions were effective, ineffective, or had no significant effect.

The NCJMM "provides a systematic, evidence-based framework for measuring whether nurse licensure candidates demonstrate at least minimal competence with respect to clinical judgment and decision making" (NCSBN, 2019). It is an assessment model, meaning it is used for developing test items that measure the six cognitive skills. Students will see these new test item formats throughout this text; however, that will not be fully implemented in NCLEX until at least 2023.

Questions may be based on single-episode client situations or unfolding case studies. Single episode questions present new client data for each question and may require any of the cognitive skills. Unfolding case studies are based on an evolving client situation with a series of questions that test multiple cognitive skills. Below are examples of testing formats used to assess each clinical judgment skill:

- Recognize Cues:
  - A client scenario is presented and a list of assessment data is provided. The student is asked to select the data that require attention.
  - A client scenario is presented and a list of laboratory results is provided. The student is asked to select those changes in lab values that would be expected in the client situation.
- Analyze Cues: A client scenario is presented and a list of assessment data is provided. Several statements have blanks that must be filled from a list based on the data. The item might be related to understanding of the client data, priorities of specific data, explanation of client signs and symptoms, or nursing actions related to the data.
- Prioritize Hypotheses: A client scenario (either single-episode or part of an unfolding case) is presented, and the student must select potential complications from a list provided.
- Generate Solutions: A client scenario (either single-episode or part of an unfolding case) is presented. A set of client questions is provided along with potential nurse responses. The student must identify the appropriate response to each question.
- Take Action: A client scenario (either single-episode or unfolding case) is presented, and a list of teaching points or nursing actions is provided. The student must decide if each point is indicated, contraindicated, or nonessential.
- Evaluate Outcomes:
  - A scenario based on a single-episode or an unfolding case is presented along with a list of assessment data. The student must decide whether each piece of data indicates effective nursing care, ineffective nursing care, or is unrelated to expected outcomes.
  - A scenario based on a single-episode or an unfolding case is presented along with a list of assessment data. Lists of nursing actions and potential complications are provided. The student must decide which nursing action is appropriate for each complication.

GET READY FOR THE NCLEX® EXAMINATION!

Key Points

- The roles that LVNs/LPNs may assume are specified in their state Nurse Practice Act.
- Medical-surgical nursing employs an array of knowledge and skills to provide care for adult patients with a variety of conditions requiring medical and/or surgical management.
- The standards for nursing practice for LVN/LPNs are specified in each state Nurse Practice Act.
- Medical-surgical practice requires knowledge of an array of medical-surgical conditions including the related pathophysiology, manifestations, complications, treatments, nursing interventions, and expected patient responses.
- Ethical dilemmas are perplexing situations because ethics does not prescribe one right answer.
- Principles of ethics include autonomy (respect individual rights), beneficence (act in the patient's best interests), justice (consider fairness, equity, appropriateness), nonmaleficence (do no harm), confidentiality (protect patient privacy), and veracity (be truthful, honest).
- Nurses are obliged to know their legal functions and limitations to protect both their patients and themselves.
- A tort is a civil wrong against a person or property such as restraining or medicating a patient against their wishes.
- Criteria for malpractice include the following: the nurse owed a duty to the patient, the nurse did not carry out that duty, the patient was injured, and the injury was caused by the nurse's failure to carry out that duty.
- Nursing students are held to the same standard of care as are licensed nurses.
- The role of the LVN/LPN in delegation depends on the state in which the LVN/LPN practices.
- An LVN/LPN who makes assignments or delegates tasks to other providers is accountable not only for their own actions but also for the actions of the staff they are directing.
- A leader creates a vision that, when combined with unifying values, creates a mission for the group to work toward.
- The role of the manager is to focus on the day-to-day work of the organization.
- SBAR (situation, background, assessment, recommendation) is a systematic communication tool that facilitates the exchange of important information between professionals.
- When a conflict occurs, it creates stress and negative feelings that can adversely affect the work situation.
- The stages of conflict are frustration, conceptualization, action, and outcomes.
- Approaches to conflict resolution include accommodation, collaboration, compromise, competition, and avoidance.
- Safety requires that all health care agency staff understand the procedures to follow in case of disasters in addition to everyday safety related to handling equipment, using proper procedures, and working with potentially dangerous drugs.

- The six cognitive skills that are essential for appropriate clinical judgment are: Recognize Cues, Analyze Cues, Prioritize Hypotheses, Generate Solutions, Take Action, and Evaluate Outcomes.

Additional Learning Resources

SG Go to your Study Guide for additional learning activities to help you master this chapter content.

Go to your Evolve website (http://evolve.elsevier.com/Linton/medsurg) for the following learning resources and much more:
- Fluid & Electrolyte Tutorial
- Review Questions for the NCLEX® Examination

Clinical Judgment and Next-Generation NCLEX® Examination-Style Questions

1. **What is the best source of information regarding the roles of the LVN/LPN in a medical-surgical setting?**
   1. The Human Resources department of the employing agency
   2. The State Board of Nursing
   3. Other staff members working on the same unit
   4. Medical-surgical nursing textbooks

   NCLEX Client Need: Safe and Effective Care Environment: Coordinated Care

2. **Which of the following are characteristics of an effective leader and manager? (Select all that apply.)**
   1. Is a role model for staff
   2. Has a graduate nursing degree
   3. Focuses on team development
   4. Motivates and empowers others
   5. Uses only an autocratic approach in decision making

   NCLEX Client Need: Safe and Effective Care Environment: Coordinated Care

3. **When preparing to administer medications, the nurse carefully confirms the drug order and the patient's identity. This is an example of which ethical principle?**
   1. Nonmaleficence
   2. Veracity
   3. Autonomy
   4. Justice

   NCLEX Client Need: Safe and Effective Care Environment: Coordinated Care

4. **A nurse uses their cell phone to take a photograph with a celebrity patient. The nurse posts the photograph on social media. This may be considered:**
   1. Malpractice
   2. Negligence
   3. Assault
   4. Tort

   NCLEX Client Need: Safe and Effective Care Environment: Coordinated Care

5. **Essential elements of effective delegation by the LVN/LPN include which of the following? (Select all that apply.)**
   1. Knowledge of each patient's condition
   2. Compliance with state and institutional policies
   3. Determination of tasks that can be safely delegated
   4. Direct supervision of tasks assigned to others
   5. Evaluation of the patient's response to the care

   NCLEX Client Need: Safe and Effective Care Environment: Coordinated Care

6. **Using the Clinical Judgment Model, the nurse has done a focused assessment on a postoperative patient. The patient's heart rate and blood pressure are slightly above normal. The nurse compares the patient's data to the preoperative assessment and reviews the postoperative orders. Which cognitive skill is the nurse demonstrating at this time?**
   1. Recognize cues
   2. Analyze cues
   3. Prioritize hypotheses
   4. Generate solutions
   5. Take action
   6. Evaluate outcomes

   NCLEX Client Need: Safe and Effective Care Environment: Coordinated Care

7. **In performing a focused assessment of a new postoperative patient, the nurse collects the following data:**
   1. BP 80/60
   2. IV fluids flowing at prescribed rate
   3. Heart rate 110 beats per minute
   4. Respirations 26 breaths per
   5. Alert and oriented
   6. Urine output 100 mL in last hour

   Which data require additional assessment by the nurse?

   NCLEX Client Need: Safe and Effective Care Environment: Coordinated Care

Medical-Surgical Practice Settings

2

http://evolve.elsevier.com/Linton/medsurg

Objectives

1. Describe the role of the licensed vocational nurse/licensed practical nurse (LVN/LPN) in community health, community-based care, home health care, rehabilitation facilities, and long-term care settings.
2. Differentiate community health nursing and community-based nursing.
3. Describe the types of specialty care that may be provided in home health care.
4. Explain the requirements for Medicare coverage of home care and implications for the LVN/LPN.
5. Describe the role of the nurse in home health care.
6. Explain the definition of *skilled nursing care* in the context of home health nursing.
7. Describe the key concepts and goals of rehabilitation.
8. Discuss the impact of legislation on individuals with disabilities.
9. Describe the types of long-term care facilities.
10. Discuss the effects of institutionalization on the individual.
11. Describe the principles of nursing care in long-term residential facilities.

Key Terms

disability
domiciliary care
handicap
impairment
rehabilitation

Chapter 1 briefly introduced the most common settings in which health care is delivered. Throughout this book, the care of patients in acute care settings is covered in detail. As the health care system changes, however, licensed vocational nurses/ licensed practical nurses (LVNs/LPNs) are finding a variety of opportunities for employment in community, rehabilitation, long-term care, and other settings. This chapter provides a more complete description of the more common employment settings where medical-surgical nurses work.

COMMUNITY AND HOME HEALTH NURSING

Community health nursing and home health nursing are specialized areas of nursing practice that are often considered as being similar. This viewpoint probably comes from defining community health nursing as anything that occurs outside the hospital setting. However, despite sharing common historic roots, these two practice areas have significant differences.

COMMUNITY HEALTH NURSING

For both humane and economic reasons, keeping people healthy is better than waiting until disease or disability occurs. Traditional community health nursing focuses on (1) improving the health status of communities or groups of people (called *aggregates*) through public education, (2) screening for early detection of disease, and (3) providing services for people who need care outside the acute care setting.

Community Health Nursing Roles

The following example demonstrates typical community health nursing roles.

A community health nurse notices a rise in blood pressure, an increase in weight, and a general lack of fitness in members of a senior citizen high-rise in her district. Her assessment shows that no recreational facilities are available nearby, the meals served at the high-rise tend to be high in fat and sodium, and social activity is generally lacking at the facility. On the positive side, a residents' organization exists, although it has never been very active. By working with the residents' organization and a local church, the nurse initiates a group exercise program to improve the strength, cardiovascular fitness, and weight control of the residents. By working with the management of the high-rise and the residents' association, the nurse gets the building manager to serve healthier meals. The nurse also asks a local school of nursing to hold a monthly blood pressure and health education clinic for the residents.

In this example, the community health nurse not only gave direct service to individual clients but also worked with three existing community groups to provide a significant number of services designed to enhance the health of the senior citizen group. Community health nurses often work with many different individuals and groups to create or modify systems of care to improve the health of a defined group. This function requires the nurse to assume several roles to accomplish care goals. The roles listed in the example include case finder, care manager, teacher, advocate, and coalition builder. To perform all aspects of the community health nurse role requires at least a bachelor's degree in nursing. However, the LVN/LPN is increasingly visible in community health settings such as clinics, retirement/senior centers, and schools.

Community-Based Nursing

The term *community-based nursing* has been used in several contexts but should not be confused with community health nursing. Community-based nursing may be described as the delivery of health care services that meet the needs of citizens at various levels of wellness and illness based on identified community needs. In a more general sense, the term is sometimes used to describe the provision of various levels of care in traditional and nontraditional community settings.

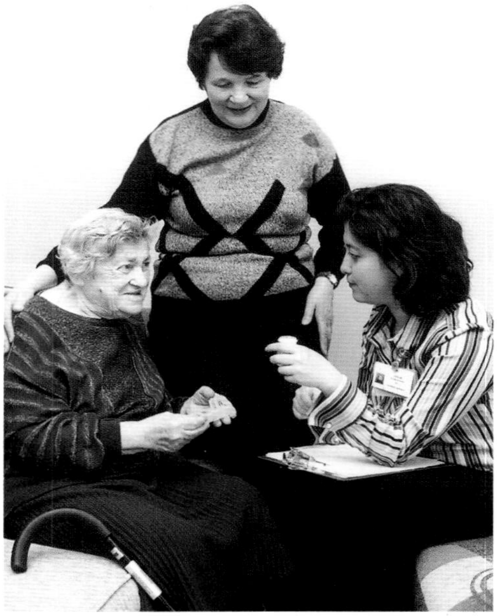

Fig. 2.1 Home health agencies deliver the services of a variety of professionals. (From Maurer FA, Smith CM: *Community/public health practice*, ed 5, St. Louis, 2013, Saunders.)

HOME HEALTH NURSING

Home health nursing blends direct nursing care and community health nursing. The main difference between home health nursing and traditional public health nursing is that home health nursing provides more direct care to patients. The main difference between home health nursing and nursing in an institution is the increased emphasis on the family and the environment in the home.

Medical-surgical nurses working in home health must adapt their knowledge and skills to this new setting. Home health nursing requires careful consideration of the family and its role in the care of the ill family member. Although giving direct care to an individual is an important part of home health care, a more important nursing role is to teach the patient and family to care for themselves (Fig. 2.1). This important role is similar to that of the rehabilitation nurse, for whom the goal is the independent functioning of the patient and family. The LVN/LPN who works in home health settings must be aware of the legal scope of practice in their state, as well as agency policies. LVNs/LPNs must recognize their limitations and inform the supervisor if they are not prepared to perform the tasks or activities required in a particular patient's home.

The environment in which home health nursing is practiced is very different from the hospital practice environment. Homes often have only a fraction of the resources of the hospital. Small bedrooms, low beds, inadequate climate control, and limited space are common. Maintaining asepsis can be challenging because of inconvenient or absent hand-washing facilities and the lack of biohazard disposal devices. Families are often overwhelmed by the task of caring for ill loved ones. They need instruction not only in the care of the patient, but also in how to perform the care in a home that was not designed for that purpose, while continuing to function as a family.

Home health nurses must collect data for the plan of care about the patient, the family, and the environment. Ongoing data collection is critical, because the home health nurse often sees the patient more frequently than other care providers and can detect problems early. For example, the observation of weight gain and ankle edema alerts the nurse to possible heart failure in the cardiac patient. Prompt intervention may prevent serious consequences. The use of technology in the delivery of health care to patients is increasingly common. Examples include e-mail, videoconferencing, patient examination cameras, video otoscopes, and remote electrocardiogram (ECG) and vital sign monitoring. The nurse must become familiar with tools that permit patient communication and assessment from the home. The COVID-19 pandemic forced the use of telemedicine making it much more widely used and accepted. Medicare now covers telehealth in certain circumstances for office visits, psychotherapy, consultations and other medical and health services (Medicare and You, 2021).

To illustrate the importance of collecting data about the family and the environment, consider the patient who requires wound care. In the home setting, decisions that need to be made include: Who can do the care? What does that person need to know? What supplies are needed and where can they be obtained? What is the best way to dispose of soiled dressings? Addressing these questions requires the home health nurse to be resourceful, knowledgeable, skillful, and creative.

Reimbursement Realities in Home Health Nursing

Medicare, although not the sole source of home health care funding, is probably the most important source. Reimbursement by the Medicare program depends on documentation that four basic conditions have been met: (1) the physician or other health care provider (e.g., nurse practitioner) orders skilled nursing care for a specific condition; (2) the patient needs intermittent skilled nursing care, or physical or speech-language therapy; (3) the patient is homebound; and (4) the agency providing the care is Medicare certified (Department of Health and Human Services, 2019). The number of hours per day and days per week that Medicare will cover are limited. Medicare will not pay for 24-hour care at home; meals delivered to the home; homemaker services such as shopping, cleaning, or laundry; or personal care given by home health aides if this is the only care needed. Medical social services may be provided as directed by the physician if the service is intended to help with social and emotional concerns that might affect recovery. Medical supplies are covered when the physician orders them as part of the care. Durable medical equipment, if ordered by the physician, may be provided separately from the home health service. The patient may be required to pay a portion of the cost (usually 20%) of Medicare-covered medical equipment such as oxygen equipment, a wheelchair, or walker. Private insurance companies may have different eligibility requirements and benefits for home care.

Physician must certify need for care, authorize a plan of care, and review it regularly

All home care treatment must be authorized by a physician who has seen the patient within 90 days for the condition requiring home care. A plan of care must include pertinent diagnoses, results of mental status evaluations, identification of the types of services needed, the supplies and equipment required, frequency of visits, prognosis, rehabilitation potential, functional limitations, nutritional requirements, medications, and treatments. This plan also must include safety measures to protect against injury and plans for discharge from home care.

In practice, the initial referral usually includes the patient's name, address, and telephone number, as well as the major medical diagnoses and a list of medications and treatments—not unlike a physician's orders in a hospital. On the first visit, the admitting nurse usually formulates the plan of care, adding all other required elements. This plan is sent to the physician for review and signature. Because the care provided in the home is predominately nursing care, it is appropriate that the nurse has a major role in developing the plan of care. The role of the LVN/LPN is to participate in patient data collection and contribute to the development and revision of the care plan. If assistive personnel are involved in the home care, the LVN/LPN may assign appropriate tasks, verify the staff member's abilities and limitations, and evaluate the staff member's performance. Disabled and frail persons may not be able to defend themselves and may have little contact with others besides the health care team. Therefore the home nurse must report evidence of abuse, neglect, and violation of rights according to agency policy.

Care must be skilled, intermittent, reasonable, and necessary

Medicare reimburses nursing care in the home provided that the care given is "skilled." This stipulation means that the care delivered must be the kind that only a nurse trained in that kind of care could be expected to do. However, not all care provided by a nurse qualifies as skilled care. Skilled nursing care is discussed subsequently with the types of home health services.

Nursing is one of three primary home health care services considered to be skilled. The others are physical therapy and speech therapy. Occupational therapy may be considered skilled, depending on the complexity of the patient's problems. Social work and home health aide services are not considered skilled in themselves but may be reimbursed if the patient has qualified for one of the three primary skilled services. These home care services are discussed in more detail later in this chapter.

The preceding definition of skilled care is an interpretation of the Medicare law. Some nursing activities that require the skill of a nurse may not be recognized as skilled under Medicare. Medicare law does not prevent nurses from giving the care they judge necessary; it only defines what care is reimbursable under that law.

Medicare reimbursement requires that the nursing visits be intermittent in nature, meaning that visits occur periodically and usually do not exceed 28 hours per week. Under normal circumstances, the patient is not seen daily. However, situations exist in which daily visits are justified. These situations usually indicate the need for family members to be trained in daily procedures such as diabetic care or wound care and dressing changes. Under these circumstances, Medicare may reimburse daily visits for 2 or 3 weeks. These instances are considered special cases, and reimbursement depends on clear and accurate documentation of the need for daily visits. Otherwise, visiting frequency can range from 3 to 4 times per week to monthly.

To demonstrate that care is reasonable and necessary, objective clinical evidence clearly justifying the type and frequency of services is required. The nurse must clearly document functional losses and goals for care. Ongoing progress or lack of progress toward treatment goals must be documented. Poor documentation not only jeopardizes patient care but also often results in denial of the agency's claim for payment because the documentation did not prove that the care given was "reasonable and necessary."

Patient must be homebound

This criterion does not mean that the patient must be bedridden. It does mean, however, that the patient must exert considerable effort to leave the home. Medicare also requires that absences from the home be infrequent and of short duration. According to Medicare regulations, if patients are well enough to leave home frequently, they are able to visit a physician's office for treatment and therefore are not in need of home care.

Home health agency must be medicare certified

Medicare-certified home health services can be identified by visiting www.medicare.gov. Click on Find Care Providers and provide the zip code of the desired location. A list of area services will be provided. When you select a specific service/agency, you can view a file that includes date of original certification and latest renewal. A home health agency can decline to accept a patient if it cannot meet the patient's needs.

Types of Home Health Services

The primary skilled services in home health care are (1) nursing, (2) physical therapy, and (3) speech therapy. Secondary services include occupational therapy (which may be primary under certain conditions), social work services, and home health aide services.

Skilled nursing

According to Medicare regulations, skilled nursing includes skilled observation and assessment, teaching, and performing skilled procedures.

Skilled observation and assessment. The phrase *skilled observation and assessment* implies that the skills of a nurse are required to observe a patient's progress, to assess the importance of signs and symptoms, and to decide on a course of action. For example, good assessment skills and judgment are needed to detect the signs and symptoms of congestive heart failure early enough to prevent rehospitalization. LVNs/LPNs commonly perform focused assessments, meaning that they collect specified data related to specific health areas. The information obtained by the LVN/LPN can become part of the registered nurse's comprehensive assessment and help guide the nursing care plan.

Teaching. Teaching is considered a skilled task because to teach effectively the nurse must identify the patient's and the family's current level of knowledge, determine their learning style, relay information at an appropriate level and pace, and evaluate the results of the teaching.

Teaching is the most important skill in home care. Much care in the home must be done by the patient and caregiver. Good patient teaching should begin in the acute care setting, but newly discharged patients may need considerable teaching to manage their care at home. When high-technology therapies are involved, teaching is even more important.

Families that have difficulty understanding complex medical issues or high-technology equipment may be anxious when the nurse is not there to help or to answer their questions immediately. Skilled nurses understand this problem and ensure that their teaching is thorough and addresses precisely what the family needs to know to care successfully for their loved one at home. To accomplish this task, the nurse must identify the exact nature of the problem. A family member's difficulty in administering an injection may arise from a lack of knowledge of the procedure, a fear of needles, an inability to read the markings on the syringe, or a denial of the disease process. Identifying the specific learning need is critical to successful patient teaching. In teaching high-technology care, keeping instructions as simple and specific as possible is especially important. Each step in the procedure should be written down and reviewed with the patient and caregiver. The skill should be demonstrated several times, asking the family caregiver to cue the nurse for each step. After this task is performed a few times, the caregiver should perform a return demonstration of the skill.

Family caregivers must understand exactly what should be done in an emergency. Any questions about the family's ability to manage their portion of the care should be immediately referred to the home care nurse responsible for establishing the care plan and managing the case.

Performing skilled procedures. Skilled procedures include dressing changes, Foley catheter insertions, and venipunctures. However, after certain nursing procedures are taught to the family, they are no longer considered skilled procedures and are not reimbursable under Medicare. For example, injecting insulin is not considered skilled because most diabetics can inject insulin themselves. Teaching how to draw up the insulin and inject it properly, however, is considered skilled because teaching is considered a skilled activity. Once the injection skill is learned, the injection itself is no longer a skilled activity according to the Medicare definition. Also, procedures such as enema administration, unsterile dressing changes, care of small wounds, and administration of eye drops are not usually considered skilled because they can be performed safely by most people.

Specialty Home Care

The number of high-technology cases in the home has increased dramatically with patients who need intravenous therapy or are ventilator dependent.

Intravenous therapy

Rising hospital costs and the development of reliable intravenous pumps have stimulated the growth of intravenous therapy in the home. The most common intravenous therapies provided in the home are hydration, antibiotics, pain control, total parenteral nutrition, and chemotherapy. Many different types of intravenous lines may be used (see Chapter 16). Nurses should be familiar with the devices commonly used in their communities. Chemotherapy drugs are almost always given through central lines by registered nurses. LVNs/LPNs must know their role and limitations in relation to all intravenous therapy.

High-technology therapies add to the complexity of home health care. Home care may be more cost effective than a hospital stay, but it also significantly increases the risk to the client and the liability of the home health agency. Agency policies and procedures should be current and specific enough to guide the nurse in managing the provision of intravenous therapy in the home. These policies protect not only the agency and the patient, but also the nurse.

The safe and successful provision of any high-technology therapy in the home depends on the commitment of everyone involved. Families must be capable of understanding what is required and have the time to participate fully in the patient's care. Nurses delivering this type of care must be thoroughly trained in the procedures and use of equipment required in these therapies. Agencies must have appropriate staff to provide care at any time if needed, including days, evenings, nights, holidays, and weekends. The pharmacy or intravenous therapy company must provide high-quality products and support to both the nurse and the family. Finally, physicians must be closely involved and available to respond to emergency problems.

The nurse's role in the delivery of high-technology care in the home includes skilled observation and assessment, the performance of skilled procedures, and teaching. Skilled observation and assessment in the delivery of intravenous therapy includes determining the adequacy of the home environment and the patient's and the family's knowledge regarding care procedures. The intravenous access site must be inspected for swelling and redness. Any side effects of the treatment should be noted, along with the family's level of comfort with performing specific procedures.

Skilled procedures with home intravenous therapy include changing access site dressings and performing venipunctures. Because home care nurses are not instantly available 24 hours a day, some procedures must be taught to the family.

Ventilator therapy

Ventilator-dependent patients are increasingly being cared for in the home setting. This type of care is complex and should be provided only by nurses and caregivers specifically trained in the use of necessary equipment and procedures. In many instances, the care of ventilator-dependent patients in the home is coordinated by the respiratory therapist. The home care nurse seeing the patient should be aware of policies and procedures followed by the respiratory therapy company, be familiar with respiratory therapy equipment, and be certified in cardiopulmonary resuscitation.

Initial assessment of the home environment includes an assessment of all factors important in other high-technology therapies, with the addition of an assessment of the electrical and structural condition of the home. This information is important to ensure proper functioning of the equipment and necessary backup generators.

As with intravenous therapy, committed family members or other caregivers must be available. In this case, the commitment is for around-the-clock observation. Physicians and respiratory therapists must be on call for any problems.

Communication Among Home Health Care Team Members

The importance of the team approach in home health care cannot be overemphasized. Quality home care requires the collaboration of several disciplines. Because these disciplines may provide their services in the home at different times, communication among health care team members is necessary if effective collaboration is to occur. Interdisciplinary communication is accomplished through clear, detailed documentation and case conferences.

Documentation

In any interdisciplinary work, the actions of one discipline often depend on the actions of another. A nurse's discovery of an unused walker in the corner of a room may prompt the physical therapist to recommend strengthening exercises and gait training. A social worker's attempts to find funding for a patient's medications may reveal that the patient is fearful of taking pain medications, which can be addressed by the nurse. If these concerns are not communicated, however, they will not be addressed. Most quality-of-care problems in home health care can be attributed to failure to communicate patient care problems. Most of the time, these problems result from either incomplete documentation or failure to keep the nursing case manager informed. Documentation of nursing care should be accurate, complete, and submitted in a timely manner.

As mentioned earlier, reimbursement for home health nursing visits depends on clear documentation of the patient's homebound status, the skilled nature of the services provided, and the medical need for the services. Failure to provide such documentation often results in denial of reimbursement by Medicare. Denials of reimbursement have serious consequences for the patient, family, and home health agency; when excessive, denials have resulted in agencies going out of business.

Case conferences

Clear documentation of interdisciplinary case conferences can go a long way toward preventing reimbursement denials based on lack of medical necessity. These conferences often provide detailed information about the complexity of problems that justifies increased visits.

Usually, a home health nurse must report to a patient's case manager, who is responsible for admitting the patient, establishing the plan of care (including visit frequencies), and coordinating the efforts of other disciplines. The case manager schedules periodic formal case conferences in which all disciplines work together to solve clinical problems. The details of these conferences are documented in the patient's record.

In addition to these regularly scheduled conferences, the case manager should be kept informed of any changes in the response of the patient or family to the plan of care. For example, significant changes in vital signs, weight, and wound parameters are important physiologic indications for a call to the case manager. A change in the home environment, such as an absence of family caregivers, deterioration in sanitation, or signs of patient neglect or abuse, should also prompt a call to the case manager.

Communication by the case manager is also important. Field nurses have the right to expect clear and current information regarding recent changes in physicians' orders, current laboratory information, and the availability of documentation by other nurses and disciplines. High-quality patient care cannot be accomplished without meticulous communication from all disciplines involved in the care of the patient.

REHABILITATION

The acute phase of many illnesses is often followed by a prolonged chronic phase, which may last from days to years and may involve the delivery of a number of health care services in a variety of settings, such as rehabilitation centers, long-term care facilities, outpatient facilities, group residential homes, and, increasingly, the patient's own home. Rehabilitation focuses on restoring maximal possible function after illness or injury.

REHABILITATION CONCEPTS

Rehabilitation is a Process of Restoration

Rehabilitation is the process of restoring an individual to the best possible health and functioning after a physical or mental impairment. The type of assistance provided allows people to care for themselves as much as possible. Inherent in this process is a commitment by the caregiver to provide the care and support that foster the client's independence.

Impairment is a Disturbance in Functioning

Impairment refers to a disturbance in functioning that may be either physical or psychologic. An example of physical impairment is paralysis of an arm or leg as the result of a stroke. Mental impairment such as loss of memory may occur as a result of Alzheimer disease. In either case, a loss of function occurs.

Disability is a Measurable Loss of Function

The term **disability** generally refers to a measurable loss of function and is usually delineated to indicate a diminished capacity for work. For example, individuals with an injured back may be classified as 50% disabled, meaning that they are incapable of doing 50% of their jobs. This type of measurable loss of function allows for specific reductions in work responsibility or may indicate the compensation to which a worker may be entitled.

Handicap is an Inability to Perform Daily Activities

The term **handicap** means that an individual is not able to perform one or more normal activities of daily living (ADLs) because of a mental or physical disability. For example, the person who experienced a stroke may be handicapped in driving a car because of the related paralysis.

Remember that disability and handicap are not the same things. A person can be moderately disabled but still manage to perform routine daily activities. People who were born without arms are often able to perform all essential ADL by using their feet and certain assistive devices. Although these people are disabled, they are not handicapped. Impairments and their resulting disabilities may not be reversible, but handicaps often can be prevented or reduced with modifications of the environment and a community attitude that seeks to promote the abilities of the disabled (see the Cultural Considerations box.)

Cultural Considerations

What Does Culture Have to Do With Disabilities?

Research shows that minority groups in the United States are more vulnerable to health problems, including disabilities. Health care providers and agencies are working to raise awareness and to learn more about the physical health of minorities with disabilities, their ability to access health care, the process of becoming disabled among people in minority groups, and barriers to using rehabilitation facilities and other resources.

LEVELS OF DISABILITY

According to the Americans with Disabilities Act (ADA), "individuals with disabilities are defined as those with a physical or mental impairment that substantially limits one or more major life activities" (ADA, 1990). An effort has been made to quantify the degree or extend of disability.

A disability is often classified by level to determine its impact on an individual's quality of life and appropriate levels of compensation:

- Level I: slight limitation in one or more ADL; usually able to work
- Level II: moderate limitation in one or more ADL; able to work but the workplace may need modifications
- Level III: severe limitation in one or more ADL; unable to work
- Level IV: total disability characterized by nearly complete dependence on others for assistance with ADL; unable to work

GOALS OF REHABILITATION

Rehabilitation aims to return the disabled individual to the highest possible level of functioning. The specific goals are to promote self-care, maximize independence, restore and maintain optimal function, prevent complications, and encourage adaptation. The rehabilitation team must treat the "whole" patient, meaning that it must consider not just the patient's physical condition but also the emotional state and psychologic and social needs of both the patient and the family.

Return of Function

The goal of return of function includes the restoration of as much function as possible in traditional ADL, such as bathing, dressing, eating, toileting, and walking. Ideal functioning includes independence in the instrumental activities of daily living (IADLs) as well, such as preparing meals, shopping, doing laundry, and using the telephone. The ultimate goal of rehabilitation is to live independently. Full independence implies a return to employment status. Not all patients can be restored to their previous state, but they can learn to adapt to the changes they have experienced, which requires emphasis on abilities rather than disabilities. Instead of focusing on what is lost, the patient and the care providers must focus on what remains.

Prevention of Further Disability

Rehabilitation also involves the prevention of further disability (secondary disability) that may potentially be caused by the patient's primary disability. Examples include prevention of problems in stroke patients such as pneumonia, pressure injuries, and limb contractures, which are often caused by lack of mobility. Attention to safety concerns also reduces the risk of further disability. For example, a walker and environmental modifications may be advised for a poststroke patient who is at risk for falls and fractures. The nurse plays a key role in the prevention of secondary disability.

Rehabilitation is a long-term process that requires the commitment of both the patient and the family. The process is often difficult and marked by periods of progress followed by occasional relapses in functional disability. These relapses can be frustrating to everyone involved and require determination on the part of the family, as well as patience and understanding by the nurse. The rehabilitation process can place additional burdens on family members when roles once filled by the disabled family member must be filled by other family members. Attention is frequently focused on the disabled member, leaving other family members feeling neglected. Ongoing family problems may intensify during this time, making the rehabilitation process even more difficult.

An important aspect when caring for a disabled patient is to be aware of the attitudes and behaviors of all family members. In many instances, families can be assisted in adjusting to role changes that occur during the rehabilitation process. The more consistently patients and family are involved in the process, the more likely it is that success will occur. Involvement in goal setting and a clear explanation of patient and family roles in daily rehabilitation activities help families to understand better the challenges of the process. This approach gives a sense of control and increases family strength.

LEGISLATION

Public attitudes toward people with disabilities play a significant role in the degree of handicap experienced by the disabled. Lack of knowledge about a disability often causes the public to react negatively to people who appear disabled. Individuals who are blind are sometimes treated as though they are deaf as well. People with conditions such as cerebral palsy that affect speech and muscle control are often treated as though they have cognitive impairment. Some employers are reluctant to hire disabled workers, fearing an increase in insurance rates or negative reactions from their customers (see the Health Promotion box).

Health Promotion

Help Disabled Patients Understand Their Employment Rights Under the Americans With Disabilities Act

- Nurses and other providers should understand basic laws that affect their patients' well-being even after they leave the health care setting. One of the most important pieces of health care legislation to be passed in recent decades is the Americans with Disabilities Act of 1990.
- Title 1 of the Act prohibits private employers with 15 or more employees, state and local governments, employment agencies, and labor unions from discriminating against qualified individuals with disabilities. An employer is required to accommodate the disability of a qualified applicant or employee if doing so would not impose an undue hardship on the employer's business. However, an employer is not required to lower quality or production standards to make an accommodation. The employer is also not obligated to provide personal use items such as glasses and hearing aids.
- Employers may not ask job applicants about the existence, nature, or severity of a disability. They are allowed to ask applicants about their ability to perform specific job functions. A job offer may be made on the condition that the applicant passes a medical examination but only if the examination is required for all newly hired employees in similar jobs. These medical examinations must be job related and consistent with the employer's business needs. To learn more, visit the website for the Equal Employment Commission at www.eeoc.gov.

The federal government has passed laws over the years to protect the rights of the disabled. The first law passed to aid the rehabilitation of World War I servicemen was the Vocational Rehabilitation Act of 1920. This law provided job training for injured veterans.

The Social Security Act of 1935 provided additional aid to states for both direct relief and vocational rehabilitation. The Rehabilitation Act of 1973, however, provided a comprehensive approach to problems experienced by the disabled. This Act not only expanded available resources for vocational training, but also defined services to be included in rehabilitation programs. It also began affirmative action programs to assist in the employment of the disabled and prohibited discrimination against the disabled in programs receiving federal funds. In 1990 the Americans with Disabilities Act was passed. This law extended the protection given to the disabled in the public sector by the Rehabilitation Act of 1973 to the private sector as well. It was designed to give the disabled full access to housing, employment, transportation, and communications. As a result of this law, any business endeavor designed to serve the public must ensure that its services are accessible to the disabled. In many cases, this requirement involves the installation of wheelchair ramps, the construction of restrooms that can accommodate wheelchairs, and the provision for communication services for the hearing and speech impaired. Public transportation authorities must ensure that buses, train cars, and concession shops are all accessible to the disabled. Businesses with fewer than 15 employees are currently exempt from many of the law's provisions. This law has prompted significant progress toward improving the quality of life of many disabled people.

REHABILITATION TEAM

Nurses who care for disabled clients must consider the whole person when planning interventions. Difficulties in physical functioning may affect many aspects of a person's life and require the coordinated services of a significant number of health care professionals to enable the individual to stay well and prevent complications or injuries.

The case of Mr. T. provides a good example of the kinds of expertise and the number of services that may be required during rehabilitation.

Mr. T., age 82 years, suffered a left-sided brain hemorrhage 3 weeks ago. Because of this injury, he was unable to speak or use his right arm or leg. He was also incontinent of urine and exhibited some right-sided facial paralysis. After 5 days in the hospital, care providers determined that Mr. T.'s condition had stabilized, and he was transferred to a rehabilitation facility to continue the rehabilitation process. At this time, his speech had returned but was slurred and halting. He had minimal movement in his right arm and leg but was still unable to walk or feed himself. The incontinence of urine persisted, and he had several reddened areas on his right hip and coccyx. Before his injury, Mr. T. had been living with only his wife of 55 years, who also was in poor health. They had no family living in the state, and she was quite concerned about how she would care for him once he was sent home.

When trying to comprehend all that is involved in helping Mr. T. to return to full functioning (if that is possible), the nurse should first imagine a typical day in the T. household and identify all the ADL and IADL competencies required to get through the day. Next, the types of people and services that may be necessary to prevent further injury and to increase functioning should be considered. At a minimum, the rehabilitation team will consist of the patient's wife, personal physician, rehabilitation physician, and rehabilitation nurse. Other likely members include the physical therapist, who assists the patient in all aspects of mobility from regaining strength and function in the extremities to the use of assistive devices such as crutches and walkers; the occupational therapist, who assists the patient with regaining fine-motor skills necessary for dressing, eating, and grooming; the speech therapist, who assists the patient in regaining swallowing or speaking functions; and the social worker, who may assist with coordinating resources for placement in the home or a convalescent facility after discharge. In other situations, the rehabilitation team might also include a clinical nurse specialist in rehabilitation nursing, a psychologist, a recreational therapist, and a vocational counselor.

The nurse's concern at this time should be that of becoming an effective member of the rehabilitation team. The successful resolution of rehabilitation problems often depends on the ability of health care workers to consider how the individual functions within the family and to work closely with other health professionals toward a common goal. If this goal is to be achieved, good communication skills are essential, which entail clear, specific documentation of the patient's functional deficits and abilities and active participation in multidisciplinary conferences to resolve patient problems.

APPROACHES TO REHABILITATION

Perhaps the most important goal of successful rehabilitation of a disabled person is independence. This fact is sometimes forgotten when a caregiver sees the slow, agonizing attempts to move an arm or a leg. The tendency is to do for patients that which is difficult for them to accomplish on their own. Occasionally, patients need to be helped to complete a task, especially when they become increasingly frustrated. However, caregivers who intervene too soon encourage dependence and delay rehabilitation. Rehabilitation patients should be cheerfully encouraged to do as much as possible for themselves. Praise for accomplishing a task should be given promptly and caregivers should reflect continuing optimism about the patient's progress.

Health professionals sometimes plan comprehensive programs of rehabilitation without much thought as to how the program will be implemented once the patient returns home. To be effective, the program should commence immediately after an injury and should involve the patient and family from the outset.

Failure to involve the family in establishing goals and strategies often produces family dependence, just as doing too many things for the patient produces individual dependence.

Rehabilitation nurses undertake several roles, all designed to assist the patient and family in returning to a high level of functioning. These roles include care planner, teacher, caregiver, counselor, coordinator, and advocate. As in-home health care, the medical-surgical nurse brings a wealth of knowledge and skill but must learn to make adaptations consistent with the rehabilitation approach.

In the home setting, nurses can best assist patients and families by helping them to adjust their activities to accommodate the disability (Fig. 2.2). Even though families may have been taught care routines in a previous setting, routines must often be adapted to the new setting and prioritized differently. In this role, the nurse is an expert caregiver and teacher. Problem-solving sessions often identify ways in which care routines can be adapted to the realities of the home setting. Caregivers may not have thought through changes in sleeping arrangements, how they will transport the patient for follow-up office visits, or how to plan for periodic relief from their caregiver role. Nurses can help families to anticipate these predictable stress points and plan realistically for how they will handle them.

Nurses should also be prepared to handle a wide variety of patient and family emotions, ranging from extreme optimism to depression. At these times, families need a great deal of support and may need the assistance of outside community support systems. Local support groups can often be very effective in helping families to respond appropriately to the stresses of a disabled family member. Professional organizations such as the Association of Rehabilitation Nurses can be an invaluable resource to nurses working in the rehabilitation field.

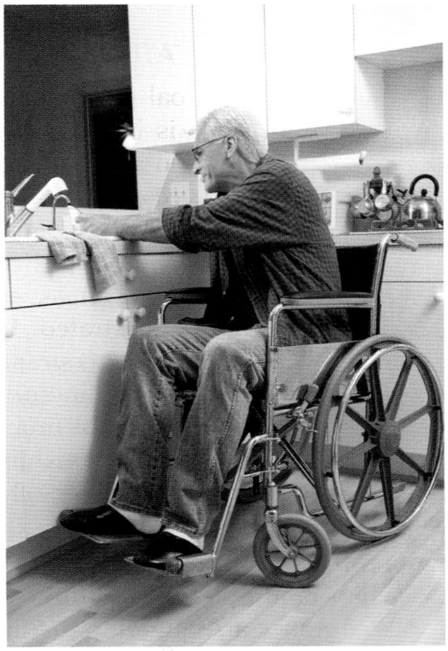

Fig. 2.2 An important nursing role in home health care is to teach patients to care for themselves. (Copyright © Jupiterimages/Stockbyte/Thinkstock.com.)

LONG-TERM CARE

Long-term care is provided in a variety of settings, such as personal homes, board and care homes, supportive housing facilities, assisted living centers, continuing care retirement communities (CCRCs), and nursing homes. In the United States, approximately 16,000 nursing homes have been certified by both Medicare and Medicaid to provide residential skilled nursing care. The great majority of these are freestanding facilities, with the others being hospital-based entities. Several thousand other nursing facilities exist that are not certified or are certified only by either Medicaid or Medicare. After an acute care hospitalization of at least 3 days, Medicare covers 100 days per event in a skilled nursing facility.

The United States population in certified nursing homes is approximately 1.4 million people. Many people think only of older persons in institutional settings when they think of long-term care settings. Long-term care services, however, are required by people of all ages who are temporarily or permanently unable to function independently. Approximately 15% of nursing home residents are younger than 65 years. Thus long-term care refers to a range of services that address the health, personal care, and social needs of all people who lack some ability necessary for self-care. The number of older adults who live in institutions actually comprises a relatively small percentage of older adults; many more live with extended families or by themselves. Unfortunately, a significant number of older adults who live alone are poor and live in inadequate housing, often without adequate heat, ventilation, food, or telephones. Eventually, problems with mobility and mental functioning force many older adults into long-term care.

RISKS FOR INSTITUTIONALIZATION

With nearly 50 million U.S. citizens over the age of 65 years, only about 4.2% are residing in a nursing home at any given time. The main reason for institutionalization, however, is not age. The best indicator of who will need nursing home placement is ADL dependency. As the number of ADL limitations increases, the likelihood of residing in a nursing home rises; half of older adults with five or six ADL limitations reside there. This figure highlights the fact that if home care services were available to assist older adults in meeting more ADL needs, costly residential care might be delayed. Individual characteristics associated with increased risk of nursing home residency include age 85 years and older, female gender, Caucasian race, cognitive impairment, functional dependence, and reliance on Medicaid. The long-term care resident today has more medical diagnoses and functional limitations than in the past. This trend has important implications for staffing these facilities. Among long-term care residents, the most common medical diagnoses are heart disease, stroke, diabetes mellitus, depression, and dementia.

Other factors bearing on who requires nursing home care include financial resources, whether the person lives alone or with family, the presence of mental illness, the type of disease process, and the degree of social support.

LEVELS OF CARE

Modern long-term residential care consists of four levels: (1) domiciliary care, (2) personal care homes, (3) intermediate care, and (4) skilled care. In many instances, one type of facility will offer more than one level of care (usually skilled and intermediate); however, in most states, institutions must have approval for whatever levels of care they plan to provide.

Domiciliary Care Homes

Facilities providing basic room, board, and supervision are sometimes called **domiciliary care** homes. In this arrangement, 24-hour care is not provided, and residents usually come and go as they please. The Domiciliary Care Program in the Department of Veterans' Affairs provides not only living quarters but also a variety of rehabilitation and treatment services.

Personal Care Homes

Personal care homes provide medically ordered medications and treatments, supervise residents in self-medication, and provide three or more personal services. Two types of personal care homes have been established. A personal care home with nursing (nursing care home) must employ at least one registered or licensed nurse; no more than one half of the residents receive nursing care. A personal care home without nursing has no residents who are receiving nursing care.

Intermediate Care Facilities

Intermediate care facilities provide custodial care at a level usually associated with nursing homes. Patients at this level often need assistance with two to three ADL (Fig. 2.3). Facilities offering this level of care must have personnel available 24 hours a day. They are not considered by the government to be medical facilities and thus receive no reimbursement under Medicare. Many of these facilities do, however, receive the bulk of their financing under Medicaid. Federal regulations require a registered nurse to serve as director of nursing and an LVN/LPN to be on duty for at least 8 hours a day.

Skilled Nursing Facilities

Skilled nursing facilities must have skilled health professionals present around the clock. The care of patients in skilled nursing facilities must be supervised by a physician and requires the services of a registered nurse, physical therapist, or speech therapist.

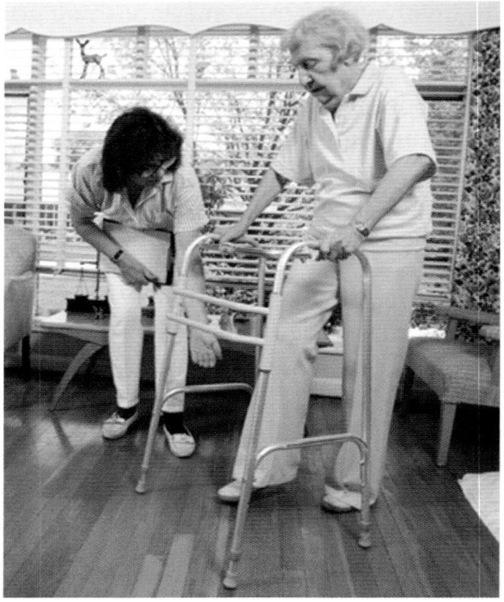

Fig. 2.3 Patients in intermediate care facilities often need assistance with activities of daily living. (From Potter P, Perry A, Stockert P, Hall A, editors: *Fundamentals of nursing*, ed 8, St. Louis, 2013, Mosby Elsevier.)

IMPACT OF RELOCATION

Relocation to a long-term care facility is rarely easy. In the best of circumstances, patients, families, and health professionals anticipate the possible future need for long-term care, set aside funds for that purpose, and make plans that are acceptable to everyone involved. Then when patients cannot make sound decisions for themselves, families seek help from extended family members and professionals in making decisions for long-term care placement. More commonly, however, the situation is quite different. A crisis situation often precipitates the decision. A sole caregiver may become ill, leaving the care of the disabled elder to the extended family members who may be either unable or unwilling to continue care. Patients may suddenly become physically or mentally incapable of caring for themselves or making their own decisions. Family members frequently feel guilty for considering institutional care. Few know very much about modern long-term care facilities and have not investigated potential placement.

In this situation, home health nurses, social workers, and other health professionals must work closely with the family to defuse the crisis situation and provide realistic options from which the family may choose. This time is when families need the utmost support and acceptance. Simply clarifying the situation, affirming the family's caring and concern, and pointing out realistic options will often return a family to effective functioning.

If relocation to a long-term care facility is the only logical choice, the patient and family must be prepared for the move. Research has shown that the more prepared the patient is, the better the adjustment will be. Preparation includes providing as much choice as possible for the patient and responding to patient questions and concerns. If possible, choices of facility, room location, types of personal belongings, and room decor are helpful, as are tours of the facility before entering. Also helpful is a professional staff member who can check on the new patient frequently during the first few weeks. Patients should be introduced to other residents with similar interests and invited or assisted to participate in appropriate activities.

EFFECTS OF RELOCATION TO A LONG-TERM CARE FACILITY

The response to moving into a long-term care facility varies with the individual resident. Positive effects can include improved nutrition, socialization, and management of medical problems. With support and assistance, the resident's overall function may improve. Other effects of institutionalization are predictable and must be considered in helping the new nursing home resident adjust to the surroundings. Frequently observed effects include depersonalization, indignity, redefinition of "normal," regression, and social withdrawal.

Depersonalization

Depersonalization plays a major part in long-term care settings. Caregivers often know little of a resident's life history and therefore treat individual residents in light of their diagnosis or dysfunctional behavior patterns. The case study (Box 2.1) about Herman and Kristina illustrates this point.

One way to help see the resident of a long-term care facility as a whole person with past relationships, accomplishments, and interests is to ask family members to bring in photographs. The photographs may have been taken on significant occasions, such as on graduation or wedding days, or they may be simple family pictures that depict the older person's place in the family or community. The photographs can be mounted on poster board or placed on a bulletin board in the resident's room. This effort helps caregivers to see more than a frail, weak, older person and can open up conversation that encourages reminiscing, which is a therapeutic means of dealing with one's past life and preparing for death.

Indignity

Indignity is another effect of institutionalization. Residents may have to request help with routine activities such as toileting and obtaining food and drink. The prompt fulfillment of the request sometimes depends on the relationship between the patient and the caregiver. Residents of long-term care facilities may be exposed unnecessarily, especially when caregivers enter rooms without knocking. Simple courtesies such as using a person's title and last name, knocking before entering the room, and draping during care activities help the resident to maintain dignity. A useful exercise would be to consider: "How would I want to be treated if I were weak and frail and could not do the things that I can do for myself now?"

Assistive personnel are important members of the nursing care team in long-term care. Because they provide much personal care, the LVN/LPN should know what tasks can be assigned to them. Also the

Box 2.1 Case Study

I don't think I truly understood what depersonalization was until I met Herman. Herman and his wife, Kristina, lived alone in a small house in a northwestern city. Herman was 62 years old and had Alzheimer disease. I met them while working as a home health nurse. I was asked to look into respite services to help relieve Kristina of the strain of caring for Herman. I remember my first impression of Herman, formed after reading his chart and talking to the staff nurse about his care problems. He was starting to neglect his personal appearance. The staff nurse said he often put soup on the stove for lunch then went out to the garden to tend his flowers, forgetting about the soup. This and other images of his functioning created in me a picture of an incompetent and helpless old man.

Over a period of weeks, Kristina shared many stories with me about who this man was, what he cared about, how they had met, and her deep devotion to her husband of 35 years. Gradually, I was able to see the distorted image I held. Herman was an Olympic gold medal skier from Austria who came to this country as a young man. He held several jobs as a ski instructor and repaired ski equipment until he met and married Kristina and moved to the northwestern United States to become the owner and manager of a small ski resort. He was tall and muscular, with an easy smile and a kind word for everyone. He was admired by many in the community for his skill as a skier and his friendliness. He was a good father and family man who was known as "the rock" because all of his family and friends relied on him for advice and assistance.

Over a period of 5 years, Herman had become more and more forgetful, less talkative, and often preoccupied with household tasks that he would start but not complete. He also failed to recognize many of his close friends and, at times, would wander off downtown without knowing why or where he was going. Throughout this, Kristina remained fiercely devoted to Herman, although the strain of the caregiver role was beginning to affect her health. "He cared for us for so many years. Now it is my turn to care for him."

I was surprised at how my view of Herman changed as I learned more about him. I was seeing him as dependent, helpless, and a burden to his small and frail wife—a view created by my observations of his behavior and what I knew of the Alzheimer disease process. A view that changed radically once I knew more about Herman. I doubt I will ever minimize the importance of learning about the whole patient again.

LVN/LPN must verify the skills of assistive personnel, provide guidance as needed, and participate in their evaluation.

Redefinition of "Normal"

Behaviors that were considered normal in one's home may be labeled abnormal or be unacceptable in a long-term care facility. Watching television at 3:00 AM, loud singing, or sexual activity may be frowned upon, depending on the residence's rules and routines. Although consideration of others is important, giving residents of long-term care facilities some flexibility and some measure of control in their daily lives is also important.

Regression

Over time, a resident's physical, mental, and social abilities may be lost because of disuse. If people are left in bed for a greater part of the day, it soon becomes impossible for them to walk. If visits from friends and relatives are few, the skill of conversation may also be lost. Encouraging independence and social interaction as much as possible is important. Avoid infantilizing older patients. Although simplifying language and activities for those who are cognitively impaired may be necessary, avoid baby talk.

Social Withdrawal

If a resident never leaves the nursing home or if family visits are few and include little discussion of the outside world, the institution can become a barrier, cutting off interest and participation in the outside world. If this situation is allowed to continue, life in the facility becomes, for many patients, their entire world. They tend to withdraw into the boundaries of their own room (see the Cultural Considerations box). Nurses can help by conversing with residents about events inside and outside the nursing home. When you know your patients well, you can bring up news that you expect will be of interest to them. Discussion of current events in small groups can broaden the resident's horizons.

Cultural Considerations

What Does Culture Have to Do With Social Withdrawal?

Most facilities are dominated by a single culture that is reflected in mealtimes, social mores, religious services, and holiday traditions. Consider how a person from a different culture might feel in this setting.

PRINCIPLES OF LONG-TERM RESIDENTIAL CARE

Long-term residential care has been called *custodial care*. By definition, custodial care refers to personal care that provides assistance with ADLs; it is not covered by Medicare. The term custodial care invokes passive images such as maintenance, warehousing, or waiting to die. Some people have called such facilities "heaven's waiting rooms." Publicized abuses by some nursing homes are at least partly responsible for negative stereotypes of long-term residential care. However, long-term care facilities in general have changed substantially in recent years. Although some continue to provide care of questionable quality, many excellent facilities do exist.

Modern facilities care for individuals with a wide array of medical and surgical problems. People who reside in long-term care facilities are commonly referred to as *residents* rather than patients. Not all residents are admitted for permanent stays in the facility. In many communities, the nursing home has become a convalescent hospital for older persons who have recently undergone surgical procedures, such as repair of a fractured hip. These acute cases often strain already limited resources. Many individuals are admitted for short stays that are prompted by care demands that temporarily overwhelm the family. Illness of a family caregiver also can result in temporary admission to the facility. When the home situation has stabilized, these residents often return home. Increasingly, those admitted for long stays are older adults with mental health problems. In these cases, the family has exhausted most of its physical, emotional, and financial resources and home care is no longer feasible.

When a person is admitted to a long-term care facility, the care delivered should be based on three principles: (1) promotion of independence, (2) maintenance of function, and (3) maintenance of autonomy.

Put On Your Thinking Cap!

If you have a clinical experience in a long-term care facility, interview a resident there. Specifically, ask:

1. What circumstances brought you here to live?
2. What are the benefits and disadvantages of living in this type of facility?
3. What advice would you give to a new resident here?
4. What can nurses do to make adjustment to living here easier?

Discuss the resident's responses in relation to the effects of institutionalization and implications for nurses.

Promotion of Independence

Successful relocation to a long-term care facility depends, in part, on the ability of patients to do things for themselves and on the involvement of families to keep the family member in contact with the outside world. Feeding residents rather than spending time encouraging residents to feed themselves may be tempting for institutional caregivers. When the workday is a never-ending series of tasks, doing things quickly often takes priority over promoting independence. Watch for this type of behavior and try to restructure assignments of nursing assistants to reward the promotion of independence. This effort can be accomplished by setting specific goals for each resident that encourage independent functioning. Then, explain to the staff members how their efforts can contribute to the goal. Involvement of staff in this way often produces results.

Maintenance of Function

In many cases, loss of function prevents an older person from staying at home. Health professionals who are disease oriented often concentrate on the disease process at the expense of a functional assessment. An incontinent resident may be incorrectly perceived as having a complication of the aging process. This kind of thinking fosters an emphasis on maintenance care, leading to efforts to prevent skin breakdown by frequent changes of clothing and linens. A more thorough assessment would begin with the determination of possible causes of the incontinence. A functional assessment explores factors that might be responsible for the incontinence. Immobility may be the basic problem. Questions to ask include: Is the resident normally mobile? If so, does the room have a light that facilitates locating the bathroom? Is the resident able to manage clothing for independent toileting? Viewing this problem as a functional problem may lead to simple solutions, such as placing a light in the room at night or a urinal next to the bed. Interventions, whenever possible, should focus on restoring and preserving function.

Maintenance of Autonomy

Most people value control over their lives. Successful relocation to a long-term care facility depends on preserving as much autonomy as possible. Older adults who participate in selecting the facility adjust better than those who have no choice in the matter.

Allowing as much flexibility as possible in establishing a routine for the new resident is also important. Choices in activities, such as when to have a bath or how late to watch television, go a long way toward preserving the autonomy and self-esteem of the resident. As much as possible, encourage the resident to assist in establishing care goals. For example, the frequency and duration of exercise and goals for weight loss or gain require the facility resident's commitment. Mutually established goals are more likely to be achieved than those selected for the resident.

Families also have a role in maintaining autonomy in the resident. Autonomy depends on knowing one's place in the world and what roles one still holds in the family structure. Families who relate to their older adult members by stressing their importance in the family and keeping them up to date on family happenings and decisions reinforce the idea that the person remains a valued family member who simply resides at another address.

Put On Your Thinking Cap!

Identify one thing you can do to achieve each of the following: (1) maintain autonomy, (2) maintain function, and (3) promote independence in:

1. The long-term care facility resident
2. The hospitalized patient
3. The homebound patient

ASSISTED LIVING

Assisted living facilities provide an alternative to nursing home care. These facilities are residences that provide self-contained living units for individuals who live independently but have on-site access to support if needed at any time. Typical services include congregate meals, recreation, housekeeping and laundry, social services, transportation, help with ADL (but not full-time nursing care), and some health-related services such as medication management. Medicare and Medicaid do not pay for assisted living care.

CONTINUING CARE RETIREMENT COMMUNITIES

CCRCs usually have various living options ranging from independent quarters, to assisted living, to skilled nursing units. As residents age, they may need to move from one level of care to another. In most CCRCs, residents pay an entry fee as well as monthly fees that may vary as the level of care changes. Medicare and Medicaid do not pay for CCRCs, except in the skilled nursing areas.

SUPPORTIVE HOUSING PROGRAMS

The federal and state governments have programs that offer low-cost housing to low-income older adults. The range of services varies but may include housekeeping, laundry, and shopping. With these supports, some older adults can continue to live independently despite some medical conditions and functional impairments.

OTHER PATIENT CARE SETTINGS

The settings addressed in this chapter represent many of those that traditionally employ licensed nurses. Other employment settings include clinics, physicians' offices, and schools, as well as adult day centers, respite care, hospices, and correctional facilities. Each setting presents unique experiences and challenges. In some of these settings, the LVN/LPN may be the only licensed nursing professional on site. Therefore the nurse's responsibilities must be clearly defined and consistent with legal functions.

Get Ready for the NCLEX® Examination!

Key Points

- The changing health care system has greatly increased the number and types of health care settings.
- Medical-surgical nurses have the knowledge and skills to work in numerous settings.
- Community health nurses work with individuals and aggregates (groups) to improve the health of the entire community.
- Traditional community health nursing focuses on (1) improving the health status of communities or groups of people (called *aggregates*) through public education, (2) screening for early detection of disease, and (3) providing services for people who need care outside the acute care setting.
- Public health is concerned with promoting and protecting the health of populations.
- The main difference between home health care nursing and public health nursing is that home health care is more focused on providing direct care to patients.
- A major nursing function in home health care is teaching patients and families to care for themselves so as to promote independent functioning.
- Medicare is a major source of home health care funding.
- To receive Medicare reimbursement for home health care, four conditions must be met: (1) the physician has determined the need for home care and has made or authorized a plan for home care; (2) the patient needs intermittent skilled nursing care, or physical or speech-language therapy; (3) the patient is homebound; and (4) the agency providing the care is Medicare certified.
- Specialty home care services include high-technology interventions (the provision of intravenous therapy and ventilator therapy), hospice services, pediatric care, and mental health care.
- The most common intravenous therapies provided in the home are hydration, antibiotics, pain control, total parenteral nutrition, and chemotherapy.
- The role of the LVN/LPN in planning home health care is to participate in patient data collection, contribute to the development and revision of the care plan, and to assign and evaluate assistive personnel.
- The LVN/LPN who works in home health settings must be aware of the legal scope of practice in their state, as well as agency policies.
- After certain nursing procedures such as insulin injection are taught to the family, they are no longer considered skilled procedures and are not reimbursable under Medicare.
- In addition to regular scheduled conferences, the case manager should be kept informed of any changes in the response of the patient or family to the plan of care.
- Rehabilitation focuses on restoring maximal possible function after illness or injury.
- Impairment is a disturbance in functioning; disability is a measurable loss of function; and handicap is an inability to perform daily activities.
- The Americans with Disabilities Act of 1990 is designed to protect the rights of persons with disabilities in employment situations.
- Perhaps the most important goal of successful rehabilitation of a disabled person is independence.
- Rehabilitation is the process of restoring an individual to the best possible health and functioning following a physical or mental impairment and the prevention of further disability.
- Caring for disabled patients requires the coordinated services of a large number of health care professionals to help patients stay as healthy as possible and prevent complications or injuries.
- As an effective member of a multidisciplinary rehabilitation team, the nurse is a care planner, teacher, caregiver, counselor, coordinator, and advocate.
- Health care workers must consider the way in which a disabled individual functions within the family, and the patient and family should be involved from the outset in determining the plan of care.
- Dependence in ADL is the best indicator of who will need nursing home placement.
- Modern long-term residential care exists in four levels: (1) domiciliary care, (2) personal care homes, (3) intermediate care, and (4) skilled care.
- Alternatives to nursing home care include assisted living facilities, supportive housing programs, and continuing care retirement communities.
- Frequently observed effects of relocation to a long-term care facility include depersonalization, indignity, redefinition of "normal," regression, and social withdrawal.
- The key principles of long-term care are: (1) promotion of independence, (2) maintenance of function, and (3) maintenance of autonomy.
- The responsibilities of the LVN/LPN must be clearly defined and consistent with legal functions regardless of the employment location.

Additional Learning Resources

SG Go to your Study Guide for additional learning activities to help you master this chapter content.

Go to your Evolve website (http://evolve.elsevier.com/Linton/medsurg) for the following learning resources and much more:

- Interactive Prioritization Exercises
- Fluid and Electrolyte Tutorial
- Pharmacology Tutorial
- Review Questions for the NCLEX® Examination

Online Resource

http://www.medicare.gov/publications

Clinical Judgment and Next-Generation NCLEX® Examination-Style Questions

1. **A home health nurse performed all the following activities listed with Medicare patients. Which activities are reimbursable? (Select all that apply).**
   1. Used sterile technique to clean and dress a large wound
   2. Took a frail older couple for a short walk to provide exercise
   3. Performed a venipuncture to obtain a blood sample for laboratory tests
   4. Taught a patient with recently diagnosed diabetes how to inject insulin
   5. Removed outdated food from the refrigerator and pantry

   NCLEX Client Need: Safe and Effective Care Environment: Coordinated Care

2. **Which nursing activity might commonly be provided by community health nurses but not by home health nurses? (Select all that apply).**
   1. Conducting health education programs in a senior citizen residence
   2. Monitoring the recovery of a postoperative patient at home
   3. Arranging blood pressure screening at a community shopping center
   4. Seeing patients in a clinic to monitor problems related to chronic illness
   5. Administering influenza vaccines at a public location

   NCLEX Client Need: Safe and Effective Care Environment: Coordinated Care

3. **LVN/LPN students are discussing the difference between community health nursing and community-based nursing. They correctly identify an example of community-based nursing as:**
   1. Meeting with residents of low-income housing to identify their health needs
   2. Telephoning patients at home after discharge from the hospital
   3. Asking nurses to identify the health services lacking in their communities
   4. Developing a hospital-based home health care service

   NCLEX Client Need: Safe and Effective Care Environment: Coordinated Care

4. **The LVN/LPN in a long-term care facility is caring for a patient who is unable to feed or dress herself independently because of a neurologic disease. Her status is most accurately described as:**
   1. Impaired
   2. Handicapped
   3. Disabled
   4. Disadvantaged

   NCLEX Client Need: Physiological Integrity: Basic Care and Comfort

5. **A nurse who has been diagnosed with a chronic illness, a nursing school applicant with hearing impairment, and a patient with cancer are all protected from discrimination in employment because of their health problems by the:**
   1. Social Security Act
   2. Americans with Disabilities Act
   3. Rehabilitation Act of 1973
   4. Vocational Rehabilitation Act

   NCLEX Client Need: Safe and Effective Care Environment: Coordinated Care

6. **A patient who is being discharged from a rehabilitation facility is applying for Medicare coverage for home health nursing care. The LVN/LPN knows that Medicare will reimburse nursing care in the home only if the care meets which criteria? (Select all that apply).**
   1. Short-term
   2. Necessary
   3. Skilled
   4. Reasonable
   5. Intermittent

   NCLEX Client Need: Safe and Effective Care Environment: Coordinated Care

7. **A patient who has suffered a head injury is feeding herself with considerable difficulty. In terms of rehabilitation, what is the most appropriate nursing response?**
   1. Offer to feed her so that she will not be embarrassed by her handicap
   2. Order a liquid diet so that she will not have to use eating utensils
   3. Point out that the sooner she can feed herself, the sooner she can go home
   4. Ensure that her food is accessible and compliment her efforts at self-feeding

   NCLEX Client Need: Physiological Integrity: Basic Care and Comfort

8. **A patient's record indicates that he is able to perform only 25% of his usual job activities since his motorcycle accident. This information is a measure of the extent of his:**
   1. Handicap
   2. Disability
   3. Incapacity
   4. Impairment

   NCLEX Client Need: Physiological Integrity: Physiological Adaptation and Psychosocial Integrity

9. **A nursing home resident has his name printed neatly on the door to his room. The interior of the room is decorated in masculine colors. One wall is covered with pictures of the resident at various occasions in his personal and professional life. In one corner is a leather recliner with a reading lamp and table. This room best reflects an effort to:**
   1. Prevent depersonalization
   2. Maintain the resident's dignity
   3. Prevent regression
   4. Prevent social withdrawal

   NCLEX Client Need: Psychosocial Integrity

10. **The nursing staff at a long-term care facility want to prevent depersonalization in the residents' environment. Which of the below actions that are being considered might help to achieve the goal of depersonalization? (Select all that apply.)**
    1. Have residents' names on their room doors
    2. Encourage residents to wear facility pajamas or gowns
    3. Invite families to bring photos of the residents at various life events
    4. Offer a variety of bedspreads for the residents to select
    5. Recommend only neutral colors in residents' rooms because they have a calming effect

    NCLEX Client Need: Psychosocial Integrity

11. **At a health class for older adults, one participant comments: "I guess we will all end up in a nursing home one day." The LVN/LPN can inform the group that the best indicator of who will need nursing home placement is:**
    1. The medical diagnosis
    2. The availability of family caregivers
    3. Dependence in ADL
    4. Financial resources

    NCLEX Client Need: Safe and Effective Care Environment: Coordinated Care

Medical-Surgical Patients: Individuals, Families, and Communities

3

http://evolve.elsevier.com/Linton/medsurg

Objectives

1. Discuss the roles and practice settings of the medical-surgical nurse.
2. Provide examples of primary, secondary, and tertiary prevention.
3. Explain cultural influences on the interactions of patients and families with the health care system.
4. Discuss considerations in providing culturally sensitive nursing care.
5. Discuss concepts related to health promotion, disease prevention, and health maintenance.
6. List the developmental tasks for each stage of adulthood.
7. Identify health problems common to the young, middle, and older adult.
8. Discuss the family from a developmental perspective.
9. Describe roles and communication patterns within families.
10. Describe adaptive and maladaptive mechanisms that families use to cope with various stressors.
11. Describe the role of the nurse in dealing with families experiencing various stresses.
12. Identify community resources that may help meet the family's needs.

Key Terms

dysfunctional communication
functional communication
primary prevention
secondary prevention
tertiary prevention

Chapter 2 described the varied settings in which medical-surgical nurses practice. This chapter explores the diverse patient populations that they serve: individuals, families, and communities; the sick and the well; from diverse cultures; across the adult life span. Medical-surgical patients include individuals at every point on the health-illness continuum. Their nurses engage in health promotion, prevention of disease and injury, management of acute and chronic health deviations, prevention of complications, and support at end of life. Regardless of the employment setting, medical-surgical nurses encounter patients and families from all corners of the earth. They must be sensitive to cultural differences, seeking to provide optimal care to all. Medical-surgical nurses work with the entire spectrum of adult patients, from late adolescents to centenarians. Some settings such as long-term care serve a limited age cohort, whereas others offer practice with young, middle, and older adults. Medical-surgical nurses in acute care settings work primarily with individual patients. Interactions with families often are limited even though the role they play in the patient's life is significant. In community and home settings, however, the nurse enters the patient's social network and has much greater opportunity to care for the family as a unit.

HEALTH-ILLNESS CONTINUUM

Despite the perception that medical-surgical nurses work primarily in acute care, opportunities abound for them to care for patients all along the health-illness continuum. Much care that once was provided only in hospital settings is now available in outpatient clinics, urgent care clinics, and day surgery facilities. In part, this is possible because home health nurses can follow up during convalescence, monitoring and documenting recovery, teaching, and communicating with the health care team about the patient's status. Care of these patients requires expert medical-surgical skills and judgment.

Nursing and residential care facilities employ the largest percentage of licensed vocational nurses/licensed practical nurses (LVNs/LPNs) in the United States. Patients in long-term care are at various points on the health-illness continuum. About 20% of long-term care residents are admitted for rehabilitation or recovery from acute events that no longer require hospitalization. The medical-surgical nurse is well prepared to manage convalescing and chronically ill residents, but the focus is not just on health deviations. Their nurses promote safety and the highest level of functioning possible. Chronically ill patients are at risk for acute events and require monitoring for physiologic and behavioral changes suggestive of disease processes, as well as adverse responses to treatments.

Residents in retirement centers range from highly functioning to very frail. The medical-surgical nurse aims to keep these patients as independent as possible for as long as possible. That requires skillful health teaching, helping the patient to manage existing health deviations, and monitoring for changes from the patient's usual state.

Home health care gives the medical-surgical nurse exposure to a broad range of patients. They may be recovering from joint replacement surgery, learning to manage an ostomy, or dealing with a slow-healing wound. Some patients will return to complete independence; others may be hoping to spend their final days in the home setting. Family teaching is a vital part of the nurse's role in home health. With adequate instruction and support, some families care for patients who are completely dependent. Home-based hospice is specifically for individuals who have a limited life expectancy. The focus is on comfort and support for the patient and the family. Nursing care at end of life is covered in Chapter 19.

Physician's offices and outpatient clinics, which employ about 13% of LVNs/LPNs, treat patients of all ages whose conditions can be managed outside the hospital. The medical-surgical nurse may assist with data collection for the assessment, reinforce physician or nurse practitioner orders, administer parenteral medications, provide comfort and reassurance, and document data collected and care provided.

HEALTH PROMOTION, DISEASE PREVENTION, AND HEALTH MAINTENANCE

Health promotion activities are directed toward maintaining or enhancing well-being as a protection against illness. Through public education, Americans have become increasingly health conscious, and many are beginning to take more responsibility for maintaining healthy lifestyles.

LEVELS OF PREVENTION

Disease or illness prevention behavior is action taken by individuals to decrease the threat of illness and its harmful consequences. The three levels of prevention are primary, secondary, and tertiary. **Primary prevention** seeks to prevent illness and injuries. **Secondary prevention** occurs when an illness or injury has occurred and is directed to minimizing complications and promoting maximum possible return to health. **Tertiary prevention** addresses the long-term effects of the health problem and helps the patient learn to manage them (Box 3.1).

Box 3.1 Examples of Activities at Each Level of Prevention

Primary: Teaching healthy lifestyle, encouraging preventive measures, promoting a safe care environment
Secondary: Providing direct care to patients during the acute phase of illness or injury or during related medical procedures
Tertiary: Providing direct care to convalescing patients and patients living with the effects of illness or injury

CULTURAL AWARENESS AND COMPETENCY

As an LVN/LPN, you must be able to accept a wide diversity of beliefs, practices, and ideas about health and illness, including many that are different from your own. The more sensitive you are to cultural differences, the more effective your nursing care will be. Failure to provide culturally sensitive care can cause additional stress and could prolong the patient's recovery time.

To contribute to the plan of care, you need to collect data to help you understand the patient's needs. A complete cultural assessment of each patient would be very time consuming and therefore impractical. All nurses should have a ready resource that provides information about various cultures. Several nursing guides are available that provide essential information such as health care beliefs, sick-care practices, relationship with health care providers, food practices, family roles, birth and death rites, and pain reactions. Accessing this information prepares you for what you may find when working with the patient and family. You can then collect data specific to that patient and family. Most of us have contact with a limited number of cultures, so it is imperative to acquire more in-depth knowledge of those cultures.

CULTURAL INFLUENCES ON INTERACTIONS WITH THE AMERICAN HEALTH CARE SYSTEM

In all health care settings, patients of different cultures may exhibit behaviors that are not understood by health care providers in the dominant culture. Culturally different patients may be labeled complaining, difficult, uncooperative, or noncompliant when in reality, they are struggling to adapt to a culture that is foreign to them. Culturally congruent care that is in harmony with the patient's values, beliefs, and practices is urgently needed.

MEDICAL-SURGICAL PATIENTS FROM VARIOUS CULTURES

Working in a variety of settings from acute care to community clinics and patient homes provides the medical-surgical nurse the opportunity to work with many diverse cultures. Culture can influence the patient's attitudes, beliefs, and practices in relation to health care. For example, many cultures have strong extended family units and family ties. When a person is hospitalized, family members visit frequently. Some cultures have traditionally cared for their elders in a home setting rather than placing them in residential facilities. Nurses should understand how one's cultural background influences behavior. A nursing fundamentals text often provides more detail about specific cultures. The biggest risk in learning "typical" behavior of people of different cultures is stereotyping. With increased worldwide travel and immigration, many countries have become very diverse. Whereas some immigrants assimilate readily into a new society, others do not. It is easy to make assumptions about a person's beliefs and practices based on appearance or surname. The best way to provide culturally appropriate nursing care is to collect data from the individual and adapt care accordingly.

RELIGION

Religious beliefs and practices can influence perceptions of health and illness, hospitalization, and death and dying. Some patients may observe specific dietary rules and others may have particular practices regarding dress, modesty, daily living habits, or medical interventions. Religious differences also occur in relation to observation of the Sabbath, baptism, the sacrament of the sick, and last rites.

COMMUNICATION

Certain cultural or ethnic groups speak different languages, making communication almost impossible. The speed at which people speak and their tone and inflections vary according to cultural background. Even within the United States, regional accents, words, and slang can affect communication. Anatomic and medical terms may be "foreign" to patients regardless of their language skills.

Nonverbal communication is also culturally based. Personal space, eye contact, gestures, displays of emotions, and the amount and meaning of touch that are acceptable are culturally determined. Some cultures find emotional display more acceptable than others. Some are more comfortable with silence than others.

Subtle forms of miscommunication may occur because of differences between and within groups. Communication should take place in language that patients understand, without talking down to them. Federal regulations require health care providers who receive federal funding to provide appropriate services to persons with limited English proficiency and those who are deaf or hard of hearing.

EDUCATIONAL BACKGROUND AND ECONOMIC STATUS

Patient teaching is a critical nursing skill. However, regardless of the care setting, the nurse must recognize the impact of education, experience, and economic status on a patient's comprehension of health teaching. Large differences in educational background exist in the United States. Millions of Americans have literacy skills below the eighth-grade level, meaning that they have difficulty with reading and writing. One aspect of literacy is health literacy, which refers to the ability to obtain and understand basic information needed to make health decisions. Health literacy has been found to be highest among women, White and Pacific Islander adults, and adults under 65 years of age. The nurse can collect data about a person's health literacy by asking the patient what they know about their condition. Start where the patient "is" and build on that knowledge to fill in the gaps and correct misconceptions.

Educational level attained is strongly tied to economic background. School dropout rates appear to be higher among adolescents living in poverty areas. Ethnic groups that are found in large numbers in poverty areas tend to have high dropout rates.

Educational background and economic levels affect the ways in which people perceive the world, health and illness, and the health care system. Teaching about health becomes a challenge because many people with low literacy levels have difficulty reading the materials presented and understanding health care jargon. In addition, people from economically deprived backgrounds may live in crowded, unsafe housing and have inadequate diets. Such conditions make health promotion and disease prevention difficult.

As mentioned in relation to culture, be careful not to stereotype patients based on their education or economic status. Many people are very knowledgeable about their health status as a result of self-study and experience. It is not uncommon for older adults to have limited formal education but a lifetime of informal learning.

HEALTH AND ILLNESS BELIEFS

Of great concern to the nurse is the impact of patient beliefs related to health and illness. Some groups believe illness is expected as part of life and is beyond one's control. Different belief systems attribute illness to punishment for sins, imbalance between the hot and cold parts of the body, or lack of harmony with nature. Western cultures generally approach illness as being treatable once the cause is identified. They also believe the risk of illness can be reduced by a healthy lifestyle. It is easy to see how these varied beliefs affect the approach a person takes toward health and illness management.

Many ethnic groups use healers who practice health care outside of the formal health care delivery system. Patients may visit a folk healer or use folk remedies, such as potions and plants, along with or in place of conventional treatment. When individuals perceive mainstream health care to be too expensive or inconvenient, or when it fails to meet their psychosocial needs, they may turn to traditional healers.

DIMENSIONS OF CULTURE IN THE UNITED STATES

Despite the diverse subcultures in the United States, certain characteristics are generally true of the American culture. Americans are very time oriented and value being on time, multitasking, and "time saving" measures. Eager to get tasks done, American health care providers may not take the time to establish rapport with patients. Americans typically embrace change, including the newest technologies and treatments. They are likely to believe that people have control over their own destiny rather than attributing outcomes to fate or karma. Self-sufficiency and individualism are highly valued. Reflecting the value of equality and rejection of a social hierarchy, Americans tend to be informal, even with strangers. Americans are described as direct or low-context communicators, meaning that they rely mostly on words and less on nonverbal messages. Indirect communication assigns equal importance to verbal messages and words. The direct speech used by many Americans may seem abrupt or rude to others. Nurses with traditional American backgrounds need to recognize how their beliefs and behaviors can affect the nurse-patient relationship.

TRADITIONAL HEALTH HABITS AND BELIEFS OF MAJOR ETHNIC GROUPS IN THE UNITED STATES

Although stereotyping individual members of any culture or subculture is inappropriate, various ethnic groups in the United States may retain unique traditional health care beliefs and practices. Great variations in beliefs and practices exist not only between but also within ethnic and subcultural groups. First- and second-generation residents of the United States often have more characteristics associated with their ethnic groups than people who have been in the United States for several generations. Many resources provide information about traditional health care beliefs and practices. Remember that these examples are included to show a range of possible health customs for selected ethnic groups. They cannot be generalized to all members of the ethnic group or subculture.

> **Put On Your Thinking Cap!**
>
> Considering your own race or ethnicity, identify three cultural beliefs related to health that are held by your family. For example, how are you expected to respond to illness or stress? When do you seek medical care and what kind of provider do you see? Do you use any complementary or alternative therapies? What activities are believed to promote health or prevent disease?

HOSPITAL HEALTH CARE

The hospital environment can be frightening, even to people who are familiar with it. For individuals who do not speak English, have different eating preferences, and view health and illness differently, adapting to the hospital environment can be overwhelming. Hospital personnel become authority figures who expect patients to conform to policies and accept directions. Patients may feel stripped of their dignity when told to wear hospital gowns that barely cover private body parts. Modesty may be ignored, causing humiliation and anxiety.

Not only do people find themselves in a totally new environment, but they must also endure separation from family and friends. Their support systems topple when visiting policies are strictly enforced. In some cultures, families expect to advocate for the patient, help with nursing care, or at least sit with sick people to keep them company and provide support. Hospital personnel may be uncomfortable with this infringement on their territory.

Language barriers greatly complicate the provision of care. The patient's language proficiency should be documented at the initial contact by asking what language is spoken at home and how well the person speaks English. Unless the patient reports speaking English very well, an interpreter should be offered. Even though nonmedical personnel and family members may help with everyday conversations, they may not correctly relay information between the nurse and the patient. Therefore an official interpreter should be used to convey health information or obtain informed consent. Even bilingual nursing staff should receive training in the skill and ethics of interpretation. Failure to use interpreters has been identified as one factor in errors that are made in the health care system. Options for oral language assistance include trained staff interpreters, professional contract interpreters, employee language banks of bilingual individuals, community interpreter banks that maintain lists of trained interpreters, telephone interpreter services, and remote simultaneous interpretation in which the nurse's statements are translated by an interpreter who conveys the information to the patient via a headset.

CULTURE SHOCK

Culture shock associated with hospitalization occurs in three phases. During the first phase, the patient asks questions regarding the hospital routine and the hospital's expectations of the patient. In the second phase, the patient becomes disenchanted with the whole situation and is frustrated, hostile, and then depressed and withdrawn. In the final phase, the patient begins to adapt to the new environment and is even able to maintain a sense of humor during interactions with others.

COMMUNITY AND HOME HEALTH CARE

LVNs/LPNs are increasingly visible in community and outpatient settings. Community settings in which culturally different individuals may interact with the health care system include physicians' offices, outpatient clinics, mental health centers, home health care, hospices, and adult day care centers. People from different cultural backgrounds may use both the formal health care system and traditional healers and practices, as described earlier.

Many people have difficulty navigating the maze of health care services either because of language differences or because of negative attitudes toward health care providers based on previous experiences. Individuals with limited financial resources are frequently clinic patients who must wait hours to see a provider only to receive a cursory assessment from the physician or nurse. Because of language barriers, their questions about their condition may be left unanswered, resulting in failure to follow directions for care.

When entering a patient's home, notice symbolic objects that may indicate cultural identity. Shrines, religious pictures or statues, and special candles are examples of symbols. Remember that many immigrant families fully embrace Western medicine while continuing to find comfort in symbols and traditional practices. Ask about your patient's health beliefs and practices that are affected by culture. Patients and their families may have magical, religious, biomedical, or holistic beliefs. If the patient does not speak English, a family member is sometimes able to interpret. Although this is not ideal, it may be the only option at the time. See the earlier section on interpreters.

HEALTH CARE IN LONG-TERM CARE

The majority of residents in long-term care facilities are White women. Traditionally, some ethnic groups including Black, Latino, and Asian Americans are reluctant to admit older relatives to residential care and prefer to provide care at home. However, changes in family structure are having an impact on these cultures. Women from all cultures are more likely to work outside the home, so they are not able to provide full-time caregiving. Also extended families are often scattered geographically, so fewer family members may be available to help with the person needing care.

Residents in long-term care facilities typically suffer from one or more functional impairments. Individuals from different cultural groups may have the added strain of communication problems and extreme changes in lifestyle and dietary practices. These differences may contribute to confusion, disability, and incontinence. For example, the resident who speaks little English may have difficulty asking for help with toileting. Because older people tend to have limited time between the urge to void and the actual voiding experience, urinary incontinence can occur.

THERAPEUTIC RELATIONSHIPS

Because all nursing care takes place in the framework of the nurse-patient relationship, an environment of acceptance and respect for the beliefs and behaviors of culturally different patients should be established. For patients to trust the nurse, they must feel safe, respected, and accepted.

Maintain an open, inquiring, and respectful attitude regarding cultural differences. Patients of another culture may initially be quiet, polite, conforming, or shy. The behavior may reflect a guarded or cautious response because patients are not sure what is expected of them and how the interaction will go. A good rule of thumb during an initial encounter is to speak softly and in an unhurried manner to put them at ease. Once you understand the lifestyle of the patient, you can work with the registered nurse (RN) to tailor the care plan as needed. The patient should be involved in the care plan by identifying familiar ways of coping with an illness and adaptations that recognize the person's culture.

Conflicts between the patient's health practices and beliefs and those of the health care system may arise. However, the cultural values of patients and their families must be given full consideration. Changes in health practices often require some major changes in lifestyle. Try to understand what prescribed changes mean from the viewpoint of the patient, family, and community. Only then can effective modifications in health practices take place.

BASIC PHYSIOLOGIC NEEDS

Cultural attitudes may affect patients' perceptions of personal hygiene and the role of the nurse in assisting with basic bodily needs. Some patients do not bathe routinely. Others may be extremely modest about having the body exposed to others. As with all patients, show sensitivity to these feelings by knocking on the door before entering and asking permission before touching or assisting with personal hygiene.

During the bath, do not remove a patient's charms, crosses, medals, or other objects without permission. These objects usually have special meaning to the patient. If the patient wishes, family members may assist with the bath, oral hygiene, bed making, ambulation, and other caregiving. Including significant others helps to alleviate stress and fulfill cultural expectations for both patients and family members. Nutrition is an aspect of care affected by culture. Diet is often culturally based and, to be successful, modifications in diet must take culture into account.

DRUG THERAPY

We are just beginning to understand how ethnicity influences the way people react to drugs. Factors that contribute to the differing responses can be categorized as environmental, cultural, and genetic. Environmental factors related to drug absorption, distribution, metabolism, and elimination include diet, smoking, and alcohol use. For example, diets that are high in sodium may reduce the effectiveness of some antihypertensive drugs.

Table 3.1 Erikson's Adult Developmental Tasks

DEVELOPMENTAL STAGE	DEVELOPMENTAL TASK	NURSING ASSESSMENT DATA
Young adulthood	Intimacy versus isolation	Meaningful, intimate relationships now and in the past Support systems
Middle adulthood	Generativity versus self-absorption and stagnation	Employment status Leisure or recreation Typical daily routine if not employed Signs of depression, such as excessive sleeping and decreased appetite
Older adulthood	Ego integrity versus despair	Daily routine Family and other relationships If lonely, note signs of depression

From Ignatavicius DD, Workman, ML, Mishler, M: *Medical-surgical nursing: a nursing process approach,* ed 3, Philadelphia, 1999, Saunders.

Cultural factors can affect drug response by influencing the patient's expectations, adherence to prescribed drugs, and willingness to report problems to the prescriber. In addition, some culturally based traditional remedies can interact with prescribed drugs to increase or decrease their effects.

Perhaps the greatest influence of ethnicity related to drug therapy is that liver enzymes are controlled by genetic factors. Liver enzymes determine the rate and extent of drug metabolism. People who metabolize a particular drug slowly are at greater risk for drug toxicity than those who metabolize that drug rapidly. For example, Black Americans with hypertension respond better than White Americans to diuretic therapy alone. Conversely, Black Americans are less responsive to monotherapy with beta blockers or angiotensin-converting enzyme inhibitors than White Americans. The implication of such differences is that you must monitor patient responses to drugs, knowing that they may be different from the expected response.

PATIENT TEACHING

Teaching patients from different cultures may be difficult. They may not be able to understand health and illness information even if they have some command of the English language. Much of the language of health care is confusing and unfamiliar. The nurse needs to develop trust so that people will feel free to ask questions and seek clarification of information they do not understand. Sometimes patients and family members nod their head in agreement even though they have little comprehension of the material.

Using both oral and written communication can help to reinforce what has been taught. Written material in the patient's native language greatly improves understanding. Have them demonstrate skills you have taught to confirm that learning has occurred. Consider requesting a trained interpreter if there is reason to believe the patient is not comprehending essential information.

STAGE OF DEVELOPMENT

Reaching adulthood is a significant milestone; however, it is not the end of the development process. Erik Erikson introduced the idea that each stage of life is associated with specific developmental tasks to be achieved to advance to the next stage. Erikson divided adulthood into young, middle, and older stages. This framework provides a useful way to understand the needs of adult patients at any age. Because medical-surgical nurses work primarily with adults, they need to consider the patient's stage of adulthood, developmental tasks, and related health implications (Table 3.1).

YOUNG ADULTS

According to Erikson, individuals in their 20s, 30s, and 40s are young adults. This is the time when most adults establish their own home, settle into a job, find an intimate partner, and raise a family.

Health Problems

Young adults, especially those in their 20s and early 30s, have relatively few health problems. The four most common causes of death in young adults are unintentional injury, homicide, suicide, and malignant neoplasms. Among the youngest members of this age group, the most common cause of unintentional injury is motor vehicle accidents, followed by poisoning (drug overdose, carbon monoxide, etc.). After 25 years of age, unintentional poisoning causes more deaths than motor vehicle accidents. As young adults progress into their late 40s, the primary causes of death are malignancies and heart disease, followed by accidents and suicide.

Typical health problems are related to stress on the job or in social interactions, lifestyle, and childbearing. These problems include depression; anxiety; complications of pregnancy; cervical and breast cancer; and back, hip, and limb injuries. By 30 years of age, half of adults have gum disease. In the quest for meaningful social relationships and a career that will gain them independence and success, young adults may experience tension and stress and may lack the time to attend to health promotion activities such as a proper diet, exercise, and rest. They may work hard and party enthusiastically. Meals may be eaten on the run and the diet may rely heavily on fast foods. The total number of calories needed is less than during adolescence, given that the young adult has completed physical growth.

Table 3.2 **Harmful Practices, Effects on Health in the Later Years, and Preventive Measures**

HARMFUL PRACTICE	POSSIBLE EFFECTS ON HEALTH	PREVENTIVE MEASURES
Lack of physical activity	Diabetes, osteoporosis, heart disease, cancer, obesity, stroke, depression	Increase moderate daily physical activity and reduce sedentary lifestyle
Obesity	Heart disease, hypertension, type 2 diabetes mellitus, degenerative joint disease, cancer, stroke, atherosclerosis	Maintain ideal weight; maintain low-cholesterol, low-fat, nutritious diet with plenty of vegetables, fruits, and grain products
Cigarette smoking	Heart disease; cancers of the lung, larynx, pharynx, oral cavity, esophagus, pancreas, and bladder; chronic bronchitis and emphysema	Stop smoking or do not start smoking
Alcohol and drug abuse	Malnutrition, cirrhosis of the liver, brain damage, mental status changes, homicide, suicide, motor vehicle fatalities	Limit alcohol intake and stop using drugs or do not start; participate in rehabilitation program
Stress	Stress-related conditions such as hypertension and heart disease	Recognize and modify stressors; use a stress management program such as exercise or biofeedback

Modified from U.S. Department of Health and Human Services: *Healthy people 2010, vol 1, With understanding and improving health, vol 2, Objectives for improving health*, ed 2 (Publication No. [PHS] 99-1256), Washington, DC, 1999, U.S. Government Printing Office.

Smoking and alcohol or drug abuse are common. These practices may have a direct bearing on health in the later years (Table 3.2).

In their 30s and early 40s, young adults typically are focused on raising a family and furthering their careers. This age may be a time to reassess their lives and careers, and often major changes are made. Factors that contribute to health problems are stress related to work, marital problems, and stress related to managing a household. Couples who have postponed childbearing may have difficulties with conception and pregnancy.

Health Care Needs

Health care needs are related to promoting optimal health. Having at least one thorough physical examination during the 20s is recommended. The examination should include tests for sexually transmitted infections, hepatitis C, hypertension, and elevated blood lipids. Several types of health screening should be initiated and repeated at regular intervals. See Chapter 7 for American Cancer Society screening guidelines. Note that guidelines are exactly that; more or less frequent screening may be recommended based on a person's personal and family history.

A tetanus booster should be given if persons have not received one in the past 10 years. The hepatitis B vaccine is recommended for adults at risk of exposure to blood and body fluids. Routine dental and eye examinations should be scheduled. Women who wish to perform breast self-examinations (BSE) should be instructed in the proper technique. They should also be informed that BSE does not replace periodic professional examinations or mammograms. Young men should be taught to do testicular self-examinations.

Health counseling in the 20s should focus on health promotion behaviors. Programs may be established to include topics such as nutrition; exercise and leisure; rest and sleep; human sexuality and family planning; stress management; and the effects of smoking, drugs, and alcohol.

In the years between 30 and 45 years of age, especially after 35 years of age, young adults should begin to think about the prevention of chronic illness, particularly cancer and heart disease. Periodic physical examinations should include tests for hypertension, anemia, elevated serum lipids, and a cervical Pap test for women. Experts suggest that people in this age group examine their skin and mouth periodically for precancerous lesions. Preventive dental checkups are usually recommended every 6 months to 2 years.

Health promotion and disease prevention programs have a similar focus as for people in their 20s. Stress management, effective parenting, proper diet and nutrition, exercise, drug and alcohol awareness, and smoking cessation are appropriate topics for health teaching and counseling.

MIDDLE-AGE ADULTS

The years from 45 to 65 years of age are considered middle age. Americans who fall into this category earn most of the money, pay most of the taxes, and have most of the power in business and government. Middle age is a time of relatively good health for most. People experience a new personal freedom and enjoy maximal command of themselves. Many people in their middle years belong to a group called the "sandwich generation" because they still have adolescents and young adults at home and also have older parents who need care. Many women work outside the home and have important careers. Taking on the care of one or more aged parents along with existing responsibilities can create a great deal of conflict and stress.

Health Problems

Most people in their middle years continue to be relatively healthy, and the same factors that contribute to the deterioration of health habits in the young adult apply to those in middle age. The most common cause of death is malignancy followed by heart disease, unintentional injury, and chronic respiratory disease. Respiratory conditions are a frequent cause of absence from work for women; injuries are a frequent cause among men.

Women usually enter a perimenopausal period between 45 and 50 years of age. Bone mass begins to decrease in the middle years. Women lose calcium from bone tissue after menopause, leading to an increased risk of osteoporosis. Muscle mass is reduced as a result of decreased muscle fibers. In the 40s, changes in vision typically begin. Age-related farsightedness (*presbyopia)* develops as a result of decreasing elasticity in the lens. The clue to developing presbyopia is that the individual begins to hold reading material at a distance to focus on it better. *Presbycusis* (i.e., the common loss of hearing acuity associated with aging) may begin to appear.

Put On Your Thinking Cap!

Mrs. J., 55 years of age, is diagnosed with a life-threatening illness. She is married to a dentist and works as a nurse manager on a medical-surgical hospital unit. Her youngest child, 20 years of age, is in college and living at home. She has two young adult children who live independently, and two grandchildren. Her mother, 87 years of age, lives nearby and relies on Mrs. J. for assistance with personal care and transportation. What are the effects of this diagnosis on family, job, and other roles?

Health Care Needs

The health care goals in middle age are the same as for younger adults: health promotion and disease prevention to preserve and prolong the period of maximal energy and optimal mental health and social activity. During the middle years, regular assessment of health status is important for maintaining good health. Good management of existing conditions and early diagnosis of illnesses help to prevent later complications. A complete physical examination every 3 years is recommended. It should include blood pressure screening and tests for serum glucose and cholesterol levels. The patient's dentist should determine the frequency of dental visits based on the oral assessment. Various cancer screening tests may be ordered depending on the patient's history. The recommendations of the American Cancer Society and other specialty organizations are commonly followed. See Chapter 7 for recommended screenings and schedules.

During the perimenopausal period, a gradual decrease in estrogen occurs, accompanied by a gradual decrease in menstrual flow. Pregnancy remains a possibility until the menstrual cycle ceases completely—usually between 45 and 55 years of age. Menopausal symptoms (hot flashes, perspiration, fatigue, etc.) may be treated with estrogen, depending on the patient's history. However, estrogen alone increases the risk of endometrial cancer. Therefore a combination of estrogen and progesterone is safer for the postmenopausal woman who still has her uterus. After menopause, any vaginal bleeding should be reported, as it may be a sign of endometrial cancer.

Health promotion activities during middle age are the same as for young adults. The focus is on proper nutrition, exercise, stress management, and the reduction or elimination of smoking, drug use, and alcohol use.

OLDER ADULTS

Age 65 years is commonly considered the beginning of old age. However, many people in their 60s and older do not consider themselves old and continue to live healthy, productive lives. People are entering old age in better health than in the past. In the United States today, 8 in 10 people will live past their 65th birthday. Markers that may be more meaningful than chronologic age to define older age are biologic age, psychologic age, and social age. Biologic age focuses on the functional capabilities of the body systems. Many older people, especially those who engage in exercise and other health promotion activities, continue to function well whereas others seem to be prematurely ill and frail. Psychologic age refers to the capacity of the person to adapt to changing environmental demands. Factors that affect psychologic age include memory and the ability to learn. Social age refers to the roles and habits of a person in relation to other members of society. Individuals of the same chronologic age may differ in biologic, psychologic, and social age. Also the three ages are not necessarily the same in an individual. The important thing for the nurse to know is that older adults are a very heterogeneous group. Nurses must avoid stereotyping based on age and assess each person as a unique individual. Chapter 10 provides detailed descriptions of the changes that occur with aging.

Health Problems

The major causes of death in older age are heart disease and cancer followed by chronic respiratory disease, cerebrovascular disease, Alzheimer disease, diabetes, influenza and pneumonia, and nephritis. Unintentional injuries rank among the top ten causes of death in this age group. The most common health problems are arthritis, heart disease, diabetes, and cancer. Benign or malignant enlargement of the prostate is common in older men; breast cancer is common in older women.

Health Care Needs

The health care goals of the older age group are to manage chronic illnesses and to maintain and prolong the period of optimal physical, mental, and social activity. Helping older adults to maintain their independence for as long as possible in the event of one or more chronic illnesses is important.

Physical examinations should be performed annually and include the same assessment as indicated for middle-aged adults. However, depending on individual risk factors, some screenings can be discontinued after 65 or 70 years of age, or when life expectancy reaches certain limits. Women who have had a total hysterectomy do not require an annual Pap test. Dental examinations and treatment should also continue in older age. Periodic evaluation and treatment by a podiatrist are recommended to promote mobility.

Annual influenza immunizations are recommended. Two forms of the pneumococcal vaccine exist: pneumococcal conjugate vaccine (PCV13) and pneumococcal polysaccharide vaccine (PPSV23). The shingles vaccine is administered in two doses. Adults who were not vaccinated as teenagers for tetanus, diphtheria, and pertussis should be given one dose of Tdap vaccine followed by the Td booster every ten years. Individuals with health deviations should discuss their specific immunization needs with their health care provider.

Health promotion activities should continue into older age. These activities can increase quality of life and, in many cases, prevent many of the chronic illnesses common in older age. Proper nutrition (low-fat, high-fiber diet with a large amount of complex carbohydrates) helps to promote intestinal motility and decrease susceptibility to some chronic illnesses. Exercise can benefit older adults, even the very old who begin an exercise program for the first time. Walking is the ideal exercise. One hundred and fifty minutes of walking each week can help maintain weight, blood pressure, coordination, and mobility and create a positive outlook on life. See Box 4.4 in Chapter 4 for more detailed exercise/activity recommendation. Older people can also benefit from counseling for alcohol and drug abuse and smoking cessation.

SOCIAL NETWORK

The importance of a patient's personal support network cannot be overestimated. Family and friends can provide encouragement, advocate for the patient, reinforce health teaching, assist with care, and relieve the patient of some responsibilities. On the other hand, sometimes family or individual issues can add to the patient's stress. Not all members are supportive or helpful. Traditionally, we have considered "legal" relatives to be the patient's family. As the modern family has evolved, we have expanded our definition of the family. Many families today vary from the traditional formula of mother, father, and children. More and more family units are composed of single parents or step-parent families. In addition, friends or partners of the same or opposite sex now are often considered family or extended family.

Therefore it makes sense for patients to define their family according to their own criteria, and to determine how those family members will participate in care and decision making. When patients are admitted for care, they usually are asked who may be given information about their health status. With that in mind, this chapter will use the term *family* to include all of those that the patient views as family. Regardless of the setting, medical-surgical nurses often work closely with their patients' significant others.

FAMILY AND CULTURE

In the United States, many variations in cultural patterns are found among families. Traditional cultural practices were discussed earlier in this chapter. Cultural diversity may occur even within ethnic groups. Immigrants are in varying stages of assimilation and acculturation, especially among various generations. To avoid stereotyping, the best way to determine the specific cultural patterns of a family is to get the information from the family itself.

Cultural Considerations

What Does Culture Have to Do With Families?

Culture influences most aspects of family function, including communication, child rearing, diet, and health practices.

FAMILY DEVELOPMENTAL THEORY

Families go through predictable stages of growth and development, just as individuals do. However, because not all families fit into the traditional nuclear family model, variations among stages are found depending on the makeup of the family. Responsibilities for growth (developmental tasks) must be met at each developmental stage to meet biologic needs, cultural demands, and goals. Table 3.3 summarizes the stages of the family life cycle and developmental tasks of the two-parent nuclear family.

Divorced Family and Step-Parent Family Life Cycle and Developmental Tasks

With approximately half of all marriages in the United States ending in divorce, the single-parent family is common. The stages and developmental tasks in single-parent families are essentially the same as in two-parent families. However, the divorced parent who maintains the home with children shoulders more responsibilities alone. Issues confronting divorced families may include financial problems, lack of a mother or father role model, and the loss of the child's relationship with the absent parent. The introduction of a step-parent or unmarried partner requires a period of adjustment that typically lasts 2 to 3 years. Once the new structure has stabilized, the new family can progress developmentally.

Table 3.3 Stages of the Family Life Cycle of the Two-Parent Nuclear Family

STAGE	DEVELOPMENTAL TASK
Beginning families	Establish mutually satisfying marriage Work out satisfactory relationship with spouse's family Make decisions about parenthood
Families with young children	Set up young family as a stable unit Develop parental roles to meet changing needs of children Maintain satisfying marital relationship Socialize children Maintain and expand relationships with extended family, adding parenting and grandparenting roles Maintain healthy relationships outside the family
Families with adolescents	Balance freedom with responsibility in adolescents Refocus on the marital relationship Communicate openly between parents and children
Launching children and moving on	Expand family circle to include new family members acquired by marriage of children Continue to renew and readjust in the marital relationship Assist aging and ill parents of the husband and wife
Families in later life	Maintain satisfying living arrangement Adjust to reduced income Maintain marital relationship Adjust to loss of a spouse Maintain intergenerational family ties Continue to make sense of one's existence

Gay and Lesbian Family Life Cycle and Developmental Tasks

Gay and lesbian marriage was ruled legal in the United States in 2015. With or without legal sanction, gay or lesbian couples who live together and have an intimate relationship, with or without children, may consider themselves a family. Same-sex families who fear discrimination and lack of social acceptance may conceal their relationship from others. Like other types of families, same-sex families go through developmental stages.

FAMILY RESPONSE TO PATIENT ILLNESS OR INJURY

Factors that affect the way the family responds to a member's illness depend on many factors, including role structure, family interactions, communication patterns, coping skills, and resources.

Family Role Structure

Each member of the family has a role. Through these roles, family functions are carried out. A family member who is ill or injured may be temporarily or permanently unable to perform his/her usual roles. A healthy family may be able to shift roles to other members so that the family can continue to function adequately.

In the traditional nuclear family, roles can also be characterized as formal or informal. Formal roles consist of a limited number of positions in the family that are explicitly defined, such as wife-mother, husband-father, son-brother, and daughter-sister. Each of the formal roles has certain role expectations, such as wage earner, homemaker, financial manager, cook, and so on, and these roles are usually given to the person who has the skills necessary to carry them out. Smaller families and single-parent families have fewer people to take on the various roles, so individuals may play several roles at different times. Single parents may engage extended family members to help with role fulfillment. In a nontraditional family, role expectations may be negotiated more based on skills than on typical male-female division of labor.

Whereas formal roles are explicit roles that each family role structure contains, informal roles are often not as apparent and usually meet the emotional needs of individuals or maintain the family's equilibrium. Informal roles have different requirements that are based on the personality attributes of individual members rather than on age or sex. Effective performance of informal roles can strengthen the performance of the formal roles. Some of the roles enhance the well-being of the family whereas others can interfere with family functioning.

Family roles may be classified as performance oriented or emotional. For example, performance-oriented roles could include breadwinner, homemaker, handyman or handywoman, or gardener. Emotional roles could be leader, nurturer, protector, healer, or rebel. Members may fill more than one role, and any member can satisfactorily fill any role in either category.

Common informal roles include encourager (praises others' contributions to the family), harmonizer (mediates differences among other members), initiator-contributor (suggests new ideas and initiates action), blocker (opposes and rejects all ideas), martyr (sacrifices everything for the sake of the family), family scapegoat (family emotional ills blamed on this member; labeled as the "problem" member), family caretaker (nurtures and cares for other members in need), family go-between (the family "switchboard"—transmits and monitors communication within the family), and family coordinator (organizes and plans family activities). The scapegoat usually assumes or is assigned this role to preserve the family and maintain homeostasis. The role generally serves to divert attention from family issues such as conflict between the spouses. The go-between is usually the mother, who monitors all communications and is in charge of settling all disputes. When the conflicts are not resolved, the go-between is often blamed. This type of interaction is sometimes considered dysfunctional because it interferes with direct communication among family members.

Family Interaction

Family interaction is a unique form of social interaction based on a set of intimate and continuing relationships. It is the sum of all family roles being actualized within a family at a given time. Family functions and tasks are carried out through the process of interaction. One of the most important influences on family interaction is the self-esteem of each member. Adult members who have adequate self-esteem are able to provide the love and nurturing that children need to develop self-esteem, belonging, and acceptance. Adults who lack self-acceptance and self-respect are unlikely to be loving spouses or parents. In a healthy family, the members love and respect one another.

Family Communication Patterns

Families continually exchange communication to provide information, correct misinformation, solve problems, and resolve misunderstandings. Family communication patterns depend on the family power structure, the closeness of relationships, and the popularity of individual members. As noted earlier, many routes of information may go through one person, who assumes the role of go-between. Communication in the family may be functional or dysfunctional. However, communication patterns are not totally one way or the other. They exist on a continuum from functional to dysfunctional, with the patterns of most families falling somewhere in between the polar extremes.

Functional communication

Functional communication is the clear transmission of a message that enables the receiver to understand the intent of what the sender transmits. Communication in healthy families is a dynamic two-way process such that both the sender and the receiver are active participants in the communication. Communication patterns in a functional family demonstrate acceptance of individual differences, openness, honesty, acknowledgment of feelings, and recognition of the needs and emotions of one another. A functional family uses communication to create and maintain mutually beneficial relationships.

Functional patterns of communication include emotional and affective communication. Emotional communication deals with the expression of emotions or feelings, such as anger, hurt, sadness, happiness, affection, and tenderness. A healthy, functional family demonstrates a wide range of emotions and feelings. For family members to be able to enjoy one another, their responses to each other should be fresh and spontaneous rather than controlled, repetitious, and predictable. Affective communication involves verbal messages of caring and nonverbal, physical gestures of touching, caressing, holding, and looking. Families with functional communication patterns value openness, spontaneity, self-disclosure, and a mutual respect for each other's feelings, thoughts, and concerns. They usually can discuss most personal issues and concerns and resolve conflicts.

Dysfunctional communication

Dysfunctional communication is the opposite of functional communication. It is the unclear transmission of a message so that the receiver cannot understand the sender's intent. The primary reason for dysfunctional communication is low self-esteem among the family members. Communications become confusing, vague, indirect, secretive, and defensive because the individuals lack the ability to appreciate differences, thoughts, and feelings of other family members and are unable to deal with conflict. Children growing up in this environment are often unable to recognize and interpret a variety of feelings and experiences.

Dysfunctional patterns of communication may be subtle, and the intent of the communication is not clear. For example, individuals in an interaction may constantly restate their own issues without really listening to others' points of view or acknowledging their needs. Another example is the inability to focus on one issue. Each individual in the interaction rambles from one issue to another instead of resolving any one problem. Unwritten rules may specify subjects that are allowed for discussion; dysfunctional families have more forbidden subjects than functional families (see the Cultural Considerations box). Sometimes, dysfunctional families avoid discussing meaningful issues or expressing feelings by using superficial conversation; they talk about unimportant daily occurrences rather than the meaningful issues of family life.

Cultural Considerations

What Does Culture Have to Do With Communication?

Cultural aspects of family communication must be considered when determining whether a family is functional or dysfunctional. Some cultures are more open and communicative whereas others are less likely to discuss various topics or to show feelings or emotions.

Family Coping

Family coping refers to a positive response that families use to resolve problems or reduce stress. Family coping processes and strategies are essential for the family to maintain its necessary functions. The processes of coping with stress and adaptation are the same for families as they are for individuals (see Chapter 4). How a family adapts to stress and change affects family health and functioning. If adaptation to stress is negative, the family functions less effectively than if adaptation to stress is positive.

If a family is handling stress poorly or using ineffective adaptive strategies, it may be in crisis. A family crisis occurs when the stressors are overwhelming, and the family is unable to cope and resolve problems. You, in concert with the RN, may be in a position to determine whether the family's problem is being adequately managed by family members, whether a crisis state exists, or whether the current problem is part of a chronic inability to solve issues. Adaptive strategies include defense mechanisms, coping strategies, and mastery. Defense mechanisms are usual ways of responding to stress. They are usually avoidance behaviors, meaning that people avoid facing problems or stressors. Although defense mechanisms may reduce anxiety, they are generally considered to be negative responses, especially when used excessively or inappropriately (see Chapter 4). Coping strategies are behaviors or efforts used for effective problem solving and are generally considered to be positive responses. With effective coping strategies, problems are solved competently and the family functions in a healthy manner.

Coping strategies

The coping strategies that families use to respond to stressors change over time with the particular demands or stressors being experienced. One effective strategy is to deal with the cause of the problem by altering or eliminating it. For example, a family that suddenly becomes homeless because of a major disaster takes steps to find temporary quarters. Another way of coping is to attach meaning to a problem. For example, one family may be devastated by a house fire that resulted in their becoming homeless whereas another may find meaning in the situation by saying that at least the family escaped safely. A third coping strategy occurs when families support and comfort one another rather than taking action to remedy the situation. The use of multiple coping strategies is generally more effective than using a single coping mechanism for every circumstance.

Coping responses include internal and external coping strategies. Families use internal coping strategies when they pull together and respond to problems as a cohesive unit. Successful internal coping requires positive family communication patterns. External coping strategies refer to the use of social support systems to solve problems. Knowledge of resources in the community and willingness to accept outside help are important for successful external coping. Specific types of internal and external family coping strategies are listed in the Health Promotion box.

Health Promotion

INTERNAL AND EXTERNAL FAMILY COPING STRATEGIES

Internal Family Coping Strategies

- Family group reliance: becoming more reliant on its own resources
- The use of humor: relieving anxiety and tension with humor
- Maintaining cohesiveness: sharing feelings, thoughts, and experiences to maintain a cohesive family unit
- Controlling the meaning of the problem: interpreting events in a positive way
- Joint family problem solving: all members working together to solve problems
- Role flexibility: changing roles as needed
- Normalizing: maintaining as normal a life as possible in the face of stressors

External Family Coping Strategies

- Seeking information: obtaining information about a situation to maintain control
- Maintaining active linkages with the community: participating in clubs or community organizations, using societal resources and information as an adjunct to serve family members' needs
- Seeking social support: using informal and formal support systems and support groups
- Seeking spiritual support: obtaining spiritual support for coping with stress

From Friedman MM: *Family nursing: theory and practice*, ed 3, Norwalk, CT, 1992, Appleton & Lange.

Family members frequently provide support for patients. They may also need a great deal of support for themselves during a loved one's illness. Consider the needs of family members, especially in cases in which a serious illness or threat of death occurs. Providing information can reduce anxiety and fear of the unknown (Fig. 3.1). Just as assessment is the first step in individual patient care, it is also an important part of family nursing care. The LVN/LPN collects meaningful data about the family that can contribute to the

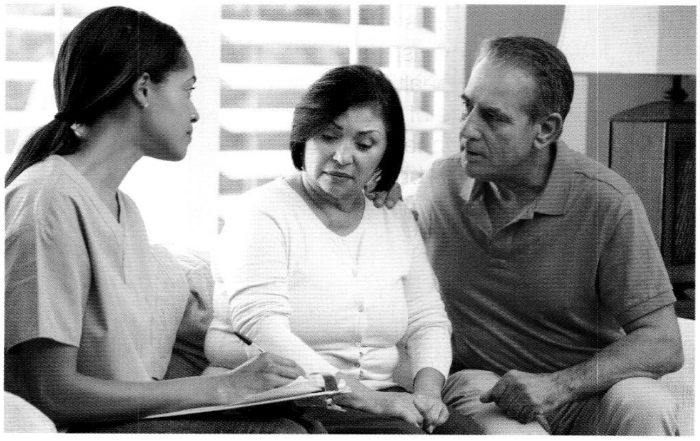

Fig. 3.1 Family members need information and reassurance. (Copyright © https://www.istockphoto.com)

complete assessment and plan of care. When collecting data about families and their coping strategies, first determine what stressors are being experienced by the family, what kinds of coping strategies are used, and how well the family is coping with stress. Knowing how well the family communicates and whether it is a functional or dysfunctional unit is important.

Understanding the relationships among the patient and other family members is also important. Families can add to the patient's burdens, provide considerable support, or serve as a mixed blessing. You should determine whether family members are supportive or detrimental in the recovery process. The nursing care plan should also consider the family's influence on individual members. Including family members in the patient's care and the decision-making process, with the patient's permission, helps to maintain the self-esteem of both patients and families.

Put On Your Thinking Cap!

Recall a patient whose family was present when you took care of the patient. Discuss how the family members and the patient interacted with each other and how the family members interacted with health care providers. What needs of family members could you identify? How can nurses help to meet the needs of families?

Community resources

Referral to community resources can help families to cope with health care problems. Nurses should be well acquainted with both informal and formal community resources. Informal resources usually consist of family members or friends who supply long-term support, comfort, and nurturing. Formal resources include community agencies that provide ongoing services.

Information provided through written and online sources can educate families about an illness or condition and its management. Online resources, social agencies, and support groups allow families to know that they are not alone and share coping strategies. Formal support systems help by assisting with problems such as home, institutional, and long-term care; finances; transportation; and social support. Many community agencies can help families dealing with stress or those in crisis. When complex family situations are encountered, the LVN/LPN should share data gathered with the supervising RN so that a plan of care can be developed.

Get Ready for the NCLEX® Examination!

Key Points

- Medical-surgical patients include individuals, across the health-illness continuum, from many cultures, in a variety of settings, and across the adult life span.
- Nursing and residential care facilities employ the largest percentage of LVNs/LPNs in the United States.
- Medical-surgical patients are found in acute care facilities, outpatient facilities, community settings, and long-term care.
- Primary prevention seeks to prevent illness and injury; secondary prevention is directed toward minimizing complications of an existing illness/injury and promoting maximum return to health; tertiary prevention addresses the long-term effects of a health deviation and helps the patient learn to manage them.
- Health literacy is the ability to obtain and understand basic information needed to make health decisions.
- The major types of families are nuclear, extended, step-parent, single-parent, and nontraditional.
- Cultural values and attitudes influence how a family interacts, carries out activities of daily living, and views health and health care.
- The best way to provide culturally appropriate nursing care is to collect data from the individual and adapt care accordingly.
- Religious beliefs can affect perceptions of health and illness, hospitalization, and death and dying.
- Health care providers receive federal funding to provide appropriate interpreter services to persons with limited English proficiency and those who are deaf or hard of hearing.
- Beliefs about health and illness affect the approach a person takes toward health and illness management.
- Including family members in patient care can help to alleviate stress and fulfill cultural expressions for both the patient and the family.
- A patient's response to a specific drug can be affected by genetic factors.
- The most common causes of death among young adults are unintentional injury, homicide, suicide, and malignant neoplasms.
- Members of the "sandwich generation" are caring for both children and adult parents.
- Older adults are very heterogeneous; avoid stereotyping based on chronological age.
- Patients should be able to define "family" by their own criteria, and to determine how those family members will participate in their care.
- Each of the stages of adulthood have developmental tasks that need to be accomplished.

- A family's response to a member's illness depends on role structure, family interactions, communication patterns, coping skills, and resources.
- Each family member has a role that defines expected behavior in given situations.
- Family roles may be classified as performance-oriented or emotional, and as formal or informal.
- When a family's emotional ills are blamed on one member, that person is called the scapegoat.
- Family functions and tasks are carried out through the process of interaction.
- Families have unique communication styles or patterns.
- Functional communication occurs when the receiver understands the sender's message as intended; with dysfunctional communication, the meaning is not understood as intended.
- Families use a variety of coping strategies to adapt to stressors.
- The inclusion of family members in a patient's care and the decision-making process helps to maintain the self-esteem of both patients and families.
- When working with families, the nurse identifies stressors, coping strategies, family communication, and resources.

Additional Learning Resources

SG Go to your Study Guide for additional learning activities to help you master this chapter content.

Go to your Evolve website (http://evolve.elsevier.com/Linton/medsurg) for the following learning resources and much more:
- Fluid & Electrolyte Tutorial
- Review Questions for the NCLEX® Examination

Clinical Judgment and Next-Generation NCLEX® Examination-Style Questions

1. **Analysis of family interactions reveals that some individuals are frequently labeled as scapegoats. What function does scapegoating serve in the family?**
   1. Diverts attention from family problems
   2. Brings attention to the family member who contributes the least
   3. Tests the bonds of loyalty within the family
   4. Motivates children to compete with siblings

   NCLEX Client Need: Psychosocial Integrity

2. **After a tornado, survivors are being interviewed. A common statement made by the survivors is: "We lost everything but each other. This has taught us what is really important in life." This statement is an example of what type of coping strategy?**
   1. Dealing directly with the cause of the problem
   2. Comfort to each other
   3. Denying the seriousness of the situation
   4. Attaching meaning to the experience

   NCLEX Client Need: Psychosocial Integrity

3. **The family of a critically ill patient is comforted by visits from their minister and church members. The family members pray often for their loved one's recovery. This situation is an example of:**
   1. An internal family coping strategy
   2. Anticipatory grieving
   3. An external family coping strategy
   4. Unrealistic thinking

   NCLEX Client Need: Psychosocial Integrity

4. **A husband and wife, 66 and 67 years of age, are seen in the Wellness Clinic. The couple has three grown children who have their own homes and families. The nurse knows that the developmental tasks for the traditional two-parent family in later life include: (Select all that apply.)**
   1. Communicating openly between parents and children
   2. Maintaining a satisfying living arrangement
   3. Adjusting to a reduced income
   4. Reorganization of the family into a continuing unit
   5. Maintaining intergenerational family ties

   NCLEX Client Need: Psychosocial Integrity

5. **A family assessment reveals which members fill the roles of leader, nurturer, and protector. These are examples of what type of role?**
   1. Performance oriented
   2. Emotional
   3. Developmental
   4. Maternal

   NCLEX Client Need: Psychosocial Integrity

6. **Common values among Euro-Americans (White Americans) include which of the following? (Select all that apply.)**
   1. Individual decision making
   2. Individualism
   3. Personal space
   4. Harmony
   5. Privacy

   NCLEX Client Need: Psychosocial Integrity

7. **The nurse at a university health clinic has initiated a program to encourage students to exercise regularly. This is an example of which level of prevention?**
   1. Primary
   2. Secondary
   3. Tertiary

   NCLEX Client Need: Psychosocial Integrity

8. **The developmental task "Ego Integrity Versus Despair" applies to which group?**
   1. Adolescents
   2. Young adults
   3. Middle adults
   4. Older adults

   NCLEX Client Need: Psychosocial Integrity

9. SLO/Objective: Describe roles and communication patterns within families.

NGN Item Type: Cloze

Cognitive Skill: Analyze cues

A LVN/LPN who is a home health nurse makes an initial visit to a family that has been referred for care. The nurse's assessment data include:

1. Ben, the 45 y.o. father, has a degenerative muscular condition that recently required him to take early retirement at a reduced salary.
2. Ben is distressed that he can no longer support his family although he still manages the budget
3. Angela, the 43 y.o. mother, is a full-time daycare worker and the primary caregiver for her husband.
4. Ron, 19 y.o. son, is a college student living at home
5. Anne, 16 y.o. daughter, is a high school junior
6. Barry, age 12, and Gary, age 5, are students
7. Angela states
8. She has trouble "making ends meet"
9. She does not discuss family problems with Ben to avoid stressing him
10. The children are not helpful and she is exhausted
11. Ron needs to set an example for the other children but he has always been "spoiled" and "self-centered."
12. When she tries to talk with Ron, it ends in a shouting match
13. If Ron would delay college and get a job, the family would be fine
14. Anne wants to drop out of school to get a job to help with expenses

Fill in the blanks in the paragraph below using options listed in this table.

OPTIONS
Wage earner
Homemaker
Financial manager
Caregiver
Harmonizer
Martyr
Encourager
Functional
Impaired
Dysfunctional

The nurse recognizes that Ben's illness has resulted in changes in the family role structure. Roles that are being shifted to Angela are ____________ and ____________. Angela has cast son Ron in the role of ____________ because he is identified as the source of many family problems. The communication style between Angela and Ron is ____________.

4 Health, Illness, Stress, and Coping

http://evolve.elsevier.com/Linton/medsurg

Objectives

1. Describe the dimensions of the healthy person in relation to physical and mental well-being.
2. Describe the five basic human need categories according to Maslow.
3. Explain illness behavior, the sick role, and the impact of illness on the family.
4. Describe Selye's general adaptation syndrome.
5. Discuss the concepts of adaptation and homeostasis.
6. Explain the factors that contribute to a person's response to illness.
7. Discuss illness as a stressor.
8. Describe the personal factors that impact the response to stress.
9. Describe factors that affect coping with illness.
10. Provide examples of adaptive and maladaptive coping strategies.
11. Define defense mechanisms that may be used to cope with stress or anxiety.
12. Identify conscious strategies used to deal with unfamiliar situations.
13. Describe these maladaptive coping strategies: helplessness, powerlessness, and denial.
14. Describe the purpose of Healthy People 2030.
15. Identify nursing interventions to promote maximum possible health along the health-illness continuum.

Key Terms

acute illness
adaptation
anxiety
chronic illness
coping
crisis
defense mechanisms
disease
exacerbation
fear
health
helplessness
illness
maladaptive coping
personality
remission
self-concept
self-esteem
stress
stressor

A person is a living being with physical, cognitive, affective, behavioral, and social dimensions who interacts with the environment to achieve a chosen life purpose. The *physical dimension* includes the biologic and physiologic aspects of a person. The physical dimension includes the person's internal environment and how it is integrated with cognitive, affective, behavioral, and social dimensions. The *cognitive dimension* involves an individual's ability to formulate thoughts, process information, and solve problems. The *affective dimension* involves an individual's ability to experience and express feelings and emotions. The *behavioral dimension* reflects a person's individuality and involves integration of the physical, cognitive, and affective dimensions. The *social dimension* involves an individual's skills in living as a member of a family and community. Together these dimensions form a complete or total person.

Environment typically refers to everything outside a person; however, it is more accurate to think of environment as having two dimensions: (1) the external environment and (2) the internal environment. The external environment includes the physical and social elements that are external to and interactive with an individual. In a health care setting, you are a part of the external environment. Environment can also refer to the internal environment of a person. An individual's internal environment refers to physical, biologic states inside the individual, such as fluid and electrolyte balance, body temperature, and nutritional status. Each of these elements affects an individual's overall health. **Health** may be viewed as the ability to express the full range of one's physical and mental potential within one's environment. A healthy person maintains stability and comfort by adapting physically, mentally, emotionally, and socially to internal and external events.

Mental health is a dynamic process in which a person's physical (internal environment), cognitive, affective, behavioral, and social dimensions interact functionally with one another and the external environment. Mentally healthy individuals are able to perceive reality accurately, manage the way that emotions are experienced and expressed, think clearly and logically, communicate effectively, anticipate events and solve problems, initiate and maintain meaningful relationships, develop a positive self-concept, and generally behave in ways that promote personal growth and development.

The understanding of human needs, both psychologic and physical, is central to all aspects of the nursing process, because nurses seek to promote or restore personal growth and development. The American psychologist Abraham Maslow was among the first to describe and define human needs in the form of a hierarchy. Maslow's theory evolved to be known as *Maslow's hierarchy of needs* (Fig. 4.1).

Maslow's theory identifies a hierarchical set of five basic human needs that motivate humans and allow for growth toward what Maslow describes as *self-actualization*. Maslow points out that human consciousness is able to reach toward attaining higher goals once more basic goals, or needs, are met. The most basic of the five needs includes physiologic needs such as food, water, air, shelter, sex, and other basic needs for general survival. Once met, the individual may seek to satisfy safety needs such as security, stability, protection, and freedom from fear, anxiety, and chaos. Safety needs also include the need for order, structure, and limits.

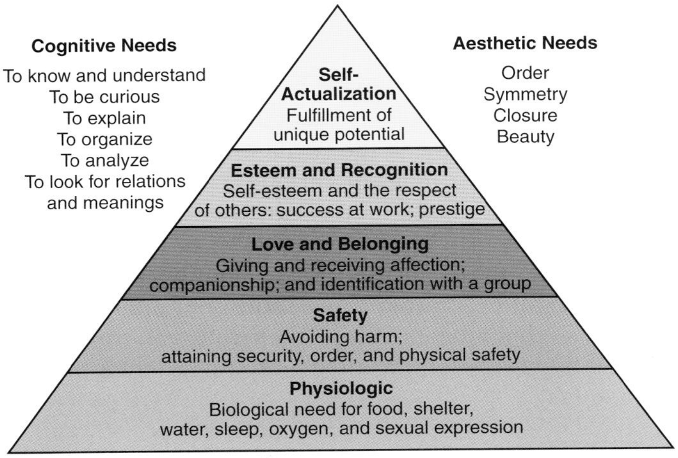

Fig. 4.1 Maslow's hierarchy of needs. Needs must be met in ascending order. For example, safety and security must be achieved before love and belonging needs can be met. (From Gaylor LJ: *The administrative dental assistant*, ed 4, St. Louis, 2017, Elsevier.)

The third set of needs is grouped as belongingness and love needs, including the need for love, affection, a sense of belongingness, and family, friends, groups, and community. Esteem needs follow as the fourth set and include the need for self-esteem, self-confidence, esteem of others, achievement, recognition, appreciation, and dignity and mastery over one's self and one's environment. Self-actualization is achieved when one meets the needs of self-mastery, gains a desire to help others, has the ability to direct one's own life, has rich emotional experiences, and develops a sense of meaning to one's life.

Nursing has a unique appreciation of Maslow's hierarchy of needs because threats to homeostasis as the result of stress and illness can impair an individual's ability to satisfy even the most basic of needs. Throughout the nursing process, you will apply Maslow's hierarchy of needs to understand your patient's needs and develop the most appropriate interventions designed to meet these needs based on your assessment of unmet needs along the hierarchy. Disturbances in health or homeostasis represent potential threats to the patient's ability to meet their needs across the hierarchy (Box 4.1).

HEALTH, DISEASE, AND ILLNESS

Health and illness are viewed as relative states along a continuum. Individuals have neither absolute health nor absolute illness. They are in an ever-changing state of being, ranging from peak or high-level wellness to extremely poor health, with death being imminent.

Each person's state of health integrates factors beyond biologic fitness. Personal, psychosocial, and spiritual values and beliefs influence how a person views health and illness.

In American culture, disease is regarded as a disruption of biologic function or psychologic function, or both. **Disease** is a condition that can be recognized through objective findings such as fever, the presence

Box 4.1 Characteristics of the Healthy, Self-Actualized Person According to Maslow

- An accurate perception of reality
- The ability to accept oneself and others
- The ability to be spontaneous
- The ability to solve problems
- A need for privacy
- Independence or autonomy
- The ability to express the self emotionally
- A frequency of "peak experiences" (i.e., happy moments that produce a sense of worth, hope, and love of life)
- Identification with humankind
- The ability to maintain satisfactory relationships
- A sense of ethics
- Some sense of resistance to conformity

of bacteria, or an individual's inability to function. **Illness** has a broader definition than disease because it incorporates personal, interpersonal, and cultural perceptions of and reactions to disease. Illness is a deviation from a healthy state that may occur acutely or as a series of long-term events. Acute and chronic illnesses are experienced and viewed differently.

Acute illness is an illness or disease that has a relatively rapid onset and short duration. The condition usually responds to a specific treatment and ends in full recovery. Examples of acute illnesses are the common cold, influenza, appendicitis, and urinary tract infections.

Chronic illness usually involves a permanent change in health status that requires long-term rehabilitation and medical or nursing treatment. Examples of chronic illnesses are coronary artery disease, chronic obstructive pulmonary disease, hypothyroidism, and diabetes mellitus. Some chronic illnesses, such as rheumatoid arthritis and asthma, are characterized by periods of **remission** and **exacerbation**. During remissions, the patient is free of acute symptoms. During episodes of exacerbation, acute symptoms recur.

ILLNESS BEHAVIOR

Reactions to illness vary among individuals. Some people take action whereas others may do nothing. Those who take action may seek the help of health care providers; others may seek help from friends or family members or use "home remedies." Among some cultures in the United States, people may seek help from folk healers or herbalists. The actions taken by individuals are influenced by the availability and affordability of health care, the individual's perception of the problem, others' perceptions of the problem, and the outcome of self-prescribed treatment.

People who take no action may wait to see whether the symptoms go away without treatment. Others may deny that something is wrong and refuse to admit that they are ill. People who take no action may be influenced by the same factors that affect those who take action.

Some individuals take counteraction in response to illness. Counteraction means that they engage in activities that should be avoided just to prove to themselves that the symptoms are not serious or do not exist. For example, a person with symptoms of chronic bronchitis may continue to smoke, regardless of the impaired breathing and coughing that the smoke may cause. Failure to follow proper health practices or treatment regimens may be labeled as *noncompliance* or *nonadherence*. Such behaviors can have harmful effects on health and self-esteem and can lead to death. When this occurs, rather than judging the patient, try to understand the basis of the patient's behavior and intervene in a positive way. For example, a patient may not take their antihypertensive drug because it makes them dizzy. You can teach the patient how to minimize and manage this drug side effect.

Box 4.2 Sick Role Behaviors

1. Exemption from normal activities
2. Recognition that the sick person is not responsible for causing the condition
3. Expectation that the sick person wants to get well
4. Obligation to seek competent help

Sick Role

When people become ill, they frequently adopt a "sick role." The sick role allows individuals time to recover from their disease. When they cannot get well on their own, others must care for them. They are temporarily exempt from social responsibilities so that they can concentrate on getting well. Society assumes that people who are sick want to get well and therefore should seek the help of health professionals and cooperate with prescribed health care regimens. However, some people are reluctant to give up the sick role because of the attention they get or because they wish to avoid work. Box 4.2 summarizes sick role behaviors.

IMPACT OF ILLNESS ON THE FAMILY

Illness affects not only the individual, but also the entire family. An illness may affect the roles of family members, the daily activities carried out, and the family's economic stability.

Three factors influence the effect of illness on the family. The first factor is the identity of the member of the family who is ill. For example, if the head of the household and chief breadwinner is sick, the financial resources may be threatened. If the person who normally cares for the home and children becomes ill, others have to pitch in to help. If an older member of the family becomes ill, grown children may have to provide care. The reversal in the parent-child roles may be difficult for both parents and children.

The second factor influencing the effect of illness on the family is the seriousness and duration of the disease. An acute illness does not produce the long-term effects of a chronic disease. Family members are able to change roles temporarily to manage an acute illness; however, a chronic illness has a long duration, and family relationships may become strained.

The third factor is the social and cultural customs of the family. Families of various cultures have different attitudes toward illness, caregiving, and changing family roles.

All of these factors affect family functioning. Feelings of frustration, anger, and grief must be managed so that all members of the family can function at their highest potential while providing care for the sick member.

STRESS

Part of being human is the need to cope with different types of stressors at different times of life. Individual coping strategies are influenced by many factors, such as personal beliefs and values as well as one's family, cultural practices, and community resources. Patients and their families may experience a wide range of feelings in response to illness. To promote adaptation to illness and to minimize maladaptive behaviors, you need to be well acquainted with the range of responses that individuals can experience during illness. The nursing process provides a systematic approach to individualized care based on careful assessment and understanding of human behavior.

The word *stress* has different meanings depending on the context or science in which it is used. In the science of physics, for example, **stress** refers to the internal distribution of forces exerted on a material body or structure. Think of a bridge crossing over a river. The bridge must be able to bear weight (i.e., stress) sufficiently to maintain its structural integrity. The word *stress* was first used in biology by the endocrinologist Hans Selye, who investigated the physiologic responses of living organisms to changes in the internal environment (physical) and external environment. The term *stress* was later broadened to refer to real and perceived challenges (i.e., stressors) and responses experienced by human beings.

Stressors can originate in any or all of the dimensions of the self. At any given moment, individuals are adapting to a variety of stressors from each of the five dimensions. Thus a person's level of health is directly related to the ability to adjust to a variety of internal and external stressors. A **stressor** can be anything, positive or negative, that necessitates an adaptive response on the part of the individual. Stress is necessary for growth and development. Mild stress produces mild anxiety and enables people to use energy focused exclusively on the problem. The result can be successful problem solving, which in turn promotes self-esteem. However, prolonged or chronic stress poses a serious threat to physical and emotional health. As the duration or intensity of stress or the number of stressors increases, a person's ability to adapt effectively decreases. Examples of potentially harmful stressors are the loss of a job or the death of a family member (Table 4.1).

Table 4.1 Examples of Stressors

PHYSIOLOGIC	EMOTIONAL/PSYCHOLOGIC
Skin burn	Diagnosis of cancer
Chronic pain	Marital problems
Hypothermia	Failing an examination
Infectious disease	Inadequate financial resources
Excessive noise	Grieving loss of spouse
Starvation	Caring for a disabled child
Running a marathon	Winning or losing an athletic event
Birth of a baby	Winning the lottery

From Lewis SL, Dirksen SR, Heitkemper MM, Bucher L, Camera IM: *Medical-surgical nursing: assessment and management of clinical problems*, ed 8, St. Louis, 2011, Elsevier-Mosby, p. 100.

ADAPTATION

Adaptation refers to a person's biologic and psychologic efforts to respond to a stressor and affects the whole organism. For example, the normal stress associated with physical activity and exercise results in maintaining or building muscle mass, circulation, and joint flexibility. If a person becomes immobilized, the lack of stress (i.e., exercise) may result in the muscles beginning to atrophy, joints becoming rigid and inflexible, and so on, until all systems of the body are affected. So it is with mental health. The dimensions of the person—physical, cognitive, affective, behavioral, and social—are not separate entities. These dimensions interact, resulting in the development of a unique human being.

HOMEOSTASIS

Stress, response, and adaptation can be thought of as a process aimed at maintaining homeostasis or equilibrium. If stressors are relatively mild, and the person is able to respond and adapt, mental health is maintained. However, if the person is overwhelmed by many stressors or does not have sufficient coping behaviors or problem-solving strategies to maintain equilibrium, illness, or crisis may ensue. A **crisis** results in inner tension and anxiety, which may affect an individual's ability to function.

PSYCHOLOGIC RESPONSES TO ILLNESS

Responses to illness are as unique as patients themselves. Individual responses to illness are related to the individual's personality, life experiences, self-concept, perceptions, values, cultural perspectives, and spiritual beliefs, to name a few. The individual's ability to adapt to stress (i.e., adaptation) is also an important factor in how they will respond to illness.

COPING WITH ILLNESS

Most people see illness as a distressing, abnormal state of being. This state of distress demands that individuals draw from their inner resources to cope. These resources may come from any or all of the following dimensions: physical, cognitive, affective, behavioral, social, and spiritual. For some, the inner strengths drawn from these various dimensions may be sufficient to cope effectively with illness. For others, however, attempts to cope may be ineffective or maladaptive. Nursing intervention is essential in fostering healthy adaptation and coping during times of illness.

A caring attitude is basic to helping a patient cope with illness. Through the trust developed in a therapeutic nurse-patient relationship, the nurse can help the patient to cope with stressors precipitated by illness (see the Patient Teaching box).

Patient Teaching

Helping Patients and Their Families to Cope With a Serious Diagnosis

Research shows that patients who are more involved in their health care tend to get better results and be more satisfied. Share with patients the following steps to help them deal effectively with the initial diagnosis and make the best possible decisions for themselves and their families:

- *Step 1: Take the time you need.* Do not rush important decisions about your health. In most cases, you will have time to carefully examine your options and decide what is best for you.
- *Step 2: Get the support you need.* Look for support from family and friends, people who are going through the same thing you are, and those who have "been there." They can help you to cope with your situation and make informed decisions.
- *Step 3: Talk with your doctor.* Good communication with your doctor can help you to feel more satisfied with the care you receive. Research shows it can even have a positive effect on things such as symptoms and pain. Getting a second opinion may help you to feel more confident about your care.
- *Step 4: Seek out information.* When learning about your health problem and its treatment, look for information that is based on a careful review of the latest scientific findings published in medical journals.
- *Step 5: Decide on a treatment plan.* Work with your doctor to decide on a treatment plan that best meets your needs.

Modified from Agency for Healthcare Research and Quality, Department of Health and Human Services: *Next steps after your diagnosis*. https://www.ahrq.gov/patients-consumers/diagnosis-treatment/diagnosis/diaginfo/index.html. Accessed October 18, 2020.

To assess an individual's potential for coping with an illness effectively, you need to understand that the ability to cope is affected by various factors. Among these factors are age, cultural beliefs, spirituality, self-concept, family and community resources, emotions, stress, fear, anxiety, loss, grief, and mourning.

Factors That Affect Coping With Illness

Age and stage of development

Age affects the coping ability of children and adults alike. The developmental process continues throughout the life span. Illness can interfere with developmental progress, and the patient's developmental stage can influence how they respond to illness. Much stress may be experienced when illness interferes with development. Illness can interfere with a number of adult roles. New or existing relationships, careers, family responsibilities, and a host of other roles may be affected by the onset of illness. An illness can be especially traumatic if a family breadwinner is self-employed or has insufficient health insurance.

When collecting data about the patient's ability to cope with illness, you need to understand that illness is a stressful, disruptive experience regardless of age. It not only disrupts the developmental process of the individual but also has a traumatic effect on spouses, children, and other loved ones. You will play an essential role in helping patients and their loved ones to cope with an illness and the changes that result.

Personality

Individuals' personalities affect their reactions to stress and illness. Although there are many different theories of **personality**, it is generally accepted that personality consists of the characteristic patterns of thoughts, feelings, and behaviors that make a person unique. Personality is made up of permanent traits that give consistency and individuality to a person's behavior. Thus people generally respond to and act in the same or similar ways in a variety of situations.

Cultural beliefs

Culture is a system of symbols shared by a group of humans. Culture is transmitted from each generation to the next and is influenced by other social contexts as well. Culture brings organization and security to people's lives. It provides many of the underlying values and beliefs on which behavior is based. Culture can affect attitudes toward health and illness, diet and eating practices, reaction to pain, and values concerning death and dying. *Ethnicity* is a broader term that denotes a group's affiliation because of shared language, race, and cultural values.

For individuals to be seen as unique, their cultural and ethnic backgrounds must be considered (see the Cultural Considerations box). This becomes especially important when trying to determine whether patients need assistance in coping with the stresses of illness. Remember, however, that not all people who look as if they belong to a specific cultural or ethnic group because of language, surname, or physical characteristics necessarily identify with any specific group. Effective nursing interventions can be determined only when we understand the patient as a unique individual, not only as White American, Black American, or Latino; man or woman; gay or straight.

Cultural Considerations

What Does Culture Have to Do With Illness?

Culture shapes attitudes toward health and illness, nutrition, pain, and death and dying.

When helping patients to cope with illness, you need to recognize that your own racial and cultural background may affect your ability to intervene effectively. This is especially true if the patient's cultural values and your own values differ greatly. It is important to respect the patient, regardless of your own personal beliefs, values, and culture. A judgmental attitude on your part interferes with delivering the best nursing care possible.

The nursing plan of care should consider whether the nursing approach being suggested is relevant to the patient's individual needs. Does the nursing care help patients to deal with stress or does it contribute to stress? Effective care is individualized according to the patient's needs, values, and beliefs.

Spirituality

During the crisis of illness, patients often turn to their spiritual beliefs and values to find meaning in the experience. Patients who perhaps had not thought of themselves as being religious may suddenly have a need to visit with a spiritual counselor. Many patients experience spiritual distress when under the stress of an illness. They may feel that the illness is unfair and that God has betrayed or abandoned them. Sometimes people feel that the illness is a punishment from God for some transgression they believe they have made.

Spiritual distress can be characterized by the following: (1) patients question the meaning of suffering or existence; (2) patients experience a sense of conflict between their personal beliefs (or desires) and their relationship with their God; or (3) patients experience symptoms such as nightmares, sleep disturbances, and alterations in behavior and mood.

To determine whether spirituality is an asset or a liability to the patient's ability to cope with illness, you must understand that all individuals are experts on their own spiritual needs and paths. Patients need an opportunity to express their feelings in a therapeutic and nonjudgmental environment. Simply put, your role is to listen, support, and care. Effective therapeutic nursing interventions enhance the healing process by supporting patients as they work through their spiritual distress and by shoring up their relationship with their spiritual connectedness.

Self-concept

Self-concept refers to the notions, beliefs, and convictions that persons hold about themselves. It is related to self-esteem and influences a person's relationship with others. **Self-esteem** develops from individuals' own evaluations of their competence and of the value others place on them. Body image refers to the combination of conscious and unconscious attitudes that people have about their own bodies. Past and present perceptions of the body and the person's feelings about their body's size, shape, function, appearance, and potential make up the body image.

Self-concept can be affected by changes in self-esteem and body image. Patients' perception of these changes and their ability or inability to cope with the changes may result in stress, fear, and anxiety. Age and developmental levels may directly affect the patient's self-esteem and body image. Adolescents are especially vulnerable to changes in body image because they have a strong need to look like their peers. Certain changes in body image can be quite traumatic at this developmental stage. Adults also can be vulnerable.

People such as actors, models, or professional football players, who rely on their physical characteristics to make a living, may not be able to cope well with an illness or injury that affects body image. A disfiguring or disabling injury could have a devastating effect on body image and self-esteem. Their personal strengths and weaknesses would determine how well they are able to cope with the threat that illness imposes on the self-concept.

Some patients, through their life experiences, have developed coping styles that allow them to confront problems effectively. Others may require more external resources such as friends, family, and the community to cope with the stress of illness.

Emotions

When a serious illness occurs, patients and their families must adapt to many changes. Some of these changes may involve permanent alterations in lifestyle, frequent visits to health care providers, frequent hospitalizations, financial problems, and increased social isolation. For those in crisis, coping can be difficult at best and seemingly impossible at worst.

This section discusses a broad range of feelings and emotions that people may experience. Many of these feelings are normal and to be anticipated. However, times exist when the coping methods being used by patients and families are maladaptive. It is important to differentiate adaptive from maladaptive coping mechanisms.

Stress. Perceptions of stress and coping mechanisms are highly individualized. People subjected to prolonged stressors eventually became totally exhausted. Individuals who cannot cope adequately with stress may experience a threat to their emotional well-being. They may find their perceptions of reality skewed, their ability to solve problems considerably compromised, and their stress consequently increased. In other words, without effective coping strategies, individuals can be caught in a vicious cycle of ineffective coping and increased stress that will stop only at the point of total exhaustion and may result in death.

You must learn to recognize individuals whose coping skills are ineffective and who consequently are caught in a downward spiral of debilitating exhaustion. Without effective nursing interventions to reverse this downward spiral, serious impairment will result.

Fear. The words *fear* and *anxiety* are often used interchangeably. However, fear generally denotes a response to a specific threat, and anxiety is often a response to a nonspecific threat. The body's physiologic reaction to fear is similar to its response to anxiety. The person experiencing the crisis of illness has much to fear: pain, financial ruin, disfigurement, loss of self-esteem, and not being able to return to a previous lifestyle.

Fears vary according to the developmental status and age of the individual. For example, toddlers may fear separation from their mothers whereas adolescents may fear threats to their body image. Terminally ill patients may be struggling with fears of death and dying.

You can be very helpful in assisting patients and families to cope with fear. Sometimes just providing an opportunity to express fear helps to lessen the stress caused by fear. Providing information about tests or nursing procedures may empower clients to begin to cope with fear. However, too much information can also be very stressful. In deciding how much information to provide, you must determine the patient's current understanding of the situation and any anticipated procedures they may be about to face. Providing basic information and then following up by answering the patient's questions is usually best.

Anxiety. **Anxiety** is a vague and sometimes intense sense of impending doom or apprehension that may appear to have no clearly identifiable cause. Anxiety is often an early response to illness. The degree of anxiety may vary with the severity of the illness. Anxiety may lead to physical and psychologic stress and may be caused by real or imagined fear resulting from loss. As people develop, they learn to cope with this painful emotion. The fight-or-flight response actually provides the physiologic ability for one to either fight or flee. Individuals continually regulate their behavior based on their level of perceived anxiety. When anxiety intensifies to an excessive level, the perception of reality becomes focused solely on the crisis.

Loss. Loss is an experience usually related to the involuntary separation of the self from someone or something loved or treasured. It may involve a separation from a person or object, relationship, personal attribute, hope, dream, desire, role, functional ability, or potential. Perceived loss of control, sense of worth, and loss of health are also types of loss.

Actual loss can be recognized by others as well as by the patients. Examples of actual loss include the loss of a spouse or the loss of a limb. *Anticipatory loss* is a sense of loss experienced before the actual loss occurs. Families may experience anticipatory loss during the terminal stages of a loved one's illness.

Loss can be a significant stressor that precipitates feelings of fear and anxiety. The fears associated with loss can be stressful enough to compromise the ability of an individual to recover from illness. One of the first psychologic steps that must be taken to begin the process of coping is to permit oneself to experience the full emotional effect of the loss. This emotional response is known as *grief* or *mourning*.

The experience of loss is related to the individual's self-concept. The extent of loss depends on how strongly the individual's sense of self was connected to that which was lost.

Grief and mourning. Grief is the subjective, emotional response that evolves from a sense of loss. Mourning is the process through which grief is faced and ultimately resolved or altered over time. Mourning occurs when a person is forced to relinquish original hopes. The process of mourning prepares the individual to reappraise values and to accept substitutions for hope.

Individuals who are experiencing grief may be under a great deal of stress and that stress may make them even more vulnerable to disease. They may become irritable and difficult to get along with; sometimes they may experience a sense of guilt. Some people blame themselves for whatever they have lost. They may perceive their illness and subsequent loss as a punishment from God for not having been a better person, a better parent, or a better spouse.

To alter the loss that grief causes, the self must change. The process of change is unique to each individual and each circumstance. One individual's need for change may require only a change in exercise and dietary habits. Another person's need for change may encompass a career, a lifestyle, or the development of better strategies to cope with stress. Most changes in a person's life are stressful. The greater the change, the greater the resulting stress. To cope with stress, the individual may mobilize psychologic resources known as *coping mechanisms*. Adaptive coping mechanisms can be effective, therapeutic ways of dealing with stress. **Maladaptive coping** behaviors, however, can be detrimental and decrease the ability to cope with illness. Chapter 19 addresses loss and grief in detail.

Family and Community Resources

The basic functions of the family include providing for physical needs, giving love, providing a sense of belonging, and strengthening the self-esteem of its members. Functional families may provide optimal support for a patient facing the stress of illness. However, the family's ability to provide support for the patient depends on many factors, including the quality of relationships among family members and the family's ability to access needed resources.

Because of increasing stresses on the family unit, many families are not able to provide as much support as the patient may need. The stress of illness in a family member may overburden a family that was already only marginally coping. Illness may have precipitated such stressors as changes in family roles, economic pressures, and geographic isolation that may make it difficult to access medical and other needed resources.

Many of the functions once provided by families increasingly are assumed by social institutions within the community. Like families, communities vary in their ability to assist their members. Some communities are well equipped to assist the family with many challenges that it may face (e.g., financial, physical, legal, spiritual, emotional). Other communities are less able to meet those same needs. This is especially true if the patient lives in an impoverished, underserved, or rural community. Your knowledge of available resources can be invaluable to patients and families. Throughout a hospital stay, you must anticipate the patient's needs before discharge. Providing contact information and creating links for patients in the community to help meet the needs of the patient outside the institution are essential parts of preparing the patient and their family for discharge. Local, state, and national organizations can be very helpful resources that may keep a family from succumbing to the pressures of a catastrophic illness.

COPING MECHANISMS AND STRATEGIES

Coping is the process of responding to stress, such as illness, or a potential stressor. Coping with stress is a self-regulatory process by which people manage their responses to stress and thus relieve the tension related to the stressor. Coping strategies can be conscious or unconscious behaviors. Unconscious coping strategies are referred to as **defense mechanisms**.

Defense Mechanisms

According to Freud, the ego may devise strategies or defense mechanisms to cope with stress or anxiety. Defense mechanisms are used to diminish anxiety; however, when used excessively or inappropriately, they can hinder the developing personality. Defense mechanisms used to protect against anxiety include the following:

- *Compensation*—an attempt to make up for real or imagined weakness. For example, an adolescent perceived as unattractive becomes an outstanding athlete.
- *Denial*—a refusal to acknowledge a real situation. For example, a woman who finds a suspicious lump in her breast does not keep an appointment for a breast biopsy.
- *Displacement*—transferring the associated feelings from one source to another that is considered less threatening. For example, a boy who is angry with a teacher comes home and yells at his dog.
- *Identification*—the emulation of admirable qualities in another to enhance one's self-esteem. For example, a child dresses and uses mannerisms similar to those of a rock star.
- *Rationalization* or *intellectualization*—the use of logic, reasoning, and analysis to avoid unacceptable feelings. For example, a student fails to complete an assignment correctly and rationalizes subsequent feelings of incompetence by complaining about the teacher's expectations for the assignment.
- *Introjection*—internalizing or taking on the values and beliefs of another person. For example, a child takes on the values and beliefs of a parent.
- *Isolation*—the separation of emotion from an associated thought or memory. For example, a man appears apathetic as he discusses a firefight in which he participated in Vietnam.
- *Projection*—transferring unacceptable feelings or impulses to another. For example, a partner who is jealous of her significant other accuses the partner of being jealous.
- *Reaction formation*—avoiding unacceptable thoughts and behaviors by expressing opposing thoughts or behaviors. For example, a patient who unconsciously hates his father continuously says how great his father is.
- *Regression*—withdrawing to an earlier level of development to benefit from the associated comfort levels of the previous level. For example, a child starts sucking her thumb when her new brother comes home from the hospital.
- *Repression*—an unconscious defense mechanism in which unacceptable ideas, impulses, and memories are kept out of consciousness. For example, a woman cannot remember a sexual assault.
- *Somatization*—the transfer of painful feelings to body parts, so that the person's feelings are expressed in the form of a physical symptom. For example, a woman who has experienced intolerable internal conflict develops a physical complaint of pain in the wrist that cannot be explained by diagnostic means.
- *Sublimation*—the transformation of unacceptable impulses or drives (e.g., aggressiveness, anger, sexuality) into constructive or more acceptable behavior. For example, a person who has aggressive tendencies becomes a jackhammer operator.
- *Suppression*—(a conscious mechanism) a conscious or voluntary inhibition of unacceptable ideas, impulses, and memories. For example, a child who fails an algebra class puts that event out of their mind.
- *Undoing*—actually or symbolically attempting to cancel out an action that was unacceptable. An example is sprinkling salt over one's left shoulder to prevent bad luck after spilling salt on the table.
- *Substitution*—replacing a highly valued, unattainable object with a less-valued, attainable object. For example, the person who has a strong unconscious sexual attraction to a parent marries someone who resembles that parent.
- *Conversion*—turning an emotional conflict into a physical symptom, which provides the individual with some sort of benefit (secondary gain). For example, the individual who witnesses a murder then experiences sudden blindness without an organic cause.

Individuals adapt defense mechanisms as protective measures to allow the ego relief from anxiety. One factor that enhances the development of ego is an environment with experiences that match the child's capacity to adapt. Ideally, unhealthy defense mechanisms are shed and replaced by more realistic and efficient methods of adaptation as the individual matures.

Put On Your Thinking Cap!

Recall two incidents when you recognized a defense mechanism being used to cope. Describe the behavior, label the mechanism, and indicate the positive and negative outcomes of the mechanism. Share and discuss this with your classmates.

Conscious Coping Strategies

Conscious coping strategies are purposeful behaviors that are used to make an unfamiliar situation into one that is perceived as more controllable and predictable. Coping strategies and mechanisms vary from individual to individual. What all these behaviors have in common is that they are attempts to help people feel less stressed and anxious about their illness. Some of these methods provide only temporary relief while others provide more permanent results. It is important for you to identify and evaluate the effectiveness of coping mechanisms used by the patient.

Some techniques that can be used to help patients cope are known as *relaxation techniques.* Relaxation techniques include interventions such as imagery, relaxation strategies, therapeutic touch, and music therapy. Relaxation techniques elicit the relaxation response that reduces the effects of stress and decreases anxiety. These techniques can provide clients with self-control during moments of stress. Relaxation techniques are taught only when patients are not in acute discomfort, because the exercise will be ineffective if the patient cannot concentrate. *Imagery* is the use of the imagination to develop sensory images that focus the mind away from the stressful experience and emphasize other sensory experiences and pleasant memories. Relaxation strategies include biofeedback, meditation, deep-breathing exercises, yoga, and Zen practices. *Therapeutic touch* is a process by which the therapist acts as a channel for environmental and universal energy through the therapist's mental concentration.

Music therapy is another relaxation technique that may help the patient to cope by enhancing the relaxation response and facilitating positive imagery. Musical selections should match a patient's mood and musical taste. Earphones with audio CDs or cassettes help the patient to avoid annoying others and allow them to concentrate on the music. This coping method provides only temporary relief of stress; however, use of such techniques can help to establish a therapeutic environment in which you can begin to discuss the real sources of the patient's concerns, fears, and anxieties.

Tapping into the spiritual dimension can also be a very effective way of coping with the stress of illness. You can talk with patients about their spiritual needs without relying on traditional religious language. The opportunity to discuss beliefs about a higher power or the search for meaning in suffering proves to be an effective way of coping for many patients.

Health Promotion

Examples of Conscious Coping Strategies

STRATEGY	DESCRIPTION	HOW TO IMPLEMENT
Aromatherapy	Use of essential oils (fragrant molecules from plants) for inhalation or topical application Variety of essential oils including lavender, peppermint, rosemary, eucalyptus, sandalwood, etc.	Place 5–8 drops in a full bath and agitate water before bathing Place a few drops in a tissue or in a diffuser or vaporizer
Art therapy	Allows an individual to nonverbally express and communicate feelings, emotions, and thoughts Can assist an individual to reduce stress, relax, and process experiences Based on the belief that the creative process is healing and life enhancing	Close your eyes and draw a line on a piece of paper. Open your eyes, continue to build on that line, draw whatever comes to mind Get a piece of paper and doodle. Do not edit Get a coloring book and crayons and just start coloring
Exercise	Can take the form of any form of movement, especially aerobic movement. Results in improved circulation, increased release of endorphins, and an enhanced sense of well-being	Walk, swim, garden, bicycle, dance, climb stairs, participate in group exercises
Humor	Can take the form of laughter, cartoons, funny movies, videos, riddles, comic books, and joke books. Humor carts have been set up in many clinical settings to be used by patients and families	Keep a "tickler" scrapbook with funny photos, cartoons, etc. Humor carts can be set up in many clinical settings to be used by patients and families
Journaling	Allows an individual to express self in written form. This may include such things as personal events, thoughts, feelings, memories, and perceptions.	Use a journaling notebook or computer to write down thoughts, feelings, memories, and perceptions
Pet therapy	Use of animals as a form of treatment Improves a patient's social, emotional, or cognitive function	Pet therapist or family member or friend brings a pet with which patient can socialize
Social support	May take the form of organized support and self-help groups, relationships with family and friends, and professional help	Get together with family and friends on a regular basis Join a support group that specifically helps to meet needs (e.g., grief support group)

From Lewis SL, Bucher L, Heitkemper MM, Harding MM: *Medical-surgical nursing: assessment and management of clinical problems*, ed 10, St. Louis, 2017, Elsevier-Mosby, p. 82.

Maladaptive Coping Mechanisms and Strategies

In an effort to reduce the stress and anxiety that is precipitated by the crisis of an illness, an individual may sometimes engage in thinking patterns or behaviors that are ineffective or even self-destructive. These ineffective coping mechanisms may evolve from a sense of helplessness or powerlessness.

Helplessness

Helplessness typically occurs when individuals have had repeated exposure to events they perceive as being uncontrollable. This leads to loss of motivation, feelings of despair or anxiety, and cognitive impairment. The individual may begin to express anger as a means of diminishing feelings of helplessness. This anger may take the form of a personal attack on you and other caregivers. The expression of anger is really not aimed at you but is simply an attempt to cope with feelings of loss of control. Helplessness can be prevented by allowing individuals to control as many events as possible within the constraints imposed by treatment and their energy level.

Powerlessness

Powerlessness is a feeling that one's actions cannot affect an outcome or that one lacks personal control over certain events or situations. Characteristics of powerlessness include nonparticipation in care of decision making when opportunities are provided, reluctance to express feelings, passivity, submissiveness, apathy, feelings of hopelessness, and expressions of having no control or influence over a situation or outcome. When people are not ready to cope with the threat of illness, unconscious defense mechanisms of avoidance, such as denial, may be used. These avoidance defense mechanisms protect individuals from having to confront and deal with the threat of illness.

Denial

Denial is the subconscious blocking out of emotional experiences. Denial can take several forms: (1) verbal denial, (2) minimizing the severity of the illness, (3) displacing symptoms onto another organ system, and (4) engaging in behaviors contrary to medical advice. The outcome of denial may be positive or negative. Denial can lead to negative consequences if people fail to engage in appropriate problem-focused behaviors. Patients who claim that they were never afraid or insist that nothing is wrong with them are engaging in denial. Denial is maladaptive when the patient's behavior interferes significantly with obtaining appropriate care. Arguing with patients about their denial only reinforces the inappropriate behavior.

When working with people in denial, make a special effort to accept them even though it may be uncomfortable to care for individuals who deny their illnesses. You may need to allow the individual to deny the illness and at the same time ask for cooperation. Once an effective therapeutic nurse-patient relationship has been established, patients may be better able to lower unconscious defenses and begin to discuss true feelings of fear and anxiety.

NURSING CARE TO PROMOTE COPING WITH ILLNESS

In this section, the various steps of the nursing process are discussed to help you collect relevant data and plan nursing interventions that will facilitate the patient's task of dealing with the crisis of illness.

FOCUSED ASSESSMENT

An individual's ability to cope with an illness varies from moment to moment and from situation to situation. Therefore assessment must be an ongoing process. To determine the effectiveness of individual coping strategies, the following questions could be posed to the individual:

- How well do you think you are coping with your illness?
- Do you have the information you need to care for yourself at this time?
- How well are you able to care for yourself?
- What resources are available to you in dealing with your illness?
- Do you follow the plan prescribed by your health care provider?
- How has your illness affected your life and that of your family?
- Has your illness required you and your family to change roles and responsibilities?
- How are you dealing with the changes required by your illness?
- Have you been able to maintain a sense of hope in spite of the demands of the illness?
- Do you feel that the important relationships in your life remain intact?

Data collected by licensed vocational nurse/licensed practical nurse (LVN/LPN) can help answer these questions. The term *focused assessment* is sometimes used to describe the data relevant to a specific patient need or problem.

PATIENT PROBLEMS

The LVN/LPN focuses on the patient's needs or presenting problems that would benefit from nursing interventions. Examples of patient problems that the LVN/LPN might identify when a patient is struggling to cope with illness include inadequate coping, denial, decreased socialization, inadequate family coping, altered self-concept, and ineffective management of the condition.

NURSING GOALS AND OUTCOME CRITERIA

The overall goal of nursing care is to help people manage and successfully cope with their illness. More specific goals depend on the patient problems identified. The LVN/LPN continually collects data

Box 4.3 Healthy People 2030 Topics

1. Health Conditions
   a. Addiction
   b. Arthritis
   c. Blood disorders
   d. Cancer
   e. Chronic kidney disease
   f. Chronic pain
   g. Dementia
   h. Diabetes
   i. Foodborne illness
   j. Healthcare-associated infections
   k. Heart disease and stroke
   l. Infectious disease
   m. Mental health and mental disorders
   n. Oral conditions
   o. Osteoporosis
   p. Overweight and obesity
   q. Pregnancy and childbirth
   r. Respiratory disease
   s. Sensory or communication disorders
   t. Sexually transmitted infections
2. Health Behaviors
   a. Child and adolescent development
   b. Drug and alcohol abuse
   c. Emergency preparedness
   d. Family planning
   e. Health communication
   f. Injury prevention
   g. Nutrition and healthy eating
   h. Physical activity
   i. Preventive care
   j. Safe food handling
   k. Sleep
   l. Tobacco use
   m. Vaccination
   n. Violence prevention
3. Populations
   a. Adolescents
   b. Children
   c. Infants
   d. LGBTQI+
   e. Men
   f. Older adults
   g. Parents or caregivers
   h. People with disabilities
   i. Women
   j. Workforce
4. Settings and Systems
   a. Community
   b. Environmental health
   c. Global health
   d. Health care
   e. Health insurance
   f. Health information technology
   g. Health policy
   h. Hospital and emergency services
   i. Housing and homes
   j. Public health infrastructure
   k. Schools
   l. Transportation
   m. Workplace
5. Social Determinants of Health
   a. Economic stability
   b. Education access and quality
   c. Health care access and quality
   d. Neighborhood and built environment
   e. Social and community context

From DHHS, 2020. https://health.gov/healthypeople/objectives-and-data/browse-objectives. Confirmed October 6, 2021.

to determine whether the desired patient outcomes have occurred. When effective coping strategies are used, patients can manage their illness and adapt to a new lifestyle that incorporates healthy behaviors and realistic goals. In addition, patients should emerge from the process with a positive self-concept and self-esteem.

People with chronic, debilitating illnesses may have difficulty acquiring and maintaining coping skills for long periods of time. Individuals may be able to cope with their illness today, but tomorrow may bring a whole new set of challenges. This is especially true in terminal stages of illness, when physical deterioration is on an accelerated course and every day brings new losses that need to be mourned and coped with by the patient and family.

Nursing Interventions Across the Health-Illness Continuum

Although this chapter has focused on understanding and providing care for people who are ill, this section discusses nursing interventions for promoting maximum possible wellness for patients across the health-illness continuum.

Prevent Health Problems

The U.S. Department of Health and Human Services has outlined goals for the year 2030 in a document called *Healthy People 2030* . *Healthy People 2030* is a national health promotion and disease prevention initiative that aims to increase the quality and years of healthy life and to eliminate health disparities. Some 62 topics have been categorized as Health Conditions, Health Behaviors, Populations, Settings and Systems, or Social Determinants of Health. Each topic has a link to a website with specific objectives and strategies (Box 4.3).

Specific activities that are generally thought to promote health are as follows:

- Adequate nutrition based on the MyPlate concept (see Chapter 15). MyPlate is an individualized approach to healthy eating and exercise that focuses on consuming fewer calories, making informed food choices, and being physically active.

Box 4.4 Recommendations for Physical Activity

The U.S. Department of Health and Human Services (DHHS) has released physical activity guidelines for all Americans 3 years of age and older.

The "2018 Physical Activity Guidelines for Americans" advise that regular physical activity improves health. People are encouraged to be as active as possible.

The guidelines recommend the types and amounts of physical activity that children, adults, older adults, and other groups should do. The guidelines also provide tips for how to fit physical activity into your daily life.

The information below is based on the DHHS guidelines.

KEY GUIDELINES FOR ADULTS

The guidelines advise that:

- Adults should move more and sit less throughout the day. Some physical activity is better than none. Adults who sit less and do any amount of moderate-to-vigorous physical activity gain some health benefits.
- For substantial health benefits, adults should do 150–300 min a week of moderate-intensity, or 75–150 min a week of vigorous-intensity aerobic physical activity, or an equivalent combination of moderate- and vigorous-intensity aerobic activity. Preferably, aerobic activity should be spread throughout the week.
- Additional health benefits are gained by engaging in physical activity beyond the equivalent of 300 min of moderate-intensity physical activity a week.
- Adults should also do muscle-strengthening activities of moderate or greater intensity and that involve all major muscle groups on 2 or more days a week, as these activities provide additional health benefits.

KEY GUIDELINES FOR OLDER ADULTS

The key guidelines for adults also apply to older adults. In addition, the following key guidelines are just for older adults:

- As part of their weekly physical activity, older adults should do multicomponent physical activity that includes balance training as well as aerobic and muscle-strengthening activities.
- Older adults should determine their level of effort for physical activity relative to their level of fitness.
- Older adults with chronic conditions should understand whether and how their conditions affect their ability to do regular physical activity safely.
- When older adults cannot do 150 min of moderate-intensity aerobic activity a week because of chronic conditions, they should be as physically active as their abilities and conditions allow.

KEY GUIDELINES FOR ADULTS WITH CHRONIC HEALTH CONDITIONS AND ADULTS WITH DISABILITIES

- Adults with chronic conditions or disabilities, who are able, should do 150–300 min a week of moderate-intensity, or 75–150 min a week of vigorous-intensity aerobic physical activity, or an equivalent combination of moderate- and vigorous-intensity aerobic activity. Preferably, aerobic activity should be spread throughout the week.
- Adults with chronic conditions or disabilities, who are able, should also do muscle-strengthening activities of moderate or greater intensity and that involve all major muscle groups on 2 or more days a week, as these activities provide additional health benefits.
- When adults with chronic conditions or disabilities are not able to meet the above key guidelines, they should engage in regular physical activity according to their abilities and should avoid inactivity.
- Adults with chronic conditions or symptoms should be under the care of a health care provider. People with chronic conditions can consult a health care professional or physical activity specialist about the types and amounts of activity appropriate for their abilities and chronic conditions.

KEY GUIDELINES FOR SAFE PHYSICAL ACTIVITY

To do physical activity safely and reduce risk of injuries and other adverse events, people should:

- Understand the risks, yet be confident that physical activity can be safe for almost everyone.
- Choose types of physical activity that are appropriate for their current fitness level and health goals because some activities are safer than others.
- Increase physical activity gradually over time to meet key guidelines or health goals. Inactive people should "start low and go slow" by starting with lower intensity activities and gradually increasing how often and how long activities are done.
- Protect themselves by using appropriate gear and sports equipment, choosing safe environments, following rules and policies, and making sensible choices about when, where, and how to be active.
- Be under the care of a health care provider if they have chronic conditions or symptoms. People with chronic conditions and symptoms can consult a health care professional or physical activity specialist about the types and amounts of activity appropriate for them.

Data from U.S. Department of Health and Human Services: Physical activity guidelines for Americans, 2018. https://health.gov/paguidelines/guidelines/default.aspx. https://health.gov/our-work/nutrition-physical-activity/physical-activity-guidelines/previous-guidelines/2008-physical-activity-guidelines

It is based on the U.S. Department of Agriculture's *2015–2020 Dietary Guidelines for Americans*. To learn more about these guidelines, go to www.ChooseMyPlate.gov.

- Moderate exercise on a routine schedule. (See Box 4.4.)
- Seven to 9 hours of sleep every 24 hours for adults; 7 to 8 hours for older adults.
- Healthy lifestyle, especially no smoking.
- Limited consumption of alcohol. Maximum average drink of 1 per day for women and 2 per day for men (1 drink = 12 ounces beer, 5 ounces wine, 1.5 ounces of 80 proof distilled spirits or liquor).
- Balance of work and recreation.

Nurses can help people to engage in healthier lifestyles to prevent disease. Education enables patients to make informed decisions regarding their health care practices. The teaching plan should include:

- Healthy diet, exercise, and rest requirements
- Diseases for which the patient is at risk
- Consequences of the disease for which the patient is at risk
- Measures the patient can take to reduce their risk for the disease

When teaching patients and their families, keep in mind that most health promotion and disease prevention measures require a change in lifestyle. Consider the biophysical, psychologic, sociocultural, spiritual, and environmental dimensions of family life and structure and be realistic in your expectations for change.

Put On Your Thinking Cap!

Make a personal plan to promote your own health while you are a nursing student.

Put On Your Thinking Cap!

Identify three factors that are threats to your health and then identify ways to deal with each of them.

Help to Satisfy the Patient's Unmet Basic Human Needs

For people to maintain the highest levels of health and wellness, basic human needs must be met. According to modern nursing pioneer Virginia Henderson (1966, p. 15), "The unique function of the nurse is to assist the individual, sick or well, in the performance of those activities contributing to health or its recovery (or to a peaceful death) that he would perform unaided if he had the necessary strength, will, or knowledge. And to do this in such a way as to help him gain independence as rapidly as possible."

Henderson identified 14 basic human needs: normal breathing, eating and drinking adequately, eliminating body wastes, maintaining desirable posture, sleeping and resting, selecting suitable clothing (dressing and undressing), maintaining normal body temperature, keeping the body clean, avoiding dangers in the environment, communicating with others, worshiping, working to achieve a sense of accomplishment, playing, and learning. The nurse assists with those needs that the patient cannot meet alone. These needs are closely related to Maslow's hierarchy of human needs in that the first eight components address physiologic needs. Other components refer to safety needs, to love and belonging needs, and to self-esteem and self-actualization needs. Henderson's work provides a useful way to identify human needs that must be met for optimal health.

Increase Adaptability

To help patients increase their adaptability, first identify what the patient perceives as stressful and how stressful it is. One way to determine the degree of stress is to ask patients to name the worst possible stressor and then compare the present stressor with that one. The second step is to ask about past methods of coping with stress that have been successful for the patient. Applying past coping strategies to new situations may then be helpful. To collect data about internal coping strategies, ask: "What kind of things do you do when you are stressed?" "Do you eat more or less?" "Do you drink alcohol?" "Do you smoke more?" "Do you sleep more or less?" Questions that help to determine external coping strategies include: "To whom do you turn when you are feeling stressed?" "Do you talk with others or do you keep things inside?" "Do you contact any professionals such as social workers, nurses, physicians, or social agencies when you have a problem?"

Older persons may have particular difficulty coping with stress and adapting to new situations. When any type of stressor occurs, getting back to their previous level of functioning takes longer and is much harder than when they were young. Fortunately, people who have lived a long time have experienced many stresses throughout life and generally have developed a wide range of coping mechanisms and skills for adapting to change. Help older patients use past successful coping mechanisms to deal with new stressors. Emphasize strengths rather than limitations.

During hospitalization, you can help patients and families to cope with the stress of a new environment, illness, and uncertainty. Some patients and families benefit from detailed information about the disease and the hospital procedures; others prefer not to know. Allowing patients to have as much control as possible helps to reduce stress. Even people who are very dependent on hospital personnel need to feel that they have some control over their lives. Other measures that may help to relieve stress and promote coping and adaptation are biofeedback, progressive muscle relaxation, meditation, massage therapy, and guided imagery. These strategies, which require specialized training, generally focus attention inward on the patient's own mind and body and reduce either physical or emotional tension.

Foster Independence

In acute illness, recovery is often speedy and people return quickly to their previous lifestyles. However, individuals with chronic illnesses must spend a lifetime managing symptoms. Many older adults have one or more chronic illnesses and may need some type of assistance in their daily lives. The goal is to maintain the highest level of independence possible and prevent further disability. The following tasks have been identified for chronically ill individuals: prevent and manage crises, carry out prescribed regimens, manage symptoms, reorder time, adjust to changes in the course of the illness, prevent social isolation, and attempt to normalize social interactions.

Prevent and manage crises

When symptoms flare up, a crisis situation may arise. Nurses can help patients and families to anticipate and recognize the onset of a crisis so it can be averted or managed.

Carry out prescribed regimens

Chronically ill individuals may need to take many medications, eat special foods, or restrict some activities. Having a restricted lifestyle day in and day out is very difficult, especially when symptoms are not always apparent. Nursing interventions include teaching patients about the need to carry out regimens, providing moral support and encouragement, and finding ways to make carrying out regimens easier. You can increase patient compliance by forming "alliances" with them so they understand that they are important participants in developing their own health regimen. Of course, when the situation involves lifestyle changes, only the patient can control them.

Manage symptoms

Chronically ill individuals need to learn to manage symptoms to continue desired activities. Gear nursing interventions toward helping patients learn about the pattern of symptoms (typical onset, duration, and severity) and the limits of their ability to control symptoms. Arrange daily routines so that more demanding activities are carried out when symptoms are least troubling and periods of rest are taken when symptoms are most acute.

Reorder time

People with chronic illness may find that they have either too much or too little available time. Forced retirement may increase the amount of free time; conversely, carrying out regimens to manage symptoms may be extremely time consuming for patients and caregivers. In both situations, the chronically ill and their family members may become frustrated and depressed. The nurse can assist patients and caregivers to develop a daily schedule that allows time for desired activities while managing the regimens of the chronic illness.

Adjust to changes in the course of the illness

Chronic illnesses often have unpredictable courses. To achieve their highest potential, chronically ill individuals need support to learn to live with the ups and downs of the disease.

Prevent social isolation

Chronically ill individuals and their families often become socially isolated. The ill person may withdraw from others, or others may feel uncomfortable and withdraw. Support groups are helpful for providing a social outlet with others in the same situation. Individuals with limited mobility may be able to maintain connections with the outside world through the internet. Adult day care can provide socialization for the patient and respite for the caregiver.

Attempt to normalize social interactions

Chronically ill people need to maintain as normal a lifestyle as possible despite having to manage symptoms, adapt to changes in appearance or function caused by the illness, or use adaptive equipment or prostheses. Encourage them to live as independently as possible in spite of their illness.

Identifying the support systems for the chronically ill person is important. Families are the major support systems for persons with chronic illnesses. Formal support systems include social service agencies, health care providers, and community agencies. If family members are unavailable or unable to provide support, formal services may be needed.

Help Family Members Deal With the Patient's Illness

Families provide the bulk of support for the chronically ill and the burden of caregiving is heavy for them. Healthy members of the family must take on more physical work because of the need to assist with activities of daily living, deal with changes in the progress of the disease, cope with feeling psychologically and physically overwhelmed, and adapt to changes in their own social roles and identities, as well as those of the ill family member. In some cases, a family caregiver also may have a chronic illness that must be managed or they may develop a physical illness or disability as a result of the burden of caregiving. This consequence is especially true for older caregivers.

Health care providers need to assist patients and their family members in developing a collaborative plan of care. In some cases, relief or respite can be obtained to ease the caregiving responsibility. Many communities have adult day centers for older adults or persons with particular chronic illnesses. These centers enable both the older or chronically ill individuals and their caregivers to have a more normal lifestyle, with social interaction and structure. Formal support services should be used whenever they are needed to assist families in caring for their chronically ill loved ones.

Assist Terminally Ill Patients to a Peaceful Death

Sooner or later, everyone must die. Nurses are often the health care providers who have the most intimate relationship with people who are terminally ill. When death comes unexpectedly, little or no time is available to prepare for death. However, when disease is chronic, patients and families often need to make difficult decisions regarding death.

With today's sophisticated technology, terminally ill patients can be kept alive longer than was ever possible in the past. Patients and families are confronted with decisions about the setting in which the terminally ill person is cared for, whether technology will be used to maintain physiologic functions, and when life-sustaining measures should be discontinued. More than anyone else, family members have to live with the memory of their loved ones and the events surrounding their death.

Nurses should be supportive of decisions made by patients and families. Dying patients and their loved ones should be informed of the options for care and their consequences. The living will and durable power of attorney for health care are legal documents called *advance directives*. They allow patients to designate, in advance, what treatments they would want in specific situations (living will) or to appoint one person to make treatment decisions when they are not able to make those decisions (durable power of attorney). Open communication and an acknowledgment of different attitudes toward terminal illness and death are extremely important. The nurse should have knowledge of the dying process and the needs of the dying person to provide compassionate care, promote comfort, and make the pain and physical treatment bearable. See Chapter 19 for more detailed information on caring for terminally ill patients (see the Sample Nursing Care Plan: Inadequate Coping With Illness).

Sample Nursing Care Plan Inadequate Coping With Illness

Patient Problem	Goal and Outcome Criteria	Interventions
Inadequate coping related to feelings of powerlessness, as evidenced by the patient's verbalization, "I don't know if I can live through this."	Patient will demonstrate more effective coping, as evidenced by verbalization that they feel more capable of dealing with the demands of the illness.	Give the patient an opportunity to verbalize feelings of powerlessness by approaching patient care in an unhurried manner. Determine the patient's and family's current coping strategies and behaviors. Conduct teaching sessions with the patient and family to enhance their coping skills and empower the patient to begin self-care. Provide community resource information and encourage the patient to ask for help from others. Implement stress reduction strategies (e.g., music therapy) to help the patient cope with stressful moments.

Get Ready for the NCLEX® Examination!

Key Points

- Health may be viewed as the ability to express the full range of one's physical and mental potential within one's environment.
- Maslow's hierarchy of needs model demonstrates that once basic needs are met, the individual may seek to satisfy progressively higher needs.
- Stress is necessary for growth and development.
- A stressor is anything, positive or negative, that causes the individual stress.
- Adaptation, the biologic and psychologic efforts to respond to a stressor, affects the entire organism.
- Illness or crisis may ensue if individuals are overwhelmed by many stressors or do not have the coping behaviors or problem-solving strategies necessary to maintain equilibrium.
- A crisis is the point at which the individual may move toward illness on the continuum between illness and health; it can result in inner tension and anxiety, which may affect an individual's ability to function.
- Anxiety is a painful emotion that results from one's perception of danger, and individuals continually regulate their behavior based on the level of perceived anxiety.
- Defense mechanisms are strategies used to diminish anxiety; however, when unconscious defense mechanisms are used excessively, they can hinder the developing personality.
- Each person's response to illness is unique and is based on such subjective experiences as self-concept, perception of threat to body image, and spiritual and cultural values.
- Illness produces a stressful state that requires individuals to draw on their innate resources or inner strengths.
- Some people have enough inner strength to cope effectively with illness; others may have ineffective or maladaptive coping abilities.
- Factors that influence an individual's ability to cope with illness are age/stage of development, personality, cultural beliefs, spirituality, self-concept, emotional responses to illness, and family and community resources.
- Specific emotional responses to illness include stress, fear, anxiety, loss, and grief and mourning.
- Coping is the process of responding to stress or a potential stressor.
- Coping strategies are conscious, purposeful behaviors that are used to make an unfamiliar situation into one that is perceived as more controllable and predictable.
- Ineffective coping mechanisms may evolve from a sense of helplessness or powerlessness.
- Conscious coping strategies, such as relaxation and music therapy, are used to make an unfamiliar situation into one that is perceived as more controllable and predictable.

- Examples of maladaptive coping mechanisms and strategies include helplessness, powerlessness, and denial.
- Nursing interventions may be used to promote health, prevent illness, manage illness, restore health, or support a peaceful death.
- Healthy People 2030 is a national health promotion and disease prevention initiative that aims to increase the quality and years of healthy life and to eliminate health disparities.
- A nurse's caring and nonjudgmental attitude is basic to helping a client cope with illness.

Additional Learning Resources

SG Go to your Study Guide for additional learning activities to help you master this chapter content.

Go to your Evolve website (http://evolve.elsevier.com/Linton/medsurg) for the following learning resources and much more:
- Fluid and Electrolyte Tutorial
- Review Questions for the NCLEX® Examination

Clinical Judgment and Next-Generation NCLEX® Examination-Style Questions

1. **The statement "Sometimes I feel so overwhelmed and sad" reflects which dimension of a human being?**
   1. Cognitive
   2. Affective
   3. Behavioral
   4. Social

   NCLEX Client Need: Psychosocial Integrity

2. **Which of the following is/are recommended in a plan for healthy living? (Select all that apply)**
   1. Use MyPlate for meal planning
   2. Engage in intense exercise for 1 hour daily
   3. Sleep at least 6 hours each night
   4. Avoid smoking
   5. Limit alcohol to three drinks per day

   NCLEX Client Need: Physiological Integrity: Physiological Adaptation

3. **Which of the following are characteristic of stress? (Select all that apply)**
   1. Requires the individual to adapt
   2. May be a negative or positive experience
   3. Increases with ineffective coping
   4. Affects all dimensions of the individual
   5. Can affect a single human dimension

   NCLEX Client Need: Psychosocial Integrity

4. **Which of the following is the primary difference between fear and anxiety?**
   1. Anxiety is much more disabling than fear
   2. Anxiety indicates that the patient has poor coping skills
   3. Anxiety interferes with effective problem solving more than fear does
   4. Anxiety is evoked by a nonspecific threat rather than a specific threat

   NCLEX Client Need: Health Promotion and Maintenance

5. **Which of the following is the basic function of defense mechanisms?**
   1. To enhance self-esteem
   2. To avoid reality
   3. To disguise true feelings
   4. To reduce anxiety

   NCLEX Client Need: Psychosocial Integrity

6. **A 9-year-old girl likes to wear her 14-year-old sister's nail polish and tries to fix her hair like her older sister's. This is an example of which defense mechanism?**
   1. Regression
   2. Introjection
   3. Identification
   4. Projection

   NCLEX Client Need: Psychosocial Integrity

7. **A patient who has a chronic disease is in a period of exacerbation. This means that:**
   1. Symptoms have returned
   2. The disease has been cured
   3. Symptoms will soon reappear
   4. The terminal stage of the disease has begun

   NCLEX Client Need: Physiological Integrity: Physiological Adaptation

8. **The LVN/LPN is assisting the RN with a care plan. The RN suggests using Maslow's hierarchy of human needs to set priorities. Using Maslow, which problem would be the first priority?**
   1. Low self-esteem
   2. Shortness of breath
   3. Unstable gait
   4. Impaired speech

   NCLEX Client Need: Physiological Integrity, Psychosocial Integrity

9. **A 50-year-old husband and father has been diagnosed with a degenerative disorder that will lead to disability. Which nursing intervention is most appropriate to help the patient and his family to deal with this stressful situation?**
   1. Limit teaching to what the patient asks about
   2. Do not require that the patient make any decisions
   3. Discourage the use of complementary and alternative therapies
   4. Identify the patient's previously successful coping strategies

   NCLEX Client Need: Physiological Integrity: Physiological Adaptation

10. A nurse in a retirement community offers classes on healthy living for residents. The topics to be addressed include:

1. Nutrition
2. Physical activity
3. Sleep and rest
4. Tobacco use
5. Alcohol consumption
6. Stress management

Using the options provided below, fill in the blanks.

Before initiating a new activity program, the inactive older adult should (1)________. To promote physical fitness, the active older adult should engage in 150 minutes of (2)________ each week. In addition, (2)__________ exercises should be done 2 days each week. Adults should limit sleep to (3) _____ hours per night. Alcohol intake should not exceed 2 drinks per (4)______. The USDA provides current dietary guidelines using the (5)________ concept.

OPTION 1	OPTION 2	OPTION 3	OPTION 4	OPTION 5
Enroll in a physical therapy program	Low-intensity	**6**	Week	MyPlate
Consult a physician	Muscle-strengthening	**7**	Day	Food pyramid
Monitor heart rate and BP	Moderate intensity	**8**	Month	RDA table
	Bone-strengthening	**9**	Year	
	High-intensity	**10**		

NCLEX Client Need: Physiological Integrity: Physiological Adaptation

Immunity, Inflammation, and Infection

5

http://evolve.elsevier.com/Linton/medsurg

Objectives

1. Describe physical and chemical barriers.
2. Describe the immune response.
3. Identify the organs involved in immunity.
4. Compare natural and acquired immunity.
5. Describe how inflammatory changes act as bodily defense mechanisms.
6. Identify the signs and symptoms of inflammation.
7. Discuss the process of repair and healing.
8. Differentiate infection from inflammation.
9. Discuss the actions of commonly found infectious agents.
10. Describe the ways that infections are transmitted.
11. Identify the signs and symptoms of infection.
12. Compare community-acquired and health care–associated infections.
13. Discuss the nursing care of patients with infections.
14. Describe the Centers for Disease Control and Prevention (CDC) Standard Precautions guidelines for infection prevention and control.
15. Describe the CDC guidelines for Airborne, Droplet, and Contact (Transmission-Based) Precautions.
16. Describe the CDC isolation guidelines for a Protective Environment.
17. Differentiate between humoral (antibody-mediated) and cell-mediated immunity.
18. Describe the nursing care of patients with immunodeficiency and of those with allergies.
19. Describe the process of autoimmunity.

Key Terms

allergen (ĂL-ĕr-jĕn)
antibodies (ĂN-tĭ-bŏ-dēs)
antigen (ĂN-tĭ- jĕn)
autoimmunity (ăw-tō-ĭ-MYŪ-nĭ-tē)
communicable disease (kŏ-MYŪ-nĭ-kă-b'l dĭ-ZĒZ)
contamination
health care–associated infection (HAI)
immunity
immunodeficiency (ĭ-myū-nō-dē-FĬSH-ĕn-sē)
infection
inflammation (ĭn-flă-MĀ-shŭn)
medical asepsis (ā-SĔP-sĭs)
multidrug-resistant organism (MDRO)
surgical asepsis (SŬR-jĭ-kăl ā-SĔP-sĭs)

Imagine you were being attacked. How would you defend yourself? Perhaps you would shout or sound an alarm. You might even text or call for assistance to help you fight off the attacker, telling them the most direct route to your location. You would probably surround yourself with some sort of barrier either to shield yourself from further harm or to keep the attacker in the area so that they would not escape and harm someone else. Then, after the battle was over, you would likely enlist the help of some friends to clean up the debris and return your situation to normal.

Remarkably, at a cellular level, the human body protects itself in much the same way. The body relies on many effective barriers to protect itself from injury and disease. However, if these barriers are compromised, several sophisticated processes are triggered to isolate and eliminate the offender. This chapter describes how the body defends itself from injury and disease, what happens when defenses fail, and how good nursing care helps the processes.

PHYSICAL AND CHEMICAL BARRIERS

Intact skin and mucous membranes are the body's first line of defense. They act as a protective covering and secrete substances that inhibit the growth of microorganisms. The sweat glands secrete lysozyme, an antimicrobial enzyme. Sebaceous glands secrete sebum, which has antimicrobial and antifungal properties. Acidic secretions from the skin and the mucosa of the gastrointestinal and genitourinary systems inhibit the growth of many pathogenic organisms. Secretions from the mammary glands and the respiratory and gastrointestinal tracts contain the antibody immunoglobulin A, as well as cleanup phagocytes. In addition, skin and mucous membrane surfaces are colonized by "normal" bacterial flora, which prevent pathogens (disease-causing organisms) from gaining access to the body. The cilia in the respiratory tract, the motility of the gastrointestinal tract, and the sloughing of dead skin cells all work to distribute and remove microorganisms, preventing their overgrowth and invasion.

The second line of defense involves two processes: phagocytosis and inflammation. Phagocytosis, the process of enveloping and destroying foreign matter, helps to rid the body of invading microorganisms and debris. White blood cells (leukocytes) are colorless blood cells that have the ability to phagocytose (ingest) bacteria that can cause **infection** when they invade the body. There are five types of leukocytes: neutrophils, monocytes, eosinophils, basophils, and lymphocytes. Neutrophils fight bacterial infections. Monocytes circulate in the blood for approximately 1 day before they enter tissue, where they are called *macrophages*, and ingest many foreign antigens. Eosinophils fight parasitic infections and increase during allergic reactions. Basophils initiate the inflammatory response and release histamine. Measuring the number of these cells gives an indication of the severity of infection and inflammation in the body. B lymphocytes produce antibodies and T lymphocytes increase the body's immune response. Therefore lymphocyte counts provide a measure of immune function. Reticuloendothelial cells are found in the blood, connective tissue, liver, spleen, bone marrow, and lymph nodes. Some reticuloendothelial cells protect the body by digesting and absorbing foreign material, such as old red blood cells, bacteria, and colloidal particles. These cells may also be called *tissue macrophages*.

This chapter provides an overview of physiologic processes that play a role in many disorders. A more complete description of blood and components of the immune system may be found in Chapters 29 and 31. More detailed information, including nursing care of people with hematologic and/or immunologic disorders is provided in Chapters 30 and 32.

IMMUNITY

The immune system is the body's defense network against infection. **Immunity** provides the body with resistance to invading organisms and enables it to fight off invaders once they have gained access. The body is constantly exposed to microorganisms capable of causing disease. If the immune system is intact and functioning properly, adequate protection from most infections and diseases is provided in a healthy individual. When the immune system is not functioning properly, the potential for overwhelming infection exists. Many factors can compromise the immune system, such as disease states, congenital defects, aging, stress, and therapeutic interventions (e.g., drugs, radiation therapy). Understanding the normal immune response and the common immune system disorders will help you to assess patients at risk for infection and provide appropriate interventions.

Any substance that is capable of stimulating a response from the immune system is called an **antigen**. In most cases, the antigen is foreign to the body and the body recognizes the antigen as different from itself ("nonself"). Antigens can be microorganisms (bacteria, viruses, fungi, parasites), abnormal or mutated body cells, transplanted cells (from blood transfusions, organ transplants), noninfectious substances from the environment (pollens, insect venom, foods), or foreign molecules from drugs such as penicillin. When healthy, the body protects what it recognizes as self and attempts to destroy that which is nonself. Tissue that is normally recognized as self may be seen as nonself by the immune system if the tissue undergoes change (mutation), is in an abnormal location, or changes structure. Once the body recognizes a substance as an antigen, natural and acquired defenses are put into action to destroy the invader and prevent disease.

Antibodies, also known as *immunoglobulins*, are proteins that are created in response to specific antigens. The formation and function of antibodies are discussed in the "Antibody-Mediated (Immediate) Immunity" section of this chapter.

INNATE (NATURAL) VERSUS ACQUIRED IMMUNITY

Innate (natural) immunity is present in the body at birth and is not dependent on a specific immune response or previous contact with an infectious agent. It may be specific to a species, a race, or an individual. For instance, humans are not as susceptible to distemper as dogs and cats are. Factors such as nutritional status, stress, and environment may influence natural immunity. Nonspecific defense mechanisms that include physical and chemical barriers to infection, phagocytosis, and the inflammatory process contribute to natural immunity.

An individual develops acquired immunity after birth as a result of the body's natural immune responses to antigens. Acquired immunity depends on the proper development and functioning of B and T lymphocytes, which are white blood cells that fight infection.

Active acquired immunity is developed after direct contact with an antigen through illness or vaccination. Vaccinations may be prepared by a variety of methods: (1) using dead or weakened organisms that can no longer cause disease, but still trigger the immune response; (2) inactivating bacterial toxins that act as antigens, (3) making the vaccine with just one part of an organism, and (4) using the virus genetic code including mRNA, and vectored viruses. The Pfizer and Moderna vaccines for COVID-19 are manufactured with mRNA technology. The Johnson & Johnson and AstraZenaca vaccines are vector virus vaccines. Once the body has been exposed to an antigen through illness or vaccination, antibodies develop and retain memory for the antigen. If the body is exposed to the same antigen later, the antibodies can react quickly to fight off disease.

When people are injected with immune globulin or antiserum (made from human or animal blood) that contains antibodies to a specific agent, such as for the emergency treatment of snakebite, rabies, or exposure to hepatitis, they receive antibodies or lymphocytes that were produced by another individual. This type of immunity, called *passive acquired immunity*, is temporary and is the type of immunity that newborns receive from their mothers through the placenta or through ingestion of breast milk (especially colostrum).

Both natural and acquired immunity are necessary for a healthy individual to have protection from disease. Innate and acquired immunity are discussed further in Chapter 31.

CELLS AND ORGANS INVOLVED IN IMMUNITY

A variety of cells work together to provide the body with an adequate defense against injury or disease. Leukocytes (white blood cells) play a key role in immune responses to infectious organisms and other antigens. The two categories of white blood cells are granulocytes and nongranulocytes. Blood cells involved in immune disorders are described in Chapter 29.

Although all parts of the body work together as a whole to resist and fight off disease, several organs are vital to a functional immune system. These organs include the thymus, bone marrow, lymph nodes, spleen, and liver (Fig. 5.1). The thymus and bone marrow participate in the formation and maturation of immune system cells. Located throughout the body, the lymph nodes attack antigens and debris in the interstitial fluid and produce and circulate lymphocytes. The spleen acts as a filter to remove dead cells, debris, and foreign molecules from the blood. The liver filters the blood and plays a part in the production of specific immunoglobulins and other chemicals involved in the immune response.

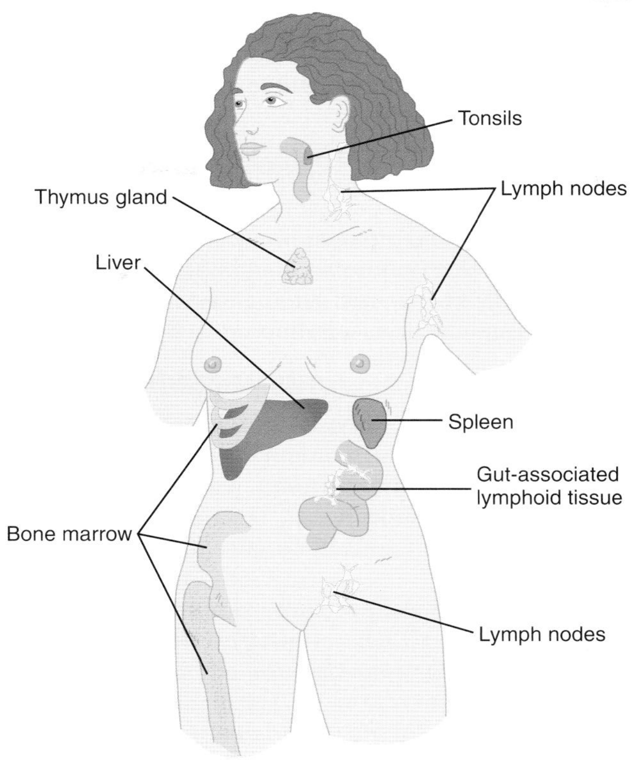

Fig. 5.1 Organs involved in immunity. (From Black JM, Hawks JH: *Medical-surgical nursing: clinical management for positive outcomes*, ed 8, St. Louis, 2009, Saunders.)

NONSPECIFIC DEFENSES AGAINST INFECTION

Innate (natural) immunity consists of physical and chemical barriers to invasion of the body as well as processes and substances that protect and repair tissues and stimulate the body to fight off disease. Physical and chemical barriers, inflammation, and phagocytosis are nonspecific defenses against infection.

Other nonspecific defenses against infection that protect the body include complement, pyrogen, and interferon. Complement is a series of proteins that enhance the inflammatory process and the immune response. Chemotaxis, phagocytosis, and the activity of antibodies are stimulated by complement. Pyrogen (an eicosanoid) is a substance released in inflammation that causes body temperature to increase. Fever is thought to inhibit the growth of pathogens and slow enzymatic reactions that occur in infectious processes. Another substance, interferon, is produced in viral infections and acts to inhibit the replication of viruses. Interferon (a cytokine) also affects the function of T lymphocytes and is used in the treatment of selected malignancies. Eicosanoids and cytokines are discussed in Chapter 31.

SPECIFIC DEFENSES AGAINST INFECTION: IMMUNE RESPONSE

The immune response is the process by which antigens are recognized as foreign, processed, and destroyed. The two types of immune responses—antibody-mediated (immediate or humoral) and cell-mediated (delayed) responses—function interdependently to provide the immune response.

ANTIBODY-MEDIATED (HUMORAL) IMMUNITY

Antibody-mediated (humoral) immunity is immediate and the first line of defense. It is called humoral because it involves substances found in the humors or body fluids. Humoral immunity involves B lymphocytes and the production of antibodies in response to specific antigens. The humoral immune response is initiated when an antigen binds to a special receptor on a B lymphocyte. This binding results in the production of antibodies that seek out and "stick to" specific antigens in the body. This combination forms antigen-antibody complexes, which are then targeted for cleanup by neutrophils and macrophages. Formation of these complexes activates complement and intensifies T-lymphocyte activity. Because circulating antibodies bind with antigens as soon as they are recognized, the chemical process is triggered immediately.

Antibodies (immunoglobulins [Ig]) are divided into five classes: IgG, IgM, IgA, IgE, and IgD. IgG is the most abundant immunoglobulin; it crosses the placenta to provide passive immunity for the newborn. IgM is the first antibody to appear in a response to initial exposure to an antigen. IgA plays a crucial role in the immune function of mucous membranes. IgE is important in allergic reactions and in parasitic infections. IgD is co-expressed with IgM in immature B lymphocytes.

CELL-MEDIATED (DELAYED) IMMUNITY

Cell-mediated immunity is a delayed immune response to injury or infection that does not involve antibodies. It involves the activation of phagocytes, T lymphocytes, and the release of substances that enhance the immune response and influence the destruction of antigens.

T cells include helper cells, suppressor cells, and killer cells. Helper T cells enhance humoral immunity; suppressor T cells help to "turn off" the humoral response. Disease may occur when the normal ratio of helper to suppressor cells (2 : 1) is altered. In acquired immunodeficiency syndrome (AIDS), for instance, the number of helper T cells is diminished. When the number of suppressor T cells is too high, infections, allergies, or immune diseases develop. Killer T cells directly destroy antigens.

Cellular immunity fights most viral or bacterial infections and hinders the growth of malignant cells. This process also launches an attack on transplanted tissue or organs in the body.

INFLAMMATORY PROCESS

The inflammatory process is a series of complex cellular changes that signal the body's response to injury or infection. Although infection is a common cause of inflammation, this complex phenomenon may be caused by trauma from (1) physical agents (excessive sunlight, x-rays), (2) chemical stimuli (insect venom, other chemicals), and (3) biologic agents (bacteria, viruses). The function of inflammation is to eliminate the initial cause of the cell injury, clear out dead cells and damaged tissues, and start tissue repair.

The word **inflammation** means literally "the fire within." This descriptive phrase illustrates the five signs that indicate local inflammation: (1) rubor (redness), (2) calor (heat), (3) tumor (swelling), (4) dolor (pain), and (5) loss of function. Thinking about the appearance of an insect bite and recalling the redness, warmth, swelling, and pain that it produces would be helpful. These signs are the direct result of several related actions that occur when the inflammatory process is initiated. The actions involve cardiovascular (hemodynamic) changes, increased permeability of membranes, chemical mediators, and hormonal factors.

ACTIONS IN THE INFLAMMATORY PROCESS

Cardiovascular Changes

The first actions of the inflammatory process are the hemodynamic changes (changes in blood vessel diameter). The body initially responds to an injury or infection with dilation of the capillary bed. This dilation brings increased blood flow to the area. The increase in blood flow is responsible for the characteristic warmth and redness at the site of inflammation.

Increased Permeability

The second action is an increased capillary permeability (Fig. 5.2). After the increased blood flow brings leukocytes into the area, chemical mediators cause leukocytes to line the small blood vessel walls near the site of inflammation. This process is called *pavementing*. Gradually, these cells pass through the vessel walls and inhabit the inflamed area. These cells, largely neutrophils and monocytes, are drawn to the site of injury or infection, where they ingest and carry away bacteria and other foreign substances (phagocytosis) (Fig. 5.3). The permeability of these vessels causes protein-rich fluid to flow through the vessel walls into the interstitial space. Some red blood cells may pass through into this area as well. This collection of fluid is responsible for the swelling that is noted when the inflammation site is close to the surface of the skin. This swelling may also produce pain.

Chemical Mediators

The hemodynamic changes and vascular permeability occur with the help of several chemical mediators, including prostaglandins, histamine, and leukotrienes. These powerful substances are found in various body tissues and are liberated during the inflammatory process. Cytokines and eicosanoids cause blood and blood vessel changes. The kinin system produces bradykinin, which also mediates blood vessel dilation and permeability. It also produces pain, another classic sign of inflammation. In some severe allergic reactions, the inflammatory response is excessive. These reactions cause a massive release of histamine and other substances that produce marked vasodilation, vascular permeability, and smooth-muscle contraction. These cellular changes produce the classic signs of anaphylactic shock: hypotension, swelling, and bronchoconstriction.

Antiinflammation

Cortisol, a hormone produced by the adrenal cortex, is an antiinflammatory substance that slows the release of histamine, stabilizes lysosomal membranes, and prevents the influx of leukocytes. The end result of these actions is to impede the inflammatory process. By limiting the inflammatory process, cortisol protects the body from the effects of excessive or prolonged inflammation. Drugs (e.g., corticosteroids) that mimic the action of cortisol are often used in the treatment of inflammatory conditions.

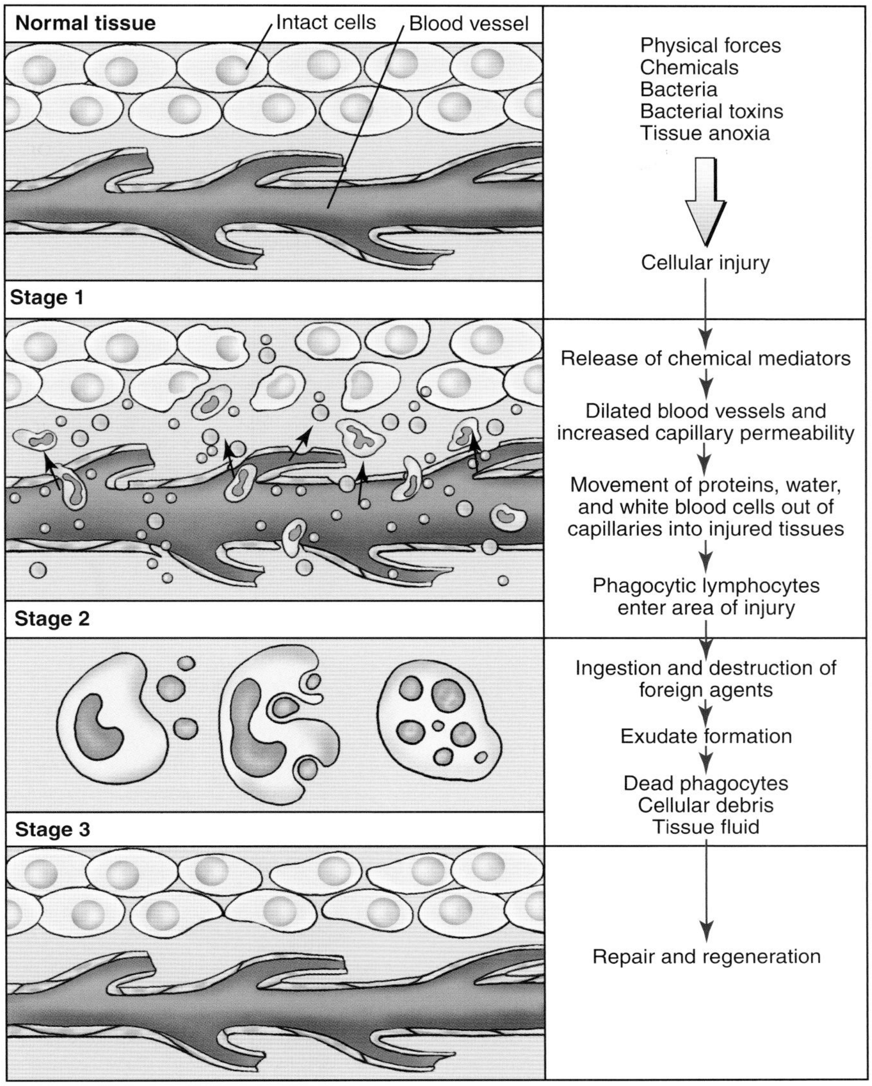

Fig. 5.2 The inflammatory response after tissue injury. (From Monahan FD, Drake DT, Neighbors M, editors: *Medical-surgical nursing: foundations for clinical practice*, ed 2, Philadelphia, 1998, Saunders.)

CLINICAL MANIFESTATIONS OF INFLAMMATION

The signs and symptoms of inflammation vary, depending on whether the reaction is local or systemic. Local inflammation generally produces the classic signs of heat, swelling, redness, and pain, all of which result in loss of function.

Systemic inflammation produces somewhat different reactions. Swelling, redness, and local warmth may not be visible; however, signs of the effects of the chemical mediators may be recognized in other ways. Fever is a common sign of systemic inflammation, probably caused by pyrogens (fever-producing substances) or defense mechanisms that are liberated during phagocytosis, or by bacterial endotoxins, antigen-antibody complexes, and certain viruses. Other symptoms of systemic inflammation include headache, muscle aches, chills, and sweating.

Leukocytosis, a defensive reaction that provides abundant white blood cells for the inflammatory response, is another sign of systemic inflammation. If infection is not present, inflammatory leukocytosis disappears within a few hours.

WOUND HEALING

Repair and regeneration of tissue are set in motion from the very beginning of the inflammatory process. The speed at which this process takes place depends on the type of tissue injured, the severity of the wound, the presence of infection, and the health of the host. At the outset, macrophage cells are produced to clean up inflammatory debris. Fibroblasts begin the repair process by laying down elastin and collagen at the edges of the wound; these substances gradually migrate to the base, forming granulation tissue. Epithelial cells migrate over the wound and under the scab (usually formed of dried blood and fibroblasts). After a few days, the scab falls off. Damaged cells are replaced by new cells of their own composition by the process of

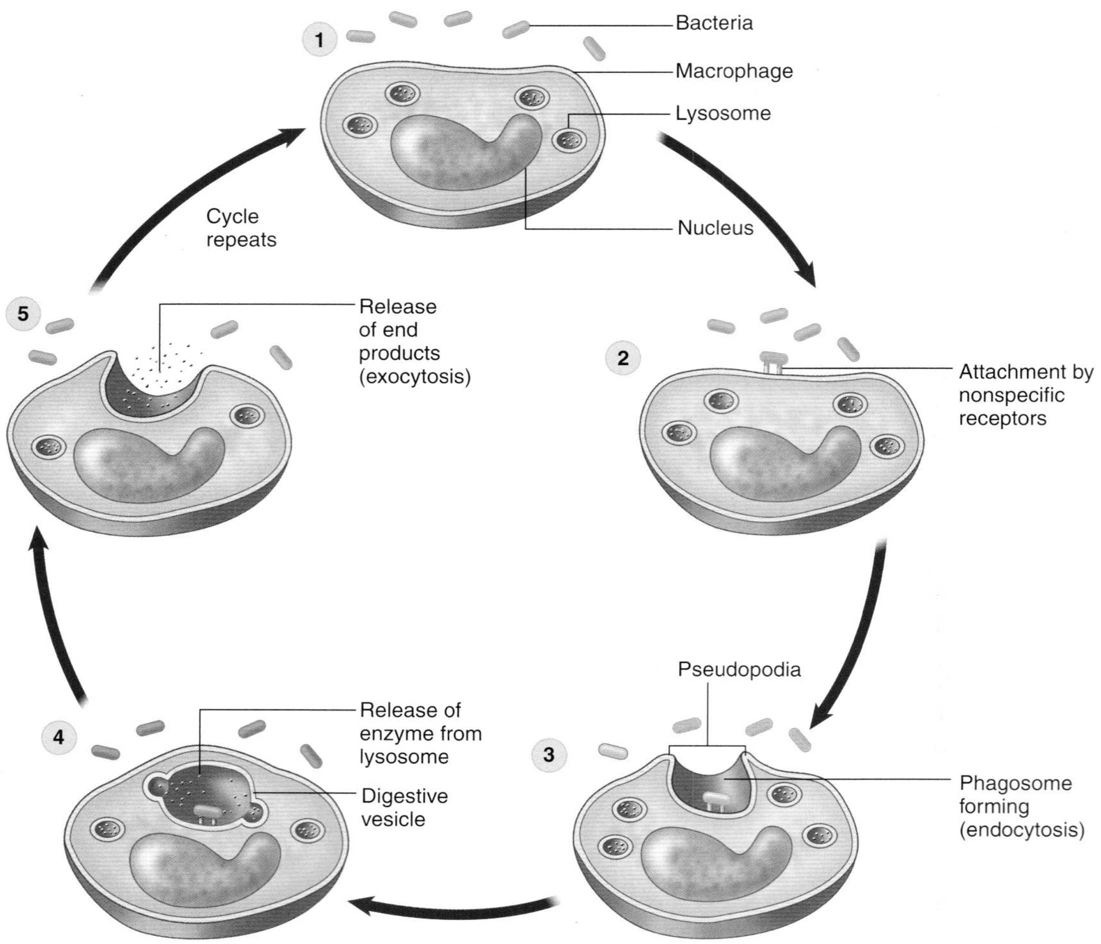

Fig. 5.3 Phagocytosis. (1) Macrophages migrate to an inflammatory site by chemotaxis. (2) Bacteria attach to macrophages by nonspecific receptors. (3) A phagosome or phagocytic vacuole forms around the microorganisms. (4) Lysosomes attach to the phagosome and release their enzymes, which destroy the microorganisms. (5) Breakdown products of phagocytosis are released. (From Patton KT, Thibodeau GA: *Human body in health & disease*, ed 7, St. Louis, 2018, Elsevier.)

regeneration. Some tissue regenerates well whereas other tissue must undergo repair, which may involve the replacement of injured cells with connective tissue that will eventually create a scar. In fact, both types of tissue repair occur in most wounds.

The age and general health of the person affect how rapidly the regeneration and repair processes occur. The healing process can be delayed in the older adult as a result of decreased tissue elasticity and decreased blood supply. Deficiencies of vitamin C, zinc, and other important vitamins and minerals can also delay the regeneration and repair processes.

A wound occasionally becomes infected or ulcerated, resulting in tissue loss. Granulation tissue and capillary buds form at the margins of the wound and eventually fill the wound with granulation tissue. The wound bed is sometimes too large for the granulation tissue to fill. In this case, the wound may be cleaned and debrided to enhance healing. The term *delayed primary closure* is used when the wound is sutured closed after the infection has resolved.

INFECTION

Infection is a process involving the invasion of body tissues by microorganisms, the multiplication of the invading organisms, and the subsequent damage of tissue. Infection is different from inflammation in that inflammation is a nonspecific reaction by the body to tissue injury whereas infection refers to a specific process that causes tissue injury. Infection nearly always results in inflammation, but inflammation may be caused by processes other than infection. Inflammation precedes infection. Infection is usually the end result of the invasion by organisms. Infection may be caused by a wide variety of microorganisms.

INFECTIOUS AGENTS

The major infectious agents are bacteria, viruses, fungi, protozoa, rickettsiae, and helminths (worms). A limited number of animal and human diseases are caused by prions.

Bacteria

Bacteria are one-celled microorganisms capable of multiplying rapidly within a susceptible host. Bacteria are classified by shape, cluster pattern, whether or not they need oxygen, and their ability to take up and retain stains. Bacteria may be round or rod shaped. Round bacteria are called *cocci;* they are further classified according to how they group or cluster together. Groups of two are called *diplococci* and clusters of cocci are called *staphylococci.* Chains of these microorganisms are called *streptococci.* Rod-shaped organisms, called *bacilli*, can be obligate aerobes or facultative anaerobes.

Bacteria may also be classified according to their ability to grow in the presence of oxygen. Those that grow in the presence of oxygen are classified as *aerobes;* those that do not grow in the presence of oxygen are labeled *anaerobes.*

Bacteria are classified as either gram positive or gram negative, depending on their ability to take up and retain a violet-colored solution called Gram stain. Gram-positive bacteria have a thick covering that retains the stain whereas gram-negative bacteria can be decolorized and counterstained pink. The acid-fast stain is used to identify bacteria such as *Mycobacterium tuberculosis.* Immunofluorescent stains reveal complexes composed of various antigens (bacteria, viruses, fungi, protozoa) and antibodies when exposed to ultraviolet light.

These classifications have a very important purpose. Each classification highlights a characteristic of a microorganism that is considered in the design of an antimicrobial drug to kill or retard the growth of the organism. For example, antimicrobials synthesized to fight gram-positive microorganisms interfere with the formation of that covering, causing the cell wall to be destroyed. Other antimicrobials used to treat aerobic bacteria rely on the ability of the bacterial cell to take up oxygen to produce its effects.

Viruses

Viruses are very small microorganisms that cause significant morbidity (disease) in humans. Viruses cannot be seen with ordinary microscopes but are visible with electron microscopy. They contain a strand of either ribonucleic acid (RNA) or deoxyribonucleic acid (DNA), which determines whether they are classified as either DNA or RNA viruses. Viruses are surrounded by a protein capsule but have no cell wall. They replicate only inside the living cells of other organisms. Viruses cause a variety of illnesses, including the common cold, measles, chickenpox, and several forms of hepatitis. Some viral infections in pregnant women may cause abnormal development of their fetus. Zika virus infection of pregnant women can result in microcephaly (abnormal brain development causing smaller than normal head), severe malformation, and other birth defects in the child. The RNA virus that causes human immunodeficiency virus (HIV) is a retrovirus.

Because replication of the virus occurs within the host cell, killing the virus without harming the host cell is a challenge. This property explains the relatively few antiviral drugs that are available. Current antiviral and antiretroviral drugs suppress viral reproduction or growth so that they decrease the severity or duration of the infection, but they are not curative. Antibiotics do not affect viruses. Prevention (immunizations, hygiene) is still the best way to combat viral illness.

COVID-19 is a new (novel) infection caused by a virus called SARS-CoV-2. It first emerged in China in 2019 and rapidly spread around the globe. As of late 2021, over 236 million cases had been confirmed worldwide with more than 4 million deaths. In the United States, more than 44 million cases had been confirmed and more than 700,000 people had died. Several effective vaccines are now available. A number of treatments are being studied including an antiviral drug and corticosteroids; however, no definitive cure has been found.

Fungi

Fungi are vegetable-like organisms that exist by feeding on organic matter. Mushrooms and molds are fungi. Most fungi are not dangerous, but some types can be harmful to health. Fungal infections are called *mycoses.* Many of these infections are superficial skin infections that can look like a rash and are very common. Ringworm (tinea corporis) and athlete's foot (tinea pedis) are two examples. However, systemic fungal infections caused by *Cryptococcus* and *Aspergillus* species can be life-threatening. Patients who have conditions that affect their immune system (e.g., those infected with HIV) are at especially high risk of acquiring opportunistic fungal infections. Because fungi tend to form spores that are resistant to many antiseptics and disinfectants, they are difficult to treat. Both systemic and topical antimycotic drugs are used to treat fungal infections.

Protozoa

Protozoa make up a large group of one-celled organisms. Ones that produce disease in humans include the *Plasmodium* species (malaria), *Entamoeba histolytica* (amoebic dysentery), *Giardia lamblia* (giardiasis, characterized by diarrhea), and *Trypanosoma brucei gambiense* (sleeping sickness). Infections are often spread by food or water that is contaminated by human or animal feces. Pneumocystic pneumonia caused by *Pneumocystis jiroveci* is another protozoal infection that was relatively rare before the onset of the HIV/AIDS epidemic. Lowered immunity with HIV infection is responsible for the dramatic rise in pneumocystic pneumonia.

Rickettsiae

Rickettsiae are microorganisms that are between bacteria and viruses in size. They may appear as rods, cocci, or pleomorphic (varied) shapes. These organisms multiply in the cells of animal hosts, such as rats and squirrels, and are transmitted to humans through the bites of fleas, mites, lice, and ticks. Diseases produced by these microorganisms include Rocky Mountain spotted fever and typhus. Diseases caused by rickettsiae tend to be more prevalent in areas in which sanitation is poor and rodent and insect populations are not well controlled.

Helminths

Helminths are parasitic worms. These parasites are generally transmitted from hand to mouth by eggs present in human feces, which contaminate the soil and water in areas where sanitation is poor. Infections occur commonly in the gastrointestinal tract and may produce mild abdominal pain and bloating, or they may be asymptomatic. Pinworms are most common, especially in children, and often produce rectal irritation. Tapeworms can be found in the gastrointestinal tract. Weight loss and abdominal pain and bloating may be early signs and symptoms. Hookworms often enter an individual through the soles of the feet and migrate throughout the body, including to the heart and the lungs. Most people infected have no symptoms. However, infected children are often physically, nutritionally and cognitively impaired. Some have respiratory symptoms during the migration of the hookworm through the lungs. Others have gastrointestinal symptoms and anemia caused by blood loss when the hookworm attaches to the intestinal wall.

Prions

A prion is a type of protein that can trigger normal proteins in the brain to fold abnormally. It does not contain any nucleic acids (either RNA or DNA). Although not actually alive, a prion can reproduce by hijacking the functions of living cells. Once transmitted, it can cause brain damage and progressive degenerative diseases of the nervous system. Prion diseases can affect humans and animals and are sometimes spread to humans by infected meat products. The most common form of a prion disease that affects humans is Creutzfeldt-Jakob disease (CJD); this form of bovine spongiform encephalopathy ("mad cow" disease) primarily affects cattle but has been transmitted to humans. Prions typically have a very long incubation period but advance rapidly once the infection becomes active. Prions are extremely resistant to standard methods of disinfection; proper cleaning and sterilization of medical equipment may prevent the spread of the disease. People who may have CJD or were potentially exposed to infected cattle may not donate blood, other tissues, and organs.

TRANSMISSION OF INFECTION

Infection is possible only when several factors are present. These factors must occur in sequence for human infectious disease to occur. They include (1) a causative agent, (2) a reservoir, (3) a portal of exit, (4) a mode of transfer, (5) a portal of entry, and (6) a susceptible host. This sequence is known as the *chain of infection.*

Causative Agent

Causative agents are the microorganisms (bacteria, viruses, protozoa, etc.) that are present in sufficient number and virulence to damage human tissue.

Reservoir

Areas in which organisms can pool and reproduce are called *reservoirs.* Reservoirs may be human or animal tissues, as well as any substance such as soil or animal feces, in which microorganisms can pool and multiply. When a reservoir of microorganisms occurs in the tissues of a human, the human is called a *host.*

Portal of Exit

Portal of exit refers to the route by which the infectious agent leaves one host and travels to another. A common route is the gastrointestinal tract, through which bacteria or viruses may escape an infected host. The nose and mouth also are common portals of exit for organisms spread by droplet **contamination** through sneezing or coughing. Fecal-oral transmission also occurs; hepatitis A virus is acquired by ingesting the virus in water contaminated with feces or by direct fecal-oral transmission.

Mode of Transfer

Mode of transfer refers to the means by which a microorganism is transported to a host. Person-to-person transfer may take place in either a direct or an indirect manner. Direct contact refers to the transfer of microorganisms directly, as occurs in sexually transmitted infections. Indirect contact occurs when pathogens are spread through droplets expelled during a sneeze or a cough or through inanimate objects (e.g., eating utensils on which microorganisms can be transported [fomites]). Common vehicle transmission occurs when water, food, blood, or air currents contaminated with a pathogen are shared by many people. Air currents, for example, are often the common vehicle for transmission of *Legionella,* the organism responsible for Legionnaires disease. Vector transmission occurs when microorganisms are transported into a host by a living organism such as a fly or mosquito. Fomites are any items that have been touched or cross-contaminated by the host, such as bed linen, side rails, or hygiene items.

Portal of Entry

Portals of entry are the ways in which the infectious agent enters a host. Influenza and cold viruses often enter the body through the mucous membranes of the nose and mouth. Other portals of entry often accessed by bacteria are the gastrointestinal tract and the urethra. Open wounds, intravenous access devices, urinary catheters, and drains also can be portals of entry for bacteria.

Susceptible Host

The susceptibility of a host depends on genetic or constitutional factors, specific immunity, and nonspecific factors that affect an individual's ability to resist infection or to limit the severity of the infection. Populations adequately immunized against rubella, for example, are not susceptible to measles. Similarly, individuals who have had chickenpox have developed immunity to the virus and do not become ill if exposed a second time.

CLINICAL MANIFESTATIONS OF INFECTION

Once an individual becomes infected with a pathogen, symptoms may or may not be apparent. In many instances, a period of subclinical infection or an incubation period occurs during which few, if any, symptoms are present. During this period, asymptomatic persons may be more contagious than those who are exhibiting symptoms. This is especially the case with people infected with such viruses as measles and many cold viruses. Persons recently infected with HIV may feel well but are highly contagious. Persons who have illnesses such as tuberculosis (TB) may remain relatively well. Still, other persons may remain contagious throughout their convalescence. Asymptomatic carriers, such as patients recovering from typhoid, may go back to their communities and unknowingly infect others.

Signs and symptoms of localized infections, such as bacterial infection of a wound, are essentially the symptoms of inflammation: redness, pain, warmth, and swelling. In addition, pus may form.

Patients with generalized infections may not show all of the signs that are apparent with localized infections. Redness, for example, may not be visible. Pain may be moderate to severe, depending on the location of the infection. Swelling of infected tissues may produce symptoms ranging from mild to severe, depending on its location. Swelling in a large organ, such as the liver, may produce a dull ache whereas swelling in a small structure, such as an infected appendix, may produce severe discomfort. Warmth is generally expressed as fever in a generalized infection as pyrogens are produced as part of the inflammatory process. Other symptoms that often are present in generalized infections include malaise, anorexia, and prostration.

In some cases, infections in the extremities such as the hands or feet exhibit a faint red line as infection extends upward along the lymphatic channels. Lymph nodes in this chain also are swollen and tender. Prompt antimicrobial treatment is necessary in these cases.

TYPES OF INFECTIONS

Two types of infections are (1) community-acquired and (2) health care–associated infections.

Community-Acquired Infections

Community-acquired infections are acquired in day-to-day contact with the public. Many viral infections are pervasive in society and occur at predictable times of the year. Childhood illnesses are common in September, when children take to school all of the new viruses to which they were exposed during the summer. This sharing of microorganisms is made easier when 20 to 40 children occupy the same classroom. During the fall and winter, people share more indoor activities, thus increasing the likelihood that they will share microorganisms with one another.

Poverty, low immunization rates, overcrowding, unsanitary living conditions, and resistant strains of pathogens are at least partially responsible for the increase in infectious diseases that were once well controlled. The resurgence of TB is an example. This increase was attributed to poverty, the HIV/AIDS epidemic, an increase in the number of infected immigrants, declining public health resources, and the emergence of strains of bacteria that are resistant to multiple drugs. Effective treatment of active TB, particularly if it is caused by a drug-resistant strain, may require several drugs at once for many months.

Foodborne illness is a common community-acquired infectious disease. It is more common in the summer when picnics and hot weather bring the possibility of food poisoning from *Staphylococcus* and *Salmonella* organisms. Periodic outbreaks of hepatitis A are possible at any time of the year and are the result of poor hygiene by food handlers.

Sexually transmitted infections such as gonorrhea, syphilis, and HIV also are spread in the community. These diseases and many others are required to be reported to public health authorities. The reports are important because they facilitate disease control, make possible the evaluation of disease control programs, and keep track of emerging disease patterns.

Certain communicable diseases must be reported to state health departments. Local laws vary regarding which diseases must be reported. A list of reportable diseases can be obtained from https://www.ndc.services.cdc.gov/search-results-year.

Prevention and control. Prevention and control of **communicable diseases** are possible in several ways. Some childhood infectious diseases can be prevented by ensuring that childhood immunizations are completed. Indifference toward childhood immunizations, as well as parental fear about side effects of vaccination, false information, and belief in alternative medicine, has resulted in the reemergence of several childhood diseases that were once well controlled. Although state laws that require certain immunizations before a child starts school have improved the picture somewhat, large groups of children from 2 to 5 years of age remain susceptible to serious illness. In addition, repeat vaccinations of older schoolchildren may be required to prevent illnesses such as measles. Adult immunizations also help to prevent and control communicable diseases. Immunization schedules for children and adults are available at the

Centers for Disease Control and Prevention (CDC) website: www.cdc.gov/vaccines/schedules/.

Although the solution to this problem defies easy answers, barriers in the health care system are at least part of the problem and result in missed opportunities to immunize individuals who are most susceptible. Barriers include factors such as cost and inconvenient access. In addition to health departments, schools, primary care providers' offices, shopping malls, and neighborhood health fairs are places where large numbers of children and parents may present themselves for immunization.

Transmission of infectious agents can be interrupted in several ways. First, education of food handlers regarding the importance of hand washing and proper food handling and refrigeration techniques decreases the spread of foodborne illness. Second, diseases such as TB can be detected through screening and treated early to prevent their spread. Isolation separates the infected individual from the public, thereby breaking the chain of infection. Other examples of measures aimed at interrupting transmission are control of vectors (spraying for mosquitos), administration of antimicrobials to children exposed to *Neisseria* meningitis, and the prompt treatment of streptococcal pharyngitis (strep throat). Sanitation of water supplies helps to prevent the occurrence of waterborne diseases. Cooking meat, eggs, and poultry until well done kills bacteria that can cause serious illness and, in some cases, death.

Personal measures to control the spread of communicable disease include proper hygiene, especially hand washing, and the use of personal barriers such as condoms. Deciding to stay home when symptoms of an infectious disease are present also can help to break the chain of infection.

Health Care–Associated Infections

Health care–associated infections (HAIs) were previously called nosocomial infections. HAIs are an important cause of increased morbidity, prolonged hospitalization, and higher health care costs. These infections occur within a health care facility and may affect both the patient and the health care worker. HAIs are much more serious than those acquired in the community because strains of bacteria in the hospital are usually more virulent and often are resistant to antimicrobials. In addition, the patient's resistance is already compromised from the disorder that led to hospitalization. Recent changes in health care in the United States have seen Medicare and other insurance companies not reimbursing institutions for HAIs such as catheter-associated urinary tract infections and surgical site infections.

A growing number of pathogenic bacteria that are no longer susceptible to previously effective antimicrobials are found in hospital patients. Vancomycin-resistant *Enterococcus* (VRE) is one example; the incidence of vancomycin resistance in patients with health care–associated enterococcal infection has increased steadily since its emergence in 1986. The CDC has emphasized the importance of the careful use of antimicrobials and infection prevention and control measures in preventing the spread of VRE. In health care agencies where antimicrobials may be overused or misused, an increase in bacterial resistance is found. Antimicrobials alter the body's normal flora so that resistant strains of enterococci replace susceptible strains.

Bacteria use a variety of mechanisms to develop resistant strains. Bacterial cells normally develop mutations to survive. Antimicrobials suppress normal forms of the bacteria, but the mutations often survive. Chromosomal mutation also permits some bacteria to produce enzymes that deactivate the antimicrobial. Some bacteria are able to alter their metabolic cycles to prevent destruction by antimicrobials. Finally, mutation alters bacterial cell membranes, making antimicrobial penetration more difficult. Newer antimicrobials are then developed to counteract the most resistant strains. As these antimicrobials in turn become more frequently used, resistance again develops, and the cycle is repeated.

Microorganisms that are resistant to one or more classes of antimicrobial agents are called **multidrug-resistant organisms (MDROs)**. Examples include methicillin-resistant *Staphylococcus aureus* (MRSA), VRE, extended spectrum beta-lactamase (ESBLs) producing enterobacteria, some gram-negative bacilli such as *Escherichia coli* and *Klebsiella pneumoniae*, *Acinetobacter baumannii*, and others. Especially among persons with poor resistance, these organisms can produce life-threatening infections. The ability of viruses to adapt and survive is illustrated in the emergence of new variants of the COVID-19 virus over time. The new variants may not respond to the same vaccines and treatments that may have worked in the earlier versions of the virus.

General practices that can help to impede the development of resistant pathogens include vaccinations for communicable diseases and appropriate use of antimicrobial drugs. Antimicrobials should be reserved for serious bacterial infections. The most appropriate antimicrobial can be selected if based on laboratory studies of infected specimens (wound drainage, body fluids such as urine or blood). Culture and sensitivity tests identify the microorganism and the antimicrobial most likely to be effective. This practice allows the most appropriate therapy to be administered and delays the onset of resistant strains. Efforts are also made to limit the use of antimicrobials that are effective against resistant strains. This practice provides fewer opportunities for the development of strains resistant to the drug. Tables 5.1 and 5.2 present the CDC steps to prevent antimicrobial resistance among hospitalized adults, long-term care residents, and surgical patients.

HAIs are more serious for the hospitalized patient who may have low resistance. These infectious organisms also have been exposed to many antimicrobials, so they are more likely to resist therapy. Patients with compromised immune systems are much more susceptible to hospital-acquired infections. These groups include patients with AIDS and patients with cancer who

Table 5.1 The 12 Steps to Prevent Antimicrobial Resistance: Hospitalized Patients

STRATEGIES	STEPS
Prevent infection	1. Vaccinate 2. Get the catheters out
Diagnose and treat effectively	3. Target the pathogen 4. Access the experts
Use antimicrobials wisely	5. Practice antimicrobial control 6. Use local data 7. Treat infection, not contamination 8. Treat infection, not colonization 9. Know when to say "no" to vanco 10. Stop treatment when infection is cured or unlikely
Prevent transmission	11. Isolate the pathogen 12. Break the chain

CDC, Centers for Disease Control and Prevention; *vanco*, vancomycin.
From CDC: *CDC campaign to prevent antimicrobial resistance in healthcare settings*, 2017: www.cdc.gov/getsmart/healthcare/. Accessed August 20, 2017.

are receiving chemotherapy. Common sites for HAIs in hospitalized patients include surgical wounds, the urinary tract, and the respiratory tract. Patients who have an indwelling urinary catheter are at risk for urinary tract infection. The risk for this infection can be reduced by using proper techniques for catheter insertion and care. Health care workers are also at risk for HAIs. Hepatitis B, for example, may be transmitted through needle punctures. Small, open wounds on the upper extremities may come in contact with resistant strains of *Staphylococcus* or *Pseudomonas* and become infected. In addition, health care workers and patients have developed Legionnaires disease when *Legionella* was spread through the facility on air currents from air conditioning systems that became contaminated with infected water. CDC recommendations to prevent transmission of MDROs in health care settings are summarized in Box 5.1.

Iatrogenic infections are caused by the treatment given to the patient. For example, iatrogenic infections

Table 5.2 Nursing Considerations Related to Centers for Disease Control and Prevention Recommendations to Prevent Antimicrobial Resistance in Health Care Settings

HOSPITALIZED ADULTS	LONG-TERM CARE RESIDENTS	SURGICAL PATIENTS
Prevent Infection		
1. Encourage patients to have an annual influenza vaccination. 2. Use proper technique for catheter insertion and care.	1. Encourage patients to have a pneumococcal vaccination (usually a one-time vaccination) as well as an annual influenza vaccination. 2. Prevent aspiration and pressure injuries. 3. Promote good hydration. 4. Use proper technique for catheter insertion and care.	1. Monitor blood glucose and body temperature. 2. Prepare skin with appropriate antiseptic agent and hair removal technique. 3. Use proper technique for insertion and care, such as with urinary catheters and drains. 4. Elevate head of bed 30 degrees or as ordered to reduce risk of health care–associated pneumonia. Avoid contamination of respiratory equipment and medications.
Diagnose and Treat Infection Effectively		
1. Carefully collect specimens for culture to prevent contamination. 2. Consult the agency protocol and infection preventionist for proper precautions and care.	1. Carefully collect specimens for culture to prevent contamination. 2. Promptly report diarrhea in patients on antimicrobials. Cause may be *Clostridioides difficile.* 3. Consult the agency protocol and infection preventionist for proper precautions and care. 4. See patient's previous laboratory studies for history of colonization or infection.	1. Carefully collect specimens for culture to prevent contamination. 2. Administer antimicrobials on schedule. 3. Consult the agency protocol and infection preventionist for proper precautions and care as needed.
Use Antimicrobials Wisely		
1. Teach patients that antimicrobials are not always necessary or appropriate for infections. 2. When antimicrobials are prescribed, explain why the entire course should be completed.	1. Question long-term antimicrobial therapy. 2. Document signs and symptoms of infection.	1. Administer preoperative prophylactic antimicrobials within 1 hour before incision is made as ordered.

Continued

Table 5.2 Nursing Considerations Related to Centers for Disease Control and Prevention Recommendations to Prevent Antimicrobial Resistance in Health Care Settings—cont'd

HOSPITALIZED ADULTS	LONG-TERM CARE RESIDENTS	SURGICAL PATIENTS
Prevent Transmission		
1. Use Standard Infection Prevention and Control Precautions for all. 2. Use Airborne, Droplet, and Contact Precautions as needed. 3. Explain precautions to patients, nursing assistants, and visitors. 4. Practice hand hygiene. 5. Stay home when *you* are sick.	1. Use Standard Infection Prevention and Control Precautions for all. 2. Follow specific precautions for patients with multidrug-resistant organisms. 3. Use Airborne, Droplet, and Contact Precautions as needed. 4. Explain precautions to patients, nursing assistants, and visitors. 5. Practice hand hygiene. 6. Stay home when *you* are sick.	1. Use Standard Infection Prevention and Control Precautions for all. 2. Use Airborne, Droplet, and Contact Precautions as needed. 3. Practice hand hygiene. 4. Do not wear artificial nails, tips, wraps, or nail jewelry. Keep nails no longer than 1/4 inch from fingertips.

CDC, Centers for Disease Control and Prevention.
Modified from CDC: *CDC campaign to prevent antimicrobial resistance in healthcare settings*, 2017: www.cdc.gov/getsmart/healthcare/. Accessed August 20, 2017.

Box 5.1 Infection Prevention and Control Precautions to Prevent Transmission of Multidrug-Resistant Organisms in Health Care Settings

- Follow Standard Precautions (SP) in all health care settings.
- Use of Contact Precautions (CP):
  - In acute care settings, implement CP for all patients known to be colonized or infected with target multidrug-resistant organisms (MDROs).
  - In long-term care facilities, consider the individual patient's clinical situation and facility resources in deciding whether to implement CP. Consult with the infection preventionist for expert direction.
  - In ambulatory and home care settings, follow SP.
  - Masks are not recommended for routine use to prevent transmission of MDROs from patients to health care workers. Use masks according to SP when performing splash-generating procedures, when caring for a patient with an open tracheostomy with potential for projectile secretions, and when evidence has been found for transmission from heavily colonized sources (e.g., burn wound).
- Patient placement in hospitals and long-term care facilities:
  - When single-patient rooms are available, assign priority for these rooms to patients with known or suspected MDRO colonization or infection.
  - Give highest priority to specific patients who have conditions that may facilitate transmission (e.g., uncontained secretions or excretions).
  - When single-patient rooms are not available, cohort patients with the same MDRO in the same room or patient care area.
  - When possible, cohort staff to minimize the spread of MDROs among patients.

CDC, Centers for Disease Control and Prevention.
From Centers for Disease Control and Prevention: *CDC management of multidrug-resistant organisms in healthcare settings, 2006*: https://www.cdc.gov/infectioncontrol/guidelines/MDRO/index.html. Last updated February 15, 2017. Accessed August 29, 2017.

may be caused by giving immunosuppressive drugs to prevent rejection of a transplanted organ, resulting in an infection. Another form of iatrogenic infection can be caused by the treatment of a primary infection. Antimicrobial therapy for one microorganism can permit the overgrowth of a second microorganism that can also cause illness. The term for this process is *superinfection*. It is especially common with treatment using broad-spectrum antimicrobials. An example of this phenomenon is the occurrence of a bowel infection after treatment with oral broad-spectrum antimicrobials. The organism *Clostridioides difficile* resides in the gastrointestinal tract of many individuals. It is kept in check by the normal bacterial flora of the gastrointestinal tract. Broad-spectrum antimicrobials can kill enough of the normal flora to allow *C. difficile* to grow out of control, producing severe colitis and diarrhea.

CARE OF PATIENTS WITH INFECTION

Just as controls must be instituted to stop the spread of infections acquired in the community, so must a process be put in place to keep hospitalized patients from acquiring HAIs. The key to preventing the spread of infection is effective medical and surgical asepsis.

MEDICAL ASEPSIS

Medical asepsis means limiting the spread of microorganisms as much as possible. This practice is often called *clean technique* and refers to practices such as changing bed linen, sanitizing bedpans, using personal equipment for each patient, and frequent hand hygiene.

Hand Hygiene

Soiled hands are the primary mode of transmission of HAIs. Although everyone agrees in principle with the need for frequent hand hygiene, problems arise when nurses are busy. For example, suppose that a nurse is passing medications and is asked by a patient with pulmonary secretions to hand her the box of tissues. At the same time, the patient's roommate asks the nurse to fill her water glass. After performing this task, the nurse hurries out of the room to pass medications to other patients. This example illustrates how a chain of infection begins. Unless the nurse interrupts the chain with effective hand hygiene, infection is easily spread from one patient to another.

The most basic and effective method of hand hygiene includes hand washing with soap and water, use of waterless antiseptic with at least 60% alcohol, or a surgical scrub. Good hand-washing technique includes the use of running water, soap, and friction. The lathered hands should be rubbed together for at least 20 seconds and longer if the nurse works in a high-risk area. To keep time, the CDC recommends humming the "Happy Birthday" song from beginning to end twice. The use of antimicrobial soaps is also recommended when working with patients who are more susceptible to infection, such as premature infants or immunocompromised patients. A waterless antiseptic is dispensed into one palm and then the hands are rubbed together to cover all surfaces until the hands are dry (Fig. 5.4). The antiseptic is appropriate for use before and after patient contact. The surgical scrub is reserved for assisting with operative procedures (Fig. 5.5).

SURGICAL ASEPSIS

Surgical asepsis, or sterile technique, refers to the elimination of microorganisms, through physical or chemical sterilization, from any object that comes in contact with the patient. It is important to remember the most important principle for sterile technique: sterile items remain sterile only when touched by other sterile items. Techniques are observed to prevent unsterile surfaces from coming in contact with the patient, such as during surgery or dressing changes.

STANDARD PRECAUTIONS

A set of infection prevention and control guidelines has been developed for hospitals and other health care agencies by the Hospital Infection Control Practices Advisory Committee (HICPAC) and the CDC. The current guidelines are called *Standard Precautions* and are used for the care of all patients in hospitals regardless of their health or medical status. *Transmission-Based Precautions* are disease-specific isolation techniques that are implemented to prevent the spread to others within the agency.

Use Standard Precautions when you perform procedures in which you will have contact with a patient's blood, body fluids, secretions (except sweat), excretions, broken skin, and mucous membranes; when you have contact with materials that are soiled or contaminated with body fluids or blood; and with all patients, no matter what their diagnosis or infectious status may be. Guidelines for the use of Standard Precautions are listed in Box 5.2.

Some guidelines under Standard Precautions address specific situations such as patient protection. These precautions are guidelines for Respiratory Hygiene/Cough Etiquette, safe injection practices, and use of masks for insertion of catheters or injections by way of lumbar puncture procedures.

Respiratory Hygiene/Cough Etiquette emphasizes education of staff, patients, and visitors to cover the mouth and nose with tissues when coughing, dispose of used tissues promptly, wash the hands after contact with respiratory secretions and contaminated objects and materials, and maintain a distance greater than 3 feet from others. Health care providers should wear a mask when giving direct care to patients with a respiratory infection. Health care providers with a respiratory infection should avoid direct patient contact; if unavoidable, the provider should wear a mask. Key points from Safe Injection Practices are noted in Table 5.3.

Put On Your Thinking Cap!

For one clinical day, note everything you did that represents the use of Standard Precautions.

TRANSMISSION-BASED (ISOLATION) PRECAUTIONS

To prevent the spread of infection in a health care facility, infected patients are sometimes isolated from other patients. Examples of illnesses requiring implementation of Transmission-Based Precautions are listed in Box 5.3. The extent of the isolation depends on the type of infection. The Transmission-Based Precautions were developed to reduce the risk of airborne, droplet, and contact transmission in hospitals.

Airborne Infection Isolation Precautions

Use Airborne Infection Isolation Precautions when caring for patients who have diseases that are spread through the air. Examples of diseases that are spread through the air are pulmonary TB, severe acute respiratory syndrome (SARS), varicella (chickenpox), and rubeola (measles). Patients with these conditions are placed in an airborne infection isolation room (AIIR), where the ventilation system provides a negative pressure and exhausts directly to the outside or through high-efficiency particulate absorption (HEPA) filtration. If AIIR is not available, the patient can be placed in a private room with the door closed. Respiratory protection for health care personnel, provided by wearing properly fitted N95 or higher respirators, is indicated when entering the patient's room. In addition, patients with infections spread by airborne transmission must wear surgical masks when leaving their rooms. Surgical masks filter expired air; respirators such as the N95 respirator filter inspired air.

Droplet Precautions

Use Droplet Precautions when taking care of patients with infections that are spread by droplets or dust particles containing the infectious agent. Droplets are spread primarily during coughing, sneezing, or talking, and during certain procedures such as suctioning and bronchoscopy. Because droplets usually travel only approximately 3 feet before falling from the air, special air handling and ventilation are not required to prevent

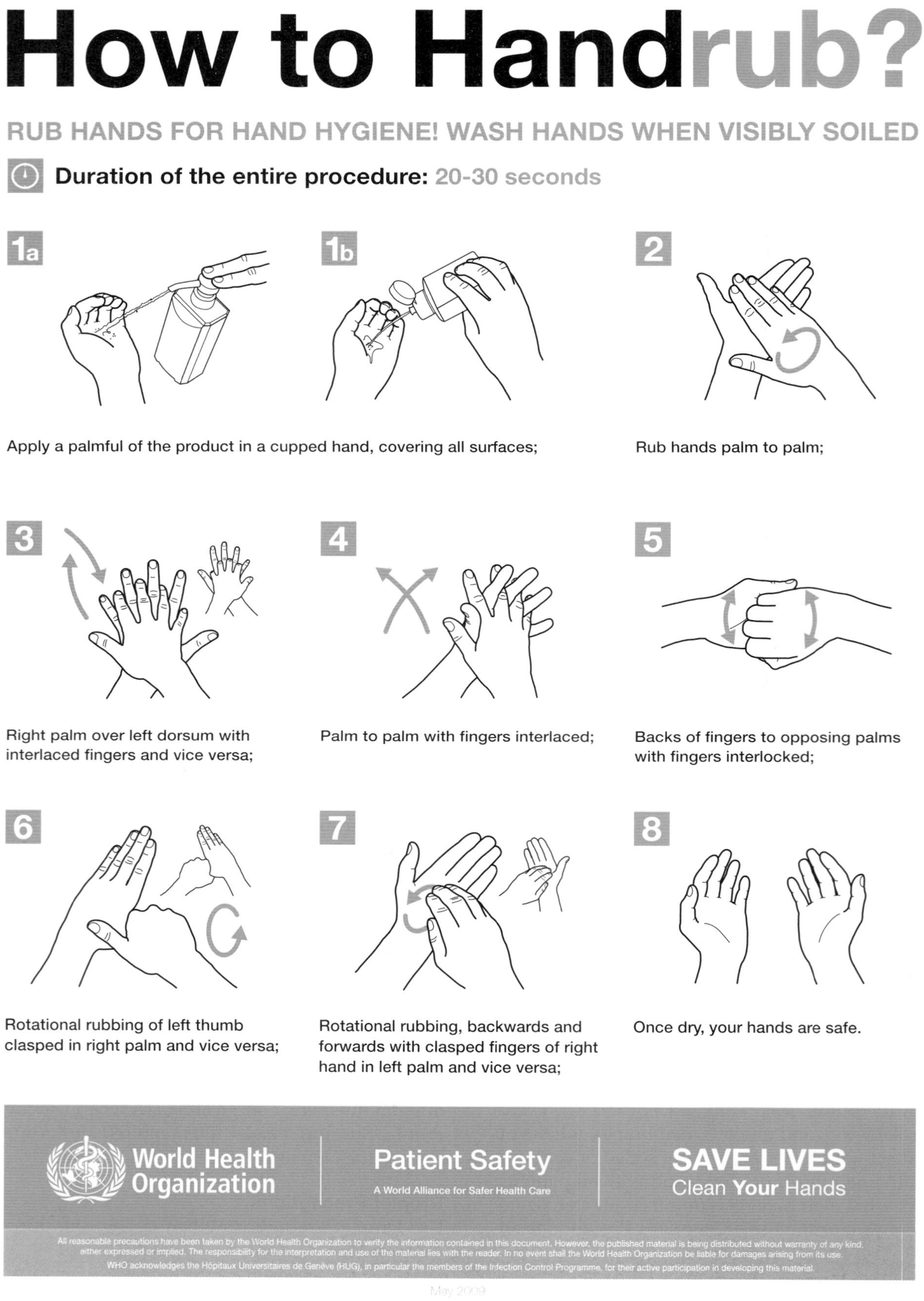

Fig. 5.4 Hand hygiene is the most basic and effective way to prevent cross-contamination and includes basic hand washing and use of waterless antiseptic. (From World Health Organization, 2009. http://www.who.int/gpsc/5may/How_To_HandRub_Poster.pdf. Accessed October 9, 2017.)

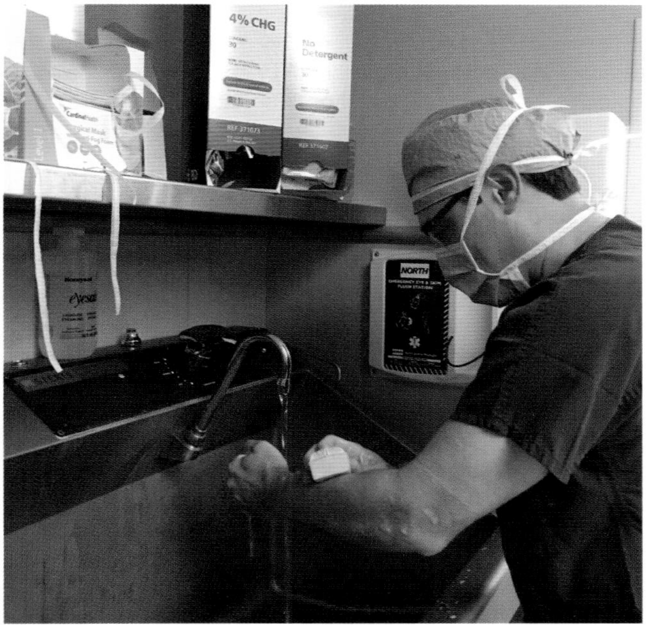

Fig. 5.5 The surgical scrub uses a topical antiinfective cleanser, takes longer, and is performed in a specific sequence that is different from basic hand washing. (Copyright from Lapiz-Bluhm, 2017.)

droplet transmission, as is the case with Airborne Precautions. The door to the room may be left open. Diseases transmitted by droplets include COVID-19, rubella, mumps, diphtheria, and influenza. Patients should be placed in private rooms. Staff and visitors must wear a surgical mask when within 3 feet of the patient for protection from contaminated droplets.

Contact Precautions

Use Contact Precautions when you are caring for patients who are infected by microorganisms that are transmitted by direct (skin-to-skin) or indirect contact with contaminated equipment. Needles, dressings, stethoscopes, bed rails, and doorknobs may become contaminated. The patient is placed in a private room. Disposable or dedicated patient-care equipment is used. Wear gloves when entering the infected patient's room; before leaving the patient's room, remove your gloves and wash your hands. Wear a gown if your clothing will come in contact with the patient, contaminated equipment, or environmental surfaces in the patient's room. A gown is also recommended if the patient is incontinent or has wound drainage. Remove

Box 5.2 Guidelines for Use of Standard Precautions

Standard Precautions should be followed for the care of all patients even when the presence of an infectious agent is not apparent or is thought to be minimal.

Standard Precautions entail:

- Hand hygiene before and after contact with every patient, regardless of whether gloves are also used. (See 'Hand hygiene' below.)
- Use of gloves, gowns, and eye protection in situations in which exposure to blood or body secretions is possible.
- Use of respiratory hygiene/cough etiquette by patients or health care workers with cough or respiratory secretions; this includes covering the nose and mouth when coughing, disposing of used tissues promptly, and practicing hand hygiene after contact with respiratory secretions. Use of a mask and spatial separation of patients with respiratory symptoms in waiting areas is also warranted.
- Safe injection practices and safe disposal of needles and sharp instruments in impervious containers.

Hand hygiene: Hand hygiene refers to hand washing with soap and water or the use of alcohol-based hand disinfection. Hand hygiene is the single most important measure to reduce transmission of microorganisms from one person to another or from one site to another on the same patient. The primary challenge associated with hand hygiene efficacy is laxity of practice, not a paucity of good products.

The SAVE LIVES: Clean Your Hands initiative is part of a major global effort led by the World Health Organization (WHO); it includes "My Five Moments for Hand Hygiene," which define the key moments when health care workers should perform hand hygiene:

- Before touching a patient
- Before clean/aseptic procedures
- After body fluid exposure/risk
- After touching a patient
- After touching patient surroundings

Most hospitals and clinics emphasize hand hygiene at the time of room entry and exit and before any procedure.

Either soap and water or alcohol-based hand disinfection (AHD) may be used. In most circumstances, we favor AHD because it is more efficient than handwashing with soap and water. Handwashing with soap and water should be used in association with care of patients with known or suspected norovirus or *Clostridioides* (formerly *Clostridium*) *difficile* infection because alcohol does not kill *C. difficile* spores or norovirus.

Health care worker compliance with hand hygiene is a longstanding challenge. Most studies have shown that hand hygiene compliance improves with monitoring and immediate feedback, although this approach is time and resource consuming. Electronic- and video-based monitoring have been employed to monitor compliance, but such monitoring has not gained widespread use because of multiple barriers.

Soap and water: Hand hygiene with soap and water should be performed as follows:

- When washing hands with soap and water, wet hands first with water, apply an amount of product recommended by the manufacturer to hands, and rub hands together vigorously for at least 20 seconds, covering all surfaces of the hands and fingers. Rinse hands with water and dry thoroughly with a disposable towel. Use towel to turn off the faucet.
- Liquid, bar, leaflet, or powdered forms of plain soap are acceptable when washing hands with soap and water. When bar soap is used, small bars of soap and soap racks that facilitate drainage should be used.

Continued

Box 5.2 Guidelines for Use of Standard Precautions—cont'd

- Multiple-use cloth towels of the hanging or roll type are not recommended for use in health care settings.

Alcohol-based hand disinfection: Hand hygiene with an alcohol-based hand rub should be performed as follows:

- Apply product to palm of one hand and rub hands together, covering all surfaces of hands and fingers, until hands are dry. Follow the manufacturer's recommendations regarding the volume of product to use.

AHD is an effective, inexpensive, and practical alternative to soap and water. AHD is faster and easier to perform than hand washing with soap and water; it should be performed at every room entry and exit and before any procedure. The use of AHD has been associated with improved hand hygiene compliance rates and reductions in nosocomial infections.

AHD products have rapid antimicrobial effects and are as effective as chlorhexidine against gram-positive and gram-negative organisms as well as viral pathogens, including influenza. AHD products do not have activity against norovirus or spore-forming bacteria, including C. *difficile.* The United States Centers for Disease Control and Prevention (CDC) endorses a three-step method for AHD (apply sanitizer and rub both palms together, cover all surfaces, and rub until dry, see above), whereas the WHO endorses a six-step method (apply sanitizer and specifically rub six different aspects of the hands and fingers. We continue to favor the three-step CDC AHD method because it is practical and the difference in the bacterial count reduction is of uncertain clinical significance.

Prohibiting artificial nails: Health care workers with direct patient contact should have fingernails that are short, clean, and free from false nails and nail polish. There is an increase in periungual colonization with a variety of pathogens when fingernails are long and when artificial fingernails are worn. Artificial fingernails and inadequately cleaned native fingernails have been epidemiologically linked to outbreaks of infection in intensive care unit patients, neonates, and patients undergoing surgery.

Gloves: Gloves should be worn by health care workers in situations in which exposure to blood or body secretions is possible; they provide a protective barrier for the health care worker as well as the patient. Nonsterile examination gloves are typically used.

Gloves are also a component of contact precautions; in such circumstances, they reduce the likelihood of health care worker colonization with microorganisms from a patient who is colonized or infected with pathogenic organisms. Wearing gloves does not replace the need for hand hygiene. Gloves may have unapparent tears, and hands predictably become contaminated during glove removal.

Gloves should be changed between patient encounters; in some cases, it may be necessary to change heavily contaminated gloves while caring for a single patient to prevent cross-contamination of body sites or contamination of medical equipment.

Masks: Masks should be worn by health care workers caring for patients in the following categories:

- Patients with respiratory secretions, to protect health care workers from patients' infectious material (such as aerosols containing blood or body fluids).
- Patients undergoing sterile procedures (including central line insertion, invasive spinal procedures), to protect patients from respiratory aerosols generated by health care personnel performing the procedure.

In addition, masks should be worn by patients with respiratory secretions who are coughing if they leave their hospital rooms, to limit spread of infectious secretions to other patients and to health care workers.

Masks should not be confused with particulate respirators that are used to prevent transmission by airborne droplet nuclei of infectious agents such as *Mycobacterium tuberculosis*.

Extracted from Anderson DJ (last updated March 11, 2020). Infection prevention: Precautions for preventing transmission of infection. *UpToDate.* Retrieved October 27, 2020 from https://www.uptodate.com/contents/infection-prevention-precautions-for-preventing-transmission-of-infection?search=standard%20precautions&source=search_result&selectedTitle=1~150&usage_type=default&display_rank=1.

Table 5.3 Safe Injection Practices

DOS	DO NOTS
• Use aseptic technique when handling sterile injection equipment. • Discard needles, syringes, and cannulas after a single use. • When possible, use single-dose vials for parenteral medications. • If a multidose vial must be used, use sterile equipment (needle/cannula, syringe) every time a dose is accessed. • Discard any multidose vial or injection equipment if sterility is questionable.	• Do not reuse syringes, needles/cannulas; these items are considered contaminated once used to enter or connect a patient's intravenous infusion bag or administration set. • Never use intravenous bags, tubing, and connectors for multiple patients. • Do not keep multidose vials in the immediate patient treatment area. • Do not use containers of intravenous fluids as a common source of supply for multiple patients. • Do not give medications from single-dose vials or ampules to multiple patients. • Do not combine leftover contents of single-dose vials or ampules.

Modified from Centers for Disease Control and Prevention: *Injection safety 2016*: https://www.cdc.gov/injectionsafety/index.html. Accessed August 21, 2017.

Box 5.3 Guidelines for Use of Transmission-Based Precautions

AIRBORNE PRECAUTIONS

Use Airborne Precautions for patients known or suspected to be infected with pathogens transmitted by the airborne route (e.g., tuberculosis, measles, chickenpox, disseminated herpes zoster).

- See Guidelines for Isolation Precautions for complete details
- **Ensure appropriate patient placement in an airborne infection isolation room (AIIR)** constructed according to the Guideline for Isolation Precautions. In settings where Airborne Precautions cannot be implemented because of limited engineering resources, masking the patient and placing the patient in a private room with the door closed will reduce the likelihood of airborne transmission until the patient is either transferred to a facility with AIIR or returned home.
- **Restrict susceptible health care personnel from entering the room of patients** known or suspected to have measles, chickenpox, or smallpox if other immune healthcare personnel are available.
- **Use personal protective equipment (PPE) appropriately**, including a fit-tested NIOSH-approved N95 or higher level respirator for health care personnel.
- **Limit transport and movement of patients** outside of the room to medically necessary purposes. If transport or movement outside an AIIR is necessary, instruct patients to wear a surgical mask, if possible, and observe Respiratory Hygiene/Cough Etiquette. Health care personnel transporting patients who are on Airborne Precautions do not need to wear a mask or respirator during transport if the patient is wearing a mask and infectious skin lesions are covered.
- Immunize susceptible persons as soon as possible following unprotected contact with vaccine-preventable infections (e.g., measles, varicella or smallpox).

DROPLET PRECAUTIONS

Use Droplet Precautions for patients known or suspected to be infected with pathogens transmitted by respiratory droplets that are generated by a patient who is coughing, sneezing, or talking.

- See Guidelines for Isolation Precautions for complete details
- **Source control:** put a mask on the patient
- **Ensure appropriate patient placement** in a single room if possible. In acute care hospitals, if single rooms are not available, use the recommendations for alternative patient placement considerations in the Guideline for Isolation Precautions. In long-term care and other residential settings, make decisions regarding patient placement on a case-by-case basis considering infection risks to other patients in the room and available alternatives. In ambulatory settings, place patients who require Droplet Precautions in an examination room or cubicle as soon as possible and instruct patients to follow Respiratory Hygiene/Cough Etiquette recommendations.
- **Use PPE appropriately.** Don mask upon entry into the patient room or patient space.
- **Limit transport and movement of patients** outside of the room to medically necessary purposes. If transport or movement outside of the room is necessary, instruct patient to wear a mask and follow Respiratory Hygiene/Cough Etiquette.

CONTACT PRECAUTIONS

Use Contact Precautions for patients with known or suspected infections that represent an increased risk for contact transmission.

- **Ensure appropriate patient placement** in a single patient space or room if available in acute care hospitals. In long-term and other residential settings, make room placement decisions balancing risks to other patients. In ambulatory settings, place patients requiring contact precautions in an examination room or cubicle as soon as possible.
- **Use PPE appropriately** including gloves and gown. Wear a gown and gloves for all interactions that may involve contact with the patient's environment. Donning PPE upon room entry and properly discarding before exiting the patient room is done to contain pathogens.
- **Limit transport and movement of patients** outside of the room to medically necessary purposes. When transport or movement is necessary, cover or contain the infected or colonized areas of the patient's body. Remove and dispose of contaminated PPE and perform hand hygiene before transporting patients on Contact Precautions. Don clean PPE to handle the patient at the transport location.
- **Use disposable or dedicated patient-care equipment** (e.g., blood pressure cuffs). If common use of equipment for multiple patients is unavoidable, clean and disinfect such equipment before use on another patient.
- **Prioritize cleaning and disinfection of the rooms** of patients on contact precautions ensuring rooms are frequently cleaned and disinfected (e.g., at least daily or before use by another patient if outpatient setting) focusing on frequently touched surfaces and equipment in the immediate vicinity of the patient.

PROTECTIVE ENVIRONMENT

Use a Protective Environment to reduce the risk of fungal infections for vulnerable patients.

- **Patient placement.** Room should have HEPA filtration of incoming air, directed room air flow, positive air pressure in the room as compared with the corridor, and a ventilator system that changes the room air at least 12 times each hour, and be sealed to prevent air flow from the outside. The room should be easily cleaned (e.g., tile vs. carpet) and may not contain potted plants or live or dried flowers.

CDC, Centers for Disease Control and Prevention; *HEPA*, high-efficiency particulate absorption.
From Centers for Disease Control and Prevention: *CDC guidelines for isolation precautions preventing transmission of infectious agents in healthcare settings, 2007* (updated October 2017). https://www.cdc.gov/infectioncontrol/guidelines/isolation/index.html. Accessed August 28, 2017.

the gown before leaving the patient's room. Contact Precautions are used for conditions such as fecal incontinence; infections of the gastrointestinal tract, respiratory tract (including respiratory syncytial virus), and skin (e.g., impetigo, scabies); or wound infections with significant drainage, especially if the infection agent is resistant to multiple antimicrobials. Special contact precautions apply to patients with infections caused by MDROs such as VRE and MRSA. Rooms of patients on contact precautions must be frequently cleaned and disinfected at least daily or before use by another patient, focusing on frequently touched surfaces and equipment in the immediate vicinity of the patient. Types of precautions and patients with whom precautions must be used are summarized in Box 5.4.

Note that recommended care of COVID-19 patients continues to evolve. As of October 2021, it is thought that droplet transmission, especially in contact with the face, appears to be most dangerous. Agencies may still be requiring airborne, droplet, contact, and standard precautions for COVID-19 patients. Nurses must follow recommendations as they evolve.

PERSONAL PROTECTIVE EQUIPMENT FOR HEALTH CARE PERSONNEL

Various precautions include the use of equipment designed to protect health care providers from infections. These items include gloves; isolation gowns; face protection including masks, goggles, and face shields; and respiratory protection. Personal protective equipment (PPE) is used along with other types of precautions.

Health care personnel should wear gloves when a possibility exists of exposure to potentially infectious material. When gloves are used in addition to other PPE (gown, mask), the gloves should be put on last. Contaminated gloves must be carefully removed to prevent contamination with the bare skin; hand hygiene should be performed to remove any contaminated material that might have been transferred to the hands.

Isolation gowns protect the health care worker's exposed skin and clothing from contamination by infected material. Gowns, if indicated, are donned before other PPE. They should be discarded in the patient care area to prevent contaminating the environment.

Box 5.4 Types of Precautions and Patients With Whom Precautions Must Be Used

STANDARD PRECAUTIONS

Use Standard Precautions for the care of all patients.

AIRBORNE PRECAUTIONS

In addition to Standard Precautions, use Airborne Precautions for patients known or suspected to have serious illnesses transmitted by airborne droplet nuclei. Examples of such illnesses include the following:

- Measles
- Severe acute respiratory syndrome (SARS)
- Tuberculosis
- Varicella (including disseminated zoster)

DROPLET PRECAUTIONS

In addition to Standard Precautions, use Droplet Precautions for patients known or suspected to have serious illnesses transmitted by large-particle droplets. Examples of such illnesses include the following:

- Invasive *Haemophilus influenzae* type b disease, including meningitis, pneumonia, epiglottitis, and sepsis
- Invasive *Neisseria meningitidis* disease, including meningitis, pneumonia, and sepsis
- Other serious bacterial respiratory infections spread by droplet transmission, including:
  - Diphtheria (pharyngeal)
  - Mycoplasma pneumoniae
  - Pertussis
  - Pneumonic plague
  - Streptococcal (group A) pharyngitis, pneumonia, or scarlet fever in infants and young children

SERIOUS VIRAL INFECTIONS SPREAD BY DROPLET TRANSMISSION

- Adenovirus (also Contact Precautions)
- Influenza
- Mumps
- Parvovirus B19
- Rubella

CONTACT PRECAUTIONS

In addition to Standard Precautions, use Contact Precautions for patients known or suspected to have serious illnesses easily transmitted by direct patient contact or by contact with items in the patient's environment. The following are examples of such illnesses:

- Gastrointestinal, respiratory, skin, or wound infections or colonization with multidrug-resistant bacteria judged by the infection prevention and control program, based on current state, regional, or national recommendations, to be of special clinical and epidemiologic significance
- Enteric infections with a prolonged environmental survival, including *Clostridioides difficile*
- For diapered or incontinent patients:
- Enterohemorrhagic *Escherichia coli* 0157:H7, *Shigella*, hepatitis A, or rotavirus
- Respiratory syncytial virus, parainfluenza virus, or enteroviral infections in infants and young children
- Skin infections that are highly contagious or that may occur on dry skin, including:
- Diphtheria (cutaneous)
- Herpes simplex virus (neonatal or mucocutaneous)
- Impetigo
- Major (noncontained) abscesses, cellulitis, or decubitus
- Pediculosis
- Ritter disease (scalded skin syndrome)
- Scabies
- Staphylococcal furunculosis in infants and young children
- Herpes zoster (disseminated or in the immunocompromised host)
- Viral/hemorrhagic conjunctivitis
- Viral hemorrhagic infections

From Centers for Disease Control and Prevention: *CDC guidelines for isolation precautions preventing transmission of infectious agents in healthcare settings, 2007* (last update October, 2017). https://www.cdc.gov/infectioncontrol/guidelines/isolation/index.html. Updated October 2017. Accessed August 27, 2017.

Masks, face shields, and goggles are used to prevent contamination of the mouth, nose, and eyes when a risk exists of facial exposure to infectious materials. They also protect the patient during sterile procedures from infectious material carried in the health care worker's mouth or nose. Personal eyeglasses and contact lenses do not provide adequate protection from infectious material. Before removing a mask, face shield, or goggles, the gloves should be removed and hand hygiene performed. Avoid touching the front of the PPE because doing so is considered contamination.

Respiratory protection from inhalation of infectious particles requires a respirator with N95 or higher filtration. The device must fit the wearer's face securely to prevent air leakage. N95 or higher-level respirators are recommended when working with patients who have suspected or confirmed TB, SARS, COVID-19, and smallpox. Certain procedures may also mandate the use of a respirator. A single health care worker can reuse a respirator when working with a patient who has TB as long as the device is clean, uncontaminated, undamaged, and fits properly.

PROTECTIVE ENVIRONMENT

A Protective Environment (PE) is needed to reduce the fungal spore count in the air and to reduce the risk of invasive environmental fungal infections for vulnerable patients. Components of a PE include HEPA filtration of incoming air, directed room air flow, positive air pressure in the room as compared with the corridor, sealed rooms that prevent air flow from outside, and a ventilator system that changes the room air at least 12 times each hour. In addition, the room should be easily cleaned (e.g., tile vs. carpet) and may not contain potted plants or live or dried flowers.

BIOTERRORISM

Bioterrorism is the intentional release of viruses, bacteria, toxins, or other harmful agents to cause illness or death to people, animals, or plants. Methods used to spread agents of bioterrorism are varied and might include powders, aerosols, or contamination of food or water. Among the pathogens considered potential biologic weapons are those that cause anthrax, botulism, plague, smallpox, tularemia, and Ebola. In addition to pathogens, bioterrorists may use toxins such as ricin, chemicals such as sarin, and radioactive material released in small explosions ("dirty bombs"). Nurses should be aware of their employing agency's plans for dealing with public exposure to bioterrorism agents, including decontamination procedures and PPE and safety procedures (CDC, 2016).

IMMUNOCOMPROMISED PATIENTS

Immunocompromised patients have decreased immunity to infection and are at increased risk for bacterial, fungal, parasitic, and viral infections. Patients receiving chemotherapy and other patients with low white blood cell counts are at increased risk of infection. Leukemia and aplastic anemia are two examples of disorders that cause low white blood cell counts. The use of Standard Precautions for all patients and of Transmission-Based Precautions for specific situations should reduce the risk of acquiring infections from other persons and from the environment. See Chapter 31 for a discussion of precautions to be used with immunocompromised patients.

NURSING CARE OF THE PATIENT WITH AN INFECTION

Patients with generalized infections easily become dehydrated because of fever and anorexia. Urge the patient to consume adequate fluids, especially water. For the average adult, fluid intake should be at least 2 L per day to replace fluids lost through perspiration and respiration. Fluid intake is also important in the transportation of nutrients to the cells to fight infection. Nutrition is very important. Encourage patients to consume a high-protein, high-vitamin diet. Vitamin C is important for wound healing and to promote resistance to future infections. The patient with a poor appetite may benefit from a consultation with a dietitian.

If a patient's infection requires isolation, remember that effective isolation techniques may also isolate the patient from normal human contact. You may be tempted to hasten your work to minimize your chance of becoming infected. Forced seclusion can cause patients, particularly children, to feel lonely, rejected, and depressed. Engage the patient in conversation while giving direct care. Discussing subjects other than the patient's disease may lessen the feeling of being unclean or rejected. Encourage the patient to move about as much as possible to increase stimulation.

Under the current CDC guidelines, some infections and conditions fall into two categories because the microorganisms are transmitted in more than one way. For example, chickenpox can spread through both airborne and contact routes, requiring both Airborne and Contact Precautions.

Laboratory tests used to screen patients for infection include the following:

- White blood cell count—increased in infection
- Erythrocyte sedimentation rate—elevated with inflammation
- Iron level—decreased in chronic infection
- Cultures of urine, blood, sputum, and specimens obtained from the throat or a wound surface. The specimen is placed in a medium that supports growth of microorganisms. Laboratory identification of the organisms that grow in the culture allows the primary care provider to select the most appropriate antimicrobial treatment.
- White blood cell differential count (neutrophils, lymphocytes, monocytes, and eosinophils)—increased; types of increased cells help to differentiate causes of infection.

Examples of patient problems for patients with infections or who are vulnerable to infections include potential for infection, potential for injury, disrupted tissue integrity, decreased socialization, altered body image, and ineffective management of condition. The primary goals in caring for patients with infection are recovery from the infection and prevention of the spread of infection to others.

Antimicrobial drug therapy is the cornerstone of treatment for many infections. Early hospital discharges mean that patients are frequently discharged on a regimen of oral antimicrobial drugs. Many people stop taking antimicrobials once they begin to feel better. This failure to take complete prescribed antimicrobials permits surviving organisms to develop resistance and to thrive, possibly causing a recurrence of illness. Therefore caution patients not to stop taking the medication when they start feeling better. They should continue their antimicrobials until the entire course has been completed or until their primary care provider specifically orders them to stop taking the medication. The emergence of antimicrobial resistance is one important reason why antimicrobial therapy for bacterial infections may fail. Increasingly, bacteria are becoming resistant, often because of the widespread or inappropriate use of antimicrobials, which leads to the killing of susceptible bacteria and allows more resistant strains to multiply. In 2017, the CDC and the American Nurses Association issued a white paper that defined the role of the nurse in antibiotic stewardship. Antibiotic stewardship refers to a set of coordinated strategies to improve the use of antibiotic medications to enhance patient health outcomes, reduce resistance to antibiotics, and reduce unnecessary costs.

Hyperbaric oxygen therapy is an intervention that is used to treat some infections. Breathing 100% oxygen at higher-than-atmospheric pressure in a closed chamber increases the amount of dissolved oxygen transported in plasma. The oxygen-rich environment improves leukocyte phagocytic activity and kills anaerobic bacteria (see Patient Teaching box).

During hyperbaric oxygen therapy, the patient must be monitored for the following complications: ear or sinus pain (from pressure buildup), respiratory problems (as a result of oxygen toxicity), seizures (a central nervous system symptom of oxygen toxicity), and bradycardia (reflex response to oxygen toxicity).

Patient Teaching

Hyperbaric Oxygen Therapy

Before undergoing hyperbaric oxygen therapy, the patient must be advised on the following:

- Do not smoke for several hours before and after treatment to decrease lung irritation.
- Do not take items that create spark or flame such as lighters or battery-powered devices.
- Do not wear, or remove, hair or skin products that are petrolatum based, which are potential fire hazards.
- Wear 100% cotton clothing in the hyperbaric oxygen chamber to prevent static electricity.
- Prevent pressure buildup in the ears by swallowing.

Earlier hospital discharges mean that substantial therapy may continue in the home after discharge. Home health care is frequently ordered for infected patients for several reasons. The patient has fewer opportunities to acquire an HAI, opportunities for infection to be spread to other hospitalized patients are reduced, and patients often do better in their own surroundings. If therapy is to be continued at home, teach the patient and other family members how to manage the care. Close coordination between members of the health care team is important to ensure good continuity of care. (Guidelines for infection prevention and control in the home are given in the Patient Teaching box.)

Patient Teaching

Infection Prevention and Control When the Patient is Treated in the Home

Infection control in the home setting is based on Standard Precautions. In the home, adapt the guidelines to the equipment and supplies available.

- **Equipment:** List for the family the activities that require the use of gloves and identify the proper gloves to use. Instruct caregivers to use an apron if clothing is likely to become contaminated and to wear gloves when changing dressings.
- **Hand hygiene:** Demonstrate good hand-washing technique and the use of waterless antiseptics to all household members. Tell family members that proper hand hygiene is the most important action they can take to prevent the spread of infection and inform them when hand washing or the use of antiseptics is appropriate.
- **Sharps disposal:** If a sharps container is not available, tell the family to use a puncture-resistant container such as a detergent bottle or coffee can with the lid securely taped until local regulations on sharps disposal can be initiated.
- **Bandages and linens:** Instruct household members to seal soiled dressings tightly in a plastic bag and dispose of dressings in the trash bag. Clothing and linens with body fluids should be stored in a plastic bag until they are laundered, at which time they should be washed in water as hot as the fabric will tolerate. One cup of bleach is added to the detergent in each load.
- **Spills:** Instruct household members to wear gloves to wash contaminated surfaces with detergent and water and then wash the surfaces with a freshly made solution of 1 : 10 household bleach. Disposable towels should be used and discarded in a plastic bag.
- **Dishes:** Leftover portions of uneaten food should not be saved. If a dishwasher is available in the home, it should be used for the patient's dishes. Otherwise, soiled dishes should be washed in detergent and hot water immediately after use.

IMMUNODEFICIENCY

CAUSES AND RISK FACTORS

When the body's self-defenses against foreign invasion fail to function normally, a state of immunodeficiency (immunosuppression) exists. In this state, known as an *immunocompromised* or *immunosuppressed state*, the body is unable to launch an adequate immune response, increasing the risk for infection. Immunodeficiencies can be congenital or, more commonly, acquired and can result from problems with humoral immunity, cell-mediated immunity, vital mediators such as complement, or the process of phagocytosis. The primary clinical clue to **immunodeficiency**, whatever the cause, is the tendency to develop recurrent infections.

In congenital immunodeficiencies, some part of the immune system fails to develop properly. The result is a defect in the B or T lymphocytes, phagocytes, or complement.

Acquired immunodeficiencies result from factors outside the immune system that render a previously functional immune system inadequate. Some causes of acquired deficiencies are infections, malignancies, autoimmune diseases (systemic lupus erythematosus, rheumatoid arthritis), chronic diseases (diabetes mellitus, renal disease), drugs, aging, stress, and malnutrition. See Chapter 32 for a more comprehensive discussion of autoimmune diseases.

Stress, whether physical or emotional, alters the body's response to disease. Although the mechanism is not fully understood, the release of hormones plays a part. Stressors include such factors as serious illness, job loss, and divorce; even noise and cold play a part.

The nutritional state of the patient also affects immunity. The malnourished patient is much more susceptible to infection, especially when a protein deficiency exists. People with chronic conditions such as diabetes and renal disease may become debilitated and unable to resist infection fully. Trauma victims, especially those with burns, have diminished immune responses. Many malignant disorders alter the functioning of the immune system. Infectious diseases also cause immunodeficiencies, especially acute viral infections.

Many treatments and interventions aimed at helping patients cause immunodeficiency. Medications often place patients at risk for infection; corticosteroids, antineoplastic drugs (used to treat cancer), and immunosuppressive drugs (used for transplant recipients) are a few of such medications.

Surgery, anesthesia, and irradiation for cancer can also alter immune function. In addition, invasive procedures such as urinary catheterization and venipuncture for intravenous therapy or blood work bypass the patient's first line of defense. In the hospitalized patient, all of these factors come into play; disease, stress, nutritional alterations, medications, and invasive procedures all set up the patient for infection.

MEDICAL TREATMENT

Congenital immunodeficiencies are usually treated with replacement therapy of the deficient immune component. Bone marrow transplants or fetal thymus tissue transplants may be used in some cases. Treating an acquired immunodeficiency entails correcting the underlying condition that is causing the problem, such as reducing stressors, correcting malnutrition, and discontinuing medications that alter immunity.

NURSING CARE OF THE IMMUNOSUPPRESSED PATIENT

The primary nursing responsibility in cases of immunodeficiency is to prevent infection. Proper hand hygiene by personnel, visitors, and patients themselves is the single most important measure in prevention. Vital signs should be assessed regularly. However, in an immunosuppressed or immunocompromised patient, signs and symptoms of infection are often atypical, masked, or absent. Be aware that a small increase in body temperature in these patients can be significant and should be reported. Avoid rectal thermometers if possible because of the potential for damage to the rectal mucosa. Encourage adequate nutritional intake. Perform effective skin, mouth, perineal, wound, and intravenous site care, with continuous assessment for signs of infection. Encourage patients to turn, cough, and breathe deeply. Protective (compromised host) isolation may be necessary. Flowers or plants may be prohibited because they provide a reservoir for bacterial growth. Fresh produce may be eliminated from the diet if the white blood cell count is too low. Disposable equipment is preferred.

Patient education concerning the risks for and signs of infection should be reinforced. Provide a supportive listening environment, because these patients may have anxiety, as well as a high stress level, and feelings of powerlessness are often overwhelming.

HYPERSENSITIVITY AND ALLERGY

CAUSES AND RISK FACTORS

The term *allergy* (or *hypersensitivity*) describes an atypical immune response that is activated by a foreign substance that normally is inoffensive. Although immune responses are usually beneficial, hypersensitivity can be harmful and even deadly. Estimates indicate that 20% to 25% of the U.S. population suffers from allergies of some sort, with allergic rhinitis (hay fever) and asthma occurring most often. Other allergic disorders include allergic contact dermatitis, angioedema (localized swelling that affects the airway if it involves the mouth or tongue), dermatitis, anaphylaxis (severe allergic reaction), gastrointestinal allergies, and urticaria (hives). The tendency to develop an allergy is inherited, although the type of allergy may vary. Someone who is prone to allergies may be called *atopic*. Hypersensitivity as an immune disorder is discussed in Chapter 32.

Table 5.4 Common Allergies and Their Triggers

ALLERGIC REACTION	STIMULUS
Allergic rhinitis	Pollens, dust, molds, animal dander
Asthma	Pollens, dust, molds, cigarette smoke, air pollutants, animal dander
Allergic eyes (conjunctivitis)	Pollens, dust, molds, animal dander, cigarette smoke
Anaphylaxis	Antimicrobials (penicillin) Insect venom (bee, wasp stings) Blood transfusions
Hives (urticaria)	Foods, drugs
Atopic dermatitis (eczema)	Soaps, cosmetics, chemicals, fabrics
Allergic contact dermatitis	Plants (poison ivy) Metals (nickel) Chemicals, cosmetics Latex gloves
Gastrointestinal allergies	Foods, drugs

An antigen that causes a hypersensitive reaction is called an ***allergen***. Any substance can act as an allergen to a susceptible person, but some of the more common ones are house dust, animal dander, pollens, molds, foods, pharmacologic agents, cigarette smoke, feathers, and insect venoms. Table 5.4 lists common allergies and triggers.

The allergic response begins with sensitization. The first encounter with a specific allergen results in only a small amount of antibody production. With subsequent exposure, however, the body steps up its defense by producing large amounts of antibodies, which circulate in the bloodstream and travel to the affected tissues. This buildup triggers the release of histamine and other chemical agents. Neutrophils arrive at the scene to engulf and destroy the antigens. A cascade of reactions occurs that produces the symptoms typical of an allergic response, although they vary according to the area affected. Local manifestations of allergic reactions include urticaria, pruritus, conjunctivitis, rhinitis, laryngeal edema, bronchospasm, dysrhythmia, gastrointestinal cramps and malabsorption, and angioedema.

MEDICAL TREATMENT

The medical treatment of patients with allergies varies, depending on the specific allergy. However, in any case, care of the airway must be the priority. In general, antihistamines are used to reduce the symptoms caused by histamine release. Many people suffer side effects from antihistamines, such as dry mouth, nausea, blurred vision, dizziness, and drowsiness. Antihistamines sometimes cause confusion in older patients. For asthma sufferers, bronchodilators, corticosteroids, or both may be prescribed to improve air movement and decrease inflammation in the lungs; oxygen and breathing treatments may also be ordered. Besides antihistamines, topical lotions and ointments may be prescribed to relieve itching associated with urticaria, atopic dermatitis, or allergic contact dermatitis.

Long-term medical treatment of allergies involves testing to determine specific allergens. Testing is performed by injecting small amounts of allergen under the skin (intradermally) or by pricking the surface of the patient's skin and monitoring for the degree of wheal and flare reaction. After the specific agents have been identified, the patient may be desensitized by injections of tiny quantities of the allergen, with the dose gradually increased over a prolonged period. Desensitization is aimed at increasing tolerance to the offending agent and decreasing the severity of the allergic response.

❖ NURSING CARE OF THE PATIENT WITH ALLERGIES

When dealing with the hospitalized patient with allergies, the most important nursing intervention is to document all allergies, the symptoms they cause, and any treatment currently used. Allergies should be posted on the patient's record, on all medication records, on the nursing care plan, and on a patient identification band. Never administer any drug to which the patient reports a previous allergic reaction.

Alert the pharmacy and dietary departments to drug and food allergies. Notify the primary care provider of any allergies that may determine which medications to avoid. For instance, a patient who is allergic to shellfish should not receive drugs containing iodine because an anaphylactic reaction may result. Ensure that patients who have been taking allergy medication, such as inhaler treatments, continue to take these medications when admitted to the hospital. Many patients, as well as health care providers, are reporting latex allergies, necessitating the use of nonlatex gloves.

Patient education is important for all patients with allergies. This area includes knowledge of specific allergens, limiting exposure to or avoiding allergens, the proper use of medications such as inhaled bronchodilators, and the actions and side effects of drugs. Patients who are at risk for life-threatening (anaphylactic) reactions should wear a medical alert bracelet that identifies their allergies. Individuals with insect sting allergies should obtain an emergency sting kit and be taught how to self-inject epinephrine. This kit should be kept readily available at all times.

Nurses should avoid the overuse of perfumes and scented cosmetics while working with patients. Live plants and flowers should not be allowed in the patient's room.

ANAPHYLAXIS

CAUSES AND RISK FACTORS

In most cases, people with allergies develop mild to moderate symptoms such as watery eyes, runny nose, or rash. However, exposure to an allergen can cause a life-threatening allergic reaction called *anaphylaxis.* Anaphylaxis can quickly deteriorate into shock, coma, and death. Histamine released in anaphylaxis causes bronchospasm, vasodilation, and increased capillary permeability throughout the body, which causes fluid to leave the circulation and enter the tissues, causing shock from hypovolemia. Signs and symptoms of anaphylaxis include anxiety, wheezing and difficulty breathing, cyanosis (bluish skin color), hives, facial edema, arthralgia (joint pain), dizziness, hypotension (low blood pressure), and cardiac arrest.

Anaphylaxis is an emergency situation, and the patient's life depends on rapid intervention. The most common cause of anaphylaxis is the use of antimicrobials, especially penicillin. Other causes include the use of medicines or serum from animal sources, insect venom (especially from bees and wasps), iodinated radioactive contrast media, local anesthetic, and blood products. The Be S.A.F.E. action guide was created to help patient with allergies to remember steps to take during and after an allergic emergency.

- **S**eek immediate medical help—Call 911 and get to the nearest emergency facility at the first sign of anaphylaxis.
- Identify the **A**llergen—Identify what you might have eaten or come in contact with that triggered the allergic reaction.
- **F**ollow-up with a specialist—Ask for a referral to an allergist/immunologist for testing, diagnosis and ongoing management.
- Carry **E**pinephrine for emergencies—Carry with you at all times a kit containing fast-acting, self-administered epinephrine. Educate your family and friends of your condition, triggers, and how to use the epinephrine. Consider wearing an emergency medical bracelet or necklace identifying you at risk for anaphylaxis.

MEDICAL TREATMENT

In anaphylaxis, oxygen is given in addition to intravenous epinephrine. Other drugs that might be given are dopamine or a volume expander (or both) to raise the patient's blood pressure, a nebulized bronchodilator to relax the bronchi and improve ventilation, diphenhydramine for antihistamine effects, and corticosteroids to decrease the inflammatory response. Endotracheal intubation, tracheostomy, and mechanical ventilation may be necessary to maintain adequate blood oxygenation.

❖ NURSING CARE OF THE PATIENT WITH ANAPHYLAXIS

The best care is to prevent anaphylaxis whenever possible by obtaining a history of allergies and taking precautions to protect the patient from substances (often drugs) that may trigger this reaction. However, when anaphylaxis occurs, prompt recognition is vital because it is a life-threatening situation. In some settings, nurses have protocols for administering subcutaneous epinephrine in the event of allergic reactions. Nursing interventions are aimed at minimizing the patient's anxiety and, once medical care is initiated, administering prescribed drugs, including oxygen, and monitoring intravenous fluids. Monitor respirations, color, heart rate, and oxygen saturation until the patient is fully recovered.

AUTOIMMUNE DISEASES

CAUSES AND RISK FACTORS

Immune tolerance is the process by which the immune system does not attack an antigen. The body's ability to determine self from nonself is called *natural or self-tolerance.* When tolerance is disrupted, the immune system reacts against and destroys its own tissues. This breakdown in tolerance and subsequent damage to self is termed ***autoimmunity***. An autoimmune process may be initiated when injury to tissues, infection, or malignancy occurs. The exact causes and pathologic nature of most autoimmune diseases are poorly understood, but many of these disorders cause severe illness and death.

Genetic factors appear to be involved because autoimmune diseases tend to be familial. Women—particularly Black American, Hispanic American, and Native American women—have higher risk for some autoimmune diseases. Some autoimmune disorders have apparent causes, such as drug-induced anemia or a low-platelet count (thrombocytopenia). Infection is often present before the onset of an autoimmune disease, leading to the conclusion that the disease results as a complication (sequela) of the infection. Autoimmune diseases cause injury in three ways: (1) by the effect of antibodies on cell surfaces, (2) through the deposit of antigen-antibody complexes (particularly in capillaries, joints, and renal tissue), and (3) through the action of sensitized T cells.

Autoimmunity can involve any tissue or organ system. In multiple sclerosis, the white matter of the brain and spinal cord is affected and the myelin sheath that protects nerve fibers is destroyed. Rheumatoid arthritis affects the lining of the joints. In type 1 diabetes mellitus, the pancreatic cells that secrete insulin are attacked. Table 5.5 lists some of the more common autoimmune disorders and the tissues they affect. One of the more familiar of the autoimmune disorders is

Table 5.5 Autoimmune Disorders and Their Targets

DISORDER	TISSUE AFFECTED
Endocrine System	
Hyperthyroidism (Graves disease)	Thyroid
Autoimmune thyroiditis	Thyroid
Type 1 diabetes mellitus	Pancreas
Addison disease	Adrenal gland
Central Nervous System	
Multiple sclerosis	Brain and spinal cord
Myasthenia gravis	Neuromuscular junctions
Cardiovascular System	
Rheumatic fever	Heart
Cardiomyopathy	Heart
Gastrointestinal System	
Ulcerative colitis	Colon
Crohn disease	Ileum
Connective Tissue	
Rheumatoid arthritis	Joints
Systemic lupus erythematosus	Multiple tissues
Scleroderma	Multiple tissues
Hematologic System	
Autoimmune hemolytic anemia	Red blood cells
Autoimmune thrombocytopenic purpura	Platelets
Idiopathic neutropenia	Neutrophils
Idiopathic lymphopenia	Lymphocytes
Respiratory and Renal Systems	
Goodpasture syndrome	Lung, kidney
Skin	
Pemphigus vulgaris	Skin
Psoriasis	Skin

Modified from McCance KL, Huether SE: *Pathophysiology: the biologic basis for disease in adults and children*, ed 6, St. Louis, 2009, Mosby-Elsevier.

systemic lupus erythematosus, which affects multiple organs.

MEDICAL TREATMENT

Medical interventions vary depending on the specific autoimmune disease and the tissues affected as well as on the symptoms. In general, corticosteroids and nonsteroidal antiinflammatory drugs are used to treat inflammation. Immunosuppressive therapies may be tried to moderate the autoimmune response.

❖ NURSING CARE OF THE PATIENT WITH AN AUTOIMMUNE DISORDER

Nursing interventions vary according to the specific disorder. Adequate rest, maintenance of optimal hydration and nutritional status, and prevention of infection are vital in preventing complications in these patients. In addition, a supportive, caring atmosphere is important to enhance the patient's coping skills and promote emotional health. Specific autoimmune disorders are addressed in Chapter 32 and with appropriate systems in this textbook.

Put On Your Thinking Cap!

In your clinical site, locate everything you would need if a patient had an anaphylactic reaction to a drug. What procedure should you use to alert other personnel?

Get Ready for the NCLEX® Examination!

Key Points

- Physical and chemical barriers that shield the body from disease or injury include the skin, the mucous membranes, and various blood cells.
- Many types of leukocytes, especially neutrophils and monocytes, act as nature's cleanup mechanism by migrating to infected or inflamed areas and engulfing and destroying antigens through a process known as *phagocytosis.*
- Reticuloendothelial cells, or tissue macrophages, found in the blood, connective tissue, liver, spleen, bone marrow, and lymph nodes protect the body by digesting and absorbing foreign material such as old red blood cells, bacteria, and colloidal particles.
- The five signs of inflammation are rubor (redness), calor (heat), tumor (swelling), dolor (pain), and loss of function.
- Wound healing begins at the same time that the inflammatory process begins.
- The process of wound healing includes the production of macrophage cells to clean up inflammatory debris, the initiation of the repair process by fibroblasts, the formation of capillaries to provide circulation and nutrients to the new tissue, and the migration of epithelial cells under the scab to form a scar.
- Age and general health affect how rapidly wound healing occurs. Older adults heal more slowly as a result of a decreased blood supply to the tissues, a decrease in tissue elasticity, and poor or inadequate nutrition.
- The major infectious agents are bacteria, viruses, fungi, protozoa, rickettsiae, and helminths.

- Infection, or the invasion of the body by microorganisms, is possible only when a causative agent, a reservoir, a portal of exit, a mode of transfer, a portal of entry, and a susceptible host are present.
- Signs and symptoms of generalized infection are moderate to severe pain, swelling, fever, malaise, anorexia, and prostration.
- Two types of infections are (1) community-acquired infections, acquired through daily contact with the public, and (2) health care–acquired infections (HAIs).
- The most basic and effective method of preventing the spread of infection is hand hygiene.
- The CDC recommends the use of Standard Precautions for all patients, especially those cared for in settings in which exposure to blood or other body fluids is common.
- To reduce MDROs in health care settings, the use of Contact Precautions with infected or colonized patients is recommended.
- In hospitals and long-term care facilities, patients with MDROs should be in single rooms or rooms with others who have the same MDRO.
- The immune system is the body's defense network against infection; it provides the body with resistance to invading organisms and enables it to fight off invaders once they have gained access.
- Antigens are substances that stimulate a response from the immune system. Antibodies, also known as *immunoglobulins*, are proteins that are created in response to specific antigens.
- Innate (natural) immunity is present in the body at birth whereas acquired immunity develops after birth as a result of the body's immune responses to antigens.
- Acquired immunity depends on the proper development of B and T lymphocytes, which are white blood cells that fight infection.
- The two types of immunity—antibody-mediated (humoral) and cell-mediated immunity—function interdependently to provide the immune response.
- Immunodeficiency occurs when the body is unable to launch an adequate immune response, resulting in risk for infection.
- When a normally inoffensive foreign substance stimulates an atypical immune response, allergy or hypersensitivity occurs.
- Anaphylaxis is a life-threatening immune response that requires immediate intervention.
- Autoimmunity occurs when the body fails to recognize itself and the immune system reacts by destroying the body's own tissues.

Additional Learning Resources

SG Go to your Study Guide for additional learning activities to help you master this chapter content.

Go to your Evolve website (http://evolve.elsevier.com/Linton/medsurg) for the following learning resources and much more:

- Fluid & Electrolyte Tutorial
- Review Questions for the NCLEX® Examination

Clinical Judgment and Next-Generation NCLEX® Examination-Style Questions

1. A physician has just told a patient that he has an autoimmune condition. What is the correct term for this type of condition?

1. The patient's immune system is not adequate to prevent infection.
2. The patient has acquired an infection in the health care facility.
3. The patient's immune system is attacking his own tissues.
4. The patient has tissue inflammation caused by an infection.

NCLEX Client Need: Physiological Integrity: Physiological Adaptation

2. The nurse inspects for inflammation at an intravenous infusion site. Which of the following are classic signs of local inflammation? (Select all that apply.)

1. Heat
2. Drainage
3. Redness
4. Fever
5. Swelling

NCLEX Client Need: Physiological Integrity: Physiological Adaptation

3. In the first phase of the inflammatory process, capillary permeability increases. What purpose does this increase serve?

1. Reduces pain in the inflamed tissue by diluting bradykinin.
2. Draws excess fluid out of inflamed tissue to reduce swelling.
3. Allows monocytes and neutrophils to pass into the inflamed tissue.
4. Counteracts bronchoconstriction in antigen-antibody reactions.

NCLEX Client Need: Physiological Integrity: Physiological Adaptation

4. Why have numerous antibacterial drugs but relatively few antiviral drugs been developed?

1. Viruses have a more advanced ability to develop resistance to drugs.
2. Making antibacterial drugs is more profitable because only a few viruses exist.
3. Very few chemicals that are capable of killing viruses have been developed.
4. The virus lives inside the host cell and drugs that harm viruses often harm host cells as well.

NCLEX Client Need: Physiological Integrity: Pharmacological Therapies

5. Characteristics of the incubation period of the infectious process include which of the following?

1. The infected person is often very contagious.
2. Signs and symptoms are most severe.
3. A high fever is usually the only symptom present
4. The patient is in the recovery phase of the infection.

NCLEX Client Need: Physiological Integrity: Physiological Adaptation

6. Each patient on an infectious disease unit has one of the infections listed. Which is/are health care–associated infection(s)? (Select all that apply.)

1. Gonorrhea
2. Hepatitis A
3. Tuberculosis
4. Vancomycin-resistant *Enterococcus*
5. Streptococcal pharyngitis

NCLEX Client Need: Physiological Integrity: Physiological Adaptation

7. Nurses on an infectious disease unit want to implement measures to reduce bacterial resistance to antibiotics. Which measure(s) will help to prevent the development of bacterial resistance? (Select all that apply.)

1. All infections are promptly treated with broad-spectrum antimicrobials.
2. Antimicrobial selection is based on the results of culture and sensitivity tests.
3. Antimicrobials are discontinued as soon as symptoms resolve.
4. Antimicrobials are prescribed only for serious infections.
5. Vaccinations for infectious diseases are encouraged.

NCLEX Client Need: Physiological Integrity: Pharmacological Therapies

8. The primary mode of transmission of health care–associated infections is:

1. Soiled caregiver hands
2. Direct contact between patients
3. Organisms brought in by visitors
4. Faulty sterilization procedures

NCLEX Client Need: Physiological Integrity: Physiological Adaptation

9. Which statement is true regarding the need to use Standard Precautions?

1. Standard Precautions are required only when caring for patients who have open wounds.
2. Standard Precautions are required when caring for any patient in any setting.
3. Standard Precautions are required only when caring for patients with tuberculosis, hepatitis, or HIV infection.
4. Standard Precautions are required only when caring for patients who are highly susceptible to infection.

NCLEX Client Need: Health Promotion and Maintenance

10. The advantage of using HEPA filter respirators rather than surgical masks is that:

1. Surgical masks are too expensive for routine use
2. HEPA filter respirators protect the caregiver by filtering inspired air
3. Surgical masks protect the caregiver against tuberculosis but no other infections
4. HEPA filter respirators protect the patient but not the caregiver

NCLEX Client Need: Health Promotion and Maintenance

11. After vaccination for measles, a person will not become ill if exposed to the measles virus. The patient's ability to resist the measles virus is called:

1. Innate immunity
2. Nonspecific defense mechanism
3. Active acquired immunity
4. Passive acquired immunity

NCLEX Client Need: Physiological Integrity: Physiological Adaptation

12. Nursing care of the immunosuppressed patient should include which of the following?

1. Take rectal temperatures every 4 hours to detect low-grade fever.
2. Encourage consumption of fresh fruits and vegetables to increase vitamin intake.
3. Encourage the family to bring in live plants to increase oxygen in the room.
4. Emphasize the need for proper hand washing by patients, visitors, and staff.

NCLEX Client Need: Health Promotion and Maintenance

13. A nurse has just completed an assessment of a patient who is immunosuppressed. Of the data collected, which items require follow-up by the nurse? (Select all that apply.)

1. Thirst
2. Difficulty voiding
3. Temperature of 100°F
4. Redness around IV insertion site
5. Fatigue
6. Complaints of feeling cold
7. Headache

NCLEX Client Need: Physiological Integrity: Physiological Adaptation

Fluid, Electrolyte, and Acid-Base Balance

6

http://evolve.elsevier.com/Linton/medsurg

Objectives

1. Describe the extracellular and intracellular fluid compartments.
2. Describe the composition of the extracellular and intracellular body fluid compartments.
3. Discuss the mechanisms of fluid transport and fluid balance.
4. Identify the causes, signs and symptoms, and treatment of fluid imbalances.
5. Describe the major functions of the major electrolytes: sodium, potassium, calcium, magnesium, and chloride.
6. Identify the causes, signs and symptoms, and treatment of electrolyte imbalances.
7. List data to be collected for the focused assessment of fluid and electrolyte status.
8. Discuss the medical treatment and nursing management of persons with fluid and electrolyte imbalances.
9. Explain why older persons are at increased risk for fluid and electrolyte imbalances.
10. List the four types of acid-base imbalances.
11. Identify the major causes of each acid-base imbalance.
12. Explain the medical treatment and nursing management of acid-base imbalances.

Key Terms

acid
acid-base balance
active transport
base
diffusion (dĭ-FYŪ-zhŭn)
electrolyte (ĕ-LĔK-trō-līt)
extracellular fluid (ĕks-tră-SĔL-ū-lăr)
filtration (f ĭl-TRĀ-shŭn)
fluid volume deficit
fluid volume excess
homeostasis (hō-mē-ō-STĀ-sĭs)
intracellular fluid (ĭn-tră-SĔL-yū-lăr)
osmolality (ŏz-mō-LĂL-ĭ-tē)
osmolarity (ŏz-mō-LĀR-ĭ-tē)
osmosis (ŏz-MŌ-sĭs)
selectively permeable membrane (sĕ-LĔK-tĭv-lē PĔR-mē-ă-b'l MĔM-brān)

Maintaining the correct amount and distribution of body fluids and electrolytes and the correct pH of body fluids is essential for survival. The body constantly makes adjustments to maintain this balance. Unfortunately, many disease processes and medical interventions pose actual or potential threats to patients' fluid and electrolyte balances. Therefore, nurses must understand the basic principles of fluid and electrolyte and acid-base balance to maintain homeostasis and to detect and correct imbalances. This chapter offers a review of key concepts.

HOMEOSTASIS

Approximately 50% to 60% of the human body is composed of water. To maintain internal balance, the body must be able to regulate the fluids within it. The tendency to maintain relatively constant conditions as in the fluid compartments is called ***homeostasis***. All organs and structures of the body are involved in the maintenance of homeostasis.

Homeostasis is necessary for cells to be able to carry out their work. Body fluids are in constant motion, maintaining healthy living conditions for body cells. The process of homeostasis involves the delivery of essential elements such as oxygen and glucose to the cells and the removal of wastes such as carbon dioxide from the cells. When the body does not maintain homeostasis, the cells cannot function properly and illness or death results.

BODY FLUID COMPARTMENTS

Body fluids are classified as intracellular or extracellular, depending on their location. **Intracellular fluid** is fluid within a cell and **extracellular fluid** is fluid outside the cell. Most of the body's fluids are found within the cell.

Extracellular fluids are found in the blood vessels in the form of plasma or serum (called *intravascular fluid*); in the fluid surrounding the cells (called *interstitial fluid*), including lymph fluid; and elsewhere, such as in digestive

Table 6.1 Total Body Fluids

	MEN (%)	WOMEN (%)	INFANT (%)
Intracellular	40	36	40
Extracellular	20	18	35
Total body fluids	**60**	**54**	**75**

secretions, sweat, and cerebrospinal fluid. Extracellular fluid is mainly responsible for the transport of nutrients and wastes throughout the body. The distribution of total body fluids varies by age and gender (Table 6.1).

COMPOSITION OF BODY FLUIDS

WATER

Water makes up the largest portion of the body weight. The percentage of body weight that is water is affected by age, sex, and amount of body fat. A person's percentage of body water usually decreases with advancing age. Women have a lower percentage of body water than do men throughout the adult years because women have more fat than men and fat cells contain less water than other cells. Obese people have a relatively lower percentage of body water because of their increased number of fat cells.

SOLUTES

In addition to water, body fluids contain solutes (dissolved substances) such as electrolytes and nonelectrolytes.

Electrolytes

An **electrolyte** is defined as a substance that develops an electrical charge when dissolved in water. Examples of electrolytes are sodium, potassium, calcium, chloride, bicarbonate, and magnesium. When these substances are dissolved in water, they break up into small particles called *ions*, which have either a positive (+) or a negative (−) charge. Ions that have a positive electrical charge are called *cations*. Examples of cations are sodium (Na^+), potassium (K^+), calcium (Ca^{2+}), and magnesium (Mg^{2+}). Ions that have a negative charge are called *anions*. Examples of anions are chloride (Cl^-), bicarbonate (HCO_3^-), and phosphate (HPO_4^-).

Electrolytes maintain a balance between positive and negative charges. For every positively charged cation, a negatively charged anion can be found. In every fluid compartment of the body, the cations and anions combine to balance one another. This process keeps the body cells in homeostasis.

The concentration of an electrolyte in a solution or body fluid compartment is measured in milliequivalents per liter (mEq/L). Milliequivalents indicate the chemical activity or combining power of ions. Hydrogen is used as a standard for comparing chemical activities of electrolytes. One milliequivalent of an electrolyte has the same chemical combining power as 1 mEq of hydrogen.

Table 6.2 Electrolyte Composition of Extracellular and Intracellular Fluids

ELECTROLYTE	EXTRACELLULAR FLUID (mEq/L)	INTRACELLULAR FLUID (mEq/L)
Sodium (Na^+)	130–145	14
Potassium (K^+)	3.5–5.1	140
Chloride (Cl^-)	98–107	4–6
Bicarbonate (HCO_3^-)	24	12
Calcium (Ca^{2+})	5	1–8
Magnesium (Mg^{2+})	1.5–2.5	6–30
Phosphate (HPO_4^-)	2	40–95

Electrolytes can move from one fluid compartment to another. However, the normal concentration of specific electrolytes is different in the two compartments (Table 6.2).

Sodium

Sodium (Na^+) is the most abundant electrolyte in the body and the primary electrolyte in the extracellular fluid. It plays a major role in the regulation of body fluid volumes, muscular activity, nerve impulse conduction, and acid-base balance. To remember the role of sodium in water distribution, think "water goes where sodium is." For example, a person whose sodium level is too high will retain water. We can promote the elimination of excess water by giving a diuretic that promotes excretion of sodium.

Potassium

Potassium (K^+) is found mainly in the intracellular fluid and is the major intracellular cation. Because it is so abundant within the cell, it plays an important role in maintaining fluid osmolarity and volume within the cell. Potassium is essential for normal membrane excitability, a critical factor in the transmission of nerve impulses. It is also needed for protein synthesis, for the synthesis and breakdown of glycogen, and to maintain plasma acid-base balance.

Chloride

Chloride (Cl^-) is an extracellular anion that is usually bound with other ions, especially sodium or potassium. Its major functions are to regulate osmotic pressure between fluid compartments and to assist in regulating acid-base balance.

Calcium

Calcium (Ca^{2+}) is usually combined with phosphorus to form the mineral salts of the bones and teeth. Of the total calcium in the body, 99% is concentrated in the bones and teeth and 1% is in the extracellular fluid. Calcium is ingested through the diet and absorbed through the intestine. Calcium and phosphorus have a reciprocal relationship, meaning that if one falls, the other typically rises; if one rises, the other falls.

In addition to maintaining strong teeth and bones, calcium promotes normal transmission of nerve impulses and helps to regulate normal muscle contraction and relaxation. Constant regulation of calcium levels takes place in the body. If the serum calcium level falls, additional calcium is absorbed in the intestine, reabsorbed through the kidneys, or taken from the bones. If more calcium is needed in the bones, it is taken from the bloodstream and also reabsorbed through the kidneys.

Magnesium

Magnesium (Mg^{2+}) is a cation that is found in bone (50%–60%), intracellular fluid (39%–49%), and extracellular fluid (1%). After potassium, magnesium is the most abundant cation in intracellular fluid; therefore it is vital to cellular function. Magnesium plays a role in the metabolism of carbohydrates and proteins, the storage and use of intracellular energy, and neural transmission. Magnesium is important in the functioning of the heart, nerves, and muscles.

Approximately 30% to 40% of magnesium ingested through the diet is absorbed, mainly through the small intestine. Magnesium is excreted through the kidneys, and the rate of excretion is regulated by sodium and calcium excretion, extracellular fluid volume, and parathyroid hormone.

Nonelectrolytes

Although most of the solutes in the body are electrolytes, other substances are dissolved in the body fluids as well. Examples are urea, protein, glucose, creatinine, and bilirubin. These solutes do not carry an electrical charge and are measured in milligrams per deciliter (mg/dL).

TRANSPORT OF WATER AND ELECTROLYTES

MEMBRANES

The intracellular and extracellular fluid compartments are separated by **selectively permeable membranes** that control movement of water and certain solutes. Selective permeability maintains the unique composition of each compartment of the body while allowing for the transport of nutrients and wastes to and from cells. For example, selectively permeable membranes surround cells to separate fluid in the cells from fluid in the tissues. Some solutes cross membranes more easily than others. Small molecules and water move freely across membranes whereas larger molecules such as protein move less readily.

TRANSPORT PROCESSES

Water and solutes are transported between intracellular and extracellular fluid compartments by one or more of the following processes: (1) diffusion, (2) active transport, (3) filtration, and (4) osmosis.

Diffusion

Diffusion is the random movement of particles in all directions. The natural tendency is for a substance to move from an area of higher concentration to an area of lower concentration. One example is the movement of oxygen from the alveoli to the pulmonary capillaries. The concentration of oxygen in the alveoli is greater than in the capillaries, therefore oxygen diffuses into the capillaries and is transported through the bloodstream to other parts of the body. The term *facilitated diffusion* is used when a carrier protein transports the molecules through membranes toward an area of lower concentration. This process does not require energy.

Active Transport

Carrier proteins can transport substances from an area of lower concentration to an area of equal or greater concentration. This process, which requires expenditure of energy, is called **active transport**. Many solutes, such as sodium, potassium, glucose, and hydrogen, are actively transported across cell membranes. An example of active transport is the sodium pump. The concentration of sodium is highest in extracellular fluid. Therefore excess sodium cannot leave the cell by diffusion. Active transport "pumps" the excess sodium out of the cell into the extracellular fluid.

Filtration

Filtration is the transfer of water and solutes through a membrane from an area of high pressure to an area of low pressure. This pressure is known as *hydrostatic pressure* and is a combination of pressures from the force of gravity on the fluid and the pumping action of the heart. Filtration is a necessary process for moving fluid out of the capillaries into the tissues and for filtering plasma through the kidneys.

Osmosis

Osmosis is the movement of water across a membrane from a less concentrated solution to a more concentrated solution. It involves the movement of water only, but sometimes the force of movement across the membrane carries some solutes along. If a fluid compartment has less water and more sodium, water from another compartment moves to the more concentrated compartment by osmosis to create a better fluid balance.

OSMOLALITY

Osmolality refers to the concentration of a solution determined by the number of dissolved particles per kilogram of water. A higher osmolality means that the concentration of salt, or any other solute, is higher in the water because the solution contains less water. Osmolality controls water movement and distribution in body fluid compartments by regulating the concentration of fluid in each compartment. When solutes such as electrolytes are added to water, the volume is expanded to include both the water and the solutes.

The osmolality of intracellular fluid and extracellular fluid tends to equalize because of the constant shifting of water. A change in osmolality of intracellular fluid affects the osmolality of extracellular fluid and vice versa. The osmolality of intracellular fluid is maintained primarily by potassium and the osmolality of the extracellular fluid is maintained primarily by sodium. The normal range of osmolality of the body fluids is between 280 and 294 milliosmoles per kilogram (mOsm/kg). You will see the term ***osmolarity*** also used to refer to the concentration of particles in body water. Osmolarity refers to the concentration of particles per liter of solution. For the study of body fluids, measuring liters of fluid is more practical than measuring kilograms; therefore you will see clinical studies of fluids using the term *osmolarity* rather than osmolality.

REGULATORY MECHANISMS

Regulation of fluid balance requires the constant adjustment of fluid volume, distribution, and composition. This process is accomplished by the kidneys and circulatory system, which are influenced by the sympathetic nervous system, specific hormones, and the thirst center.

KIDNEYS

The kidneys are the main regulators of fluid balance. They control extracellular fluid by adjusting the concentration of specific electrolytes, the osmolality of body fluids, the volume of extracellular fluid, blood volume, and pH. Kidney function is delicately controlled by hormones and other coordinating mechanisms (see Chapter 41 for a review of renal structure and function).

The nephron is the functioning unit of the kidney. Each nephron is made up of a glomerulus and tubules. The glomerulus is the filtering portion of the nephron and the tubule is responsible for secretion and reabsorption. The nephrons conduct the work of the kidney through the processes of filtration, reabsorption, and secretion.

Filtration

A primary activity of the kidney is filtration. Blood plasma entering the kidney via the renal artery is delivered to the glomerulus. Approximately 20% of the plasma is filtered into the glomerular capsule. This fluid is called *filtrate.* Most of the remaining plasma leaves the kidney through the renal vein. The filtrate then moves through the tubules, where it is transformed into urine by the processes of tubular reabsorption and secretion.

Tubular Reabsorption

Tubular reabsorption is a process by which most of the glomerular filtrate is returned to the circulation. Water and selected solutes move from the tubules into the capillaries. Waste products remain in the tubules for excretion whereas most water and sodium are reabsorbed into the bloodstream. Tubular reabsorption is important for adjusting the volume and composition of the filtrate and for preventing excessive fluid loss through the kidneys.

Tubular Secretion

Tubular secretion is the last phase in the work of the kidneys. During this phase, the filtrate is transformed into urine. Various substances, among them drugs, hydrogen ions, potassium ions, creatinine, and histamine, pass from the blood into the tubules. This process eliminates some excess substances to maintain fluid and electrolyte balance as well as metabolic waste products.

HORMONES

Hormones that have a major effect on fluid volume and balance are renin, aldosterone, antidiuretic hormone (ADH), and atrial natriuretic factor (ANF). Renin is a hormone that is secreted when blood volume or blood pressure falls. Renin activates angiotensinogen, a substance secreted by the liver, to form angiotensin I. Angiotensin-converting enzyme then converts angiotensin I to angiotensin II. Angiotensin II is a potent vasoconstrictor that also stimulates the release of aldosterone, with subsequent sodium and water retention.

Aldosterone is released by the adrenal glands in response to the hormone renin. Aldosterone acts on the kidney tubules to increase the reabsorption of sodium and decrease the reabsorption of potassium. Because the retention of sodium causes water retention, aldosterone acts as a volume regulator. The release of aldosterone from the adrenal gland is stimulated by many factors, including increased potassium levels and decreased sodium levels in the blood.

ADH is produced by the hypothalamus and is secreted into the general circulation by the posterior pituitary gland. It causes the capillaries to reabsorb more water so that urine is more concentrated and less volume is excreted. An increase in plasma osmolality (plasma is more concentrated) stimulates the release of ADH into the bloodstream to replenish needed fluid in the body. Other factors that stimulate the release of ADH are related to stress situations such as hypotension, pain, surgery, and certain medications.

ANF is a hormone released by the atria in response to stretching of the atria by increased blood volume. ANF stimulates excretion of sodium and water by the kidneys, decreased synthesis of renin, decreased release of aldosterone, and vasodilation. The effect of these actions is to reduce blood volume and to lower blood pressure.

THIRST

An additional regulatory mechanism is thirst, which regulates fluid intake. Increased plasma osmolality stimulates osmoreceptors in the hypothalamus to trigger the sensation of thirst. In other words, more sodium and less water in the body make a person thirsty. Additional fluids are consumed and the kidneys conserve water until plasma osmolality returns to normal.

FLUID GAINS AND LOSSES

In a healthy adult, the 24-hour fluid intake and output are approximately equal (Table 6.3). Fluids are gained by drinking and eating and are lost through the kidneys, skin, lungs, and gastrointestinal tract. The usual adult urine volume is between 1 and 2 liters per day (L/day), or 1 milliliter per kilogram of body weight per hour. In the kidneys, water loss varies largely with the amount of solute excreted and with the level of ADH.

Water and electrolyte (sodium, chloride, and potassium) losses through the skin occur by sweating. Water loss through the lungs occurs by evaporation at a rate of 300 to 400 milliliters per day (mL/day). In a hot, dry environment, water loss via the skin and lungs increases. In the gastrointestinal tract, the usual loss of fluid is approximately 100 to 200 mL/day. The bulk of fluid secreted into the gastrointestinal tract is reabsorbed in the small intestine. Water loss through the skin, lungs, and intestinal tract is referred to as *insensible loss*. Fig. 6.1 diagrams the regulation of body fluid volume.

Table 6.3 24-Hour Intake and Output of Body Fluids

FLUID GAINS	AMOUNT (mL)	FLUID LOSSES	AMOUNT (mL)
Liquids	1000	Lungs	400
Food (solid)	1200	Skin	400
H_2O of oxidation (metabolic production)	300	Kidneys (urine)	1500
Daily total intake	**2500**	Intestines (feces)	200
		Daily total output	**2500**

AGE-RELATED CHANGES AFFECTING FLUID BALANCE

Multiple factors place the older person at risk for fluid and electrolyte imbalances. The aging kidney is slower

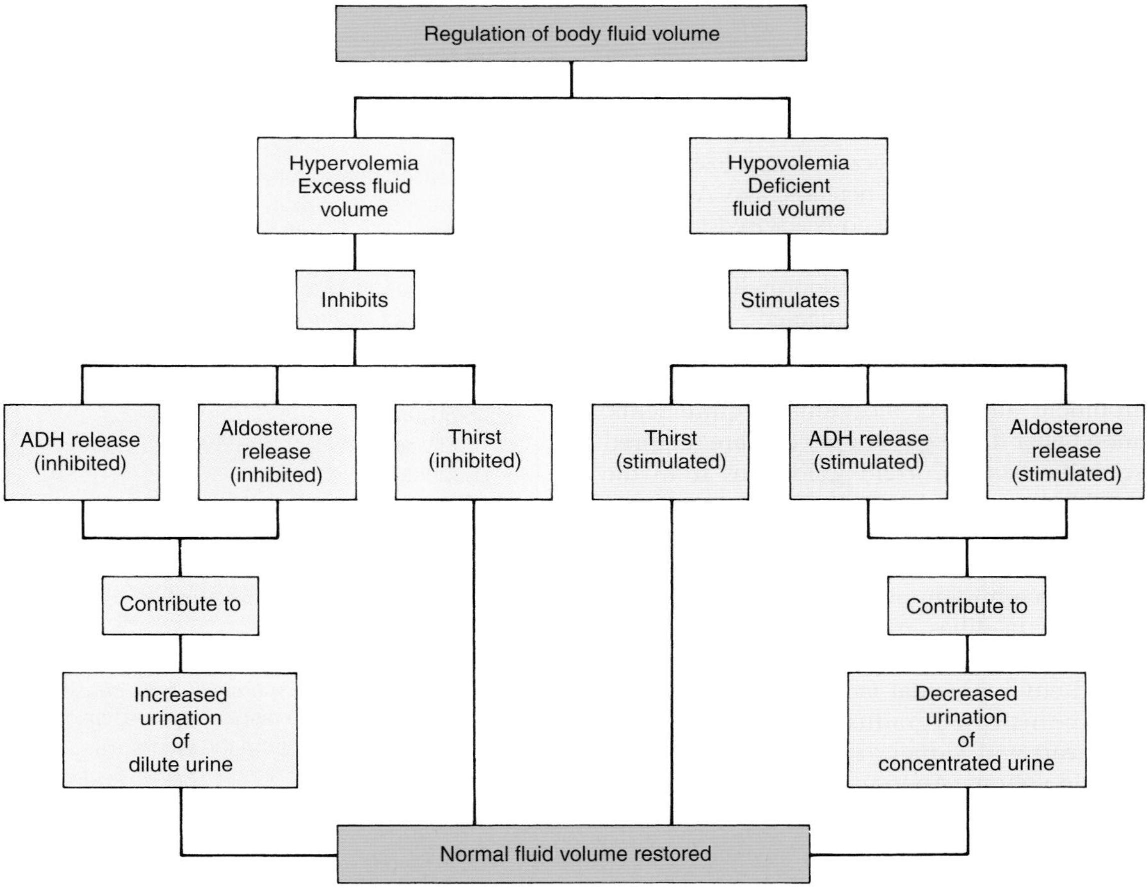

Fig. 6.1 Regulation of body fluid volume depends on aldosterone, antidiuretic hormone (*ADH*), and thirst. (From Black JM, Hawks JH, Keene AM: *Medical-surgical nursing: clinical management for continuity of care*, ed 8, Philadelphia, 2009, Saunders.)

to adjust to changes in acid-base, fluid, and electrolyte balance. The older adult often has a reduced sense of thirst and therefore may be in a state of chronic dehydration because of inadequate fluid intake. Total body water declines with age, with the greatest loss being from the intracellular fluid compartment. Therefore an older person has limited reserves with which to maintain fluid balance when abnormal losses occur.

You must monitor fluid status in the older person and be alert for signs and symptoms of imbalances, including disorientation, confusion, constipation, and falls resulting from postural hypotension. The health history may reveal many chronic conditions, such as heart failure and renal insufficiency, which are more common among older adults and place them at risk for fluid and electrolyte imbalances. Drugs such as antihypertensives, diuretics, and antacids used to treat these and other conditions can also contribute to imbalances. In addition, chronic conditions that affect mobility or mental status may interfere with adequate fluid intake. Some factors that contribute to acute fluid deficits are trauma, infection, fever, influenza or cold, NPO (nothing by mouth) status, and drug therapies (diuretics, antidepressants, sedatives). In addition to the general assessment data, it is especially important to document fluid intake patterns, medications, mental status, and recent weight changes.

Components of the physical examination are described later in this chapter. Note that skin turgor is a less reliable indicator of fluid status in older persons than in younger individuals, because some loss of skin elasticity normally occurs with increased age. Assessing turgor on the sternum or forehead is advised for better accuracy in the older person. Serum electrolytes should be the same for all adults, so any abnormalities of such in the older person should be investigated.

No prescription for a specific daily fluid intake exists because body weight, health state, activity level, and environment all affect individual requirements. The common belief that 8 glasses per day are required has no scientific basis. Current guidelines from the Institute of Medicine advise that adult men should take in 3 L/day, and adult women should take in 2.2 liters daily. Some sources recommend an intake of 30 mL/kg/day with a minimum of 1.5 L/day. Residents at long-term care facilities are at high risk for inadequate fluid intake because of physiologic, functional, cognitive, and environmental factors. However, fluid intake should be increased gradually in the older adult, because the heart and kidneys adapt more slowly to changes in fluid volume. An individual with cardiac or renal disease sometimes has fluid restrictions because of fluid retention.

Put On Your Thinking Cap!

Measure your fluid intake and output for 24 hours. If they are not equal, list possible explanations for the difference.

FOCUSED ASSESSMENT OF FLUID AND ELECTROLYTE BALANCE

HEALTH HISTORY

A complete health history helps to determine whether patients have any conditions that may contribute to fluid or electrolyte imbalances. Conditions that have great potential for disrupting fluid balance are vomiting, diarrhea, kidney diseases, diabetes, salicylate poisoning, burns, congestive heart failure, cerebral injuries, ulcerative colitis, and hormonal imbalances. Other risk factors include the intake of drugs such as diuretics and cathartics and medical interventions such as gastric suctioning. Anticipate fluid and electrolyte imbalances in patients who are at risk. Patient complaints that may be associated with fluid imbalances are fatigue, palpitations, dizziness, edema, muscle weakness or cramps, dyspnea, and confusion. Because electrolyte disturbances produce nonspecific symptoms, they can be confirmed only with laboratory tests.

PHYSICAL EXAMINATION

Vital Signs

Assessment of pulse, respiration, temperature, and blood pressure can detect indicators of changes in both fluid and electrolyte balance, as shown in Box 6.1.

Box 6.1 Vital Sign Changes With Fluid and Electrolyte Imbalances

PULSE

- Increased rate with fluid volume deficit, sodium deficit, or magnesium deficit.
- Decreased rate with magnesium excess or potassium deficit.
- Weak quality, irregular rhythm, and rapid rate suggest severe potassium excess or sodium deficit.
- Bounding quality with fluid volume excess, which often results in circulatory overload.

RESPIRATION

- Fluid volume excess can cause pulmonary edema with dyspnea and tachypnea.
- Changes in respiratory function are noted also with acid-base imbalances. Slow, shallow respirations with intermittent periods of apnea occur in severe metabolic alkalosis. Deep, rapid respirations indicate metabolic acidosis.

TEMPERATURE

- Fever increases the metabolic rate, causing fluid loss; it also increases the respiratory rate, which increases loss of water vapor from the lungs.
- Temperature may be subnormal with fluid volume excess.

BLOOD PRESSURE

- A fall in systolic pressure of more than 20 mm Hg when the patient changes from the lying to the standing position or from the lying to the sitting position usually indicates fluid volume deficit.
- Fluid volume excess that expands blood volume raises the blood pressure.

Body temperature variations can be associated with excess or deficit fluid volume. Also fever poses a risk of water and electrolyte loss associated with sweating and an increased metabolic rate. Blood pressure is directly related to blood volume. The pulse rate and quality may change in response to blood volume alterations. Because electrolytes affect the conduction of impulses, electrolyte changes can affect heart rate and rhythm. Respirations are minimally affected by electrolyte changes. However, rapid respirations increase water loss. Also excess fluid volume can lead to heart failure and pulmonary edema with shortness of breath. Measuring blood pressure with the patient lying, sitting, and standing can detect positional differences that may reflect inadequate blood volume.

Intake and Output

An accurate record of intake and output is essential to determine whether the patient's intake is equal to output. All fluids entering or leaving the body should be noted, as explained in Box 6.2. A changing urine output may reflect attempts by the kidneys to maintain or restore balance or it may reflect a problem that causes fluid disturbances. In addition to urine volume, urine characteristics also give clues to fluid balance. Clear, pale urine in a healthy person suggests the excretion of excess water whereas dark, concentrated urine indicates that the kidneys are retaining water.

Body Weight

Measurement of body weight is a good indicator of fluid loss or retention (Box 6.3). One liter of fluid weighs 2.2 lb. Therefore, retention of 1 liter of fluid is reflected as a weight gain of 2.2 lb (1 kg). A patient can accumulate up to 10 lb (4.5 kg) of fluid before pitting edema is evident. To monitor fluid status, weigh the patient daily on the same scale, at the same time of day, and wearing the same type of clothing.

Box 6.2 Focused Assessment of Intake and Output

- Many serious fluid and electrolyte imbalances can be averted by carefully monitoring records of fluid intake and output.
- If the total intake is substantially less than the total output, the patient is in danger of fluid volume deficit.
- If the total intake is substantially more than the total output, the patient is in danger of fluid volume excess.
- Intake should include all fluids taken into the body: oral fluids, foods that are liquid at room temperature, intravenous fluids, subcutaneous fluids, fluids instilled into drainage tubes or irrigants, tube feeding solutions, water given through feeding tubes, and enema solutions.
- Output measures include urine, vomitus, diarrhea, drainage from fistulas, drainage from suction machines, excessive perspiration, and drainage from excisions; normal adult urine output is 40–80 mL/h.

Skin

Skin characteristics

Skin color, moisture, turgor, and temperature all reflect fluid balance. Dry, flushed skin is associated with dehydration. Pale, cool, clammy skin is associated with the severe fluid volume deficit that occurs with shock. Moist, edematous tissue, especially in dependent areas, may be seen with excess fluid volume.

Facial characteristics

The patient who is severely dehydrated usually has a pinched, drawn facial expression. Soft eyeballs and sunken eyes accompany a severe fluid volume deficit. Puffy eyelids and fuller cheeks suggest excess fluid volume.

Skin turgor

Skin turgor is best measured by pinching the skin over the sternum, the inner aspects of the thighs, or the forehead. In patients who are dehydrated, skin flattens more slowly after the pinch is released. The term *tenting* is sometimes used to describe skin that does not flatten promptly after being gently pinched into a tent shape. The skin of older people generally has a slower return to normal, so assuming a fluid deficit based only on poor skin turgor would be inappropriate in the older person.

Edema

Edema reflects water and sodium retention, which can result from excessive reabsorption or inadequate excretion of sodium, as may occur with kidney failure. Inspect and palpate the skin for edema. Test for edema by pressing the skin that lies over the tibia, fibula, sacrum, or sternum. Edema is described as *pitting* if a depression remains in the tissue after pressure is applied with a fingertip. Pitting edema is evaluated on a four-point scale, ranging from 1+ edema (barely detectable pit) to 4+ edema (deep and persistent pit that is approximately 1 inch or 2.54 cm deep).

Edema can be so severe that pitting is not possible. The tissue becomes so full that fluid cannot be displaced when pressed. Edematous tissue that feels hard is known as *brawny edema*. After a radical mastectomy,

Box 6.3 Focused Assessment of Body Weight

The use of body weight as an accurate index of fluid balance is based on the assumption that the patient's dry weight remains relatively stable. Even under starvation conditions, an individual loses no more than ⅓ to ½ lb dry weight per day.

A rapid loss of body weight occurs when the total fluid intake is less than the total fluid output.

A rapid gain of body weight occurs when total fluid intake is more than the total fluid output.

	MILD	MODERATE	SEVERE
Rapid loss	2%	5%	8% = deficit
Rapid gain	2%	5%	8% = excess

Rapid gain or loss of 1 kg (2.2 lb) of body weight is approximately equivalent to the gain or loss of 1 liter of fluid.

brawny edema commonly occurs because the removal of axillary nodes allows fluid to accumulate in the affected arm.

Mucous Membranes

Tongue turgor

In a normal person, the tongue has one longitudinal furrow. A person with deficient fluid volume has additional longitudinal furrows, and the tongue is smaller as a result of fluid loss. Sodium excess causes the tongue to appear red and swollen.

Moisture of the oral cavity

A dry mouth may be the result of deficient fluid volume or mouth breathing. Normally, saliva is pooled in the area where the cheek and the gum meet. Dryness in this area usually indicates a true fluid volume deficit. However, dry mouth is a common side effect of many medications.

Veins

The appearance of the jugular veins in the neck and the veins in the hands can suggest either a deficient or excess fluid volume.

Neck vein distention

Distention of the jugular veins can indicate excess fluid volume. Inspect the neck veins by having the patient recline with the head of the bed elevated at a 30- to 45-degree angle. If the jugular veins can be seen more than 3 cm above the sternal angle, then excess fluid volume is most likely present.

Deficient fluid volume may be detected by examining the jugular neck veins with the patient lying down. If no distention occurs, then deficient fluid volume is most likely present.

Hand veins

Observation of hand veins can also be helpful in evaluating the patient's fluid volume. Elevate the hands and then note how long it takes for the veins to empty. Veins usually empty in 3 to 5 seconds. Next, place the hands in a dependent position and note the time needed for the veins to fill. Veins usually fill in 3 to 5 seconds. If the volume is decreased, veins take longer than 3 to 5 seconds to fill. When the fluid volume is increased, veins take longer than 3 to 5 seconds to empty. The nursing assessment of fluid and electrolyte status is summarized in Box 6.4.

DIAGNOSTIC TESTS AND PROCEDURES

A variety of laboratory tests may be performed to assess fluid and electrolyte status and to determine whether they are within the normal range (Table 6.4). Various references report slightly different ranges of normal. Clinical laboratories typically report the normal range along with patient results, therefore you do not need to memorize these ranges.

Box 6.4 Focused Assessment of Fluid and Electrolyte Status

HEALTH HISTORY

Present Illness
Vomiting, diarrhea, burns, head injury

Past Health History
Renal or cardiac disease, diabetes, inflammatory bowel disease, adrenal or thyroid disease

Current Drugs
Diuretics, salicylates, antacids, potassium or calcium supplements

Family History
Diabetes, cardiac disease

Review of Systems
Fatigue, palpitations, dizziness, edema, dyspnea, confusion

Functional Assessment
Change in activity tolerance, mental alertness

PHYSICAL EXAMINATION

General Survey: Alertness, orientation, posture
Vital Signs: Pulse rate/rhythm/quality; respiratory rate/pattern; blood pressure in lying, sitting, and standing positions; temperature
Weight: Present compared with usual
Skin: Color, moisture, turgor, temperature
Facial Characteristics: Expression, firmness of eyeballs, edema of eyelids or cheeks
Edema: Presence, location, pitting, or brawny
Mucous Membranes: Tongue turgor, moisture of the oral cavity
Veins: Jugular vein distention, hand vein emptying and refilling time

Urine Studies

Urine pH

The kidneys can change the acidity or alkalinity of the urine by excreting hydrogen (H^+) ions. Urine pH is a measure of hydrogen ions in the urine. It is useful for determining whether the kidneys are responding appropriately to metabolic acid-base imbalances. The normal range is 4.5 to 8.0; however, fresh urine is usually acidic (~6.0). Urine tends to be most acidic in the morning (after a fast) and more alkaline after meals. Diet is a factor in that a person who consumes large amounts of citrus fruits and vegetables tends to have alkaline urine whereas a person who eats a lot of meat tends to have acidic urine. A urine specimen that is not tested within 4 hours of collection may become alkaline, therefore urine pH should be measured within 1 to 2 hours of collection. If the specimen cannot be tested promptly, it should be refrigerated.

Urine specific gravity

Urine specific gravity (SpG) is a measure of urine concentration. In most instances, normal urine SpG is between 1.016 and 1.022 in adults.

Table 6.4 **Normal Values Related to Fluid and Electrolyte and Acid-Base Balance**

URINE		BLOOD	
Urine pH	4.6–6.8	Arterial blood pH	7.35–7.45
Urine specific gravity	1.016–1.022	NA	
Urine osmolality (random specimen)	250–1200 mOsm/kg H_2O	Serum osmolality	285–300 mOsm/kg
Urine sodium	40–220 mEq/24 h or SI = 40–220 mmol/24 h	Serum sodium	136–145 mEq/L
Urine potassium	25–125 mEq/24 h	Serum potassium	3.5–5.1 mEq/L
Urine chloride	40–220 mEq/24 h or SI: 40–220 mmol/24 h	Serum chloride	98–107 mEq/L
Urine phosphorus	0.4–1.3 g/24 h	Serum phosphorus	2.8–4.5 mg/dL
Urine magnesium	6.0–10.0 mEq/L or SI: 3–5 mmol/day	Serum magnesium	Age 21–59 years: 1.6–2.6 mg/dL Age 60–90 years: 1.6–2.4 mg/dL
Urine creatinine	Male: 1–2 g/day Female: 0.8–1.8 g/day	Serum calcium (total)	Ages 18–60 years: 8.6–10.0 mg/dL Ages 60+ years: 8.8–10.2
		Serum creatinine	Female: 0.6–1.1 mg/dL Male: 0.7–1.3 mg/dL
		Serum bicarbonate	
		Arterial	21–28 mEq/L
		Venous	24–28 mm Hg or SI: 24–28 mmol/L

From Malarkey, LM, McMorrow, ME: *Saunders nursing guide to laboratory and diagnostic tests*, ed 2, St. Louis, 2012, Elsevier-Saunders.

SpG is a good indicator of fluid balance. A high SpG indicates that the urine is highly concentrated, usually as a result of deficient fluid volume. A low SpG indicates that the urine contains a large amount of water in relation to solutes, usually as a result of excess fluid volume. The SpG also reflects renal function. If the kidneys are not functioning properly, they may fail to concentrate or dilute urine as needed to maintain extracellular fluid balance. The presence of x-ray dyes, glucose, or protein in the urine can cause an increased SpG that may be misleading; that is, the patient may not really have a deficient fluid volume. As people age, their kidneys are less efficient at conserving water by concentrating urine. Therefore the older person may produce relatively dilute urine (low or normal SpG) even when they are dehydrated.

Urine osmolality

Osmolality measures the number of dissolved particles in a solution. This information provides a more precise measurement of the kidney's ability to concentrate urine than does the SpG. For the most accurate interpretation, a serum osmolality should be done simultaneously with the SpG.

Dilute urine has a low osmolality and generally reflects renal excretion of excess water. Low osmolality is also apparent when kidneys are unable to conserve water by concentrating urine. Concentrated urine has a high osmolality and generally indicates renal conservation of water. It can also be present when the kidneys are failing because the volume of urine secreted declines.

Urine creatinine clearance

Urine creatinine clearance tests are used to detect glomerular damage in the kidney. A 24-hour specimen is required. The patient is instructed to void, discard the specimen, record the time, and start collecting all urine thereafter for 24 hours. The specimen must be refrigerated.

During the specimen collection period, the patient should maintain good hydration, should not engage in vigorous exercise, and should avoid high-protein foods, coffee, tea, and cola drinks. Be aware that many drugs, including cephalosporin antibiotics, can alter test results. For best interpretation, serum creatinine clearance should be assessed as well. Also the laboratory needs to know the patient's height, weight, and age. The normal creatinine clearance for men is 85 to 125 mL/min/1.73 m^2 of body surface area; for women, it is 75 to 115 mL/min/1.73 m^2 of body surface area. The range decreases with age.

Urine sodium

Urine sodium reflects sodium intake and fluid volume status. When the intake of sodium is high, the kidneys will increase the excretion of sodium in the urine. When large amounts of fluids are taken in or sodium intake is restricted, the urine is more dilute, thus the urine sodium falls. The urinary excretion of sodium is normally highest during the day. The normal urine sodium is 75 to 200 mEq/L. If collected over a period of 24 h, the normal range is 40 to 220 mEq/24 hours or SI = 40 to 220 mmol/24 h.

Urine potassium

Urine potassium is a measure of renal tubular function. A 24-hour specimen is most meaningful because the urinary excretion of potassium is highest at night and lowest during the day. Therefore a random sample would not truly represent function of the renal tubules. The normal value is 25 to 125 mEq/24 hours.

Blood Studies

Serum hematocrit

The hematocrit is the percentage of blood volume that is composed of red blood cells. An increased hematocrit is seen with deficient fluid volume and dehydration because the blood is more concentrated. A low hematocrit is consistent with excess fluid volume because of dilution. The normal range for hematocrit is 40% to 54% for men and 38% to 47% for women.

Serum creatinine

Creatinine is a metabolic waste product. The serum creatinine level is a better indicator of renal function than the blood urea nitrogen. A high level of creatinine in the blood indicates poor renal function. The normal range is 0.6 to 1.1 mg/dL for females and 0.7 to 1.3 mg/dL for males. Even small changes in the serum creatinine can be significant.

Blood urea nitrogen

Blood urea nitrogen (BUN) provides a measure of renal function. Normal is 5 to 20 mg/dL for adults under 60 years of age and 8 to 23 mg/dL for adults over 60 years of age. A high BUN is associated with deficient fluid volume and possibly impaired renal function; conversely, a low BUN is associated with excess fluid volume.

Serum osmolality

Serum osmolality is a measure of blood concentration. High serum osmolality is related to a deficient fluid volume, and low serum osmolality is related to excess fluid volume. The normal range is 285 to 300 mOsm/kg.

Serum albumin

Albumin is a plasma protein that helps to maintain blood volume by creating colloid osmotic pressure. The normal range for serum albumin is 3.5 to 5.5 g/dL. Low serum albumin allows water to shift into the interstitial compartment, which reduces blood volume and creates edema.

Serum electrolytes

Normal values for serum sodium, potassium, chloride, and calcium are shown in Table 6.4.

FLUID IMBALANCES

FLUID VOLUME DEFICIT

Fluid volume deficit occurs when water is less than normal in the body. The two types of fluid volume deficits are isotonic extracellular fluid deficit (hypovolemia) and hypertonic extracellular fluid deficit (dehydration). A fluid volume deficit may result from decreased intake, abnormal fluid losses, or both. Examples of abnormal fluid losses are the loss of water as a result of excessive bleeding, severe vomiting and diarrhea, and severe burns.

The signs and symptoms of fluid volume deficit vary depending on how suddenly the deficit develops and how severe it is. Symptoms are not as apparent with deficits that are mild and have a gradual onset but are quite dramatic when the loss is severe and the onset is abrupt. In general, the body attempts to compensate for fluid volume deficits by decreasing urine output. The heart rate increases to maintain blood flow to body tissues. The blood pressure may fall because of the reduced blood volume.

Treatment varies somewhat according to the cause of a fluid volume deficit and the severity of symptoms. Nursing care should be based on specific patient problems, which might include the following:

- Fluid volume deficit/loss, potential for fluid volume deficit related to inadequate fluid intake, excessive fluid loss, high blood glucose, inadequate ADH production or effect, high fever, altered capillary permeability
- Acute confusion related to decreased cerebral tissue perfusion
- Constipation related to excessive reabsorption of water from stool in the colon
- Decreased activity tolerance related to decreased blood volume, decreased tissue perfusion
- Hyperthermia related to infectious process, decreased fluid volume
- Potential for injury related to decreased level of consciousness
- Potential for disrupted tissue integrity related to poor tissue turgor
- Inadequate circulation related to decreased cardiac output secondary to decreased blood volume

The characteristics, causes, assessment findings, treatment, and nursing care for each type of fluid volume deficit are outlined in Table 6.5.

FLUID VOLUME EXCESS

An increase in body water is called ***fluid volume excess***. The two types of fluid volume excess are extracellular fluid excess (isotonic fluid excess) and intracellular water excess (hypotonic fluid excess). Fluid volume excess may result from renal or cardiac failure with retention of fluid, increased production of ADH or aldosterone, overload with isotonic intravenous fluids, or the administration of 5% dextrose in water (D_5W) after surgery or trauma. The body attempts to compensate for fluid volume excess by increasing the filtration and excretion of sodium and water by the kidneys and decreasing the production of ADH.

As with fluid volume deficit, the severity of the symptoms in fluid volume excess depends on how quickly the condition develops. Severe fluid volume excess can cause or aggravate heart failure and pulmonary edema.

Nursing care varies somewhat according to the cause of a fluid volume excess and the severity of symptoms. Care should be based on appropriate patient problem statements, which might include the following:

- Fluid volume excess related to fluid retention, excess or hypotonic intravenous fluid administration
- Acute confusion related to cerebral edema
- Activity intolerance, inadequate oxygenation related to pulmonary edema

Table 6.5 Fluid Volume Deficit

	ISOTONIC EXTRACELLULAR FLUID DEFICIT (HYPOVOLEMIA)	HYPERTONIC EXTRACELLULAR FLUID DEFICIT (DEHYDRATION)
Definition	Deficiency of both water and relative electrolytes	Deficiency of water without electrolyte deficiency
Etiology	Decreased fluid intake related to inability to obtain or ingest fluids Excessive fluid loss related to vomiting, diarrhea Shifting of fluid into interstitial space (third spacing) related to increased capillary permeability	Increased water loss related to high blood glucose as in uncontrolled diabetes mellitus, inadequate ADH production or renal response to ADH, high fever, excessive sweating Decreased fluid intake with continued intake of electrolytes, as with concentrated tube feedings
Focused Assessment Findings		
Blood pressure	Hypotension	Hypotension
Pulse	Weak, rapid	Weak, rapid
Respirations	Rapid	Rapid
Temperature	Decreased	Increased
Weight	Loss	Loss
Tissue turgor	Normal or edema	Poor
Mucous membranes	Moist	Dry
Blood cells	Hgb, Hct, RBCs increased	Hgb, Hct, RBCs increased
Urine output	Decreased	Decreased or increased
Thirst	Normal	Thirsty
Treatment	Correction of underlying cause. Water and electrolyte replacement. Antiemetics, antidiarrheals. Oral and intravenous fluids.	Correction of underlying cause. Water replacement. Oral and intravenous fluids. Hypoglycemic agents, ADH, antipyretics.
Nursing care	Protect edematous tissue with third spacing. Assist with rising and ambulating if patient is dizzy. Keep hourly records of intake and output; expect intake to exceed output at first. Be alert for fluid excess (rising pulse and blood pressure, dyspnea) caused by excessive fluid replacement.	Monitor blood glucose if patient has diabetes. Assist with oral hygiene. Assist with rising and ambulating if patient is dizzy. Keep hourly records of intake and output; expect intake to exceed output at first. Be alert for fluid excess (rising pulse and blood pressure, dyspnea) caused by excessive fluid replacement.

ADH, Antidiuretic hormone; *Hct*, hematocrit; *Hgb*, hemoglobin; *RBCs*, red blood cells.

- Potential for injury related to decreased level of consciousness
- Potential for disrupted skin tissue integrity related to edema
- Inadequate circulation related to reduced cardiac output with heart failure

The causes, assessment findings, treatment, and nursing care of the patient with fluid volume excess are outlined in Table 6.6.

ELECTROLYTE IMBALANCES

The two electrolytes that cause the majority of problems when an imbalance exists are sodium and potassium.

HYPONATREMIA (SODIUM DEFICIT)

Hyponatremia is lower-than-normal sodium in the blood serum. It can be an actual deficiency of sodium or an increase in body water that dilutes the sodium excessively. Causes include excessive intake of water without sodium; excessive loss of sodium, as with vomiting, diarrhea, or diaphoresis with only water replacement; the use of distilled water to irrigate body cavities; and excessive secretion of ADH. Increased ADH secretion is associated with severe stress, some head injuries, and a condition called *syndrome of inappropriate antidiuretic hormone secretion* (SIADH). Other disorders that put the patient at risk for hyponatremia include congestive heart failure, liver cirrhosis, and nephrotic syndrome.

Sodium normally holds water in the extracellular compartment. When serum sodium is low, water can enter cells more freely. This shift of fluids is most significant in relation to brain cells. The accumulation of fluid in brain cells produces the most important physiologic effects of hyponatremia.

Focused Assessment

If hyponatremia is suspected or the patient is at risk, monitor for signs and symptoms, which include headache, muscle weakness, fatigue, apathy, confusion, abdominal cramps, and orthostatic hypotension. Take blood pressure readings with the patient lying or sitting and then standing to determine whether a drop

Table 6.6 Fluid Volume Excess

	EXTRACELLULAR FLUID EXCESS	INTRACELLULAR WATER EXCESS
	Isotonic Fluid Excess	*Hypotonic Fluid Excess*
Definition	Excess of both water and electrolytes. Major symptoms are caused by increased blood volume.	Excess of body water without excess electrolytes. Major symptoms are caused by cerebral edema.
Etiology	Retention of water and electrolytes related to kidney disease; overload with isotonic IV fluids.	Overhydration in presence of renal failure; administration of D_5W after surgery or trauma.
Focused Assessment Findings		
Blood pressure	Increased	Increased systolic
Pulse	Bounding, increased rate	Decreased rate
Respirations	Increased rate, crackles, dyspnea	Increased rate
Weight	Gain	Gain
Edema	Extremities: dependent, pitting Puffy eyelids	Cerebral
Neck veins	Distended	Normal
Mucous membranes	Moist	Moist
Blood	Hgb, Hct, RBCs decreased by dilution	Hgb, Hct, RBCs normal or decreased
Mental status	Irritability, confusion, lethargy	Irritability, confusion, lethargy
Hand vein engorgement	Present	Absent
Pupils	Sluggish response to light with cerebral edema	Sluggish response to light with cerebral edema
Treatment	Correction of underlying cause. Restriction of water and sodium intake. Diuretics to promote fluid elimination, digitalis to improve cardiac output. Renal dialysis if kidney failure is a factor.	Correction of underlying cause. Restricted water intake. IV and oral fluids with electrolytes. Demeclocycline (Declomycin) to decrease kidney response to ADH.
Nursing care	Give drugs and IV fluids as ordered. Monitor for excess diuresis. Explain and enforce fluid restriction. Offer ice chips; use small fluid containers, let patient help design plan for fluid intake. If patient is not confused, allow to swish fluids in mouth and spit out without swallowing. Explain salt restriction; obtain dietary consult for teaching (see Box 6.5). Protect edematous tissue: turn and reposition q2h. Inspect for signs of skin breakdown. If dyspneic: Elevate head of bed 30 degrees or for comfort, loosen restrictive clothing, oxygen as ordered.	Give drugs and IV fluids as ordered. Explain and enforce fluid restriction. Offer ice chips, provide oral hygiene, serve only fluids allowed with meal trays, let patient design plan for fluid intake. If patient is not confused, allow to swish fluids in mouth and spit out without swallowing. If confused, take safety precautions: side rails up, bed in low position, call light in reach, check often. Seizure precautions per agency policy.

ADH, Antidiuretic hormone; *D_5W*, dextrose 5% in water; *Hct*, hematocrit; *Hgb*, hemoglobin; *IV*, intravenous; *q2h*, every 2 hours; *RBCs*, red blood cells.

in pressure is significant. A drop in systolic blood pressure of more than 20 mm Hg indicates orthostatic hypotension.

Medical Treatment

The usual treatment for hyponatremia is restriction of fluids while the kidneys excrete excess water. Intravenous normal saline or Ringer's lactate may be ordered. If sodium falls below 115 mEq/L, hypertonic sodium may be ordered. The diuretic furosemide (Lasix) may be ordered because of its ability to promote water loss that exceeds the sodium loss. A balanced diet usually provides adequate sodium, but patients with moderate or severe hyponatremia may need sodium replacement therapy.

If the patient has SIADH, which can be chronic or acute, an effort is made to determine and correct the cause. In addition to fluid management and diuretic therapy, drugs such as tolvaptan (Samsca) and conivaptan (Vaprisol), which block the action of ADH, or demeclocycline may be ordered.

◆ NURSING CARE OF THE PATIENT WITH HYPONATREMIA

You can help to prevent hyponatremia in patients with feeding tubes by using normal saline rather than water for irrigation. For patients with hyponatremia, administer prescribed medications and intravenous fluids and monitor the response to these. Measure fluid intake and output, assess mental status, and monitor laboratory test results. If the patient is confused, take safety measures to prevent injury. If the patient who has hyponatremia has low blood pressure or postural hypotension, assist with ambulation.

Box 6.5 Guidelines for Sodium Restriction

Salt substitutes containing potassium chloride should be recommended only if approved by the physician. Potassium is generally contraindicated for patients with renal disease. Salt-free, herb-based seasoning products are readily available in most grocery stores and should be suggested instead.

- Instruct patients/clients on reading the Nutrition Facts food label for sodium content of foods.
- Encourage patients to prepare food at home without adding salt and to limit eating in restaurants.
- Recommend baked products, using sodium-free baking powder, potassium bicarbonate (instead of sodium bicarbonate or baking soda), and salt-free shortening in place of those containing sodium.
- Avoid obviously salted foods such as bouillon, soup and gravy bases, canned soups and stews; bread and rolls with salt toppings, salted crackers; salted nuts or popcorn, potato chips, pretzels, and other salted snack foods. Avoid buying vegetables prepared in sauce.
- Avoid smoked or cured meats, such as bacon, bologna, cold cuts, other processed meats, chipped or corned beef, frankfurters, ham, koshered or kosher-style meats, and canned meat poultry.
- Avoid salted and smoked fish such as cod, herring, and sardines.
- Avoid sauerkraut, olives, pickles, relishes, kimchi, and other vegetables prepared in brine, tomato, and vegetable cocktail juices.
- Avoid seasonings such as celery salt, garlic salt, Worcestershire sauce, fish sauce and soy sauce. Reduced sodium versions of items like soy sauce can still be very high in sodium.
- Serve cheeses in limited amounts. Swiss cheese and cream cheese are relatively low in sodium.
- Monitor the sodium content of various medications, including over-the-counter brands.

The front of the food package can be used to identify foods that may contain less sodium, but it is important to understand terminology such as salt/sodium-free (<5 mg per serving), very low sodium (<36 mg per serving), low sodium (<141 mg per serving), reduced sodium (25% less sodium than original product), light in sodium or lightly salted (at least 50% or less sodium added than in the regular product), and no-salt added or unsalted (not necessarily sodium-free).

Seasoning without salt: Flavorings or seasonings will make food more appetizing. For example:

- Fish, meat, vegetables: lemon, vinegar
- Meat: onion, garlic, green pepper, nutmeg, ginger, dry mustard, sage, cumin, marjoram, and curry without salt
- Meat and poultry: cranberry sauce, applesauce, jelly
- Vegetables: onion, mint, ginger, mace, dill seed, parsley, green peppers, fresh mushrooms
- Unsalted cottage cheese: minced onion, chopped chives, raw green pepper, grated carrots, chopped parsley, crushed pineapple

From Mahan LK, Raymond JL: *Krause's food and the nutrition care process*, 14th ed, St. Louis, 2017, Elsevier, 1037–1038.

HYPERNATREMIA (SODIUM EXCESS)

Hypernatremia refers to a higher-than-normal concentration of sodium in the blood. It is a very serious imbalance that can lead to death if not corrected. Hypernatremia can occur alone or in combination with extracellular fluid volume deficit. The high level of sodium in the serum and other extracellular fluids causes water to shift out of the cells, which creates cellular dehydration. Hypernatremia occurs when loss of water or retention of sodium is excessive. Some causes of hypernatremia are vomiting, diarrhea, diaphoresis (profuse sweating), and insufficient ADH. Signs and symptoms of hypernatremia are thirst, a flushed skin, dry mucous membranes, a low urine output, restlessness, an increased heart rate, convulsions, and postural hypotension.

Medical Treatment

Medical intervention focuses on oral or intravenous replacement of water to restore balance. The aim is to restore the fluid balance slowly to prevent cerebral edema resulting from excessive dilution of extracellular fluid. If the patient has an extracellular fluid volume deficit as well, intravenous fluids with decreasing amounts of sodium may be ordered. A low-sodium diet is often prescribed.

◆ NURSING CARE OF THE PATIENT WITH HYPERNATREMIA

Encourage patients with hypernatremia to drink water for hydration. Closely monitor the infusion of intravenous fluids, especially when the patient's cardiac or renal function is abnormal. Patient education is important. Teach the patient with hypernatremia to track daily intake and output and to recognize the signs and symptoms of fluid retention or depletion. Advise patients of any dietary restrictions. If a low-sodium diet is prescribed, patients should avoid foods that are high in sodium: ketchup, monosodium glutamate (Accent), mustard, pickles, olives, ham, most canned foods, artificial sweeteners, laxatives, cough medications, and some antacids. Box 6.5 provides guidelines for patients who need to restrict their sodium intake.

HYPOKALEMIA (POTASSIUM DEFICIT)

Hypokalemia is low serum potassium. Causes include vomiting, diarrhea, nasogastric suction, inadequate dietary intake of potassium, diabetic acidosis, excessive aldosterone secretion, and drugs such as potassium-wasting diuretics and corticosteroids. Because potassium is necessary for normal cellular function, deficiencies may result in gastrointestinal, renal, cardiovascular, and neurologic disturbances. Most important is the effect on myocardial cells, which tends to cause abnormal, and potentially fatal heart rhythms.

Signs and symptoms of hypokalemia are anorexia, abdominal distention, vomiting, diarrhea, muscle cramps, weakness, dysrhythmias (abnormal cardiac rhythms), postural hypotension, dyspnea, shallow respirations, confusion, depression, polyuria (excessive urination), and nocturia.

Medical Treatment

The physician will attempt to identify and correct the underlying problem. Potassium replacement by the intravenous or oral route may be prescribed.

◆ NURSING CARE OF THE PATIENT WITH HYPOKALEMIA

When a patient has hypokalemia, monitor for decreased bowel sounds, a weak and irregular pulse, decreased reflexes, and decreased muscle tone. Monitoring the heart rate and rhythm of patients taking digitalis is especially important because hypokalemia increases the risk of digitalis toxicity. Cardiac monitors may be used to detect dysrhythmias.

Administer prescribed oral potassium supplements with a full glass of water or fruit juice to prevent gastrointestinal irritation. Instruct patients to sip slowly. Encourage dietary sources of potassium, particularly fruits and vegetables, such as bananas and oranges or orange juice. A chart of foods high and low in potassium is found in Box 6.6.

Administer intravenous potassium as ordered. Potassium is always diluted and never given in concentrated form. A concentration of 40 mEq/L or less is recommended. Ideally, potassium is administered through a central venous catheter; otherwise, the potassium may not be adequately diluted by blood before it reaches the heart. The infusion rate generally should not exceed 10 mEq/h in adults. Closely monitor the rate of intravenous infusion because of the risk of cardiac arrest with rapid infusion. Also inspect the infusion site because potassium salts can cause inflammation of the veins. *Note that potassium is never given by intravenous push.*

Check the patient's urine output before starting an intravenous infusion of potassium. When the urine output is low, intravenous fluids without potassium may be given until the urine output is acceptable and then fluids with potassium are started. If you were to administer the intravenous potassium before normal urinary output was restored, the patient could develop hyperkalemia. Urinary output should be no less than 30 mL/h. If it is less than 30 mL/h for 2 consecutive hours, alert the physician, who may order a stop of the infusion.

Pharmacology Capsule

Potassium is always diluted before intravenous administration. It is never administered by intravenous push. Rapid infusion of potassium can cause cardiac arrest.

Box 6.6 Potassium Content in Common Foods

LOW (0–100 mg/SERVING*)

Fruits
Applesauce
Blueberries
Cranberries
Lemon, ½ medium
Lime, ½ medium
Pears, canned
Pear nectar
Peach nectar

Vegetables
Cabbage, raw
Cucumber slices
Green beans, frozen
Leeks
Lettuce, iceberg, 1 cup
Water chestnuts, canned
Bamboo shoots, canned

VERY HIGH (>300 mg/SERVING*)

Fruits
Avocados, ¼ small
Banana, 1 small
Cantaloupe, ¼ small
Dried fruit, ¼ cup
Honeydew melon, ⅛ small
Mango, 1 medium
Papaya, ½ medium
Prune juice

Vegetables
Artichoke, 1 medium
Bamboo shoots, fresh
Beet greens, ¼ cup
Corn on the cob, 1 ear
Chinese cabbage, cooked
Dried beans
Potatoes, baked, ½ medium
Potatoes, French fries, 1 oz
Spinach
Sweet potatoes, yams
Swiss chard, ¼ cup
Tomato, fresh, sauce or juice; tomato paste, 2 tbsp
Winter squash

Miscellaneous
Bouillon, low sodium, 1 cup
Cappuccino, 1 cup
Chili, 4 oz
Coconut, 1 cup
Lasagna, 8 oz
Milk, chocolate milk, 1 cup
Milkshakes, 1 cup
Molasses, 1 tbsp
Pizza, 2 slices
Salt substitutes, ¼ tsp
Soy milk, 1 cup
Spaghetti, 1 cup
Yogurt, 6 oz

*One serving equals ½ cup unless otherwise specified.
Modified from Mahan LK, Escott-Stump SE, Raymond JL: *Krause's food and the nutrition care process,* 14th ed, 2017, St. Louis, Saunders, 94.

HYPERKALEMIA (POTASSIUM EXCESS)

Hyperkalemia is high serum potassium. Potassium is plentiful in common foods, so taking in adequate amounts is easy for people on normal diets. However, the kidneys do not readily conserve potassium, so continuous replacement is necessary. Patients at risk for hyperkalemia are those with decreased renal function, people in metabolic acidosis, and people taking potassium supplements. Also, patients who have had severe traumatic injuries may develop hyperkalemia because of the loss of potassium from damaged cells into the extracellular fluid.

Hyperkalemia is a serious imbalance because of the potential for life-threatening dysrhythmias. Elevated potassium typically causes first bradycardia, then tachycardia. A risk of cardiac arrest is also present. In the gastrointestinal system, hyperkalemia can cause explosive diarrhea and vomiting. Neuromuscular effects are muscle cramps and weakness and paresthesia (a tingling sensation). Other signs and symptoms of hyperkalemia include irritability, anxiety, abdominal cramps, and decreased urine output.

Medical Treatment

Hyperkalemia is treated by correcting the underlying causes and restricting potassium intake. Intravenous calcium gluconate or calcium chloride may be given if the patient is having cardiac arrhythmias caused by the effects of potassium on the myocardium. A variety of other drugs that may be used include intravenous insulin and glucose and inhaled beta-adrenergic agonists. Sodium polystyrene sulfonate (e.g., Kayexalate), a drug that can be given orally or rectally, promotes excretion of excess potassium through the intestinal tract. Two newer drugs that may be ordered for hyperkalemia are patiromer (Veltassa) and zirconium cyclosilicate.

◆ NURSING CARE OF THE PATIENT WITH HYPERKALEMIA

Patients with low urine output or those taking potassium-sparing diuretics must be monitored carefully for signs and symptoms of hyperkalemia, because decreased renal function can cause hyperkalemia. To prevent hyperkalemia in patients receiving potassium supplements, especially intravenously, special attention is warranted. Carefully monitor the flow rate of intravenous fluids, which should not exceed 10 mEq/h of potassium chloride through peripheral veins. Examine the infusion site because potassium is very irritating to subcutaneous tissues. Extravasation can cause serious tissue damage.

Screen the results of laboratory studies. Because serum potassium levels greater than 5.0 mEq/L can cause cardiac arrest, immediately report the results to the physician and anticipate an order for the patient to be placed on cardiac monitoring and a change in the potassium supplement order. Monitor patients who take potassium supplements for signs and symptoms of abnormal potassium levels. Explain to the patient the importance of frequent blood tests to monitor potassium levels.

CHLORIDE IMBALANCE

Because chloride is usually bound to other electrolytes, chloride imbalances accompany other electrolyte imbalances. High serum chloride, known as *hyperchloremia*, is usually associated with metabolic acidosis. Low serum chloride, known as *hypochloremia*, usually occurs when sodium is lost because chloride is most frequently bound with sodium. Hypochloremia may be caused by vomiting and uncontrolled diabetes.

CALCIUM IMBALANCE

Calcium in the blood is regulated by the parathyroid glands, which secrete parathyroid hormone (PTH). A low serum level of calcium (hypocalcemia) stimulates PTH secretion. PTH enhances calcium retention and phosphate excretion by the kidneys, promotes calcium absorption in the intestines, and mobilizes calcium from the bones to raise the serum calcium level.

Hypocalcemia results from diarrhea, inadequate dietary intake of calcium or vitamin D, multiple blood transfusions (banked blood contains citrates that bind to calcium), and some diseases, including hypoparathyroidism. The most prominent sign of hypocalcemia is neuromuscular irritability manifested by a tingling sensation in the face and hands, muscle twitches, and progressively severe muscle cramps that typically affect the hands, feet, and legs first. Assessment for hypocalcemia is discussed more fully in Chapters 47 and 49 (see Fig. 47.4).

Hypercalcemia is the abnormally increased level of calcium in the serum. Causes of hypercalcemia include a high calcium or vitamin D intake, hyperparathyroidism, and immobility that causes stores of calcium in the bones to enter the bloodstream; it is also a complication of certain types of cancer.

MAGNESIUM IMBALANCE

Hypomagnesemia is a lower-than-normal concentration of magnesium in the blood resulting from decreased gastrointestinal absorption or excessive gastrointestinal loss, usually from vomiting and diarrhea, or from increased urinary loss. Hypomagnesemia often is associated with hypocalcemia and hypokalemia.

A higher-than-normal concentration of magnesium in the bloodstream is known as *hypermagnesemia*. It occurs most often with the excessive use of magnesium-containing medications or intravenous solutions in patients with renal failure or preeclampsia of pregnancy.

ACID-BASE DISTURBANCES

Acid-base balance refers to homeostasis of the hydrogen ion concentration in the body fluids. A solution containing a higher number of hydrogen ions is an **acid**, and a solution containing a lower number of hydrogen ions is an alkaline or **base**. The symbol used to indicate hydrogen ion concentration is pH. pH is reported on a scale of 1 to 14, with 1 to 6.9 being acidic, 7 being neutral, and 7.1 to 14 being alkaline.

The hydrogen ion concentration in extracellular fluid is indicated by the pH of the blood. The normal pH of blood is between 7.35 and 7.45, which is slightly alkaline. The normal acid-base balance is maintained by three primary, complex mechanisms: (1) buffers, (2) respiratory control of carbon dioxide, and (3) renal regulation of HCO_3^-. The principal buffers in renal tubular fluid are the carbonic acid/bicarbonate system, ammonia, and phosphate. Other substances that function as buffers are proteins and hemoglobin. Buffer systems comprise a weak acid and a salt. To maintain body fluids in the normal pH range, the blood buffers circulate throughout the body in pairs, acting as sponges to soak up hydrogen ions. One of the buffers takes away a hydrogen ion if a fluid is too acid and one of the buffers gives an ion if the fluid is too alkaline.

The lungs and kidneys are the next line of defense after the blood buffers for maintaining acid-base balance. The lungs are primarily responsible for the regulation of carbon dioxide in the blood, which is controlled by the rate and depth of respirations. Carbonic acid in the alveolar capillaries breaks down into water and carbon dioxide, which is eliminated through exhalation. Deep, rapid breathing eliminates excess carbon dioxide, thereby reducing extracellular fluid acidity. Shallow, slow respirations reduce the loss of carbon dioxide, thereby increasing extracellular acidity. If the pH of the blood becomes too high or too low, the respiratory center in the brain sends signals to the lungs to increase or decrease respirations to either "blow off" or retain the appropriate amount of carbon dioxide.

The kidneys act as the metabolic regulators of pH by excreting acids or bases as needed. Renal regulation of bicarbonate and excretion of hydrogen ions are the chief means of regulating acid-base balance through the kidneys. Bicarbonate is a major acid buffer in the blood and is reabsorbed and produced through the kidneys.

If the regulatory mechanisms fail, acid-base imbalances occur. The four major types of acid-base imbalances are (1) respiratory acidosis, (2) respiratory alkalosis, (3) metabolic acidosis, and (4) metabolic alkalosis.

FOCUSED ASSESSMENT OF ACID-BASE STATUS

Health History

Note a history of renal, endocrine, or respiratory disease. A history of diabetes mellitus is especially important because acidosis is a complication of diabetes. Data that contributes to the complete nursing assessment focuses on symptoms of acid-base imbalance, which could include very deep or rapid respirations (or both), anxiety, confusion, dizziness, light-headedness, seizures, and change in weight. List any medications the patient is taking.

Box 6.7 Focused Assessment of Acid-Base Balance

HEALTH HISTORY

Signs and Symptoms: Dyspnea, anxiety, confusion, dizziness, seizures, changes in weight, muscle weakness, abnormal sensations (numbness, tingling)

Medical Conditions: Respiratory impairment, diabetes mellitus, adrenal disorders, cardiac disorders, renal failure

Current Medications

PHYSICAL EXAMINATION

Height and Weight: Current compared with previous measurements

Vital Signs: Pulse rate and rhythm; respiratory rate, depth, and rhythm

Neurologic Function: Muscle strength, sensation in extremities, mental status

Measures of Oxygenation: Arterial blood gases

Physical Examination

Observe the patient's general appearance in terms of responsiveness. Look for signs of anxiety or other distress. Take the vital signs and weigh the patient. Pay special attention to the rate, depth, and rhythm of respiration. Test muscle strength and sensory function in the extremities. Evaluate mental status.

In addition to collecting data for the nursing assessment, as described in Box 6.7, note the results of arterial blood gas measurements (Table 6.7).

RESPIRATORY ACIDOSIS

Respiratory acidosis occurs when the respiratory system fails to eliminate the appropriate amount of carbon dioxide to maintain the normal acid-base balance. Carbon dioxide is retained, with a resultant accumulation of carbonic acid and a decrease in blood pH. The body responds to respiratory acidosis by stimulating respirations to eliminate excess carbon dioxide. If that mechanism cannot restore balance, renal compensation begins. The kidneys attempt to help by reabsorbing more bicarbonate to balance the amount of carbonic acid in the blood.

Acute respiratory acidosis is caused by respiratory diseases such as pneumonia, drug overdose, head injury, chest wall injury, obesity, asphyxiation, drowning, or acute respiratory failure. People with chronic pulmonary disease may have elevated carbon dioxide levels but a normal pH as a result of renal compensation. Common clinical signs and symptoms include rapid heart rate, headache, sweating, lethargy, and confusion.

Table 6.7 Arterial Blood Gas Values With Uncompensated Respiratory and Metabolic Acidosis and Alkalosis

CONDITION	CAUSE	pH (7.35–7.45)	HCO_3^- (21–28 mEq/L OR SI 21–28 mmol/L)	$PaCO_2$ (35–45 mm Hg OR SI 4.7–5.3 kPa)
Respiratory acidosis	Hypoventilation	↓	Normal	↑
Respiratory alkalosis	Hyperventilation	↑	Normal	↓
Metabolic acidosis	Diabetic ketoacidosis Lactic acidosis Diarrhea Renal insufficiency	↓	↓	Normal
Metabolic alkalosis	Vomiting HCO_3^- retention Volume depletion K^+ depletion	↑	↑	Normal

HCO_3^-, Bicarbonate; *kPa*, kilopascals; *$PaCO_2$*, partial pressure of carbon dioxide in arterial blood.

Medical Treatment

Interventions for respiratory acidosis are geared toward improving ventilation, which in turn restores the partial pressure of carbon dioxide in arterial blood ($PaCO_2$) to normal. Underlying respiratory conditions are treated to eliminate the cause of respiratory acidosis. Antibiotics, bronchodilators, and specific breathing treatments such as noninvasive ventilation (NIV) with a nasal mask, face mask, or nasal plug may be prescribed. In some cases, intubation and mechanical ventilation are necessary (see Chapter 25). Sodium bicarbonate in 5% dextrose in water may be given cautiously in selected circumstances.

◆ NURSING CARE OF THE PATIENT WITH RESPIRATORY ACIDOSIS

Focused Assessment

The most accurate method of assessing for respiratory acidosis is the measurement of the $PaCO_2$ level. The $PaCO_2$ directly reflects the degree of respiratory dysfunction. In addition, observe the patient for signs and symptoms of respiratory distress, including restlessness, anxiety, confusion, and tachycardia. Monitor oxygen saturation. Frequently note the rate, depth, and rhythm of respirations. Respiratory rate and depth vary with the situation. For example, the patient with a head injury or drug overdose may have slow respirations that contribute to carbon dioxide retention. The patient with pneumonia may have rapid respirations to eliminate carbon dioxide that has accumulated as a result of impaired gas exchange. Monitor the level of consciousness, including orientation to person, place, and time, to detect changes in mental status.

Interventions

Encourage fluid intake as appropriate to loosen secretions and keep mucous membranes moist. Position patients with the head elevated 30 degrees to promote comfort and ensure optimal gas exchange. Monitor confused patients frequently and attempt to anticipate their needs. Because confused patients may fall as they try to get to the bathroom, they should be assisted to the bathroom every 2 hours, especially if fluids are increased. Constant reassurance and reorientation are helpful.

RESPIRATORY ALKALOSIS

Respiratory alkalosis is marked by low $PaCO_2$ with a resultant rise in pH. The most common cause of respiratory alkalosis is hyperventilation. Hyperventilation is characterized by rapid or deep respirations that cause excessive amounts of carbon dioxide to be eliminated through the lungs. When the body fluids become alkaline, ionized extracellular calcium decreases and the patient develops symptoms of hypocalcemia.

One cause of hyperventilation leading to respiratory alkalosis is anxiety. Other causes are conditions that result in decreased oxygen in the blood, such as pneumonia, adult respiratory distress syndrome, anemia, severe blood loss resulting from trauma, and congestive heart failure. Fever, pain, drugs (aspirin overdose), head trauma, and gram-negative septicemia also may contribute to respiratory alkalosis. The body attempts to compensate for respiratory alkalosis by eliminating excess bicarbonate through the kidneys. Clinical signs and symptoms include increased respiratory and heart rates, an anxious appearance, irritability, dizziness, lightheadedness, muscle weakness, and tingling or numbness of the fingers. In extreme respiratory alkalosis, confusion, fainting, and seizures may occur. Assessment of the rate and depth of respirations is the key observation for this condition.

Medical Treatment

The major goal of therapy is to treat the underlying cause of the condition. Sedation may be ordered for the anxious patient.

NURSING CARE OF THE PATIENT WITH RESPIRATORY ALKALOSIS

Focused Assessment

The general assessment of patients with acid-base imbalances was described earlier in this chapter. With respiratory alkalosis, a description of respiratory status is especially important.

Interventions

To relieve anxiety, give sedatives as ordered and reassure the patient. Encourage the patient to breathe slowly, which will retain carbon dioxide in the body. Breathing slowly into a paper bag raises the $PaCO_2$ because the patient rebreathes exhaled carbon dioxide. When breathing stabilizes, allow the patient to have uninterrupted rest, because hyperventilation can result in fatigue.

METABOLIC ACIDOSIS

Metabolic acidosis occurs when the body retains too many hydrogen ions or loses too many bicarbonate ions. With too much acid and too little base, the pH of the blood falls. Metabolic acidosis leads to hyperventilation because the lungs try to compensate by blowing off carbon dioxide and lowering $PaCO_2$ levels, which raises the pH.

Causes of metabolic acidosis are starvation, dehydration, diarrhea, shock, renal failure, and diabetic ketoacidosis. Signs and symptoms vary according to the underlying cause and the severity of the acid-base disturbance. However, patients may experience changing levels of consciousness, ranging from fatigue and confusion to stupor and coma, headache, vomiting and diarrhea, anorexia, muscle weakness, and cardiac dysrhythmias.

Medical Treatment

The primary intervention for metabolic acidosis is treatment of the underlying disorder. Mechanical ventilation may be necessary, especially in patients who are comatose. Once corrective measures have been initiated, oral or intravenous sodium bicarbonate might be ordered based on arterial blood gas results. An alternative to sodium bicarbonate is Tromethamine (THAM).

NURSING CARE OF THE PATIENT WITH METABOLIC ACIDOSIS

Focused Assessment

Assessment of the patient in metabolic acidosis should focus on vital signs, mental status, and neurologic status.

Interventions

Nursing care is geared toward emergency measures to restore acid-base balance. Administer drugs and intravenous fluids as prescribed. Reassure and orient confused patients. Patients receiving intravenous fluids must be closely monitored. Rapid infusions can cause metabolic alkalosis and/or hypernatremia.

METABOLIC ALKALOSIS

Metabolic alkalosis is the opposite of metabolic acidosis. It results from an increase in bicarbonate levels or a loss of hydrogen ions. Loss of hydrogen ions may be caused by prolonged nasogastric suctioning, excessive vomiting, diuretics, and electrolyte disturbances. Retention of bicarbonate may result from the administration of bicarbonate or massive blood transfusions.

Clinical signs and symptoms may include headache, irritability, lethargy, changes in level of consciousness, confusion, changes in heart rate, slow and shallow respirations with periods of apnea, nausea and vomiting, hyperactive reflexes, and numbness of the extremities.

Medical Treatment

As with other acid-base imbalances, treatment depends on the underlying cause and severity of the condition.

NURSING CARE OF THE PATIENT WITH METABOLIC ALKALOSIS

Focused Assessment

Take vital signs and daily weight measurements of the patient and monitor heart rate, respirations, and fluid gains and losses. Keep accurate intake and output records, including the amount of fluid removed by suction. Assess motor function and sensation in the extremities and monitor laboratory values, especially pH and serum bicarbonate levels.

Interventions

To prevent metabolic alkalosis, use isotonic saline solutions rather than water for irrigating nasogastric tubes, because the use of water for irrigation can result in a loss of electrolytes. Provide reassurance and comfort measures to promote safety and well-being.

Put On Your Thinking Cap!

Recall a patient who either had or was at risk for fluid and electrolyte imbalances.

1. Explain why the patient was at risk.
2. List the assessment data that were or should have been collected.
3. Identify measures to treat or prevent the imbalances.

Get Ready for the NCLEX® Examination!

Key Points

- Approximately 50% to 60% of the human body is composed of water. To maintain homeostasis, the body must be able to regulate the fluids within it.
- The process of homeostasis involves delivery of nutrients and oxygen to the cells and removal of wastes, including carbon dioxide, from the cells.
- Body fluids are classified based on location in body compartments: (1) intracellular fluid (fluid within the cell), and (2) extracellular fluid (fluid outside the cell). Most of the body's fluids are found within the cell.
- Extracellular fluid is mainly responsible for the transport of nutrients and wastes throughout the body.
- Electrolytes, which are substances that develop an electrical charge when dissolved in water, maintain a balance between positive and negative charges to keep the body in homeostasis.
- Total body water decreases in older adults, with the greatest decline in intracellular fluid.
- The fluid compartments of the body are separated by selectively permeable membranes that control movement of water and certain solutes.
- Water and solutes move between intracellular and extracellular fluid compartments by one or more of the following processes: (1) diffusion, (2) active transport, (3) filtration, and (4) osmosis.
- The kidneys are the primary regulators of fluid balance in the body, and the nephrons conduct the work of the kidneys through the processes of filtration, reabsorption, and secretion.
- Hormones that have a major effect on fluid balance include renin, aldosterone, ADH, and ANF.
- Renin is secreted when blood volume or blood pressure falls. It stimulates release of aldosterone and helps to produce angiotensin I, which is converted to angiotensin II, a potent vasoconstrictor.
- Aldosterone is secreted by the adrenal glands and promotes sodium retention. ADH, produced by the hypothalamus and secreted by the posterior pituitary gland, promotes water retention.
- ANF is secreted when stretch receptors in atria detect an increase in blood volume. It promotes excretion of water and sodium, decreases renin synthesis, inhibits release of aldosterone and ADH, and causes vasodilation.
- The thirst center creates a desire to drink fluids when extracellular fluid becomes concentrated.
- In a healthy adult, the 24-hour fluid intake and output are approximately equal.
- The body attempts to compensate for fluid volume deficit by increasing the heart rate and conserving water in the kidneys.
- The body attempts to compensate for fluid volume excess by increasing urine output.
- The kidneys are the primary regulators of electrolytes in the blood.
- Two electrolytes that cause the majority of problems when there is an imbalance are sodium and potassium.
- Change in body weight is a good indicator of fluid loss or retention.
- Edema reflects sodium retention, which can result from excessive reabsorption or inadequate secretion because of failing kidney function.
- Potassium excess or deficit can lead to life-threatening cardiac dysrhythmias.
- Because older adults often have a reduced thirst sensation and may not conserve water efficiently, they are at risk for fluid volume deficit.
- Acid-base balance is the homeostasis of the hydrogen ion concentration in the body fluids.
- Mechanisms that maintain acid-base balance are blood buffers, respiratory control of carbon dioxide, and renal regulation of bicarbonate.
- Acid-base imbalances occur when an imbalance in the functioning of the lungs, kidneys, or both exists. The four major acid-base imbalances are (1) respiratory acidosis, (2) respiratory alkalosis, (3) metabolic acidosis, and (4) metabolic alkalosis.

Additional Learning Resources

SG Go to your Study Guide for additional learning activities to help you master this chapter content.

Go to your Evolve website (http://evolve.elsevier.com/Linton/medsurg) for the following learning resources and much more:
- Fluid and Electrolyte Tutorial
- Review Questions for the NCLEX® Examination

Clinical Judgment and Next-Generation NCLEX® Examination-Style Questions

1. **What is fluid surrounding the cells called?**
   1. Interstitial fluid
   2. Extracellular fluid
   3. Intracellular fluid
   4. Circumcellular fluid

   NCLEX Client Need: Physiological Integrity: Basic Care and Comfort

2. **The largest portion of a person's body weight is contributed by:**
   1. Water
   2. Fat
   3. Bone
   4. Muscle

   NCLEX Client Need: Physiological Integrity: Basic Care and Comfort

3. **The movement of water across a membrane from a less concentrated solution to a more concentrated solution defines:**
   1. Diffusion
   2. Osmosis
   3. Filtration
   4. Active transport

   NCLEX Client Need: Physiological Integrity: Basic Care and Comfort

4. **A hormone with physiologic effects that decrease blood pressure is:**
   1. ADH
   2. Renin
   3. Aldosterone
   4. ANF

   NCLEX Client Need: Physiological Integrity: Basic Care and Comfort

5. **A 79-year-old nursing home patient develops severe diarrhea. To plan appropriate care, which of these statements should the nursing staff understand best describes the risk of fluid and electrolyte imbalances in the older adult?**
   1. Most older adults can maintain fluid and electrolyte balance just as well as younger adults.
   2. Older adults have limited reserves to maintain fluid balance when abnormal losses occur.
   3. Body water increases with age, putting the older adult at risk for excess fluid volume.
   4. The amount of extracellular fluid declines, leaving the patient with reduced fluid stores.

   NCLEX Client Need: Physiological Integrity: Physiological Adaptation

6. **A patient is receiving diuretics to eliminate excess fluid that has been retained in body tissues. In 2 days, the patient lost 4.4 lb (2 kg) in body weight. This represents how many liters of fluid loss? ________.**

   NCLEX Client Need: Physiological Integrity: Pharmacological Therapies

7. **You gently pinch the skin over a patient's sternum. The skin does not flatten right away, leading you to suspect:**
   1. Recent weight loss
   2. History of excessive sun exposure
   3. Dehydration
   4. Need for increased diuretics

   NCLEX Client Need: Physiological Integrity: Reduction of Risk Potential

8. **When reviewing a patient's laboratory results, the nurse notes that the patient has a potassium imbalance. Which of the following nursing assessments is most important for this patient?**
   1. Auscultate bowel sounds
   2. Evaluate muscle strength
   3. Monitor heart rate and rhythm
   4. Assess reflexes

   NCLEX Client Need: Physiological Integrity: Reduction of Risk Potential

9. **Arrange the mechanisms that maintain acid-base balance in the correct order of occurrence.**
   1. Renal regulation
   2. Buffers
   3. Respiratory regulation

   NCLEX Client Need: Physiological Integrity: Physiological Adaptation

10. **What is the physiologic function of deep, rapid respirations in metabolic acidosis?**
    1. Eliminates excess carbon dioxide that is formed in the presence of acidosis.
    2. Raises the arterial oxygen level, which reduces the pH of the blood.
    3. Supplies additional oxygen needed because of the increased metabolic rate.
    4. Reduces the $PaCO_2$, resulting in a rise in blood pH and correction of acidosis.

    NCLEX Client Need: Physiological Integrity: Physiological Adaptation

11. **A patient who is being treated for severe vomiting and diarrhea has blood drawn to assess their fluid and electrolyte status. If the patient's serum potassium is low, the nurse should anticipate which signs and symptoms? (1) _______, (1)________, and (1) __________.**

    If intravenous potassium replacement is ordered, nursing responsibilities should include (2) ________, (2) ________, and (2) ________,

OPTION 1	OPTION 2
Irregular heart rate	Assess infusion site for extravasation
Abdominal distention	Monitor the heart rate and rhythm
Muscle cramps	Administer intravenous fluid as rapidly as possible
Numbness in extremities	Monitor infusion rate
Muscle weakness	Stop the infusion if urine output falls

The Patient With Cancer

7

http://evolve.elsevier.com/Linton/medsurg

Objectives

1. List the most common sites of cancer in men and women.
2. Explain the differences between benign and malignant tumors.
3. Define terms used to name and classify cancer.
4. Describe measures to reduce the risk of cancer.
5. List nursing responsibilities in the care of patients having diagnostic tests to detect cancer.
6. Explain the nursing care of patients undergoing each type of cancer therapy: surgery, radiation, chemotherapy, and biotherapy.
7. Assist in developing a nursing care plan for the terminally ill patient with cancer and the patient's family.

Key Terms

adjuvant (ĂJ-ă-vănt)
alopecia (ă-lō-PĒ-shă)
alternative therapy
antineoplastic (ăn-tī-nē-ō-PLĂS-tĭk)
benign (bĕ-NĪN)
biotherapy
carcinogens (kăr-SĬN-ō-jĕn)
chemotherapy (kē-mō-THĔR-ă-pē)
complementary therapy
extravasation (ĕks-tră-vă-SĀ-shŭn)
gray
malignant (mă-LĬG-nănt)
metastasis (mĕ-TĂS-tă-sĭs)
neoadjuvant (nē-ō-ĂJ-ă-vănt)
neoplasms (NĒ-ō-plăsm)
neutropenia (nū-trō-PĒ-nē-ă)
radiotherapy
xerostomia (zē-rō-STŌ-mē-ă)

WHY STUDY CANCER?

Specific cancers are discussed with every body system in this text. Why, then, is a separate chapter devoted to the subject? The American Cancer Society defines cancer as a large group of diseases characterized by uncontrolled growth and spread of abnormal cells. More than 100 diseases are classified as cancer. They share some common characteristics, progress in similar ways, and respond to similar types of treatments. To reduce repetition throughout the text, this chapter addresses the common features of diseases known as cancer.

Health statistics often group all types of cancer together. Not surprisingly, cancer is listed as the second most common cause of death in the United States. Almost everyone has been touched by cancer. It is estimated that 1 in 3 Americans will develop cancer during their lifetime. The most common sites of cancer in men and in women are shown in Fig. 7.1. Because so many die of cancer, many people assume that a diagnosis of cancer is a death sentence. In reality, almost 17 million Americans with a history of cancer are alive today.

Some cancers can be prevented by avoiding or limiting exposure to chemicals and lifestyle behaviors associated with the development of cancer (see the Nutrition Considerations box). Early diagnosis has been found to make a significant difference in survival with many types of cancer, and advances in treatment have prolonged the lives of many cancer patients.

Nutrition Considerations

1. *Diet and lifestyle* choices associated with an increased risk of cancer include:
   - Diets high in salt-cured, smoked, and nitrate-cured foods are associated with esophageal and stomach cancers.
   - Obesity is associated with cancers of the colon, breast, prostate, gallbladder, ovary, and uterus.
   - Cancers of the breast, colon, and prostate may be associated with high-fat diets.
   - High alcohol intake is associated with cancers of the oral cavity, larynx, pharynx, esophagus, liver, colon, rectum and breast.
2. To *reduce the risk* of cancer, the American Cancer Society recommends the following:
   - Consume adequate fruits and vegetables (five or more servings each day).
   - Consume adequate grains, rice, pasta, and beans (several servings each day).
   - Limit consumption of fats.
   - Engage in moderate physical activity of at least 30 minutes or more on most days and maintain a healthy weight.
   - Limit alcohol consumption (or do not drink any alcohol).

Leading Sites of New Cancer Cases and Deaths—2017 Estimates

Estimated New Cases

Male			Female		
Prostate	161,360	19%	Breast	252,710	30%
Lung & bronchus	116,990	14%	Lung & bronchus	105,510	12%
Colon & rectum	71,420	9%	Colon & rectum	64,010	8%
Urinary bladder	60,490	7%	Uterine corpus	61,380	7%
Melanoma of the skin	52,170	6%	Thyroid	42,470	5%
Kidney & renal pelvis	40,610	5%	Melanoma of the skin	34,940	4%
Non-Hodgkin lymphoma	40,080	5%	Non-Hodgkin lymphoma	32,160	4%
Leukemia	36,290	4%	Leukemia	25,840	3%
Oral cavity & pharynx	35,720	4%	Pancreas	25,700	3%
Liver & intrahepatic bile duct	29,200	3%	Kidney & renal pelvis	23,380	3%
All sites	**836,150**	**100%**	**All sites**	**852,630**	**100%**

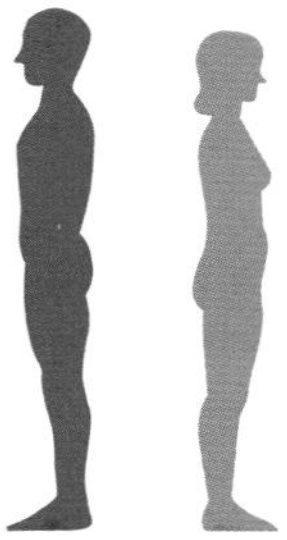

Estimated Deaths

Male			Female		
Lung & bronchus	84,590	27%	Lung & bronchus	71,280	25%
Colon & rectum	27,150	9%	Breast	40,610	14%
Prostate	26,730	8%	Colon & rectum	23,110	8%
Pancreas	22,300	7%	Pancreas	20,790	7%
Liver & intrahepatic bile duct	19,610	6%	Ovary	14,080	5%
Leukemia	14,300	4%	Uterine corpus	10,920	4%
Esophagus	12,720	4%	Leukemia	10,200	4%
Urinary bladder	12,240	4%	Liver & intrahepatic bile duct	9,310	3%
Non-Hodgkin lymphoma	11,450	4%	Non-Hodgkin lymphoma	8,690	3%
Brain & other nervous system	9,620	3%	Brain & other nervous system	7,080	3%
All sites	**318,420**	**100%**	**All sites**	**282,500**	**100%**

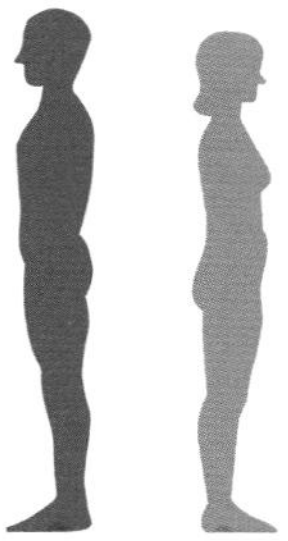

Estimates are rounded to the nearest 10, and cases exclude basal cell and squamous cell skin cancers and in situ carcinoma except urinary bladder.

Fig. 7.1 American Cancer Society estimates, 2021: Leading site of new cancer cases and deaths. *Cancer facts and figures.* (Copyright 2021, American Cancer Society, Inc., Surveillance Research.)

Nurses use their teaching and assessment skills in the prevention and detection of cancer. They also care for patients undergoing diagnostic procedures and treatments for cancer. In almost any specialty, nurses work with patients who are being treated for or have survived cancer.

WHAT IS CANCER?

NORMAL BODY CELLS

A normal cell has the following characteristics:

- A distinct, recognizable appearance typical of all cells from a particular tissue ("tissue of origin"); has a single small nucleus
- The ability to perform a specific function when mature
- The production of substances that hold cells from the same type of tissue closely together
- The ability to recognize other cells and identify the other cells' tissue of origin
- The ability to reproduce in a controlled manner to produce additional identical cells only as needed for growth and replacement
- The ability to inhibit cell replication if there is inadequate space or insufficient nutrients to support growth
- The ability to remain in their tissue of origin (except for blood cells, which migrate)

Cells that reproduce abnormally and in an uncontrolled manner form **neoplasms** or tumors. Such cells may be benign or malignant.

BENIGN TUMORS

Benign tumors are relatively harmless, primarily because they do not spread to other parts of the body. However, benign tumors present problems if they create pressure on or obstruct body organs. Because of this, surgical removal of benign tumors may be indicated.

MALIGNANT TUMORS

The presence of **malignant** cells is the basis for a diagnosis of cancer. Characteristics of cancer cells include the following:

- Change in appearance from normal cells of tissue of origin (said to be *undifferentiated* if tissue of origin cannot be determined); large nucleus or multiple nuclei
- Inability to properly perform the function of the tissue of origin; may assume functions of other cells
- Cells not readily recognized by other cells
- May have abnormal proteins (called *tumor markers*) on cell surface
- Random, disorganized, uncontrolled growth pattern

Table 7.1 A Comparison of Benign and Malignant Tumors

CHARACTERISTIC	BENIGN	MALIGNANT
Growth rate	Usually slow and encapsulated	Usually rapid but may be slow
Growth mode	Enlarges and expands	Invades surrounding tissue
Cell structure and differentiation	Cells closely resemble those of tissue of origin	Tissue of origin may not be readily identifiable
Recurrence after removal	Unlikely	Common
Metastasis	No	Yes
Tissue destruction	Usually none unless compression or obstruction occurs	Can cause necrosis, ulceration, perforation, tissue sloughing; effects can be fatal

Table 7.2 Steps in Transformation of Normal Cells to Malignant Cells

STEP	PROCESS	EFFECTS ON CELLS AND TISSUE
Initiation	Deoxyribonucleic acid (DNA) exposed to a carcinogen	Cell appears somewhat abnormal
	Irreversible changes occur in DNA	Continues to function normally
Promotion	Sufficient exposure to an agent (a promoter) to encourage or enhance cell growth	Latent period before increased growth forms tumors (early detection period)
Progression	Accelerated growth rate Enhanced invasiveness Altered appearance and biochemical activity	Tumor development Cells mutate so that they are not all identical and have differing sensitivities to treatment
Metastasis	Tumor develops internal blood vessels Tumor cells produce enzymes that dissolve substances that hold normal cells together Tumor penetrates capillaries, other body structures, and cavities Tumor cells transported throughout the body; most destroyed by body's defenses Tumor cells trapped in capillary bed and form a fibrin meshwork that prevents detection by immune system Enzymes dissolve lining of blood vessels; cells invade surrounding tissue Cells attempt to establish blood supply to support development of metastatic colony	Transformed cells relocate by direct extension, invasion, establishment of remote sites

- May continue dividing even when no need exists for additional cells, inadequate space exists for new cells, or nutrients are inadequate to support growth of new cells
- Ability to migrate from one tissue or organ to another

As they grow, malignant tumors cause some of the same problems as benign tumors. They press on normal tissues and compete with normal cells for nutrients. Malignant growths are more threatening, however, because they can invade nearby tissues or "seed" malignant cells to colonize distant parts of the body. *Regional invasion* is the term used to describe the movement of cancer cells into adjoining tissue. The process by which cancer spreads to distant sites is called ***metastasis***. Tumor cells found away from the original site of malignant cells are called *metastases*. The most common sites of metastases are liver, brain, bone, and lungs. Once metastasis has occurred, cancer treatment is more limited and less likely to be curative.

A comparison of the features of benign and malignant cells is presented in Table 7.1.

MALIGNANT TRANSFORMATION

Environmental factors associated with the transformation of normal cells to malignant cells include chemical exposure, radiation exposure, increasing age, diet, hormones, and chronic inflammation. Malignant transformation occurs when normal cells are exposed to substances (called ***carcinogens***) that damage cell deoxyribonucleic acid (DNA), from genetic changes inherited from parents, or from accumulated mutations in the DNA that cells are unable to repair. The transformation occurs in four steps as outlined in Table 7.2.

CLASSIFICATION OF TUMORS

Tumors are classified by anatomic site, stage, and cell appearance and differentiation. The term *differentiation* refers to how cells are different from their parent cells ("tissue of origin"). When it is difficult to recognize the original type of tissue from which tumor cells came, they are described as *poorly differentiated cells.* When cells are well differentiated, the tissue of origin is recognizable.

Anatomic Site

The suffix *-oma* means "tumor." Technically, a tumor is a swelling. However, the word is most commonly used to refer to a malignant or benign neoplasm. Tumors are named according to the type of tissue from which they developed originally. Examples may be found in Table 7.3.

Additional prefixes are sometimes used to designate the exact type of malignant tissue. For example, a sarcoma could be an osteosarcoma or a chondrosarcoma. An osteosarcoma is a tumor of the bone whereas a chondrosarcoma is a cartilage tumor. Many other combinations of terms are used to describe tumors precisely by origin and location.

Staging System for Cancer

Because cancers tend to grow and spread in predictable ways, their progress can be described in stages. Specific stages exist for most types of cancer. Staging is evaluated at the time of diagnosis and at intervals during and after treatment. Such staging is helpful in planning treatments and in predicting long-term survival.

One method of describing the extent of cancer is shown in Table 7.4. A second, more specific system is the TNM staging system (Table 7.5), which specifies the status of the primary tumor, regional lymph nodes, and distant metastases. In the TNM system, *T* refers to the tumor, *N* to regional lymph nodes, and *M* to distant metastases. To illustrate, a patient whose primary tumor has grown and spread to regional lymph nodes but not to distant sites would be staged *T2, N1, M0.* Based on the combinations of scores for each component, a stage is determined.

Put On Your Thinking Cap!

You are assigned to care for a patient who has cancer. The cancer has been staged T4, N3, M1. How would you interpret this information?

RISK FACTORS

A single, specific cause of cancer has not been identified. Genetic and environmental factors appear to increase the risk for development of cancer. Changes in genetic information of a normal cell can cause

Table 7.3 Tumor Names by Anatomic Site

TYPE OF TUMOR BY ANATOMIC SITE	TISSUE OF ORIGIN
Benign Tumor	
Fibroma	Fibrous connective tissue
Lipoma	Fat tissue
Leiomyomas	Smooth muscle tissue
Malignant Tumor	
Carcinoma	Skin; glands; linings of digestive, urinary, and respiratory tracts
Sarcoma	Bone, muscle, other connective tissue
Melanoma	Pigment cells in the skin
Leukemia and lymphoma	Blood-forming tissues: lymphoid tissue, plasma cells, and bone marrow

Table 7.4 Staging Classification for Cancer

STAGE	DESCRIPTION
Stage I	The malignant cells are confined to the tissue of origin. No invasion of other tissues takes place.
Stage II	Limited spread of the cancer occurs in the local area, usually to nearby lymph nodes.
Stage III	The tumor is larger or has spread from the site of origin to nearby tissues (or both). Regional lymph nodes are likely to be involved.
Stage IV	The cancer has metastasized to distant parts of the body. The term *advanced* is also used to describe Stage IV.

Table 7.5 TNM Staging System for Cancer

T (PRIMARY TUMOR)	N (REGIONAL LYMPH NODES)	M (DISTANT METASTASIS)
TX—primary tumor cannot be assessed	NX—lymph nodes cannot be assessed	
T0—no sign of tumor after treatment	N0—no regional lymph nodes involved	M0—no distant metastasis
Tis—malignancy in epithelial tissue but not basement membrane	N1—minimal regional lymph node involvement	M1—distant metastasis present*
T1[a]—minimal size and extension	N2—increased involvement of regional lymph nodes	
T2[a] T3—progressively increasing size and extension	N3—extensive involvement of regional lymph nodes	
T4—large size and extension		

[a]Complete document has sub-categories.

Box 7.1 Common Carcinogens

VIRUSES AND CHEMICALS
Tar
Soot
Asphalt
Aniline dyes
Hydrocarbons
Crude paraffin oils
Nickel
Arsenic
Benzene
Cadmium

PHYSICAL AGENTS
Radiation
Asbestos
Tobacco smoke
Hormonal Agents
Synthetic estrogens
Androgenic anabolic steroids

IMMUNOSUPPRESSANT AGENTS
Antimetabolites
Corticosteroids
Alkylating agents
Antilymphocyte serum

CYTOTOXIC DRUGS
Phenylalanine mustard
Cyclophosphamide

alterations that lead to malignancies. Cancer-causing agents, called *carcinogens*, include a variety of chemicals, radiation, and viruses. Box 7.1 shows a partial list of carcinogens. Carcinogens such as cigarette smoke, asbestos, and nitrites are commonly found in the environment. Drugs that may act as carcinogens include diethylstilbestrol, androgenic steroids, and high-dose unopposed synthetic estrogens.

Other factors thought to be associated with cancer development are increasing age, heredity, and hormones. Cancers that appear at a higher rate than expected in one family are called *familial cancers*. In these situations, no single genes have been identified to explain the frequency. Hereditary cancers, on the other hand, have clearly predictable patterns of inheritance based on identified gene mutations. For people with family histories of familial or hereditary cancers, genetic counseling can direct the person to appropriate screening and lifestyle changes and serve as a basis for making decisions about reproductive options.

Pharmacology Capsule

Some drugs are carcinogenic, meaning they can cause cancer. Examples are diethylstilbestrol, androgenic steroids, high-dose unopposed synthetic estrogens, and some antineoplastic drugs used to treat cancer.

SEVEN WARNING SIGNS

The signs and symptoms of cancer vary with the location and severity of the disease. The American Cancer Society has identified seven warning signs that are associated with many common types of cancer. They can serve to guide the nurse and the public in identifying signs and symptoms that require medical evaluation. The first letters of the warning signs spell out *CAUTION*, making it easier to remember them (see Health Promotion box: Warning Signs of Cancer).

Health Promotion

Warning Signs of Cancer

Change in bowel or bladder habits
A sore that does not heal
Unusual bleeding or discharge
Thickening or lump in a breast or elsewhere
Indigestion or difficulty swallowing
Obvious change in a wart or a mole
Nagging cough or hoarseness

PREVENTION AND EARLY DETECTION

There are a number of ways to reduce the risk of developing cancer or to detect it in the early stages. These include (1) general measures to promote health, (2) avoidance of known carcinogens, (3) identification of high-risk individuals, and (4) cancer screening.

Health Promotion

Many behaviors associated with good health may reduce the risk of some cancers. The recommended diet is low in fat, calories, and preservatives and high in fiber, with at least five servings of various fruits and vegetables daily. Alcoholic beverages and foods that are salt cured, smoked, or nitrite preserved should be consumed in limited quantities. Appropriate calorie intake to maintain or attain normal body weight is also important because obesity is a risk factor for some cancers. A balanced program of activity and rest with stress management may enable the body to resist diseases, including cancer (see Health Promotion box: Healthy Choices).

Avoidance of Carcinogens

Some specific carcinogens were mentioned earlier. They include cigarette smoke, alcohol, intercourse with multiple partners, a variety of chemicals and drugs, and lifestyle behaviors such as excessive sun or ultraviolet radiation exposure. Public education has focused attention on carcinogens, and people are becoming more aware of their contribution in cancer prevention.

For example, smoking tobacco has long been considered a risk factor for developing certain cancers. Over the past 50 years, antismoking programs have had a significant effect on tobacco use. The fact that 1 million people quit smoking each year demonstrates that public education is making a difference. On a broader scale, legal restrictions on public smoking are reducing the exposure of nonsmokers to so-called secondhand smoke. Since 2006, smokers in the United States have had the option to choose e-cigarettes that create a vapor that is inhaled. The long-term health effects are unknown at this time. Also, some people use them as a first step toward smoking cessation; however, the effectiveness in smoking cessation has not been determined.

Health Promotion

Healthy Choices

You can reduce your risk of getting cancer by making healthy choices such as:

- **Avoiding tobacco:** Lung cancer is the leading cause of cancer death, and cigarette smoking causes almost all cases. Compared with nonsmokers, current smokers are about 25 times more likely to die from lung cancer. Smoking causes about 80%–90% of lung cancer deaths. Smoking also causes cancer of the mouth and throat, esophagus, stomach, colon, rectum, liver, pancreas, larynx (voice box), trachea, bronchus, kidney and renal pelvis, urinary bladder, and cervix. Adults who are exposed to secondhand smoke at home or at work increase their risk of developing lung cancer by 20%–30%. Concentrations of many cancer-causing and toxic chemicals are higher in secondhand smoke than in the smoke inhaled by smokers. Visit https://smokefree.gov/ to learn how you can quit smoking.
- **Protecting your skin:** Skin cancer is the most common kind of cancer in the United States. Exposure to ultraviolet (UV) rays from the sun and tanning beds appears to be the most important environmental factor involved with developing skin cancer. To help prevent skin cancer while still having fun outdoors, protect yourself by seeking shade, applying sunscreen, and wearing sun-protective clothing, a hat, and sunglasses.
- **Limiting the amount of alcohol you drink:** Drinking alcohol raises the risk of some cancers. Drinking any kind of alcohol can contribute to cancers of the mouth and throat, larynx (voice box), esophagus, colon and rectum, liver, and breast (in women). The less alcohol you drink, the lower the risk of cancer. Studies around the world have shown that drinking alcohol regularly increases the risk of getting mouth, voice box, and throat cancers. A large number of studies provide strong evidence that drinking alcohol is a risk factor for primary liver cancer, and more than 100 studies have found an increased risk of breast cancer with increasing alcohol intake. The link between alcohol consumption and colorectal cancer has been reported in more than 50 studies.
- **Keeping a healthy weight:** Research has shown that being overweight or having obesity raises a person's risk of getting some cancers, including endometrial (uterine), breast in postmenopausal women, and colorectal cancers. Overweight is defined as a body mass index (BMI) of 25–29, and obesity is defined as a BMI of 30 or higher.
- **Getting tested for hepatitis C:** Hepatitis is inflammation of the liver, which is most often caused by a virus. In the United States, the most common type of viral hepatitis is hepatitis C. Over time, chronic hepatitis C can lead to serious liver problems including liver damage, cirrhosis, liver failure, or liver cancer. The CDC recommends that anyone who was born between 1945 and 1965 get tested for hepatitis C.

From Centers for Disease Control and Prevention. (August 9, 2018; last reviewed July 29, 2020). http://www.cdc.gov/cancer/ and http://www.cdc.gov/.

A harmful effect associated with use of smokeless tobacco (e.g., chewing tobacco, snuff) is the increased risk of oral cancers. Alcohol consumption also increases the risk of cancers of the mouth, head and neck, liver, breast, colon, and rectum. Many industrial products are recognized as carcinogens as well. Their use is regulated by the Occupational Safety and Health Administration and published in guidelines for the safety of workers and consumers. Unprotected sun exposure is a risk factor for skin cancers, including the deadliest type—melanoma. Increased awareness of the dangers of excessive sun exposure has boosted the use of sunscreens.

Identification of High-Risk Individuals

Identifying individuals or populations at risk for development of specific cancers serves several purposes. It helps researchers and health care providers to recognize factors that may contribute to the development of various cancers. In addition, individuals who are known to fall into high-risk categories can be monitored closely to detect cancer early (see the Cultural Considerations box). Examples of people at risk for specific cancers are those with familial rectal polyposis, those with family histories of breast cancer, and those with Down syndrome, who are at increased risk for leukemia.

Cultural Considerations

What Does Culture Have to Do With Cancer?

Of all racial and ethnic groups, Black American men have the highest rates of cancer deaths. Although White women have the highest rates of breast cancer, Black American women are more likely to die from breast cancer. Nurses should encourage individuals of all ethnicities who are at higher risk than the general population to participate in screenings and to seek early treatment for warning signs of cancer.

Put On Your Thinking Cap!

1. What are possible reasons that minorities in the United States have higher rates of several types of cancer and are more likely to die from cancer?
2. How can you use your knowledge of culture to intervene?

Screening for Cancer

When cancer does occur, early diagnosis and treatment may improve the chances of a cure. Public education should emphasize the following:

- The value of early detection and treatment
- The seven warning signs of cancer
- How to do self-examinations (skin, testicular)

Table 7.6 Recommended Cancer Screening Tests

TYPE OF CANCER	RECOMMENDED SCREENING
Screening means checking your body for cancer before you have symptoms. Getting screening tests regularly may find breast, cervical, and colorectal (colon) cancers early, when treatment is likely to work best. Lung cancer screening is recommended for some people who are at high risk.	
Recommended Screening Tests: CDC supports screening for breast, cervical, colorectal (colon) cancer as recommended by the U.S. Preventive Services Task Force. Because screening recommendations are updated at intervals, see cancer.org or ht tp://www.uspreventiveservicestaskforce.org/) for the latest information.	
Breast	Mammograms are the best way to find breast cancer early when it is easier to treat.
Cervical	The Pap test can find abnormal cells in the cervix, which may turn into cancer. The HPV test looks for the virus (human papillomavirus) that can cause these cell changes. Pap tests also can find cervical cancer early, when the chance of being cured is very high.
Colorectal (Colon)	Colorectal cancer almost always develops from precancerous polyps (abnormal growths) in the colon or rectum. Screening tests can find precancerous polyps, so they can be removed before they turn into cancer. Screening tests also can find colorectal cancer early when treatment works best.
Lung	The U.S. Preventive Services Task Force recommends yearly lung cancer screening with low-dose computed tomography (LDCT) for people who have a history of heavy smoking (≥30 pack year history), and smoke now or have quit within the past 15 years and are between 55 and 74 years old.
Screening for the cancers listed below has not been shown to reduce deaths from those cancers.	
• Ovarian • Pancreatic • Prostate • Testicular • Thyroid	

From Centers for Disease Control and Prevention. Screening tests. (May 2, 2018; last updated July 29, 2020). Retrieved October 3, 2020 from https://www.cdc.gov/cancer/dcpc/prevention/screening.htm.

- The importance of periodic examinations by a health care professional for common cancers

The current recommended screening activities can be accessed at www.cancer.org. See Table 7.6 for a list of recommended cancer screening tests.

DIAGNOSIS OF CANCER

The health history and physical examination often provide the first clues to the presence of cancer. Diagnostic procedures may be used when cancer is suspected, when high-risk individuals are screened, or to determine the extent of known disease. Diagnostic procedures rely on tissue examinations, imaging studies, endoscopic procedures, and laboratory tests. Combinations of procedures may be indicated for cancers that are difficult to locate or to determine whether more than one site exists. It is important to note that many laboratory tests are nonspecific for cancer. Abnormal laboratory results can have many causes but, combined with other data, they assist in the diagnostic process. In addition, the same diagnostic tests and procedures may be used during and after cancer treatment to assess treatment effectiveness. Table 7.7 presents examples of tests and procedures that might be used in the diagnostic process.

MEDICAL TREATMENT OF CANCER

Methods of treating cancer include surgery, radiotherapy, chemotherapy, biotherapy, transplantation of hematopoietic (blood-forming) stem cells, and hormone therapy. Various complementary therapies may be used as well. One treatment or a combination may be recommended, depending on the type and location of the cancer.

SURGERY

Surgery is performed in the majority of patients to diagnose and stage the cancer, relieve symptoms, maintain function, effect a cure, or reconstruct affected structures. Although not common, surgery is sometimes done prophylactically for individuals who are at very high risk for developing specific cancers. For example, those with familial polyposis may have a portion of the colon removed to prevent colon cancer. Surgery is commonly used in the treatment of cancer, often in combination with other therapies. Surgery for cancer may be extensive or simple. A thorough preoperative diagnostic evaluation enables the surgeon to plan the most appropriate procedure.

Surgery is most likely to be curative when tumors are detected early, are slow growing, are confined to

Table 7.7 Diagnostic Tests and Procedures: Cancer

TEST OR PROCEDURE	EXAMPLES OF USES
Tissue Examination	
Specimens of body fluids, secretions, or tissues are obtained and examined microscopically to detect the presence of malignant cells.	Papanicolaou (Pap) test detects cancer cells in cervical smear.
Fluids and secretions can be obtained by swabs or smears, by venipuncture, or by withdrawal of fluids from body structures.	Blood cells are examined to diagnose leukemias and lymphomas.
Tissue samples are obtained by biopsy. Specimen may be entire growth, sample cut from the growth, or cells drawn from the growth with a needle.	Samples can be taken from any accessible growth. Tissue is examined for cancer cells.
Imaging Studies	
Plain radiographs Images produced result from the different absorption rates of different tissues. Calcium in bones absorbs x-rays the most; therefore bones look white on the radiograph. Fat and other soft tissues absorb less and look gray. Air absorbs the least and therefore lungs look black.	Chest radiographs detect changes in lung tissue and bones. Can reveal organ size, position, abnormal structures and shapes. Mammography detects potentially malignant breast calcifications before they can be felt.
Contrast radiographs Contrast media given orally or intravenously to outline hollow organs. Shadows of abnormal structures can be visualized.	Used primarily to detect cancers of the digestive and urinary tracts.
Computed tomography (CT) Provides cross-sectional, three-dimensional views of body tissue (Fig. 7.2). Details are much clearer than radiographs. Can be done with or without contrast media.	Used to detect cancers of the head and trunk, spine, joints, and soft tissue. Also useful in staging bronchogenic and gastrointestinal (GI) tumors.
Positron emission tomography (PET) PET is a nuclear scan that reveals patterns of tissue metabolism.	Used to detect solid tumors in the brain and breast and to assess the effects of cancer treatment.
Magnetic resonance imaging (MRI) Radiofrequency waves are used in the presence of a strong magnetic field. Energy changes are measured and converted to computer images. Does not expose patient to radiation.	Used to detect cancers of the central nervous system, spinal column, neck, bones, joints, lungs, kidneys, and others.
Radionuclide Scans Radionuclides are radioactive substances that are taken up by specific body tissues. The patient is given a radionuclide, usually intravenously, and is then scanned to study the pattern of uptake of the radionuclide in target tissues. The radionuclide accumulates in target tissue, with greater uptake in abnormal tissue.	Used to detect tissue abnormalities. For example, technetium tagged with phosphorus is used for bone scans because technetium is absorbed in increased amounts in bone tissue where abnormal activity or increased metabolism is evident. Other radionuclides are used to detect cancers of the thyroid, liver, lung, and breast as well as lymphoma and melanoma.
Endoscopic Procedures Lighted tubes are inserted into hollow organs or body cavities to visualize and take specimens of suspicious tissue for examination.	Examples of endoscopic procedures and the areas they examine include: • Bronchoscopy (bronchi) • Colonoscopy (colon) • Cystoscopy (urinary bladder) • Laparoscopy (abdominal cavity)
Laboratory Tests	
Oncofetal Antigens Oncofetal antigens are substances found on fetal cells and the surface of cancer cells. They are called *tumor markers* because elevations are associated with certain cancers. Can be elevated by nonmalignant conditions also, yielding a false-positive result for cancer. Often used to monitor response to cancer treatments. If treatment is successfully destroying the cancer, the antigen level goes down.	The following are examples of oncofetal antigens and the types of cancers with which they are associated: • Carcinoembryonic antigen (CEA): digestive tract, breast; also elevated in heavy smokers • Alpha-fetoprotein (AFP): liver, testicle

Table 7.7 Diagnostic Tests and Procedures: Cancer—cont'd

TEST OR PROCEDURE	EXAMPLES OF USES
NOTE: Elevated oncofetal antigens can have causes other than cancer. For example, oncofetal antigens may be elevated with cirrhosis of the liver and ulcerative colitis.	• CA-125: ovary, breast, cervix, colon, endometrium, fallopian tube, GI tract, liver, lung, lymphoma, non-Hodgkin lymphoma, pancreas • Prostate-specific antigen (PSA): prostate • CA-19-9: pancreas, liver, lung, colon, rectum • Pancreatic oncofetal antigen: pancreas and lung • CA 15-3: breast, liver, lung, prostate • Bladder tumor antigen (BTA): urinary bladder • Human chorionic gonadotropin (HCG): testicle
Other Studies	
Other laboratory studies of body fluids do not specifically diagnose cancer but may suggest possible malignancies.	The following are examples of other useful laboratory tests: • Serum alkaline phosphatase: elevated with metastatic bone cancer, hyperparathyroidism • Serum acid phosphatase: elevated with metastatic bone cancer, hairy cell leukemia, prostate cancer • Serum and urine calcium: elevated with bladder, breast, kidney, lung, endocrine cancer, leukemia, lymphoma • Thyroid antithyroglobulin antibody: elevated with thyroid cancer NOTE: Elevations can be caused by numerous other, nonmalignant conditions.

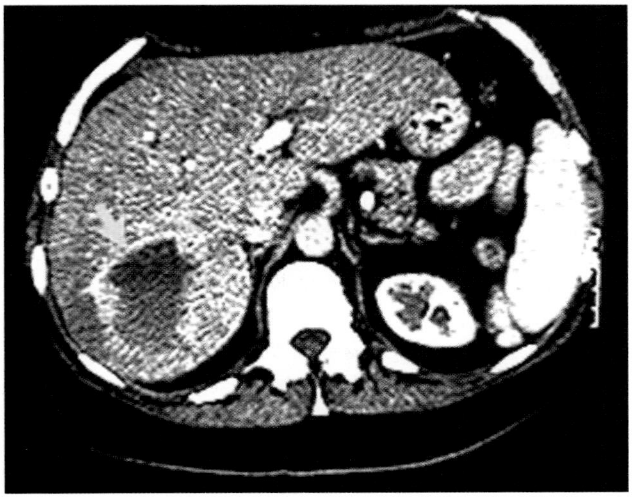

Fig. 7.2 Computed tomography (CT) provides cross-sectional, three-dimensional views of body tissue. This upper abdominal CT scan shows a blood vessel tumor (hemangioma) (*arrow*) in the liver. (Courtesy National Institutes of Health.)

one area, and do not invade vital body structures. Surrounding tissues, including lymph nodes, are often removed to explore whether or not malignant cells have escaped the tumor mass, indicating that the individual is at higher risk for metastatic disease. When surgery is extensive, it is often referred to as a *radical procedure.*

The preoperative and postoperative care of the surgical cancer patient varies with the specific surgery. General care of the surgical patient is detailed in Chapter 17. Specific surgeries are discussed in individual chapters. After surgery, other therapies may be recommended. The recommended treatment is based on the type of cancer, its unique characteristics, its location, the staging, and the extent of metastasis. The surgeon often consults with a radiologist and medical oncologist (a physician who specializes in treating patients who have cancer) to determine the best therapy.

Adjuvant and **neoadjuvant** therapies are relatively recent approaches to cancer treatment. Adjuvant therapy may be used when a patient has had surgery or radiotherapy and is free of signs of disease but has a high likelihood of recurrence. Such patients may be given chemotherapy to eradicate any remaining undetected cells. Adjuvant therapy is often used in the treatment of breast cancer. In neoadjuvant therapy, chemotherapy is administered to reduce the size of the tumor before surgery or radiotherapy.

RADIOTHERAPY

Radiotherapy is the use of ionizing radiation in the treatment of disease. The unit of measure for radiation doses is the **gray (Gy)**. Radiation is used to treat cancer because malignant cells are more sensitive than normal cells to radiation. Radiation has immediate and delayed effects on cells. The immediate effect is cell death because of damage to the cell membrane. The delayed effect is alteration of DNA, which impairs the cell's ability to reproduce. Types of cancer cells vary in their sensitivity to radiation. A tumor is considered radiosensitive if the cancer cells can be killed by radiation at a dose that is tolerated by surrounding normal tissue.

Radiotherapy may be given internally or externally. Internal radiation requires the introduction of the radioactive substance into the body. External radiation is given by way of a beam directed at the tumor.

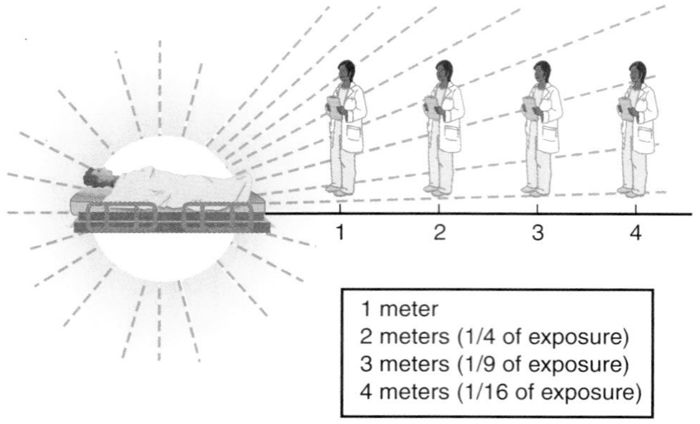

Fig. 7.3 Radiation exposure decreases as distance from the source increases. (From Black JM, Hawks JH: Medical-surgical nursing: clinical management for positive outcomes, ed 8, St. Louis, 2009, Saunders.)

Caregiver Safety

To work with radiation safely, the medical professional must understand it. The amount of radiation received by those who come in contact with the patient depends on the type of radiation and time of exposure, the distance from the radiation source, and the amount of shielding between the caregiver and the source. For example, the less time spent near the patient with a radiation implant, the less exposure incurred. Doubling the distance from the source decreases the exposure to one fourth. When the distance from the source is tripled, the exposure is reduced to one-ninth (Fig. 7.3). Unless direct care is being given, nurses and caregivers should remain at least 6 feet from the source. There should be time limits for visitors when a radiation implant is in place. As a precaution, most hospitals do not allow pregnant women or children younger than 18 years of age to visit patients who have a radiation implant. Visitors need to check with the staff before they enter the room. For their protection, visitors may be instructed to stay at least 6 feet from the patient and visit for less than 30 minutes each day while the patient is undergoing treatment. Effective shielding depends on the type of rays being emitted. In general, the denser the material composing the shield, the better protection it provides. Therefore lead is more protective than concrete or wood. Because shielding is awkward and cannot provide complete protection during patient care, many agencies rely more on time and distance along with shielding to limit exposure.

External Radiation

Procedure. With external radiation therapy, the source of the radioactivity is located outside the body. A special type of x-ray machine is used to deliver a beam of radiation to the area being treated. Beams may be directed from several different angles to provide the greatest dose to the tumor and minimal exposure of other tissues. The number of treatments given is based on the radiation oncologist's recommendation. It is not unusual for a patient to be treated five times a week for 2 to 8 weeks. A variation of this therapy is intraoperative radiation therapy, a technique in which the tumor or tumor bed is radiated directly during surgery.

Patient preparation. Before the first radiation treatment, the patient goes through a treatment simulation to determine the exact location to be treated. The patient is positioned in various ways while radiographs are taken. The radiation therapist then marks the skin over the area to be treated (radiation field). The markings are usually made with waterproof ink; however, tiny permanent markings are sometimes made. The markings must remain visible throughout the course of radiation. It is important to instruct the patient not to remove the markings until given permission to do so by the physician. For the actual treatments, various devices may be used to shield healthy tissue in the radiation treatment field.

Internal Radiation

Internal radiation involves the introduction of a radiation source into the body. Sources of radiation used for therapy include radioactive forms of iodine, phosphorus, radium, iridium, radon, and cesium. The source may be either sealed or unsealed. The term brachytherapy refers to the implantation of radioactive sources such as seeds or needles into or adjacent to the tumor. In general, patients being treated with internal radiation emit radiation and do pose a threat to others until the source is removed or excreted. An exception is the patient who has small radioactive beads permanently implanted to treat localized prostate cancer or inoperable lung cancer.

Sealed-source radiation. Sealed-source radiation is inserted in the body in a sealed container. One example of sealed-source radiation is cesium, which is contained in a sealed applicator that is inserted into body cavities to treat cancer of the prostate, mouth, tongue, vagina, and cervix. Sealed-source radiation may also be placed in threads, beads, needles, or seeds and implanted in body tissues or may be enclosed in a mold and applied externally. The radiologist determines how long the source is left in place. The patient's body fluids, as well as objects the patient touches, are not radioactive because the radiation source is closed. However, because radiation is emitted from the source while it is in the patient, the following safety measures are necessary in most cases to protect all visitors and nurses from excessive exposure to radiation:

1. The patient is placed in a private room, preferably one that is lined with lead or isolated in one corner of the unit.
2. A sign is placed on the door to the patient's room indicating that the room is a radiation area. A standard

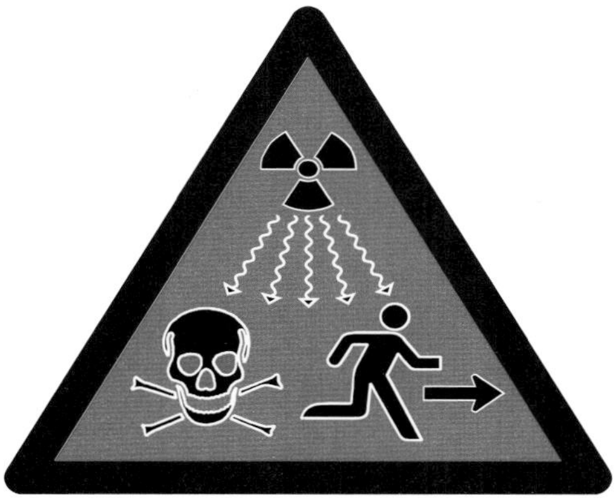

Fig. 7.4 The radiation sign alerts others to the dangers of radiation.

sign is usually available for this purpose (Fig. 7.4) and should indicate that radiation is in use and requires precautions.

3. Anyone who might enter the room for any reason is informed of the proper precautions to take. People younger than 18 years of age and pregnant women should not enter the room. This restriction applies to staff as well as to others. Exposure to radiation is potentially harmful to a fetus.
4. The amount of radiation exposure is reduced by limiting time spent in the room and by working as far as possible from the radiation source (distance) and using the appropriate shielding, such as a portable lead shield, to protect the caregiver during direct care. Institutional policies prescribe the time restrictions for implants. Nursing personnel who regularly spend time with this patient population should wear film badges to monitor their cumulative radiation exposure. As noted earlier, nurses and visitors who are pregnant as well as young children and adolescents should not enter the room.
5. Work must be organized efficiently to minimize exposure. For most patients, care can be provided in a total of 30 minutes per shift. A lead apron used for routine x-rays is not effective in this situation. Portable lead shields can be used to provide some protection.
6. Recognize that sealed sources can be dislodged accidentally. The placement of the source is selected to exert the direct effects of radiation on the area being treated. Specific positions may be ordered for the patient to decrease the risk of displacing the source. Check bedpans and linens for any dislodged source before disposal. If the source moves out of position, immediately notify the physician and the radiation safety personnel. If the source comes out of the patient's body, do not touch it with bare hands. Forceps and a lead container (called a *pig*) that are routinely placed in the room are used to retrieve and contain the source.

Unsealed-source radiation. When unsealed sources are used, additional considerations exist. Because body fluids may be contaminated, you must wear gloves when working with the patient. Contaminated fluids, dressings, and the like may require special care, as outlined in the agency policy. Disposable utensils are recommended. Equipment used in the room will need to be checked for radioactivity before it can be removed from the room. The radiologist can advise the staff on specific precautions and their duration.

Side Effects

The ideal radiation treatment destroys the tumor with the least harm to surrounding cells. Because cells that regenerate rapidly are more susceptible to radiation, cancer cells and some normal cells may be harmed. Normal cells that are most sensitive to radiation include those of the hair follicle, bone marrow, lining of the digestive and urinary tracts, ovaries, testes, and lymph tissue. Radiation damage to these cells explains many of the side effects of the therapy. Depending on the area being irradiated, the following side effects may occur: bone marrow suppression; alopecia (hair loss); anorexia; dry mouth; nausea and vomiting; diarrhea; and inflammation of the skin, esophagus (esophagitis), lungs (pneumonitis), and bladder (cystitis). Regardless of the site treated, radiation therapy commonly causes skin changes and fatigue. Side effects are usually not evident until at least 1 week after treatments are started. These side effects are slow to start and slow to subside. Some people tolerate therapy well whereas others become very ill. Factors that influence the severity of side effects include the area being treated, total and daily radiation doses, volume of tissue treated, method of treatment, and individual factors.

Bone marrow suppression. In healthy people, the bone marrow produces red blood cells (RBCs), white blood cells (WBCs), and platelets. Depending on the treatment site, total area irradiated, and daily radiation dose, radiation treatment can suppress the production of these cells. Anemia results from a deficiency of RBCs. Without adequate WBCs, the patient's ability to resist infection is reduced. Without adequate platelets, the patient is at risk for bruising and bleeding. Bone marrow suppression is most common among patients whose treatment area involves a large area of hematopoiesis, such as the pelvis and the sternum.

Blood counts are usually ordered every other week during radiation therapy, depending on the treatment area, to detect excessive bone marrow suppression. If blood counts are too low, transfusions may be required. The radiation treatments may need to be temporarily held until the bone marrow recovers. WBC and platelet counts usually recover in 2 to 6 weeks. When radiation treatments are used in combination with chemotherapy treatments, an increased chance of bone marrow suppression exists. Growth factors for WBCs may be used to help the blood cell counts recover sooner.

Table 7.8 Side Effects of Radiation Therapy and Nursing Implications

SITE	SIDE EFFECTS	NURSING IMPLICATIONS
Skin	Erythema (redness), desquamation (peeling), permanent darkening	Skin is easily injured. Avoid exposure to sun, trauma, harsh chemicals, or soaps. Until therapy is completed, no lotions or topical medications should be applied. Do not remove markings.
Scalp	Partial or complete alopecia (hair loss); may be permanent	New hair may be different color and texture. Cover scalp with wig, cap, or scarf if patient desires. Refer to American Cancer Society for assistance with hairpieces and help with styling and care.
Digestive tract	Anorexia, inflammation and dryness of the mouth, decreased or altered sense of taste	Schedule small, frequent feedings. Respect patient preferences. Promote frequent oral hygiene. Suggest artificial saliva and ice chips. Monitor weight to assess nutritional state.
	Dental caries	Encourage good dental care. Conduct mouth care per protocol.
	Painful swallowing	Provide antacids and viscous lidocaine as ordered.
	Nausea, vomiting	Provide antiemetics as ordered. Monitor intake.
	Diarrhea	Provide antidiarrheals as ordered. Encourage good perianal care.
Urinary tract	Cystitis	Increase fluid intake.
	Contracted bladder	Have patient empty bladder often.
	Crystalluria	Keep intake and output records.
Bone marrow	Suppressed production of red blood cells, white blood cells, and platelets	Schedule activities to prevent overtiring. Protect patient from infection and injury. Watch for excessive bruising or bleeding. Check results of blood tests. Report fever. Encourage use of soft toothbrush and electric razor.
Lungs	Pneumonitis	Encourage coughing and deep breathing to prevent pneumonia. Use humidifier if ordered. Protect patient from respiratory infections. No one with an elevated temperature or children should visit.
Reproductive organs	Harm to embryo or fetus; sterility, impotence	Advise patient not to become pregnant during therapy or for specified time afterward. Physician may counsel male patient about banking sperm.

Alopecia. Because the cells in the hair follicles are very sensitive to radiation, radiation of the head often produces partial or complete **alopecia** (loss of hair). Whether the hair grows back depends on the radiation dosage. If the hair does grow back, it may be different in color or texture than it was before treatment.

Anorexia. Anorexia is a loss of appetite. Factors that may cause the patient undergoing radiation therapy to experience anorexia include inflammation of the mouth and tongue, altered taste perception, and nausea. Anorexia is a significant problem because it can lead to inadequate nutrition and weight loss. It is especially problematic for patients undergoing treatment for cancer of the esophagus, stomach, neck, or oral cavity. Depression may contribute to anorexia in the patient undergoing radiation therapy.

Dry mouth. Dry mouth, called ***xerostomia***, is a special problem with radiation of the head and neck. The production of saliva decreases, putting the patient at risk for infections of the teeth and gums. Diseased teeth are often extracted before radiation of the head or neck because the risk of osteoradionecrosis is so great. Osteoradionecrosis is the destruction of bone caused by radiation. It is a debilitating complication of head and neck radiation. Medication is available that can help to protect the salivary glands as well as any mucus-producing tissue. These medications are called *radioprotectors* and are given before radiation treatment on a daily basis or as ordered by the physician.

Effects on reproduction. Radiation is potentially harmful to reproductive cells as well as to the developing fetus and embryo. Therefore radiotherapy is not recommended during pregnancy, and patients are advised to avoid becoming pregnant during the therapy. The major side effects of radiation are summarized in Table 7.8.

CHEMOTHERAPY

Chemotherapy is the use of chemical agents in the treatment of disease. Chemical agents specifically used to treat cancer are called ***antineoplastic*** or *anticancer drugs*. The terms *chemotherapy*, *anticancer*, and *antineoplastic drugs* are used interchangeably in this chapter, just as they are in common practice. These drugs act in a variety of ways and may be used alone or in combination

Table 7.9 Cytotoxic Drugs

CLASS AND MECHANISM OF ACTION	EXAMPLES
Alkylating agents: cell cycle phase-nonspecific agents damage DNA by causing breaks in the double-stranded helix. If repair does not occur, cells will die immediately (cytocidal) or when they attempt to divide (cytostatic).	bendamustine (Treanda), busulfan (Myleran), chlorambucil (Leukeran), cyclophosphamide, dacarbazine (DTIC-Dome), ifosfamide (Ifex), mechlorethamine (Mustargen), melphalan (Alkeran), temozolomide (Temodar), thiotepa
Nitrosoureas: cell cycle phase-nonspecific agents like alkylating agents, break DNA helix, interfering with DNA replication. Cross blood-brain barrier.	carmustine (BiCNU, Gliadel, lomustine (Gleostine), streptozocin (Zanosar)
Platinum Drugs: cell cycle phase-nonspecific agents bind to DNA and RNA, miscoding information and/or inhibiting DNA replication, and cells die.	carboplatin, cisplatin (Platinol-AQ), oxaliplatin (Eloxatin)
Antimetabolites: cell cycle phase-specific agents mimic naturally occurring substances, thus interfering with enzyme function or DNA synthesis. Primarily act during S phase. Purine and pyrimidine are building blocks of nucleic acids needed for DNA and RNA synthesis. 1. Interfere with purine metabolism 2. Interfere with pyrimidine metabolism 3. Interfere with folic acid metabolism 4. Interfere with DNA synthesis	1. cladribine, clofarabine (Clolar), fludarabine, mercaptopurine (Purixan), nelarabine (Arranon), pentostatin (Nipent), thioguanine 2. capecitabine (Xeloda), cytarabine (ara-C [Cytosar-U, DepoCytl]), floxuridine, 5-fluorouracil (5-FU), gemcitabine (Gemzar) 3. methotrexate (Trexall), pemetrexed (Alimta), 4. hydroxyurea (Hydrea, Droxia)
Antitumor antibiotics: cell cycle phase-nonspecific agents bind directly to DNA, thus inhibiting the synthesis of DNA and interfering with transcription of RNA.	bleomycin, dactinomycin (Cosmegen), daunorubicin (Cerubidene, DaunoXome), doxorubicin (Doxil), epirubicin (Ellence), idarubicin, mitomycin, mitoxantrone, valrubicin (Valstar)
Mitotic inhibitors: cell cycle phase specific agents: **1. Taxanes** **2. Vinca alkaloids** **3. Others**	1. albumin-bound paclitaxel (Abraxane), docetaxel (Taxotere), paclitaxel (Taxol) 2. vinblastine, vincristine, vinorelbine (Navelbine) 3. estramustine (Emcyt), ixabepilone (Ixempra), eribulin (Halaven)
Topoisomerase inhibitors: cell cycle phase-specific agents inhibit topoisomerases (normal enzymes) that function to make reversible breaks and repairs in DNA that allow for flexibility of DNA in replication.	etoposide, innotecan (Camtosar), teniposide (Vumon), topotecan (Hycamtin)
Miscellaneous 1. Enzyme derived from the yeast Erwina used to deplete the supply of asparagine (amino acid) for leukemic cells that are dependent on an exogenous source of this amino acid. Inhibits protein synthesis 2. Causes changes in DNA in leukemia cells and leads to death 3. Suppresses mitosis. Appears to alter DNA, RNA, and protein	1. Erwina asparaginase, L-asparaginase (Elspar) 2. arsenic trioxide (Trisenox) 3. procarbazine (Matulane)

Data from Lewis SL, Bucher L, Heitkemper MM, Harding MM. *Medical-surgical nursing: Assessment and management of clinical problems*, 10th ed. St. Louis: Elsevier; 2017.

with other forms of treatment. In some cases, chemotherapy is curative. In other circumstances, it may reduce the number of cancer cells, causing symptoms to decrease and often prolonging life.

Types of Antineoplastic Drugs

Types of antineoplastic drugs now commonly used in chemotherapy include cytotoxic agents, hormones and hormone antagonists, biotherapy, immunotherapy, targeted drugs and others. With a growing number of anticancer drug classes and hundreds of specific agents, it is beyond the scope of this book to list them all. Instead, Table 7.9 and Table 7.11 list the classes and a few examples. A current drug handbook is essential to keep up with specific drugs that you encounter in your practice. Cytotoxic drugs, as the name implies, are able to kill cancer cells; however, they are harmful to healthy cells as well. The term *targeted drugs* applies to those that promote cell death by binding with specific targets on cancer cells. Proteasome inhibitors, signal transduction inhibitors, and angiogenesis inhibitors are examples of targeted anticancer drugs.

Various types of cancer are sensitive to different drugs or drug combinations. Combinations are sometimes used to attack cells at different stages of development or to target different cellular mechanisms. Drugs that are effective only during a particular phase of cell development are said to be *cell cycle phase specific.*

Table 7.10 Side Effects of Antineoplastic Therapy and Nursing Implications

SITE	SIDE EFFECTS	NURSING IMPLICATIONS
Bone marrow	Suppressed production of red blood cells, white blood cells (WBCs), and platelets	Monitor blood test results. Balance activity and rest. Prevent overtiring and stress. Protect from infection. Report fever. Watch for excessive bruising or bleeding. Apply pressure to injection sites. Avoid rectal temperatures if WBC count is low. Use soft toothbrush and electric razor.
Digestive tract	Nausea and vomiting	Give antiemetics as ordered. Assess for dehydration. No fluids with meals. Pleasant environment. Respect food preferences.
	Anorexia	Schedule small, frequent feedings and frequent oral hygiene. Monitor weight. Give supplements as ordered.
	Xerostomia	Increase fluid intake. Recommend artificial saliva, sugarless gum or hard candy, and ice chips. Moisten dry food.
	Stomatitis	Encourage dental care and mouth care as ordered or per protocol. Assess for lesions.
	Diarrhea	Administer antidiarrheals as ordered. Encourage good perianal care.
	Constipation	Encourage fluids and high-fiber foods and exercise as tolerated. Give laxatives, stool softeners, enemas as ordered.
Heart	Cardiomyopathy Heart failure	Monitor for dyspnea, edema, increasing pulse pressure. Request electrocardiograms as ordered.
Lungs	Inflammation, fibrosis	Encourage turning, coughing, and deep breathing to prevent pneumonia. Use humidifier as ordered. Elevate head if dyspneic. Protect from respiratory infections. Monitor activity tolerance.
Nerve tissue	Numbness, tingling, loss of deep tendon reflexes	Assess sensation. Protect affected areas from injury.
Scalp	Alopecia	Cover scalp with hairpiece, scarf, or turban if patient wishes. Refer to American Cancer Society for assistance with hairpieces and help with grooming.
Veins	Phlebitis at infusion site	Watch for possible necrosis of surrounding tissue with extravasation. Monitor infusion carefully. Protect infusion site. Report signs of extravasation immediately.
Reproductive cells	Harm to developing embryo or fetus Sterility, impotence with some agents	Discourage pregnancy while on therapy and for specified period thereafter. (Physician may discuss banking sperm with male patients.)

Drugs that are effective during any phase of cell development are said to be *cell cycle phase nonspecific*.

A physician or a nurse who has had specialized education administers chemotherapy. Some drugs are most often given in an outpatient setting; others must be given in an inpatient setting. The route may be oral, topical, intramuscular, intravenous, intracavity, or intrathecal. Intracavity means that the drug is instilled in a body cavity such as the bladder. Intrathecal chemotherapy is given in the subarachnoid space.

Chemoembolization is a technique in which the drug is injected directly into an artery supplying the tumor. Chemoembolization has been used in the treatment of metastatic liver cancer. The goal of this approach is to stop liver tumors from growing or cause them to shrink.

Pharmacology Capsule

The most dangerous adverse effect of antineoplastic drugs used in chemotherapy is bone marrow suppression.

Side Effects

Like radiotherapy, antineoplastic drugs act on normal cells and malignant cells. The major systemic side effects of antineoplastic drugs are the same as those of radiation: bone marrow suppression, nausea and vomiting, and alopecia. Depending on the specific antineoplastic agent, the patient is also at risk for toxic effects to the heart, lungs, nerve tissue, kidneys, and bladder. These problems and related nursing interventions are discussed in "Nursing Care of the Patient Who Has Cancer" and are summarized in Table 7.10.

Although bone marrow suppression is the most dangerous side effect, nausea and vomiting are likely to be the most distressing. Antineoplastic drugs simultaneously irritate the lining of the digestive tract and stimulate the vomiting center in the brain. Some agents have toxic effects on the heart that may lead to heart failure. Others are neurotoxic, with effects manifested most often by numbness and tingling of extremities, paralytic ileus, and loss of deep tendon reflexes. Hypersensitivity reactions can occur with many

Table 7.11 BIOTHERAPY: Hormonal Agents, Targeted Drugs, and Other Noncytotoxic Anticancer Drugs

AGENTS AND ACTIONS	EXAMPLES
Hormonal Agents mimic or control the action of endogenous (natural) hormones	
1. Antiestrogens: block receptors for estrogen	1. tamoxifen, toremifene
2. Aromatase inhibitors: inhibit estrogen synthesis	2. anastrozole, letrozole
3. GnRH agonists suppress production of androgens by the testes	3. leuprolide
4. GnRH antagonists: suppress production of androgens by the testes, but not by the adrenals and the prostate tumor	4. degarelix
5. Androgen receptor blockers: suppress production of androgens by the testes, but not by the adrenals and the prostate tumor	5. flutamide
6. CYP17 inhibitor: inhibit androgen production by the adrenals and the prostate tumor	6. abiraterone
Targeted Therapy targets cell cancer cells without affecting normal cells.	
1. Angiogenesis inhibitors: block formation of new blood vessels that support cancer cells	1. bevacizumab, necitumumab
2. Monoclonal antibodies recognize specific targets on cancer cells tagging them for destruction by the immune system or enhance immune function	2. alemtuzumab, trastuzumab, cetumimab
3. Protease inhibitors: kill cancer cells by disrupting normal functions	3. bortezomib carfilzomib
4. Signal transduction inhibitors: change actions of cancer cells by disrupting cell signals	4. imatinib
Cancer Immunotherapy uses parts of the human immune system to fight cancer by stimulating natural defenses or using lab-created products that act like immune system components.	
1. Checkpoint inhibitors: help immune system recognize and attack cancer cells	1. ipilimumab
2. Chimeric antigen receptor (CAR) T-cell therapy: treats the patient's T-cells so they can find, attach to, and kill cancer cells	2. CD19 chimeric antigen receptor T cells
3. Cytokines: use small proteins that carry messages between cells to stimulate immune cells to attack cancer cells	3. interleukin, interferon
4. Immunomodulators: boost the immune system	4. interferon beta, et al.
5. Cancer vaccines: boost the immune system to treat certain types of cancer	5. sipuleucel-T
6. Monoclonal antibodies: man-made immune system proteins designed to attach a specific part of the cancer cell	6. gemtuzumab, rituximab
7. Oncolytic viruses: modified viruses that infect and kill certain tumor cells	

From Burchum JR, Rosenthal LD. *Lehne's pharmacology for nursing* care, 10th ed. St. Louis: Elsevier; 2019.

chemotherapeutic agents that require vigilant assessment, especially during the initial stage of infusion. Like radiation, antineoplastic drugs are hazardous to reproductive cells and some cause erectile dysfunction and sterility.

Some antineoplastic drugs can also cause very serious tissue injury to the vein during administration. If the agent leaks out of the vein, surrounding tissue destruction may occur. When **extravasation** is suspected, stop the infusion immediately and notify the provider. The physician or advanced practice provider may use various interventions to limit potential harm done by a particular agent.

Pharmacology Capsule

Tissue destruction can result from a group of intravenous antineoplastic drugs classified as *vesicants.* Extravasation is leakage of these intravenous drugs into surrounding tissues which may lead to serious damage requiring surgery.

BIOTHERAPY

Agents that work by affecting biologic processes (referred to as ***biotherapy***) include a variety of drugs and hormones (see Table 7.11). Because antineoplastic drugs suppress the bone marrow, colony stimulating factors (CSFs) may be used as supportive care in patients receiving aggressive regimens that can suppress the bone marrow. CSFs do not directly affect cancer cells, but stimulate the bone marrow to produce platelets, RBCs, and WBCs in patients receiving chemotherapy. This reduces the risk of infection by shortening the period of **neutropenia**, which is characterized by low WBCs. Examples of CSFs are filgrastim (Neupogen) and pegfilgrastim (Neulasta). Chapter 29 provides additional information about CSFs. With CSFs, higher doses of chemotherapy can be given for longer periods of time or at a more frequent schedule.

Surgery, radiotherapy, and chemotherapy work by destroying malignant cells and thereby reduce the size of the tumor. It is hoped that the body's natural defenses will then destroy the remaining malignant cells. Certain immunotherapies are intended to boost the body's existing defenses. Interleukins and interferons are naturally occurring proteins in the body that act as chemical messengers to stimulate immune responses. When given in very high doses, these agents act directly on malignant cells or stimulate the immune system to act against them. These therapies are most effective if the immune system is functioning adequately.

Because some tumors are affected by hormones, various treatments may be used to suppress natural

Table 7.12 Common Side Effects of Biotherapy and Nursing Implications

SITE	SIDE EFFECTS	NURSING IMPLICATIONS
Generalized	Flulike symptoms: fever, chills, muscle aches, severe fatigue, malaise, headaches, tachycardia	Side effects may mask signs and symptoms of infection, so assess carefully. Give acetaminophen as ordered (meperidine is sometimes ordered for severe chills). Help patient plan for adequate rest.
Heart	Serious dysrhythmias, myocardial infarction	Monitor heart rate and rhythm. Report abnormal findings.
Capillaries	Increased permeability, pulmonary and dependent edema, hypotension	Assess for edema. Monitor blood pressure. Have patient change positions slowly; avoid prolonged standing, hot baths, and showers. For hypotension, give colloids or vasopressors as ordered.
Bronchi and lungs	Anaphylaxis with bronchial constriction Pulmonary edema	Note signs of allergy: rash, wheezing, itching. For anaphylaxis, give epinephrine or steroids as ordered. Maintain airway. Assess lungs for crackles. Position for comfort (head elevated).

NOTE: many other side effects occur with individual biotherapies. these include nausea, diarrhea, anorexia, weight loss, skin redness or rash, pruritus, desquamation, bone pain, renal toxicity, anemia, thrombocytopenia, leukopenia, leukocytosis, altered mental status, and liver toxicity. the nurse should identify the specific effects and implications for the specific agents the patient is receiving.

hormone secretion, block hormone actions, or provide supplemental hormones. For example, hormones may be used to block the male sex hormones in the treatment of prostate cancer and female hormones in the treatment of breast cancer.

In antibody therapy, large numbers of antibodies are made in a laboratory rather than by a person's own immune system; these are called *monoclonal antibodies* (mAbs) because the antibody is replicated from a single clone. Scientists can now produce mAbs designed to recognize very specific targets, or antigens that are present on certain types of cancer cells, tagging them for destruction by the body's immune system. The first mAbs were made entirely from mouse cells. One problem with this is that the human immune system can see these antibodies as foreign (because they are from a different species) and can mount a response against them. In the short term, this can sometimes cause allergic-type reactions. Over time, researchers have learned how to replace some parts of these mouse antibody proteins with human parts. Depending on how much of the mAb is human, these are called *chimeric* or *humanized* antibodies. Some mAbs are now fully human, which means that they are likely to be safer and may be more effective than older mAbs. Some monoclonal antibodies, such as ipilimumab used to treat melanoma, help inhibit certain immune system pathways, called checkpoints, allowing the immune system to recognize the cancer cell and boost the patient's immune response to the tumor cell.

The most common side effects are extreme fatigue, headache, muscle aches, chills, and fever. Side effects are more common in older people and in people who are dehydrated, anemic, and malnourished. Previous cardiac, neurologic, gastrointestinal (GI), hepatic, or renal disease also increases the risk of side effects. The patient should be told to report a rash, a blister, or pain at the injection site or a fever. Since 1997 the U.S. Food and Drug Administration (FDA) has approved several mAbs for the treatment of certain cancers. Clinical trials of mAb therapy are also in progress for people with almost every type of cancer. As researchers have found more cancer-associated antigens, they have been able to make mAbs against more and more cancers.

In T-cell therapy, T lymphocytes are engineered to recognize certain cell surface proteins on tumor cells, targeting them for destruction. An example of T-cell therapy is CD19 chimeric antigen receptor T cells that target the tumor cells in patients with non-Hodgkin lymphoma. Finally, vaccines have been developed to treat cancer. Cancer vaccines activate T cells to recognize specific cancer types, targeting them for destruction by the immune system. The first cancer vaccine, sipuleucel-T, was approved in 2010 for the treatment of metastatic prostate cancer. Table 7.11 lists examples of biologic agents used to combat cancer. Side effects of biotherapy are summarized in Table 7.12.

Pharmacology Capsule

Biotherapy mobilizes the body's natural defenses to combat malignant cells.

HEMATOPOIETIC STEM CELL TRANSPLANTATION

Hematopoietic stem cell transplantation is most often used in the treatment of leukemia and lymphoma. Hematopoietic stem cell transplantation can also be used to treat the destruction of the bone marrow caused by too high doses of chemotherapy and radiotherapy. Transplantation of bone marrow or peripheral blood stem cells is done to restore the blood-manufacturing cells and, in diseases such as leukemia, to replace the diseased blood-forming cells with healthy donor cells.

If a patient donates their own stem cells or bone marrow before therapy, it is classified as an *autologous transplant.* If a patient receives cells from a sibling or other relative, it is classified as an *allogeneic transplant;* if the cells are donated from an unrelated donor, it is classified as a *matched unrelated donor transplant.* See Chapter 29 for additional discussion of CSFs and hematopoietic stem cell transplants.

COMPLEMENTARY AND ALTERNATIVE THERAPIES

Some patients choose to use nontraditional treatments such as relaxation techniques, guided imagery, music, meditation, herbal remedies, and acupuncture (see Complementary and Alternative Therapies box). If a nontraditional therapy is used with conventional treatment, it is called ***complementary therapy***. The term ***alternative therapy*** is used if the patient uses nontraditional therapy in place of traditional treatment. The National Center for Complementary and Alternative Medicine, part of the National Institutes of Health, is conducting research to determine the therapeutic value of nontraditional therapies.

Complementary and Alternative Therapies

The American Cancer Society identifies some complementary therapies that can help to relieve symptoms or side effects, ease pain, and increase enjoyment of life. These include the following:

- Aromatherapy
- Art therapy
- Biofeedback
- Massage therapy
- Music therapy
- Prayer, spiritual practices
- Tai chi
- Yoga

Many patients with cancer or other chronic conditions use alternative therapies, including herbal remedies, and many are "secretive" about their use. It is important for patients to report all herbal products used to their physician and to consider their use carefully. In general, very few clinical trials take place evaluating the true safety and efficacy of these products. In addition, some affect the action of prescribed medications.

UNPROVEN METHODS OF CANCER TREATMENT

It is important for health care providers to incorporate clear assessment strategies to ascertain the type of complementary and alternative medicine (CAM) the patient is using or plans to use. The American Cancer Society discourages the use of treatments that have not been studied and found to be safe and effective. Alternative therapies can be harmful and may delay treatment with potentially effective conventional therapies (see Patient Teaching box and Complementary and Alternative Therapies box). The National Center for Complementary and Integrative Health (NCCIH, 2017) reported that almost 12% of children are involved in some sort of CAM therapy. The safety and efficacy of CAM in children requires further research. The nurse can direct patients to the American Cancer Society for further information about questionable therapies. Special considerations about the use of herbs as therapy can be found in Box 7.2.

Patient Teaching

Herbal Therapy

- "Natural" does not always mean safe.
- Discuss herbal products with your physician before use.
- Try to research the product thoroughly.
- Use products with a single component or ingredient (additional ingredients add to the potential toxicity).
- Use products from a reputable manufacturer. The label should have the manufacturer's address and expiration date.
- Look for products that have a drug identification number (DIN). The DIN guarantees that the specified medicinal components will be present. For example, Tanacet 125 guarantees that an exact amount of tanacet, the medicinal component of feverfew, is present and that the product is quality controlled.

Complementary and Alternative Therapies

Myth: Herbs are natural products and therefore are safe.

Truth: Many herbs have serious side effects, including liver toxicity and even death.

Plants are composed of many different chemicals; some are medicinal and others are poisonous.

NURSING CARE OF THE PATIENT WHO HAS CANCER

When working with someone who has cancer, it is easy to focus on the cancer and forget the person. However, medical professionals can do many things that can significantly affect the patient's quality of life (see Nursing Care Plan: Patient With Cancer. Assessment of the patient who has cancer is discussed, along with nursing care for each phase of illness: diagnostic phase, treatment phase, rehabilitation, and recurrence of terminal illness).

DIAGNOSTIC PHASE

People who develop one of the common signs of cancer are often unaware of the seriousness of the condition. Out of fear, some ignore the signs until the disease is advanced. When people seek evaluation of the signs, they are likely to be very worried. Patients often say that "not knowing" is the hardest part. They go through tests and procedures, some uncomfortable, and then wait for the final word. Cancer is often what they fear most.

Box 7.2 Herbs: A Few Things to Think About

The following are common problems with herb use:

- The quantity and quality of any medicinal components in an herbal product can vary considerably. Herbal products are not regulated by the U.S. Food and Drug Administration (FDA). Safety and effectiveness do not have to be demonstrated before these products are marketed.
- No legal standards are applied to herbs' growing conditions, harvesting, processing, or packaging. The possibilities of poor quality, adulteration, contamination, and varying strengths must be kept in mind when evaluating them (e.g., sprayed with pesticides, grown in contaminated soil). The country of origin in which the herb is grown is often not known.
- If the product label has *whole plant* listed, the amount of active medicine or chemical in the product is not known and can vary considerably. This can make dosing difficult or inaccurate. If the label indicates the chemical in *total weight*, this can be considered a specific amount of that product. See information about drug identification number in Patient Teaching box.
- Finding herbs in the wild can be dangerous. For example, wild parsley looks very similar to poison water hemlock; poisonous mushrooms are (virtually) indistinguishable from edible ones.
- Many herbs interfere with prescription medications.
- Some natural products such as thymus are derived from animal sources and could be contaminated by prions, which can cause Creutzfeldt-Jakob disease (the human equivalent of mad cow disease). Another example: products that contain thyroid can alter the body's natural balance of thyroid hormone.
- Some herbal products *decrease* the risk of cancer; others may *increase* the risk of cancer or increase cancer growth.
- The American Cancer Society website includes information about complementary and alternative cancer therapies. .
- Internet resources concerning herbs are as follows:
  - FDA and Center for Food Safety and Applied Nutrition (CFSAN)
  - FamilyDoctor.org—Herbal Products and Supplements (www.familydoctor.org)

Nursing Care Plan Patient With Cancer

FOCUSED ASSESSMENT

Health History

A 63-year-old Black American man was recently diagnosed with lung cancer that is being treated with radiotherapy and chemotherapy. He reports a chronic, nonproductive cough but denies dyspnea or hemoptysis. He states that he has been fatigued and weak since starting his therapy. He has had mild nausea, anorexia, and occasional diarrhea. He complains of dry mouth and is having some dysphagia. The skin over the area being radiated is tender. He is married, is the father of three grown children, and is an insurance salesperson. He smoked one pack of cigarettes a day for 30 years until he quit smoking in 1996. He continues to work part time and expresses concern about his financial situation. He states that he has excellent insurance coverage.

Physical Examination

Vital signs: blood pressure 176/92 mm Hg, pulse 72 beats per minute, respiration 18 breaths per minute, temperature 98°F (37°C) measured orally. Height 5′9″, weight 175 lb. Patient is alert and oriented but does not initiate conversation. Mucous membranes are dry, and lips are cracked. Skin on the upper chest and neck is more darkly pigmented. A central venous catheter is in place; the insertion site is free of swelling and drainage. Respirations are not labored, and breath sounds are clear throughout lung fields. Abdomen is soft and bowel sounds are present. Extremities are warm, with strong peripheral pulses. No edema is seen. Patient is unable to distinguish warm and cold or sharp and dull sensations in lower legs.

Patient Problems	Goals and Outcome Criteria	Interventions
Anxiety related to effects of treatment and uncertain outcomes	Patient will experience reduced anxiety as evidenced by patient statements and by objective observation of decreased anxiety.	Encourage the patient to talk about his illness and his feelings about it. Listen attentively and use touch to convey concern. Help the patient identify sources of anxiety and strategies to deal with it, such as teaching, counseling, spiritual guidance, and support groups.
Inadequate coping related to multiple stressors	Patient will identify stressors and strategies to deal with them to improve coping.	Help the patient to set priorities during therapy. Provide information about management of therapy side effects. Encourage self-care as much as possible. Emphasize his strength. Teach relaxation techniques. Refer the patient to the American Cancer Society for information about support services in the community.

Nursing Care Plan Patient With Cancer—cont'd

Patient Problems	Goals and Outcome Criteria	Interventions
Inability to manage self-care related to lack of knowledge of the prescribed therapy, effects, and precautions	Patient will correctly describe his disease, treatment, the effects of therapy, and the precautions needed.	Determine what the patient already knows and what additional information he wants. Reinforce pretreatment teaching. Remind him not to wash off skin markings until the radiologist gives permission to do so and not to apply lotion to irritated skin. Recommend cotton clothing over irritated skin. Provide information about specific drugs used in his chemotherapy. Refer the patient to the Cancer Information Service (CIS) (1-800-4-CANCER) if he is interested (available in English and Spanish).
Potential for injury related to side effects of therapy	Patient will have no injuries related to therapy, as evidenced by absence of bleeding, dyspnea, skin lesions, or bruises.	Monitor for excessive bruising or prolonged bleeding, edema, dyspnea, and impaired sensation. Report blood in stool, urine, or sputum. Handle gently. Apply pressure for 5 minutes after venipunctures or injections. Instruct the patient to use a soft toothbrush and an electric razor and to protect his feet and legs from trauma. Inspect daily for injury. Advise the patient to wear shoes whenever out of bed.
Potential for infection related to decreased white blood cells, venous access devices	Patient will remain free of infection, as evidenced by normal body temperature and absence of swelling or warmth at central line insertion site.	Teach basic infection preventions such as hand washing, avoiding raw foods that have high bacteria possibility, and avoiding crowds and people with infections. Report fever, foul wound drainage, or confusion to physician promptly. Teach the patient proper care of central venous catheter and have him return demonstration.
Inadequate nutrition related to anorexia and nausea	Patient will maintain adequate nutrition, as evidenced by body weight within 10 lb of usual (180 lb).	Emphasize the importance of good nutrition. Request a dietary consult. Consider frequent feedings. Respect preferences and aversions. Suggest soft diet eaten slowly for dysphagia. Tell the patient not to drink alcohol while receiving chemotherapy. Advise him not to drink fluids with meals and to decrease intake of sweets and fatty foods. Create a pleasant environment without offensive odors. Suggest mild exercise before meals and rest afterward. Give ordered antiemetics as necessary. Additional protein in the form of shakes is often well tolerated.
Disrupted oral tissue integrity related to decreased salivation, inflammation	Patient will report successful management of dry mouth and oral mucous membranes will be intact.	Tell the patient to do frequent, gentle mouth care. Recommend artificial saliva for dryness. Encourage increased fluids, sugarless gum or candies, and ice chips. Suggest moistening food before eating. When the mouth is inflamed, avoid acidic, salty, or spicy foods.
Fatigue related to anemia, effects of cancer	Patient will report adaptations in lifestyle that reduce fatigue.	Determine the patient's need for assistance and schedule activities to conserve energy.
Altered family dynamics related to illness and therapy	Patient and family will discuss need to alter roles and relationships during treatment.	Include the family in patient teaching. Encourage them to plan with the patient for accomplishment of family tasks and responsibilities. Acknowledge family stress and fears. Refer to American Cancer Society, National Cancer Institute, and Oncology Nursing Society resources for help as needed. Ask the social worker to assist with financial arrangements.

CRITICAL THINKING QUESTIONS

1. How could you find out what the patient already knows about his disease and what he wants to know?
2. How might the patient's emotional reaction to the diagnosis of cancer affect his prognosis or treatment?
3. Identify safety threats and specific nursing interventions to maintain safety for this patient.

Focused Assessment

When a patient is having diagnostic procedures related to an actual or potential diagnosis of cancer, collect data needed for the planning and provision of care. A complete list of data follows. The data collected by the licensed vocational nurse/licensed practical nurse (LVN/LPN) depend on individual state requirements, agency policy and individual training.

Health history

Reason for seeking care. Begin with the reason the patient is seeking care. The patient may report pain, lesions, lumps, or changes in some body functions. Elicit a complete description of the problem and the related signs and symptoms.

Past health history. Document chronic illnesses, serious injuries, surgeries, and hospitalizations.

Family history. Inquire about the incidence of cancer and other serious diseases in the patient's immediate family.

Review of systems. In the review of systems, record any of the following signs and symptoms, if present: pain, lumps, fatigue, activity intolerance, lesions of the skin or mucous membranes, easy bruising or bleeding, headache, vision or hearing disturbances, hoarseness, cough, dyspnea, hemoptysis, loss of appetite, difficulty swallowing, digestive disturbances, blood in the urine or stool, and change in bowel pattern.

Functional assessment. Ask the patient about their diet, use of alcohol and tobacco, safe sex practices, activity, and sleep routines. Document the patient's occupation and describe a usual day. Document health practices, including frequency of breast self-examination, testicular examination, and medical checkups. Identify the patient's concerns about living conditions and location. Ask about sources of stress and of support and usual coping strategies.

Physical examination. The physical examination begins with measurement of vital signs, height, and weight. Note whether there has been a change in weight. Inspect the face, scalp, and oral mucosa for lesions. Palpate the neck for enlarged lymph nodes. Throughout the examination, inspect the skin for color, lesions, edema, and bruising. Auscultate breath sounds and observe respiratory effort. Inspect the breasts for symmetry, dimpling, and abnormal skin color and palpate for lumps or thickened areas. Inspect the abdomen for distention, auscultate for bowel sounds, and palpate for masses. Inspect the genitalia for lesions.

Patient Problems, Goals, and Outcome Criteria: Diagnostic Phase

Patient Problems	Goals and Outcome Criteria
Denial related to fear of diagnosis of cancer, medical evaluation, and treatment	Acceptance and seeking out of medical evaluation and treatment by patient
Anxiety related to threat of or change in health status	Reduced anxiety: patient states anxiety reduced, demonstrates calm manner
Inability to manage self care related to inadequate knowledge of diagnostic tests and procedures	Patient prepares appropriately for tests and procedures: patient correctly describes tests and procedures and follows directions related to them

Interventions

Denial. When people detect possible signs or symptoms of cancer, they may be so anxious that they cannot cope with their fears. Instead, they deny the seriousness of the situation and do not seek medical care. Such delays may allow the disease to progress, making treatment more difficult and less likely to be successful. Encourage individuals to learn the warning signs of cancer and to report them promptly. Emphasize that these signs may be caused by conditions other than cancer, but medical evaluation is needed for a correct diagnosis. Stress the fact that many cancers are curable, especially in the early stages.

Anxiety. During the diagnostic phase, the patient needs encouragement, support, and honest information. Be careful to remain hopeful yet not give false reassurance ("I'm sure it will not be cancer."). Clichés are not helpful either ("Everything has a purpose."). It is helpful to recognize what the patient seems to be feeling (e.g., "You seem to be very worried."). Information about tests and procedures allows the patient to prepare mentally.

Remember that patients who are being evaluated for cancer are under stress. They may show this stress through anger, irritability, fear, or depression. All of these reactions are normal under the circumstances and should be accepted with understanding (Fig. 7.5).

The physician reports findings to the patient and informs the patient of the diagnosis. In the past, it was not uncommon for the diagnosis of cancer to be kept from the patient. Now, most patients are told of their diagnoses. This change has come about because patients are better informed, cancer treatment has improved the odds of survival, and the patient's right to know is recognized. Nevertheless, you should know what the patient has been told, to avoid giving the patient conflicting messages. At times, you may need to help patients to communicate their needs and questions to the physician.

Once a diagnosis of cancer has been made, the patient needs support to adapt to the situation. Even at this phase of the illness, the patient may show various responses related to grief. Responses could include

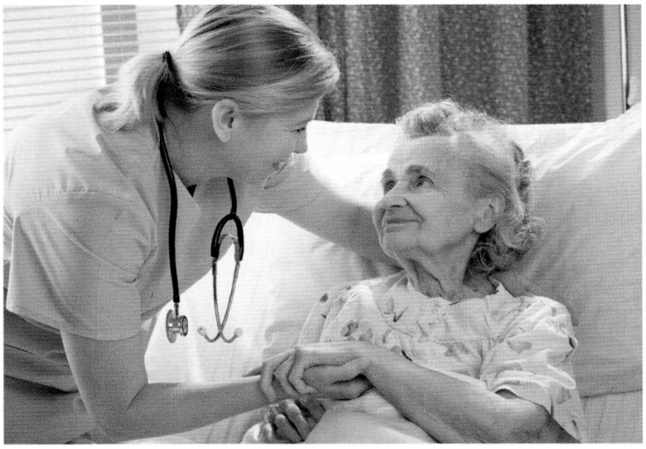

Fig. 7.5 Listening and touching convey acceptance and caring. (Copyright © www.istock.com)

denial, shock and disbelief, anger, depression, bargaining, and acceptance. It is useful to understand and recognize how to help the grieving patient. Chapter 19 discusses nursing care of the grieving patient.

Patients struggle to adjust to the knowledge that they have cancer. For many, this is the first time they have seriously considered the possibility of their own deaths. They are typically preoccupied with what will happen to them. Patients' understanding of their illness and their prognosis is vital to ensuring that they are able to make informed decisions about treatment that align with their own personal beliefs and values.

People have different ways of coping with a diagnosis of cancer. Poor coping is sometimes related to lack of information about the disease and its treatment. In that case, a trained oncology nurse may be consulted to provide patient education. Some coping styles are more effective than others. In a study exploring coping and prognostic awareness in patients with advanced cancer, Nipp and colleagues (2017) found that adoption of positive coping strategies including positive reframing, seeking emotional support, and active and acceptance coping were associated with better quality of life and less depression in patients who acknowledged that they were diagnosed with incurable cancer. Research by Franks and Roesch (2007) found that individuals with cancer who appraise their illness as a threat are likely to use more problem-focused coping strategies, those who appraise their cancer as harm or loss are likely to use more avoidance coping strategies, and those who appraise their cancer as a challenge are likely to use approach coping strategies. Factors found to modify the relationship between appraisals and coping included age of the participant, time since diagnosis, and type of cancer (Franks & Roesch, 2007).

In the diagnostic phase of cancer care, patients typically use their usual methods of dealing with stress. When coping is not effective, a referral to a psychiatric clinical nurse specialist or a mental health counselor may be in order.

Inadequate self-care. Tell the patient about diagnostic tests and procedures, including preparation, what the procedure is like, and any specific postprocedure care.

TREATMENT PHASE

Focused Assessment

During the treatment phase, specific assessments depend on the type and site of cancer and the prescribed treatment. Information obtained in the initial assessment provides baseline data. Frequently and systematically collect data to determine changes related to the disease process and for effects and side effects of therapy. Areas of ongoing data collection are presented here.

Health history. Note the patient's diagnosis and treatment plan. Take the past health history to reveal other acute and chronic conditions that require attention during cancer therapy. Obtain a complete drug profile and record allergies prominently. Review the systems to detect significant symptoms related to cancer or the treatment, including fatigue, weakness, headache, sore or dry mouth, dyspnea, palpitations, altered taste sensations, nausea, diarrhea, constipation, blood in stools, change in urinary frequency, hematuria or dysuria, sexual dysfunction, numbness, and tingling sensations. In the functional assessment, determine the effects of the illness and therapy on the patient's daily functioning. Explore the patient's knowledge, fears, concerns, and coping strategies and level of distress. Also explore adaptations made by the patient and family during this phase.

Physical examination. Note the patient's general appearance, level of consciousness, posture, and gait. Be alert for clues to the patient's mental and emotional state (e.g., eye contact, mannerisms, tone of voice). Measure weight and vital signs and compare with previous measurements. Inspect the skin for lesions and bruises. Inspect the scalp for hair loss. Inspect the oral mucous membranes for lesions and inflammation. Observe the patient's respiratory effort and auscultate the lung fields for atelectasis or abnormal breath sounds. Inspect the abdomen for distention and auscultate bowel sounds. Inspect and palpate the extremities for color, edema, and peripheral pulses. Test reflexes and sensation in the extremities.

Assessment of the patient with cancer during the treatment phase is summarized in Box 7.3.

Patient Problems, Goals, and Outcome Criteria: Cancer Treatment Phase

Patient Problems	Goals and Outcome Criteria
Anxiety related to effects and outcomes of treatment	Reduced anxiety: patient states less anxiety, demonstrates relaxed manner

Continued

Patient Problems	Goals and Outcome Criteria
Inadequate coping related to multiple stressors or overwhelming threat to self	Effective coping: patient identifies and uses strategies that decrease distress
Potential for injury related to adverse effects of therapy	Absence of serious adverse effects: patient has no signs/symptoms of injuries associated with therapy
Potential for infection related to decreased white blood cell count and invasive procedures/devices	Decreased risk/presence of infection: precautions in place to avoid exposure to infectious agents; patient has normal body temperature; absence of redness, drainage from wounds, or venous access sites
Inadequate nutrition related to anorexia, nausea, vomiting	Adequate nutrition: patient's body weight remains stable
Disrupted oral tissue integrity related to decreased salivation and/or inflammation	Decreased oral discomfort: patient states they are more comfortable, moist mucous membranes
Constipation related to decreased activity, drug side effects	Normal bowel elimination: soft, formed stool passed at least every 3 days
Fatigue related to anemia or effects of cancer	Adaptation to decreased energy level: patient completes essential activities without exhaustion
Altered body image related to alopecia, surgical scars, loss of function, stoma	Adaptation to change in body: patient demonstrates acceptance of hair loss and scars or conceals them; adapts to functional changes; adjusts to stoma and learns self-care
Grief related to loss of body part or altered appearance or function	Patient recognizes losses and moves toward resolving grief: patient discusses feelings of loss, touches affected body parts
Altered family dynamics related to illness and therapy	Adjustment of family roles and relationships: reassignment within family
Inability to manage self-care related to lack of knowledge and feelings of hopelessness	Effective management of treatment program: patient describes and carries out plan and self-care measures

Interventions

Anxiety. The thought of having surgery or of receiving cancer therapy may be very frightening to the patient. Suspect anxiety when a patient seems tense, apprehensive, or helpless. The patient may have poor eye contact, increased pulse and respirations, perspiration, and trembling. Tactfully share your observations and offer the patient an opportunity to talk. Encourage the patient to express feelings and identify the source of the anxiety. Listening and touch can be very effective in reducing anxiety. Recognize the need for patient teaching or for referrals.

Inadequate coping. The patient may need help in setting priorities and in coping with the side effects of therapy. Strategies to promote coping include teaching, encouraging self-care within the patient's limitations, treating physical signs and symptoms, emphasizing abilities, coaching in relaxation strategies, and encouraging the use of coping strategies that have been effective in the past.

Support groups may be most effective at this phase. People who have been through the same treatments as the patient can be especially informative and supportive. The local chapter of the American Cancer Society can provide information about services in the patient's community. Some agencies can arrange transportation for therapy and medical care. The Reach for Recovery program trains women who have had mastectomies to counsel others in undergoing treatment for breast

Box 7.3 Focused Assessment of the Patient With Cancer in the Treatment Phase

HEALTH HISTORY

Reason for Seeking Care
Diagnosis, prominent symptoms related to disease or treatment

Past Health History
Acute and chronic conditions, previous surgeries and hospitalizations, drug profile, allergies

Review of Systems
Fatigue, weakness, headache, sore mouth, dyspnea, palpitations, altered taste sensations, nausea and vomiting, diarrhea, constipation, blood in stools or urine, urinary frequency, dysuria, numbness or tingling sensations, sexual dysfunction

Functional Assessment
Effects of illness and treatment on functioning, patient knowledge and concerns, stresses and coping strategies, family adaptation

PHYSICAL EXAMINATION

General Survey: Level of consciousness, posture and gait, eye contact, mannerisms, tone of voice
Height and Weight: Present and previous weight
Vital Signs: Present and previous readings, fever, tachypnea, tachycardia, hypotension, hypertension
Skin: Lesions, bruises, darkened or irritated areas
Scalp: Hair loss
Mouth: Condition of mucous membranes, dryness
Thorax: Respiratory effort, breath sounds
Abdomen: Distention, bowel sounds
Extremities: Color, edema, peripheral pulses, reflexes, sensation

cancer. Groups are also available to help patients with ostomies resulting from cancer of the colon, bladder, or larynx.

When a patient must be isolated physically (as when receiving internal radiotherapy), it is difficult to provide emotional support. Remember to check on the patient frequently. Intercom conversations let the patient know that they have not been forgotten.

Potential for injury. The patient may exhibit various signs and symptoms of tissue injury associated with cancer therapy. Specific nursing measures are described as follows for some of the injurious effects of cancer therapy.

Pneumonitis and pulmonary fibrosis. Encourage patients with pneumonitis to do coughing and deep-breathing exercises to reduce the risk of pneumonia. Protect the patient from exposure to people who have upper respiratory infections. If the patient has dyspnea, elevate the head and schedule care to allow adequate rest and avoid exhaustion. If the patient is not able to adequately oxygenate, report this finding to the registered nurse (RN).

Cardiac toxicity. Patients receiving potentially cardiotoxic drugs such as doxorubicin (Adriamycin) and BRMs (interferon, interleukin-2, and trastuzumab) may show signs of heart failure, so monitor for dyspnea, increasing pulse pressure, and edema. Notify the RN promptly if these signs occur. Care of the patient with heart failure is covered in Chapter 34.

Neurotoxicity. The patient who has neurotoxic effects of chemotherapy has special needs as well. Patients may experience metabolic changes from the chemotherapy that may cause them to be somnolent, confused or agitated. Drugs such as fluorouracil (5-FU) and vincristine are associated with peripheral neuropathies. Extremities that lack normal sensation (neuropathy) are prone to injury and should be protected. These patients may be at an increased risk for falls. Certain drugs such as cytarabine can cause issues with balance. Notify the RN of any reported or observed changes in gait, difficulty walking, or performing activities of daily living.

Cystitis and diarrhea. If the patient is receiving certain chemotherapies that can cause cystitis, such as cyclophosphamide (Cytoxan), or if the abdomen or lower back is irradiated, encourage the patient to increase fluid intake and empty the bladder often because of the risk of cystitis. Ask the patient to immediately report any symptoms of cystitis such as burning or painful urination or blood in their urine. Assessments of tissue turgor and mucous membrane moisture help to detect dehydration. Diarrhea may require the administration of antidiarrheal drugs and special perianal care.

Thrombocytopenia. Radiation and chemotherapy can suppress the production of platelets. When a patient has a low platelet count (thrombocytopenia), the blood does not clot promptly. Gentle handling is necessary to avoid trauma and bruising. Minimize invasive procedures, including rectal temperatures. After venipunctures or injections, apply pressure for 5 minutes to control oozing. Instruct the patient to use a soft toothbrush and an electric razor to prevent trauma to the oral tissues or the skin.

Immediately report any blood in the stool, urine, or sputum to the physician. Signs and symptoms of internal bleeding include increased pulse and respirations, restlessness, pallor, decreased urine output, and falling blood pressure (a late sign).

Anemia. Anemia is common after repeated cycles of chemotherapy, so patients should have hemoglobin and hematocrit testing done. Anemia is treated with packed RBCs and, for select patients, erythropoietin (epoetin alfa). A diet high in iron is recommended. Tell the patient to report palpitations, pallor, and excessive fatigue to the physician.

Reproductive cells. Because of the potential for harm to the developing embryo or fetus, women are usually advised not to become pregnant during and immediately following chemotherapy or while receiving radiotherapy until cleared by their physician. Female patients of childbearing age should discuss specific guidelines with their physicians. Because sperm production is reduced, male patients are counseled about the advisability of banking sperm before beginning therapy with certain drugs. Both males and females should use birth control while undergoing cancer treatment.

Potential for infection. Patients with low WBC counts because of radiation or chemotherapy must be protected from infection. They should avoid crowds and close contact with others who have infectious diseases. Promptly report any signs of infection (elevated temperature, foul wound drainage, confusion).

If the WBC count is very low, compromised host precautions (or neutropenic precautions) may be needed to protect the patient. Such precautions include a private room and strict hand washing by all who enter the room. Fresh flowers are not allowed in the room because they harbor potentially harmful organisms. Additional details on compromised host precautions are presented in Chapter 31.

Patients who receive chemotherapy may have a venous access device placed to permit frequent intravenous access without repeated venipunctures. An access device also delivers the antineoplastic drug into a large vein with turbulent blood flow. This decreases the local tissue injury caused by the drug. The venous access device presents a potential portal for infection. Most agencies have standard procedures for care of the device. Because the device usually remains in place for the entire treatment period, the patient or a helper must know how to care for it at home. Care of venous access devices is discussed in Chapter 16.

Inadequate nutrition. Anorexia is common with cancer therapy, but maintaining good nutrition is essential. The patient is advised to eat a high-protein, high-calorie diet. Small, frequent feedings are sometimes easier to take than three large meals a day. Light exercise before meals may stimulate the appetite. If patients have specific food preferences and aversions, these should be respected. Many patients find that red meat and some other foods taste bitter when on chemotherapy. Use of plastic utensils may decrease the bitter taste. Nutritional supplements (e.g., Carnation Instant Breakfast, Ensure, Boost), enteral feedings, or both may be ordered if the patient has excessive weight loss (see Nutrition Considerations box).

Nutrition Considerations

1. Impaired nutrition in patients with cancer can result from the disease itself or from the various treatment modalities, such as chemotherapy and radiation.
2. Cancer cachexia is a complex metabolic problem characterized by weight loss, anemia, and abnormalities in fat, protein, and carbohydrate metabolism.
3. The goals of nutritional care for patients with cancer are to prevent or correct nutritional deficiencies and to minimize weight loss.
4. Interventions for common problems associated with cancer therapy (nausea and vomiting, food aversions, anorexia, dry mouth, diarrhea, constipation) should be geared toward individual needs.
5. Immunotherapy indirectly affects nutrition by causing fatigue, chills, fever, and flulike symptoms, which may affect appetite.
6. Diets for cancer patients must be individualized depending on their baseline nutritional status, symptoms, and therapy side effects.
7. If oral intake is inadequate, enteral tube feedings or parenteral nutrition is considered.

Nurses should be familiar with the specific antineoplastic drugs so that the patient can be advised of any specific food restrictions. For example, patients taking procarbazine (Matulane) may have severe hypertensive reactions if they consume foods containing tyramine while on this drug. Foods rich in tyramine are produced by fermentation or decay. Foods that are spoiled, pickled, aged, smoked, fermented, or marinated, such as aged beef or cheeses and alcoholic beverages, have a higher tyramine level. Other foods that contain tyramine are avocados, bananas, beverages containing caffeine, eggplants, figs, pineapple, red plums, raspberries, yogurt, Brazil nuts, coconuts, peanuts, and liver. Patients taking procarbazine should not consume alcohol.

Persistent nausea and vomiting can lead to dehydration and malnutrition. Various combinations of antiemetics and sedatives can be tried as ordered to obtain relief, as outlined in Table 7.13. Newer antiemetic drugs such as palonosetron (Aloxi), dolasetron (Anzemet), ondansetron (Zofran), and granisetron (Kytril) have greatly improved the management of nausea and vomiting associated with chemotherapy and have fewer side effects.

Contrary to common belief, not all patients with cancer have problems with weight loss. Some patients with cancer may gain weight during therapy, possibly because they eat often to settle their stomachs. The important point for the nurse is to assess and treat each patient individually.

While antineoplastic drugs are being administered, sedatives are sometimes ordered so that the patient can sleep. Nursing measures to manage nausea and vomiting are detailed in Chapter 38. The following are additional suggestions for patients from the American Cancer Society (2013):

1. Take your antinausea medicine. Call your doctor or nurse if the medicine is not working.
2. Stay away from some foods. Eat less greasy, fried, salty, sweet, or spicy foods if you feel sick after eating them. If the smell of food bothers you, ask others to cook for you. Eat food at room temperature.
3. Have enough to eat and drink. Take small sips of water during the day.
4. On days you get treatment, talk with your nurse to learn about ways to relax if you feel sick before treatment.
5. Learn the best time for you to eat and drink. Some people feel better when they eat a little before treatment and others feel better when they do not eat before treatment.
6. After treatment, wait at least 1 hour before eating or drinking.

Food and beverages that are helpful for patients with nausea and vomiting are listed in Box 7.4.

Pharmacology Capsule

Many newer drugs are in oral formulation. Patients may feel that taking pills will produce fewer side effects than intravenous medications. However, the actual emetic potential of a drug, not necessarily the route of administration, determines the degree of chemotherapy-induced nausea and vomiting. Patients who are receiving oral medicines need as much education as those receiving intravenous drugs. It is vital that they receive the appropriate antiemetics to take at home.

Impaired oral tissue integrity. A number of measures are helpful when the patient has xerostomia. Patients should try frequent, gentle mouth care and artificial saliva to increase comfort. Several commercial products on the market moisten the mouth. Various protocols for mouth care can be used. For example, the patient can rinse the mouth with normal saline, a solution of 1 tablespoon of hydrogen peroxide in a glass of water, or a solution of $^1/_2$ teaspoon of bicarbonate of soda in a glass of water. Encourage the patient to increase fluid intake, chew sugarless gum or candies, suck on ice chips, and moisten dry food before eating. Lemon and

Table 7.13 Medication Therapy: Commonly Prescribed Antiemetics

CLASSIFICATION	SPECIFIC DRUGS	SIDE EFFECTS
Phenothiazines	prochlorperazine maleate (Compazine)	Sedation, hypotension, extrapyramidal symptoms
	promethazine hydrochloride (Phenergan)	
Antihistamines	diphenhydramine (Benadryl)	Sedation, dry mouth, constipation
Butyrophenones	haloperidol lactate (Haldol)	Extrapyramidal symptoms (such as akathisia, dystonia, pseudoparkinsonism, and dyskinesia) Sedation, hypotension
Corticosteroids	dexamethasone (Decadron)	Fluid retention
Hypnotics or sedatives	diazepam (Valium)	Sedation, ataxia
	lorazepam (Ativan)	Amnesia, sedation, dizziness
Cannabinoid	dronabinol (Marinol)	Visual hallucinations, somnolence, ataxia, hypotension
5-HT_3 Receptor Blockers	ondansetron hydrochloride (Zofran)	Constipation, diarrhea, headache
	granisetron (Kytril)	Headache, constipation, somnolence, diarrhea, asthenia, fever, taste disorders
	dolasetron (Anzemet)	Headache, bradycardia
	palonosetron (Aloxi)	Headache, constipation, diarrhea, dizziness
Miscellaneous agents	metoclopramide hydrochloride (Reglan)	Sedation, diarrhea, dizziness, extrapyramidal symptoms
	aprepitant (Emend)	Abdominal pain, fatigue, dehydration, dizziness

Box 7.4 Recommended Food and Beverages for the Patient With Nausea and Vomiting

SOUPS
- Clear broth, such as chicken, beef, and vegetable

BEVERAGES
- Clear soda such as ginger ale
- Cranberry or grape juice
- Oral rehydration solution drinks
- Tea
- Water

MEALS AND SNACKS
- Chicken—broiled or baked, without the skin
- Cream of Wheat or Cream of Rice cereal
- Crackers or pretzels
- Oatmeal
- Pasta or noodles
- Potatoes—boiled, without the skin
- White rice
- White toast

FRUITS AND SWEETS
- Bananas
- Canned fruit such as applesauce, peaches, and pears
- Gelatin (Jell-O)
- Popsicles and sherbet
- Yogurt (plain or vanilla)

glycerin swabs are no longer recommended because lemon juice dehydrates oral tissues and glycerin provides a medium for bacterial growth.

Mucositis is inflammation of the mucosa, and it may extend from the mouth and affect the entire intestinal tract. It is a painful condition that can interfere with adequate food intake. The patient who has stomatitis should continue mouth care as prescribed, eat soft foods, and avoid foods that are acidic, salty, or spicy. A soft-bristled or foam toothbrush should be used. Normal saline alone or with sodium bicarbonate makes a soothing mouthwash and should be used at least four times a day.

Constipation. Some patients are constipated while on cancer therapy because of reduced activity, opioid analgesics, and the effects of some antineoplastic drugs. Monitor the patient's bowel movements to detect constipation. The physician may prescribe a high-fiber diet, stool softeners, laxatives, and enemas to prevent or treat constipation.

Fatigue. Fatigue is a common symptom in the patient with cancer. In addition, side effects of therapy may cause the patient to tire easily. Determine the patient's need for assistance and schedule activities to conserve energy. In addition, encourage the patient to prioritize activities and ask others to assume less important ones. Daily naps and mild exercise may be helpful.

Altered body image. The effects of cancer and cancer treatments can alter physical appearance and function. For example, patients receiving chemotherapy may have hair loss. Surgical interventions may result in visible scars, altered functioning, loss of body structures, and ostomies.

Be sensitive to the patient's concern about hair loss. At first, the patient may just note extra hair in the brush or comb. Later, hair often comes out in clumps. Hair loss may be partial or complete. Typically, hair begins to grow back soon after the completion of chemotherapy and 4 to 6 months after the completion of radiotherapy. It is not unusual for the new hair to be a different color or texture. After large doses of radiation to the head, hair in the treated area may not return. Although some patients take this in stride, others may wish to use wigs, scarves, or hats to cover the head. Some insurance companies cover the price of wigs; others do not. The American Cancer Society gives wigs to patients free of charge. The society also sponsors the "Look Good … Feel Better" program to assist patients in looking their best during therapy.

Whereas hair usually grows back, other effects of cancer treatment are often permanent. Patients need time and support to incorporate those changes into their body images and to regain a healthy self-concept.

Grief. Treatment of cancer often results in temporary or permanent changes in body appearance or function. Changes or losses often trigger a grief response. The patient may be sad or tearful or verbalize feelings about the loss. Listen in an accepting way that lets the patient know that the feelings are understood. Behaviors that suggest that the patient is beginning to accept the loss or change include talking about the loss and looking at or touching the affected part. Support the patient as needed and provide practical information about adapting to the loss. Participation in a support group may help the patient to learn new coping strategies and begin to resolve the grief process.

Altered family dynamics. While undergoing treatment for cancer, the patient may be concerned with meeting responsibilities at home and at work. Some treatments extend over many months and make it difficult to maintain one's usual activities. Side effects of the treatment may make the patient feel tired and discouraged. Family and friends need to understand what the patient is going through and what they can do to help. Encourage them to remain involved with the patient. Family members may need help in handling their own responses to the patient's illness.

Financial concerns may be very serious for the patient and family. Obtain a social work consultation if necessary to assist them with insurance and disability claims and financial assistance referrals.

Inability to perform self-care. A pretreatment teaching plan informs the patient of what the prescribed therapy involves and what the experience will be like. Know what the physician has told the patient and reinforce that teaching. One source of information is the National Cancer Institute's Cancer Information Service (CIS). Booklets on cancer, cancer therapy, and coping can be obtained by calling CIS at 1-800-4-CANCER. A variety of materials is available from the American Cancer Society that can be accessed by calling 1-800-227-2345 (or at www.cancer.org).

Chemotherapy and biotherapy. If chemotherapy or biotherapy is prescribed, the teaching plan includes a description of the drugs to be administered, the potential side effects, and related precautions. Provide written information to supplement the verbal teaching. Explore what the patient has heard about chemotherapy and correct any misconceptions. Many patients have heard horror stories about drug side effects, especially nausea and vomiting. Inform the patient of measures that can be taken that usually make the side effects more tolerable. Key teaching points for the patient who is receiving chemotherapy or radiation therapy are summarized in the Patient Teaching boxes.

Patient Teaching

External Radiation Therapy

- Having the treatment is much like having a radiograph (x-ray). You are positioned on a table and the machine is adjusted to direct the beam appropriately. During the treatment, you are alone in the room, but closed-circuit television permits the staff to see you. In addition, a two-way intercom allows you and the therapist to talk as needed during the procedure.
- The treatment is not painful. In fact, no sensations at all are felt related to the radiation. The machine that houses the radiation is controlled by a radiotherapist. You will hear whirring or clicking sounds as the machine operates.
- These treatments do not cause you to be radioactive. The radioactive material remains in the machine. Only the rays emitted by the material come in contact with you. When the machine is turned off, no radiation exposure occurs.
- The skin markings made by the therapist are used to direct the radiation to the treatment site. Do not wash the marks off until the physician gives you permission to do so.
- Skin over the area being treated may become irritated. Keep irritated skin clean and dry but do not apply lotions. Cotton clothing may feel more comfortable over irritated skin. Antiperspirants should not be applied to a treatment site, but cornstarch can be used to absorb moisture. Special lotions are available from your radiation nurse or physician, who will instruct you on how and when to use them.

Patient Teaching

Internal Radiation Therapy

- The radioactive material is given orally, injected into a vein, or implanted by a physician.
- You are placed in a private room for a specified period of time for the treatment.
- Visitors and staff are restricted in the amount of time they can spend in your room, to limit their exposure to radiation. They also will maintain some distance from you when they are in the room.
- If a sealed source is to be placed in a body cavity, you may be required to maintain a certain position to keep the source positioned correctly.

RECOVERY AND REHABILITATION

If the outcome of treatment appears to be a cure, the patient and family are usually overjoyed. However, some patients become excessively concerned with their bodies, constantly monitoring for new evidence of cancer. Periodic checkups are essential but may be dreaded because the patient realizes that complete or permanent recovery cannot be guaranteed. If any signs of a possible recurrence appear, patients are understandably concerned.

As patients recover from the effects of cancer and cancer therapy, rehabilitation may be needed to restore them to the highest possible level of functioning.

Put On Your Thinking Cap!

You are assigned to two patients who are being treated for cancer. One is receiving external radiation; the other is receiving chemotherapy.

1. Identify patient problems that might appear in the care plans of both of these patients.
2. Identify one adverse effect that occurs with radiation but not with chemotherapy.
3. Identify one adverse effect that occurs with chemotherapy but not with radiation.

TERMINAL ILLNESS

Although increasing numbers of people are surviving cancer, it is still the second leading cause of death. If treatment is unsuccessful, the patient eventually begins to decline. Patients need to know what resources are available to them and to their families. Provide information about home health care, palliative and hospice care, and voluntary and charitable organizations whose services might be needed. For patients who wish to die at home, hospice provides the support and teaching needed for this to be honored. The focus of hospice is to keep the patient's symptoms, especially pain, under control during the final period of the illness. In addition, hospice staff provides bereavement care after the patient's death.

To work effectively with these patients, you must be aware of your own feelings about dying. You can help these patients in many ways. Continue to be attentive and accepting. New nurses often fear that patients will ask them questions they cannot answer. It is all right to admit that you do not know, but acknowledge the patient's concerns. Listening carefully is more important than talking. Guide patients to claim their accomplishments and find peace with their failures. Chapter 19 discusses care of the dying patient in more detail.

People with terminal cancer often express fear of having great pain as the disease progresses. Although cancer is usually painless in the early stages, advanced disease often causes pain. Cancer pain can be caused by pressure on nerves, interference with circulation, obstruction of hollow structures (e.g., ureter, bowel, bronchi), and local tissue destruction.

General medical and nursing measures for the management of pain are discussed in Chapter 8. An especially good resource is the Agency for Healthcare Research and Quality (AHRQ—formerly AHCPR) publication on management of cancer pain. A variety of approaches should be tried to keep the patient as comfortable as possible. With severe, chronic pain, it is appropriate to medicate the patient at fixed intervals rather than on request. The patient may have pain at specific times or during certain activities despite the routine analgesic. This is referred to as *breakthrough pain*. If that happens, there may be an order for the additional as-needed (PRN) use of a short-acting drug with a rapid onset of action. Do not withhold ordered opioids out of concern about causing addiction. Analgesics that may be ordered include long-acting opioids (morphine sulfate [MS-Contin, Roxanol], fentanyl patches) that may be supplemented with short-acting opioids for breakthrough pain. Combinations of drugs, including opioids, a stimulant, and an antiemetic, may be effective for the patient with cancer. These "cocktails," although not used as much as they once were, often control pain when given regularly without causing excessive sedation. Advise the RN or physician if pain control is not achieved.

ONCOLOGIC EMERGENCIES

Patients with cancer sometimes develop conditions that require emergency intervention as a result of the disease process or the therapy. Some of the conditions requiring prompt recognition and action are hypercalcemia, syndrome of inappropriate antidiuretic hormone (ADH), disseminated intravascular coagulation (DIC), superior vena cava syndrome, and spinal cord compression. Characteristics of these conditions and related interventions are described in Table 7.14.

Put On Your Thinking Cap!

A patient who is receiving outpatient chemotherapy for cancer tells you that he is using natural vitamins and herbal products to help combat his cancer. He says, "They are all natural products, so they can't be harmful, right?"

1. How should you answer him?
2. What should you advise him to do?

Table 7.14 Oncologic Emergencies

EMERGENCY	RISK FACTORS	SIGNS AND SYMPTOMS	TREATMENT	NURSING CARE
Hypercalcemia	Multiple myeloma, metastatic bone cancer; cancer of lung, breast, or kidney; prolonged immobility	Fatigue, confusion, weakness, constipation, polyuria, hypertension, tachycardia, poor muscle tone If untreated, possible renal failure, coma, cardiac dysrhythmias, or death	IV normal saline and furosemide (Lasix) Drugs to promote excretion of calcium: plicamycin, calcitonin, etidronate disodium	Monitor fluid status. Give IV fluids and drugs as ordered. Record intake and output.
Syndrome of inappropriate antidiuretic hormone	Thoracic or mediastinal tumors, thymoma, lymphomas, pancreatic cancer, cyclophosphamide (Cytoxan) or vincristine (Oncovin) therapy	Water intoxication and dilutional hyponatremia because of water retention: nausea and vomiting, anorexia, weakness Lethargy at first, followed by confusion, psychosis, loss of deep tendon reflexes, seizures, coma, and death	Fluids restricted to 500 mL/d; demeclocycline (Declomycin); IV fluids and diuretic agents administered only in late stage	Explain and enforce fluid restriction. Monitor vital signs. Keep intake and output records. Do not give demeclocycline with food or dairy products.
Disseminated intravascular coagulation	Septicemia, transfusion reaction Some drugs: vincristine, methotrexate, mercaptopurine, prednisone, asparaginase	Normal clotting process exaggerated, which depletes clotting factors Early signs: petechiae, ecchymoses, prolonged bleeding from venipuncture Late signs: signs of vascular obstruction, tachycardia, dyspnea, gastrointestinal bleeding, heart failure, and shock	Platelets, fresh frozen plasma, other blood components; heparin may be prescribed	Avoid trauma. Handle gently. Give blood products and heparin as ordered. Monitor vital signs. Look for bleeding.
Superior vena cava syndrome	Breast or lung cancer, lymphoma, Kaposi's sarcoma, or metastatic testicular cancer that puts pressure on the superior vena cava; central venous catheter placement	Redness and edema of face, conjunctiva; distended neck and thoracic veins; dyspnea, cough, tachypnea, tachycardia, cyanosis progressing to increased intracranial pressure	Radiation therapy, stent placement, diuretic agents, steroidal agents	Give medications as ordered. Elevate head and arms but not legs. Tell patient not to bend forward. Reassure patient that symptoms usually subside in 2–3 days.
Spinal cord compression	Lung and breast cancers, lymphomas	Tumor in epidural space presses on spinal cord, causing intense pain, weakness, altered sensation in arms or legs, impaired bowel and bladder function	High-dose radiation, corticosteroid agents, chemotherapy for chemosensitive tumors, surgery to relieve pressure	Give analgesic agents as ordered. Assess for full bladder, constipation. Do neurologic checks on affected extremities.

IV, Intravenous.
From Lewis MA, Hendrickson AW, Moynihan TJ: Oncologic emergencies: pathophysiology, presentation, diagnosis, and treatment, *CA Cancer J Clin* 61(5):287–314, 2011.

Get Ready for the NCLEX® Examination!

Key Points

- Cancer is the second most common cause of death in the United States.
- Early diagnosis and treatment increase the chances of survival with many types of cancer.
- The risk of developing certain types of cancers, and dying from some cancers, varies with race and ethnicity.
- Cells that reproduce abnormally and in an uncontrolled manner form neoplasms that can be benign or malignant.
- Benign neoplasms do not spread to other parts of the body whereas malignant neoplasms invade nearby tissues and can form metastases in distant parts of the body.
- Tumors are classified by anatomic site, cell appearance and differentiation, and staging.
- Carcinogens are factors that appear to increase the risk for development of cancer.
- The seven warning signs of cancer are change in bowel or bladder habits, a sore that does not heal, unusual bleeding or discharge, thickening or a lump, indigestion or difficulty swallowing, obvious change in a mole or wart, and a nagging cough or hoarseness.
- A diagnosis of cancer is based on tissue studies, laboratory tests, endoscopic examinations, and radiologic and imaging procedures.
- Surgery is a common treatment for malignant tumors.
- Internal or external radiotherapy is used to treat cancer because malignant cells are more sensitive than normal cells to radiation.
- Chemotherapy is the use of chemical agents in the treatment of disease.
- Radiotherapy and chemotherapy have serious side effects and adverse effects, including bone marrow suppression, anorexia, alopecia, nausea and vomiting, and local inflammation.
- Most patients who receive internal radiation emit rays that can be harmful to others.
- Biotherapy acts directly on malignant cells and promotes the body's natural defenses against cancer.
- Patients who have suspected or confirmed cancer are under great stress and may respond with anger, irritability, fear, denial, or depression.
- In addition to helping with specific physical problems, nursing care of the patient with cancer addresses potential for injury, inability to manage self-care, inadequate coping, anxiety, grieving, altered family dynamics, altered body image, impaired oral tissue integrity, constipation, fatigue, and inadequate management of condition.

Additional Learning Resources

SG Go to your Study Guide for additional learning activities to help you master this chapter content.

Go to your Evolve website (http://evolve.elsevier.com/Linton/medsurg) for the following learning resources and much more:

- Fluid & Electrolyte Tutorial
- Review Questions for the NCLEX® Examination

Clinical Judgment and Next-Generation NCLEX® Examination-Style Questions

1. **Benign and malignant tumors are alike in that both:**
   1. Press on normal tissues and compete with normal cells for nutrients
   2. Usually grow very rapidly
   3. Invade nearby tissues or disperse cells to colonize distant parts of the body
   4. Contain cells that closely resemble the tissue of origin

   NCLEX Client Need: Physiological Integrity: Physiological Adaptation
2. A chemical, viral, or radioactive substance that can cause cancer is called a(n) ______________________.

   NCLEX Client Need: Health Maintenance: Disease Prevention
3. **The nurse is teaching a class on healthy living. Select the dietary recommendation(s) believed to reduce the risk of some cancers that should be included in the lesson plan. (Select all that apply.)**
   1. Limited alcohol consumption
   2. No dairy products or red meat
   3. High fiber, low fat, and low calories
   4. A variety of fruits and vegetables
   5. Limited smoked and nitrate-preserved foods

   NCLEX Client Need: Health Promotion and Maintenance: Disease Prevention
4. **A patient's blood level of the oncofetal antigen CA-125 has continued to rise during 6 months of chemotherapy for ovarian cancer. What is the most likely explanation?**
   1. The chemotherapy is effectively destroying the cancer cells.
   2. The patient is having an adverse response to the chemotherapy.
   3. The cancer is continuing to grow despite chemotherapy.
   4. The patient's immune system has been strengthened.

   NCLEX Client Need: Physiological Integrity: Reduction of Risk Potential
5. **When working with a patient who has an internal radiation source, safety precautions include which of the following? (Select all that apply.)**
   1. Always wear a lead apron when providing direct care to the patient with internal radiation.
   2. If the radiation source comes out of the patient's body, gloves should be worn to pick it up.
   3. When not providing direct care, stay at least 3 feet from the source.
   4. No pregnant visitors or staff should enter the patient's room.
   5. The patient must be in a private room.

   NCLEX Client Need: Safety and Infection Control: Handling Hazardous and Infectious Materials

6. **Adverse effects of radiation therapy commonly affect the bone marrow, hair follicles, and GI tract. What makes these tissues especially sensitive to the effects of radiation?**
   1. They have inadequate defenses against harmful substances.
   2. These tissues attract radioactive substances.
   3. These tissues have very poor circulation.
   4. These tissues regenerate rapidly.

   NCLEX Client Need: Pharmacological Therapies: Adverse Effects

7. **A patient asks why she is receiving a CSF as part of her cancer treatment. Which replies by the nurse are accurate? (Select all that apply.)**
   1. CSFs stimulate the production of WBCs by the bone marrow.
   2. With CSFs, the dosage of chemotherapy drugs can be reduced.
   3. CSFs reduce the risk of anemia that commonly occurs with chemotherapy.
   4. CSFs eliminate the need for bone marrow or stem cell transplantation.
   5. CSFs reduce the nausea and vomiting associated with chemotherapy.

   NCLEX Client Need: Pharmacological Therapies: Expected Effects

8. **To monitor patients who are taking antineoplastic drugs, the nurse must be aware that the *most dangerous* adverse effect is:**
   1. GI bleeding
   2. Increased intracranial pressure
   3. Bone marrow suppression
   4. Nausea and vomiting

   NCLEX Client Need: Pharmacological Therapies: Adverse Effects

9. **Which of the following describes the action of biotherapy (BRMs)?**
   1. Treat mental depression that is common during cancer treatment.
   2. Promote the body's natural defenses against cancer cells.
   3. Immunize patients against some types of cancer.
   4. Prevent the spread of cancer cells before metastasis occurs.

   NCLEX Client Need: Pharmacological Therapies: Pharmacological Actions

10. **Three patients at a urology clinic received diagnoses of prostate cancer. All were in an early stage and had similar expectations of cure. Mr. A. asked many questions and started to plan his work schedule around his treatments. Mr. B. stalked out of the office and slammed the door, saying that he would rather die than give up sex. Mr. C. was stunned and seemed unable to take in any more information at that time. Which of these patients' responses would be considered "normal" in this situation?**
    1. Mr. A.'s
    2. Mr. B.'s
    3. Mr. C.'s
    4. They are all normal reactions to grief.

    NCLEX Client Need: Psychosocial Integrity: Coping Mechanisms

11. **SLO/Objective:** Apply knowledge of anatomy and physiology and pathophysiology to determine which assessment data require follow-up from the nurse.

    NGN Item Type: Enhanced Hot Spot

    Cognitive Skill: Recognize Cues
    The home health nurse is visiting a patient who is being treated for lung cancer with chemotherapy and radiation. The focused assessment collected the data listed below. Highlight or place a check mark next to the assessment findings that require follow-up by the nurse.
    1. Blood pressure 176/92 mm Hg
    2. Pulse 72 beats per minute
    3. Respirations 18 breaths per minute
    4. Dry mouth
    5. Fatigue and weakness
    6. Darkly pigmented skin on upper chest and neck
    7. Strong peripheral pulses
    8. Lack of sensation in lower legs
    9. Nausea and anorexia
    10. Occasional diarrhea

    NCLEX Client Need: Pharmacological Therapies: Adverse Effects

12. **SLO/Objective:** Apply knowledge of side effects of radiation and chemotherapy to determine which laboratory values may be affected.

    NGN Item Type: Extended Multiple Response

    Cognitive Skill: Analyze Clues
    A cancer patient is being treated with chemotherapy and radiation. Which lab test results would the nurse expect to see? (Select all that apply.)
    1. Elevated white blood cells
    2. Increased oxygen saturation level
    3. Decreased hemoglobin
    4. Decreased red blood cells
    5. Decreased platelet count

    NCLEX Client Need: Pharmacological Therapies: Adverse Effects

13. **SLO/Objective:** Prioritize nursing care for patients receiving chemotherapy and radiation.

    NGN Item Type: Cloze

    Cognitive Skill: Prioritize Hypotheses
    A 42-year-old Hispanic woman is receiving chemotherapy after a right mastectomy for breast cancer. Assessment data include:
    1. Blood pressure 110/70 mm Hg
    2. Pulse 82 beats per minute
    3. Respirations 18 breaths per minute
    4. Dry mouth
    5. Fatigue and weakness
    6. Stomatitis
    7. Numbness and tingling of both legs
    8. Nausea and vomiting
    9. Bruises on arms and shins
    10. Decreased fluid intake
    11. Anorexia

    Choose the *most likely* options for the information missing from the statements below by selecting from the list of options provided.

The nurse recognizes that _____________ and ___________ are complications of chemotherapy and need to be closely monitored. Failure to recognize these conditions can most likely lead to ____________.

Options
Anorexia
Fatigue and weakness
Nausea and vomiting
Liver damage
Kidney failure
Dehydration

NCLEX Client Need: Pharmacological Therapies: Adverse Effects

14. **SLO/Objective:** Plan actions for clients for patients experiencing treatment for lung cancer.

NGN Item Type: Matrix

Cognitive Skill: Generate Solutions

A 56-year-old female is being treated with immunotherapy for metastatic cancer. The assessment data are as follows:

1. Blood pressure 130/70
2. Heart rate 80 beats per minute
3. Respirations 20
4. Temperature 101°F
5. Recent episodes of nausea and vomiting
6. Fatigue
7. Chills
8. Muscle aches and pains
9. Anxiety

Determine whether each nursing action below is indicated, contraindicated, or nonessential.

NURSING ACTION	INDICATED	CONTRA-INDICATED	NONESSENTIAL
Encourage patient to express feelings			
Suggest daily naps and mild exercise			
Advise antiemetics as ordered			
Encourage fluids as tolerated			
Apply ice packs to lower temperature			
Install elevated toilet seat			
Explore options for nursing home care			

NCLEX Client Need: Physiological Integrity: Basic Care and Comfort, Psychosocial Integrity: Stress Management, and Therapeutic Communication; Physiological Adaptation

15. **SLO/Objective:** Evaluate the effectiveness of nursing and collaborative interventions for patients experiencing end stage cancer.

NGN Item Type: Matrix

Cognitive Skill: Evaluate outcomes

A 76-year-old male diagnosed with end-stage cancer has elected not to continue curative treatment. He is being visited by a home health nurse who has recommended him for hospice care.

For each assessment finding, use an X to indicate whether the interventions were effective (helped to meet the expected outcomes), ineffective (did not help to meet expected outcomes), or unrelated (not related to the expected outcomes).

ASSESSMENT FINDING	EFFECTIVE	INEFFECTIVE	UNRELATED
Advance directive completed			
Pain under control			
Opioids discontinued to prevent addiction			
Family referred for bereavement care			
BMI – 18			

8 Pain

http://evolve.elsevier.com/Linton/medsurg

Objectives

1. Define pain.
2. Explain the physiologic basis for pain.
3. Explain the relationships between past pain experiences, anticipation, culture, anxiety, and a patient's response to pain.
4. Identify differences in the duration of pain and patient responses to acute and chronic pain.
5. Identify situations in which patients are likely to experience pain.
6. Explain the special needs of the older adult patient with pain.
7. List the data collected in assessing pain.
8. Describe interventions used in the management of pain.
9. Describe the nursing care of patients receiving opioid and nonopioid analgesics for pain.
10. List the factors that should be considered when pain is not relieved with analgesic medications.

Key Terms

acute pain
addiction
analgesia (ăn-ăl-JĒ-zē-ă)
analgesi (ăn-ăl-JĒ-zĭk)
anesthesia (ăn-ĕs-THĒ-zhă)
chronic pain
neuropathic (nŭ-rō-PĂTH-ĭk)
nociceptive (nō-sĕ-SĔP-tĭv)
nociceptor (nō-sĕ-SĔP-tĕr)
pain
pain threshold
pain tolerance
physical dependence
referred pain
tolerance (TŎL-ĕr-ăns)

Pain is one of the most complex experiences to understand and treat. It is also the most common problem that nurses encounter. Research about pain, **analgesics** (therapeutic agents for pain relief), and the mind-body influence is just beginning to filter down to nursing practice. Still, many questions about pain remain unanswered.

Pain is influenced by many variables: the individual experiencing it, the cause of the pain, and the environment. Pain may arise from a new source, from an old injury, or from nerve injury. The cause is sometimes unknown. Pain relief rests primarily with the nurse, who must assess the patient and implement appropriate interventions.

Nurses have many categories of pain-relieving interventions from which to choose, yet they frequently administer only analgesic drugs. Most nurses believe that pain is easily managed with analgesic drugs; however, patients often report that pain remains moderate to severe despite these medications. Research has found that nurses fail to assess pain, tend to under medicate for pain, and have inadequate knowledge of pain relief measures. Because of these findings, The Joint Commission published standards for the management of pain for all patients. Specific standards apply to various care settings. Health care facilities are expected to comply with these standards, which include (1) prioritizing pain assessment and pain management, including safe opioid prescribing, (2) involving staff in improvement activities related to quality of care and patient safety, (3) assessing and managing patient's pain while minimizing risks of treatment, and (4) collecting and analyzing data related to pain interventions. The purpose of this chapter is to enable the nurse to understand pain, assess pain, and provide the most effective interventions for pain relief.

DEFINITION OF PAIN

Pain is defined in many ways. The International Association for the Study of Pain (IASP) defines it as an unpleasant sensory and emotional experience associated with actual or potential tissue damage. IASP further states patient reports of pain not objectively attributable to tissue damage is still considered as pain. Margo McCaffery, a nurse and leader in the pain management field, has a more useful definition for nurses. She says, "Pain is whatever the person experiencing it says it is and exists whenever he says it does" (McCaffrey & Beebe, 1989, p. 7).

PHYSIOLOGY OF PAIN

Nociceptive pain occurs in response to various stimuli on pain receptors. The perception of pain involves afferent pathways, the central nervous system, and efferent pathways. Afferent (ascending) pathways are nerves that carry messages to the brain for interpretation. Efferent (descending) pathways are nerves that carry messages away from the brain to the rest of the body via the spinal cord.

Afferent pathways are activated by pain receptors called ***nociceptors***. These pain receptors are unevenly distributed in muscles, tendons, subcutaneous tissue, and the skin. This distribution may explain why parts of the body are more sensitive to pain than other parts. Pain receptors are sensitive to chemical changes, temperature, mechanical stimuli, and tissue damage. Some receptors are sensitive to more than one type of stimulus. When subjected to repeated stimuli, pain receptors may continue to react even after the stimuli are removed. With repeated stimulation to receptors over time, physical and chemical changes can occur in the pain pathways; therefore pain is still perceived after the original painful event or stimulus is removed.

When pain receptors are stimulated, impulses are transmitted to the spinal cord. The impulses then travel up the spinal cord to the brain. In the brain, the cortex interprets the impulses as pain and identifies the location and qualities of the pain. Other structures involved in the interpretation of pain signals activate the stress response and produce the unpleasant qualities associated with pain, such as fear. Once pain is transmitted to the spinal cord and brain, the descending pathway is activated and several substances (e.g., endorphins, serotonin, norepinephrine, gamma-aminobutyric acid, enkephalins) that can inhibit pain transmission to the spinal cord are released.

Endorphins and enkephalins are the body's natural opioid-like substances that block the transmission of painful impulses to the brain. Differences in the amount of endorphins in individuals may explain why some people seem to experience more pain than others. Research suggests that prolonged stress and pain, as well as the prolonged use of morphine and alcohol, decrease endorphin levels. Factors that increase endorphin levels include brief stress and pain, laughter, exercise, acupuncture, transcutaneous electrical nerve stimulation (TENS), massive trauma, and sexual activity.

The nature of neuropathic pain is different in that it is caused by a lesion or disease of the somatosensory nervous system. Numerous diseases may be involved with similar signs and symptoms. Pathophysiology is not fully understood at this time. Diabetic neuropathy is one of the more common types.

GATE CONTROL THEORY

Although many theories have been proposed to explain pain, none fully describes the pain experience. One of the best-known theories is Melzack and Wall's gate control theory. It assumes that the pain experience reflects both physical and psychosocial factors. Painful impulses are transmitted to the spinal cord through small-diameter nerve fibers in the afferent pathway. When these small-diameter fibers are stimulated, the gating mechanism opens in the spinal cord, which permits the transmission of impulses from the spinal cord to the brain. Consequently, the patient perceives pain. Factors that cause the gate to open include tissue damage, a monotonous environment, and fear of pain. These small-diameter fibers end in the spinal cord along with large-diameter fibers. The stimulation of large-diameter fibers can close the gate and interfere with impulse transmission between the spinal cord and the brain. This interference causes diminished pain perception. Large-diameter nerve fibers are stimulated by cutaneous (skin) stimulation through massage, position change, and heat or cold applications. Sensory input such as distraction, guided imagery, and preparatory information also may close the gate. Fig. 8.1 shows the structures and mechanisms associated with the gate control theory.

FACTORS INFLUENCING RESPONSE TO PAIN

Consider the following example: Miss Smith and Mrs. Johnson are roommates in Room 200. Miss Smith, 39 years of age, and Mrs. Johnson, 67 years of age, underwent the same surgical procedure on the previous day. The nurses discussed the difference in the behavior of each patient:

> *Miss Smith constantly wants more pain medication. She moans and groans all the time. She won't even turn, cough, or breathe deeply for more than 10 seconds. She always rates her pain as a 9 or a 10 on the pain scale. On the other hand, look at Mrs. Johnson. She's already ambulating. She rarely rates her pain as more than a 2 or a 3 on the pain scale. She usually just complains of aching and she sure doesn't ask for as much pain medication as Miss Smith. You'd never guess they had undergone the same procedure.*

This example illustrates that although people may have the same injury or insult (in this case, surgery), they may respond differently. This difference exists because many physical and psychosocial factors affect the response to pain. Health professionals should be nonjudgmental and avoid comparing one individual in pain with another individual in pain.

PHYSICAL FACTORS

Many physical factors influence the pain experience, including the individual's pain threshold, pain tolerance, age, physical activity, nervous system integrity, and, in cases of surgery, the type of surgery performed and the type of **anesthesia** (agents that induce a loss of sensation) used.

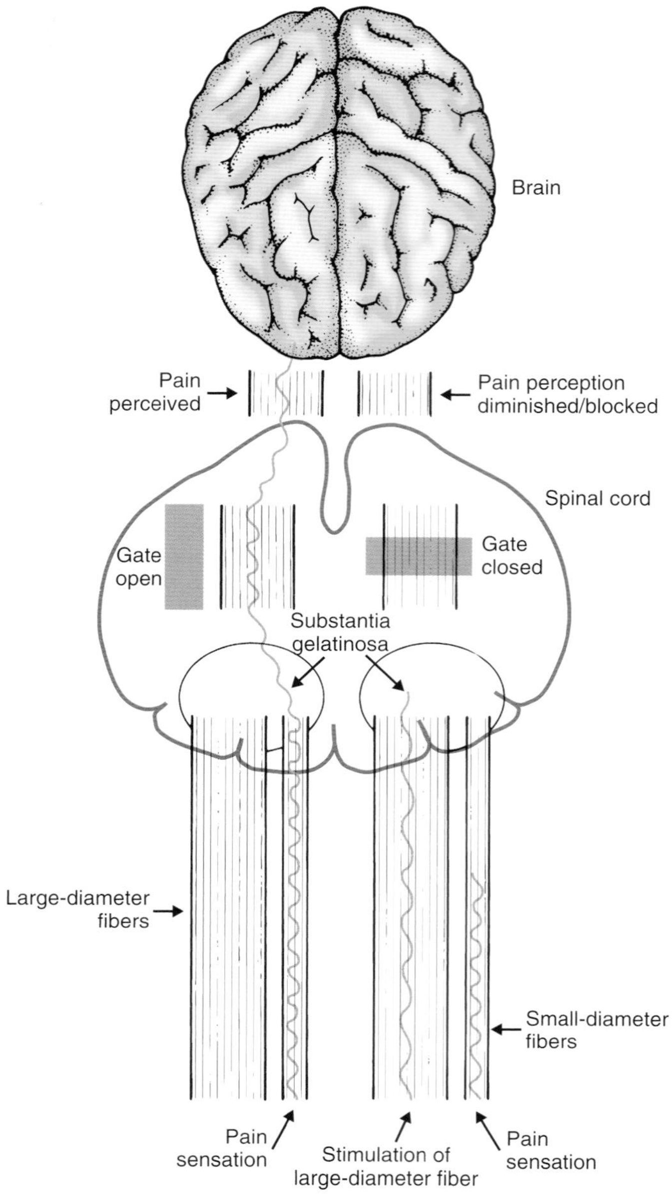

Fig. 8.1 The gate control theory of pain. (From Ignatavicius DD, Workman ML: *Medical surgical nursing: patient-centered collaborative care*, ed 6, St. Louis, 2010, Saunders-Elsevier.)

Pain Threshold

The **pain threshold** is the point at which a stimulus causes the sensation of pain. Anger, fatigue, anxiety, insomnia, depression, and uncontrolled pain all lower the pain threshold. With a lower threshold, the person experiences pain more readily with less stimuli. During hospitalization or illness, a patient may experience anxiety, fatigue, or loss of sleep, all of which can lower the pain threshold or cause the patient to experience pain more easily.

Pain Tolerance

Pain tolerance refers to the intensity of pain that a person will endure. It is another factor influencing response to pain. Pain tolerance varies among patients and varies for an individual patient, depending on the situation. Increasing or prolonged pain may lower the pain tolerance because the patient fears that the pain will not be relieved. Low pain tolerance or high pain tolerance must be respected and must not interfere with adequate pain management.

Age

Age may also influence response to pain. At times, older patients do not report their pain, or they report that their pain is much less severe than it really is. Some do not report pain because they are stoic, or they have been told incorrectly that pain is a normal part of aging. Some older patients may not want to bother the nurse, or they may fear rejection from the caregiver. Pain is not a normal part of aging, although older adults often suffer from chronic conditions such as arthritis, cancer, and bone fractures that are associated with pain.

Physical Activity and Nervous System Integrity

Physical activity and the integrity of the nervous system can also influence the reaction to pain. Physical activity may aggravate or precipitate pain. However, with some patients, physical activity may be used to relieve pain. Because pain is perceived and interpreted within the nervous system, the integrity of the system affects the response to pain. For example, patients with diabetic neuropathy may have peripheral nerve damage caused by high glucose levels. As a result, these patients may lose sensation in the extremities and may not feel pain, or they may feel burning sensations in their feet and legs at rest or with activity.

Surgery and Anesthesia

In surgical patients, the type of surgery and the type of anesthesia used can influence the response to pain. Surgery on the upper thoracic and abdominal regions of the body is thought to be the most painful because of the numerous tissues traumatized during the procedure. Within this group are cardiac, pulmonary, gastric, and gallbladder procedures. The type of anesthetic agent used can influence postoperative pain. For example, ketamine has analgesic and anesthetic properties. Some anesthetic agents injected at the operative site may prolong **analgesia** for 12 to 24 hours after surgery. When these types of agents are used, patients may experience much less pain after surgery than those who do not receive these anesthetic agents.

Surgery or invasive procedures may be performed to relieve pain that is severely debilitating; however, pain relief from these procedures may not be permanent because nerve tissue regenerates. These surgical procedures have been replaced by nerve-deadening procedures performed with localized heating (radiofrequency lesioning) or freezing techniques (cryoanalgesia) by pain specialists, usually done in outpatient settings. The goal of these procedures is to provide prolonged pain relief, and patients may report tingling or buzzing sensations instead of pain. Nerve blocks or injections of drugs into specific tissues or joints can reduce pain and improve function for acute pain and chronic pain. Drugs are injected to block the transmission of pain signals. For example, femoral anesthetic nerve blocks may be performed before hip replacement surgery to reduce postoperative pain up to 24 hours after surgery is completed, or a small catheter connected to a container with the anesthetic drug may be placed into the surgical wound before closure to provide continuous pain relief in the immediate postoperative period. Acupuncture is another invasive technique that produces anesthesia or analgesia. It is an ancient Chinese practice in which tiny needles are inserted into the skin or subcutaneous tissues at specific points on the body. This technique may be used to relieve acute and chronic pain such as headache, menstrual cramps, and low-back pain.

PSYCHOLOGIC FACTORS

Along with physical factors, several psychologic factors can influence the response to pain, including culture, religion, past experiences with pain, anxiety, and situational factors.

Culture, Ethnicity, and Gender

Although studies have been conducted to determine the effect of culture, ethnicity, and gender on people's reaction to pain, you should avoid making judgments based on how you think a person should react or behave. Some persons may deny pain, remain calm and unemotional, or withdraw. Other persons may cry, moan and groan, and involve their families in the painful experience. Be aware of the different ways of expressing pain and respect individual variations in the response to pain.

Religious Beliefs

Religious beliefs may also have an impact on reaction to pain. Some patients may pray and believe that divine intervention will help them to endure the pain. Others may view pain as a punishment for sins. Some individuals believe that suffering is required before pain relief can be obtained.

Past Experiences and Anxiety

Past experiences and anxiety may affect a person's response to current pain. A person may have developed positive coping strategies to deal with previous painful experiences. If, however, previous coping strategies were unsuccessful, the patient may be very anxious and overwhelmed by another painful experience.

Situational Factors

Finally, situational factors may influence response to pain. If the pain is associated with a serious illness such as cancer, the pain may have a greater impact on mood and activity than if the pain were associated with a less serious condition. The pain associated with childbirth is relatively short lived and usually results in a beautiful outcome, whereas cancer pain may be chronic and increasing and may be associated with progression of the disease and death.

Box 8.1 Autonomic Nervous System Responses to Pain

SYMPATHETIC NERVOUS SYSTEM RESPONSES
- ↑ Blood pressure
- ↑ Pulse rate
- ↑ Respiratory rate
- Dilated pupils
- Perspiration
- Pallor

PARASYMPATHETIC NERVOUS SYSTEM RESPONSES
- Constipation
- Urinary retention

Cultural Considerations

What Does Culture Have to Do With Pain?

The way a person behaves in response to pain is determined, in part, by cultural norms. Thus, people from some cultures quietly endure pain whereas people from other cultures loudly express their pain. As nurses, we must accept each response and assess and intervene to promote maximal comfort.

RESPONSES TO PAIN

AUTONOMIC NERVOUS SYSTEM

The pain signal is interpreted by the brain as a stressor. The autonomic nervous system activates the fight-or-flight response and certain physiologic responses are initiated. Box 8.1 indicates some of the responses that occur and the associated effects. The patient in pain may exhibit these physiologic responses, along with behaviors such as grimacing, moaning, and verbalizing pain or withdrawing. The nervous system responses can be measured by an increased heart rate, respiratory rate, and blood pressure. These reactions are possible responses to acute pain; however, the pain responses and behaviors will vary from individual to individual and are not reliable indicators of pain. Acute pain and chronic pain elicit different kinds of responses. Table 8.1 lists some differences between acute pain and chronic pain.

ACUTE PAIN

Most pain experienced in the hospital is **acute pain**. Acute pain follows the normal pathway for pain from nociceptor activation to the brain. Examples of nociceptive pain are postoperative pain from incisions, renal colic pain from kidney stones, bone fractures, and pain in childbirth. Acute pain is temporary, and its cause is known and treatable; it also serves as a

Table 8.1 Differences in Acute Pain and Chronic Pain

CHARACTERISTIC	ACUTE	CHRONIC
Time	Limited, short duration	Lasts 3–6 months, longer duration
Purpose	Sign of tissue injury	No purpose
Verbal	Reports pain, focuses on pain	No report of pain unless questioned
Behavioral	Restless, thrashing, rubbing body part, pacing, grimacing, and other facial expressions of pain	Tired looking, minimal facial expression, quiet, sleeps, rests, attention on other things
Physiologic	Increased heart rate, blood pressure, respiratory rate	Normal heart rate, blood pressure, respiratory rate
Interventions	Responds to analgesics	Less responsive to analgesics
	Standard doses effective for pain relief	Higher doses needed for pain relief
	Parenteral or oral route used	Oral route preferred
	Additional drugs (adjuvant) seldom needed to manage pain	Additional drugs often needed to manage pain

Table 8.2 Classification of Pain

CLASS	EXAMPLES
Acute pain	Appendicitis Kidney stone Tendonitis
Chronic noncancer pain	Low-back pain Rheumatoid arthritis Phantom limb pain Fibromyalgia
Cancer-related pain	Cancer pain syndromes (direct effect of tumor or cancer treatment), postchemotherapy pain, postradiation pain, spinal cord compression

warning of tissue damage and subsides when healing takes place. Nurses observe behavioral and physiologic signs of acute pain when the patient guards or rubs a body part, wrinkles the brow, bites the lip, and has changes in the heart rate, blood pressure, and respiratory rate. These responses may be absent or lessened in chronic pain.

CHRONIC PAIN

Chronic pain is usually defined as pain that persists or recurs for more than 3 to 6 months; it may last a lifetime. Chronic pain may be nociceptive like osteoarthritis or neuropathic pain, which follows an abnormal pathway for processing pain. Review Fig. 8.1. Nerve damage resulting from a wide variety of anatomic and physiologic conditions and underlying diseases is neuropathic pain. It causes unusual sensations such as burning, shooting pain, and abnormal sensations that occur when no painful stimulus is present. The cause of this pain is often unknown. Treatment may or may not be helpful in relieving the pain. Chronic pain has many classifications. Some chronic pain examples are shown in Table 8.2. Chronic pain is associated with a variety of diagnoses, including cancer, arthritis, peripheral vascular diseases, and traumatic injuries. It usually occurs daily and is not life threatening. Intractable pain is another term used to describe pain that cannot be relieved and has no known effective treatment.

Chronic noncancer pain is also defined as persistent pain that interferes with sleep and function, resulting in possible disability and loss of health and normal lifestyle. Although injury often initiates chronic pain, other factors may contribute to ongoing or persistent pain over time. This type of pain is usually best treated by pain specialists and multidisciplinary health care teams.

Many conditions common in older adults may be associated with chronic pain. Phantom limb pain, in which the patient still feels sensations and pain in the amputated limb, is an example of chronic neuropathic pain. It can be extremely debilitating if it is not recognized and treated early. Phantom limb pain may occur in any related body part that has been amputated or traumatized (e.g., amputation of the breast or leg). Several therapies may be used to reduce this type of pain (e.g., drugs, nerve block, surgical revision, physical therapy). Research indicates serotonin and norepinephrine reuptake inhibitors ([SNRIs], e.g., duloxetine venlafaxine), antiepileptics (e.g., gabapentin, pregabalin) and tricyclic antidepressants (e.g., amitriptyline) are most effective for reducing neuropathic pain. Second line drugs are lidocaine patches, tramadol, and capsaicin 8% patches. The third line options are strong opioids. Some other options for chronic pain include surgically implanted pumps for drugs, and epidural stimulators that can block pain impulses in the spinal cord.

CANCER-RELATED PAIN

Cancer-related pain may be considered acute and chronic pain. Cancer pain may be chronic pain if it lasts longer than 3 to 6 months. Cancer may also cause the development of new nociceptive pain when the cancer causes pressure or damage to tissue or nerves. This type would be acute pain. Pain related to cancer can be very complex because it may include a variety of

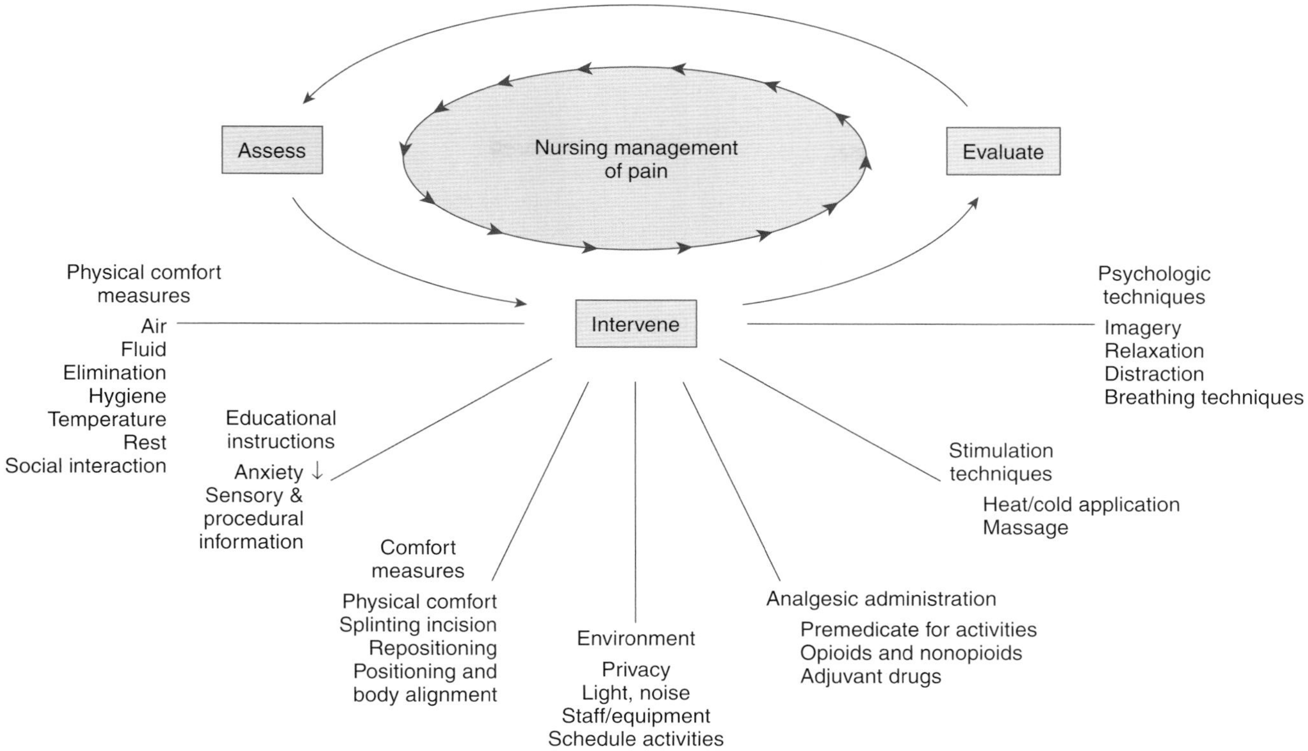

Fig. 8.2 Nursing management of pain.

pain problems that can be nociceptive or neuropathic (or both) and it may be caused by the treatment.

COMPARISON OF ACUTE PAIN AND CHRONIC PAIN

In contrast to acute pain, which warns of tissue damage and trauma, chronic pain serves no useful purpose. It can have a debilitating and destructive effect on a person's life. Chronic pain can lead to depression, marital difficulties, loss of self-esteem, immobility, and isolation. The patient in chronic pain often does not report pain and shows little facial expression or few physical signs of pain. When pain is chronic, adaptation may occur. The sympathetic nervous system adapts. The heart rate, blood pressure, and respiratory rate may not be elevated, and the patient may rest, sleep, or turn attention to other activities despite severe pain.

The nurse may underestimate the severity of the pain or undermedicate a patient with chronic pain. Nursing assessment of pain is essential to identify (1) the characteristics and intensity of pain, (2) whether the pain is chronic or acute, and (3) whether the patient has both acute pain and chronic pain at the same time. The patient who reports pain but shows no pain behaviors or physical symptoms experiences pain, but the patient may have learned other ways to deal with the pain, or the patient may be taking other medications that block the response of the sympathetic nervous system to pain. For example, some cardiac medications block increases in heart rate and blood pressure.

❖ NURSING CARE OF THE PATIENT IN PAIN

Pain management continues to be a challenge for every nurse. Every individual experiences pain differently and reacts to pain with a variety of physiologic and behavioral responses. Based on an accurate assessment of pain, the physician prescribes treatment and the nurse provides nonpharmacologic and pharmacologic measures together to provide pain relief. The nurse plays a key role by assessing, intervening, and evaluating the patient in pain. Fig. 8.2 shows the variety of interventions you can use to relieve pain.

FOCUSED ASSESSMENT

Assessment is the first step in pain management. Data collected by the licensed vocational nurse/licensed practical nurse (LVN/LPN) contribute to the complete and ongoing assessment. Assessment of pain should be performed on admission and on a regular basis. Anticipate pain as a result of procedures, surgery, or progression of a disease. Accurately record the assessment data and compare with previous information. This process permits evaluation of the pattern of pain and or the effectiveness of an intervention.

Assessing pain in some patients, especially older adults, can be difficult. Visual, speech, hearing, and motor impairments may limit the ability of older patients to communicate pain or to use scales to rate pain. Patients with cognitive impairment may be unable to report pain or recall pain sensations. Pain can

Box 8.2 Six Steps in Pain Assessment

1. Accept the patient's report.
2. Determine the status of the pain.
3. Describe the pain:
   a. Location
   b. Quality
   c. Intensity
   d. Aggravating and alleviating factors
4. Examine the site.
5. Identify coping methods.
6. Record the assessment, interventions, and evaluation of interventions.
   (Reassessment after interventions is important to document effectiveness.)

also cause confusion, irritation, and depression in older adults. Consider these aspects when assessing the older adult.

When the patient cannot communicate verbally, they may be able to point to or direct your attention to a location on a body diagram or pain intensity scale. You may also have to use family observations and patient behaviors to assess pain and pain relief in this type of situation. When the patient cannot report pain, you may have to perform a different assessment that includes observing for usual or unusual behaviors that may indicate pain. These behaviors are not specific to pain; therefore other causes of discomfort, such as fecal impaction or bladder infection, should be assessed as well.

The six steps in pain assessment are listed in Box 8.2 and are discussed in the following sections.

Accept the patient's report. The first step in pain assessment is to establish rapport with the patient and accept what the patient says about the pain. When possible, all information about pain should be obtained directly from the patient. The person in pain is the only authority on the pain; no one else can really describe how the pain feels. Accept the report in a nonjudgmental and caring manner. Obtain specific details about the pain and respond positively that action will be taken to relieve the pain.

The assessment of pain requires excellent therapeutic communication skills. Important attitudes are conveyed through verbal and nonverbal behaviors. Listen patiently without interruption, use eye contact, touch the patient, and repeat and clarify information in an unhurried manner to establish trust and obtain information. Do not compare one patient's report of pain with another's report because pain is an individual experience.

Determine the status of the pain. The second step in pain assessment is to determine whether the pain is a new occurrence or has been experienced before. Ask the patient if they have had this pain before and whether it was diagnosed by a health care provider. Based on the patient's responses and history, decide whether the pain is chronic in nature or acute pain that needs immediate treatment. For example, a patient who is recovering from a prostatectomy may suddenly have chest pain. The patient identifies this discomfort as the typical angina pain for which he has taken medication in the past. A similar patient with chest pain and no previous cardiac history should be seen by a health care provider immediately because this pain is a new pain that the patient has not had before. Although both patients need to be evaluated by a health care provider, an accurate nursing assessment is essential to determine the difference between these two types of pain and consequently the action to be taken.

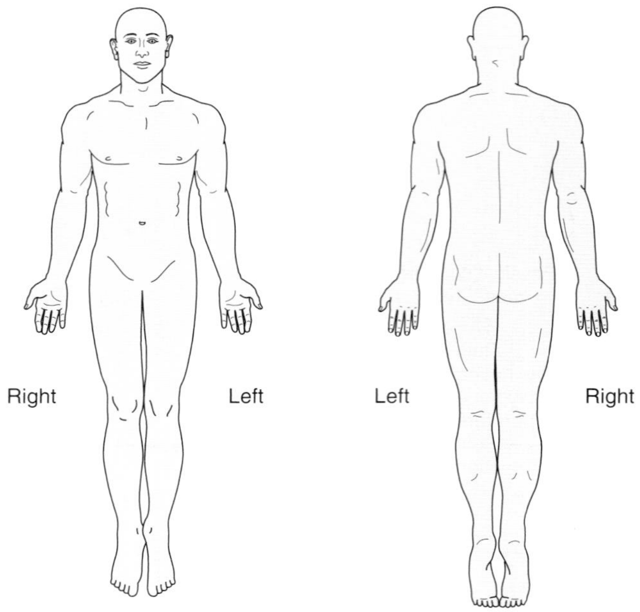

Fig. 8.3 Body diagram.

Describe the pain. The third step in pain assessment is to describe the pain in terms of its location, quality, intensity, and aggravating and alleviating factors.

Location. Have the patient describe where the pain is and point to the exact location with one finger. If more than one location of pain is described, use a body chart, as shown in Fig. 8.3. When possible, have the patient shade in or mark an X at the locations of pain. Then number the various locations on the body chart so that you can refer to the number rather than writing the exact location each time. Also, determine whether the pain is confined to one area or whether it starts at one place and moves to another.

The location identified as painful does not always correspond with the disease or operative site. For example, patients may experience back and neck spasms after surgical procedures. Another example is referred pain. **Referred pain** is often experienced in a location different from its source (Fig. 8.4). To illustrate, pain from appendicitis is usually felt around the umbilicus and is of the aching, cramping type. The pain impulses come from an inflamed appendix

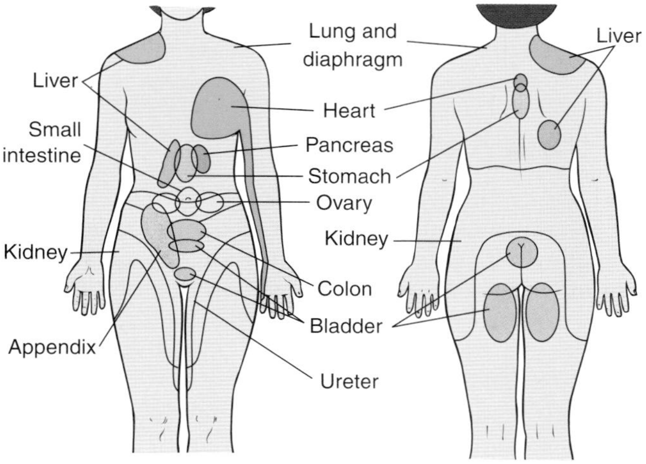

Fig. 8.4 Anterior and posterior referred pain sites. (From Heuther SE, McCance KL: *Understanding pathophysiology*, ed 5, St. Louis, 2012, Mosby-Elsevier.)

in the right lower quadrant of the abdomen, where sharp pain also may be experienced. Anginal pain is another type of referred pain. It is caused by lack of blood flow to the heart muscle and may be experienced as pain in the jaw, arm, and neck, as well as in the chest.

Quality. Ask the patient: "What words do you use to describe your pain?" or "What would you do to me to have me feel the pain you have?" If the patient has difficulty describing the pain, suggest words. Commonly used words are *sharp, dull, cramping, aching, gnawing, burning, heavy, tender,* and *throbbing*. However, allowing the patient to use their own words is best, and these exact words should be recorded in the medical record.

Intensity. Because pain is a subjective experience, nurses must have some way to measure the severity of pain. The purpose of asking about intensity is to put the patient's description into an objective term or number. To determine intensity, use one of the scales shown in Fig. 8.5. A simple descriptive scale uses words of varying intensity (e.g., mild, moderate, or severe). Some patients have difficulty with these words, and using words such as "a little pain," "a lot of pain," or "too much pain" may be better. A numeric scale can be 0 to 10 or 0 to 5, with 0 meaning "no pain" and the highest number meaning "the worst pain experienced." A "faces" scale with numbers rating intensity can also be used, and some adults prefer to use this type of scale. For example, the Wong-Baker FACES Pain Rating Scale was designed for children but can be used by older adults, some of whom are cognitively impaired. Because it has been translated into several languages, it may be appropriate for patients of various cultures as well.

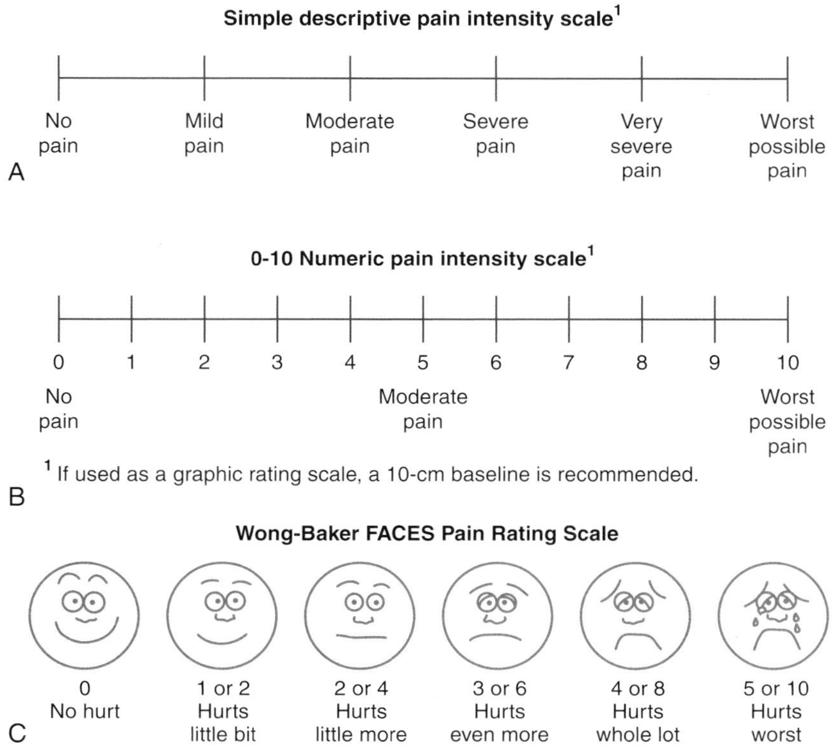

Fig. 8.5 Examples of pain intensity scales. (A) Simple descriptive pain intensity scale. (B) 0–10 numeric pain intensity scale. (C) Wong-Baker FACES Pain Rating Scale. (A and B, From Acute Pain Management Guidelines Panel: *Acute pain management: operative and medical procedures and trauma. Clinical practice guidelines* [AHCPR Publication No. 92-0052], Rockville, MD, 1992, Agency for Health Care Policy and Research, Public Health Service, U.S. Department of Health and Human Services. C, from Hockenberry MJ, Wilson D: *Wong's nursing care of infants and children*, ed 8, St. Louis, 2015, Mosby. Used with permission. Copyright Mosby.)

Explain the selected scale to the patient and ask, "Where would you rate your pain right now?" The scale used should make sense to the patient, be easy to use, and be consistently used with the same words or numbers. Remember to explain the scale to the patient each time that pain intensity is assessed. The advantage of using a scale is that it provides a personal measure of the patient's pain and allows evaluation of pain relief using a consistent measure. A scale that is meaningful to the patient and that can be used repeatedly requires less effort for the patient in pain.

For example, a 42-year-old man with multiple fractures in the right arm used the numeric scale from 0 to 10 for rating pain. The patient complained of throbbing in his right arm and a backache. He rated the intensity of both pains at 7 on the scale at 8:00 PM. The nurse applied heat to the lower back as ordered, massaged his back, and administered 10 mg of morphine orally. At 9:00 PM, the patient rated the intensity of both pains at 2 and stated that the pain was slowly going away. The nurse recorded this information and identified that the interventions were effective in relieving the pain in both locations because the pain intensity had decreased from 7 to 2 on the 0-to-10 scale. The nurse also noted that she would reassess the patient's pain every 2 hours. Pain that is not relieved should be reported to the nurse in charge.

Since 2001 The Joint Commission has published standards to improve pain management. This resulted in some hospital policies that set a number or "comfort goal" that automatically triggers pain intervention. For example, any pain rating 4 or above on the pain scale requires a nursing intervention for pain relief, because research has shown that a pain rating of 4 or above interferes with function and recovery. Reports after the initial 2001 standards revealed an overly aggressive pattern of pain interventions (particularly the increased use of opioids), resulting in serious adverse reactions. The American Society for Pain Management Nursing specifically denounces medicating based solely on pain scale intensity. The Joint Commission issued new recommendations for pain interventions in January 2021. The standards include recommendations that health care professionals (1) involve the patient in pain management discussions, (2) develop strategies for pain reduction that may include pharmacologic and nonpharmacologic interventions, (3) establish realistic and measurable goals with the patient, and (4) provide pain management education for health care professionals.

Aggravating and alleviating factors. Ask if any event or activity causes the pain or makes it better or worse. Ask: "What were you doing when the pain occurred?" Aggravating factors are those that make the pain worse. Certain positions, temperatures, or times of day or night may cause the pain to be more severe. Similarly, alleviating factors might include specific positions; application of heat, cold, or menthol; or physical activities that reduce pain in specific areas.

Patients can usually identify factors that aggravate or reduce pain and what specific pain relief methods have worked in the past. For example, four patients having abdominal surgery may have arthritic shoulder pain and have four different methods of reducing the pain. The first patient obtained relief with elevation and rest of the right arm. The second applied an analgesic balm, a menthol ointment. The third patient used a heating pad on the area, and the fourth increased the antiinflammatory drug dose as prescribed by the primary care provider.

Examine the Site of the Pain

The fourth step in the assessment of pain is to examine the location that the patient states is painful. Assess the area for heat, redness, swelling, tenderness, abnormal position, or other factors that may be causing local irritation.

Patients may identify a location of pain that is not expected as part of their medical problem. This pain location may be the result of a complication or an injury that was sustained during a procedure or hospitalization. For example, one patient who had undergone orthopedic surgery on the ankle had also sustained a large burn on his back at some time during the procedure. When the nurse examined the pain location, the burn was discovered. Another example is a patient who had undergone abdominal surgery and complained of pain in the right calf. Examination of the right calf revealed a red, firm, painful area that was reported to the health care provider and diagnosed as thrombophlebitis. When the exact location of the pain was examined, the correct cause of the pain could be identified.

Identify Coping Methods

The fifth step in pain assessment is to identify the patient's coping methods. People develop coping methods to increase control over pain or to relieve pain. Nurses should become aware of the methods that patients use to cope with pain and should support these coping methods. Some patients actively deal with pain. For example, they may complain and get up and move around or perform some other activity. Some patients cope by staying quiet, praying, sleeping, or withdrawing.

Nurses must emphasize to patients and their families that their cooperation and information are critical to achieving pain relief. Some patients expect nurses to know that they are experiencing pain and to know what to do about it. Confirm how the patient copes with pain by discussing observations of the patient's behavior with them. You can also suggest other coping methods that could be used to relieve pain (e.g., changing positions, imagery, distraction). Pain in older adults, especially those with cognitive deficits, can be difficult to evaluate. Boxes 8.3 and 8.4 offer guidelines for evaluating pain in cognitively impaired adults and

Box 8.3 Evaluating Pain in Cognitively Impaired Older Adults and Observing Pain Behaviors

- Ask the patient about pain first. Many patients who appear cognitively impaired may be able to answer yes/no questions about pain or complete a simple descriptive or numeric pain intensity scale.
- Ask family members and caregivers what particular behaviors indicate pain for the patient.
- Review the medical record to identify a past history of pain or diagnoses that are associated with pain.
- Examine the patient physically to identify potential sources of pain or common problems causing pain.
- Observe behaviors that may indicate pain for the patient. Observe the behaviors at rest and with activity. Note whether the behaviors change or improve when pain medication is administered. Assess, intervene, and evaluate behaviors again after intervention.

Box 8.4 Common Pain Behaviors in Cognitively Impaired Older Adults

FACIAL EXPRESSION
Frown, grimace, rapid blinking, wince, clenched teeth, narrowed eyes

SOUNDS
Sighing, moaning, groaning, calling out, noisy breathing, cursing during movement

BODY MOVEMENT
Rigid, tense body posture, fidgeting, pacing, gait changes, rocking, rubbing affected area

CHANGES IN INTERACTIONS WITH OTHERS
Aggressive, striking out, resisting care, withdrawn, decreased social interactions

CHANGES IN ACTIVITY PATTERNS OR ROUTINES
Refusing food, appetite changes, sleep or rest pattern changes, increased wandering

MENTAL STATUS CHANGES
Crying, increased confusion, irritability, distress

list common pain behaviors that are likely to be observed in such patients.

Document Assessment Findings and Evaluate Interventions

The sixth and last step in the pain assessment is to record the information in the patient's medical record so that this information can be conveyed to nurses on other shifts and to other health care professionals. Record the location, quality, and intensity of the pain; related factors; and how the patient copes with pain. Document the interventions provided and their effectiveness. Include the intensity of the pain after the intervention. If the nursing intervention was not effective in relieving the pain or reducing pain to an acceptable comfort goal, record what intervention was performed and report this to the charge nurse. This reassessment of pain after intervention is an important step in complying with The Joint Commission's standard about pain management.

Among the patient problems that often accompany pain are:

- Immobility
- Anxiety
- Constipation (especially if taking an opioid)
- Sleep disturbance
- Fatigue
- Discomfort

Put On Your Thinking Cap!

Think of one of your patients who had pain. Discuss with your classmates how you knew that the patient had pain. Compare and contrast how different patients expressed pain, the interventions that were used for pain control, and the effectiveness of these interventions.

Patient Problems, Goals, and Outcome Criteria: Patients in Pain

Patient Problems	Goals and Outcome Criteria
Acute pain related to tissue injury (e.g., surgery, laceration, contusion)	Pain relief: Patient states pain is relieved, has relaxed manner
Chronic pain related to condition (e.g., arthritic joint inflammation, spinal injury, cancer)	Pain reduction or relief: Patient states pain is lessened or relieved, has relaxed manner

INTERVENTIONS

Nonpharmacologic Interventions

Nonpharmacologic interventions are those that do not use drugs. They include a wide range of physical and psychologic interventions for pain relief (Table 8.3). Physical interventions usually involve comfort measures, adjusting the patient's environment, and cutaneous application techniques such as heat or cold. Psychologic interventions include unconditionally accepting the patient's pain report and providing information about pain, analgesics, and procedures or psychologic strategies such as relaxation and imagery. These types of interventions should be used along with analgesics to obtain optimal pain relief.

Physical comfort measures. These nursing interventions focus on the patient and the environment. Comfort may increase pain tolerance and the patient may experience less pain. Because adequate air, food and fluid, elimination, mobility, hygiene, temperature, and rest and sleep are essential to comfort, monitor these areas for potential problems. For example, patients who are sleep deprived or fatigued may have

Table 8.3 Nonpharmacologic Interventions for Acute Pain

INTERVENTION	COMMENTS
Physical	
Heat, cold, massage, transcutaneous electrical nerve stimulation (TENS)	Increase pain threshold, reduce muscle spasm, and decrease congestion in injured area. Effective in reducing pain and improving physical function. Some techniques require skilled personnel and special equipment. May be useful as adjuncts to drug therapy.
Psychologic	
Relaxation	
Jaw relaxation Progressive muscle relaxation	Effective in reducing mild to moderate pain and as an adjunct to analgesic drugs for severe pain.
Simple imagery	Use when patients express an interest in relaxation. Requires 3–5 minutes of staff time for instructions.
Music	Both patient-preferred and "easy listening" music are effective in reducing mild to moderate pain.
Imagery	Effective for reduction of mild to moderate pain. Requires skilled personnel.
Educational instruction	Effective for reduction of pain. Should include sensory and procedural information and be aimed at reducing activity-related pain. Requires 5–15 minutes of staff time.

Modified from Acute Pain Management Guidelines Panel: *Acute pain management: operative and medical procedures and trauma. Clinical practice guidelines* (AHCPR Publication No. 92-0032), Rockville, MD, 1992, Agency for Health Care Policy and Research, Public Health Service, U.S. Department of Health and Human Services.

increased pain. Therefore, providing for uninterrupted sleep and periods of rest can enhance pain relief.

For some patients in pain, progressive exercise or immobility may be prescribed as a treatment for pain. The patient with an injury or incision should be moved carefully so that further trauma is avoided. Turning the patient carefully from side to side or supporting an affected extremity during activity can reduce pain. The patient can usually describe which movements or positions increase or decrease the pain.

Assist and teach patients how to splint abdominal and thoracic wounds to minimize pain when deep breathing, coughing, and ambulating. A change of bed linen and sheets free of wrinkles can be refreshing and reduce irritation of the skin. Apply ointment to cracked lips and provide ice chips for a dry mouth. Any tubes or equipment attached to the patient should be secure but should not produce tension on the skin. Correct body alignment and frequent changes of position will relieve monotony, increase circulation, and prevent muscle contractures and spasms, which aggravate pain.

Environmental control. Each patient has individual preferences that affect comfort. Some patients prefer an active environment in which they can be distracted from pain. Listening to audio recordings or music on the radio, browsing internet sites, watching television, working with the hands, walking around, or visiting with others allows a person to focus attention on stimuli other than the pain sensation. On the other hand, the lights, noise, and constant activity of the hospital environment often cause sensory overload for the patient in pain, which can increase pain. In this event, coordinate with staff to promote a quiet environment with nonglaring lights and scheduled rest and activity periods that meet the patient's needs.

Stimulation techniques. Stimulation of the skin and underlying tissues relieves pain. Various types of skin or cutaneous stimulation can be applied and each type has variable effects. These techniques are not curative; rather, they can decrease the intensity of pain or change the sensation so that it is more acceptable. The exact mechanism for pain relief is unknown, but the belief is that superficial stimulation may block the transmission of pain impulses to the brain. Applications of heat, cold, massage, and TENS are examples of cutaneous stimulation. TENS applies external electrical stimulation of the skin and underlying tissues through electrodes attached to a small unit that the patient can carry around. The electrodes are placed over, above, or below painful sites and attached to a battery-operated device that delivers low-voltage electrical currents to block the pain signals. Numerous other products are sold as pain relief devices. Patients should consult their health care provider to select appropriate and safe devices with evidence of effectiveness. Products that use stimulation tend to be most effective for mild to moderate pain, well-localized pain, and acute and chronic pain. The effects of these therapies last as long as or slightly longer than the application.

The application of heat or cold may be prescribed for pain. Heat or cold is used to reduce muscle spasm and decrease congestion or swelling in an injured area. Either therapy may be applied to the painful site, at a location beyond the site, between the site and the brain, or on the opposite side of the body. These therapies should be applied intermittently, not continuously. Heat and cold may be alternated. Both therapies should be applied at a temperature that is comfortable for the patient, and the patient's skin and circulation should be monitored frequently.

Cold may be applied with ice packs or cooling pads to decrease initial tissue injury and swelling (e.g., with musculoskeletal sprains or orthopedic procedures). Cold is contraindicated for patients with peripheral vascular disease or heart disease because it may cause further vasoconstriction of blood vessels and thus decrease circulation. Cold application should be limited to 15 minutes per session to prevent tissue injury or frostbite.

Moist or dry heat can be applied with heating pads, hot-water bottles, towels, gel packs, or warm tub baths or showers. Superficial heat has been shown to be effective for gastrointestinal cramps and muscle and joint pain. Treatment should be limited to 30 minutes to prevent tissue injury. Heat should not be applied to a site of malignancy, to areas of decreased sensation or circulation, or to patients who cannot communicate their discomfort.

Massage involves rubbing, kneading, manipulating, and applying pressure and friction to the body. Rubbing or massaging an area is a natural response when one has an injury or ache. Massage may be used to promote relaxation and relieve muscle cramps. Massage is commonly applied to the back, neck, and large leg muscles; however, massage of the hands and feet is more easily performed and perhaps more effective. Massage should not be applied to areas with injury, phlebitis, or skin lesions or to patients with bleeding problems.

Cold, heat, and massage are easy to apply, inexpensive, effective, and simple for the patient or family to learn. For each therapy, evaluate whether the method or location of application is effective and monitor for any side effects.

Psychologic Interventions

Anxiety reduction. Anxiety, fear of the unknown, and feelings of loss of control may be related directly to the level of pain experienced. The patient who is anxious and uncertain will tend to rate pain high. If the nurse can increase the predictability and control of painful stimuli, pain may be reduced. An important aspect of relieving anxiety associated with pain is the relationship between the nurse and the patient. The nurse can be with the patient, assure the patient that everything possible is being tried, and provide timely and appropriate interventions for pain relief.

Several strategies are used to decrease anxiety and increase control. Telling the patient about events and providing descriptions of the sensations or feelings that may accompany the event can reduce anxiety. However, some patients may prefer not to know this information, and their wishes should be respected. Allowing the patient to choose physical comfort measures and the time for treatments also provides control.

Preoperative teaching should include skills to help patients cope with their pain, such as breathing, relaxation, or imagery techniques. Providing strategies to help the patient cope with pain and anxiety also provides the patient with a sense of control. The Health Promotion box describes a sample relaxation exercise, one of the psychologic interventions used for pain relief.

Health Promotion

Sample Relaxation Exercise: Slow, Rhythmic Breathing

1. Breathe in slowly and deeply.
2. As you breathe out slowly, feel yourself beginning to relax; feel the tension leaving your body.
3. Now breathe in and out slowly and regularly at whatever rate is comfortable for you. You may wish to try abdominal breathing. If you do not know how to do abdominal breathing, ask your nurse for help.
4. To help you focus on your breathing and to breathe slowly and rhythmically, do the following:
   a. Breathe in as you say silently to yourself, "in, two, three."
   b. Breathe out as you say silently to yourself, "out, two, three."
   c. Each time you breathe out, say silently to yourself a word such as "peace" or "relax."
5. You may imagine that you are doing this in a position and a place you have found very calming and relaxing, such as lying on a beach in the sun.
6. Perform steps 1 through 4 only once or repeat steps 3 and 4 for up to 20 minutes.
7. End with a slow, deep breath. As you breathe out, say to yourself, "I feel alert and relaxed."

ADDITIONAL POINTS

If you intend to perform this exercise for more than a few minutes, try to get into a comfortable position in a quiet environment. You may close your eyes or focus on an object. This technique has the advantage of being very adaptable in that it may be used for only a few seconds or for up to 20 minutes.

Modified from McCaffery M, Beebe A: *Pain: clinical manual for nursing practice*, St Louis, 1989, Mosby.

Distraction. Distraction refers to focusing on stimuli other than pain. Distraction may help the patient to gain a sense of control, as well as increase pain tolerance, decrease pain intensity, and alter the quality of pain, but it does not eliminate pain. Because the pain is not eliminated, the patient will usually need analgesics and other methods of pain relief. A patient using distraction such as watching a movie or interacting on social media apps may not appear or behave as if in pain, which may cause other people to doubt that the pain exists. After a patient has used a distraction technique, they may once again focus on the pain and experience a heightened awareness of pain.

Distraction techniques are often most helpful with mild to moderate pain or during brief periods of pain associated with painful procedures such as dressing changes, intramuscular injections, and venipunctures. Examples of distraction methods include rhythmic breathing, listening to music, laughing, counting, watching television, reading, exercising, resting, talking on the telephone, and visiting with others. Older adults may find reminiscing (relating past experiences) to be an effective distraction technique. Including several distraction techniques in the plan of care is helpful so that the patient can choose the methods most effective for their individual pain relief.

Relaxation. Patients should be aware that relaxation is one of the options for pain relief. Patients may already know this technique or may be taught relaxation techniques. Be aware that the patient is using relaxation, know the rationale for using relaxation, and know the effects of relaxation.

Relaxation is a cognitive approach to pain management. It is a self-hypnotic technique that may, but does not always, produce the relaxation response. The relaxation response counteracts the stress response. It is characterized by decreased muscle tension, a decreased heart rate, a decreased respiratory rate, and normal or decreased blood pressure. Relaxation decreases mental stress and physical tension; this exercise is helpful because pain is often accompanied by increased anxiety and muscle tension. Relaxation is usually more effective for mild to moderate pain than for severe pain.

Rhythmic breathing is a relaxation technique that focuses on just breathing, as described in the Health Promotion box. Relaxation techniques that focus on body relaxation require the patient's active participation. Progressive muscle relaxation techniques suggest that each part of the body is deliberately relaxed, usually in an orderly sequence, such as head to toe or vice versa. Relaxation often involves breathing exercises combined with other methods to promote freedom from anxiety and muscle tension. Methods may include yoga, meditation, and music.

The patient may be taught relaxation through coaching by the nurse, the use of a script, or an audio relaxation exercise. Emphasize to patients that the use of relaxation does not indicate that the pain is thought to be psychologic or that the patient must substitute relaxation for analgesics. Relaxation is a technique to be used in addition to analgesics to enhance pain control and reduce anxiety that contributes to pain.

Imagery. Imagery is another cognitive approach to pain control that encourages physical and mental relaxation. Imagery uses a person's imagination to help control pain. Besides promoting relaxation, imagery may be used for distraction or may help the patient to imagine pain relief.

Patients are asked to describe the quality of pain they are experiencing. Based on this description, imagery can be used to modify the patient's experience. For example, if the pain is described as "burning," an image of something cool may help to reduce pain intensity. As with relaxation, the use of imagery does not mean that medical personnel view the pain as imaginary. In both relaxation and imagery, a script or a recorded tape may be used to guide the patient through the experiences. Encourage the patient to practice relaxation or imagery, or both, to evaluate their potential effectiveness.

Complementary and Alternative Therapies

Massage and relaxation with music or imagery are examples of complementary therapies that can be used with analgesics to obtain optimal pain relief.

Pharmacologic Interventions

Drug therapy continues to be the mainstay of pain management. Although the medication orders include analgesics, the nurse is responsible for assessing the pain to decide which analgesic and how much to administer and evaluating the drug's effectiveness.

When administering analgesics, you need to use a preventive approach to pain management. When pain is predictable, such as with postoperative pain and cancer pain, analgesics are more effective when given around the clock (ATC) rather than as needed (PRN). An ATC schedule maintains therapeutic blood levels of the analgesics. With a PRN schedule, the patient may have frequent periods of unrelieved pain and more significant and frequent side effects, such as sedation. If an analgesic is ordered every 3 to 4 hours PRN, you should assess the patient's pain at least every 3 to 4 hours to determine the need for the analgesic. This avoids gaps in pain relief experienced by the patient on a PRN schedule.

When pain is unpredictable, administering analgesics on a PRN basis may be appropriate. In these situations, instruct the patient to request medication as soon as the pain begins rather than wait for the pain to become more severe. Patients often report that they wait to call for analgesics, thinking that the pain will decrease with time. Unfortunately, waiting often results in pain reaching an intensity level that is difficult to control.

The three categories of drugs that are used to relieve pain are (1) nonopioid analgesics, (2) opioid analgesics, and (3) adjuvant drugs. Fig. 8.6 shows how these categories of drugs are used by themselves or in combination to relieve mild, moderate, and severe pain.

Nonopioid analgesics. Nonopioid analgesics include aspirin, acetaminophen, and nonsteroidal antiinflammatory drugs (NSAIDs) such as ibuprofen. The nonopioids are generally the initial treatment choice for mild pain. These analgesics may also be combined with opioids to control moderate to severe pain.

Nonopioid analgesics act mostly on the peripheral nervous system and are used for pains such as arthritic pain, backache, headache, dysmenorrhea, postoperative pain, cancer pain, and bone pain. Nonopioids may

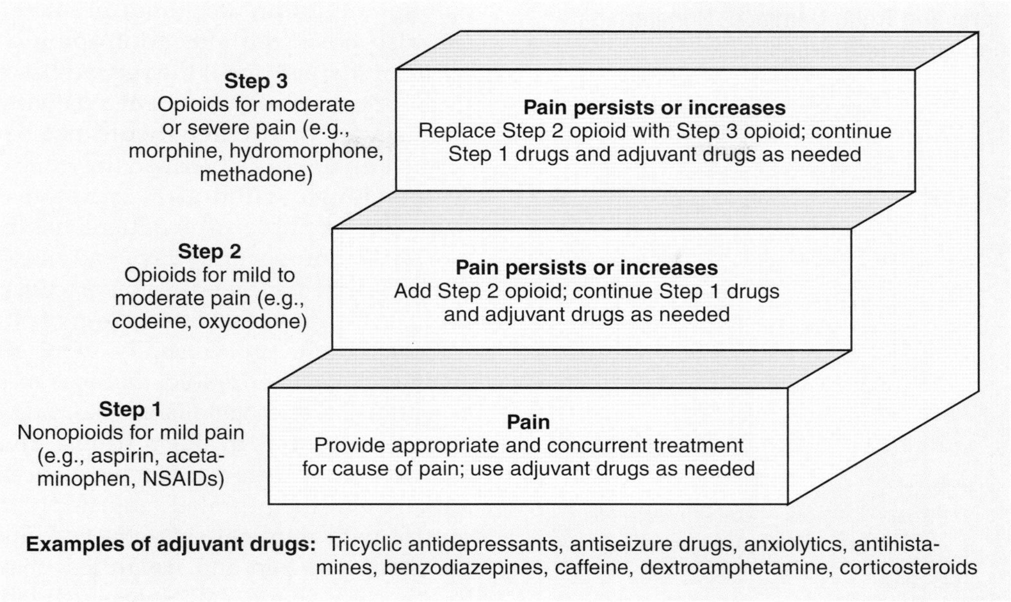

Fig. 8.6 The three-step analgesic ladder for cancer pain. *NSAID*, Nonsteroidal antiinflammatory drug. (From Lewis SM, Heitkemper MM, Dirksen SR: *Medical-surgical nursing: assessment and management of clinical problems*, ed 5, St. Louis, 2000, Mosby-Elsevier.)

have antipyretic (fever-reducing), analgesic (pain-reducing), or antiinflammatory (inflammation-reducing) properties. This range of actions makes them especially useful for many conditions.

Most of the nonopioids are oral preparations, but a few are available for rectal administration. Transdermal patches (diclofenac, ketoprofen, capsaicin) may be used for acute musculoskeletal pain. A parenteral NSAID, ketorolac (Toradol), also is available. It is generally used for the short-term management of postoperative pain. Ketorolac has a longer duration of action than many of the opioid analgesics and, as with other NSAIDs, can cause nausea and possibly bleeding.

The nonopioids, unlike the opioids, have a ceiling effect on analgesia. This property means that, beyond a certain dose, improved analgesia will not occur and toxicity may occur. The NSAIDs have side effects, including stomach irritation, fluid retention, increased bleeding time, and increased risk of cardiovascular events (heart attack and stroke). Therefore, they are usually not recommended for patients with heart disease, liver or kidney disorders, thrombocytopenia, or neutropenia (thrombocytopenia is a deficiency of platelets in the blood. Neutropenia is a decreased percentage of neutrophils, the white blood cells that respond to inflammation.) Some nonopioids should be used cautiously in patients with congestive heart failure or hypertension because they cause fluid retention, which may aggravate these conditions. Because nonopioids have many side effects, you should assess the patient's history and present condition before administering prescribed analgesics. Some patients have better pain relief with certain types of nonopioids compared with others. You should ask which nonopioids work best to relieve their pain.

Table 8.4 identifies commonly used NSAIDs and some considerations to keep in mind when administering these drugs. Older adults may be more sensitive to NSAIDs and may experience more side effects. Carefully monitor each patient's reaction to the analgesic. Older adults especially should be monitored for signs of increased bleeding time, gastrointestinal irritation, and unusual drug reactions such as confusion, constipation, and headaches. Experts agree that some drugs should be avoided in older adults because of the high risk of side effects (e.g., propoxyphene, meperidine, indomethacin, ketorolac, and promethazine).

Many nurses forget to administer nonopioids because they fail to recognize the importance of using these drugs for the types of mild to moderate pain mentioned previously. The nonopioids can be administered along with opioids and may be as effective as lower doses of opioids. Nonopioids tend to block pain transmission peripherally whereas opioids block pain transmission in the central nervous system. Administering both for pain relief is advantageous.

Pharmacology Capsule

The adverse effects of nonsteroidal antiinflammatory drugs include stomach irritation, fluid retention, and increased bleeding time.

Opioid analgesics. Opioid analgesics are generally used for moderate to severe acute pain, chronic cancer pain, and some other types of pain. The opioids vary in potency and duration of action.

Table 8.4 Generic and Trade Names of Nonsteroidal Antiinflammatory Drugs

GENERIC NAME	TRADE NAMES
Salicylates	
Aspirin	Many
Propionic Acid Derivatives	
Fenoprofen	Nalfon
Flurbiprofen	Generic
Ibuprofen	Advil, Motrin, others
Ketoprofen	Generic
Naproxen	Aleve
Oxaprozin	Daypro
Others	
Diflunisal	Dolobid
Diclofenac	Voltaren, Cambia, Cataflam, Arthrotec (combination with misoprostol)
Etodolac	Generic
Indomethacin	Indocin
Ketorolac	Generic
Meclofenamate	Generic
Mefenamic acid	Ponstel, Ponstan
Meloxicam	Mobic, Mobicox
Nabumetone	Generic
Piroxicam	Feldene
Sulindac	Clinoril
Tolmetin	Generic
COX-2 Inhibitors	
Celecoxib	Celebrex

From Burchum JR, Rosenthal LD: *Pharmacology for* nursing *care*, ed 10, St. Louis, 2019, Elsevier.

Currently, the two types of opioid analgesics are:

- Pure opioid agonists. Examples include codeine, methadone (Dolophine), hydromorphone (Dilaudid), meperidine (Demerol), morphine, and fentanyl.
- Opioid agonist-antagonists. Examples include buprenorphine (Buprenex), nalbuphine, butorphanol, and pentazocine (Talwin).

Both types of opioids relieve pain at the level of the central nervous system. Agonist drugs fit into receptor sites on the cell to "turn on" the site and produce the drug effect. Antagonists are drugs that block drug effects at the receptor sites. Opioid agonists bind to opioid receptors to produce analgesia but also bind to other receptors to produce unwanted side effects such as decreased respiration, drowsiness, and nausea. Opioid agonist-antagonists are drugs designed to produce analgesia and block certain side effects. The agonist-antagonists block some of the effects of the pure opioid agonists in much the same way that naloxone (Evzio, Narcan) acts to block or reverse the effects of opioids. Drugs classified as agonist-antagonists (e.g., pentazocine, nalbuphine, buprenorphine) produce analgesia but can also block the effects of opioids such as morphine or meperidine if the patient has been receiving these drugs. Thus, a patient receiving pure opioid agonists for pain relief should not be given opioid agonist-antagonists because they may block analgesia, precipitate withdrawal symptoms, and increase pain. For example, if a patient has been receiving morphine for several days, administering nalbuphine would not be advisable because it may block some of the analgesic effects of morphine.

Older adults are generally more sensitive to the analgesic effects of opioids because of delayed excretion and slower metabolism. Also, side effects may be more pronounced in older adults. Thus, the recommended adult dose should be reduced 25% to 50% initially and then titrated (adjusted) for optimal pain control with minimal side effects. Some older adults are small and thin and weigh less than 100 pounds. In this case, charts with recommended opioid doses for adults and children weighing less than 50 kg or less than 110 pounds are available. When patients are changed from parenteral to oral opioids, the prescriber must adjust the dosage. Oral doses must be larger than parenteral doses of the same drug to achieve the same effect, largely because oral opioids must pass through the liver after absorption, which reduces the amount of medication absorbed.

Meperidine (Demerol) use for moderate to severe pain has declined because it may cause central nervous system toxicity. You should be aware that one of the products of meperidine metabolism is normeperidine, which is a central nervous system stimulant. When this metabolite accumulates in the body, the patient may exhibit anxiety, twitching, tremors, muscle jerking, and generalized seizures. This opioid is contraindicated for long-term administration, specifically over 48 hours, and for patients who have diminished renal function. Meperidine should be avoided in older adults because they often have decreased renal function.

Nonpharmacologic therapy and nonopioid pharmacologic therapies are both preferred for the treatment of acute pain and chronic pain unrelated to cancer, palliative care, or end-of-life care. Frank discussions between the patient and the prescriber are needed to establish realistic goals for pain relief before beginning opioid therapy. If an opioid is prescribed, a plan for monitoring both prescription and illicit drug use must be in place. The plan must also include strategies to reduce the use of opioid medications and a time frame for discontinuing them. When opioids are used for acute pain, no more than 3 to 7 days of medication should be prescribed. Again, nonpharmacologic therapies and nonopioid pharmacologic therapies are effective pain relief interventions and serve an additional role as effective means to avoid opioid misuse and addiction.

Box 8.5 Characteristics of Tolerance, Physical Dependence, and Addiction

TOLERANCE
- Physiologic changes that occur from repeated doses of opioids
- *Result*: Higher doses are needed to achieve pain relief.

PHYSICAL DEPENDENCE
- Physiologic changes that occur from repeated doses of opioids
- *Result*: Withdrawal symptoms (e.g., irritability, chills, sweating, nausea) may occur if the opioid is stopped abruptly.

ADDICTION
- Psychologic dependence characterized by continued craving for opioid for other than pain relief
- *Result*: Compulsive and continued use for psychic effects despite harm.

NOTE: Risk of addiction is not a concern in treating acute pain or cancer pain.

Pharmacology Capsule

Older adults are more sensitive to opioid analgesics and should be monitored frequently for side effects.

Misconceptions about opioid analgesics. When discussing opioid analgesics, a few terms should be reviewed that are often misunderstood, resulting in undertreatment of pain. Patients, families, nurses, and physicians have misconceptions about **addiction**; therefore, the term must be defined and differentiated from ***tolerance*** and ***physical dependence***. Box 8.5 contains information about these terms. Tolerance and physical dependency may occur when patients are prescribed opioids over an extended period of time for chronic pain related to cancer, palliative care, or end-of-life care. The patient who is tolerant requires higher doses of a drug to achieve an analgesic effect. The patient who is physically dependent on an opioid will experience unpleasant withdrawal symptoms when the opioid is stopped. Both tolerance and physical dependence are commonly encountered responses to continued opioid administration for chronic pain relief; they do not lead to a craving for the drug for its mind-altering effects.

Patients who are at a higher risk for substance misuse (taking a substance in a way other than intended) or patients who have a history of addiction still require nonjudgmental treatment for pain. Patients who are younger, experience major depression, and are prescribed psychotropic medications along with opioids are at a higher risk of misusing opioids. Patients in these categories are best managed by a team that includes a pain management specialist.

Routes of administration. The opioids can be administered through various routes, depending on the needs of the patient. If tolerated, the oral route is preferred, especially for patients with chronic pain. Oral opioids can control severe pain when given in adequate dose levels.

Although not the recommended route, the intramuscular route may be used to administer opioids for breakthrough pain, that is, pain that occurs between regularly scheduled doses of pain medication. Breakthrough pain would require immediate-acting or short-acting analgesic medication, such as morphine. Consider the drug being administered when selecting appropriate needle-gauge size and administration site for intramuscular medication. For example, to administer morphine intramuscularly, you may need to use at least a 1.5-inch needle to reach the muscle, depending on the patient's size. Some drugs are more irritating to muscle tissue and should be administered deep into the muscle with the Z-track method. You can use the ventrogluteal, deltoid, and vastus lateralis muscles. The intramuscular route is impractical for repeated injections. Absorption is often unpredictable with intramuscular injections, particularly in older adults, who have reduced muscle mass. This route is also painful. An accessible and appropriate site for the intramuscular injection of analgesics is the ventral gluteal muscle, especially in older adults.

A limited number of opioids, such as morphine, hydromorphone, and oxymorphone, may be administered rectally. This route is useful when the patient is nauseated or has difficulty swallowing (e.g., when a patient is dying).

Opioids may also be administered sublingually (under the tongue). Intermittent bolus injections, continuous infusions, and patient-controlled analgesia (PCA) are methods of administering medications subcutaneously. These methods may be used in patients in whom the oral and rectal routes cannot be used and who also have poor intravenous access.

The intravenous route is another method of administering opioids. Intravenous PCA is commonly used postoperatively. With PCA, the patient is able to self-administer doses of analgesics to control pain. Opioids when administered intravenously have a rapid onset but shorter duration of action than when given by any other route. Although the registered nurse (RN) is usually responsible for the PCA, the LVN/LPN may be responsible for monitoring the patient's response and the effectiveness of the medication. Side effects should be reported to the RN or charge nurse. See the Patient Teaching box.

Opioids can also be administered via the spinal route epidurally (in the epidural space) or intrathecally (in the subarachnoid space). The epidural or intrathecal route may be selected in patients with postoperative pain and chronic cancer pain. The LVN/LPN may participate in monitoring the patient. Side effects such as itching, hypotension, nausea, urinary retention, sedation, and respiratory depression may occur more frequently in patients receiving opioids epidurally or intrathecally than by other routes of administration. The older adult who has received a spinal opioid infusion is at increased risk for respiratory depression. If anesthetics such as bupivacaine are used with spinal opioids, the nurse must be alert for the side effects of numbness and motor weakness. Side effects, as well as any adverse effects, should be reported promptly. A sedation assessment scale should be used with patients receiving spinal opioid infusions. Sedation is usually seen before signs of respiratory depression.

Patient Teaching

Patient-Controlled Analgesia

Safety features: The pump has a delay feature and a lockout interval that prevents the patient from receiving more than the prescribed amount of medication. Only the patient should push the patient-controlled analgesia (PCA) button.

Patient instructions: Press the PCA button when pain begins to return; then put it down and wait 10 to 15 minutes to evaluate pain relief. If pain returns, push the PCA button again and repeat the process until the pain is relieved.

If pain is not relieved: Notify the registered nurse, who can then recommend changes in the opioid, bolus amount, or lockout interval to the physician to achieve satisfactory pain relief.

Other routes of administration of opioids are also available. Liquid morphine may be administered sublingually. Intranasal butorphanol is available and may be used preoperatively for sedation and postoperatively for analgesia. Package inserts should be reviewed for doses, precautions, and administration guidelines. Duragesic or fentanyl transdermal patches are used to treat cancer and chronic pain by producing constant delivery of the opioids for 72 hours through the skin surface. Fentanyl patches can be used only for patients who have developed opioid tolerance. They are applied to a hairless area of the upper torso and pressed for 30 seconds to assure adherence. External heat will increase absorption, so the patient should be instructed not to apply heat in any form over the patch. Used fentanyl patches still contain a significant amount of the drug, which is particularly dangerous to children and small pets if they come in contact with them. The U.S. Food and Drug Administration (FDA) recommends folding the patch in half so the adhesive sides adhere to each other, then flushing the patch down the toilet. The FDA states the risk of accidental exposure to the used patches outweighs the potential risks associated with flushing the patch.

Side effects. Regardless of the route of administration, opioid analgesics have specific side effects. A common side effect is constipation. Tolerance for this side effect does not develop. Ask the patient about bowel movements daily and assess the patient for abdominal distention, cramping, and abdominal pain. Stool softeners and laxatives, along with increased fluid intake, exercise, and bulk-containing foods, may prevent this side effect.

Box 8.6 Sedation Scale

S Sleeping but easy to arouse when called or stimulated
1 Awake and alert
2 Slightly drowsy but easily aroused
3 Frequently drowsy, arousable but drifts off to sleep during conversation—alert the registered nurse
4 Somnolent, minimal or no response to physical stimulation—emergency

Opioids may also cause nausea, with or without vomiting. Some patients develop a tolerance for nausea but may require antiemetic therapy until tolerance develops. At times, the order may need to be changed to a different opioid to relieve this problem.

Sedation is another side effect that may occur initially with opioids, but it usually subsides in a few days. In patients who have had unrelieved pain for some time and have been sleep deprived, sudden pain relief may allow the patient to sleep, which may be misinterpreted as sedation. When sedation is noted, however, the dose of the opioid may need to be titrated to a level that does not cause sedation but still provides pain relief. Box 8.6 illustrates a sedation scale that should be used each time an opioid is administered. Patients receiving opioids should be at 1 or 2 on the sedation scale. If a nurse rates the patient as 3 on the sedation scale, notify the RN because the opioid dose should be reduced to prevent progression to respiratory depression. Respiratory depression can occur but does not occur as frequently as commonly thought. If a patient is easily arousable, respiratory depression is highly unlikely. If severe respiratory depression occurs (fewer than 6 to 8 respirations per minute) and physical stimulation does not awaken the patient, this situation is an emergency. Stay with the patient and call for help. The RN may administer naloxone (Evzio, Narcan) intravenously if prescribed to reverse the opioid. Be aware that drugs such as promethazine (Phenergan) or lorazepam (Ativan) may be ordered to be given with opioids. These drugs, when given with an opioid, may contribute to sedation, respiratory depression, and hypotension.

Other side effects may be noted with the use of opioid analgesics. These include confusion, hypotension (especially orthostatic), dizziness, itching, and urinary retention. Nonopioid analgesics given with opioids may allow a decrease in the opioid dose to one that maintains pain control with fewer opioid side effects.

Placebos. Placebos are inactive substances (e.g., saline) used in research or clinical practice to determine the effects of a legitimate drug or treatment. Placebos are appropriately used in studies in which patients consent to participate in the study. Many professional health care organizations take the position that placebos should not be used to assess or manage pain. Nurses have an ethical obligation to ensure that patients are not deceived and that institutional policies related to placebos are followed.

Complementary and Alternative Therapies

The use of complementary and alternative therapies, also referred to as *integrative medicine*, is becoming more prominent in health care. Traditional Chinese medicine (TCM) and acupuncture are often used to treat pain. TCM includes acupressure, herbal medicine, cupping (deep-tissue massage involving suction), and meditative movements such as Tai Chi. Mind-body techniques are also increasing in popularity because they are easily accessible for most people. Mind-body techniques include meditation, yoga, abdominal breathing, guided imagery, and biofeedback. Mind-body techniques have been proven useful in the treatment of rheumatoid arthritis, osteoarthritis, headaches, stress, and procedural pain. Manual therapies such as massage and chiropractic manipulation have become more widely accepted in the United States to reduce pain. Other complementary and alternative therapies include art or music therapy, Reiki (manipulation of energy by a trained practitioner), and the use of herbals or nutritional supplements. As a nurse, you must ask your patients about the use of any complementary and alternative therapies and monitor for adverse reactions or contraindications. Chapter 20 provides additional information about complementary and alternative therapies.

Put On Your Thinking Cap!

Ask five people (patients, friends, strangers) what helps when they have pain. Compile a list with your classmates and sort the treatment measures into pharmacologic and nonpharmacologic. Include home remedies and herbal remedies.

Pharmacology Capsule

Oral analgesics are preferred for the treatment of chronic pain.

Adjuvant analgesics and medications. Drugs that are not usually classified as analgesics may relieve pain in certain situations. For instance, a patient who has undergone back surgery may complain more about muscle spasms than incisional pain. A muscle relaxant may be more effective in relieving pain than an analgesic alone. Specific pain syndromes, especially neuropathic pain syndromes, may be controlled with drugs other than the commonly known analgesics. Table 8.5 lists some of the adjuvant drugs and the conditions they treat effectively.

Pharmacology Capsule

The adverse effects of opioid analgesics include constipation, nausea, sedation, respiratory depression, confusion, hypotension, dizziness, itching, and urinary retention.

Problem solving with pain medication. Nurses often encounter patients whose prescribed analgesic drugs do not relieve pain. In these situations, use all the information presented here. Ask questions about the analgesic drug and the "five rights" (right dose, right patient, right time, right route, right analgesic) to determine why the patient is not getting adequate pain relief. Box 8.7 provides a nursing plan of care checklist. Box 8.8 describes a method for problem solving when analgesic drugs do not provide effective pain relief.

The administration of analgesics is simply one intervention in the nursing care of a patient in pain. Nurses should provide many interventions along with analgesics to relieve pain. The Coordinated Care box also includes the expected patient outcomes and guidelines for nursing care.

Coordinated Care

Delegation of Pain Assessment

Pain assessment is one of the most important responsibilities for which the nurse is accountable. According to the American Pain Society, one-half of all hospitalized patients experience moderate to severe pain during the last days of their lives. Of the 70% of patients with cancer and with significant pain, fewer than one-half receive adequate relief. Pain may also be caused by postoperative wounds, sickle cell disease, arthritis, and many other conditions.

Pain assessment cannot be delegated to an unlicensed person. However, unlicensed personnel must understand the importance of informing the nurse of any reports of pain from the patient. Although a licensed practitioner with prescribing authority is ultimately responsible for adjusting dosages, both the LVN/LPN and the RN must be able to assess the patient's pain to implement range dose orders. Working within their scope of practice and adhering to applicable organizational policy, nurses must draw on their knowledge, skills, abilities, and experience to execute the pain management plan. They must be aware of the following:

- The medication to be administered
- Dosage and route of administration
- Potential interactions with other medications, foods, and herbal or nutritional supplements
- Time to onset and peak effect
- Duration of action
- Potential side effects

If the patient experiences an unacceptable level of pain or has troublesome side effects, the nurse should document the finding and report it to the prescriber so that appropriate pharmacologic or nonpharmacologic interventions can be implemented. Ideally, the patient will take part in achieving safe, effective pain management. Good communication among all members of the health care team is essential to ensure the patient's optimal comfort and well-being.

Table 8.5 Adjuvant Drugs and Pain Treatment

DRUG CLASSIFICATON WITH GENERIC AND BRAND NAME EXAMPLES	EXAMPLES OF PAIN AND PAIN-RELATED PROBLEMS
Antidepressants	Neuropathic pain; dull, aching pain
Amitriptyline (Elavil)	Various neuropathic pain syndromes, pain associated with herpes zoster (shingles), headache
Bupropion (Wellbutrin)	Painful diabetic neuropathy, headache, fatigue
Duloxetine (Cymbalta)	Painful diabetic neuropathy, fibromyalgia, depression-associated pain
Muscle Relaxants	Muscular pain, spasms, anxiety
Methocarbamol (Robaxin)	Acute traumatic sprains or strains, myofascial pain syndromes, low-back or neck pain
Cyclobenzaprine (Flexeril)	Acute traumatic sprains or strains, myofascial pain syndromes, low-back or neck pain
Antihistamines	Nausea, anxiety
Hydroxyzine (Vistaril)	Nausea, anxiety
Corticosteroids	Pain syndromes associated with cancer, spinal cord or nerve compression
Methylprednisolone (Medrol)	Bone pain, pain related to metastasis
Dexamethasone (Decadron)	Preradiation therapy
Anticonvulsants/Antiepileptics	Neuropathic pain; sharp, shooting, stabbing pain
Carbamazepine (Tegretol)	Neuropathic pain, trigeminal neuralgia
Topiramate (Topamax)	Headache pain, migraine
Gabapentin (Neurontin)	Acute, chronic, and neuropathic pain; acute perioperative pain
Pregabalin (Lyrica)	Acute, chronic, and neuropathic pain; fibromyalgia
Local Anesthetics	Acute, chronic, and neuropathic pain
Lidocaine	Local analgesia, local or regional anesthesia for acute pain
Lidocaine (topical Lidoderm 5% patch)	Pain associated with herpes zoster, painful diabetic neuropathy, arthritis, back pain
2.5% lidocaine and prilocaine topical cream (EMLA)	Anesthetize tissue before needle insertion or superficial skin surgery
Bupivacaine	Local or regional anesthesia for surgery; wound infiltration
Other Adjuvants	
Clonidine (Catapres)	Pain from spinal cord injury, phantom limb pain, peripheral nerve injuries
Capsaicin (Zostrix)	Arthritis pain, postmastectomy pain, myofascial pain, back pain, peripheral nerve pain, painful diabetic neuropathy
Ketamine (Ketalar)	Acute pain, chronic pain
Baclofen (Lioresal)	Pain/spasm from spinal cord injury, multiple sclerosis

Box 8.7 Southwest Texas Methodist Hospital Nursing Plan of Care: Pain

PATIENT PROBLEM
Pain related to:
Date/initials
Disease processes/illness
Surgery
Injury/trauma
Diagnostic procedures

PAIN ASSESSMENT
Type of pain scale
Verbalization of pain/discomfort
Verbalization of spasms (specify bladder, back, muscle)
Facial grimacing
Tense body posture
Rubbing/guarding of body parts
Inability to concentrate
Increased vital signs
Restlessness/difficulty sleeping
Crying, moaning
Withdrawal
Change in appetite
Decreased activity

PAIN EVALUATION/GOALS/REASSESSMENT OF INTERVENTIONS
Patient will verbalize/demonstrate minimal discomfort or absence of pain as evidenced by:
- Statements of pain relief and effectiveness of pain medications and/or other interventions
- Decreased need for pain medication
- Relaxed facial expression and body part

Box 8.7 Southwest Texas Methodist Hospital Nursing Plan of Care: Pain—cont'd

- Increase in voluntary movement, ambulation, and ADL
- Increased ability to concentrate
- Stable vital signs
- Statements or demonstrations of coping behaviors and/or factors that reduce or eliminate discomfort or pain
- Able to sleep/rest
- Increased appetite

NURSING ASSESSMENT

Accept patient's level/tolerance of pain.

Assess pain characteristics to include location, intensity, duration, type, precipitating factors.

NURSING INTERVENTIONS

Provide the patient with prescribed medication as ordered.

Provide and teach alternative methods of pain relief based on individual needs and/or physician orders:

- Positioning
- Back rub
- Massage
- Application of heat
- Application of cold
- Diversion/distraction
- Relaxation/imagery
- Exercise/ambulation
- Range of motion
- Other
- Consults

Teach patient and/or significant other pain management strategies:

- Use of PCA
- Medications

Explain procedures to decrease/relieve anxiety.

EVALUATION

Validate patient's understanding/coping.

Evaluate effectiveness of interventions and reintervene as necessary.

ADL, Activities of daily living; *AEB*, as evidenced by; *PCA*, patient-controlled analgesia.

Box 8.8 Problem Solving With Pain Medication

When the analgesic medication prescribed for pain is not effective in relieving pain, the nurse should take the following steps to solve the problem.

1. Check the analgesic order.
   a. Right dose: Is the dose prescribed a recommended starting dose for analgesia or is the dose prescribed less? If a dose range of medication is prescribed, has the maximum dose been administered? *Solution:* Review dosing with the prescriber or pharmacist to confirm the prescribed dose falls in the recommended dosing range for your patient. Administer the maximum dose prescribed and closely monitor for sedation or other undesired side effects. Notify the prescriber if the dose is ineffective in relieving pain.
   b. Right patient: Is the patient experiencing side effects of the analgesic at the present dose? Can the patient tolerate the increase in dose with few side effects?
   c. Right time: What are the onset, peak, and duration of the analgesic? Is the analgesic administered around the clock based on the duration or properties of the drug? *Solution:* Evaluate pain intensity periodically to see if correct timing of drug is more effective in relieving pain.
   If the patient's pain is still not relieved, the following steps should be taken.
2. Consider an alternative prescription.
   a. Right patient: What is the diagnosis or source of pain and what analgesic is most effective for this type of pain? What are patient characteristics to consider (e.g., age, liver or renal problems, NPO status)?
   b. Right route: Which route is most appropriate for the patient's condition, severity of pain, and medication prescribed (e.g., IV, IM, PO, or topical administration)?
   c. Right analgesic: Which analgesic or adjuvant drug is best for this type of pain? Which analgesic has proven effective for the patient in the past or in a similar condition? Can the opioid or nonopioid prescribed be switched to another drug in the class that may provide more effective pain relief? Have both opioids and nonopioids been prescribed to increase pain relief?
   d. Right dose: Has the dose of opioid been titrated up or adjusted to a higher dose to reduce the pain? Has the patient been receiving opioids over time, and does the patient require increased doses of opioids to control pain because of the development of tolerance? If switching opioid drugs, is the correct equianalgesic dose calculated to make sure you have the approximate same level of analgesia?
   e. Right time: What is the time interval at which the analgesic should be administered or evaluated given its duration of action and patient?
3. Collaborate with the patient, other nurses, pharmacist, and family.
   a. Collect information.
   b. Establish credibility with facts about the patient, analgesics, and written references (articles or drug guides).
   c. Anticipate questions.
   d. Be assertive and keep trying.
   e. Always use other nursing interventions in addition to the analgesic to relieve pain.

IM, Intramuscularly; *IV*, intravenously; *NPO*, nothing by mouth; *PO*, orally; *PRN*, as needed.

Modified from Walker M, Wong D: A battle plan for patients in pain, *Am J Nur* 91(6):32–36, 1991. Used with permission.

Get Ready for the NCLEX® Examination!

Key Points

- Pain is the most common problem that nurses encounter.
- "Pain is an unpleasant sensory and emotional experience associated with actual or potential tissue damage or described in terms of such damage" (International Association for the Study of Pain, 1994).
- When nociceptors (pain receptors) are stimulated, impulses are transmitted to the spinal cord and then to the brain, where the cortex interprets the signals as pain.
- Endorphins are natural opioid-like substances that block the transmission of painful impulses to the brain.
- According to the gate control theory, stimulation of large-diameter fibers in the spinal cord interferes with the transmission of painful impulses to the brain.
- Physical factors that influence the pain experience are pain threshold, pain tolerance, age, physical activity, nervous system integrity, and, in surgical patients, the type of surgery and anesthesia.
- Psychologic factors that influence the pain experience include culture, religion, past experiences with pain, anxiety, and situational factors.
- Based on the duration and cause, pain is classified as acute, chronic, and cancer-related pain.
- Most chronic pain is neuropathic because of nerve damage.
- Assessment is the first step in pain management.
- Pain can be described in terms of location, quality, intensity, and aggravating and alleviating factors.
- Assessment findings and the effects of pain interventions must be documented.
- Patient problems for the patient in pain may include pain, decreased activity tolerance, anxiety, fatigue, sleep disturbance, and discomfort.
- Examples of nonpharmacologic interventions are comfort measures, control of environmental factors, stimulation techniques, and measures to reduce anxiety.
- Predictable pain is best controlled by ATC analgesics rather than PRN medication.
- The categories of drugs used to relieve pain are nonopioid analgesics, opioid analgesics, and adjuvant drugs.
- Placebos are inactive substances such as saline that are used as a control to determine the effects of a legitimate drug or treatment.
- Most professional health care organizations take the position that placebos should not be used to assess or manage pain.
- Opioid side effects to monitor and treat include constipation, nausea, sedation, and respiratory depression.

Additional Learning Resources

SG Go to your Study Guide for additional learning activities to help you master this chapter content.

Go to your Evolve website (http://evolve.elsevier.com/Linton/medsurg) for the following learning resources and much more:

- Fluid & Electrolyte Tutorial
- Review Questions for the NCLEX® Examination

Clinical Judgment and Next-Generation NCLEX® Examination-Style Questions

1. **Pain is *best* defined by the:**
   1. Patient
   2. Nurse
   3. Physician
   4. Physiologist

   NCLEX Client Need: Physiological Integrity: Basic Care and Comfort

2. **When you cut your finger, which of the following represents the steps involved in your experiencing pain?**
   1. Afferent pathways activate nociceptors, which transmit information to the spinal cord for interpretation.
   2. Nociceptors are stimulated, and afferent pathways send impulses to the spinal cord and then to the brain.
   3. Efferent pathways stimulate nociceptors, which transmit impulses to the brain.
   4. The brain stimulates nociceptors, which trigger efferent pathways to send impulses to the spinal cord.

   NCLEX Client Need: Physiological Integrity: Basic Care and Comfort

3. **Mr. A. and Mr. B. both had back surgery yesterday. Mr. A. has used his PCA regularly. He says that he is "pretty comfortable" and he sleeps most of the time. Mr. B. has used the maximal analgesic permitted by his PCA and has required an additional analgesic twice while continuing to complain of some discomfort. Of the following, which is the most likely explanation for the difference in the pain experience of these two patients?**
   1. Mr. B. is a complainer who is seeking attention.
   2. Mr. B. has higher pain tolerance than Mr. A.
   3. Mr. B. has a lower pain threshold than Mr. A.
   4. Mr. B. is more anxious, which has raised his pain threshold.

   NCLEX Client Need: Physiological Integrity: Basic Care and Comfort

4. **Autonomic nervous system responses to pain include which of the following? (Select all that apply.)**
   1. Decreased respiratory rate
   2. Constipation
   3. Urinary frequency
   4. Increased heart rate
   5. Constricted pupils

   NCLEX Client Need: Physiological Integrity: Basic Care and Comfort

5. **A patient says that she has pain whenever she bends over. Which aspect of the pain assessment is she describing?**
   1. Location
   2. Alleviating factor
   3. Quality
   4. Aggravating factor

NCLEX Client Need: Physiological Integrity: Basic Care and Comfort

6. **A frail, older adult patient who is being cared for by her family at home says that she finds a heating pad soothing to stiff joints. What patient or family teaching is needed for safe and effective heat therapy? (Select all that apply.)**
    1. "It is more effective to use the heating pad intermittently rather than continuously."
    2. "Do not apply heat to any area that lacks normal sensation or circulation."
    3. "Set the heating pad at the highest temperature that the patient can tolerate."
    4. "Heat application is not a safe or effective strategy for pain management."
    5. "Limit heat application to 15 minutes."

    NCLEX Client Need: Physiological Integrity: Reduction of Risk Potential

7. **Which statement correctly describes a nonpharmacologic approach to pain control?**
    1. Imagery is the use of the patient's imagination to help control pain.
    2. Distraction is most effective in the management of chronic pain.
    3. Relaxation therapy requires that the nurse must be able to hypnotize the patient.
    4. Patient education is usually all that is needed to reduce anxiety.

    NCLEX Client Need: Physiological Integrity: Basic Care and Comfort

8. **When preparing to give an NSAID, the nurse notes that the patient also takes drugs for hypertension. The nurse knows that NSAIDs must be used cautiously in patients with hypertension because the drugs cause:**
    1. Peripheral vasoconstriction
    2. Potassium loss
    3. Sleep disturbances
    4. Fluid retention

    NCLEX Client Need: Physiological Integrity: Reduction of Risk Potential

9. **The medication nurse has several patients who take NSAIDs in addition to the drugs listed below. The nurse should question the NSAID order for a patient who is also taking:**
    1. Antibiotics
    2. Decongestants
    3. Anticoagulants
    4. Hormone replacements

    NCLEX Client Need: Physiological Integrity: Reduction of Risk Potential

10. **When patients take opioid analgesics, the nurse's first priority is to monitor which of the following?**
    1. Bowel elimination
    2. Hydration
    3. Respiratory status
    4. Urinary elimination

    NCLEX Client Need: Physiological Integrity: Reduction of Risk Potential

9 Shock

http://evolve.elsevier.com/Linton/medsurg

Objectives

1. List the types of shock.
2. Describe the pathophysiologic features of each type of shock.
3. List the signs and symptoms of each stage of shock.
4. Explain the first-aid emergency treatment of shock outside the medical facility.
5. Identify general medical and nursing interventions for shock.
6. Explain the rationale for medical-surgical treatment of shock.
7. Assist in developing care plans for patients in each type of shock.

Key Terms

coagulopathy
epistaxis
ischemia (ĭs-KĒ-mē-ă)
metabolic acidosis (mĕt-ă-BŎL-ĭk ă-sĭ-DŌ-sĭs)
multiple organ dysfunction syndrome
sepsis (SĔP-sĭs)
shock
systemic inflammatory response syndrome

DEFINITION OF SHOCK

Shock is a syndrome characterized by inadequate tissue perfusion resulting in impaired cellular metabolism. Inadequate tissue perfusion deprives cells of essential oxygen and nutrients, forcing cells to rely on anaerobic (without oxygen) metabolism. As a result, a reduced amount of energy is produced and lactic acid, a byproduct of anaerobic metabolism, causes tissue acidosis and subsequent organ dysfunction. Several types of shock have been identified, each with a different cause that requires specific interventions. Although some aspects of treatment may be appropriate for treating the effects of all types of shock, patient needs and responses will vary; therefore, continual and astute nursing assessments and prompt interventions are required.

TYPES OF SHOCK

Historically, shock has been classified into one of four types based on the etiology or cause: hypovolemic (inadequate circulating volume), cardiogenic (decreased myocardial contractility), obstructive (inadequate circulatory blood flow caused by a physical impairment or obstruction), and vasogenic or distributive shock (widespread vasodilation). Distributive shock further encompasses anaphylactic, septic, and neurogenic shock (Anderson & Watson, 2013; Gaieski & Mikkelsen, 2016). When a specific cause cannot be identified immediately, the shock is said to be undifferentiated. Also, patients can have more than one type of shock at the same time.

HYPOVOLEMIC SHOCK

Hypovolemic shock is the most common type of shock and occurs when the circulating blood volume is inadequate to maintain the supply of oxygen and nutrients to body tissues. It can result from loss of blood, plasma volume loss of more than 20% of circulating volume, or extreme dehydration. Intravascular or circulating volume deficits can occur from external or internal losses. Rapid blood loss is the most frequent cause of hypovolemic shock. The source of hemorrhage may be traumatic (e.g., major vessel injury with external blood loss or bleeding into a body cavity, long bone fracture) or nontraumatic (e.g., gastrointestinal bleeding, **epistaxis** [nosebleed], hemorrhagic pancreatitis, aneurysm rupture, ectopic pregnancy, postpartum, **coagulopathy** [reduced ability of the blood to clot]).

Causes of hypovolemic shock from fluid loss include gastrointestinal losses from severe diarrhea or vomiting, excessive diuresis (urination) from diabetes insipidus or diuretics, excessive diaphoresis (perspiration), diabetic ketoacidosis, or aggressive fluid removal during dialysis. Excessive shift of plasma out of the vascular compartment can result in hypovolemic shock and is associated with conditions such as burns, pancreatitis, and intestinal obstruction (Strickler, 2013; Nickson, 2017).

Table 9.1 Obstructive Shock

CAUSE	DEFINITION AND SYMPTOMS	CAUSES
Tension pneumothorax	Complete collapse of a lung, causing increase in intrathoracic pressure and compression of the vena cava and resulting in decreased preload and cardiac output	Blunt or penetrating trauma, barotraumas, central venous catheter placement, chest compressions during cardiopulmonary resuscitation
Cardiac tamponade	Fluid collects within the pericardial sac, causing compression of the myocardium and resulting in reduced cardiac output and myocardial ischemia	Malignancies, uremia, idiopathic pericarditis, infectious diseases
Pulmonary embolism	A blockage of the pulmonary artery or one or more of its branches, resulting in shortness of breath and hemodynamic compromise	Deep vein thrombosis; air, fat, or tissue emboli resulting from surgery or trauma
Abdominal compartment syndrome	Increase in pressure within the confined anatomic space of the abdominal cavity, resulting in vascular or organ compression and decreased blood flow	Abdominal surgery, fluid resuscitation, ileus, intraperitoneal bleeding, ascites, peritonitis
Superior vena cava syndrome	Obstruction of the superior vena cava, resulting in facial or chest edema, shortness of breath, tachycardia, and hypotension	Malignancies, tuberculosis, indwelling central venous catheters, pacemaker wires

CARDIOGENIC SHOCK

Cardiogenic shock occurs when the heart fails as a pump. A decrease in myocardial contractility results in decreased cardiac output and impaired tissue perfusion. This type of shock is one of the most difficult to treat and usually results when diseased coronary arteries cannot meet the demand of the working myocardial cells, such as occurs in acute myocardial infarction (MI). Although only 5.5% to 6% of patients with an MI develop cardiogenic shock during hospitalization, mortality rates of 70% to 90% have been reported in the absence of aggressive, experienced care (Hochman & Reventovich, 2020). Other causes of cardiogenic shock are conditions that result in ineffective myocardial cell function, such as dysrhythmias, cardiomyopathy, myocarditis, valvular disease, and structural disorders such as ventricular septal defects. These specific conditions are discussed in detail in Chapter 34.

OBSTRUCTIVE SHOCK

In obstructive shock, blood flow is reduced and prevented from entering or leaving the heart by a mechanical obstruction. The lack of blood flow results in circulatory arrest, causing the heart to stop pumping blood through the body. Causes of obstructive shock include tension pneumothorax, compression of the vena cava (superior vena cava syndrome, tumor compressing the inferior vena cava), cardiac tamponade, atrial tumor, or clot (Moya, 2013; Table 9.1).

DISTRIBUTIVE SHOCK

In distributive shock, the problem is not loss of blood but rather excessive dilation of blood vessels or decreased vascular resistance, causing the blood to be improperly distributed. To demonstrate this point, imagine pouring 5 mL of water into a test tube and another 5 mL into a mixing bowl. The water would nearly fill the test tube, exerting even pressure against the walls of the tube. The water in the mixing bowl, however, might just barely cover the bottom of the bowl. The diameter of the mixing bowl is so large that the water exerts pressure primarily against the container bottom. This example is similar to what happens in the vascular system when the diameter enlarges because of dilation. Fluid pools in the dependent areas of the body and is not returned to the arterial circulation to supply critical cellular metabolic needs. Distributive shock can be complicated by increased capillary permeability, which permits plasma to leak into the interstitial compartment, thereby decreasing intravascular blood volume. The three types of distributive shock are (1) anaphylactic, (2) septic (most common), and (3) neurogenic (Lessnau, 2015).

Anaphylactic Shock

Anaphylactic shock occurs when a person has a severe allergic reaction that results in the release of chemicals that dilate blood vessels and increase capillary permeability. Fluid leaks out of the capillaries into the tissues. Pooling of blood in peripheral tissues and the shift of fluid out of the capillaries cause venous return and cardiac output to fall. In addition, the allergic reaction causes constriction of the bronchi and airway obstruction. People can be allergic to many substances, including drugs, vaccines, contrast media, insect bites and stings, foods and food additives, pet dander, molds, and pollens. Insect stings present the greatest number of cases of anaphylaxis. The onset of anaphylaxis is typically sudden and dramatic after exposure to a substance to which the patient has developed antibodies. If untreated, anaphylaxis can result in a shock state with cardiac, renal, pulmonary, and multisystem organ failure.

Septic Shock

Sepsis is a systemic inflammatory response to a documented or suspected infection. Sepsis can progress to septic shock, which is hypotension unresponsive to fluid resuscitation along with signs of inadequate tissue perfusion such as metabolic acidosis, acute encephalopathy, oliguria, or coagulation disorders. Septic shock develops when pathogenic organisms (e.g., bacteria, fungi, viruses, rickettsiae) release toxic substances that cause blood vessels to dilate, thereby decreasing vascular resistance and increasing capillary permeability. The increased permeability results in leakage of plasma proteins and reduced intravascular volume, preload, and cardiac output that contributes to inadequate tissue perfusion and oxygenation as in other shock states. This process is more complex in sepsis, however, as microvascular thrombosis and maldistribution further compromises perfusion to tissues and cells (Miranda, 2016).

The incidence, hospitalization, and mortality rates of patients diagnosed with sepsis makes sepsis one of the leading causes of morbidity and mortality worldwide. Although these statistics are alarming, proof that evidence-based interventions decrease sepsis-related mortality is growing. Initiatives such as the Surviving Sepsis Campaign (SSC), which involves adherence to guidelines and implementing "sepsis bundle" components, can improve patient outcomes (Rhodes et al., 2017). The committee of the SSC is composed of international experts from 30 organizations who published updated guidelines in 2016 designed to increase the early recognition and treatment of sepsis. Additional information on these guidelines and sepsis bundles can be found at www.survivingsepsis.org/.

Several assessment tools are available to detect early sepsis. The qSOFA (quick Sequential Organ Failure Assessment) tool consists of three components:

- Respiratory rate equal to or greater than 22 breaths per minute
- Altered mentation
- Systolic blood pressure equal to or less than 100 mm Hg

A patient who has two or more of these components is thought to be at increased risk for death associated with sepsis. Although no assessment tool is perfect, prompt recognition and reporting of these components may permit intervention to decrease the risk of sepsis-related mortality.

Neurogenic Shock

Neurogenic shock occurs when a disruption in the nervous system affects the vasomotor center in the medulla. Normally, the vasomotor center initiates sympathetic stimulation of nerve fibers that travel down the spinal cord and out to the periphery where they cause the smooth muscles of the blood vessels to constrict. In neurogenic shock, disruption of sympathetic nerve impulses results in vasodilation or loss of vascular resistance. The most common cause of neurogenic shock is spinal cord injury from trauma (with the injury usually occurring above the level of T4) or regional anesthesia (Moya, 2013). Other causes of neurogenic shock are disease of the upper spinal cord, depression of the vasomotor center from certain drugs, and adrenal insufficiency. The patient will have signs and symptoms similar to those just described in the distributive shock syndromes, including pooling of blood in peripheral tissues with subsequent decreased venous return and cardiac output. The classic signs of shock may be absent in neurogenic shock because of the alteration in sympathetic tone resulting in bradycardia and skin that is warm, dry, and pink below the level of spinal cord injury (Chinn, 2013).

EFFECTS OF SHOCK ON BODY SYSTEMS AND FUNCTIONS

- Respiratory system: tissue hypoxia and anoxia, respiratory failure, acute respiratory distress syndrome
- Acid-base balance: metabolic acidosis
- Cardiovascular system: myocardial depression
- Neuroendocrine system: release of catecholamines (epinephrine and norepinephrine), mineralocorticoids (aldosterone and desoxycorticosterone), glucocorticoids (hydrocortisone), and antidiuretic hormone; decreased level of consciousness when cerebral blood flow falls
- Hematologic system: disseminated intravascular coagulation—activation of the clotting cascade, leading to microthrombi in the microvasculature of various organs and **multiple organ dysfunction syndrome (MODS)**, as well as depletion of clotting factors with a predisposition to bleeding (Levi, 2016); peripheral ischemia and necrosis of digits and extremities
- Integumentary system: cyanosis may be present, but it is a late, unreliable sign; central cyanosis of mucous membranes, nose; cyanosis of nails and earlobes
- Immune system: depressed immune response
- Gastrointestinal system: decreased peristalsis, ischemia of intestinal submucosa, impaired liver function
- Renal system: reduced glomerular filtration, inadequate renal perfusion, tubular necrosis, renal ischemia

STAGES OF SHOCK

Shock has long been identified as a continuum, initiated by an inciting event. However, over recent years, literature no longer describes such phenomena as warm shock and cold shock; previously referenced stages such as initiation, compensatory, progressive, and refractory are no longer used. More recently identified stages of shock include: (1) preshock, (2) shock, and (3) end-organ dysfunction (Gaieski and Mikkelsen, 2020).

Table 9.2 Compensatory Mechanisms in Shock

MECHANISM	RESPONSE	BENEFITS
Baroreceptors activate the sympathetic nervous system	Increased heart rate	Speeds delivery of oxygen and nutrients to tissues
	Peripheral vasoconstriction	Shunts blood to vital organs, helps maintain BP
	Constriction of renal arteries	Activates renin-angiotensin-aldosterone system
	Renin-angiotensin-aldosterone system activation (angiotensin is a potent vasoconstrictor)	Vasoconstriction shunts blood to vital organs and helps maintain BP
	Aldosterone causes the kidneys to retain sodium, which induces ADH secretion and water retention	Fluid retention increases blood volume by decreasing urine output
Chemoreceptors in the carotid arteries respond to acidic blood pH and increased arterial carbon dioxide by stimulating the respiratory center	Increased respiratory rate and depth	Helps eliminate the excess carbon dioxide and normalize the blood pH; takes in additional oxygen

ADH, Antidiuretic hormone; *BP*, blood pressure.

PRESHOCK

In this stage, compensatory mechanisms respond to decreased delivery of oxygen, inadequate extraction of oxygen, or both, depending on the type of shock compensated. Physiologic responses such as tachycardia and peripheral vasoconstriction may maintain a normal blood pressure. Mild to moderate elevations in lactic acid levels, tachycardia, and slight increases or decreases in blood pressure may be the only clinical signs detectable. With prompt intervention, progressive deterioration may be prevented.

SHOCK

In this stage, signs and symptoms of organ dysfunction become apparent as compensatory mechanisms become overwhelmed.

Physiology of the Early Phases of Shock (Preshock, Shock) and Associated Signs

Neural, endocrine, and chemical compensatory mechanisms are activated in an effort to overcome the consequences of anaerobic metabolism and maintain blood flow to vital organs. During this stage, the following responses may become apparent but can be reversed if interventions are begun:

1. Activation of baroreceptors in the carotid arteries and the aorta stimulates the sympathetic nervous system.
2. Sympathetic stimulation causes increased heart rate, constriction of peripheral blood vessels, and reduced blood flow to the kidneys, lungs, muscles, skin, and gastrointestinal tract.
3. Decreasing renal blood flow triggers the release of renin and a sequence of events that produces angiotensin II, a potent vasoconstrictor.
4. The adrenal cortex secretes aldosterone, which promotes sodium retention by the kidneys.
5. Antidiuretic hormone is released by the posterior pituitary, resulting in additional retention of water by the kidneys.
6. Falling blood pH and increasing arterial carbon dioxide are detected by chemoreceptors in the carotid arteries that stimulate the respiratory center. Increased respiratory rate and depth help to eliminate excess carbon dioxide and normalize the blood pH.

Assessment findings may include the following:

- Mental status: anxiety, restlessness
- Blood pressure: possibly normal initially, decreasing pulse pressure later
- Pulse: slight increase in rate progressing to tachycardia; decreased rate (bradycardia) that may be present in neurogenic shock as a result of loss of sympathetic stimulation
- Respirations: increased rate and depth
- Urine output: decreased to less than 0.5 to 1.0 mL/kg/h
- Skin: cool and pale; exception: warm and dry with septic shock
- Abdomen: decreased bowel sounds; decreased perfusion and ischemic injury can result in movement of bacteria from the intestine to the circulation with subsequent development of sepsis
- Blood glucose: increased
- Other: thirst
- The licensed vocational nurse/licensed practical nurse (LVN/LPN) who recognizes these signs and symptoms in a patient must inform the RN or health care provider immediately. Early interventions can be implemented that may avoid progression to more severe shock.

Table 9.2 summarizes the compensatory mechanisms activated in the first two stages of shock.

END-ORGAN DYSFUNCTION

If the cause of shock is not corrected or if compensatory mechanisms continue without reversing the shock, irreversible organ damage, multiple organ failure, and death ensue. Even though the neural, endocrine, and chemical compensatory mechanisms worked together in the earlier stages, they now begin to function independently and in opposition. In this decompensated stage of shock, the systemic circulation continues to constrict in the attempt to maintain blood flow to vital organs. The decrease in peripheral blood flow, however, leads to weak or absent pulses and **ischemia** of the extremities. As intravascular blood volume decreases, the blood becomes increasingly viscous (or thick), causing clumping of red blood cells, platelets, and proteins. Deprived of adequate oxygen, cells resort to anaerobic metabolism, which produces lactic acid and results in **metabolic acidosis**, which has a depressant effect on myocardial cells (Gaieski & Mikkelsen, 2020).

Typical assessment findings at this stage are as follows:

- Mental status: listlessness, confusion, loss of consciousness
- Blood pressure: hypotension
- Pulse: weak and thready, tachycardia, dysrhythmias
- Respirations: increased, deep, crackles on auscultation
- Temperature: increased or subnormal
- Urine output: decreased, renal failure
- Skin: cold, pale, clammy, slow capillary refill, cyanosis
- Other: dry mouth, thirst, sluggish pupillary response, peripheral edema, muscle weakness

Box 9.1 Focused Assessment and Interventions in First Aid for the Patient in Shock

DATA COLLECTION

Pulse

Rapid and weak, "thready"

Respirations

Normal or increased initially; air hunger, then shallow

Blood Pressure

Stable initially, then decreased

Skin

Cool and moist at first; diaphoresis; later, cyanosis of lips and nail beds

Mental Status

Restless, then listless; confused; unconscious

Thirst

Increased

Interventions

- Summon medical assistance.
- Establish or maintain patent airway.
- Control external bleeding with direct pressure or pressure dressing.
- Maintain blood flow to the brain.
- Keep patient calm and prevent unnecessary movement.
- Position flat; legs may be elevated unless the shock is caused by heart failure, the head or neck is bleeding, head injury is possible, intracranial pressure is increased, or the patient has dyspnea.
- Protect the patient from cold but do not overheat (patient should not shiver or perspire).
- Even if the patient complains of thirst, withhold oral fluids in case surgical intervention is needed.
- Tell the patient what actions are being taken; provide assurance that someone will stay with them, and that help is coming.

DIAGNOSIS

A diagnosis of shock is based on the health history and physical examination and a variety of other data sources. Tests and procedures that help to establish the type of shock, the stage, and the cause include blood and urine studies, measurement of hemodynamic pressures, chest radiographs and other imaging procedures, electrocardiographic and continuous cardiac monitoring, pulse oximetry and arterial blood gases, and urine output.

FIRST AID FOR SHOCK OUTSIDE THE MEDICAL FACILITY

Treatment that is provided to patients in shock before medical care is available can have a significant impact on the chances of survival. The overall goal of treatment is restoration and maintenance of oxygen delivery to the tissues. Essential to this process is a systematic approach to patient assessment to determine life-threatening issues with initial interventions based on these findings. Beginning with a primary survey, immediate life-threatening conditions are identified and addressed immediately (Richards & Wilcox, 2014). Box 9.1 describes emergency first-aid care.

GENERAL MEDICAL TREATMENT

General medical interventions for the patient in shock are directed toward maintaining perfusion of vital organs until the cause is found and treated. Care is directed toward correcting or reversing the altered circulatory component or components, including blood volume, myocardial contractility, blood flow, and vascular resistance, in addition to improving oxygen delivery to the cells. Interventions to increase oxygen delivery are a combination of fluid, pharmacologic, and mechanical therapies are implemented to maintain tissue perfusion.

OXYGENATION

Maintaining a patent airway and improving tissue oxygenation are priorities. Proper head position is maintained and use of appropriate airways including intubation may be indicated, depending on the patient's condition. Oxygen is administered by methods ranging from nasal cannula to mechanical ventilation. In addition to standard assessment of respiratory rate, pattern, and quality of breath sounds, adjuncts such as pulse oximetry, end-tidal carbon dioxide monitoring, and positive end expiratory pressure may be used to determine and enhance adequate oxygenation. Low tidal volume breaths on the ventilator are established at 6 mL/kg and plateau pressures with each breath are kept at or below 30 cm water to prevent damage to the lungs until mechanical ventilation is no longer needed (Kalil, 2017). Prompt treatment of pain, agitation, fever, or other underlying causes of unnecessary oxygen consumption is essential. Paralytics, sedatives, and analgesics may be ordered to decrease oxygen requirements.

FLUID REPLACEMENT

Shock results in major alterations in fluid balance. Patients experiencing hypovolemic or distributive shock require administration of intravenous (IV) fluids to restore intravascular volume and adequate tissue perfusion. In general, aggressive fluid administration is not routinely indicated for patients in cardiogenic shock, as large volumes of fluid may further compromise a failing heart.

After IV access is established, a *fluid challenge* consisting of rapid administration of 250 mL of a crystalloid solution may be administered to assess the patient's hemodynamic response to fluid administration. Nursing responsibilities at this time may include obtaining hemodynamic measurements, administering the fluid challenge, and assessing the patient's response.

The administration of additional fluids depends on the cause of volume deficit, the patient's status, and the physician's preference. Isotonic solutions such as normal saline, Plasma-Lyte, or Lactated Ringers may be administered initially. Subsequent fluids may include additional crystalloids and colloids depending on the situation. The optimal choice of resuscitation fluid in the critically ill is constantly debated. Crystalloids (normal saline, Ringer's lactate) provide replacement water and electrolytes for all fluid compartments. Colloids, such as albumin, remain in the vascular system and draw fluid into the bloodstream, thereby increasing circulatory volume.

Patient response must be monitored closely during fluid replacement to ensure adequate but not excessive replacement. Fluid replacement is best determined by monitoring pulmonary artery wedge pressure, cardiac output, lactic acid levels, and urine output. In general, volume replacement continues until a mean arterial pressure of 60 mm Hg or greater is attained and evidence of adequate tissue perfusion is noted. Once sufficient fluids have been administered, an inotropic agent may be ordered to increase myocardial contractility, or a vasopressor agent to maintain vascular tone, depending on the type of shock being treated.

PHARMACOLOGIC THERAPY

Pharmacologic interventions for the patient in shock are based on management of the cardiovascular dynamics: contractility, preload, afterload/systemic vascular resistance, and heart rate. See Chapter 33 for a review of these concepts. Although no single drug will provide nutrients and oxygen to the cells, several agents have been developed that assist in manipulation of the dynamics listed earlier, thus improving the availability of these vital components (Table 9.3).

MECHANICAL MANAGEMENT

The management of shock may also include the use of mechanical devices that assist in the restoration of cellular perfusion (Fig. 9.1). These devices are listed in Table 9.4.

Put On Your Thinking Cap!

Three patients are in the emergency department. All of them are in shock. Patient A is in hypovolemic shock. Patient B is in cardiogenic shock. Patient C is in septic shock.

1. What assessment finding would you expect in Patient C but not in Patient A or B?
2. For which patient or patients would crystalloid intravenous fluids be preferred over colloids? Why?
3. Which patient would you expect to have a history of:
   a. Coronary artery disease
   b. Severe vomiting and diarrhea
   c. Urinary tract infection

NURSING CARE OF THE PATIENT IN SHOCK

Patients in shock are treated in emergency or intensive care settings. The role of the LVN/LPN in these settings depends on the State Practice Act and individual training for such care. However, patients in any setting may experience shock, requiring the LVN/LPN to understand the condition and act appropriately when it occurs.

FOCUSED ASSESSMENT

Assessment of the patient who is at risk for shock should include continuous monitoring of cardiac rate and rhythm; blood pressure; body temperature; hemodynamic values; respiratory rate, rhythm, and depth; and arterial blood gases. In the routine nursing assessment, observe the color of the skin and palpate for skin warmth and moisture. Note pupil size, equality, and response to light. Describe the patient's level of consciousness and response to commands and assess reflexes. Auscultate heart, lung, and bowel sounds. Observe the movement of the chest wall with respirations. Inspect and palpate the abdomen for distention. Palpate for bladder distention and note the appearance of urine and the hourly output. Inspect the extremities for color and palpate for temperature, peripheral pulses and edema. Inspect IV infusion sites for pallor, swelling, or coolness that suggests extravasation.

Table 9.3 Drugs Commonly Used in Shock

DRUG	ACTION	USE	SIDE/ADVERSE EFFECTS	NURSING IMPLICATIONS
epinephrine	Vasoconstriction in skin, viscera, and mucus membranes Relaxation of bronchi	Anaphylactic shock, hypotension Bronchial constriction	Hypertensive crisis, cardiac dysrhythmias, angina pectoris, tissue necrosis with extravasation, hyperglycemia in people with diabetes mellitus	Monitor heart rate and rhythm and BP Inspect infusion site for extravasation
norepinephrine	Vasoconstriction, increased heart rate and myocardial contractility, increased cardiac output	Hypotension, cardiac arrest	Hypertensive crisis, cardiac dysrhythmias, angina pectoris, tissue necrosis with extravasation	Monitor cardiovascular status continuously Inspect infusion site for extravasation
dopamine	Increased cardiac output, vasoconstriction At low dose: renal and mesenteric vasodilation	Cardiogenic shock, septic shock, heart failure	Anginal pain, dysrhythmias, tachycardia, tissue necrosis with extravasation	Monitor heart rate and BP Assess infusion site
dobutamine	Increased myocardial contractility, increased cardiac output	Heart failure	Tachycardia, dysrhythmias, anxiety	Monitor heart rate, rhythm, and BP
vasopressin	Vasoconstriction, retention of water by kidneys Improved blood flow to heart and brain during cardiac arrest	Septic shock, cardiogenic shock	Chest pain, myocardial infarction, nausea, vomiting	Monitor heart rate, rhythm, and BP

To prevent tissue necrosis after extravasation, infiltrate area with phentolamine as ordered.
From Burchum JR, Rosenthal LD: *Lehne's pharmacology for nursing care*, ed 10, St. Louis, 2013, Elsevier.

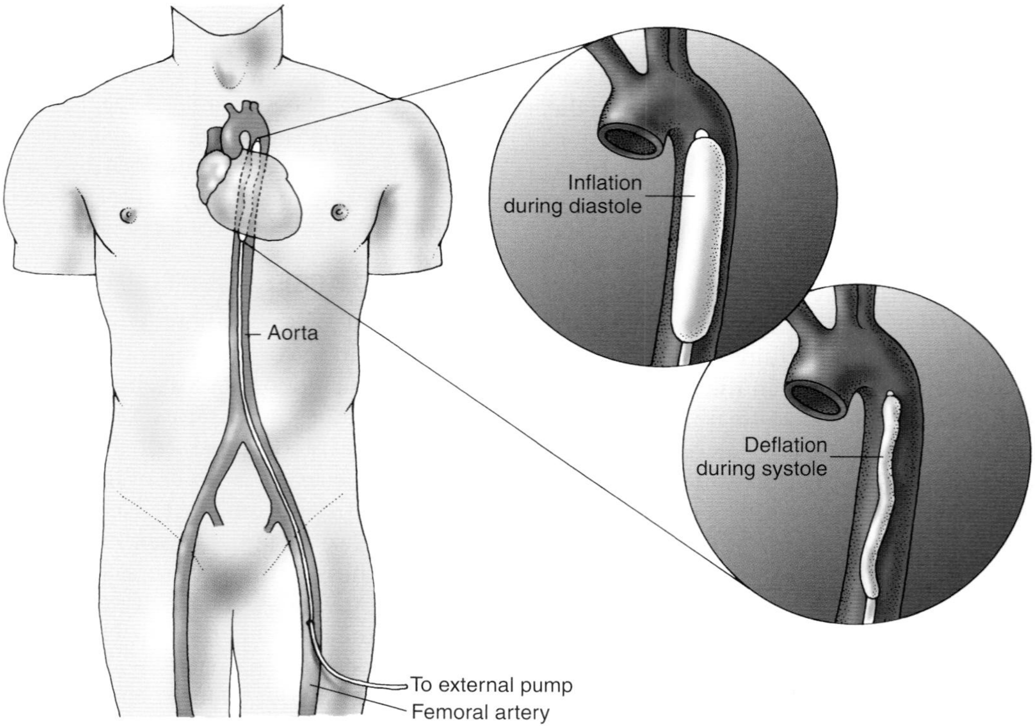

Fig. 9.1 An intraaortic balloon pump is inserted in the femoral artery and advanced to the ascending aorta. The catheter is connected to an external pump that inflates the balloon during diastole and deflates it during systole. (From Black JM, Hawks JH, Keene AM: *Medical-surgical nursing: clinical management for continuity of care*, ed 10, Philadelphia, 2001, Saunders.)

Table 9.4 Mechanical Devices Used in the Treatment of Shock

DEVICE	DESCRIPTION	PURPOSE
Hypothermic devices—Thermo Suit	Maintains body temperature at 91.4°F; circulates ice water in direct contact with patient's skin.	May improve neurologic recovery after cardiac arrest of cardiac origin.
Intraaortic balloon pump (IABP)	A balloon-tipped catheter is inserted into the descending thoracic aorta. The balloon inflates during diastole and deflates just before systole.	Reduces preload with cardiogenic shock. Heart pumps more efficiently; increases cardiac output.
Ventricular assist devices (VADs)	Various devices include pulsatile and nonpulsatile pumps, external and implantable devices, right and left VADs.	Decreases myocardial workload and oxygen demand. Supports circulation until the heart recovers or is replaced.
Extracorporeal membrane oxygenation (ECMO)	Blood is removed from the inferior or superior vena cava, oxygenated, and returned via the femoral artery.	Used for short-term stabilization.

Patient Problems, Goals, and Outcome Criteria: Shock (General)

The primary problem for all patients in shock is inadequate peripheral tissue perfusion. This problem may be related to alterations in circulating blood volume, myocardial contractility, blood flow, and/or vascular resistance.

Patient Problems	Goals and Outcome Criteria
Inadequate peripheral tissue perfusion related to decreased blood volume (hypovolemic shock); decreased myocardial contractility (cardiogenic shock); impaired circulatory blood flow (obstructive shock); widespread vasodilation (distributive shock)	Normal tissue perfusion: urine output at least 0.5 mL/kg/h, patient alert and oriented, normal heart rate and rhythm, normal blood pressure, active bowel sounds, extremities warm with palpable pulses
Decreased cardiac output related to hypovolemia, peripheral vasodilation, myocardial disorders	Improved cardiac output: normal hemodynamic values, vital signs consistent with patient norms, mental alertness
Acute confusion related to inadequate cerebral perfusion, metabolic acidosis	Improved orientation: patient alert and oriented, responds to commands appropriately, behaves appropriately
Fluid volume deficit related to hemorrhage, inadequate fluid intake, excessive fluid loss	Normal fluid volume: vital signs consistent with patient norms, capillary refill in 3–5 seconds
Anxiety related to hypoxia, life-threatening situation	Reduced anxiety: patient calm, states is less anxious
Potential for injury related to confusion, adverse effects of drugs, invasive treatments	Absence of injury: no trauma
Potential for infection related to trauma, invasive therapeutic procedures	Absence of infection: body temperature within normal range, normal white blood cell count
Inadequate family coping related to anxiety, uncertainty of patient's outcome	Effective coping: family members are supportive of the patient and each other and indicate that they have adequate resources to cope with present situation

INTERVENTIONS

Inadequate Peripheral Tissue Perfusion

Your continuous assessment must include all body systems because shock, if not corrected, eventually results in failure of all major organs. Specific organ failures are addressed here under other patient problems.

Decreased Cardiac Output

Administer IV fluids as ordered and assess for both fluid volume deficit and fluid volume excess. With cardiogenic shock, monitoring hemodynamic parameters is especially important. Administer inotropic, antidysrhythmic, and vasopressor agents as ordered (see Table 9.3). Continuous cardiac monitoring enables you to assess the effectiveness of these drugs. You can reduce oxygen requirements by managing pain and anxiety, handling the patient gently, and coordinating care to allow for rest. Maintain adequate body heat to prevent shivering, which also increases metabolic (and circulatory) demands. Fever may be treated with acetaminophen or nonsteroidal antiinflammatory drugs. In some situations, a cooling blanket is ordered.

Acute Confusion and Anxiety

As patients progress through the stages of shock, they may become anxious, then confused and disoriented, and finally unconscious. For the anxious patient, you must remain calm and give simple explanations of what actions are being taken. Remember that the intensive care environment is foreign and frightening to most people. As much as possible, protect the patient from constant, excessive noise and light.

Protect confused patients from harm. Repeat orientation, instructions, and reassurance often. While in the presence of unconscious patients, remember that they may hear even when they cannot respond. Continue to speak to the patient and beware of negative comments made in the patient's presence.

Fluid Volume Deficit

Monitor for hypovolemia (tachycardia, hypotension, tachypnea, decreased urine output, decreased central venous pressure and pulmonary artery wedge pressure). Administer IV fluids cautiously while assessing output of urine. Notify the physician if urine output falls below 0.5 mL/kg/h because low urine output may signal inadequate fluid replacement or renal failure, or both. Assess for fluid overload, especially with renal impairment. Signs and symptoms of overload include full, bounding pulse; dilute urine; increased respiratory rate; abnormal lung sounds; dyspnea; and edema.

Potential for Injury

In addition to the risk for injury related to changes in consciousness, the patient in shock can be harmed by the therapeutic measures being used. For example, antidysrhythmics can depress cardiac activity, anticoagulants can permit excessive bleeding, and extravasation of vasopressors (drugs that raise blood pressure by vasoconstriction) can cause local tissue necrosis. Therefore you must closely monitor the patient for both therapeutic and adverse effects of drugs used to treat the patient in shock.

Because of poor peripheral tissue perfusion and the need to minimize activity, the patient in shock is at high risk for complications of immobility. Institute measures to prevent prolonged pressure on susceptible sites. Pressure injuries can develop very rapidly. In addition, personal hygiene may be limited by the patient's tolerance of such activity. A partial bath and gentle range-of-motion activities may be provided if the patient is stable enough. Mouth care provides some comfort and helps to prevent cracking of the lips and dryness of the oral mucosa. Apply water-soluble lubricant to the lips and moisten the mouth with normal saline. Brushing teeth with a soft toothbrush is recommended.

Put On Your Thinking Cap!

Why would a vasopressor be harmful to surrounding tissues if it leaked out of the vein?

Potential for Infection

Indwelling urinary catheters, IV lines, chest tubes, airways, cardiac assist devices, and other equipment provide avenues for infection in the patient in shock. The potential for infection is greatest in very young, very old, and immunocompromised patients. To reduce the risk of infection, wash your hands thoroughly between patients. Follow agency guidelines for care of IV and urinary catheters. Use aseptic technique when inserting these devices, caring for insertion sites, and providing wound care. Monitor for signs of infection (elevated body temperature and white blood cell count; redness, swelling, and warmth of wounds and tube insertion sites; purulent drainage; abnormal breath sounds; and yellow or green sputum). When antibiotics are ordered, administer them on schedule to maintain a therapeutic blood level. Oral care with chlorhexidine mouth rinses twice per day is essential to reduce the accumulation and colonization of dental plaque that can result in pneumonia in intubated patients (Brooks, 2014).

Inadequate Family Coping

The patient in shock may often have one or more family members present. Members of the health care team should be sensitive to the family's needs for information and support (see the Cultural Considerations box). You can explain the nursing care and encourage family members to ask questions. Offer the services of a counselor or patient representative.

Table 9.5 summarizes the interventions for each type of shock.

Cultural Considerations

What Does Culture Have to Do With Shock?

When a patient is critically ill, family expectations and behavior may be influenced by culture. For example, some families expect to participate in patient care or to remain at the bedside. Extended families may gather to be near the patient and to support one another. In some cultures, important decisions may be deferred to male relatives. Culturally based rituals related to illness and death may be very important to the patient and the family.

SYSTEMIC INFLAMMATORY RESPONSE SYNDROME

Inflammation is a normal response to tissue injury. However, in certain clinical situations, generalized inflammation that threatens vital organs occurs. This state is called ***systemic inflammatory response syndrome (SIRS)***. Some of the conditions that can lead to SIRS are multiple transfusions, trauma, burns, pancreatitis, and infection (Kaplan, 2017).

The effects of SIRS include damage to the endothelium of blood vessels and a hypermetabolic state. Damaged endothelium increases capillary permeability, allowing fluid to leak into body tissues. Hypotension, microemboli, and shunting of blood flow compromise organ perfusion. The hypermetabolic state is

Table 9.5 Medical Management for Each Type of Shock Based on Causation

CAUSE	CLINICAL SITUATION	INTERVENTION[a]
Hypovolemic		
Blood loss	Massive trauma Gastrointestinal bleeding Ruptured aortic aneurysm Surgery Erosion of vessel from lesion, tubes, or other devices DIC	Stop external bleeding with direct pressure, pressure dressing, tourniquet (as last resort) Reduce intraabdominal or retroperitoneal bleeding or prepare for emergency surgery Administer lactated Ringer solution or normal saline Transfuse with fresh whole blood, packed cells, fresh-frozen plasma, platelets, or other clotting factors if significant improvement does not occur with crystalloid administration Conduct autotransfusion if appropriate Use of nonblood plasma expanders or colloids remains controversial
Plasma loss	Burns Accumulation of intraabdominal fluid Malnutrition Severe dermatitis DIC	Administer low-dose cardiotonics (dopamine, dobutamine) Administer lactated Ringer's solution or Plasma-Lyte Use of 5% albumin, fresh-frozen plasma, and dextran are possible
Crystalloid loss	Dehydration (e.g., diabetic ketoacidosis, heat exhaustion)	Administer isotonic or hypotonic saline with electrolytes as needed to maintain normal circulating volume and electrolyte balance
Cardiogenic		
Myocardial disease or injury	Acute myocardial infarction Myocardial contusion Cardiomyopathies	Fluid challenge with up to 300 mL of normal saline solution or lactated Ringer solution to rule out hypovolemia, unless heart failure or pulmonary edema is present Vasodilators (e.g., sodium nitroprusside, nitroglycerin, calcium channel blockers, morphine) Diuretics (e.g., mannitol or furosemide) Cardiotonics (e.g., digitalis) Beta blockers (e.g., propranolol) Intraaortic balloon pump, ventricular assist device, or extracorporeal life support may be used Reperfusion interventions, including percutaneous transluminal angioplasty or coronary artery bypass graft Thrombolysis for treatment of myocardial infarction depends on timely drug delivery to the clot
Valvular disease or injury	Ruptured aortic cusp Ruptured papillary muscle Ball thrombus	Same as myocardial disease or injury above; if rapid response does not occur, prepare for prompt cardiac surgery
Cardiac dysrhythmias	Tachydysrhythmias Bradydysrhythmias Pulseless electrical activity	Treat dysrhythmias; be prepared to initiate CPR, cardiac pacing
Obstructive (See Also Table 9.1)		
External pressure on heart interferes with heart filling or emptying	Pericardial tamponade caused by trauma, aneurysm, cardiac surgery, pericarditis Massive pulmonary embolus Tension pneumothorax Hemoperitoneum Mechanical ventilation	Relieve tamponade with ECG-assisted pericardiocentesis; surgical repair if it recurs Thrombolytic (streptokinase) or anticoagulant (heparin) therapy; surgery for removal of clot Relieve air accumulation with needle thoracostomy or chest tube insertion Relieve fluid accumulation with paracentesis Reduce inspiratory pressure

Continued

Table 9.5 Medical Management for Each Type of Shock Based on Causation—cont'd

CAUSE	CLINICAL SITUATION	INTERVENTION[a]
Distributive		
Anaphylaxis	Allergy to food, medicines, dyes, insect bites, stings, or latex	Prepare for surgical management of airway Decrease further absorption of antigen (e.g., stop IV fluid, place tourniquet between injection or sting site and heart if feasible) Epinephrine (1 : 100) per inhalation *or* Epinephrine (1 : 1000) subcutaneously, *or* Epinephrine (1 : 10,000) IV infusion IV fluid resuscitation with isotonic solution Diphenhydramine HCl or H_1-receptor antagonist IV Theophylline IV drip for bronchospasm Steroids IV Vasopressors (e.g., norepinephrine, metaraminol bitartrate, high-dose dopamine) Gastric lavage for ingested antigen Ice pack to injection or sting site Meat tenderizer paste to sting site
Sepsis	Often gram-negative septicemia but also caused by other organisms in debilitated, immunodeficient, or chronically ill clients	Identify origin of sepsis; culture all suspected sources Vigorous IV fluid resuscitation with normal saline Empirical antibiotic therapy until sensitivities are reported Administer vasopressors (e.g., norepinephrine, epinephrine, vasopressin, dopamine [only in selected patients as alternative to norepinephrine]) Dobutamine may be used in selected patients Corticosteroid use in selected patients IV insulin to maintain serum glucose at or less than 180 mg/dL DVT prophylaxis with low-molecular-weight heparin in severe sepsis Temperature control (both hypothermia and hyperthermia are noted) Platelet administration considered in severe sepsis when counts <10,000/mm^3
Nervous system disruption (Neurogenic/spinal shock)	Spinal anesthesia Spinal cord injury	Normal saline to restore volume Treat bradycardia with atropine Vasopressors (e.g., norepinephrine, metaraminol bitartrate, high-dose dopamine, and phenylephrine) may be given Place client in modified Trendelenburg position Place client in a head-down or recumbent position
Vasovagal reaction	Severe pain Severe emotional stress	Place client in a head-down or recumbent position Atropine if bradycardia and profound hypotension; eliminate pain

[a]Assumes that airway management and cardiac monitoring are ongoing.
CPR, Cardiopulmonary resuscitation; *DIC*, disseminated intravascular coagulation; *DVT*, deep vein thrombosis; *ECG*, electrocardiography; *IV*, intravenous.

characterized by increased serum glucose, which eventually depletes carbohydrate, fat, and protein stores.

Although there is some controversy over the SIRS criteria, a commonly used definition states that a diagnosis of SIRS is made when a patient exhibits two or more of the following symptoms:

- Temperature less than 97°F (36°C) or more than 101.3°F (38.5°C)
- Tachycardia: heart rate greater than 90 beats per minute
- Tachypnea: respiratory rate more than 20 breaths per minute or arterial pressure of carbon dioxide less than 32 mm Hg
- White blood cell count less than 4000 cells/mcL or more than 12,000 cells/mcL or more than 10% immature (band) neutrophils (Singer et al., 2016; Kaplan, 2017).

These criteria are easily assessed and may enable the health care provider to intervene before the condition progresses. Manifestations of SIRS range from mild to severe. When more than one organ begins to fail as a result of SIRS, the patient is said to have MODS (Kaplan, 2017). Various prognostic scoring systems are available, but MODS is always associated with a high mortality rate.

The term *SIRS* is now more commonly associated with organ dysfunction or refractory hypotension related to an ischemic or inflammatory process rather than to an infectious etiology.

MEDICAL TREATMENT AND NURSING CARE

Prevent and Treat Infection

Prevention and early identification of sepsis may enable prompt treatment and prevention of progression to MODS. The following have been identified as priority prevention measures: monitor potential infection sites and assess for signs and symptoms of infection; maintain strict asepsis with invasive procedures and equipment; exercise scrupulous hand washing; provide frequent oral care including tooth brushing (decontamination with oral chlorhexidine gluconate is suggested to reduce the risk of ventilator-associated pneumonia in patients with severe sepsis); position the patient in the semirecumbent position, if tolerated, as this may reduce ventilator-associated pneumonia; administer antimicrobials as ordered; and administer enteral feedings as ordered to enhance perfusion of the gastrointestinal tract (Kleinpell et al., 2013).

Maintain Tissue Oxygenation

Administer sedatives and analgesics as ordered to reduce oxygen requirements. Monitor the patient on mechanical ventilation. Administer drugs to improve cardiac output and tissue perfusion as ordered. Plan care to minimize physical demands on the patient.

Provide Nutritional and Metabolic Support

Provide enteral or parenteral nutrition as ordered (see the Nutrition Considerations box). Monitor blood glucose and weight.

Support Failing Organs

Examples of measures to support failing organs include mechanical ventilation for respiratory distress syndrome and replacement therapy for renal failure.

Nutrition Considerations

1. Hypermetabolism in shock causes protein-calorie malnutrition.
2. Early enteral feedings for all patients who are unable to consume adequate calories orally is thought to (a) prevent and treat shock, (b) improve perfusion of the gastrointestinal tract, and (c) reduce the movement of bacteria through the intestinal walls into the bloodstream (translocation).
3. Nutritional status of the patient in shock is assessed by monitoring serum protein, nitrogen balance, blood urea nitrogen, serum glucose, and serum electrolytes.

Get Ready for the NCLEX® Examination!

Key Points

- Shock is a state of acute circulatory failure and impaired tissue perfusion.
- Untreated shock progresses to SIRS and then to MODS or death.
- The types of shock are hypovolemic, cardiogenic, obstructive, and distributive.
- Hypovolemic shock results from inadequate circulating blood volume.
- Cardiogenic shock occurs when the heart fails as a pump.
- Obstructive shock occurs when physical impairment prevents adequate circulation of blood.
- Distributive shock results from the excessive dilation of blood vessels or decreased vascular resistance that causes blood to be improperly distributed.
- The three types of distributive shock are anaphylactic, septic, and neurogenic.
- Compensatory responses to shock represent neurologic, endocrine, and chemical stimulation intended to maintain blood flow to vital organs.
- The final stage of shock is marked by irreversible changes in vital organs; death is imminent.
- Because brain cells begin to die within 4 minutes without oxygen, a priority in the first-aid treatment of shock is to maintain blood flow to the brain.
- Positioning of the patient is dependent on the type of shock identified and is somewhat controversial.
- Except for cardiogenic shock, all types of shock may require significant fluid volume replacement.
- Normal saline is often administered first, followed by various crystalloids. Administration of colloids remains controversial, but they may be used.
- The physician should be notified if urine output falls below 0.5 mL/kg/h.
- Focused assessment of the patient in shock includes monitoring of vital signs, hemodynamic values, respiratory status, and arterial blood gases.
- General problems encountered when a patient is in shock include inadequate tissue perfusion, acute confusion, anxiety, fluid volume deficit, potential for injury, potential for injury, potential for infection, and inadequate family coping.
- SIRS is generalized inflammation that damages the lining of blood vessels and creates a hypermetabolic state.
- Failure of more than one organ as a result of SIRS is called MODS; failure of three or more organs presents a very poor prognosis.
- The goals of care with SIRS and MODS are to prevent and treat the cause, maintain tissue oxygenation, provide nutritional and metabolic support, and support individual failing organs.

Additional Learning Resources

SG Go to your Study Guide for additional learning activities to help you master this chapter content.

Go to your Evolve website (http://evolve.elsevier.com/Linton/medsurg) for the following learning resources and much more:
- Fluid and Electrolyte Tutorial
- Review Questions for the NCLEX® Examination

Clinical Judgment and Next-Generation NCLEX® Examination-Style Questions

1. **A patient has developed peritonitis after a traumatic injury to the abdomen. The nurse knows that this patient is at greatest risk for which type of shock?**
   1. Cardiogenic
   2. Anaphylactic
   3. Neurogenic
   4. Hypovolemic

   NCLEX Client Need: Physiological Integrity: Reduction of Risk Potential

2. **A patient is admitted to the emergency department in distributive shock. Which of the following factors can lead to distributive shock? (Select all that apply.)**
   1. Bacterial infection
   2. Blood or fluid loss
   3. Dilation of blood vessels
   4. An antigen-antibody reaction
   5. Failure of the heart as a pump

   NCLEX Client Need: Physiological Integrity: Physiological Adaptation

3. **What do anaphylactic shock, septic shock, and neurogenic shock have in common?**
   1. Infection
   2. Allergic reactions
   3. Vasodilation
   4. Heart failure

   NCLEX Client Need: Physiological Integrity: Physiological Adaptation

4. **Which acid-base disturbance should the nurse anticipate when a patient is in shock?**
   1. Metabolic alkalosis
   2. Respiratory alkalosis
   3. Metabolic acidosis
   4. Respiratory acidosis

   NCLEX Client Need: Physiological Integrity: Reduction of Risk Potential

5. **The nurse is concerned about cerebral perfusion in a patient who is in shock. Which assessment provides the best indicator of cerebral perfusion?**
   1. Presence of reflexes
   2. Level of consciousness
   3. Emotional state
   4. Mean arterial pressure

   NCLEX Client Need: Physiological Integrity: Physiological Adaptation

6. **Even though aggressive fluid administration is often required for patients in shock, which type of shock could be made WORSE by large volumes of intravenous fluids?**
   1. Cardiogenic
   2. Neurogenic
   3. Septic
   4. Obstructive

   NCLEX Client Need: Physiological Integrity: Pharmacological Therapies

7. **What is the most common cause of cardiogenic shock?**
   1. Pancreatitis
   2. Anaphylaxis
   3. Acute myocardial infarction
   4. Gastrointestinal bleed

   NCLEX Client Need: Physiological Integrity: Physiological Adaptation

8. **A patient in shock has been given blood, crystalloids, and colloids. The nurse's assessment reveals: pulse rate 80 beats per minute, bounding, regular; respiratory rate 30 breaths per minute; blood pressure 140/86 mm Hg; dyspnea and crackles throughout lung fields. Which complication would the nurse suspect?**
   1. Sepsis
   2. Multiple organ failure
   3. Pneumonia
   4. Circulatory overload

   NCLEX Client Need: Physiological Integrity: Physiological Adaptation

9. **Which interventions reduce the risk of SIRS and MODS in a patient with pancreatitis? (Select all that apply.)**
   1. Maintain strict asepsis with invasive procedures
   2. Provide frequent oral care with chlorhexidine gluconate
   3. Position the patient in high Fowler position
   4. Practice scrupulous hand washing
   5. Administer enteral feedings as ordered

   NCLEX Client Need: Physiological Integrity: Basic Care and Comfort

10. **SLO Objective: List the signs and symptoms of each stage of shock. Identify general medical and nursing interventions for shock.**

    NGN Item Type: Cloze

    Cognitive Skill: Recognize Cues, Analyze Cues
    A patient comes to the Urgent Care Clinic with chills and fever. A blood sample is taken for a stat complete blood count. Their assessment data includes the following:

- Oral temperature 38.9º C
- Heart rate 104 beats per minute
- Respirations 26 breaths per minute
- BP 96/60
- No pain
- Alert and oriented to person, place, and time
- History of peptic ulcer disease
- Elevated white blood cells
- Normal hemoglobin and hematocrit

Choose the *most likely* options for the information missing from the statements below by selecting from the list of options provided.

The nurse recognizes that this patient has (1) ______and a BP of 96/60 which are components of the qSOFA criteria. Identifying that the patient is at risk for (2)_________, the nurse would immediately report these symptoms to the health care provider.

OPTION 1	OPTION 2
Temperature greater than 100ºF	Appendicitis
Heart rate greater than 100 beats per minute	Peptic ulcer perforation
Respiratory rate of 22/min or more	Septic shock
Elevated white blood cell count	Heart failure

10 The Older Adult Patient

http://evolve.elsevier.com/Linton/medsurg

Objectives

1. Describe the roles of the gerontological nurse.
2. Determine the extent to which selected myths and stereotypes about older adults are factual.
3. Describe biologic and psychosocial factors associated with aging.
4. Explain the importance of assessing activities of daily living and instrumental activities of daily living.
5. Explain why drug dosage adjustments may be needed for older persons.

Key Terms

ageism (ĀJ-ĭzm)
aging
cataract (KĂT-ă-răkt)
conduction deafness (kŏn-DŬK-shŭn DĔF-nĕs)
gerontological nurse
gerontology (jĕr-ŏn-TŎ-lŏ-jē)
glaucoma (glăw-KŌ-mă)
kyphosis (kī-FŌ-sĭs)
presbycusis (prĕz-bĕ-KYŪ-sĭs)
presbyopia (prĕz-bē-Ō-pē-ă)
sensorineural deafness (sĕn-sō-rē-NYŪ-răl)

The care of older adults can be a richly rewarding experience. As the over 65 years of age population has continued its unprecedented growth, the need for nurses with expertise in the care of older people has grown rapidly. Nursing care of older adults requires specialized knowledge and skills. Indeed, maintaining the best possible quality of life in the presence of aging changes and pathologic processes requires a high level of knowledge, skill, and compassion. This chapter provides an overview of the aging process and the needs of older persons. Nursing care of patients with specific medical conditions is addressed in subsequent chapters.

DEFINITIONS

Aging is the process of growing older or more mature. It is an ongoing developmental process that begins at conception and ends at death (Box 10.1). Defining old age is not as simple as it might seem. A child or teenager may define "old people" as persons in their 30s, 40s, or 50s whereas people in their 50s may define old as "at least 10 years older than I am." Most gerontologists agree that old age is not measured in years. Although the age of 60 to 65 years is commonly used to indicate the onset of older age, this number is clearly arbitrary and a function of social policy.

Gerontology, the study of aging, encompasses social, cultural, psychological, cognitive, and biological aspects of growing old.

Geriatrics is the biomedical science of old age and the application of knowledge of aging to the prevention of disease and immunity, diagnosis, treatment, and care of older persons.

ROLES OF THE GERONTOLOGICAL NURSE

In 2018, 16% of the U.S. population was 65 years of age and over. By 2060 estimates predict that 95 million or 23% of the population will be 65 years of age and older. Average life expectancy in the United States has increased from 68 years in 1950 to 78.6 years in 2017. The difference in life expectancy between men and women has narrowed from seven years in 1990 to five years (76.1 years versus 81.1 years) in 2017. These older adults will need health care services to help them maintain their health, prevent disabling and life-threatening diseases and conditions, and manage chronic illnesses. Nurses have always been involved in the care of the aged. Whereas geriatric nursing is the care of sick older adults, gerontological nursing focuses on care of older persons across the health-illness continuum. "Gerontological nursing involves the care of aging people and emphasizes the promotion of the

Box 10.1 An Old Lady's Poem

What do you see, nurse, what do you see?
What are you thinking when you're looking at me?
A crabby old woman, not very wise,
Uncertain of habit, with faraway eyes?
Who dribbles her food and makes no reply
When you say in a loud voice, "I do wish you'd try!"
Who seems not to notice the things that you do,
And forever is losing a stocking or shoe…
Who, resisting or not, lets you do as you will,
With bathing and feeding, the long day to fill…
Is that what you're thinking? Is that what you see?
Then open your eyes, nurse; you're not looking at me.
I'll tell you who I am as I sit here so still,
As I do at your bidding, as I eat at your will.
I'm a small child of ten … with a father and mother,
Brothers and sisters, who love one another.
A young girl of sixteen, with wings on her feet,
Dreaming that soon now a lover she'll meet.
A bride soon at twenty—my heart gives a leap,
Remembering the vows that I promised to keep.
At twenty-five now, I have young of my own,
Who need me to guide and a secure happy home.
A woman of thirty, my young now grown fast,
Bound to each other with ties that should last.
At forty, my young sons have grown and are gone,
But my man's beside me to see I don't mourn.
At fifty once more, babies play round my knee,
Again we know children, my loved one and me.
Dark days are upon me, my husband is dead;
I look at the future, I shudder with dread.
For my young are all rearing young of their own,
And I think of the years and the love that I've known.
I'm now an old woman … and nature is cruel;
'Tis jest to make old age look like a fool.
The body, it crumbles, grace and vigor depart,
There is now a stone where I once had a heart.
But inside this old carcass a young girl still dwells,
And now and again my battered heart swells.
I remember the joys, I remember the pain,
And I'm loving and living life over again.
I think of the years … all too few, gone too fast,
And accept the stark fact that nothing can last.
So open your eyes, nurses, open and see,
… Not a crabby old woman; look closer … see ME!

From Anonymous. Attributed to an elderly woman who died in a geriatric ward in Scotland. Available at www.carepathways.com.

highest possible quality of life and wellness throughout the life span" (Eliopolous, 2014, p. 73).

The term ***gerontological nurse*** typically refers to professional nurses and advanced-level practitioners, such as nurse practitioners, clinical specialists, and nurses who hold national certification in the specialty of gerontological nursing. However, some nursing personnel have also demonstrated competencies as a result of on-the-job training. Registered nurses with appropriate knowledge and experience can seek credentialing as a certified gerontological nurse through the American Nurses Credentialing Center. Employment settings for licensed vocational nurses/licensed practical nurses (LVNs/LPNs) have shifted from primarily traditional hospital-bound positions to include a range of community-based, long-term care, and home health care positions. LVN/LPN programs are responding by increasing content and learning experiences to prepare students for this change. Laurie Gunter and Carmen Estes describe gerontological nursing as a health service that incorporates basic nursing methods and specialized knowledge about the aged to establish conditions within the patient and within the environment that (1) increase healthy behaviors in the aged, (2) minimize and compensate for health-related losses and impairments of aging, (3) provide comfort and sustenance through the distressing and debilitating events of aging, including dying and death, and (4) facilitate the diagnosis, care, and treatment of disease in the aged. Dr. Charlotte Eliopolous, a leader in the field, lists the roles of the gerontological nurse as healer, caregiver, educator, advocate, and innovator. Table 10.1 gives examples of the LVN/LPN functions in relation to each of these roles.

AGEISM: MYTHS AND STEREOTYPES

Gerontology is a relatively new science, so we are only beginning to understand aging processes and the lives of older people. In the absence of facts, people rely on "common knowledge" that may or may not be accurate. Many of these "facts" are actually myths that are widely accepted beliefs that have not been proven. Some myths have an element of truth. For example, it is a myth that most old people live in nursing homes. Some old people do live in nursing homes but most do not. When we take a fact about some older people and assume that it applies to all or most older people, we are guilty of stereotyping. When we stereotype, we make assumptions without assessing the individual. Nurses must be knowledgeable about aging and older adults to dispel myths and avoid stereotyping.

Ageism is the systematic stereotyping of and discrimination against people because of their age, most often directed toward older adults. For example, older people may be labeled senile, "set in their ways," asexual, and old-fashioned. Ageism denies the older person's uniqueness. Like other prejudices, ageism influences the behavior of its victims. An older person who believes that retired people are nonproductive may not seek meaningful activity in retirement. Other older adults refuse to conform to this stereotype and seek new interests, activities, or even employment.

MYTHS AND FACTS ABOUT AGING

If myths about aging were true, older people would be unable (or unwilling) to learn, childlike, nonproductive, disengaged, inflexible, and lonely. Even if they were interested in sex, it is assumed that they probably would not be able to perform sexually. Retirement would be a sad state spent in a rocking chair, living in poverty or in a nursing home, and waiting to die. Let's examine these perceptions and see what the facts are.

Table 10.1 The Licensed Vocational Nurse/Licensed Practical Nurse in Gerontological Nursing Settings

ROLE	LICENSED VOCATIONAL NURSE/LICENSED PRACTICAL NURSE ACTIVITIES
Healer	Consider the individual's physical and psychologic needs. Embrace the philosophy that individuals at every stage of life can have meaning and purpose. Recognize that the physical and emotional environments affect the individual's functioning and well-being. Consider wellness needs even in the frail older person or one with multiple chronic conditions.
Caregiver	Learn about aging and the special needs of older adults. Seek knowledge to provide care based on science rather than tradition. Participate actively in the development of nursing care plans. Because of the amount of time spent with the patient, the LVN/LPN may have information or insights that the RN does not have. Encourage older persons to participate actively in their care and to maintain as much independence as possible.
Educator	Include patient education in care plans. Consider what the older person and/or the significant others want and need to know about health, aging, and management of chronic conditions. Share knowledge about gerontological nursing with colleagues. Explain and demonstrate to assistive personnel appropriate strategies for working with older adults.
Advocate	Participate in organizations that advance causes important to older persons. The National Gerontological Nursing Association welcomes LVN/LPN memberships. Participate in community initiatives that benefit older persons. Speak up for the rights of older adults in your care. Encourage families and other caregivers to hear and consider the patient's wishes.
Innovator	Maintain a questioning attitude. Ask if there is a better way to carry out nursing activities. When you encounter a challenge, engage others in developing novel solutions. Be open to suggestions of others, including patients.

Some cognitive decline occurs with old age; however, it does not normally impair everyday functions. There is some evidence that educational and intellectual experiences actually build cognitive reserve. A person who has built a cognitive reserve through the years can continue to function at a higher level despite some decline. Individuals with minimal education and intellectual development will show the effects of decline sooner because they lack cognitive reserve.

Not all cognitive functions decline equally with normal aging. The speed and efficiency of processing and storing information decline. The older person is more readily distracted and less able to focus attention. These changes explain the problem that many healthy older people report with short-term memory. Normal aging does not cause intelligence to plummet. However, there are differences in types of intelligence. Functions related to factual knowledge are retained. On the other hand, the ability to solve complex or novel problems declines.

Dementia is a progressive decline in cognitive function. It is not part of normal aging. Only 5% to 7% of persons older than 60 years of age have dementia, with the greatest incidence after 85 years of age. Among the many causes of reversible cognitive changes are drug effects, hypoxemia, fluid and electrolyte imbalance, infection, and sensory deficits.

Health Promotion

Mental Acuity in Older Age

Encouraging middle-aged and older adults to engage in mentally challenging activities may build cognitive reserve, which provides some protection against future cognitive losses.

Many people, including some older adults, expect sexual interest to fade with age. The idea of older people engaging in sex is a source of endless comedy. That perception may be changing as the baby boomers strive to stay active, view sex as healthy and natural at any age, and seek treatment for sexual dysfunction. In general, older people who have enjoyed sexual activity throughout their lives are likely to retain that interest. Those who were never very interested in sex will probably remain disinterested in later years. Some older people remain interested in sexual activity but either lack a partner or have a partner who is not interested or capable of sexual activity. No doubt, some have been influenced by the stereotype and expect to give up sex in later years.

Older people typically engage in sexual activity less often than younger people. Physical and psychosocial factors may explain this change. The sexual response is slower and less intense in both men and women. Although erectile dysfunction (ED) is not part of normal aging, it occurs more often in older men. Factors that contribute to ED include diabetes, atherosclerosis, endocrine disorders, and drug therapy. Problems that women often encounter after menopause include vaginal atrophy and dryness, sleep disturbances, and "mood swings." Sexual dysfunction can occur at any age and is usually evidence of some disorder or a result of medication side effects. Baby boomers who grew up with "a pill for every ill" expect medical science to find treatments for everything, including sexual dysfunction.

What really happens when older people retire and no longer have child-rearing roles? First, many people continue to work beyond 65 years of age. In 2018, 24% of men and about 16% of women aged 65 years and older worked in the labor force. By 2026, the levels are projected to increase to 26% for men and 18% for women. More older persons are divorced compared with previous generations. The number of divorced women over age 65 years increased from 3% in 1980 to 14% in 2018 and in men over age 65 from 4% to 11%. In 2012, about 8 million older women and 3 million older men lived alone. Over 26% of women aged 65 to 74 years lived alone in 2018, while the number jumped to 39% in those aged 75 to 84 years, and 55% in those aged 85 and older. In 2012 institutional settings were home to 1% of persons aged 65 to 74 years, 3% of persons aged 75 to 84 years, and 11% of those aged 85 years and over. There likely will be an increase in Americans over age 65 years requiring nursing home care from about 1.2 million in 2017 to about 1.9 million in 2030. A steep projected rise in the incidence of dementia among older adults from 5.8 million today to 13.8 million by 2050 may contribute to the demand for increased elder care. These numbers will generate an increase in Medicare and Social Security expenditures from a combined 8.7% of gross domestic product today to 11.8% by 2050.

The older population is becoming more racially and ethnically diverse. The proportion of the older population that is non-Hispanic white is projected to drop from 75% to 55% between 2018 and 2060. Although the poverty rate has dropped sharply during the past 50 years, 17% of Latinos and 19% of Black Americans lived in poverty in 2017, more than twice the rate of non-Hispanic Whites.

Education levels are increasing among people over age 65. In 1965 only 5% had completed a bachelor's degree or more. By 2018, the proportion had risen to 29% (Population Reference Bureau (PRB) July 15, 2019; Office of Disease Prevention and Health Promotion, et al. n.d.).

The examples cited are only some of the myths and facts that exist about aging and older people. Rather than accepting information as common knowledge, seek the facts from professional sources. Armed with knowledge, you as a nurse can help dispel many misconceptions.

BIOLOGIC AND PHYSIOLOGIC FACTORS IN AGING

The search for immortality has been a recurrent theme in human history. Medical science has not escaped this quest. Although it has made great strides in conquering many ills, thereby allowing more people to live longer, the life span has changed little. Most experts believe that the maximal attainable age is between 115 and 125 years.

How and why do humans age? Why is individual aging so varied? Which of the many theories of aging are valid? Each of these questions represents a fascinating area for scientific exploration. However, despite intense interest in longevity by so many cultures, scientists do not agree on precisely why or how humans age. Knowledge of the underlying mechanisms of aging may enable scientists to slow the aging process. Even if the maximum life span cannot be extended, science may be able to help us remain healthier in the years that we have.

THEORIES OF BIOLOGIC AGING

At this time, no one theory of biologic aging is entirely explanatory or universally accepted. Many experts believe that aging cannot be explained by a single theory but represents multiple processes working simultaneously. Thus theories about aging continue to evolve in an effort to shed light on this process.

PHYSIOLOGIC CHANGES IN BODY SYSTEMS

Aging occurs slowly and is a complex and dynamic process involving many internal and external influences. It affects every system, organ, and cell in the body to varying degrees. With increasing age, the ability to maintain physiologic functions in the face of challenges is reduced. Common age-related changes are discussed here. However, these changes do not occur at the same rate or to the same extent in all people. For example, wrinkling of the skin is common among older persons, but individuals who have had much sun exposure have much more wrinkling. Nurses should consider the implications of common aging changes in planning and providing nursing care.

NERVOUS SYSTEM

Some neurologic changes were discussed earlier in the section titled "Myths and Facts about Aging." Brain size is thought to decrease with age because of the loss of neurons (brain cells) that begins in the early 30s. The conduction of impulses slows. This may result in slower responses, problems with short-term memory, and altered learning. Nevertheless, functional ability may not be affected significantly because reserve cells are able to compensate. In the absence of disease, most aged people maintain normal intellectual capability, sound judgment, and creativity.

Atherosclerosis reduces the supply of oxygen to the brain, which may affect the ability to store new information. Short-term memory loss is a frequent complaint of the aged, although long-term memory may remain intact. It may be that old memories are preserved as permanent changes in the structure of the neurons. Consequently, the aged person may experience difficulty remembering planned events for the day but may easily recall childhood experiences. Momentary lapses in memory, such as forgetting a name or misplacing an item, are common examples of normal memory changes.

People who have more persistent memory problems with otherwise normal cognitive function are said to have mild cognitive impairment (MCI). An estimated

40% to 50% of people who develop MCI most likely will develop dementia within 3 years; others do not progress to more serious impairment.

Other neurologic functions that are affected by age-related changes include temperature regulation, pain perception, and tactile sensation. The aged individual usually has a low tolerance for extremes in temperature. Changes that may affect maintenance of normal body temperature include deterioration in vascular tone, changes in hypothalamic temperature control, and loss of subcutaneous tissue. Some researchers have found dulling of pain and tactile sensation in older persons, but these findings are not consistent. Many diseases and medications can alter sensory perception.

The neurologic changes associated with aging occur gradually; therefore the aging person compensates for these changes by using adaptive strategies and modifying behavior. For example, the person may avoid temperature extremes, approach tasks at a slower pace, and attend to one task at a time. Mnemonics and repetition are two strategies that may be used to cope with memory problems. Mnemonics (pronounced *nee-mon-icks*) connects known and unknown information. For example, a person might remember that her grandchildren are named Amy, Brian, and Carl by associating their names with the ABCs. However, stressors such as illness, relocation, or a loss may overwhelm the person's ability to compensate, resulting in a decline in function.

RESPIRATORY SYSTEM

Tests of pulmonary physiology have shown several age-related alterations. Tidal volume is relatively stable with aging; however, residual volume (RV) increases. Forced vital capacity (FVC), forced expiratory capacity in 1 second (FEV_1), forced expiratory volume (FEV), maximal voluntary ventilation (MVV), and vital capacity (VC) are thought to decrease progressively with aging. These alterations are related to atrophy and weakening of the respiratory muscles and changes in the rib cage and spine. Increased curvature of the thoracic spine, called kyphosis, is common. Osteoporosis causes the vertebrae to become more fragile and prone to fracture. The cartilage between the ribs stiffens, which limits chest expansion. Alterations in the lungs include a decreased number of capillaries, thickened capillary walls, and fewer capillaries surrounding the alveoli. The changes in the capillaries affect pulmonary diffusion so that gas exchange is impaired. Pulmonary secretions are handled less effectively. Ciliary action, which normally sweeps secretions from the airway, is less efficient. The cough reflex is frequently less effective because of decreased sensitivity to stimuli and decreased muscle tone. These factors make the older person more susceptible to and less able to recover from respiratory infections. Even though vaccinations and antibiotics are available, pneumonia is one of the leading causes of death of Americans 65 years of age and older. Chronic pulmonary disease is the third leading cause of death in this age group.

Despite these changes, the healthy older adult usually maintains adequate oxygenation with moderate activity. Problems arise when increased demands are placed on the body, as occurs during periods of extreme exertion or respiratory illness. Exertional dyspnea (shortness of breath with exertion) is a frequent complaint of the older adult. The ability to perform prolonged strenuous work decreases with aging.

Put On Your Thinking Cap!

Considering the many changes in the respiratory system, what nursing care would be especially important when caring for a hospitalized older person?

CARDIOVASCULAR SYSTEM

Resistance to blood flow in many organs increases as people age. In the absence of cardiovascular disease, heart size remains unchanged or decreases slightly. Whitish patches, fibrosis, and sclerosis develop in the endocardium, the inner layer of the heart. The heart becomes increasingly rigid and myocardial contractility is compromised. Coronary blood flow in the aged person may be reduced by as much as 35% because of changes in the vessels. Aortic and pulmonic valves stiffen. If they do not close completely, murmurs result. Aging heart cells have a decreased capacity to use oxygen, which may help to explain the aged person's reduced tolerance for physical work.

The blood vessels of the heart and the systemic circulation, particularly the arteries, undergo age-related changes that may begin as early as the teen years. By 20 years of age, thickening and calcification of the intimal layer of the coronary arteries and aorta are evident. Arteries dilate, lengthen, and become more rigid. The pulse tends to increase in force and the pulse pressure widens. Vascular changes increase the risk for myocardial infarction ("heart attack") and heart failure. In fact, heart disease is the leading cause of death among older adults.

By 70 years of age, the systolic blood pressure commonly increases to approximately 150 mm Hg and the diastolic blood pressure increases to 90 mm Hg for many people. Because of the current guidelines for diagnosis of hypertension, older persons are more likely than younger people to be treated for a blood pressure reading that once was considered normal.

Another cardiovascular change related to aging is a decrease in resting cardiac output, which is the amount of blood pumped by the heart each minute. Between 25 and 65 years of age, resting cardiac output falls 30% to 40%. This reduced cardiac output reflects a decreased heart rate and a decreased stroke volume. Despite the diminished cardiac output, cerebral blood flow is maintained. However, blood supply to other body systems, notably the liver and kidneys, is diminished.

Nevertheless, these organs usually maintain adequate function, partly because of reduced demands.

RENAL SYSTEM

The renal system of healthy older people functions adequately; however, in the event of injury, disease, or disability, the additional demands may cause the kidneys to fail. By the seventh decade, the number of nephrons in each kidney is reduced by one-half to two-thirds, with corresponding changes in the glomeruli. The renal filtration rate, plasma flow rate, and tubular reabsorption and secretion all decrease. Blood urea nitrogen tends to increase. The tubules of the aging kidneys are less able to conserve base and eliminate excess hydrogen. Thus the regulation of acid-base balance is less efficient.

Total body water decreases with age. This is important because it means that the older adult can become dehydrated quickly. The older person's kidneys are less able to compensate for deficient fluid balance by concentrating urine. Alternatively, older persons excrete excess fluid more slowly, so they are at risk for overload if given large volumes of fluids quickly.

Additional changes are noted in the ureters, bladder, and urethra as a result of loss of muscle tone. The bladder capacity may be reduced by one-half, resulting in frequent trips to the toilet. Furthermore, response to the stretch receptors in the bladder wall that signal the need to void may be delayed until the pressure is high and the bladder is almost full. This condition results in an urgency to urinate, which may be especially problematic for older adults with visual and motor impairment. Urge incontinence, the involuntary passage of urine shortly after the urge to void occurs, is a major health concern for older adults. Poor muscle tone may lead to incomplete emptying of the bladder. The urine that remains after voiding (residual volume) favors bacterial growth, putting the older person at risk for urinary tract infections. Other types of incontinence may appear as a symptom of upper or lower urinary tract dysfunction. For several of these conditions, behavioral treatment may be helpful. Behavioral treatments include scheduled or prompted voiding, environmental adaptation, and pelvic muscle exercises (Kegel exercises). Interventions for incontinence are discussed in Chapter 14.

INTEGUMENTARY SYSTEM

Changes related to aging of the skin include dryness, loss of elasticity, wrinkles, uneven pigmentation and brown spots, roughness, looseness, thinness, and the development of various skin lesions.

One of the first signs of aging is the development of wrinkles. Wrinkles occur when the deep layer of the skin loses moisture and elasticity. Tiny creases and folds are formed. The extent and timing of these wrinkles are determined by genetics and sun exposure. Men and persons in certain ethnic groups that have thicker, oilier skin wrinkle at a slower rate. Skin that is exposed to the sun most often, such as the face, hands, and back of the neck, wrinkles quickly. Older people are encouraged to use sunscreens to prevent excessive dryness and to reduce the risk of skin cancer, which is more common in older persons. The American Academy of Dermatology recommends using a sunscreen with a sun protection factor (SPF) of at least 30.

Pruritus (itching) related to loss of oils in the skin is a common complaint of older persons. Hot baths, harsh soaps, and vigorous scrubbing contribute to dryness. If the patient has generalized itching, inform the registered nurse (RN) or the physician because it may be a symptom of illness such as diabetes, cancer, kidney disease, gallbladder disease, or liver disease.

Most older people can expect some hair loss, hair thinning, and color changes in the hair and nails. Both men and women experience graying and thinning of the hair on the scalp, axilla, and genitalia. Men are more likely to grow bald to varying degrees. Facial and nasal hairs may increase. Gray hair is caused by a slowing of pigment production in the hair follicles. Graying is determined by genetics and tends to be irreversible. Nails tend to become thicker and brittle with longitudinal striations. The most common benign lesions of aging are seborrheic dermatitis, acne, contact dermatitis, drug reactions, pressure injuries, stasis ulcers, pruritus, herpes zoster, onychomycosis and tinea pedis, and impetigo. Skin cancer is also more common in older people. New lesions or changes in existing lesions should be examined by the physician or nurse practitioner. These conditions are discussed in Chapters 56 and 57.

GASTROINTESTINAL SYSTEM

Changes in gastrointestinal functions occur with normal aging. Changes in the oral cavity include deterioration of the teeth and possibly a decrease in the number or sensitivity of taste buds. The commonly reported dry mouth is probably related to medications, inadequate hydration, and illness states rather than normal aging. Saliva becomes more alkaline and contains less amylase and ptyalin. The muscles associated with chewing weaken, so the patient may avoid foods that require more chewing. These changes may interfere with an older person's ability and desire to eat a nutritious meal.

Muscle contractions of the esophagus weaken which may explain complaints of reflux symptoms. Gastric emptying of liquids is also slower in older people than in the young. Decreased hydrochloric acid secretion is common in older adults but it is now thought to be caused by *Helicobacter pylori* infection rather than normal aging. With advanced age, calcium and zinc absorption is reduced. This is significant because a calcium deficiency contributes to loss of bone mass. Gallbladder function may decline with aging as well.

Collectively, the changes in the gastrointestinal system caused by aging increase the older person's risk for anorexia, bloating, indigestion, gas, and diarrhea or constipation. Constipation is one of the most frequent gastrointestinal complaints of older adults. Experts tend to agree that constipation is more likely caused by lack of dietary bulk and roughage, disease states, immobility, and drug effects rather than aging changes. Digestive complaints can be signs of more serious disorders. Symptoms that may suggest possible illness are decreased appetite, unexplained weight loss, excessive thirst, blood in the stool, or a change in the usual pattern of bowel movements.

The usual frequency for a bowel movement may range from as many as three movements per day to as few as one bowel movement every 7 days. However, most people have a bowel movement at least every 3 days. The most important factors are the person's usual pattern and whether the stool is passed easily. Constipation may be caused by lack of dietary fiber, inactivity, and dehydration rather than normal aging. See Chapter 39 for additional discussion about constipation.

MUSCULOSKELETAL SYSTEM

Of the multiple changes associated with an aging musculoskeletal system, changes affecting mobility are most significant. Age-related changes include decreased muscle strength, endurance, joint range of motion, coordination, bone density, and elasticity and flexibility of connective tissue.

Arthritis is the most prevalent chronic disease in men. However, it is more severe in women and is the leading cause of disability in old age. Osteoarthritis, the most common form of arthritis, is caused by damage to the inner surface of the joint. Age is the primary risk factor for arthritis, with heredity and obesity contributing to its development. The large weight-bearing joints (knees, hips, and spine) are most affected by arthritis. **Kyphosis** is the term applied to the curvature of the thoracic spine and gives rise to the bent-over appearance of some older adults. The loss of bone mass (osteoporosis) increases the risk of fractures, with the most common sites being the forearm, vertebrae, humerus, pelvis, and hip. Postural instability and low-body weight increase the risk of fractures.

Changes in muscle tissue include a gradual decrease in mass accompanied by an even greater decline in strength. The term *sarcopenia* is used to describe the loss of muscle strength. Weight-bearing exercises, particularly resistance strength training, may minimize sarcopenia. Walking, bicycling, and stair climbing also help to maintain bone and muscle mass. Assistive devices such as a walker can help a person to avoid falls if the person is unstable (Fig. 10.1).

SENSORY SYSTEM

Hearing

Because we depend on our five senses for almost everything we do, any loss of sensory ability can greatly affect our quality of life, function, and general well-being.

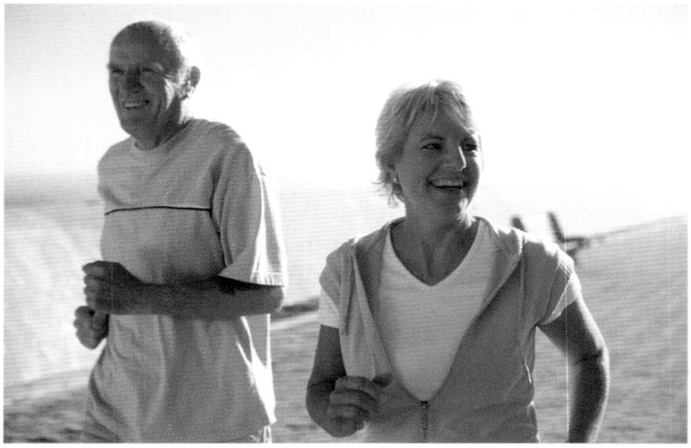

Fig. 10.1 Regular exercise is an important part of health promotion for the older adult. (Copyright Pixland/Thinkstock.com.)

Sensory changes in the older adult also place them at risk for injury and weaken self-confidence.

Presbycusis is the term for hearing loss associated with old age. Age-related causes of presbycusis include atrophic changes in the cochlea, auditory nerve, auditory brainstem pathways, and temporal lobe of the brain.

Basically, two types of hearing loss have been identified. **Conduction deafness** is a blockage of the ear canal caused by impacted cerumen (excessive earwax accumulation), abnormal structures, or infection. This type of loss may be easily treated. The other type of hearing loss is **sensorineural deafness**. It results from damage to nerve tissue as a result of exposure to loud noises, disease, and certain drugs. Hearing aids can often provide significant improvement. Tinnitus, an annoying ringing or buzzing in the ear, is a sensorineural disorder. Some cases of tinnitus can be caused by the use of aspirin or certain antibiotics or diuretics, or by tumors.

Some 25% of adults over 69 years of age and as many as one-half of adults over 85 years of age are hard of hearing. Older men tend to experience greater hearing loss than women. Many older adults are less able than younger people to hear high-pitched sounds and consonants, particularly ch, f, g, s, sh, t, th, and z. They can generally hear a lower voice tone better than a high-pitched voice. Not all older adults experience this type of loss and causes other than old age may be involved (e.g., noise exposure, ototoxic drugs). Regardless of the cause, hearing impairment creates a barrier to communication and is often associated with depression and isolation.

Vision

Common vision complaints reported by older persons include floaters, flashers, and dry eyes. Floaters are bits of debris floating in the vitreous humor that appear as spots moving in the field of vision. Traction on the retina causes the perception of flashing lights, or flashers. Although floaters and flashers are not in themselves harmful, they should be evaluated by a vision specialist as they may be related to serious conditions. Dry eyes occur because of decreased tear production. They can be treated with topical moisturizers.

The most common age-related change in vision is a condition called ***presbyopia***, which results from changes in the lens. The shape of the lens is controlled by muscles in the eye. By changing its shape, the lens allows us to change focus when looking from objects that are near to objects that are far. With age, the lens becomes more rigid and less able to change shape. Consequently, reading and other types of close work become difficult. Presbyopia is easily corrected by reading glasses or multifocal lenses. Furthermore, adapting to changes in lighting is also a function of the lenses. Maintaining good lighting in the home, particularly in hallways and around walkways, can help to prevent falls and other accidents. Whether the older person is a candidate for vision-correcting surgeries such as Lasik must be assessed individually.

Whereas presbyopia is considered a normal change, there are pathologic eye conditions that are common in older persons. The leading cause of new cases of blindness in older people is age-related macular degeneration. This condition affects the macula, the part of the eye that is responsible for sharp central vision. The two types are atrophic ("dry") and exudative ("wet") macular degeneration. There is no known treatment for the atrophic form. For the exudative form, repeated injections of a monoclonal antibody into the vitreous compartment of the eye are often effective in slowing the progression of macular degeneration. In some cases, a significant improvement in visual acuity has been achieved. Laser surgery offers some benefits but is not the first-line treatment.

Another serious eye disorder that occurs with aging is cataract. **Cataract** is clouding or opacity of the normally transparent lens within the eye. Cataracts are caused by changes in structural lens proteins, by damage to the lens as a result of high levels of blood glucose in people with diabetes, or by other factors. Cataract is treated by surgical removal of the clouded lens. Some type of lens replacement is required. Surgery is highly successful, and vision is usually restored in 90% to 95% of cases.

The leading cause of blindness in the United States is glaucoma. **Glaucoma** is characterized by atrophy of the optic nerve, usually associated with elevated pressure of the fluid in the eye. The optic nerve carries visual impulses from the eye to the brain. Thus damage to the nerve can result in progressive vision loss, described as "tunnel vision."

At present, glaucoma is not curable but is treatable with drugs or surgery. Early detection and effective treatment can slow or halt the disease process and save remaining eyesight. Older adults should receive annual eye examinations and a test for glaucoma.

Taste and Smell

Disorders of the senses involving taste and smell are called *chemosensory disorders*. More than 10 million Americans are affected by these types of disorders. Most of these disorders occur after 60 years of age and involve the ability to detect and differentiate scents. Men tend to be more affected than women and many causes exist, including nasal obstruction, allergies, and the use of certain drugs. The decline in the sense of smell may be caused by a decrease in olfactory nerve fibers.

Taste perception declines with age, possibly because of changes in the number or sensitivity of taste buds. The ability to detect sweet seems to remain intact while the ability to detect salty and bitter tastes declines. Major changes in the ability to taste are usually caused by diseases or are the side effects of certain drugs. Dentures, decreased saliva, hormonal changes, medications, and changes in chemicals needed to transmit taste are all potential causes of the older person's diminished sense of taste. This loss can affect changes in appetite.

Sensory losses are more than a minor nuisance for older adults. Poor vision and hearing increase a person's risk for falls and other accidents, which are leading causes of accidental death and disability in people over the 65 years of age. Furthermore, the inability to smell smoke, poisons, or other noxious odors endangers the lives of many older people. Decreased ability to taste food puts the older person at risk for malnutrition. Sensory changes greatly reduce the quality of life. To summarize, many of the physiologic changes associated with aging may reflect the presence of age-related diseases more than aging itself. Research is rapidly expanding and changing our knowledge of aging. Conditions once thought to represent normal aging are now known to be the product of disease. Many of the conditions can be prevented or controlled by good health practices and competent nursing care.

PSYCHOSOCIAL THEORIES OF AGING

Just as biologic changes occur with aging, so do psychosocial changes. Older adults are the products of decades of living that produce unique personalities, coping mechanisms, challenges, and growth. The social network is influential in the aging process and can support the individual in adapting to age-related changes (Fig. 10.2).

The fact that a person has survived to old age is one marker of successful adaptation. The survival of large numbers of relatively healthy older people is a new experience for humankind. The vast majority of older people have adapted adequately. These individuals are able to function independently and maintain a sense of well-being.

Maturity is defined as an optimal psychologic, social, and biologic adaptation achieved at some point

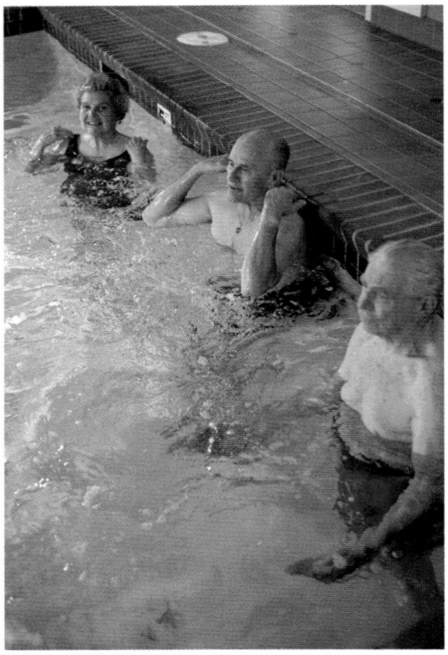

Fig. 10.2 Most older adults are active and independent. (Copyright Keith Brofsky/Photodisc/Thinkstock.com.)

during the midlife years, arbitrarily set between 45 and 65 years of age. Current thinking asserts that midlife crisis occurs, in part, when the individual in midlife becomes fully aware of their mortality.

ERIKSON'S DEVELOPMENTAL TASKS

As explained in Chapter 3, Erik Erikson developed one of the first developmental theories in the area of aging. Erikson identified the developmental task of old age as ego integrity versus despair. Ego integrity is attained when individuals review their lives and gain a feeling of accomplishment and fulfillment. They remain concerned with life in the face of death and begin to experience the wisdom that they have gained. The opposite of ego integrity is feelings of despair, in which people feel bitter about their lack of accomplishments in life and tend to regret life as they have lived it. Many people say that they have more regrets about the things they have not done or the risks they have not taken than the mistakes they have made.

Old age involves much more than a psychologic waiting station before death. It represents an important stage of development and coping that occurs between the high points and accomplishments of the middle years and the concerns that are involved as the end of life approaches. Movement toward ego integrity is facilitated when the older person:

- Recognizes and accepts changes in physical and mental capabilities
- Gives up some roles and develops new ones
- Develops new activities that can be carried out successfully with aging
- Develops a different self-concept
- Revises life goals
- Adapts to new lifestyles

In the final stage of development, older persons are faced with a variety of internal and external losses that require coping and adaptation using diminished biologic, psychologic, and social resources. The challenge is to maintain performance in the face of adverse circumstances. A complete discussion of adult developmental tasks is found in Chapter 3.

DISENGAGEMENT, ACTIVITY, AND CONTINUITY THEORIES

Various scientists have studied the way in which social life changes in later years. Disengagement theory predicts the gradual withdrawal of society and older people from each other. The process is described as mutually beneficial, relieving the older person of social responsibilities and making way for younger people to fill the gap. Disengagement theory has lost favor because it has failed to demonstrate mutual appeal and is viewed as disenfranchising older people who still have much to give. Activity theory describes successful aging as remaining mentally and physically active. It assumes that activity is better than inactivity, that happiness is better than unhappiness, and that the older person must decide how successful their aging is. In a sense, it actually encourages people to continue their middle-age lifestyle for as long as possible. Continuity theory provided an alternative to disengagement and activity theories. It asserts that old age is part of the life cycle and that old people behave in later years much as they did throughout life. A person who has always been sociable is likely to remain sociable in later years. The individual who preferred a more solitary lifestyle would continue to prefer that lifestyle when older. Other theories that attempt to explain aging from a social perspective include subculture theory, age stratification theory, and person-environment fit theory.

COPING AND ADAPTATION

Old age has been described as the season of losses, including loss of roles, status, and physical abilities, and deep personal losses through the deaths of friends and the disruption of family networks. Loss, whether real, threatened, or imaginary, is a stressor that requires adaptation, flexibility, and resiliency if a person is to cope successfully.

In most respects, older people cope in much the same way as younger people. Differences are largely the result of the different types of stressors experienced. Older people tend to experience more negative and irreversible types of stressors. Given the many losses associated with old age as potential stressors, the older person may cope with these losses in a positive or negative manner. Positive adaptation might include rational action, perseverance, positive thinking (e.g., the lost loved one is now out of pain), intellectual denial (e.g., "I don't want to think about it now."), restraint, drawing strength from adversity, and humor.

Unfortunately, some older individuals are unable to cope effectively with their losses. They lose their sense of personal identity and fulfillment and suffer from deterioration in self-esteem, an altered self-concept, and a loss of meaningfulness in life. A small percentage of older people become seriously depressed. They may lose motivation for working, playing, and living. Depression resulting from loss is a factor in approximately two-thirds of the suicides among older people. Suicide is most common among White men 85 years of age and older.

FAMILY

With an aging population that needs support and assistance, kinship networks take on added importance. Most of the older persons in the United States occupy a variety of family roles and come from multigenerational units. It is common for a person at 65 years of age to be married, have at least one living adult child, have at least one living sibling, be a grandparent, and be a great-grandparent. The person over 65 years of age may also be a child of a much older parent. The kinship network may also include cousins, nieces, and nephews. Of all these roles and relationships, marital relationships and the relationships between parent and child seem to be most important.

In an era when the aged are sometimes labeled as burdens, an important point to recognize is that more financial support flows from the old to the young in the family than in the reverse direction. Although family responsibility is respected by most people, laws exist in many states that can require children to provide financial support for needy parents. However, what is most needed and most often given is emotional support and help in times of illness and disability. Home care for the frail older adult is most often given by a spouse or a child. Typically, the caregiver is a daughter, and almost half of these women are also rearing children.

Informal caregivers experience enormous stress and encounter various levels of emotional, physical, financial, and family strain. Caregivers frequently report symptoms of depression, anxiety, helplessness, low morale, and emotional exhaustion. In part because of caregiver stress, more than 1 million older persons are thought to be abused physically and psychologically or are neglected each year by their caregivers. When working with these families, health care providers should acknowledge the stressful impact of caregiving and work with them to identify ways to minimize the burdens on the individuals and the family.

You are in an excellent position to recognize stress, depression, and abuse among caregivers and care recipients. Nurses are obligated to report suspected abuse. The LVN/LPN should work with the RN or other supervisor to handle reporting and interventions in abuse situations. Education for learning positive adaptive behaviors can assist both caregivers and care recipients. Caregivers who feel knowledgeable, useful, productive, and appreciated are usually happier, less stressed, and less prone to be abusive. Nursing care should treat the patient and family as a unit and seek to determine the needs and resources of all members.

FUNCTIONAL ASSESSMENT

Ongoing functional assessments are essential as the needs of the older patient evolve. Although a diagnosis may give you a general idea about a patient's abilities, it does not tell you how well the patient is functioning with that diagnosis. For example, one patient with a medical diagnosis of coronary artery disease might be independent and active whereas another patient might be homebound and on oxygen. The functional assessment should describe both basic and instrumental activities of daily living, noting the amount of assistance, if any, needed to carry out each activity. Activities of daily living include grooming, bathing, dressing, eating, elimination, and mobility. Instrumental activities of daily living (IADL) include the ability to prepare a meal, shop for groceries, use the telephone, negotiate transportation, take medications, and maintain housekeeping and laundry tasks. IADL are less important in institutional settings but are essential for a person to continue or return to independent living.

The LVN/LPN contributes to the functional assessment by collecting data about activities of daily living as well as environmental, financial, family, economic, and community resources.

A variety of tools are available for comprehensive assessments. The Duke Older Americans Resources and Services (OARS) Multidimensional Functional Assessment Questionnaire (MFAQ) is a widely used comprehensive guide for assessing the overall personal functional status and the need for services. A content summary is provided in Box 10.2. In most instances, the nursing home Minimum Data Set incorporates all components of a quality functional assessment. SPICES is a convenient tool that includes six key assessment areas for the older adult patient and can be used for routine focused assessments (Box 10.3).

Put On Your Thinking Cap!

Discuss the importance of functional assessments of older adults who receive home health care. What functions would an older adult need to manage self-care in the home?

DRUG THERAPY AND OLDER ADULTS

ABSORPTION, DISTRIBUTION, METABOLISM, AND EXCRETION

Medication use by older adults in the United States is extremely common. Some sources estimate that 44% of men and 57% of women 65 years of age and over

Box 10.2 Content Areas of the Duke Older Americans Resources and Services Multidimensional Functional Assessment Questionnaire

PART A: FUNCTIONAL ASSESSMENT	PART B: SERVICES
Social	Transportation
Living arrangements	Social/recreational
Contact with others	Employment
Social help from family and kin	Sheltered employment
Economic	Educational, employment related
Employment status	Remedial training
Income source, amount, adequacy	Mental health
Home ownership	Psychotropic drugs
Mental	Personal care
Cognitive and psychiatric status	Nursing care
Mental well-being	Medical services
Physical	Supportive devices/prostheses
Prescribed medications used	Physical therapy
Physical conditions with impairment levels	Continuous supervision
Activities of Daily Living	Checking
Physical and instrumental activities of daily living	Relocation and placement
Demographics and Administrative	Homemaker-household
Age, gender, race, education	Meal preparation
Location, length of interview	Administrative legal and protective
Information source	Systematic multidimensional evaluation
	Financial assistance
	Food, groceries
	Housing
	Coordination, information, referral

Modified from Fillenbaum GG. *Multidimensional functional assessment of older adults: The Duke Older Americans Resources and Services Procedures.* Erlbaum, Hillsdale, NJ; 1988; updated 1996 (available only from Center for the Study of Aging and Human Development, Duke University Medical Center, Durham, NC).

Box 10.3 SPICES Assessment Tool

Sleep disorders
Problems with eating or drinking
Incontinence
Confusion
Evidence of falls
Skin breakdown

may take five or more prescription and/or over-the-counter (OTC) medications each week. Some 12% of both genders take 10 or more medications each week. Imagine the potential for errors and drug interactions with so many medications! Age-related changes affect patterns of drug use and drug effects (Table 10.2). The most important changes involve body composition, the cardiovascular and nervous systems, renal function, tissue sensitivity to drugs, and blood pressure reflex sensitivity.

Table 10.2 Association Between Age-Related Physiologic Changes and Drug Effects

AGE-RELATED CHANGES	DRUG EFFECTS
Increased body fat	Increased storage of fat-soluble drugs
Decreased body water	Increased drug/active concentration
Decreased hepatic blood flow	Decreased drug metabolism
Decreased lean muscle mass	Increased drug tissue concentration
Decreased renal function	Decreased drug elimination
Decreased serum albumin	Increased concentration of free drug molecules that bind to protein

With aging comes a reduction in body size, with a decrease in lean body mass and body water content and an increase in fat. The serum albumin concentration is reduced, which tends to make additional free drug molecules available to tissues or to permit increasingly rapid elimination of the drug. A gradual decrease in blood flow to the liver and kidneys reduces drug clearance. Drug characteristics also affect distribution of drug molecules in the tissues. For example, a water-soluble drug may result in increased blood concentrations of that drug. However, a highly fat-soluble drug might bind to the increased fat in the aged body and may be stored longer before excretion.

The liver prepares drugs for elimination in the urine or in feces. Age-related changes in the liver, which include decreased size, reduced blood flow, and reduced enzyme activity, affect the metabolism (inactivation) of drugs. When drug metabolism is impaired, drug concentrations in the blood increase and elimination of the drug may be delayed. Because of changes in the kidneys, drugs that are eliminated primarily in the urine may accumulate and have adverse effects. Thus lower dosages or longer intervals between doses are often indicated to avoid harm.

Put On Your Thinking Cap!

A 75-year-old woman was diagnosed as having a progressive brain disease after she developed urinary incontinence, general mental deterioration, and an inability to walk. She had been taking the fat-soluble drug diazepam (Valium) daily for at least 1 year to treat anxiety. After the drug was discontinued, the patient recovered completely. What might explain this sequence of events?

ADVERSE DRUG REACTIONS

Adverse drug reactions are more common in older people partly because they use more drugs. The risk of adverse drug reactions increases with the number

Table 10.3 Drugs Commonly Associated With Adverse Drug Reactions in Older Persons

DRUG CLASS	EXAMPLE	PROBLEM
Analgesics	meperidine	Confusion
Antibiotics	streptomycin	Nephrotoxicity
Anticoagulants	warfarin	Hemorrhage
Antidepressants	amitriptyline	Sedation
Antihypertensives	verapamil	Hypotension
Antiparkinsonians	benztropine	Confusion, psychotic-like symptoms
Antipsychotics	haloperidol	Orthostatic hypotension, sedation, extrapyramidal effects
Diuretics	spironolactone	Hyperkalemia
Nonsteroidal antiinflammatory drugs (NSAIDs)	aspirin, ibuprofen	Bleeding, peptic ulcers
Sedatives/hypnotics	flurazepam	Ataxia, excessive sedation

of drugs consumed, dose level, duration of treatment, and severity of illness. Adverse effects may also result when the patient does not take drugs as prescribed.

Some of the common signs and symptoms of adverse drug reactions in the older person are restlessness, falls, depression, confusion, loss of memory, constipation, and urinary incontinence. Older persons tend to be more sensitive than the young to drugs that act on the central nervous system. Thus drugs for anxiety, pain, or sleep may produce excessive drowsiness and respiratory depression. When patients experience unpleasant side effects, they may not follow the prescribed regimen. Starting new drugs at low doses usually reduces side effects and increases patient cooperation. Some drugs commonly associated with adverse drug reactions in older adults are listed in Table 10.3.

Nurses who work with older adults should be familiar with the Beers Criteria for Potentially Inappropriate Medication Use in Older Adults. This source identifies drugs that are generally problematic in older persons and has a second listing of drugs that are problematic in the presence of specific conditions. Inclusion of a drug in the Beers Criteria does not mean that the drug is absolutely contraindicated, but the prescriber should be aware that the drug poses specific risks for the older patient. Although the LVN/LPN does not select drugs, they should question any drug order that might be harmful and share resources such as the Beers Criteria with other professionals.

Pharmacology Capsule

Copies of the Beers Criteria tables can be obtained at AGS Beer Criteria for Potentially Inappropriate Medication Use in Older Adults. AmericanGeriatrics.Org.

Because older adults experience a greater number of drug reactions and interactions than younger people and are believed to be more sensitive to some medications, their drug regimens should be monitored carefully. Home care patients should maintain records of data relevant to their medications (e.g., blood pressure, pulse, respiration, drug effect, state of alertness). Such a record could be helpful in making necessary changes. Changing a drug, reducing the dose level, or lengthening the intervals between doses may be necessary to minimize the risk of adverse drug reactions. The nurse is very often in the best position to minimize adverse effects by careful monitoring and notifying the prescriber of concerns. Baseline and continual assessments should include the following:

- The amount, frequency, and purpose of all medications taken
- The older person's ability and willingness to take recommended medications
- The potential for drug interactions and adverse drug reactions
- The effectiveness of the medication over time
- Whether any of the drugs taken can be discontinued or decreased in dose

Assessment of drug effects and adverse reactions must be documented.

A problem that is sometimes overlooked is the potential for drug interactions between OTC medications and prescription medications taken by older adults. Examples include the use of aspirin, which enhances the effect of anticoagulants, or the use of large amounts of sodium bicarbonate, which counteracts diuretic actions. Botanicals can also interact with prescription and OTC drugs. A second problem is that the older adult may mix older prescription medications with newer ones and fail to discontinue and discard older drugs. Hoarding of medications may be viewed as future savings by an older adult. Having the patient bring all medications to office visits provides an opportunity to review the drugs and identify problems, duplications, or misunderstandings.

THE NURSE AND THE OLDER PATIENT

Nurses who work with older adults have the opportunity to maintain or improve quality of life by providing holistic care that addresses their physiologic and psychosocial needs. The challenges are sometimes daunting, but the rewards are huge. This chapter has provided an overview of the aging process and the health care implications of the many changes that occur. Throughout this book, the special needs of older persons will be reinforced. Specific interventions for various health deviations will be addressed in appropriate chapters that cover disease processes in each body system.

Put On Your Thinking Cap!

Recall an older adult who has been discharged from the hospital with some physical or cognitive impairments. What instrumental activities of daily living are likely to be affected in this person?

Get Ready for the NCLEX® Examination!

Key Points

- Aging is an ongoing developmental process that begins at conception and ends at death.
- Gerontology is the study of aging.
- Geriatrics is the biomedical science of old age and the application of knowledge of aging to the prevention, diagnosis, treatment, and care of older persons.
- The roles of the gerontological nurse include healer, caregiver, educator, advocate, and innovator.
- Gerontological nursing aims to increase healthy behaviors in the aged; minimize and compensate for health-related losses and impairments of aging; provide comfort and sustenance through the events of aging; and facilitate the diagnosis, care, and treatment of disease in the aged.
- Health care providers can dispel myths about the older adult and aging that result in stereotyping of and discrimination against older people.
- Aging occurs slowly and is a complex and dynamic process involving many internal and external influences.
- Physiologic changes that are common with aging may reflect the presence of age-related diseases and lifestyle more than the process of aging itself.
- The older adult shows cumulative developmental effects that produce unique personality styles, coping mechanisms, challenges, and growth, all of which occur in a societal context.
- Age-related changes that increase the risk of adverse drug effects include a decreased ability to metabolize and eliminate drugs through the liver and renal system, increased sensitivity to some drugs, and altered body composition.

Additional Learning Resources

SG Go to your Study Guide for additional learning activities to help you master this chapter content.

Go to your Evolve website (http://evolve.elsevier.com/Linton/medsurg) for the following learning resources and much more:

- Fluid & Electrolyte Tutorial
- Review Questions for the NCLEX® Examination

Clinical Judgment and Next-Generation NCLEX® Examination-Style Questions

1. The nurse educator in a retirement community is preparing an orientation for new staff about working with older adults. Which statement should be included in the lesson plan?

1. Many older people continue to enjoy sexual activity.
2. Older people generally lack family and other support networks.
3. Almost 50% of people over 65 years of age have dementia.
4. About 25% of the older population resides in nursing homes.

NCLEX Client Need: Psychosocial Integrity

2. Neurologic changes commonly found in the healthy older adult include: (Select all that apply.)

1. Impaired short-term memory
2. Inability to learn new material
3. Decline in intellectual function
4. Easy distraction from tasks
5. Loss of creative abilities

NCLEX Client Need: Health Promotion and Maintenance and Physiological Integrity: Physiological Adaptation

3. Mr. J. had been a healthy 90-year-old man until he developed pneumonia. While acutely ill with pneumonia, he showed signs of early heart and renal failure. He became weak and his tolerance for physical activity declined. Even though the pneumonia resolved, several months passed before he returned to his previous level of functioning. How would you explain this delay?

1. At 90 years of age, immune function is severely impaired.
2. He probably did not seek treatment for his pneumonia soon enough.
3. Acute illness overwhelmed his already limited cardiac and renal function.
4. He wanted to continue getting the attention he received when he was acutely ill.

NCLEX Client Need: Health Promotion and Maintenance

4. **Which of the following statements should be included when teaching a group of active older people about skin care? (Select all that apply.)**
   1. Sunscreens are recommended to reduce the risk of skin cancer.
   2. Changes in existing skin lesions should be reported to the nurse or physician.
   3. To remove dead skin, take hot baths followed by vigorous towel drying.
   4. Generous use of moisturizers and minimal use of soap prevent skin drying.
   5. Generalized itching may be a symptom of a serious illness.

   NCLEX Client Need: Health Promotion and Maintenance

5. **You observe that an older patient's thoracic spine is curved, causing her to bend forward. The term used to describe this condition is ______________________.**

   NCLEX Client Need: Physiological Integrity: Physiological Adaptation

6. **When a patient has presbycusis, which of the following nursing interventions is most important?**
   1. Ensure that room lighting is adequate
   2. Lower the pitch of your voice
   3. Monitor the patient's blood pressure
   4. Implement body fluid precautions

   NCLEX Client Need: Physiological Integrity: Physiological Adaptation

7. **Which of these statements by older adults reflects movement toward ego integrity?**
   1. "Since I cannot drive now, I rarely get out or see other people."
   2. "After my children grew up and my husband died, I just wasn't needed anymore."
   3. "In my day, when you got married, you stayed married, no matter how bad it was."
   4. "I can't run marathons anymore, but I still enjoy a brisk walk around the neighborhood."

   NCLEX Client Need: Psychosocial Integrity

8. **Instrumental activities of daily living include which of the following? (Select all that apply.)**
   1. Bathing
   2. Cooking
   3. Shopping
   4. Eating
   5. Elimination

   NCLEX Client Need: Physiological Integrity: Basic Care and Comfort

9. **An older postoperative patient is receiving pain medications that depress the central nervous system. Based on your knowledge of drug therapy and aging, what adverse effect is most likely?**
   1. Respiratory depression
   2. Difficulty sleeping
   3. Vomiting and diarrhea
   4. Agitation

   NCLEX Client Need: Physiological Integrity: Pharmacological Therapies

10. **SLO/Objective: Apply knowledge of anatomy and physiology and pathophysiology to determine which assessment data require follow-up by the nurse.**

    NGN Item Type: Enhanced Hot Spot

    Cognitive Skill: Recognize Skills

    An 85-year-old woman is residing in a long-term care facility (LTC) because of her inability to care for herself. She is frequently **incontinent** of urine and needs assistance to use the bathroom for bathing and toileting. The patient moves from the bed to a wheelchair with assistance. Highlight or place a checkmark next to the assessment finding that requires follow-up by the nurse.
    1. Blood pressure 120/80 mm Hg sitting, 100/68 mm Hg standing
    2. Heart rate 88 beats per minute
    3. Respiration rate 20 per minute
    4. Urge incontinence
    5. Needs assistance with ADLs (toileting, bathing, dressing, eating)
    6. Oriented x3

11 Falls

http://evolve.elsevier.com/Linton/medsurg

Objectives

1. Define falls.
2. State the incidence of falls.
3. Describe factors that increase the risk of falls.
4. Discuss the relationship between restraint use and falls, types of restraints, and regulations for restraint use.
5. Describe fall prevention techniques in acute care and long-term care and the home.
6. Describe nursing interventions to use when a fall occurs.
7. Explain what is meant by *least restrictive* interventions for fall prevention.

Key Terms

chemical restraint
extrinsic factors
fall
intrinsic factors
Omnibus Budget Reconciliation Act (OBRA)
physical restraint

If several people were asked whether they had fallen in the past 6 months, the chances are that many would say "yes." The chances are even greater that those who have fallen, particularly the young and healthy adults, have not sustained a significant injury. Although falls do not necessarily result in serious physical injuries or death, many older people who have fallen become less confident in their ability to function independently. Those who fear falling may tend to restrict their physical and social activities, become more dependent, and have an increased need for long-term care (LTC). In addition, caregivers tend to restrict older persons' activities out of the concern that ill or frail people, who have been weakened from sickness, hospitalization, or inactivity, may fall and be injured.

DEFINITION OF FALLS

The World Health Organization (WHO, 2016) defines a **fall** as an event that results in a person coming to rest inadvertently on the ground or floor or other lower level. The American Nurses Association further defines falls as an unplanned descent to the floor (or extension of the floor, e.g., trash can or other equipment) with or without injury to the patient. All types of falls are to be included, whether they result from physiologic reasons (fainting) or environmental reasons (slippery floor).

INCIDENCE AND RISK FACTORS

Although falls and fall-related injuries occur at every age, the greater severity of injuries in old age, combined with longer recovery periods, makes a fall a particularly serious threat to the health and functioning of older people. Falls are the leading cause of injury, both fatal and nonfatal, among the older population. The incidence of falls increases with age and setting. In 2018, 27.5% of people aged 65 years and older reported at least one fall in the past year, increasing to 34% in those 85 years and older. Approximately 50% of older adults in long-term care settings fall every year (Moreland et al., 2020).

Falls are the most frequent cause of accidental injury and death among older adults, and the risk of injury from falls is highest in people over 75 years of age. Among community-dwelling older persons, approximately 30% fall every year, compared with 50% to 75% of those living in residential care facilities. In most incidents, no injuries occur; however, approximately 5% to 10% of falls result in serious injury, including head trauma, major lacerations and fractures. In nursing home residents, the incidence rises to 10% to 30%.

The U.S. Public Health Service (USPHS) has estimated that two-thirds of deaths as a result of falls are preventable. Potentially avoidable environmental factors cause about half of fatal falls. According to the USPHS, adequate medical evaluation and treatment for underlying medical conditions probably could prevent most of the remaining fatal falls.

Falling is not a normal part of aging. However, older adults are at particular risk for accidents because of predisposing and precipitating factors that are more common in older adults. Falls occur because of two major factors: (1) **intrinsic factors**, or factors related to the functioning of the individual; and (2) **extrinsic factors**, or environmental factors. Intrinsic factors enhance the possibility of falling whereas extrinsic factors enhance the opportunity to fall.

Intrinsic factors related to falls include sensory impairments such as reduced vision and hearing, changes in posture and gait, confusion, depression, lack of exercise leading to weakness, urge or stress urinary incontinence, acute infections, neurologic conditions that affect balance, and overestimation of abilities. In addition, the medications that many older adults take for various chronic illnesses may cause dizziness or drowsiness.

Extrinsic factors may differ according to the setting. For example, potential hazards in the home environment include low-lying and poorly visible tables, trailing electrical wires, pets, steep and unlit stairs, loose carpeting, throw rugs, unsafe walking aids, and inconvenient bathroom or kitchen arrangements. Falls occurring in the institutional setting as a result of various environmental factors are often related to changes in position, such as transferring to and from a bed or chair; toileting procedures; unstable and defective equipment (e.g., nonfunctioning brake locks on wheelchairs); wet or excessively waxed floors; use of assistive devices; and obstructions in hallways. In addition, falls may result from imposed immobility. Patients who spend much of their time in a bed or chair weaken and develop problems with balance. Falls often occur during periods of high activity when staff members are busy.

The cost of falls is greater than simply the billions of dollars spent in required treatments; the loss of independence and confidence, as well as the loss of life, must be considered. To address this important problem, the Joint Commission (2015) recommended actions to help health care organizations prevent falls and fall-related injury. The goal is to achieve risk reduction and continuous improvement within specific settings and among specific populations (Box 11.1). (See the Nursing Care Plan).

Put On Your Thinking Cap!

Assess one of your patients in the clinical setting to identify intrinsic and extrinsic risk factors for falling. Develop nursing interventions to prevent falls in this specific situation.

RESTRAINTS

Restraints restrict an individual's movement and are classified as either *physical* or *chemical*. A **physical restraint** can be anything that restricts movement and that cannot be removed by the patient. Examples of physical restraints are side rails; chairs with trays; and vest, waist, wrist, or ankle ties. Physical restraints are sometimes classified as safety restraint devices (SRDs). A **chemical restraint** is a drug that is given to subdue agitated or confused patients.

Box 11.1 The Joint Commission Recommended Actions to Prevent Falls and Fall-Related Injuries

1. Lead an effort to raise awareness of the need to prevent falls resulting in injury.
2. Establish an interdisciplinary falls injury prevention team or evaluate the membership of the team in place.
3. Use a standard, validated tool to identify risk factors for falls.
4. Develop an individualized plan of care based on identified fall and injury risks and implement interventions specific to a patient population or setting.
5. Standardize and apply practices and interventions demonstrated to be effective including:
   - A standardized hand-off communication process for communicating patient risk for falls with injury between caregivers.
   - One-to-one education of each patient at the bedside by trained health professionals.
6. Conduct post-fall management, which includes: a post-fall huddle; a system of honest, transparent reporting; trending and analysis of falls that can inform improvement efforts; and reassess the patient.

Preventing falls and fall-related injuries in health care facilities. The Joint Commission Issue 55, September 28, 2015, Sentinel Event Alert, 2020.

SAFETY RESTRAINT DEVICE

Older patients, particularly those who are confused, are more likely to be physically restrained than younger patients, probably because they are at greater risk of falling. The most common reasons given for using safety restraint devices (SRDs) with older patients in hospitals or LTC facilities are to (1) protect the patient or others from harm or prevent tampering with medical devices (e.g., feeding tube, catheter), (2) prevent falls from the bed or chair, and (3) prevent wandering. The most common incidents precipitating the use of restraints involve attempts to get out of bed or resistance to treatment while confused or disoriented.

It is difficult to justify the use of restraints to prevent injuries because research has shown that restraints actually cause injuries. Physical restraints can tear the skin and impair circulation and joint mobility. Accidental strangulation has occurred when patients slide down while secured to a chair or bed by a vest or strap restraint. Nurses have long been taught to raise side rails so that vulnerable patients will either stay in bed or call for help. The wisdom of using side rails to keep a person in bed is now in question. Although properly installed modern bed rails should be safe, patients have been injured, sometimes fatally, after crawling over side rails or becoming trapped between side rail bars or between the side rails and the mattress. It has been found that many patients who had fallen out of bed had raised side rails. Half-rails may be safer than full rails.

Restraints likely have damaging psychologic effects on older patients. Patients may experience anger, discomfort, resistance, and fear in response to physical

Nursing Care Plan Patient With a History of Falling

FOCUSED ASSESSMENT

Health History

A 75-year-old woman resides in a long-term care (LTC) facility because of chronic health problems that include hypertension, emphysema, and mild dementia. She has a history of several falls at home, including one that resulted in a wrist fracture that led to her admission to the LTC facility. She can walk but requires assistance because her balance is poor, she becomes short of breath, and she experiences dizziness with position changes. The nursing staff frequently reminds her to call for help and often checks on her but she continues to get up unassisted when unsupervised. In the past, she enjoyed daily walks but gave them up when she began to have trouble breathing and sometimes had dizzy spells. Her only activity since admission has been attendance at religious services and bingo games. She enjoys reading large-print romance novels.

Physical Examination

Vital signs: blood pressure 144/76 mm Hg, pulse 90 beats per minute; respiration 22 breaths per minute; oral temperature 97°F (35°C). Height 5′1″, weight 98 lb. Skin is warm and dry. Wheezing is noted on expiration. The patient is oriented to person, time, and place.

Patient Problems	Goals and Outcome Criteria	Interventions
Potential for injury related to falls because of weakness, dizziness, and poor balance	Patient will remain free from injury	Ask the patient whether she is concerned about falling. Explain the fall risk and need to call for assistance. Provide the nurse call button and respond quickly to her calls. Discuss possible physical therapy consultation to evaluate the use of cane or walker and to recommend appropriate strengthening and balance exercises. Advise her to wear supportive, nonslip shoes. Provide the patient's glasses or hearing aid.
Potential for injury related to falls owing to environmental hazards		Assess the patient and environment for possible hazards. Discuss possible environmental hazards and measures to reduce risks. Consider rearranging furniture to provide clear pathways. Keep her bed at its lowest level. Consult with the patient about providing a bedside commode if she has difficulty getting to the toilet.
Potential for injury related to falls owing to postural hypotension		Consult with a registered nurse about drugs that may be causing postural hypotension; a change may be indicated. Suggest elastic stockings to improve venous return. Teach the patient to change positions slowly and to exercise her legs before rising. Determine usual fluid intake and encourage adequate fluids to prevent dehydration.

CRITICAL THINKING QUESTIONS

1. How could glasses and a hearing aid reduce the risk of falls?
2. When in a clinical site, examine the patient's room to identify possible hazards in the patient's environment that might contribute to falls.

restraint. Other possible outcomes include poor self-image, growing dependency, increased confusion and disorientation, regressive behavior, and withdrawal.

The many negative effects of physical restraints prompted passage of the **Omnibus Budget Reconciliation Act (OBRA)** of 1987, which included policies to protect patients from unnecessary restraint in LTC facilities. The law specified that patients have the right to be free from restraint used for purposes of discipline or convenience and that is not required to treat patients' medical symptoms. Restraint use requires a physician's order that specifies the duration and circumstances under which the restraint may be used. Although the number of falls rose as restraint use declined, most of those incidents did not result in serious injury. In fact, the most serious injuries occurred among patients who were restrained.

According to OBRA regulations, the only people who are candidates for restraints are those who:

- Have a history of severe falls or are at extremely high risk of taking a fall that is life threatening;
- Are neurologically, orthopedically, or muscularly impaired and need postural support for safety or comfort, or both;
- Experience any number of mental dysfunctions that may cause them to be a serious hazard to themselves, objects, or others; or
- Have medical symptoms that are life threatening and require the temporary use of a restraint to provide necessary treatment.

When restraints are used, data indicating the need for restraints must be documented in the patient record. If a physical restraint is used, the least restrictive device is best. For example, use a mitt rather than a wrist restraint that limits movement. Check the patient frequently, at least every 15 to 30 minutes. A patient who is agitated or combative must be monitored continuously. Ensure that the restraint is used properly and is providing adequate protection and comfort without impeding circulation or breathing. Remove and release physical

Box 11.2 Alternatives to Physical Restraint

1. Anticipate needs.
2. Provide companionship and supervision by involving family, friends, or volunteers, especially at night.
3. Distract attention with television, radio, CD player, or other activities that interest patient.
4. Arrange environment for easy access to equipment and personal items (e.g., call bell, water, bedside commode).
5. Change forms of treatment contributing to restraint use (e.g., substitute oral feedings for intravenous or nasogastric tubes, remove catheters).
6. Redesign furniture (e.g., lower beds, place mattress on floor, remove wheels from furniture).
7. Use bed and chair alarms to alert caregiver that patient is up.
8. Use exit alarms on exterior doors. Disguise exit doors or doorknobs to discourage exiting (e.g., shower curtain or drape over door). Install slide lock near bottom of door.
9. Enroll patient in Safe Return program that includes identification device with contact information.

restraints every 2 hours for 10 minutes to provide for range of motion, toileting, nourishment, and comfort measures. Document ongoing assessments while the patient is restrained.

Identify patients at risk for restraint so that you can try alternatives. Several alternatives to physical restraint are participating in physical therapy, engaging the patient in group activities, sitting and talking with patients for short periods of time, recruiting family members or volunteers to spend time with the patient, and assigning staff to be responsible for high-risk patients in small blocks of time. Box 11.2 lists more alternatives to physical restraint. In addition, patients, family members, or both should be involved in the decision to use or not to use physical restraint. Special units for the care of persons with dementia typically are designed so that wanderers can move about freely without fear of leaving the premises.

Put On Your Thinking Cap!

When in the clinical setting, observe the methods used as alternatives to physical restraint. Could other steps be taken?

CHEMICAL RESTRAINTS

The same guidelines that apply to the use of physical restraints apply to chemical restraints. Never use psychotropic drugs for the purposes of discipline or convenience. They should be used only when the danger of self-injury or injury to others exists. The administration of a psychotropic drug requires a physician's written order that specifies the duration and circumstance under which the medication is to be used. Always document the patient assessment before giving a psychotropic drug and after administering the drug.

Psychotropic drugs, including antidepressants, sedatives/hypnotics (e.g., benzodiazepines), and antipsychotic drugs, are the most commonly prescribed chemical restraints. All can have serious adverse effects, such as greater confusion, agitation, postural hypotension, and an increased number of falls in older persons. Other drugs that increase the risk of falls because of postural hypotension are some of the antihypertensives and diuretics, both commonly used by older persons. Avoid the use of psychotropic drugs if at all possible. The same alternatives to physical restraints apply to chemical restraints (see Box 11.2).

NURSING ASSESSMENT AND INTERVENTION

FALL PREVENTION

The most important intervention for falls is prevention. The best prevention is education of patients, families, and caregivers about the ways to prevent falls. Prevention is aimed toward minimizing both the intrinsic and the extrinsic factors that cause falls and increase the potential for injury.

The first step in preventing falls and injury is to determine who is at risk. People who are at greatest risk for falls and injury are those who have fallen before and those who have multiple intrinsic risk factors. Table 11.1 lists intrinsic risk factors for falling and possible interventions. The more risk factors a person has, the greater the risk of falling. Several tools for the assessment of fall risk exist, including the Hendrich II Fall Risk Model for use in acute care settings. A simple screening tool for fall risk is to have the patient sit in an armless chair, rise, walk, return, and sit back down in the chair. Patients who have difficulty with this task should be assessed in greater detail. Be ready to assist if the patient is unsteady. Other related tools assess gait, balance, and fear of falling (Box 11.3). One strategy that can be used to alert staff to patients at risk for falling is the use of a yellow wristband. It is important for staff to include information about fall risk and known effective interventions when patients are transferred to other units or settings.

Fall prevention strategies are carried out in the home and in institutional environments (Fig. 11.1). Evidence-based interventions that are likely to be effective include muscle strengthening and balance training, tai chi, modification of the home environment, withdrawal of psychotropic medications and drugs that cause hypotension, and cardiac pacing for selected patients. Effective interventions need to be individualized based on the specific factors that create a fall risk for the individual patient. Fall prevention guidelines for the home are listed in the Patient Teaching box; those for use in institutional settings are listed in Box 11.4. Finally, the Health Promotion box offers general tips for preventing falls.

Table 11.1 Intrinsic Risk Factors for Falling and Possible Interventions

RISK FACTORS	INTERVENTIONS
Impaired Vision	
Reduced visual acuity	Ensure that the individual wears glasses, if appropriate. Keep glasses clean. Encourage regular eye examinations. Paint last step a lighter color.
Impaired dark adaptation	Maintain adequate lighting, reduce glare from shiny floors, and allow time to adjust to light levels (e.g., as patient moves from a dark room to the outside). Wear sunglasses in sunlight. Use a night-light in the bedroom and bathroom.
Impaired Hearing	
Impacted cerumen (earwax)	Remove earwax.
Presbycusis	Speak slowly, use a low voice, and decrease background noise. Encourage the use of a hearing aid. Advise to scan environment while walking.
Balance and Gait Problems	
Musculoskeletal disorders	Encourage balance and gait training and muscle-strengthening exercises.
Balance disorders	Encourage balance exercises. Provide and educate the patient on the use of assistive devices. Avoid alcohol.
Peripheral neuropathy	Encourage the patient to use correctly sized footwear with firm soles.
Foot disorders	Trim toenails. Encourage patient to wear appropriate footwear. Advise podiatry for foot care.
Cardiovascular Disease	
Postural hypotension	Encourage dorsiflexion exercises. Use pressure-graded stockings. Elevate the head of the bed before rising. Teach the patient to get up from a chair or bed slowly. Advise patient not to tip the head backward.
Neurologic Disease	
Stroke	Place the call bell in the visual field and within reach of an unaffected arm. Anticipate needs for toileting, dressing, eating, and bathing. Assist with transfer. Provide active and/or passive range-of-motion exercises to improve functional ability.
Slowed reaction time	Encourage patient to avoid rushing and to assess pathway ahead for uneven surfaces and barriers.

Patient Teaching

Fall Prevention Guidelines for the Home: Instructions for the Patient

LIGHTS AND LIGHTING

1. Eyes tire quickly in improper lighting. Illuminate reading material or the object worked on. Illuminate steps, entranceways, and rooms before entering. Use 70- or 100-watt bulbs, not 60-watt bulbs.
2. Avoid glaring light caused by highly polished floors or large expanses of uncovered glass. Use sunglasses to avoid the glare of highway driving but use light tints or photo-ray lenses.
3. Allow more time to adjust to changes in light levels. When entering a light room from a dark area or vice versa, allow 1 to 2 minutes for the eyes to accommodate to the change in light before proceeding.
4. Dirty glasses or outgrown prescription lenses inhibit vision. Schedule regular eye examinations to identify changes in vision and to get new glasses when needed. If possible, do not use bifocals when walking because the ground cannot be seen clearly. Keep glasses clean.
5. Ability to see up, down, and sideways decreases with age. Observe the "lay of the land"; learn to look ahead at the ground to spot and avoid hazards such as cracks in the sidewalks. Use canes, walking sticks, and walkers that are prescribed.
6. At night, keep a night-light on in the bedroom and bathroom. When getting out of bed at night, turn the light on and wait 1 to 2 minutes for the eyes to adjust before getting up. Have a telephone in the bedroom so you do not have to get out of bed to answer the telephone. Before leaving in the evening or late afternoon, turn on a light for your return.

ACTIVITY

1. Get up from a chair slowly.
2. When getting out of bed, sit up and then wait 1 to 2 minutes. Move to the side of the bed, exercise the legs, and wait another minute. Stand after sitting for a few minutes.
3. If you are dizzy, sit down immediately. Sit on a step or a chair or ease yourself to the sidewalk if you are outdoors.
4. Avoid tipping the head backward (extending the neck). Activities to avoid (because they extend the neck) include washing windows, hanging clothes, and getting things from high shelves.
5. Use shelves at eye level. Avoid rapid turning of the head.
6. If weather is rainy and windy, avoid going out.
7. Use alcohol and tranquilizers with caution.
8. Exercise programs help your flexibility, balance, and strength. Enroll in a senior exercise program if your physician approves.

Patient Teaching—cont'd

Fall Prevention Guidelines for the Home: Instructions for the Patient

9. Shoes and slippers should be low-heeled with rubber soles. Avoid clothing such as long robes and loose-fitting garments that may catch on furniture or doorknobs.

AROUND THE HOUSE

1. Avoid scatter rugs and small bathroom mats that can slide. Repair loose, torn, wrinkled, or worn carpet.
2. Avoid slick, glossy polish on floors.
3. Put things in easy reach and avoid reaching to high shelves.
4. Use nonskid treads on stairs and nonskid mats in the bathtub.
5. Install grab rails in the bath, in the shower, and also by the toilet.
6. Install handrails on both sides of the stairs. Paint stair edges in a bright contrasting color.
7. Remove door thresholds.
8. Remove low-lying objects, such as coffee tables and extension cords.
9. Wipe up spills immediately.
10. Watch for pets underfoot and scattered pet food.
11. Check for even, nonglare lighting in every room with easily accessible light switches.
12. Avoid floor coverings with complex patterns.
13. Avoid clutter in living areas.
14. Select furniture that provides stability and support, such as chairs with arms.
15. Check walking aids routinely, such as rubber tips on canes and screws on walkers.

Modified from Chenitz WC, Stone JT, Salisbury SA, eds. *Clinical gerontological nursing*, Philadelphia, 1991, Saunder.

Health Promotion

Strategies for Preventing Falls

In summary, basic strategies for reducing all types of falls include the following:

- Increase physical activities that enhance and maintain muscular strength, endurance, balance, and flexibility.
- Increase regular, moderate physical exercise.
- Reduce visual impairments.
- Teach and encourage proper use of aids (e.g., cane, walker) for ambulation.
- Increase health care provider review of prescribed and over-the-counter medications.
- Increase health care provider screening and referral for alcohol and drug problems.
- Modify the environment to reduce or eliminate factors that can cause falls or to minimize injury if a fall occurs.

REDUCING FEAR

Even if all recommended measures are taken, the older adult may restrict activity out of fear of falling. Part of patient education is helping the patient to view fall risks as controllable. Just as a good driver practices defensive driving, a safe walker recognizes risks and makes adaptations to reduce their risks. When people have the facts about falling and proactive measures, they are empowered to remain active.

REDUCING FALL-RELATED INJURIES

Some falls will occur no matter what precautions are taken. In some societies, falls are viewed as indicators of greater activity and independence. Health care providers generally accept an increased number of falls as an inevitable risk that is outweighed by the benefits of physical activity and rehabilitation. Evidence is growing to support exercise interventions to improve balance, thereby reducing the risk of falls. Recommended exercises include walking; balance, coordination, and functional exercises; muscle strengthening; and multiple exercise types. Individuals at risk for falling can also be taught how to fall in a way that reduces the risk for hip injury. The patient is less likely to sustain a fracture if they can rotate forward or backward to avoid falling sideways. Measures to prevent osteoporosis may reduce the risk of fractures associated with falls. These measures are discussed in Chapter 44. Because persons with low vitamin D levels have been found at greater risk for fractures, some physicians recommend calcium and vitamin D supplementation for susceptible patients. The use of hip protectors is one strategy that accepts the risk of falling but aims to decrease the severity of fall-related injuries. Overall, research has not found a significant reduction in hip fractures when the protectors are worn in institutional settings or by persons living in the community. Many patients who have been offered hip protectors decline to wear them, citing discomfort and not liking the way they look.

Put On Your Thinking Cap!

A patient who fell near the bathroom door was found to be wet with urine. What intervention might reduce future falls for this patient?

WHEN A FALL OCCURS

When a fall occurs in a hospital or LTC facility, determine the circumstances of the fall and any injuries sustained. Document the fall according to the agency protocol. Note what the patient was doing at the time of the fall, the patient's mental and emotional status, and environmental factors that may have contributed

Box 11.3 Hendrich II Fall Risk Model™

RISK FACTOR	RISK POINTS	SCORE
Confusion/disorientation/ impulsivity	4	
Symptomatic depression	2	
Altered elimination	1	
Dizziness/vertigo	1	
Gender (male)	1	
Any administered antiepileptics (anticonvulsants): (carbamazepine, divalproex sodium, ethotoin, ethosuximide, felbamate, fosphenytoin, gabapentin, lamotrigine, mephenytoin, methsuximide, phenobarbital, phenytoin, primidone, topiramate, trimethadione, valproic acid)[a]	2	
Any administered benzodiazepines:[b] (alprazolam, chloridiazepoxide, clonazepam, clorazepate dipotassium, diazepam, flurazepam, halazepam[c], lorazepam, midazolam, oxazepam, temazepam, triazolam)	1	
GET-UP-AND-GO TEST: "RISING FROM A CHAIR"		
If unable to assess, monitor for change in activity level, assess other risk factors, document both on patient chart with date and time		
Ability to rise in single movement—no loss of balance with steps	0	
Pushes up, successful in one attempt	1	
Multiple attempts but successful	3	
Unable to rise without assistance during test	4	
If unable to assess, document this on the patient chart with the date and time		
(A score of 5 or greater = high risk)	**TOTAL SCORE**	

[a]Levetiracetam (Keppra) was not assessed during the original research conducted to create the Hendrich Fall Risk Model. As an antiepileptic, levetiracetam does have a side effect of somnolence and dizziness which contributes to its fall risk and should be scored (effective June 2010).
[b]The study did not include the effect of benzodiazepine-like drugs because they were not on the market at the time. However, because of their similarity in drug structure, mechanism of action and drug effects, they should also be scored (effective January 2010).
[c]Halazepam was included in the study but is no longer available in the United States (effective June 2010).

to the fall. When the cause of the fall is determined, take steps to remove or correct the cause. After a fall, the patient should be examined for injury. Inspect the extremities for deformity or trauma. Inspect and palpate the head for bleeding or swelling and collect data for a mental status assessment. Describe the nature and severity of any pain that the patient reports. Have the patient begin ambulating as soon after the fall as possible and at least several times a day to prevent the hazards of bed rest and to restore confidence. Table 11.2 lists the information to include in fall incident reports in institutions.

Dealing with falls in the home requires the cooperation of the person who is at risk, the family, and possibly neighbors. A plan of action for when a fall occurs should include information about getting up and seeking help.

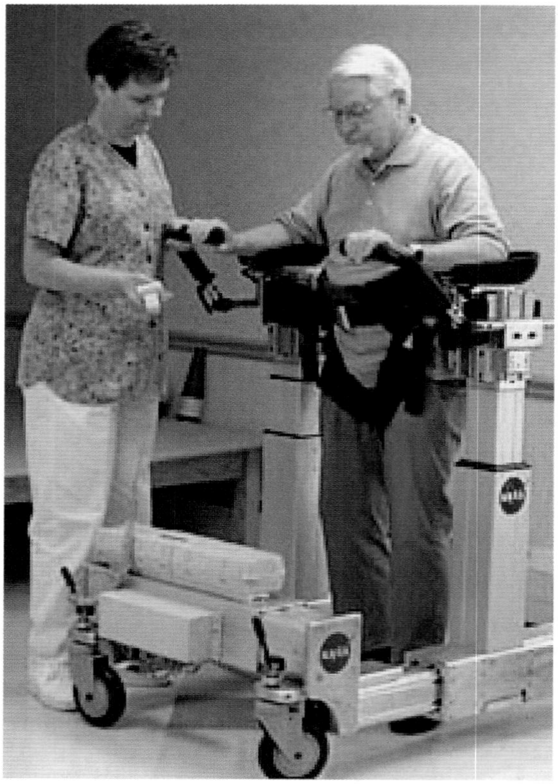

Fig. 11.1 The National Aeronautics and Space Administration has developed a secure ambulation mode that allows patients to ambulate safely and securely as they regain the ability to walk after a traumatic injury or receive physical therapy for a degenerative disease. A unique harness supports the patient's body weight without restricting hip movement. (Courtesy National Aeronautics and Space Administration.)

Several ways to get up after a fall in the home are described in the Patient Teaching box. These techniques should be practiced by the potential faller to ensure confidence in managing the problem. If none of the methods is possible, the person at risk for falling would be wise to have a call system to obtain help from others. Devices worn around the neck that can send signals to a control center are effective and provide a feeling of well-being for the potential faller. A cellphone attached to the waist also provides a means of calling for help. In addition, having a person or agency call every day can provide reassurance.

Box 11.4 Fall Prevention Techniques Used in Hospitals and Long-Term Care Facilities

PATIENT-ORIENTED TECHNIQUES
- Encourage exercise to strengthen muscles and improve balance. Use electronic alarm devices such as Bed-Check or Ambularm.

MEDICATIONS
- Monitor effects of drugs that cause sedation or orthostatic hypotension.
- Inform physician of adverse drug effects so that alternatives might be considered.
- Administer diuretics and laxatives in the morning to reduce nighttime toileting.

ACTIVITIES OF DAILY LIVING
- Assist the patient to the toilet at regular intervals.
- Check for proper footwear (e.g., nonskid footwear).
- Keep the patient's belongings close to the bed; consider on which side of the bed to place items based on patient's abilities.
- Request referrals for rehabilitation training by physical therapy and/or occupational therapy to improve function.

ENVIRONMENT-ORIENTED TECHNIQUES
- Relocate the patient at high risk for falling to rooms close to the nurses' station. Place the nurse call light system within reach (e.g., pinned to pillow); assess ability to use.
- Use the bed rails judiciously; half rails are best.
- Keep the bed in the low position (ideally, 14 to 20 inches above the floor, including the mattress).
- Keep the room light on during waking hours; illumination should be bright and even without glare.
- Keep the rooms and hallways free of clutter.
- Carpet all hard surfaces.
- Clean up spills.
- Lock all equipment with wheels.
- Keep equipment on one side of hallway.
- Use night-lights in rooms during sleeping hours.
- Place safety (grab) bars in the bathroom and hall.
- Install high-seated toilets or use bedside commodes. Remove wheels from bedside commodes.

PATIENT EDUCATION
- Hand out safety brochure to patient and family on admission.
- Teach the patient about proper use of room equipment and assistive devices.
- Encourage the patient to request help.
- Encourage the use of the bathroom and corridor handrails.
- Teach the patient how to transfer from the bed to the chair.
- Teach the patient to rise slowly and pump ankles before standing.

NURSING ASSESSMENT
- Perform assessment at admission and throughout the hospital stay.
- Apply agency protocol for "Fall Risk" based on assessment.
- Check hourly and offer fluids, assistance to toilet, etc.

OTHER
- Monitor falls, watch for trends, and conduct in-service training when a trend emerges.
- Have staff move slowly around ambulatory, unsteady patients.

Table 11.2 Information to Include in Falls Incident Reports in Institutions

EXAMPLES OF INFORMATION		REASON TO COLLECT THIS INFORMATION
Reporting factors	Witnessed/not witnessed	Make a clear distinction between what was seen or heard and the patient's account of what happened.
	Outcome of investigations recorded	When patients are reported as having x-rays or other investigations after a fall, the results of the x-ray or other investigations should be included in the report.
	Type of injury	Be specific, for example, "fractured tibia," not broken leg.
Environmental factors	Buzzer/bell available within reach before fall	Highlight whether there is an issue about accessing call bells.
	If a fall from bed, whether or not bedrails were in use	Help assess how bedrail use is affecting falls or injuries.
	Floor wet/dry/talcum powder	Reflect on cleaning regimen and need for nonslip surfaces.
	Footwear	If problems with missing or unsuitable footwear are highlighted, organizations could develop systems for providing alternatives.
	Walking aid in use/in reach	It may highlight bedside storage issues or access to walking aids for patients admitted in the evenings or on the weekend.
Patient factors	Mental status	Identify those patients most vulnerable to falls because of sedation, dementia or delirium.
	First fall this admission or repeat fall	Balance resources between preventing initial falls and secondary prevention.
	Days since admission	Ensures timescales for assessing and preventing falls are tailored to when falls are most likely to occur.
	Medication affecting risk of falls	Sedative and psychotropic medication, or medications with drowsiness as a side effect, may contribute to falls.

Preventing falls in hospitals: Tool 5A: Information to include in incident reports. Agency for Healthcare Research and Quality (AHRQ), DHHS, 1, 2013, Rockville, MD.

Patient Teaching

Methods for Getting Up After a Fall: Instructions for the Patient

ROLL

1. Roll onto your right side.
2. Bend the right knee.
3. Lever upward to the kneeling position by pressing down on the right forearm.
4. Reach out with the left arm to a nearby chair or bed.
5. With a twist of the trunk, pull yourself into a sitting position.
6. Sit on the chair or bed to recover.

CRAWL

1. Roll to a prone position.
2. Get up on all fours.
3. Crawl to a sturdy couch, chair, or bed and place your hands on it.
4. Bring one foot forward, putting the foot flat on the floor.
5. Pull yourself up to a standing position.
6. Sit on the chair or bed to recover.

SHUFFLE

1. Pull yourself to a sitting position on the floor.
2. Shuffle on the buttocks to a nearby piece of furniture.
3. Pull yourself up onto your knees directly in front of the item of furniture.
4. Stand up.

STAIR SHUFFLE

1. Pull yourself to a sitting position on the floor.
2. Shuffle on the buttocks to the stairs.
3. Gradually move up and backward to a stair height suitable for standing.
4. Grab on to the handrail and pull up.

From Chenitz WC, Kussman HL, Stone JT. Preventing falls. In: Chenitz WC, Stone JT, Salisbury SA, editors. *Clinical gerontological nursing*, Philadelphia, 1991, Saunders.

Put On Your Thinking Cap!

Practice the methods for getting up after a fall described in the Patient Teaching box. Consider the limitations on patients with restricted movements. Which methods would work best for patients you have seen?

Get Ready for the NCLEX® Examination!

Key Points

- The risk of injury from falls is highest in people over 75 years of age, and falls are the most frequent cause of accidental injury and death among older adults.
- The USPHS estimates that two-thirds of the deaths as a result of falls are preventable.
- Falls occur in older adults because of intrinsic factors (i.e., factors related to the functioning of the individual, such as weakness, drug side effects, or physical illness) and extrinsic factors (i.e., environmental factors).
- In an institutional setting, falls often occur during periods of high activity when the staff is busy.
- Serious injuries occur in 20% to 30% of all falls; fractures occur in approximately 1% to 5% of all reported falls.
- People who are at greatest risk for falls and injury are those who have fallen before and those who have multiple intrinsic risk factors.
- Older patients, particularly those who are confused, are more likely to be physically restrained than younger patients.
- SRDs (physical restraints) seldom eliminate the risk for injury and may actually cause or worsen problems.
- The OBRA of 1987 was enacted to protect patients from unnecessary restraint in LTC facilities.
- A physician's order is required for restraint use and the order must specify the duration of use and the circumstances under which the restraint may be used.
- Remove restraints for at least 10 minutes every 2 hours, assess the skin and mental status, and reapply, if indicated. Document.
- Alternatives to using physical restraint include physical therapy, sitting and talking with patients for short periods, and asking staff to be responsible for wanderers in small blocks of time.
- Special care units for persons with dementia allow patients to wander in a safe environment.
- The most important intervention for falls is prevention and the first step in preventing falls and injury is to determine who is at greatest risk.
- When a fall occurs in a hospital or LTC facility, nurses should assess the circumstances of the fall and any injuries sustained and report the fall according to the protocol of the institution.
- When the cause of a fall is determined, steps should be taken to remove or correct the cause.
- Because most people who fall have multiple risk factors, fall prevention usually requires individualized care plans.

Additional Learning Resources

SG Go to your Study Guide for additional learning activities to help you master this chapter content.

Go to your Evolve website (http://evolve.elsevier.com/Linton/medsurg) for the following learning resources and much more:

- Fluid & Electrolyte Tutorial
- Review Questions for the NCLEX® Examination

Clinical Judgment and Next-Generation NCLEX® Examination-Style Questions

1. **The nurse in a retirement center is conducting a fall prevention program. She explains to the residents that fractures occur in what percentage of falls among older adults?**
   1. Less than 10%
   2. 15%
   3. 40%
   4. 65%

   NCLEX Client Need: Safe and Effective Care Environment: Safety and Infection Control

2. **The health history of a resident of an assisted living facility includes the data below. Which is the strongest predictor of falling for this resident?**
   1. History of falling
   2. Diagnosis of heart disease
   3. Recent weight loss
   4. Urinary incontinence

   NCLEX Client Need: Safe and Effective Care Environment: Safety and Infection Control

3. **Part of the orientation for new nurses in a LTC facility includes information about restraint devices. Which statement should be included in the orientation?**
   1. Anything that restricts movement and cannot be released by the patient is a restraint.
   2. Physical restraints greatly reduce the risk of injury.
   3. Side rails have been found to be the safest means of preventing falls.
   4. Restraints must be removed once each shift for exercise and to assess skin and circulation.

   NCLEX Client Need: Safe and Effective Care Environment: Safety and Infection Control

4. **A patient who has fallen twice is being given a psychotropic drug to control agitation. The nurse recognizes that psychotropic drugs may contribute to falls because they often cause which of the following?**
   1. Hallucinations and delusions
   2. Constipation
   3. Postural hypotension
   4. Insomnia

   NCLEX Client Need: Physiological Integrity: Pharmacological Therapies

5. **The home health nurse is conducting a fall risk assessment. Which of these are *intrinsic* risk factors for falling? (Select all that apply.)**
   1. Confusion
   2. Inadequate lighting
   3. Weakness
   4. Poor vision
   5. Broken wheelchair brakes

   NCLEX Client Need: Safe and Effective Care Environment: Safety and Infection Control

6. **A newly admitted patient has an order for restraints. Under OBRA, the physician's order for the use of restraints should include which of the following? (Select all that apply.)**
   1. Duration that restraints may be used
   2. Circumstances under which restraints may be used
   3. Nursing assessment data to be recorded
   4. Measures to be taken to prevent injury
   5. Patient consent to be restrained for safety reasons.

   NCLEX Client Need: Safe and Effective Care Environment: Coordinated Care

7. **A restraint device is applied to a confused postoperative patient who is pulling on her intravenous tubing and surgical dressing. How often must the restraint be released?**

   NCLEX Client Need: Safe and Effective Care Environment: Safety and Infection Control

8. **Classes of drugs that may be used as chemical restraints include which of the following? (Select all that apply.)**
   1. Antipsychotic drugs
   2. Sedatives and hypnotic drugs
   3. Antidepressants
   4. Analgesics
   5. Skeletal muscle relaxants

   NCLEX Client Need: Physiological Integrity: Pharmacological Therapies

9. **Which of the following nutritional supplements may reduce the risk of fall-related fractures? (Select all that apply.)**
   1. Vitamin C
   2. Iron
   3. Vitamin D
   4. Calcium
   5. Vitamin B_{12}

   NCLEX Client Need: Health Promotion and Maintenance

10. **The nurse is encouraging regular exercise for residents of a retirement center. The nurse should explain that physical training can help to prevent falls by improving which of the following? (Select all that apply.)**
    1. Muscle strength
    2. Balance
    3. Flexibility
    4. Alertness
    5. Bone mass

    NCLEX Client Need: Health Promotion and Maintenance

11. **Cognitive Skill:** Recognize Cues

    A 75-year-old woman resides in a long-term care facility (LTC) because of chronic health problems that include hypertension, emphysema, dizziness, poor balance and mild memory loss. She is receiving metoprolol and hydrochlorothiazide to treat hypertension and bronchodilators to treat emphysema. She fails to ring for assistance with going to the bathroom and sometimes goes unattended.
    Highlight or place a check mark next to the assessment findings that require follow-up by the nurse.

    1. Blood pressure = 120/76 mm Hg sitting; 100/60 mm Hg standing

2. Pulse = 84 beats per minute
3. Respirations = 22 breaths per minute
4. Height 5′1″, weight 126 lb
5. Dizziness
6. Mild memory loss
7. Ambulates with assistance
8. Shortness of breath
   • Poor balance

12. **SLO/Objective: Apply knowledge of pathophysiology of falls to determine which assessment data are characteristic of falling.**

    NGN Item Type: Extended Multiple Response

    Cognitive Skill: Analyze Cues

    A 75-year-old woman resides in a long-term care facility (LTC) because of chronic health problems that include hypertension, emphysema, dizziness, poor balance and mild memory loss. She is receiving medications to treat hypertension and emphysema.

    1. Blood pressure = 12.76 mm Hg sitting; 100/60 mm Hg standing
    2. Pulse = 84 bpm
    3. Respirations = 22 breaths per minute
    4. Height 5′1″, weight 126 lb
    5. Dizziness
    6. Mild memory loss
    7. Ambulates with assistance
    8. Shortness of breath
    9. Poor balance
    10. Altered sleep patterns

    Choose the most likely options for the information missing from the statements below by selecting from the list of options provided.

    Based on the patient's assessment data, the nurse determines that the patient's vital sign findings are attributed to (1) ______, and (1)______. Factors that have contributed to her fall history are (2)______, (2)______, and (2)______.

OPTION 1	OPTION 2
Hypertension	Drug side effects
Emphysema	Postural hypotension
Incontinence	Mild memory loss
Memory loss	Wandering
Altered sleep patterns	Disorientation
Obesity	Poor balance

13. **SLO/Objective: Prioritize nursing care for patients with falls.**

    NGN Item Type: Extended Multiple Response

    Cognitive Skill: Prioritize Hypotheses

    A 75-year-old woman resides in a long-term care facility (LTC) because of chronic health problems that include hypertension, emphysema, dizziness, poor balance and mild memory loss. She is receiving medications to treat hypertension and emphysema.

    When planning care for this patient, for which *priority* potential complications would the nurse monitor. (Select all that apply.)

    1. Dementia
    2. Urinary incontinence
    3. Pulmonary embolism
    4. Head injury
    5. Pneumonia
    6. Joint contractures

14. **SLO/Objective: Plan actions for patients experiencing falls.**

    NGN Item Type: Matrix

    Cognitive Skill: Generate Solutions

    A 75-year-old woman resides in a long-term care facility (LTC) because of chronic health problems that include hypertension, emphysema, dizziness, poor balance and mild memory loss. She is receiving metoprolol and hydrochlorothiazide to treat hypertension and bronchodilators to treat emphysema. She fails to ring for assistance with going to the bathroom and sometimes goes unattended.

    Use an X for the nursing actions listed below that are *Indicated* (appropriate or necessary), *Contraindicated* (could be harmful), or *Nonessential* (makes no difference or not necessary for the patient's care at this time).

NURSING ACTION	INDICATED	CONTRAINDICATED	NONESSENTIAL
Provide assistance with ambulating			
Discuss possible physical therapy			
Place in restraints to prevent walking unassisted			
Remove environmental hazards			
Establish a routine toileting schedule			
Have patient change positions slowly			
Consult with a registered nurse about drugs that cause postural hypotension			
Increase social activities			

15. **SLO/Objective: Evaluate the effectiveness of nursing and collaborative interventions for patients experiencing a fall.**

    NGN Item Type: Matrix

    Cognitive Skill: Evaluate Outcomes

    Two weeks later the patient in questions 11–14 remains in a long-term care facility.

    Indicate in the right hand column which of the nursing actions listed in the far-left column are indicated, contraindicated, or nonessential for the potential complications of a patient experiencing a fall.

NURSING ACTION	POTENTIAL COMPLICATION	APPROPRIATE NURSING ACTION FOR COMPLICATION
1. Immobilize injured extremity	Fracture	
2. Maintain elevation of head	Head Injury	
3. Clean and dress head wound	Bleeding	
4. Monitor mental status	Hypotension	
5. Assist with position change	Delirium	
6. Elevate feet above	////////////////////	
7. Prepare to administer a thrombolytic agent	///////////////////	

16. **SLO/Objective: Evaluate the effectiveness of nursing and collaborative interventions for patients experiencing a fall.**

NGN Item Type: Matrix

Cognitive Skill: Evaluate Outcomes

Following a fall, x-rays revealed a Colles fracture of a patient's left wrist. A cast is applied and pain medications administered. The patient's head injury is being further evaluated. The patient is disorientated to time and place. His BP has remained stable at 126/72 after the physician changed his medication.

For each assessment finding, use an X to indicate whether the interventions were *Effective* (helped to meet expected outcomes), *Ineffective* (did not help to meet expected outcomes), or *Unrelated* (not related to the expected outcomes).

ASSESSMENT FINDING	EFFECTIVE	INEFFECTIVE	UNRELATED
Capillary refill is 2 seconds in fingers of left hand			
No swelling or discoloration of left hand			
Denies difficulty with urination			
Dressings on sutured head wound are clean and dry			
Blood pressure stabilizing on new medications			
No dizziness with position changes			
Right radial pulse 3+			
Pupils equal and reactive to light			
Persistent pain in left wrist			

12 Immobility

http://evolve.elsevier.com/Linton/medsurg

Objectives

1. Describe common problems associated with immobility.
2. Discuss the impact of exercise and positioning on preventing complications related to immobility.
3. Identify the risk factors for pressure injuries.
4. Describe the stages of pressure injuries.
5. Describe methods of preventing and treating pressure injuries.
6. Discuss measures to manage the effects of immobility on respiratory status, nutrition, elimination, and circulation.

Key Terms

active exercise
contracture (kŏn-TRĂK-shŭr)
erythema (ĕr-ĭ-THĒ-mă)
immobility
isometric exercise (ī-sō-MĔT-rĭk)
passive exercise
pressure injury
range-of-motion exercises
shearing forces

Immobility (the inability to move) is a restriction imposed on all or part of the body. Immobility is the enemy of function. The human body, regardless of age, is designed for movement, but without an active lifestyle, our bodies and minds will deteriorate. Older persons may spend lengthy periods sitting in their favorite chairs, but inactivity brings with it many potential health risks. People become immobilized by physical factors such as joint disease, paralysis, or pain, or psychologic factors such as depression or fear.

Sometimes immobilization is prescribed for beneficial purposes. Therapeutic outcomes of immobility include (1) pain relief and prevention of further injury of a part, as in a fractured bone, (2) reduced workload of the heart in a cardiac condition, (3) healing and repair, and (4) reversal of the effects of gravity, as in abdominal hernias and prolapsed organs. But immobility promotes muscle weakness, with muscle mass dropping 1.5% to 2% per day in the first 2 to 3 weeks of bedrest. After 10 days in bed, healthy older adults lose 2.2 pounds of muscle mass from the legs, impacting the person's ability to walk.

Immobility can also have a profound impact on both the mind and the body. Psychosocial effects may include depression, fear, anxiety, social withdrawal, apathy, loss of independence, and a feeling that life has no meaning. Almost every body system can be affected by immobility, depending on the extent and duration of the immobilization. The physiologic effects of immobility are summarized in Table 12.1

Common aging changes, combined with common medical conditions, place older people at risk for immobility and its consequences. Examples of age-related physical changes that affect mobility are decreased flexibility and strength and changes in posture and gait. Chronic medical conditions such as arthritis, stroke, Parkinson disease, cardiovascular disease, anemia, pulmonary disease, and foot deformities can lead to decreased mobility. Pain also may be a factor that leads to immobility in older adults. Drugs that cause drowsiness, hypotension, or dizziness can affect mobility as well.

PSYCHOSOCIAL

Geriatric psychiatry will assume greater importance because the population is aging in the 21st century at a rate unprecedented in human history, and this will place substantial pressure on health systems with concurrent rises in chronic diseases, depression, and immobility. Age-related cognitive decline, dementia, and geriatric depression will rise with serious consequences. Innovative prevention and treatment strategies are needed. Some promising advances in geriatric psychiatry include preventive public awareness campaigns, resilience building, alternative therapies such as yoga, tai chi, meditation, and brain stimulation techniques. Telepsychiatry and internet-based interventions are also promising mechanisms to enhance access to therapies and limit costs.

Table 12.1 Consequences of Immobility of Body Systems

BODY SYSTEM	CONSEQUENCES
Musculoskeletal	Thickening of joint capsule; loss of smoothness of cartilage surface; decreased flexibility of connective tissues; changes similar to osteoarthritis—joint contractures, demineralization of bone, bone loss; atrophy and shortening of muscle; decreased muscle strength; decreased muscle oxidative capacity; decline in aerobic capacity
Pulmonary	Arterial oxygen desaturation; increased hypostatic pooling; increased risk of atelectasis and infection
Cardiovascular	Decreased cardiac output and stroke volume; increased peripheral resistance; net loss of total body water and total blood volume; stasis of blood in veins of legs may allow blood clots to form (deep vein thrombosis [DVT])
Integumentary	Pressure injuries
Gastrointestinal	General weakening of muscles, causing altered colonic motility; constipation
Urinary	Increased levels of nitrogen, phosphorus, total sulfur, sodium, potassium, and calcium excretion; renal insufficiency; decreased glomerular filtration rate; loss of ability to concentrate urine; low creatinine clearance
Metabolic	Decreased basal metabolic rate; increased storage of fat or carbohydrates; negative nitrogen and calcium metabolic balance as a result of decreased protein and calcium intake; decreased glucose tolerance; metabolic alkalosis
Sensory	Decreased sensory stimulation (kinesthetic, visual, auditory, tactile); decreased social interaction; changes in affect, cognition, and perception

(Modified from Chenitz WC, Stone JT, Salisbury SA. *Clinical gerontological nursing*. Philadelphia: Saunders; 1991.)

Psychosocial factors that can impair mobility include depression, dementia, bereavement, lack of motivation, fear of falling, isolation, and loss of friends. The older person's environment can also promote or hinder mobility. An unsafe home setting, hospitalization, or institutionalization, for example, may be associated with reduced activity. The older person who is hospitalized may quickly become debilitated and dependent as a result of the combined effects of inactivity, pain, drugs, various therapies such as bed rest or traction, and an unfamiliar environment.

The impact of immobilization depends on the duration, degree, and type of mobility limitation. Temporary immobilization can begin a vicious cycle that leads to an ever-increasing loss of independence for patients. As patients become less able to move, they become more dependent. As they become more dependent, they are less able to care for themselves, which in turn leads to an increasing number of adverse effects from immobility.

Whatever the reason for resting a part or all of the body, measures must be taken to manage the adverse effects of immobility. You can prevent the vicious cycle of events from the beginning by helping patients to maintain normal functioning as much as possible and for as long as possible (see the Nursing Care Plan). Before patients begin to suffer the ill effects of immobilization, therapeutic interventions must be implemented. The health care team must work together to develop a plan of care that includes preventive and therapeutic measures that address the individual's needs. The patient and family, as central members of the health care team, should participate in care planning if able. The Health Promotion box discusses how the family and health care team can collaborate to support the patient's self-care as they regain independence.

Health Promotion

Promoting Independence in Self-Care Activities

Regaining independence in self-care activities requires the collaboration of all members of the health care team. Following a thorough assessment, the team designs a rehabilitation plan. Each discipline then develops the parts of the plan for that discipline. The overall goal is for the patient to reach the highest level of wellness possible to achieve an acceptable quality of life. Rehabilitation seeks to help patients relearn lost skills and compensate for temporary or permanent losses. Family members need to be included in all teaching so that they understand how to support independence rather than dependence. Given adequate time, most motivated patients with moderate impairments can relearn the skills needed for basic activities of daily living.

Assistive devices can play a major role in regaining independence with eating, dressing, and other activities of daily living (ADLs). Nurses or therapists should instruct patients and families in the proper use and care of these devices. Any measures that simplify tasks can improve independence. For example, slip-on shoes, Velcro closures, loose pullover shirts, and elastic-waist pants can promote independence in dressing and toileting. Encourage patients to dress in simple workout-type clothes, rather than in pajamas and gowns, as soon as active rehabilitation is started.

Nursing Care Plan Preventing Hazards of Immobility

FOCUSED ASSESSMENT

Health History

A 90-year-old retired general lives alone in the assisted living section of a senior retirement community. He has multiple medical conditions and has become increasingly frail. He has fallen three times, with the last fall resulting in a serious knee injury. While recovering from this injury, he has been instructed to use a walker or wheelchair and to avoid full weight-bearing activities. Therefore he was moved to the nursing home area until he can again care for himself. In the nursing home, he has been irritable and insists on caring for himself. He attempts to transfer himself without assistance by bearing weight on one leg. On several occasions he has been unable to delay urination until he could get help. He eats very little other than toast at breakfast and he is drinking little fluid.

Physical Examination

Vital signs: blood pressure 94/52 mm Hg, pulse 88 beats per minute; respirations 18 breaths per minute, temperature 97° F orally. Height 5′10″, weight 140 lb. All extremities exhibit muscle atrophy and weakness. Reddened areas are noted on the elbows and sacrum. Urine is dark with a strong odor.

Patient Problems	Goals and Outcome Criteria	Interventions
Potential for falls related to weakness	Patient will remain safe from falls during his recovery.	Ask the patient to request help with transferring. Arrange his room for easy movement in a wheelchair. Assist with active range-of-motion exercises for unaffected limbs. Suggest physical therapy referral to strengthen upper body and his weight-bearing leg.
Potential for infection (urinary) related to stasis of body fluids associated with low fluid intake	Patient's daily fluid intake will be at least 1200 mL. The patient's urine will be clear and light in color.	Explain the need to increase fluid intake to prevent urinary tract infections. Determine preferred liquids and make them available. Instruct the CNA to offer 3 ounces (90 ml) of fluids hourly while the patient is awake, for a total of 40 ounces or 1200 mL/day, and to record intake. Report foul urine odor. Provide urinal. Assure easy access to toilet.
Potential for disrupted skin tissue integrity related to prolonged pressure while sitting.	Patient's skin will remain intact throughout the recovery period.	Obtain pressure-reducing pad for wheelchair. Teach patient to shift weight every 15 min. Plan periods of bed rest to prevent constant pressure on sacrum. Keep sacral area clean and dry.
Inadequate coping related to loss of independence, situational crisis, uncertainty.	The patient will adapt to temporary dependence by participating in rehabilitation efforts. The patient will resume self-care activities by discharge to his home.	Explain the benefits of rehabilitation activities in relation to regaining independence. Stress goal of returning to his former residence and need to avoid further injuries. Encourage self-care within limitations. Compliment efforts. Arrange for him to attend social function in previous living section. Request consult for occupational therapist to improve self-care abilities.

CRITICAL THINKING QUESTIONS

1. How do age-related changes increase the risk of complications of immobility for this patient?
2. Why is it important to consider both physical and emotional needs of the patient with reduced mobility?

CNA, Certified nursing assistant.

Pharmacology Capsule

Drugs that cause drowsiness, hypotension, or dizziness can impair mobility.

NURSING ASSESSMENT AND INTERVENTION

A thorough assessment of the patient's abilities and limitations is essential to planning interventions. Data collected by the licensed vocational nurse/licensed practical nurse (LVN/LPN) make an important contribution to the assessment. Although the health care provider may order specific activities or therapies related to immobility, there are many measures the nurse can implement independently to prevent the adverse effects of immobility. Nursing interventions focus on promoting exercise and maintaining adequate respiratory status, food and fluid intake, normal elimination, skin integrity, joint mobility, and circulation (Box 12.1).

EXERCISE

Exercise has the potential to lessen the development of depressive symptoms in older adults experiencing acute stressors associated with aging. Regardless of the severity of their condition, most people can engage in some form of exercise. For example, patients with fractures can tighten and relax muscles in an immobilized extremity; debilitated patients can gradually increase their range of movement, number of movements, or resistance against movement; and patients in pain can coordinate activity with pain medication and adapt their pace or intensity for comfort.

Exercises may be **active** (performed by the patients themselves) or **passive** (movement of the patient's

Box 12.1 Case Study: Immobility

Mrs. Smith is an 84-year-old woman who has resided in an intermediate care facility for 2 years. She was admitted to the facility because she had been living at home alone and had become unable to shop and cook for herself or to dress herself after sustaining a broken wrist as a result of a fall. She was incontinent of urine and mildly confused.

Mrs. Smith had previously been quite active in the community, but in the residential home she remained confined to her room and was not interested in interacting with other people. Her daughter visited her 2 or 3 times a week.

Because Mrs. Smith preferred to stay in bed or in a chair most of the time, the nurses and other members of the interdisciplinary team were concerned about the consequences of her immobility. She had fallen many times, usually on the way to the dining room to eat. She had reached the point where she stayed in a wheelchair most of the time because she had become too weak to walk.

The team held a case conference and identified problems associated with her immobility: (1) continued falling, (2) incontinence, and (3) isolation and perhaps depression. They formulated a plan to get her up and moving while at the same time avoiding falls. The nurses walked with Mrs. Smith three times daily. The first week they walked around the bed. The second week they walked to the door and back. The third week they walked a few feet outside the door to her room. As the weeks progressed, Mrs. Smith was able to walk to the dining room at the end of the hall without falling. The nurses encouraged in-bed and in-chair exercises to further build up her strength.

Eventually, Mrs. Smith was able to walk to the bathroom independently. The nurses worked with her to develop a regular schedule of toileting so that the number of "accidents" decreased. Because she was slightly confused and disoriented, the nurses provided gentle reminders for her to go to the bathroom. After a meal, they would guide her back to her room to use the bathroom. At other times they would stop by her room, look in, and suggest that she goes to the bathroom.

With all of the increased activity, Mrs. Smith became more outgoing and involved in activities. She sat with the same group at meals and developed friendships with others around her. The nurses found that taking small steps with a walking program can have many benefits for a person of any age in any condition.

body by another person). Active and passive exercises may be performed in bed, in a chair, or standing. The exercises can be performed while giving other care, such as during a bed bath or while grooming. Examples of bed and chair exercises are listed in the Health Promotion box.

Range-of-Motion Exercises

Range-of-motion exercises are effective in preventing some disabilities of the musculoskeletal system. Each of the joints of the body has a range of motion, meaning the limits to which it may be safely moved. Muscular activity maintains range of motion by allowing the joint to remain flexible and functional.

Health Promotion

Sample Bed and Chair Exercises

IN-BED EXERCISES	IN-CHAIR EXERCISES
• Deep breathing (slow inhalation and full exhalation) • Head rolls (neck forward flex, backward extend, lateral flex, rotate) • Knee to chest (on back or side, bring one knee to chest, wrap arms around, hold and breathe, straighten leg slowly) • Pelvic tilts (on back, knees bent, feet flat, tuck in tummy, relax) • Bridging (on back, feet flat on bed, raise hips, lower slowly) • Head raising in prone and supine positions • Unilateral leg lifts • Foot dorsiflexion • Rolling • Prone lying • Arms straight over head of bed in supine position • Arms out to sides, palms up, in supine position • Hands behind head, elbows bent • Hands at lower back	• Deep breathing • Head rolls (neck forward flex, backward extend, lateral flex, rotate) • Knee to chest • Head to knees • Shoulder rolls (forward and back) • Weight shifts (hip to hip) • Hands on head, elbows out and in, lateral trunk flex-extension, trunk rotation • Leg lifts • Ankle rotation and dorsiflexion • Ankle on knee (external hip rotation, place ankle on opposite knee and lower the bent leg) • Push down on legs as if to stand, lean forward, bear weight

From Giduz BH, Snow TL, Wildman DL, McConnell ES: *Geriatric first aid kit*, Chapel Hill, NC, 1986, Program on Aging–University of North Carolina.

When little or no movement of a joint occurs, its structures change. Normal muscle tissue is replaced by fibrous tissue. Muscles shorten and lose their elasticity. Shortening of muscles and tendons creates a **contracture** that is defined as "a lack of full active or passive range of motion because of joint, muscle, or soft tissue limitations" (Wagner et al., 2008). A contracture can severely and permanently limit joint movement.

The purpose of range-of-motion exercises is to put each joint that is at risk for loss of motion through its full range of motion to the highest degree possible. These exercises may be active or passive. Range-of-motion exercises should be initiated early in immobile patients to prevent contractures.

Isometric Exercises

Isometric exercises maintain muscle tone without moving the joint. The muscle is contracted and held in that position for several seconds. The muscle is then relaxed briefly and contracted again. This type of exercise is especially helpful in maintaining muscle strength after a fracture.

POSITIONING

Proper positioning in a bed or chair is extremely important for preventing many of the side effects of immobility (see the Coordinated Care box). The patient's position should be changed at least every 2 hours to prevent prolonged pressure on the skin. If redness from pressure persists after 2 hours, the interval between repositioning needs to be shortened. Maintain joints in their functional positions so that they are not abnormally flexed or extended. Use pillows, trochanter rolls, footboards or positioning boots, and splints to maintain proper positioning for patients lying in bed. Footboards and positioning boots keep the feet at right angles to the legs so that foot drop is avoided. Splinting the limbs keeps them straight. For example, a firm splint in the hands prevents the fingers from curling up into a tight fist. Avoid positioning the patient with the knees and hips flexed. Imagining how a person looks while standing helps to achieve that position while the patient is lying down. Patients who are seated in chairs should be encouraged to shift their weight every 15 minutes.

Coordinated Care

Effects of Immobility

Educate certified nursing assistants (CNAs) about the importance of turning, positioning, exercise, and hydration to prevent complications of immobility. Explain how turning and proper positioning relieve pressure on sensitive or painful areas.

Monitor care to ensure that patients are being repositioned on schedule and that fluids are being provided. Show CNAs what the early signs of pressure injuries look like and stress the importance of promptly reporting such observations. Ask CNAs to report constipation, incontinence, or diarrhea, if it occurs, so that corrective measures can be taken.

SKIN INTEGRITY

Immobility can lead impaired skin integrity. Skin becomes easily damaged in pressure areas such as hips, heels, and sacrum. Pressure injuries affect approximately 3 million adults. The cost of treatment of a pressure injury is two and a half times the cost of prevention. Nurses hold an indispensable role in pressure injury management. Management includes identifying at-risk persons and implementing specific prevention measures. Nurses must embrace the new trends in the management of pressure injuries to reduce costs, period of hospital stays, as well as to avoid litigation.

Pressure injuries are localized areas of tissue necrosis (tissue death) that develop when soft tissue is compressed between a bony prominence and an external surface or when pressure occurs in combination with shearing force or friction or both. *Pressure points* are areas over bony prominences such as the elbows, hips, shoulders, and sacrum (Fig. 12.1). The most frequent sites of skin breakdown are the sacrum (35%), ischial tuberosities (16%), heels (11%), trochanters (7%), ankles (3%), and scapulae (2%). The term *pressure injuries* is preferred for what are commonly called "*bedsores*," "*decubitus ulcers*," or "*decubiti*." The word *decubitus* means "lying down," and an ulcer is a lesion produced by the sloughing of necrotic, inflammatory tissue (Fig. 12.2). Thus a decubitus ulcer is an open wound that is associated with lying in bed. However, skin breakdown can just as easily develop in patients who are sitting for a long period because of pressure against blood vessels.

Preventing Pressure Injuries

The first step in the prevention of pressure injuries is to identify patients who are at risk for developing them. The Norton scale is a useful instrument for identifying those at risk (Fig. 12.3). The scores in all five categories of the scale are added. If the total score is greater than 14, little risk exists for developing pressure injuries. If the score is less than 14, a significant risk exists for developing pressure injuries. Any patient with a score of less than 14 needs a formal pressure injury prevention program started as soon as the risk is recognized. The skin of patients "at risk" should be assessed and documented every day.

A pressure injury prevention protocol consists of the following:

Skin care: Once the skin becomes injured, it becomes a higher risk for further damage. Regular skin inspection includes looking for reddened or darkened areas. Skin should be kept clean and dry. Use nonirritant moisturizers if needed. Do not rub reddened areas. Keep fluid away from skin through use of barrier creams, incontinence systems, and prompted voiding where possible.

Pressure reduction: Taking pressure off patients' bony areas will depend on their own capabilities. For patients who are mobile, encourage them to walk, swim, or whatever activity is possible. Persons who are wheelchair bound may be able to shift their positions frequently. Regular movement stimulates blood flow and reduces risks of pneumonia and immobility.

- Static devices include foam, water, gel, air mattresses, or mattress overlays.
- Dynamic devices include alternating pressure mattresses that can lower ulcer incidence by 60% compared with a regular mattress. Newer technology provides sensors that send out an alarm when there is too much pressure for too long under a bony prominence.
- Head of the bed elevation should be no more than 30 degrees to prevent sliding and shearing.
- Protect bony areas by positioning and cushioning. Cushions should be used to support the front and back and to relieve pressure between knees, ankles, and heels.

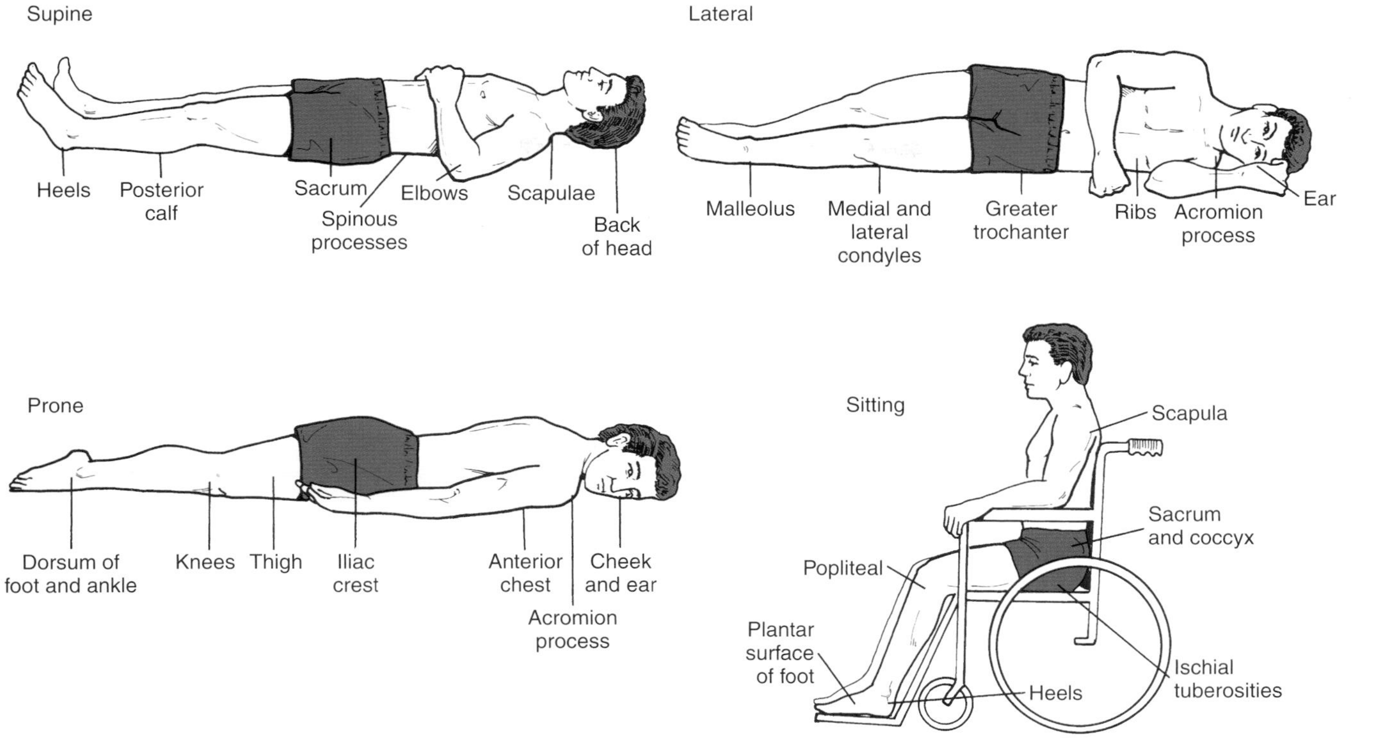

Fig. 12.1 Possible locations of pressure injuries.

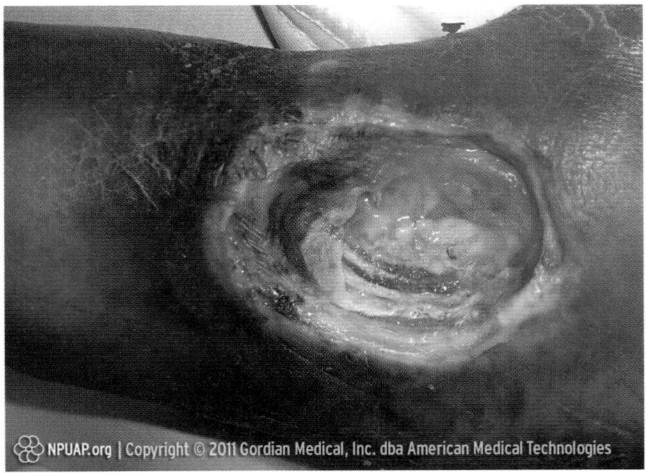

Fig. 12.2 Stage IV pressure injury with full-thickness involvement of all soft tissue. (Used with permission of National Pressure Ulcer Advisory Panel, January 2017.)

Accessible and adequate support: Patients may need more intensive support services or caregivers may need more training or assistance with lifting and turning.

Improve mobility: Patients who cannot move themselves must be repositioned. Repositioning should occur every 2 hours. The nurse needs to use proper repositioning techniques and body mechanics to ensure both nurse and patient are not injured.

- Repositioning devices such as an overhead trapeze may enable patients to reposition themselves. Using a draw sheet to lift or turn a patient reduces friction and shearing.

Adequate nourishment: Adequate nutrition is the cornerstone of not only healing ulcers but for prevention as well. The patient needs adequate calories, protein, hydration, and vitamins and minerals. A nutritional consult is recommended for any patient who has difficulty consuming adequate nutrition. Adequate hydration is important for maintaining healthy skin. Watch for signs of poor hydration such as decreased urine output, darker urine, dry mouth, thirst, dry skin, and constipation. Offer at least 3 or 4 ounces of fluids every waking hour.

Education: The more education and learning that patients, caregivers, staff members, and families receive about the prevention of pressure injuries, the more successful they will be at preventing them. The human body has a built-in alarm system through pain. This alarm system may not work for patients who have decreased cognition, but these are the patients at higher risk for pressure injuries.

Effective communication: Communication within the care team is vital. Reduced rates of pressure injuries can only occur if the culture of the facility is changed, not by changes in one area or isolated activities. Everyone needs to get involved and support the prevention process.

The best preventive measure is frequent position change. Do not massage pressure points. Any type

NORTON SCALE

		PHYSICAL CONDITION	MENTAL CONDITION	ACTIVITY	MOBILITY	INCONTINENT	
		Good 4 Fair 3 Poor 2 Very bad 1	Alert 4 Apathetic 3 Confused 2 Stupor 1	Ambulant 4 Walk/help 3 Chairbound 2 Bedrest 1	Full 4 Slightly limited 3 Very limited 2 Immobile 1	Not 4 Occasional 3 Usually/urine 2 Doubly 1	TOTAL SCORE
Name	Date						

Fig. 12.3 Norton scale for the identification of those at risk for the development of pressure injuries. (From Norton D, McLaren R, Exton-Smith AN: *An investigation of geriatric nursing problems in the hospital*, London, 1986, Centre for Policy on Ageing. Reproduced with permission from the Centre for Policy on Ageing [formerly NCCOP], London, UK.)

of massage around or on a reddened area of skin can damage fragile capillaries. In addition, rubber rings should not be used to elevate heels or sacral areas. Rings cause a concentrated area of pressure that places patients at a higher risk for developing pressure injuries. Remember: no massage on reddened skin and no rings! Another important factor that must be considered is the patient's nutritional status. Adequate nutrients are essential to maintain or restore skin integrity. Additional information regarding pressure injuries can be found in Chapter 57.

RESPIRATORY STATUS

Even after small periods of immobility, the effects on the lungs can be quite severe. Chest muscles weaken resulting in shallow breathing. The major risk is pneumonia. Oxygen and carbon dioxide are exchanged in the thin, moist mucous membrane that lines the airway passages and the alveoli. Most healthy people take between six and eight deep, sighing breaths every hour. Sighs help to keep the lungs expanded and move secretions upward along the air passages. When a person remains immobile or does not take deep breaths, thick secretions can accumulate and pool in the lower respiratory structures. These secretions interfere with the normal exchange of gases, can cause areas of the lung to collapse (atelectasis), and can provide an environment for growth of pathogens. A lung infection associated with immobility is called *hypostatic pneumonia*.

Individuals who are at risk for impaired gas exchange related to immobility include those who:

- Are given drugs that depress respirations, such as general anesthetic agents, opioids, or sedatives
- Have tight binders or bandages that limit chest expansion
- Have abdominal distention from gas, fluid, or feces
- Lie in one position for extended periods

Older adults are also at risk for respiratory problems related to immobility because age-related changes reduce lung expansion and breathing capacity (see the Patient Teaching box).

Patient Teaching

Coughing and Deep Breathing

- Coughing and deep breathing are most effective in a sitting position.
- If you have a chest or abdominal surgical incision, support the area with a pillow to minimize discomfort.
- Use the abdominal muscles and diaphragm to expand the lower chest. Inhale deeply through the nose, hold the breath for 1 to 3 seconds, and exhale slowly while pursing your lips. Focus on how much air you can exhale rather than on the force with which you exhale it.
- After 4 to 6 deep breaths, cough deeply. Some sources recommend taking a single deep breath followed by three consecutive coughs, trying to clear all air from the lungs with each cough.

Nursing interventions for patients at risk for respiratory complications include frequent turning and position changes and coughing and deep-breathing exercises. These interventions must be performed every 2 hours to be effective. Coughing and deep-breathing exercises are done at the same time to allow for periods of rest and to obtain the best results.

Effective coughing may be difficult for patients, especially for those who are in pain from a surgical incision or for those who have chronic coughs and are worried that the coughing may trigger a long, exhausting coughing experience. The objective of coughing is to move the secretions gradually upward and to cough them out a little at a time. Teach patients how to cough and to deep breathe effectively (see the Patient Teaching box). Incentive spirometry is widely used; however, by itself, it is not adequate to prevent complications. The patient must use the spirometer correctly and practice coughing and deep breathing as well.

To evaluate the effectiveness of nursing interventions, monitor the patient's respiratory status. Count the respiratory rate, observe the respiratory effort and chest movement, check the oxygen saturation if oximetry is used, and listen for crackles in the lung fields.

FOOD AND FLUID INTAKE

Careful attention should be paid to dehydration, malnutrition, and weight loss. In relation to food and fluid intake, the most common problem associated with immobility is anorexia (loss of appetite). Factors that contribute to anorexia are worry, depression, anxiety about dependence on others, and decreased metabolic needs resulting from inactivity. Hypoproteinemia (protein deficiency) can develop in patients who are immobilized.

Immobilized patients may also have inadequate fluid intake. Getting up for a drink of water may be too difficult and time consuming for inactive individuals, or they may not think to drink liquids regularly. Older people are particularly prone to becoming dehydrated from an inadequate fluid intake, resulting in complications such as confusion, constipation, or urinary tract infection.

Maintain accurate records of patients' dietary and fluid intakes. Small, frequent meals may be more acceptable than three large meals for patients with anorexia. Dietary supplements that are high in protein content may also be encouraged. Offer fluids, even small sips of water, juice, or other liquids, at least every hour while awake. Fluids need to be within reach so that patients may have easy access to them if they are able to drink without help. Encourage family members to offer fluids while they are visiting.

ELIMINATION

Constipation

Constipation is one of the most common problems associated with immobility. As the gastrointestinal system slows down, more water is removed from the fecal mass. Contributing factors in the immobile patient include changes in the usual routine and environment, inability to defecate on a bedpan because of embarrassment or discomfort and weakened muscle tone. In addition, many medications cause constipation by slowing intestinal motility. Constipated individuals may strain to defecate, causing an increase in intraabdominal pressure. This pressure is called the *Valsalva maneuver* or vasovagal reflex and it can lead to cardiovascular alterations and even to light-headedness and fainting. The vasovagal reflex can be especially problematic in the older person whose circulation may be somewhat impaired.

Confused patients may ignore the normal urge to have a bowel movement. If the impulse is ignored for a considerable time, the natural urge to defecate can diminish and eventually disappear.

Long-standing constipation can result in a fecal impaction. Fecal impaction is the presence of hardened or puttylike feces in the rectum and sigmoid colon. If the condition is not relieved, intestinal obstruction can occur. Symptoms of a fecal impaction include painful defecation, a feeling of fullness in the rectum, abdominal distention, and sometimes cramps and watery stool. The presence of diarrhea does not mean that a fecal impaction has been removed, because the liquid fecal material may flow around the hardened mass.

When an impaction develops, the mass of feces must be broken up with a gloved finger (a physician's order is usually needed). Before digital removal of the mass, giving an oil retention enema to soften the mass may be helpful. In addition, an analgesic may be given 1 hour before digital removal of an impaction.

Inactivity, medications, decreased fluid intake, and lack of adequate fiber in the diet all contribute to constipation. A vicious cycle may begin when immobility promotes inactivity, decreased fluid intake, and poor appetite. Patients become weaker, more immobile, and less likely to eat and drink adequately. Encouraging proper foods with adequate roughage, fluids, and as much activity as possible can help to prevent or relieve constipation. Whenever possible, patients should use a bedside commode or be taken to the bathroom to defecate rather than try to use a bedpan. Laxatives should be used sparingly; however, stool softeners may be helpful if the stools are hard and difficult to pass. Patients with long-established laxative dependence may require continued laxative therapy during the period of immobility.

Put On Your Thinking Cap!

With pencil and paper in hand, note the time. Now, sit perfectly still for 10 minutes. At the end of that time, note what sensations and thoughts you experienced. When the time was up, what was the first thing you did? Discuss what a nurse could have done to make you more comfortable. Compare your experience with that of a patient who is immobilized.

Urinary Incontinence

The urinary system functions best when the body is upright. Physical activity and gravity help to drain urine from the kidneys to the bladder. Immobility can cause a build-up of urine in the kidneys. Urine flows downward from the kidney by gravity. When the body is in a reclining position, the kidney must force urine into the ureters against the pull of gravity. Urine is continually being formed in the kidney, but the peristaltic action of the ureters is not strong enough to maintain a constant flow of urine. If the body remains in a supine (lying down) position for even a few days, the flow becomes sluggish and the urine pools, which sets the stage for the development of a urinary tract infection.

Lying in bed can also cause a loss of control of the urinary sphincter muscles and result in incontinence. Without the downward pressure of the full bladder against the sphincter muscles, awareness of the need to void is less. The result can be bladder distention with an overflow or a dribbling of urine that the patient cannot control.

Older persons who have problems with mobility may have functional incontinence because they are unable to respond to the urge to void in time. The bladder is usually fuller when the urge to void occurs; consequently, less time is available to get to the bathroom. In addition, they may not be able to move quickly enough because of the slowed reaction time associated with older age or chronic illness.

The most effective way to prevent urinary incontinence associated with immobility is to set up a toileting program. Patients should have scheduled toiletings with adjustments in schedule based on the patients' voiding patterns. If voiding patterns cannot be assessed, patients should, at the very least, be taken to the bathroom or commode or offered a bedpan every 2 hours during waking hours. Some individuals restrict fluids at certain times of the day, especially after dinner and through the night to avoid nighttime incontinence. However, studies have been inconclusive regarding the effectiveness of limiting fluids. Incontinence is covered in greater detail in Chapter 23.

CIRCULATORY EFFECTS

Immobility is a key risk factor for the formation of blood clots in the deep veins of the pelvis and legs. Deep vein thrombosis (DVT) may be manifested by edema, warmth, and tenderness in the affected area. However, about half of patients with DVT have no symptoms. The most serious complication of DVT is pulmonary embolism (PE). Patients considered to be at risk for DVT may be treated with preventive anticoagulants. Other preventive measures include positioning to maintain circulation, range-of-motion exercises, and good hydration. Treatment of DVT is discussed in Chapter 35, and treatment of PE is covered in Chapter 27.

NEUROLOGIC

Immobility affects the nervous system, resulting in lack of coordination and balance, increasing the risk of falling. Longer periods of immobility can result in anxiety, anger and confusion. Older adults often can suffer from "learned dependency syndrome," when they seek help for the most trivial of tasks. Encouraging social interaction and as much self-dependence as possible is key.

Put On Your Thinking Cap!

Observe a person during class, church, a movie, or other situation where people are expected to stay seated. Note the number of movements by that person in a 5-minute period. Identify the therapeutic value of those motions.

Get Ready for the NCLEX® Examination!

Key Points

- The psychologic effects of immobility may include depression, fear, anxiety, social withdrawal, apathy, loss of financial and personal independence, and lack of meaningful existence.
- Among the complications of immobility are pressure injuries, respiratory problems, impaired nutrition, constipation, urinary tract infection and incontinence.
- Exercise is the best medicine for immobility.
- Exercises may be active (performed by the patient) or passive (movement of the patient's body performed by another person without assistance from the patient).
- Pressure injuries are expensive to treat, extend hospital stays, increase the likelihood of placement in a long-term care facility, and increase mortality.
- The best preventive measure for pressure injuries is frequent position changes.
- Especially in older adults, immobility can contribute to respiratory problems, including impaired gas exchange, atelectasis, and hypostatic pneumonia.
- Factors that contribute to respiratory complications of immobility include drugs that depress respirations and dry secretions; tight binders or bandages that limit chest expansion; abdominal distention from gas, fluid, or feces; and lying in one position for extended periods.
- Frequent turning and position changes and encouraging coughing and deep-breathing exercises help to prevent respiratory complications of immobility.
- Anorexia (loss of appetite) is the most common nutritional problem associated with immobility.
- Immobility contributes to constipation by causing a change in the usual routine and environment, an inability to defecate on a bedpan because of embarrassment or discomfort, and a weakening of muscle tone.
- Immobility can promote a loss of control of the urinary sphincter muscles, resulting in incontinence.
- The most effective way to prevent urinary incontinence associated with immobility is to set up a toileting program.
- Urinary stasis increases the risk of urinary tract infections.
- Anticoagulants may be prescribed to prevent DVT in the immobilized patient.

Additional Learning Resources

SG Go to your Study Guide for additional learning activities to help you master this chapter content.

Go to your Evolve website (http://evolve.elsevier.com/Linton/medsurg) for the following learning resources and much more:
- Fluid & Electrolyte Tutorial
- Review Questions for the NCLEX® Examination

Clinical Judgment and Next-Generation NCLEX® Examination-Style Questions

1. **A patient who sustained a head injury has not regained consciousness. The nurse moves the patient's joints through their normal movements twice a day. This exercise intervention is called:**
   1. Isometric
   2. Active
   3. Passive
   4. Isotonic

   NCLEX Client Need: Physiological Integrity: Basic Care and Comfort

2. **The home health nurse is teaching family members how to move a patient up in bed by using a draw sheet to prevent which of the following?**
   1. Tissue trauma from shearing force
   2. Strain on the caregiver
   3. Disturbing the bed linens
   4. Extension contractures of the spine

   NCLEX Client Need: Physiological Integrity: Basic Care and Comfort

3. **The nursing care plan for an immobilized patient includes the following interventions. Which one is specifically intended to maintain skin integrity?**
   1. Keep joints in functional positions
   2. Reposition the patient at least every 2 hours
   3. Perform range-of-motion exercises twice daily
   4. Give at least eight 8-ounce glasses of fluids each day

   NCLEX Client Need: Physiological Integrity: Basic Care and Comfort and Reduction of Risk Potential

4. **During a bed bath, you observe a reddened area over the sacrum. You should:**
   1. Document erythema and instruct nursing assistants to keep the patient off his back
   2. Gently massage the reddened area with skin lotion to provide protective moisture
   3. Place a round inflatable cushion under the patient's buttocks to relieve pressure on the sacrum
   4. Position the patient on one side and use a heat lamp to stimulate circulation to the area

   NCLEX Client Need: Physiological Integrity: Basic Care and Comfort

5. **Instructions in effective coughing for the patient after abdominal surgery should include which of the following?**
   1. Try not to use the abdominal muscles during coughing and deep-breathing exercises
   2. Assume a comfortable position on your side to reduce strain on the incision
   3. Exhale as forcefully and for as long as you can
   4. Take one deep breath and then cough three times, trying to clear all air from the lungs

   NCLEX Client Need: Physiological Integrity: Reduction of Risk Potential

6. **A postoperative patient reports that she was straining to have a bowel movement when she became light-headed. You should suspect which of the following?**
   1. Valsalva maneuver
   2. Internal hemorrhage
   3. Dehydration
   4. Wound dehiscence

   NCLEX Client Need: Physiological Integrity: Physiological Adaptation

7. **What is the effect of immobility on the urinary tract?**
   1. Decreased urine production by the kidneys
   2. Pooling of urine in the urinary system
   3. Increased blood flow to kidneys
   4. Increased bladder sensitivity to fullness

   NCLEX Client Need: Physiological Integrity: Reduction of Risk Potential

8. **SLO/Objective: Apply knowledge of immobility to determine which assessment data require follow-up from the nurse.**

   NGN Item Type: Enhanced Hot Spot

   Cognitive Skill: Recognize Cues

   A 68-year-old male resides in a long-term care facility because he is unable to care for himself. He has a history of heart disease, peripheral vascular disease, falls and early stage dementia. He is out of bed with assistance to a wheelchair. The nurse documents the assessment findings below. Highlight or place a check mark next to the assessment findings that require follow-up by the nurse.

   - Blood pressure 134/80 mm Hg
   - Pulse 86 beats per minute
   - Respirations 18 beats per minute
   - Muscle atrophy
   - Weak peripheral pulses
   - Occasional functional urinary incontinence
   - Reddened areas on sacrum and elbows
   - Disoriented to time and place
   - States he wants to go home

13 Delirium and Dementia

http://evolve.elsevier.com/Linton/medsurg

Objectives

1. Describe the neurocognitive disorders (NCDs): delirium and dementia (mild and major NCD).
2. Describe the subtypes of mild and major NCDs.
3. Identify the common causes of delirium.
4. Explain the differences between delirium and dementia.
5. Identify drugs used to treat delirium and dementia.
6. Discuss nursing assessment and interventions related to delirium and dementia.

Key Terms

delirium (dĕ-LĒ-rē-ŭm)

dementia (dĕ-MĔN-shēă)

The loss of independence is one of the greatest fears of older age. Significant disturbances in cognition can impair the ability to care for oneself, thus diminishing the capacity to live independently. Fortunately, a decline in cognitive ability is not a part of normal aging, despite some changes in information processing described in Chapter 10. Nevertheless, older age is a risk factor for various conditions that may cause cognitive impairment.

Altered mental function develops suddenly or gradually depending on the underlying pathology. Some causes can be treated, resulting in a return to usual cognition, whereas other causes are not reversible. Altered cognitive states are commonly diagnosed as delirium or dementia depending on the onset, duration, contributing factors, response to intervention, and progression. It is possible to have both conditions at the same time.

The *Diagnostic and Statistical Manual of Mental Disorders*, 5th edition (DSM-5) published by the American Psychiatric Association, provides guidelines for the diagnosis and classification of mental disorders. Neurocognitive disorders (NCDs) include delirium, and mild and major neurocognitive disorders. The term *delirium* is used to describe a state of impaired cognition that occurs suddenly and usually resolves when the underlying problem is corrected. Examples of factors that may cause delirium in the older adult are infection, fever, and drug effects.

The term *dementia* is commonly used to refer to mild and major neurocognitive disorders. Neurocognitive disorders are described as those with "a significant impairment of cognition or memory that represents a marked deterioration from a previous level of function."

Each of the neurocognitive disorders affects one or more domains of cognitive function. These domains are complex attention, executive function, learning and memory, language, perceptual-motor function, and social cognition. Complex attention disorders result in difficulty staying on task and sorting through multiple stimuli. Executive function allows people to plan, make decisions, carry out plans, and evaluate activities. Thus a person with impaired executive function has difficulty with multitasking and carrying out multiple steps. Disorders of learning and memory may affect short-term and long-term memory, which can affect all aspects of functioning. A person might forget appointments, leave food on a hot stove, be unable to dress or shop, or become lost. Language disorders can affect the ability to understand or use words. Perceptual-motor disorders can affect the ability to perform usual activities, such as driving a car. Various defects in vision may be present. Social cognition is concerned with recognizing emotions. When social cognition is disturbed, people may say or do socially inappropriate things. They may have personality changes and become insensitive to the feelings of others. These disturbances can be mild or major (Table 13.1).

DELIRIUM

Delirium is a decline from an individual's orientation to the environment. In addition to disorientation, the patient can experience altered awareness, memory deficits, or language or perceptual problems. There may be difficulty with focusing or paying attention, causing patients to be easily distracted. Engaging in a conversation can be trying so that questions must be repeated. Delirium develops over a short period of time and tends to vary in severity throughout the day. Speech may be slurred and disjointed with aimless repetitions.

Table 13.1 Cognitive Domains and Effects of Dementia

DOMAINS OF COGNITIVE FUNCTION	EFFECTS OF DEMENTIA
Complex Attention	Difficulty staying on task and sorting through multiple stimuli
Executive Function	Difficulty with making decisions, carrying out plans, and evaluating activities
Learning and Memory	Impairment of long-term and short-term memory
Language	Inability to understand or use words
Perceptual-Motor Function	Inability to perform usual activities, such as driving a car
Social Cognition	Saying or doing inappropriate things; personality changes; insensitivity to others' feelings

Individuals may misinterpret what is happening in the environment and may develop delusional thinking and experience hallucinations. For example, they may think that the banging of a door is a gunshot. A common delusion is that someone is trying to steal from them. Sleep-wake disturbances are common. A delirious person may be hyperactive, hypoactive, or alternate between the two. The level of consciousness may fluctuate from drowsiness to stupor or coma. At the other extreme, the individual may be extremely alert and agitated.

For a diagnosis of delirium, evidence must exist that the symptoms can be explained by a medical condition, substance intoxication or withdrawal, exposure to a toxin, or multiple causes. Examples of medical conditions that can cause delirium are infections, liver or kidney failure, fluid and electrolyte imbalances, and hypoxia. Among the many drugs that can cause delirium are alcohol, opioids, cannabis, hallucinogens, sedatives, anti-anxiety drugs, amphetamines, and cocaine. Withdrawal after regular use of these and other drugs can cause substance withdrawal delirium. Anticholinergics have been found to contribute to delirium among older persons. In addition to drugs and some medical conditions, immobility and boredom also are risk factors for delirium. Although delirium can occur at any age, it is more prevalent in older adults. Examples of factors that can contribute to delirium are listed in Box 13.1.

Delirium typically responds to treatment, with the patient returning to the previous level of cognitive function. The medical management of delirium includes managing the symptoms and treating or removing the cause. For example, if delirium is the result of a drug or drug interaction, medication orders need to be changed. If delirium occurs with an infection, antimicrobial medications are ordered. If the patient is so severely agitated that essential care cannot be given or the patient poses a danger to self or others, an antipsychotic drug may be ordered. Examples of antipsychotic drugs are low-dose haloperidol (Haldol), risperidone (Risperdal), aripiprazole (Abilify), quetiapine (Seroquel), and olanzapine (Zyprexa). However, because antipsychotic drugs increase the risk of death in older adult patients, they should be used with great caution. Some antipsychotics can cause serious reactions in patients with Lewy body dementia or Parkinson disease dementia. Benzodiazepines should be avoided in older persons because they are more likely to cause oversedation or worsen confusion.

Box 13.1 Systemic and Central Nervous System Causes of Delirium

SYSTEMIC CAUSES

Cardiovascular Disease
Congestive heart failure
Dysrhythmias
Cardiac infarction
Hypovolemia (deficient fluid volume)
Aortic stenosis

Infections
Pneumonia
Urinary tract infections
Bacteremia
Septicemia

Medications
Alcohol
Amphetamines
Analgesics
Anticholinergics
Antidepressants
Antihistamines
Antiparkinsonian agents
First-generation H2-receptor blockers (e.g., cimetidine [Tagamet])
Diuretics
Neuroleptics (e.g., haloperidol [Haldol])
Sedatives or hypnotic agents (benzodiazepines [e.g., diazepam {Valium}, barbiturates])

Metabolic Conditions
Electrolyte and fluid imbalance
Hepatic, renal, or pulmonary failure
Diabetes, hyperthyroidism, hypothyroidism, or other endocrine disorders
Nutritional deficiencies
Hypothermia and heat stroke

Poisons
Heavy metals
Solvents
Pesticides
Carbon monoxide

Trauma
Head injury
Burns
Hip fracture

Other Systemic Causes
Neoplasm
Postoperative state

CENTRAL NERVOUS SYSTEM CAUSES

Infections
Meningitis
Encephalitis
Septic emboli
Neurosyphilis
Brain abscess
HIV

Neoplasm
Primary intracranial
Metastatic

Trauma
Subdural hematoma
Extradural hematoma
Contusion

Vascular Incidents
Transient ischemic attack
Stroke
Chronic subdural hematoma
Vasculitis
Arteriosclerosis
Hypertensive encephalopathy
Subarachnoid hemorrhage

Seizures
Ictal and postictal states

HIV, Human immunodeficiency virus.
From Zisook S, Braff DL. Delirium: recognition and management in the older patient, *Geriatrics* 1986;41(6):67–78.

Table 13.2 **Major Neurocognitive Disorder (Dementia) Subtypes**

DEMENTIA ETIOLOGIC SUBTYPE	USUAL FEATURES
Alzheimer disease	Insidious onset. Gradual, steady progression in cognitive and behavioral symptoms. Decline in memory and learning and at least one other cognitive domain. Depression and apathy common in early stage. Irritability, agitation, combativeness, delusions, hallucinations, and wandering may occur in later stages. Final stage marked by gait disturbance, dysphagia, incontinence, muscle spasms, and possible seizures. Patient becomes mute and totally dependent for care.
Frontotemporal lobar degeneration	Insidious onset. Progression is gradual but faster than AD. Two variants (forms) exist: behavioral and language. Behavioral symptoms: disinhibition, apathy, loss of sympathy or empathy, repeated or compulsive behavior, excessive eating. Persons with behavioral form also decline in social cognition and executive function. Individuals with language form decline in speech production, word finding, object naming, grammar, or word comprehension.
Lewy body disease	Insidious onset and gradual progression. Often seen with AD or vascular disease. Attention and awareness fluctuate. May have auditory hallucinations, orthostatic hypotension, and incontinence. Repeated falls and syncope (fainting) are common, as are Parkinson symptoms (tremor, slow movement, shuffling gait). Cognitive symptoms appear around the same time as motor symptoms. Patients are very sensitive to antipsychotic drugs.
Vascular disease	Onset is related to a cerebrovascular event. Primary decline is in complex attention and executive function. Personality and mood changes, depression, emotional lability, and psychomotor slowing are common.
Parkinson disease	Insidious onset and gradual progression. Established diagnosis of Parkinson disease. May have apathy, depression, anxiety, hallucinations, delusions, personality changes, REM sleep behavior disorder, and excessive daytime sleepiness.

AD, Alzheimer disease; *NCD*, neurocognitive disorder; *REM*, rapid eye movement.
From Mayo Clinic: *Alzheimer's disease*. Accessed June 5, 2014 from http://www.mayoclinic.org/diseases-conditions/alzheimers-disease/indepth/alzheimers-stages/art-20048448?pg=2&p=1; Mayo Clinic: *Frontotemporal dementia*. Accessed June 5, 2014 from http://www.mayoclinic.org/diseases-conditions/frontotemporal-dementia/basics/definition/con-20023876?p=1; Mayo Clinic: *Lewy body dementia*. Accessed June 5, 2014 from http://www.mayoclinic.org/diseases-conditions/lewy-body-dementia/basics/definition/con-20025038?p=1; Mayo Clinic: *Parkinson's disease*. Retrieved June 5, 2014 from http://www.mayoclinic.org/diseases-conditions/parkinsons-disease/basics/definition/con-20028488?p=1; Mayo Clinic: *Vascular dementia*. Accessed June 5, 2014 from http://www.mayoclinic.org/diseases-conditions/vascular-dementia/basics/definition/con-20029330?p=1.

MILD NEUROCOGNITIVE DISORDER

Mild NCD is a modest decline from one's usual function in one or more cognitive domains, but the individual functions well enough to live independently. The disorder can be caused by various types of dementia described later in the section on major NCD as well as to other medical conditions. Patients may or may not exhibit behavioral symptoms such as agitation, apathy, sleep disturbances, depression, anxiety, hallucinations, and delusions.

Nursing care with mild NCD focuses on compensating for the functions that are declining. For example, numerous strategies can be used to cope with impaired memory. A medication container with daily dividers can help the person to take the correct drugs each day and avoid double dosing. Written "to do" lists can provide reminders of activities or chores. If executive function is impaired, the person can be helped to focus on a single task at a time and to break tasks into smaller steps that can be readily done.

MAJOR NEUROCOGNITIVE DISORDER (DEMENTIA)

Major NCDs (dementias) are characterized by a "significant cognitive decline from a previous level of performance in one or more of the cognitive domains" (DSM-5). **Dementia** is not a disease in itself; it is a clinical syndrome, a collection of symptoms that can occur with many types of diseases. The onset and progression vary with the subtype. Features of the major subtypes are described in Table 13.2 (see also the Cultural Considerations box). The most prevalent types of dementia are caused by Alzheimer disease (AD), vascular disease, frontotemporal dementia (FTD), Lewy body disease, and Parkinson disease. Other conditions that are associated with dementia include traumatic brain injury, substance use and medication effect, human immunodeficiency virus (HIV) infection, prion disease, Huntington disease, and specific or multiple medical conditions. People can have more than one type of dementia at the same time and can also have delirium in addition to dementia.

The cause of AD is unknown, but characteristic changes in the brain include deposits of amyloid (a protein), neurofibrillary tangles (i.e., tangled microtubules in neurons) associated with altered tau protein, and a deficiency of neurotransmitters, especially acetylcholine. Neurotransmitters are chemicals that transmit signals in the brain. These changes affect the structure and function of the neurons in the brain. *Vascular dementia* results from damage to brain cells caused by inadequate blood supply. Patients with vascular dementia often have had a series of small strokes that cause progressive damage. *Lewy body disease* is characterized by the presence of a protein called *synuclein*, first seen in the substantia nigra and later in the cerebral cortex. *Parkinson disease* is associated with a deficiency of dopamine. *Frontotemporal dementia* is manifested by behavioral symptoms and/or language disorders, depending on the areas of the brain affected. Atrophy of the frontal lobes is associated with behavioral changes, whereas problems with language are the result of temporal lobe changes. At this time there is no "cure" for dementia, which is generally considered irreversible. The medical treatment offered depends on the type of dementia. Several drugs are available for patients with AD. The response to these drugs is highly variable; a small percentage of individuals have significantly improved function, whereas most others do not. Most AD drugs act to increase the amount of acetylcholine in the brain. They are most effective in the early to middle stages of AD. These include donepezil (Aricept), rivastigmine (Exelon), and galantamine (Razadyne). Memantine (Namenda) is used in mid- to late-stage dementia. It prevents the effects of galantamine, a harmful substance released by AD-damaged cells, and prevents excess calcium entry into the neurons. None of the AD drugs is curative, and eventually the patient will decline despite drug therapy. All of these drugs have significant side effects that some patients may not be able to tolerate, primarily gastrointestinal symptoms (e.g., nausea, vomiting, diarrhea). Taking the medications with meals helps to lessen the gastrointestinal side effects. Antidepressant and antipsychotic medications are sometimes prescribed as well; however, antipsychotic drugs increase the risk of death, so their use requires careful consideration. If antidepressants are used, selective serotonin reuptake inhibitors (SSRIs) such as citalopram or sertraline are recommended. If sleep is disturbed, mirtazapine or trazodone is recommended. Treatment of cerebrovascular disease and Parkinson disease is discussed in other chapters of this book.

Cultural Considerations

What Does Culture Have to Do With Dementia?

Tests used in the diagnosis of dementia may not be appropriate for individuals with less than high school education or those whose primary language is not English. Caregivers from lower socioeconomic families are more likely to be caring for older parents at an earlier age, when the caregiver is employed or still has children at home.

NURSING CARE OF THE PATIENT WITH A NEUROCOGNITIVE DISORDER

FOCUSED ASSESSMENT

The first step in collecting data about a person with an NCD is to observe the behavior and to collect data about mental status. Licensed vocational nurses/licensed practical nurses (LVNs/LPNs) may use standardized tools, such as the Folstein Mini-Mental State Examination (MMSE) (Folstein & Folstein, 1975), for a focused assessment of cognition, orientation, and memory. Orientation is commonly based on the patient's ability to state their name, location, and date and time. The inability to accurately report one's name, location, and time labels a person disoriented or confused. However, for patients in long-term care, uncertainty about days of the week and dates is not unusual. Note the patient's response to questions and instructions to determine use of language. If a change in cognitive status is recent, note any events surrounding the change (i.e., infection, relocation, major loss). Also record other symptoms such as depression, apathy, agitation, restlessness, and wandering. If the patient has exhibited aggression or agitation, ask what factors trigger these behaviors. In the community, the patient or family may be able to supply information about acute or chronic illnesses and current medications. In long-term care settings, the health care provider's health history should give this information. Be alert for medications that most often cause confusion in older adults. These include anticholinergic drugs, digoxin, H2 receptor blockers, benzodiazepines, nonsteroidal antiinflammatory drugs (NSAIDs), and many antidysrhythmic and antihypertensive drugs (see Box 13.1). Also ask about any drugs prescribed for neurocognitive symptoms.

Of greatest importance for nursing care is a description of the patient's usual routine, preferences, use of assistive devices, including eyeglasses and hearing-aids, and ability to carry out activities of daily living. Note patterns of activity and rest, dietary needs, mobility, and elimination. If the patient lives independently, it is important to assess the ability to prepare meals, shop, use the telephone, manage finances, and maintain the living environment. With delirium, self-care should improve as confusion diminishes. The person with dementia will need increasingly more assistance as the condition progresses.

Determining when confusion started and whether it has been constant or intermittent can help to differentiate delirium and dementia. Some major differences between the clinical features of delirium and dementia are described in Table 13.3. Nursing care of delirium and dementia is addressed separately, although there are some common interventions. The Coordinated Care box offers tips on helping certified nursing assistants (CNAs) to provide nursing care for patients with delirium and dementia.

Table 13.3 Clinical Features in Delirium and Dementia

FEATURE	DELIRIUM	DEMENTIA
Onset	Sudden onset	Months to years
Duration	Hours to days	Long term or lifetime
Mood	Labile, suspicious, mood swings	Fluctuating, depressed, apathetic, uninterested
Behavior	Variable; hyperactive or hypoactive	Variable; psychomotor retardation or agitation
Cognition		
Orientation	Impaired; variable severity	Slow decline over time
Alertness	Lethargic or hypervigilant	Generally normal
Memory	Impaired recent memory	Initially, impaired recent memory; later, remote memory also impaired
Thought processes	Poor concentration; disorganized, fragmented thinking	Impaired abstract thinking; difficulty finding words; impaired judgment
Perception	Possible visual, auditory, and tactile hallucinations or delusions	Hallucinations and delusions may occur
Speech and language	Slurred, forced, or rambling	Disordered

Modified from Kazer MW. Cognitive and neurologic function. In: Meiner SE, editor. *Gerontological nursing*, 4th ed., St. Louis, Elsevier-Mosby, 2011.

Patient Problems, Goals, and Outcome Criteria: Delirium

The following patient problems are only a few that might apply to the patient with delirium. Depending on the situation, different priorities will present themselves (see Nursing Care Plan 13.1: Patient with Delirium).

Patient Problems	Goals and Outcome Criteria
Impaired cognition related to drugs, infection, dehydration, unfamiliar setting, sensory overload or deprivation	Improved thought processes: orientation to person, place, and time; calm behavior, no combative actions
Sleep disturbance related to agitation, mood alterations, drug effects	Restoration of patient's usual sleep pattern: fewer nighttime awakenings, patient reports feeling rested
Potential for injury related to agitation, disorientation, unfamiliar setting	Safety maintained: absence of injury

INTERVENTIONS: DELIRIUM

When managing the patient with delirium, a health care provider focuses on identifying and treating the cause of the problem. The nurse focuses on supporting the patient to maintain safety and comfort and to reduce anxiety. Nursing care can be more effective than drugs in managing confusion.

Impaired Cognition

Delirium may develop during hospitalization or may be a reason for hospitalization. If possible, the patient should be in a private room with continual supervision. Keep the room quiet and uncluttered to avoid agitation caused by extraneous stimuli. Lighting should be soft and diffuse to avoid shadows that may be misinterpreted and add to the patient's fears. Familiar objects such as photographs, a clock, and a large calendar placed in the room may help orient the patient to time and person. Encourage patients who normally wear hearing aids and glasses to use them.

Communication with a confused patient should be simple and direct. Anyone dealing with a delirious patient should be calm, warm, and reassuring. Speak before touching the patient and always explain what you are doing. It is helpful if the same personnel are assigned to care for the patient from day to day. Handle the patient gently when providing care.

Patients with delirium may have frightening hallucinations that cause them to strike out, cry, or scream. The best response is to orient the patient to the reality of being sick and hospitalized and to explain that the hallucinations are not real even though they seem to be. You might say, "You are sick in the hospital and what you are seeing is part of the illness." Hallucinating patients in a delirious state need one-to-one nursing observation and repeated verbal reorientation. They need to be assured that the medical and nursing staff are helping them and keeping them safe.

Frequent orientation to the surroundings and the situation is important for patients with delirium. Orienting phrases such as "here in the hospital" or "now that it is evening" can be woven into conversation. Keep choices to a minimum. Simple, direct statements ("Now it is time to take your bath") are better than questions ("When would you like to take a bath?"). All communication and nursing care should

Nursing Care Plan 13.1 Patient With Delirium

FOCUSED ASSESSMENT

Health History

An 81-year-old man was admitted for hip replacement surgery 2 days ago. He lived alone and cared for himself before his surgery. He was active, alert, and independent. However, because of his surgery he has been confused and at times combative with the nurses. His physician believes that he is suffering from delirium related to the anesthesia and other drugs and that it should resolve within a few days.

Physical Examination Vital signs: blood pressure 165/95 mm Hg, pulse 98 beats per minute with slight irregularity, respiration 20 breaths per minute, temperature 97.4° F (35.3° C) orally. Height 5′7″, weight 178 lb. Is alert; disoriented to time, place, and sometimes person, is combative. Awakens during the night. Dark circles around the eyes. Refuses food and oral fluids.

Patient Problems	Goals and Outcome Criteria	Interventions
Impaired cognition related to confusion after surgical procedure	Confusion will resolve as evidenced by orientation to time, place, and person and absence of combative behavior.	Place in a private room with minimal stimuli, soft lighting. Request that a family member stay with the patient. Maintain consistency with the nursing staff caring for the patient. Approach and communicate with the patient in a calm, reassuring manner. Have patient use a hearing aid or glasses if previously used. Reorient frequently and consistently. Place familiar objects in the room: pictures, clock, calendar. Music may be soothing.
Sleep disturbance related to agitation and mood alterations	Will have adequate sleep and rest, as evidenced by fewer awakenings during the night, absence of dark circles around the eyes, and no complaints of fatigue.	Provide a back rub or offer milk at bedtime. Engage in soothing conversation to relax the patient. Plan activities to allow long periods (at least 2–4 hours) of uninterrupted sleep.
Inadequate nutrition related to confused state and poor food intake	Will have adequate fluid and food intake, as evidenced by eating meals as offered and maintaining normal body weight.	Assist the patient with meals. Offer small, light meals more frequently. Ask a family member to stay with the patient during meals.
Potential for injury related to agitation, confusion, and aggressive behavior	Will be free of injuries as evidenced by no falls, bruises, breaks in the skin, or fractures.	Adapt the environment to decrease stimuli: bed in the low position, television off or at low volume, limited number of people in room at the same time. Calm approach. Encourage a family member to stay with the patient. Consider sources of discomfort such as untreated pain or constipation that may be a factor in the confusion. Administer prescribed analgesics as appropriate. If nonpharmacologic interventions fail and severe agitation persists, administer neuroleptic drug as ordered.

CRITICAL THINKING QUESTIONS

1. Assuming that the patient's delirium is indeed related to the anesthesia and other drugs, explain how the patient's age might have played a role in his current state.
2. What factors in addition to anesthesia might be contributing to the patient's confusion?
3. The patient's daughter, who lives out of town, arrives for a visit. She is distressed by her father's behavior. What information would be helpful to her?

be carried out in a way that conveys respect and preserves the patient's dignity.

Sleep Disturbance

Sleep deprivation can cause or contribute to disorientation and confusion. Nursing measures such as giving a back rub, providing a glass of warm milk, and having a soothing conversation may help the patient to relax and fall asleep. Encourage the patient to void before bedtime. Schedule medications or treatments at times that do not interrupt nighttime sleep. The presence of a family member may help to calm an agitated and confused patient (Fig. 13.1).

Potential for Injury

The patient with delirium may pull on tubes, try to get out of bed unassisted, or attempt to leave the setting. Protecting the patient from harm without imposing excessive restrictions can be challenging. Avoid physical restraints, which tend to increase anxiety and agitation in confused patients and often result in injuries. Instead, ask a family member to remain with the patient or assign a staff member to do so. Use common sense. Position tubes out of sight. Place the bed in the low position. Postpone activities that are flexible. If the confused patient does not need to stay in bed, allow them to sit in a chair or even to "visit" the nurses'

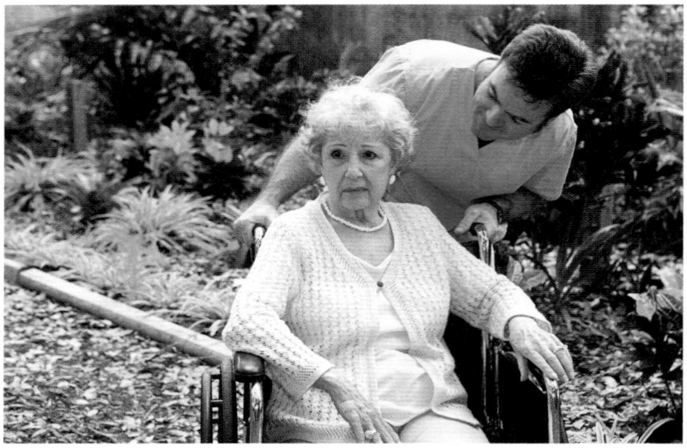

Fig. 13.1 Presence of a family member may help to calm a confused patient. (Copyright Pixland/iStock.com.)

station in a wheelchair. Avoid arguing with delirious patients. Give a gentle explanation of what is being done and the reason why it is being done.

Patient Problems, Goals, and Outcome Criteria: Dementia

Patient Problems	Goals and Outcome Criteria
Impaired performance of activities of daily living (ADLs) related to impaired thinking, sensory and motor dysfunction	Maximum possible independence in activities of daily living: patient participates in bathing, grooming, feeding, and toileting with assistance as needed.
Inadequate nutrition related to difficulty with self-feeding, inattention	Adequate nutrition: weight is stable (within 5 pounds of the ideal weight).
Sleep disturbance related to neurologic changes, altered perceptions	Adequate sleep: patient rests at night and remains physically active and awake during the day.
Potential for injury related to poor judgment, physical decline, sensorimotor changes	Absence of injuries: patient has no falls, suffers no bruises, cuts, or fractures.
Behavioral disturbances/ inability to communicate effectively related to memory loss, altered perception, impaired judgment, anxiety	Cooperative behavior: patient is calm; no combative or dangerous behavior is demonstrated. Effective communication: caregivers recognize patient needs.

INTERVENTIONS: DEMENTIA

Most people with dementia suffer from chronic, debilitating, progressive illness. The goal for individuals with dementia is to maintain the highest level of functioning possible as their abilities gradually diminish (see Nursing Care Plan 13.2: Patient with Dementia).

Coordinated Care

Working With Patients With Dementia

Working with patients with dementia can be frustrating for CNAs. The best thing the LVN/LPN can do is to model good interactions with patients. In addition, give the following explanations to CNAs:

- Rudeness and uncooperative behavior are symptoms of dementia and are best managed with kindness and patience.
- Memory impairments with dementia make it necessary for information and instructions to be repeated at intervals.
- Resisting care may occur with dementia patients; let the LVN/LPN know and try a different approach later.

Impaired Activities of Daily Living

As with patients with delirium, the first priority for patients with dementia is to meet their basic needs. Adequate nutrition, fluid and electrolyte balance, sleep, elimination, and hygiene must be maintained. Patients with dementia have varying levels of competence when it comes to carrying out these functions. Determine the patient's level of functioning and then provide whatever assistance is needed for bathing, dressing, eating, and toileting. Patients may be able to participate in self-care if tasks are broken down into individual steps to be performed one at a time. For example, instead of instructing a patient to get dressed, lay out clothing in the order it should be put on: underclothing, socks or hose, pants or skirt, shirt or blouse, belt, and shoes. Then prompt the patient to put on each item in order. Allow time for the patient to complete each step before giving another direction. Praise the completion of each task. Assist if the patient becomes frustrated.

Patients with severe dementia may be incontinent of urine and feces. Frequent, routine toileting helps to reduce incontinence episodes. Document stools and signs of constipation (e.g., straining, abdominal distention, poor appetite, passage of liquid stool). Avoid laxatives if possible; high-fiber foods in the diet are more effective for promoting regular bowel movements. If constipation cannot be managed with diet, fluids, and exercise, a bulk-forming stool softener may be needed. However, bulk-forming softeners can actually cause impaction if the patient cannot take adequate fluids.

Inadequate Nutrition

People with dementia eventually may need help with eating. Assistance with meals may mean cutting up food or total feeding. Foods that can be managed with a single utensil may facilitate self-feeding. Finger foods high in protein and carbohydrates allow patients to feed themselves more easily. Because of the patient's short attention span, they may actually consume more if given small, frequent meals. Remove distractions from the eating area. Group meals may be helpful because patients often imitate the behaviors of others. Offer fluids frequently during the day.

Nursing Care Plan 13.2 Patient With Dementia

FOCUSED ASSESSMENT

Health History

A 75-year-old woman is admitted to a long-term care facility by her daughter because she has been unsafe living alone at home. Her daughter reports that her mother had been in good health. However, during the past 5 years, she has gradually had more and more problems with her memory; during the past year, she has resisted taking a bath or changing her clothes. Lately, she has had times when she has not known her daughter. At times, she has been unable to find the bathroom and has been incontinent of urine. She often forgets to eat and, when she does eat, she prefers sweet snacks. She has recently begun "wandering." She was found at a local park not knowing who she was or where she lived. Her physician has diagnosed probable AD.

Physical Examination Vital signs: blood pressure 170/95 mm Hg, pulse 88 beats per minute, respiration 22 breaths per minute, temperature 98.2°F (36.78°C). Height 5′3″, weight 126 lb. Is disoriented to time, place, and person.

Patient Problems	Goals and Outcome Criteria	Interventions
Impaired activities of daily living related to impaired thinking, sensory and motor dysfunction	Patient will perform activities of daily living (ADLs) as independently as possible, as evidenced by participation in bathing and dressing with the assistance of the nurse as needed.	Determine whether the patient can perform her own ADLs. Allow the patient to perform as many ADLs as possible. Remain with the patient while she performs ADLs to maintain safety. Establish a routine toileting schedule and encourage the patient to go to the toilet at regular intervals.
Inadequate nutrition related to difficulty with self-feeding, inattention	Patient will maintain adequate nutrition, as evidenced by staying within 5 pounds of her ideal weight.	Remove distractions from the table. Cut food into small portions. Offer finger foods. Offer foods high in protein and carbohydrates. Offer small, frequent meals and snacks. Offer fluids frequently. Stay with the patient while she eats.
Sleep disturbance related to neurologic changes, altered perceptions	Patient will have adequate sleep, as evidenced by quiet restfulness at night and remaining physically active and awake during the day.	Try to keep her awake during the day and encourage her to sleep only at night. Minimize activities late in the day to allow her to "wind down" by bedtime. Have a quiet hour in the evening with soft music. If she awakens during the night and becomes confused or agitated, reassure in a soft, soothing manner to avoid precipitating extreme agitation and loss of control. Try gently stroking and singing to her. Provide a comfort object if she has one (e.g., blanket, doll).
Potential for injury related to poor judgment, physical decline, sensorimotor changes	Absence of injuries: patient has no falls, suffers no bruises, cuts, fractures.	Provide a safe environment: no clutter, no medications or dangerous chemicals within reach. Avoid use of restraints. Provide opportunities for safe, supervised walking. Monitor exits to prevent wandering from the premises.
Behavioral disturbance/inability to communicate effectively related to altered perception, impaired judgment, anxiety	Patient will remain calm and free of combative behavior as evidenced by a calm, cooperative manner during nursing care.	Speak to the patient in a calm, reassuring manner. Avoid confrontations with the patient. Break down tasks into steps to be performed one at a time. Provide consistency in nursing care. Attempt to understand what the patient is communicating verbally and nonverbally.

CRITICAL THINKING QUESTIONS

1. Why is it important to stay with the resident while she completes her ADLs and while she feeds herself?
2. What strategies might you use to minimize the incidents of urinary incontinence in the resident who has dementia?

Sleep Disturbance

Sleep and awakening hours are often reversed in patients with dementia. Providing stimulation to keep them awake during the day may help them to sleep at night. Schedule tests and treatments during the morning and early afternoon to allow the patient time to wind down by bedtime. Some caregivers have found that a quiet hour in the evening with soft music playing promotes sleep at night. However, sometimes the patient persists in nighttime awakening. When that occurs, assist the patient to the toilet, offer fluids and/or a snack, and provide comfort measures. Offer reassurance in a soft, soothing manner. The patient may go back to sleep afterward. Avoid regular use of sedatives; however, prolonged periods of wakefulness can lead to delirium. If a sleeping aid is needed, trazodone (Oleptro) is preferred.

Potential for Injury

A safe, structured environment is essential for the person with dementia. Nothing harmful should be left around. Falls and injuries may be prevented with environmental modifications, careful observation, muscle strengthening, and a fall prevention program (see Chapter 11). Avoid restraints, if possible; they may aggravate agitation and have been associated with injuries such as skin tears, obstructed circulation, and even strangulation. Arrange furniture for easy access to toilets from the patient's bed or chair. Use nightlights to illuminate the path to the bathroom. Lights that turn on in response to detected motion may be used as well.

Behavioral Disturbances and Inability to Communicate Effectively

Communication usually becomes increasingly difficult. Patients with dementia are disoriented and their thinking ability is impaired. They are confused by what is going on around them. Communication should be simple and direct. Approach them gently, calmly, and quietly. They tend to copy the behavior of people around them; consequently, a caregiver who is anxious or upset can easily convey these feelings to a patient. Nonverbal communication is extremely important. Cues from the patient's actions and facial expressions are important because patients are frequently unable to express their needs verbally. When patients resist activities such as bathing or dressing, avoid confrontations, which only provoke agitation and possible violence. Instead, come back at another time. A consistent schedule of care given by the same caregivers provides security for the patient with dementia.

Whereas frequent reality orientation is helpful for the patient with delirium, such orientation is not effective for the patient with dementia. Clocks, calendars, constant mention of the date and time, and other such orientation reminders used to be a staple of care for patients with dementia. However, reality orientation may agitate people with dementia. Furthermore, patients may not be able to use clocks and calendars. Assisting them in a nonconfrontational manner and redirecting activities without constantly reminding them of their deficits is a better approach.

Put On Your Thinking Cap!

A patient's daughter is distressed because her mother does not seem to recognize her at times. What could you say to help the daughter? What suggestions could you give her to promote communication with her mother?

GUIDELINES FOR WORKING WITH PATIENTS WITH DEMENTIA

Two important concepts are helpful to keep in mind when taking care of patients with dementia: (1) they usually forget things relatively quickly and (2) they are usually unable to learn new things. For example, if persons with dementia start to become agitated, it may be effective to divert their attention somewhere else. They may be gently guided to another activity; usually within a relatively short period they will forget what was bothering them and focus on the new activity. Sometimes agitation indicates pain, hunger, stress, fear, or the need for toileting. Investigate whether any of these problems are present. Take advantage of the fact that patients with dementia are usually slow or unable to learn new things. For example, putting new locks on the doors in new places may prevent wandering patients from opening exit doors. Using these two concepts as a basis for care allows the caregiver to be creative in the care of patients with dementia.

The cognitive developmental approach (CDA) can also guide care for patients with dementia. The CDA adapts interventions based on the patient's cognitive abilities. Eliminating unrealistic expectations and allowing the patient to do as much as they are able is believed to reduce patient stress and frustration. Some principles derived from the CDA that can be applied are as follows:

- Accept that the patient with dementia may no longer be able to make adult decisions and behave as a healthy adult would. Offer limited choices to simplify decision making.
- Adapt the environment to the patient rather than the patient to the environment. For example, create a safe environment for wandering instead of trying to keep the patient from wandering.
- Encourage self-care at whatever level the patient can function. If the patient can eat independently with their hands but not with utensils, provide finger foods.
- Recognize irrational fears such as a fear of the bathtub; arrange for alternative ways to give personal care.
- Accept that, in advanced dementia, patient behaviors and thinking are not typical of a healthy adult. Some strategies that work with children often work with dementia patients.
- Recognize that the patient deserves to be treated with dignity, regardless of abilities or behaviors. Even the most impaired patient can probably sense compassion in a caregiver.

Get Ready for the NCLEX® Examination!

Key Points

- NCDs include delirium, mild NCD, and major NCD.
- The domains of cognitive function that may be affected by NCDs are complex attention, executive function, learning and memory, language, perceptual-motor function, and social cognition.
- Patients who are not oriented to person, place, and time are said to be disoriented or confused.
- Delirium is a rather sudden decline from a person's usual attention and awareness (orientation to the environment) that is usually reversible.
- Symptoms of delirium may include memory deficit, disorientation, delusions, hallucinations, and a language or perceptual problem.
- Delirium is usually caused by some underlying medical condition such as infection, liver or kidney failure, fluid and electrolyte imbalances, hypoxia, substance intoxication or withdrawal, exposure to a toxin, or multiple causes.
- Dementia is chronic, progressive, and generally considered irreversible.
- Dementia exists on a spectrum from mild to major neurocognitive dysfunction.
- Dementia is characterized by a "significant cognitive decline from a previous level of performance in one or more of the cognitive domains" (DSM-5, p. 602). Dementia is not a disease entity in itself; it is a clinical syndrome, a collection of symptoms that may be caused by a variety of conditions.
- The most common types of dementia are AD, vascular dementia, FTD, Lewy body dementia, and Parkinson disease dementia.
- The first step in the focused assessment of a cognitively impaired person is to observe the patient's behavior and to evaluate mental status.
- Determine how long the symptoms have been present and how and when they started.
- In caring for a patient with delirium, provide safety and comfort measures, as well as frequent orientation to the surroundings and situation.
- The goal for patients with dementia is to maintain the highest level of functioning possible as their abilities gradually diminish.
- A safe, structured environment is essential for patients with dementia, and tasks should be broken down into steps that can be performed one at a time.
- When patients with dementia resist activities such as bathing or dressing, avoid confrontations and divert their attention elsewhere.
- The cognitive developmental approach (CDA) adapts interventions to the patient's cognitive level.

Additional Learning Resources

SG Go to your Study Guide for additional learning activities to help master this chapter content.

Go to your Evolve website (http://evolve.elsevier.com/Linton/medsurg) for the following learning resources and much more:

- Fluid & Electrolyte Tutorial
- Review Questions for the NCLEX® Examination

Clinical Judgment and Next-Generation NCLEX® Examination-Style Questions

1. What is the primary difference between delirium and dementia?

1. Delirium is typically reversible; dementia is usually irreversible.
2. Agitation is constant with delirium but intermittent with dementia.
3. The onset of delirium is gradual; the onset of dementia is typically rapid.
4. Delirium usually lasts only a few minutes; dementia lasts weeks to months.

NCLEX Client Need: Physiological Integrity: Physiological Adaptation

2. A delirious patient repeatedly cries out for her daughter in the middle of the night. What is the best intervention?

1. Check to see whether she has an order for a sedative.
2. Call the daughter and ask her to come see the patient.
3. Calmly tell her where she is and that her daughter is not there.
4. Tell her she needs to be quiet because she is disturbing other patients.

NCLEX Client Need: Physiological Integrity: Basic Care and Comfort

3. A patient with AD wanders away from the table during meals, leaving most of his food uneaten. What should you do?

1. Consult with the dietitian about providing finger foods.
2. Restrain the patient in his seat during meals.
3. Tell him he must sit down and finish his meal.
4. Ask another patient to try to keep him at the table.

NCLEX Client Need: Physiological Integrity: Basic Care and Comfort

4. When addressing a person who has dementia, which message is most appropriate?

1. "You need to be dressed for church in 30 minutes."
2. "Put your arm in the sleeve of your shirt."
3. "Put your shirt on."
4. "What would you like to wear today?"

NCLEX Client Need: Physiological Integrity: Basic Care and Comfort

5. A new nurse on the special care unit for patients with AD repeatedly asks patients what time it is and if they know where they are. What information should you share with her?

1. If a patient cannot answer the questions correctly, wait 5 minutes and ask again.
2. Consistently tell patients the time, date, and place to keep them oriented.
3. Frequent attempts at orientation tend to agitate patients with AD.
4. Ask the patient to repeat the date, time, and place after you say them.

NCLEX Client Need: Psychosocial Integrity

6. **If you applied the principles of the CDA to the care of a patient with dementia, you would:**
   1. Consistently use the same interventions for all patients with dementia.
   2. Have patients confront irrational fears so they can be overcome.
   3. Insist that the patient behave as a mature adult at all times.
   4. Adapt expectations and interventions to the patient's abilities.

   NCLEX Client Need: Psychosocial Integrity

7. **Which type of dementia is most common?**
   ____________________.

   NCLEX Client Need: Physiological Integrity: Physiological Adaptation

8. **Most drugs used to treat AD work by increasing the amount of which neurotransmitter in the brain?**
   ____

   NCLEX Client Need: Physiological Integrity: Pharmacological Therapies

9. **When a patient and her family are informed that the patient probably has early AD, the patient says, "Don't they have drugs to cure this disease?" To explain drug therapy for AD, the health care provider should include which statements? (Select all that apply.)**
   1. Drugs are curative only if started early in the course of the disease.
   2. Drugs currently used for the treatment of AD have no side or adverse effects.
   3. There are no drugs for moderate dementia.
   4. Benefits gained from taking AD drugs vary greatly among individuals.
   5. A combination of drugs usually arrests the progression of AD.

   NCLEX Client Need: Physiological Integrity: Pharmacological Therapies

10. **Your home health patient has become confused over the past week. He is taking all of the drugs listed subsequently. Which of these can cause confusion? (Select all that apply.)**
    1. Digoxin for heart failure
    2. Antacid for heartburn
    3. First generation H2 receptor blocker for peptic ulcer disease
    4. Anticholinergic for seasonal allergies
    5. NSAID for arthritis

    NCLEX Client Need: Physiological Integrity: Pharmacological Therapies

11. **SLO/Objective: Apply knowledge of anatomy and physiology and pathophysiology to determine which assessment data require follow-up from the nurse.**

    NGN Item Type: Enhanced Hot Spot

    Cognitive Skill: Recognize Cues

    An 81-year-old man was admitted for left hip replacement surgery two days ago. He lived alone and cared for himself before his surgery. He was active, alert and independent. However, because of his surgery he has been confused and at times combative with the nurses. The patient is being treated with hydrocodone for pain in his left hip. His physician believes that he is suffering from delirium related to the anesthesia and other drugs and that it should resolve within a few days.

    Highlight or place a check mark next to the assessment findings that require follow up by the nurse.

    - Blood pressure 94/52 mm Hg
    - Pulse 98 beats per minute
    - Respirations 20 breaths per minute
    - Two days postop
    - Hydrocodone for pain in operative hip
    - Disoriented to time, place, person
    - Combative
    - Refuses food and fluids
    - Sleeplessness

12. **SLO/Objective: Apply knowledge of pathophysiology of delirium to determine which laboratory values may be affected.**

    NGN Item Type: Extended Multiple Response

    Cognitive Skill: Analyze Cues Which lab values may be affected in a patient with delirium. Check all that apply.

    ____ A. Elevated urine specific gravity
    ____ B. Decreased oxygen saturation
    ____ C. Elevated red blood cells
    ____ D. Decreased hematocrit
    ____ F. Decreased serum sodium
    ____ G. Increased platelet count

13. **SLO/Objective: Prioritize nursing care for patients with immobility.**

    NGN Item Type: Cloze

    Cognitive Skill: Prioritize Hypotheses

    An 81-year-old man was admitted for left hip replacement surgery two days ago. He lived alone and cared for himself before his surgery. He was active, alert and independent. However, because of his surgery he has been confused and at times combative with the nurses. The patient is being treated with hydrocodone for pain in his left hip. His physician believes that he is suffering from delirium related to the anesthesia and other drugs and that it should resolve within a few days.

- Blood pressure 94/52 mm Hg
- Pulse 98 beats per minute
- Respirations 18 breaths per minute
- Disorientation
- Agitation
- Dehydration
- Anorexia

Choose the *most likely* options for the information missing from the statements below by selecting from the list of options provided.

The patient is experiencing confusion and disorientation most likely caused by delirium. His acute confusion is most likely the result of ______, ______, and _________ and needs to be closely monitored. Failure to recognize these conditions can lead to _______ and harm to self and others.

Pain
Dehydration
Confusion
Drug effects
Infection
Weakness
Harm to Self and Others
Falls

14. **SLO/Objective: Plan actions for patients experiencing delirium.**

    NGN Item Type: Matrix

    Cognitive Skill: Generate Solutions

    An 82-year-old man is residing in a nursing home after discharge from a hospital after being treated for hip fracture after a fall. He is often confused and disoriented to time and place and is combative at times. He's refusing to eat or drink fluids. He is receiving PT and is gradually walking with a walker. The patient repeatedly says he wants to go home. Vital signs: BP 130/70; P 100 beats per minute, Respirations 22 breaths per minute, Temperature 99.8°F.

NURSING ACTION	INDICATED	CONTRAINDICATED	NONESSENTIAL
Provide urinal within reach			
Maintain minimum fluid intake of 1200 mL/24 h			
Place in restraints when combative to protect self and others			
Reorient frequently and consistently			
Implement fall prevention regimen			
Turn, cough and deep breathe every 2 hours			

15. **SLO/Objective: Determine appropriate nursing actions for patients experiencing delirium.**

    NGN Item Type: Extended Drag and Drop

    Cognitive Skill: Take Action

    The patient has been residing in a rehab center after hospitalization for assistance after sustaining a broken hip from a fall. While in the nursing home, he reports painful urination. The urine is dark and cloudy. He sustained a fall while trying to get to the bathroom by himself. Fluid intake remains limited.

    Indicate in the right-hand column which nursing action listed in the far left column is appropriate for the potential complications of a patient experiencing a fall.

NURSING ACTION	POTENTIAL COMPLICATION	APPROPRIATE NURSING ACTION FOR COMPLICATION
1. Keep bed in high position with bedrails	Urinary tract infection	
2. Maintain minimum daily fluids at 1200 mL	Dehydration	
3. Monitor type and frequency of stools	Delirium	
4. Collect urine specimen for analysis	Falls	
5. Assist with ambulation	//////////////////////	
6. Orient to environment	//////////////////////	

16. **SLO/Objective: Evaluate the effectiveness of nursing and collaborative interventions for patients experiencing delirium.**

NGN Item Type: Matrix

Cognitive Skill: Evaluate Outcomes

Two weeks later the patient in Question 15 remains in a rehab center. A repeat urinalysis and mental status examination were conducted. Intake and output were measured. A fall assessment was conducted.

For each assessment finding, use an X to indicate whether the interventions were *Effective* (helped to meet expected outcomes), *Ineffective* (did not help to meet expected outcomes), or *Unrelated* (not related to the expected outcomes).

ASSESSMENT FINDING	EFFECTIVE	INEFFECTIVE	UNRELATED
Denies pain with urination			
Urine output is amber and clear			
Occasional confusion at night, otherwise oriented x3			
Fluid intake averaged 800 mL/day			
Pupils equal and reactive to light			
Ambulating without falls			

16. **SLO/Objective: Apply knowledge of dementia to determine which assessment data require follow-up from the nurse.**

NGN Item Type: Enhanced Hot Spot

Cognitive Skill: Recognize Cues

A 75-year-old woman is admitted to a memory care unit by her daughter because she has been unsafe at home. Her daughter reports that her mother had been in good health. However, during the past 5 years, her memory has continued to decline. During the past year, she has resisted taking a bath or changing her clothes. Lately, she has had times when she has not known her daughter. At times, she has been unable to find the bathroom and has been incontinent of urine. She often forgets to eat and, when she does eat, she prefers sweet snacks. She has recently begun "wandering" and sleeping during the day. She was found at a local park not knowing who she was or where she lived. Her physician has diagnosed probable Alzheimer disease.

Highlight or place a check mark next to the assessment findings that require follow-up by the nurse.

- Blood pressure 170/95 mm Hg
- Pulse 88 beats per minute
- Respirations 22 breaths per minute
- Impaired ability to carry out ADLs independently
- Resists care
- Disoriented to time, place, person
- Wandering
- Urinary incontinence
- Altered sleep patterns

17. **SLO/Objective: Apply knowledge of pathophysiology of dementia to determine which assessment data are characteristic of dementia.**

NGN Item Type: Extended Multiple Response

Cognitive Skill: Analyze Cues

- Blood pressure 170/95 mm Hg
- Pulse 88 beats per minute
- Respirations 22 breaths per minute
- Impaired ability to carry out ADLs independently
- Resists care
- Disoriented to time, place, person
- Wandering
- Urinary incontinence
- Altered sleep patterns

Choose the most likely options for the information missing from the statements below by selecting from the list of options provided.

The patient is experiencing confusion and disorientation probably caused by dementia. Factors that contribute to her confusion are most likely (1) ______, and (1)_________, and (1)________. Based on assessment data, the nurse identifies risk for injury owing to (2)________ and (2)_________.

OPTION 1	OPTION 2
Altered perception	Resisting care
Impaired judgment	Wandering
Impaired thinking	Malnutrition
Urinary incontinence	Urinary tract infection
Hypertension	Dehydration

18. **SLO/Objective: Prioritize nursing care for patients with dementia.**

NGN Item Type: Extended Multiple Response

Cognitive Skill: Prioritize Hypotheses

A 75-year-old woman continues to reside in a memory care unit. After three weeks her blood pressure has decreased because of treatment with metoprolol and HCTZ.

- Blood pressure 150/95 mm Hg
- Pulse 88 beats per minute
- Respirations 22 breaths per minute
- Impaired ability to carry out ADLs independently
- Resists care
- Disoriented to time, place, person
- Wandering
- Urinary incontinence
- Altered sleep patterns

When planning care for this patient, for which *priority* potential complications would the nurse monitor. Select all that apply.

a. Stroke

b. Sleep deprivation
c. Malnutrition
d. Skin breakdown
e. Joint contractures
f. Urinary tract infection
g. Pneumonia

19. **SLO/Objective: Plan actions for patients experiencing dementia.**

NGN Item Type: Matrix

Cognitive Skill: Generate Solutions

A 75-year-old woman has been residing in a memory care unit with a diagnosis of dementia for the past two weeks. Her memory has continued to decline. She has resisted taking a bath or changing her clothes. At times, she has been unable to find the bathroom and has been incontinent of urine. She sometimes refuses to eat, and when she does eat, she prefers sweet snacks. She continues to wander and sleeps fitfully.

Use an X for the nursing actions listed below that are *Indicated* (appropriate or necessary), *Contraindicated* (could be harmful), or *Nonessential* (makes no difference or not necessary) for the patient's care at this time.

NURSING ACTION	INDICATED	CONTRAINDICATED	NONESSENTIAL
Administer prescription for Haloperidol for behavioral disturbances			
Avoid confrontations with patient			
Place in restraints to prevent agitation			
Offer small frequent healthy meals and snacks			
Establish a routine toileting schedule			
Provide memory exercises			
Break down bathing and dressing tasks into steps to be performed one at a time			

20. **SLO/Objective: Evaluate the effectiveness of nursing and collaborative interventions for patients experiencing dementia.**

NGN Item Type: Matrix

Cognitive Skill: Evaluate Outcomes

Two months later, the patient in Questions 16 to 19 remains in a memory care unit.

For each assessment finding, use an X to indicate whether the interventions were *Effective* (helped to meet expected outcomes), *Ineffective* (did not help to meet expected outcomes), or *Unrelated* (not related to the expected outcomes).

ASSESSMENT FINDING	EFFECTIVE	INEFFECTIVE	UNRELATED
Decreased incidences of incontinence			
Maintained body weight within 5 pounds of admission weight			
Agitation escalated when restrained			
Remained safely in memory care unit			
Cooperates with bathing and dressing			
Memory decline continues			

14 Incontinence

http://evolve.elsevier.com/Linton/medsurg

Objectives

1. Describe the scope and consequences of incontinence.
2. Identify common therapeutic measures used for the patient with incontinence.
3. List the types of urinary and fecal incontinence.
4. Explain the pathophysiology and treatment of specific types of incontinence.
5. Recognize nursing assessment data needed to assist in the evaluation and treatment of incontinence.
6. Assist in developing a nursing care plan for the patient with incontinence.

Key Terms

anorectal incontinence (ā-nō-RĔK-tăl ĭn-KŎN-tĭ-nĕns)
Credé technique (kră-DĀ)
overactive bladder
bowel incontinence
fecal incontinence
functional incontinence
micturition (mĭk-tŭ-RĬSH-ŭn)
mixed incontinence
neurogenic bladder (nū-rō-JĔN-ĭk)
neurogenic incontinence
overflow urinary incontinence
persistent incontinence
stress incontinence
transient incontinence (TRĂN-zē-ĕnt)
urge incontinence
urinary incontinence
void

Incontinence is the term used to describe the involuntary passage of urine (**urinary incontinence**) or feces (fecal or bowel incontinence). Many conditions and situations can cause either temporary or permanent incontinence. Incontinence deserves special attention because of the toll it takes on an older individual. A person who is troubled by incontinence faces physical, psychosocial, and financial burdens. The management of incontinence in patient care settings also requires many hours of nursing care.

The goals of treatment for an incontinent person include the restoration or improvement of control for treatable incontinence, the management of irreversible incontinence, and the prevention of complications.

URINARY INCONTINENCE

PREVALENCE AND COSTS

Statistics on urinary incontinence vary greatly depending on the gender, age, type of incontinence, and setting (community versus institution) of the individuals studied. Exact figures are difficult to obtain because people often do not report the problem to health care providers. General surveys of adults in the United States have found that 5% to 25% note leakage at least once a week and 5% to 15% experience it daily or most of the time. Among U.S. women who live in the community, 15% to 69% are affected by urinary incontinence, with 5% to 24% having severe leakage. The prevalence of urinary incontinence is twice as high among women as among men. Estimates indicate that approximately 17% of men older than 60 years of age report urinary incontinence. Among men who have had a radical prostatectomy, as many as 30% report some degree of incontinence.

In addition to the emotional costs, urinary incontinence exerts a heavy financial toll. The cost of care related to incontinence in the United States is estimated to be more than $20 billion per year. This figure is compounded by the cost of supplies such as absorbent pads and briefs, medications, surgery, and management of complications such as skin breakdown and urinary tract infections. Health care providers need to recognize the economic and personal value of aggressively treating incontinence. Nurses play an important role in educating people about the need for evaluation and treatment. Although urinary incontinence is more common in older people, it should not be considered normal. Incontinence can often be improved or cured, regardless of age. However, individuals may not seek treatment for incontinence because of embarrassment, misunderstanding that it comes with aging, lack of knowledge about treatment, or the view that incontinence is more of an inconvenience rather than a health problem. These barriers can be addressed by proactive nursing that includes asking about bowel and bladder concerns, assessing urinary status, providing education, implementing effective strategies, and providing referral for further medical evaluation.

PHYSIOLOGY OF URINATION

Terms used to describe the passage of urine are *urination*, **micturition**, and *voiding*. The terms **void** and *voiding* are used in this chapter because they are common in medical settings.

Normal controlled voiding requires a healthy bladder muscle (detrusor muscle), a patent (open) urethra, normal transmission of nerve impulses, and mental alertness. Alterations in any of these factors may result in incontinence.

Urine continually drains from the kidneys to the bladder, where it is stored until it can be eliminated. When 200 to 250 mL of urine collects in the bladder, stretch and tension receptors in the muscular bladder wall are stimulated. The bladder muscles relax to allow for bladder expansion to hold urine and the internal sphincter contracts to retain urine in the bladder. As the bladder fills, messages are sent to the brain, making the person aware of bladder fullness and the need to void. Because the act of voiding is normally voluntary, voiding can be delayed until a convenient time. When the individual determines an appropriate time to void, the external sphincter relaxes, and the bladder then contracts, permitting urine to flow out through the urethra (Fig. 14.1). Age-related changes in the urologic system that impact normal urinary elimination are described in Table 14.1.

RISK FACTORS FOR URINARY INCONTINENCE

Although urinary incontinence is prevalent among middle-aged and older individuals, identification of risk factors can guide prevention and treatment. Risk factors for incontinence that are intrinsic and not modifiable include older age, gender, pregnancy- and childbirth-associated factors, and medical conditions. Extrinsic and potentially modifiable factors include lifestyle behaviors and habits. Risk factors are listed in Box 14.1.

DIAGNOSTIC TESTS AND PROCEDURES

Measurement of residual urine volume, stress tests, imaging procedures (computed tomography or magnetic resonance imaging), cystoscopy, renal ultrasound, and urodynamic studies may be used to identify underlying anatomic and physiologic abnormalities. Urodynamic procedures assess the neuromuscular function of the lower urinary tract. These procedures include uroflowmetry, which measures voiding duration and the amount and rate of urine voided. Cystometry is used to evaluate the neuromuscular function of the bladder. Cystoscopy involves the insertion of a scope through the urethra to visualize the urethra and bladder. The

Box 14.1 Risk Factors for Urinary Incontinence

INTRINSIC FACTORS

Older age
Immobility
Chronic degenerative joint disease
Parkinson disease, diabetes, stroke, multiple sclerosis, spinal cord injury
Surgery: hysterectomy, prostatectomy
Pelvic radiation
Impaired cognition: delirium, dementia
Depression
Medications
Estrogen deficiency
Pregnancy, vaginal delivery, episiotomy, heavy birthweight

EXTRINSIC FACTORS

Obesity
Smoking
Chronic cough
Constipation, fecal impaction
Malnutrition
Low-fluid intake
Caffeine intake
High-impact physical exercise, weight lifting

Table 14.1 Age-Related Changes in the Urinary System

AGE-RELATED CHANGE	IMPLICATION
Decreased bladder tone and elasticity	Total bladder capacity decreases to about 300 mL from 600 mL
Loss of bladder holding capacity	Voiding frequently at smaller urine volumes
Urge to void occurs at lower bladder volumes	Urinary frequency and nocturia
Increased urine production at night	Nocturia
Changes in collagen content and sensitivity of muscle receptors	Increased bladder contractions and urge to void at smaller bladder volumes
Less muscle tone and elasticity	Weakened contractions during bladder emptying and increased postvoid residual urine volume

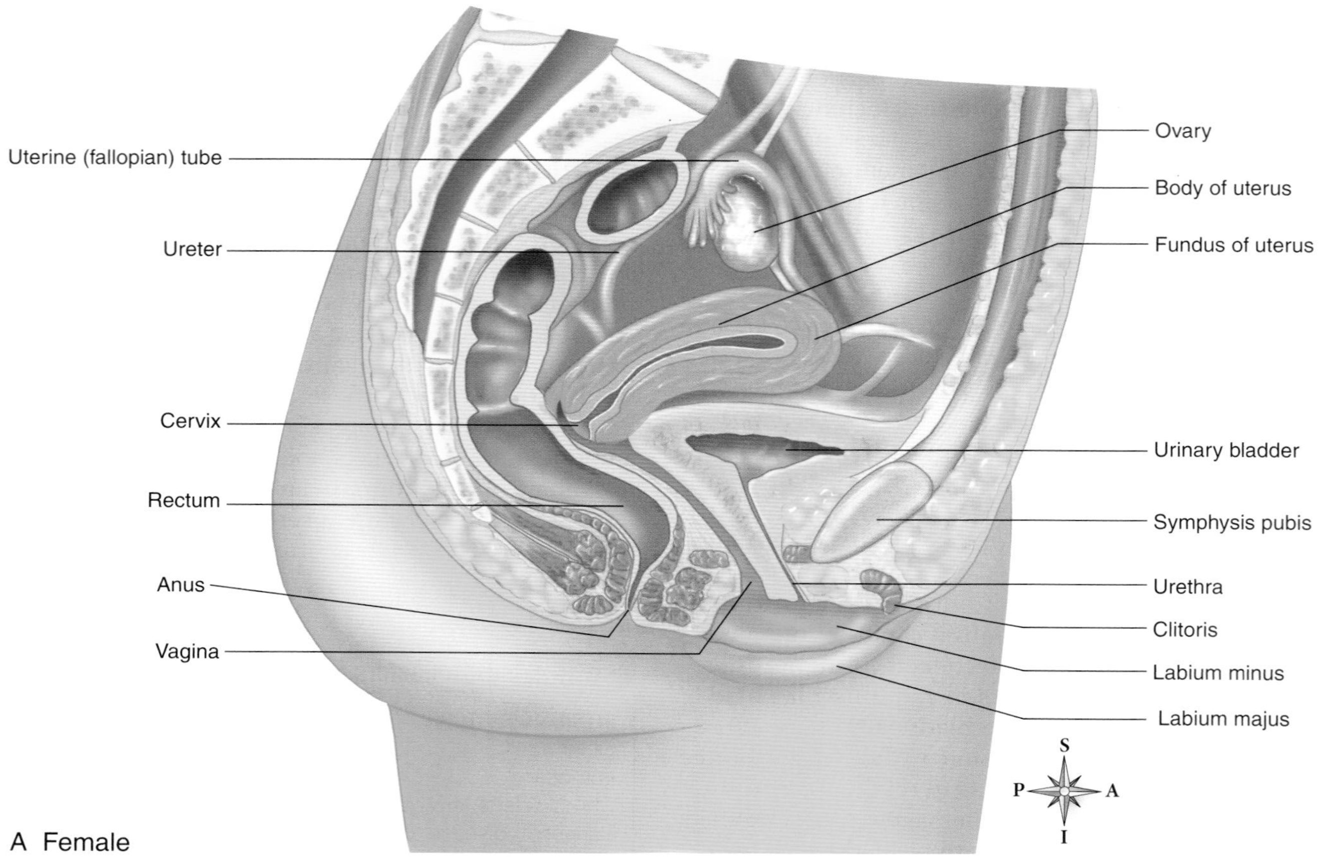

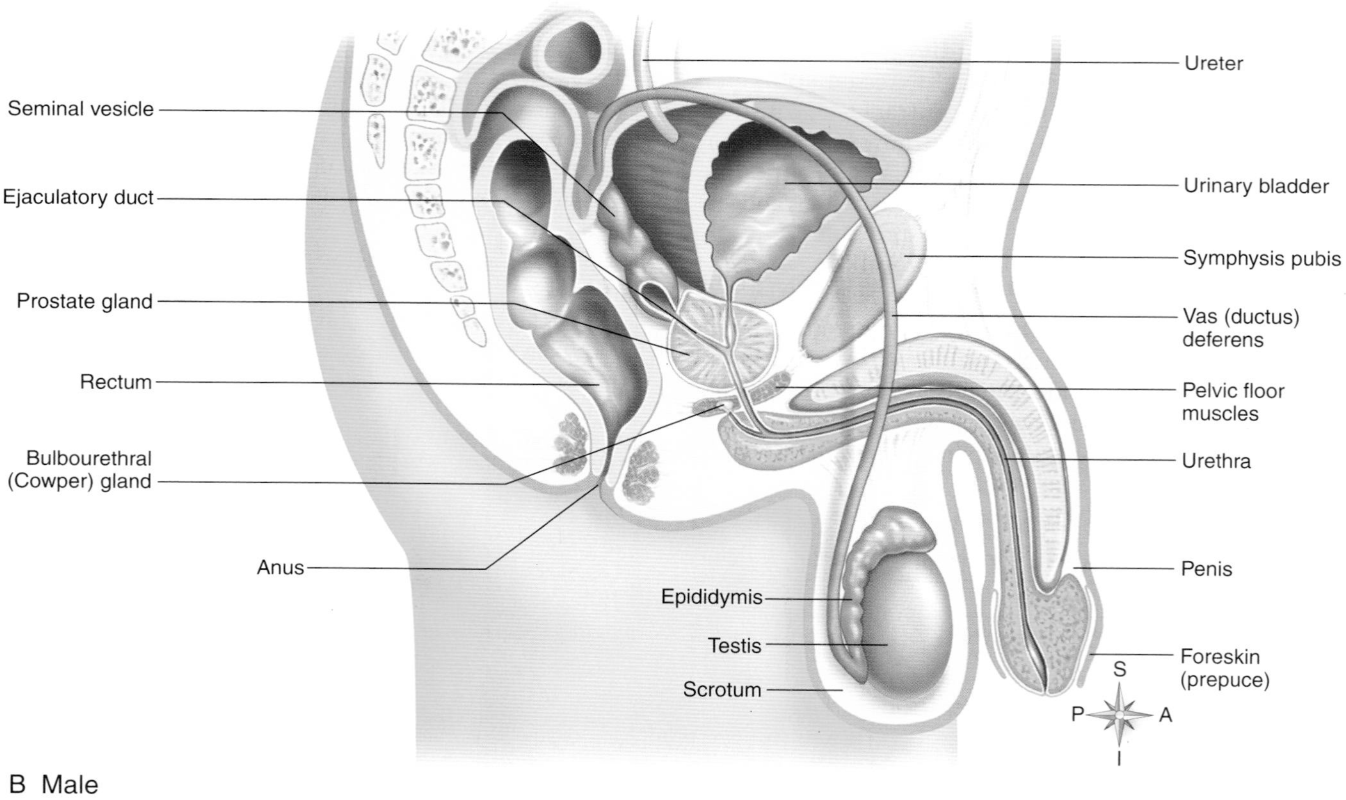

Fig. 14.1 The bladder, urethra, and adjacent structures. (A) Female patient. (B) Male patient. (From Patton K, Thibodeau G: *The human body in health and disease*, ed 7, St. Louis, 2018, Elsevier.)

results help to identify the type of incontinence, which in turn guides treatment decisions. Details of these and other urologic tests are presented in Chapter 41.

LABORATORY TESTS

A blood sample may be analyzed for specific gravity, pH, blood urea nitrogen, creatinine, glucose, A1C, and calcium. A clean-catch urinalysis with culture and sensitivity testing is usually ordered to assess the urine for abnormalities. External collection devices such as straight catheterization can be used for persons with cognitive or mobility problems that make obtaining a clean urine specimen difficult. The specimen is studied for bacteria, red blood cells, white blood cells, protein, and glucose. Sometimes bacteria are found in the urine when there are no symptoms of infection. Such asymptomatic bacteriuria usually does not require treatment and treatment may not improve bladder control.

POSTVOID RESIDUAL VOLUME

Determining whether the patient is emptying the bladder completely is an important part of assessment. Postvoid residual (PVR) volume is the amount of urine remaining in the bladder within 15 minutes of voiding. Several methods are used to determine the PVR volume. The preferred method uses a noninvasive portable ultrasound device. Although there is no risk for urinary tract infection with this method, accuracy may be affected by the skill of the user, calibration of the machine, and characteristics of the patient such as abdominal adiposity and anatomic displacement of the bladder. The second method, which is more accurate but is associated with risk for infection, involves urethral catheterization of the patient. Normally less than 50 mL of urine remains in the bladder after voiding, but in older adults a PVR volume up to 200 mL may be acceptable.

Put On Your Thinking Cap!

Why is it better to use portable bladder ultrasound to assess PVR volume instead of catheterizing the patient?

COMMON THERAPEUTIC MEASURES

Depending on the type of urinary incontinence, a number of therapeutic measures may be implemented. These measures are generally classified as *behavioral*, *pharmacologic*, or *surgical* treatments. Despite the variety of treatments available, many people do not seek medical care for urinary incontinence. Some individuals manage incontinence with practices such as limiting activities outside the home, emptying the bladder frequently, restricting fluids, and avoiding activities that induce leakage, such as exercise. Unfortunately, these strategies can have negative consequences. For example, inadequate fluid intake can lead to dehydration and urinary tract infection and giving up social and recreational activities for fear of embarrassment because of visible leakage or odor can lead to social isolation, loneliness, and depression.

BEHAVIORAL INTERVENTIONS

Behavioral interventions include toileting programs such as bladder training, habit training, and prompted voiding, pelvic muscle exercises, urge suppression, and hydration management. These techniques are low risk and are often effective in decreasing the frequency of incontinent episodes. In general, these interventions require patient cooperation or the assistance of a caregiver.

Toileting Programs

Bladder training. Bladder retraining uses patient education, scheduled toileting, and positive reinforcement. The teaching plan includes information about normal urinary function and the bladder retraining program. With scheduled toileting, the patient is encouraged to delay voiding and void only at scheduled times. Initially voiding is usually scheduled every hour while the patient is awake. Urge suppression is used to delay voiding (see instructions later). The length of time between voiding is gradually increased, with the goal of every 2 to 3 hours. If the patient voids ahead of schedule, the next voiding may be rescheduled at the prescribed interval. Another approach is to ignore the unscheduled voiding and have the patient void again at the previously scheduled time. The patient's efforts and improvement are positively reinforced and feedback provided indicating reduction in the volume and/or frequency of incontinent episodes.

Habit training. Habit training is also called *timed voiding* and is similar to bladder training in that the patient is encouraged to void at scheduled intervals. The voiding schedule is developed based on a voiding diary kept for 3 to 5 days to determine voiding patterns. For example, voiding frequency may be increased in the morning when the patient takes a diuretic and decreased in the afternoon and evening.

Prompted voiding. Prompted voiding is used with people who are dependent or cognitively impaired. The caregiver checks the patient for wetness at regular intervals and asks the patient to state whether they are wet or dry. The caregiver then encourages the patient to try to use the toilet. The caregiver praises the patient for trying to use the toilet and for remaining dry. This process is intended to help the patient increase their ability to recognize the signal to void, to hold urine, to maintain continence, and to ask for or accept assistance from caregivers with toileting. The voiding interval can vary between 2 and 3 hours.

Pelvic Muscle Rehabilitation

Pelvic muscle rehabilitation strengthens the pelvic muscles and includes pelvic muscle exercises with or without biofeedback, pelvic floor electrical stimulation, and vaginal weight training. Pelvic muscle exercises, commonly called *Kegel exercises,* are described in the Patient Teaching box. They actively exercise the pubococcygeus muscle, which helps to close the urethra and strengthen muscles of the pelvic floor to prevent urine leakage.

Patient Teaching

Instructions for Pelvic Muscle (Kegel) Exercises

Uncontrolled loss of urine is commonly caused by a weakness in the perineal muscles that normally control urination. Strengthening perineal muscles, which are located around the vagina and rectum, can improve urinary control. To identify the correct muscles you need to exercise, practice tightening the perineal muscles as if you were trying to control the passage of intestinal gas. To improve muscle strength and endurance, two types of exercises should be done:

- Short (2–5 seconds), firm contractions, followed by a brief period of relaxation, improves strength.
- Long (6–12 seconds) contractions, followed by relaxation for 6 to 12 seconds, improves endurance.
- Perform both exercises several times a day starting with just three to five repetitions and build up to 10 to 15 repetitions.
- Gradually work up to a total of 40 to 50 of short and long contractions each day.
- You may notice improvement in urinary control after 3 weeks; however, it may take 6 to 8 weeks before improvement is noticed.
- Continue the exercises indefinitely to maintain control.
- You can perform these exercises anywhere: at your desk, while driving, or while standing in line at the grocery store. No one will notice!

Biofeedback may be used in conjunction with other pelvic muscle exercises. Electronic or mechanical sensors are used to help the patient isolate the appropriate pelvic muscles to contract while keeping the abdominal muscles relaxed. Electrical stimulation of the muscles of the pelvic floor can also be used along with pelvic muscle exercises to provoke a pelvic muscle contraction and to increase its strength.

Vaginal weights (cones) may be used with pelvic muscle training in women. The cones are ceramic devices of various weights that are inserted into the vagina. The patient begins with the lightest cone, inserts it, and tries to retain it for up to 15 minutes twice daily. Repeated pelvic muscle contractions keep the cone in the vagina. When the lightest cone is successfully retained, the heavier cones are then used in succession. Vaginal weight training can accelerate progress of pelvic muscle rehabilitation.

Urge Suppression

Urge suppression is used to gain control of the bladder to prevent leakage. When a bladder urge is felt, the natural tendency is to rush to the bathroom to void. This action tends to make the bladder more unstable and likely to leak urine. By interrupting the bladder urge and gaining control, incontinence is prevented. The following urge suppression procedure can be used with every urge to gain control, prevent urine leakage, and delay voiding:

- When you have the strong urge to void, stop what you are doing. Sit down or stand quietly.
- Quickly tighten the pelvic floor muscles several times without resting between squeezes.
- Breathe slowly in and out while contracting the pelvic floor muscles.
- Visualize suppressing the urge to void.
- Wait until the urge passes.
- While continuing to squeeze the pelvic floor muscles, walk to the bathroom at a normal pace.

DRUG THERAPY

Drug therapy is most effective in the management of urge incontinence. Classifications of drugs most commonly used are anticholinergic and muscarinic receptor antagonist (antispasmodic) medications. Alpha-adrenergic agonists and serotonin-norepinephrine reuptake inhibitors may be helpful for stress incontinence. However, side effects of alpha-adrenergic agonists such as tachycardia and hypertension limit their use in many older adults. Postmenopausal women with urge or stress incontinence may obtain improvement using intravaginal estrogen cream or tablets. Examples of these and other types of drugs, their side effects, and nursing considerations are presented in Table 14.2. Suburethral bulking agents such as glutaraldehyde cross-linked collagen (Contigen), silicone microimplants in gel (Macroplastique), or zirconium oxide beads (Durasphere) may be injected into the tissues around the urethra. The substance adds bulk to the bladder neck, thereby increasing resistance to urine outflow. This procedure, called *periurethral bulking,* is helpful in certain situations for both men and women. The effects may last only 2 to 3 years, and patients may elect to have the procedure repeated.

Skin care is needed to prevent development of rashes and dermatitis related to moisture and urine on the skin. Barrier ointments provide a protective coating to the skin that minimizes maceration. Some ointments include antifungal medication to resist yeast infections. Cornstarch or talcum powder is not recommended because they promote the development of yeast infections between folds of skin.

URINE COLLECTION DEVICES

Indwelling Catheters

An indwelling catheter may be ordered to control urinary incontinence when all other measures have failed and skin integrity is endangered. A catheter may also be needed temporarily if urine is coming in contact with a wound. Use of indwelling catheters for the management of incontinence is not

Table 14.2 **Medications for Treating Urinary Incontinence**

DRUG	USE	ACTION	NURSING INTERVENTIONS
Cholinergic Medications			
bethanechol (Urecholine)	Overflow incontinence (atonic bladder)	Bladder contraction	Common side effects: sweating, flushing, GI distress, headache, visual disturbances Toxicity: nausea, dyspnea, irregular pulse, headache Antidote: atropine Contraindications: bladder or intestinal obstruction, asthma, hyperthyroidism, ulcer, cardiac disease, parkinsonism Works within 1 hour; ensure bedpan or toilet is accessible
Muscarinic Receptor Antagonists (Blockers)			
oxybutynin chloride (Ditropan) darifenacin (Enablex) solifenacin (VESIcare)	Urge incontinence	Bladder relaxation	Side effects: dry mouth, constipation, tachycardia, drowsiness, urinary retention, insomnia, blurred vision (less with tolterodine)
tolterodine (Detrol)		Increased bladder capacity Delayed urge to void	Administer 1 hour before meals; provide oral care; potentiates other CNS depressants
trospium (Sanctura)		Bladder relaxation	Administer 1 hour before meals on empty stomach; no CNS side effects
Serotonin-Norepinephrine Reuptake Inhibitors			
duloxetine (Cymbalta)	Stress incontinence (off-label use)	Sphincter contraction	Common side effects: dry mouth, constipation, drowsiness, dizziness, trouble sleeping, low energy, excessive sweating, loss of appetite, nausea, diarrhea
Adrenergic Receptor Blockers			
doxazosin (Cardura) terazosin (Hytrin) tamsulosin (Flomax)	Overflow incontinence	Relaxation of internal sphincter	Side effects: postural hypotension (especially in older adults), tachycardia, headache, dizziness, nasal congestion
phenoxybenzamine hydrochloride (Dibenzyline)			After the first dose, patient should lie down for 2 hours to prevent fainting; elastic stockings may help During dose adjustments, monitor blood pressure; most side effects decrease over time
Bulking Agents			
glutaraldehyde cross-linked (GAX) collagen (Contigen)	Stress incontinence	Adds bulk to sphincter to increase resistance to urine	Injected around urethra by physician Monitor voiding and assess bladder for distention
5-Alpha Reductase Inhibitors			
finasteride (Proscar)	Used to treat overflow incontinence associated with prostate enlargement	Inhibit a male hormone that is thought to cause prostate enlargement	Adverse effects include impotence, decreased libido, decreased volume of ejaculate
dutasteride (Avodart)		Shrinking the enlarged prostate allows urine to flow through the urethra more easily	Inform patients that pregnant women and women who may become pregnant should not come in contact with this drug or the semen of a man taking the drug

Continued

Table 14.2 Medications for Treating Urinary Incontinence—cont'd

DRUG	USE	ACTION	NURSING INTERVENTIONS
Beta Agonists			
mirabegron (Myrbetric)	Used to treat urge incontinence; overactive bladder	Relaxes smooth muscles in the urinary tract, increases bladder capacity	Common side effects: Headache, nose and throat irritation, dry mouth, flu-like symptoms, back pain, dizziness, joint pain, constipation, hypertension, tachycardia Regularly monitor BP and pulse. Watch for swelling of the lips, face, tongue, dyspnea

CNS, Central nervous system; *GI*, gastrointestinal.

considered appropriate. Criteria for the use of indwelling urinary catheters include acute urinary retention or bladder outlet obstruction, need for continuous bladder irrigation, accurate measurement of urinary output, intermittent decompression for neurogenic bladder, and to improve comfort for end-of-life care if needed. Inappropriate use of indwelling catheters includes their use as a substitute for nursing care of the patient with incontinence, as a means for obtaining urine for culture or other tests when the patient can voluntarily void, and for prolonged postoperative duration without an appropriate indication. Care of the patient with an indwelling catheter is discussed in Chapter 41.

External Devices

External catheters should be considered as an alternative to indwelling urethral catheters in patients without urine retention or bladder outlet obstruction. External urine collection devices are useful for men who do not have retention or bladder outlet obstruction. Latex sheaths, sometimes referred to as *condom catheters,* are secured to the penis and allow urine to drain into a bag that is secured to the leg. These devices are effective in maintaining dryness, but the adhesive may cause skin irritation on the penis. The directions for applying a condom catheter must be followed carefully. The patient and all caregivers should know not to encircle the penis with tape. To do so can restrict circulation and can lead to ischemia and injury. Elastic tape should be used and wrapped in a spiral pattern. External adhesive urine collection devices are available for women to use while lying in bed or seated in a chair. These devices are adhered to the perineum like an ostomy bag; thus skin shaving and preparation is needed. An external urinary catheter is also available that uses a flexible, contoured catheter that is positioned at the urethra and connected to a vacuum device that wicks away urine.

Intermittent Self-Catheterization

Intermittent catheterization is a preferred alternative to urethral catheterization because it is associated with lower risk of urinary tract infection. Some patients are quite successful at using intermittent self-catheterization, but its use requires dexterity, adequate vision, and the ability and motivation to learn. Clean, aseptic technique rather than a sterile technique is taught in the home setting. Initially, the bladder is drained every 4 hours. Urine production may vary throughout the day; therefore catheterization schedules may vary. For example, if more than 500 mL of urine is obtained, the time interval is shortened, and if less than 200 mL is obtained, the time interval is extended. Individual schedules can be adjusted to accommodate this variation. Hand hygiene, prevention of constipation, and adequate fluid intake are important to prevent urinary tract infection.

GARMENTS AND PADS FOR INCONTINENCE

A variety of incontinence products are available that help to absorb urine and maintain dryness and ensure social continence, or the preservation of dignity and ability to remain socially engaged without embarrassment as a result of visible urine leakage or odor. A wide variety of disposable and reusable briefs, pull-ups, inserts, and pads are readily available in pharmacies and grocery stores. Bladder control products are designed to absorb urine faster and wick it away from the skin, with a fabric-type layer that stays dry to minimize moisture on the skin and maceration. Full incontinent briefs are more suitable for individuals with more limited mobility who spend most of the time in the bed or chair and have moderate to large volumes of urine loss, whereas pull-up-type briefs may be preferred by persons with this amount of leakage who are ambulatory. Women and men may be conscious of the bulkiness of incontinence briefs and pads; however, there are pad and brief designs that are nonbulky and absorbent. Incontinence pads that are designed like menstrual pads and fit inside the undergarment may be used for mild to moderate leakage. Menstrual pads are used by some women because they are less expensive, but their absorptive ability is poor for moderate leakage, and skin irritations can develop if not changed

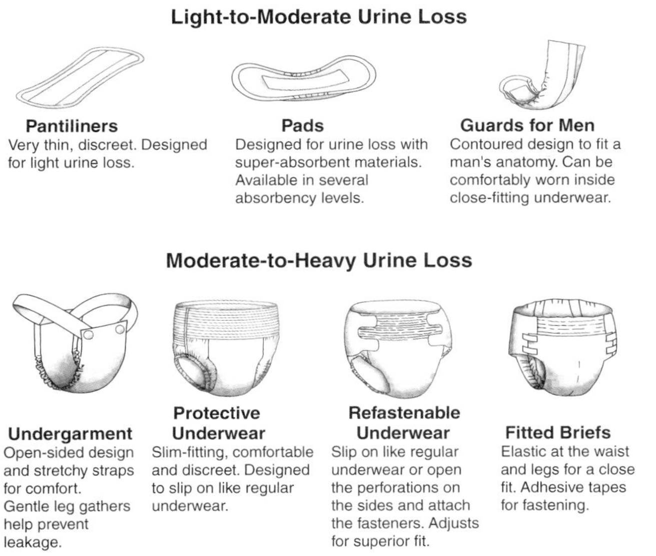

Fig. 14.2 Types of absorbent products for light/moderate and moderate/heavy urine loss. (Modified from Newman DK: *Managing and treating urinary infection,* Baltimore, MD, 2002, Health Professions Press.)

often enough. Feminine mini-pads may be helpful for women with small volume leakage. Men with urinary dribbling may find that absorbent pouches designed like a condom and adhere to undergarments are discrete and do not add bulkiness to clothing. Fig. 14.2 illustrates different types of products for light/moderate and moderate/heavy urine loss.

Social stigma about incontinence products may discourage their use based on the belief that using these products encourages patients to void in their clothing. Incontinence products may give a person the confidence to be socially active without the risk of having an embarrassing accident. When trying to restore control, use briefs that can be removed easily for toileting. For patients who are unlikely to ever be continent, these products are an acceptable management tool.

For the immobile patient, an absorbent pad with a waterproof backing may be used instead of briefs. These pads can also be placed under the buttocks of a bedridden patient who wears briefs in case leakage occurs. One factor to remember is that multiple layers of padding interfere with special beds or mattresses designed to prevent pressure injuries. Some paper pads stick to the skin and become lumpy when wet; thus they should be checked frequently for wetness and immediately changed. Never place the patient directly on a plastic surface; doing so keeps the skin wet from perspiration and urine.

PENILE COMPRESSION DEVICE

The penile compression (penile clamp) is a device that is applied to the penis to compress the urethra and prevent the passage of urine. A small amount of leakage may persist, requiring a pad to protect the clothing. To prevent neurologic and circulatory impairment and pressure injuries, the clamp must be removed and repositioned frequently. Use of the penile clamp is controversial because it can cause injury if not used correctly. The patient must be mentally and physically capable of managing the device.

PELVIC ORGAN SUPPORT DEVICES

A pessary is a device similar to a diaphragm that is inserted into the vagina that lifts and holds the pelvic organs in place. It may be used to treat stress incontinence in women with relaxation and prolapse of the pelvic structures. Once placed, the patient must be reexamined within 24 hours to ensure proper placement and to rule out urinary obstruction. The device must then be removed periodically for cleansing and replacement. Document that the patient has a pessary to ensure that it will not be forgotten.

For women with stress incontinence, a bladder neck support prosthesis may be helpful. When the silastic device is fitted into the vagina, it supports the area where the urethra connects to the bladder, thereby reducing the incidence of involuntary urine loss. Another device used to prevent leakage is the urethral insert, a small plastic device that creates a mechanical barrier to urine loss.

SURGICAL TREATMENT

Surgical intervention may be recommended to address underlying conditions that cause urinary incontinence. Specific surgical procedures may be performed to remove obstructions, treat severe bladder overactivity, implant an artificial sphincter, reposition the sphincter unit, improve perineal support, and inject substances that increase urethral compression (suburethral bulking agents). Electrostimulation is the use of electrodes that stimulate the pelvic floor muscles. Electrodes can be surgically implanted in the vagina or rectum. Retropubic urethropexies and pubovaginal slings are surgical procedures most often used for stress urinary incontinence in women. A sling procedure for men creates a support system for the urethra so that it does not open inappropriately. Nursing care of the patient undergoing surgery on the urinary tract is described in Chapter 42.

The artificial sphincter (Fig. 14.3) consists of an inflatable cuff, a reservoir of fluid that fills the cuff, and a pump. The cuff is positioned around the urethra or bladder neck. The reservoir is placed in the abdomen and the pump is positioned in the scrotum or labia. Fluid fills the cuff, applying pressure to the urethra to prevent urine passage. To void, the patient squeezes the pump, which deflates the cuff by transferring fluid from the cuff to the reservoir and allowing urine to pass through the urethra. After voiding, the cuff is then reinflated.

TYPES OF URINARY INCONTINENCE

Incontinence is classified as either transient (acute) or established and persistent. **Transient incontinence**

Table 14.3 Types of Urinary Incontinence

TYPE	DESCRIPTION	CAUSES	NURSING CARE	TREATMENTS
Urge	Loss of urine that usually follows a strong desire to void	Nervous system disorder Urinary tract infection Bladder obstruction	Schedule toileting Limit fluids 2 hours before bedtime Administer drugs as ordered to control bladder contractions (see Table 14.2) Keep incontinence record	Behavior modification Drug therapy: anticholinergics Surgical procedures to increase bladder capacity or to decrease bladder contractions
Overflow	Loss of urine associated with a full bladder Frequent voiding Volume usually small Reflex incontinence: loss of urine as a result of reflexive contraction	Urethral obstruction Disorders of bladder, nerves, or muscles Spinal cord injury Post anesthesia Spinal cord injury Radiation cystitis	Catheterize as ordered; teach self-catheterization as appropriate Administer drugs as ordered to stimulate the bladder and to relax the internal sphincter (see Table 14.2) Cutaneous triggers; teach stimulation techniques	Surgery to relieve obstruction Drug therapy to stimulate the bladder and to relax the sphincter Catheterize as necessary
Stress	Loss of urine during physical exertion	Relaxation of pelvic floor muscles Urethral trauma Sphincter injury	Teach Kegel exercises Advise patient to void frequently Administer drugs as ordered to stimulate the sphincter (see Table 14.2)	Surgical correction Bladder suspension Artificial sphincter Drug therapy to improve sphincter contraction
Functional	Bladder functions normally but patient voids inappropriately	Dementia Head injury Cerebrovascular accident (stroke)	Schedule toileting Reinforce appropriate behavior Remove environmental barriers	

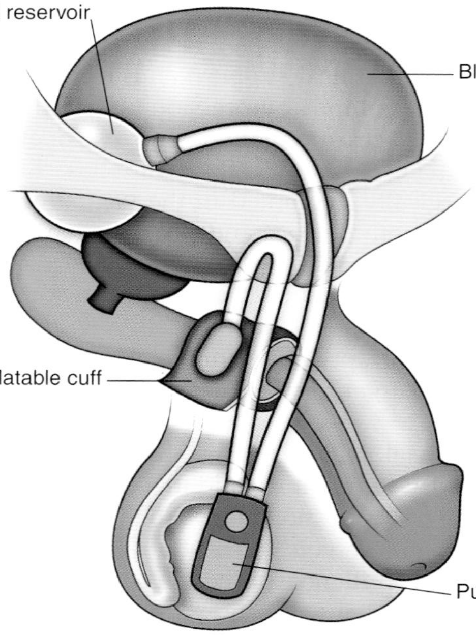

Fig. 14.3 An artificial urinary sphincter in place. (From Wein AJ, Kavoussi L, Partin A, Peters C: *Campbell-Walsh urology*, ed 11, Philadelphia, 2016, Elsevier.)

typically has a sudden or more recent onset and is associated with treatable factors that can be remembered by the acronym DRIP (Box 14.2).

Established **(persistent) incontinence** is determined after reversible causes of incontinence have been addressed and is categorized into the following types: (1) stress urinary incontinence (UI), (2) urge UI, (3) overflow UI, (4) mixed UI (stress and urge), and (5) functional UI. Table 14.3 describes the defining characteristics of the types of urinary incontinence.

Box 14.2 DRIP

D: Delirium, dehydration
R: Restricted mobility
I: Infection, impaction
P: Polyuria, polypharmacy, pain

STRESS INCONTINENCE

Description

Stress incontinence is the involuntary loss of small amounts of urine during physical activity that increases abdominal pressure. Coughing, laughing, sneezing, and lifting are examples of activities that often result in urine loss. In women, stress incontinence is usually caused by a relaxation of the pelvic floor muscles and the ureterovesical junction as a result of pregnancy, childbirth, obesity, and aging. Urethral trauma, sphincter injury, congenital sphincter weakness, urinary infection, neurologic disorders, and stress can cause stress incontinence in men and women. It may

Nursing Care Plan Patient With Stress Urinary Incontinence

FOCUSED ASSESSMENT

Health History

Mrs. Seigel is an 85-year-old resident in a long-term care facility. She complains of having trouble "holding my urine." She is unable to control urination if she strains, coughs, or laughs. She is the mother of five children, all born at home. She reports no other physical complaints except for arthritis in her hips and knees, and hypertension. Her medications are acetaminophen, 325 mg, three times daily, and hydrochlorothiazide, 25 mg daily. Fear of losing control of her urine has caused her to avoid leaving her room except for meals. She is wearing perineal pads to keep her clothing dry.

Physical Examination Vital signs: blood pressure 130/86 mm Hg, pulse 72 beats per minute, respiration 16 breaths per minute, temperature 98°F (36.67°C) orally. Height 5′3″, weight 179 lb. Heart and breath sounds are normal. Abdomen is rounded and soft. No bladder distention is noted. Faint urine odor is present. Rises with some difficulty. Walks slowly with walker. Has limited range of motion in the knees and hips.

Patient Problems	Goals and Outcome Criteria	Interventions
Stress urinary incontinence related to weak pelvic muscles and high intraabdominal pressure	Improved urinary control: patient will report fewer incidents of stress incontinence.	Explain to the patient how weak perineal muscles cause stress incontinence. Instruct her how to do Kegel perineal exercises (see *Patient Teaching* box). Advise the patient to empty her bladder every 2 hours while awake. Encourage the intake of normal amounts of fluid but discourage liquids with diuretic effects (e.g., coffee, tea, alcohol). Explain that obesity increases intraabdominal pressure and contributes to stress incontinence. Explore her interest in weight loss and refer her to a dietitian.
Potential for disrupted skin integrity related to prolonged contact of urine with skin	Reduced potential for disrupted skin integrity: skin is kept clean and dry; remains intact and free of excessive redness.	Inspect the perineal area and buttocks and report signs of irritation (e.g., redness, breaks in the skin). Apply skin protectants as ordered or per agency protocol. Teach the patient the importance of good perineal care to remove urine from the skin. Encourage her to cleanse the area with mild soap, rinse, and gently dry twice daily. Perineal pads or other incontinence pads should be changed promptly if they are wet.
Decreased socialization related to fear of embarrassment as a result of incontinence	Increase social interaction: patient resumes usual social activities.	Identify activities that the patient would like to resume. Discuss strategies to decrease embarrassment about incontinent episodes: (1) empty bladder before leaving room; (2) wear perineal pads or special incontinence pads to absorb urine and protect clothing and furniture. Avoid any comments that could humiliate the patient, such as references to "diapers." Avoid discussing her problem in front of others.

CRITICAL THINKING QUESTIONS

1. What are the possible contributing factors to stress incontinence in this resident?
2. How would you teach the resident the importance of perineal care?

occur after prostatectomy or radiation therapy. Cough caused by smoking or chronic bronchitis and other respiratory conditions contribute to weakening of pelvic floor muscles and urine leakage. Straining to have a bowel movement also weakens the pelvic muscles.

Management

First-line treatment of stress incontinence are behavioral methods such as toileting programs (including scheduled voiding and bladder training) and pelvic muscle exercises (see the Nursing Care Plan: Patient With Stress Urinary Incontinence). Topical estrogen may be given to improve vaginal dryness and urethral irritation in postmenopausal women. Surgical interventions include retropubic urethropexies, pubovaginal slings, and collagen injections.

URGE INCONTINENCE

Description

Urge incontinence is the involuntary loss of urine associated with a strong, sudden urge to void. It most often results from an overactive detrusor (bladder) muscle. Urge incontinence is associated with ingestion of caffeinated products such as coffee and tea, urinary tract infection, fecal impaction, dehydration, neurologic disorders such as stroke, Parkinson disease, multiple sclerosis, and spinal cord lesions; however, the cause cannot always be identified. **Overactive bladder** is the most common cause of incontinence in older adults. Use of tobacco products is associated with urge incontinence because the tobacco by-products that are metabolized and excreted in the urine are irritating to the bladder.

Management

Treatment of urge incontinence is aimed at correcting the cause and includes fluid hydration, caffeine elimination, smoking cessation, antibiotics for infection, and removal of fecal impaction. Behavioral techniques such as toileting programs, pelvic muscle exercises, and urge inhibition, drug therapy, or surgical intervention may be used. Anticholinergic and muscarinic antagonists (antispasmodics) are the medications most commonly used for urge incontinence. Anticholinergic drugs may cause confusion and agitation that might be mistaken for dementia in the older patient. They should be used with caution and the patient should be evaluated for side effects. (Frequently prescribed drugs include oxybutynin [Oxytrol, Ditropan], tolterodine [Detrol], darifenacin [Enablex], trospium [Sanctura], and solifenacin [VESIcare]). Botulinum toxin injected into the detrusor may improve symptoms for as long as 9 months. If behavioral techniques and medications do not work, surgical procedures may be recommended. Sacral neuromodulation involves the implantation of a nerve stimulator to improve nerve function in the pelvic floor.

MIXED INCONTINENCE

Description

Mixed incontinence indicates the co-occurrence of stress and urge incontinence. With aging, the prevalence of mixed incontinence increases in women. Management includes interventions previously identified for these conditions.

OVERFLOW INCONTINENCE

Description

Overflow incontinence is the involuntary loss of urine associated with an overdistended bladder. Small amounts of urine are expelled from the overfilled bladder, especially during episodes of increased intraabdominal pressure such as with movement or coughing. The overfilled bladder also leads to increased pressure within the bladder, which may cause backflow of urine from the bladder into the ureters and kidneys and lead to hydronephrosis, damage to the nephrons, and kidney injury. Patients who have normal sensation usually feel uncomfortable because of bladder distention. Factors that contribute to overflow incontinence are urethral obstruction caused by an enlarged prostate in men or cystocele in women, an underactive bladder muscle caused by neurologic conditions, or medications with anticholinergic effects. Patients who have undergone anesthesia are also at risk for urine retention and overflow incontinence because of the effects of anesthesia and other medications on the bladder.

These patients are not aware of bladder fullness and the bladder becomes overdistended. Urinary retention with overflow is also common after general anesthesia, childbirth or after the removal of an indwelling catheter. Medications that may cause urinary retention include anticholinergics, antihistamines, epinephrine, calcium-channel blockers, and theophylline (Table 14.4). **Neurogenic bladder** is bladder dysfunction caused by neurologic dysfunction associated with a spinal cord injury, pelvic radiation, or surgery.

Management

The medical treatment of overflow incontinence depends on the cause. A common reason for urethral obstruction in men is prostate enlargement. Surgical removal of all or part of the prostate gland often restores normal emptying of the bladder. Other management options include sphincterotomy, in which an incision is made in the sphincter, and sacral neuromodulation.

Table 14.4 Medications That Cause Urinary Retention or Incontinence

CLASS	EXAMPLE
Urinary Retention	
Anticholinergics	atropine sulfate
Antihistamines	diphenhydramine hydrochloride (Benadryl)
Alpha-adrenergic agonists	epinephrine hydrochloride (Adrenalin)
Xanthine	theophylline (Theo-Dur)
Incontinence	
Alpha-adrenergic blockers	prazosin hydrochloride (Minipress)
Anticholinergics	atropine sulfate
Antihistamines	diphenhydramine hydrochloride (Benadryl)
Antiparkinsonian drugs	levodopa (Dopa), trihexyphenidyl hydrochloride (Artane)
Antipsychotics	chlorpromazine (Thorazine)
High ceiling diuretics	furosemide (Lasix)
Opiate agonists	morphine sulfate (Epimorph)
Sedatives or hypnotics	phenobarbital sodium (Luminal Sodium), diazepam (Valium)
Sympathomimetics	phenylephrine hydrochloride (Neo-Synephrine), isoproterenol hydrochloride (Isuprel)

In some cases, intermittent or indwelling catheterization is necessary. For the neurogenic bladder, drugs to stimulate the bladder (e.g., bethanechol chloride [Urecholine]) and relax the internal sphincter (e.g., prazosin hydrochloride [Minipress]) may be ordered. Postoperative and postpartum patients may require short-term intermittent catheterization before normal bladder function returns. The indwelling catheter is considered the measure of last resort in the management of overflow incontinence. Self-catheterization using clean technique may be taught to patients who are able to perform it in the home setting. Intermittent self-catheterization is preferred over indwelling urethral catheterization as this technique is associated with lower risk for urinary tract infection.

Another technique that may be used to empty the bladder is the **Credé method**, which involves using the open hand to gently press on the abdomen over the bladder to promote urine passage. Ask the physician about the safety of this procedure for individual patients. These techniques and others are described more fully in rehabilitation texts.

For patients who have incontinence because of neurologic conditions, bladder drainage must be maintained! Bladder overdistention may trigger a serious reaction called *autonomic dysreflexia,* in which the blood pressure rises to life-threatening levels. This can be prevented by emptying the bladder often enough to prevent overdistention. Monitoring for urine retention can be done using bladder diaries recording urine output, portable bladder ultrasound, and straight urethral catheterization. Another technique that may be used to stimulate bladder emptying is the cutaneous triggering method, which involves tapping the suprapubic area and stroking the inner thigh. Other techniques are more fully described in texts on rehabilitation. The Credé method is not used for these patients. Chapter 24 discusses in detail the care of the patient with spinal cord injury.

FUNCTIONAL INCONTINENCE

Description

Functional incontinence is the term used when a person is incontinent because of an inability to get to the toilet as a result of physical or cognitive impairments, the inability to manage the mechanics of toileting, or environmental barriers.

Management

The treatment of functional incontinence depends on the cause. Arrange the environment to permit independent toileting and provide assistive devices that enable the immobile patient to void appropriately. The use of assistive devices to facilitate getting to the toilet such as a wheelchair or walker, the use of a toilet substitute such as a bedside commode or urinal, or measures to increase safety when using the toilet such as grab bars and a raised toilet seat may be especially useful. The confused patient may respond well to scheduled or timed voiding and periodic orientation to toilet facilities. In all care contexts, promoting the attitude that incontinence usually can be improved or effectively managed to promote dignity and socialization without embarrassment, even in physically and cognitively impaired patients is an important role of the nurse.

NURSING CARE OF THE PATIENT WITH URINARY INCONTINENCE

FOCUSED ASSESSMENT

The presence of urinary incontinence is determined based on the history, physical examination, and various diagnostic tests and procedures.

Reason for Seeking Care

Determine the patient's concerns about incontinence and the impact on functioning.

Present Health

Determine the pattern of incontinent voiding, urine volume, any related symptoms and psychosocial impact.

Pattern. Ask the patient how often incontinent episodes occur and whether they are associated with particular activities, such as sneezing or laughing, or coughing. A voiding diary is a helpful tool in identifying the pattern of urinary incontinence. Many patients are able to keep their own diaries. If the patient is unable to maintain an accurate record, a caregiver must do so for the patient.

Bladder (voiding) diary
- Record for 3 to 5 days voiding and incontinent episodes, if urge present, fluids, activity
- Absorbent pad or brief count and weight, total per day

Fluid intake pattern
- Usual fluid intake over 24 hours
- Types and volume of fluid consumed, including caffeinated and alcoholic beverages

Bowel pattern
- Timing, frequency, amount, consistency, odor, straining
- Use of laxatives or other aids

Volume. If a patient is incontinent, measurements of urine can only be estimated, but the patient can probably describe the amount voided as being large, moderate, or small. If pads or briefs are used, record the number used and the degree of saturation. Weighing wet pads and subtracting the dry weight of the pad is more precise but not very practical in the home setting. When the patient resides in a long-term care facility or hospital, measure and record the amount of urine passed with continent voiding as well. Note if the urine is strong-smelling as this can be an indication of dehydration and urinary tract infection.

Box 14.3 Screening Questions for Patients With Incontinence

- "During the past 12 months, have you leaked or lost control of even a small amount of urine with activity like coughing, lifting, or exercise?"
- "During the past 12 months, have you leaked or lost control of even a small amount of urine with an urge or pressure to urinate, and you could not get to the toilet fast enough?"
- "During the past 12 months, have you leaked or lost control of even a small amount of urine during nonphysical activities?"
- "Do you ever use pads, tissue, or cloth in your underwear to catch urine/water?"
- "If you have leaked urine, how much does it bother you?"
- "Do you ever have pain or burning with urination?"
- "Is it hard for you to begin voiding or to complete emptying of the bladder?"

Related symptoms. Ask whether the patient has had dysuria (painful voiding or burning with voiding) or pain in the suprapubic area (the lower abdomen where the bladder is located). Urinary obstruction because of enlarged prostate gland in men or cystocele in women is associated with obstructive voiding symptoms that include hesitancy or difficulty starting the urine stream, straining to void, intermittent stream, prolonged time needed to empty bladder, the sensation of incomplete bladder emptying, and postvoid dribbling.

To assess the degree and severity of the problem, specific screening questions are useful for accurately describing the problem of incontinence (Box 14.3).

Past Health History

Past problems that might be related to incontinence include urologic, gynecologic, neurologic, and endocrine conditions. Specifically ask whether the patient has diabetes mellitus. People who have diabetes may develop neurologic problems that affect the bladder. In addition, a person with poorly controlled diabetes may produce large volumes of urine that quickly fill the bladder.

Document all abdominal disorders, surgeries, and trauma. Record the number of pregnancies and types of deliveries, episiotomy, and heavy infants' birthweight. Inquire about current and recent medications because many drugs can affect kidney or bladder function. Drugs that might contribute to urinary incontinence are diuretics, major tranquilizers, antihistamines, decongestants, some sedatives or hypnotics, and antiparkinsonian drugs. Anticholinergics, which are used to treat some types of incontinence, may cause overflow incontinence in persons with neurologic conditions that result in poor bladder contractility or in persons with urinary outflow obstruction such as prostatic enlargement in men and cystocele in women. Other drugs that can disrupt normal voiding are epinephrine, theophylline, isoproterenol, and prazosin.

Pharmacology Capsule

When urinary incontinence is of recent onset, check the patient's drug profile for drugs known to contribute to incontinence.

Review of Systems

The review of systems may offer clues by identifying conditions that contribute to incontinence. For example, the patient with severe arthritis in the hands or severely impaired vision may have difficulty managing toileting independently. Constipation is a common problem that can contribute to incontinence.

Measure vital signs, height, and weight. Be alert for fever, tachycardia, edema, and weight gain. Note the patient's level of awareness and appropriateness of responses.

Sometimes incontinence is first recognized when an odor of urine is detected during the examination or when providing care. Palpate the abdomen for masses, tenderness, fullness, or distention. A distended bladder or abdominal distention associated with constipation is an important finding. A health care provider performs a pelvic examination on the female patient to assess for prolapse of pelvic organs, to evaluate perineal muscle tone, and to examine the skin for abnormalities, irritation, or infection. A rectal examination is performed to determine sensation, sphincter tone, presence of fecal impaction, and ability to voluntarily contract the pelvic muscles. In male patients, the prostate is palpated for size, contour, and consistency.

Functional Assessment

A description of the patient's usual activities and habits provides clues about possible contributing factors and about the effect of incontinence on the individual. Assess time to ambulate to the toilet, ability to manage clothing and hygiene, and ability to hold urine once the urge is felt. In addition, the environment must be assessed, including toilet accessibility, grab bars, lighting, and availability of toileting options (e.g., urinals, commode chairs).

Assessment of the patient with urinary incontinence is outlined in Box 14.4.

Patient Problems, Goals, and Outcome Criteria: Urinary Incontinence

Patient problems and goals for the patient with urinary incontinence may include the following.

Patient Problems	Goals and Outcome Criteria
Altered urinary elimination related to inadequate knowledge of causes of urinary incontinence and corrective measures	Patient accurately describes and participates in the treatment plan

Patient Problems, Goals, and Outcome Criteria: Urinary Incontinence—cont'd

Patient Problems	Goals and Outcome Criteria
Functional urinary incontinence related to physical, cognitive, or environmental barriers	Fewer episodes of functional urinary incontinence
Overflow urinary incontinence related to obstruction or neurologic impairment accomplished with minimal involuntary leakage	Fewer episodes of involuntary urinary leakage
Stress urinary incontinence related to weak pelvic structures, increased intraabdominal pressure	Improved control of urine flow: fewer episodes of involuntary voiding when under stress
Urge urinary incontinence related to decreased bladder capacity or bladder spasms	Ability to hold increasing volume of urine: time between voiding increases without leakage
Decreased socialization related to fear of embarrassment	Decreased social isolation: patient participates in usual social activities
Altered self-concept related to inability to control voiding	Improved self-concept: patient demonstrates positive self-image (confidence, pride in appearance)
Potential for disrupted skin tissue integrity related to the presence of urine on the skin	Reduced potential for skin breakdown: skin kept clean, dry, and free of urine or feces
Potential for infection related to chronic bladder distention or catheterization	Absence of urinary tract infection: normal body temperature and white blood cell count

INTERVENTIONS

Nursing interventions for various types of incontinence may overlap. Thus interventions are discussed in general terms here.

General Strategies for Bladder Health Promotion

Promoting healthy bladder habits can improve quality of life and function and reduce the risk for urinary incontinence and urinary tract infection. Tips for bladder health promotion are found in Box 14.5.

Altered Urinary Elimination

Patient and caregiver education are key elements in the management of urinary incontinence. Do not assume that improvement is not possible, even in frail older adults. In fact, improvement or restoration of continence is possible for most people. Sometimes the incontinent patient is very discouraged and reluctant to try retraining techniques. Thus remain positive, encourage the person to take small steps, and praise the patient's attempts and successes.

Box 14.4 Focused Assessment of Patients With Urinary Incontinence

HEALTH HISTORY

Reason for Seeking Care

Concern about incontinence and its impact

Present Health

Pattern of continent and incontinent voiding behaviors or activities associated with incontinence; amount of urine passed with continent and incontinent voiding; awareness of need to void; ability to hold urine once urge to void, dysuria

Symptoms: urgency/frequency/nocturia, obstructive voiding symptoms: hesitancy or difficulty starting the urine stream, straining to void, intermittent stream, prolonged time needed to empty bladder, the sensation of incomplete bladder emptying, and postvoid dribbling

Urinary incontinence symptom profile: when incontinence started and severity; how managed, what makes it better or worse

Past Health History

Urologic, gynecologic, neurologic, urologic, and endocrine problems; abdominal, urologic, and gynecologic surgery; trauma; mental status and dementia; stroke, paralysis

Review of Systems

Constipation or motor or sensory dysfunction that could affect continence

Functional Assessment

Ability to transfer, manual dexterity for clothing

Reach and use the toilet

Orientation and ability for self-care, hygiene

Physical Examination

Height, Weight, and Body Mass Index: Weight gain

Vital Signs: Fever, tachycardia

Level of Consciousness: Orientation

Abdomen: Masses, tenderness, fullness, distension

Male Genitalia: Abnormalities of foreskin, glans penis, perineal skin

Female Genitalia: Redness, irritation

Rectum: Sensation, sphincter tone, fecal impaction

Box 14.5 Bladder Health Promotion

- Void before and after meals and at bedtime
- Aim to drink 6 to 8 glasses of water a day
- Get regular physical exercise
- Practice pelvic muscle exercises daily
- Practice urge suppression to control urine when a toilet is not available
- Avoid caffeinated beverages if urgency and urinary frequency develop
- Maintain ideal body weight and avoid obesity
- Ensure bowel regularity and avoid constipation

The teaching plan should explain how the bladder works, the type of incontinence the patient is experiencing, and the recommended treatment. Supplement verbal information with written material and inform the patient that improvement takes time and to not expect immediate results. Praise the patient's participation in the treatment plan and interest in working toward continence.

Decreased Socialization

The person with urinary incontinence may curtail social activities out of fear of having embarrassing accidents. In addition, access to toilets in public places is often limited, so patients who cannot delay voiding may be afraid to venture far from home. If continence is unlikely or not yet established, a variety of incontinence products are available that may permit the patient to venture out without fear of wetness or odor. Specially designed pads and undergarments as well as some external urine collection devices may be used. As mentioned earlier, effective external collection devices for men are readily available. The patient can also be encouraged to maintain the voiding schedule during the social outing. If the patient has an incontinent episode, those responsible for their care should be careful not to show disapproval.

Altered Self-Concept

The ability to control elimination is an important childhood accomplishment. Adults who become incontinent may be so embarrassed that they are reluctant to tell anyone about it. Nurses often discover that a newly admitted patient has concealed incontinence from family and physicians. Some older people do not seek help for incontinence because they think it is caused by old age and cannot be corrected.

You can help patients learn to manage incontinence and see that it is not a barrier to achieving a full life. Your attitude toward the patient and toward incontinence influences how the patient deals with the change in body function. Caregivers must be committed to efforts to help patients avoid incontinence. The following situation should not be allowed to happen:

A stroke patient in a long-term care facility calls out, "I need to go to the bathroom!"

A busy nursing staff member rushes by, pats the patient on the hand, and says, "That's all right. You have a diaper on. Go ahead and pee."

Encourage patients to attend to dress and grooming to promote a more positive self-image. The patient who takes an active role in carrying out the treatment plan may feel less helpless and better able to cope with incontinence. Advise caregivers not to refer to incontinence pads and undergarments as *diapers* because this term is demeaning as it is associated with infants.

Potential for Disrupted Skin Integrity

A major problem for the incontinent patient is the risk of skin breakdown. Urine and feces, if left in contact with the skin, may contribute to development of a rash or yeast infection, especially in persons with diabetes mellitus. Continuous moisture causes the skin to lose its oily protective barrier, and skin breakdown may follow. The key to preventing breakdown is to keep the skin clean, dry, and free of urine or feces and protected with a barrier ointment. If a patient is incontinent and unable to report voiding, check hourly for wetness. Remove wet garments and linens immediately and wash the patient's skin with mild soap and warm water, rinse, and gently pat dry. Inspect the genitals, perineum, thighs, and buttocks for redness and skin breakdown. In addition, apply a protective ointment as ordered or according to agency policy. If skin breakdown does occur, notify the registered nurse or physician and provide treatment as ordered or according to agency policy.

Potential for Infection

The patient who is incontinent of urine is at risk for urinary tract infection and urinary calculi (bladder or kidney stones). These complications are most likely to occur in patients with urine retention and in those who restrict their fluids. Retained urine is a good medium for bacterial growth and the overstretched bladder wall is susceptible to bacterial colonization and infection. Patients may restrict fluid intake to try to reduce the frequency of incontinence. However, concentrated urine is a risk factor for infections and calculi. Patients with indwelling catheters are at increased risk for urinary tract infections.

To reduce the risk of urinary tract infection, encourage the patient to empty the bladder as scheduled, provide adequate fluids, and use strict aseptic techniques during catheterization. Keep the perineal area clean and encourage an intake of 1500 to 3000 mL of fluid per day unless contraindicated. Details of catheter care are covered in Chapter 42.

Put On Your Thinking Cap!

Four of the patients you have cared for in the past week have had diagnoses of "urinary incontinence."

- Mrs. A., 55 years of age, was admitted for treatment of her asthma. She has five adult children and often babysits for two toddlers. She says that she loses a small amount of urine when she coughs or picks up a toddler.
- Mr. B., 72 years of age, had a prostatectomy 2 weeks ago. His catheter has been removed but he was readmitted with a urinary tract infection. He complains of constant dribbling of urine that requires him to wear incontinence pads.
- Mrs. C., 25 years of age, had an appendectomy. The day after the procedure, she voided 25 to 60 mL of urine at frequent intervals for a total of 200 mL over 12 hours. Her bladder was distended, and she complained of a feeling of fullness and constant urge to void.
- Mr. D., 85 years of age, was admitted with pneumonia. He has a diagnosis of moderate dementia. On two occasions, he was found out of bed and urine was found on the floor. On another occasion, he urinated in the wastebasket.

Decide which type of incontinence each patient probably had and fill in the subsequent chart with the probable cause or causes for the specific patient, the recommended treatment, and the appropriate nursing interventions for each patient related to incontinence.

PATIENT	TYPE OF INCONTINENCE	PROBABLE CAUSE	TREATMENT	NURSING CARE
Mrs. A.				
Mr. B.				
Mrs. C.				
Mr. D.				

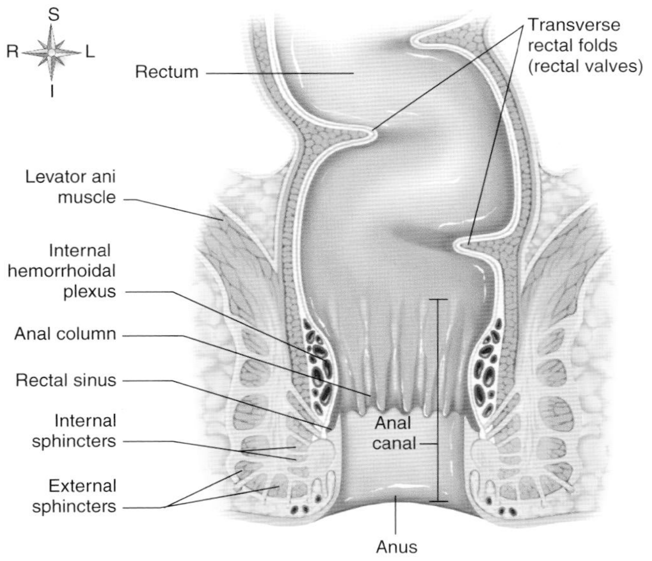

Fig. 14.4 The anal sphincters and musculature. (From Patton K, Thibodeau G: *Anatomy & physiology*, ed 8, St. Louis, 2013, Mosby.)

BOWEL (FECAL) INCONTINENCE

Bowel incontinence (fecal incontinence) is less common than urinary incontinence, but it can be very distressing for patients who are affected by it. It is believed to affect 20% of community-dwelling older persons and 50% of long-term care residents. Bowel incontinence is usually related to anal sphincter dysfunction caused by anal surgery, trauma during childbirth, Crohn disease affecting the anus, diabetic neuropathy, and laxatives. Some patients experience temporary incontinence with sudden onset of severe diarrhea and the inability to reach the toilet in time. Incontinent diarrhea may also be present with fecal impaction. Diminished muscle strength associated with aging may also be a factor. Liquid stool is more difficult to manage, and a goal of treatment is to normalize stool consistency.

PHYSIOLOGIC PROCESS OF DEFECATION

The structures that maintain bowel control are the internal and external sphincters and the puborectal muscle. The muscles of the pelvic floor and the external sphincter are under voluntary control (Fig. 14.4). The bowel has its own nerve network that stimulates peristalsis when distended. Thus disorders of the central nervous system and spinal cord do not impair bowel control as much as they do bladder control.

The fecal mass enters the rectum by mass movement. The presence of feces in the rectum creates a desire to defecate. Defecation occurs when the anal sphincter relaxes and the rectum contracts. Tightening of the diaphragm and abdominal muscles promotes defecation by increasing pressure in the abdomen. If defecation does not occur soon after this pressure is felt, the sensation of needing to defecate soon fades. People who often ignore or delay defecation tend to become constipated.

DIAGNOSTIC TESTS AND PROCEDURES

Evaluation of fecal incontinence may include assessment of rectal sphincter tone, laboratory examination of a stool specimen for blood or pathogens, and endoscopic or radiologic procedures to detect underlying problems. Diagnostic tests and procedures for the lower gastrointestinal system are presented in detail in Chapter 37.

COMMON THERAPEUTIC MEASURES

ENEMAS

Enemas may be necessary to stimulate emptying of the bowel in the patient with fecal impaction. Removing retained stool is imperative before starting a bowel program that includes increased fiber and fluids. In general, frequent use of large-volume enemas is not advised because it overstretches the bowel and may contribute to loss of muscle tone. A patient with poor anal sphincter tone may have difficulty retaining enema solutions. An adapter can be placed on the enema tubing and inserted into the anus. The nipple-like adapter helps the patient to retain the solution.

RECTAL TUBES AND POUCHES

Rectal tubes with containment bags can be inserted to collect loose stools and protect the skin. Similarly, plastic pouches, much like ostomy bags, may be applied to the perianal area and held in place with adhesive. They are helpful for patients who have frequent stools because the digestive enzymes, bacteria, and other waste products in the feces are highly irritating to the skin and can very quickly lead to skin breakdown. Because they are bulky and uncomfortable, pouches are not practical for ambulatory patients. Another disadvantage is the skin irritation caused by the adhesive. When the pouch is changed, provide meticulous skin care. An alternative to the pouch is an adult incontinent brief or (for bed patients) linen protectors. Application of a barrier ointment for skin protection is crucial.

DRUG THERAPY

Types of drugs used to prevent or treat fecal incontinence because of fecal impaction include laxatives and stool softeners. Antidiarrheal drugs may be used for loose stools, depending on the cause of the incontinence. For patients with *Clostridium difficile*, antidiarrheal medications are contraindicated. These drugs are discussed in Chapter 39.

Put On Your Thinking Cap!

When would a patient with fecal incontinence need laxatives?

What is a primary concern regarding the patient with diarrhea and fecal incontinence?

Table 14.5 Types of Bowel Incontinence

TYPE	DESCRIPTION	CAUSES	NURSING CARE
Overflow	Uncontrolled, frequent passage of small, semisoft stools Fecal impaction may be present	Constipation in which entire colon is full of fecal matter	Administer laxatives and enemas as ordered. Increase fluids and fiber as appropriate.
Anorectal	Uncontrolled passage of stool several times a day	Weak pelvic muscles Loss of anal reflexes Poor rectal sphincter tone Rectal prolapse	Teach Kegel exercises. Prepare for surgery, if planned.
Neurogenic	Formed stools passed after meals Usually seen in dementia patients	Gastrocolic reflex stimulates defecation Patient does not delay until appropriate time	Ensure scheduled toileting.
Symptomatic	Incontinent stools, usually diarrhea Not related to other types of fecal incontinence	Colon or rectal disease	Provide comfort measures and proper skin care. Prepare for diagnostic tests and procedures.

SURGICAL TREATMENT

Surgical options include repair of anal muscles, implanting electrodes to stimulate and strengthen the perineal muscles, and placement of an artificial sphincter. The artificial sphincter functions like the urinary artificial sphincter described earlier. A fluid-filled chamber around the anus maintains continence. The patient deflates the chamber by pressing a reservoir in the scrotum or labia to allow bowel movements. Infection and other complications may require removal of the device.

BIOFEEDBACK

Patients who are motivated and able to follow directions and whose external anal sphincter is capable of responding to rectal distention may achieve bowel control with biofeedback. A balloon is inserted into the rectum and inflated. A manometer creates a tracing of the normal response of the sphincter to rectal pressure. The patient tries to consciously reproduce the pattern by contracting the muscles that delay defecation. The size of the balloon is progressively decreased to help the patient recognize and respond to the amount of rectal distention expected with normal stool volume. Pelvic muscle strengthening exercises, as described with urinary incontinence, can also be used to increase anal sphincter tone and strength. Biofeedback-assisted pelvic muscle exercises have been effective for many patients but have not proven useful for treatment of fecal incontinence associated with diabetes, spinal cord injury, rectal trauma, or radiation injury.

DIETARY CHANGES

The patient can be advised to avoid foods that stimulate the anal sphincters to relax. These include chocolate, coffee, tea, and other caffeinated beverages. Raw fruits, fruit juices (especially prune and grape juice), raw vegetables, cabbage, sweets, alcohol, and highly spicy foods stimulate stool production. Conversely, foods that thicken the stool (as well as potentially contribute to constipation) include bananas, rice, white bread, processed foods, fried foods, potatoes, red meat, dairy products (milk, cheese, yogurt), oatmeal, wheat bran and oat bran, and pasta. Alcohol and caffeine both can have a diuretic effect and contribute to dehydration and constipation. A diet high in fiber will help normalize loose stools. For women, the goal is 25 grams of fiber per day and for men, 38 grams of fiber per day. Until fecal incontinence is corrected, the patient may also wish to avoid foods that cause odor and gas. Odor-causing foods include cabbage-family vegetables, beans, garlic, eggs, fish, and turnips. Beans, beer, carbonated beverages, cucumbers, cabbage, broccoli, dairy products, and corn produce gas.

TYPES OF BOWEL (FECAL) INCONTINENCE

The four types of bowel incontinence are overflow, neurogenic, symptomatic, and anorectal. Table 14.5 summarizes the features of each type.

OVERFLOW INCONTINENCE

Description

Overflow incontinence is caused by constipation in which the rectum is constantly distended. The fecal mass backs up until the entire colon is full. A fecal impaction may or may not be present. The patient passes semisolid stools frequently. This condition may be related to a long-standing dependence on laxatives or enemas.

Medical Treatment

Medical management of bowel overflow incontinence is concerned with immediate relief of the constipation and long-term control of the problem. The first step is to cleanse the colon. Phosphate enemas and suppositories may be ordered to empty the rectum. Daily enemas for 7 to 10 days are then needed to empty the entire colon.

Instead of the enemas, the physician may order oral laxatives such as bisacodyl, polyethylene glycol, or mannitol. If hard masses of stool are present, they can be softened with oil retention enemas and then removed digitally.

Once the colon has been cleansed, regular evacuation is essential. Increased fluids and fiber may be helpful, but some patients need regular aids to elimination. The physician may order enemas or suppositories twice a week or daily laxatives. For older patients, senna or lactulose is preferred by many geriatric specialists. Mineral oil should be avoided because it interferes with absorption of fat-soluble vitamins and because it may be aspirated, causing lipid pneumonia.

NEUROGENIC INCONTINENCE

Description

Many people report having a bowel movement shortly after breakfast. Bowel activity is stimulated by the gastrocolic reflex. When food enters the stomach, it stimulates peristalsis throughout the digestive tract and causes the movement of the fecal mass into the rectum. Patients who are unable to voluntarily delay defecation are said to have bowel **neurogenic incontinence**. This occurs most often in patients with dementia. These patients may have one or two formed stools daily after meals.

Medical Treatment

Neurogenic incontinence is usually treated with scheduled toileting based on the patient's usual time of defecation. If this is not successful, some physicians order a constipating drug (e.g., anticholinergic) each morning and a laxative (e.g., senna, milk of magnesia) each night. This routine results in a controlled bowel movement each morning and avoids later accidents.

ANORECTAL INCONTINENCE

Description

Anorectal incontinence is associated with nerve damage that causes the muscles of the pelvic floor to be weak. Rectal abnormalities may be present, including loss of anal reflex and loss of anal sphincter tone. Patients typically have several incontinent stools a day.

Medical Treatment

Anorectal incontinence is initially treated with pelvic muscle exercises with or without biofeedback. If these techniques are ineffective, surgical repair of the anal sphincter may be advised.

NURSING CARE OF THE PATIENT WITH BOWEL INCONTINENCE

FOCUSED ASSESSMENT

The data the licensed vocational nurse/licensed practical nurse (LVN/LPN) collects contributes to a thorough nursing assessment that can help to determine the type and cause of bowel incontinence and guide the selection of treatment.

Bristol Stool Chart

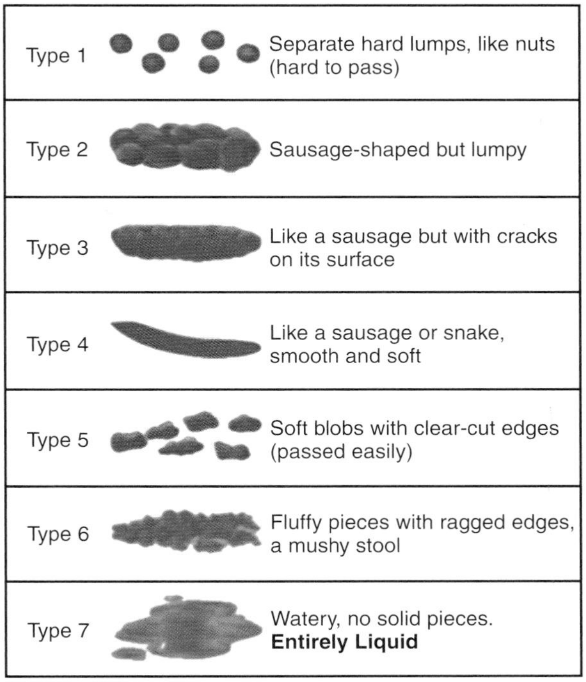

Fig. 14.5 The Bristol Stool Chart. (From Kliegman RM, Stanton BF, St Geme W III, Schor NF: *Nelson textbook of pediatrics*, ed 20, Philadelphia, 2016, Elsevier.)

Reason for Seeking Care

Elicit the individual's primary concerns about bowel function and its impact on their life.

Present Health

When a patient has bowel incontinence, determine the usual bowel pattern, changes, stool characteristics, and related symptoms such as pain or cramping.

Bowel pattern. Document the patient's usual frequency of bowel movements. Regarding incontinent episodes, ask if the patient is aware of the sensation to defecate. For dementia patients, a caregiver may be able to detect clues that the patient is about to have a bowel movement (e.g., restlessness, trying to remove clothing). If the patient is confused, initiate a record of times and circumstances when defecation occurs.

Characteristics of stools. Describe the amount, consistency, color, odor, and constituents of the patient's stools. The Bristol Stool Scale characterizes the shapes and types of stool for seven categories. The ideal stool is generally type 3 or 4, easy to pass without being too watery, type 1 or 2 is considered *constipated*, and types 5, 6, and 7 tend toward *diarrhea*. Fig. 14.5 illustrates the different types of stools on the Bristol Stool Chart. Other terms used to describe consistency include *liquid, watery, pasty, tarry, semi-formed, formed*, and *hard*. Most of these terms are self-explanatory. Tarry is used to describe stools that are shiny, sticky, and black. Stool is normally brown in color. Abnormal colors are black, red, green, and white. Abnormal stool constituents might include blood, mucus, or undigested food.

Past Health History

Document chronic illnesses, past acute illnesses, and surgeries or trauma to the abdomen or rectum. Neurologic conditions, including stroke, spinal cord injury, and dementia, are significant. List recent and current medications and all allergies. It is especially important to determine the use of laxatives, enemas, or suppositories. Because these are often purchased without a prescription, the patient may not mention them when reporting medications. Record the obstetric history of female patients, including the number of pregnancies, types of deliveries, and complications of childbirth.

Review of Systems

The review of systems identifies problems that may be related to bowel incontinence, such as motor, sensory, or cognitive impairments.

Inspect and palpate the abdomen for distention and auscultate for bowel sounds. In addition, inspect the perianal area for irritation or breakdown. The physician or nurse practitioner may perform a rectal examination and test the strength of the rectal sphincter.

Functional Assessment

The functional assessment focuses on habits that may be related to bowel function, including diet, fluid intake, and exercise or activity pattern. Determine whether the patient has the mobility and dexterity needed to manage toileting independently. Recent travel to other countries may be significant because travelers sometimes acquire uncommon intestinal infections.

Assessment of the patient with bowel incontinence is outlined in Box 14.6.

Patient Problems, Goals, and Outcome Criteria: Fecal Incontinence

Patient problems and goals for the patient with fecal incontinence may include the following:

Patient Problems	Goals and Outcome Criteria
Loss of bowel control related to impaction, cognitive impairment, neurologic impairment, environmental barriers, or impaired mobility	Controlled bowel elimination: regular voluntary bowel evacuation of soft, formed stool
Potential for disrupted skin tissue integrity related to contact of feces with skin	Normal skin integrity: no redness or skin breakdown
Altered self-concept related to loss of control of elimination	Positive self-concept: patient's comments and behavior reflect positive view of self (e.g., confidence, takes pride in appearance)

Box 14.6 Focused Assessment of Patients With Bowel Incontinence

HEALTH HISTORY

Reason for Seeking Care

Bowel pattern changes, stool characteristics (consistency, color, constituents), awareness of need to defecate, symptoms associated with passage of incontinent stool

Past Health History

Chronic illnesses, past acute illnesses, abdominal or rectal trauma or surgery, abdominal radiotherapy, recent and current medications, dementia, allergies

Review of Systems

Motor, sensory, or cognitive dysfunction that could affect continence

Functional Assessment

Diet, fluid intake, exercise or activity pattern, foreign travel

Physical Examination

Abdomen: Distention, bowel sounds

Perianal Area: Irritation, breakdown

INTERVENTIONS

Loss of Bowel Control

Continued monitoring is an essential part of the nurse's role in caring for the patient with bowel incontinence. Documentation of the patient's usual bowel pattern provides a guideline for scheduled elimination and for setting realistic goals. To establish a bowel program, take the patient to the toilet at the usual time of defecation, commonly 30 minutes after eating. If suppositories or enemas are ordered, administer as ordered and document the results and the patient response.

When enemas or laxatives are prescribed on a routine basis for overflow incontinence, caregivers often fear creating laxative or enema dependency. For these patients, however, normal bowel function may not be a realistic goal. They may do better with a program that promotes regular bowel evacuation.

Explain normal bowel physiology and interventions for incontinence to the patient. Advise the patient to consume adequate fluids and fiber to prevent constipation and impaction. A fluid intake of at least 1500 mL/day is recommended if not contraindicated. Instruct the patient that fresh fruits and vegetables and high-fiber foods provide bulk that keeps the stool soft. Encourage ambulation if the patient is able to walk. Toileting should occur sitting upright to facilitate peristalsis and complete evacuation of stools. If pelvic muscle exercises are prescribed, encourage the patient to practice contracting the muscles that control defecation to prevent leakage.

Potential for Disrupted Skin Tissue Integrity

After each incontinent stool, cleanse the perianal area thoroughly and apply protective ointments as ordered or per agency policy. Incontinence undergarments may be needed to prevent soiling and embarrassment; be sure to check frequently so that stool does not remain in contact with the skin. Fecal pouches may be used, but care must be taken to perform skin prep as ordered to prevent irritation caused by the adhesive.

Altered Self-Concept

Loss of bowel control can be devastating for the patient. Express understanding of the patient's distress and encourage the patient to strive for as much improvement as possible. In addition, praise the patient for participation in the treatment program and for decreased frequency of incontinent stools. Encourage the patient to practice good grooming and to maintain social activities. It is important to help patients to coordinate their social schedule with their bowel programs.

Get Ready for the NCLEX® Examination!

Key Points

- Incontinence is the inability to control the passage of urine or feces.
- Normal controlled voiding requires healthy bladder muscle, a patent urethra, normal transmission of nerve impulses, and mental alertness.
- Data collection relevant to urinary incontinence includes recording the voiding pattern, urine volume, associated signs and symptoms, medications, medical history, and physical findings.
- The types of urinary incontinence are urge, stress, overflow (including reflex), and functional.
- Transient incontinence is caused by reversible conditions and is often corrected by treatment of the underlying problem.
- Urge urinary incontinence (involuntary loss of urine after a strong urge to void) may be corrected by treating the cause with behavior modification (toileting programs, pelvic muscle exercises, biofeedback, urge suppression, caffeine elimination) and drug therapy.
- Overflow urinary incontinence (involuntary loss of urine associated with a full bladder) may be corrected by treating the cause (e.g., enlarged prostate) or by using drugs that stimulate the bladder and relax the internal sphincter.
- Stress urinary incontinence (the involuntary loss of urine during physical exertion and coughing and sneezing) may be improved by strengthening the perineal muscles, biofeedback, surgical intervention, or placement of an artificial sphincter.
- Functional urinary incontinence is loss of urine because of environmental barriers (lack of available toilet or toilet substitute), functional impairments, or cognitive deficits.
- Assessment of bowel incontinence includes recording the usual bowel pattern, stool characteristics, related symptoms, activity, diet, fluid intake, medications, and use of aids to help elimination, as well as performing an abdominal assessment.
- Types of bowel incontinence include overflow, anorectal, neurogenic, and symptomatic.
- Fecal overflow incontinence is caused by constipation in which the rectum is constantly distended and is treated by relieving the constipation and preventing future episodes.
- Anorectal incontinence is caused by abnormalities in the pelvic muscle, anus, or rectum and may be treated with pelvic floor muscle exercises or surgery.
- Neurogenic bowel incontinence is automatic defecation seen in people (e.g., dementia) who are unable to voluntarily delay defecation; it may be corrected by scheduled toileting.
- Symptomatic bowel incontinence results from colorectal disease and requires correction of the basic problem.
- Nursing care of the patient who is incontinent may address measures to correct the specific type of incontinence, to prevent skin breakdown, to improve situational low self-concept, and to improve ability to manage the treatment program.
- Bowel training may be accomplished by scheduled toileting, stimulation techniques, or both.

Additional Learning Resources

SG Go to your Study Guide for additional learning activities to help you master this chapter content.

Go to your Evolve website (http://evolve.elsevier.com/Linton/medsurg) for the following learning resources and much more:
- Fluid & Electrolyte Tutorial
- Review Questions for the NCLEX® Examination

Clinical Judgment and Next-Generation NCLEX® Examination-Style Questions

1. **Habit training is being used to treat a patient with urinary incontinence. What should the nurse instruct the nursing assistant to do? (Select all that apply.)**
   1. Check the patient for wetness every 2 hours and ask the patient to state whether they are wet or dry.
   2. Encourage the patient to void every 2 hours on a schedule based on the patient's usual pattern.
   3. Encourage the patient to delay voiding and to void only at scheduled times.
   4. Have the patient practice pelvic muscle exercises by contracting perineal muscles as if holding back gas.

   NCLEX Client Need: Safe and Effective Care Environment: Coordinated Care

2. **The nurse is teaching a patient to perform pelvic muscle exercises. Instructions should include which of the following? (Select all that apply.)**
   1. You should contract perineal muscles for 30 seconds, then relax for 30 seconds.
   2. You will notice improvement within 1 week after starting exercises.
   3. Strengthening perineal muscles can improve urinary control.
   4. To do these exercises correctly, you must be in a sitting position.
   5. You will need to continue the exercises indefinitely to maintain control.

   NCLEX Client Need: Health Promotion and Maintenance

3. **The nurse is preparing to discharge a patient who will be doing self-catheterization at home. How does intermittent self-catheterization in the home setting differ from that in an institution?**
   1. Clean technique may be used at home but not in a hospital.
   2. Sterile technique must be used regardless of the setting.
   3. Clean technique may be used anywhere as long as the patient performs the procedure.
   4. Clean technique can be used in long-term care facilities because patients live there.

   NCLEX Client Need: Safe and Effective Care Environment: Safety and Infection Control

4. **A clinic patient has had a pessary inserted because of urinary incontinence. Care of this patient includes:**
   1. Evaluation of placement position within 1 week after insertion
   2. Documentation of pessary placement so it will not be forgotten
   3. Monitoring for signs of bowel obstruction
   4. Removal for cleansing each time perineal care is done

   NCLEX Client Need: Safe and Effective Care Environment: Safety and Infection Control

5. **An older adult patient has been diagnosed with urge urinary incontinence. Her husband asks what this means. Which statements accurately describe this diagnosis? (Select all that apply.)**
   1. A strong, abrupt urge to urinate occurs shortly before involuntary urine loss.
   2. Urge incontinence is often caused by anticholinergic drugs.
   3. Urge incontinence is commonly the result of an overactive bladder muscle.
   4. In urge incontinence, the bladder overfills so that small amounts of urine are passed to relieve pressure.
   5. Medications are often effective in reducing bladder overactivity.

   NCLEX Client Need: Physiological Integrity: Physiological Adaptation

6. **Autonomic dysreflexia is a very serious complication of which type of incontinence?**

   NCLEX Client Need: Physiological Integrity: Physiological Adaptation

7. **Which statement should be included when teaching a woman about stress urinary incontinence?**
   1. It is usually caused by relaxation of the pelvic floor muscles.
   2. You should limit fluid intake to 1000 mL/day.
   3. Fluids containing caffeine stimulate contraction of perineal muscles.
   4. The only effective treatment for stress incontinence is surgical repair.

   NCLEX Client: Physiological Integrity: Physiological Adaptation

8. **A patient in the independent living unit of a retirement home reports that she has had several incidents of bowel incontinence. The nurse's assessment reveals that the patient consumes all of the items listed subsequently. Which one might be related to the patient's fecal incontinence?**
   1. Bananas
   2. Alcohol
   3. Pasta
   4. Cheese

   NCLEX Client Need: Physiological Integrity: Physiological Adaptation

9. **A bedridden patient with no history of bowel incontinence has been involuntarily passing liquid stools for 2 days. What additional data should the nurse collect?**
   1. Last formed bowel movement
   2. Urine output
   3. Temperature
   4. Usual mental status

   NCLEX Client Need: Physiological Integrity: Basic Care and Comfort

10. **SLO/Objective:** Prioritize nursing care for patients with urinary incontinence.

    NGN Item Type: Cloze

    Cognitive Skill: Prioritize Hypotheses

    A 73-year-old woman residing in assisted living reports burning on urination; cloudy, dark urine; and episodes of urge incontinence. She is receiving medication for hypertension and NSAIDS for chronic osteoarthritis. She usually drinks 3–4 cups of coffee per day and 1–2 glasses of wine in the evening. She smokes ½ pack of cigarettes on her patio every day.
    - BP = 130/76 mm Hg
    - Heart rate = 82 beats per minute
    - Respirations = 20 beats per minute
    - Temperature = 100.0°F.
    - Metoprolol 50 mg po qd
    - HCTZ 25 mg po qd
    - Ibuprofen 400 mg q4h

    Choose the *most likely* options for the information missing from the statements below by selecting from the list of options provided.

    Her urge incontinence is *most likely* the result of (1) ____________, (1)____________, or (1)____________. The nurse would monitor (2)____________, (2)____________, (2)____________.

OPTIONS FOR 1	OPTIONS FOR 2
Orthostatic hypotension	BP sitting and standing
Weakness	Mental status
Medication effects	Daily weights
Urinary tract infection	Intake and Output
Coffee intake	Urinalysis results
Cigarette smoking	Temperature

Nutrition

15

http://evolve.elsevier.com/Linton/medsurg

Objectives

1. List data included in the nutritional assessment.
2. Describe the changes in nutrient needs as a person ages.
3. Explain factors that are thought to contribute to obesity and current approaches to treatment.
4. Discuss the issues involved in changing eating habits.
5. Discuss methods of nutritional support for patients who cannot consume adequate nutrients orally.
6. Describe common therapeutic diets.

Key Terms

cognitive restructuring
complete protein
ketosis
obesity
satiety
stimulus control

To support and maintain life or fight disease, the body requires an ongoing supply of the proper nutrients. Nutrition is the cornerstone of the healing process. This chapter provides an overview of the nutritional needs of adult and older adult patients, guidelines for dietary planning, the assessment of nutritional status, modified nutrient delivery approaches, medical nutrition therapy, common therapeutic dietary regimens, nutrition issues for the older adult, and nutrition therapy based on medical diagnoses.

NUTRITIONAL REQUIREMENTS OF HEALTHY ADULTS

Every five years the U.S. Departments of Health and Human Services and of Agriculture publish *Dietary Guidelines for Americans*. The 2020–2025 guidelines focus on choosing healthy foods and beverages rich in nutrients and within a recommended limit of calories. The theme for this edition is "Make every bite count with the Dietary Guidelines." Overarching guidelines (2020) are:

- Follow a healthy dietary pattern at every life stage.
- Customize and enjoy nutrient-dense food and beverage choices to reflect personal preferences, cultural traditions, and budgetary considerations.
- Focus on meeting food group needs with nutrient-dense foods and beverages, and stay within calorie limits.
- Limit foods and beverages higher in added sugars, saturated fat, and sodium, and limit alcoholic beverages.

Nutrient dense foods are advised to make every bite count. These are foods that "provide vitamins, minerals, and other health promoting components and have little added sugar, saturated fat, and sodium" (U.S. DHHS and Department of Agriculture, 2020, p. 95). Specifically, added sugars and saturated fats should contribute less than 10% of total daily calories. The maximum daily sodium intake should be limited to 2300 mg/day. Alcohol intake should be limited to two drinks per day for men and one drink per day for women.

DIETARY REFERENCE INTAKES

In 1941 nutritionists coined the term *recommended daily allowances* (RDAs) to describe daily nutrient requirements. The RDAs were used as a basis to evaluate and plan healthy meals. This familiar system for identifying nutritional needs was changed in the 1990s to dietary reference intakes (DRIs). The four types of DRIs are RDAs, estimated average requirements, adequate intake, and tolerable upper intake level. These new values were meant to prevent nutrient deficiencies and to reduce the risk of chronic diseases such as cardiovascular disease. Resources for detailed DRI information are listed under Additional Learning Resources at the end of this chapter.

Recommended Dietary Allowance/Dietary Reference Intake for Carbohydrates

The RDA for carbohydrates for adults is 130 g/day. The best sources of carbohydrates are whole grains, beans, peas, vegetables, and fruits, especially those high in fiber. Grains include all foods made from wheat, rice, oats, cornmeal, and barley. Of all grains consumed, one half should be whole grain. Added sugars should be limited to less than 10% of daily calories. Product labels are being revised to include the amount of added sugar per serving.

Insufficient intake of carbohydrates can lead to ketosis. **Ketosis** is a condition caused by lack of adequate glucose that causes an excessive breakdown of tissue protein, loss of sodium and other cations, and involuntary dehydration.

The mean fiber intake for adults in the United States is estimated to be only 14 to 15 g/day. Several groups have recommended that Americans increase their intake of dietary fiber and that this increase should come from a wide variety of whole-grain products, fruits, vegetables, and legumes. The National Academy of Sciences, Engineering, and Medicine recommends 25 to 28 g of fiber per day for adult women and 31 to 34 g/day for adult men. After 50 years of age, the goal for fiber intake decreases to 22 g for women and 28 g for men.

Recommended Dietary Allowance/Dietary Reference Intake for Fats

The 2020–2025 Dietary Guidelines for Americans recommends that less than 10% of daily calories should come from saturated fats. People should also try to eat unsaturated fats rather than saturated fats to minimize the risk of heart disease. Studies have shown that Americans tend to consume too much fat, which can contribute to the development of cardiovascular disease and diabetes mellitus. Therefore, health promotion efforts have centered on teaching people how and why to limit the dietary intake of fat, particularly saturated fat.

Recommended Dietary Allowance/Dietary Reference Intake for Protein

The recommended DRI for protein is 56 g/day for men and 46 g/day for women. Protein should contribute 10% to 35% of the macronutrients in the adult diet.

A protein is a chain of amino acids that can form many different configurations and can combine with other substances. Twenty-two common amino acids have been identified, but only nine are essential amino acids. The nine essential amino acids must be obtained from the diet and are cysteine, proline, leucine, isoleucine, valine, tryptophan, phenylalanine, methionine, and histidine. The body can manufacture adequate amounts of the other amino acids from the essential amino acids. A protein that contains all nine essential amino acids in sufficient quantity and ratio for the body's need is called a **complete protein**.

The body cannot store protein; therefore, protein needs to be eaten each day. Nitrogen in the urine is a good indicator of protein levels in the body. If protein intake is inadequate, nitrogen will be conserved by the kidneys, causing the urine nitrogen to be low. When this adaptive process is no longer adequate, evidence of protein deficiency appears. The signs and symptoms include edema, wasting of body tissues, fatty liver, dermatosis (thickening and hardening of the skin), diminished immune response, weakness, and loss of energy.

Box 15.1 Comparative Kcal of Energy Per Gram

Carbohydrates: 4
Fats: 9
Proteins: 4

Kilocalories of Macronutrients

The kilocalories per gram for carbohydrates, fats, and proteins are noted in Box 15.1.

Recommended Dietary Allowance/Dietary Reference Intake for Vitamins and Minerals

The recommendations for vitamins and minerals include DRIs, RDAs, adequate intake, and tolerable upper intake. National Institutes of Health Tables of these values can be accessed at https://ods.od.nih.gov/Health_Information/Dietary_Reference_Intakes.aspx.

GUIDELINES FOR DIETARY PLANNING

MYPLATE

Over the years, various guidelines have been established in the United States to help in planning for optimal nutrition. The newest program, based on the U.S. Departments of Health and Human Services and Agriculture's 2015–2020 Dietary Guidelines for Americans and endorsed in the 2020–2025 guidelines, is MyPlate. The MyPlate icon is a placemat with a simple plate divided into four sections and a glass. The glass represents a dairy serving and the plate divisions represent the recommended proportions of fruits, vegetables, grains, and protein (Fig. 15.1). Its intent is to remind Americans to make better food choices. Specific information about food choices is available at https://www.myplate.gov. See Box 15.2 for key dietary recommendations.

The licensed vocational nurse/licensed practical nurse (LVN/LPN) can promote healthy eating by educating patients and families about sources of accurate information. Individuals can obtain personal dietary plans based on the 2020–2025 Dietary Guidelines for Americans using. You can create a personal eating plan based on your age, height, weight, and activity level using the tools on the *MyPlate website.* Fig. 15.2 provides a sample plan created for an individual (http://ChooseMyPlate.com/).

NUTRITION LABELS

With the increase in public awareness of health and nutrition, many people want information to help them make good food choices. Most foods are labeled so that the average person can make determinations about the quality and quantity of the nutrients consumed. Because of the lack of space available on a package label, the Nutrition Facts table is abbreviated to include essential information to describe the number of nutrients per serving (Fig. 15.3). In addition to calories, calories from fat, and grams of specific nutrients, the

USDA
United States Department of Agriculture

10 tips
Nutrition
Education Series

MyPlate MyWins

Based on the Dietary Guidelines for Americans

Choose MyPlate

Use MyPlate to build your healthy eating style and maintain it for a lifetime. Choose foods and beverages from each MyPlate food group. Make sure your choices are limited in sodium, saturated fat, and added sugars. Start with small changes to make healthier choices you can enjoy.

1 Find your healthy eating style
Creating a healthy style means regularly eating a variety of foods to get the nutrients and calories you need. MyPlate's tips help you create your own healthy eating solutions—"MyWins."

2 Make half your plate fruits and vegetables
Eating colorful fruits and vegetables is important because they provide vitamins and minerals and most are low in calories.

3 Focus on whole fruits
Fruits
Choose whole fruits—fresh, frozen, dried, or canned in 100% juice. Enjoy fruit with meals, as snacks, or as a dessert.

4 Vary your veggies
Vegetables
Try adding fresh, frozen, or canned vegetables to salads, sides, and main dishes. Choose a variety of colorful vegetables prepared in healthful ways: steamed, sauteed, roasted, or raw.

5 Make half your grains whole grains
Grains
Look for whole grains listed first or second on the ingredients list—try oatmeal, popcorn, whole-grain bread, and brown rice. Limit grain-based desserts and snacks, such as cakes, cookies, and pastries.

6 Move to low-fat or fat-free milk or yogurt
Dairy
Choose low-fat or fat-free milk, yogurt, and soy beverages (soymilk) to cut back on saturated fat. Replace sour cream, cream, and regular cheese with low-fat yogurt, milk, and cheese.

7 Vary your protein routine
Protein
Mix up your protein foods to include seafood, beans and peas, unsalted nuts and seeds, soy products, eggs, and lean meats and poultry. Try main dishes made with beans or seafood like tuna salad or bean chili.

8 Drink and eat beverages and food with less sodium, saturated fat, and added sugars
Limit
Use the Nutrition Facts label and ingredients list to limit items high in sodium, saturated fat, and added sugars. Choose vegetable oils instead of butter, and oil-based sauces and dips instead of ones with butter, cream, or cheese.

9 Drink water instead of sugary drinks
Water is calorie-free. Non-diet soda, energy or sports drinks, and other sugar-sweetened drinks contain a lot of calories from added sugars and have few nutrients.

10 Everything you eat and drink matters
The right mix of foods can help you be healthier now and into the future. Turn small changes into your "MyPlate, MyWins."

Center for Nutrition Policy and Promotion
USDA is an equal opportunity provider, employer, and lender.

Go to ChooseMyPlate.gov for more information.

DG TipSheet No. 1
June 2011
Revised October 2016

Fig. 15.1 U.S. Department of Agriculture Center for Nutrition Policy and Promotion.

Box 15.2 2020–2025 Dietary Guidelines for Americans: Key Recommendations

BALANCING CALORIES TO MANAGE WEIGHT

The Dietary Guidelines' advise us to make every bite count by following these recommendations:

1. Follow a healthy dietary pattern at every life stage to meet nutrient needs, help achieve a healthy body weight, and reduce the risk of chronic disease.
2. Customize and enjoy nutrient-dense food and beverage choices to reflect personal preferences, cultural traditions, and budgetary considerations. A healthy dietary pattern can benefit all individuals regardless of age, race, or ethnicity, or current health status. The Dietary Guidelines provides a framework intended to be customized to individual needs and preferences, as well as the foodways of the diverse cultures in the United States.
3. Focus on meeting food group needs with nutrient-dense foods and beverages and stay within calorie limits. An underlying premise of the Dietary Guidelines is that nutritional needs should be met primarily from foods and beverages; specifically, nutrient-dense foods and beverages. Nutrient-dense foods provide vitamins, minerals, and other health-promoting components and have no or little added sugars, saturated fat, and sodium. A healthy dietary pattern consists of nutrient-dense forms of foods and beverages across all food groups, in recommended amounts, and within calorie limits. The core elements that make up a healthy dietary pattern include:
   - Vegetables of all types: dark green, red and orange; beans, peas, and starchy, and other vegetables
   - Fruits, especially whole fruits
   - Grains, at least half of which are whole grain
   - Dairy, including fat-free or low-fat milk, yogurt, and cheese, and/or lactose-free versions and fortified soy beverages and yogurt as alternatives
   - Protein foods, including, lean meats, poultry, and eggs; seafood; beans, peas, and lentils; and nuts, seeds, and soy products
   - Oils, including vegetable oils and oils in food, such as seafood and nuts
   - Saturated fats and *trans* fats, added sugars, and sodium
4. Limit foods and beverages higher in added sugar, saturated fat, and sodium; and limit alcoholic beverages. At every life stage, meeting food group recommendations—even with nutrient-dense choices—requires most of a person's daily calorie needs and sodium limits. A healthy dietary pattern doesn't have much room for extra added sugars, saturated fat, or sodium—or for alcoholic beverages. A small amount of added sugars, saturated fat, or sodium can be added to nutrient-dense foods and beverages to help meet food group recommendations, but foods and beverages high in these components should be limited. Limits are:
   - Added sugars: Less than 10% of calories per day starting at age 2 years. Avoid foods and beverages with added sugars for those younger than age 2 years.
   - Saturated fat: Less than 10% of calories per day starting at age 2 years.
   - Sodium: Less than 2300 mg/day—and even less for children younger than age 14 years.

Alcoholic beverages: Adults of legal drinking age can choose not to drink, or to drink in moderation by limiting intake to 2 drinks or less in a day for men and 1 drink or less in a day for women. Drinking less is better for health than drinking more. There are some adults who should not drink alcohol, such as women who are pregnant.

Physical activity: In tandem with the earlier recommendations, Americans of all ages—children, adolescents, adults, and older adults should meet the *Physical Activity Guidelines for Americans* to help promote health and reduce the risk of chronic disease. See Box 4.4 for a summary of the physical activity guidelines.

Body weight: Americans should aim to achieve and maintain a healthy body weight. The relationship between diet and physical activity contributes to calorie balance and managing body weight.

From U.S. Departments of Health and Human Services and of Agriculture. *2020–2025 dietary guidelines for Americans: Executive summary.* https://www.dietaryguidelines.gov/sites/default/files/2020-12/DGA_2020-2025_ExecutiveSummary_English.pdf. Retrieved December 30, 2020.

label also specifies daily values (DVs). A DV of 10% means that one serving of the product provides 10% of the recommended daily intake of that nutrient based on a 2000-calorie diet. A recent change requires labels to include the amount of added sugars and potassium in the product.

VEGETARIAN DIETS

Vegetarian diets are not new but have only gradually gained acceptance as a balanced nutritional option in the United States. Many Americans who call themselves vegetarians eat all foods except red meat, although some exclude poultry and fish as well. A lacto-vegetarian diet includes milk, cheese, and other dairy products but excludes meat, fish, poultry, and eggs. A lacto-ovo-vegetarian diet includes dairy products and eggs but excludes meat, fish, and poultry. A person who consumes no foods of animal origin is said to be a *vegan.* Only the vegan is at real risk for nutritional deficiencies if the diet is not carefully planned.

Some evidence suggests that vegetarian diets have distinct health benefits, including reduced risks of type 2 diabetes mellitus, breast and colon cancer, and cardiovascular and gallbladder disease. Vegetarians generally consume less protein than do nonvegetarians, but most still exceed the RDA for protein. Tips for healthy eating for vegetarians are summarized in Box 15.3.

NURSING ASSESSMENT OF NUTRITIONAL STATUS

The areas covered in a nutritional assessment include a dietary history, anthropometric data, laboratory data (if available), and physical examination data.

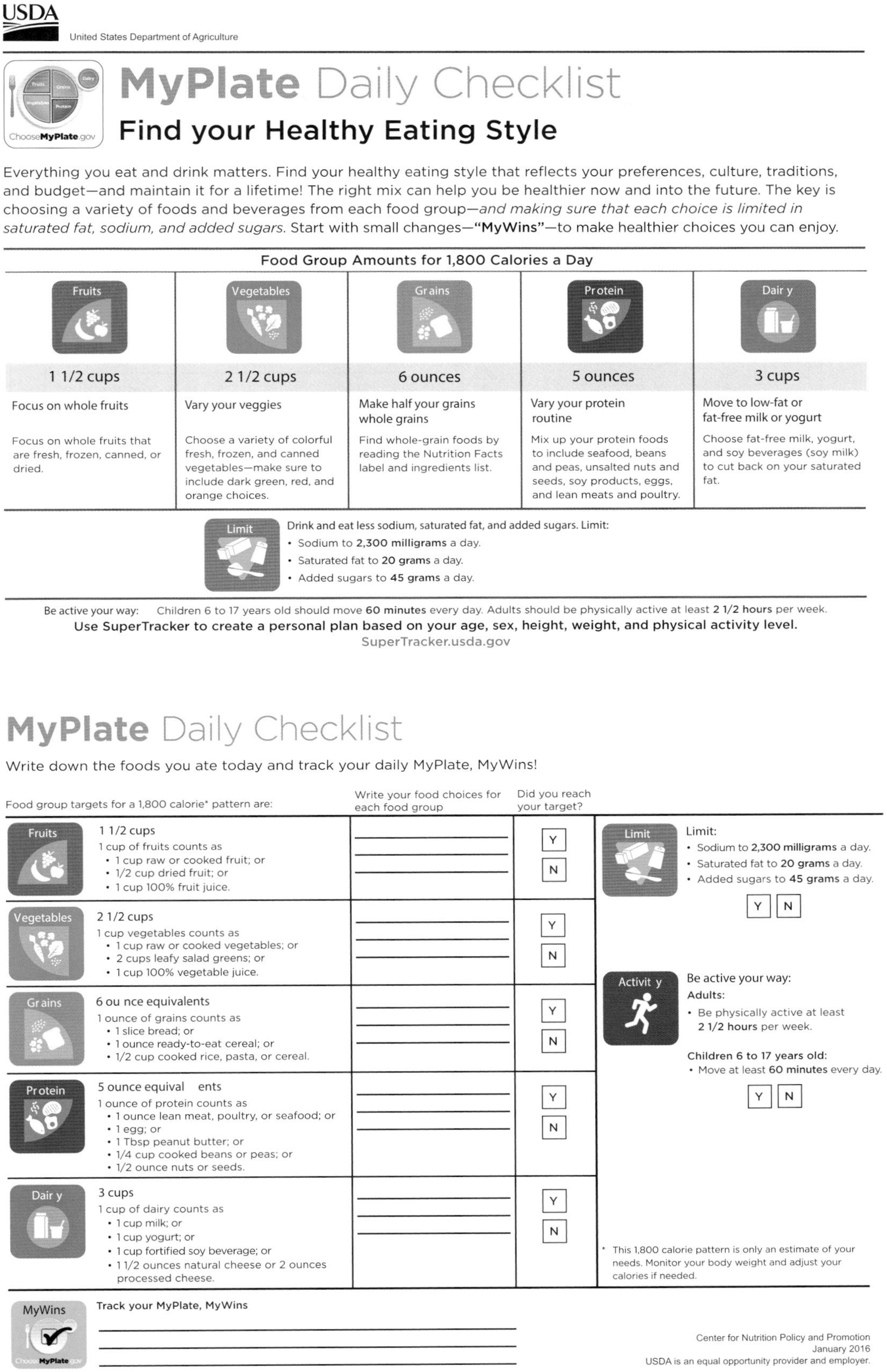

USDA
United States Department of Agriculture

MyPlate Daily Checklist

Find your Healthy Eating Style

Everything you eat and drink matters. Find your healthy eating style that reflects your preferences, culture, traditions, and budget—and maintain it for a lifetime! The right mix can help you be healthier now and into the future. The key is choosing a variety of foods and beverages from each food group—*and making sure that each choice is limited in saturated fat, sodium, and added sugars.* Start with small changes—**"MyWins"**—to make healthier choices you can enjoy.

Food Group Amounts for 1,800 Calories a Day

Fruits	Vegetables	Grains	Protein	Dairy
1 1/2 cups	2 1/2 cups	6 ounces	5 ounces	3 cups
Focus on whole fruits	Vary your veggies	Make half your grains whole grains	Vary your protein routine	Move to low-fat or fat-free milk or yogurt
Focus on whole fruits that are fresh, frozen, canned, or dried.	Choose a variety of colorful fresh, frozen, and canned vegetables—make sure to include dark green, red, and orange choices.	Find whole-grain foods by reading the Nutrition Facts label and ingredients list.	Mix up your protein foods to include seafood, beans and peas, unsalted nuts and seeds, soy products, eggs, and lean meats and poultry.	Choose fat-free milk, yogurt, and soy beverages (soy milk) to cut back on your saturated fat.

Limit

Drink and eat less sodium, saturated fat, and added sugars. Limit:
- Sodium to **2,300 milligrams** a day.
- Saturated fat to **20 grams** a day.
- Added sugars to **45 grams** a day.

Be active your way: Children 6 to 17 years old should move **60 minutes** every day. Adults should be physically active at least **2 1/2 hours** per week.

Use SuperTracker to create a personal plan based on your age, sex, height, weight, and physical activity level.
SuperTracker.usda.gov

MyPlate Daily Checklist

Write down the foods you ate today and track your daily MyPlate, MyWins!

Food group targets for a 1,800 calorie* pattern are:		Write your food choices for each food group	Did you reach your target?
Fruits	1 1/2 cups 1 cup of fruits counts as • 1 cup raw or cooked fruit; or • 1/2 cup dried fruit; or • 1 cup 100% fruit juice.		Y N
Vegetables	2 1/2 cups 1 cup vegetables counts as • 1 cup raw or cooked vegetables; or • 2 cups leafy salad greens; or • 1 cup 100% vegetable juice.		Y N
Grains	6 ounce equivalents 1 ounce of grains counts as • 1 slice bread; or • 1 ounce ready-to-eat cereal; or • 1/2 cup cooked rice, pasta, or cereal.		Y N
Protein	5 ounce equivalents 1 ounce of protein counts as • 1 ounce lean meat, poultry, or seafood; or • 1 egg; or • 1 Tbsp peanut butter; or • 1/4 cup cooked beans or peas; or • 1/2 ounce nuts or seeds.		Y N
Dairy	3 cups 1 cup of dairy counts as • 1 cup milk; or • 1 cup yogurt; or • 1 cup fortified soy beverage; or • 1 1/2 ounces natural cheese or 2 ounces processed cheese.		Y N

Limit

Limit:
- Sodium to **2,300 milligrams** a day.
- Saturated fat to **20 grams** a day.
- Added sugars to **45 grams** a day.

Y N

Activity

Be active your way:
Adults:
- Be physically active at least **2 1/2 hours** per week.

Children 6 to 17 years old:
- Move at least **60 minutes** every day.

Y N

* This 1,800 calorie pattern is only an estimate of your needs. Monitor your body weight and adjust your calories if needed.

MyWins

Track your MyPlate, MyWins

Center for Nutrition Policy and Promotion
January 2016
USDA is an equal opportunity provider and employer.

Fig. 15.2 An example of an individualized MyPlate Daily Checklist created on the Choose My Plate website. (Courtesy U.S. Food and Drug Administration. Retrieved December 30, 2020 from MyPlate.gov/eat-healthy/what-is-myplate.)

Side-by-side comparison

Original label

Nutrition facts
Serving size 2/3 cup (55g)
Servings per container 8

Amount per serving	
Calories 230	Calories from fat 70
	% daily value*
Total fat 8g	**12%**
Saturated fat 1g	**5%**
Trans fat 0g	
Cholesterol 0mg	**0%**
Sodium 160mg	**7%**
Total carbohydrate 37g	**12%**
Dietary fiber 4g	**16%**
Sugars 12g	
Protein 3g	
Vitamin A	10%
Vitamin C	8%
Calcium	20%
Iron	45%

* Percent daily values are based on a 2,000 calorie diet. Your daily value may be higher or lower depending on your calorie needs.

	Calories:	2,000	2,500
Total fat	Less than	65g	80g
Sat fat	Less than	20g	25g
Cholesterol	Less than	300mg	300mg
Sodium	Less than	2,400mg	2,400mg
Total carbohydrate		300g	375g
Dietary fiber		25g	30g

New label

Nutrition facts
8 servings per container
Serving size 2/3 cup (55g)

Amount per serving	
Calories	**230**
	% daily value*
Total fat 8g	**10%**
Saturated fat 1g	**5%**
Trans fat 0g	
Cholesterol 0mg	**0%**
Sodium 160mg	**7%**
Total carbohydrate 37g	**13%**
Dietary fiber 4g	**14%**
Total sugars 12g	
Includes 10g added sugars	**20%**
Protein 3g	
Vitamin D 2mcg	10%
Calcium 260mg	20%
Iron 8mg	45%
Potassium 240mg	6%

* The % daily value (DV) tells you how much a nutrient in a serving of food contributes to a daily diet. 2,000 calories a day is used for general nutrition advice.

FDA

Fig. 15.3 Example of a nutrition label. (Courtesy U.S. Food and Drug Administration. fda.gov/food/food-labeling-nutrition/changes-nutrition-facts-label. Retrieved December 30, 2020.)

DIETARY HISTORY

While collecting data for the dietary history, observe the patient's physical appearance for obesity, signs of malnutrition, and other factors that may indicate nutritional deficits. The well-nourished person should have shiny and healthy-looking hair, bright and clear eyes, smooth facial skin, smooth lips and tongue, and healthy teeth and gums. Signs of malnutrition include dull, thin, and sparse hair; pale conjunctiva; a swollen face; swollen lips and tongue; teeth with cavities or missing teeth; and bleeding or receding gums.

The dietary history includes physical, psychologic, social, and medical data that may have an impact on nutritional status. Box 15.4 summarizes information you should obtain in the dietary history. Commonly used tools to collect retrospective ("after the fact") data about dietary patterns include the 24-hour recall and the food frequency record. For a 24-hour recall, ask the patient to recall everything eaten during the past 24 hours, usually from the time of awakening until the next morning. Note everything consumed, including meals, snacks, drinks (especially water), and seasonings (especially salt). The food frequency record uses a

Box 15.3 Ten Tips: Healthy Eating for Vegetarians

1. Think about protein. Your protein needs can easily be met by eating a variety of plant foods. Sources of protein for vegetarians include beans and peas, nuts, and soy products (such as tofu, tempeh). Lacto-ovo-vegetarians also get protein from eggs and dairy foods.
2. Bone up on sources of calcium. Calcium is used for building bones and teeth. Some vegetarians consume dairy products, which are excellent sources of calcium. Other sources of calcium for vegetarians include calcium-fortified soymilk (soy beverage), tofu made with calcium sulfate, calcium-fortified breakfast cereals and orange juice, and some dark green leafy vegetables (collard, turnip, mustard greens, and bok choy).
3. Make simple changes. Many popular main dishes are or can be vegetarian—such as pasta primavera, pasta with marinara or pesto sauce, veggie pizza, vegetable lasagna, tofu-vegetable stir-fry, and bean burritos.
4. Enjoy a cookout. For barbecues, try veggie or soy burgers, soy hot dogs, marinated tofu or tempeh, and fruit kabobs. Grilled veggies are great too!
5. Include beans and peas. Because of their high nutrient content, consuming beans and peas is recommended for everyone, vegetarians and nonvegetarians alike. Enjoy some vegetarian chili, three-bean salad, or split pea soup. Make a hummus-filled pita sandwich.
6. Try different veggie versions. A variety of vegetarian products look—and may taste—like their nonvegetarian counterparts but are usually lower in saturated fat and contain no cholesterol. For breakfast, try soy-based sausage patties or links. For dinner, rather than hamburgers, try bean burgers or falafel (chickpea patties).
7. Make some small changes at restaurants. Most restaurants can make vegetarian modifications to menu items by substituting meatless sauces or nonmeat items, such as tofu and beans for meat, and adding vegetables or pasta in place of meat. Ask about available vegetarian options.
8. Nuts make great snacks. Choose unsalted nuts as a snack and use them in salads or main dishes. Add almonds, walnuts, or pecans instead of cheese or meat to a green salad.
9. Get your vitamin B_{12}. Vitamin B_{12} is naturally found. only in animal products. Vegetarians should choose fortified foods such as cereals or soy products, or take a vitamin B_{12} supplement if they do not consume any animal products. Check the Nutrition Facts label for vitamin B_{12} in fortified products.
10. Find a vegetarian pattern for you. Go to www.dietaryguidelines.gov and check appendices of the *2020–2025 Dietary guidelines for Americans* for vegetarian adaptations of the U.S. Department of Agriculture food patterns

From U.S. Department of Agriculture, Center for Nutrition Policy and Promotion: *DG TipSheet No. 8*, June 2011: www.ChooseMyPlate.gov. Accessed July 8, 2017.

Box 15.4 Dietary History Data

Food and Nutrition	
Appetite	Good, poor, any changes Factors that affect appetite Changes in sense of taste or smell
Attitude toward food and eating	Interest in eating Ideas about food, eating, or body weight Parental interest in child's eating
Allergies, intolerances, or food avoidances	Foods avoided and reason Problems caused by foods
Nutrition problems	Concerns perceived by patient and family
Weight pattern and history	Recent loss or gain: how many pounds and over what length of time? Intentional or unintended?
Psychosocial	
Occupation and background	Type of work, hours/week, shift, energy expenditure Educational background
Culture	Influence of culture on eating habits Religious practices, holiday rituals Health beliefs related to food
Home life and meal patterns	Number in household (eat together?) Who does shopping? cooking? Food storage and cooking facilities?
Physical activity, stress, leisure time, rest	Exercise: type, amount, frequency Relaxation and leisure activities: type, amount, frequency Sleep: uninterrupted hours per day Stress: amount, frequency, chronic?
Environment and toxin exposure	Exposure to known toxins: when, amount, duration, effects
Economics	Perceived food security: adequate income Public assistance: eligible? enrolled?

Continued

Box 15.4 Dietary History Data—cont'd

Medical

Dental and oral health	Problems with chewing, swallowing., salivation, choking
Gastrointestinal factors	Problems with digestion and elimination
Chronic disease	Dietary modifications
	Physical limitations/Handicaps
Medications	Medications: prescribed, over-the-counter, routine, PRN
Supplements, herbal remedies	Vitamin and mineral supplements, herbal remedies

Modified from Mahan LK, & Raymond JL.(2017). *Krause's Food and the Nutrition Care Process*, 14th ed. St. Louis MO. Elsevier.

list of foods from all food groups to assess how often the patient consumes specific foods. Because neither tool provides perfectly accurate data, using both of them is probably best. From these assessments, general dietary deficits and excesses can be determined.

ANTHROPOMETRIC DATA

Anthropometric data include height, weight (including weight patterns), and body composition. Height and weight measurements should be performed correctly to complete an accurate assessment of the patient. Box 15.5 gives guidelines on the proper way to perform these measurements.

Body composition is related to the ratio of fat to lean muscle mass. Determining a person's body composition requires taking several measurements. These measurements include skinfold thickness and hydrostatic weighing. Skinfold thickness is measured by means of calipers that pinch skin over areas of the body that seem to reflect best the fat content of the subcutaneous tissue. These sites include areas over the triceps, over the biceps, below the scapula, above the iliac crest, and on the upper thigh (Fig. 15.4).

A variety of other methods of measuring body composition are available, including bioelectrical impedance analysis, air displacement plethysmography, dual-energy x-ray absorptiometry, and hydrostatic (underwater) weighing. However, these procedures require specific equipment and training, so they are not practical for routine assessments.

Body mass index (BMI) is a way to evaluate the weight of an adult. BMI is obtained by using the following formula. A value of 20 to 25 is optimal.

$$\text{BMI} = \text{Weight (in pounds)} \times 703 \div (\text{Height [in inches]})^2$$

Put On Your Thinking Cap!

Calculate your BMI and determine whether it falls in the optimal range.

A body shape index (ABSI) formula uses weight, height, and waist circumference to assess body weight and the risk for weight-related complications. The addition of waist measurement makes ABSI a better predictor of mortality than BMI alone.

Box 15.5 Recommendations for the Measurement of Height and Weight

HEIGHT

- Height should be measured without shoes.
- Feet should be together with the heels against the wall or measuring board.
- The subject should stand erect, neither slumped nor stretching, looking straight ahead, without tipping the head up or down. The top of the ear and outer corner of the eye should be in a line parallel to the floor.
- A horizontal bar, a rectangular block of wood, or the top of the stadiometer should be lowered to rest flat on the top of the head.
- Height should be read to the nearest ¼ inch or 0.5 cm.

WEIGHT

- Use a beam balance scale, not a spring scale, whenever possible.
- Periodically calibrate the scale for accuracy, using known weights.
- Weigh the subject in light clothing without shoes.
- Record weight to the nearest 1/2 pound or 0.2 kg. Measurements above the 90th or below the 10th percentile warrant further evaluation.

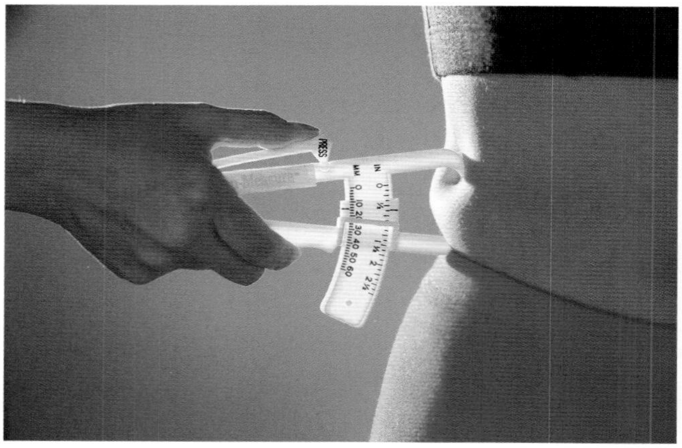

Fig. 15.4 Skinfold calipers measure in millimeters the thickness of the subcutaneous fat tissue, which gives a rough measurement of adiposity. (Copyright Comstock www.istock.com.)

BIOCHEMICAL ASSESSMENT: LABORATORY DATA

Among the laboratory tests that are helpful in assessing nutritional status are:

- Serum albumin: Protein depletion is one reason for low serum albumin. The normal serum albumin level is 3.5 to 5.0 g/dL.
- Total lymphocyte count (TLC): Protein and calorie deficits interfere with immune function, resulting in a low TLC. The normal lymphocyte count is 2500 mm^3. A count of less than 1500 mm^3 is consistent with protein/calorie malnutrition.
- Urine creatinine/height index: Expected urine creatinine, based on the patient's height, provides an estimate of skeletal muscle mass.
- Nitrogen balance: Nitrogen balance exists when nitrogen intake and excretion are equal. A patient who is in a state of starvation will excrete more nitrogen in the urine than consumed, creating a negative nitrogen balance.
- Mean corpuscular volume (MCV): MCV measures the size of red blood cells (RBCs). With different types of anemia, RBC size varies. Therefore when anemia is present, MCV helps to determine the type of anemia.
- Transferrin saturation: Transferrin is a protein that transports iron. Transferrin saturation is normally between 30% and 50%; less than 30% indicates anemia; more than 50% indicates iron overload.

DISORDERS ASSOCIATED WITH FOOD CONSUMPTION

OVERWEIGHT AND OBESITY

The prevalence of overweight and obesity is increasing in developed nations. Approximately one-third of adults in the United States are considered obese. The highest age-adjusted obesity rates are among non-Hispanic Black, followed by Hispanic, non-Hispanic White, and non-Hispanic Asian peoples. The rate of obesity is highest among adults 40 to 59 years of age.

A person with a BMI of 25.0 to 29.9 is considered overweight whereas **obesity** is defined as having a BMI of 30 or higher. Obesity is associated with coronary artery disease, stroke, lipid disorders, and type 2 diabetes mellitus. It is also considered a risk factor for some kinds of cancer and is associated with joint disease, gallstones, and respiratory problems. Some genes that predispose a person to obesity have been identified. It is possible that lifestyle factors activate these genes. Scientists are studying various other factors that might play a role in obesity.

Box 15.6 lists those factors that research has shown may contribute to obesity. This range of factors makes it clear that the prevention and treatment of obesity is extremely complex. It also helps to explain why most approaches that act on only one factor often fail to achieve significant weight loss.

The goal of treatment for obesity is to attain the best weight possible in the context of overall health. Patients tend to have unrealistic goals and may need encouragement to work toward a more modest goal

Box 15.6 Factors Under Study in Relation to Obesity

- Genetics
- Inadequate physical activity
- Inflammation
- Drugs such as steroids and antidepressants
- Sleep deprivation and disrupted circadian rhythms
- Stress
- Taste, **satiety** (feeling of fullness after eating) and excessive portion sizes
- Disruption of normal lipid metabolism by obesogens
- Some pathogens
- Gut microflora and diet

From Mahan LK, Raymond J: *Krause's food and the nutrition care process*, ed 14, St. Louis, MO, 2017, Elsevier.

of 5% to 10% body weight loss. For a person with a BMI of 27 to 35, the recommended goal is a weekly loss of 0.5 to 1.0 pounds for a period of 6 months followed by 6 months of maintenance. Individuals with a BMI greater than 35 should aim for a loss of 1 to 2 lb/week.

Management of Obesity

Weight management requires balancing energy intake and energy expenditure. Elements of a weight loss program are lifestyle modifications, dietary modification, and physical activity. Lifestyle modifications focus on the patient's environment, nutritional intake, and physical activity. In general, reduction in body fat is best achieved with adequate protein intake and a reduction of saturated fats, refined sugar, and calories along with an increase in physical activity.

Lifestyle Modifications. Strategies for modifying a person's lifestyle include goal setting, stimulus control, cognitive restructuring, problem solving, and relapse prevention. The patient must accept responsibility for making the changes. **Stimulus control** focuses on the settings or chain of events that precede eating, the kinds of foods consumed, and the consequences of eating. Patients are encouraged to eat slowly, perhaps putting the utensil down between bites or chewing each bite a specific number of times. This allows time for the patient to perceive and recognize satiety cues.

Problem solving for weight loss is much like the nursing process. Problems with food intake are identified, possible interventions in the form of new behaviors are generated, then implemented. The outcome of the intervention is evaluated and may be continued or replaced by another.

Because negative thoughts often undermine weight loss efforts, **cognitive restructuring** is used to teach patients to identify, challenge, and correct those thoughts. A journal noting place and time of eating, food intake, accompanying thoughts and feelings, and physical activity can be helpful in understanding how all of these factors are related. Structured behavioral therapy programs can be effective; however, long-term follow-up is usually needed to maintain results. Ongoing contact with the therapist can occur via telephone, mail, e-mail, or texting. Technology is gaining acceptance as a professional communication tool.

Dietary Modifications. Food choice changes are vital for weight loss. Combined with lifestyle changes and exercise, it may be sufficient for some obese people to lose weight. Others may require the addition of drug therapy or, for morbidly obese persons, surgical intervention.

A balanced, restricted-calorie diet must be individualized but generally consists of

- 50% to 55% carbohydrates from vegetables, fruits, beans, and whole grains
- 15% to 25% protein
- Extra fiber
- 30% or less fat
- Limited alcohol and foods high in sugar

Artificial sweeteners can be used if desired. Vitamin and mineral supplements are needed in males with an intake of less than 1800 calories and females with a daily intake of less than 1200 calories.

Physical Activity. A minimum of 30 minutes of moderate activity each day is recommended. Moderate activity is defined by the 2020–2025 Dietary Guidelines for Americans as activity equivalent to walking 1.5 to 3 miles/day at 3 to 4 miles/h in addition to activity involved in activities of daily living.

Drug Therapy. Patients with a BMI of 30 or higher or those with significant risk factors or disease may be prescribed drug therapy along with the lifestyle, dietary, and activity modifications. In general, drug benefits are described as "modest." Weight loss drugs have a discouraging history of new drugs being introduced and then withdrawn because of adverse effects. For that reason, you may see some of these drugs discontinued and new ones approved. Several prescription antiobesity drugs are available as of 2020: orlistat (Alli, Xenical), naltrexone/bupropion (Contrave), diethylpropion, phentermine, phentermine with topiramate (Osymia), and liraglutide (Saxenda). Information about these drugs is summarized in Table 15.1. Surgical options to treat obesity are addressed in Chapter 39.

UNDERWEIGHT

The underweight person is one whose weight is 15% to 20% or more below accepted weight standards. This circumstance may be caused by food intake insufficient to meet activity needs, excessive activity, poor

Table 15.1 Drug Table: Antiobesity Drugs

DRUG	ACTION	ADVERSE EFFECTS	COMMENTS
orlistat (Xenical, Alli)	Reduces absorption of fat in the digestive tract by inhibiting enzymes that break down fats	Oily rectal leakage, flatulence with discharge, fecal urgency, fatty or oily stools. Rarely, severe liver damage, acute pancreatitis, kidney stones.	Affects absorption of fat soluble vitamins so supplements may be needed. Supplement should be taken at least 2 hours apart from orlistat. Can intensify anticoagulant effect of warfarin.
naltrexone/ bupropion (Contrave)	Weight loss mechanism not known	Nausea, vomiting, constipation, headache, dizziness, insomnia. Suicide risk.	Contraindicated in patients taking other products containing bupropion. Not recommended for eating disorders.
diethylpropion, phentermine	Stimulate CNS to suppress appetite	Increased alertness, nervousness, insomnia, tachycardia, angina pain, hypertension.	Some risk for abuse. Tolerance may occur. Phentermine is Pregnancy Category Risk X.
phentermine with topiramate (Qsymia)	Suppresses appetite and induces sense of satiety	Dry mouth, constipation, altered taste, nausea, blurred vision, dizziness, insomnia, numbness and paresthesia in limbs. Can cause birth defects, acidosis, hypertension, and tachycardia.	Increased risk of hypoglycemia with insulin. May be prescribed for long-term use.
liraglutide injection (Saxenda)	Works on area of the brain that regulates appetite; reduces hunger	Most serious side effects: possible thyroid tumors (including cancer), pancreatitis, gallbladder problems, hypoglycemia in people taking drugs for type 2 diabetes, tachycardia, kidney failure, serious allergic reactions, depression, thoughts of suicide. Numerous other common side effects.	Should be used with a reduced-calorie meal plan and increased physical activity. Be aware of drug-drug interactions. Contraindicated in pregnancy and people with specific medical diagnoses.

Data for orlistat, diethylpropion and phentermine, naltrexone/bupropion, and phentermine with topiramate from Burchum JR, Rosenthal LD: *Lehne's pharmacology for nursing care*, ed 10, St. Louis, 2019, Elsevier. Data for liraglutide injection retrieved from https://www.saxenda.com/learn-about-saxenda/how-it-works.html.

Table 15.2 Nutrition Support Indications and Methods

CONDITION REQUIRING NUTRITIONAL SUPPORT	FEEDING METHODS
Enteral Nutrition	
Inability to eat Inability to eat enough Impaired digestion, absorption, metabolism	Nasogastric tube Nasoduodenal tube Nasojejunal tube Gastrostomy Jejunostomy
Parenteral Nutrition	
Gastrointestinal incompetency Critical illness with poor enteral tolerance or accessibility	Peripherally inserted central catheter "Tunneled" long-term catheter

absorption and use of food consumed, a wasting disease, or psychologic or emotional stress.

NUTRITIONAL DELIVERY METHODS FOR FEEDING PROBLEMS

NUTRITIONAL SUPPORT WITH SUPPLEMENTAL FEEDINGS

The preferred method of meeting nutritional requirements is through eating a balanced diet. However, when a person's nutritional needs cannot be met by oral feeding, some type of nutritional supplement is required. These supplements can be formulated using liquid or powdered milk, powdered whole eggs, and powdered egg albumin as concentrated protein sources. Commercially prepared products like Ensure and Boost can provide extra nutrients in a convenient way. Liquid feedings can meet the nutritional requirements of patients who are unable to take solid food. Table 15.2 summarizes the situations that might require artificial feeding. Nursing care of patients receiving enteral and parenteral feedings is addressed in Chapter 37.

Enteral Tube Feedings

Patients who are unable to take in supplemental liquid feedings orally may require enteral tube feedings. Enteral feedings bypass the mouth and deliver nutrients directly into the stomach or small intestine through an inserted tube or catheter. Conditions that interfere with taking in liquids orally include oral surgery, gastrointestinal (GI) surgery, dysphagia (difficulty swallowing), unconsciousness, anorexia, or esophageal obstruction. The tubes can be inserted into the stomach, duodenum, or jejunum through the nose or through the abdominal wall (Fig. 15.5).

A variety of formulas are used for enteral feedings. The standard formula provides for the nutritional requirements of most people. Special formulas are available for individuals who require less volume, require extra protein for healing, have poor kidney function or pulmonary disease, or are in critical care. Enteral tube

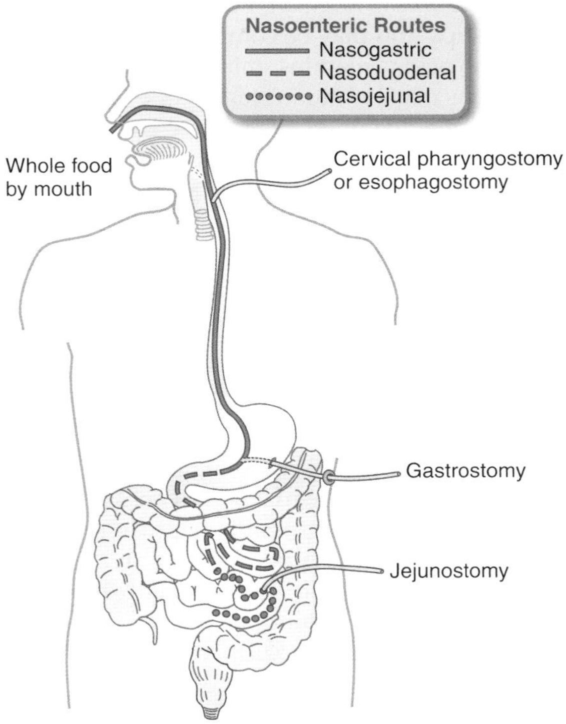

Fig. 15.5 Diagram of the placement of enteral feeding tubes. (From Mahan LK, Raymond JL: *Krause's food and the nutrition care process*, ed 14, St. Louis MO, 2017, Elsevier.)

feedings may cause complications such as nasal irritation and erosion, sinusitis, pharyngeal or vocal cord paralysis, nausea or vomiting, diarrhea, GI bleeding, aspiration pneumonia, hyperkalemia (excessive serum potassium), hyponatremia (serum sodium deficit), hyperglycemia (elevated blood glucose), or nutritional deficiencies. Dumping syndrome may occur when hypertonic fluid enters the jejunum; water is drawn into the lumen of the intestine to dilute the fluid, causing a drop in circulating blood volume. Tube blockage can occur, most likely caused by viscous formulas with inadequate flushing, crushed medications, and incompatible medications that form clumps. Enteral feedings are generally preferred over parenteral nutrition (described next) which poses more risks of complications and is more expensive.

Parenteral Nutrition

Another method of administering nutrients is through parenteral nutrition, in which nutrients are delivered directly into the bloodstream. The two major types of parenteral nutrition are (1) peripheral parenteral nutrition (PPN) and (2) central parenteral nutrition (CPN) or total parenteral nutrition (TPN). PPN is given through the peripheral veins in the arms and legs and may use a peripheral venous catheter or a peripherally inserted central catheter. CPN or TPN is given through a central vein, with the catheter usually in the superior vena cava. This method is used for nutrition only if the GI tract cannot be used; it can be lifesaving.

Peripheral parenteral nutrition. PPN is the standard intravenous therapy and may be composed of dextrose (5%–10%), amino acids, vitamins, minerals, and electrolytes. Fat emulsions may be administered peripherally as well. Total nutritional requirements usually are not met with PPN therapy and at most it supplies 1800 kcal/day. It is used primarily for short-term nutritional support.

Total parenteral nutrition. CPN or TPN feedings are used for patients who are unable to obtain adequate nutrition enterally or with PPN. They are usually debilitated and malnourished, with a weight loss of 10% of body weight or more.

TPN can meet the high-energy and high-protein needs of burn patients. It can also be used for patients with cancer who have become malnourished as a result of oncologic treatments. TPN can supply up to 4000 kcal/day, which is possible because the solution is administered into the superior vena cava, where the hypertonic solution can be diluted rapidly by the large, fast-flowing volume of blood.

Patients who are being fed parenterally should be monitored closely for any signs of complications. Potential complications include pulmonary complications, injury to the veins and arteries surrounding the TPN catheter site, air embolism, infection, electrolyte imbalance, mineral deficiencies, hyperglycemia, and, if treatment is ended suddenly, rebound hypoglycemia.

TRANSITIONAL FEEDING

When patients are ready to be changed from one of these feeding methods to another, they are ready for transitional feeding. Transitional feeding can be from parenteral nutrition to enteral tube feeding or oral intake, from enteral tube feeding to oral formula or food, or a combination of these.

Transitional feeding should be done gradually and with specific principles in mind. If patients who have been without adequate food for an extended period are given food too quickly, they may develop nutritional recovery syndrome. This syndrome causes hypophosphatemia (deficiency of phosphates in the blood) from the shift of phosphorus from the plasma into the cells. This shift may also affect potassium as it moves into cells with the glucose during refeeding.

Refeeding of the malnourished patient disrupts the adaptive state of starvation and therefore must proceed slowly with close patient monitoring. The ideal early feeding appears to be moderate in carbohydrates, low in sodium, lactose free, and supplemented with phosphorus and potassium.

When moving from parenteral to oral or enteral feeding, continuing the parenteral feeding is important, which allows for maintenance of adequate nutrient and fluid intake as tolerance of enteral feedings is assessed. As the patient is able to tolerate the oral or enteral feedings, the parenteral feedings can be tapered off.

When moving from enteral to oral feedings, the patient may complain of a poor appetite. In making this transition, changing the enteral feeding from a continuous drip to an intermittent feeding may be helpful. In this way, the patient has a chance to get hungry between feedings and desire for food may increase.

MEDICAL NUTRITION THERAPY

The relationship between nutrition and disease prevention and treatment has become increasingly clear. Medical nutrition therapy (MNT) encompasses assessment, nutrition diagnosis, interventions, and evaluation of persons with established disease. Whereas nurses are accustomed to categories of diets that are commonly

Box 15.7 Diet Progression and Therapeutic Diets

Clear liquid: Clear fat-free broth, bouillon, coffee, tea, carbonated beverages, clear fruit juices, gelatin, fruit ices, popsicles

Full liquid: As for clear liquid, with addition of smooth-textured dairy products (e.g., ice cream), strained or blended cream soups, custards, refined cooked cereals, vegetable juice, pureed vegetables, all fruit juices, sherbets, puddings, frozen yogurt

Pureed: As for clear liquid, with addition of scrambled eggs; pureed meats, vegetables, and fruits; mashed potatoes and gravy

Mechanical soft: As for clear and full liquid and pureed, with addition of all cream soups, ground or finely diced meats, flaked fish, cottage cheese, cheese, rice, potatoes, pancakes, light breads, cooked vegetables, cooked or canned fruits, bananas, soups, peanut butter, eggs (not fried)

Soft/low residue: Addition of low-fiber, easily digested foods such as pastas, casseroles, moist tender meats, and canned cooked fruits and vegetables; desserts, cakes, and cookies without nuts or coconut

High fiber: Addition of fresh uncooked fruits, steamed vegetables, bran, oatmeal, and dried fruits

Low sodium: 4-g (no added salt), 2-g, 1-g, or 500-mg sodium diets; vary from no-added salt to severe sodium restriction (500-mg sodium diet), which requires selective food purchases

Low cholesterol: 300 mg/day cholesterol, in keeping with American Heart Association guideline for serum lipid reduction

Diabetic: Nutrition recommendations by the American Diabetes Association: focus on total energy, nutrient and food distribution; include a balanced intake of carbohydrates, fats, and proteins; varied caloric recommendations to accommodate patient's metabolic demands.

Regular: No restrictions, unless specified

From Stockert PA: Nutrition. In: Potter PA, Perry AG, Stockert PA, Hall AM, editors: *Fundamentals of nursing*, ed 9, St. Louis, Elsevier/Mosby.

Table 15.3 System Changes in the Older Adult That Affect Nutrition

SYSTEM/FUNCTION	CHANGES
Sensory	Senses of taste, smell, sight, hearing, and touch are diminished. There are a decreased number of taste buds and a decreased sensitivity to sweet and salty tastes. Patient may experience glossodynia (pain in the tongue).
Gastrointestinal	Changes in appetite response contribute to anorexia. Ill-fitting dentures and periodontal disease make eating painful. Decreased salivary secretion decreases the ability to chew and swallow foods. Decreased acid secretion causes an overgrowth of the bacteria of the gut. Lack of intrinsic factor leads to decreased absorption of vitamin B_{12}. There is an increased incidence of gallbladder disease; decreased motility of intestines leads to constipation.
Metabolic	Decreased tolerance to glucose leads to an increase in plasma glucose levels. Basal metabolic rate decreases by 20% caused by decrease in lean body mass.
Cardiovascular	Blood vessels become less elastic. Total peripheral resistance increases. There is an increased risk for hypertension.
Renal	Kidney function diminishes and the acid-base response to metabolic challenges is slowed. There is increased difficulty in handling excessive amounts of protein waste products.
Musculoskeletal	Progressive replacement of lean body mass by fat and connective tissue. Body protein is decreased by 30% to 40%. More fat is deposited on the trunk and around the visceral organs. Bone density is diminished and there is shortening of the spinal column.
Immunocompetence	The immune function declines with age. There is a diminished ability to fight infection.
Psychosocial	Many experience depression as a result of a sense of loss or of loss of loved ones, productivity, a sense of worth, mobility, income, and body image.

ordered in health care facilities (Box 15.7), diets for many conditions are more specific. Nutrition plans that might be ordered for individuals with various common disorders are discussed in the Disorders chapters.

NUTRITION FOR THE OLDER ADULT

AGE-RELATED CHANGES RELEVANT TO NUTRITION

Healthy eating is a lifelong commitment that pays particular benefits in the later years of life. Maintaining a good diet can help middle-aged and older people to maintain a high level of function and reduce the risks of chronic disease. Table 15.3 summarizes changes occurring with aging that are relevant to nutrition. Table 15.4 provides daily nutritional goals for age-sex groups based on DRIs and dietary guidelines recommendations.

ENERGY

Because of the normal decline in metabolism and common decrease in physical activity, energy needs are reduced with age. Therefore the older person often reduces the calories taken in per day. This reduction can result in an inadequate intake of other essential nutrients. The recommended daily energy intake for light to moderately active older adults is 30 kcal/kg of body weight. This level reflects a reduction of 600 kcal/day for older men and 300 kcal/day for older women. However, the lifestyle and health status of older adults vary widely, and these figures may need adjustment for each individual. Nutrients such as proteins, carbohydrates, lipids, vitamins, minerals, and water may need adjustment for the older person (Table 15.5). Persons who are less active require less than the usual recommended amounts of thiamine, riboflavin, and niacin. Some experts recommend daily multivitamin-mineral supplements because the average American diet often lacks sufficient amounts of these nutrients. Contrary to popular belief, vitamin supplements do not provide energy or slow the aging process. However, there is evidence that patients with macular degeneration and colorectal polyps can benefit from specific supplements. Otherwise, there is not sufficient evidence to claim that supplements prevent various chronic diseases.

Psychosocial factors also may lead to poor nutrition in the older person. Depression, cognitive impairment, and loneliness can affect appetite and the intake of food. The term *failure to thrive* has been applied to older adults who are undernourished, depressed, and declining physically and cognitively. Failure to thrive has been attributed to organic and nonorganic factors. This phenomenon is the subject of study to determine how to identify reversible conditions and how best to intervene.

NUTRITIONAL CARE OF THE OLDER ADULT

Dietary Planning

Dietary planning for the older adult is no different from planning for a younger adult. Meals need to be appealing, taking into consideration individual likes and dislikes, and should be tasteful and filling. Planning may be different for older adults with special needs. Some prefer four or five small meals over three large ones. In addition, problems such as difficulty swallowing, dentures that do not fit properly, and arthritis, which makes using utensils uncomfortable, must be considered.

Table 15.4 Dietary Guidelines for Americans Daily Nutritional Goals for Age-Sex Groups Based on Dietary Reference Intakes and Dietary Guidelines Recommendations

MACRONUTRIENTS, MINERALS & VITAMINS		AGE-SEX GROUPS												
		M/F 2-3	F 4-8	F 9-13	F 14-18	F 19-30	F 31-50	F 51+	M 4-8	M 9-13	M 14-18	M 19-30	M 31-50	M 51+
Calorie Level Assessed	Source of Goal[a]	1,000	1,200	1,600	1,800	2,000	1,800	1,600	1,400	1,800	2,200	2,400	2,200	2,000
Macronutrients														
Protein (% kcal)	AMDR	5-20	10-30	10-30	10-30	10-35	10-35	10-35	10-30	10-30	10-30	10-35	10-35	10-35
Protein (g)	RDA	13	19	34	46	46	46	46	19	34	52	56	56	56
Carbohydrate (% kcal)	AMDR	45-65	45-65	45-65	45-65	45-65	45-65	45-65	45-65	45-65	45-65	45-65	45-65	45-65
Carbohydrate (g)	RDA	130	130	130	130	130	130	130	130	130	130	130	130	130
Fiber (g)	14g/1,000 kcal	14	17	22	25	28	25	22	20	25	31	34	31	28
Added Sugars (% kcal)	DGA	<10	<10	<10	<10	<10	<10	<10	<10	<10	<10	<10	<10	<10
Total lipid (% kcal)	AMDR	30-40	25-35	25-35	25-35	20-35	20-35	20-35	25-35	25-35	25-35	20-35	20-35	20-35
Saturated Fatty Acids (% kcal)	DGA	<10	<10	<10	<10	<10	<10	<10	<10	<10	<10	<10	<10	<10
18:2 Linoleic acid (g)	AI	7	10	10	11	12	12	11	10	12	16	17	17	14
18:3 Linoleic acid (g)	AI	0.7	0.9	1.0	1.1	1.1	1.1	1.1	0.9	1.2	1.6	1.6	1.6	1.6
Minerals														
Calcium (mg)	RDA	700	1,000	1,300	1,300	1,000	1,000	1,200	1,000	1,300	1,300	1,000	1,000	1,000[b]
Iron (mg)	RDA	7	10	8	15	18	18	8	10	8	11	8	8	8
Magnesium (mg)	RDA	80	130	240	360	310	320	320	130	240	410	400	420	420
Phosphorus (mg)	RDA	460	500	1,250	1,250	700	700	700	500	1,250	1,250	700	700	700
Potassium (mg)	AI	2,000	2,300	2,300	2,300	2,600	2,600	2,600	2,300	2,500	3,000	3,400	3,400	3,400
Sodium (mg)	CDRR	1,200	1,500	1,800	2,300	2,300	2,300	2,300	1,500	1,800	2,300	2,300	2,300	2,300
Zinc (mg)	RDA	3	5	8	9	8	8	8	5	8	11	11	11	11
Vitamins														
Vitamin A (mcg RAE[d])	RDA	300	400	600	700	700	700	700	400	600	900	900	900	900
Vitamin E (mg AT[d])	RDA	6	7	11	15	15	15	15	7	11	15	15	15	15
Vitamin D (IU[d])	RDA	600	600	600	600	600	600	600	600	600	600	600	600	600
Vitamin C (mg)	RDA	15	25	45	65	75	75	75	25	45	75	90	90	90
Thiamin (mg)	RDA	0.5	0.6	0.9	1.0	1.1	1.1	1.1	0.6	0.9	1.2	1.2	1.2	1.2
Riboflavin (mg)	RDA	0.5	0.6	0.9	1.0	1.1	1.1	1.1	0.6	0.9	1.3	1.3	1.3	1.3

Table 15.4 Dietary Guidelines for Americans Daily Nutritional Goals for Age-Sex Groups Based on Dietary Reference Intakes and Dietary Guidelines Recommendations—cont'd

MACRONUTRIENTS,		AGE-SEX GROUPS												
MINERALS & VITAMINS		**M/F**	**F**	**F**	**F**	**F**	**F**	**F**	**M**	**M**	**M**	**M**	**M**	**M**
Niacin (mg)	RDA	6	8	12	14	14	14	14	8	12	16	16	16	16
Vitamin B-6 (mg)	RDA	0.5	0.6	1.0	1.2	1.3	1.3	1.5	0.6	1.0	1.3	1.3	1.3	1.7
Vitamin B-12 (mcg)	RDA	0.9	1.2	1.8	2.4	2.4	2.4	2.4	1.2	1.8	2.4	2.4	2.4	2.4
Choline (mg)	AI	200	250	375	400	425	425	425	250	375	550	550	550	550
Vitamin K (mcg)	AI	30	55	60	75	90	90	90	55	60	75	120	120	120
Folate (mcg DFE[d])	RDA	150	200	300	400	400	400	400	200	300	400	400	400	400

[a]AI = Adequate Intake, CDRR = Chronic Disease Risk Reduction Level, DGA = *Dietary Guidelines for Americans, 2020-2025* , RDA = Recommended Dietary Allowance.
[b]Calcium RDA for males ages 71+ years is 1,200 mg.
[c] Vitamin D RDA for males and females ages 71+ years is 800 IU.
[d]AT = alpha-tocopherol, DFE = Dietary Folate Equivalent, IU = International Units, RAE = Retinol Activity Equivalents.
Sources: Institute of Medicine. *Dietary Reference Intakes: The Essential Guide to Nutrient Requirements.* Washington, DC: The National Academies Press; 2006. Institute of Medicine. *Dietary Reference Intakes for Calcium and Vitamin D.* Washington, DC: The National Academies Press; 2011. National Academies of Sciences, Engineering, and Medicine. *Dietary Reference Intakes for Sodium and Potassium.* Washington, DC: The National Academies Press; 2019.

Table 15.5 Changes in the Nutritional Requirements for the Older Adult

NUTRIENT	CHANGES IN NEEDS	SPECIAL PROBLEMS
Protein	Need unchanged (0.8 g/kg) unless ill. Needs may increase with infection, altered gastrointestinal function, or chronic diseases that affect metabolism. Tend to rely mostly on meat, poultry, and eggs. Varied protein sources would provide additional vitamins, minerals, and fiber.	Protein-calorie undernutrition may be a special problem for older men who live alone.
Carbohydrate	Need less sugar, more complex carbohydrates. Complex carbohydrates should contribute 55% of calorie intake.	Reduced glucose tolerance, lactose intolerance.
Lipid	Same as younger adult (not more than 30% of total kilocalories).	Serum cholesterol levels in men tend to peak during middle age and then drop slightly; levels in women continue to rise with increasing age.
Minerals	The needs for trace elements may be reduced owing to decreased lean body mass; calcium intake of 1000–1500 mg/day for postmenopausal women.	Hypertension is common, which results in the need to decrease sodium and increase potassium and magnesium for those taking diuretics.
Vitamins	Vitamin A is sufficient in the older adult owing to stores in the liver; may require vitamin D supplement if patient is not exposed to sunlight; some require vitamin C supplements; vitamin B_6 and folate are maintained with normal diet; vitamin B_{12} may be deficient owing to loss of intrinsic factor.	A maintenance level multivitamin and mineral supplement may be required. Patient must be monitored closely for overdose. Check supplements for added sugars.
Water	30 to 35 mL/kg of ideal body weight. Older adults may restrict fluid intake because of problems with bladder control and mobility. Recommend unsweetened beverages and low-fat or fat-free milk.	Dehydration is the most common fluid and electrolyte disturbance. Patient must be monitored closely.

The diet should include all of the food groups. Severely restricted diets such as low-sodium and low-fat diets generally are not advised for older adults. When food is unappetizing, the older person may simply not eat enough to obtain necessary nutrients. The Patient Teaching box gives suggestions for teaching older patients about nutrition.

Patient Teaching

Nutrition for the Older Patient

In addition to general information about nutritional requirements, you should share the following with the older adult patient:

- A normal diet typically supplies adequate vitamins; however, a daily multivitamin may be recommended.
- Some dietary supplements can interact with medications.
- Megadoses (very large doses) of vitamins have not been proven to be beneficial and can be harmful.
- "Natural vitamins" are more expensive and there is no evidence that they are better than synthetic vitamins.
- Vitamins do not provide the body with more energy.

Nutrition Programs

Many community-based programs, administered by both public and private agencies, provide hot, nutritious meals to older adults. The meals are served either in a group setting or in the home. Special regulations and conditions must be met to qualify for these programs. Some other government resources are the Commodity Supplemental Food Program, Supplemental Nutrition Assistance Program (SNAP), Home Delivered Nutrition Services, and the Child and Adult Care Food Program (CACFP) that reimburses for nutritious meals and snacks for older adults in day care.

Nutritional Needs During Prolonged Illness

All people have increased nutritional needs during periods of illness. Older adults with chronic diseases such as emphysema and bronchitis, cancer, organic brain disease, cirrhosis, and maldigestion or malabsorption syndromes are at increased risk for protein deficiency and negative nitrogen balance. Individuals at risk need to be monitored very carefully for this condition, which can be prevented by increasing nutritional support. Enteral feedings or parenteral nutrition may be required to meet these increased needs.

Nutritional Care in Institutional Settings

Good nutrition can have a dramatic effect on the physical, mental, and emotional function of your older adult patients. Nurses in long-term care and home health settings must be especially vigilant in monitoring the nutritional status of older adult patients. Age-related changes, chronic and acute conditions, cognitive and emotional disorders, medications, and situational factors can contribute to inadequate nutritional intake, digestion, or elimination. Also patients who are obese have special needs. Excess body weight makes the task of controlling many chronic conditions more difficult and can greatly interfere with activities of daily living. The nutritional needs of older adults in institutional settings may change over time. Therefore periodic reassessment of nutritional status is critical to avoid imposing unnecessary diet restrictions or missing important nutritional needs.

Assisting older adult patients with meals must be a high priority. Have you ever seen a meal cart with trays that have barely been touched being returned to the kitchen? You should question why patients are not eating and implement nursing measures to improve the situation.

Put On Your Thinking Cap!

Interview an older person (a patient, family member, or other acquaintance) about how their eating habits have changed with age. Identify any changes that could lead to inadequate nutrition.

Get Ready for the NCLEX® Examination!

Key Points

- Dietary reference intakes (DRIs) include recommended daily allowances, estimated average requirements, adequate intake, and tolerable upper intake level.
- A lack of adequate carbohydrates can cause ketosis characterized by breakdown of tissue protein, loss of sodium and other cations, and dehydration.
- Less than 10% of daily calories should come from saturated fats.
- Protein must be eaten each day because the body cannot store it.
- Signs of protein deficiency include edema, wasting, thickening and hardening of the skin, diminished immune response, weakness, and lack of energy.
- A lactovegetarian diet includes dairy products but excludes meat, fish, poultry, and eggs.
- A lacto-ovo-vegetarian diet includes dairy products and eggs but excludes meat, fish, and poultry.
- A vegan consumes no foods of animal origin and must plan the diet carefully to avoid nutritional deficiencies.
- A nutritional assessment includes a dietary history, anthropometric data, laboratory data (if available), and physical examination data.
- Signs of malnutrition include dull, thin, and sparse hair; pale conjunctiva; a swollen face; swollen lips and tongue; teeth with cavities or missing teeth; and bleeding or receding gums.
- Skinfold thickness and hydrostatic weighing are done to determine the ratio of fat to lean muscle mass.
- Body mass index is calculated with the body weight and height; the ideal BMI is 20 to 25.
- A patient in a state of starvation excretes more nitrogen than consumed, creating a negative nitrogen balance.
- A person with a BMI of 25.0 to 29.9 is considered overweight whereas obesity is defined as having a BMI of 30 or higher.
- Obesity is a risk factor for numerous health problems.
- Weight loss requires lifestyle modifications, dietary modifications, and physical activity.
- Strategies for modifying one's lifestyle include goal setting, stimulus control, cognitive restructuring, problem solving, and relapse prevention.
- Weight loss drugs generally have modest benefits.
- The underweight person is one whose weight is 15% to 20% below accepted standards.
- Enteral feedings deliver nutrients directly into the stomach or small intestine for patients who cannot take oral feedings.
- Complications of enteral feedings can include nasal irritation, sinusitis, pharyngeal or vocal cord paralysis, nausea or vomiting, diarrhea, GI bleeding, aspiration pneumonia, electrolyte imbalances, hyperglycemia, and nutrition deficiencies.
- Dumping syndrome is hypotension caused by the administration of hypertonic fluid that draws water into the intestines.
- Parenteral nutrition delivers nutrients directly into the bloodstream.
- Central and total parenteral nutrition are given through a central vein; peripheral parenteral nutrition is given through a vein in the extremities.
- Peripheral parenteral nutrition is used short-term because it does not supply all nutritional requirements.
- Transitional feedings from one method to another must be done gradually to prevent nutritional recovery syndrome with hypophosphatemia and possible hypokalemia.
- Energy needs are reduced with age.
- Vitamin supplements do not increase energy or slow the aging process.

Additional Learning Resources

SG Go to your Study Guide for additional learning activities to help you master this chapter content.

Go to your Evolve website (http://evolve.elsevier.com/Linton/medsurg) for the following learning resources and much more:

- Fluid & Electrolyte Tutorial
- Review Questions for the NCLEX® Examination

Clinical Judgment and Next-Generation NCLEX® Examination-Style Questions

1. **The 2020–2025 Dietary Guidelines for Americans recommends that which nutrient(s) should be restricted to less than 10% of the daily calorie intake? (Select all that apply.)**
   1. Added sugar
   2. Saturated fats
   3. Incomplete protein
   4. Whole grains
   5. Raw vegetables

   NCLEX Client Need: Physiological Integrity: Basic Care and Comfort

2. **Which of the following nutrients yields the highest number of kilocalories per gram?**
   1. Protein
   2. Fat
   3. Carbohydrate

   NCLEX Client Need: Physiological Integrity: Basic Care and Comfort

3. **A nursing student is teaching a patient how to read the nutrition label on a canned product. The label reads: Daily value 20% Vitamin A. The patient asks what that means. Which of the following is the most accurate reply?**
   1. The contents of this can contain 20% of the recommended daily intake of vitamin A.
   2. The amount of vitamin A in the can exceeds the recommended daily amount by 20%.
   3. One serving of this product provides 20% of the recommended daily intake of vitamin A.
   4. The contents of the can do not meet standards for nutrient values.

   NCLEX Client Need: Physiological Integrity: Basic Care and Comfort

4. **Situation: The nurse is teaching older adults in the community about nutrition. Possible teaching points are listed in the table.**

   Use an X for the health teaching below that is Indicated (appropriate or necessary), Contraindicated (could be harmful), or Nonessential (makes no difference or not necessary).

   SLO/Objective: Plan content to teach older persons about their changes in nutrient needs.

   NGN Item Type: Matrix

   Cognitive skill: Generate Solutions

HEALTH TEACHING	INDI-CATED	CONTRAINDICATED	NONESSEN-TIAL
"It is best to eliminate all sodium from your diet.			
"If you are less active, you need fewer calories than when you were younger."			
"Monitor your blood pressure on a regular basis."			
"A megavitamin is recommended to meet nutritional requirements."			
"Try to maintain a BMI (body mass index) between 20 and 25."			

   NCLEX Client Need: Physiological Integrity: Basic Care and Comfort

5. **A patient reports that she is lactovegetarian. You know that her diet includes which of the following?**
   1. Eggs
   2. Fish
   3. Poultry
   4. Milk

   NCLEX Client Need: Physiological Integrity: Basic Care and Comfort

6. **When a patient is receiving total parenteral nutrition, the nurse must monitor for which of the following potential complications?**
   1. Vomiting
   2. Air embolism
   3. Hypoglycemia
   4. Aspiration

   NCLEX Client Need: Physiological Integrity: Reduction of Risk Potential

7. **A patient is being transitioned from parenteral nutrition to oral nutrition. The nurse should monitor for nutritional recovery syndrome, which is characterized by:**
   1. Hypophosphatemia
   2. Hypocalcemia
   3. Hyponatremia
   4. Hypoglycemia

   NCLEX Client Need: Physiological Integrity: Reduction of Risk Potential

8. Students have calculated their BMI. The results are listed subsequently. Which one is within the optimum range?

1. 18
2. 32
3. 28
4. 22

9. For patients trying to lose weight, cognitive restructuring may be used to:

1. Recognize triggers for overeating
2. Correct negative thoughts
3. Set attainable goals
4. Accept responsibility for eating habits

16 Intravenous Therapy

http://evolve.elsevier.com/Linton/medsurg

Objectives

1. List the indications for intravenous fluid therapy.
2. Describe the types of fluids used for intravenous fluid therapy.
3. Describe the types of venous access devices and other equipment used for intravenous therapy.
4. Given the prescribed hourly flow rate, calculate the correct drop rate for an intravenous fluid.
5. Explain the causes, signs and symptoms, and nursing implications of the complications of intravenous fluid or drug therapy.
6. Explain the nursing responsibilities when a patient is receiving intravenous therapy.
7. Identify intravenous medications that require dilution because they are vesicants or irritants.

Key Terms

cannula (KĂN-yū-lă)
embolism (ĔM-bō-lĭzm)
embolus (*pl.* emboli) (ĔM-bō-lŭs, ĔM-bō-lī)
extravasatio (ĕks-tră-vā-SĀ-shŭn)
hypertonic (hī-pĕr-TŎN-ĭk)
hypotonic (hī-pō-TŎN-ĭk)
infiltration (ĭn-fĭl-TRĀ-shŭn)
isotonic (ī-sō-TŎN-ĭk)
phlebitis (flĕ-BĪ-tĭs)
solution
thrombus (*pl.* thrombi) (THRŎM-bŭs)
tonicity (tō-NĬS-ĭ-tē)
vesicant (VĔS-ĭ-kănt)

Intravenous therapy is the administration of fluids directly into a vein. Most hospitalized patients receive some form of intravenous therapy. Home infusion of intravenous products has become common as well.

INDICATIONS FOR INTRAVENOUS THERAPY

Intravenous therapy is used to administer drugs, fluids (including nutrients), and blood or blood components. Intravenous administration of drugs may be ordered when a rapid drug effect is needed, when the drug is not available in an oral form, or when the patient is unable to take drugs by mouth. The intravenous route is also recommended when a drug must be maintained at a certain level in the blood.

In addition to drugs, intravenous fluids can provide water, normal saline, electrolytes, amino acids, lipids, vitamins, and glucose. Intravenous lines may also be used to provide continuous venous access for intermittent and emergency drug administration.

Whole blood and blood components are also given intravenously. Blood components include packed red blood cells, frozen red blood cells, platelets, and plasma proteins. Blood transfusions are discussed in Chapter 29.

TYPES OF INTRAVENOUS FLUIDS

By definition, a fluid is any liquid or gas. A **solution** is a liquid containing one or more dissolved substances. The terms *fluid* and *solution* are often used interchangeably in relation to intravenous therapy. Fluids that contain water and electrolytes and that can diffuse through a semipermeable membrane are called *crystalloids*. Fluids containing suspended substances, such as blood plasma, are called *colloids*.

TONICITY

Fluids can be classified by **tonicity**, a measure of the concentration of electrolytes in the fluid. The normal concentration of electrolytes in body fluids is approximately 285 milliequivalents per liter (mEq/L). Solutions that have the same concentration as body fluids are called **isotonic**. When the concentration of a solution is greater than 300 mEq/L, the solution is said to be **hypertonic**. **Hypotonic** solutions have a concentration of less than 280 mEq/L. The tonicity of fluids is important because it affects blood volume. Fluid that is hypertonic draws and retains water in the circulation, increasing the blood volume. Hypotonic fluid allows water to shift out of the capillaries into body tissues, resulting in decreased blood volume. See Chapter 6 for a thorough discussion of tonicity.

COMPONENTS

Many types of fluids are available for intravenous use. The health care provider selects the appropriate fluid to meet the patient's needs. The most commonly used intravenous solutions are specific combinations of water, sugar (in the form of dextrose), sodium chloride, and other electrolytes.

In most intravenous solutions, dextrose is the only source of calories. The patient receives 34 calories for each 1% of dextrose in a liter of fluid; thus 1 liter of 5% dextrose provides 170 calories ($34 \times 5 = 170$). Dextrose fluids given in a peripheral vein are 2.5%, 5.0%, or 10.0% dextrose. Fluids infused into a larger (central) vein may have a much higher percentage of dextrose.

Sodium chloride solutions are also commonly used. An isotonic solution is 0.9% sodium chloride and is called *normal saline*. It is used to supply balanced amounts of water and sodium chloride. A hypotonic solution of 0.45% sodium chloride may be ordered if the patient's body fluids are concentrated owing to excessive water loss. More concentrated hypertonic solutions are needed when the patient has had excessive losses of both sodium and chloride.

Dextrose, sodium chloride, and other electrolytes are available in numerous combinations. Some commonly used electrolyte solutions are Plasma-Lyte and lactated Ringer's solution. Dextrose 5% in Ringer's solution is a combined dextrose and electrolyte solution.

When a patient needs long-term or aggressive intravenous therapy for nutrition, total parenteral nutrition (TPN) may be indicated. A specialized catheter is placed in the distal superior vena cava for administering TPN. TPN fluids provide dextrose, water, amino acids, electrolytes, vitamins, and minerals. Fat emulsions can also be given intravenously. TPN is discussed in greater detail in Chapter 15.

Pharmacology Capsule

Always check the "six rights" when administering intravenous fluids.

TPN cannot be administered using a peripheral IV or midline IV!!!

VENOUS ACCESS DEVICES

Intravenous fluid is delivered by various types of venous access devices (Fig. 16.1). These devices include needles, over-the-needle catheters, inside-needle catheters (rarely used), subcutaneous infusion ports, and subcutaneously implanted pumps. The term **cannula** can be used to describe both a needle and a catheter. Cannula size is based on the inside diameter and is expressed as a *gauge*. The smaller the gauge is, the larger the inside diameter of the cannula is. Therefore a 14-gauge cannula is larger than a 22-gauge cannula.

The intravenous administration of fluids requires placement of the venous access device into a peripheral or central vein. Peripheral veins are located in the extremities (and in the scalp of an infant). They are used for short-term therapy, when a patient has healthy veins, and when relatively nonirritating or nonvesicant fluids are given.

Central veins, large vessels located nearer the heart, are used when long-term therapy is required, when the patient has poor peripheral veins, and when **vesicant** fluids or fluids that are irritating to vessels are administered. Central lines are inserted into the left or right subclavian or jugular or femoral veins, with the tip of the catheter resting in the superior vena cava. The line may be placed in the subclavian vein through venipuncture, inserted into a peripheral vein and advanced to the desired location, or inserted

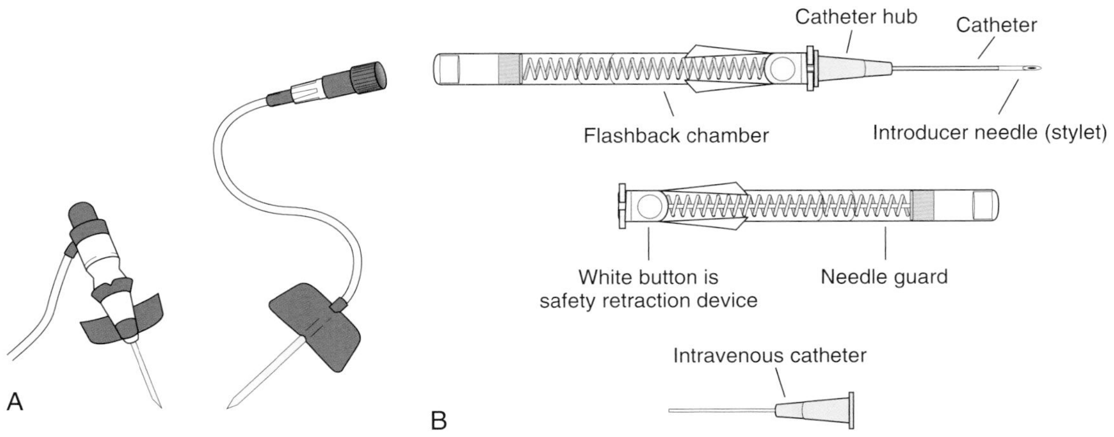

Fig. 16.1 Venous access devices. (A) Winged infusion needles. (B) Catheter. (From Potter PA, Perry AG, editors: *Fundamentals of nursing*, ed 8, St. Louis, 2013, Mosby.)

through a skin incision and tunneled under the skin and into the large vessel. Devices placed through a cutdown incision are called *percutaneous catheters*. The central line threaded through a peripheral vein is called a *peripherally inserted central catheter* (PICC). Examples of central venous tunneled catheters are the Hickman, Broviac, Groshong, Hickman-Broviac, and Raaf, and the implanted venous access ports. Fig. 16.2 shows common peripheral infusion sites for intravenous fluids.

A port is a device with a central catheter that is surgically implanted in the subcutaneous tissue. It consists of a venous catheter and a port through which fluids can be injected but it has no external parts (Fig. 16.3A). The catheter is inserted into a central vein and the port, which has a rubber septum, can be felt under the skin. A noncoring needle catheter that does not damage the septum is used to puncture the skin and access the port to deliver fluid and medications (Fig. 16.3B). A port requires less care and is less restrictive than other access devices but it does require a needle puncture for each infusion.

For therapy over a period of weeks to months, the percutaneous catheter or PICC is preferred. Midline catheters should only be used up to 29 days. Tunneled catheters, PICCs, and implanted ports are more appropriate for long-term use.

NEEDLES

One type of needle used is a winged ("butterfly") infusion needle, a short needle with two plastic wings that are held during insertion. A winged infusion needle is useful in infants when a scalp vein is used for intravenous therapy. It is also used at times in adults who have very poor or small veins, for one-time therapy, to draw blood samples, and for therapy of short duration (<24 hours).

To reduce the risk of bloodborne injuries acquired through needlesticks, various devices have been developed. One style has a self-sheathing stylet that retracts into a rigid chamber at the catheter hub after insertion; others use Luer-Lok connections rather than diaphragms that must be punctured with a needle. Concern about bloodborne pathogens has led to the development of various devices to reduce the risk of needlesticks. Among the products that make venipunctures safer for the nurse are safety needles that cover the needle after it has been used.

CATHETERS

A catheter is a small plastic tube that fits over a needle. After insertion into the vein, the needle is withdrawn, leaving the catheter in the vein. The tubing that will deliver the fluid is then connected to the plastic catheter, which remains in the vein. Catheters are less likely than needles to puncture the vein once they are in place. They come in a variety of lengths. Short catheters are only ¾ to 2 inches in length. Midline catheters are designed for therapy up to 4 weeks. Midline catheters are inserted above the antecubital region of the arm, in the middle upper section using the basilic, brachial, or

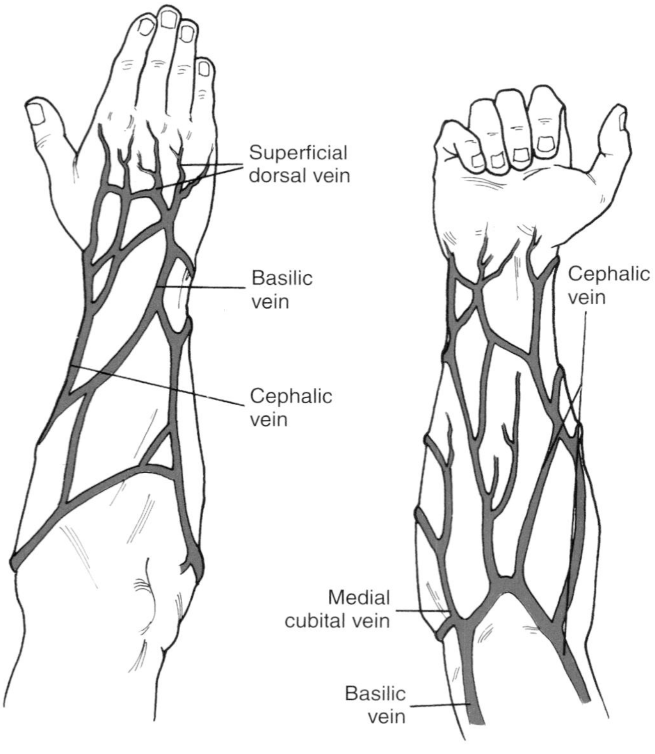

Fig. 16.2 Common peripheral intravenous infusion sites.

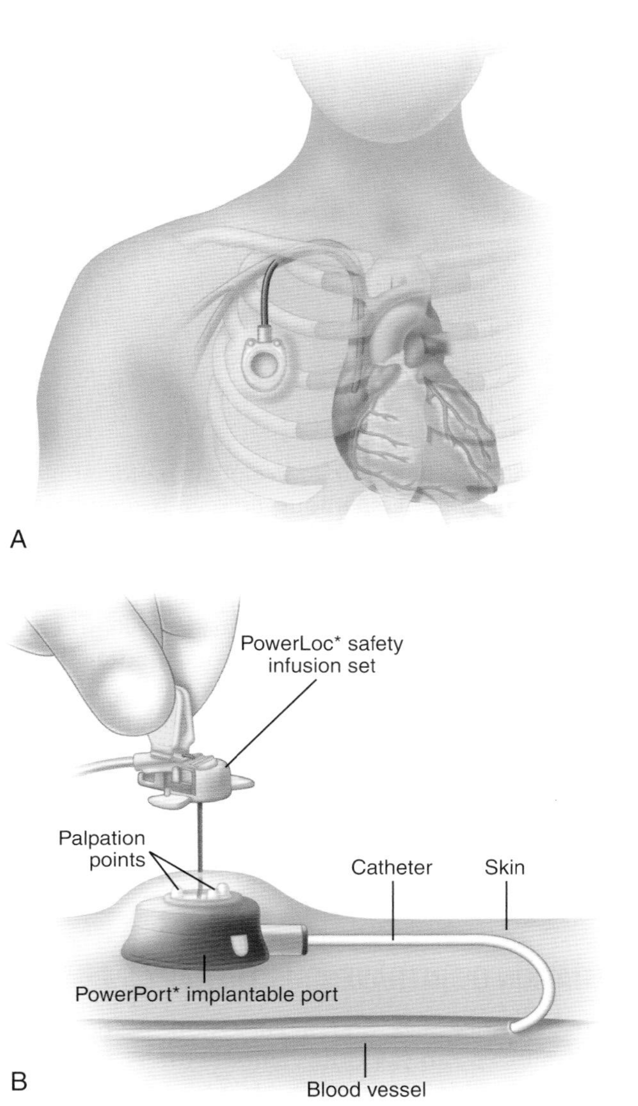

Fig. 16.3 (A) An implantable port in place. The entire unit is under the skin. (B) Injection of medication into the port. (From Ignatavicius DD, Workman ML, Blair M, et al: *Medical-surgical nursing: patient-centered collaborative care,* ed 8, St. Louis, 2016, Elsevier.)

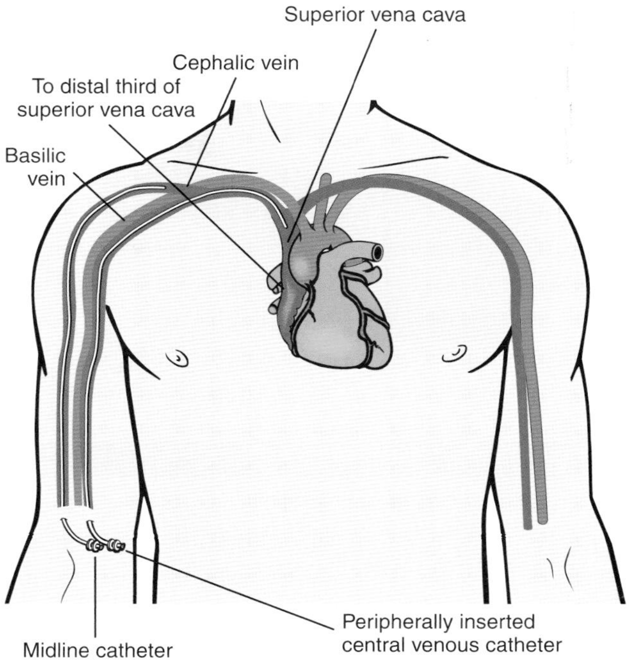

Fig. 16.4 A peripherally inserted central catheter. The exact placement depends on the type of fluid to be infused. The midline catheter extends only 3 to 10 inches into a larger vessel of the upper arm. (From Stevens A, Lowe J: *Pathology: illustrated review in color*, ed 2, London, 2000, Mosby-Elsevier.)

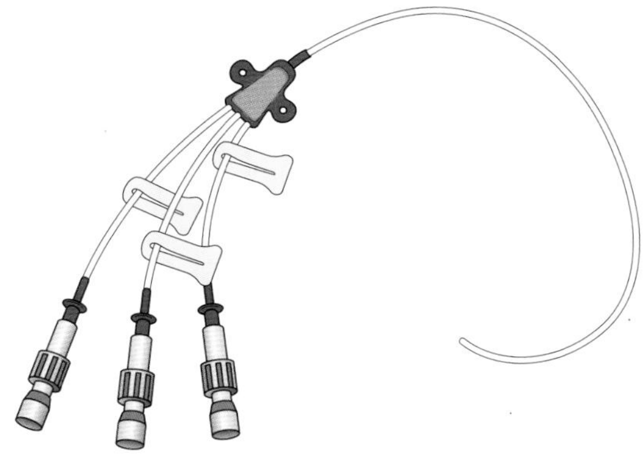

Fig. 16.5 A triple-lumen catheter.

cephalic vein, and are advanced preaxillary (Fig. 16.4). Nurses generally insert only short (¾- to 2-inch) catheters unless they receive special training.

A central catheter that can be inserted by trained nurses is the PICC (Fig. 16.4). The PICC is inserted into a vein in the middle upper arm space into the (1) basilic vein, (2) brachial vein, or (3) cephalic vein and the tip is advanced into the lower third part of the superior vena cava. Advantages of the PICC over other central catheters include easier insertion, cost savings, no risk of pneumothorax or hemothorax and very low risk of infection or air embolism. Compared with peripheral cannulas, PICCs can be left in place unless compromised (some have remained in place for more than 3 years without complication). PICCs do not restrict arm movement and are less traumatic to the vein. A variety of PICCs exist with single, dual, or triple lumens; some have combinations of regular and power lumens. A power-injectable PICC or lumen is needed for tests that require rapid (3–5 mL/s) infusion of contrast medium. A regular PICC cannot be used for such rapid infusions. Currently, most PICCs and midlines are power-injectable.

Subclavian catheters can have from one to four lumens. Fig. 16.5 depicts a triple-lumen catheter, which is essentially one catheter with three separate lumens. Each catheter has a port through which blood can be drawn. One port can be used to measure central venous pressure. The other ports can be used to administer drugs, fluids, or blood.

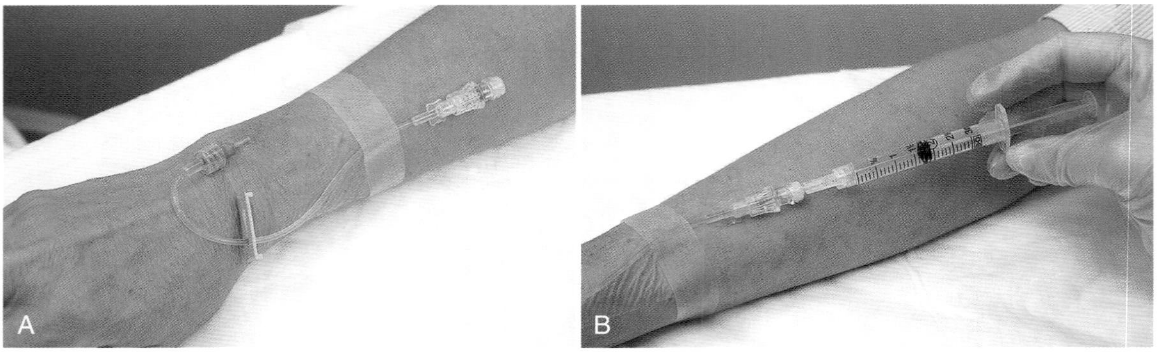

Fig. 16.6 (A.) Intravenous catheter with saline lock adapter. (B) Syringe inserted into injection port.

Put On Your Thinking Cap!

If each lumen in a triple lumen catheter is separate all the way to the end of the catheter, can noncompatible medications be administered at the same time?

IMPLANTED DEVICES

Some devices are implanted to allow immediate access to a vein without repeated, painful venipunctures. They include infusion ports, described earlier, pumps that are implanted under the skin, and external infusion pumps. Infusion ports consist of a catheter and a chamber into which fluids can be injected directly into a vein or an artery; they are also used for intraspinal infusions. The chamber is easily felt directly under the skin. Infusion pumps are filled using a noncoring needle that is inserted through the skin into the port. They dispense the fluid into the vein at a prescribed rate. Infusion pumps are always used to administer chemotherapy drugs for treating cancer and for TPN.

INTERMITTENT INFUSION DEVICES

Many patients need intravenous medications at specific intervals, such as every 4 or every 6 hours. Such drugs are often "piggybacked"; that is, the drug is given through an injection port in the tubing of a continuous infusion. An option for the patient who does not need continuous intravenous therapy is a resealable lock, sometimes called a *saline lock* or *heparin lock* (Fig. 16.6).

Pharmacology Capsule

A drug given "piggyback" is administered through the tubing of a continuous infusion using the injection port that is closest to the fluid bag. The injection port closer to the patient is used for intravenous push medications. If the patient does not need continuous fluids, an access port can be used to give the medication.

A resealable lock is a short cannula with an attached injection port. It is taped in place and medications are injected when needed through the port. It may be called either a saline lock or a heparin lock because it may be flushed with either saline or a dilute heparin solution after each use to keep clots from forming and blocking the catheter. Although research suggests that flushing with normal saline may be just as effective, less expensive, and safer than heparin, the use of heparin persists in some settings. One concern about the use of heparin is that it prolongs the time required for blood to clot whereas saline does not, avoiding, for example, heparin-induced thrombocytopenia. You must know the agency's procedure for flushing these devices and exactly what the licensed vocational nurse/licensed practical nurse (LVN/LPN) is permitted to do. Any intravenous cannula (needle or catheter) can be converted to intermittent administration by attaching a resealable, usually needleless cap, or an extension with a cap.

INITIATION OF INTRAVENOUS THERAPY

Nurse practice acts and agency policies determine which nurses can perform venipunctures, administer intravenous fluids, and give intravenous medications by various routes.

EQUIPMENT

To start intravenous fluids, gather the equipment needed to start the infusion: cannula (needle or catheter), tourniquet, alcohol swabs, skin cleansing solution, tape, dressing supplies, gloves, tubing, solution container, a pole to suspend the container, and possibly an infusion pump. The size of the cannula depends on the patient's condition and the type of fluid to be administered. Surgical patients and those receiving blood usually require an 18- or 20-gauge cannula. A 22-gauge cannula is appropriate for most adults receiving crystalloid fluids in ordinary circumstances. Smaller-gauge cannulas can be used in children, in adults with small veins, and for administration of most other nonirritating fluids. Read the product literature to identify any special requirements such as a filter or special tubing. Obtain the prescribed solution or drug using the "six rights": right solution or drug, right dose or strength, right patient, right route, right time, and right documentation. Attach tubing to the solution container, fill the drip chamber halfway, and allow some fluid to run through the tubing until the tubing is completely filled with fluid and there are no air bubbles in the tubing.

Pharmacology Capsule

The intravenous administration of nitroglycerin, blood, or fat emulsions requires special administration sets and is generally administered by RNs.

SITE SELECTION

Select the venipuncture site for the infusion. The site chosen should be the least restrictive (i.e., not over a joint or on the hand). It should have a large vein that is in good condition. A soft, straight vein is best. Avoid veins that are hard and bumpy, bruised, swollen, near previously infected areas, or close to a recently discontinued site. A transilluminator or portable ultrasound can facilitate locating a vein. The preferred site is usually the patient's nondominant arm. Begin with the most distal veins and then move proximally as needed so that you can use the same vein at a more proximal site. Venipuncture should not be performed in an arm that has impaired circulation or poor lymphatic drainage, as in a patient who has had a radical mastectomy. In addition, do not use an arm that has been affected by a stroke or has a shunt or fistula for hemodialysis. Although veins on the legs are accessible, they are not normally used in adults.

Put On Your Thinking Cap!

Why should you use the most distal site to start an intravenous infusion?

PROCEDURE

Gather all supplies and wash your hands thoroughly. Identify the patient and explain the procedure to them. Apply a tourniquet above the venipuncture site to distend the vein. Check the radial pulse to make sure that the tourniquet is not too tight thereby cutting off arterial flow. The tourniquet should be flat, at least ½-inch wide, not be so tight as to obstruct arterial blood flow, and is used on only one patient. Never place a tourniquet under clothing as it may be forgotten and left on the patient's extremity. A blood pressure cuff inflated just above the patient's diastolic pressure makes an excellent tourniquet and is less traumatic for fragile skin. After locating an appropriate vein, temporarily remove the tourniquet. Vigorously cleanse the venipuncture site in a circular pattern, first with alcohol and then with a recommended solution. Recommended cleansing solutions are different for each medical facility but may include chlorhexidine or 70% isopropyl alcohol. Chlorhexidine is considered to be the best choice and the standard in most facilities. Between 1% and 2% tincture of iodine is rarely used, but if the patient is allergic to iodine, cleanse with alcohol only. Allow the site to air dry after each cleansing step. Do not blow on the site or fan it. Reapply the tourniquet and put on gloves.

Some facilities are also using ultrasound to check the size of a vein before the tourniquet is placed on the patient. This approach, however, requires advanced training. Using ultrasound is an option worth considering, particularly with patients who have had multiple intravenous attempts and are difficult candidates for peripheral intravenous placements.

1. Perform the venipuncture using standard precautions. Carefully insert the cannula through the skin and guide it into the vein in the direction of blood flow. The first puncture through the skin will flatten the vein, moving it out of the way. After the tip of the needle has penetrated the skin, a slight upper lift evenly of the entire needle equally will bring the vein back into alignment with the needle being inserted. The even lift on the entire catheter with the needle still in the catheter will also elongate the vessel, making it less likely to pass the catheter through the entire vein. Apply traction to the vein using the nondominant hand and maintain traction until the cannula is advanced all the way into the vein.
2. After seeing the "flash" of blood, advance the needle only far enough into the site to allow the tapered tip of the cannula to be placed just inside the vein and over the needle tip and no more. Then advance the cannula, which will slide over the needle. Once the cannula has been advanced all the way to the hub, release traction on the vein and pull the needle out of the cannula and discard.
3. After threading the cannula into the vein, connect it to the infusion tubing. Check for a continuous flow of fluids first, then tape the cannula securely without restricting circulation. Be careful to avoid contaminating the open hub of the cannula. Do not apply tape to the site where the cannula enters the skin.

In accordance with your agency policies and procedures, dress the site with a clear occlusive dressing that allows inspection of the insertion site or with a sterile gauze pad. On peripheral sites, dressings are changed per facility protocol. Dressings on central lines are changed per facility protocol also. Some agencies may use antimicrobial barrier patches that fit around the cannula and under the dressing. The application of antibiotic ointment to the insertion site is controversial. Antibiotic ointments without antifungals have been associated with *Candida* infections. PICC and other central lines may have dressings that use a biopatch (e.g., BioPatch). These dressings are changed per facility protocol, usually every 7 days. Of course, if the dressing is compromised for any reason, immediate attention is required, regardless of how long the dressing has been in place.

Put On Your Thinking Cap!

What's wrong with this picture? A nurse preparing to start intravenous therapy tears strips of tape and sticks them on the edge of the bedside table. The nurse cleanses the site with chlorhexidine and blows on the site to hasten drying.

PAIN

Venipuncture and cannula placement can be painful. Clinicians are seeking measures to reduce the discomfort without making the procedure more difficult than it normally is. Drugs that have been used to decrease the pain of venipuncture include intradermal lidocaine (Xylocaine), transdermal lidocaine, and prilocaine (EMLA cream). Each of these measures has some disadvantages. Intradermal lidocaine may cause vasospasm, allergic reactions, and anaphylaxis. Both lidocaine and EMLA cream must be applied and covered with an occlusive dressing for 60 minutes to be effective. Another option is iontophoresis of lidocaine, a noninvasive system that uses an electrical current to deliver lidocaine to the skin and takes effect in approximately 10 minutes. Again, a risk of reaction to the lidocaine exists. Intradermal injection of normal saline alongside the vein also produces anesthesia. The Infusion Nurses Society does not recommend lidocaine or normal saline for this purpose.

DOCUMENTATION

Place a piece of tape on the site dressing with the date and time that the cannula was inserted, the length and gauge of the cannula, and your initials. Label every bag of fluid and tubing with the date, time that it was hung, and the fluid's expiration date.

MAINTENANCE OF INTRAVENOUS THERAPY

The health care provider orders the type of fluid and the rate at which it is to be given. The nurse is responsible for maintaining the correct rate of flow and for monitoring the patient's response to the infusion. The Coordinated Care box discusses the role of the LVN/LPN in initiating intravenous therapy.

Coordinated Care

Initiation of Intravenous Therapy

Depending on state practice acts, LVNs/LPNs with appropriate training may be able to initiate and monitor intravenous therapy. These responsibilities cannot be delegated to unlicensed assistive personnel (UAP). However, UAPs should be told how to protect the infusion while assisting the patient with basic care.

If the patient is ambulatory, attach the fluid container to a pole with wheels. Tell the patient to protect the infusion by keeping the solution container above the infusion site and to avoid pulling on the tubing or applying pressure to the infusion site.

Intravenous fluids can be allowed to flow by gravity or can be regulated by an electronic infusion control device. When gravity flow is used, the rate must be adjusted with the roller clamp or screw clamp on the tubing. The clamp should be positioned on the upper third of the tubing. The slide clamp should not be used to set the rate; it is not reliable!

Check the infusion rate hourly, even if an infusion control device is used. If the fluid is running too slowly, adjust the flow rate. Do not attempt to "catch up" by administering extra fluid rapidly. If the fluid is running too quickly, slow the rate and assess the patient for signs of fluid volume excess.

FACTORS AFFECTING INFUSION RATE

Even after the infusion rate is set, many factors can alter the rate. The main determinants of the infusion rate are the following:

- The height of the fluid container over the patient's heart. When the container is raised, the fluid flows faster. Lowering the container causes the fluid to run more slowly. The optimal height is 30 to 36 inches above the patient.
- The volume of fluid in the container. A full container causes the fluid to run faster. As the container empties, the rate decreases.
- The viscosity of the fluid. Thin fluids such as normal saline flow more quickly than thick fluids such as blood.
- Cannula diameter. Fluid flows more quickly through a large cannula than through a small cannula.
- Venting of the fluid container. Soft plastic bags collapse as they empty, but glass containers and rigid plastic containers cannot. Therefore, rigid containers must be vented to allow air to enter as fluid leaves. Without proper venting, the fluid does not flow.
- Position of the extremity. With peripheral lines, certain movements or positions may interfere with the flow of fluid. In this event, the extremity may need to be splinted with a padded armboard to limit movement, or the patient may be advised to avoid certain movements or positions.

CALCULATING THE INFUSION RATE

You should know how to calculate infusion rates, even if infusion control devices are used routinely. To calculate the infusion rate, first determine (1) how much fluid to give each hour and (2) how many drops equal 1 mL in the delivery set used (called the *drop factor*).

The health care provider's order specifies the amount of fluid to be administered in a specific time period. The instructions on the delivery set package state how many drops equal 1 mL using that set. Standard delivery sets (sometimes called *macrodrip sets*) deliver 10, 12, 15, or 20 drops per milliliter. Microdrip sets deliver 50 or 60 drops per milliliter. They are used in children and when small volumes of fluid are being given.

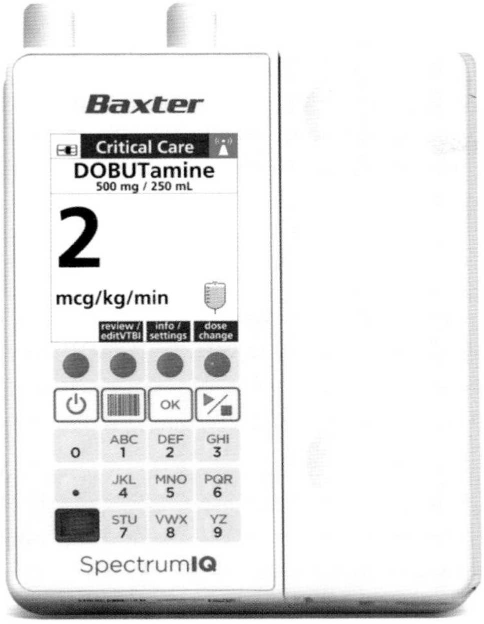

Fig. 16.7 An electronic infusion pump. (Courtesy Baxter Healthcare Corp. All rights reserved.)

Once the infusion rate per minute is known, use the roller clamp or screw clamp on a gravity infusion to adjust the flow rate until the correct number of drops per minute is infusing. Recheck the rate hourly. Common practice is to put a timed tape on the fluid container that shows where the fluid level should be each hour. This action allows a quick assessment of whether the fluid is running on schedule.

INFUSION CONTROL DEVICES

Electronic infusion control devices maintain an infusion rate that the nurse sets. The most commonly used types also have alarms that sound when the fluid bag is empty, when air is in the line, or when resistance to infusion exists. A variety of infusion control devices are available (Fig. 16.7). Ambulatory pumps are available that allow the patient to resume normal activities. You must become familiar with the type used in your work setting. Infusion control devices save time and should prevent accidental delivery of large amounts of fluid. However, they do not excuse you from monitoring the flow rate at intervals and assessing the catheter or needle insertion site. Box 16.1 gives step-by-step instructions for calculating the flow rate.

Box 16.1 Sample Flow Rate Calculation

PHYSICIAN'S ORDER

1000 mL 5% dextrose in 0.45% normal saline every 8 hours. Delivery set: 20 drops = 1 mL.

Step 1: Calculate how many milliliters should be given in 1 hour. Divide the total number of milliliters to be given by the prescribed number of hours.

$$1000 \text{ mL} \div 8 \text{ hours} = 125 \text{ mL/h}$$

Step 2: Calculate how many drops should be given in 1 hour. Multiply the number of milliliters to be given each hour by the number of drops in 1 mL using the specific delivery set.

$$125 \text{ mL} \times 20 = 2500 \text{ drops/h}$$

Step 3: Calculate how many drops should be given in 1 minute. Divide the number of drops per hour by 60 to find out how many drops should be given in 1 minute.

$$2500 \text{ drops} \div 60 \text{ min} = 41.6 \text{ or } 42 \text{ drops/min}$$

Some people prefer to use a formula to calculate the drop rate. The formula is:

(Fluid volume to be infused) × (Number of drops per mL with selected infusion set) ÷ Time (min) = Drops per minute

Put On Your Thinking Cap!

A patient is to receive an antibiotic intravenously in 100 mL of intravenous fluid. Directions are to administer the drug over 30 to 60 minutes. Drop factor: 10 drops/mL. Calculate the minimal and maximal allowable flow rates.

INTRAVENOUS INFUSION OF MEDICATIONS

Agency policies usually dictate what medications the nurse may give by piggyback or by direct injection through a cannula into the vein (intravenous push). Many states do not permit LVNs/LPNs to administer medications by intravenous push. When giving such medications, you must know how to dilute the medication and the correct rate of infusion. Improper administration of intravenous medications can be extremely dangerous. For example, potassium is *never* given by direct injection because of the risk of potentially fatal cardiac dysrhythmias.

You must also be aware that some medications and intravenous solutions are incompatible; that is, they cannot be given together.

CHANGING VENOUS ACCESS DEVICES AND ADMINISTRATION SETS

The Infusion Nurses Society recommends that administration sets be changed no more frequently than every 96 hours for continuous infusions and every 24 hours for intermittent infusions. Exceptions are for lipids and blood and blood components. Blood administration sets are changed every 4 hours. Administration sets for intravenous fat emulsion should be changed every 24 hours. Continuous parenteral nutrition without fat emulsions should be changed every 96 hours. An intravenous fluid container should not be used for more than 24 hours.

PICC lines have been in place for up to 3 years. Even though many factors influence the length of time that

PICC lines are maintained, as long as adequate care and maintenance has taken place, a hard-and-fast rule no longer exists about how long they can remain in place and be used. Ports can be left in place for years. Agency policies are generally quite specific about the schedule.

TERMINATION OF INTRAVENOUS THERAPY

To discontinue intravenous therapy with needles or short catheters, put on gloves, stop the flow of fluid, loosen or remove the tape and dressing, gently press a dry gauze pad over the site, and remove the cannula, keeping the hub parallel to the skin. Dispose of the needle or catheter according to standard precautions guidelines. Elevate the extremity, apply pressure to the puncture site with a sterile gauze pad for 2 or 3 minutes to prevent bleeding, and then secure the gauze with tape. Record the appearance of the site, the condition of the catheter, and how the patient tolerated the procedure. Removal of mid-length and long catheters requires special training. Document the length of these devices upon removal and compare it with the insertion length. Also report any signs and symptoms of infection.

PRECAUTIONS

When performing a venipuncture or handling used needles or catheters, always be aware of the risk of exposure to bloodborne pathogens. The most serious pathogens that can be transmitted by this route are the human immunodeficiency virus (HIV) and hepatitis B virus.

Several products for venipuncture and intravenous therapy that reduce the risk of needle punctures or other exposure to blood are available. Every nurse should be familiar with the agency needle puncture and body fluid exposure guidelines. In the event of an accidental needlestick, most policies require blood specimens to be drawn from the nurse and the patient to test for bloodborne infections. Drug therapy may be advised if the patient has an infectious disease. Documentation of the incident and the health status of the nurse at the time of the exposure may be very important if the nurse becomes ill as a result of the exposure.

COMPLICATIONS OF INTRAVENOUS THERAPY

Intravenous therapy is so widely used that safety is often taken for granted. Several potential complications of intravenous therapy can be very serious, however. Complications include tissue trauma, infiltration, inflammation, infection, fluid volume excess, bleeding, and embolism. Each of these complications is discussed in detail in the Nursing Care During Intravenous Therapy section.

THE OLDER PATIENT AND INTRAVENOUS THERAPY

The older patient requires special consideration during intravenous therapy. Key points include the following:

- Anchor the vein with the thumb of your nondominant hand to maintain traction until the catheter is inserted to the hub.
- When performing the venipuncture, you may be able to distend the vessel by simply pressing on or touching the vein. If a tourniquet is needed, protect fragile skin by using the sleeve of the patient's gown or wrapping a washcloth under the tourniquet, or use a blood pressure cuff inflated just above the patient's diastolic pressure. In some cases, a tourniquet is not used at all because it may cause the vein to rupture when punctured.
- Special adhesives or dressings may be needed to prevent damage to the skin. A skin polymer solution can be applied to protect the skin from adhesives.
- If the hand or arm is secured to an armboard, the armboard must be padded; apply another piece of tape or gauze to the back of the tape to prevent direct contact of the adhesive with the skin.
- Because older people have less subcutaneous tissue than do younger patients, infiltrated fluid may drain away from the cannula insertion site. For example, if the hand is elevated, fluid may collect in the elbow area.
- If the patient is confused or restless, protect the infusion site and tubing with a commercial securement device or conceal the site under long sleeves or an ACE wrap.
- If a soft wrist immobilizer is justified, secure the immobilizer to the armboard, and then secure the arm with the infusion to the armboard.
- Never apply an immobilizer over an infusion site; the immobilizer must be below the site.
- Confusion during acute illness is common. Reassure the confused patient, use a calm and gentle approach, and frequently reinforce instructions.
- With dementia patients, who have dementia, distraction may take their attention away from the intravenous apparatus. Keeping the infusion equipment out of sight may reduce attempts to handle it.
- Monitoring for fluid volume excess is especially important because older people often have less efficient cardiac and renal function.

NURSING CARE DURING INTRAVENOUS THERAPY

FOCUSED ASSESSMENT

When a patient is receiving intravenous therapy, frequent assessment is needed to ensure that the correct fluid is infusing at the correct rate and that the patient is not suffering any complications from this therapy (see the Nursing Care Plan: Patient Receiving Intravenous Therapy box).

Nursing Care Plan Patient Receiving Intravenous Therapy

FOCUSED ASSESSMENT

Health History

A 77-year-old patient was admitted for nausea and vomiting of 3 days' duration. He reported fluid intake of only water and cola in the previous 2 days and complained of dizziness and fatigue. Intravenous fluids were started at a rate of 150 mL/h using a 21-gauge cannula.

Physical Examination Lethargic but oriented. Vital signs: blood pressure 96/58 mm Hg, pulse 102 beats per minute, respirations 22 breaths per minute, temperature 101.6°F (38.6°C) orally. Mucous membranes dry and sticky; urine dark yellow; intravenous infusion site: no swelling or redness.

Patient Problems	Goals and Outcome Criteria	Interventions
Potential for injury related to trauma, infiltration	The patient will experience minimal trauma, as evidenced by absence of bruising, bleeding, swelling.	Use gentle technique to start the infusion. Inspect the infusion site for swelling and bleeding. Palpate for warmth or coolness. Anchor the tubing securely. Exercise caution to prevent movement of the cannula. Stop the infusion if signs of infiltration (swelling near infusion site, pain, slow infusion rate) and restart.
Potential for infection related to disruption of skin integrity, presence of cannula in vein	The patient will remain free of infection at infusion site, as evidenced by absence of redness, swelling, edema, or drainage.	Use strict aseptic technique when starting the infusion and handling the site. Monitor for signs of inflammation and infection: redness, swelling, warmth, purulent drainage, fever. Report signs to physician. Administer antibiotics and apply warm compress to inflamed site as ordered.
Fluid volume excess related to rapid fluid infusion	The patient's fluid status will be normal, as evidenced by normal vital signs and fluid intake approximately equal to output.	Monitor rate of fluid infusion and maintain correct rate of flow. Measure all fluid intake and output. Monitor for signs and symptoms of fluid volume excess (hypervolemia): increasing blood pressure, bounding pulse, dyspnea. If patient is hypervolemic, slow infusion rate, elevate patient's head, and notify physician.
Decreased cardiac output related to blood loss	The patient will have no bleeding at infusion or tubing connections.	Check connections to be sure they are secure. Tape tubing to prevent accidental disconnection.
Impaired peripheral circulation related to obstruction of blood flow by embolus	The patient will maintain normal circulation, as evidenced by usual skin color and absence of respiratory distress.	Do not irrigate obstructed cannula. Aspirate gently or administer thrombolytic if permitted per agency protocol. Document and report any signs of respiratory distress.
Impaired ability to perform self-care (bathing, dressing, feeding, toileting) related to restricted movement of infusion site and connection to fluid delivery system	The patient will accomplish self-care activities without disruption of intravenous therapy.	Provide assistance with meals, hygiene, dressing, and toileting as needed. Provide gown that unfastens at the shoulder. Assure the patient that they can move with the infusion.
Lack of knowledge of intravenous therapy management related to lack of exposure to information	The patient will demonstrate ability to protect and manage the infusion.	Tell the patient the purpose of the infusion and what symptoms should be reported: pain, bleeding, swelling. Assure the patient that movement is possible with the infusion as long as it is protected and the tubing is not disconnected.

CRITICAL THINKING QUESTIONS

1. What is the importance of telling the patient the purpose of the infusion and possible symptoms?
2. What type of aseptic technique should be used in this situation in the initiation, maintenance, and discontinuance of intravenous infusion? Explain your answer.

Check the health care provider's order to ensure that the correct intravenous solution is infusing. Determine the prescribed rate of flow and assess the actual flow rate. Inspect the infusion site for edema, pallor or redness, bleeding, and drainage. Palpate the infusion site for edema and warmth or coolness. Ask the patient if the infusion site is painful.

Many people believe that the infusion is not infiltrating if blood flows into the tubing when the fluid container is lowered. This test is not accurate because blood may return even when fluid is escaping into the tissue. Notably, the lack of blood return does not necessarily mean that the needle is out of the vein. Therefore this time-honored test for needle placement is not reliable. Inspection and palpation of the infusion site remain the best means of evaluating for infiltration.

Assess the patient's vital signs and compare the readings with previous findings to detect increased pulse and blood pressure. Measure and record the fluid intake and output and auscultate the patient's lungs for crackles.

Patient Problems, Goals, and Outcome Criteria: Intravenous Therapy

When a patient is receiving intravenous therapy, patient problems address the risk for complications, the need for assistance with activities of daily living, and the need for patient teaching. Specific patient problems and related goals are as follows.

Patient Problems	Goals and Outcome Criteria
Potential for injury related to trauma, infiltration, inflammation	Absence of trauma, inflammation, infiltration: no bruising, bleeding, edema, pallor, redness, or drainage at infusion site
Potential for infection related to disruption of skin integrity or presence of a cannula in a vein	Absence of infection: normal body temperature, no purulent drainage or redness at venipuncture site
Potential for fluid volume excess related to rapid fluid infusion	Normal fluid volume: fluid output approximately equal to intake, no dyspnea or edema
Decreased cardiac output related to blood loss through disrupted intravenous line	Normal cardiac output: pulse and blood pressure within normal limits, skin warm and dry, tubing connection intact
Inadequate peripheral tissue perfusion related to obstruction of blood flow by an embolus	Unobstructed blood flow: normal skin color and warmth in extremities
Impaired ability to manage self-care related to restricted movement of infusion site and connection to fluid delivery system	Patient's performance of self-care activities: activities completed without disruption of intravenous therapy

INTERVENTIONS

Potential for Injury

Trauma. The insertion of a cannula is traumatic to the skin and underlying tissues. Tape may irritate or tear the skin. If a dressing such as Tegaderm is in place, excess tape will prevent loss of moisture under the dressing and it will loosen. Use gentle technique when performing the venipuncture and anchor the cannula to reduce tissue trauma. Apply a commercial site protector, if available, to shield the intravenous site.

Infiltration. Infiltration is the collection of infused fluid in the tissue surrounding the cannula. The term **extravasation** is often used interchangeably with **infiltration**, but extravasation specifically refers to leakage of fluid from a blood vessel. Infiltration can be caused by leakage at the point where the cannula enters the vein or by puncture of a second site in the vein by the cannula. Drugs that are especially toxic to subcutaneous tissues are called *vesicants*. Common vesicants are vasopressors, potassium chloride, and antineoplastic agents.

Frequently inspect the site for signs and symptoms of infiltration. When the infusion is infiltrated, the patient may report pain or a burning sensation in the area. On inspection, the site may be pale and puffy. If an excessive amount of fluid is in the tissue, it may feel hard and cool. When evidence of infiltration is noted, stop the infusion and restart it in a different vein; otherwise the patient may not be receiving the drug or fluid as intended. Tissue that is edematous with infiltrated fluid is fragile, so handle it gently. Elevate the affected arm on a pillow to promote reabsorption of excess fluid.

Because many medications harm subcutaneous tissue, the physician should be notified if a solution containing a vesicant infiltrate. When administering vesicants, selecting a large, soft vein is especially important. Use the smallest appropriate cannula, ensure cannula placement before giving the vesicant, and flush the cannula after the vesicant is given. Examples of fluids and medications that are irritants or vesicants or that have a pH less than 5 or more than 9 or osmolarity above 500 mOs are 10% dextrose in water (D10W), calcium gluconate, dobutamine (Dobutrex), and amphotericin B (Fungizone, Abelcet).

Put On Your Thinking Cap!

A patient complains of pain at an intravenous insertion site. The site feels cool and is slightly swollen. When the intravenous fluid container is lowered, blood flows back into the tubing. Do you think the infusion is infiltrated? What should you do?

Potential for Infection

Inflammation of the vein is called **phlebitis**. With intravenous fluid therapy, phlebitis may be caused by irritation by the cannula or by medications. Redness, swelling, warmth, and tenderness near the insertion site suggest phlebitis. The inflammation may be mild or severe and carries the possibility of the formation of blood clots in the vein (thrombophlebitis). If a venipuncture site is infected, there may be purulent drainage in addition to redness and swelling and the patient may have a fever.

To reduce the risk of inflammation and infection, use a strict aseptic technique when starting and handling intravenous infusions. Agency policy describes specific site care, including the frequency of dressing changes.

If the infusion site appears to be inflamed or infected, stop the infusion and restart it in another site. If agency policy permits, a warm compress can be applied to the inflamed site. If evidence of infection is noted, notify the health care provider. Antibiotic therapy may be ordered.

Pharmacology Capsule

Drugs that are toxic to body tissues are called vesicants. They can cause phlebitis or tissue necrosis.

Potential for Fluid Volume Excess

The patient's blood volume may increase excessively when fluid is delivered directly into the bloodstream. This situation is most likely to happen when large volumes of fluid are infused, especially in patients who have impaired renal or cardiac function.

Signs and symptoms of fluid volume excess include rising blood pressure, bounding pulse, and edema. Severe fluid volume excess produces heart failure and pulmonary edema (discussed in Chapter 34).

The risk of fluid volume excess is reduced by controlling the rate of fluid infusion. If the infusion falls behind schedule, correct the rate as noted previously but do not increase it to make up for the slow infusion. Normally, fluid intake and output are approximately equal. When the heart or kidneys are unable to handle excess blood volume, heart failure may develop. Young children and older adults must be monitored closely for fluid volume excess because they do not adapt to fluid changes as readily as a young adult. If indications of fluid volume excess (increasing blood pressure, bounding pulse, dyspnea) appear, slow the infusion rate, elevate the patient's head, and notify the health care provider.

Pharmacology Capsule

Rapid intravenous administration of drugs or fluids may cause fluid volume excess, leading to heart failure.

Decreased Cardiac Output

Bleeding may occur if the cannula is moved excessively after insertion. Even more serious bleeding is possible if the tubing becomes disconnected from the cannula, allowing blood to flow freely from the vein.

To prevent bleeding, make sure that all connections in the infusion set are secure. Tape tubing so that it cannot be pulled loose easily. Protect the infusion site and tubing when the patient moves. If a large amount of blood is lost, assess the patient's vital signs and notify the physician. Institute emergency measures if the patient is in shock.

Inadequate Peripheral Tissue Perfusion

An **embolus (pl. emboli)** is an unattached blood clot or other substance in the circulatory system. An embolus can have serious, even life-threatening effects if it lodges and obstructs blood flow in a critical blood vessel. The obstruction created by a trapped embolus is called an **embolism**.

Intravenous therapy presents risks of emboli from blood clots, air, and broken catheters. A blood clot, or **thrombus (pl. thrombi),** can develop in intravenous needles or catheters. Air can enter the bloodstream if the infusion system is opened. As little as 10 mL of air can cause serious complications. The risk of air embolism with peripheral lines has been greatly reduced by the use of plastic rather than glass fluid containers. The danger is greatest with central venous lines such as the subclavian, Hickman-Broviac, and triple-lumen catheters. If a port is disconnected, air may be drawn into the bloodstream. The patient experiences shortness of breath, hypotension, and possibly shock and cardiac arrest.

A rare occurrence is a catheter embolus. This event occurs when a piece of the catheter breaks off in the vein. Broken catheters may be caused by defects in the catheter, reintroduction of the needle into the catheter, accidental cutting with scissors, or forceful flushing of an intravenous (IV) or PICC line.

Chest discomfort may be caused by a catheter embolism and should be reported to the health care provider immediately. If a catheter breaks in a peripheral vein, keep the patient calm with the head elevated, and notify the physician. A radiograph will be ordered to locate the broken catheter, usually in the right ventricle or pulmonary artery. The fragment may be removed with a snare that is passed through the femoral vein.

When the cannula seems to be obstructed, blood clots may have formed in it. Irrigation of the cannula is not recommended because it may force clots into the bloodstream. Depending on agency policy, gentle aspiration may be attempted to remove the obstruction. Alteplase may be ordered to dissolve clots that are obstructing the cannula.

Exercise extra caution to prevent an air embolism when a patient has a central line. The chance of this event happening with PICC lines that have valves is greatly reduced. The infusion set must remain closed. When hanging new bags of fluid, clamp the catheter port to prevent air entering the bloodstream. When a central catheter is inserted or removed, instruct the patient to take a deep breath and bear down. This action helps to prevent air entering the bloodstream. If air accidentally enters the line, close the leak immediately. Turn the patient on the left side with the head lowered. This position traps the air in the right atrium, where it can be absorbed gradually. Air in the bloodstream is an emergency situation in which cardiac arrest is possible; thus close monitoring is vital. Notify the health care provider immediately and keep the emergency supply cart close at hand.

One-hundred percent oxygen with a nonrebreather mask may be ordered.

Impaired Ability to Perform Self-Care

Provide assistance as needed with eating, dressing, toileting, and hygiene. Dressing may be easier if the patient is provided with a gown or shirt that unfastens at the shoulder. These garments are simpler to remove than garments that must be removed over the arm. Some patients are fearful of moving with an intravenous infusion. Explain what restrictions, if any, are needed to protect the infusion (see the Patient Teaching box). If a commercial intravenous shield is available, consider using one to reduce the risk of trauma at the insertion site.

Patient Teaching

Intravenous Therapy in the Home

When intravenous therapy is ordered outside the acute care setting, explain what will be performed and why. Teaching should begin well before discharge so that the patient's ability to perform the care can be assessed. With long-term therapy, teaching the patient (and family, if appropriate) the following is especially important:

- Infusion site care
- Proper administration of fluids or drugs
- Signs that should be reported to the physician or home health nurse
- How to flush infusion ports if appropriate
- Care of central lines or implanted infusion ports

  Details depend on the situation.

Get Ready for the NCLEX® Examination!

Key Points

- Intravenous therapy is used to administer drugs, fluids including nutrients, and blood or blood products.
- The terms *fluid* and *solution* are used interchangeably in relation to intravenous therapy.
- Tonicity is a measure of the concentration of electrolytes in a fluid.
- Hypertonic intravenous solutions tend to increase blood volume whereas hypotonic intravenous solutions tend to decrease blood volume.
- A patient receives 34 calories for each 1% of dextrose in a liter of fluid.
- Devices used to deliver intravenous fluids include needles, over-the-needle catheters, inside-needle catheters, subcutaneous infusion ports, and subcutaneously implanted pumps.
- Central veins are large veins located nearer the heart that are used for long-term therapy, when the patient has poor peripheral veins, and when irritating or vesicant medications or fluids are administered.
- Peripheral veins in the extremities and scalp are used for short-term therapy, when a patient has healthy veins, and when relatively nonirritating fluids are given.
- Nurse practice acts and agency policies govern who can perform venipuncture and who can administer intravenous fluids and intravenous medications.
- Cannula size is selected based on the patient's vein size and general condition and the type of fluid to be administered.
- Use the "six rights" when administering intravenous fluids as well as drugs.
- Administration sets are changed every 24 hours for intermittent infusions, parenteral nutrition, and fat emulsion; for continuous infusions other than blood or blood products or lipids, sets are changed every 96 hours.
- On the site dressing, record the date and time that the cannula was inserted, the length and gauge of the cannula, and your initials.
- When an infusion flows by gravity, the rate is influenced by the height of the fluid container, fluid volume in the container, fluid viscosity, cannula diameter, venting of the fluid container, and position of the extremity.
- If your state permits you to administer drugs per intravenous push, you must know how to dilute the medication, the correct rate of infusion, and whether the drug is compatible with the infusing fluid.
- Use standard precautions when starting infusions, providing site care, discontinuing infusions, and making dressing changes.
- Complications of intravenous therapy are tissue trauma, infiltration, inflammation, infection, fluid volume excess, bleeding, and embolism.
- Monitor for fluid volume excess in the older person who is receiving intravenous fluids.
- When a cannula appears to be obstructed, irrigation is not recommended because you may force blood clots into the bloodstream.
- With central lines, take precautions to prevent air entering the line, which can cause an air embolism—a potentially fatal complication.

Additional Learning Resources

SG Go to your Study Guide for additional learning activities to help you master this chapter content.

Go to your Evolve website (http://evolve.elsevier.com/Linton/medsurg) for the following learning resources and much more:

- Fluid & Electrolyte Tutorial
- Review Questions for the NCLEX® Examination

Review Questions for the NCLEX® Examination

1. Which intravenous cannula is largest?

1. 12 gauge
2. 14 gauge
3. 18 gauge
4. 22 gauge

NCLEX Client Need: Physiological Integrity: Pharmacological Therapies

2. **A patient is receiving an intravenous infusion of 0.45% sodium chloride. The nurse knows that this solution is:**
   1. Isotonic
   2. Hypotonic
   3. Hypertonic
   4. Concentrated

   NCLEX Client Need: Physiological Integrity: Pharmacological Therapies

3. **Solutions that have the same concentration of electrolytes as body fluids are called ________________ solutions.**

   NCLEX Client Need: Physiological Integrity: Pharmacological Therapies

4. **When intravenous fluid is given to increase blood volume, the tonicity of the solution should be ________________.**

   NCLEX Client Need: Physiological Integrity: Pharmacological Therapies

5. **A central line is preferred over a peripheral line under which of the following conditions? (Select all that apply.)**
   1. Irritating intravenous fluids are to be administered.
   2. The patient is an infant.
   3. Short-term therapy is required.
   4. The patient has poor peripheral veins.
   5. Antibiotics will be infused.

   NCLEX Client Need: Physiological Integrity: Pharmacological Therapies

6. **A patient is to receive 1000 mL of intravenous fluid every 8 hours at a rate of 34 drops/min. If the infusion has slowed so that he has received only 700 mL near the end of one 8-hour shift, the correct action is to:**
   1. Quickly infuse an additional 300 mL before the end of the shift.
   2. Increase the infusion rate to deliver an additional 300 mL over the next shift.
   3. Notify the physician to determine what action should be taken.
   4. Reset the infusion rate at 34 drops/min to continue the infusion.

   NCLEX Client Need: Physiological Integrity: Pharmacological Therapies; Reduction of Risk Potential

7. **An older patient is receiving intravenous fluids to treat dehydration. When she complains of shortness of breath, your assessment reveals a 20-point increase in her systolic blood pressure and a heart rate of 100 beats per minute. The most likely cause of these findings is:**
   1. Shock caused by deficient fluid volume
   2. Anxiety associated with hospitalization
   3. Fluid volume excess related to fluid overload
   4. Renal failure caused by circulatory collapse

   NCLEX Client Need: Physiological Integrity: Reduction of Risk Potential

8. **SLO/Objective:** **Plan actions for older patients receiving intravenous therapy.**

   NGN Item Type: Matrix

   Cognitive Skill: Generate Solutions

A 90-year-old man is admitted after he fell when working in his garden. He sustained several deep cuts including one to the back of his head. The wounds were sutured under local anesthesia in the ED. He is admitted for observation and hydration. The nurse prepares to start a peripheral infusion to administer fluids and antibiotics.

Use an X for the nursing actions listed below that are ***Indicated/Anticipated*** **(appropriate or necessary),** ***Contraindicated*** **(could be harmful),** ***Nonessential*** **(makes no difference or not necessary) for the patient's care at this time.**

NURSING ACTION	INDICATED/ ANTICIPATED	CONTRAINDICATED	NONESSENTIAL
Pad the armboard, if used			
Minimize contact of adhesive tape with the skin			
Provide pain medication before venipuncture			
Apply an immobilizer over the infusion site			
Use a blood pressure cuff rather than a tourniquet to distend the vein			
Release traction on the skin as soon as the cannula pierces the skin			

NCLEX Client Need: Physiological Integrity: Reduction of Risk Potential

9. **A PICC line is inserted into a vein and advanced into the ________________________.**

   NCLEX Client Need: Physiological Integrity: Pharmacological Therapies; Therapeutic Procedures

10. **The greatest danger of irrigating an obstructed intravenous line is:**
    1. Embolism
    2. Trauma to the blood vessel
    3. Rupture of the cannula
    4. Infusion site irritation

    NCLEX Client Need: Physiological Integrity: Reduction of Risk Potential

17 Surgery

http://evolve.elsevier.com/Linton/medsurg

Objectives

1. State the purpose of each type of surgery: diagnostic, ablative, palliative, reconstructive or restorative, procurement for transplant, constructive, and cosmetic.
2. List data to be included in the nursing assessment of the preoperative patient.
3. Identify the patient problems, goals and outcome criteria, and interventions during the preoperative phase of the surgical experience.
4. Outline a preoperative teaching plan.
5. List the responsibilities of each member of the surgical team.
6. Explain the nursing implications of each type of anesthesia.
7. Explain how the nurse can help to prevent postoperative complications.
8. List data to be included in the nursing assessment of the postoperative patient.
9. Identify patient problems, goals and outcome criteria, and interventions for the postoperative patient.
10. Explain patient needs that should be considered in discharge planning.

Key Terms

ablative surgery
anesthesiologist (ăn-ĕs-thē-zē-Ŏ-lō-jĭst)
anesthetic (ăn-ĕs-THĔ-tĭk)
constructive surgery
cosmetic surgery
dehiscence (dē-HĬS-ĕns)
evisceration (ē-vĭs-ĕr-Ā-shŭn)
nurse anesthetist
palliative surgery
paralytic ileus
procurement for transplant
reconstructive or restorative surgery
sanguineous (săn-GWĬN-ē-ŭs)
serosanguineous (sĕ-rō-săn-GWĬN-ē-ŭs)
serous (SĔ-rŭs)

Surgical procedures have been performed since early times. However, until fairly recently, surgery was considered the last resort, to be used only when more conservative measures had failed or for emergency life-saving care. Twentieth-century advances brought antibiotics, safe anesthesia, refined surgical techniques, and improved diagnosis and treatment of illness and injury. Through these advances, surgery became safer than ever before and it is now almost commonplace (Fig. 17.1).

Surgical procedures are performed in physicians' offices, clinics, ambulatory surgery centers, and full-service hospitals. Over recent years, cost control measures resulted in a tremendous shift toward ambulatory surgery centers for many procedures. In all of these settings, nurses play important roles. Nurses who care for patients before, during, and after surgery are called *perioperative nurses.* They admit surgical patients, perform initial assessments and prepare them for surgery, coordinate and assist in the procedures, and provide immediate postoperative care. Because hospital stays for surgical procedures have shortened dramatically and many procedures are performed in ambulatory settings, nurses are challenged to provide adequate preoperative and postoperative teaching. Verbal instructions to patients and their significant others should be supplemented with written materials. Follow-up phone calls provide a chance to answer questions, reinforce instructions, and assess postoperative status (pain, nausea, wound healing, etc.).

PURPOSES OF SURGERY

Surgery may be performed for a variety of reasons. Surgical procedures classified by purpose include diagnostic, ablative, palliative, reconstructive or restorative, procurement for transplant, constructive, and cosmetic.

Diagnostic surgery is done to make an accurate diagnosis. It often involves the removal and study of tissue, as with a biopsy of a skin lesion or the removal of a lump in breast tissue. More extensive procedures require opening a body cavity to diagnose and to find out the extent of a disease process. A common example is an exploratory laparotomy, in which the abdomen is opened to find the cause

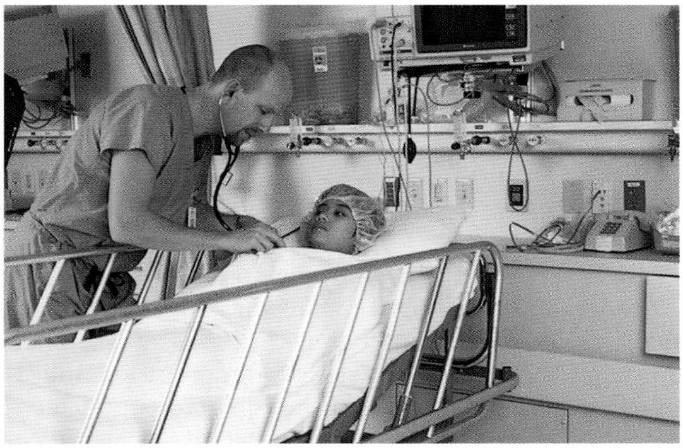

Fig. 17.1 The nurse provides continuity of care for the surgical patient. (From Harkreader H, Hogan MA: *Fundamentals of nursing: caring and clinical judgment*, ed 3, St. Louis, 2007, Saunders.)

of unexplained pain. Some exploratory surgery can be performed using specialized scopes inserted into the body through small incisions.

Ablative surgery is performed to remove diseased tissue such as an inflamed gallbladder.

Palliative surgery relieves symptoms or improves function without correcting the basic problem. For example, palliative surgery may be performed just to remove a malignant tumor obstructing the intestine even if cancer is widespread elsewhere in the body.

Reconstructive or restorative surgery restores function or structure to damaged or malfunctioning tissue. Breast reconstruction after mastectomy or total knee replacement are examples.

Procurement for transplant refers to the removal of organs (e.g., heart, lungs, liver) from a living donor or a deceased person for transplantation into another person.

Constructive surgery restores function lost because of congenital defects such as a cleft palate.

Cosmetic surgery is performed to improve a person's appearance. It is often chosen because the patient wants to change a physical feature. Common cosmetic procedures are performed to change the shape of facial features, remove wrinkles, flatten the abdomen, and change the size or shape of the breasts.

VARIABLES AFFECTING SURGICAL OUTCOMES

Among the variables that must be considered when caring for surgical patients are age, nutritional status, fluid and electrolyte balance, medical diagnoses, comorbidities, drugs, and habits.

AGE

Health care providers and older adults themselves often believe that surgery is dangerous for older people; however, with today's surgery techniques, safe surgery can be performed for patients in their 90s. Modern surgical techniques can restore lost functions and often can greatly improve the patient's quality of life. Improved monitoring, less invasive procedures, and better drugs have made surgery safer for everyone. People over 70 years of age who are frail or have cardiovascular disease, renal disease, or diabetes are at increased risk for surgical complications. Hospitalization and surgery may disrupt control of chronic conditions, leading to impaired healing and recovery. However, older adults who are in good health may do just as well in surgery as younger people.

As a general rule, inactivity is not good for anyone; it is especially bad for the older person, who takes longer to regain strength. An old adage is that 1 day in bed equals 3 days of recovering strength. One other important consideration is that older people may respond differently to drugs because of age-related changes in liver and kidney function and multiple drug interactions.

Surgical risks for the older adult can be greatly reduced if chronic conditions are well controlled, drug therapy is carefully evaluated and documented, and the patient is well hydrated and nourished before surgery. For this reason, emergency procedures carry greater risks for older patients than scheduled procedures.

NUTRITIONAL STATUS

Patients who are overweight or underweight require special care when surgery is indicated. The patient who is malnourished is at risk for poor wound healing and infection. In severely malnourished patients, surgery may be delayed and enteral feedings used to improve the nutritional status. Obese patients are generally in surgery longer and are more likely to have postoperative respiratory and wound complications than patients of normal weight. Effective deep-breathing exercises are limited by the excess weight. Because adipose tissue has poor blood supply, the healing process is slower than normal. The obese patient may also need additional time to recover from anesthesia because the drug tends to remain longer in adipose tissue than in other tissue.

FLUID AND ELECTROLYTE BALANCE

Fluid and electrolyte status can have a significant bearing on the outcome of surgery. Adequate fluids are necessary to maintain blood volume and urine output. However, excess body fluid can overload the heart, aggravating the stress of surgery. Sudden changes in fluid volume are especially dangerous for the older patient who cannot adapt as efficiently as a younger person. Electrolyte imbalances may also predispose the patient to dangerous cardiac dysrhythmias. Diuretics (e.g., Lasix) can play a part in balancing fluid overload; they can also play a part in creating electrolyte imbalances, including potassium deficit. Many older patients take diuretics on a regular basis. Physicians usually order laboratory tests to measure serum electrolytes along with other laboratory tests before surgery. Fluid and electrolyte imbalances can then be corrected preoperatively.

MEDICAL DIAGNOSES

A significant number of medical conditions increase surgical risks or require special attention in the perioperative period. Patients with bleeding disorders or those who are taking anticoagulants are at risk for excessive bleeding and must be monitored closely. People with heart disease are at risk for cardiac complications related to anesthesia and the stress of surgery. Chronic respiratory disease increases the risk of pulmonary complications as a result of anesthesia or hypoventilation. Obstructive sleep apnea increases the risk for postoperative airway obstruction, especially if opioids are given. A patient who has liver disease may have impaired wound healing and impaired blood clotting and may experience drug toxicity arising from the inability to metabolize drugs effectively. Disorders of the immune system and chemotherapy or immune-suppressing drugs place the patient at risk for infection and delayed wound healing. Patients with uncontrolled blood sugar because of diabetes mellitus also heal more slowly and are at greater risk for infection than patients who do not have diabetes. Surgeons usually attempt to regulate blood sugar before and during surgery to prevent these complications. The control of chronic conditions may be disrupted by surgery, which then mandates adjustments in therapy. In addition, patients who undergo surgery in life-threatening or traumatic situations are at increased risk of complications.

DRUGS

Many drugs, especially those that depress the central nervous system (CNS), have the potential to interact with anesthetics. Serious adverse effects may result. The effects of surgery and drugs used during surgery may also require dosage adjustments in drugs that the patient had been taking routinely. Over-the-counter self-medication such as aspirin and herbal drugs can also affect recovery and must be documented. It is vital to document all drugs, prescriptions, and other, that the patient has been taking preoperatively.

Pharmacology Capsule

Drugs that should be held or modified before surgery include anticoagulants, nonsteroidal antiinflammatory drugs (NSAIDs), aspirin, and herbal products, including ginger, ginkgo, and ginseng. See Table 17.1.

HABITS

Habits that alert the nurse to the possibility of specific perioperative complications are smoking and the use of recreational drugs, herbal medications, and alcohol. Smoking increases the risk of pulmonary complications because smokers have more copious and tenacious secretions and their ciliary activity is less effective compared with nonsmokers. Smoking also delays wound healing because of capillary constriction from the nicotine. Most surgeons ask that patients stop or cut down on smoking at least a week before surgery. Recreational drugs, such as cocaine and methamphetamine, can increase the heart rate, alter cardiac function, and increase the need for higher-than-usual doses of anesthesia. If withdrawal problems are anticipated, intraoperative and postoperative drugs can minimize complications. Withdrawal symptoms can occur within 24 hours in the postoperative period. Herbal medication is thought to interact with certain medications, and experts recommend that they be discontinued before surgery (Table 17.1). Alcohol interacts with many drugs. In addition, patients who use alcohol excessively may need a higher-than-normal dose of anesthetic agent because of increased drug tolerance. If liver damage has occurred, the metabolism of drugs, including anesthetics, can be impaired. In addition, patients with liver disease are at increased risk for bleeding.

PREOPERATIVE PHASE

PREOPERATIVE NURSING CARE

The preoperative phase begins when a decision is made to perform a surgical procedure and ends when the patient enters the operating room. During the

Table 17.1 Herbs That May Pose Risks for Surgical Patients

HERB	EFFECTS	WHEN TO DISCONTINUE BEFORE SURGERY
Ephedra	May increase risk of heart attack and stroke	At least 24 hours
Garlic	May increase bleeding	At least 7 days
Ginkgo	May increase bleeding risk	At least 36 hours
Ginseng	Lowers blood glucose, may increase bleeding risk	At least 7 days
Kava	May increase sedative effect of anesthetics; has been associated with fatal hepatotoxicity	At least 24 hours
St. John's wort	May diminish effects of several drugs	At least 5 days
Valerian	May increase sedative effect of anesthetics; associated with symptoms like benzodiazepine withdrawal	Best tapered over several weeks
Echinacea	Associated with allergic reactions and immune stimulation	Unknown

From Muluk V, Cohn SL, Whinney C: *UpToDate*. October 15, 2020. From https://www.uptodate.com. Retrieved November 12, 2020.

preoperative phase, the goals of nursing care are for the patient to know what to expect in the surgical experience and to have minimal anxiety.

Focused Assessment

When nonemergency surgery is scheduled, a thorough assessment is made that starts with the patient's health history and physical examination. Although not responsible for the total patient assessment as described here, the licensed vocational nurse/licensed practical nurse (LVN/LPN) often assists by collecting specific, relevant data. This assessment is usually performed before admission to the nursing care unit. If not done before admission, laboratory studies of blood and urine, blood grouping and crossmatching, chest radiography and other imaging procedures, pulmonary function tests, and electrocardiography (ECG) may be ordered. A nasal swab test may be done to rule out methicillin-resistant *Staphylococcus aureus* (MRSA).

Most surgical facilities have standardized forms for assessing the newly admitted patient. The nursing assessment should obtain important data needed to plan preoperative, intraoperative, and postoperative care; it also provides baseline data for monitoring the patient's status. Box 17.1 shows the elements of the preoperative assessment. For outpatient surgery, obtaining some information in advance is especially important because the time available for a comprehensive assessment will be limited.

Box 17.1 Focused Assessment of the Preoperative Patient

HEALTH HISTORY

Identifying Data
Age

History of Present Illness
Problem being treated surgically

Past Medical History
Acute and chronic conditions, previous hospitalizations and surgeries, allergies, recent and current medications (to include recreational and herbal medications)

Review of Systems
Disabilities and limitations: hearing or vision loss, paralysis, stiffness, weakness, cognitive impairment; any current health deviations

Functional Assessment
Occupation, roles, responsibilities, diet and fluid intake, activity/exercise, tobacco and alcohol use, sources of stress and support, coping strategies, expectations of surgery

PHYSICAL EXAMINATION

General Survey: Emotional state, ability to communicate, response to directions

Height and Weight

Vital Signs

Skin: Color, lesions, bruises, warmth, turgor, moisture

Thorax: Respiratory pattern and effort, breath sounds, apical pulse

Abdomen: Distention, scars, bowel sounds

Extremities: Color, hair distribution, lesions, deformities, range of motion, crepitus, pain, weakness

Prostheses: Hearing aids, eyeglasses, contact lenses, dentures, artificial limbs, other devices

Health history

Identifying data. Record identifying data, including the patient's age.

History of present illness. Describe the problem that is being treated surgically.

Past health history. Include acute and chronic conditions, hospitalizations, surgeries, allergies, and drug history. Record all chronic health problems such as diabetes, heart failure, pulmonary disease, sleep apnea, or liver or kidney disease. Note if any family member has had complications with anesthesia.

Document any known allergies (food, drug, tape, latex, chemical) according to agency policy. Place an allergy alert bracelet on the patient's wrist if any allergies are found. A large number of drugs are routinely given to surgical patients. During and immediately after surgery, the patient is unable to report allergies; therefore if an emergency should arise, any allergies can be determined promptly by checking the patient's allergy alert bracelet.

Compile a complete list of medications and complementary and alternative therapies that the patient is taking or has recently taken. Knowledge of the patient's drug history enables the health care team to anticipate possible effects of drug interactions.

Pharmacology Capsule

Long-term drug therapy with agents such as anticoagulants and hypoglycemics may require dosage adjustments before and after surgery, determined by physician's orders preoperatively.

Review of systems. Collect data about each body system, noting any abnormalities. Record any disabilities or limitations. Include the presence of acute problems (e.g., a cold, a urinary tract infection, a bout of diarrhea) that could necessitate delay of a surgical procedure. In addition to the conditions identified in the past medical history, document problems that may be significant during the surgical experience, such as vision or hearing loss, partial paralysis or joint stiffness, weakness, or cognitive impairment. Strategies such as bracelets may be used to alert staff to these issues.

Functional assessment. Describe the patient's usual activity pattern, including occupation, roles, and responsibilities. Determine the usual diet and fluid intake, as well as the use of tobacco, recreational drugs, herbal medications, over-the-counter drugs, and alcohol. Note exercise and rest patterns. Ask about sources of stress and support, usual ways of coping, and specific fears or concerns about this surgery. Although some anxiety is normal, be alert for indications of excessive anxiety (e.g., tearfulness, trembling, tachycardia).

Physical examination. Throughout the physical examination, be alert to the patient's emotional state, ability to communicate, and ability to understand directions.

Height and weight. Measure height and weight. Unless the patient is very ill or malnourished, the admission weight provides a goal weight to be maintained after surgery.

Vital signs. Vital signs assessed shortly after admission provide a baseline for evaluating readings during and after surgery. If the patient's pulse and blood pressure are slightly higher than expected on admission, the cause may be anxiety. After allowing the patient to rest, reassess the vital signs. If they remain abnormal, notify the physician.

Skin. Inspect the skin for color, lesions, and bruises. Palpate to determine texture, warmth, turgor, and moisture. Assess older skin carefully because it may be fragile and tear or bruise easily upon moving from stretcher to bed. Document any findings such as discoloration, bruises, and cuts preoperatively so postoperative care providers can identify if injuries are new or preexisting.

Thorax. Observe the patient's respiratory rate, pattern, and effort. Auscultate the lungs to assess breath sounds. Assess the apical heartbeat for rate and rhythm.

Abdomen. Inspect the abdomen for distention and scars and auscultate bowel sounds.

Extremities. Inspect the extremities for skin color, hair distribution, lesions, edema, and deformities. Assess range of motion while checking for edema and noting pain or weakness.

Prostheses. Note the presence of any prosthetic devices, including hearing aids, contact lenses, eyeglasses, dentures, artificial limbs, or other devices used to maintain appearance or function.

Patient Problems, Goals, and Outcome Criteria: Preoperative Nursing Goals

Some of the patient problems and goals that might be made during the preoperative phase are as follows. More specific diagnoses and goals are made based on individual patient data and specific surgical procedures.

Patient Problems	Goals and Outcome Criteria
Anxiety related to uncertain outcome of surgery, anticipated pain, potential disfigurement, or loss of function	Patient's anxiety is reduced: patient is calm, states that anxiety is reduced.
Inadequate coping related to lack of knowledge about the surgical experience	Patient understands the surgical experience: patient describes preoperative and postoperative routines, what to expect.

Interventions

Anxiety. Most patients are somewhat anxious and some are very fearful about surgery. Determine the presence and the level of anxiety, the contributing factors, and the need for intervention. The patient's previous experiences, if any, with hospitalization and surgery can be especially important. If a patient admitted for heart surgery had an acquaintance who died after similar surgery, the patient might be understandably frightened. However, a person whose previous experiences have been positive is more likely to expect this procedure to go well. If the patient seems excessively nervous or fearful about the surgery, report this behavior to the surgeon or to the anesthesia personnel. Extreme fear is associated with surgical complications; thus it should be controlled with preoperative medication and other therapeutic interventions. In some cases, surgery is postponed until anxiety is reduced.

Inadequate coping. Patient teaching may be done in the physician's office, in the clinic, during the preadmission workup, or after admission to the hospital. Ideally, patient teaching is not left until shortly before surgery, when many activities are scheduled and the patient may be distracted. A cost-saving routine is to admit patients very early in the morning on the day of surgery. In this case, the burden of preoperative teaching rests heavily on the physician, the office nurse, the admission nurse, or the clinic nurse.

Preoperative teaching should include the patient and those who will be with the patient during the recovery period. The patient will need to identify who is allowed to receive information about their condition during hospitalization. An attentive family member or companion can reinforce instructions and help to reassure the patient. Telling the patient and family or friends what to expect in the immediate postoperative phase can prevent unnecessary stress. An appropriate teaching plan is based on an assessment of what the patient already knows, wants to know, and needs to know (Fig. 17.2). Verbal instructions should be supplemented with written material or media.

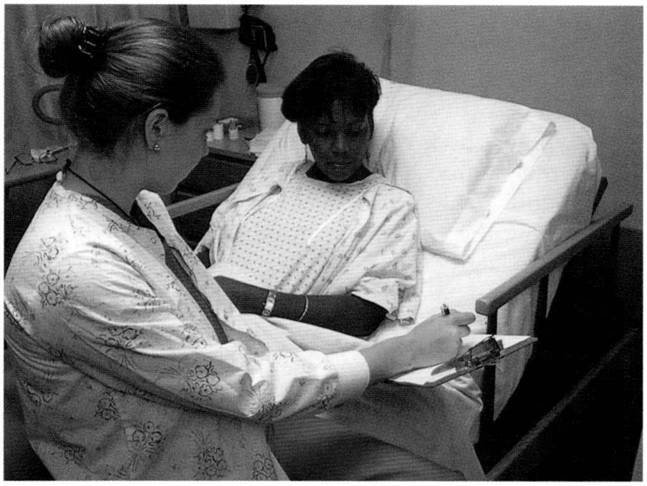

Fig. 17.2 Preoperative teaching prepares the patient for the surgical experience. (From Harkreader H, Hogan MA: *Fundamentals of nursing: caring and clinical judgment*, ed 3, St. Louis, 2007, Saunders.)

Teaching methods. The teaching methods selected depend on the situation. Direct patient teaching that the nurse provides is probably used most often. This method has advantages in that the teaching plan can be individualized and the patient can ask questions freely. The main disadvantage of one-to-one instruction is that it is time consuming.

Some hospitals have group classes for all preoperative patients. The main advantage of group classes is economy of time. In addition, some people like talking to others who are having similar procedures. Group classes have several disadvantages. Scheduling times that are accessible to multiple patients before admission may be difficult. Some patients are less likely to ask questions or express fears in a group setting. In addition, information presented to mixed groups of patients is necessarily rather generalized.

Written material, media, and computer-based products are available for patient use. Unfortunately, many patient teaching materials are appropriate only for a limited audience. The reading level may be above the patient's ability or too many technical terms may be used. Many people in the United States do not speak or read English well enough to learn from these materials. If foreign language materials are not available, the services of a professional translator should be obtained. Although media can be very helpful, do not depend on them completely for patient teaching. Personal follow-up allows the nurse to assess the patient's understanding of the material and to answer questions (see the Patient Teaching box).

Patient Teaching

Preoperative Patient

Most people need basic information and simple explanations without technical details. The family members or significant others will probably want to know the expected time of surgery, where to wait for the patient, and how they will be informed when the procedure is over. The teaching plan should include an orientation to the upcoming experience. and the following information preoperatively:

- In preparation for surgery, there may be specific preparations based on the specific surgical procedure, agency protocols, and physician's orders. If you are an ambulatory surgery patient, these will usually be provided by the physician's office.
- Be sure that all preoperative instructions have been followed. For example, if you have had anything to eat or drink before surgery, it can be canceled.
- The nurse will start an intravenous infusion and you will be visited by the anesthesia care provider, and usually the surgeon.
- All jewelry will be removed and locked in a secure place, or given to a relative or significant other. Wedding rings can be taped so they won't fall off and get lost. Any body jewelry, such as nose and body rings, will be removed to prevent potential damage and infection.
- The following information regarding the operating room (OR) is usually appreciated by the patient.
- You will be transported on a gurney (stretcher) and moved to the OR bed.
- Restraints may be placed when you are on the OR table to protect you and keep you safe.
- The room will be cold, so extra warming blankets or special heating pads may be given to you to keep you comfortable. You can ask for this.
- The lights will be very bright.
- Everyone in the OR will have special gowns on.
- Information regarding the postanesthesia care unit (PACU; sometimes called the *recovery* room) includes:
- You may have tubes, dressings, or equipment in place. You may have a clip on your finger that monitors your blood oxygen level.
- Nurses will check your pulse and blood pressure often and perform other procedures specific to your surgery.
- You will be coached to deep breathe, cough, turn, and exercise your legs (as practiced preoperatively) to help you eliminate the anesthetic and to prevent complications.
- You may be asked to respond to various commands, depending on your surgery.
- You need to report pain so that measures can be taken to provide pain relief. You will be asked to rate your pain on a scale of 1 to 10, with 1 being "no pain" and 10 being "the worst pain imaginable."
- When the nurses and physicians deem you are awake enough, you will be discharged to home or the floor unit.
- If you are an outpatient surgery patient, you must have someone to drive you home, regardless of the type of surgery you have.

Preparation for surgery. Preparation of the patient for surgery starts before or shortly after admission. Patients admitted for emergency surgery may not have the benefit of preoperative teaching.

Informed consent. Before surgery, a patient must sign a legal document called a *consent form* (Fig. 17.3). It states that the patient has been informed about the procedure to be performed, the alternative treatments, the risks involved, and that the patient agrees to the procedure. Written consent is also required for blood or blood products to be used. The purpose of written consent is to protect the patient from unwanted procedures; it also protects the health care facility and caregivers. Explaining the procedure and risks to the patient is the physician's responsibility, but the nurse may obtain and witness the patient's signature on the form if agency policy allows. If the patient has questions or seems to be in doubt, contact the registered nurse (RN) or the physician.

Because the consent form is a legal document, the patient must be fully alert and aware of what it contains when signing it. If the patient is a minor, a parent or guardian must sign the form. The age at which a person is considered an adult varies from state to state. Know the law in the state in which you practice.

A patient who is confused, mentally incompetent, or under the influence of drugs (including preoperative intravenous drugs) cannot give informed consent. For this reason, the consent form is always signed before the patient is given preoperative medications.

The patient should sign the consent form in the presence of a witness who also signs the form. The nurse who witnesses the consent is confirming that the signature is authentic, consent was given voluntarily, and the patient appeared to be competent at the time. Nursing students should not serve as witnesses. The consent form becomes part of the patient's record.

Preparation of the digestive tract. The extent of bowel preparation, if any, depends on the type of anesthesia and the type of surgery planned. For surgery on the lower abdomen or the digestive tract, laxatives and

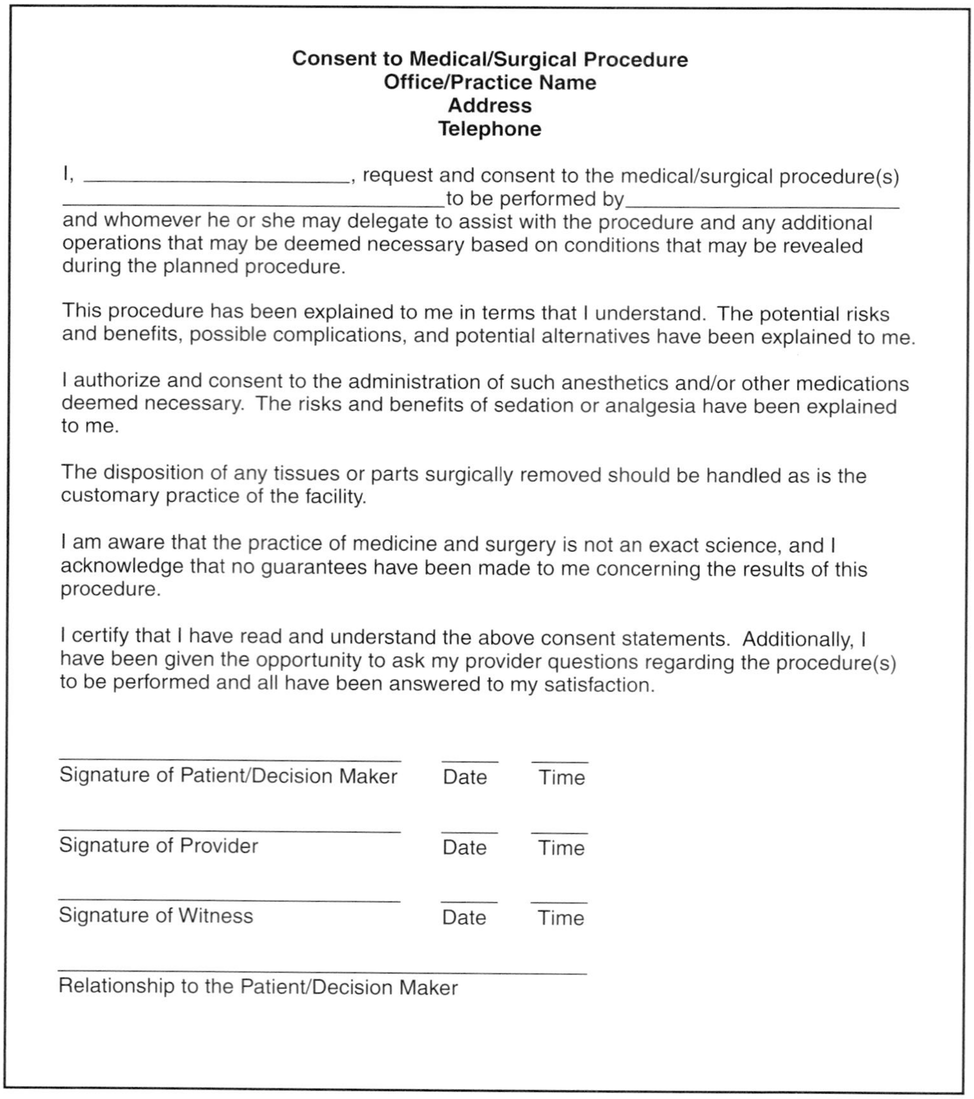

Consent to Medical/Surgical Procedure
Office/Practice Name
Address
Telephone

I, ______________________, request and consent to the medical/surgical procedure(s) ________________________________to be performed by______________________ and whomever he or she may delegate to assist with the procedure and any additional operations that may be deemed necessary based on conditions that may be revealed during the planned procedure.

This procedure has been explained to me in terms that I understand. The potential risks and benefits, possible complications, and potential alternatives have been explained to me.

I authorize and consent to the administration of such anesthetics and/or other medications deemed necessary. The risks and benefits of sedation or analgesia have been explained to me.

The disposition of any tissues or parts surgically removed should be handled as is the customary practice of the facility.

I am aware that the practice of medicine and surgery is not an exact science, and I acknowledge that no guarantees have been made to me concerning the results of this procedure.

I certify that I have read and understand the above consent statements. Additionally, I have been given the opportunity to ask my provider questions regarding the procedure(s) to be performed and all have been answered to my satisfaction.

Signature of Patient/Decision Maker Date Time

Signature of Provider Date Time

Signature of Witness Date Time

Relationship to the Patient/Decision Maker

Fig. 17.3 Surgical consent form.

enemas may be given to empty the bowel. In some instances, patients are instructed to take a cathartic to empty the bowel at home before being admitted to the hospital.

Bowel cleansing serves three purposes. First, it reduces the risk of contamination from fecal matter during the operation. Second, it helps to prevent postoperative distention until normal bowel function returns. Third, it prevents constipation and straining in the postoperative period. Straining can create pressure on the surgical wound. Surgery may be canceled if bowel preparation is inadequate.

Food and fluid restriction. Even if bowel cleansing is not ordered, ingestion by mouth of fluids and foods is restricted for a specific period. The evening meal before the day of surgery may be restricted to fluids. This precaution is used to reduce the risk of vomiting and aspiration during or after anesthesia. The American Society of Anesthesiologists recommends minimal fasting times, depending on the type of food and liquid taken (Table 17.2). If a patient routinely takes an oral medication that is considered essential (e.g., antihypertensive drugs, asthma inhalers), it may be ordered early on the morning of surgery with a few sips of water or given parenterally.

Skin preparation. When an incision is made in the skin, microorganisms can enter the wound. Skin preparation is intended to reduce the number of organisms near the incision site. The process usually includes scrubbing and sometimes removing hair from a wide margin around the planned surgical site. The exact skin preparation is ordered by the physician or outlined in a procedure manual.

A typical procedure requires the patient (if able) to shower and wash with an antiseptic soap the evening before the surgery and again the next morning. The physician, perioperative nurse, or operating room technician scrubs the operative site when the patient arrives in the OR and is asleep. If the patient's skin is very hairy or if the hair might interfere with the surgical procedure or dressing, it can be removed by clipping with electrical surgical clippers in the preoperative holding area. Shaving with a straight razor is not done today because it opens nicks or portals for infection. Therefore if shaving is done at all, it is best delayed until shortly before surgery to allow less time for organisms to multiply.

Dress and grooming. On the morning of surgery, provide a clean gown and instruct the patient to remove all undergarments unless agency policy dictates otherwise. All jewelry should be removed, which includes body piercings. If a ring cannot be removed or the patient refuses to remove it, it can be secured in accordance with agency policy. Because jewelry often has considerable sentimental value, as well as monetary value, handle it carefully. The patient may leave jewelry with a relative or friend; it should not be left at the bedside or accepted by the nurse for safekeeping. Most hospitals have a process for valuables to be collected, signed for, and stored in a safe place until the patient asks for them to be returned. Document the disposition of eyeglasses, jewelry, dentures, and hearing aid, if not worn, in the patient's chart.

Braid or secure long hair with a rubber band. Remove hairpins or clips. Provide a cap to cover the hair. Traditionally, dentures have been removed and placed in a denture cup and stored in a safe place. In some cases, the anesthesiologist or nurse anesthetist may prefer that dentures be left in. Institutional policies should be specific about this situation.

Remove nail polish to permit assessment of nail beds for circulation and to permit use of a pulse oximeter. If the patient has acrylic nails, consult with the anesthesiologist or perioperative nurse about the need to remove them. Makeup, including mascara, may also be removed. Oils or creams or Vaseline should not be left on the face or body because it could be flammable with the oxygen in the OR.

A patient identification band must be in place on the patient's wrist on admission. Other wristbands are placed to indicate allergies and specific precautions. Before surgery, ensure that all bands are in place. Allergies must be clearly identified on a wristband and in the patient's chart because the anesthetized patient cannot report them to the surgical staff.

Prostheses. Prostheses are usually removed, marked, and secured before surgery to prevent them from being lost or damaged and to prevent them from causing injury during anesthesia. Nonremovable prostheses such as orthopedic metal or pacemakers must be documented and clearly identified to the surgical team. Be sure that the devices are returned to the patient as soon as possible after surgery. If the patient is very stressed

Table 17.2 Preoperative Fasting Recommendations of the American Society of Anesthesiologists

LIQUID AND FOOD INTAKE	MINIMAL FASTING PERIOD (HOURS)
Clear liquids (e.g., water, clear tea, black coffee, carbonated beverages, and fruit juice without pulp)	2
Breast milk	4
Nonhuman milk, including infant formula	6
Light meal (e.g., toast and clear liquids)	6
Regular or heavy meal (may include fried or fatty food, meat)	8

For healthy patients of all ages undergoing elective surgery (excluding women in labor).
From American Society of Anesthesiologists: Practice guidelines for preoperative fasting and the use of pharmacologic agents to reduce the risk of pulmonary aspiration: application to healthy patients undergoing elective procedures: an updated report by the American Society of Anesthesiologists Committee on Standards and Practice Parameters, *Anesthesiology* 126:5, 2017.

about having to go to surgery without the prosthesis, consult with the perioperative nurses about making an exception to the rule. A patient who is hard of hearing and does not have a hearing aid may be anxious or unable to cooperate with postoperative care; therefore hearing aids often are left in place for surgery. False teeth may also sometimes be left in if the anesthesia care provider gives permission.

Circulation. To reduce the risk of thrombi (blood clots) forming in the deep veins of the legs and pelvis during and after surgery, compression hose and devices may be applied. Depending on the patient's general condition and the nature of the procedure, drugs to reduce clotting may be ordered. Options are low-molecular-weight heparin, low-dose unfractionated heparin, and fondaparinux. Drug therapy may be started shortly before surgery or afterward. (See Chapter 33 for additional information.)

Pharmacology Capsule

Preoperative medications usually consist of a combination of an antianxiety, sedative-hypnotic, opioid analgesic, antiemetic, and anticholinergic drugs.

Preoperative medications. A preoperative medication may be given when the patient is in a holding area. Preoperative medication may include an opioid to decrease anxiety and promote sedation, an antiemetic to control nausea and vomiting, and an anticholinergic drug to prevent bradycardia and decrease secretions. Examples are listed in Table 17.3.

Table 17.3 Drug Table: Perioperative Medications

DRUG CLASS AND EXAMPLES	PERIOPERATIVE USE
Benzodiazepine • midazolam (Versed)	• Decrease anxiety • Promote amnesia
Opioids • morphine • fentanyl	• Decrease pain
Sedative • dexmedetomidine (Precedex)	• Maintain general anesthesia
Anticholinergic • atropine	• Prevent bradycardia • Reduce pulmonary secretions
Neuromuscular blocking agent • pancuronium (Pavulon)	• Relax skeletal muscle to prevent movement during surgery • Facilitate intubation
Hypnotic • etomidate (Amidate)	• Induce anesthesia
Intravenous anesthetics • Ketamine (Ketalar)	• Sedation • Control pain • Cause amnesia • Immobility
Sedative-hypnotic • propofol (Diprivan)	• Induce anesthesia • Maintain anesthesia

The timing of preoperative medications is important because they interact with the anesthetic agent. They may also be given to have the optimal dosage in the body during surgery. For example, preoperative antibiotics are very time specific and are usually ordered 1 hour before surgery. For safety reasons, the patient is asked to void before the preoperative medication is given. Tell the patient that the medications will cause drowsiness and dry mouth. Raise side rails, place the call bell within reach, and instruct the patient not to get up.

Preoperative checklist. Most agencies have a preoperative checklist that must be completed and signed before the patient leaves the unit. Ensure that all laboratory and radiology reports are with the chart; that jewelry, prostheses, and nail polish have been removed; that the patient has voided; that premedication has been given if ordered; that vital signs have been recorded; and that the consent form has been signed (Fig. 17.4).

The Joint Commission requires that agencies develop guidelines to "hand off" a patient from one patient care unit to another. The mnemonic "I pass the baton or situation, background, assessment, recommendation" (SBAR) is frequently used. The Joint Commission further requires a medical facility to develop, define, and implement a method to communicate pertinent patient information between nursing units. The information communicated for a surgical patient should include, at a minimum, the patient's diagnosis, surgical procedure to be performed, any relevant medical history, any medication given, any blood administered, latest vital signs, any drains (e.g., Foley catheter), and any intravenous access lines. A "hand off" is considered a transfer of primary responsibility of care from one health care provider to another.

Pharmacology Capsule

Because preoperative medications have a sedative effect, the surgical consent form must be signed before medications are given. After the medications are given, raise side rails, provide the call bell, and instruct the patient to remain in bed to prevent falls.

Put On Your Thinking Cap!

What observations would lead you to think that a patient is excessively anxious before surgery? What are some interventions that might reduce the patient's anxiety?

INTRAOPERATIVE PHASE

OR personnel transfer the patient from the ambulatory preparation unit or nursing unit to the surgical suite. They assist the patient onto a gurney (wheeled stretcher) and take the patient and the medical record to the surgical area.

Planned Procedure: ______________________

____

____

______________ Date of procedure

COMPONENT #1 VERIFICATION PROCESS

Mark all that apply ***indicates required field*	Sending Unit	Prep & Holding	Unit Doing Procedure
Name and date of birth confirmed**			
Patient/decision maker verbalizes planned procedure			
Schedule confirms planned procedure			
Consent confirms planned procedure**			
History and physical confirms planned procedure			
Diagnostic study confirms planned procedure			
Progress record/consult confirms planned procedure			
Site marking required (*go to component 2*)			
Site marking not required			
Date/time:			
Initial:			

COMPONENT #2 SITE MARKING (if required)

After verification has been completed, the patient if able will write " **Yes**" with a permanent marker on or as near the site as possible:

☐ Right ______________ ☐ Left ______________

Side marked by:

☐ Patient ☐ Family member (Relationship): ______________ ☐ Healthcare provider

Initial: ______________ Time: ______________

Initials	Signature/Title	Print Name

COMPONENT #3 TIME OUT

The entire procedure team has performed a Time Out and all members have verbally agreed.

Time out included the verification of:	1st	2nd	3rd
Correct patient identity			
Agreement on procedure to be done			
Correct site and side			
Diagnostic study confirmation of site and side			
Availability of implants			
Availability of special equipment			

1st Time out: Time: __________ Initial: __________

2nd Time out: Time: __________ Initial: __________

3rd Time out: Time: __________ Initial: __________

FIRE RISK ASSESSMENT

Procedure site or incision above the xiphoid	1 (Yes)	0 (No)
Open oxygen source (face mask/nasal cannula)	1 (Yes)	0 (No)
Ignition source (cautery, laser, fiberoptic light source)	1 (Yes)	0 (No)

Score 1 or 2: ☐ Initiate routine protocol
Score 3: ☐ Initiate high risk fire protocol (see side 2 for specifics)

Initial: __________

Total score: __________

Initials	Signature/Title	Print Name

21020 S(36590)(0307)C

Fig. 17.4 The preoperative checklist must be completed before the patient goes to surgery. (From Rothrock JC, McEwan DR: *Alexander's care of the patient in surgery,* ed 14, St. Louis, 2011, Mosby.)

The patient may be taken directly to an OR or to a holding room first. In the holding room, skin preparation may be performed and intravenous fluids started, if these procedures were not performed earlier. The patient who knows what to expect will feel more secure in the surgical area. When moved into the OR, the patient will see many pieces of equipment, bright lights, and various people. The patient is helped to move to the OR table and safety straps are applied carefully because of the risk of impaired circulation or nerve damage caused by pressure. Comfort and warmth are maintained while the patient is awake (Fig. 17.5). The anesthetic agent is then administered and is maintained throughout the procedure. The patient is then positioned in a specific way such as side-lying or lithotomy depending on the type of surgery being performed. Measures must be taken to assure that the correct procedure is performed on the correct site. An overview of the guidelines to prevent wrong site and wrong procedure surgery is presented in Box 17.2.

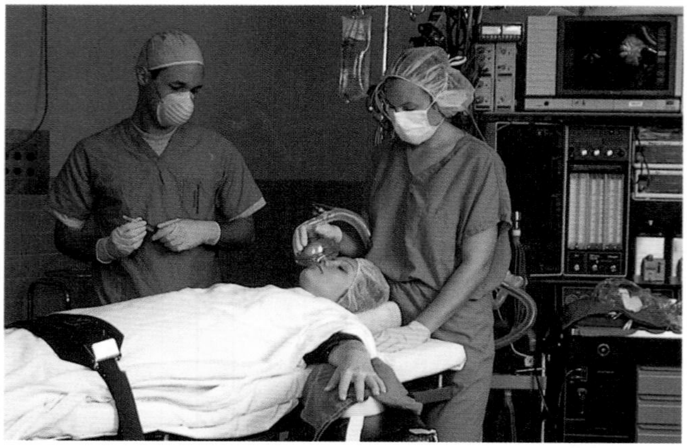

Fig. 17.5 The nurse ensures the patient's safety on the operating table. (From Harkreader H, Hogan MA: *Fundamentals of nursing: caring and clinical judgment*, ed 3, St. Louis, 2007, Saunders.)

Box 17.2 The Universal Protocol for Preventing Wrong Site, Wrong Procedure, and Wrong Person Surgery Principles

1. Conduct a preprocedure verification process: confirm procedure, patient, site, availability of all items and documents needed for the procedure. Involve the patient if possible. Address missing information or discrepancies before starting the procedure.
2. Mark the procedure site when possible for the procedure. The surgeon usually does this in the preoperative area. Perform a "time-out" in the operating room. The procedure is not started until all questions or concerns are resolved. It must be done before an incision is made, involve active members of the procedure team, confirm the patient identity, site, and procedure; and be documented.

From The Joint Commission: The universal protocol for preventing wrong site, wrong procedure, and wrong person surgery: guidance for health care professionals, 2013: http://www.jointcommission.org/standards_information/up.aspx. Accessed July 6, 2013.

Before the procedure begins, all the surgical team performs a final "time-out." The total surgical procedure is reviewed by the whole team, using a check list that includes the right patient, right procedure, and right site. The Joint Commission has published protocols in *National Patient Safety Goals Effective January 2021 for the Hospital Program* which is available at jointcommission.org and provides additional details. The Association of periOperative Registered Nurses has used the Joint Commission and World Health Organization guidelines to issue a *Comprehensive Surgical Checklist.* This document is available at aorn.org. When all is confirmed to be correct, the surgery begins.

SURGICAL TEAM

On arrival in the surgical suite, the patient is greeted by the nurse, the physician, the anesthesiologist, or the **nurse anesthetist**. A large number of people participate in the intraoperative period. Depending on the procedure, they may include the following:

- The surgeon who actually performs the procedure.
- An assistant surgeon, a registered nurse first assistant (RNFA), or a physician assistant (PA), who assists the surgeon in the procedure.
- The RN in the circulating role. This nurse is responsible for assessing the patient, planning intraoperative nursing care, functioning as patient advocate, and maintaining patient safety. This person oversees the OR. Responsibilities include seeing the room and equipment is set up correctly, monitoring and maintaining aseptic technique, assisting in positioning, monitoring the patient, preparing the skin, providing needed supplies and equipment, and documenting nursing care (Fig. 17.6).
- An RNFA works collaboratively with the surgeon and has advanced training for specific duties such as suturing and handling tissue with instruments.
- An RN, LVN/LPN, or surgical assistant scrubs and handles instruments within the sterile field and monitors the sterility of the surgical field.
- The anesthesia care provider (ACP) can be a certified registered nurse anesthetist (CRNA) or anesthesiologist. The ACP administers anesthetics and monitors the patient's status throughout the procedure. A CRNA is an advanced practice registered nurse (APRN) with special training in anesthesia and a graduate degree. An **anesthesiologist** is a physician who specializes in anesthesia.
- Other technical personnel have specialized jobs. For example, a perfusionist operates the heart bypass machine during open heart surgery.

ANESTHESIA

Although surgery has been performed since prehistoric times, anesthesia has been used only for approximately 150 years. **Anesthetics** are used to alter sensation so that surgical procedures can be performed painlessly

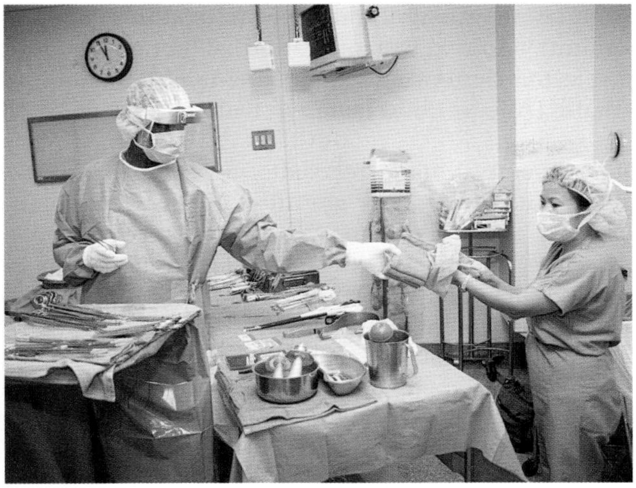

Fig. 17.6 The nurse sets up the operating room. (From Ignatavicius DD, Workman ML: *Medical-surgical nursing: patient-centered collaborative care*, ed 8, St. Louis, 2016, Saunders.)

and safely. Agents used for anesthesia include local, regional, and general anesthetics.

Local and Regional Anesthesia

Examples of local anesthetics are lidocaine hydrochloride (Xylocaine), bupivacaine hydrochloride (Marcaine HCl), tetracaine (Pontocaine), and ropivacaine (Naropin). These agents are commonly used for dental procedures, eye surgery, cosmetic surgery on the face, repair of lacerations, childbirth, and other procedures in which general anesthesia is not needed or desired by the patient. Local anesthetics are often the agents of choice for older adult patients because of other medical conditions.

Local anesthetics may be administered topically, by local infiltration, and by nerve-blocking techniques. Topical anesthetics are applied directly to the area to be anesthetized. For local infiltration, the anesthetic agent is injected into and under the skin around the area of treatment.

Regional anesthesia is achieved by using local anesthetics that block the conduction of nerve impulses in a specific area. These anesthetics do not cause the patient to lose consciousness. For some procedures, intravenous sedatives are given in addition to the local anesthetic.

A nerve block is administered by injecting an anesthetic agent around a nerve to block the transmission of impulses. Epidural anesthesia and subarachnoid anesthesia are examples of regional nerve blocks. Both methods are achieved by injecting the anesthetic agent into the area around the spinal nerves. Motor and sensory functions are blocked below the level of the anesthetic administration. This anesthesia is especially useful for surgical procedures on the lower abdomen and legs. Regional nerve blocks may be done to control postoperative pain in some procedures.

As a rule, spinal and epidural anesthesia pose less risk for respiratory, cardiac, and gastrointestinal (GI) complications than does general anesthesia. However, if the level of spinal or epidural anesthesia rises higher in the spinal cord than intended, a risk of respiratory and cardiovascular depression increases. The level of anesthesia—that is, how much of the body from legs to chest is affected from the anesthesia process—is controlled by the amount of the drug injected and the position of the patient on the operating table.

One complication of spinal anesthesia is postspinal headache, which is thought to be caused by the leaking of cerebrospinal fluid at the puncture site. Postspinal headache can be severe and may last for several weeks. It is relieved while lying flat. Postspinal headache is more common in women, especially postpartum women, than in men. The belief that keeping the patient flat for a specified period after spinal puncture reduces the risk of headache has not been supported by research (Bateman et al., 2020). Always check the postoperative orders, however, for any positioning or activity restrictions. Forcing fluids in the postoperative period, if allowed, may help.

Severe spinal headache may be treated by injecting a small amount of the patient's blood into the epidural space at the site of the previous subarachnoid puncture. The blood clot forms a "blood patch" that prevents further leaking. The procedure can be repeated if it is unsuccessful the first time. A successful patch relieves the headache immediately. Postanesthesia headache should not occur with epidural anesthesia.

As the effect of a regional anesthetic wears off, the patient often reports that the affected limbs feel numb and heavy. You should assure the patient that this feeling is normal and that movement and sensation gradually return to normal. Passive range-of-motion exercises, compression hose, and sequential compression devices (SCDs) help to prevent thrombus (clot) formation until mobility returns. Typically, motor function returns before sensory function. At this time, the patient is susceptible to injury resulting from trauma or pressure because movement is possible but pain is not perceived.

Complications of local anesthesia include toxic effects caused by overdose, local tissue damage, and allergic responses. Initial signs and symptoms of toxic effects are excitement and CNS stimulation followed by depression of the CNS and the cardiovascular system. Local tissue effects may be inflammation and edema. Abscesses and necrosis sometimes develop at the injection site. This circumstance is thought to be caused by poor technique rather than by the anesthetic agent.

General Anesthesia

General anesthesia acts on the CNS, causing loss of consciousness, sensation, reflexes, pain perception, and memory. Combinations of drugs are used to achieve these effects without excessive CNS depression. This use of multiple drugs, known as *balanced anesthesia*, allows lower dose levels of each drug, which reduces the risks of adverse effects. General anesthetics are most often given by inhalation or intravenous infusion. Although the intramuscular and rectal routes can be used to administer anesthetics, the use of these routes is uncommon.

Near the end of procedures performed under general anesthesia, the anesthetist or anesthesiologist administers drugs to reverse the effects of the anesthetic. When the procedure is completed, a member of the surgical team escorts the patient to the PACU and hand-off information is given. Careful monitoring is maintained until the patient recovers from the anesthesia according to protocols.

Inhalation agents. Inhalation agents include isoflurane (Forane), sevoflurane (Ultane), enflurane (Ethrane), desflurane (Suprane), and nitrous oxide. For most procedures using inhalation agents, the patient is first induced with a short-acting intravenous agent that causes rapid loss of consciousness. An endotracheal tube is then inserted into the patient's trachea to permit administration of the maintenance inhalation anesthesia and to control mechanical ventilation. A cuff on the endotracheal tube is inflated to prevent leakage during mechanical ventilation and aspiration of gastric contents while the patient is unconscious (Fig. 17.7). The laryngeal mask airway (LMA) is an alternative to the endotracheal tube.

Intravenous agents. The most commonly used intravenous agents for induction of anesthesia include ketamine hydrochloride (Ketalar), propofol (Diprivan),

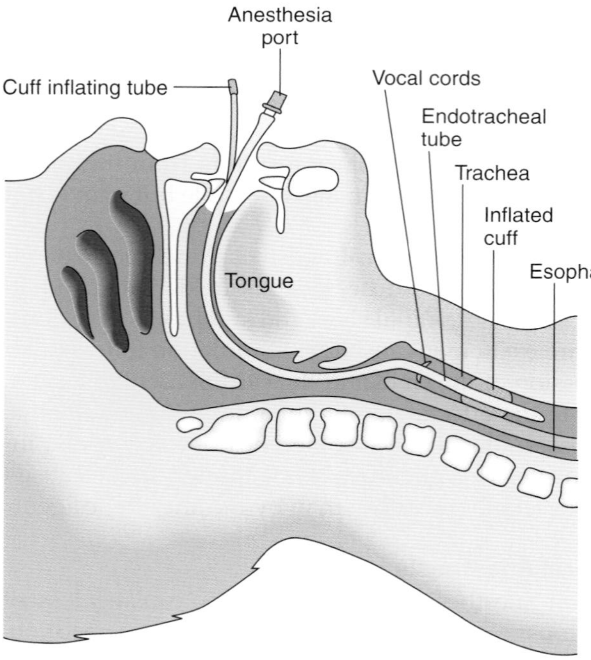

Fig. 17.7 Inhalation anesthetic is given through an endotracheal tube. (From Ignatavicius DD, Workman ML, Mishler MA: *Medical-surgical nursing across the health care continuum*, ed 3, Philadelphia, 1999, Saunders.)

etomidate (Amidate), methohexital sodium (Brevital Sodium), and midazolam (Versed). Other agents used in selected circumstances are sufentanil (Sufenta), alfentanil (Alfenta), and fentanyl (Duragesic).

Other agents. Muscle relaxants, opioids, benzodiazepines, and antiemetics are often given with the anesthetics. A muscle relaxant such as succinylcholine (Anectine, Quelicin), pancuronium, (and cisatracurium (Nimbex) may be used to ease intubation and to prevent movement of muscles during the surgical procedure. Opioids supplement anesthetics and support postoperative pain management. Benzodiazepines may be used to induce and maintain anesthesia, for moderate sedation, and to sedate patients during local or regional anesthesia. Antiemetics help to prevent vomiting during surgery. Using combinations of drugs allows for a lower and safer dose of the inhalation anesthetic.

Complications. Inhalation anesthetics and the endotracheal tube itself can cause irritation of the respiratory tract and the larynx. Swallowing must be closely monitored, and no fluids given by mouth until it is assured the awake patient can swallow without choking. Oxygen and carbon dioxide levels are also closely monitored to prevent disturbances of acid-base balance in case of inadvertently aspirating secretions. Individual agents may have the potential to cause serious adverse effects such as cardiac dysrhythmias, seizures, liver damage, nausea and vomiting, and death.

Malignant hyperthermia. Malignant hyperthermia is a rare but life-threatening complication that occurs in response to certain drugs. Susceptibility to this response is inherited. It is characterized by increasing body temperature and metabolic rate, tachycardia, hypotension, cyanosis, and muscle rigidity. Immediate measures must be taken to cool the patient. Oxygen is administered, and the patient is given dantrolene (Ryanodex), furosemide (Lasix) or mannitol, and sodium bicarbonate. There should be a separate crash cart available for this crisis, so the nurse should know where it is and how to obtain it quickly.

Moderate Sedation

Moderate (or procedural) sedation was previously called conscious sedation. It refers to the use of intravenous drugs to reduce pain intensity or awareness without loss of reflexes. It is used with some diagnostic and therapeutic procedures, including cardiac catheterization and endoscopy. Only patients who meet specific psychologic and physiologic criteria are candidates for moderate sedation. RNs with specialized training may administer the drugs used for moderate sedation. During the procedure, the patient's vital signs, oxygen saturation, airway, level of consciousness, and ECG readings must be closely monitored. Documentation must include assessment data; interventions such as oxygen therapy; and the time, dose level, route, and effects of all drugs administered. Complications include respiratory depression and apnea, hypotension, excessive sedation approaching that of general anesthesia, and agitation and combativeness.

After procedures using moderate sedation, the patient may be discharged home with a responsible person when the following conditions are met: stable vital signs, patent airway, intact motor function and reflexes, satisfactory surgical site, no nausea or vomiting, and the patient is alert and able to void.

INTRAOPERATIVE NURSING CARE

Intraoperative nursing care (called *perioperative nursing*) is a specialty and is beyond the scope of this chapter. Perioperative nursing focus is on patient care (preventing hypothermia, infection and positional injuries), aseptic technique, equipment and product safety, and sterilization and disinfection. Only selected patient problems and goals are listed here. For further information on perioperative nursing go to https:/www.aorn.org.

Patient Problems, Goals, and Outcome Criteria: Intraoperative Nursing Care

Patient Problems	Goals and Outcome Criteria
Potential for injury related to the effects of anesthesia, positioning, use of restraints, wrong surgery or site error, hypothermia	Absence of physical injury: infection control, complete recovery from anesthesia, no pressure on nerves or traumatic tissue damage associated with positioning or restraints. The Joint Commission guidelines to confirm site, procedure, and patient verified and documented. Body temperature of 96.8°F (36°C) (normothermia).
Inadequate oxygenation related to the effect of anesthesia and immobility	Adequate gas exchange: normal arterial blood gases.
Decreased cardiac output related to drug effects or blood loss	Adequate cardiac output: heart rate and blood pressure consistent with patient norms.
Potential for fluid volume deficit related to blood loss, insensible loss of water, NPO status	Normal fluid volume: balanced intake and output, pulse and blood pressure consistent with patient norms.

NPO, Nothing by mouth.

POSTOPERATIVE PHASE

When the surgical procedure is completed, the patient is usually transferred to the PACU (also known as the *recovery room*) or the critical care unit before returning to the nursing unit or being discharged to home. Exceptions are patients who have undergone minor procedures with only local anesthesia. The information communicated from the perioperative nurse to the PACU nurse should include patient diagnosis, surgical procedure performed, any relevant medical history, how the procedure was tolerated by the patient, medication given and times, blood loss, any blood given, latest vital signs, drains present and outputs, and any peripheral or central infusion lines. This formal sharing of information is known as the hand off.

SURGICAL COMPLICATIONS

The postoperative patient is at risk for a significant number of complications. These complications may be related to the surgical procedure itself, to the drugs used before and during the procedure, or to immobility during and after the procedure. The types of postoperative complications vary depending on the length of time that has elapsed since the surgical procedure. For example, shock and hypoxia are most likely to occur in the immediate recovery period. Wound infection, however, does not appear until several days after surgery. Complications in the immediate and later postoperative periods are described in Table 17.4. Prevention, recognition, and nursing implications are discussed in the section on nursing care.

Pharmacology Capsule

Opioid analgesics given before the effects of general anesthesia wear off may cause a drop in blood pressure and slow respirations.

Shock

Shock is inadequate tissue perfusion, which is most likely to occur as an effect of anesthesia or loss of blood. If opioid analgesics are given before the anesthesia wears off, they may contribute to a drop in blood pressure.

Shock may also result from low blood volume (hypovolemic shock). Bleeding is an obvious cause of low blood volume, but other factors may contribute as well. Dehydration without adequate fluid replacement or fluid losses through wounds and suction can explain low blood volume.

"Bloodless" surgical procedures use a variety of strategies to reduce the need for blood replacement necessitated by excessive blood loss. Such strategies include drug therapy to stimulate production of red blood cells; the use of Gamma Knife radiosurgery, electrocautery and laser beam coagulation; and the collection of the patient's own blood before or during the procedure, with reinfusion during the procedure.

Hypoxia

Hypoxia refers to inadequate oxygenation of body tissues. The patient is at risk for hypoxia in the immediate

Table 17.4 Surgical Complications

COMPLICATIONS	PREVENTION	TREATMENT
Shock related to deficient fluid volume	Inspect wound dressing Report excessive drainage or bleeding Monitor vital signs every 15 minutes until stable Note early changes in vital signs Report tachycardia, tachypnea, hypotension Monitor input and output Keep intravenous fluid rate on schedule Evaluate respirations before giving opioids	Fluid or blood replacement Vasopressors (drugs to raise blood pressure) as ordered Additional surgery may be needed to control bleeding
Hypoxia related to ineffective airway clearance, ineffective breathing pattern	Keep airway in place until patient awakens Position unconscious patient on side, if not contraindicated Suction as necessary Monitor vital signs every 15 minutes until stable Encourage deep breathing	Position to promote effective ventilation Suction as necessary Administer oxygen Encourage deep breathing and coughing
Wound complications related to impaired wound healing and/or infection Dehiscence Evisceration Infection	Provide adequate fluids and nutrition Splint incision during activity, coughing, and deep breathing Good hand washing; sterile or clean technique or wound care as appropriate	Cover open wound with sterile dressing If organs protrude, saturate dressing with normal saline and cover wet dressing with dry, sterile dressing; notify physician Keep patient still and quiet with knees flexed Anticipate return to surgery; withhold opioids until consent form signed
Inadequate oxygenation related to pneumonia Atelectasis	Change position at least every 2 hours Assist to cough and deep breathe hourly Incentive spirometry	Rest Administer oxygen and antibiotics as ordered
Digestive disturbances Nausea and vomiting	Withhold oral fluids until nausea subsides Give antiemetics to prevent vomiting as soon as nausea is reported	Administer antiemetic drugs as ordered
Altered elimination Urine retention Kidney failure Abdominal distention "Gas" pains Constipation	Provide privacy; offer warm bedpan; position comfortably; take to bathroom or bedside commode chair if allowed; pour warm water over the perineum; let tap water run Promptly report urine output of less 30 mL/h Nothing by mouth until bowel sounds return Encourage ambulation as allowed Encourage fluids, food, and ambulation as ordered; use stool softeners as ordered	Catheterize as ordered Use heat to abdomen, bisacodyl suppositories as ordered Position on right side Initiate nasogastric intubation with suction as ordered Ambulate frequently when permitted Administer laxatives or enemas, or both, as ordered
Thrombophlebitis	Avoid pressure on blood vessels Encourage leg exercises every 1 to 2 hours Early, frequent ambulation as ordered Elastic or automatic compression stockings	Bed rest Administer anticoagulant therapy as ordered
Fluid and electrolyte imbalances	Monitor intravenous fluid rate Provide a variety of oral fluids when permitted; treat vomiting promptly Recognize signs of imbalances (see Chapter 6)	Give intravenous fluids as ordered Encourage oral intake when allowed

postoperative phase for several reasons. First, general anesthetics depress respirations such that the patient's breathing efforts may be inadequate initially. Second, when the patient is unconscious, the tongue may fall back and block the airway. Third, anesthesia depresses the cough and swallowing reflexes. Until these reflexes return, vomitus and saliva can enter the airway. A fourth reason that hypoxia may occur in the immediate postoperative period is the risk of laryngospasm or bronchospasm. Spasm of the larynx or bronchi narrows the airway and obstructs airflow. Postoperatively, oral fluids are withheld until the patient can swallow safely. Spasms of the larynx can be life-threatening. Because they are at increased risk for hypoxia, patients with sleep apnea may be treated with continuous positive airway pressure (CPAP) in the PACU.

Pharmacology Capsule

Regional anesthesia blocks sensation and movement; as a result, the affected body part is at risk for injury.

Injury

Immediately after surgery, the patient is at risk for injury because of the decreased level of consciousness and self-protection associated with general anesthesia or other sedatives. If regional anesthesia was used, the affected body part may be injured because it lacks sensation.

Pharmacology Capsule

General anesthetics and opioid analgesics depress respirations.

Pneumonia and Atelectasis

Drug effects and immobility place the surgical patient at risk for pneumonia and atelectasis. Patients who are most prone to these complications are older adults, the obese, those with chronic pulmonary disease, and those who have undergone chest or abdominal surgery. General anesthetics and opioid analgesics depress respiratory function. Anticholinergics cause pulmonary secretions to be drier and thicker than normal.

Immobility limits lung expansion and allows fluids to pool in the lungs. Fluid provides a medium for infectious organisms to grow. An infection of the lungs associated with immobility is called *hypostatic pneumonia*.

As secretions accumulate, they begin to block off branches of the respiratory tree. When gases can no longer enter or leave the affected alveoli, they collapse. *Atelectasis* is the term used to describe collapse of alveoli, which may affect a portion or an entire lobe of the lung. Because atelectasis impairs the exchange of gases, it can be very serious.

WOUND COMPLICATIONS

Complications in wound healing include infection, dehiscence, or evisceration. All of these complications are, to some extent, preventable.

Infection

The risk of wound infection is greatest in cases of traumatic injuries, wounds that were not treated promptly, and wounds that were infected before surgery. Obese patients and those with diabetes mellitus or immune suppression are also at increased risk for slow or nonhealing wounds.

Dehiscence and Evisceration

Dehiscence is the reopening of the surgical wound. It involves one or more layers of tissue. Dehiscence is most likely to happen when strain on the suture line is excessive. Factors that increase the risk of dehiscence include wound infection, malnutrition, obesity, dehydration, and extensive abdominal wounds or injuries. Dehiscence is most likely to occur between the fifth and twelfth postoperative days. **Evisceration** is the term used when body organs protrude through the open wound. Dehiscence and evisceration are illustrated in Fig. 17.8.

GASTROINTESTINAL DISTURBANCES

The primary GI problems that follow surgery are nausea, vomiting, impaired peristalsis, and constipation. Nausea and vomiting are most common in the early postoperative period. Causative factors include

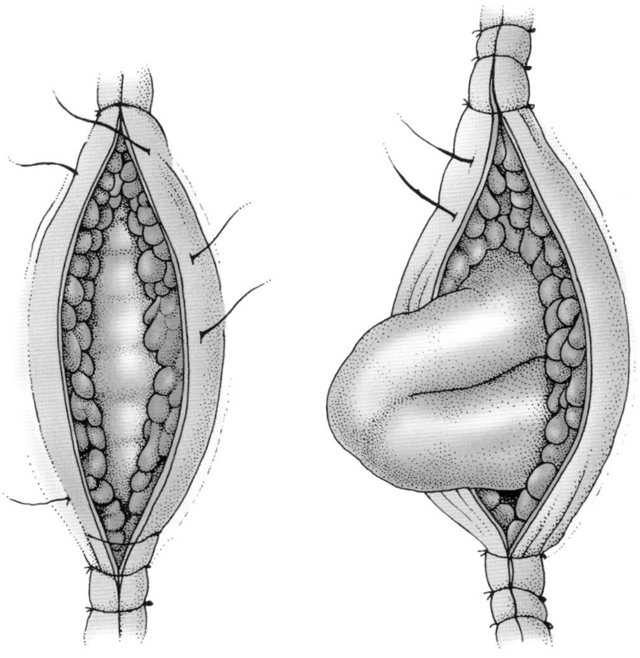

A Dehiscence B Evisceration

Fig. 17.8 Complications of wound healing. (A) Dehiscence. (B) Evisceration. (From Ignatavicius DD, Workman ML, Mishler MA: *Medical-surgical nursing across the health care continuum*, ed 3, Philadelphia, 1999, Saunders.)

anesthesia, pain, opioids, decreased peristalsis, and resuming oral intake too soon.

Factors that cause peristalsis to be impaired after surgery include anesthesia, immobility, opioid analgesics, and handling of the bowel during surgery. Patients who develop metabolic imbalances, respiratory problems, or shock are also at risk for GI disturbances.

The effects of slowed peristalsis can be mild or severe. Gas normally forms in the digestive tract. When peristalsis is slow, the gas builds up and causes cramping pain and distention. Mild effects are generally experienced as gas pains that typically occur on the second or third postoperative day. Constipation is also related to slow peristalsis.

If peristalsis stops completely, the patient is said to have a **paralytic ileus**. The patient with a paralytic ileus has abdominal distention that may be severe enough to impair lung expansion and decrease blood return from the legs, causing cardiac output to fall. Distention also causes strain on an abdominal incision.

URINARY RETENTION AND RENAL FAILURE

With urinary retention, the kidneys produce urine but the patient is unable to empty the bladder. Urinary retention can be caused by the effects of anesthesia or opioids, trauma to the urinary tract, or anxiety about voiding. Urine volume may also be decreased because of dehydration or blood loss.

With kidney failure, the kidneys are unable to produce enough urine to remove wastes from the body. Urine production falls dangerously low.

Put On Your Thinking Cap!

Use the stress response (discussed in Chapter 4) to explain the signs and symptoms of fluid volume deficit during the immediate postoperative period.

THROMBOPHLEBITIS

The risk of hemorrhage and shock decreases after the immediate postoperative period. A more common circulatory problem in the later period is thrombophlebitis. Thrombophlebitis is the inflammation of veins with the formation of blood clots. It occurs most often in the legs after a period of immobility. Patients who have very lengthy surgical procedures or who must be immobilized are at greatest risk for thrombophlebitis and frequently will come to PACUs or nursing units with an SCD in place as a preventive measure.

Clots that cling to the walls of blood vessels are called *thrombi*. Thrombi that break loose and flow with the blood are called *emboli*. Emboli formed in the legs are most likely to pass through the heart and lodge in the pulmonary circulation. They can also lodge in the heart, leading to a life-threatening incident. If they lodge in the lungs, the patient will develop severe respiratory distress. Clots or emboli can also go to the brain and cause a stroke.

IMMEDIATE POSTOPERATIVE NURSING CARE IN THE POSTANESTHESIA CARE UNIT

FOCUSED ASSESSMENT

When the patient is admitted to the PACU, determine the medical diagnosis and the surgical procedure and other assessment data listed earlier. Promptly assess the patient's status (level of consciousness, vital signs, pain) and inspect the wound or dressing. Check and set up equipment, such as suction devices, wound drains, oxygen, urinary drainage, and intravenous lines, as needed. When the patient returns to the nursing unit, a more complete assessment will be performed.

Patient Problems, Goals, and Outcome Criteria: Immediate Postoperative Care

Depending on the specific surgical procedure, patient problems and goals for the patient immediately after surgery may include the following.

Patient Problems	Goals and Outcome Criteria
Decreased cardiac output related to excessive loss of blood and other body fluids or the effects of drugs	Normal cardiac output: pulse and blood pressure consistent with patient norms, normal skin color.
Inadequate oxygenation and/or ineffective airway clearance related to effects of anesthetics or pain	Adequate oxygenation: respiratory rate, effort, and pattern consistent with patient norms; normal arterial blood gases; breath sounds clear; SpO_2 of 95% to 100%.
Acute pain related to tissue trauma or to positioning during surgical procedures	Decreased pain: relaxed expression, patient statement of pain relief.
Acute confusion related to the effects of anesthetics	Absence of confusion; orientation to person and place.
Potential for injury related to decreased level of consciousness or loss of sensation and movement as effect of anesthesia	Patient remains safe during recovery period: no falls, bruises, trauma when under effects of anesthesia.

SpO_2, Oxygen saturation.

INTERVENTIONS

Decreased Cardiac Output

Be alert to the possibility of shock. To detect impending shock, the patient's vital signs are monitored every 5 to 15 minutes in the PACU. Signs and symptoms of impending shock include a rapid, thready pulse; restlessness; decreasing blood pressure; and decreasing urine output. Use the patient's preoperative vital signs to evaluate whether postoperative vital signs are normal. An increasing pulse usually precedes a fall in blood pressure. Monitor intravenous fluid intake and urinary output. When blood volume is low (hypovolemia), the kidneys reduce urine production. Continuous cardiac monitoring is usually used to identify early signs of hypovolemia or potentially dangerous changes in cardiac rhythm.

Measures to reduce the risk of shock include prompt recognition and treatment of bleeding, replacement of lost fluids, and the cautious use of opioid analgesics. Frequently inspect wound dressings and drains for the color and amount of drainage. The amount of bleeding expected varies with different surgical procedures.

An open intravenous route must be maintained during the early postoperative period. This access permits the infusion of fluids, blood, and emergency medications if needed. Therefore check the venipuncture site to ensure that the fluid is infusing properly. The intravenous fluid infusion rate is ordered by the physician, but the nurse regulates the rate. If the rate falls behind, the patient may not receive adequate fluids to replace losses during surgery. If given too rapidly, intravenous fluids can overload the circulatory system, causing heart failure. Make sure infusion pumps are correctly set up and functioning properly.

Inadequate Oxygenation

To detect early signs of hypoxia in the PACU, monitor the patient's respiratory status. Assess respiratory depth, rate, and effort. Listen for abnormal breath sounds that suggest breathing difficulty. In addition, be alert for changes in the pulse rate because an increasing pulse rate is often an early indicator of poor oxygenation. The oximeter is a device with a wire that clips to a finger or an earlobe and provides a continuous reading of blood oxygenation as SpO_2.

The patient's color, especially in the nail beds and lips, provides a clue to oxygenation. Because cyanosis is a late sign of hypoxia, however, you should detect problems long before color changes develop.

Take measures to reduce the risk of hypoxia during the immediate postoperative period. An airway is inserted to keep the air passages open until the patient begins to awaken. Position the unconscious patient (if permitted) on one side to reduce the risk of aspiration. Suction if necessary to remove secretions or vomitus. When the gag reflex returns, the airway can be removed.

Acute Pain

Decisions to medicate for pain in the early postoperative phase are based on physician's orders and nursing judgment. If opioid analgesics are given too early, their effects when combined with the effects of the anesthesia may lead to shock. However, severe pain may also cause shock. Pain is what the patient says it is, not what the nurse thinks it should be! Never ignore a patient complaint of pain. Monitor and report the effect of the drug on pain after 30 to 60 minutes. Use of nonopioid drugs may control pain as well as opioid analgesics.

Acute Confusion

As patients begin to regain consciousness, they may move around and touch dressings and drains. Tell patients where they are, that the surgery is over, and what is happening. Simple explanations and gentle reminders are often sufficient to calm and reassure them. The amnesic effects of drugs used in surgery may cause the patient to forget what was said, making it necessary to repeat information. Often after surgery, older patients may be "labeled" as someone who is permanently cognitively impaired, when it is a temporary occurrence caused by drugs. Preoperative cognition should be compared with postoperative status if this happens.

Potential for Injury

Patients who have had local anesthesia may be sent to the PACU postoperatively or they may be returned directly to the nursing unit or the ambulatory surgery unit. In the immediate postoperative period, patients are usually drowsy because preoperative and intraoperative sedatives typically have been given.

When regional block anesthesia is used, remember that sensation in that area is impaired. Take care therefore to prevent injury to the anesthetized body region.

After spinal anesthesia, the patient regains the ability to move the legs before sensation returns. Chart the times that the patient regains both movement and sensation. Assess the bladder for distention because the patient is unable to feel pressure. Patients may be kept flat for a specific time period in the belief that it may help to prevent spinal headache.

PATIENT'S FAMILY

The time between the patient leaving the nursing unit and returning can be 3 or 4 hours, even with relatively simple procedures. This period may seem like a very long time for family and friends who are waiting. Most hospitals have some system for communicating the patient's status to those who wait. These visitors are usually relieved to know when the patient is in the recovery room. Many surgeons take time to speak with the family shortly after the surgery is completed. When problems arise, offer visitors privacy and the services of a patient representative or a spiritual counselor.

DISCHARGE FROM THE POSTANESTHESIA CARE UNIT

Most patients remain in the PACU for 1 to 2 hours, although the time varies considerably. The patient's progress in the

Box 17.3 Modified Aldrete Score

CRITERIA	SCORE
ACTIVITY	
Able to move four extremities voluntarily or on command	2
Able to move two extremities voluntarily or on command	1
Unable to move extremities voluntarily or on command	0
RESPIRATORY	
Able to breathe deeply and cough freely	2
Dyspnea or limited breathing	1
Apneic	0
CIRCULATION	
BP 20% of preanesthetic level	2
BP 20% to 49% of preanesthetic level	1
BP 50% of preanesthetic level	0
CONSCIOUSNESS	
Fully awake	2
Arousable on calling	1
Not responding	0
OXYGEN (O_2) SATURATION	
Able to maintain O_2 saturation >92% on room air	2
Needs O_2 inhalation to maintain O_2 saturation >92%	1
O_2 saturation <90% even with O_2 supplement	0
TOTALS: POSSIBLE SCORE RANGE OF 0–10	

CRITERIA	SCORE
For patients in ambulatory surgical settings, the Aldrete score is derived by assessing the earlier criteria plus these indices:	
DRESSING	
Dry and clean	2
Wet but marked and not increasing	1
Growing area of wetness	0
PAIN	
Pain free	2
Mild pain handled by oral medication	1
Severe pain requiring parenteral medication	0
AMBULATION	
Able to stand up and walk straight[a]	2
Vertigo when erect	1
Dizziness when supine	0
FASTING-FEEDING	
Able to drink fluids	2
Nauseated	1
Nausea and vomiting	0
URINE OUTPUT	
Has voided	2
Unable to void but comfortable	1
Unable to void and uncomfortable	0
TOTALS: POSSIBLE SCORE RANGE OF 0–20	

[a]May be substituted by Romberg test, or by picking up 12 paper clips in one hand.

Note: Total score must be at least 18 for the patient to be discharged to the home; a lower score is allowed if the patient was unable to walk or move the extremities before surgery.

BP, Blood pressure.

Modified from Aldrete JA: Modifications to the post anesthesia score for use in ambulatory surgery, *J Perianesth Nurs* 13(3):148, 1998; Aldrete JA, Kroulik D: A post-anesthesia recovery score, *Anesth Analg* 49:924, 1970)

PACU is carefully monitored. Patients who are unstable or who need very close observation may be transferred to a critical care unit. Several systems of scoring have been used to determine when recovery is adequate and the patient can be transferred. The modified Aldrete score is used to assess patients at intervals while in the PACU (Box 17.3). For inpatients, only the first five criteria are included and a total score of 8 or more is required for the patient to be discharged from the PACU. Patients in ambulatory care settings are assessed on all 10 criteria and indices and must have a score of 18 to be discharged.

POSTOPERATIVE NURSING CARE ON THE NURSING UNIT

When the patient is transferred to the nursing unit, the PACU nurse reports on the patient to the nurse who will be caring for that patient, again using a hand-off procedure like SBAR. Several people are usually necessary to move the patient safely from the gurney to the bed. Be careful to prevent pulling or dislodging tubes and to prevent a shearing force on the skin. Hang intravenous fluids and set infusion at the ordered rate. Connect nasogastric suction tubes to suction equipment. Identify and arrange drains to avoid obstruction. For safety, raise the side rails, lower the bed, place the call bell within reach, and instruct the patient not to get up without assistance (see Nursing Care Plan: Postoperative Patient).

FOCUSED ASSESSMENT

Health History

Review the patient's preoperative assessment (as outlined in Box 17.1), noting long-term conditions, disabilities, prostheses, drugs, and allergies. When the patient is able to respond, ask about significant symptoms, including pain, nausea, and altered sensations (as explained in Box 17.4).

Nursing Care Plan Postoperative Patient

FOCUSED ASSESSMENT

Health History

Ms. M, 37 years old, was admitted for an abdominal hysterectomy and surgical excision of endometriosis implants. She is a secretary, married, and the mother of a 3-year-old child. On day 1 after the surgery: Complains of moderate abdominal and incisional pain (7 on a scale of 1–10); has been out of bed three times since surgery; ambulated well with assistance; has not voided since Foley catheter removed 3 hours ago; intravenous fluids infusing at 100 mL/h; no nausea but nothing by mouth (NPO) until noon, when 550 mL of clear liquids were taken and retained.

Physical Examination Patient is alert and oriented. Vital signs: temperature 99.4°F orally; pulse 90 beats per minute, respirations 16 breaths per minute, blood pressure 130/86 mm Hg. (Admission vital signs were temperature 98°F orally; pulse 84 beats per minute, respirations 20 breaths per minute, blood pressure 126/82 mm Hg.) Breath sounds diminished in lower lobes; abdomen soft; no bladder distention; wound covered with dry dressing; bowel sounds present but hypoactive.

Patient Problems	Goals and Outcome Criteria	Interventions
Acute pain related to tissue trauma	Patient will report pain relief and appear more relaxed.	Assess nature, location, and severity of pain. Evaluate effectiveness of analgesia. Assure patient that opioids can be taken safely for acute pain for a limited time. Assist to change positions at least every 2 hours. Give back rub. Coach in relaxation exercises and mental imagery. Assess anxiety and explore causes. Be available. Reassure.
Disrupted tissue integrity related to surgical incision	Patient's wound edges will remain clean and closed until discharge.	Check dressing hourly for bleeding first 24 hours then twice each shift. Report bleeding to physician. Protect wound by supporting during respiratory exercises. Treat nausea promptly.
Potential for infection related to break in skin, invasive devices, and procedures	Patient will remain free of infection, as evidenced by oral temperature less than 100°F, decreasing redness of incision; no purulent drainage; clear breath sounds; no dysuria; no phlebitis.	Monitor vital signs every 4 hours. Report increasing temperature. Assess wound for increasing redness, edema, or drainage each shift. Inspect for purulent drainage. Exercise good hand washing. Use aseptic technique for wound care. Monitor and encourage fluid intake. Collect specimens for culture if ordered. Teach patient how to care for wound after discharge.
Inadequate oxygenation related to stasis of pulmonary secretions	Patient's breath sounds will remain clear and respiratory rate will be between 12 and 20 breaths per minute without dyspnea.	Help patient to support incision and turn, cough, and deep breathe or use incentive spirometry at least every 2 hours. Teach to take 10 deep breaths each hour. Auscultate breath sounds for crackles or atelectasis every 2 hours. Encourage fluid intake. Assist out of bed to walk as tolerated.
Urinary retention related to effects of anesthesia	Patient's urine output will be approximately equal to fluid intake; no bladder distention.	Measure all fluid intake and output. Palpate for distended bladder every 2 hours. Provide privacy and try to stimulate voiding. Catheterize using sterile technique as ordered if patient is unable to void.
Constipation related to effects of drugs, immobility, bowel manipulation during surgery	Patient will have bowel sounds and pass flatus before discharge.	Assess bowel sounds and ask patient to report passage of flatus (gas). Count and document gurgles per minute in each quadrant of abdomen. Encourage frequent ambulation as allowed. Position the patient on the right side. Report distention.
Potential for fluid volume deficit related to blood loss, wound drainage, NPO status	Patient's fluid intake and output will be approximately equal; serum electrolytes will remain within normal limits.	Measure fluid intake and output. Assess fluid status: tissue turgor, mucous membranes, pulse quality. Administer antiemetics promptly for nausea or vomiting. Offer fluids as prescribed.
Impaired motor function related to weakness, tissue trauma	Patient will gradually increase activity and assume more self-care.	Assist out of bed until patient can do so alone. Teach patient importance of ambulation to promote healing and prevent complications.
Altered body image related to abdominal wound	Patient will state any concerns about appearance of wound.	Observe patient's reaction to the incision. Elicit any patient questions or concerns. Answer questions honestly or refer to surgeon. Tell the patient the incision will fade, and the edema will diminish.
Inability to perform self-care related to lack of knowledge of postoperative needs	Patient will correctly describe postoperative self-care during hospitalization and after discharge.Patient will identify complications that should be reported to the physician.	Reinforce physician's instructions for wound care and activity limitations. Encourage consideration of adaptations needed in work or home roles and responsibilities. Stress need for good nutrition. Explain any drugs being prescribed: dose level, schedule, side effects, and adverse effects that should be reported to the physician. Include husband in teaching.

CRITICAL THINKING QUESTIONS

1. In addition to your desire to ensure that the patient is comfortable, why is collecting data about postoperative pain necessary?
2. Members of the health care team often repeat and reinforce one another's instructions when talking to the patient. List at least three reasons to explain the importance of doing so.

Physical Examination

Vital signs. Take vital signs and compare the results with the preoperative readings. Note the respiratory rate, depth, and effort. Take the pulse, noting rate, rhythm, and quality. Record the blood pressure. Document patient's rating of pain. Measurements are usually repeated every 15 minutes until the vital signs stabilize.

Box 17.4 Focused Assessment of the Postoperative Patient

HEALTH HISTORY

Reason for surgery, name of procedure, medical diagnosis, disabilities, prostheses, drugs, allergies, intravenous (IV) fluids, dressings, drains, tubes

Presence of pain, nausea, altered sensations

PHYSICAL EXAMINATION

Vital Signs

Neurologic Status: Level of consciousness; pupil size, equality, response to light; sensation; spontaneous movement, response to commands

Skin: Color, temperature, incision or dressing appearance, amount and appearance of drainage on dressing and in closed drainage systems; appearance of IV insertion site

Thorax: Chest expansion, symmetry, breath sounds

Heart: Apical pulse

Abdomen: Contour, bowel sounds, bladder distention, tenderness

Extremities: Color, capillary refill, pulses, edema, warmth, redness

Neurologic status. The assessment of neurologic status includes level of consciousness and pupil size, equality, and reaction to light. Evaluate sensation in affected body areas. Note spontaneous movements and the patient's ability to move affected parts on command. For example, when a cast has been applied to a fractured arm, test the patient's ability to move the fingers. Compare precognition to postcognition and awareness, especially in older adults.

Skin. Inspect the skin color and palpate for temperature. Inspect the surgical area. If the wound is visible, assess the incision for intactness of the wound margins, drainage, and excessive redness or swelling. If a dressing covers the incision, inspect the dressing for bleeding or other drainage. If closed drains are in place, observe the amount and appearance of the drainage (Table 17.5).

Thorax. Observe chest expansion with respirations. Chest movement should be symmetric. Auscultate for breath sounds to detect atelectasis, crackles, and wheezes.

Table 17.5 Expected Drainage From Tubes and Catheters

SUBSTANCE	DAILY AMOUNT	COLOR	ODOR	CONSISTENCY
Indwelling catheter: urine	800–1500 mL first 2 hours; minimal expected output: 0.5 mL/kg/h	Clear, yellow	Ammonia	Watery
Nasogastric tube/ gastrostomy tube: gastric contents	Up to <1500 mL/day	Pale, yellow-green Bloody after gastrointestinal surgery	Sour	Watery
Open drains (e.g., Penrose)	Varies with procedure May decrease over hours or days	Varies with procedure Initially may be sanguineous or serosanguineous, changing to serous	Same as wound dressing. Little or no odor. Foul odor may indicate infection	Thin, watery
Closed suction drains (Hemovac, Jackson-Pratt): wound drainage	Varies with procedure; may decrease over hours or days	Variable with procedure; initially, may be sanguineous or serosanguineous, changing to serous	Little or no odor Foul odor may indicate infection	Thin, watery
T-tube: bile	500 mL	Bright yellow to dark green	Acid	Thick
Mediastinal chest tube: wound drainage postcardiothoracic surgery	Varies with procedure Should decrease over several hours postoperatively	Sanguineous or serosanguineous	N/A	Thin
Pleural chest tube fluid that collected in the pleural space	Varies with procedure Decreases over hours or days 100 mL/h is considered excessive	Varies with indication for insertion and fluid collected in the pleural spaces	N/A	Varies with indication for insertion

From Hoch CR: Postoperative care. In: Lewis SM, Bucher L, Heitkemper MM, Harding MM, editors: *Medical-surgical nursing: assessment and management of clinical problems*, ed 10, St. Louis, 2017, Elsevier.

Heart. Auscultate the apical pulse if the peripheral pulse is weak or irregular or if the patient has heart disease.

Abdomen. Inspect the abdomen for distention and auscultate for bowel sounds. Light palpation may also be performed to assess bowel and bladder distention and tenderness. Check the patency of GI tubes and note the characteristics of any output.

Extremities. Assess the color and capillary refill of nail beds and the presence and quality of peripheral pulses in affected extremities. Note the presence of edema or excessive warmth or redness. Simultaneously compare the color and temperature of both arms and then both legs to detect differences.

Patient Problems, Goals, and Outcome Criteria: Postoperative Nursing Care

Once the immediate postoperative phase has passed, the types of potential complications change somewhat. The risks of shock and hypoxia lessen. The nurse's attention turns toward other patient problems and goals, which are detailed in this chart.

Patient Problems	Goals and Outcome Criteria
Acute pain related to tissue trauma	Reduced pain: relaxed expression, patient statement of pain reduction or relief
Disrupted tissue integrity related to poor wound healing	Normal wound healing: intact wound margins
Potential for infection related to break in skin or invasive devices and procedures	Absence of infection: minimal redness, clear drainage, no purulence; no fever
Inadequate oxygenation related to stasis of pulmonary secretions, thrombosis, or emboli	Adequate oxygenation: respiratory rate and effort consistent with patient norms, normal arterial blood gases Absence of thrombophlebitis: no redness or swelling in legs
Urinary retention related to the effects of anesthesia or restricted position	Normal bladder emptying: urine output approximately equal to fluid intake, no bladder distention
Constipation related to the effects of drugs, immobility, or bowel manipulation during surgery	Normal bowel function: bowel sounds present, passage of flatus, bowel movement
Potential for fluid volume deficit related to wound drainage, inadequate intake, vomiting, or gastrointestinal decompression	Normal hydration: approximately equal fluid intake and output, normal serum electrolytes, pulse and blood pressure consistent with patient norms
Inadequate nutrition related to nausea and vomiting or medical restriction of intake	Adequate nutrition for metabolic demands: retention of oral food and fluids, stable body weight
Impaired motor function related to weakness, tissue trauma, or medical activity restrictions	Improved physical mobility: gradual increase in mobility to preoperative level
Altered body image related to change in body appearance and function	Adaptation to changes in body image: patient looks at and touches affected area, patient verbalizes acceptance of physical changes

INTERVENTIONS

Acute Pain

Pain is expected in the early postoperative phase. Pain receptors are stimulated because tissues are cut and stretched during surgery. Muscle spasms in the area around the incision add to the patient's discomfort. Many surgeons now inject the areas around the incision with a local anesthetic so incisional pain may not be evident for several hours. The pain is usually most severe during the first 48 hours after surgery. During this time, an intravenous opioid analgesic such as morphine is most appropriate. Patient-controlled analgesia (PCA) may be used to provide prompt relief of pain and to maintain a more stable blood level of the drug. PCA is discussed in Chapter 8. By the third postoperative day, most patients require less narcotic medication for pain relief. The dose level or frequency may be reduced, or the order may be changed to an oral analgesic such as acetaminophen with codeine on an as-needed basis. Nonnarcotic agents are used more often today to ease pain, especially with ambulatory surgery patients. The patient's response to any analgesic should be assessed within 30 to 60 minutes to judge the effectiveness on lowering pain.

When postoperative patients complain of pain, determine the exact nature of the complaint. Where is the pain located? An easy assumption would be that the pain is incisional when, in fact, the patient may have a headache or a backache. Chest pain, leg pain, or gas pain requires additional assessment and interventions. How severe is the pain? Ask the patient to rate the severity of the pain on a scale of 1 to 10, with 1 being no pain and 10 being the worst pain imaginable. This system provides a means for evaluating response to comfort measures.

During the first few days after surgery, promptly medicate the patient for pain. Pain is controlled better if it is treated before it becomes severe. Some physicians will order routine (rather than as-needed) analgesics for the first 24 to 36 hours, which maintains consistent therapeutic blood levels of the analgesic and reduces episodes of acute pain. Pain medication can also be given before activities that normally cause pain. Some patients are afraid that they will become addicted to opioids. Assure them that the short-term use of opioids for acute pain relief generally has not been associated with addiction.

A patient whose pain is controlled adequately is better able to participate in the exercises necessary to prevent postoperative complications. Schedule turning, coughing, deep breathing, and even walking to take advantage of periods when the patient is most comfortable. Of course, a medicated patient must be closely supervised when out of bed.

Although drugs are the mainstay of pain management in the early postoperative phase, other nursing measures can be used to help reduce pain. Position changes and back rubs can be very soothing. Relaxation exercises and mental imagery are often very effective alone or in combination with other nursing measures.

One source of discomfort in the postoperative patient is singultus, commonly known as *hiccups*. Hiccups are caused by intermittent spasms of the diaphragm. They are uncomfortable and may put stress on the incision, disrupt rest, and interfere with the intake of food and fluids. If hiccups persist, notify the physician.

Anxiety seems to intensify discomfort. Measures to decrease anxiety may therefore enhance the effects of pain relief measures. Recognize when the patient is tense and try to discover the source of the anxiety. Patients need to feel safe and need reassurance about what is happening to them.

Pain management in older adults can pose special challenges. The older patient may be stoic, reluctant to request analgesics, and fearful of addiction and overdose. Nurses who are concerned about the increased risk of adverse drug effects or who believe that the older person experiences less pain than younger patients may fail to treat the older person adequately. Good management of postoperative pain in the older person can often be attained with NSAIDs or acetaminophen in combination with opioids at somewhat reduced dose levels. The rule of thumb with opioids is to start with a low dose and gradually increase it. Drugs that are likely to have increased adverse effects in the older person are meperidine (Demerol) and long-acting benzodiazepines such as diazepam (Valium). Regardless of age, well-prepared patients can participate in pain management by describing and rating their pain, informing the nurse of the effects of treatment, and using PCA when appropriate.

The management of pain in cognitively impaired older adults is especially difficult. You may have to rely on your observations of patient behavior or family perceptions to recognize pain. Inappropriate behaviors such as pulling at tubes, striking out, and yelling may be manifestations of pain. Some impaired older adults can use pediatric pain rating scales, which provide you with some measure of pain intensity. After procedures that are known to be painful, it is reasonable to assume that the patient has pain. Provide analgesics in combination with other comfort measures.

Disrupted Tissue Integrity

Various techniques are used to close the wound after surgery. The patient's incision may be closed with sutures, staples, surgical skin glue, or tape, as shown in Fig. 17.9. When the patient returns to the nursing unit, a dressing probably covers the wound. After some procedures such as rectal, vaginal, nasal, or ear surgery, the operative site may be packed with gauze. In some situations, wounds are left open and covered with a dressing.

In healthy people, surgical wounds begin to heal immediately. By the third or fourth day, the healing process is increased. Although the wound appears to be healed after approximately 10 days, complete healing may take as long as a year.

Clean sutured incisions heal by first (primary) intention. Because the wound edges are closed, tissue bonds with little scarring. An infected wound is left open to heal from the bottom up. This method is called *healing by secondary intention*. Some sources refer to healing by *tertiary intention* when the wound is initially left open and later closed. Fig. 17.10 illustrates these three types of healing.

For the first 24 hours, check the dressing hourly for bleeding or drainage. If dressings become saturated, reinforce them using aseptic technique. Depending on physician preference and agency policy, reinforcement may be accomplished several ways. One method is simply to place dry dressings over the wet ones. Another method is to remove bulky outer layers of the wet dressing and replace them with dry dressings. A variety of wound dressings are available. After the first 24 hours, check the dressing once or twice each shift. Bleeding should be minimal and should stop within a few hours after the wound is closed. Report continued or excessive bleeding to the physician.

Some wounds have drains in a "stab" wound close to the incision (Fig. 17.11). Drains remove fluids from the operative site. Fluid accumulation in a wound interferes with healing. A Penrose drain is a soft tube that permits passive movement of fluids from the wound. The drainage is absorbed by the wound dressing.

Other types of drains are attached to collection devices that create suction to draw fluid from the wound. This type of drain is called an *active drain*. Examples of low-suction active drains are the Hemovac and the

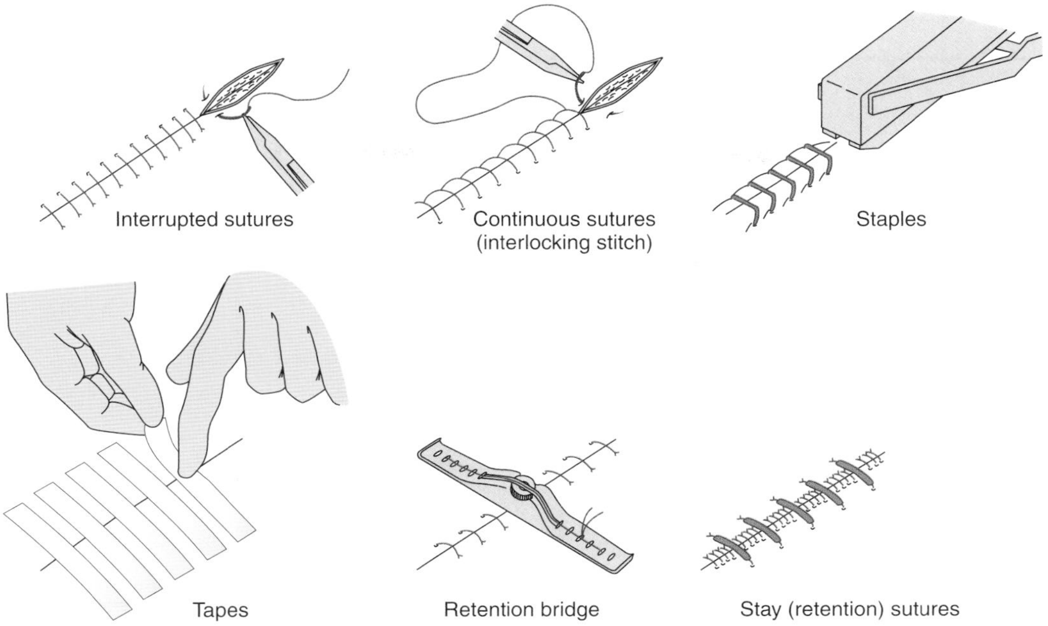

Fig. 17.9 Methods of wound closure. (From Ignatavicius DD, Workman ML: *Medical-surgical nursing: patient-centered collaborative care*, ed 8, St Louis, 2016, Saunders.)

Jackson-Pratt drain. Both create negative pressure when they are compressed. As they fill with fluid, the collection devices expand. They must be emptied and recompressed ("recharged") using aseptic technique to maintain their effectiveness. The frequency of emptying depends on the amount of drainage and the physician's orders. Wound drains may also be connected to a suction device. Record drainage as output. Vacuum-assisted closure devices are used to apply negative pressure to certain open wounds.

In the immediate postoperative phase, wound drainage is often bright red (**sanguineous**). As the amount of blood in the drainage decreases, the fluid becomes pinkish (**serosanguineous**). It should become progressively lighter in color and thinner until it is straw colored and clear (**serous**). At the same time that the color is changing, the amount of drainage should steadily decrease. Negative pressure wound therapy (NPWT), also called vacuum-assisted wound closure, is another type of dressing that accelerates wound healing.

Take care to reduce the risk of wound complications: infection, dehiscence (separation of wound margins), evisceration (protrusion of abdominal organs thorough an open wound). Although dehiscence is not expected in a clean wound, always avoid strain on the suture line. Teach the patient to support the incision during coughing and when getting in and out of bed (Fig. 17.12). Patients who have had abdominal surgery should not use trapeze bars to move themselves. Promptly treat nausea to avoid the stress of retching and vomiting. Because many surgical patients go home within a few days, they need verbal and written instructions about safe activities. The exact type of surgery that was performed determines the restrictions. Consult with the physician about correct instructions.

Wounds that are healing normally are unlikely to undergo dehiscence. If infection develops under surgical sutures, the sutures dissolve too soon. Fluid accumulates in the wound and the wound dehisces. A sudden increase in wound drainage may precede wound dehiscence. When the suture line ruptures, the patient may feel as though the wound is "pulling apart."

If dehiscence occurs, keep the patient in bed and in a position to decrease strain on the wound and decrease the risk of evisceration. For example, the patient with an abdominal wound should be in semi-Fowler position with the knees flexed. If dehiscence or evisceration occurs, the usual practice is to cover the wound with sterile dressings saturated with normal saline and to notify the physician. The saline is thought to prevent damage from drying of the exposed organs. However, some authorities are concerned that moisture increases the risk of wound contamination by promoting bacterial movement through the dressings. Covering the saline-soaked gauze with a dry dressing may prevent this complication. After inspecting the wound, the physician may order an abdominal binder. Anticipate a possible return to surgery and do not administer opioid analgesics until surgical consent is obtained. Infected wounds may be allowed to heal by secondary intention.

Potential for Infection

Continuously assess the patient for indications of infection. Signs and symptoms of wound infection usually do not develop until the third to fifth day after the operation; they may appear as late as a week after surgery. The classic signs and symptoms of wound infection include pain, fever, redness, swelling, and purulent drainage. Surgical pain should decrease as the

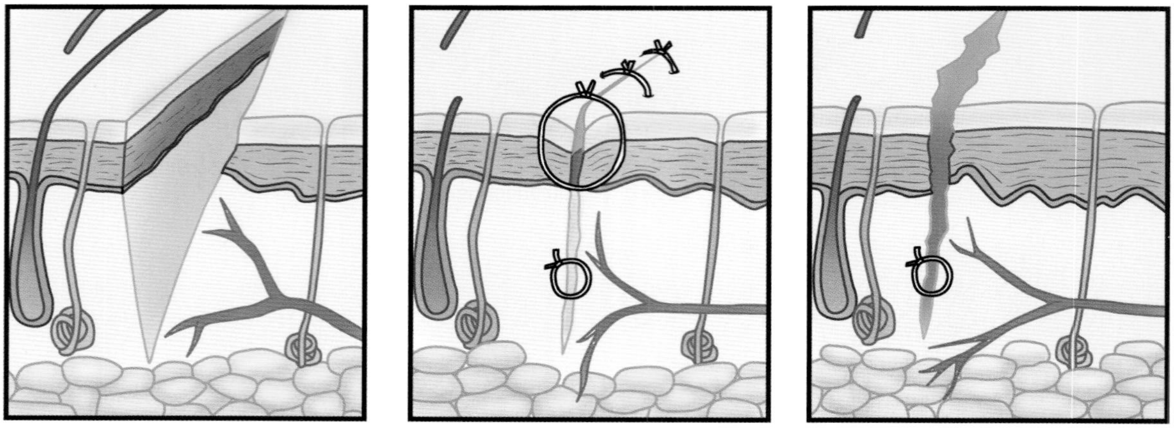

An aseptically made wound with minimal tissue destruction and minimal tissue reaction begins to heal as the edges are approximated by close sutures or staples. No open areas or dead spaces are left to serve as potential sites of infection.

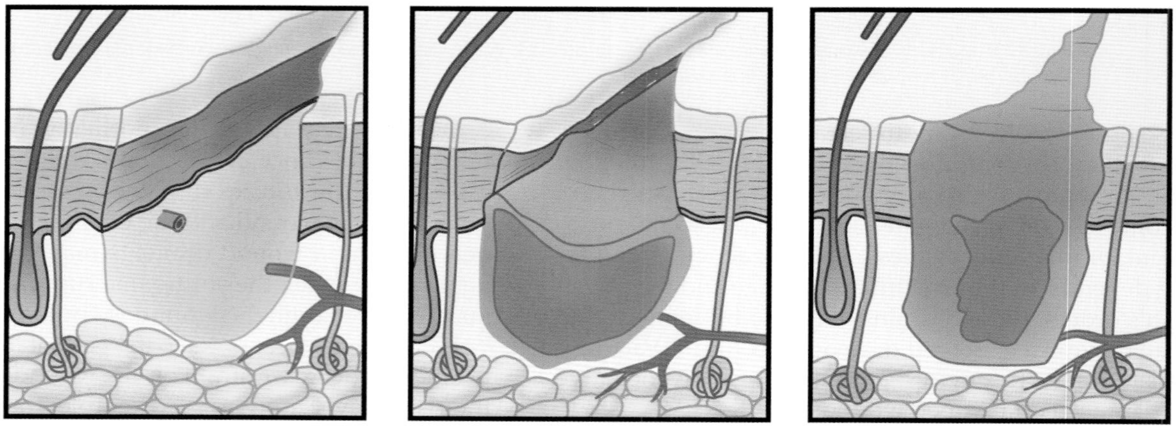

An infected or chronic wound or one with tissue damage so extensive that the edges cannot be smoothly approximated is usually left open and allowed to heal from the inside out. The nurse periodically cleans and assesses the wound for healthy tissue production. Scar tissue is extensive, and healing is prolonged.

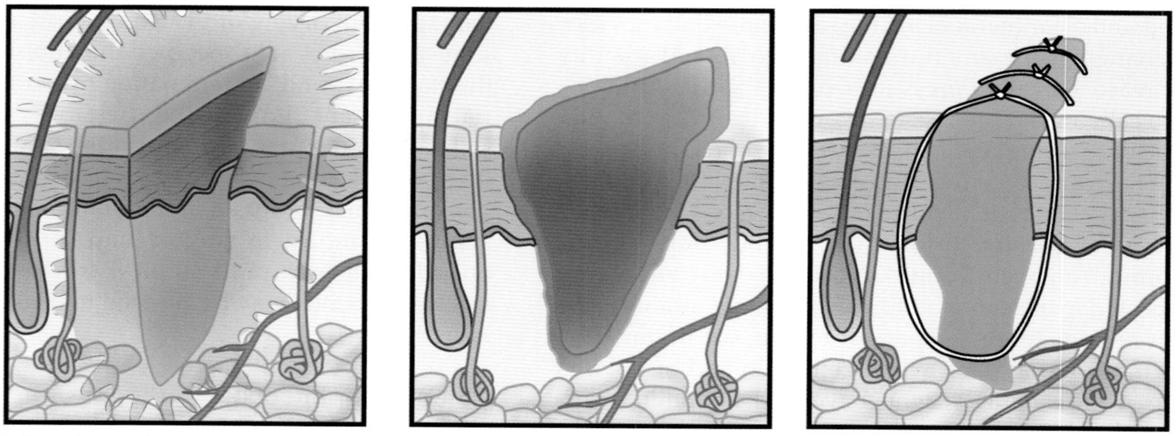

A potentially infected surgical wound may be left open for several days. If no clinical signs of infection occur, the wound is then closed surgically.

Fig. 17.10 Wound healing. (From Rothrock JC: *Alexander's care of the patient in surgery*, ed 15, St. Louis, 2015, Mosby.)

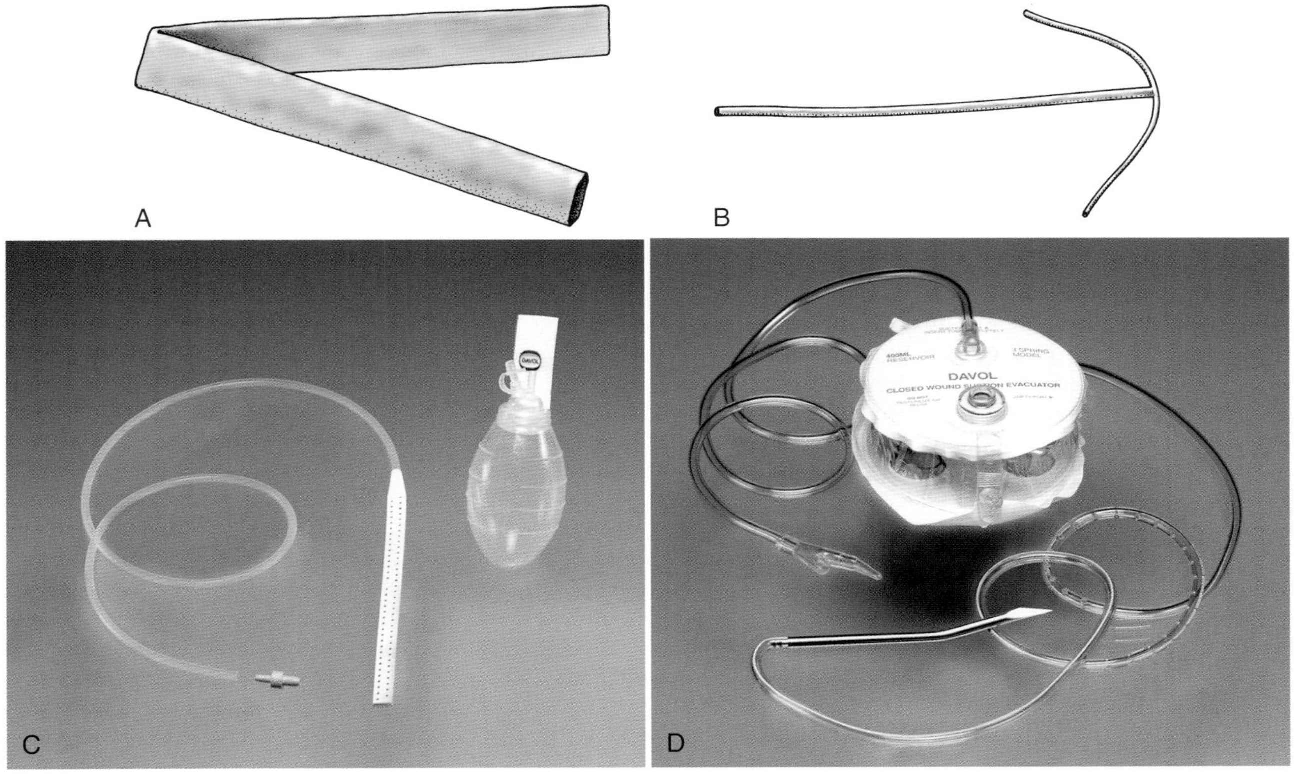

Fig. 17.11 Types of surgical drains used to remove fluid from wounds. Passive or gravity drains include (A) the Penrose the Jackson-Pratt drain and (D) the Hemovac. (T-tube and Hemovac are less commonly used now.) (A and B, From Rothrock JC: *Alexander's care of the patient in surgery*, ed 15, St. Louis, 2015, Mosby. C and D, Copyright 2014 C.R. Bard, Inc. Used with permission.)

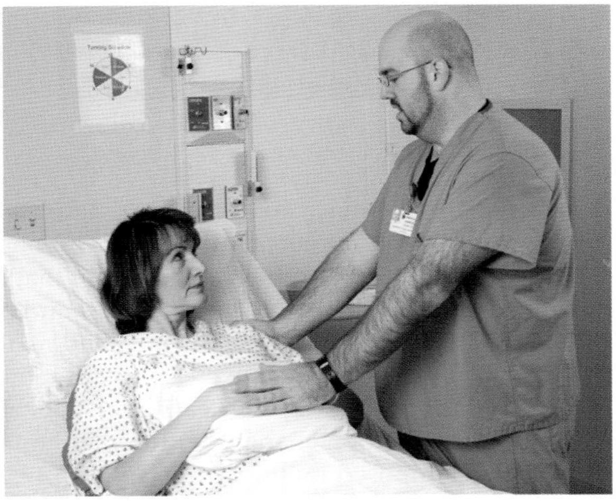

Fig. 17.12 Splinting supports the incision during coughing. (From Potter P, Perry A, et al: *Fundamentals of nursing*, ed 8. St. Louis, 2013, Mosby.)

days go by. Continued or increasing pain suggests the possibility of infection. A low-grade fever is common during the first 2 postoperative days because of the normal inflammation stage of healing. However, if the temperature is higher than 100.4°F (38°C) or lasts more than 2 days, infection may be present. Early signs of infection are sometimes hard to detect in older surgical patients because these patients typically do not develop high fevers even with serious infections. Some redness is expected at the wound suture line and around the sutures or staples. Increasing redness or redness that spreads to surrounding tissue is not normal.

Prevention of wound infection requires decreasing the exposure to microorganisms and maintaining the patient's resistance to infection. Good hand washing, the use of sterile or clean gloves (as appropriate), aseptic dressing changes, and diligent wound care prevent the introduction of infectious organisms. Good hydration and nutrition support the patient's healing and resistance to infection.

If infection is suspected, a culture of any drainage may identify the infectious organism or organisms. Cultures should be taken before administering any antibiotics. The antibiotics that are most likely to be effective can then be prescribed. While awaiting results of the culture and sensitivity tests, the physician often orders a broad-spectrum antibiotic. Various wound care procedures may also be ordered. The patient may need to be isolated from other patients to prevent transfer of the organisms. The presence of highly contagious organisms such as MRSA requires patient isolation. Personal protective equipment (PPE) should be used by the nurse for any procedure involving touching the patient or their body secretions.

Because infection may develop after the patient is discharged, patient teaching should include signs and symptoms of infection that should be reported to the physician. The patient should also know whether the wound requires any special treatment. If wound care is needed at home, ensure that the patient or a family member is able to perform wound care before the patient leaves the hospital.

Inadequate Oxygenation

Document the patient's respiratory status every hour for the first 24 hours and once or twice per shift after that. Signs and symptoms of pneumonia include dyspnea, fatigue, fever, cough, purulent or bloody sputum, and "wet" breath sounds. When gas exchange is impaired, as with pneumonia or atelectasis, the pulse rate generally increases and the arterial blood oxygen saturation (SaO_2) falls. Breath sounds are absent in areas of atelectasis.

The most important nursing measures to prevent pneumonia and atelectasis are frequent position changes and coughing and deep-breathing exercises. Initially, assist the patient to turn at least every 2 hours. Patients are often assisted out of bed on the day of surgery. They are usually ambulated several times daily, beginning on the second day. Early ambulation has been found to greatly reduce the respiratory complications of surgery.

Deep breathing inflates the lungs fully and coughing removes secretions. Help the patient to cough and deep breathe every hour. Instruct the patient to take in a deep breath through the nose and gradually blow out through the mouth. After taking several deep breaths, a cough should be attempted to bring up secretions.

The incentive spirometer is a device used to promote lung expansion (Fig. 17.13). It consists of a tube through which air is inhaled and a cylinder containing a ball. The ball rises in the cylinder as the patient inhales through the tube. The more air that is taken in, the higher the ball moves. Markings on the cylinder indicate the volume of air taken in, which gives the patient a measurable goal toward which to work while using the spirometer.

Deep breathing and coughing are painful for the patient who has had abdominal or chest surgery. To reduce discomfort, coordinate the exercises with analgesics and splint the incision. The patient can splint by holding a pillow firmly over the surgical area while coughing.

The best course of action is to teach the patient about turning, deep breathing, coughing, and using the incentive spirometer before surgery. A patient who is in pain or drowsy from anesthesia is not in the best condition for learning. Instances in which coughing is contraindicated are few. They include surgeries for hernias and cataracts as well as brain surgery.

If the patient develops pneumonia, treatment includes rest, oxygen, and antibiotics. Care of the patient with pneumonia is discussed in Chapter 27.

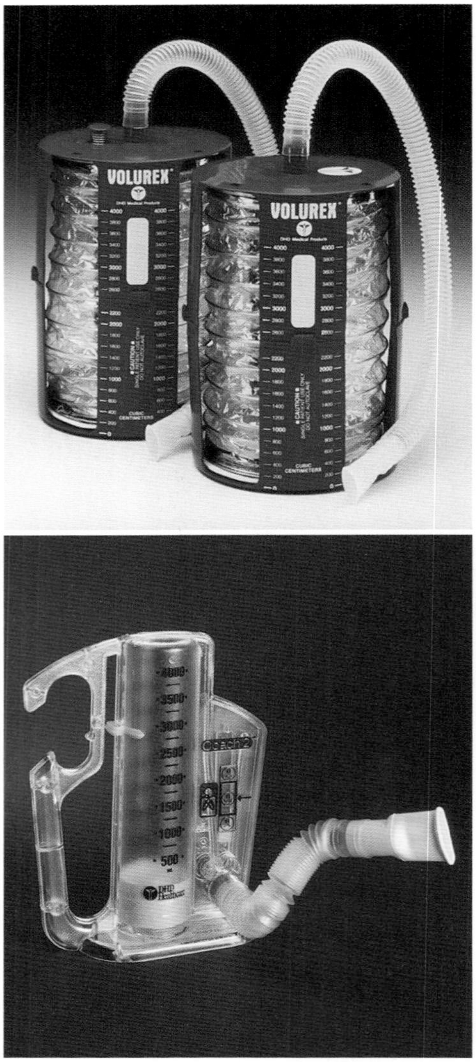

Fig. 17.13 The incentive spirometer is used to promote lung expansion. (Courtesy Smiths Medical, Dublin, OH. All rights reserved.)

Another factor that may cause severe, sometimes fatal respiratory complications is pulmonary embolism. Pulmonary emboli usually arise from thrombi that develop in veins, especially the veins of the legs and pelvis. Measures to prevent thrombophlebitis and related pulmonary emboli include leg exercises, early ambulation, drug therapy as described earlier in the chapter, and frequent position changes within the limits of any restrictions imposed by the physician (Fig. 17.14). Antiembolic stockings such as thromboembolic disorder (TED) hose or an SCD may be ordered. Signs and symptoms that alert the nurse to possible pulmonary embolism are dyspnea, tachypnea, chest pain, and hemoptysis. If the embolus is very large, the patient may become cyanotic and go into shock. Emboli may be treated with heparin, thrombolytics, or both.

Pharmacology Capsule

Anesthesia, anticholinergics, and opioid analgesics can contribute to urinary retention.

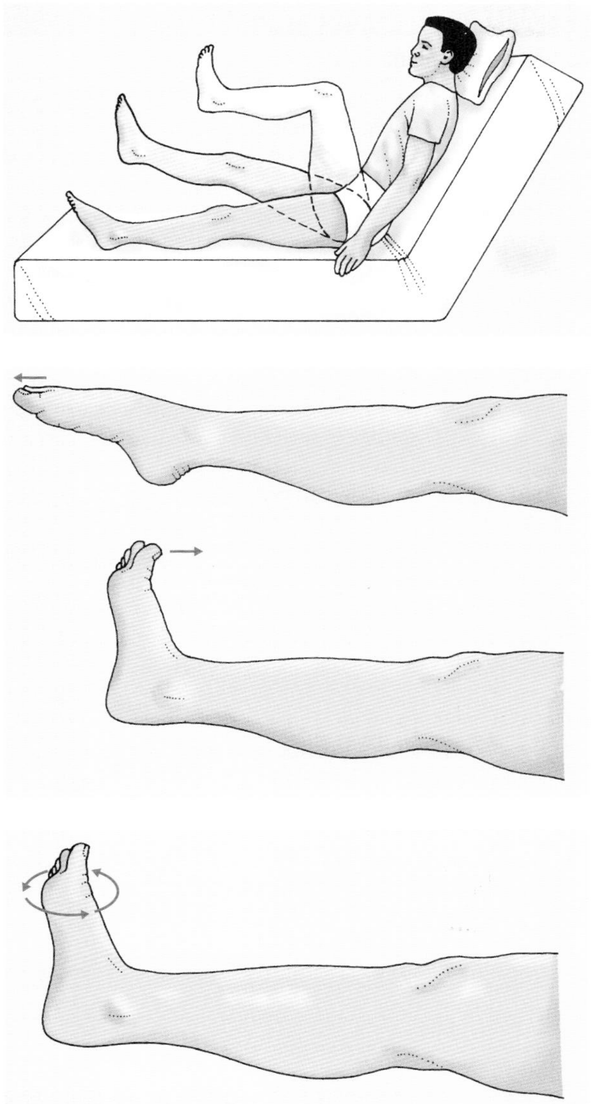

Fig. 17.14 Postoperative leg exercises promote venous return. (From Ignatavicius DD, Workman ML, Mishler MA: *Medical-surgical nursing across the health care continuum*, ed 3, Philadelphia, 1999, Saunders.)

Urinary Retention

Carefully monitor urinary output after surgery. Normal urine output is about 30 mL/h. In the first 24 hours, urinary output is typically reduced because of the stress response. Be aware, however, of the possibilities of urine retention or kidney failure in the early postoperative phase. Monitor urinary function by measuring intake and output. Bladder distention can be detected by palpation and by use of a bladder scanner. If the patient does not void within 6 to 8 hours, catheterization is usually performed to empty the bladder.

Patients who have had perineal or abdominal surgery are most likely to have difficulty voiding. They often have indwelling catheters inserted before or during surgery. The patient with urinary retention usually reports feelings of fullness and pressure over the lower abdomen. Some patients are unable to void at all. When a patient passes small amounts of urine frequently without feeling relief of fullness, suspect urine retention with overflow. The bladder releases just enough urine to reduce the pressure but does not empty completely. Gentle palpation of the lower abdomen usually reveals the smooth, rounded, full bladder. Distention can be confirmed with the scanner. If the patient is unable to void, catheterization is necessary. Because catheterization can cause urinary infection, it should be performed only if other interventions fail. Interventions must take the physician's activity orders into consideration. The patient should be provided with privacy while attempting to void. The toilet is preferred if the patient can go to the bathroom. If a bedpan must be used, raise the head of the bed, if permitted, to create a normal position for voiding. Men who need to stand to void should be assisted to do so if not contraindicated.

Sensory stimuli help some people to overcome difficulty voiding. The sound of running water or the sensation of warm water poured over the perineum or hands may encourage voiding. Use a measured amount of the water so it can be subtracted from the urine output.

If all independent measures fail, a physician's order is required for catheterization. In most instances, an "as-necessary" order is given to empty the bladder with a catheter if the patient does not void within 6 to 8 hours after surgery.

If the patient has to be catheterized several times, the physician may order the insertion of an indwelling catheter. Catheterization and the care of the patient with a catheter are discussed in Chapter 41.

If the bladder is not distended but little or no urine output occurs, the patient may be in kidney failure. The minimal urine output is considered to be 30 mL/h. Failure to produce at least 30 mL/h should be reported promptly to the physician. The diagnosis and treatment of kidney failure are discussed in Chapter 42.

Constipation

GI function is disrupted by surgery, especially surgery on GI structures. Postoperatively, inspect and palpate for abdominal distention and auscultate for bowel sounds. Document the passage of flatus and the first bowel movement. The patient may not realize the significance of passing flatus and may wonder why it should be reported. Explain that passing flatus means that the digestive tract is beginning to function again. Most patients pass flatus approximately 48 hours postoperatively. After GI surgery, a normal diet can usually be resumed once the patient passes flatus.

Early, frequent ambulation is the best way to prevent GI discomfort. The intake of oral fluids and ingestion of a normal diet also help to stimulate peristalsis.

Oral intake is usually withheld, however, until bowel sounds return (normally 24–48 hours after surgery).

Measures to promote the passage of flatus may be ordered, including early ambulation, application of heat to the abdomen, positioning the patient prone or on the right side, and insertion of bisacodyl suppositories.

If the patient develops a paralytic ileus, a nasogastric tube may be ordered to permit decompression of the intestines. If the surgical procedure is one that often causes GI problems, the nasogastric tube may be inserted during surgery to prevent problems.

The patient should have a bowel movement within a few days after resuming the intake of solid foods. In some instances, a suppository or an enema is necessary to stimulate emptying of the bowel.

Pharmacology Capsule

Antiemetic drugs control postoperative nausea and vomiting.

Fluid Volume Deficit and Inadequate Nutrition

Depending on the type of surgery performed, fluid and nutrition needs are met in a variety of ways. Some patients are given regular diets on the evening of surgery; others receive nothing by mouth for several days. Most patients return from the PACU with intravenous infusions. Patients are traditionally given clear liquids at first and then full liquids. If liquids are retained, the diet is advanced to include soft foods and then regular foods. Physiologically, no reason has been found to delay the introduction of solids once GI function has returned and a few oral liquids are retained, but this practice persists in many settings.

When the patient is able to tolerate liquids well, the intravenous infusion is usually discontinued unless it is needed for the administration of medication. Monitor the flow rate and the patient response. Nursing care of the patient receiving intravenous fluids is discussed in Chapter 16.

To promote healing, the patient's diet must provide adequate carbohydrates, protein, zinc, iron, folate, and vitamins C, B_6, and B_{12}. Alternative methods of feeding may be ordered if the patient is unable to resume oral intake for a long time. These methods are discussed in Chapter 37.

Fluid intake and output are usually measured for several days after surgery. In addition, laboratory studies of serum electrolytes often are ordered.

Nausea and vomiting interfere with the intake of food and fluids and can cause considerable fluid loss. Antiemetics (drugs used to control nausea and vomiting) are usually ordered as necessary (see the Patient Teaching box). General nursing measures for the patient with nausea and vomiting are discussed in Chapter 38.

Patient Teaching

Postoperative Patient

Patient teaching in the postoperative phase emphasizes recovery from the surgical experience and preparation for return to maximal possible function. Discharge planning should be started when the patient is admitted for surgery and revised as needed during the course of hospitalization. Topics to include in the discharge teaching plan are the following:

- Take your prescribed drugs as directed but notify the physician if you have adverse effects (specify drug, dose level, schedule, side effects, and adverse effects).
- Wound care: You will need to continue your wound care as I have demonstrated and you have practiced. Notify your physician if you have symptoms of infection (fever, increasing redness, swelling, pain, drainage at the incision site). Wash your hands before and after touching your wound.
- When regular activities can be resumed, do not lift anything heavier than specified by your physician.
- If you need assistance, community services are available. (Specify services for patient needs.)
- If the physician advises specific fluids and nutritional requirements, you need to follow this special diet and/or take the prescribed amounts of fluids.
- You will need some specialized equipment and supplies. (Tell the patient how to obtain and use assistive devices, special equipment, and supplies.)
- Can you identify any adaptations that will be needed in your home environment before you are discharged?
- You need to keep medical appointments to ensure that you are healing properly.

Pharmacology Capsule

Discharge teaching includes information about drug therapy.

Put On Your Thinking Cap!

Observe the room of a recent postoperative patient and identify four ways in which the environment can be modified to promote safety.

Impaired Motor Function

After general anesthesia and invasive surgical procedures, patients are usually weak and tire quickly. The physician prescribes measures to increase the patient's activity level (progressive ambulation in most cases). Assist the patient out of bed the first few times until the patient can safely get up alone. Help the patient to sit on the bedside, press the feet on the floor, stand, and then walk increasingly greater distances. Monitor for weakness and dizziness associated with orthostatic hypotension. Emphasize the physical benefits of early ambulation to the patient.

Altered Body Image

The effects of surgery (scars, loss of body parts or organs, altered physical functions) can be very traumatic.

A sense of loss can be demonstrated by anger, depression, or even denial. Understand and accept these responses. Nursing care of the grieving patient is discussed in detail in Chapter 19. Surgery can also produce positive changes in body image when it improves appearance or function or relieves symptoms.

Get Ready for the NCLEX® Examination!

Key Points

- Surgical procedures classified by purpose are diagnostic, ablative, palliative, reconstructive or restorative, procurement for transplant, constructive, or cosmetic.
- Variables that affect surgical outcomes are age; nutritional status including weight, fluid, and electrolyte balance; medical diagnoses; drugs; and habits such as use of tobacco and alcohol.
- The phases of the surgical experience are preoperative, intraoperative, and postoperative.
- Nursing measures to reduce patient anxiety and increase knowledge about the surgical experience may actually decrease complications.
- Preoperative teaching should include surgical preparation; what to expect in the surgical suite and the PACU; what tubes, dressings, or equipment may be in place after surgery; and how patient participation can promote recovery.
- Before surgery, the patient or legal guardian must sign a legal consent form. Consent from the patient must be obtained before preoperative medications are given.
- Preparation for surgery may involve bowel cleansing, food and fluid restriction, skin scrubbing and hair removal, securing and covering hair, and administering preoperative medications as ordered. Clothing, jewelry, nail polish, and prostheses are usually removed.
- After preoperative medications are given, the patient should remain in bed with the call bell in reach and the side rails up.
- The surgical team can consist of nurses who circulate, nurses or assistants who scrub, a RNFA, one or more surgeons, an anesthesiologist or a nurse anesthetist, and other technical personnel.
- Several types of drugs are used for general anesthesia; combined drug effects induce unconsciousness, alter sensation, and prevent movement so that surgical procedures can be performed painlessly and safely.
- The patient problems in the intraoperative phase may include potential for injury, inadequate oxygenation, decreased cardiac output, and potential for fluid volume deficit.
- Postoperative surgical complications may include shock, hypoxia, wound infection, wound dehiscence and evisceration, injury, pneumonia, atelectasis, nausea and vomiting, impaired peristalsis, urinary retention, renal failure, and thrombophlebitis.
- Possible patient problems in the immediate postoperative period are decreased cardiac output, inadequate oxygenation, pain, confusion, and potential for injury.
- Confirm the person or persons who the patient has approved to be given information about the patient and inform visitors where to wait and how they will be notified of the patient's status.
- Patient problems after recovery from anesthesia may include pain, disrupted tissue integrity, potential for infection, inadequate oxygenation, urinary retention, constipation, potential for fluid volume deficit, inadequate nutrition, impaired motor function, and altered body image.
- Patient teaching for discharge emphasizes drug therapy, wound care, activity limitations, fluid and nutrition needs, equipment and supplies needed, adaptation of the home environment, and the importance of follow-up care.

Additional Learning Resources

SG Go to your Study Guide for additional learning activities to help you master this chapter content.

Online Resource

Go to your Evolve website (http://evolve.elsevier.com/Linton/medsurg) for the following learning resources and much more:

- Fluid & Electrolyte Tutorial
- Review Questions for the NCLEX® Examination

Clinical Judgment and Next-Generation NCLEX® Examination-Style Questions

1. **An older adult who is scheduled for a surgical procedure expresses fear that he is too old for surgery and asks what you think. Your response should be based on the knowledge that:**
   1. Older adults are twice as likely to have surgical complications as younger people.
   2. An older adult in good health is likely to do just as well in surgery as a younger person.
   3. For most older adults, the risks of surgery are too great to justify any possible benefits.
   4. Older adults who have chronic health problems are poor candidates for surgery.

   NCLEX Client Need: Physiological Integrity: Physiologic Adaptation

2. **New LVNs/LPNs are being oriented to an ambulatory surgical center. The educator should explain that the nurse's responsibility when obtaining a patient's signature on a surgical consent form includes:**
   1. Explaining the surgical procedure to the patient
   2. Obtaining the signature before the patient is given sedatives
   3. Informing the patient of possible risks associated with the procedure
   4. Assessing which alternative options the patient has explored

   NCLEX Client Need: Safe and Effective Care Environment: Coordinated Care

3. **A patient is recovering from a surgical procedure that was done using spinal anesthesia. The PACU nurse assesses whether the patient has sensation and movement in his legs. Why is this data especially important?**

1. Regional anesthesia can impair blood flow to the extremities, causing gangrene.
2. The patient cannot move the extremities despite feelings of pain or pressure.
3. The extremities are susceptible to injury because movement returns before sensation.
4. The effects of regional anesthesia may persist for several weeks.

NCLEX Client Need: Physiological Integrity: Pharmacologic Therapies

4. **Complications that are most likely to occur during the immediate postoperative period include which of the following? (Select all that apply.)**
   1. Wound infection
   2. Pneumonia
   3. Shock
   4. Hypoxia
   5. Thrombophlebitis

   NCLEX Client Need: Physiological Integrity: Physiological Adaptation

5. **In the PACU, a patient's vital signs are as follows: temperature 98°F (36.66°C), pulse 66 beats per minute and regular, respirations 14 breaths per minute, blood pressure 100/56 mm Hg. Which other piece of information is most important to allow the nurse to evaluate these vital signs?**
   1. Medications given during surgery
   2. Length of time under general anesthesia
   3. Whether the patient is having pain
   4. Patient's preoperative vital signs

   NCLEX Client Need: Physiological Integrity: Physiologic Adaptation

6. **A patient with an abdominal incision reports that his dressing is soaked with drainage and that he felt a pulling sensation when getting out of bed. On inspection, the nurse observes that a loop of intestine is protruding from the open wound. The appropriate action is to:**
   1. Have the patient lie flat in bed.
   2. Gently reapply the surgical dressing and call the physician.
   3. Administer a dose of prescribed opioid analgesic for pain.
   4. Apply saline-soaked gauze and cover with a sterile, dry dressing.

   NCLEX Client Need: Physiological Integrity: Reduction of Risk Potential

7. **After surgery, a patient voids 10 to 20 mL of urine at frequent intervals. You should suspect:**
   1. Urinary retention with overflow
   2. Damage to the bladder during surgery
   3. Fluid volume excess
   4. Kidney failure

   NCLEX Client Need: Physiological Integrity: Reduction of Risk Potential

8. **During the shift hand-off, the nurse is informed that a postoperative patient reportedly has a paralytic ileus. The nurse should anticipate which of the following? (Select all that apply.)**
   1. The patient will be unable to walk.
   2. A nasogastric tube and suction may be in place.
   3. Bowel sounds should be auscultated.
   4. The patient will be limited to a liquid diet.
   5. Blood transfusions will probably be needed.

   NCLEX Client Need: Physiological Integrity: Reduction of Risk Potential

9. **Preoperative medications typically include: (Select all that apply.)**
   1. Sedative-hypnotic agent
   2. Opioid analgesic
   3. Antiemetic agent
   4. Anticholinergic drug
   5. Nonsteroidal antiinflammatory drug

   NCLEX Client Need: Physiological Integrity: Pharmacologic Therapies

10. **Guidelines to prevent wrong-site surgery include: (Select all that apply.)**
    1. Confirm that the operative site is marked before giving any sedating drugs.
    2. Verify that the appropriate equipment is available for the procedure.
    3. Confirm that the surgical consent form has been signed and witnessed.
    4. Verify with the patient the procedure that is expected to be performed.
    5. Conduct a time out before the first incision to resolve any concerns.

    NCLEX Client Need: Safe and Effective Care Environment: Coordinated Care

Unfolding Case Test Items: Postoperative Care

Phase I

Question 1: Recognize cues using enhanced hot spot test item type

SLO/Objective: Apply knowledge of anatomy, physiology, and pathophysiology to determine which assessment data requires follow up by the nurse

Patient situation: A 70-year-old woman required repair of a right hip fracture sustained in a fall. She is a heavy smoker with a history of pneumonia last year. She takes levothyroxine for hypothyroidism. Otherwise, she has been healthy and active. She is one day postop. The nurse's assessment data includes the following:

- Alert and oriented
- dressing on right hip is dry and intact
- pain in operative hip rated 8 on a 0-10 pain scale
- BP 126/76
- Heart rate: 72
- IV fluids infusing in left hand
- Temperature: 99° F
- Productive cough
- Crackles on auscultation of lungs
- Out of bed to chair with assistance tolerated well

Highlight or place a check mark next to the assessment findings that require follow up by the nurse.

Question 2: Analyze cues using Cloze Test Item

Patient situation: A 70-year-old woman required repair of a right hip fracture sustained in a fall. She is a heavy smoker with a history of pneumonia last year. She takes levothyroxine for hypothyroidism. Otherwise, she has been healthy and active. She is two days postop. The nurse's assessment date includes:

- Alert and oriented
- Dressing on right hip is dry and intact
- Pain in operative hip rated 4 on a 0 to 10 pain scale
- BP 126/76 mm Hg
- Heart rate: 72 beats per minute
- IV fluids infusing in left hand
- Temperature: 99°F
- Productive cough
- Crackles on auscultation of lungs
- Out of bed to chair with assistance tolerated well

Choose the most likely options for the information missing from the statements below by selecting from the lists of options provided.
The nurse recognizes that (1)__________, (1)__________, and (1)__________ may indicate a postoperative complication. Failure to address these findings most likely will lead to (2)__________. Nursing measures to decrease the risk of these complications include (3)__________, (3)__________, and (3)__________.

OPTIONS FOR 1	OPTIONS FOR 2	OPTIONS FOR 3
Temperature – 99° F	Pain	Maintain alignment of hip
Pain rating 4 on 1–10 scale	Incisional infection	Turn, cough, deep breath every 2 hours
Productive cough	Pneumonia	Administer oxygen at 5 Liters/min
Blood pressure 126/76 mm Hg	Respiratory arrest	Encourage increased fluid intake
Coarse crackles in both lungs	Heart failure	Incentive spirometry
Strong peripheral pulses in both legs	Delayed bone healing	Enforce bedrest

Phase II

Question 3: Prioritize hypotheses using extended multiple response test items

Patient situation: A 70-year-old woman required repair of a right hip fracture sustained in a fall. This is her third postoperative day. She is a heavy smoker with a history of pneumonia last year. She is anxious for a cigarette. She takes levothyroxine for hypothyroidism. Physical therapy has been arranged for her after discharge.

When planning care for this patient, for which priority potential complications would the nurse monitor? Select all that apply:

a. Pneumonia
b. Deep vein thrombosis
c. Myocardial infarction
d. Urinary tract infection
e. Chronic pain syndrome
f. Pulmonary embolus

Question 4: Generate solutions using extended drag and drop test items

A 70-year-old woman required repair of a right hip fracture sustained in a fall. This is her third postoperative day. She is a heavy smoker with a history of pneumonia last year. She is anxious for a cigarette. She takes levothyroxine for hypothyroidism. Physical therapy has been arranged for her after discharge.

Indicate which nursing response listed in the far left column is appropriate for each patient question. Note that not all responses will be used.

NURSE'S RESPONSES	PATIENT QUESTIONS	APPROPRIATE NURSE'S RESPONSE FOR EACH PATIENT QUESTION
1. Physical therapy is usually continued for several weeks after discharge.	Is it safe to bear weight on my right leg?	
2. You can resume usual activities when you feel like it.	Will I always have to use a walker?	
3. You will gradually be able to bear weight on your right leg as you can tolerate it.	Will I need physical therapy after discharge from the hospital?	
4. You can use the walker until you feel confident without it.	When will I be able to shower?	
5. You can shower as long as you keep your incision dry.	Will I be able to ride my bicycle in the future?	
6. It is best if you only take tub baths from now on.		
7. You will always need the walker because you will not be able to bear weight on your right leg.		

Phase III

Question 5: Take action using matrix test item

A 70-year-old woman required repair of a right hip fracture sustained in a fall. This is her third postoperative day. She is a heavy smoker with a history of pneumonia last year. She is anxious for a cigarette. She takes levothyroxine for hypothyroidism. Physical therapy has been arranged for her after discharge.

Use an X for the health teaching below that is *Indicated* (appropriate or necessary), *Contraindicated* (could be harmful), or *Nonessential* (makes no difference or not necessary) before the patient's discharge at this time.

HEALTH TEACHING	INDICATED	CONTRAIN-DICATED	NONES-SENTIAL
Notify your physician in your incision becomes red, has drainage, or the margins separate.			
The physical therapy exercises will help you resume usual activities.			
Ask the home health nurse about an elevated toilet seat.			
If the surgical scar bothers you, you could see a plastic surgeon about possible revision.			
Place a pillow under your knees when lying down.			
Smoking delays healing. If you are interested in smoking cessation, I can provide some resources.			
You can reduce trips to the bathroom by decreasing your fluid intake.			

Question 6: Evaluate outcomes using matrix test item

A 70-year-old woman required repair of a right hip fracture sustained in a fall. She will be discharged home in 2 days. She is a heavy smoker with a history of pneumonia last year. She is anxious for a cigarette. She takes levothyroxine for hypothyroidism. Physical therapy has been arranged for her after discharge.

For each assessment finding, use an X to indicate whether nursing and collaborative interventions were *Effective* (helped to meet expected outcomes), *Ineffective* (did not help to meet expected outcomes, or *Unrelated* (not related to the expected outcomes).

ASSESSMENT FINDING	EFFECTIVE	INEFFECTIVE	UNRELATED
Ambulating well with walker			
Fluid intake and output approximately equal			
Margins of surgical wound are closed; no redness or drainage			
Goes outside to smoke several times each day		x	
Reports a pain level of 2 on a ten point scale.			

The Patient With an Ostomy

18

http://evolve.elsevier.com/Linton/medsurg

Objectives

1. List the indications for ostomy surgery to divert urine or feces.
2. Describe nursing actions/interventions to prepare the patient for ostomy surgery.
3. Explain the types of procedures used for fecal diversion.
4. Assist in developing a nursing plan of care for the patient with each of the following types of fecal diversion: ileostomy, continent ileostomy, ileoanal reservoir, and colostomy.
5. Explain the types of procedures used for urinary diversion.
6. Assist in developing a nursing plan of care for the patient with each of the following types of urinary diversion: incontinent (ileal conduit), continent (internal reservoir), and orthotopic neobladder.
7. Discuss content to be included in teaching patients to learn to live with ostomies.

Key Terms

colonic or sigmoid conduit
colostomy (kŏ-LŎS-tō-mē)
ileal conduit
ileostomy (ĭ-lē-ŎS-tō-mē)
neobladder
nephrostomy (nĕ-FRŎS-tō-mē)
ostomy (ŎS-tō-mē)
reanastomosis
stoma (STŌ-mă)
ureterostomy (yŭ-rĕ-tĕr-ŎS-tō-mē)
vesicostomy (vĕ-sĭ-KŎS-tō-mē)

Ostomy is the term used to describe an artificial opening into a body cavity. The site of the opening on the skin is called a **stoma**. An ostomy in the digestive tract may be a gastrostomy, jejunostomy, duodenostomy, ileostomy, or colostomy. The gastrostomy is an opening through the abdominal wall into the stomach that is used for long-term tube feedings. Duodenostomies and jejunostomies are openings through which tubes are also placed for feeding or drainage. Ileostomies and colostomies are created to drain fecal matter from the intestines. Examples of stomas in the urinary tract are the ureterostomy, ileal or colonic conduit, vesicostomy, and continent internal reservoir. Ostomies of the urinary tract drain urine from the kidney, ureters, or bladder. Ostomies are sometimes described as a means of urinary or fecal diversion. The term *ostomate* refers to a person who has an ostomy. However, many people prefer to be thought of as *individuals with ostomies* rather than as *ostomates*. This chapter describes the care of patients with ostomies created to divert urine or feces.

INDICATIONS AND PREPARATION FOR OSTOMY SURGERY

Ostomy surgery is done for a number of reasons. A temporary ostomy may be indicated after surgery or trauma or when severe inflammation or infection exists. The ostomy bypasses the affected portion of the bowel or urinary tract, giving it time to heal. Permanent ostomies are usually necessitated by cancer of the bladder or colon or severe inflammatory bowel disease. Pouches are external appliances that are used with most ostomies to collect drainage. Whether ostomies are temporary or permanent, patients require considerable assistance as well as educational and psychologic support while learning to manage them.

Ideally the patient is prepared for the ostomy before surgery. The physician informs the patient of the need or possible need for the ostomy, what it is, and whether it will be temporary or permanent. Sometimes the procedure is done in emergency situations, as when treating acute bowel obstruction, perforation, or trauma. In these situations, the ostomy may come as a great shock to the patient.

An important resource for the nurse and the patient is the wound, ostomy, continence nurse (WOC nurse). The WOC nurse is a registered nurse (RN) who has special training in stoma care. The WOC nurse may be a certified ostomy care nurse (COCN) or a certified wound, ostomy, continence nurse (CWOCN). The WOC nurse is the appropriate person to assess and teach the ostomy patient. However, this does not relieve the staff nurse of all teaching responsibility. The staff nurse follows up and reinforces the instructions of the WOC nurse. In settings in which specialists are not available, the responsibility for teaching may fall primarily on the staff nurse.

The exact placement of the stoma is very important. The WOC nurse often consults with the surgeon regarding the ideal site. Two factors must be considered: (1) secure pouch placement and (2) ease of self-care. To provide a good seal, the site must not be too close to the umbilicus, bony prominences, scars, folds, or creases. If the pouch does not fit smoothly around the stoma, liquid stool or urine may leak around or beneath it. The stoma is placed below the waistline if possible. If it can be placed within the margins of the rectus muscle, the muscle will help to prevent peristomal hernias. Ideally, the stoma must also be placed where it can be seen and touched by the patient. A patient cannot learn to care for a stoma that is located where it cannot be viewed or reached.

NURSING CARE OF THE PATIENT HAVING OSTOMY SURGERY

General preoperative nursing care is discussed in detail in Chapter 17. This section emphasizes only those aspects that are unique to the patient with an ostomy.

FOCUSED ASSESSMENT

Before ostomy surgery, you should be especially concerned with determining the patient's expectations, understanding of the procedure, information desired, fears, and misconceptions. The health history reveals the reason for the procedure. The medical history documents other acute and chronic conditions that will require management before and after surgery. (Note drug therapy and allergies.) During the physical examination, expect to see a mark on the abdominal skin where the stoma will be created. See Chapter 17 for other details of the preoperative assessment.

Patient Problems, Goals, and Outcome Criteria: Ostomy Surgery: Preoperative Phase

The patient problems and goals that require particular attention are as follows.

Patient Problems	Goals and Outcome Criteria
Anxiety and grieving related to perceived threat to self-image, anticipated changes in body appearance and function	Reduced anxiety: patient states anxiety is reduced; relaxed manner Grieving: verbalizes reality of impending loss
Inadequate knowledge of what to expect after surgery in relation to the stoma related to lack of exposure to information	Patient understands postoperative routines and procedures in relation to ostomy surgery: patient correctly describes what to expect before and after surgery

INTERVENTIONS

Anxiety and Grieving

Be accepting of the patient's anxiety and try to help the patient identify exactly what their concerns are. Some patients may be concerned about appearance and others about how their jobs or family lives might be disrupted. The anticipated loss of normal function and change in self-image triggers the grief response. Encourage patients to talk and use coping strategies that have been effective in the past. In addition, inform them about support groups and psychologic counseling that may be helpful at this time. Because moderate or severe anxiety interferes with learning, try to reduce anxiety before teaching.

Inadequate Knowledge

Basic aspects of ostomy care should be taught before surgery. The patient's responses and questions guide you as to how much detail is appropriate. However, preoperative teaching requires repetition and reinforcement after surgery.

In addition to the WOC nurse, an important resource is a volunteer from an organization such as the American Cancer Society or the United Ostomy Associations of America (UOAA). Volunteers are people with ostomies who have been trained to counsel other patients about adjustment to their ostomies. Their personal experiences in everyday ostomy management can make them very effective role models. Another good reason for using these volunteers is that the patient has a chance to meet a person who is living fully with an ostomy. When a patient is referred to an ostomy group (with the patient's permission, of course), the organization tries to send a volunteer who is similar in age, gender, occupation, and type of ostomy.

FECAL DIVERSION

Intestinal ostomies divert fecal matter through a surgically created opening in the abdomen. Although the various types of ostomies (e.g., ileostomy, colostomy) have much in common, differences exist and should be noted. The characteristics of the fecal material vary with the location of the ostomy within the intestine and influence the type of care needed. Normally the colon absorbs water from the fecal mass as it moves toward the rectum so that it becomes progressively more solid. When the mass is diverted from the colon, it may be liquid, semisolid, or formed depending on the section of the colon where the ostomy is created. Fecal matter in the ileum is liquid. The closer the ostomy is to the rectum, the more formed the fecal matter will be (Table 18.1).

Depending on the way an ostomy is constructed, it is described as an end (single-barreled) stoma, a double-barreled stoma, or a loop stoma (Fig. 18.1). An end stoma is constructed from the proximal end of the

Table 18.1 Comparison of Ileostomy and Colostomy

		COLOSTOMY		
CHARACTERISTIC	ILEOSTOMY	ASCENDING	TRANSVERSE	SIGMOID
Stool consistency	Liquid to semiliquid	Semiliquid	Semiliquid to semiformed	Formed
Fluid requirement	Increased	Increased	Possibly increased	No change
Bowel regulation	No	No	No	Yes (if there is a history of a regular bowel pattern)
Pouch and skin barriers	Yes	Yes	Yes	Dependent on regulation
Irrigation	No	No	No	Possibly every 24–48 hours (if patient meets criteria)
Indications for surgery	Ulcerative colitis, Crohn disease, diseased or injured colon, familial polyposis, trauma, cancer	Perforating diverticulum in lower colon, trauma, rectovaginal fistula, inoperable tumors of colon, rectum, or pelvis	Same as for ascending	Cancer of the rectum or rectosigmoid area, perforating diverticulum, trauma

From Lewis SM, Bucher L, Heitkemper MM, Harding MM: *Medical-surgical nursing: assessment and management of clinical problems*, ed 10, St. Louis, 2017, Elsevier.

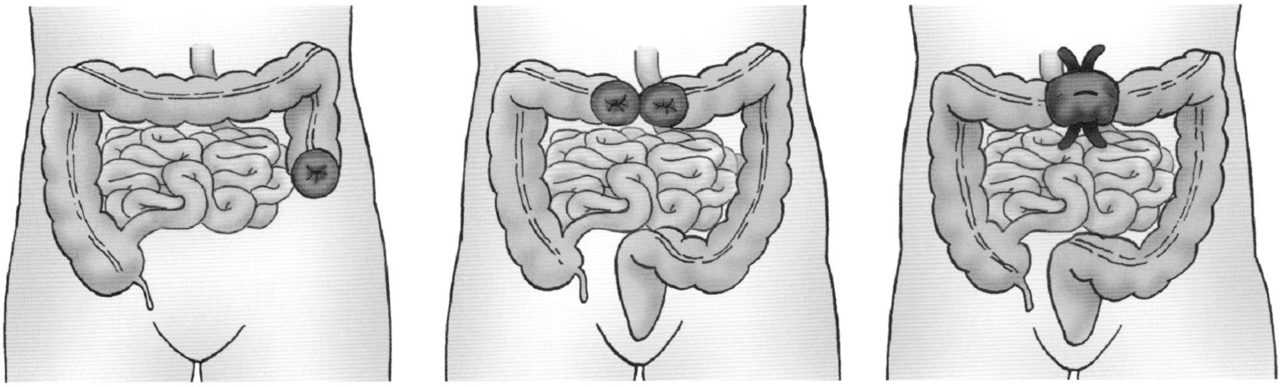

Fig. 18.1 Types of fecal stoma construction: Single-barreled (end) locations vary. Double-barreled stomas may be adjacent or several inches apart. Loop ostomies are temporary or palliative. (From Black JM, Hawks JH: *Medical-surgical nursing: clinical management for positive outcomes*, ed 8, St. Louis, 2009, Saunders-Elsevier.)

resected portion of bowel. The distal bowel may be removed or closed and left in place inside the abdomen (Hartmann pouch) (Fig. 18.2). If left in place, it is possible for the ends of the bowel to be reconnected, a procedure called **reanastomosis**. A double-barreled stoma has two stomas but they are no longer attached (i.e., the bowel is completely divided). The proximal stoma, which is continuous with the upper intestinal tract, drains fecal matter. The distal stoma is nonfunctional; it is referred to as a *mucus fistula*. A loop stoma is created by bringing a loop of bowel to the abdominal surface and opening it so that fecal matter can drain. The posterior wall of the bowel remains connected so that the loop stoma has two openings: one to the proximal bowel and one to the distal bowel (Fig. 18.3). Both loop and double-barreled ostomies are usually temporary.

Before fecal diversion, a low-fiber diet may be prescribed for several days. This would require the patient

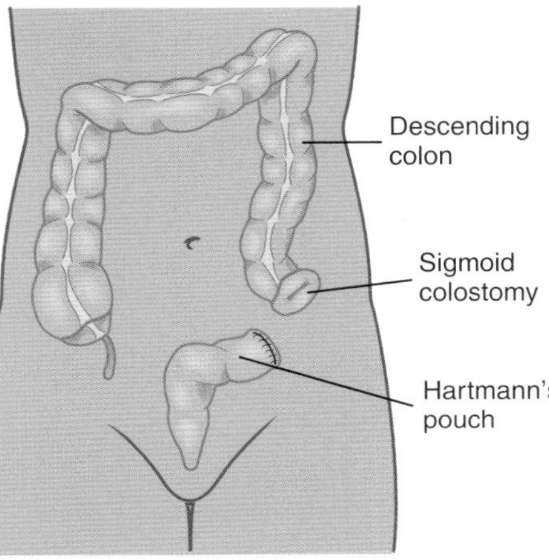

Fig. 18.2 Sigmoid colostomy. Distal bowel is oversewn and left in place to create a Hartmann pouch. (From Lewis SM, Bucher L, Heitkemper MM, Harding MM: *Medical-surgical nursing: assessment and management of clinical problems*, ed 10, St. Louis, 2017, Elsevier.)

to avoid consuming whole grains and most fruits and vegetables. Antibiotics that are not absorbed but pass through the intestinal tract may be given to reduce the bacterial flora in the intestines. Cathartics and laxatives are usually ordered to empty the digestive tract. Clearing feces and reducing the bacteria in the bowel aims to lower the risk of bacterial contamination of the abdominal cavity when the bowel is opened surgically.

ILEOSTOMY

An **ileostomy** is an opening in the ileum. The ileum is the distal portion of the small intestine that empties into the large intestine. An ileostomy is necessary when the entire colon must be bypassed or removed. Conditions that require colon bypass include congenital defects, cancer, inflammatory bowel disease, bowel trauma, and familial conditions such as multiple polyposis. Multiple polyposis is characterized by the presence of many polyps in the colon. Because these polyps often become malignant, removal of the colon may be recommended.

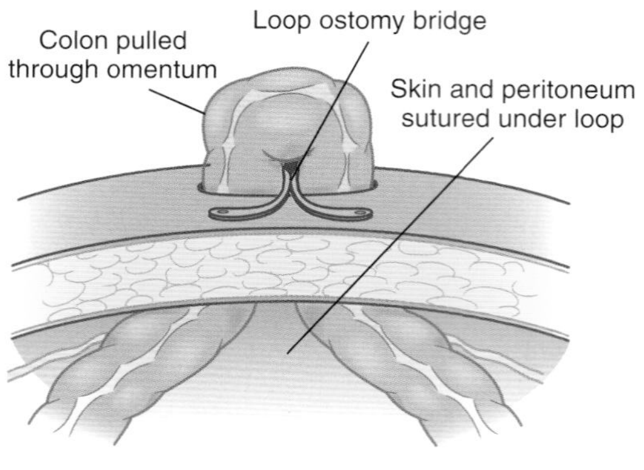

Fig. 18.3 Loop colostomy. (From Lewis SM, Bucher L, Heitkemper MM, Harding MM: *Medical-surgical nursing: assessment and management of clinical problems*, ed 10, St. Louis, 2017, Elsevier.)

Procedure

A surgical incision is made in the abdomen and a loop or the end of the ileum is brought out through a second abdominal incision. The edges of the loop or the end of the ileal segment are everted and sutured to the abdominal skin to create a stoma. Loops may be supported with a device such as a rod or bridge instead of being sutured to the skin.

The physician applies a disposable pouch or a fluffy dressing to absorb drainage in the operating room. The pouch collects fecal drainage to keep it from contaminating the surgical incision and to protect surrounding skin. The incontinent ileostomy frequently or intermittently drains liquid to pasty stool, so the patient will always have to wear a pouch. The stool output may be as high as 2000 mL per day initially. The small bowel gradually adapts, and the output will decrease and thicken over time.

The first continent ileostomy, created in 1975, was the Kock pouch (Fig. 18.4), which creates a reservoir for the liquid stool so that it can be drained from a stoma at intervals with a tube. The Barnett continent intestinal reservoir is a modification of the Kock procedure. A number of variations on the Kock pouch have since been developed, including the ileal pouch anal anastomosis (IPAA) (Fig. 18.5). This essentially creates a new rectum from the terminal ileum. This procedure allows for nearly normal bowel evacuation. This type of surgery involves several different versions of reconstructed bowel, which are named after the letters they resemble, including J, S, W, or H pouches. The patient may have a temporary loop ileostomy while the pouch heals. Laparoscopic procedures are relatively new but promise a more rapid postoperative recovery, lower infection risk, and better cosmetic outcome.

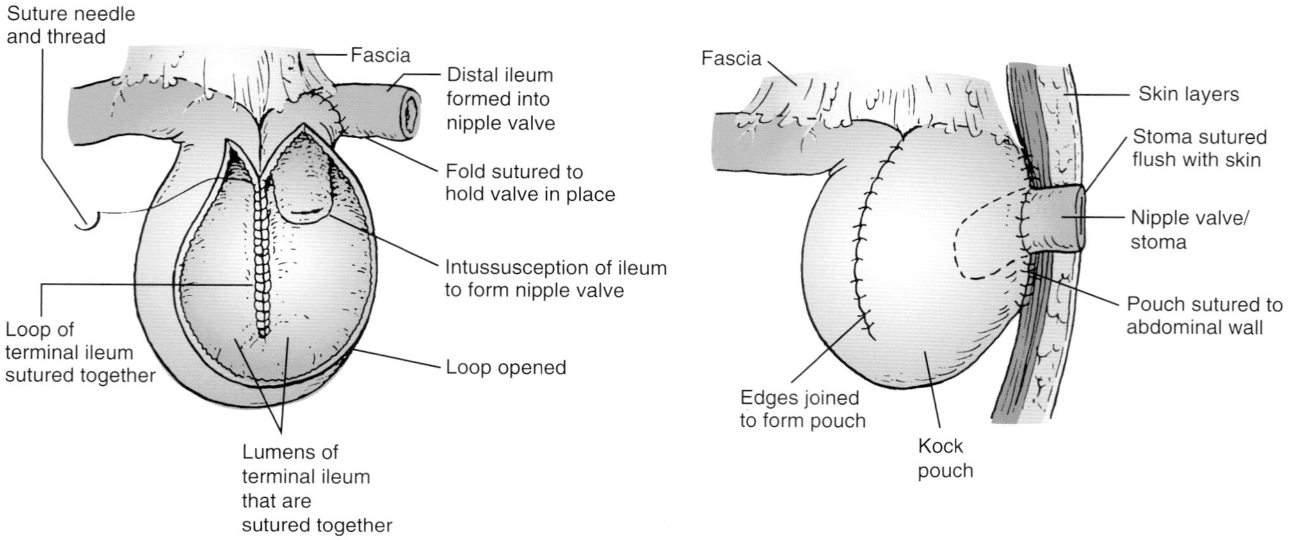

Fig. 18.4 Continent ileostomy (Kock pouch). The pouch to hold fecal matter is created from a loop of ileum folded back on itself. (From Black JM, Hawks JH: *Medical-surgical nursing: clinical management for positive outcomes*, ed 8, St. Louis, 2009, Saunders-Elsevier.)

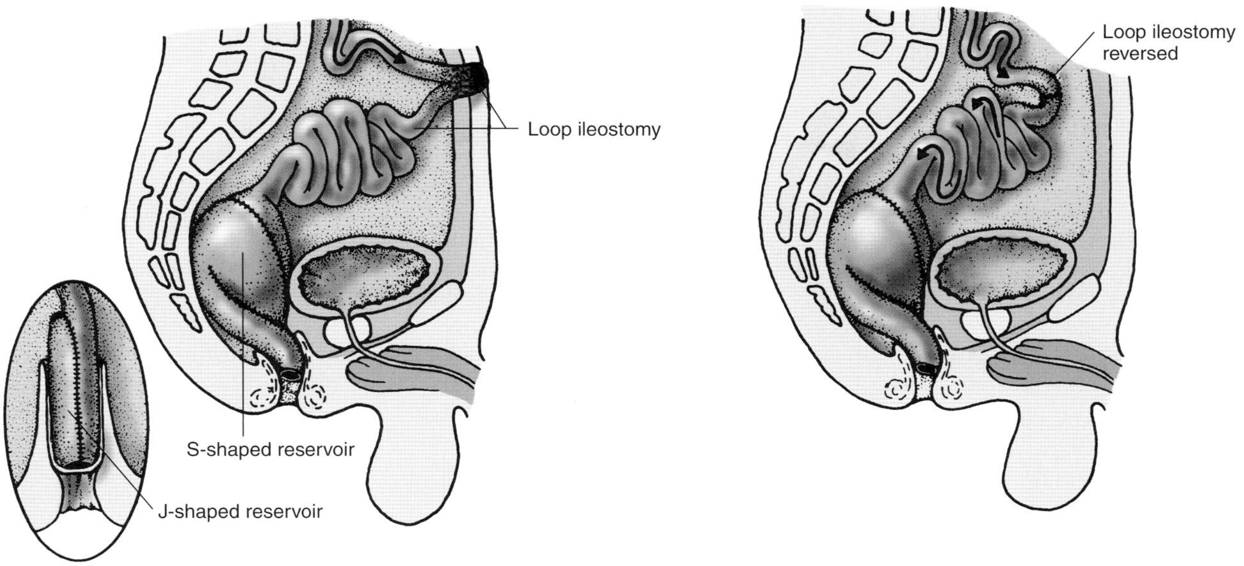

Stage 1.
After removal of the colon, a temporary loop ileostomy is created and an ileo anal reservoir is formed. The reservoir is created in an S-shaped reservoir (using three loops of ileum) or a J-shaped reservoir (suturing a portion of ileum to the rectal cuff, with an upward loop).

Stage 2.
After the reservoir has had time to heal–usually several months–the temporary loop ileostomy is reversed and stool is allowed to drain into the reservoir.

Fig. 18.5 Creation of an ileoanal reservoir. Stage 1: The colon is removed, a temporary loop ileostomy is created, and an ileoanal reservoir is formed. The reservoir may be J-shaped or S-shaped, depending on the technique used. Stage 2: After the reservoir heals (usually several months), the temporary loop ileostomy is reversed and stool drains into the reservoir for storage until it is eliminated through the rectum. (From Ignatavicius DD, Workman ML: *Medical-surgical nursing: patient-centered collaborative care*, ed 7, St. Louis, 2013, Saunders.)

Pharmacology Capsule

Ileostomy patients are usually not given timed-release capsules or enteric-coated tablets because they are likely to be eliminated before they can dissolve or be absorbed.

POSTOPERATIVE NURSING CARE OF THE PATIENT WITH AN ILEOSTOMY

The immediate postoperative care of the patient with an ileostomy is like that of most other patients having abdominal surgery. The patient may have a nasogastric tube attached to low intermittent suction. Intravenous fluids are ordered for several days, after which oral intake is gradually increased.

General care of the surgical patient is discussed in Chapter 17. This section emphasizes only the special needs of the ileostomy patient beyond the immediate recovery period.

Focused Assessment

Health History. After surgery, document significant symptoms such as pain, anorexia, nausea, vomiting, weakness, thirst, and muscle cramps in the review of systems. The functional assessment reveals how the patient is reacting to the surgery and how they think it will affect usual functioning. In addition, determine what stressors the patient perceives, as well as their usual coping strategies and sources of support. Finally, determine the patient's understanding of ileostomy care and lifestyle implications.

Physical examination. Begin the physical examination with observation of the patient's general status: level of consciousness, orientation, posture, and expression. Take vital signs and weight and compare them with preoperative findings. Inspect the skin color, and palpate for warmth and turgor; inspect oral tissues for moisture. Observe respiratory effort and auscultate breath sounds. In addition, examine the abdomen for distention and bowel sounds.

Inspect the stoma for color and bleeding. A new stoma created from a segment of bowel should be beefy red. When healed it should be rose red, somewhat darker than the color of the oral mucosa. A very pale, bluish, or black stoma has impaired circulation and must be reported to the RN or physician immediately. Prompt surgical intervention may be needed to restore circulation and prevent tissue necrosis.

Swelling of the stoma is expected initially, after which it shrinks during a period of 6 to 8 weeks. Inspect the base of the stoma for redness, skin separation, and purulent drainage. A small amount of bleeding around the base of a new stoma is not unusual. In fact, it may be a positive sign indicating an adequate blood supply. If edema occurs later, it is probably caused by pressure created by an improperly fitting collection appliance. The

Box 18.1 Postoperative Focused Assessment of the Patient With an Ostomy

HEALTH HISTORY

Reason for Seeking Care
Type of ostomy procedure done and reason

Past Health History
Acute and chronic conditions, prescribed drugs, allergies

Review of Systems
Pain, anorexia, nausea, vomiting, abdominal cramping or pain, weakness, thirst, muscle cramps

Functional Assessment
Response to surgery, anticipated effects on lifestyle, sources of stress and support, usual coping strategies

PHYSICAL EXAMINATION

General Survey: Level of consciousness, orientation, posture, expression
Skin: Color, warmth, turgor
Mouth: Moisture
Thorax: Respiratory effort, breath sounds
Abdomen: Distention, bowel sounds
Stoma: Color, bleeding, edema; condition of skin at base of stoma
Characteristics of Drainage: Amount, color, odor, blood, mucus
Extremities: Warmth, peripheral pulses
Neuromuscular Status: Trembling, twitching, cramping, change in mental status

appliance should be removed and replaced with one that has a correctly sized opening. (Note the characteristics of draining fluid or fecal matter.) The presence of some blood and mucus in the drainage is normal at first.

Record urine appearance and volume. Palpate extremities for warmth and peripheral pulses. It is important to observe for neuromuscular symptoms such as trembling, twitching, or cramping, which may indicate electrolyte imbalances.

General postoperative assessment of the patient with an ostomy is summarized in Box 18.1.

Patient Problems, Goals, and Outcome Criteria: Ileostomy

The patient problems and goals common to most postoperative patients (pain, potential for airway obstruction, potential for infection, inadequate circulation, and urinary retention) are discussed in Chapter 17. Additional diagnoses specific to the ileostomy patient in the immediate postoperative phase are as follows.

Patient Problems	Goals and Outcome Criteria
Potential for fluid volume deficit (dehydration) related to nothing by mouth (NPO) status, nasogastric suction, passage of liquid stool	Normal fluid balance: pulse and blood pressure consistent with patient norms, moist mucous membranes, urine output approximately equal to fluid intake, absence of neuromuscular symptoms.
Potential for inadequate tissue perfusion of stoma	Effective stoma perfusion: stoma is beefy red.
Potential for disrupted skin tissue integrity related to adhesive, fecal drainage, leaking appliance	Normal skin integrity: skin intact with minimal redness around stoma.
Altered body image related to presence of stoma, altered body function, loss of fecal continence	Adjustment to change in body image: patient makes positive statements about ability to adapt, learns and takes over ostomy care.
Potential for impaired sexual function related to altered body structure and function or reactions to those changes	Fulfilling sexual expression: patient reports making adaptations as necessary for satisfying sexual expression.
Inability to manage self-care related to lack of knowledge of ostomy management, failure to accept ostomy, lack of resources for proper care	Patient effectively manages ostomy: patient accepts responsibility for self-care, demonstrates proper care of ostomy, obtains necessary supplies.
Potential for injury related to obstruction of the ileum	Absence of injury: ostomy remains patent, drainage is continuous or frequent.

Interventions

Potential for fluid volume deficit. The loss of fluids and electrolytes through nasogastric suction and the passage of liquid stool can lead to deficient fluid volume and electrolyte imbalances. Administer intravenous fluids as ordered, with careful monitoring of hydration status. Maintain accurate intake and output records including urine, gastric contents, and fecal drainage. Monitor serum electrolytes closely and watch for signs and symptoms of imbalances: changes in mental status (confusion, anxiety), changes in neuromuscular status (twitching, trembling, weakness), poor tissue turgor, edema, and dry mucous membranes.

When the patient resumes oral intake, advise a daily fluid intake of 2 to 3 L. During hot weather or illness, additional fluids may be required. It is best to consume a variety of fluids, rather than plain water, to obtain electrolytes. The loss of bicarbonate in ileostomy drainage can result in metabolic acidosis. To prevent this, the physician may order bicarbonate replacement.

Potential for inadequate tissue perfusion of stoma. As noted earlier, a healthy stoma is beefy red during the postoperative period. As it heals, the color becomes more rose red. If blood flow to the stoma is impaired, the stoma may appear pale, bluish, or even black. Unless adequate circulation is restored quickly, the tissue will become necrotic. The surgeon must be informed immediately because surgical intervention may be needed to restore blood flow.

Potential for disrupted skin tissue integrity. Check the pouch hourly at first to detect leakage. When the pouch is emptied or changed, try to keep fecal matter from contaminating the primary incision. Digestive enzymes present in the liquid stool are especially harmful to the abdominal tissue. Cleanse the skin around the stoma gently but thoroughly. Maintaining skin integrity is an ongoing problem for the patient with an intestinal ostomy. The presence of fecal matter on the skin provides a medium for bacterial, fungal, and yeast infections. In addition, the materials used to hold the pouch securely can cause traumatic injuries and allergic responses.

A protective barrier must be maintained to prevent skin breakdown. A pouch is used to collect fecal drainage. A good pouch is one that protects the skin, contains wastes and gas, is odor proof, permits freedom of movement, provides security for the patient, and is not noticeable. Many kinds of pouches are available, but their features are basically the same. Some type of adhesive is needed to secure the pouch around the stoma. The pouch has an opening at the bottom that allows for emptying and rinsing. Some have gas filters that allow gas to escape while minimizing odor. Disposable pouches are used primarily, but reusable pouches are still available. The WOC nurse is a good resource person to help the patient find the right appliance.

Periodically (about every 3 to 7 days) remove the appliance for thorough cleansing of the skin surrounding the stoma. Gently peel the skin barrier (wafer) off the skin. Rough handling and frequent changes contribute to skin breakdown. Commercial adhesive removers are available if needed. After removing the skin barrier, clean the stoma and the area around it with water. If soap is used, it should be nonoily and must be rinsed off thoroughly. Then pat or fan the skin dry. The patient may be surprised to find that the stoma itself has no sensation, although the surrounding skin may be tender.

A protective barrier may be applied before the pouch can be replaced. Skin sealants that come in the form of gels, wipes, sprays, liquids, and roll-ons may be applied to the skin. Sealants protect the skin; they do not hold the pouch in place. Next, products that improve the seal may be applied. Commonly used products include powders, pastes, wafers, rings, or strips. If the skin around the stoma is broken, ostomy powder may be applied followed by a special coating material or hydrocolloid dressing. Dust away excess powder before the wafer is applied. Wafers and rings may be precut or may require cutting or stretching to fit around the stoma. The opening should be no more than ⅛ inch larger than the stoma because a larger opening permits more fecal matter to come in contact with the skin. If a paste, barrier ring, or strip is used, apply it around the stoma or on the cut edge of the wafer. Place the wafer over the stoma and press down. Some pouching systems have the pouch preattached to the wafer (one piece); other systems consist of a wafer that is placed around the stoma and a separate pouch that attaches to the wafer (two-piece). Some patients have an uneven skin surface around the stoma, making it difficult to create a seal. In that case, a caulking material such as barrier strips or rings can be applied around the stoma to create a smooth surface. Clamp or close the pouch tail after it is securely placed. Initially, the pouch opening will probably need to be custom cut. As the stoma heals and shrinks, precut appliances may work well. Custom-cut pouches can be ordered for stomas of unusual size or shape. Patients whose barriers quickly erode and those with very flush or retracted stomas can obtain special barriers to maintain good fit. Once the stoma and surgical incision heal, some patients will prefer to cleanse the peristomal skin in the shower.

Altered body image. Establishment of bowel control is an important developmental task of childhood. The patient who has an ileostomy is no longer able to control the passage of fecal matter and must learn to manage bowel elimination in a new way. This can be very distressing to the adult who fears spillage and exposure.

Inability to control odor associated with passage of gas through the stoma is another concern for the patient with an intestinal ostomy. The characteristic odor of stool is generally considered unpleasant. Because the ostomy patient may have fecal matter draining intermittently, the source of odor is almost always present.

Assure the patient that odor is normal when the pouch is being changed or emptied but that it can be controlled at other times. Causes of odor include certain foods and poor hygiene. Foods that produce gas or stimulate bowel activity are most likely to contribute to odor problems. These generally include spicy foods, onions, garlic, some vegetables, such as cabbage and beans, and high-fiber foods such as whole grains and fresh fruits and vegetables. Reactions to specific foods depend on the individual. Therefore advise the patient to delete and reintroduce various foods to find those that are most troublesome. Because flatus is usually evident several hours after eating gas-forming foods, the patient can eat those foods selectively at times when flatus would not be embarrassing.

Good hygiene also helps to control odor. Most pouches today are odor proof and disposable. Any reusable collection pouches should be washed with soap and water. Rinsing with a vinegar solution neutralizes odors that cling to the pouch. Commercial pouch deodorizers are available as well.

Potential for impaired sexual function. One area that often worries patients with an ostomy is sexuality. Encourage patients to ask questions about how the ostomy might affect sexual function or behavior. Patients may feel unattractive or fear rejection by their partner. Some men have erectile dysfunction or disruption of ejaculation, especially if they have had nerve damage associated with perineal surgery. Women may experience vaginal dryness and discomfort during intercourse. The surgeon and the WOC nurse counsel these men about options, which may include penile implants. Affected women are counseled to try vaginal lubricants. Other patients have problems because of psychologic factors, which may improve with counseling or medications prescribed by the health care practitioner.

Some practical suggestions may help the patient to resume sexual activity. The pouch should be emptied and taped down before sexual intercourse. Pouch covers and specialized undergarments are available to conceal the appliance and its contents. The partner wearing the pouch should experiment with positions that are most comfortable. Female patients should know that ostomy surgery does not interfere with pregnancy or delivery.

Inability to manage self-care. After surgery, some teaching should be included every time stoma care is done. At first, you may simply tell the patient what is being done and why. Then encourage the patient to take over more and more of the procedure. Ask the patient to demonstrate and practice as much as possible before discharge.

Some patients adjust more easily than others to an ostomy. A first step in accepting the stoma is looking at it. (Note when the patient begins to watch stoma care.) Patients should be encouraged but not forced to participate in the care. If a patient does not begin to show some interest in learning self-care after a few days, consider seeking help from supportive resources, such as the WOC nurse or an ostomy association volunteer. You may feel frustrated if patients seem unwilling to learn self-care (see the Patient Teaching box). You must be sensitive to the patient's feelings. An ostomy requires adjustments in body image and self-concept. Patients also have a grief response to this type of surgery.

Patient Teaching

After Ostomy Surgery

The staff nurse, WOC nurse, or both must help the patient to plan for discharge. General topics to include in the teaching plan after ostomy surgery are outlined below. Specifics must be individualized to the patient and the surgical procedure.

- Stoma and skin care: Explain recommended procedures and supplies with written care instructions and some temporary supplies when the patient is discharged.
- Appliances: Provide a list of the supplies needed and where they can be purchased.
- Irrigation (if appropriate) or drainage: Explain about the frequency, procedure, and supplies needed.

Other helpful points include the following:

- You can bathe or shower with the appliance in place because the pouch and the seal are waterproof.
- Wear regular clothing but avoid direct pressure over the stoma.
- Learn to recognize foods that cause excess gas or odor so that these can be avoided.
- Maintain a fluid intake of at least 2000 mL daily unless contraindicated.
- Avoid heavy lifting and strenuous activities at first; usually no restrictions are made after approximately 3 months; ask your physician about specific activities and contact sports.
- Adaptations for sexual activity can include concealing the pouch and experimenting with positions.
- Contact your physician or the WOC nurse if you observe skin breakdown, prolapse (bulging out) of the stoma, or obstruction (output absent or markedly decreased).
- Resources for information about living with an ostomy include the American Cancer Society (www.cancer.org), United Ostomy Associations of America (www.ostomy.org), Crohn's and Colitis Foundation of America (www.ccfa.org), Wound Ostomy and Continence Nurses Society (www.wocn.org), and home health agencies.
- Ostomy surgery does not interfere with traveling. Tips on traveling include the following:
- Take adequate supplies.
- If flying, keep the supplies in a hand-carried bag. This could prevent problems if luggage is lost or delayed.
- Include sealable plastic bags to dispose of used supplies.
- Exercise caution with new foods that may cause diarrhea or gas.
- If visiting a country where drinking the water is not advised, do not irrigate a colostomy with the water. Use only water that is safe for drinking.

Potential for injury. The lumen (interior diameter) of an ileostomy is less than 1 inch; therefore, it can easily become obstructed. To reduce the risk of obstruction, the patient is initially given a low-fiber diet. High-fiber foods are then added gradually. Certain foods such as dried fruit, mushrooms, olives, celery, nuts, coleslaw, popcorn, Chinese vegetables, and foods with skins must be chewed very thoroughly and taken with fluid so that they do not create an obstruction in the ileum.

Put On Your Thinking Cap!

Locate a resource in the area where you live that provides information for people with an ostomy. Share this with classmates.

CONTINENT (POUCH) ILEOSTOMY

The continent ileostomy has an internal pouch created from a loop of ileum for storing fecal matter. The advantage of this type of ileostomy is that the patient does not have continuous drainage and so does not have to wear a pouch.

Not all patients are candidates for the continent ileostomy. The patient must be capable of draining the pouch with a catheter, and the ileum must be sufficient for the valve to be constructed. People with ulcerative colitis are candidates for the continent ileostomy but patients with Crohn disease are usually not eligible.

Procedure

To create a continent ileostomy, a loop of the ileum is sutured together and then opened. A portion of the distal end of the ileum is inverted within itself to create a nipple valve. The valve prevents the leakage of fluid from the pouch. The looped section of the ileum is then closed, leaving a pouch capable of expanding and storing fecal matter. The distal end of the ileum is brought through the abdominal wall and sutured into place to create a stoma (see Fig. 18.4). During surgery, a catheter is placed through the stoma into the pouch and sutured in place. The catheter is connected to low intermittent suction to keep the pouch empty. This prevents stress on the suture lines while the pouch heals.

POSTOPERATIVE NURSING CARE OF THE PATIENT WITH A CONTINENT ILEOSTOMY

In general, postoperative nursing care is like that described for the patient with an ileostomy. This section provides information on additional nursing measures that are specific to the patient with a continent ileostomy.

Focused Assessment

Postoperative assessment of the patient who has a continent ileostomy is essentially the same as that of the patient with an ileostomy. When the patient has a continent ileostomy, it is especially important to assess for continuous drainage because obstruction of the catheter may occur. Absence of drainage or patient complaints of a feeling of fullness in the pouch suggests obstruction. The drainage from the catheter is bloody at first and then brownish.

Patient Problems, Goals, and Outcome Criteria: Continent Ileostomy

The patient problems, goals, and outcome criteria in addition to those previously listed are as follows.

Patient Problems	Goals and Outcome Criteria
Potential for injury related to obstruction of the pouch drainage	Absence of injury: patient's pouch drains readily
Inability to perform (stoma) self-care related to lack of knowledge of technique for draining pouch and caring for stoma and pouch	Patient understands pouch and stoma care: patient demonstrates proper pouch drainage and stoma care

Interventions

Potential for injury. In the initial postoperative period, the patient is given only intravenous fluids, then sips of water until gas and liquid stool pass through the catheter. The catheter is removed after 2 to 3 weeks, which allows the pouch to heal and peristalsis to resume. At first, the pouch can hold only 70 to 100 mL of fluid. Later it can hold as much as 500 mL. Initially the patient is taught to drain the pouch every 2 hours during the day by inserting the catheter through the stoma/bowel. At night, the catheter can be placed to gravity drainage. During the next few weeks to months, the interval between catheterizations is gradually lengthened as the pouch capacity increases. Eventually the patient will need to drain the pouch only 2 to 4 times a day. As the patient's body adapts to the ileostomy, the drainage gradually becomes thicker and the color of normal stool.

Inability to perform (stoma) self-care. Key points in draining the continent ileostomy are as follows:

1. Have the patient sit or lie down for the procedure.
2. Gather supplies: lubricant, 28 to 32 Fr catheter, drape, basin, irrigating syringe, irrigating solution, gauze dressing.
3. Lubricate the catheter and insert it gently into the stoma.
4. Resistance will be felt when the catheter reaches the nipple valve (approximately 2 inches past the stoma). Instruct the patient to bear down and then roll the catheter between your fingers and advance it into the pouch.
5. As soon as the catheter is in the pouch, gas and fecal matter begin to be expelled. Drainage usually continues for approximately 10 minutes and produces a total volume of 50 to 200 mL.
6. If the drainage is too thick or the catheter becomes blocked, instill 30 mL of normal saline or tap water as ordered and let it drain off. Gently aspirate only if necessary because this may cause dislocation of the nipple.
7. When drainage stops, quickly remove the catheter.
8. Place a gauze dressing over the stoma to absorb any secretions.

9. Measure, describe, and discard the drainage.
10. Instruct the patient on how to perform this procedure as soon as possible.
11. Advise the patient to wear a medical alert bracelet at all times that states they have a continent diversion that must be drained.

See the Health Promotion box and the Dietary Considerations box for a review of special considerations for the patient with a continent ileostomy.

Health Promotion

Dietary Considerations for the Patient With a Continent Ileostomy

Patients with a continent ileostomy will have some dietary restrictions, and it is helpful to request a postoperative dietary consultation. The diet is intended to avoid excess gas, maintain a soft stool, and avoid obstruction of the catheter. Be sure that patients know they should avoid the following foods:

- Coffee, alcohol, and gas-forming foods (initially)
- Skins, seeds, and nuts (including corn, olives, peas, and mushrooms)
- Pineapple, berries, and fresh fruit (initially)
- Milk products (if they cause excessive gas)

Nutrition Considerations

1. The patient with an ileostomy or colostomy may eat a normal diet and simply omit foods that seem to cause problems.
2. The main concern of the patient with an ileostomy or colostomy is odor, which is caused by flatulence.
3. Patients should be encouraged to avoid foods tending to cause bad odor, especially corn, dried beans, onions, cabbage, spicy foods, and fish.
4. Fibrous vegetables should be avoided and all food should be chewed well.

ILEAL POUCH ANAL ANASTOMOSIS

An IPAA is somewhat like the continent pouch ileostomy except that fecal matter is stored and then eliminated through a surgically constructed rectum. It is an alternative to an ostomy, and information about it is included in this chapter because the patient will have a temporary ileostomy and the nursing care is similar to that of the ostomy patient.

Procedure

The ileal pouch anal anastomosis requires a complex set of surgical procedures that are done in two stages. In the first stage, the colon is removed and an internal pouch that is created from the ileum is attached to the anorectal canal. A temporary ileostomy diverts stool while healing occurs. Approximately 2 to 3 months later, the ileostomy is closed if the reservoir does not leak and stool is then eliminated through the anus (see Fig. 18.5). The procedure is not recommended for patients with Crohn disease or poor rectal sphincter control.

Complications

The major complications of the IPAA are (1) small bowel obstruction, (2) leaking of suture lines leading to peritonitis, and (3) inflammation of the reservoir.

Obstruction. Scar tissue or strictures may cause obstruction. Signs and symptoms of small bowel obstruction are abdominal distention, nausea, and vomiting, decreased bowel sounds, and a change in bowel pattern.

Peritonitis. If fecal matter leaks through the suture lines of the reservoir into the abdominal cavity, abscesses or peritonitis can develop. Signs and symptoms are increased pulse, respirations, and temperature; rigid abdomen and abdominal pain; and elevated white blood cell count.

Inflammation. Inflammation of the ileal reservoir (pouchitis) may be manifested by abdominal cramping, bloody diarrhea, urgency, and pain.

POSTOPERATIVE NURSING CARE OF THE PATIENT WITH AN ILEAL POUCH ANAL ANASTOMOSIS

Focused Assessment

The nursing assessment after surgery to create an ileoanal reservoir is the same as for the patient with an ileostomy. In addition, assess for rectal drainage and condition of the perianal skin.

Patient Problems, Goals, and Outcome Criteria: Ileal Pouch Anal Anastomosis

In addition to the patient problems, goals and outcomes for the patient with an ileostomy, the following problems may occur with an IPAA.

Patient Problems	Goals and Outcome Criteria
Potential for disrupted skin tissue integrity related to frequent passage of liquid stool through the rectum	Healthy skin: intact skin without excessive redness around the anus and the perianal area
Bowel incontinence related to inability to control passage of frequent liquid stools	Control of bowel elimination: decreasing number of incontinent episodes
Potential for injury related to possible small bowel obstruction, leaking of reservoir suture line, inflammation of reservoir	Absence of signs and symptoms of obstruction, suture leakage, or reservoir inflammation: no fever, abdominal pain or distention, or bloody stools

Interventions

Potential for disrupted skin tissue integrity. After the first surgical procedure, the patient's skin around the ileostomy stoma and in the perianal area needs special care (see the Cultural Considerations box). Ileostomy care is discussed earlier in this chapter. Until the reservoir is well healed, liquid discharge may be expelled without warning. Thorough, gentle cleansing and protective creams help to prevent skin breakdown.

Cultural Considerations

What Does Culture Have to Do With Stoma Care?

The Muslim patient is expected to perform a washing ritual and pray 5 times each day. Because the patient with a stoma may have urine or feces in the pouch, he will be concerned about obeying the rules of purity during daily prayers. The Mosque leader (Imam) can counsel the patient about a special excuse in this situation. The WOC nurse may also offer suggestions to alleviate the patient's concerns.

Bowel incontinence. Initially the patient may have as many as 20 stools a day. After 1 week, the number decreases to 8 to 10 daily. By 6 months the frequency is usually only approximately 4 to 6 a day. Nighttime control may continue to be a problem. Perineal pads or incontinence briefs may be needed to prevent soiling of clothing.

The patient must learn to strengthen the perineal muscles to restore control of fecal elimination. A recommended exercise is to tighten the anus, count to 10, and relax. This should be repeated five to six times, four times daily. In addition, drugs can be prescribed to decrease the frequency of stools and to make them less watery.

No absolute dietary restrictions exist. Advise patients to avoid fatty foods at first. The patient learns through trial and error how their body handles specific foods. Caffeine and fresh fruits and vegetables tend to cause loose, frequent stools. Pasta, boiled rice, and low-fat cheese tend to produce thicker stools.

Potential for injury. Be alert for signs and symptoms of bowel obstruction (abdominal distention, pain, no stool passage), peritonitis (pain, fever), and inflammation (pain, bloody stools), which should be reported to the physician. If obstruction occurs, the patient is given intravenous fluids and kept NPO. A nasogastric tube is inserted to decompress the bowel. If the obstruction is caused by adhesions (scar tissue), surgery may be necessary to release the restriction.

Sometimes a stricture or narrowing develops at the site where the ileum is joined to the rectum. This is most likely to happen in the fourth week after surgery. The physician may be able to stretch the tissue manually and relieve the obstruction. If an abscess or peritonitis develops, the infection is treated with antibiotic drugs. Intravenous fluids are ordered. Surgery may be necessary to drain abscesses and repair the leaking suture line.

If the inner lining of the reservoir becomes inflamed or infected, the physician may do a proctoscopic examination to identify the cause. The condition may be treated with metronidazole (Flagyl) and steroids given orally.

COLOSTOMY

A **colostomy** is an opening in the colon through which fecal matter is eliminated. The location of the colostomy affects the characteristics of the fecal drainage; the closer to the rectum it is, the more formed the stool.

Procedure

A colostomy is performed by bringing a loop or an end of the intestine through the abdominal wall and creating a stoma for the passage of fecal matter. The location of the stoma depends on the portion of the intestine removed. Colostomies are classified by location in the colon. Therefore, a patient may have an ascending, transverse, descending, or sigmoid colostomy (Fig. 18.6) (see Table 18.1). An ascending colostomy passes relatively liquid material. The drainage from a transverse colostomy is liquid to semisolid. A descending or sigmoid colostomy passes softly formed stool. The colostomy begins to function on the third to fifth postoperative day.

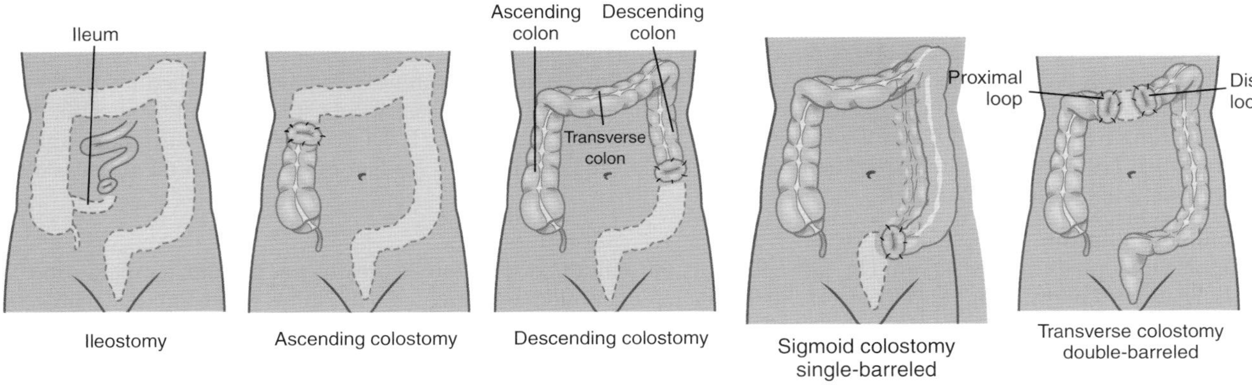

Fig. 18.6 Types of ostomies. (From Lewis SM, Bucher L, Heitkemper MM, Harding MM: *Medical-surgical nursing: assessment and management of clinical problems*, ed 10, St. Louis, 2017, Elsevier.)

A colostomy may be temporary or permanent. A temporary colostomy is done to allow healing of the intestine after surgery, trauma, or in certain disease states. Because the intestine below the colostomy is intact, the temporary colostomy may have two stomas. The stoma that drains fecal matter from the intestine is the proximal stoma. The distal stoma opens into the portion of the colon connected to the rectum. This is called a *double-barreled colostomy.* Sometimes the opening of the distal portion is brought through another location on the abdominal wall, creating a fistula through which mucus drains. If there is more than one stoma, the patient record should clarify which is the functional stoma that drains feces. An end colostomy with a Hartmann pouch for the distal segment is now more common than the double-barreled colostomy. A Hartmann pouch is created by closing the distal bowel and leaving it in place (see Fig. 18.2). The patient with a Hartmann pouch passes mucus through the rectum. In a total abdominal colectomy with ileorectal anastomosis (TAC-IRA), the pouch stores fecal matter to be eliminated through the anus. When it is necessary to remove a large part of the colon or the rectum, a permanent colostomy is made. If the colostomy is created in two stages, the patient returns from the first procedure with a loop of intestine protruding from an abdominal wound. The loop is held in place by a rod or a bridge (see Fig. 18.3). Later, the surgeon cuts the loop to create the stoma.

The main long-term complications of colostomy are prolapse and stenosis. A prolapsed stoma protrudes farther out than usual. It is caused by increased abdominal pressure, as can occur with coughing or sneezing. Other contributing factors might include an abdominal opening that is too large or a poorly attached stoma. Stenosis is the narrowing of the abdominal opening around the base of the stoma. If severe, stenosis blocks the passage of feces. Additional complications are associated with poor blood supply to the stoma, leading to necrosis and peristomal hernia. Peristomal hernia can limit bowel function, causing constipation, strangulation of the bowel, and poor results from colostomy irrigation.

POSTOPERATIVE NURSING CARE OF THE PATIENT WITH A COLOSTOMY

Focused Assessment

The postoperative care of the patient with a colostomy is essentially the same as that for the patient with an ileostomy.

Patient Problems, Goals, and Outcome Criteria: Colostomy

In addition to the patient problems and goals already identified, the following may also apply to the patient with a colostomy.

Patient Problem	Goals and Outcome Criteria
Inability to manage colostomy care related to lack of knowledge of self-care and irrigation procedure (if ordered), lack of confidence, lack of resources, failure to accept ostomy	Patient manages colostomy effectively: patient accepts responsibility for self-care, patient demonstrates ostomy care and irrigation (if ordered) correctly; uses resources as needed, obtains necessary supplies.
Potential for injury related to prolapse or stenosis	Absence of injury: no signs of prolapse, no protrusion of stoma; patent stoma with lumen of adequate diameter: regular elimination of feces through stoma.

Interventions

Most aspects of care are the same as those discussed for the patient with an ileostomy. A few points specific to the patient with a colostomy are presented here (see also the Nursing Care Plan: Patient with a Colostomy box).

Nursing Care Plan **Patient With a Colostomy**

FOCUSED ASSESSMENT

Health History

A 47-year-old Asian American had a bowel resection and permanent colostomy in the descending colon to remove a malignant tumor. He is 3 days postsurgery. He has been receiving intravenous morphine by patient-controlled analgesia and reports adequate pain control. He has had no nausea or vomiting but has a nasogastric tube attached to low suction. He is allowed nothing by mouth (NPO) and is receiving intravenous fluids at 150 mL/h. He participates in turning, coughing, deep breathing, and using incentive spirometry every 2 hours. He has discussed his fear of cancer with the nurse, stating that his mother died of stomach cancer.

Physical Examination

Vital signs: blood pressure 118/64 mm Hg, pulse 92 beats per minute, respiration 20 breaths per minute, temperature 100° F (38° C) measured orally. Height 5′5″, weight 140 lb. The patient is alert and oriented. His skin is warm and dry with good turgor. Oral mucous membranes are moist. Breath sounds are clear to auscultation. The abdomen is soft and bowel sounds are present in all four quadrants. The stoma is beefy red and edematous. A temporary drainage device is in place, and the collection pouch has approximately 100 mL of greenish-brown liquid stool. Extremities are warm with palpable peripheral pulses. No muscle twitching or cramps are noted.

Nursing Care Plan **Patient With a Colostomy—cont'd**

Patient Problems	Goals and Outcome Criteria	Interventions
Potential for fluid volume deficit related to NPO status, nasogastric suction, passage of liquid stool	Patient will maintain normal fluid balance, as evidenced by pulse and blood pressure consistent with patient's baseline, moist mucous membranes, and approximately equal fluid intake and output.	Monitor for signs of hypovolemia: tachycardia, hypotension, decreasing urine output, and dry mucous membranes. Keep accurate intake and output (i.e., urine, liquid stool, gastric fluid) records. Monitor for signs of electrolyte imbalances: confusion, anxiety, twitching, trembling, muscle weakness, and cardiac dysrhythmias. Give intravenous fluids as ordered, monitoring rate of flow carefully.
Potential for disrupted skin integrity related to stoma adhesive, fecal drainage	Skin at the base of the stoma will be intact and free of redness.	Check pouch hourly to detect leakage. When pouch is emptied, prevent fecal matter from contaminating the incision. When changing the appliance, gently remove adhesive. Cleanse skin around stoma with soap and water, rinse, and pat dry. Apply a protective skin barrier before replacing the pouch. Make the opening of the skin barrier not more than ⅛ larger than the stoma. Report rash or skin breakdown.
Altered body image related to presence of stoma, altered body function	Patient will adapt to colostomy as evidenced by self-care and ability to resume normal activities.	Provide an opportunity for the patient to share his thoughts about colostomy. Identify specific concerns such as activity limitations, stoma care, odor control, and effect on sexuality. Provide information. Be accepting of the patient's feelings. Encourage him to attend to grooming and appearance. Offer to have a volunteer from the American Cancer Society or United Ostomy Associations of America visit him. Advise the patient that services are available from a WOC nurse, a mental health counselor, and a spiritual counselor if he desires.
Inability to manage (colostomy) self-care related to complexity of ostomy care, lack of knowledge, lack of resources, failure to accept ostomy	Patient will manage ostomy care effectively: patient demonstrates proper ostomy care, uses available resources, and resumes valued activities with adaptations as needed.	During stoma care in early postoperative period, tell the patient what is being done and why. When the patient begins to watch the procedure, gradually encourage him to participate and then to take over care. Recognize the patient's need to grieve and that the patient may use denial as a coping mechanism. Develop a teaching plan that includes skin care, pouches, diet fluids, irrigation if appropriate, activity, sexuality, complications, tips on traveling, and resources.

CRITICAL THINKING QUESTIONS

1. What would be some behaviors that indicate the patient is beginning to accept the permanent colostomy?
2. Why might a patient with a new colostomy experience grief?

Inability to manage (colostomy) self care. People with a descending colostomy may be taught to irrigate it every day or two to maintain regular, controlled elimination. Many patients have regular bowel movements without irrigation. Others are unlikely to establish controlled elimination and may find the procedure not worth the trouble. Patients who have liquid stools do not benefit from irrigation because they drain fecal matter continuously. Irrigation is unlikely to establish control if the patient has diarrhea when under stress, has had radiotherapy, has a poor prognosis, or has a history of inflammatory bowel disease. The surgeon and WOC nurse will decide whether irrigation is appropriate in individual cases.

Irrigation can cause complications. The tube used to introduce irrigating fluid can perforate the bowel. A perforated bowel permits fecal matter to flow into the abdominal cavity, causing peritonitis, a very serious infection. The risk of perforation can be reduced greatly by using a cone-tipped catheter. Other complications are caused by the type, amount, or temperature of the solution used. Plain tap water may cause fluid and electrolyte imbalances if used repeatedly or in large amounts. If too much solution is used or if it is too cold, the patient may experience cramping, nausea, and dizziness. Inform the physician if weakness occurs after irrigation even after the amount and temperature of the solution are adjusted.

If irrigations are indicated, you or the WOC nurse may perform them initially. However, the goal is for the patient or significant other to learn to do the procedure, so an explanation of the process must be provided.

The following are key points to remember when irrigating a colostomy:

1. Have the patient select the time of day that is most convenient. The procedure should be done at

approximately the same time every day. The entire process takes 45 minutes to 1 hour.

2. Have the patient sit on or in front of the toilet if possible. If the patient cannot get out of bed, the procedure can be done while the patient is in bed.
3. Remove the old pouch and apply an irrigating sleeve. This device opens at the top so that the tubing can be inserted into the stoma and it opens at the bottom so that fecal matter can drain into the toilet.
4. Pour 500 to 1500 mL of lukewarm irrigating solution into an enema fluid container and hold it at the level of the patient's shoulder. Initially, 500 mL is used but adults eventually increase the fluid to 1500 mL (Landmann & Cashman, June 9, 2020).
5. Clear the air from the tubing, lubricate the tubing, and insert it gently 2 to 4 inches into the stoma. The direction to insert the tubing can be assessed by first inserting a gloved, lubricated finger into the stoma. Do not use force! If a cone-tipped catheter is used, the catheter can be inserted only approximately 1 inch. This reduces the risk of perforation.
6. Allow the solution to flow slowly into the stoma. If the patient has cramping, slow down or stop the flow for a few minutes. Remove the tubing or cone after the solution has been administered.
7. If the solution does not drain promptly, close the bottom of the sleeve so that the patient can carry out other activities. Complete emptying may take 20 to 30 minutes.
8. When elimination is complete, remove, wash, and dry the sleeve.
9. Measure the stoma before applying a new pouch, especially in the first 4 to 6 weeks, because the stoma size will change as healing occurs. The opening in the skin barrier should be just slightly larger than the stoma.
10. Apply a clean pouch if additional drainage usually occurs during the day. Some patients need only a small dressing or a stoma cap.
11. Rectal suppositories can be inserted into a colostomy stoma to stimulate evacuation.
12. Patients who have double-barreled colostomies can be given rectal medications through the distal stoma. Be sure you identify which stoma is the distal one.

Potential for injury. Be alert for indications of colostomy complications. Although a prolapsed stoma may look frightening, it is not usually serious. No reason exists for immediate action if it continues to drain feces. It can usually be gently put back in place by the surgeon or WOC nurse. If the prolapse is severe or causes fecal obstruction, surgical repair is indicated.

Inform the physician if the ostomy is not draining properly. The surgeon may be able to dilate the stoma and enlarge the opening. If dilation is not successful, surgery may be needed.

URINARY DIVERSION

When the normal route for urine elimination is disrupted, it may be necessary to divert urine out of the body in a different way. The most common type of incontinent urinary diversion is the ileal conduit, often called a urostomy. Other incontinent diversions include cutaneous ureterostomy, colonic (sigmoid) conduit, vesicostomy, and nephrostomy (Fig. 18.7). Continent urinary diversions use a segment of bowel to create an internal reservoir that is drained via an abdominal stoma at intervals (Fig. 18.8). The orthotopic bladder construction, or "**neobladder**," is a new bladder constructed from a segment of bowel. The orthotopic bladder is placed in the normal bladder location. It is attached to the urethra so that the patient voids normally. Not all patients are good

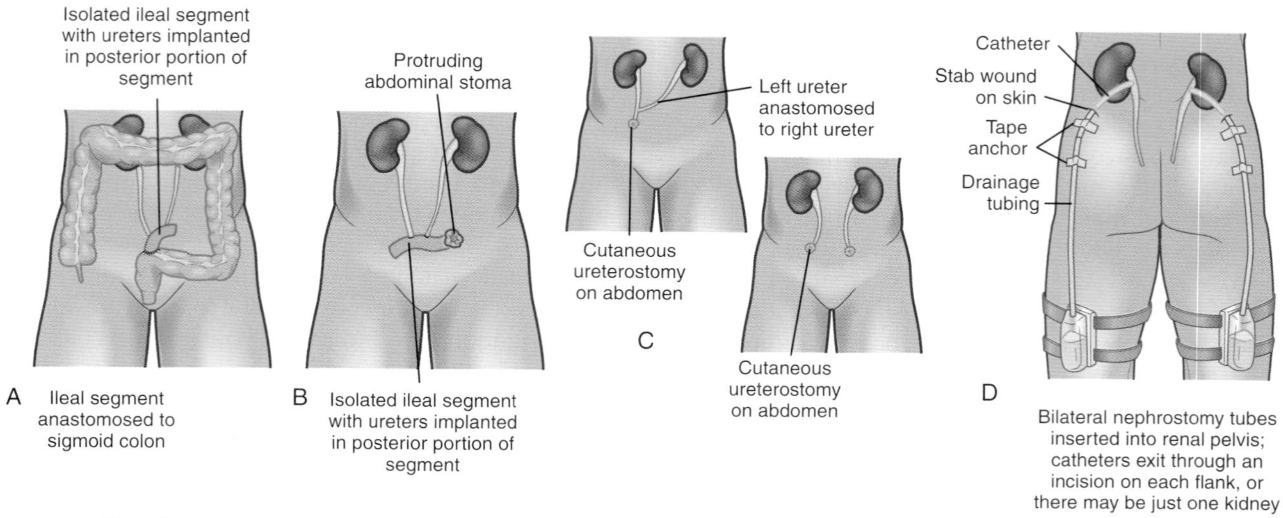

Fig. 18.7 Methods of urinary diversion. (From Lewis SM, Bucher L, Heitkemper MM, Harding MM: *Medical-surgical nursing: assessment and management of clinical problems*, ed 10, St. Louis, 2017, Elsevier.)

candidates for the neobladder. Ureterosigmoidostomy and ureteroileosigmoidostomy are older procedures that have been largely replaced by newer techniques; however, patients who have had them may still be encountered. Decisions about which procedure to use are based on the patient's ability to tolerate surgery, life expectancy, and ability to carry out the care required for the various options.

Urinary diversion may be temporary or permanent. Permanent urinary diversion is necessary when the bladder is congenitally absent or removed because of malignancy or trauma or when extensive pelvic malignancy obstructs urine flow. Temporary diversion may be used when obstruction to urine flow occurs, as might be caused by a urinary calculus, or to permit healing of the ureters or bladder.

Preparation of the patient for ostomy surgery is discussed at the beginning of this chapter. Postoperative care after each type of diversion is discussed separately.

ILEAL CONDUIT

The ileal conduit is the most common type of urinary diversion. Other names for the ileal conduit are *urostomy*, *ureteroileostomy*, *ureteroileocutaneous anastomosis*, *ileal loop*, and *Bricker procedure*.

Procedure

The **ileal conduit** is a urinary drainage system made out of a portion of small intestine. A 6- to 8-inch segment of ileum is first removed. The remaining ends of the ileum are then anastomosed (stitched) to restore bowel function. The ureters are cut from the bladder and attached to the ileal segment at an angle to prevent reflux. One end of the ileal segment is sutured closed. The other end of the ileal segment is brought through an abdominal incision and sutured to create a stoma for urine drainage. A similar procedure that uses a segment of large intestine is called a **colonic or sigmoid conduit.** The stoma of an ileal or colonic conduit is bright red because it is intestinal mucosa.

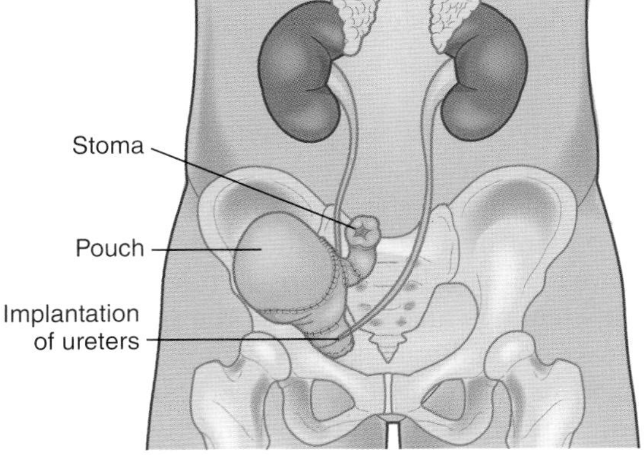

Fig. 18.8 Creation of a continent Kock urinary pouch with ureters implanted and stoma with nipple valve. (From Lewis SM, Bucher L, Heitkemper MM, Harding MM. *Medical-surgical nursing: assessment and management of clinical problems*, ed 10, St. Louis, 2017, Elsevier.)

Complications

During the postoperative period, the patient is at risk for a number of complications. Complications related to the surgical procedure include leakage of the anastomosed ureters and intestinal segments, ureteral obstruction, and separation of the stoma from surrounding skin.

Other problems include wound infection, necrosis of the stoma, and paralytic ileus. The stoma may become necrotic if the blood supply in the resected segment is inadequate. If the stoma turns gray or black, circulation is impaired; the physician should be notified at once.

Complications that may occur in the later postoperative period are infection, crystal formation, and calculi (stones). The patient may also have problems with the stoma, including retraction, prolapse, or hernia.

POSTOPERATIVE NURSING CARE OF THE PATIENT WITH AN ILEAL CONDUIT

Nursing care of the patient who has an ileal conduit is essentially the same as that for the patient with an ileostomy. Box 18.1 summarizes the nursing assessment data after ostomy surgery. A few special points should be made about the ileal conduit. This patient will have a nasogastric tube attached to suction to prevent abdominal distention and stress on the resected portion of the ileum while it heals. The patient is NPO and is given intravenous fluids until bowel sounds return. A temporary ileus (absence of bowel activity) is expected after bowel resection. Ureteral catheters or stents to drain urine may be seen in the new stoma postoperatively. If stents are present, output is monitored because obstruction can occur (Fig. 18.9). Mucus is normally present in drainage from an ileal conduit because it is produced by the lining of the bowel segment. The pouch should be emptied when it is one-third to one-half full. The pouch should be attached to a bedside drainage collection device during the night because the output may exceed the pouch capacity.

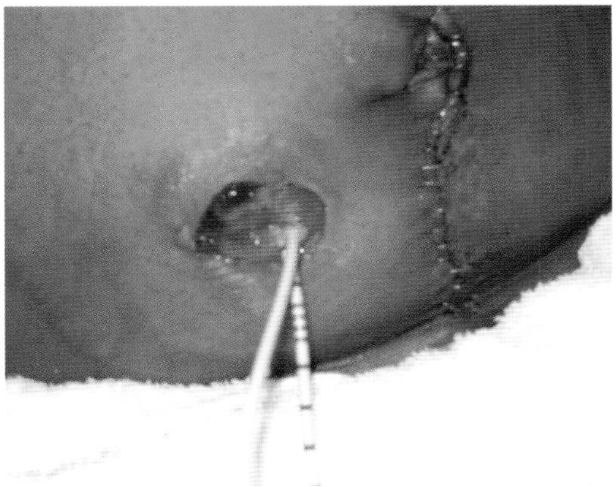

Fig. 18.9 Urostomy stoma with stents in place. (Courtesy Jane Fellows.)

Patient Problems, Goals, and Outcome Criteria: Ileal Conduit

In addition to the common problems and goals for postoperative patients (see Chapter 17), the following diagnoses may apply to the patient who has an ileal conduit/urostomy.

Patient Problems	Goals and Outcome Criteria
Potential for disrupted skin integrity related to contact of urine with skin	Normal skin around stoma: healed stoma base without redness or edema
Potential for infection related to contamination of stoma	Absence of infection: no fever or foul urine odor
Potential for injury related to obstruction of urine flow	Unobstructed urine flow: urine output approximately equal to fluid intake
Altered body image related to presence of stoma, altered body function	Adjustment in body image: patient acknowledges stoma, shows increasing interest in self-care, resumes previous sexual activity.
Inability to perform ostomy care related to lack of knowledge to manage complex therapeutic regimen	Patient assumes self-care of ostomy: patient demonstrates proper techniques of ostomy care and describes self-care with an ostomy.

Interventions

Potential for disrupted skin integrity. After an ileal conduit, the patient's urostomy pouch is usually attached to a bedside collection device to prevent pouch overfilling and leakage. Once the patient is ambulatory, the bedside collection device is only used during the night. A variety of pouches are available (Fig. 18.10). Some have antireflux valves to prevent the flow of urine back into the stoma. A skin barrier product can be used around the stoma for protection. Karaya products are used for intestinal ostomies but not for urinary drainage because urine breaks down the product. Belts can be worn with some appliances to hold them in place. Some pouches can be connected to a leg bag for urine collection.

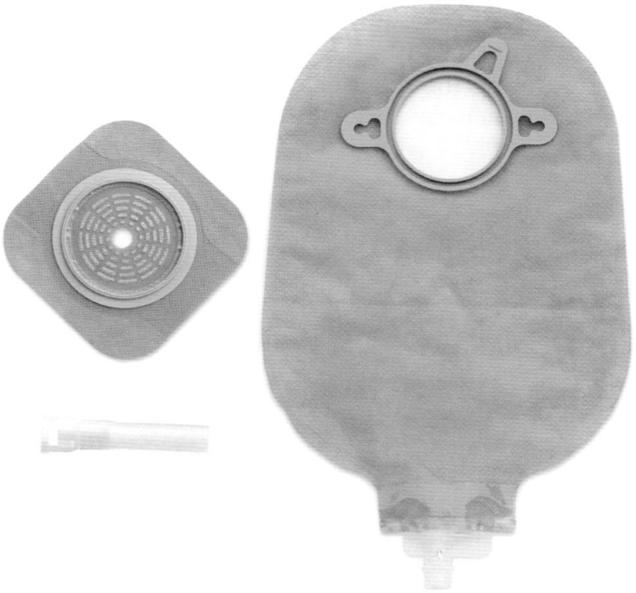

Fig. 18.10 Urostomy pouching system with adapter to connect pouch to bedside drainage bag. (Courtesy Hollister Inc., Libertyville, IL.)

The pouch is changed every 3 to 4 days or when it leaks, because frequent changes are irritating to the surrounding skin. When it is changed, gently remove any adhesive, and take care not to dislodge stents, which are usually sutured to the peristomal skin. A gauze pad, tampon, or tissue may be placed at the opening of the stoma to absorb urine. Pouch changes are usually done in the morning when urine production is lowest, but if the patient is still receiving continuous intravenous fluids, output will be increased. Steps in the application of a urinary pouch are illustrated in Fig. 18.11. Wash the peristomal area with water and pat dry. If soap is used, it should be nonoily and rinsed off thoroughly. If crystals are present, a gauze pad saturated in a dilute vinegar solution can be used to dissolve them. Urinary stoma problems are summarized in Table 18.2.

Potential for infection. The stoma serves as a portal for pathogens to enter the urinary tract, causing infection. Urinary tract infections can have serious consequences, including kidney damage and septicemia. Pouch care is treated as a clean, rather than sterile, procedure because the stoma is not sterile. However, you must still take care to avoid introducing organisms to the area.

Yeast infections that sometimes develop around the stoma are characterized by a skin rash surrounding the stoma. These are usually treated with antifungal powder applied to the peristomal skin and sealed with a skin barrier spray/wipe, then covered with the wafer.

Potential for injury. If urine does not flow readily, an obstruction is possible. Minimal urine output postoperatively should be approximately 800 mL in 24 hours. If output decreases significantly, notify the RN or surgeon immediately.

Altered body image. Adjustment to a stoma can be very difficult. The patient may be afraid of leakage and odor and may feel disfigured. Demonstrate acceptance of the patient and care for the stoma in a matter-of-fact manner. In addition, express understanding of the patient's feelings and encourage the patient to groom and dress normally. If odor is a problem, odor-proof pouches are recommended, but excessive odor can be an indicator of colonization or infection. Some foods can also cause increased odor, for example, fish and asparagus. Learning to care for the urostomy boosts the patient's self-confidence and may help to restore a more positive body image.

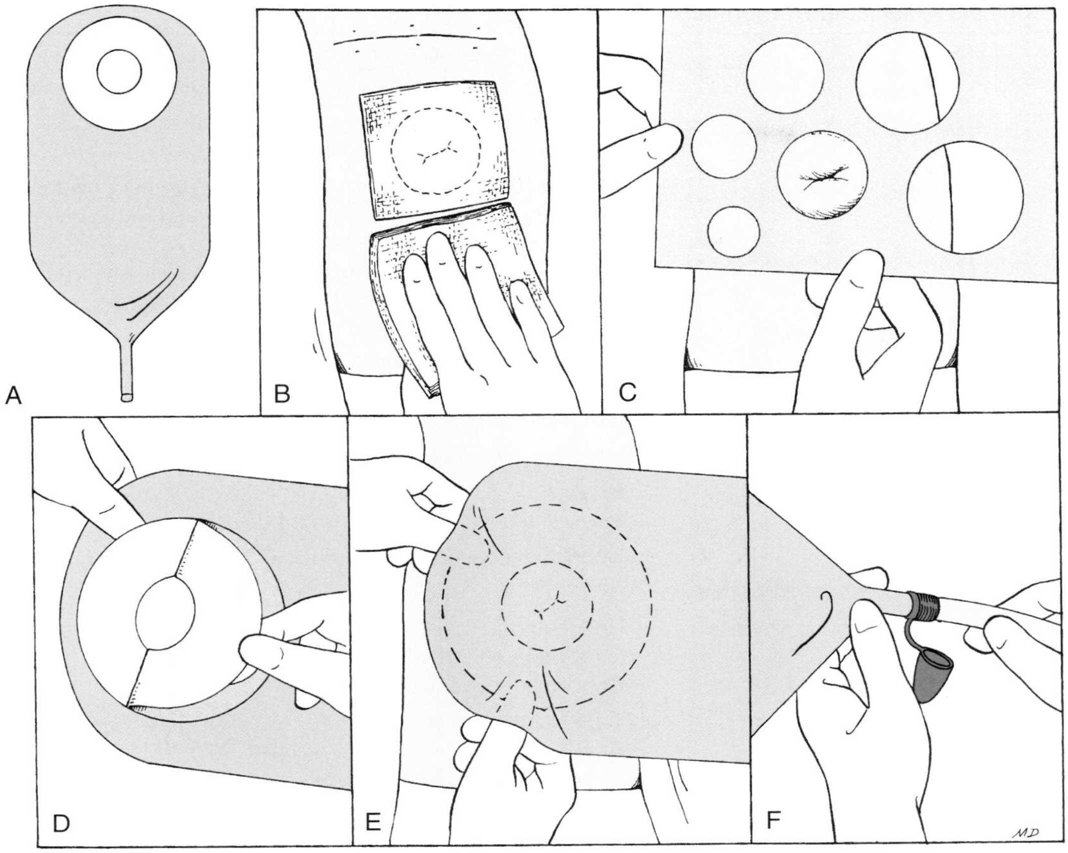

Fig. 18.11 Procedure for applying pouch. (A) Gather supplies: pouch, ostomy belt, skin barrier, stoma template, gauze pads, pouch clamp or rubber band, safety pin, and clean gloves. Wash hands and put on gloves. (B) After removing the old pouch and cleaning the area around the stoma, place a gauze square over the stoma to absorb the drainage. (C) Use a stoma template to measure the size of the stoma and then cut an opening the same size as the stoma into the skin barrier and adhesive. (D) Remove the backing from the adhesive of the new pouch. (E) Place the opening in the new pouch over the stoma and gently press into place with the pouch drain pointed toward the floor. (F) Connect the drain to the tubing or close the drain if appropriate. Secure the tubing to sheets or according to agency policy. (From Black JM, Hawks JH: *Medical-surgical nursing: clinical management for positive outcomes*, ed 8, St. Louis, 2009, Saunders-Elsevier.)

Table 18.2 Problems Associated With Urinary Stomas

PROBLEM	CAUSE	ASSESSMENT AND INTERVENTION
Stomal laceration	Pouch opening too small	Enlarge pouch opening.
	Pouch not positioned correctly	Reposition pouch. Monitor healing.
Peristomal laceration	Improperly fitting pouch	Evaluate the pouch fit with the patient in sitting, lying, and standing positions. Check the fit of the belt.
	Improper pouch removal technique	Consider the need for adhesive removers and/or specialized pouching systems.
Bleeding	Trauma	Apply a cool cloth. Cleanse gently.
Crystal formation	Urinary tract infection, stasis	Treat the infection and acidify the urine. Apply a vinegar compress to the stoma during dressing change. Use equal parts water and white vinegar. Put 1–2 oz of vinegar solution in the pouch for 20 minutes twice a day, then rinse. Use a vinyl or plastic pouch rather than a rubber one.
Stenosis	Scar formation	Dilation performed by or under direction of physician.

Continued

Table 18.2 Problems Associated With Urinary Stomas—cont'd

PROBLEM	CAUSE	ASSESSMENT AND INTERVENTION
Skin irritation	Skin barrier or wafer too small	Adjust the size of the skin barrier or wafer to cover skin around the stoma.
	Leaking appliance	Check the belt. If it is too tight, the seal can break. Replace the appliance as needed (PRN).
	Hair follicle inflammation	Use topical antimicrobial powder and skin barrier powder. Cover any lesions with nonstick dressing and with a barrier before applying the pouching system. Use adhesive remover; remove sealants gently. After the skin returns to normal, shave or cut any hair around the stoma.
	Perspiration under pouch	Dry the skin well. Apply a protective barrier. Apply powder to skin under pouch. Use a soft pouch cover.
	Allergy to pouching products	Spot test other brands to find one that does not cause irritation.
	Candida ("yeast") infection	Dry well. Apply antifungal powder as ordered.
Hernia/ prolapse	Muscle weakness Increased intraabdominal pressure	Condition requires surgical repair.
Wartlike lesions	Excessive peristomal wetness	Reduce pouch opening size or acquire custom-cut system to reduce moisture on the skin. Condition may require debridement by a physician.
Odor	Urinary tract infection	Treat infection.
	Appliance soiled or leaking	Check the seal; change the appliance. Provide deodorant tablets PRN.

Patients with ostomies commonly experience grief in response to the loss of normal function and perceived disfigurement. This may be exhibited as denial, shock, anger, bargaining, or depression. Chapter 19 offers guidance for dealing with the patient who is grieving.

The change in body image may affect the patient's sexuality. Provide opportunities for patients with an ostomy to ask questions or discuss how the ostomy might affect sexual function or behavior. Patients may feel unattractive or fear rejection by their partners. People who have had radical perineal surgeries may have physical barriers to sexual performance; other patients have problems because of psychologic factors.

The same practical suggestions identified for the patient with an intestinal ostomy may be useful to the patient with a urinary ostomy. The pouch should be emptied before sexual intercourse. Pouch covers are available to conceal the appliance and its contents. The partner wearing the pouch should experiment with positions that are most comfortable. Female patients should know that ostomy surgery does not interfere with pregnancy or delivery.

Inability to perform self-care (stoma). Many aspects of teaching the patient with a urostomy are the same as those identified for the patient with an ileostomy. The topics to include in the teaching plan are ostomy care, pouches, diet, fluids, activity, sexuality, complications, and resources. See the teaching plan in the section on Ileostomy.

From the early postoperative period, try to help the patient learn independent ostomy care. At first, patient teaching may take place each time stoma care is done by simply telling the patient what is being done and why. Encourage the patient to participate and gradually assume more responsibility for the care. Practice builds confidence and provides the patient with the opportunity to identify problems while help is available.

Some people adapt more readily to the stoma than others. You must be sensitive to the patient's feelings and encourage the patient in a kind way. A volunteer from the American Cancer Society or the UOAA can be especially helpful as a role model for the patient with a new ostomy. With the patient's and the physician's approval, the agency can be contacted about sending a volunteer to visit the patient.

The nurse, WOC nurse, or both must help the patient to plan for discharge. Provide written care instructions. The patient needs a list of supplies and places where they can be purchased. In addition, send some temporary supplies home with the patient. Finally, give the patient information (and referrals as needed) regarding resources such as home health care and community organizations.

In general, normal activities can be resumed within 3 months, but specific directions should be obtained from the physician or WOC nurse. Because the pouch and seal are waterproof, the patient can bathe or shower with the appliance in place. Regular clothing can be worn but should not apply pressure to the stoma. Pouches can be attached to a collection device at night to permit continuous drainage.

Patients with an ostomy who enjoy traveling are encouraged to continue to do so. When traveling, patients are advised to take adequate supplies, including sealable plastic bags to dispose of used materials. If the patient is flying, their supplies should be kept in a hand-carried bag to avoid problems if luggage is lost or delayed. On a long flight, a leg bag attached to the pouch may be beneficial in case the patient must remain seated because of turbulence.

CONTINENT INTERNAL RESERVOIRS

All of the methods of urinary diversion already discussed permit urine to flow steadily through a stoma. Newer procedures allow for the storage and controlled drainage of urine. Examples of these, called *continent internal reservoirs*, are the Kock, Mainz, Indiana, and Florida pouches (see Fig. 18.8). The orthotopic neobladder eliminates the need for a stoma. The neobladder is an internal urinary reservoir constructed using a resected segment of the ileum that is attached to the urethra and the ureters. Urine drains into the reservoir and is eliminated through the urethra instead of a stoma. The neobladder is used more often in men than in women. Continence varies with the neobladder, so an artificial urinary sphincter is sometimes implanted. Another option for patients who cannot achieve continence with the neobladder is intermittent self-catheterization. Even though the procedure is well received by patients, some surgeons are reluctant to spare the urethra with bladder cancer, fearing the urethra could be a site for recurrent cancer.

The Kock pouch is constructed with a segment of ileum. The ureters are implanted in one side of the ileum segment. A nipple valve is constructed from the other side and attached to the skin, where a stoma is created. The valve prevents urine from flowing from the reservoir (see Fig. 18.8). A catheter is used to drain the reservoir at 4- to 6-hour intervals. Other types of pouches are constructed from different parts of the bowel. The Indiana pouch is constructed of a tapered ileal segment and plicated (pleated) ileocecal valve. This reservoir is larger than that of the Kock pouch. The Indiana pouch is also drained with a catheter every 4 to 6 hours. The Indiana pouch and similar structures have largely replaced the Kock pouch because the Kock pouch requires a more complex surgical procedure and has more complications that require additional surgery.

Complications

Complications of the continent pouches are incontinence, difficult catheterization, and urinary reflux leading to pyelonephritis, obstruction, and bacteriuria.

POSTOPERATIVE NURSING CARE OF THE PATIENT WITH A CONTINENT URINARY DIVERSION

Box 18.1 summarized the general postoperative assessment of the patient having ostomy surgery. Some additional data unique to the continent pouches are added here. Immediately after surgery, the patient may have a drain to remove fluid from the operative site and a clear tube in place for continuous urine drainage. Irrigations may be ordered to remove clots and mucus. When the tube is removed, the pouch may be drained every 2 to 3 hours at first. Later, the patient may need to drain the pouch only every 4 to 6 hours during the day and once during the night. If the pouch functions properly, the patient does not have to wear an external appliance. A small gauze dressing may be placed over the stoma to absorb mucus drainage. Advise the patient to wear a medical alert bracelet that identifies the presence of a continent device that needs intubation to drain.

CUTANEOUS URETEROSTOMY

A cutaneous **ureterostomy** is created when one or both ureters are brought out through an opening in the abdomen or flank. Often the two ureters are joined surgically so that only one stoma is needed. In some situations, a stoma is created from each ureter.

A ureterostomy stoma is much smaller than an intestinal stoma. Immediately after surgery the urinary stoma is pink, but it quickly fades to a lighter color. Because no reservoir exists to hold it, urine drains from the stoma continuously. A pouch is needed to collect the urine and protect the skin.

Complications

Complications experienced by patients with a cutaneous ureterostomy include stenosis and urinary tract infections. Stenosis is a narrowing of the opening that interferes with the flow of urine. If the obstruction is not relieved, urine backs up in the kidney. The kidney may become swollen with urine, a condition called *hydronephrosis*, which leads to serious kidney damage. The kidneys can also be damaged by urinary tract infections.

POSTOPERATIVE NURSING CARE OF THE PATIENT WITH A CUTANEOUS URETEROSTOMY

Nursing assessment and care of the patient with a ureterostomy is essentially the same as for the patient with an ileostomy and urostomy. (See Box 18.1 for a summary of general assessment data.) A few special points should be made about the ureterostomy.

In the postoperative period, the review of systems should include questions about the presence of flank or abdominal pain, fatigue, malaise, and chills.

The ureterostomy stoma is usually much smaller than an intestinal stoma and lighter in color. Document the amount, appearance, and odor of the urine. Some blood in the urine is normal at first but it should clear gradually. Ureterostomy drainage should not contain mucus.

URETEROSIGMOIDOSTOMY AND URETEROILEOSIGMOIDOSTOMY

Ureterosigmoidostomy and ureteroileosigmoidostomy are not done as often now as in the past. However, you may care for patients who have had these diversions for some time and have adapted well to them. In a ureterosigmoidostomy, the ureters are implanted into the sigmoid colon. Urine drains into the colon and is eliminated through the rectum. In a ureteroileosigmoidostomy, a segment of the ileum is anastomosed to the sigmoid and the ureters are implanted into that part of the ileum. Neither procedure provides continence and both procedures present problems with kidney infections and urinary calculi (stones). Additional complications are caused by the colon's absorption of electrolytes from the urine. Patients are at risk for deficits in potassium and bicarbonate and for excesses in sodium, chloride, and hydrogen. These imbalances may lead to metabolic acidosis.

VESICOSTOMY

A **vesicostomy** is an opening into the urinary bladder. Several types exist. Some are drained continuously through what is commonly called a suprapubic catheter; others have a surgically constructed nipple valve and are catheterized at intervals.

NEPHROSTOMY

A **nephrostomy** tube diverts urine directly from the kidney through a tube that exits through the skin. This device may be used as a temporary or permanent method of urinary diversion. Conditions that may be treated with these tubes are discussed in Chapter 42.

Get Ready for the NCLEX® Examination!

Key Points

- An ostomy is an artificial opening into a body cavity; a stoma is the site of the opening on the skin.
- Ostomy surgery may be done to bypass a section of the digestive or urinary tract, either temporarily or permanently.
- Nurses who have specialized training in ostomy management are an important resource for staff nurses and ostomy patients. They include the certified ostomy care nurse (COCN), the certified wound ostomy nurse (CWON), and the certified wound, ostomy, continence nurse (CWOCN).
- Before ostomy surgery, it is important to determine the patient's expectations, understanding of the procedure, information desired, and fears.
- Intestinal ostomies include the ileostomy, the continent ileostomy, the ileal pouch anal anastomosis (IPAA), and the colostomy.
- The characteristics of fecal material depend on the location of the ostomy; liquid stool drains from the ileum and softly formed stool drains from the descending colon.
- The new intestinal stoma should be beefy red, and a small amount of bleeding around the base is not unusual.
- Postoperative nursing care after intestinal ostomy surgery addresses potential for fluid volume deficit, potential for inadequate tissue perfusion to stoma, disrupted skin integrity, altered body image, potential for sexual dysfunction, and inability to perform (ostomy) self-care.
- Protective barriers are applied around the stoma to fill creases and create a seal, and a pouch to collect fecal drainage is secured over the stoma with adhesive.
- Elimination of gas-forming foods, secure pouch seal, and good hygiene can help to control odor associated with an intestinal ostomy.
- The continent pouch ileostomy and the IPAA both store fecal matter, but the continent ileostomy is drained periodically with a catheter, whereas the ileoanal reservoir allows fecal elimination through the rectum.
- Routine colostomy irrigations are no longer recommended.
- The most common types of urinary diversion are ileal conduit, continent internal reservoirs, and orthotopic neobladder; other urinary diversions are cutaneous ureterostomy and colonic conduit.
- A ureterostomy stoma is pink immediately after surgery but quickly fades to a light color.
- Ureterostomies and ileal conduits drain urine continuously, so collection pouches are needed and meticulous skin care must be provided.
- A continent internal reservoir allows for storage and controlled drainage of urine through a specially constructed stoma with a one-way valve, while an orthotopic neobladder allows for storage and controlled drainage of urine through the urethra.
- Complications of urinary stomas include urinary infections, obstruction of urine flow, and skin breakdown.

Additional Learning Resources

SG Go to your Study Guide for additional learning activities to help you master this chapter content.

Go to your Evolve website (http://evolve.elsevier.com/Linton/medsurg) for the following learning resources and much more:
- Fluid & Electrolyte Tutorial
- Review Questions for the NCLEX® Examination

Clinical Judgment and Next-Generation NCLEX® Examination-Style Questions

1. **Which of the following is/are created surgically to drain fecal matter from the intestines? (Select all that apply.)**
   1. Colostomy
   2. Ileostomy
   3. Ileal conduit
   4. Vesicostomy
   5. Ureterosigmoidostomy

   NCLEX Client Need: Physiological Integrity: Physiological Adaptation

2. **Which of the intestinal stoma sites will produce the most formed stool?**
   1. Jejunostomy
   2. Duodenostomy
   3. Ileostomy
   4. Colostomy

   NCLEX Client Need: Physiological Integrity: Physiological Adaptation

3. **What color should a new intestinal stoma be on the first postoperative day?**

   NCLEX Client Need: Physiological Integrity: Physiological Adaptation

4. **The nursing team is reviewing the care plan for a patient having ileostomy surgery that day. One of the postoperative patient problems is risk for deficient fluid volume. What does the licensed vocational nurse/licensed practical nurse (LVN/LPN) know is the reason for this risk?**
   1. A significant loss of blood occurs during the surgical procedure.
   2. Patients with ileostomies often have anorexia, nausea, and vomiting.
   3. Fluid normally reabsorbed in the colon is lost through the ileostomy.
   4. Fluid intake will be restricted until the stoma heals completely.

   NCLEX Client Need: Physiological Integrity: Physiological Adaptation

5. **The LVN/LPN is reviewing stoma care with a patient before discharge. What teaching point should the nurse reinforce?**
   1. Remove the drainage appliance daily to cleanse skin around the stoma.
   2. Wash the stoma and surrounding skin with a moisturizing soap.
   3. Vigorously rub the skin surrounding the stoma to stimulate circulation and healing.
   4. Cut the opening on the wafer no more than ⅛ inch larger than the stoma.

   NCLEX Client Need: Physiological Integrity: Physiological Adaptation

6. **When teaching a new colostomy patient how to control odor, the nurse provides a list of foods that commonly cause gas. The patient says, "You mean I can't eat any of these foods?" Which of the following is the most appropriate reply?**
   1. "Gradually try them one at a time to see how you tolerate them."
   2. "That is correct. You can never eat any of these foods again."
   3. "Because flatus production is unpredictable, you never know what will happen if you eat these foods."
   4. "It would be better if you took vitamins instead of eating fresh fruits and vegetables."

   NCLEX Client Need: Physiological Integrity: Physiological Adaptation

7. **Mr. Y. had ostomy surgery 3 days ago. Which of the following is most likely to help Mr. Y. adjust to his stoma and learn how to perform self-care?**
   1. Shield the stoma from Mr. Y's sight until he asks to see it.
   2. Tell Mr. Y., "If you don't do your stoma care, then no one will do it for you."
   3. Encourage Mr. Y. to participate in care once he begins looking at the stoma.
   4. Teach a family member how to do the care.

   NCLEX Client Need: Psychosocial Integrity: Coping Mechanisms; Unexpected Body Image Changes

8. **A patient with a new continent ileostomy has abdominal distention and hypoactive bowel sounds. These observations suggest which complication?**

   NCLEX Client Need: Physiological Integrity: Reduction of Risk Potential

9. **The nurse on a urology unit has patients with each of the following types of urinary diversion. The nurse should anticipate needing to change pouches on three of the patients. The patient with which type of urinary diversion will not need to wear a pouch?**
   1. Cutaneous ureterostomy
   2. Ileal conduit
   3. Indiana pouch
   4. Ureteroileostomy

   NCLEX Client Need: Physiological Integrity: Basic Care and Comfort

10. **The surgeon has explained the advantages and disadvantages of various types of procedures that might be done for a patient who has bladder cancer. Which of the following is the main advantage of the ileum neobladder?**
    1. The patient does not have a stoma for urine drainage.
    2. Urinary continence is always maintained.
    3. Urine is eliminated through the rectum.
    4. The neobladder has to be drained only once a day.

    NCLEX Client Need: Physiological Integrity: Physiological Adaptation

Unfolding Case Test Items: Ostomy Surgery

Phase I

SLO Objective: Assist in developing a nursing plan of care for the patient with an ileostomy

NGN Item Type: Enhanced hot spot test item type

Cognitive Skill: Recognize cues

Question 1

Patient situation: A 50-year-old man required a colectomy (removal of the colon) and creation of an ileostomy. On the first postoperative day he is NPO, receiving intravenous fluids, and has a nasogastric tube in place and set on low intermittent suction. He received an intravenous analgesic 2 hours ago for abdominal pain rated 7 on a scale of 1 to 10. Assessment data include the following:

- Withdrawn and tearful
- BP = 110/64 mm Hg
- Pulse = 88 beats per minute, regular
- Respirations = 18 breaths per minute

- Temperature = 97.4°F
- Stoma beefy red and swollen
- Ileostomy pouch contains greenish-brown liquid stool
- Small amount of blood at base of stoma
- Foley catheter in place; urine is light yellow, clear
- Bowel sounds not audible
- 24 hour intake = 1800 mL; output = 2500 mL
- Looks away when nurse examines stoma and pouch

Highlight or place a check mark next to the assessment findings that require follow up by the nurse.

NCLEX Client Need: Physiological Integrity: Physiological Adaptation; Psychosocial Integrity: Coping Mechanisms

Question 2

SLO Objective: Assist in developing a nursing plan of care for the patient with an ileostomy.

NGN Item Type: Cloze

Cognitive Skill: Analyze Cues

Patient situation: A 50-year-old man required a colectomy (removal of the colon) and creation of an ileostomy. On the first postoperative day he is NPO, receiving intravenous fluids, and has a nasogastric tube in place and set on low intermittent suction. He received an intravenous analgesic 2 hours ago for abdominal pain rated 7 on a scale of 1 to 10. Assessment data include the following:

- Withdrawn and tearful
- BP = 110/64 mm Hg
- Pulse = 88 beats per minute, regular
- Respirations = 18 per minute
- Temperature = 97.4°F
- Stoma beefy red and swollen
- Ileostomy pouch contains greenish-brown liquid stool
- Small amount of blood at base of stoma
- Foley catheter in place; urine is light yellow, clear
- Bowel sounds not audible
- 24 hour intake = 1800 mL; output = 2500 mL
- Looks away when nurse examines stoma and pouch

Choose the most likely options for the information missing from the statements below by selecting from the lists of options provided.

"Fill in the blanks" statements: Based on the patient's assessment data, the nurse recognizes that the absence of bowel sounds is most likely because of (1)_________. Nursing actions related to this finding should include (2)_________, (2) _________, and (2)_________. Indications that the patient is having trouble accepting the ileostomy include (3)_________and (3)_________.

OPTIONS FOR 1	OPTIONS FOR 2	OPTIONS FOR 3
Damage to the nerves that serve the bowel	Inform the registered nurse or surgeon	Looking away during stoma care
Lack of oral intake for 2 days	Prepare the patient for a return to surgery	Increased heart rate
Manipulation of the bowel during surgery	Tell patient to report when he passes flatus	Withdrawn and tearful behavior
Removal of the large intestine	Document absence of bowel sounds	Request for pain medications
Inactivity	Auscultate abdomen with each assessment	Reluctance to get out of bed

NCLEX Client Need: Physiological Integrity: Physiological Adaptation; Psychosocial Integrity: Coping mechanisms

Phase II

Question 3

SLO Objective: Assist in developing a nursing care plan for the patient with an ileostomy

NGN Item Type: Extended multiple response

Cognitive Skill: Prioritize hypotheses

A 50-year-old required a colectomy (removal of the colon) and creation of an ileostomy. On the second postoperative day he is NPO, receiving intravenous fluids, and has a nasogastric tube in place and set on low intermittent suction. He has received an analgesic for abdominal pain every 6 hours. Two hours after his last analgesic, he says his pain level is 2 on a 1–10 pain scale. He resists position changes, spirometry, getting out of bed, and walking.

When planning care for this patient, which **priority** potential complications would the nurse monitor? (Select all that apply.)

a. Pneumonia
b. Inadequate coping, or altered body image, or threat to self-concept
c. Heart failure
d. Deep vein thrombosis
e. Fluid and electrolyte imbalances
f. Impaired circulation to stoma

NCLEX Client Need: Physiological Integrity: Physiological Adaptation

Question 4

SLO Objective: Discuss content to be included in teaching patients to learn to live with ostomies

NGN Item Type: Extended drag and drop test item

Cognitive Skill: Generate solutions

A 50-year-old man required a colectomy (removal of the colon) and creation of an ileostomy. On the fourth postoperative day he is passing flatus. The nasogastric tube was removed and oral fluids provided. With encouragement by the nurse, he is getting out of bed and walking more often. He has been visited by the WOC nurse and is showing more interest in his stoma care.

Indicate which nursing response listed in the far left column is appropriate for each client question. Note that not all responses will be used.

NURSE'S RESPONSES	PATIENT QUESTIONS	APPROPRIATE NURSE'S RESPONSE FOR EACH PATIENT QUESTION
"You will need to experiment with foods you like to see what agrees with you and what causes discomfort."	"Do you think I can learn to do this (stoma care) by myself?"	
"Some patients have problems with sexual functions; the WOC nurse can talk to you about management."	"How can I bathe with the stoma?"	
"Usually there are no restrictions after three months; ask your surgeon about sports activities."	"Will I have to change my diet?"	
"You can bathe or shower with the pouch in place."	"Will this surgery affect my sex life?"	
"Notify your physician if there is no stoma output ."		
"You will gain confidence with practice; I can recommend some resources if you need help when you go home."	"When can I resume my usual activities?"	
"Drink at least 2000 mL of fluid each day."		

Phase III

Question 5: Take action using matrix test item

SLO Objective: Discuss content to be included in teaching patients to learn to live with ostomies.

NGN Item Type: Matrix

Cognitive Skill: Generate solutions

A 50-year-old man required a colectomy (removal of the colon) and creation of an ileostomy. The nurse is teaching self-care to prepare him for discharge.

Use an X for the health teaching below that is *Indicated* (appropriate or necessary), *Contraindicated* (could be harmful), or *Nonessential* (makes no difference or not necessary) before the patient's discharge at this time.

HEALTH TEACHING	INDICATED	CONTRAIN-DICATED	NONES-SENTIAL
"After six weeks, you can resume heavy lifting and strenuous activity."			
"Notify your physician if the stoma stops draining."			
"You can wear regular clothing, but do not apply pressure over the stoma."			
"You can get pouch covers if you wish."			
"If you are traveling, always pack extra supplies and keep them with you."			

19 Palliative and Hospice Care

http://evolve.elsevier.com/Linton/medsurg

Objectives

1. Describe palliative care services for people with conditions that are life-limiting or chronic conditions that decrease quality of life.
2. Describe hospice care for a person with a limited life expectancy.
3. List the Medicare criteria for admission to hospice.
4. Describe the common fears that people experience when facing death.
5. Describe the role of the licensed vocational nurse/licensed practical nurse (LVN/LPN) in palliative care, hospice care, and end-of-life care.
6. Identify focused assessment data to be collected when providing end-of-life care.
7. Identify interventions to promote comfort for the patient and family at end-of-life.
8. Discuss legal and ethical issues related to terminal illness and end-of-life.
9. Discuss strategies to address stress experienced by family and professional caregivers providing end-of-life care.

Key Terms

bereavement
brain death
grief
hospice care
loss
mourning
palliative care

In 1965, 74-year-old Lillian had emergency surgery for severe abdominal pain. The surgeons found metastatic colon cancer and removed as much of the tumor as possible. No curative treatment was recommended. Her adult children were devastated by the findings and were adamant that Lillian not be told she had cancer. They insisted Lillian be told that she had had her gallbladder removed and implied that she would soon recover. Lillian did not question this information despite worsening symptoms over the next few months. Eventually, she confided in a friend that she had received insurance papers that listed a diagnosis of cancer, something she had suspected all along. Nevertheless, she maintained the pretense that her family wanted until she died.

Perhaps you are amazed that this actually happened. In fact, it was not unusual until the 1960s when the subjects of death and dying came out into the open. This change was partly stimulated by the publication of Elizabeth Kübler-Ross's book *On Death and Dying*. An important concept in this work was that humans facing death go through stages that ideally end in a state of acceptance and peace. This study of the human response to death and dying opened the doors for more discussion among health professionals, scientists, theologians, and the general public alike. Since those years, health care professionals have advanced their understanding of the death and dying experience and how best to care for individuals going through this final stage of life. Communication between health care providers, patients, and families has become more transparent, opening the door for patients to share their wishes, fears, and hopes. Individuals are encouraged to complete documents such as "living wills" that convey their wishes to their family and care providers.

Today it is unlikely that Lillian's diagnosis would be withheld from her. Instead of a conspiracy of silence, Lillian and her family could be supported by health care providers so that they could share their grief and support each other.

This chapter addresses responses of patients who are facing life-limiting conditions and their significant others. The grief process is reviewed, followed by a description of the physical and psychosocial changes that occur at end-of-life. Nursing care throughout this phase of life is explained with emphasis on palliative and hospice care. In addition, legal and ethical considerations related to the end-of-life are presented.

LOSS AND GRIEF

Loss may be defined as a real or potential absence of someone or something that is valued. Real losses occur when something actually happens so that valued people or possessions are no longer available. Potential losses relate to an individual's perceptions of what *might* occur if a valued person or object were lost permanently. For example, families of soldiers who are deployed to combat zones must face the potential loss of the soldier. Death may be thought of as the ultimate loss. Whatever the loss, people experience similar feelings and thoughts when it happens. Anxiety, fear, and grief are common with both real and potential losses. The intensity of feelings varies with the importance of the specific loss to each person. Changes in self-image, developmental changes, loss of possessions, and loss of significant others are common types of loss.

Grief is the normal personal response to a loss. It is an emotional reaction that serves to maintain emotional and physical well-being. The grieving process is a complex and intense experience that affects a person's thoughts, feelings, and behaviors. The grief process is usually most profound when the loss experienced is death. **Mourning** is the outward part of coping with grief. It represents a period of grieving marked by social customs. Most societies have expectations for appropriate behavior during the period of mourning. The concept of **bereavement** is broader in that it includes the total grief and mourning experience.

Working through the grief process helps the dying person and significant others to adapt to the loss. Grief that assists the person in accepting the reality of death may be called *uncomplicated grief.* Various terms are used to describe grief that does not progress in the "normal" fashion. Grief that is prolonged, unresolved, or disruptive to the person who experiences it may be termed *complicated grief.* Complicated grief may relate to a real loss or a perceived loss. It may occur when grief is not resolved from a prior experience or when the expression of grief is blocked in some way. Feelings and behaviors may become exaggerated and disruptive to a person's typical lifestyle. Specific behaviors are associated with complicated grief. Many times, distress at the loss is expressed. Unresolved issues may be identified and past experiences reviewed. Complicated grief is sometimes described as dysfunctional.

When a person's relationship to the person or lost object is not socially recognized, the survivor may experience *disenfranchised grief.* For example, when a same-sex partner dies, others may not be aware of or may not accept the relationship and fail to provide the same level of support offered to others.

Uncomplicated grief is a healthy response. When it begins before a death actually occurs or when the reality that death is inevitable is known, it is referred to as *anticipatory grief.* Anticipatory grief is usually related to an impending loss or death. Both the patient and the family members can experience anticipatory grieving.

Emotions such as anger, sadness, guilt, and denial may be present in all types of grief. Some people have difficulty expressing these feelings. The person experiencing grief may demonstrate changes in eating, sleeping, and other activities of daily living. Difficulty concentrating and making decisions may occur.

GRIEVING PROCESS

People who are facing the inevitability of death need caregivers who understand how personal attitudes affect the experience. The attitudes of the dying person, those of the significant others, and the nurse's own attitudes affect the death experience.

Understanding how culture, spirituality, family, and stage of development influence the dying person will help you to appreciate the person's needs, wants, and fears. Culture, religious beliefs, and age affect a person's understanding of and reaction to death or loss. Often, beliefs and attitudes are interrelated between culture and religion. The American work ethic is closely related to the Protestant ethic, which emphasizes independence, self-reliance, hard work, and rugged individualism. Death and dying tend to be private matters shared only with significant others. Often feelings are repressed or internalized. People who believe in "toughing it out" or "being strong" may not express themselves when they face a tragic loss.

Members of Black American and Latin cultures commonly express their feelings more openly than do White Americans. Kinship tends to be very strong within the Latino culture. Family members, both immediate and extended, provide support for one another. Expressing feelings of loss is encouraged and accepted.

Religious teachings usually include beliefs about death and life after death. These beliefs can have a powerful influence on the way a person reacts to loss and death. Most religious groups have common practices related to care of the dying person, care of the body after death, and final rites. Specific information about religious preferences should be obtained from the family.

Family members' past experiences and stages of development influence their responses to death and dying. Through experience with other losses, a generalized acceptance of dying can take place. Past experience with death of a loved one provides a frame of reference for some members of the family. Adaptive skills that have worked in the past may help individuals to cope with the loss of a loved one.

The age or stage of development also affects a person's reactions to death and dying. Children have a different understanding of loss and death than adults. Some adults believe that children should be protected from the pain associated with the death of a loved one. Often, however, children who are "protected" feel abandoned, frightened, and alone with their feelings. A child who loses a loved one through death may regress or be delayed in emotional development until the grief can be resolved.

Table 19.1 Age-Related Beliefs About Death

AGE RANGE	BELIEFS
Infancy to 5 years (preschool)	Child has little or no understanding of death. Child believes death is temporary and reversible, like sleep.
6–9 years (school age)	Child believes death is final. Child believes one's own death can be avoided. Child believes death is related to violence. Child believes that wishing or hoping for death can make it happen.
10–12 years (preadolescent)	Preadolescent believes death is an inevitable end to life. Preadolescent grasps their own mortality by discussing fear of death or life after death. Preadolescent expresses feelings of death based on adult attitudes.
13–18 years (adolescent)	Adolescent is afraid of prolonged death. Adolescent may act out defiance of death through dangerous or self-destructive acts. Adolescent has a philosophic or religious approach to death. Adolescent seldom thinks about death.
19–45 years (young adulthood)	Young adult's cultural and religious beliefs influence their attitudes about death. Young adult sees death as a future event.
45–65 years (middle adulthood)	Middle-aged adult accepts their own mortality as inevitable. Middle-aged adult faces the death of parents and peers. Middle-aged adult may experience death anxiety.
65 years and older (older adulthood)	Older adult is afraid of prolonged health problems. Older adult faces the death of family members and peers. Older adult sees death as inevitable. Older adult examines death as it relates to various meanings, such as freedom from discomfort.

Maturity contributes to understanding and accepting death. During adulthood, people must come to terms with the death of their parents and other older family members. Coping with the death of one's parents is often identified as a developmental crisis. During adulthood, people also have to confront their own mortality. The death of a spouse has a profound impact on older adults. Widowed persons reportedly have an increase in health problems during the first year after the death of the spouse. Loss of one's child at any age is an especially traumatic event. Table 19.1 identifies some common age-related attitudes associated with death.

STAGES OF GRIEVING

Various scholars have studied grief as a process that has stages. The best known among these scholars of grief is Dr. Elisabeth Kübler-Ross.

In 1969, Dr. Kübler-Ross shattered the taboo against talking about death and dying when she published a book that identified five stages of grieving that occur in response to impending death. The five stages are (1) denial, (2) anger, (3) bargaining, (4) depression, and (5) acceptance. The stages represent categories of responses to a diagnosis of a fatal illness. The term *stages* is not intended to imply sequence or mutually exclusive categories. Indeed, stages can overlap and multiple stages can exist at the same time. Kübler-Ross identified behaviors common to each stage. Not all people experience all stages and there is no predictable timetable on which the stages occur. This model is often applied to other individuals who experience significant losses, such as loss of a loved one, an amputation, loss of vision, or paralysis.

Denial

The person refuses to acknowledge the terminal diagnosis and may put forth a cheerful appearance to prolong the denial of the loss. Denial is a defense mechanism that helps the patient and others to manage anxiety evoked by the threat.

Anger

Patients express anger toward themselves or others. The anger may be directed at the health care providers, the institution, or even significant others.

Bargaining

In the bargaining stage, the person recognizes the terminal nature of their illness and seeks to "buy" more time. The individual may express feelings that the loss is a punishment for past actions and try to negotiate with a higher power to gain time. For example, the patient may pray to live through some important event, such as a child's wedding or a landmark birthday.

Depression

The depressed patient may experience many emotions, including sadness, regret, and fear. The patient needs to review their life. In this stage, the person has begun to accept the reality of impending death.

Acceptance

The individual may become somewhat emotionally detached and objective. The patient identifies the loss as inevitable and may want to make plans.

COMMON SIGNS AND SYMPTOMS OF GRIEF

Common signs and symptoms of grief are shared by the terminally ill person and those who lose a significant other. Knowledge of the signs and symptoms allows the nurse to better communicate with everyone involved.

Physical symptoms experienced during the grief process might include tightness in the chest, sensations of shortness of breath or suffocation, generalized weakness, intense tightening in the abdomen, and emptiness or churning in the stomach. These symptoms may fluctuate throughout the grief process. In general, they occur with the initial acknowledgment of death as the outcome. The patient and the family members may experience symptoms of a stress reaction (see the Cultural Considerations box). You should be aware that the stress reaction is a very real experience. Nursing intervention may be needed to assist a person in regaining a sense of physical function.

Cultural Considerations

What Does Culture Have to Do With Grief?

Culture strongly influences the way people handle grief. For example, traditional Vietnamese value stoicism, traditional Mexicans express grief openly, and traditional Swedes accept quiet or open grief. Traditional widows in Greece wear black for a long or indefinite period of time. Such characteristics and practices should not be assumed. Always collect data from individual patients.

AWARENESS OF TERMINAL ILLNESS

Awareness of terminal illness and impending death affects the dying person and the family both emotionally and physiologically. The classic work of Strauss and Glaser (1970) identified three states of awareness: (1) closed awareness, (2) mutual pretense, and (3) open awareness.

Closed Awareness

When closed awareness occurs, the family and the patient recognize that the patient is ill. They may not understand the severity of the illness and impending death.

Mutual Pretense

With mutual pretense, the patient, the loved ones, and the care providers know of the terminal prognosis. However, no one discusses the issue openly and they may make every effort to avoid the subject. Frequently the patient avoids the subject to protect the family and the caregivers from discomfort.

Open Awareness

With open awareness, the patient and others involved freely discuss the impending death. The discussions may be difficult, but they allow the patient and the family to become comfortable with the topic. Patients who wish to do so can participate in making final arrangements and wrapping up personal business. Even though health care providers should respect the individual's right to know, some people let it be known that they do not want some information. That wish should be respected. The law requires that patients identify who, if anyone, else can be informed about their condition. Nurses must be careful not to share information with anyone without the patient's permission.

PALLIATIVE CARE

The emergence of palliative care and hospice care represent major steps toward providing compassionate care for persons dealing with conditions that may be terminal.

When cure is not expected, patients may benefit from palliative care. The goal of **palliative care** is to improve quality of life for patients and their families by anticipating, preventing, and treating suffering. It may be sought by a person with a chronic condition such as heart failure, kidney disease, chronic obstructive pulmonary disease (COPD), dementia, or amyotrophic lateral sclerosis (ALS). Patients receiving palliative care can continue treatment for such conditions.

The primary issues that are addressed in palliative care include physical symptoms; emotional, coping, intellectual, social, and spiritual needs; and facilitation of patient autonomy, access to information, and choice. In addition, assistance with practical problems, such as wills and advance directives, is provided. Common physical symptoms that are addressed in palliative care include pain, dyspnea, fatigue, constipation, loss of appetite, and sleep disturbances. Emotional and coping support might be used to manage depression and anxiety.

Whereas some patients with chronic conditions live for many years with those conditions, other have a less optimistic outlook. For example, certain cancers are known to advance rapidly with little chance of survival. These patients may benefit from palliative care until they become candidates for hospice. Palliative care refocuses health care on allowing natural death in a pain- and symptom-controlled environment with psychosocial support. It can be provided in any setting. An interdisciplinary palliative care team works collaboratively to provide care and coordinate services for the patient and family. When aggressive treatment is no longer benefitting the patient, it may be discontinued and the patient transferred to hospice care.

HOSPICE CARE

Hospice care embraces palliative care with a focus on quality of life, comfort, and dignity near the end of life.

It also includes bereavement care for survivors after the death of the patient. The goal of hospice care as stated by the National Institutes of Health Clinical Center (2017) is "to work aggressively to manage symptoms of end of life and disease while maintain (sic) the person in the place they call 'home' or where they would like to spend the remainder of their life."

Hospice care most often is provided in the patient's home but is also available in free-standing centers, hospitals, nursing homes, and other long-term care facilities. Care employs a multidisciplinary team with a strong nursing component. Team members typically include the patient's personal physician, hospice physician or medical director, nurses, hospice aides, social workers, bereavement counselors, clergy or other spiritual counselors, and trained volunteers. If needed, speech, physical, and occupational therapists may be included as well.

When the patient remains at home, a family member is usually the primary caregiver. Hospice staff visit on a regular basis and are on call around the clock. Although visits are typically longer as the patient declines, 24-hour care is not provided. Respite care may be available for a short time if the patient's care becomes too difficult or if the caregiver needs a break. Hospice care is covered by Medicare, Medicaid, and most private insurance plans.

CRITERIA FOR ELIGIBILITY

Individuals are eligible for hospice care under Medicare when the patient's physician, along with a hospice physician, certifies that the patient has a life-limiting condition, and that their life expectancy is 6 months or less. This assumes that the patient's condition follows its usual course. Patients who live more than 6 months can be recertified. Sometimes the patient's condition improves unexpectedly and they can be discharged from hospice. A patient who agrees to hospice care agrees to palliative care (comfort care) instead of curative measures.

HOSPICE CARE SERVICES

According to the National Hospice and Palliative Care Organization (2020), the services that may be provided by the hospice care team includes:

- Management of pain and symptoms
- Assistance with emotional, psychosocial, and spiritual aspects of dying
- Needed drugs, medical supplies, and equipment
- Family instruction in the patient's care
- Special services like speech and physical therapy when needed
- Short-term inpatient care when symptoms are difficult to manage at home or caregiver needs respite
- Bereavement care and counseling to surviving family and friends

In addition, Medicare patients are eligible for aide and homemaker services. Short-term inpatient care can be covered if the purpose is to better manage symptoms. Volunteers are an essential component of the hospice service. In fact, Medicare requires that at least 5% of total patient care hours are contributed by volunteers. Volunteers can assist in three general areas: direct support, clinical support, and general support. Direct support entails spending time with patients and families. Clinical support includes clerical and other services that support patient care and clinical services. Examples of general support activities are fundraising, outreach and education, and service on boards.

HOSPICE USAGE IN THE UNITED STATES

Nearly 1.6 million Medicare beneficiaries received hospice services in 2018 (NHPCO, 2020). This figure represents a steady increase in patients since 2010. The average length of service in 2018 was 89.6 days. The great majority of hospice patients are 65 years of age or older and are White Americans. Cancer (the most common diagnosis), heart disease, dementia, and lung disease account for 75% of hospice patients. Half of the patients were in hospice for 14 or fewer days. Why might patients delay seeking hospice until so late in the course of their illness? Some are unaware of the option, others are concerned about costs, and still others believe that entering hospice care means that they have "given up" and will not receive needed care. This is unfortunate because earlier admission provides access to many services and sources of support that can make the last days of life easier.

> **Cultural Considerations**
>
> Medicare beneficiaries are predominately White Americans, however, in recent years, the number of Asian/Pacific Islander and Hispanic Americans has been rising.

LEGAL AND ETHICAL ISSUES RELATED TO TERMINAL ILLNESS AND DEATH

Patients and families struggle with many emotional decisions during the terminal illness and dying experience. These decisions often focus on physical and emotional comfort, such as whether to initiate artificial feeding. The decisions may involve the choice of advance directives, medical power of attorney, living wills, organ donations, and resuscitation. Advance directives are especially helpful because they specify the patient's wishes.

ORGAN DONATION

Organ donation may be made by any person who is legally competent. Any body part or the entire body may be donated. The decision to donate organs or to provide anatomic gifts may be made by a person before death. The decision to donate organs after death may be made by immediate family members.

Some people carry donor cards. Some states allow for organ donation to be marked on drivers' licenses. The names of agencies that handle organ donation vary by locale. Some common names for such an agency are *organ bank*, *organ-sharing network*, *tissue bank*, or *organ-sharing alliance.* Legal requirements and facility policy for organ donation must be followed. The physician should be notified immediately when organ donation is intended because some tissues must be used within hours after death.

CARDIOPULMONARY RESUSCITATION

Over the past 50 years, cardiopulmonary resuscitation (CPR) has become common practice in health care. CPR is initiated when patients suffer respiratory or cardiac arrest, unless a physician has given a do not resuscitate (DNR) order. A DNR order is usually written when a patient or their representative has made it clear that CPR should not be initiated. Several different types of CPR decisions can be made. Complete and total heroic measures, which may include CPR, medications, and mechanical ventilation, can be referred to as a *full code.* Some states offer DNR protocols that enable the patient to specify exactly which actions may be carried out during CPR.

The Patient Self-Determination Act was an important part of the Omnibus Budget Reconciliation Act (OBRA) of 1990. This Act requires all institutions that participate with Medicare to provide written information to patients concerning their right to accept or refuse treatment. The information must explain the patient's right to initiate advance directives. Advance directives are written statements of a person's wishes regarding medical care. The first advance directive document, developed in 1974, was called the *Living Will.*

Most states have replaced the idea of living wills with Natural Death Acts. Within many of these Acts are specific aspects related to the individual's wishes and durable powers of attorney for health care. Directives to physicians may be included. Under the Natural Death Acts, an individual can tell the physician exactly what is desired. Each state will have its own unique requirements and rules for the use of advance directives. Special forms for durable power of attorney, medical power of attorney, and directives for physicians, family members, or surrogates can be obtained from local medical associations and the internet. Specific details as to withholding or withdrawing treatments must be included. What is to be done and what is not to be done must be included in very clear terms.

A person may write a durable power of attorney or directive to physicians without special forms. Verbal directives with specific instructions may be given to physicians in the presence of two witnesses. Attorneys and notaries are not necessarily required.

In the event that the person is not capable of communicating their wishes, the family and the physician can agree on what measures will or will not be taken. The physician should document the family's decision.

Another option is the durable power of attorney for health care or medical power of attorney. This document allows individuals to select someone to make health care decisions for them if they are unable to do so for themselves. This power of attorney can be used only if the physician certifies in writing that the person is incapable of making decisions. Until the physician does this, the individual remains in control of their own decisions.

Put On Your Thinking Cap!

The durable power of attorney/medical power of attorney varies by state. Go to https://www.nhpco.org/advancedirective/ to read and download a copy for the state where you live.

In addition to advance directives, another initiative called *Five Wishes* has been put in place. Fig. 19.1 shows the first page of this document. The Aging with Dignity (www.agingwithdignity.org) organization developed *Five Wishes* to promote better care for individuals and families facing the end of life. This document focuses on a patient's needs and includes personal, medical, spiritual, and emotional needs. In most states and the District of Columbia, the *Five Wishes* document is legally recognized as an advance directive; the remaining states accept it as an attachment to another legal form.

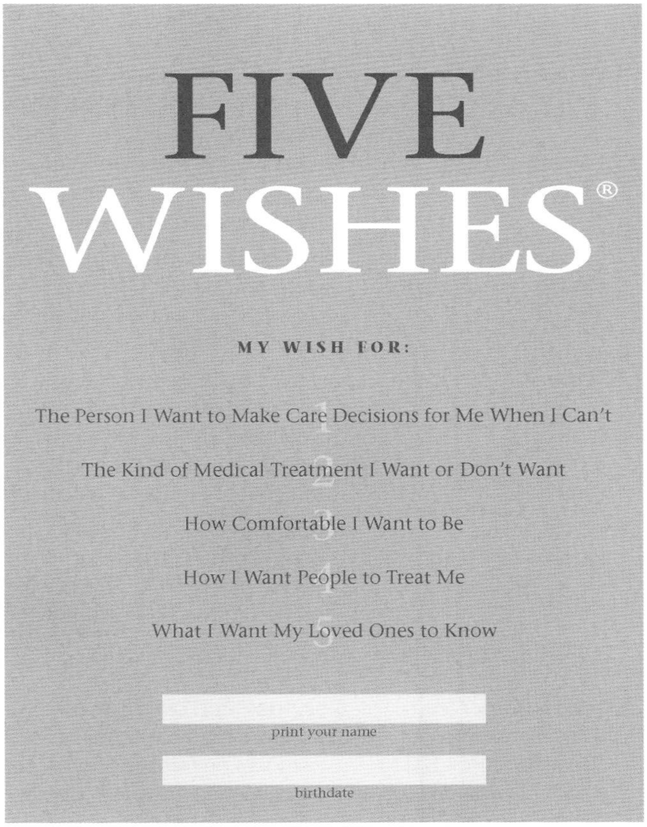

Fig. 19.1 The *Five Wishes* document (www.agingwithdignity.org) helps patients to communicate their wishes to their families and to members of the health care team. Written in language that is easily understood by those outside the medical and legal professions, the document helps people to discuss and make reasonable decisions about issues that are often difficult to face. This is the first page of the 12-page document that allows individuals to express their wishes on various issues. (Copyright Aging With Dignity, www.agingwithdignity.org.)

The *Five Wishes* document specifies how the family and the health care team are expected to treat the patient. It includes the following:

- The name of the person who will make decisions for health care if the patient cannot do it
- The type of medical care the patient wants or does not want
- The amount of comfort the patient wants
- How the patient wants to be treated
- What information the patient wants the loved ones to know

You must be aware of legal issues and the wishes of the patient. Advance directives and organ donor information should be located in the medical record and identified on the nursing care plan. All caregivers responsible for the patient need to know the patient's wishes.

Table 19.2 summarizes the documents commonly used in end-of-life care.

THE DYING PROCESS

Death occurs when all vital organs and systems cease to function. During the death process, systems and organs slow and lose their ability to maintain life. All systems are involved. Table 19.3 summarizes the clinical signs of impending death.

Table 19.2 Common Documents Used in End-of-Life Care

DOCUMENT	DESCRIPTION	SPECIAL CONSIDERATIONS
Advance Directive	General term used to describe documents that give instructions about future medical care and treatments and who should make the decisions in the event the person is unable to communicate	Should comply with guidelines established by state of residence
Allow Natural Death (AND)	Written order acknowledging that comfort measures only are being provided to patient. Used in many palliative care and hospice settings to indicate that patient wants to die naturally with dignity and comfort	In many settings may be used in conjunction with DNR terminology to ensure patient/family wishes for advance directives are followed (DNR/AND)
Directive to Physicians (DTP)	Written document specifying the patient's wish to be allowed to die without heroic or extraordinary measures	Indicates specific measures to be used or withheld
Do not resuscitate (DNR)	Written physician's order instructing health care professionals not to attempt CPR. DNR order often requested by family	Must indicate any specific measures to be used or withheld Must be signed by a physician to be valid
Power of attorney for health care (POAH)	Term used by some states to describe a document used for listing the person(s) to make health care decisions should the patient become unable to make informed decisions for self	May be the same as medical power of attorney Indicates specific measures to be used or withheld
Living will	Lay term used to describe any documents that give instructions about future medical care and treatments or the wish to be allowed to die without heroic or extraordinary measures should the patient be unable to communicate for self	Must identify specific treatments that a person wants or does not want at end of life
Medical power of attorney (MPOA)	Term used by some states to describe a document used for listing the person(s) to make health care decisions should a patient become unable to make informed decisions for self	May be the same as durable power of attorney for health care, health care proxy, or appointment of a health care agent or surrogate Person appointed may be called a health care agent, surrogate, attorney-in-fact, or proxy
Physician Order for Life-Sustaining Treatment (POLST) or Medical Order for Life-Sustaining Treatment (MOLST)	A standardized physician order guided by the patient's medical condition and based on personal preferences verbalized by patient or expressed in advance directive	Only for those whose illness may limit life to less than 12 months Guides current treatments. Differs from advance directive which guides future treatments Physician completes form based on discussion with patient or authorized representative, or in review of advance directive. Signed by physician, patient, or patient representative Printed on bright pink paper

From Upchurch LAL: Palliative care at end of life. In: Lewis SL, Bucher L, Heitkemper MM, Harding MM, editors: *Medical-surgical nursing*, ed 10, St. Louis, MO, 2017, Elsevier.

Table 19.3 Physical Manifestations of Approaching Death

FUNCTION AND SYSTEM	MANIFESTATION
Hearing	Thought to be last sense to be lost Remember that comatose patients may still be able to hear.
Touch	Decrease of sensation Decrease of pain and touch perception
Taste	Decreases as illness progresses
Smell	Decreases with disease progression Related to loss of taste
Sight	Blurring of vision Sinking and glazing of eyes Blinking stops; eyelids remain halfway open
Skin	Mottling on hands and feet Cold, clammy skin High fever because of improper functioning of thermoregulation in the brain or dehydration "Waxlike" skin appearance very near death
Respiration	Becomes rapid and deep with periods of apnea (Cheyne-Stokes respiration) Becomes irregular, gradually slowing down to terminal gasps (may be described as "guppy breathing") Grunting and noisy tachypnea (death rattle) common Families need to be reassured that these symptoms do not signal emotional or physical distress.
Urinary tract	Becomes incontinent of urine or unable to excrete or pass urine
Bowel	Slowing of digestive tract and possible cessation of function (may be enhanced by pain medications) Accumulation of gas, distention, and nausea because of diminished peristalsis Loss of sphincter control (may produce incontinence) May have a bowel movement when death is imminent
Muscle tone	Sagging of jaw because of loss of tone of the facial muscles Possible speaking difficulty because of decreased muscle coordination Possible swallowing difficulty (taking food, fluids, and medications by mouth becomes increasingly difficult) Loss of gag reflex Jerking movements (myoclonic jerking) seen in patients on large amounts of opioid agents
Circulation	Slowing and weakening of pulse Drop in blood pressure

CLINICAL SIGNS OF IMPENDING DEATH

Physical Changes

The muscular system weakens gradually. Body movements are slowed. Facial muscles lose tone, and the jaw may sag. Speech may be difficult because of decreased muscle coordination. Swallowing becomes increasingly difficult and the gag reflex is eventually lost. The functions of the gastrointestinal (GI) and genitourinary systems slow down. Peristalsis diminishes, which can lead to constipation, gas accumulation, distention, and nausea. Pain medications may enhance the GI slowing. Loss of sphincter control may result in fecal and urinary incontinence.

Vital signs reflect cardiovascular and respiratory changes that precede death. The pulse slows and weakens. Blood pressure drops. Temperature may be elevated. Respirations may be rapid, shallow, and irregular, or they may be very slow. Noisy, wet-sounding respirations, termed the *death rattle*, are caused by mouth breathing and the accumulation of mucus in the upper airways. Cheyne-Stokes respirations are irregular with periods of apnea and develop as a person nears death.

Decreased circulation causes the skin to become fragile. The extremities become mottled and cyanotic. The skin feels cool to the touch, first in the feet and legs, then progressing to the hands and arms. However, the patient may feel warm because of an elevated temperature.

Sensory changes include decreasing pain and touch perception, blurred vision, and decreasing sense of taste and smell. The sense of touch decreases first in the lower extremities as a result of circulatory changes. The blink reflex is lost eventually, and the patient appears to stare. Liquid tears may be ordered to lubricate the eyes.

Hearing is commonly believed to be the last sense lost during the death process. You should assume that the patient can hear and understand. Speaking slowly and clearly may increase the patient's understanding. Inform the patient's family and visitors that the patient may still be able to hear. Encourage family members to talk to the patient in a comforting way.

During the death process, the body gradually relaxes until all function ends. In general, the respirations cease first. The heart stops beating within a few minutes. The physician is responsible for ordering discontinuation of life support if it is in use. The physician is also responsible for pronouncement of death in most situations. In a number of states, under specific circumstances, registered nurses (RNs) are legally permitted to pronounce death. A death certificate must be completed and signed. State laws designate who can sign a death certificate. This person is usually a physician, medical examiner, or nurse practitioner. Licensed vocational nurses/licensed practical nurses (LVNs/LPNs) should know the policies and procedures in their state and their employing institution.

When life sustaining technology is in use, determination of death requires additional evidence. The Harvard criteria were developed in 1968 to standardize the criteria used to determine death. According to the Harvard criteria, the following must occur to pronounce death:

1. Unresponsiveness to external stimulation that would normally be painful
2. A complete absence of spontaneous movement and breathing
3. A total lack of reflexes that are normally found on a neurologic examination, particularly the reaction of the pupils to light
4. A flat electroencephalogram (EEG) for 24 hours, which indicates that no electrical activity exists in the brain
5. The lack of circulation to the brain for 24 hours as identified by technology

Usually the first three criteria are enough for a pronouncement of death. The EEG and other technology are generally used when life support equipment is in use. The Harvard Committee recommended that if the final two criteria are used, the tests be repeated 24 hours later to confirm results.

Another definition associated with the diagnosis of death is cerebral or brain death. Cerebral or **brain death** occurs when the cerebral cortex stops functioning or is irreversibly destroyed. The cerebral cortex, or the higher brain, is responsible for voluntary movement, actions, and thought. Some believe that cerebral cortex function *is* the individual.

Life-sustaining technology has raised many issues. Scientists ask whether cerebral or brain death occurs when the whole brain (cortex and brainstem) ceases activity or when cortical function alone stops. In 1995, the Quality Standards Subcommittee of the American Academy of Neurology recommended diagnostic criteria guidelines for clinical diagnosis of brain death in adults. The criteria include coma or unresponsiveness, absence of brainstem reflexes, and apnea as three findings in brain death. Specific assessments by a physician are required to validate each of the criteria.

Currently, legal and medical standards require that all brain function must cease for brain death to be pronounced and life support to be disconnected. Diagnosis of brain death is of particular importance when organ donation is an option.

Psychosocial Changes

As the patient approaches the end of life, they may begin to withdraw, conversing less, and showing less interest in external activities. The range of emotions that patients experience might include anxiety, fear, helplessness, or peacefulness. Some focus on saying goodbye to loved ones, reviewing their life, expressing regrets, or reinforcing their wishes. They may seek spiritual comfort and reassurance that their life has had meaning. It is not unusual for patients to have vision-like experiences where they see people, objects, or places that are not present.

PHYSICAL CHANGES AFTER DEATH

After death, many changes occur in the body as decomposition takes place. Three specific changes are (1) rigor mortis, (2) algor mortis, and (3) livor mortis.

Immediately after death, some involuntary jerking movements may take place. Within 2 to 4 hours, the body stiffens, a condition referred to as *rigor mortis*. Rigor mortis is caused by chemical changes within the body's cells that prevent muscle relaxation. It is usually fully developed in 6 to 12 hours and resolves within 36 hours.

After death, the body begins to cool. This is known as *algor mortis*. Body temperature falls until it reaches the environmental temperature in approximately 24 hours. As the body cools, the skin tends to lose elasticity and can be broken easily.

The breakdown of red blood cells after death causes a discoloration in the skin, which is called *livor mortis*. The skin may appear bruised with reddish-purple discoloration, usually in the dependent parts of the body. Livor mortis usually occurs within 30 minutes to 2 hours.

Decomposition happens faster in warmer temperatures because of bacterial growth. To slow decomposition, the body must be kept cool. Embalming reverses the process of decomposition by replacing the body's fluids with chemicals that prevent further growth of the bacteria that cause decomposition.

Put On Your Thinking Cap!

1. Write down the customs and rituals that are followed in your family in relation to deaths: care of the body, viewing, wake, spiritual counselors, services, burial or cremation, types of memorials, support for survivors.
2. Discuss your answers with others in your clinical group.
3. Consider how you reacted to others' customs and rituals. Recognize the importance of your customs and rituals to you and appreciate the need to be accepting of different practices. Do not assume that your patients will handle death in the same way you do.

NURSING CARE AT END OF LIFE

CARE OF THE GRIEVING PATIENT

Kübler-Ross's work provides a framework for anticipating and understanding the experience of the dying and their survivors.

Nursing care of patients who are terminally ill or dying must address their psychologic and physical needs. Respect, dignity, and comfort are important for the patient and the family. In addition, nurses and other care providers must recognize their own responses and needs when dealing with grief and dying. The nursing plan of care for the grieving patient must be individualized depending on individual patient data.

FOCUSED ASSESSMENT

It is useful to identify the stage of grief (denial, anger, bargaining, depression, acceptance) that the person is experiencing. Awareness of the stage permits you to react according to the individual's needs.

Patient Problems, Goals, and Outcome Criteria: The Grieving Patient

The following is an example of patient problems, goals, and outcome criteria frequently used during the process of grieving.

Patient Problems	Goals and Outcome Criteria
Grief related to an actual or perceived loss	Resolution of grief: patient expresses feelings related to grief, progresses through stages of grief resolution
Anticipatory grief related to an expected loss	Resolution of grief: patient acknowledges impending loss, demonstrates behaviors that reflect progress in grief resolution
Unresolved grief related to the inability to adapt to the loss	Resolution of grief: patient verbalizes feelings related to grief process, begins to move toward resolution of grief

INTERVENTIONS

Priority interventions for anticipatory grieving and unresolved grieving focus on providing an environment that allows the patient to express feelings. Open discussion of feelings helps the patient and family to work toward resolution of the grief process. Accept expressions of anger, fear, or guilt without judgment. Assure the patient and family that these feelings are a normal part of grieving. Demonstrate respect for the patient's privacy and need or desire to talk (or to not talk). Be honest in answering questions and giving information.

Encourage families and patients to continue their usual activities as much as possible. They need to discuss their activities and maintain some control of their lives. You might help them to identify what they can and cannot change.

Grieving relatives, friends, and significant others can provide emotional support for one another. Be sensitive to the importance of significant others who are not necessarily relatives. Provide information about resources such as community counseling and support groups that may assist some people in working through their grief. Support groups share experiences and coping strategies that can help individuals to deal with their grief.

Respect the person's right to privacy, right to have a wide range of emotions, and right to talk when they choose. Suggest a referral to a social worker if the family needs assistance with planning for the future or for the funeral. Anger is a common and normal response to grief. Recognize that the grieving person cannot be forced to accept the loss. Acknowledge and encourage the expression of feelings but at the same time realize how difficult it is to come to terms with grief. If you find yourself the target of the patient's anger, try to understand what is happening and to not react on a personal level.

Feelings of hopelessness and powerlessness are common in terminal illness and during grief. Encourage realistic hope within the limits of the situation. Allow the patient and the family to identify and deal with what is within their control and to recognize what is beyond their control. Encourage patient-identified goals to restore some sense of power.

NURSING CARE NEAR END OF LIFE

FOCUSED ASSESSMENT

Assessment of the dying patient varies with the patient's condition. In general, the assessment is limited to essential data. If the patient is admitted to an inpatient facility, document the specific event or change that brought the patient to the health care facility. Record the patient's medical diagnoses, recent medications, and allergies. If the patient is alert, briefly review the body systems to detect important signs and symptoms. In addition, document discomfort such as pain or nausea for prompt intervention. Depending on the specific terminal condition, other relevant information should be recorded. For example, if the patient has colon cancer, you would assess elimination in more detail.

The functional assessment of activities of daily living (ADLs) elicits information about the patient's abilities, food and fluid intake, patterns of sleep and rest, and response to the stress of terminal illness. It is important to determine how the patient (if able to communicate) and family are coping. You can draw inferences about the stage of grief and the coping mechanisms based on statements reflecting sorrow, anger, guilt, or denial.

The physical assessment is abbreviated and detects changes that accompany terminal illness. The frequency of assessment depends on the patient's stability but is performed at least every 8 hours. As changes occur, documentation is performed more frequently.

Neurologic assessment is especially important and includes level of consciousness, reflexes, and pupil responses. Evaluation of vital signs, skin color, and temperature detects changes in circulation. Monitor the patient's respiratory status and describe the character and pattern of respirations and breath sounds. Renal and GI functions are assessed by monitoring nutritional and fluid intake, urinary output, and bowel sounds. Skin condition must also be monitored because skin becomes very fragile and may break down. To reemphasize, it is important to be sensitive and not to impose repeated, unnecessary assessments on the dying patient. If health history data are available in the chart, you can use that resource rather than tiring the patient with an interview. However, it is important to check on the patient frequently so that they do not feel abandoned.

PATIENT PROBLEMS, GOALS, AND OUTCOME CRITERIA

Common problems for the dying patient and the family are listed below. The nursing plan of care must be individualized depending on individual patient data. Refer to Chapter 12 for additional patient problems and interventions for the immobile patient and to Chapter 8 for pain management.

Patient Problems, Goals, and Outcome Criteria: Terminally Ill and Dying Patients

Patient Problems	Goals and Outcome Criteria
Discomfort; acute pain; chronic pain related to pathologic processes	Pain relief/reduction: Patient verbalizes pain reduction or relief, improved comfort. Relaxed expression.
Fear related to the dying process and/or anxiety related to unknown threats	Reduced fear and/or anxiety: Patient verbalizes less fear, anxiety. Calm, relaxed expression.
Potential for disrupted skin integrity related to immobility, poor circulation, inadequate nutrition, anemia	Decreased risk of skin breakdown: Pressure areas are protected, minimal contact of urine and feces with skin, shearing forces are avoided.
Nausea related to drug effects or disease process	Relief of nausea: Patient verbalizes relief, no vomiting.

Patient Problems, Goals, and Outcome Criteria: Terminally Ill and Dying Patients—cont'd

Patient Problems	Goals and Outcome Criteria
Inadequate oxygenation related to retained secretions in the respiratory tract, disease process, failing circulation to brain	Patent airway: clear breath sounds.
Constipation related to immobility, opioids, dehydration; diarrhea related to muscle relaxation, fecal impaction	No acute constipation: Negative rectal examination for impaction. Cessation of diarrhea: No liquid stool passage.
Altered cognition related to drug effects, poor cerebral circulation	Safety is maintained; patient is reassured as needed.

INTERVENTIONS

During terminal illness and impending death, meeting the patient's safety and physiologic needs is the priority. Physical requirements for oxygen, nutrition, pain relief, mobility, elimination, and skin care remain throughout the life cycle. Physical care, including comfort measures and skin care, should be continued. People who are dying deserve and require the same physical care as people who are expected to recover. However, intrusive monitoring need not be continued.

Discomfort and Pain

Look for causes of discomfort such as bedding in disarray, pressure, poor positioning, wound drainage, incontinent stool or urine, kinked tubing, and so on and take corrective action. In an ideal situation, the patient would have had the opportunity to tell health care providers how they feel about pain medications. For some, pain control is a priority, whereas others may wish to remain alert as long as possible. Document the patient's pain on a scale of 1 to 10 if possible. Pain is best managed by scheduled administration of analgesics rather than waiting for the patient to request them when they can no longer bear the pain. Fears about opioid addiction are not relevant at the end of life; the priority is to relieve the pain. The possibility that opioids will hasten the patient's death is not cause for withholding drugs.

Fear and Anxiety

Fear is a common feeling experienced by people at end of life. Among the most common fears are fear of pain, fear of shortness of breath, fear of loneliness and abandonment, and fear of meaninglessness (Upchurch, 2017). Pain at the end of life is not thought to be a universal experience. However, patients can be assured that any pain they have will be treated as discussed earlier. Feelings of air hunger may occur. This can be reduced with opioids, bronchodilators, oxygen, and antianxiety drugs. Dying people often express fear of dying alone. Therefore it is important for significant others to be present if possible. Explain to them that touching and speaking to the patient can be comforting. If no one else is present, consider having a staff member sit with the patient to provide comfort. In the time leading up to the final phase of dying, patients can be encouraged to review their life and to identify the positive aspects of that life.

Disrupted Skin Integrity

It can be a challenge to maintain skin integrity in the final days of life, and this goal is not always achieved. Skin care of the immobilized patient is described in Chapter 12.

Nausea

Administer antiemetics as needed. Do not encourage the patient to eat or drink if they do not wish to. It is normal for dying patients to gradually stop eating and drinking.

Inadequate Oxygenation

Secretions accumulate in the airway and patients may be unable to clear them. Suction may be used but may be distressing for the patient. Raise the head of the bed and administer oxygen if the patient appears to be dyspneic. In the final hours of life, breathing slows and becomes irregular. Cheyne-Stokes respirations are characterized by alternating periods of apnea and deep, rapid breathing. No intervention will correct this rhythm.

Constipation and Diarrhea

Opioids and immobility make constipation a common problem at end of life. Patients who can take oral medications may be given stool softeners or laxatives as needed. Fecal impactions may develop and must be removed, usually with enemas and manual extraction. Suspect fecal impaction in the patient who has not had a recent bowel movement but has diarrhea.

Altered Cognition

As cerebral circulation falls, cognitive processes are affected. Patients' verbalizations may not make sense, and they may have hallucinations. Take precautions to avoid injuries. Offer soothing comments and gently stroke the patient. Reorient as appropriate.

CARE OF THE BODY AFTER DEATH

After death, the body must be prepared for transfer to the morgue or funeral home. Nurses are responsible for the care and preparation of the body. Dignity and privacy for the deceased and the family must be maintained. Table 19.4 identifies nursing management for preparation of the body for family viewing after death.

Legal and religious issues may affect the care required for the disposition of the body. In certain instances, an autopsy may be required. An autopsy is a postmortem examination of the deceased. It may

Table 19.4 Preparation of the Body for Family Viewing After Death

TOPIC	NURSING MANAGEMENT
Autopsy	Identification band remains on the body. Contact medical examiner/coroner if required. Consent form signed by next of kin if autopsy is requested. Follow legal requirements and agency policy.
Positioning	Place body in supine position with arms at sides or hands folded across the abdomen. Place small pillow under the head and shoulders. Close eyelids gently and hold for a few minutes or apply moist cotton balls as needed. Close mouth. Place a rolled towel under the chin as needed. Follow agency policy.
Hygiene	Wash soiled areas of the body. Apply a clean gown. Place linen savers under the buttocks. Comb hair. Apply clean top linens and cover body to shoulder level. Follow agency policy.
Personal effects	Insert dentures gently. Do not force. If dentures cannot be inserted, place them in denture container marked with appropriate identification. Secure jewelry that cannot be removed easily with tape. Inventory all valuables and possessions with the family, the funeral director, or the medical examiner/coroner staff. Clearly document the disposition of possessions. Follow agency policy.

be requested by the next of kin, suggested by the physician, or required by law. Consent for an autopsy must be given before the procedure can be performed, unless the law requires that the procedure be performed.

Each state has its own laws regarding autopsy. Under the law in most states, an autopsy is required if a person expires by suicide, by homicide, within 24 hours of admission to a health care facility, or from unknown causes. In such cases the coroner or the medical examiner must be notified.

During an autopsy, organ specimens and samples may be removed for examination. Body parts that are removed are either disposed of or preserved for burial, depending on the situation and the family's wishes. An autopsy is no more disfiguring than a surgical procedure. When the body is dressed, signs of an autopsy are not visible.

The family may wish to view the body before it is transported to the mortuary or morgue. It is important to make the environment as comfortable as possible for the family. It is your responsibility to prepare the body for viewing before the transfer (see the Cultural Considerations box).

Cultural Considerations

What Does Culture Have to Do With Care After Death?

Cultural practices related to care of the body after death must be respected. Examples of traditional practices include the following:

- Greece: Body is washed by a relative or older woman.
- Roman Catholics: Body should not be shrouded until sacraments have been performed.
- Orthodox Jews: Dying person is not left. Body is not left alone between death and burial, which must occur within 24 hours. Body must not be touched for up to 30 minutes after death. Only designated Orthodox persons or Jewish Burial Service care for the body.

Normally, after death you will place the body in the supine position with the arms at the sides or with the hands across the abdomen. Identification bands should remain in place. A single pillow is placed under the head and shoulders to prevent discoloration of the face from pooling of the blood. Avoid use of large, overstuffed pillows.

Gently holding the eyelids closed for a few seconds helps them to remain closed. If the eyelids do not remain closed after a few seconds, the application of moist cotton balls for a few minutes may help.

Dentures may be inserted gently to maintain the normal facial appearance. If the dentures cannot be inserted easily, they should not be forced. Dentures that are not in place should be stored in a denture container, marked with identification, and sent with the body to the mortuary. The mouth should be closed. A rolled towel placed under the chin helps to hold the mouth closed.

Areas of the body that are soiled should be washed. Linen savers are placed under the buttocks to absorb urine or feces that may be released as the sphincters relax. A clean gown is applied, and the hair is combed.

Depending on agency procedures, tubes that are present in the body may be removed unless an autopsy is required. Some agencies require that tubes remain in place or that they be trimmed to approximately 1 inch and taped in place. It is important to review state and agency requirements.

Jewelry is generally removed, except for wedding bands, which may be taped to the patients' fingers. If other rings cannot be removed easily, they should be taped in place.

An inventory of possessions and valuables is done with the family. Each valuable is listed and signed for by the family. If no family is available, the inventory of valuables is listed and signed for by the funeral home director. The disposition of possessions is documented in the medical record.

After the positioning and preparation of the body, top linens should be straightened and pulled up to the deceased's shoulder level. The family may view the body after preparation is complete.

Often the family needs the nurse's emotional support while viewing the body. If only one family member is present, it is wise to accompany the person who is viewing the body. Close the door to allow for privacy and allow the family as much time as desired.

When the family leaves, apply additional identification tags to the wrist and ankle or toe of the deceased. The gown is removed, and the body may be wrapped in a shroud. The shroud may be a large square or rectangle of cloth or plastic material. An identification tag is placed on the outside of the shroud. Additional identification markings may be required if the deceased had a communicable disease. The body is then transported to the morgue or removed by the mortician. Agency policy regarding the transport of a body from the room may vary. Some agencies require that all patient doors be closed before transport and that service elevators be used. Table 19.5 lists the nursing management for preparation of the body for transfer.

NEEDS OF CAREGIVERS

The nurse-patient relationship often extends over weeks or even months. Throughout the terminal illness, nurses may experience feelings of helplessness, sorrow, guilt, and frustration. Nurses who are in touch with their own feelings are better able to help patients and families deal with their feelings. When the patient finally dies, the caring nurse will experience a personal sense of loss. Grieving is the normal response. The nurse must work through the stages of grief even if their grief is less intense than that of the patient or family. It is acceptable to cry with the patient or family during the grief process.

Table 19.5 Preparation of the Body for Transfer

TOPIC	NURSING MANAGEMENT
Body identification	Identification band remains on the body. Apply additional identification tags to the wrist, ankle, or toe per agency policy. Place additional identification on the outside of the shroud. Communicable disease identification should be listed on the body and outside the shroud. Follow agency policy.
Autopsy	Tubes and medical appliances are frequently left as originally placed in accordance with agency policy and legal requirements. Follow agency policy.
Positioning	Place body in supine position with arms at sides or hands folded across the abdomen. Wrists and ankles may be bound based on agency policy. Remove gown. Apply shroud. Follow agency policy.
Personal effects	Inventory all valuables and possessions with the family, the funeral director, or the medical examiner/coroner staff. Clearly package and document the disposition of possessions. Follow agency policy.
Transport	Transport via stretcher to the morgue based on agency policy. Assist with transfer of the body to the mortician's stretcher for transport.

If possible, nurses or a representative member of the nursing staff may attend the patient's viewing or funeral. Nursing staff also need to be supportive of one another when dealing with the death of a patient. Failure to deal with the grief experience can lead to nurse burnout and a loss of sensitivity to patient needs. Some agencies have formal grief support groups for nurses. Another helpful activity is a periodic memorial service in which patients who have died recently are remembered.

Get Ready for the NCLEX® Examination!

Key Points

- Loss is the real or potential absence of someone or something that is valued.
- Mourning is the period marked by social customs associated with grief.
- Bereavement is the total grief and mourning experience.
- Loss that is not socially recognized can result in disenfranchised grief.
- The response to loss, called *grief*, is similar regardless of the nature of the loss but is usually most profound when the loss experienced is death.
- Uncomplicated grief is a healthy response to loss; unresolved grief is a prolonged or exaggerated response.
- Culture, spirituality, age, and past experiences affect a person's understanding and reaction to death.
- Kübler-Ross stages of grieving are denial, anger, bargaining, depression, and acceptance.
- Common fears associated with terminal illness and death are fear of pain, fear of shortness of breath, fear of loneliness and abandonment, and fear of meaninglessness.
- The goal of palliative care is to improve quality of life for patients and their families by anticipating, preventing, and treating suffering.
- The primary issues that are addressed in palliative care include physical symptoms; emotional, coping, intellectual, social, and spiritual needs; and facilitation of patient autonomy, access to information, and choice.
- Individuals are eligible for hospice care under Medicare when a physician certifies that the patient has a life-limiting condition, and that his or her life expectancy is 6 months or less.
- Hospice care embraces palliative care with a focus on quality of life, comfort, and dignity near the end of life. It also includes bereavement care for survivors after the death of the patient.
- Hospice volunteers can assist in direct support (i.e., spending time with patients and families), clinical support related to patient care and clinical services, and general support such as outreach and education.
- Legal documents that may be completed near end of life may include organ donation wishes, advance directives, durable power of attorney, medical power of attorney, and directives for physicians, family members, or surrogates.
- The Patient Self-Determination Act requires all institutions that participate with Medicare to provide written information to patients concerning their right to accept or refuse treatment.

- Advance directives are written statements of a person's wishes regarding medical care. The first advance directive document, developed in 1974, was called the *Living Will.*
- Clinical signs of impending death are loss of muscle tone, bradycardia, hypotension, abnormal respiratory pattern, abnormal breath sounds, cyanosis, cool skin, blurred vision, and sensory changes.
- Changes in the body after death are rigor mortis, algor mortis, and livor mortis.
- Data collection/assessment of the condition of the terminally ill or dying person varies with the person's condition but is often limited to essential data related to comfort.
- Nursing problems that may be addressed in the person who is terminally ill or dying may include: discomfort/pain, fear, anxiety, disrupted skin integrity, inadequate oxygenation, constipation, diarrhea, and altered cognition.
- The nurse is responsible for the care of the body after death.
- An autopsy (postmortem examination of the body) requires family consent unless it is required by law.
- The *Five Wishes* document records the patient's desires in relation to decision-making authority, medical care, comfort measures, treatments, and information to be shared with loved ones.

Additional Learning Resources

SG Go to your Study Guide for additional learning activities to help you master this chapter content.

Go to your Evolve website (http://evolve.elsevier.com/Linton/medsurg) for the following learning resources and much more:
- Fluid & Electrolyte Tutorial
- Review Questions for the NCLEX® Examination

Clinical Judgment and Next-Generation NCLEX® Examination-Style Questions

1. **Which of the following can result in a feeling of loss? (Select all that apply.)**
   1. A worker is required to retire after 30 years.
   2. Family records are destroyed in a house fire.
   3. An adult child accepts a job in another country.
   4. A patient's hair falls out because of chemotherapy.
   5. An electrician has an arm amputated after an injury.

   NCLEX Client Need: Psychosocial Integrity

2. **Palliative care has been recommended to a patient with advanced cancer who has decided to discontinue treatment. The patient should be told that the focus of palliative care is:**
   1. Finding alternative methods of disease treatment
   2. Providing supportive care while allowing natural death
   3. Delaying death for as long as possible by any means
   4. Hastening death when no hope for a cure exists

   NCLEX Client Need: Psychosocial Integrity

3. **When a patient was diagnosed with a terminal illness, his wife began to grieve. Which term describes this grief response?**
   1. Anticipatory grief
   2. Complicated grief
   3. Uncomplicated grief
   4. Normal grief

   NCLEX Client Need: Psychosocial Integrity

4. **A patient who has been diagnosed with terminal lung cancer tells the nurse, "If God will just let me live to see my children finish school, I will never smoke another cigarette." This illustrates which of Kübler-Ross stages of grief?**
   1. Denial
   2. Anger
   3. Bargaining
   4. Depression

   NCLEX Client Need: Psychosocial Integrity

5. **A new hospice patient reports that her pain has been getting worse. The nurse should explain that the hospice approach to pain management is guided by which of the following principles?**
   1. Pain relief is a priority
   2. Caution must be used to prevent addiction
   3. Patients should be heavily sedated
   4. Medications should be used only when pain is severe

   NCLEX Client Need: Physiological Integrity: Basic Care and Comfort

6. **During the last few days of a patient's life, family members visited her and talked about shared memories and how much the patient meant to them. How might this be helpful? (Select all that apply.)**
   1. This would probably benefit the family more than the patient.
   2. Reviewing her life can help the patient find meaning in her life.
   3. Visitors will prevent the patient from focusing on her impending death.
   4. This sharing experience helps to confirm the patient's worth.
   5. This experience reinforces that the family is in denial about the patient's illness.

   NCLEX Client Need: Psychosocial Integrity

7. **As a patient nears death, her husband says, "I wish I could do something for her." What should the nurse tell the husband?**
   1. "Unfortunately, nothing can be done at this point."
   2. "It's just a matter of time now. Why don't you take a break?"
   3. "It may be comforting if you will talk to her slowly and clearly."
   4. "She probably cannot hear you, but she may be able to feel your touch."

   NCLEX Client Need: Psychosocial Integrity

8. **A new nursing assistant leaves the room in tears the first time one of her patients dies. What is the most appropriate comment by the nurse?**
   1. "Get back in there and take care of your patient."
   2. "It hurts to lose a patient, but you will get used to it."
   3. "It is normal for you to feel upset. How can I help you?"
   4. "You really can't get so emotionally involved with patients."

   NCLEX Client Need: Psychosocial Integrity

9. **Which statement describes a power of attorney?**
   1. A document that declares whether organ donation is desired.
   2. A document that specifies who should carry out the wishes specified in the patient's will.
   3. A document that lists the measures a person wants to be initiated in the event of sudden death.
   4. A document that identifies the person(s) to make health care decisions should the patient become unable to make informed decisions for self.

   NCLEX Client Needs: Psychosocial Integrity

10. **The *Five Wishes* document specifies which of the following? (Select all that apply.)**
    1. Who will be responsible for implementing the distribution of personal property.
    2. The type of medical care the patient wants or does not want.
    3. What information the patient wants loved ones to know.
    4. The amount of comfort the patient wants.
    5. How the patient wants to be treated.

    NCLEX Client Need: Psychosocial Integrity

11. **SLO Objective: Identify interventions to promote comfort for the patient and family and family at end-of-life.**

    NGN Item Type: Matrix

    Cognitive Skill: Generate Solutions

    The hospice nurse has been called to the home of a 79-year-old patient who has a diagnosis of terminal cancer. Her husband and two daughters are present. The nurse's assessment data is as follows:
    - Patient moans and grimaces when moved
    - She has required increasing opioids to manage her pain
    - She has taken only sips of water for 2 days
    - Vital signs: BP 90/40; Pulse = 82 beats per minute, irregular; Respirations = 22 breaths per minute, irregular with period of apnea
    - Pedal pulses not palpable; feet cold; toes bluish in color

    Use an X for the nursing actions listed below that are *Indicated* (appropriate or necessary), *Contraindicated* (could be harmful), or *Nonessential* (makes no difference) for the patient's care at this time.

NURSING ACTION	INDICATED	CONTRA-INDICATED	NONES-SENTIAL
Ask the physician to order IV fluids for hydration.[			
Document vital signs every 30 minutes			
Withhold additional opioids until she is more alert			
Advise the family to touch and talk to her in a soothing manner			
Call EMS to institute resuscitation measures			
Focus on comfort measures			
Talk to family members about the dying process outside the patient's room			

20 Complementary and Alternative Therapies and Integrative Health Care

http://evolve.elsevier.com/Linton/medsurg

Objectives

1. Define complementary and alternative therapies.
2. Describe integrative health care.
3. Describe the National Center for Complementary and Integrative Health (NCCIH) categories of nonmainstream products and therapies.
4. Provide examples of possible interactions between nonmainstream and conventional products.
5. Describe the role of the nurse in educating patients about nonmainstream therapies.
6. List resources for scientifically based information about nonmainstream therapies.

Key Terms

allopathic medicine
alternative health practice
complementary health approach
integrative health care

Conventional Western medicine, also referred to as **allopathic medicine**, *biomedicine*, and *mainstream medicine*, relies strongly on science and technology in the treatment of illness. However, it is not always effective, especially in the management of stress-induced conditions, chronic symptoms, and the emotional and spiritual needs of individuals. Some symptoms have no known cause, and therefore have no specific conventional treatment.

Americans are increasingly turning to nonmainstream products and practices in place of, or along with, mainstream conventional care. Nonmainstream practices that are used along with conventional therapies are called **complementary health approaches**. For example, a patient with chronic pain might take analgesics but also practice guided imagery. If used in place of conventional treatment, nonmainstream practices are called **alternative health practices**. An example of an alternative practice is the use of relaxation therapy or acupuncture instead of analgesics to treat pain. Americans are more likely to use nonmainstream drugs and practices as complementary practices rather than alternatives. The term **integrative health care** is used when nonmainstream practices are incorporated into conventional health care. An integrative plan of care focuses on the whole person and uses various evidence-based practices determined by a team of conventional and complementary practitioners. The term *evidence-based practice*, which refers to health care practices that are based on current and valid research findings, may be applied to both conventional and nonmainstream therapies if sufficient research has been done.

NONMAINSTREAM THERAPIES

The National Center for Complementary and Integrative Health (NCCIH) classifies nonmainstream practices into two subgroups: (1) natural products, and (2) mind and body practices. However, some practices including traditional healers, Ayurvedic medicine, traditional Chinese medicine (TCM), homeopathy, and naturopathy do not fit well in either of these categories (Table 20.1).

NATURAL PRODUCTS

Among the natural products are herbs/botanicals, vitamins, minerals, and probiotics. They are often sold as dietary supplements. Under the Dietary Supplement Health and Education (DSHEA) Act of 1994, natural products are categorized as dietary supplements rather than drugs. Dietary supplements can be marketed directly to consumers. The DSHEA requires herbal products to have the following statement on the label: "This product is not intended to diagnose, treat, cure, or prevent any disease." However, the label can claim to favorably influence body structure or function. Examples of acceptable claims are: helps promote urinary tract health, supports the immune system, or reduces stress and frustration. Unacceptable label claims might include statements like "protects against cancer" or "improves symptoms of Alzheimer disease." Box 20.1 lists some common dietary supplements.

Safety and Efficacy of Dietary Supplements

Whereas drug manufacturers must present evidence of safety and effectiveness to the U.S. Food and Drug

Table 20.1 Types of Complementary and Alternative Therapies

TYPE	DESCRIPTION	EXAMPLES
Whole medical systems	Built on complete systems of theory and practice that have evolved in different cultures apart from conventional medicine	Homeopathy, naturopathy, Ayurveda, traditional Chinese medicine
Mind and body interventions	Focuses on interactions among brain, mind, body, and behavior. Uses techniques designed to enhance the mind's capacity to affect bodily function and promote health	Meditation, acupuncture, deep breathing exercises, hypnotherapy, progressive relaxation, Tai Chi, guided imagery
Manipulative and body-based practices	Based on manipulation or movement of one of more parts of the body	Osteopathic medicine, naturopathy, physical therapy, massage, chiropractic
Energy therapies	Focuses on manipulation of energy fields to affect health. (1)veritable (measurable energy) (2)biofield (fields yet to be measured)	Veritable: magnet therapy, light therapy Biofield: qi gong, reiki, healing touch
Movement therapies	Uses movement to promote physical, mental, emotional, and spiritual well-being	Pilates, Trager psychophysical integration
Natural products	Aims to affect biochemical and physiologic processes	Herbal medicines (botanicals), vitamins, minerals, fish oil, Echinacea, probiotics, microorganisms like normal gastrointestinal flora

Some therapies such as naturopathy can be classified as more than one type of therapy.
From National Center for Complementary and Alternative Medicine: *What is complementary and alternative medicine?* Washington, DC, 2006, National Institutes of Health.

Box 20.1 Commonly Used Dietary Supplements

- Black cohosh
- Coenzyme Q-10
- Cranberry juice
- Echinacea
- Feverfew
- Flaxseed
- Garlic
- Ginger root
- *Ginkgo biloba*
- Glucosamine
- Green tea
- Probiotics
- Resveratrol
- Saw palmetto
- Soy
- St. John's wort
- Valerian

Administration (FDA), manufacturers of supplements only are required to report "claims of efficacy." If claims of efficacy prove to be false or if the product proves to be harmful, the FDA can file a suit in court. The FDA can act only after a supplement has been released for marketing.

A primary concern with the use of dietary supplements is that many lack scientific evidence of safety and effectiveness. Ephedra provides an excellent example of the problems that can arise from nonregulated manufacturing. Ephedrine alkaloids have been used in China for centuries to treat colds, asthma, and nasal congestion. In the United States it was used to treat asthma in the 1940s and 1950s, and in some dietary supplements that claimed to promote weight loss, increased energy, and improved athletic performance. Reports of adverse effects (heart problems, stroke, death) eventually led the FDA to ban the sale of dietary supplements containing ephedrine alkaloids in 2004.

The Dietary Supplement and Nonprescription Drug Consumer Protection Act was passed in 2006. This Act mandates the reporting of serious adverse events, including deaths, hospitalizations, life-threatening events, persistent or significant disabilities, and birth defects. With the intent of improving manufacturing and labeling of dietary supplements, the FDA issued a set of standards in 2007—the Current Good Manufacturing Practices (CGMP). These standards aim to ensure that dietary supplements have no adulterants, contaminants, or impurities and that the label correctly states the identity, purity, quality, and strength of the contents.

Some private quality certification programs, including the U.S. Pharmacopeia (USP), are testing dietary supplements for quality. Following testing, the programs report the product's purity, identity, potency, dissolution, accuracy of labeling, and conformity with the CGMP.

Interactions of Natural Products With Conventional Drugs

Any time multiple drugs are taken, whether conventional or herbal products, the potential for interactions exists. Interactions may result in decreased or increased effects. Examples of known interactions are the following:

- St. John's wort increases an enzyme that accelerates the metabolism of numerous conventional drugs including oral contraceptives. The conventional drug is metabolized more quickly, resulting in a loss of therapeutic effects.

Table 20.2 Examples of Commonly Used Herbal Products: Uses and Drug Interactions

PRODUCT AND USE[a]	DRUG	POTENTIAL EFFECT OF INTERACTION
Black cohosh: treatment of menopausal symptoms	Antihypertensive agents, insulin and other antidiabetes drugs, estrogens	Hypotension, hypoglycemia, enhanced estrogen effects
Coenzyme Q-10: hypertension, angina, improved exercise performance	Warfarin	Interferes with effects of warfarin
Cranberry juice: UTI prevention	Warfarin	Increased risk of bleeding
Echinacea: treat cold symptoms	Immunosuppressants	May inhibit immunosuppression; can compromise drug therapy for cancer, TB, and HIV
Feverfew: migraine headache prevention, treatment of rheumatoid arthritis stiffness and pain	Antiplatelet agents and anticoagulants	Increased risk of bleeding
Flaxseed: treat laxative, treat heart disease after MI	Conventional medications	May interfere with absorption of conventional drugs if taken within 2 hours of each other
Garlic: lower cholesterol, reduce blood clotting, treat high blood pressure	Antiplatelet agents and anticoagulants	Increased risk of bleeding
Ginger root: treat nausea and vomiting of pregnancy and related to chemotherapy	Antiplatelet agents and anticoagulants	Increased risk of bleeding
Ginkgo biloba: treat claudication, treat early-stage dementia	Antiplatelet agents and anticoagulants Drugs used to control seizures	Increased risk of bleeding May lower seizure threshold
Glucosamine: treatment of osteoarthritis, especially in knees	Antiplatelet agents and anticoagulants	Increased risk of bleeding
Green tea: treat arthritis	Vasodilators, stimulants, psychoactive drugs, hepatotoxic drugs, anticoagulants	Many drug interactions, including interference with effects of warfarin
Probiotics	Antibacterial and antifungal drugs	Kill bacteria and yeasts in the probiotic product
Resveratrol: antioxidant effects that might delay aging and reduce the risk of cancer and heart disease	Anticoagulant and antiplatelet drugs. Estrogen Insulin	Intensified anticoagulant effects. Should not be given to women with estrogen-dependent breast cancer. Increased insulin sensitivity.
Saw palmetto: treatment of urinary symptoms associated with benign prostatic hypertrophy	Antiplatelet drugs	Enhanced antiplatelet effect
St. John's wort: treat depression and anxiety	Interacts with many drugs	Accelerated metabolism and elimination of some drugs; increased risk of serotonin syndrome with many antidepressants
Valerian: treat insomnia and anxiety	CNS depressants	Increased sedation

[a]Uses are reasons that people may take these products. There may or may not be scientific evidence to support the product efficacy.
CNS, Central nervous system; *HIV*, human immunodeficiency virus; *MI*, myocardial infarction; *TB*, tuberculosis; *UTI*, urinary tract infection.
From Burchum JR, Rosenthal LD: *Lehne's Pharmacology for nursing care*, 9th ed, St. Louis, 2016, Elsevier Saunders.

- Garlic and *ginkgo biloba* suppress platelet aggregation. When taken by a patient on anticoagulant or antiplatelet drugs, the risk of bleeding increases. Table 20.2 lists numerous other interactions.

Reliable Resources

When you use a drug in the United States, you can obtain information about the drug action, directions for use, safe and therapeutic dose, interactions, contraindications, and side and adverse effects. You also can be assured that the product meets government standards. This information is often not readily available for nonmainstream products. Resources that do provide factual information are the following:

- The NCCIH. Responding to the increased use of natural products and therapies, the National Institutes of Health (NIH) established the NCCIH with the mission "to define, through rigorous scientific investigation, the usefulness and safety of complementary and integrative health interventions and their roles in improving health and health care" (NCCIH, last updated November 28, 2020).

Findings are published on the NCCIH website and in professional literature.

- Cochrane Database of Systematic Reviews. An excellent source of information about research on nonmainstream products and practices is the Cochrane Review, which collects research studies, assesses the research quality, compiles the findings, and states whether the research evidence is strong enough to support or not support the use of the practice. You can obtain Cochrane Reviews online at www.cochranelibrary.com/about/about-cochrane-systematic-reviews.html.
- German Commission E. The commission has extensive information about plant-based products. Their publications provide information about the chemistry, pharmacology, toxicology, and traditional uses of herbals in addition to research data and patient case records.
- Natural Medicines Brand Evidence-Based Rating (NMBER) System. The NMBER system is a subscription service that provides evidence-based ratings of safety and efficacy for over 60,000 supplements. Each supplement is rated on a scale of 1 to 10 with 1 being the poorest rating (not recommended) and 10 being the best.
- Office of Dietary Supplements evaluates scientific information, supports research, shares research results, and educates the public about dietary supplements. It publishes *Dietary Supplements: What You Need to Know*, fact sheets, and the PubMed Dietary Supplement Subset.

MIND AND BODY APPROACHES

Conventional and nonmainstream practices are based on differing views of health and illness. Conventional medicine focuses on conditions that are treated by correcting the underlying pathologic processes with drugs, surgery, diet, and physical manipulation. Most nonmainstream therapies are based on the belief that illness is caused by lack of balance or harmony within the individual or between the individual and the environment. Therapy aims to restore balance or harmony, which puts the individual in a position such that healing can occur.

Mind-body techniques that are familiar in the United States are yoga, chiropractic and osteopathic manipulation, meditation, massage therapy, acupuncture, Tai Chi, qi gong, healing touch, hypnotherapy, relaxation therapy (breathing exercises, guided imagery, progressive muscle relaxation), and movement therapies (Pilates, Rolfing structural integration, etc.).

Some mind-body techniques, including yoga, acupuncture, spinal manipulation, and mediation, have been the focus of numerous research studies. For many other practices, research is limited or nonexistent.

Yoga

Numerous styles of yoga exist. The most commonly practiced style in the United States is hatha yoga, which emphasizes postures, breathing exercises, and meditation. Reasons for using yoga include to improve physical fitness, relieve stress, and enhance quality of life. Some people use it to address specific health conditions such as back pain, neck pain, arthritis, or anxiety. The practice of yoga is generally considered safe for healthy people under the guidance of a well-trained instructor. The risks are low, although, in rare cases, certain types of stroke as well as pain from nerve damage have occurred when practicing yoga. Modifications in some poses should be made for pregnant women and people with high blood pressure, glaucoma, or sciatica. Conclusions of selected research studies on the effects of yoga include the following:

- A carefully adapted set of yoga poses may reduce low back pain and improve function.
- Practicing yoga (as well as other forms of regular exercise) might improve quality of life; reduce stress; lower heart rate and blood pressure; help relieve anxiety, depression, and insomnia; and improve overall physical fitness, strength, and flexibility.
- Yoga may not improve asthma.
- Results of yoga and arthritis studies have been inconclusive

According to the NCCIH, many research studies of yoga have had small numbers of participants and have not been high quality studies. The NCCIH concluded that "in most instances, we can only say that yoga has shown promise for particular health uses, not that it's been proven to help" (NCCIH, last updated May 2019).

Chiropractic

Chiropractic focuses on the relationship between the body's structure and its functioning. Practitioners primarily perform adjustments (manipulations) to the spine or other parts of the body. The goal is to correct alignment problems, alleviate pain, improve function, and support the body's natural ability to heal itself (NCCIH, 2017). In addition to adjustments, other therapies that may be used by chiropractors are heat and cold, electrical stimulation, relaxation techniques, rehabilitative and general exercise, dietary supplements, and counseling about diet, weight loss, and other lifestyle factors. Joint mobilization is another type of manual therapy that may be used to increase the range and quality of motion in the area being treated.

Most chiropractic research has focused on spinal manipulation. This procedure appears to offer some benefit to people with low-back pain. Some evidence also exists for its use to treat headaches, neck pain, upper- and lower-extremity joint conditions, and whiplash-associated disorders.

A review of scientific evidence on manual therapies concluded that spinal manipulation/mobilization may be helpful for migraine and cervicogenic (neck-related) headaches, neck pain, upper- and lower-extremity joint conditions, and whiplash-associated disorders. The review also noted that spinal manipulation/mobilization did not appear to be helpful for asthma, hypertension, and menstrual pain. The evidence of effectiveness in treating fibromyalgia, mid-back pain, premenstrual syndrome, sciatica, and temporomandibular joint disorders was deemed inconclusive.

Serious complications of spinal manipulation are rare, but temporary headaches, tiredness, or discomfort in the treated parts of the body may occur. Although rare, stroke has occurred after spinal manipulation, but whether the manipulation was a causative factor is uncertain. Chiropractic care is covered by some medical insurance programs.

Meditation

Meditation is another mind and body practice used to promote calmness and physical relaxation, improve psychologic balance, cope with illness, and enhance overall health and well-being. All types of meditation have four elements in common: a quiet location with as few distractions as possible; a specific, comfortable posture (sitting, lying down, walking, or in other positions); a focus of attention (a specially chosen word or set of words, an object, or the sensations of the breath); and an open attitude (letting distractions come and go naturally without judging them). Some practices, such as yoga and Tai Chi, include meditation with movement.

Numerous studies have explored whether meditation is helpful for a variety of conditions, such as high blood pressure, certain psychologic disorders, and pain. Research has also helped explain how meditation might work and how it affects the brain. Some evidence exists that meditation may lower blood pressure and reduce symptoms of ulcerative colitis. It may also ease anxiety, depression, and insomnia. Its effectiveness in treating pain and as a smoking-cessation treatment is uncertain.

Most people can engage safely in meditation. Meditation that involves physical movement may not be appropriate for individuals with physical limitations. Although rare, people with certain psychiatric disorders have reported worsening symptoms with meditation. Therefore, individuals with mental health disorders should consult their health care provider before practicing meditation. The meditation instructor should be informed of the patient's condition.

Massage Therapy

Massage is the manipulation of soft tissue to stimulate circulation, decrease pain, and promote relaxation. Maneuvers include stroking, rubbing, kneading, or tapping with varying amounts of pressure. Various types of massage, such as acupressure or shiatsu, can be used depending on the purpose and the patient's condition.

Massage has been the target of numerous research studies. Although the results are often preliminary or conflicting, there is scientific evidence that massage may help with back pain and may improve quality of life for people with depression, cancer, and human immunodeficiency virus/acquired immunodeficiency syndrome (HIV/AIDS).

When used appropriately and provided by a trained massage professional, it appears to have few risks. The effects appear to be short term so that repeated massages are necessary to maintain the benefits.

Acupuncture

Acupuncture is one of the practices used in TCM. Practitioners insert thin needles through the skin to stimulate specific points on the body. It is based on the theory that vital energy, called *qi*, flows through the body in channels that form a system of pathways called *meridians*. If the flow of energy through the channels is blocked, needles inserted in specific areas of the channels (acupoints) can restore the flow of qi.

The use of acupuncture for back and neck pain, osteoarthritis/knee pain, and headaches has been extensively studied and appears to be helpful. However, researchers do not yet know whether acupuncture can be helpful for various other health conditions. Studies are underway that are assessing the effects of acupuncture on menopausal hot flashes and discomfort associated with chemotherapy. Scientists note that it is possible that patient expectations and beliefs may play an important role in the beneficial effects of acupuncture on pain.

When performed by an experienced, well-trained practitioner using sterile needles, acupuncture is generally considered safe. Improperly performed acupuncture can cause infection, fainting, punctured organs, collapsed lungs, and injury to the central nervous system. Before visiting an acupuncturist, you should check their credentials. Requirements vary from state to state, but most require a license, diploma, certification, or registration. Some physicians and dentists practice acupuncture as well. Before beginning treatment, the patient should ask about the number of treatments expected and the treatment costs. Insurance companies may or may not cover the costs.

Relaxation Therapy

Relaxation therapy includes a variety of techniques designed to produce the body's natural relaxation response, characterized by slower breathing, lower blood pressure, and a feeling of increased well-being. Relaxation therapy is commonly included in stress management programs. A variety of practices such as progressive relaxation, guided imagery, biofeedback, self-hypnosis, and deep breathing exercises may be used to induce relaxation. Among the health conditions that may benefit from relaxation therapy are anxiety associated with illnesses or medical procedures, insomnia, labor pain, chemotherapy-induced nausea, and temporomandibular joint dysfunction.

Relaxation techniques are generally considered safe for healthy people, although there have been a few reports of negative experiences such as increased anxiety. People with serious physical or mental health problems or a history of abuse or trauma should discuss whether they should use relaxation techniques with their health care providers. People with heart disease should ask their health care provider before doing progressive muscle relaxation.

Tai Chi and Qi Gong

Tai Chi and qi gong are ancient mind and body practices that involve certain postures and gentle movements with mental focus, breathing, and relaxation. The movements can be adapted or practiced while walking, standing, or sitting, which accommodates individual abilities.

Possible benefits of Tai Chi may be improved balance and stability in older people and in those with Parkinson disease, reduced back pain and pain from knee osteoarthritis, and improved quality of life in people with chronic illnesses. Also, it may improve reasoning ability in older people. Both Tai Chi and qi gong may ease fibromyalgia pain and promote general quality of life. Qi gong may reduce chronic neck pain; however, study results have been mixed. Tai Chi and qi gong appear to have no negative effects except minor aches and pains. Instructors are not required to have licenses. However, training and certification are available through Tai Chi or qi gong organizations.

WHOLE MEDICAL SYSTEMS

Just as conventional Western medicine has evolved, so have other forms of medicine. They include Ayurvedic medicine, homeopathic medicine, traditional healing, Naturopathic medicine, and TCM. A brief description of each of these follows. The NCCIH (2015) issues the following caution about the use of these products and practices:

- Women who are pregnant or nursing, or people who are thinking of using complementary health practices to treat a child, should consult their (or their child's) health care providers.
- Tell all your health care providers about any complementary health practices you use. Give them a full picture of all you do to manage your health. This will ensure coordinated and safe care. (NCCIH, 2015, https://nccih.nih.gov/health/homeopathy)

AYURVEDIC MEDICINE

Ayurvedic medicine originated in India more than 3000 years ago and remains one of the country's traditional health care systems. It is a holistic approach that uses herbal compounds, metals, special diets, exercise, massage, lifestyle modifications, and other unique health practices. Although some research on Ayurvedic practices has been done, there are not enough high-quality studies to confirm or deny its effectiveness.

Some products used in Ayurvedic medicine contain herbs, minerals, or metals that may be harmful, particularly if used improperly. As discussed earlier, some herbs have significant side effects or interact with conventional medicines. Also ingesting some metals, such as lead, can be poisonous. In the United States, Ayurvedic products are marketed as dietary supplements, so they do not have to prove safety and efficacy. In 2008, an NIH study of 193 Ayurvedic products purchased over the Internet found that 21% of the products contained levels of lead, mercury, and/or arsenic that exceeded the standards for acceptable daily intake. People who use Ayurvedic medicine along with conventional medicine should discuss their treatments with the physician. Women who are pregnant or breastfeeding should not use Ayurvedic products unless approved by their physician. No states in the United States license Ayurvedic practitioners.

HOMEOPATHIC MEDICINE

Homeopathy is based on two unconventional theories: "like cures like" and "law of minimum dose." "Like cures like" claims that a disease can be cured by a substance that produces similar symptoms in healthy people. The "law of minimum dose" refers to the idea that the lower the dose of the medication, the greater its effectiveness. Among the substances used in homeopathy are plants, minerals, or animals, such as red onion, arnica (mountain herb), crushed whole bees, white arsenic, poison ivy, belladonna (deadly nightshade), and stinging nettle.

There is little scientific evidence to show effectiveness of homeopathy. Although regulated by the FDA, homeopathic products are not evaluated for safety or effectiveness. Even though highly dilute products are generally safe, the consumer does not know the actual dilution of individual products. Some of the products have side effects and interact with conventional drugs. Licensing laws for homeopathic practitioners vary from state to state.

TRADITIONAL HEALING

All cultures have traditional or folk medicine practices that were used before the advent of modern medicine. Examples are curanderismo and Native American healing. Traditional healers learn their skills mostly by observing experienced healers. The ability to heal is often considered a gift. Practices are based on indigenous theories, beliefs, and experiences passed down from one generation to the next. Traditional healing might use prayer, healing touch or laying on of hands, charms, herbal teas or tinctures, magic, and rituals.

NATUROPATHIC MEDICINE

Naturopathy focuses on primary care, overall well-being, and treatment of illnesses. Treatment approaches may include dietary and lifestyle changes, stress reduction, dietary supplement, homeopathy, manipulative therapies, exercise therapy, practitioner-guided detoxification, psychotherapy, and counseling.

Naturopathic practitioners in the United States may be naturopathic physicians, traditional naturopaths, or some other health care providers (dentists, nurses, chiropractors, etc.) who include naturopathy in their practices. Naturopathic physicians are usually educated in accredited 4-year graduate degree programs. Some states required licensure, others do not. Various nonaccredited programs are used by traditional naturopaths. They are usually not eligible for licensure.

TRADITIONAL CHINESE MEDICINE

The ancient beliefs on which TCM is based include the following:

- The human body is a miniature version of the larger, surrounding universe.
- Disease results from an imbalance between two opposing yet complementary forces, called *yin* and *yang*.
- Five elements—fire, earth, wood, metal, and water—symbolically represent all phenomena, including the stages of human life, and explain the functioning of the body and how it changes during disease.
- *Qi*, a vital energy that flows through the body, performs multiple functions in maintaining health.

Among the many different practices in TCM are acupuncture, moxibustion (burning an herb above the skin to apply heat to acupuncture points), Chinese herbal medicine, cupping (applying a heated cup to the skin to create a slight suction), tui na (Chinese therapeutic massage), dietary therapy, and Tai Chi and qi gong. In the United States, the most commonly used approaches are Chinese herbal medicine, acupuncture, and Tai Chi. Acupuncture, herbal therapy, Tai Chi, and qi gong have been discussed individually.

Acupuncture, Tai Chi, and qi gong are generally considered safe when performed properly. Herbal remedies carry greater risk because they may be contaminated and can have serious side effects. They may also interact with conventional drugs. Herbal products are marketed as dietary supplements, thereby avoiding stringent FDA requirements for safety and efficacy. Allergic reactions, burns, and infections have occurred with moxibustion. Both moxibustion and cupping may mark the skin temporarily and be mistaken for signs of disease or physical abuse.

NONMAINSTREAM PRODUCTS AND PRACTICES IN THE UNITED STATES

A large NIH survey assessed the use of nonmainstream products and practices among Americans. The most common approaches used and percent of Americans using that approach were as follows: natural products (17.7%), deep breathing (10.9%), yoga, Tai Chi, or qi gong (10.1%), chiropractic or osteopathic manipulation (8.4%), meditation (8.0%), and massage (6.9%). The most commonly used natural product was fish oil. Therapies reported by 3% or less included special diets, homeopathy, progressive relaxation, and guided imagery. The practice of yoga in the United States has increased dramatically in this century.

Why is the use of nontraditional therapies becoming more common in the United States? First, many people can be self-taught or learn from practitioners whose fees, if any, are typically less than those of physicians. Botanicals and other folk remedies are available without medical prescriptions. Second, nontraditional therapies are usually noninvasive. Third, they are part of a holistic approach to health and healing rather than just focusing on the disease or injury. Fourth, many people have found these therapies to be effective. Fifth, although not always true, people generally believe that nontraditional practices are safer than medical and surgical treatment. Sixth, a perception exists that anything labeled *natural* is better, which is also not necessarily true.

Many medical and nursing publications now include nontraditional therapies. As research on nonmainstream products and practices gains support, we are seeing more scientific information to use in discussing these remedies with patients. The Health Promotion box discusses some of the pros and cons of nonmainstream therapies.

Health Promotion

Considering Nonmainstream Therapies

The role of the nurse in relation to nontraditional remedies and therapies includes the following:

- When collecting data for the patient assessment, ask questions about the use of nonmainstream remedies or therapies, or both: "Do you use any natural products with or in place of prescribed drugs?" "Do you use any activities like yoga, exercise, or meditation for health reasons?" If the patient replies in the affirmative, note specific products or practices, amount used, and frequency of use. Ask whether the approach has been helpful and if the patient notices any negative effects.
- Be open-minded about nonmainstream practices as a valid choice by some patients. Learn about these therapies and try some if you feel comfortable doing so. For example, guided imagery and relaxation techniques are useful in many situations and have no adverse effects. However, do not attempt to use techniques with patients unless you have been properly instructed in their use. Professional education courses are a good place to learn noninvasive techniques that can be used with many types of patients.
- Teach patients about any adverse effects of nontraditional remedies.
- Be aware of potentially dangerous remedies and those that can interact with prescription drugs that the patient is taking. Potentially dangerous herbs include St John's Wort, sassafras, ephedra, chaparral, borage, calamus ("sweet flag"), comfrey, germander, life root, and pokeroot.
- Caution patients about very expensive therapies, especially if they make outlandish claims.

Get Ready for the NCLEX® Examination!

Key Points

- Complementary and alternative therapies are often based on holistic beliefs about the nature of health and illness.
- Complementary therapies are used along with conventional treatment; alternative therapies are used in place of conventional therapies.
- Integrative therapy is the use of both conventional and complementary or alternative therapies.
- Natural products used for health purposes include herbs/botanicals, vitamins, minerals, and probiotics.
- The labels of DSHEA-approved herbal products must state that the product is not intended to diagnose, treat, cure, or prevent any disease.
- Manufacturers of dietary supplements are not required to show evidence of safety and efficacy.
- Many dietary supplements lack scientific evidence of their safety and effectiveness.
- The CGMP require labels of dietary supplements to correctly state the identity, purity, quality, and strength of the contents.
- Most mind and body approaches are based on the belief that illness is caused by lack of balance or harmony within the individual or between the individual and the environment.
- Chiropractic uses spinal adjustments and other techniques to correct alignment problems, alleviate pain, improve function, and support the body's ability to heal itself.
- The essential components of meditation are: quiet, distraction-free setting; a specific, comfortable posture; a focus of attention; and an open attitude.
- Acupuncture is based on the belief that needles inserted in specific locations restore the flow of vital energy called *qi* to treat various conditions.
- Relaxation therapy is used to produce the body's natural relaxation response characterized by slower breathing, lower blood pressure, and feeling of increased well-being.
- Tai Chi and qi gong use postures and gentle movements with mental focus, breathing, and relaxation to improve balance, reduce pain, and improve the quality of life.
- Ayurvedic medicine, originated in India centuries ago, uses a variety of practices as well as many potentially unsafe herbals and metals.
- Homeopathic medicine treats illnesses with very low doses of substances that create symptoms similar to the condition being treated. It lacks scientific support.
- All cultures have some form of traditional or folk medicine that persist in modern society.
- TCM is based on the belief that disease results from an imbalance between two opposing but complementary forces called *yin* and *yang.*
- The use of nonmainstream products and practices is increasing in the United States.
- Advantages of nonmainstream products are that they do not require a prescription and are often less expensive than conventional medicine.
- The nurse should be open-minded about complementary and alternative therapies and should learn about them.

Additional Learning Resources

SG Go to your Study Guide for additional learning activities to help you master this chapter content.

Go to your Evolve website (http://evolve.elsevier.com/Linton/medsurg) for the following learning resources and much more:

- Fluid & Electrolyte Tutorial
- Review Questions for the NCLEX® Examination

Clinical Judgment and Next-Generation NCLEX® Examination-Style Questions

1. **A patient with cancer has decided to treat herself with herbal remedies instead of receiving chemotherapy and radiotherapy. The use of herbal remedies in this situation is an example of:**
   1. Complementary therapy
   2. Conventional therapy
   3. Alternative therapy
   4. Integrated therapy

   NCLEX Client Need: Physiological Integrity: Physiological Adaptation, Psychosocial Integrity

2. **A patient who takes prescription medications for a chronic condition is considering the complementary therapies listed. She asks how each therapy works. Which of these uses the power of the mind and body to affect each other?**
   1. Chiropractic
   2. Guided imagery
   3. Ginkgo biloba
   4. Homeopathy

   NCLEX Client Need: Physiological Integrity: Physiological Adaptation, Psychosocial Integrity

3. **In the United States, products that are classified as dietary supplements include which of the following? (Select all that apply.)**
   1. Herbs
   2. Minerals
   3. Tai Chi
   4. Vitamins
   5. Pilates

   NCLEX Client Need: Physiological Integrity: Physiological Adaptation, Psychosocial Integrity

4. **A nonmainstream therapy that uses spinal manipulations to alleviate pain and improve function is:**
   1. Yoga
   2. Massage therapy
   3. Acupuncture
   4. Chiropractic

   NCLEX Client Need: Physiological Integrity: Physiological Adaptation, Psychosocial Integrity

5. **What is the most important information to provide people with who are considering complementary therapy for joint pain?**
    1. Nonmainstream practices are generally safer than conventional therapy.
    2. Be sure to discuss additional therapies with your health care provider first.
    3. Products sold on the internet are required to be safe and effective.
    4. Nonmainstream therapies are as effective as conventional therapy, and less expensive.

    NCLEX Client Need: Physiological Integrity: Physiological Adaptation, Psychosocial Integrity

6. **The main concern with Ayurvedic medicine products has been:**
    1. Excessive cost
    2. Contamination with toxic substances
    3. Interactions with conventional medications
    4. Unavailability of products in the United States

    NCLEX Client Need: Physiological Integrity: Physiological Adaptation, Psychosocial Integrity

7. **In general, what has research shown about acupuncture? (Select all that apply.)**
    1. It is considered safe when properly performed.
    2. Incorrect technique can injure internal organs.
    3. It appears to be helpful for neck and back pain.
    4. Patient expectations may affect the perceived benefits.
    5. Acupuncture practitioners have no professional credentials.

    NCLEX Client Need: Physiological Integrity: Physiological Adaptation, Psychosocial Integrity

8. **The most commonly used nonmainstream therapy in the United States is:**
    1. Yoga
    2. Relaxation therapy
    3. Meditation
    4. Natural products

    NCLEX Client Need: Physiological Integrity: Physiological Adaptation, Psychosocial Integrity

9. **The role of the nurse in relation to nonmainstream therapies is to: (Select all that apply.)**
    1. Document the use of any nonmainstream products and therapies.
    2. Inform patients of alternative therapies to their mainstream drugs.
    3. Discourage the use of nonmainstream products and practices.
    4. Respect the right of patient to choose conventional or nonmainstream therapies.
    5. Inform patients about resources for accurate information about nonmainstream therapies.

    NCLEX Client Need: Physiological Integrity: Physiological Adaptation, Psychosocial Integrity

10. **Magnet therapy, light therapy, and healing touch are examples of:**
    1. Movement therapies
    2. Mind and body interventions
    3. Energy therapies
    4. Body-based practices

    NCLEX Client Need: Physiological Integrity: Physiological Adaptation, Psychosocial Integrity

11. **SLO Objective: Describe the role of the nurse in educating patients about nonmainstream therapies**

    NGN Item Type: Matrix

    Cognitive Skill: Generate Solutions

    Patient Situation: A new patient in a neighborhood clinic takes a low-dose aspirin daily and medication for high blood pressure. She reports drinking cranberry juice for recurring urinary infections and glucosamine for joint pain. She also takes black cohosh for menopausal symptoms. The physical examination reveals multiple bruises but no other abnormal findings. How should the nurse respond to this information?

    Use an X for the nursing actions listed below that are *Indicated/Anticipated* (appropriate or necessary), *Contraindicated* (could be harmful), or *Nonessential* (makes no difference or not necessary) for the client's care at this time.

NURSING ACTION	INDICATED	CONTRAINDI-CATED	NONES-SENTIAL
Advise the patient to stop taking low-dose aspirin			
Inform the patient that herbal remedies are safer than prescription drugs.			
Tell the patient that her prescription drugs and herbals can have serious interactions.			
Inform the patient that aspirin, glucosamine and cranberry juice may contribute to easy bruising.			

Neurologic System Introduction

21

http://evolve.elsevier.com/Linton/medsurg

Objectives

1. Describe the anatomy and physiology of the nervous system.
2. Identify age-related changes in the neurologic system.
3. List the components of the nursing assessment of the patient with a neurologic disorder.
4. Explain the diagnostic tests and procedures used to evaluate neurologic function and the nursing responsibilities associated with each.
5. Distinguish the uses, side effects, and nursing interventions associated with common drug therapies used in patients with neurologic disorders.

Key Terms

ipsilateral (ĭp-sĭ-LĂT-ĕr-ăl)
neurotransmitter (nū-rō-TRĂNS-mĭ-tĕr)
autonomic nervous system
thoracolumbar system
contralateral
craniosacral system
axons
dendrites
depolarization
myelin
repolarization
afferent neurons
efferent neurons
interneurons
decorticate
decerebrate

Neurologic disease and injury present some of the greatest challenges in health care today. Nurses provide care for patients in both the acute and rehabilitation phases of recovery. The long-term effects of many neurologic disorders are frequently devastating to the patient and the family. An important aspect of care is assisting the patient and family to adjust physically and emotionally to the alterations that often result from neurologic dysfunction.

ANATOMY AND PHYSIOLOGY OF THE NERVOUS SYSTEM

The nervous system may be thought of as an elaborate control system that coordinates and regulates all bodily functions. It receives and interprets information from the external environment and initiates responses to the specific information internally.

The nervous system is divided into two main parts: (1) the central nervous system (CNS), made up of the brain and spinal cord; and (2) the peripheral nervous system, which comprises all nerves of the distal parts of the body, including both spinal and cranial nerves.

CENTRAL NERVOUS SYSTEM

Brain

The central structures of the brain include the cerebrum, the cerebellum, and the brainstem (Fig. 21.1). The cerebrum is composed of left and right hemispheres, which are subdivided into specific lobes. It is the largest and most highly developed part of the brain. It has many complex functions, including initiation of movements, recognition of sensory input, higher-order thinking, regulation of emotional behavior, and regulation of endocrine and autonomic functions.

The cerebrum is divided into two halves, called *hemispheres*, connected by the corpus callosum. Each hemisphere controls the opposite side of the body; that is, the right hemisphere controls the left side of the body and the left hemisphere controls the right side of the body. For most people, the left hemisphere is dominant. This hemisphere controls the more analytic mental processes such as language acquisition and use, mathematics, and reasoning powers. The right hemisphere encompasses emotional and artistic tendencies. Each hemisphere of the cerebral cortex is divided into the parietal, frontal, temporal, and occipital lobes. Each lobe has a different area of function (Fig. 21.2).

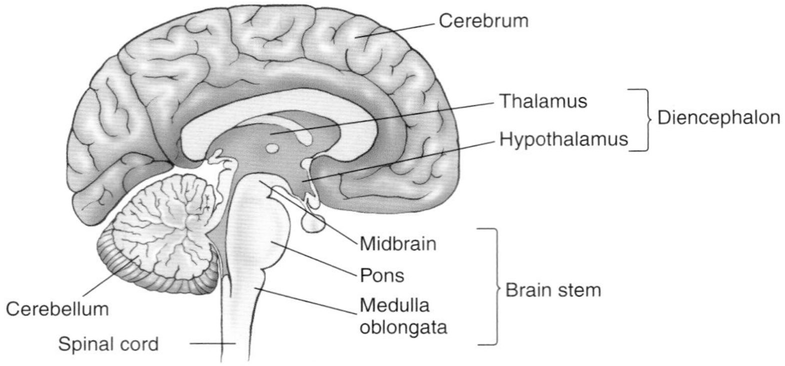

Fig. 21.1 Structures of the brain (coronal section). (From Leonard PC: *Building a medical vocabulary with Spanish translations*, ed 10, St Louis, 2018, Elsevier.)

The thalamus, hypothalamus, and basal ganglia are other important structures identified in the cerebrum.

The cerebellum is located at the back of the brain beneath the occipital and temporal lobes of the cerebrum and accounts for about 10% of the brain's volume. The cerebellum coordinates movement, balance, and posture.

The brainstem includes the midbrain, pons, medulla, and part of the reticular activating system. The brainstem controls vital basic functions, including respiration, heart rate, and consciousness. Box 21.1 lists the functions of the major parts of the brain.

Cerebrospinal fluid (CSF) is composed primarily of water, glucose, sodium chloride, and protein. It is produced in the ventricles of the brain in the arachnoid granulations. CSF circulates within the subarachnoid space, the ventricles, and the central canal of the spinal cord (Fig. 21.3). The fluid is reabsorbed in the arachnoid villi. The CSF acts as a shock absorber for the brain and spinal cord. If excess fluid forms or if fluid is not normally reabsorbed, pressure within the ventricular system increases.

Brain Circulation

The brain is rich with arterial circulation to satisfy its need for oxygen. Fig. 21.4 shows the major cerebral arteries. Although the brain comprises only 2% of the body's weight, it consumes 20% of the oxygen supply and cardiac circulation each minute. The two major arterial systems are (1) the carotid, and (2) the vertebral arteries. The carotid system begins as one common artery that later divides into the external and internal carotid arteries. The external carotid arteries divide to supply blood to the face. The internal arteries further divide into the middle cerebral artery and the anterior cerebral artery to supply blood to the brain. The vertebral arteries originate from the subclavian artery and travel up the brainstem. A second division forms the posterior cerebral artery. The internal carotid arteries and vertebral-basilar arteries unite to form the circle of Willis. Some people have anatomic differences in bold vessels that can increase the likelihood that they will sustain a cerebrovascular accident (CVA).

Spinal Cord

The spinal cord extends from the border of the first cervical vertebra (C1) to the level of the second lumbar vertebra (L2). Thirty-one pairs of spinal nerve roots exit from the spinal cord, each consisting of a *posterior sensory* (afferent) root and *anterior motor* (efferent) root (Fig. 21.5). These nerve roots, along with the 12 cranial nerves, make up the peripheral nervous system.

PERIPHERAL NERVOUS SYSTEM

Part of the peripheral nervous system, known as the **autonomic nervous system**, helps to maintain homeostasis for the body. The autonomic nervous system controls the involuntary activities of the viscera, including smooth muscles, cardiac muscle, and glands. The two major subdivisions of the autonomic nervous system are (1) the sympathetic nervous system and (2) the parasympathetic nervous system.

Stress triggers the sympathetic nervous system to increase the secretion of epinephrine and norepinephrine. These neurotransmitters increase heart rate and constrict peripheral blood vessels, causing the blood pressure to rise. This reaction to stress is called the *fight or flight response.* The sympathetic nervous system is also referred to as the **thoracolumbar system**.

Conversely, the parasympathetic nervous system mediates a rest response. Stimulation of this system results in decreased heart rate and blood pressure. The parasympathetic nervous system is also known as the **craniosacral system**. Specific effects of the stimulation of the sympathetic and parasympathetic nervous systems are outlined in Table 21.1.

The functional unit of the nervous system is the neuron (nerve cell), which conducts electrical impulses from cell to cell. The main cell body has branches called **axons** and **dendrites**. Axons conduct impulses away from the cell body and dendrites convey impulses toward the cell body. Many axons and dendrites are covered with a material called **myelin,** which enhances conduction along nerve fibers. Myelin gives the axons

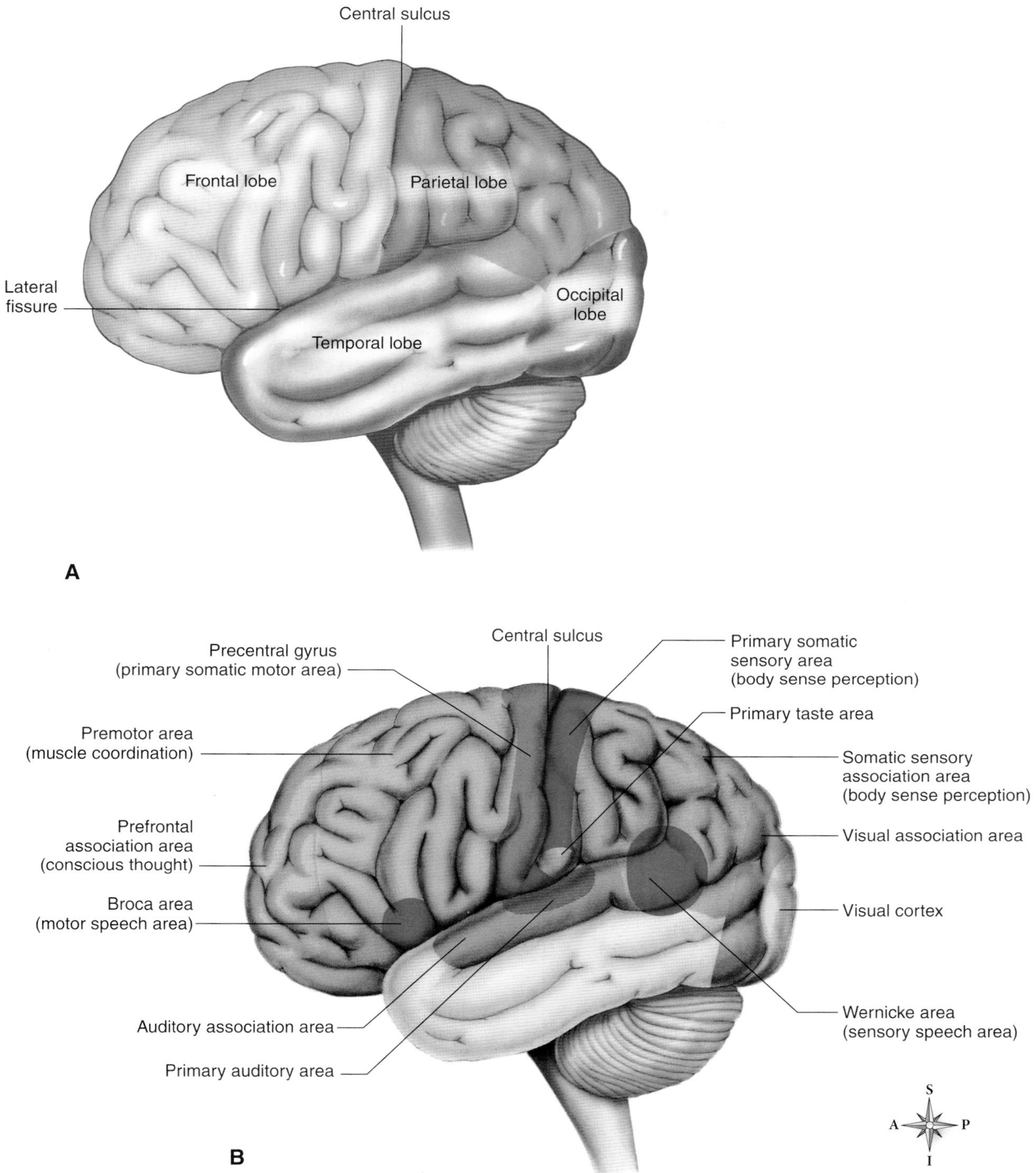

Fig. 21.2 Control zones of the brain. (A) The lobes of the cerebral cortex. (B) The areas of function in each lobe. (From Patton KT, Thibodeau GA: *Human body in health & disease,* ed 7, St. Louis, 2018, Elsevier.)

a white appearance (white matter), whereas cell bodies without myelin are gray (gray matter) (Fig. 21.6).

Coordinated, organized function is a result of a well-integrated system of impulse transmission. When the end of a dendrite is stimulated, a series of electrochemical events are initiated. At the point of stimulation, sodium and potassium ions are exchanged, resulting in a process called **depolarization**. This process continues down the dendrite to the axon, until the ions return to their resting state. This return to the resting state is known as **repolarization**.

Impulses must be able to pass from one neuron to another across the neural synapse—the space between the axons of one neuron and the dendrites of the next neuron. When an impulse reaches the end of its axon, a biochemical messenger called a **neurotransmitter** is released. Among the most understood neurotransmitters are acetylcholine, norepinephrine,

Box 21.1 Functions of the Major Parts of the Brain

BRAINSTEM AND DIENCEPHALON
Control awareness or alertness through the reticular activating system, composed of fibers scattered throughout the midbrain, pons, and medulla.

MEDULLA
Links the higher brain centers to other parts of the body through the spinal cord. Controls muscles of respiration through the respiratory reflex center. Controls the heartbeat (to some extent) through the cardiac reflex center. Constricts blood vessels to raise blood pressure through the vasomotor reflex center. Is the point of origin for some cranial nerves.

PONS
Relays messages from the medulla to the higher centers in the brain. Is a reflex center for some cranial nerves.

CEREBELLUM
Coordinates movement, balance, posture, and spatial orientation.

HYPOTHALAMUS
Controls the pituitary. Controls appetite, sleep, and some emotions. Controls much activity of the autonomic nervous system.

FOREBRAIN (CEREBRUM)
Controls the higher functions and activities: conscious mental processes, sensations, emotions, and voluntary movements.

FRONTAL LOBE
Controls the voluntary muscle movements, verbal and written speech.

PARIETAL LOBE
Contains the sensory reception areas to interpret pain, touch, temperature, distances, sizes, and shapes.

TEMPORAL LOBE
Contains the auditory center for hearing and understanding spoken language. Contains the olfactory center for smell.

OCCIPITAL LOBE
Contains the visual center for seeing and reading.

From Jacob SW, Francone CA: *Elements of anatomy and physiology*, ed 2, Philadelphia, 1989, Saunders.

epinephrine, and dopamine. The neurotransmitter crosses the synapse to the neighboring dendrite, where it stimulates an electrical impulse. The process of depolarization then continues down the length of the nerve cells.

Neurons are classified according to their particular functions. Those that transmit information from distal parts of the body or environment toward the CNS are sensory neurons, also known as **afferent** ("bearing toward") neurons. Motor information is carried from the CNS to the periphery by motor neurons, also known as **efferent** ("bearing away from") neurons. **Interneurons** also exist and are like relay stations between sensory and motor neurons.

AGE-RELATED CHANGES

With normal aging, the number of nerve cells decreases. Brain weight is reduced, and the ventricles increase in size. An aging pigment called *lipofuscin* is deposited in nerve cells, along with amyloid, a type of protein. Increased plaques and tangled fibers are found in the cerebral nerve tissue. These changes are associated with Alzheimer disease but are also seen in the brains of people who have no symptoms of dementia. Fortunately, many more nerve cells are present than are needed for normal function. Thus the majority of older people retain normal cognition and function despite the decreasing number of nerve cells.

The physical examination reveals some neurologic changes typical of aging. The pupil of the eye is often smaller and may respond to light more slowly. When asked to track (follow with the eyes) a moving object, the older person's eye movements may be jerky rather than smooth. Reflexes are usually intact except for the Achilles tendon jerk, which is often absent.

Older people frequently demonstrate some changes in functional abilities as well. Reaction time increases with aging, especially for complex reactions. Tremors in the head, face, and hands are common. Some older people develop dizziness and problems with balance. These are not considered normal age-related changes but may be related to disease or drug side effects.

Put On Your Thinking Cap!

Identify three implications for nursing care related to normal neurologic changes that occur with age.

PATHOPHYSIOLOGY OF NEUROLOGIC DISEASES

Potential causes of neurologic disorders include developmental and genetic disorders, trauma, infections and inflammation, neoplasms, degenerative processes, vascular disorders, and metabolic and endocrine disorders.

- **Developmental and genetic disorders:** Developmental disorders include structural problems such as hydrocephalus. An example of a genetic disorder is Huntington disease.
- **Trauma:** CNS injuries resulting from trauma can be life threatening or severely disabling. Physical trauma to the nervous system may follow accidental injury, violent crime, or chemical injury caused by drugs, alcohol, or other harmful substances.
- **Inflammation and infection:** Meningitis and encephalitis are examples of disease states that cause inflammation of meningeal tissue and brain tissue, respectively. Causative agents may be viruses or bacteria that can be transmitted by a variety of vectors and routes.

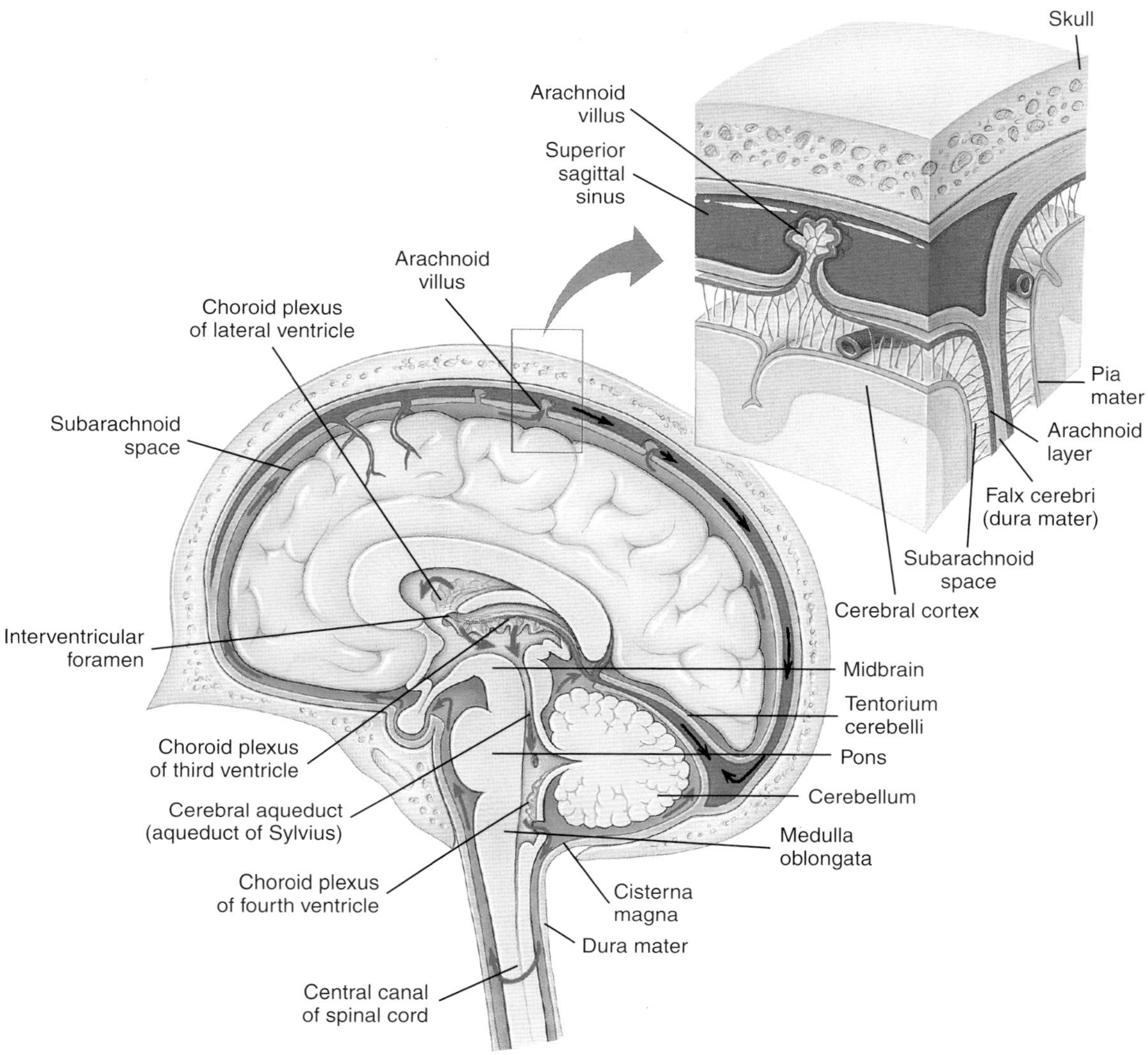

Fig. 21.3 Structures of the brainstem and cerebrospinal fluid (CSF) circulation. *Red arrows* represent the route of the CSF. *Black arrows* represent the route of blood flow. CSF is produced in the ventricles, exits the fourth ventricle, and returns to the venous circulation in the superior sagittal sinus. The inset depicts the arachnoid granulations in the superior sagittal sinus, where the CSF enters the circulation. (From Wilson SF, Giddens JF: *Health assessment for nursing practice*, ed 5, St. Louis, 2013, Mosby.)

- **Neoplasms:** CNS tumors may be primary or metastatic in origin. Although considerable progress has been made in treating these tumors, definitive therapy can be difficult to achieve, depending on the cell type involved in the tumor and the degree of invasion of surrounding tissue.
- **Degenerative processes:** The primary degenerative disease of the brain is Alzheimer disease, a progressive condition that begins with memory loss, and eventually results in severe mental and physical deterioration. Alzheimer disease is discussed in Chapter 13. Other degenerative disorders are multiple sclerosis (MS), Parkinson disease, amyotrophic lateral sclerosis (ALS, also known as *Lou Gehrig disease*), and Huntington disease.
- **Vascular disorders:** Any factor that interferes with blood flow to nervous tissue can lead to cell death, with resulting loss of function. Nerve tissue is so sensitive to hypoxia that cells begin to die after being deprived of oxygen for 4 minutes. Neurologic disorders associated with impaired blood flow include cerebrovascular accident (see Chapter 23) and vascular dementia. Vascular abnormalities, including aneurysms and arteriovenous malformations, can rupture or prevent the delivery of adequate oxygen to affected tissue.
- **Metabolic and endocrine disorders:** The brain depends on constant supplies of glucose and other nutrients. Disturbances in glucose metabolism and electrolyte imbalances can lead to deterioration in thought

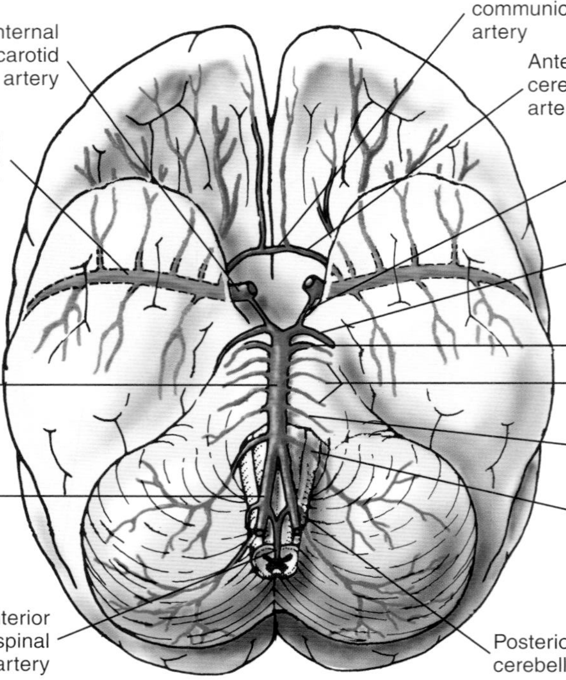

Fig. 21.4 Cerebral circulation. (From Ignatavicius DD, Workman ML: *Medical-surgical nursing: patient-centered collaborative care*, ed 7, St. Louis, 2013, Saunders, 2013.)

processes and level of consciousness. Neurologic dysfunction also can result from accumulation of toxins, as in poisoning, renal failure, and liver failure.

NURSING ASSESSMENT OF NEUROLOGIC FUNCTION

Any evaluation begins with an accurate assessment, which may be initiated by the nurse. The licensed vocational nurse/licensed practical nurse (LVN/LPN) assists with the assessment by collecting relevant data. Much of the assessment requires simply observing the patient, and then recording the findings. Box 21.2 lists components of assessment of a patient with a neurologic disorder.

HEALTH HISTORY

Reason for Seeking Care

Document the event that prompted the patient to seek medical attention and describe any injuries. A complete description of the illness includes the initial symptoms and how the symptoms progressed.

Present Health

Throughout the assessment, the patient's speech, behavior, coordination, alertness, and comprehension should be noted. Immediately begin to study the patient's ability to understand language and to respond verbally and nonverbally. Responses to simple yes-or-no commands provide a good basis for initial assessment. Evaluate verbal responses, facial expressions, and physical reactions for appropriateness. If responses are not appropriate, try to identify the source of difficulty. Does the patient have trouble finding words? Do clues help the patient to respond? Does the patient speak fluently? If the patient cannot provide the information needed, attempt to obtain it from a family member or friend. Note the name of the informant (the person who provides the history) and assess the patient's orientation to person, place, and time.

Past Health History

Past neurologic disorders and pertinent signs and symptoms are vital pieces of information. Ask about a history of head injury, seizures and previous strokes, or transient ischemic attacks (TIAs). Record past serious illnesses or conditions, including hypertension, heart disease, diabetes mellitus, liver disease, gout, and cancer. Note previous hospitalizations, operations, and injuries.

Record dates and types of immunizations, including influenza, and list current medications. In addition, record current drugs and highlight allergies according to agency policy.

Family History

Questions about the presence of neurologic disease or other diseases in the immediate family may elicit valuable information about risk factors, such as those for stroke or neuromuscular diseases. Thus ask whether any immediate family members have had heart disease, stroke, diabetes mellitus, cancer,

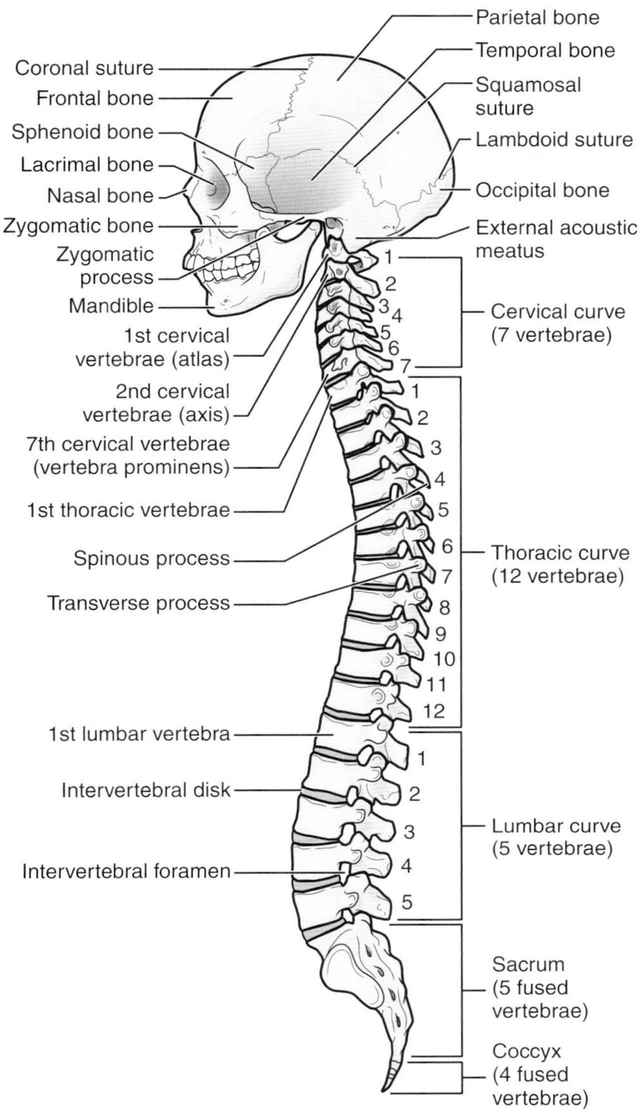

Fig. 21.5 Bony structure of the skull and vertebral column.

seizure disorders, muscular dystrophy, or Huntington disease.

Review of Systems

Ask the patient about significant problems. Important items to assess include weakness, impaired movement, pain (especially headache), dysphagia, bowel or bladder incontinence, visual disturbances, mental or emotional changes, and altered sensation.

Observe the patient's general appearance, responsiveness, and behavior and record any displays of restlessness or agitation. The patient's level of consciousness is important because subtle changes in level of consciousness such as confusion, irritability, or a decrease in level of consciousness may suggest a stroke in evolution or increasing intracranial pressure (ICP). Measure vital signs. A description of the patient's breathing pattern and effort are especially important. If possible, obtain the patient's weight and height.

Throughout the examination, inspect the skin for lesions and color change and palpate for temperature. Assess hydration status by evaluating tissue turgor and moisture of mucous membranes. Inspect the head for lesions and palpate for masses or swelling. Observe the patient's respiratory effort and auscultate breath sounds.

Inspect the face for symmetry, and assess the mouth for moisture and drooling, then evaluate the alert patient's ability to swallow. Inspect the patient's pupils for size, equality, and reaction to light. Conduct a gross vision assessment by asking the patient to read something. Inspect the patient's skin for color and palpate for moisture and turgor. Assess extremities for muscle tone and strength, sensation, and voluntary movement. Instruct the patient to move each extremity individually and observe the

Table 21.1 Effects of Sympathetic and Parasympathetic Stimulation

ORGAN	EFFECT OF SYMPATHETIC STIMULATION	EFFECT OF PARASYMPATHETIC STIMULATION
Eye		
Pupil	Dilated	Constricted
Ciliary muscle	Slight relaxation (far vision)	Constricted (near vision)
Glands: nasal, lacrimal, parotid	Vasoconstriction and slight secretion	Stimulation of copious secretions
Sweat glands	Copious sweating (cholinergic)	Sweating on palms of hands
Apocrine glands	Thick, odoriferous secretion	None
Blood vessels	Mostly constricted	Most often little or no effect
Heart		
Muscle	Increased rate	Slowed rate
	Increased force of contractions	Decreased force of contractions (especially atria)
Coronary arteries	Dilated ($beta_2$), constricted (alpha)	Dilated

Continued

Table 21.1 Effects of Sympathetic and Parasympathetic Stimulation—cont'd

ORGAN	EFFECT OF SYMPATHETIC STIMULATION	EFFECT OF PARASYMPATHETIC STIMULATION
Lungs		
Bronchi	Dilated	Constricted
Blood vessels	Mildly constricted	Dilated
Gut		
Lumen	Decreased peristalsis and tone	Increased peristalsis and tone
Sphincter	Increased tone (most times)	Relaxed (most times)
Liver	Glucose released	Slight glycogen synthesis
Gallbladder and bile ducts	Relaxed	Contracted
Kidney	Decreased output; increased renin secretion	None
Bladder		
Detrusor	Relaxed (slight)	Contracted
Trigone	Contracted	Relaxed
Penis	Ejaculation	Erection
Systemic Arterioles		
Abdominal viscera	Constricted	None
Muscle	Constricted (alpha adrenergic) Dilated ($beta_2$ adrenergic) Dilated (cholinergic)	None
Skin	Constricted	None
Blood		
Coagulation	Increased	None
Glucose	Increased	None
Lipids	Increased	None
Basal metabolism	Increased up to 100%	None
Adrenal medullary secretions	Increased	None
Mental activity	Increased	None
Piloerector muscles	Contracted	None
Skeletal muscle	Increased glycogenolysis Increased strength	None
Fat cells	Lipolysis	None

Modified from Hall JE: *Guyton and Hall textbook of medical physiology*, ed 12, Philadelphia, 2011 Saunders.

responses. Impaired movement or inappropriate response may be caused by aphasia or dyspraxia, as well as by neuromuscular damage. The patient who has aphasia has difficulty interpreting messages and may not perform the requested movement for that reason. The patient with dyspraxia may comprehend instructions but be unable to direct the body part to move. Also record any evidence of incontinence or bladder distention.

Neurologic checks consisting of evaluating level of consciousness, pupil appearance and response to light, the patient's ability to follow commands, and the movement and sensation of extremities should be conducted frequently. These checks, along with vital signs, are essential to detect increasing ICP if it is not being monitored.

PHYSICAL EXAMINATION

Basic Neurologic Examination

The neurologic examination should be completed when the patient is stable. A neurologic assessment provides baseline data to compare with ongoing assessments and serves as the basis for developing the nursing care plan. Four major components of a routine neurologic examination that provide valuable information regarding the overall integrity of the CNS are (1) level of consciousness, (2) pupillary evaluation, (3) neuromuscular response, and (4) vital signs. Look at the trends in the patient's neurologic status. A single finding considered in isolation may not provide a true picture of the patient's status. For example, one elevated blood pressure reading may not be significant but continuing increases may be associated with increased ICP.

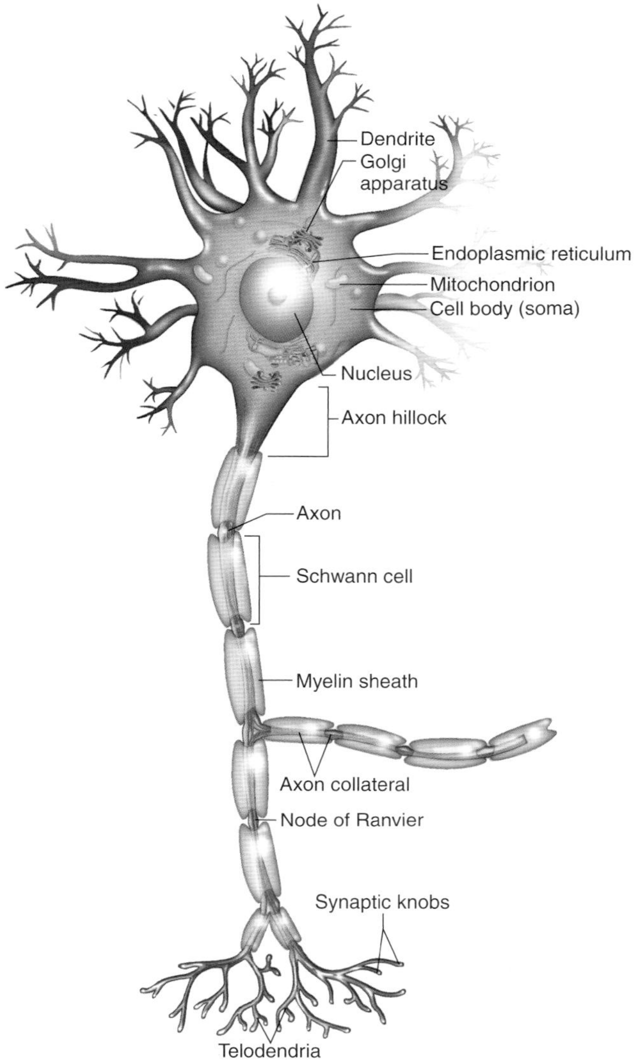

Fig. 21.6 A neuron (nerve cell). The dendrites receive incoming messages. The axons convey outgoing signals. (From Patton K: Thibodeau G. *Anatomy & physiology*, ed 8, St. Louis, 2013, Mosby.)

Box 21.2 Assessment of the Patient With a Neurologic Disorder

HEALTH HISTORY

Reason for Seeking Care
Event requiring medical attention

Present Health History
Onset and progression of condition. Reliability and ability of patient to provide information

Past Health History
Head injury, seizures, other neurologic disorders, other diseases (diabetes mellitus, hypertension, heart disease, cancer), dates of immunizations, current medications, allergies

Family History
Stroke, neuromuscular diseases, heart disease, diabetes mellitus, cancer, seizures

Review of Systems
Fatigue, weakness, headache, dizziness, vertigo, changes in vision or hearing, tinnitus, drainage from nose or ears, dysphagia, neck pain or stiffness, vomiting, bladder or bowel dysfunction, fainting, blackouts, tremors, paralysis, incoordination, numbness or tingling, memory problems, mood changes

Functional Assessment
Usual occupation and activities, effect on life, changes in sexuality, changes in activities of daily living (ADL), sources of stress, usual coping strategies, sources of support

PHYSICAL EXAMINATION

Height and Weight: If/when stable
Initial Level of Consciousness: Response to stimulation
Pupils: Size, shape, response to light, equality
Neuromuscular Status: Voluntary movement, reflexes
Vital Signs: Blood pressure, pulse, respirations, temperature
Skin: Lesions, injuries, turgor
Head: Lesions, injuries, masses, swelling
Oral Cavity: Moisture
Thorax: Respiratory effort, breath sounds
Abdomen: Distention, bowel sounds
Extremities: Injuries, abnormal positions

Level of consciousness. The most accurate and reliable indicator of neurologic status is level of consciousness. Evaluate patients for orientation to person, place, and time by asking them to state their names, where they are, and what time it is. Evaluate the degree of stimulation required to evoke a response from the patient. If the patient responds only to vigorous physical stimulation, consciousness is more impaired than if the patient responds immediately to a verbal greeting. Consider patient behavior in response to stimulation. Does the patient respond pleasantly or are they combative, agitated, or lethargic? All of these observations provide additional information regarding mental status.

Some of the common terms used to describe altered levels of consciousness are *somnolence*, *lethargy*, *stupor*, *semicoma*, and *coma*. Somnolence is unnatural drowsiness or sleepiness. Lethargy is also used to describe excessive drowsiness. Stupor suggests decreased responsiveness accompanied by lack of spontaneous motor activity. If a patient is in a stupor (stuporous) but can be aroused, the term *semicomatose* is used. A patient who cannot be aroused even by powerful stimuli is said to be in a coma, or comatose.

Because the terms related to altered levels of consciousness are open to interpretation, it is clearer to describe the patient's response to specific stimuli. The description should always begin with the mildest stimuli and stop when a response is elicited. The mildest stimulus is simply approaching the patient. This can be followed, in order, with verbal stimuli, with tactile stimuli (shaking the shoulder gently), and finally with painful stimuli. Appropriate methods of applying painful stimuli include applying pressure on the nail bed using an object such as a pen, pressing on the sternum, or pinching the trapezius muscle firmly between the thumb and forefinger and twisting.

Pupillary evaluation. The second major component of the neurologic assessment is the pupillary evaluation. To evaluate the pupils, assess and compare their size, shape, and reactivity. Pupils are normally about 3 mm in size, round, and react briskly to light. Changes in equality or reactivity from one assessment to the next may indicate neurologic deterioration.

Neuromuscular response. Assessment of neuromuscular response provides a means of evaluating cerebral and spinal cord function. All electrical impulses responsible for eliciting motor responses are initiated in the frontal lobe of the cerebral cortex. The impulses travel down the brainstem into the spinal cord. Motor spinal nerve roots then stimulate muscle movement.

Vital signs. Monitoring pulse, respirations, and blood pressure provides highly reliable information regarding neurologic well-being. However, changes in vital signs are late indicators of deterioration. The significance of these values is discussed in detail in the section entitled "Increased Intracranial Pressure." Elevated temperature may be associated with infection or with impaired thermoregulation. Fig. 21.7 is a sample assessment tool that includes the Glasgow Coma Scale. This scale is commonly used to rate the patient's eye-opening response, motor response, and verbal response. The numeric ratings are totaled for a summary score. A normal, alert person would score 15; a person in a coma would score 7 or less.

Advanced Neurologic Examination

Baseline and serial examinations are critical in the evaluation of the patient with a neurologic disorder. Cranial nerve function, coordination and balance, neuromuscular function, sensory function, and reflexes are the components that can assist the health care provider in localizing the area of injury or disease and in developing a plan of care relevant to the individual patient.

Cranial nerves. The cranial nerves mediate various motor, sensory, and autonomic functions. The cranial nerves enter and exit the brain rather than the spinal cord. The primary function of the cranial nerve is to control sensory, motor, and autonomic activities of the head and neck. The *vagus nerve* affects autonomic cardiac, respiratory, gastric, and gallbladder function. The examiner with advanced assessment skills may assess each nerve individually (Table 21.2).

Coordination and balance. Both the cerebellum and the cerebral cortex influence coordination and balance. Cerebellar dysfunction creates loss of steady, balanced posture and gait on the **ipsilateral** side (same side) as the brain lesion. Lesions of the cortex, however, cause motor dysfunction on the contralateral side (opposite side) of the lesion.

Observation of routine activity, such as ambulation, feeding, or performing activities of daily living (ADL), can provide valuable information about coordination and balance. In the assessment of balance, ask the patient to walk 10 to 20 feet away, turn, and walk back toward you. Observe the patient's gait and arm swing, then ask the patient to walk a straight line in a heel-to-toe fashion.

To perform the Romberg test, have the patient stand with feet together and arms at their sides. Instruct the patient to close their eyes and maintain that position (while you stay close by in case the patient starts to fall). Normally, the patient will display only slight swaying. To evaluate coordination of movements:

1. Ask the patient to pat their knees with the palms of the hands, and then with the backs of the hands in a rapid, alternating pattern.
2. Hold up one of your fingers, and instruct the patient to touch it with their index finger.
3. Ask the patient to touch their nose with the index finger, first with the eyes open, and then with the eyes closed.
4. Ask the patient to run the heel of one foot down the shin of the other leg, and then repeat with the opposite heel.
5. Have the patient alternate tapping with the heel, and then the toes of one foot, and then the other foot.

Normally these responses are done smoothly and rapidly.

Neuromuscular function. Muscle strength is assessed by using passive range-of-motion exercises and by testing strength against gravity and against resistance applied by the examiner. Instruct the patient to try to move the extremity against the examiner's hand. Evaluate both upper and lower extremities and compare one side to the other. Function is graded on a scale of 0 (complete paralysis) to 5 (normal strength) (Table 21.3). If the patient is unconscious, some noxious stimulus, such as pressure on the nail bed, must be applied to determine whether movement is possible.

Evaluate individual muscle groups by assessing their size, tone, and strength. Upper arm strength is evaluated by having the patient provide resistance to a movement. For example, you can ask the patient to extend the arms and bend the elbows, while alternately trying to push the examiner away or pull the examiner forward. To test the strength of the intrinsic muscles of the hand, have the patient spread the fingers apart, and then resist having them pushed together. To test the strength of hand grasp, have the patient put one finger on top of another so that a firm squeeze will not painfully press the knuckles together. Also instruct the patient to lift each hand or to raise a finger on each hand. To assess for a subtle weakness in upper arm strength, have the patient extend both arms forward with the palms up. Ask the patient to close their eyes

MISSION HOSPITAL
REGIONAL MEDICAL CENTER

ADULT NEURO FLOW SHEET

TIME

			0700	0800	0900	1000	1100	1200	1300	1400	1500	1600	1700	1800	1900	2000	2100	2200	2300	2400	0100	0200	0300	0400	0500	0600
GLASGOW COMA SCALE		Eyes open																								
		Best motor																								
		Best verbal																								
		TOTAL																								
VOLUNTARY MOTOR	Right	Upper extremity																								
		Lower extremity																								
	Left	Upper extremity																								
		Lower extremity																								
CRANIAL NERVES — PUPILS	Right	Size																								
		Reaction																								
	Left	Size																								
		Reaction																								
EOMS	Conjugate																									
	Disconjugate																									
	Tracking	Right																								
		Left																								
	Blink reflex																									
	Gag reflex																									
	Facial symmetry																									
			0700	0800	0900	1000	1100	1200	1300	1400	1500	1600	1700	1800	1900	2000	2100	2200	2300	2400	0100	0200	0300	0400	0500	0600

TIME

KEY

MOTOR
5+ Normal power
4+ Weakness
3+ Anti-gravity
2+ Not anti-gravity
1+ Trace
0 No movement

Pupil Size
B = Brisk
S = Sluggish
A = Absent

2 mm 3 mm 4 mm 5 mm

6 mm 7 mm 8 mm

, = Present
O = Absent
S = Symmetrical
A = Asymmetrical

Date

Speech patterns: ______

Comments: ______

GLASGOW COMA SCALE			
Eyes Open	4	Spontaneously
	3	To verbal command
	2	To pain
	1	No response
Best Motor Response	6	Obeys command
	5	Localize pain
	4	Flexion to pain withdraw
	3	Flexion decorticate
	2	Extension to pain (decerebrate)
	1	No response to pain
Best Verbal Response	5	Oriented
	4	Confused
	3	Inappropriate words
	2	Incomprehensible sounds
	1	No response

Unit ______

R.N. signature ______ Shift: ______

R.N. signature ______ Shift: ______

R.N. signature ______ Shift: ______

Form: 408 5/92 **Adult Neuro Flow Sheet**

ADDRESSOGRAPH

Fig. 21.7 A neurologic flow sheet is used to record the assessment of neurologic function. (Courtesy Linda R. Littlejohn, RN, BSN, CCRN, Neuro Clinician, and Mission Hospital Regional Medical Center, Mission Viejo, CA.)

and maintain the position for 10 to 20 seconds. With normal strength, the arms remain steady. In the presence of a slight weakness, the weak arm will rotate internally and drift slightly downward. This is referred to as *ulnar* or *motor drift*.

To evaluate strength of the legs, position the patient supine and ask them to raise one leg at a time. The patient with normal strength can lift the leg 90 degrees. Test the strength of other muscles as indicated (Table 21.4).

Table 21.2 Cranial Nerves

NUMBER/NAME		FUNCTION	TEST
I	Olfactory	Smell	Common odors to one nostril at a time
II	Optic	Vision	Visual acuity Visual fields Optic disc
III	Oculomotor	Movement of eye (medially, upward and inward, downward and outward, upward and outward), pupillary accommodation and constriction, raises upper eyelid	EOMs Doll's eyes (when head is moved, eyes move in opposite direction) Light examination direct and consensual; accommodation
IV	Trochlear	Movement of eye (down and inward)	EOMs Doll's eyes
V	Trigeminal	Facial sensation to hot/cold; light touch Chewing Branches: ophthalmic, maxillary, mandibular	Respective testing of three divisions. Clench jaw and check masseter and temporalis muscles; jaw and corneal reflex
VI	Abducens	Movement of eye (laterally)	EOMs Doll's eyes
VII	Facial	Facial expression; salivation; lacrimation, taste	Smile, frown, show teeth, puff out checks Taste (anterior 2/3 of tongue), close eyes
VIII	Acoustic	Hearing (cochlear) Equilibrium (vestibular)	Vestibular usually not tested
IX	Glossopharyngeal	Motor response limited; sensory on posterior tongue Innervates carotid body and sinus	Swallow on command, gag reflex Taste (posterior 1/3 of tongue)
X	Vagus	Movements of pharynx and larynx (raises the palate) Innervates organs of thorax abdomen	Gag reflex, midline elevation of uvula
XI	Spinal accessory	Movements of shoulders and neck	Shrug shoulders, and turn head against resistance
XII	Hypoglossal	Movement of tongue for speech and swallowing	Protrude tongue (deviates to affected side)

EOMs, Extraocular movements.

Table 21.3 Grading Scale for Muscle Strength

SCORE	FINDINGS
0	No movement, total paralysis
1	Weak contraction palpated or observed
2	Muscle moves when supported against gravity
3	Active muscle movement against gravity
4	Full active range of motion against gravity but with some weakness when resistance is tested
5	Full active range of motion against gravity and resistance

Sensory function. Many tests of sensory function exist, including evaluation of the patient's perception of pain, temperature, light touch, vibration, proprioception (position sense), and tactile discrimination. Apply various stimuli to the skin, and ask the patient to identify the type of stimulus perceived.

To evaluate sensory function, determine the patient's ability to perceive sharp and dull sensations and touch with the eyes closed. As with the motor evaluation, compare one side of the body with the other to assess equality. Include the hands, forearms, upper arms, trunk, thighs, lower legs, feet, and perineal area. Sensory loss is best described with the aid of a dermatome chart (Fig. 21.8). A dermatome defines an area of the skin that is innervated by a particular subcutaneous nerve root. In the initial postinjury period, frequently reassess the sensation because the injury may ascend (rise) and affect vital functions.

Pain. Pain can be evaluated by using a wooden applicator that is broken to create a sharp point. This broken applicator is used as the "sharp" stimulus, whereas the cotton end is used as a "dull" control stimulus. Ask the patient to state whether sharp or dull sensations are felt. Recognition of sharp pricks indicates ability to perceive painful stimuli.

Temperature. To test temperature perception, place test tubes containing hot or cold water against the patient's skin, and ask the patient to distinguish hot from cold.

Table 21.4 Assessment Techniques for Major Muscle Groups

NERVE ROOT	MUSCLE ACTION	ASSESSMENT TECHNIQUE
C4–C5	Abduction of shoulder	Shrug shoulder against downward pressure
C5–C6	Elbow flexion (biceps)	Arm flexed toward body against resistance
C7	Elbow extension (triceps)	Arm extended away from body against resistance
C8	Hand grasp (finger flexors)	Hands grasped around examiner's fingers with attempts to withdraw fingers from grasp
L2–L4	Hip flexion	Leg raised against resistance
L2–L4	Knee extension	Knee extended away from body against resistance
L5	Foot dorsiflexion	Foot pulled upward against resistance
L5–S1	Knee flexion	Knee flexed toward body against resistance
S1	Plantar flexion	Foot and toes pointed downward against resistance

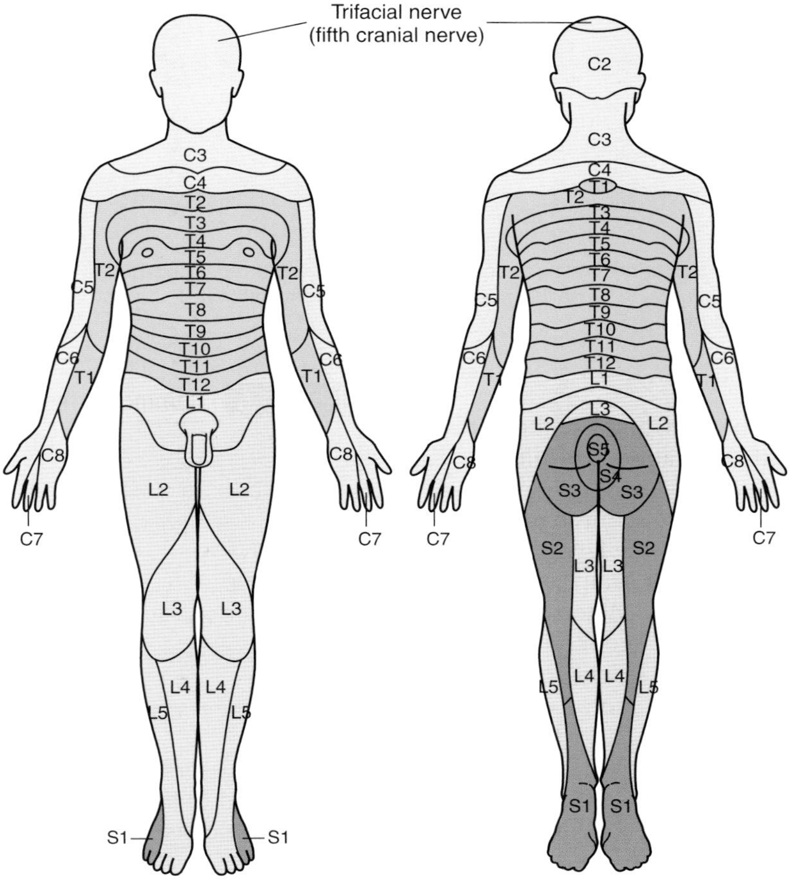

Fig. 21.8 A dermatome chart. A dermatome is an area of the skin that a particular nerve root innervates. (From Phillips NM: *Berry & Kohn's operating room technique*, ed 12, St. Louis, 2013, Mosby.)

Light touch. Brush a wisp of cotton against the skin to assess perception of light touch. Ask the patient to state when the sensation is felt.

Vibration. To test vibration, strike a tuning fork and touch the base to a joint in the great toe or a finger. Then ask the patient to report when the vibration is felt and when it stops. The examiner actually stops the tuning fork from vibrating. If the sensation is not perceived, repeat the test on a more proximal joint until the patient perceives it.

Proprioception. To test proprioception, ask the patient to close their eyes and identify the position of a toe or finger as you move it up or down.

Tactile discrimination. Tests for tactile discrimination include stereognosis, graphesthesia, and point localization. To test stereognosis, place a familiar object (e.g., paper clip, cotton ball) in the patient's hand and request identification using only one hand. Graphesthesia tests the patient's ability to recognize a number or letter "written" on the palm with a dull object. To test point

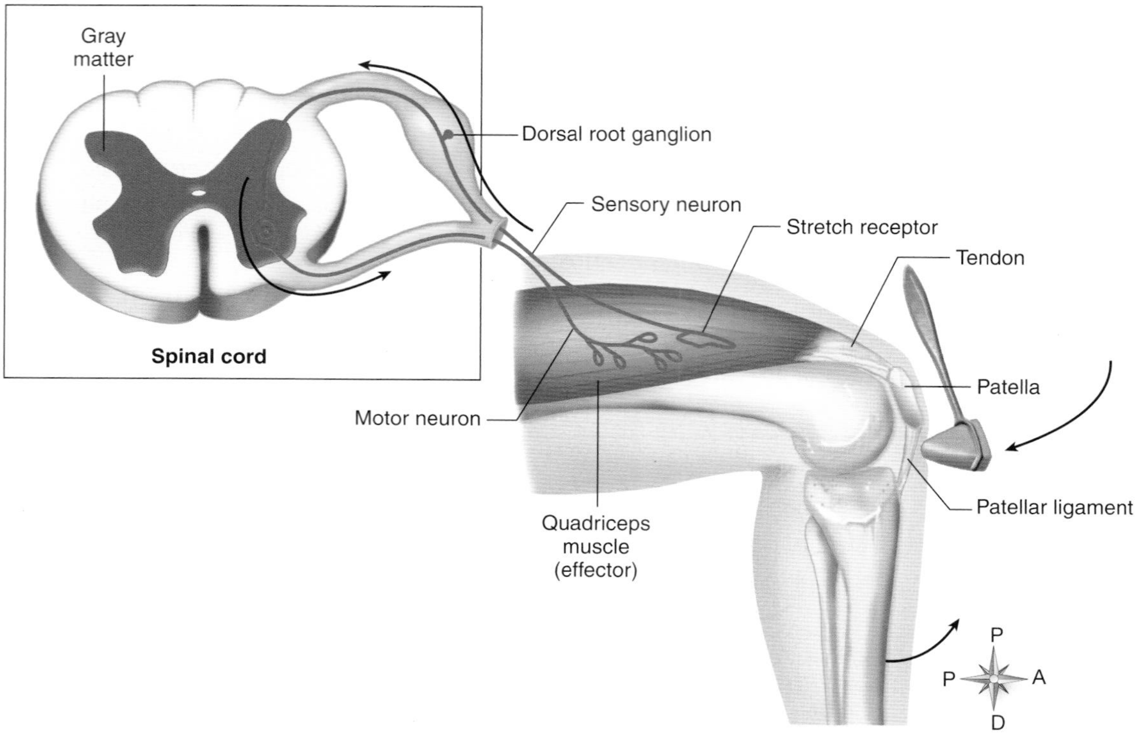

Fig. 21.9 Reflexes are elicited by stimulating a sensory nerve, which conveys an impulse to the spinal cord. An impulse is then conveyed by a motor nerve to cause the muscle to contract. (From Patton K, Thibodeau G: *Anatomy & physiology*, ed 8, St. Louis, 2013, Mosby.)

localization, briefly touch the skin, and ask the patient to touch the place where the sensation was felt.

Reflexes. A reflex is an unconscious, involuntary response that is entirely mediated at the level of the spinal cord, without input from higher brain centers. The knee jerk represents a simple reflex. When a stimulus is applied to the patella, the sensory root of the spinal nerve transmits the impulse to the spinal cord. At the cord, the impulse is relayed to the motor nerve root, which then elicits the knee jerk (Fig. 21.9). Other commonly tested reflexes are listed in Table 21.5.

Although these common reflexes are normal, others appear only with pathologic states. The Babinski reflex accompanies abnormalities in the motor pathways originating in the cerebral cortex. Assess for it by stroking the lateral side of the bottom of the foot and across the ball of the foot with a blunt object and observing the resulting movement of the toes. Normally, the toes curl downward. However, in the presence of cortical dysfunction, the big toe bends upward and the other toes fan out. Fig. 21.10 illustrates the response.

FUNCTIONAL ASSESSMENT

The functional assessment addresses the patient's usual activities and health practices. Inquire about activity level, use of adaptive equipment at home, prior disability, dietary pattern, occupation, use of alcohol and tobacco, drug use, interpersonal relationships, and current stressors. These are important elements that will be used to identify risk factors for stroke and cardiovascular disease.

Table 21.5 Commonly Tested Reflexes

REFLEX	EXPECTED RESPONSE
Biceps	Flexion of forearm
Triceps	Extension of forearm
Brachioradialis	Flexion and supination of forearm
Quadriceps	Extension of lower leg
Achilles (ankle jerk)	Plantar flexion of foot
Clonus	Repetitive movement after brisk dorsiflexion of foot

DIAGNOSTIC TESTS AND PROCEDURES

Once an initial evaluation and history have been obtained, more detailed diagnostic tests and procedures are often indicated (Table 21.6).

LUMBAR PUNCTURE

A lumbar puncture is an invasive procedure that is used most often to detect infections and other disorders of the CNS, tumors, and hydrocephalus. A local anesthetic is used to anesthetize the puncture site. Then a cannula is inserted into the subarachnoid space at the level of the fourth or fifth lumbar vertebra (Fig. 21.11). Entering at this level allows the physician to avoid

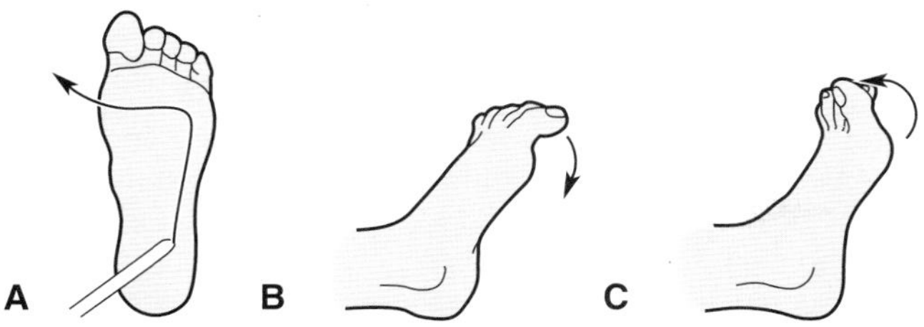

Fig. 21.10 Babinski reflex. (A) The examiner scrapes the foot as shown, using a blunt point. (B) The normal response (absence of Babinski response) is plantar flexion of the toes. (C) An abnormal response (presence of Babinski response) is characterized by dorsiflexion of the big toe and often fanning of the other toes. (From Herlihy B: *The human body in health and illness*, ed 5, St. Louis, 2014, Saunders.)

traumatizing the spinal cord, which ends at the level of the second lumbar vertebra. Once the needle is in place, a sample of CSF is collected for laboratory analysis. CSF specimens are placed in test tubes and labeled. The first specimen is usually discarded because it may contain blood from the puncture. Normal CSF has the following characteristics: pressure 50 to 175 mm H_2O; pH 7.30 to 7.40; clear, colorless appearance; fasting glucose 40 to 80 mg/dL; white blood cells 0 to 5 small lymphocytes/mm^3.

Injuries resulting from lumbar puncture are rare. However, some patients experience severe headaches resulting from a CSF leak. Leaks are sometimes treated with a blood patch, which is created by injecting a

Table 21.6 Diagnostic Tests and Procedures: Neurologic Disorders

TEST AND PURPOSE	PATIENT PREPARATION	POSTPROCEDURE NURSING CARE
Lumbar Puncture		
Lumbar puncture is used to diagnose infections, meningitis, and other CNS disorders. CSF pressure is measured. A CSF sample is taken for analysis. Also used to administer some medications such as for anesthesia.	Informed consent is required. Tell the patient a fluid sample will be taken from the spinal column. Have the patient void to reduce the discomfort of a full bladder. Anticoagulants are usually withheld. Local anesthesia is administered first. Support the patient lying on one side in a knee-to-chest position during the procedure (see Fig. 21.11). Procedure can also be performed in a prone or upright position.	The risk of headache may be reduced by lying flat for a specific period after the procedure. Encourage oral fluids. Assess for numbness, tingling, or pain in the extremities; CSF or bleeding from the puncture site; and changes in vital signs. Promptly deliver labeled specimens to the lab. The puncture site is covered with a small bandage.
Electroencephalography		
EEG is used to detect seizure activity by monitoring electrical activity in the brain.	Explain that electrodes will be applied to the scalp; patient will not feel any electrical shocks. Shampoo hair the night before EEG, but do not use conditioner. Withhold medications (anticonvulsants, sedatives, anticoagulants, stimulants, and tranquilizers) and caffeine for up to 8–12 hours before EEG as ordered.	Help patient shampoo hair to remove electrode paste.
Electromyography		
EMG is useful in diagnosing neuromuscular abnormalities such as ALS, peripheral neuropathy, myasthenia gravis, and carpal tunnel syndrome.	Signed consent is required. Tell patient procedure takes 1–2 hours. No caffeine or smoking for 3 hours before EMG.	Inspect the sites of needle electrode placement. Patient may be instructed to return within 5 days to have blood drawn for enzyme tests (AST, CK, LD).
Imaging Studies		
A brain scan depicts the pattern of distribution of a radioactive isotope that has been injected intravenously. Used to diagnose brain abscesses, tumors, contusions, vascular occlusions or hemorrhage, and hematomas.	Informed consent is required. Contraindicated during pregnancy. KCl is given several hours before the procedure. Tell patient that scan is painless and radiation exposure is minimal. An isotope will be injected, and the patient will lie on a stretcher while the scanner moves over the head. The scan will be repeated 1 hour later.	Encourage oral fluids to promote elimination of the isotope.

Continued

Table 21.6 Diagnostic Tests and Procedures: Neurologic Disorders—cont'd

TEST AND PURPOSE	PATIENT PREPARATION	POSTPROCEDURE NURSING CARE
Cerebral angioplasty uses computer-based images taken after injection of contrast medium to assess abnormalities in cerebral, carotid, and vertebral blood vessels.	Informed consent is required. Inform radiologist if patient is allergic to contrast media, shellfish, or iodine. Remove any metal from head area. Tell patient a "dye" will be injected and radiographs taken as the patient lies on a stretcher. When medium is injected, patient may feel flushed, warm, and nauseated and report a salty taste.	Apply pressure to puncture site and monitor for bleeding. Bed rest may be ordered for specified period. Extremity used to inject contrast medium may be immobilized for a specified period of time; assess circulation and neurologic function. Allergic response to contrast medium causes hives, nausea, swollen salivary glands. Treat with antihistamines as ordered.
Computed tomography (CT) shows intracranial structures. Used to diagnose tumors, inflammation, edema, hematomas, and infarctions. Distinguishes normal from clotted blood. CT may be done along with angiography.	Patient may be NPO 4–8 hours before scan if contrast medium is planned; can take prescribed medications and diabetic diet. Patient must lie still on a stretcher that fits into a donut-shaped frame that moves around the head. A mechanical sound can be heard. Procedure is painless and takes 15–20 minutes. Give sedatives as ordered for patients who cannot stay still.	No special aftercare needed. Observe patient who receives contrast medium for a delayed allergic reaction.
Magnetic resonance imaging/ magnetic resonance angiogram (MRI/MRA) creates images of intracranial structures without radiation.	Tell patient they will lie on a stretcher that passes into a tubular structure. Loud drumming noises will be heard while imager is in use. No special preparation is required. Sedation may be ordered for confused patients or those who are claustrophobic. Open MRI may be available for claustrophobic patients. Patients with some metal or electrical implants cannot be exposed to MRI because magnet can cause metal to move in the body. Special oxygen equipment, ventilators, and infusion pumps must be used.	No special aftercare needed.
Blood Flow Studies		
Doppler flow uses ultrasound (contrast enhanced, 3-dimensional, compound ultrasound) to assess carotid blood flow. Can be used with a duplex scanner to detect plaques in blood vessels.	Signed consent is required. Inform patient that test is painless and not to smoke for 30 minutes before test. Patient will need to lie supine while instrument is moved over the neck area.	No special aftercare needed unless activity restrictions are ordered.

ALS, Amyotrophic lateral sclerosis; *AST*, aspartate aminotransferase; *CK*, creatine kinase; *CNS*, central nervous system; *CSF*, cerebrospinal fluid; *EEG*, electroencephalography; *EMG*, electromyography; *KCl*, potassium chloride; Lab, laboratory; *LD*, lactate dehydrogenase; *NPO*, nothing by mouth.

small amount of the patient's blood into the lumbar puncture site. The blood clots and seals the puncture site, preventing further loss of CSF.

ELECTROENCEPHALOGRAPHY

The electroencephalogram (EEG) is a graphic representation of electrical activity in brain cells. Small electrodes are placed at various positions on the head to detect electrical signals generated from neurons located near the surface of the cerebral cortex. It is an excellent tool in the diagnosis of seizure activity (Fig. 21.12).

Some people have misconceptions about the EEG. Assure the patient that no electrical shock will be experienced, that the examiner is not able to "read the patient's mind," and that the test is not done to detect mental illness. Fatigue stresses the brain and may evoke abnormal activity not usually seen on the EEG. Thus patients may be evaluated with a sleep-deprived EEG, in which they are awakened after a short sleep period in an effort to elicit such activity during the test.

ELECTROMYOGRAPHY

Electromyography (EMG) studies the response of peripheral motor and sensory nerves to electrical stimuli. Needle electrodes are placed on several points over

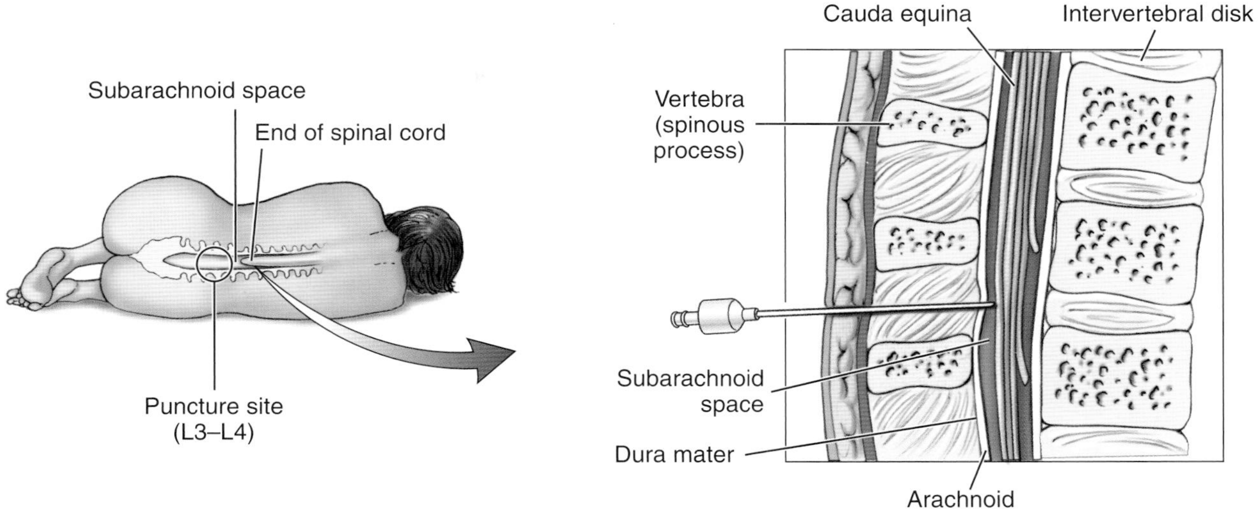

Fig. 21.11 Lumbar puncture. With the patient in a flexed position to maximize the space between vertebrae, the lumbar puncture needle is inserted between L4 and L5 or L3 and L4 to gain entry to the subarachnoid space. During the actual procedure, the patient would be gowned and draped to protect privacy. (From Shiland BJ: *Mastering healthcare terminology*, ed 5, St. Louis, 2016, Mosby.)

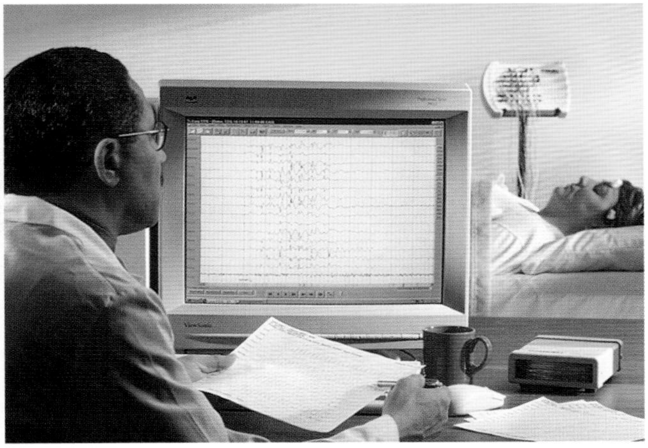

Fig. 21.12 Client undergoing an electroencephalogram. (From Black JM, Hawks JH, Keene AM: *Medical-surgical nursing: clinical management for continuity of care*, ed 6, Philadelphia, 2001, Saunders.)

a nerve and over the muscles supplied by the nerve. Stimuli are administered, and the effects are recorded on an oscilloscope.

RADIOLOGIC STUDIES

Brain Scan

The brain scan shows the pattern of distribution of a radioactive isotope injected intravenously. It is useful in detecting brain abscesses, tumors, contusions, vascular occlusion or hemorrhage, and hematomas. The patient is given potassium chloride 2 hours before the isotope is injected to prevent excessive isotope uptake. The isotope is given immediately before the scan is done. While the patient lies still on a stretcher, the scanner, which is somewhat like a radiograph machine, moves back and forth over the head. No sensation is associated with the scanning process. The scan is repeated 1 hour later.

Cerebral Angiography and Digital Subtraction Angiography

Cerebral angiography provides images of the cerebral, carotid, and vertebral blood vessels. A catheter is inserted into an artery (usually femoral) and advanced to the carotid or vertebral arteries. A contrast dye is injected, and a series of radiographs are taken. Angiography is the most definitive diagnostic test in the diagnosis of cerebral aneurysm or congenital vascular disorders, such as arteriovenous malformation. Risks include severe allergy to contrast media, embolus, hematoma, hemorrhage, renal toxicity, transient ischemic attack, infection, and loss of consciousness. Digital subtraction angiography (DSA) is a complementary, computer-assisted radiographic procedure for visualization of cerebral vessels.

Computed Tomography

The evolution of computed tomography (CT) represents one of the most significant developments in neurologic diagnostic procedures. CT is an excellent tool in the evaluation of trauma, tumors, and hemorrhage (Fig. 21.13). Enhancement of an area may be achieved by injecting contrast medium; thus any allergy to such media must be reported to the radiologist in advance. The entire scanning procedure lasts 15 to 20 minutes and generally requires no advance preparation or postprocedure care.

Magnetic Resonance Imaging

Magnetic resonance imaging (MRI), unlike CT, does not expose the patient to radiation. It is a noninvasive examination that involves placing the patient in a strong magnetic field, and then applying bursts of radiofrequency waves. Sophisticated technology converts information about the movement of

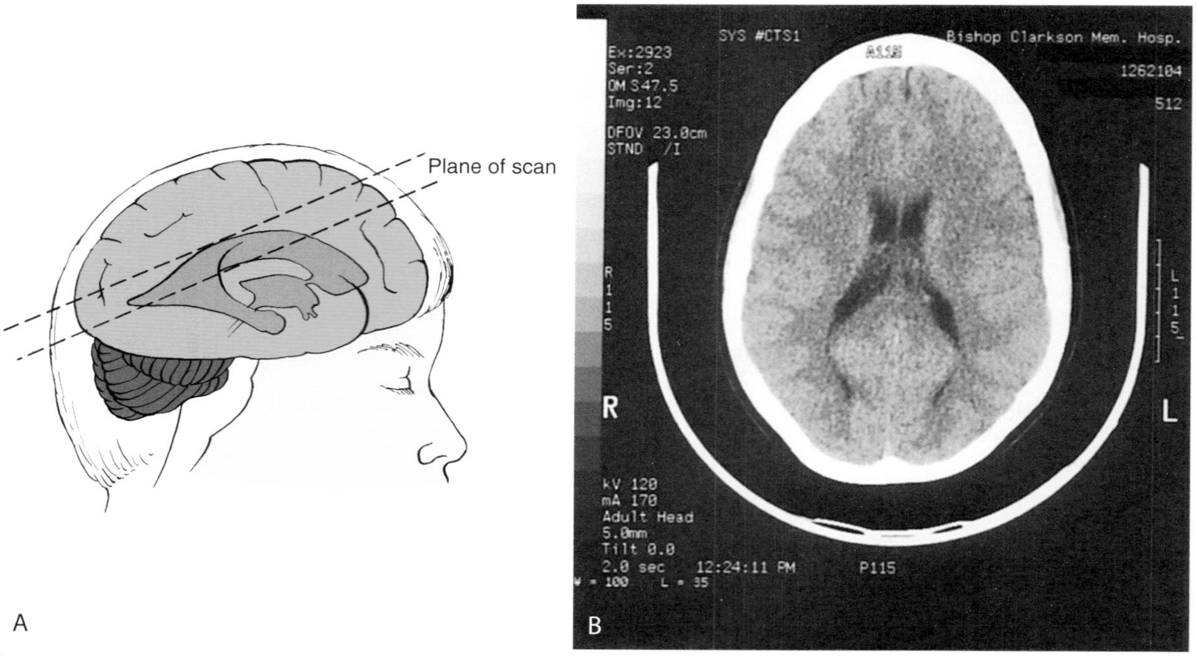

Fig. 21.13 Computed tomography scans are taken at various cross-sections of the brain. The image in (A) illustrates the cross-section used for the scan shown in (B). (From Black JM, Hawks JH, Keene AM: *Medical-surgical nursing: clinical management for continuity of care*, ed 6, Philadelphia, 2001, Saunders.)

molecules in the tissue into precise, clear images (Fig. 21.14). Magnetic resonance angiography (MRA) is a special technique that allows the measurement of flow through blood vessels. Depending on the type of equipment available, metal prostheses, pacemakers, and various implants may contraindicate MRI. This noninvasive diagnostic procedure is painless, has no known risks, and requires no preparation.

Myelography

A myelogram is obtained to visualize the spinal cord and vertebrae. A puncture is made in the lumbar area between L3 and L4. Radiopaque dye is then injected into the subarachnoid space of the spinal canal. Any obstruction that impedes the flow of the dye can be seen on radiography. Because of the invasive nature of the procedure, informed consent must be obtained. Nursing care before and after myelography is summarized in Box 21.3.

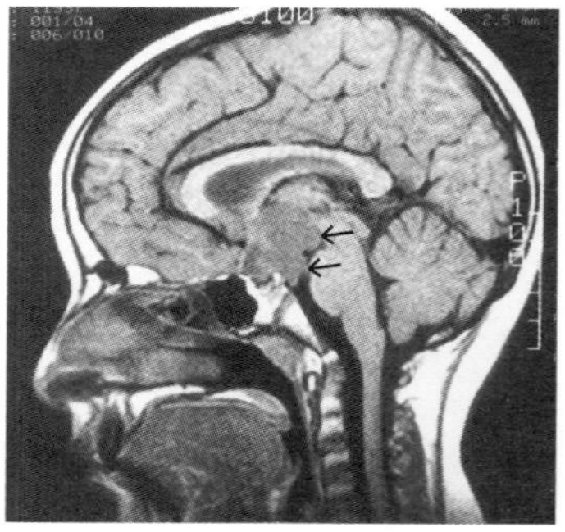

Fig. 21.14 Magnetic resonance imaging uses magnetic fields to create cross-sectional views of the brain. This sagittal section shows the cerebrum, ventricles, cerebellum, and medulla. (From Bontrager K, Lampignano J: *Textbook of radiographic positioning and related anatomy*, ed 8, St. Louis, 2014, Mosby.)

> **Pharmacology Capsule**
>
> Many drugs stimulate or depress the central nervous system (CNS). For example, caffeine is a stimulant, whereas morphine is a depressant.

COMMON THERAPEUTIC MEASURES

DRUG THERAPY

A number of drugs are used to treat neurologic disorders. They include antimicrobials, analgesics, antiinflammatory agents, corticosteroids, anticonvulsants, diuretics, chemotherapeutic agents, and dopaminergic, anticholinergic, cholinergic, and antihistamine medications. Because of the great variety of drugs used for neurologic conditions, specific drugs are discussed with individual conditions (see Chapter 22, Table 22.1 and Chapter 23, Table 23.2).

SURGERY

A craniotomy (surgical opening of the skull) may be done to treat tumors, correct defects, evacuate hematomas, and relieve pressure associated with trauma. A craniectomy is the excision of a segment of the skull, and a cranioplasty is any procedure done to repair a skull defect. General care of the surgical patient is discussed in Chapter 17, but interventions specific to neurologic surgery are emphasized here.

Box 21.3 Nursing Care of the Patient Having Myelography

PREPARATION
- Ensure that signed consent has been obtained.
- Inquire about any allergies to dye, iodine, or shellfish; inform the radiologist if the patient is allergic.
- Allow nothing by mouth (NPO) for 4 to 6 hours before the procedure, according to agency protocol.
- Administer the prescribed premedications.
- Have the patient empty the bladder if they have the ability to do so.
- Determine whether any medications should be withheld.

POSTPROCEDURE CARE
- Frequently assess the patient's vital signs and neurologic status.
- Encourage increased fluid intake to promote elimination of dye, if not contraindicated.
- Measure and record fluid intake and output.
- Position the patient as ordered: flat or head of bed elevated 30 to 45 degrees, depending on type of contrast medium used.
- Administer analgesics as ordered for headache.
- Assess the patient for back pain, increased temperature, difficulty voiding, neck stiffness, and nausea and vomiting.

Preoperative Nursing Care

Preoperatively, document the patient's neurologic status to provide a baseline for evaluating postoperative progress. Encourage the patient to ask questions and to express fears. If the patient has cerebral edema, parenteral corticosteroids may be ordered to help reduce cerebral swelling. Hair on part of the scalp is usually clipped. Because shaving the head can be very stressful for patients, they should be assured that the hair grows back. Sometimes clipping is done after the patient is anesthetized to reduce the trauma. Advise the patient's family that a craniotomy can take as long as 12 h, and that they will get progress reports during the procedure.

Postoperative Nursing Care

Postoperative craniotomy care includes monitoring level of consciousness, vital signs, movement and strength, pupil size and response to light, and speech. Signs and symptoms that may be related to complications are headache, visual disturbances, vomiting, seizures, and respiratory depression. Vital signs are recorded, and neurologic checks are done hourly until the patient is stable. Maintain intake and output records, and inspect any dressings for evidence of bleeding or CSF drainage. Note drainage from the ears or nose (if this occurs, a dressing may be placed loosely to absorb the drainage). Replace the dressing if it becomes wet because the moisture can harbor bacteria. On dressings, CSF appears as a pink stain surrounded by a lighter ring described as a *halo*. However, other fluids may produce halos as well. It is no longer recommended to check CSF with a dipstick for glucose because dipsticks are calibrated only for the specific fluids they were designed to test. Report any signs of deteriorating neurologic status to the physician immediately. The physician prescribes the patient's position and usually specifies that the head of the bed be elevated about 30 degrees.

If the patient has an external ventricular drainage system, use strict aseptic technique when changing the insertion site dressing and the drainage bag. Keep the zero-reference point of the drip chamber of the drainage bag at the level of the external auditory canal (or at the level the physician prescribes) to prevent drainage of excessive CSF. When the patient is being repositioned, clamp, and then restore the drainage tube to the correct level and unclamp it.

In addition to the usual surgical complications, the patient having a craniotomy is at risk for increased ICP, CSF leak, meningitis, and seizures. Other complications depend on the area of the brain affected and could include paralysis; memory loss; confusion; and impaired speech, vision, or hearing. Because increased ICP is a concern with cranial surgery, as well as with many neurologic disorders, it is described here.

INCREASED INTRACRANIAL PRESSURE

Increased ICP poses an extremely serious threat to the neurologic patient. Understanding the physiology, as well as the signs and symptoms will enable you to recognize the problem and respond appropriately to prevent life-threatening consequences.

PATHOPHYSIOLOGY

Anatomically, the skull is a cavity with rigid sides and an opening at the bottom. This cavity contains the brain, blood, and CSF, which are the components that exert pressure in the cranium. This pressure, or ICP, is normally 0 to 15 mm Hg.

In the course of a day, ICP fluctuates minimally because alterations are usually corrected rapidly. The Monro-Kellie hypothesis describes the adaptations that must occur in the three components (brain, blood, and CSF) for ICP to remain normal. If the volume of one component increases, ICP will rise unless a subsequent decrease occurs in the other two components. For example, if a brain tumor increases the volume of brain tissue, ICP will rise unless the volume of both blood and CSF decreases.

As ICP increases, the perfusion (delivery of blood and oxygen) to brain tissue decreases. This can be measured by calculating cerebral perfusion pressure (CPP), which is obtained by subtracting the ICP from the mean arterial pressure (MAP):

$$CCP = MAP - ICP.$$

A minimum perfusion pressure of 70 mm Hg is necessary to ensure adequate cerebral functioning. If perfusion pressure falls to 40 mm Hg, ischemia occurs. A perfusion pressure of 30 mm Hg or less is incompatible with life. To increase perfusion pressure, ICP must be decreased.

CLINICAL MANIFESTATIONS

To detect increases in ICP and assess the adequacy of perfusion, observe for specific signs and symptoms. Assess the patient's level of consciousness, pupillary characteristics, motor function, sensory function, and vital signs to detect signs of increasing ICP and initiate prompt treatment, if necessary.

Level of consciousness is the most reliable indicator of mental status because of its extreme sensitivity to oxygen levels in the cerebral blood. As ICP increases and perfusion is reduced, oxygen delivery to cerebral tissue is also reduced. Changes in level of consciousness are the earliest changes seen in ICP. These changes may be very subtle, with minimal agitation or drowsiness, or quite extreme, with profound unresponsiveness. Patients who are restless and agitated or suddenly quiet must be closely monitored, and significant changes must be reported.

Classic pupillary changes are seen with increasing ICP. As pressure rises, the pupil progresses from its normal size to a dilated state described as a *blown pupil.* The pupil becomes dilated and fixed and no longer reacts to light. These changes occur because of pressure on the oculomotor nerve (third cranial nerve). This is a late sign of increased ICP.

Another major indicator of increased ICP is altered motor function. As the motor areas of the frontal lobe are compressed by rising pressure, deficits develop on the side opposite the expanding mass. When deficits are on the opposite side from brain injury, they are said to be **contralateral** *to the injury.* For example, if a tumor exists in the right side of the brain, motor deficits will appear in the left side of the body. The deficits may involve a single extremity or an entire side. Hemiparesis (weakness on one side) or hemiplegia (paralysis on one side) may be seen.

As increased pressure becomes more extensive, abnormal posturing may be evident. As increasing pressure is exerted on the cerebral tissue above the midbrain, a pattern known as *abnormal flexion* (**decorticate**) *posturing* can be observed. The patient exhibits abnormal flexion in the upper extremities, with extension of the lower extremities. Increasing pressure affecting the midbrain or upper pons causes *extension* (**decerebrate)** *posturing.* The lower extremities remain extended, and the upper extremities are abnormally extended as well. These motor changes may occur spontaneously or may be seen only with painful stimuli (Fig. 21.15).

Hypothalamic impairment results in the loss of temperature control. As ICP compresses the tissue around the hypothalamus, it becomes ischemic and unable to regulate body temperature.

ICP elevations evoke an increase in systolic blood pressure with little or no associated increase in diastolic blood pressure. This results in a widening pulse pressure, defined as an increasing difference between systolic and diastolic blood pressure values. Initially, the heart rate may be slightly accelerated. However, as ICP compresses the center for cardiac control in the brainstem, the heart

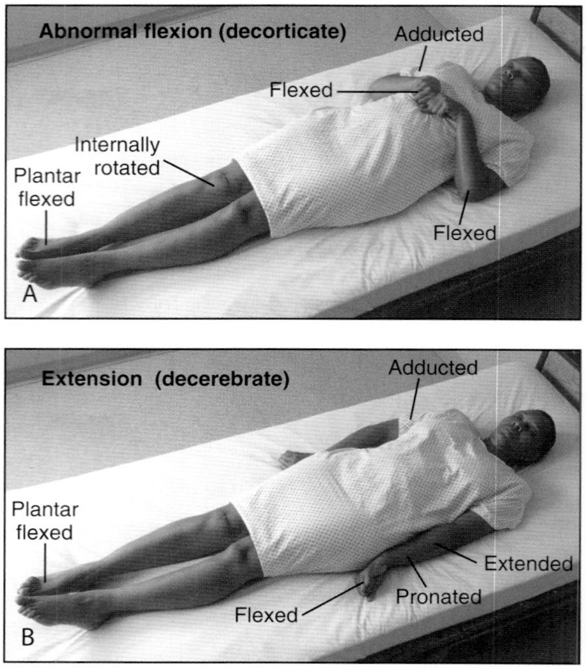

Fig. 21.15 Abnormal postures may be seen in the patient with neurologic impairment. (A) Abnormal flexion posturing (decorticate rigidity). (B) Abnormal extension posturing (decerebrate rigidity). (From Monahan FD, Neighbors M, Sands JK, et al.: *Phipps' medical surgical nursing: Health and illness perspectives,* ed 8, St. Louis, 2008, Mosby.)

rate becomes slow and irregular. Alterations in respiratory pattern are directly related to the extent of tissue compression. Fig. 21.16 illustrates areas of tissue compression (types of "herniation" syndromes).

Although it is extremely important to monitor vital signs in the neurologic patient, remember that changes in pulse, respiratory pattern, and blood pressure are late signs of increasing ICP. The combination of hypertension, bradycardia, and a widening pulse pressure is known as *Cushing's triad.* Cushing's triad is generally associated with increased ICP, but it is unreliable in determining the severity of neurologic compromise.

MEDICAL TREATMENT

Prompt treatment of increased ICP is vital for survival. Measures to lower ICP include positioning, hyperventilation, fluid management, mechanical drainage, and drug therapy.

The jugular vein is the primary route for venous outflow from the brain. It has long been thought that raising the head of the bed 30 to 45 degrees improves the flow of venous blood from the brain, thereby decreasing cerebral blood volume and ICP. However, recent research indicates that perfusion pressure may be better preserved if the head of the bed is elevated no more than 30 degrees. Further investigations may lead to some changes in current practice.

As oxygen delivery to cerebral tissue becomes more impaired, the level of carbon dioxide in the tissue increases. Increased carbon dioxide leads to dilation of cerebral blood vessels, thereby increasing

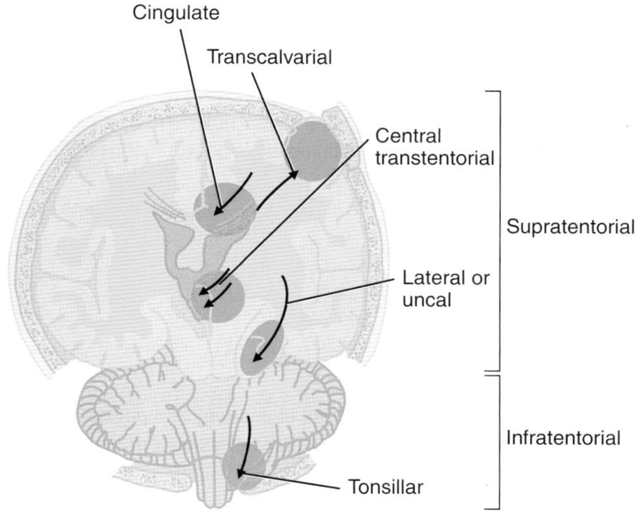

Fig. 21.16 Types of intracranial herniation. In transcalvarial herniation, edematous brain tissue is extruded through a fracture in the skull. In central transtentorial herniation, the lesion is located centrally or superior in the cranium and compression of central and midbrain structures may result. In lateral or uncal herniation, the lesion is located laterally within the cranium and can cause pressure on the midbrain. Cingulate herniation occurs between the two frontal lobes; the brain is pressed under the falx cerebri. In tonsillar herniation, the cerebellar tonsils are driven between the posterior arch of the atlas and the medulla and may be compressed. (From Black JM, Hawks JH: Medical-surgical nursing: clinical management for positive outcomes, ed 8, St. Louis, 2009, Saunders.)

the cerebral blood volume and ICP. With controlled hyperventilation, the excess carbon dioxide is eliminated, causing blood vessels to constrict and ICP to fall. Controlled hyperventilation is best achieved by mechanical ventilation. It decreases ICP within 1 to 2 minutes, but its effectiveness is diminished after 36 to 48 hours. Hyperventilation does have risks. Excessive vasoconstriction reduces cerebral oxygenation and worsens ischemia. Hyperventilation may be reserved for situations in which other treatments fail to reduce ICP. The goal is to achieve normocapnia.

The patient must have adequate fluids to maintain CPP. Fluid volumes are often increased to boost perfusion. Patients with questionable cardiac function must be monitored closely for fluid volume excess. A specialized catheter, called a *ventriculostomy catheter*, can be placed in the brain to drain excess CSF. After placement, the catheter is connected to tubing and a collection bag for gravity drainage. Drainage of CSF lowers ICP. Maintaining absolute sterility when managing this system is important to prevent contamination through the tubing to the brain.

Intravenous mannitol administration is one of the mainstays in the treatment of increased ICP. Mannitol is a hyperosmolar diuretic that draws edema fluid from the tissue spaces into the bloodstream. The mannitol and excess fluid are then eliminated through the kidneys. A rebound phenomenon may occur after administration. During administration, some of the medication crosses the blood-brain barrier. As mannitol is eliminated from the bloodstream, fluid is pulled into the brain. Other diuretics, such as furosemide, may also be used to reduce edema.

Corticosteroids, although controversial, may be used to help decrease cerebral edema and ICP. They decrease the edema, thereby lowering the elevated ICP associated with CNS tumors. Dexamethasone (Decadron) is a major agent used for patients with neurologic disorders.

Pharmacology Capsule

Diuretics used to treat increased intracranial pressure (ICP) can cause fluid and electrolyte imbalances.

1. How does increased ICP affect respirations?
2. Why would the patient lose consciousness when the ICP is elevated?

Get Ready for the NCLEX® Examination!

Key Points

- The functional unit of the nervous system is the neuron (nerve cell), which conducts electrical impulses throughout the nervous system.
- The brain and the spinal cord compose the CNS, whereas the nerves in the peripheral parts of the body compose the peripheral nervous system.
- CSF circulates through the CNS.
- The neurologic assessment includes evaluation of the level of consciousness, pupillary size and response, coordination and balance, sensory function, reflexes, and vital signs.
- Increased ICP may impair cerebral tissue perfusion, resulting in ischemia and possibly respiratory arrest.
- Signs and symptoms of increased ICP and impaired cerebral blood flow are decreasing level of consciousness, pupil dilation with no response to light, motor deficits, abnormal posture, fever, increased blood pressure, bradycardia, and respiratory depression.
- Measures to decrease ICP include positioning, hyperventilation, fluid restriction, mechanical drainage, and drug therapy.

Additional Learning Resources

SG Go to your Study Guide for additional learning activities to help you master this chapter content.

Go to your Evolve website (http://evolve.elsevier.com/Linton/medsurg) for the following learning resources and much more:

- Fluid & Electrolyte Tutorial
- Review Questions for the NCLEX® Examination

Clinical Judgment and Next-Generation NCLEX® Examination-Style Questions

1. **Neurotransmitters include which of the following? (Select all that apply.)**
   1. Acetylcholine
   2. Norepinephrine
   3. Epinephrine
   4. Dopamine
   5. Monoamine oxidase

   NCLEX Client Need: Physiological Integrity: Physiological Adaptation

2. **Which of the following statements about normal aging of the neurologic system are true? (Select all that apply.)**
   1. The number of neurons decreases.
   2. Lipofuscin and amyloid are deposited in nerve cells.
   3. Despite loss of neurons, most older people retain normal cognition.
   4. By 80 years of age, the only intact reflex is the Achilles tendon jerk reflex.
   5. Brain size decreases and ventricles enlarge.

   NCLEX Client Need: Physiological Integrity: Physiological Adaptation

3. **To evaluate neuromuscular function, the patient is instructed to raise one leg at a time while lying supine. How many degrees (at a minimum) would a patient with normal strength be able to lift each leg?**

   NCLEX Client Need: Physiological Integrity: Physiological Adaptation

4. **Which one of the following is a nursing measure used to decrease ICP?**
   1. Suction the patient frequently.
   2. Encourage isometric exercises.
   3. Avoid flexing the neck and hips.
   4. Provide continuous stimulation.

   NCLEX Client Need: Physiological Integrity: Reduction of Risk Potential

5. **A male patient who is being treated for a closed head injury is lying still and appears to be sleeping even in the noisy emergency department. When you shake his shoulder and call his name, he opens his eyes and says, "Huh?" Then he closes his eyes again. Which of the following is a term that describes his level of consciousness?**
   1. Somnolent
   2. Lethargic
   3. Stuporous
   4. Semicomatose

   NCLEX Client Need: Physiological Integrity: Physiological Adaptation

6. **SLO/Objective: Apply knowledge of anatomy and physiology and pathophysiology to determine which assessment data require follow-up by the nurse.**

   NGN Item Type: Enhanced Hot Spot

   Cognitive Skill: Recognize Cues

   A 78-year-old man was admitted to the hospital in a semi-comatose state after falling in his backyard. He had bruises and lacerations around his left eye and cheek. The nursing assessment on admission included the following:
   - Blood pressure: 150/68 mm Hg
   - Pulse 58 beats per minute
   - Respirations 16 breaths per minute
   - Difficulty breathing
   - Headache
   - Temperature 99.6°F
   - Incontinent of urine and feces

   Highlight or place a check mark next to the assessment findings that require follow-up by the nurse.

Neurologic Disorders

22

http://evolve.elsevier.com/Linton/medsurg

Objectives

1. Describe the pathophysiologic condition, signs and symptoms, complications, and medical or surgical treatment for patients with selected neurologic disorders.
2. Assist in developing a nursing care plan for the patient with a neurologic disorder.

Key Terms

amyotrophic lateral sclerosis
aura (ĂW-ră)
bradykinesia
concussion
contusion
degenerative
dysphagia (dĭs-FĀ-zhă)
encephalitis (ĕn-sĕf-ă-LĪ-tĭs)
epidural hematoma
Guillain-Barré syndrome
Huntington disease
Meningitis
myasthenia gravis
parkinsonism
postictal (pōs-TĬK-tĕl)
seizure (SĒ-zhŭr)
subdural hematoma
tumor

HEADACHE

Headache is the most common type of pain. It is a symptom, rather than a disease, that has many causes. Five common types of headaches are (1) migraine headache, (2) cluster headache, (3) tension headache, (4) headache related to disorders of the eyes, teeth, or sinuses, and (5) new daily persistent headache. For headaches associated with these and other conditions, treatment depends on the underlying cause.

MIGRAINE HEADACHE

Migraine headache results from intracranial vasoconstriction followed by vasodilation. Although no single cause is known, it may be triggered by menstruation, ovulation, alcohol, some foods, and stress.

Patients may experience depression, irritability, vision disturbances, nausea, and paresthesia before the onset of pain. The pain is usually unilateral, often begins in the temple or eye area, and is usually very intense. Tearing of the eye, and nausea and vomiting may occur. The patient is hypersensitive to light and sound and prefers a dark, quiet environment.

Mild migraines may be treated with acetaminophen or aspirin, but more severe ones may be treated with ergotamine (Cafergot) or sumatriptan (Imitrex), administered as a tablet or by autoinjector for self-injection. However, prevention should be emphasized. Medications such as beta-blockers or calcium-channel blockers may help to control the vascular influences. Identification and avoidance of triggering agents, such as particular foods (e.g., chocolate, yogurt, aged meats, cheeses), beverages (e.g., alcohol, red wine), or emotional stress, may also prove helpful. To treat chronic migraines in adults, onabotulinumtoxin A (Botox) is used for those individuals with migraine headaches greater than 14 days of the month that last more than 4 hours a day. Injections are given every 12 weeks to prevent migraine headaches before they start.

CLUSTER HEADACHE

Cluster headaches occur in a series of episodes followed by a long period with no symptoms. They are intensely painful and seem to be related to stress or anxiety. Unlike migraines, cluster headaches usually have no warning symptoms. They are also shorter in duration than migraines. Treatment may include cold application, indomethacin (Indocin), and tricyclic antidepressants.

TENSION HEADACHE

Tension headaches result from prolonged muscle contraction associated with anxiety, stress, or stimuli from other sources such as a brain tumor or an abscessed tooth. The location of the pain may vary, and the patient may have nausea and vomiting, dizziness, tinnitus, or tearing of the eyes. Tension headaches may persist for days or even years. Treatment measures include correction of known causes, psychotherapy, massage, heat application, and relaxation techniques. Analgesics, usually nonopioid drugs, may be prescribed along with other medications to reduce anxiety.

NEW DAILY PERSISTENT HEADACHE

New daily persistent headaches have a distinct and clearly remembered onset, with pain becoming continuous and unremitting within 24 hours. The pain lacks characteristic features and may be migraine-like or tension-type-like or have elements of both. The headaches may be present for more than three months. (Table 22.1).

NURSING CARE OF THE PATIENT WITH A MIGRAINE HEADACHE

FOCUSED ASSESSMENT

Nursing assessment of the neurologic patient is summarized in Chapter 21, Box 21.2.

Patient Problems, Goals, and Outcome Criteria: Migraine Headache

Patient Problems	Goals and Outcome Criteria
Acute pain related to migraine episode	Decreased pain: lower pain evaluation on pain scale
Nausea and vomiting related to acute migraine episode	Decreased nausea and vomiting: fewer episodes of nausea and vomiting; patient able to consume food and liquids
Visual disturbance related inability to tolerate light during acute migraine episode	Light tolerance: able to tolerate sunlight or well lighted room
Decreased activity tolerance related to pain caused by physical activity	Activity tolerance: able to tolerate activity without producing pain

Table 22.1 Drug Therapy: Headache Medications

DRUG	USE/ACTION	SIDE EFFECTS	NURSING INTERVENTIONS
Migraine			
NSAIDs aspirin, ibuprofen (Motrin, Advil), naproxen (Aleve)	Analgesic, antiinflammatory, antipyretic	Anorexia, GI bleeding, MI, stroke, heart failure	Take with full glass of water; sit upright after use; take with food to lessen GI effects Use cautiously in older adults Avoid use if pregnancy is planned or suspected
acetaminophen (Tylenol) (Tylenol) or in combination with aspirin and caffeine (Excedrin)	Nonopioid analgesic; antipyretic.	Headache, fatigue, anxiety, nausea, vomiting, abdominal pain; hepatotoxicity	Assess fever and type and intensity of pain. Patient and family teaching: Do not exceed recommended dosage which may result in symptoms of hepatotoxicity (liver damage), including nausea, vomiting and abdominal pain. Evaluate therapeutic response: absence of pain using pain scoring; absence of fever.
Cluster Headaches			
Triptans Sumatriptan, zolmitriptan	Serotonin agonist Vasoconstriction in cranial arteries	Tingling, hot sensation, flushing, burning, feeling of pressure, tightness, numbness, dizziness, anxiety, fatigue	Assess type of pain, aggravating factors Patient and family teaching: Report chest pain, tightness, sudden, severe abdominal pain; swelling of eyelids, face, lips: skin rash Maintain dark, quiet environment; avoid hazardous activities if dizziness, drowsiness occur; avoid alcohol, which may increase headache
Lidocaine intranasal	Produces vasoconstriction	Anxiety, restlessness, insomnia, weakness; irritation, burning of nasal passages, nausea, vomiting, anorexia	Administered ipsilateral to the pain; head extended 45 degrees and rotated toward the symptomatic side; assess for redness, swelling, pain in nasal passages
Verapamil (Calan, Verelan)	Calcium channel blocker; prevention for cluster headaches	Headache, drowsiness, edema, nausea, constipation	Patient/family teaching: Increase fluids, fiber to counteract constipation; avoid hazardous activities until dizziness is no longer a problem; limit caffeine and alcohol consumption; change positions slowly to prevent syncope; do not discontinue abruptly; report chest pain, palpitations, swelling of extremities, skin irritation, rash, tremors, weakness

Table 22.1 Drug Therapy: Headache Medications—cont'd

DRUG	USE/ACTION	SIDE EFFECTS	NURSING INTERVENTIONS
Glucocorticoids: Prednisone, dexamethasone	Preventive therapy for cluster headaches; short term use; may be given in conjunction with verapamil	Depression or euphoria, potassium depletion, hypertension, nausea, vomiting, peptic ulcer, acne	Assess intake and output, daily weights, mental status Patient/family teaching: Carry medical alert ID as a corticosteroid user at all times; do not discontinue abruptly; take with food or milk, look for bruising that may occur
Galcanezumab (Emgality)	Monoclonal antibody; prevention of cluster headaches	Infection site reaction, rash, urticaria, pruritis, erythema, dyspnea	Assess pain, location, intensity and duration of headaches in the past; assess response to preventing headaches after use of the medication Patient/family teaching: How to self-administer medication; do not double or skip doses; report injection site reaction, rash, itching that may indicate an allergic reaction
Tension Headaches			
NSAIDs aspirin, ibuprofen (Motrin, Advil), naproxen (Aleve)			Take with full glass of water; sit upright after use; take with food to lessen GI effects Use cautiously in older adults Avoid use if pregnancy is planned or suspected
acetaminophen (Tylenol) (Tylenol) or in combination with aspirin and caffeine (Excedrin)	Nonopioid analgesic; antipyretic.	Headache, fatigue, anxiety, nausea, vomiting, abdominal pain; hepatotoxicity	Assess fever and type and intensity of pain. Patient and family teaching: Do not exceed recommended dosage which may result in symptoms of hepatotoxicity (liver damage), including nausea, vomiting, and abdominal pain. Evaluate therapeutic response: absence of pain using pain scoring; absence of fever.

INTERVENTIONS

Acute Pain

Provide a quiet environment to minimize extraneous stimuli. Encourage rest. Administer pain medications as needed for pain relief. Liquids such as coffee or tea cause vasoconstriction and may help to alleviate pain. Encourage complementary therapies such as muscle relaxant techniques, guided imagery, and acupressure. Applying firm but nonpainful circular pressure to the area between the thumb and index finger using the opposite hand for 5 min, as well as warm or cold compresses to the head, may help to alleviate pain.

Nausea and Vomiting

Administer antiemetic medications. Provide ice chips and encourage fluids, if possible, to prevent dehydration. Ginger root in various forms is helpful for treating nausea.

Visual Disturbance

Provide a cool, dark environment.

Decreased Activity Tolerance

Encourage rest during a migraine attack. Position patient for maximum comfort. Slowly resume normal activities when migraine episode subsides (see the Complementary and Alternative Therapies box).

Complementary and Alternative Therapies

Complementary and alternative therapies are recommended adjuncts in the management of migraine headaches. Progressive muscle relaxation techniques, imagery, acupuncture, and electromyography (EMG) biofeedback may reduce the frequency and intensity of headaches. Home remedies that may help prevent or alleviate pain from headaches are lavender essential oils, ginger powder, butterbur, feverfew, magnesium, and B-complex vitamins.

SEIZURE DISORDER

Seizures affect approximately 8% to 10% of the population over a lifetime and account for 1% to 2% of all emergency department visits. A **seizure** is a sudden change in behavior caused by electrical hyperactivity of the neuronal networks in the cerebral cortex. The electrical impulses generated in the brain normally spread in a very organized fashion. However, in the patient with a seizure disorder, electrical impulses are conducted in a highly chaotic pattern that yields abnormal activity and behavior. Seizure activity involves many hyperactive neurons that use excessive oxygen and glucose. Thus oxygen and glucose stores may be depleted, leading to permanent neurologic damage.

Seizure activity may be related to trauma, reduced cerebral perfusion, infection, electrolyte disturbances, poisoning, tumors, epilepsy, or a genetic tendency. Other events can mimic seizures in adults, including syncope, migraine, transient ischemic attack, and psychogenic nonepileptic seizures.

MEDICAL DIAGNOSIS

Diagnostic testing for seizure activity is directed toward ruling out specific problems. An accurate history of the seizure activity can provide clues to the type of seizure disorder, possible triggering events, and the origin of activity. Unexpected seizure activity is often very frightening to the family, the nurse, or other health care provider who may be the first reliable eyewitnesses. If you observe a seizure, note the patient's behavior before, during, and after the seizure, as well as the duration of the seizure. The patient's electroencephalography (EEG) tracing, which records the electrical activity of the brain, is used to detect abnormal brain activity.

Seizure Classification

Most seizures can be categorized as either *focal* or *generalized*, depending on whether the onset of electrical activity involves a single region or both sides of the brain simultaneously. The specific seizure activity corresponds to the area of the brain affected and the amount of cortex involved. Focal seizures are further classified according to whether or not there is a loss of consciousness during the event. In addition, focal seizures may affect a sufficient number of adjacent cells so that the activity can spread throughout the cerebral hemispheres. This is known as a *focal seizure with secondary generalization.* Generalized seizures involve the entire brain from the onset and are associated with loss of consciousness.

Other classifications of seizures are *acute symptomatic* seizure and *unprovoked seizure.* An acute symptomatic seizure occurs at the same time that a cause can be identified such as a brain injury, metabolic abnormalities, drug or alcohol withdrawal, or acute neurological disorders. Unprovoked seizure refers to a seizure of unknown cause that occurs in relation to a preexisting brain lesion or nervous system disorder.

Focal Seizures. Focal seizures are described as either focal seizures with retained awareness or focal seizures with impaired awareness. Focal seizures with retained awareness (previously called simple partial seizures) vary according to the area of the cortex affected at the onset of the seizure. For example, a seizure that begins in the occipital cortex may result in flashing lights, whereas one that begins in the motor cortex may result in jerking movements of the face, arm, or leg on the side opposite to that part of the cortex affected (Jacksonian seizure).

Focal seizures with impaired awareness (previously called complex partial seizures) most commonly occur with epilepsy. Patients may appear to be awake but are not in contact with others in the environment and usually do not respond to instructions or questions. The seizures often last less than three minutes beginning with an aura that can be remembered after the seizure event. The patient may have sleepiness, confusion and headache and have no memory of the seizure other than the aura after its occurrence.

Both types of focal seizures may cause bilateral tonic-clonic seizures (previously called secondarily generalized seizures) as the neuronal electrical activity in the cortex diffuses. When this occurs, patients may have no memory of the seizure event.

Aura. A symptom that may occur at the beginning of a seizure is called a warning or *aura*. An aura is a focal seizure that affects enough of the cortex to cause symptoms, but not enough to result in unconsciousness. An aura is a sensation such as dizziness, numbness, visual or hearing disturbance, perception of an offensive odor, or pain. It occurs before loss of consciousness. The individual retains the memory of the aura and is able to recognize an oncoming seizure.

Generalized Seizures. Generalized *tonic-clonic seizures* (also called grand mal seizures, major motor seizures, or convulsions) are the most common type of generalized seizures. The *tonic phase* of the seizure lasts about one minute with the occurrence of muscle or extremity stiffness, loss of consciousness, and, sometimes, cyanosis. After the tonic phase, a rhythmic movement of the extremities called the *clonic phase* of the seizure occurs, lasting about 2 to 3 minutes. During that time the tongue may be bitten with frothy and bloody sputum coming out of the mouth. The patient may be incontinent of urine during a generalized seizure. The *postictal phase* occurs when seizure activity ceases. The patient is usually in a deep sleep, breathing deeply, waking up gradually, often with confusion and agitation. Most patients become responsive and alert within 10 to 20 minutes. These phases are illustrated in Fig. 22.1.

Other types of generalized seizures are *absence*, *clonic*, *myoclonic*, and *atonic* seizures. Absence seizures (previously called *petit mal*) are brief periods of loss of consciousness usually lasting 5 to 10 seconds in which the person may appear to be daydreaming. Absence seizures lasting more than 10 seconds may be associated with movements such as eye blinking and lip smacking. These seizures are generally identified during childhood. Clonic seizures cause rhythmic jerking muscle contractions that usually involve the arms, face, and neck. During a myoclonic seizure, the person

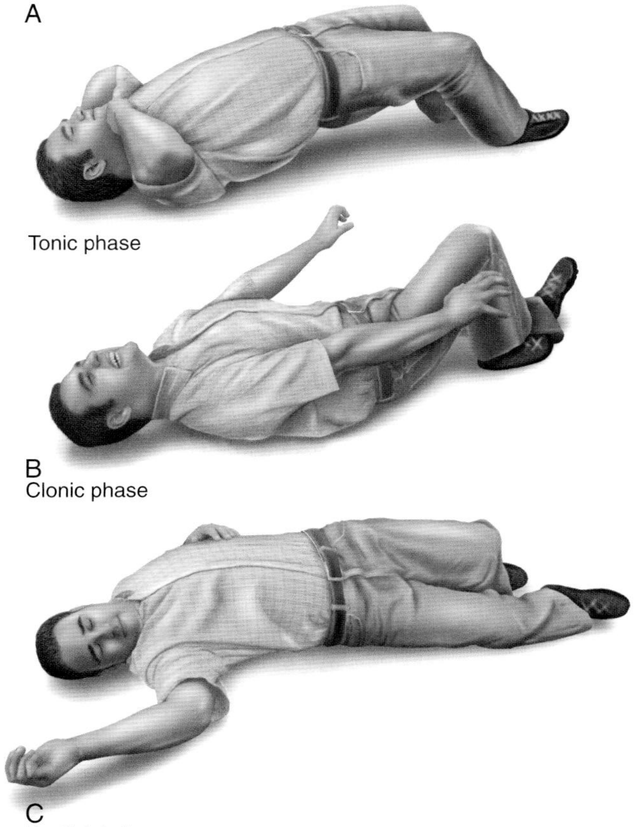

Fig. 22.1 Phases of a generalized tonic-clonic seizure. (A) Tonic phase is marked by loss of consciousness, falling, crying, and generalized stiffness. Incontinence may occur. (B) During the clonic phase, jerking of the limbs and salivary frothing occurs. (C) During the postictal phase, seizure activity has ceased. The patient is drowsy and has no memory of the seizure. (From Black JM, Hawks JH: *Medical-surgical nursing: clinical management for positive outcomes*, ed 8, St. Louis, 2009, Saunders.)

has only brief jerking or stiffening of the extremities. Atonic seizures (also known as *drop seizures*) have the opposite effect of tonic seizures because a sudden loss of muscle tone, especially in the legs, causes the patient to collapse.

Status Epilepticus

Status epilepticus is a medical emergency in which the patient has continuous seizures or repeated seizures in rapid succession for 30 minutes or more. The prolonged seizure activity depletes the brain of oxygen and glucose, which can lead to permanent brain damage.

MEDICAL TREATMENT

The most desirable treatment of a seizure disorder is the resolution of the underlying condition. For example, if a tumor causes seizure activity, surgical excision of the tumor would be the most desirable therapy. However, if a cause is not readily identifiable or correctable, medical management is implemented.

Anticonvulsant drug therapy provides satisfactory chemical control of seizure activity in about 75% of patients. A variety of drugs is available, some being more effective in certain seizure disorders than others. The selected drug is introduced, and the dose is gradually increased until a therapeutic level is achieved. If good seizure control is not accomplished with one drug, combinations of drugs may be prescribed. Examples of specific drugs used to treat epilepsy are presented in Table 22.2. Status epilepticus is treated with intravenous anticonvulsant drugs. If the patient does not respond to anticonvulsants, general anesthetics and neuromuscular blockers may be used (see the Health Promotion box).

Health Promotion

PREVENTION OF SEIZURE DISORDER

- Identify common seizure triggers or precipitating factors such as sleep deprivation, alcohol, certain medications, and infection or systemic illness
- Avoid alcohol use.
- Get adequate rest.
- Engage in stress-reducing activities such as meditation and visualization.
- Maintain general health through proper diet and exercise.

SEIZURE PRECAUTIONS

- Promote general safety behaviors by avoiding unsupervised activities such as bathing and/or swimming alone, working at heights, and operating heavy machinery.
- Take showers instead of baths to prevent seizure-induced drowning
- Restrict driving to prevent a seizure-induced accident or injury

SURGICAL TREATMENT

Patients whose seizures are poorly controlled with medication may be candidates for surgical procedures to decrease or control seizures. Procedures include removal of seizure foci in the temporal lobe and pallidotomy or implantation of a vagal nerve stimulator.

Pharmacology Capsule

Sudden discontinuance of anticonvulsant drugs can trigger seizure activity.

NURSING CARE OF THE PATIENT WITH A SEIZURE DISORDER

FOCUSED ASSESSMENT

Nursing assessment of the neurologic patient is summarized in Chapter 21, Box 21.2. With a seizure disorder, it is especially important to describe the seizure episode, including the postictal period and to document drug therapy.

Table 22.2 Drug Therapy: Antiseizure Drugs

DRUG	USE/ACTION	SIDE EFFECTS	NURSING INTERVENTIONS
Anticonvulsants			
phenytoin (Dilantin)	Reduces neuron hyperexcitability; inhibits seizure activity. Reduces pain of trigeminal neuralgia; used for focal onset seizures	Sluggishness, ataxia, slurred speech, nystagmus, constipation, nausea, vomiting, overgrowth of gingiva, and skin rashes. Hypotension with IV route. Unusual side effects include aplastic anemia and agranulocytosis.	With IV doses, monitor BP and pulse and report bradycardia. Do not exceed recommended rate of IV administration per minute. Take safety precautions if the patient becomes ataxic or drowsy. Give the drug with food to reduce GI irritation. Provide meticulous mouth care to prevent gingival overgrowth. Identify concurrent drugs to detect possible interactions that enhance or inhibit the drug's effect.
fosphenytoin (Cerebyx)	Converts to phenytoin when administered. Used for long-term suppression of seizures after status epilepticus stopped by phenothiazine.	Side effects are the same as phenytoin.	Given IV. Less irritating than phenytoin. Can be infused faster than phenytoin. Follow recommended rate of IV administration.
phenobarbital (Luminal)	Depresses CNS and raises seizure threshold.	Drowsiness, respiratory depression, nausea, vomiting, diarrhea, constipation, rash, photosensitivity, and muscle aches. Side effects with the IV route include laryngospasm, bronchospasm, and hypotension.	Safety precautions if the patient is drowsy. Monitor respiratory rate and BP, especially with IV route. Note other drugs for possible drug interactions. Tell patient not to stop taking the drug without consulting the physician and to avoid alcohol and excessive sunlight.
primidone (Mysoline)	Similar to phenobarbital.	Behavioral changes, lethargy, dizziness, and ataxia.	Safety precautions if the patient is drowsy.
carbamazepine (Tegretol)	Slows transmission of impulses in CNS; prevents seizures. Reduces pain of trigeminal neuralgia.	Drowsiness, ataxia, blurred vision, BP increase or decrease, heart failure, urinary retention, rash, hepatitis, aplastic anemia, and agranulocytosis.	Safety precautions if the patient is drowsy. Monitor BP. Teach the patient to avoid alcohol and excessive sunlight; to not change the dose or stop taking the drug without the physician's guidance; and to immediately report fever, sore throat, excessive bruising or bleeding, and jaundice.
lorazepam (Ativan)	Used for initial treatment of status epilepticus.	Drowsiness, rash, nausea, vomiting, diarrhea, constipation, respiratory depression, and psychologic and physical dependence. Side effects with the IV route include hypotension and phlebitis.	Safety precautions if the patient is drowsy. Monitor infusion site for extravasation. Monitor BP.
clonazepam (Klonopin)	Raises seizure threshold.	Drowsiness, ataxia, agitation, rash, edema, nocturia, blurred vision, dry mouth, and excitement in older adults. Toxicity causes lethargy, confusion, and coma.	Safety precautions if the patient is drowsy. Advise the patient that abrupt withdrawal may cause restlessness, insomnia, and status epilepticus.
valproic acid (Depakene, Depakote)	Mechanism of action is unknown. May increase levels of GABA.	Lethargy, dizziness, ataxia, headache, thrombocytopenia, nausea, vomiting, weight gain, tremor, and alopecia.	Monitor blood work. Safety precautions if the patient is drowsy.

Table 22.2 Drug Therapy: Antiseizure Drugs—cont'd

DRUG	USE/ACTION	SIDE EFFECTS	NURSING INTERVENTIONS
Newer Antiepileptic Drugs			
gabapentin (Neurontin)	Affects unique gabapentin-specific binding site in the brain; produces no effect on GABA system.	Somnolence, dizziness, and ataxia (particularly after initiation of therapy or dose increase). Additional side effects include weight gain and edema, dyspepsia, nausea, vomiting, constipation, rhinitis, and pharyngitis.	Safety precautions if the patient is drowsy. Give the drug with food to prevent GI distress. Notify the physician of side effects. Encourage periodic rest periods to help with fatigue.
lamotrigine (Lamictal)	Inhibits release of excitatory amino acid glutamate. Blocks sodium channels.	Dizziness, headache, insomnia, somnolence, ataxia, diplopia, nausea, and vomiting. May cause a potentially life-threatening rash.	Safety precautions if the patient is drowsy. Notify the physician of rash. Identify current drugs to detect possible interactions that enhance or inhibit the drug's effect. Monitor renal and hepatic function. Tell the patient to take the drug with food or milk. Medicate the patient for headaches.
pregabalin (Lyrica)	Mechanism of action is unknown.	Somnolence, ataxia, diplopia, arthralgias, and thrombocytopenia.	Safety precautions if the patient is drowsy. Monitor the patient's blood work.
topiramate (Topamax)	Blocks voltage-dependent sodium and calcium channels; enhances GABA activity at some GABA receptors; blocks excitatory receptors (kainite/glutamate).	Somnolence, abnormal thinking, dizziness, agitation, confusion, ataxia, nystagmus, nephrolithiasis, nausea, dyspepsia, anorexia, weight loss, dysmenorrhea, and upper respiratory tract infection.	Safety precautions if the patient is drowsy. Inform the physician of agitation, confusion, and abnormal thinking. Administer the drug with food if GI upset occurs. Caution the patient not to chew or break the tablet because of bitter taste. Maintain adequate hydration to prevent renal stones. Suggest use of barrier contraceptives because of decreased effectiveness of oral contraceptives. Encourage avoidance of alcohol because of increased CNS depression.
tiagabine (Gabitril)	Increases level of GABA by inhibiting reuptake systems.	Tiredness, dizziness, headache, nervousness, asthenia, somnolence, and difficulty concentrating. Additional side effects include GI upset, pain, and serious skin rash.	Safety precautions if the patient is drowsy. Note other drugs for possible drug interactions. Give the drug with food. Monitor the patient's weight, liver function, and neurologic status. Avoid alcohol and sleep-inducing drugs.
zonisamide (Zonegran)	Medication is a sulfonamide agent; the mechanism of action is unclear. May decrease seizure activity by inhibiting sodium and calcium channels.	Skin rash, somnolence, anorexia, dizziness, headache, nausea, and agitation/irritability. Additional side effects include renal calculi, bone marrow depression, nausea, vomiting, dry mouth, and unusual taste.	Safety precautions if the patient is drowsy. Ensure adequate hydration to prevent renal calculi. Monitor hepatic, renal, and cardiac function. Monitor the patient closely at the beginning of therapy and with dose changes.
oxcarbazepine (Trileptal)	Inhibits seizure activity by preventing sodium shift that causes neuron hyperexcitability.	Dizziness, drowsiness, double vision, fatigue, ataxia, nausea, vomiting, abdominal pain, tremor, dyspepsia, and gait abnormalities.	May be taken with or without food. Implement safety precautions if CNS effects occur. Encourage rest periods for fatigue.

Continued

Table 22.2 Drug Therapy: Antiseizure Drugs—cont'd

DRUG	USE/ACTION	SIDE EFFECTS	NURSING INTERVENTIONS
levetiracetam (Keppra)	Mechanism of action is unknown.	Somnolence, dizziness, impaired coordination, abnormal behavior, fatigue, and infection.	Safety precautions if the patient is drowsy. Give the drug with food to prevent GI side effects. Be aware of interactions with other drugs. Advise the patient to use barrier contraceptives. Implement safety precautions if CNS side effects occur.

BP, Blood pressure; *CNS*, central nervous system; *GABA*, gamma-aminobutyric acid; *GI*, gastrointestinal; *IV*, intravenous/intravenously.

Patient Problems, Goals, and Outcome Criteria: Seizure Disorder

Patient Problems	Goals and Outcome Criteria
Potential for injury related to seizure activity	Absence of injury: no bruises, breaks in skin, or fractures
Inadequate coping related to social stigma of seizure disorder or chronicity	Adequate coping: patient makes positive statements about life with seizure disorder, patient adheres to prescribed therapy
Lack of knowledge of seizure disorders, treatment, and self-care	Patient understands self-care: patient and family accurately describe condition, drug therapy, and care; demonstrate appropriate care

INTERVENTIONS

Potential for Injury

You must protect the patient from injury during and after a seizure. *Seizure precautions* include applying seizure pads to the upper side rails of the bed, ensuring that the patient has a functional intravenous (IV) line, and maintaining oxygen and suction setups. Some experts believe that padding the side rails is unnecessary, is cumbersome, and may have a negative emotional effect on the patient and visitors. However, it is a common practice used to protect the patient in the event that they strike the rails during a seizure.

If the patient has a seizure, quickly move objects away from reach. If the patient falls to the floor, the head may be cradled in your lap to prevent injury. Do not attempt to restrain the patient. In the past, it was common practice to attempt to insert a tongue blade or oral airway between the teeth to prevent biting of the tongue. However, this is no longer recommended. Attempts to force an object between clenched teeth may result in injury to the mouth and do not help if the tongue has already been bitten. The patient will not "swallow the tongue," but it may fall back and occlude the airway. Turning the patient to one side can help to maintain a patent airway. Dos and Do Nots of seizure management are listed in Box 22.1.

Box 22.1 Management of Seizures

"DOS"

DO remove any objects that could cause harm.
DO turn the person to one side if possible.
DO note the time the seizure began and how it progressed.
DO assess and document postictal (postseizure) status.
DO allow the person to rest quietly.
DO call a medical emergency if a generalized tonic-clonic seizure lasts more than 4 minutes or if seizures occur in rapid succession.

"DO NOTS"

DO NOT restrain the person unless he or she is in grave danger of severe injury.
DO NOT attempt to force anything between the person's teeth.

When seizure activity ceases, the patient is typically drowsy and needs to rest. During this postictal period, the nurse should provide quiet and privacy. Afterward, they should document the conditions and any unusual behaviors that preceded the seizure, the length of the seizure, associated patient activity, deviation of the eyes, and any incontinence. In addition, document any lingering effects and the length of time of recovery.

Inadequate Coping

Inadequate coping can be related to lack of information or misconceptions and may be reflected in noncompliance with prescribed therapy, anxiety, or social isolation. Important aspects of nursing management include not only the care of the patient during hospitalization, but also teaching the family and patient about the seizure disorder and the therapy.

Lack of Knowledge

Because a seizure disorder is often a lifelong problem, patient teaching must be directed toward helping the patient and family adjust to a chronic condition. Patients must adjust physically, psychologically, and vocationally to the changes brought on by the disorder itself, as well as to the side effects of the medications. The nurse should encourage the patient to ask questions and to express concerns. For guidelines on teaching, see the Patient Teaching box.

Patient Teaching

Seizures

- Factors that may trigger a seizure are fatigue, stress, fever, visual disturbances, alcohol, failure to take medication, and large caffeine intake.
- When an impending seizure is perceived, immediately seek a safe place.
- Know your prescribed drug names, dosages, schedules, and side effects to be reported to the physician.
- Consult your physician regarding the use of generic substitutions for your drugs.
- Never stop taking your seizure medication without direction from your physician.
- Psychologic counseling may help you to deal with stress associated with this disorder.
- Always wear a medical alert tag, which states that you have a seizure disorder, and carry a card that specifies drug therapy, physician, and individuals to be contacted in an emergency.
- A sensation that warns of an impending seizure is called an *aura*; common sensations include dizziness, numbness, visual or hearing disturbance, pain, and perception of an offensive odor.
- Therapy dogs may be available to warn of an impending seizure.
- The local chapter of the Epilepsy Foundation is an excellent resource (1-800-332-1000; www.EFA.org).

HEAD INJURY

Traumatic brain injury is a leading cause of death caused by trauma in the United States. The most common causes of head injury are motor vehicle accidents, assaults, and falls; drug and alcohol abuse are major contributing factors. Several different types of injuries can be identified.

TYPES OF HEAD INJURIES

Scalp Injuries

Scalp injuries include lacerations, contusions, abrasions, and hematomas. They may bleed profusely and may or may not be associated with skull or brain injuries.

Acute Mild Traumatic Brain Injury (Concussion)

Acute mild traumatic brain injury (TBI) occurs after an external blunt force to the head or an acceleration/deceleration injury to the head in which the brain is slapped against intracranial surfaces. **Concussion** is a term frequently used instead of mild TBI; however, it is used more specifically to describe the signs and symptoms that a person may experience after a mild TBI. The major causes are motor vehicle accidents, falls, occupational accidents, recreational accidents, and assaults. Falls are the most likely the cause of mild TBI in older adults, whereas motor vehicle accidents are more common in the young. Sports, especially contact sports such as American football, ice hockey, soccer, boxing, and rugby are frequent causes of mild TBI. In addition, soldiers in combat commonly experience mild TBI. Mild TBI is more common in males and individuals between the ages of 15 and 34 years.

Symptoms of concussion include confusion and amnesia, with or without loss of consciousness. Patients may forget events immediately before and after an injury occurs. In addition, they may experience headache, dizziness, lack of awareness of surroundings, and nausea and vomiting. In some cases, patients may have a vacant stare, a slowed response to questions, and may be easily distracted, as well as disoriented with slurred speech and memory deficits. Seizures may occur during the first week after the trauma, but primarily occur in more severe TBI and are rare in mild to moderate cases.

Individuals who are suspected of having a concussion or mild TBI, should be evaluated by a health care professional. The evaluation should include a neurological assessment and mental status testing. Some form of inpatient or at-home observation should be carried out for at least 24 hours after a mild TBI because of the risk of intracranial complications. Patient monitoring should include the following warning signs for seeking immediate medical help:

- Inability to awaken the patient at time of expected wakening
- Severe or worsening headaches
- Somnolence or confusion
- Restlessness, unsteadiness, or seizures
- Difficulties with vision
- Vomiting, fever, or stiff neck
- Urinary or bowel incontinence
- Weakness or numbness involving any part of the body

Contusion

A **contusion** is more serious than a concussion because actual bruising and bleeding exist in the brain tissue. Signs of contusion reflect the area of the brain affected and include focal neurological signs, confusion, and impaired consciousness. Brain contusions may delay recovery from a concussion.

Hematomas

A hematoma is a collection of blood, usually clotted, that may be classified as *subdural* or *epidural.*

Subdural Hematoma. A **subdural hematoma** usually results from tearing of the veins in the brain and the *dura*, the outermost meningeal covering of the brain, causing accumulation of blood in the space beneath the dura (Fig. 22.2A). The three types of subdural hematomas are (1) acute, (2) subacute, and (3) chronic. Acute subdural hematomas develop within 24 hours of the injury. Subacute subdural hematomas are seen more than 24 hours and less than 1 week after the initial injury. Chronic subdural hematomas occur within

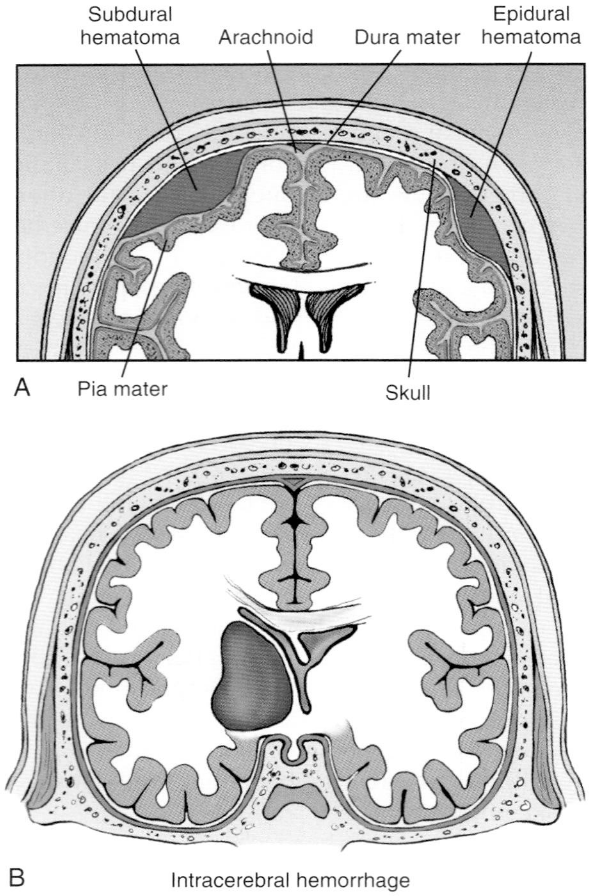

Fig. 22.2 (A) Epidural hematoma and subdural hematoma. (B) Intracerebral hemorrhage. (From Black JM, Hawks JH, Keene AM: *Medical-surgical nursing: clinical management for continuity of care*, ed 6, St. Louis, 2001, Saunders.)

weeks or even months of the original injury and are associated with low-impact injuries that cause very slow, diffuse bleeding. Because the bleeding associated with any hematoma can cause potentially serious consequences, astute assessment is needed to determine patient status. Surgical intervention is usually indicated for these types of injuries.

Epidural Hematoma. An **epidural hematoma** forms in the space between the inner surface of the skull and the outermost meningeal covering of the brain (see Fig. 22.2A). In general, epidural hematomas result from arterial bleeding secondary to a laceration and tearing of the middle meningeal artery. The patient typically has a momentary lapse of consciousness, then a period of alertness, followed by rapid deterioration. Thus you must be alert for any indication of increasing intracranial pressure (ICP), especially drowsiness progressing to coma. Surgical intervention may be necessary to relieve pressure, remove the clot, and stop the bleeding.

Intracerebral Hemorrhage

Intracerebral hemorrhages result from lesions within the tissue of the brain itself (Fig. 22.2B). These injuries may be small or large and may be accompanied by massive neurologic deficits.

Penetrating Injuries

Penetrating injuries result from sharp objects that penetrate the skull and brain tissue. In addition to the obvious brain injury, a scalp laceration exists along with a skull fracture. All penetrating injuries require prompt surgical intervention and pose an extremely high risk of infection for the patient because of the wound contamination that occurs.

SURGICAL TREATMENT

Surgical intervention for each of these types of trauma is directed at evacuating (removing) hematomas and debriding damaged tissue.

NURSING CARE OF THE PATIENT WITH A HEAD INJURY

FOCUSED ASSESSMENT

Nursing assessment of the patient with a neurologic disorder is outlined in Chapter 21, Box 21.2. (See also Nursing Care Plan: Patient With a Head Injury and the Health Promotion box.)

Patient Problems, Goals, and Outcome Criteria: Head Injury

Patient Problems	Goals and Outcome Criteria
Inadequate cerebral tissue perfusion related to ICP	Adequate cerebral tissue perfusion: patient alert and oriented
Inadequate oxygenation related to increased ICP	Normal oxygenation: respiratory rate of 12 to 20 breaths per minute with normal arterial blood gas values
Impaired mobility related to neuromuscular impairment, decreased mental alertness	Absence of complications of immobility (contractures, pressure injuries, pneumonia, atelectasis, constipation, urinary retention): intact skin, mobile joints, regular bowel movements, no bladder distention, breath sounds clear on auscultation.
Potential for injury related to decreased level of consciousness, disorientation, vision disturbances	Absence of injury: no abrasions, fractures, or severe bruising incurred after head injury
Potential for infection related to traumatic wounds or invasive procedures	Absence of infection: normal body temperature without signs of wound infection (redness, edema, purulent drainage), urinary infection (cloudiness, foul odor), or phlebitis (redness, tenderness)

Patient Problems, Goals, and Outcome Criteria: Head Injury—cont'd

Patient Problems	Goals and Outcome Criteria
Altered self-concept related to loss of function	Adaptation to altered body function: patient verbalizes way to compensate for changes in body function
Inability to perform usual roles related to neurologic impairment	Adjustment of roles and responsibilities consistent with abilities: patient assumes new roles within abilities

INTERVENTIONS

Inadequate Cerebral Tissue Perfusion

Monitor the patient closely for signs of increased ICP and impaired cerebral blood flow: decreasing level of consciousness, pupillary dilation with no response to light, motor deficits, abnormal posture, fever, increased blood pressure, bradycardia, and respiratory depression. Particularly note early signs of deterioration, including restlessness, agitation, or lethargy, and promptly report changes to the physician or the registered nurse (RN). Nursing care that can decrease ICP includes positioning to prevent neck and hip flexion, limiting suctioning, spacing nursing care, and preventing isometric muscle contraction. Elevate the head of the bed as ordered. Carefully regulate the rate of administration of intravenous fluids to prevent fluid volume excess. Also monitor urine output to assess fluid balance. If a ventriculostomy catheter is in place, inspect and measure the drainage fluid as ordered using strict aseptic technique. Administer diuretic and antiinflammatory drugs as ordered.

Inadequate Oxygenation

Closely monitor the patient's respiratory status using pulse oximetry or measurement of arterial blood gases. Immediately advise the physician for signs of respiratory depression or changes in the patient's respiratory pattern.

Potential for Injury

Observe patient for signs of dizziness, confusion, disorientation, ataxia, and lack of coordination. Assist with toileting as needed. Lower bed to prevent falls.

Potential for Infection

The patient who has suffered a head injury may have serious lacerations or abrasions that can admit pathogenic organisms. Intravenous lines and urinary catheters also place the patient at risk for infection. Use standard precautions when handling all invasive lines and when dressing wounds. In addition, monitor the patient's temperature and inspect wounds for increasing redness, swelling, or foul drainage. Administer antibiotic drugs as ordered.

Impaired Mobility

After a head injury, the patient may have temporary or permanent motor impairment. While confined to bed, the patient should be turned, repositioned, and encouraged to deep breathe at least every 2 hours. Routinely inspect the patient's skin for signs of pressure or breakdown and use antiembolism stockings if ordered. Encourage the patient to perform range-of-motion exercises and position joints in functional alignment. Assess urine and bowel elimination frequently to detect retention or constipation. As soon as permitted, help the patient out of bed and encourage as much activity as possible. Unfortunately, some head-injured patients have permanent impairments that necessitate lifelong care. Care of the immobile patient is discussed in detail in Chapter 12.

Altered Self-Concept and Inability to Perform Usual Roles

The losses associated with a serious head injury can render the patient unable to resume usual activities. The injury may also leave disfiguring scars or distorted features. Demonstrate acceptance of the patient through touch and genuine interest. Encourage the patient to ask questions, express concerns, and anticipate problems and solutions. Be realistic about the patient's disabilities while emphasizing abilities.

Patients with serious deficits usually are treated by a team that includes rehabilitation specialists. These experts help the patient to regain physical mobility, learn to carry out activities of daily living (ADL), learn new job skills, and deal with the emotional trauma of the injury and its effects.

Include the patient's family in the rehabilitation process. In many cases, family members serve as the caregivers after head injury. Activities provided by families include giving personal care, obtaining rehabilitation services, providing a safe environment, seeking reminders of the preinjury person, exploring what abilities might be regained, encouraging return to preinjury activities, encouraging active decision making, becoming active members of the rehabilitation team, and staying open to potential gains.

Health Promotion

Preventing Head Injury

Everyone should practice general safety by using the following:

- Helmets for sports activities such as football, baseball, skydiving, snowboarding, and skateboarding
- Helmets for riding bikes and motorcycles
- Seat belts while in automobiles
- Helmets on job sites for high-risk jobs such as construction and mining

Put On Your Thinking Cap!

You are caring for a patient with a head injury. The patient has been lethargic for most of the day but now seems more difficult to arouse. His vital signs and pupils are the same as they have been. What do you think is your best course of action in this situation?

BRAIN TUMORS

Brain **tumors** are classified as primary, in which the lesion arises from different cells within the central nervous system (CNS), or metastatic, in which a cancerous lesion in the brain develops from the spread of a primary cancer site somewhere else in the body. Systemic cancers that are most likely to metastasize to the CNS are lung cancer, melanoma, and breast cancer. Tumor cells can spread to the CNS through the blood and cerebrospinal fluid (CSF).

Not all brain tumors are malignant. Some tumor types, such as the meningioma, a tumorous growth of the meningeal tissue, are often benign. One might assume that benign tumor cells would suggest an excellent chance of complete recovery. However, the invasion of any kind of tumor into normal brain tissue is never insignificant. This invasion can cause significant damage that may prove fatal because of increasing ICP or surgical inaccessibility of the tumor.

CAUSES AND RISK FACTORS

The causes of brain tumors are generally unknown, but some appear to be congenital in origin, whereas others may be related to heredity. In addition, drug influences and environmental factors may play a role in the development of some brain tumors.

CLINICAL MANIFESTATIONS

The signs and symptoms of brain tumors are directly related to the area of the brain that is invaded by the tumor. Motor and sensory symptoms, visual disturbances, and headache all may be early manifestations of tumor growth. New-onset seizure activity in an adult patient may indicate the presence of a tumor. Cerebellar tumors may cause difficulties with balance and coordination. Other tumors, depending on their location, may involve cranial nerves.

DIAGNOSIS

The initial evaluation for a suspected brain tumor consists of a history and neurological examination, a brain MRI with contrast, and a systemic cancer screening for suspected metastasis; in addition, a CT scan of the chest and abdomen is performed if metastatic disease is suspected. Diagnostic tests are described in Chapter 21, Table 21.6.

MEDICAL TREATMENT

Management of the patient with a brain tumor depends on the type of cells present in the tumor. Surgery can be done to remove as much of the tumor tissue as possible. If the tumor is malignant, surgery is often followed by radiation therapy with or without chemotherapy. Medications may be given to relieve symptoms, such as seizures, that may occur with a brain tumor.

NURSING CARE OF THE PATIENT WITH A BRAIN TUMOR

Nursing care of the patient with a brain tumor depends on the specific deficits, treatment, and prognosis and may be the same as the care of the patient with a head injury. Care of the patient with cancer is discussed in Chapter 7.

FOCUSED ASSESSMENT

The complete neurologic assessment is summarized in Chapter 21, Box 21.2. The assessment is especially important before brain surgery to provide a baseline for comparing postoperative findings.

Patient Problems, Goals, and Outcome Criteria: Brain Tumor

Patient problems vary with the patient's specific symptoms and disabilities and the type of treatment used. Common patient problems and goals include the following.

Patient Problems	Goals and Outcome Criteria
Acute and/or chronic pain related to pressure of expanding tumor mass	Pain relief: patient states pain is relieved, has relaxed manner
Impaired cognition related to effects of tumor on brain tissue	Adaptation to altered thinking: improved mental orientation
Potential for injury related to impaired conduction of sensory information	Safety maintained: absence of injury associated with sensory or perceptual impairment
Decreased mobility and inability to manage self-care (bathing, dressing, feeding, toileting) related to motor disturbances, impaired cognition	Accomplishment of self-care: maximum possible patient mobility level and absence of complications of immobility (contractures, pneumonia, constipation, urinary retention)
Inadequate coping related to life-threatening disease, changes in behavior function	Effective coping: patient and family make positive statements about ability to deal with the illness

INTERVENTIONS

Acute and/or Chronic Pain

Document pain and administer analgesics as ordered. Codeine, opioids, or acetaminophen are often used. Small doses of morphine also may be used for pain relief. If pain relief is not achieved, inform the physician and assess for signs of increased ICP.

Impaired Cognition

Monitor the patient for changes in cognitive function by assessing orientation and response to instructions. Patients may demonstrate cognitive dysfunction, including impaired short-term memory, poor judgment, poor decision making, and impaired problem solving. Investigate sudden changes in mental status that may be caused by the tumor or by correctable factors such as drugs, hypoxia, and fluid and electrolyte imbalances. Listen carefully to the patient and present reality in a straightforward manner. Use devices to help the patient maintain orientation such as clocks, calendars, and seasonal decorations.

Potential for Injury

Explain to the patient that the effects of the brain tumor may cause unusual sensations and perceptual disturbances. Implement safety measures, as needed, to prevent injury caused by impaired vision, spatial perceptual problems, sensation, or seizures.

Decreased Mobility and Inability to Manage Self-Care (Bathing, Dressing, Feeding, Toileting)

Patients with brain tumors may have varying degrees of physical impairment. Assess the patient's ability to perform ADL and provide assistance as needed. Encourage the patient to remain as active as possible. If the patient's mobility is severely impaired, a high risk exists for disuse syndrome and the associated complications. Care of the immobilized patient is described in Chapter 12.

Inadequate Coping

The patient and family need assistance in dealing with a difficult diagnosis, in addition to the obvious residual physical effects. A diagnosis of a malignant brain tumor is devastating for the family, and emotional support is vital to help family members understand the nature of the disease and the anticipated problems and outcomes. Nursing care depends on the specific deficits, treatment, and prognosis and may be the same as the care of the patient with a head injury. Care of the patient with cancer is discussed in Chapter 7.

INFECTIOUS AND INFLAMMATORY CONDITIONS: MENINGITIS

Meningitis is inflammation of the meningeal coverings of the brain and spinal cord caused by either viruses or bacteria. Organisms may reach the meninges through the blood, via head wounds, or from other cranial structures such as the sinuses or inner ear. Frequently, pathogens are found on the surfaces of the nose and pharynx and are transported from person to person by direct contact through respiratory secretions.

With bacterial meningitis, most patients are quite ill and are regarded as a medical emergency. Many organisms may be responsible for bacterial meningitis, including *Neisseria meningitidis*, *Streptococcus pneumoniae*, and *Haemophilus* influenzae; *S. pneumoniae* is the most common cause of bacterial meningitis in the U.S. and globally. Before antibiotics, the mortality rate for bacterial meningitis was virtually 100%. Although current antibiotics are effective for treating meningitis, the death rate remains at 10% to 14%. Neurological complications of bacterial meningitis that may occur in about half of the patients include impaired mental status, increased ICP and cerebral edema, seizures, focal neurological deficits, cerebrovascular abnormalities, sensorineural hearing loss, and intellectual impairment.

Organisms causing viral meningitis include enteroviruses, HIV infection, herpes simplex meningitis, lymphocytic choriomeningitis virus, mumps, and various miscellaneous viruses such as encephalitis and West Nile virus. Viral meningitis is serious, but most people recover from viral meningitis within 1 to 2 weeks.

CLINICAL MANIFESTATIONS

Common signs and symptoms of meningitis include a sudden onset with fever, headache, nausea or vomiting, nuchal rigidity (stiffness in the back of the neck), mental status changes, and light sensitivity. Specific symptoms of viral meningitis often depend on the virus causing the infection, such as diarrhea, runny nose, sore throat, muscle aches, cough or rash. A rash may also occur with bacterial meningitis.

The presence of Kernig sign and Brudzinski sign is also indicative of meningeal irritation. To assess for Kernig sign (Fig. 22.3A), flex the patient's hip to a 90-degree angle and then extend the knee. In the presence of a meningeal infection, this movement produces pain in the hamstring area. Brudzinski sign (Fig. 22.3B) is flexion of both hips and knees when the examiner flexes the patient's neck.

MEDICAL DIAGNOSIS

Bacterial and viral meningitis have similar symptoms, so testing is necessary for diagnosis. A lumbar puncture is done to obtain a CSF sample for laboratory analysis. The sample is examined to detect the presence of microorganisms in the CSF and to identify the infecting organism. With bacterial meningitis, the CSF appears milky and purulent because of white blood cells suspended in the fluid. Computed tomography (CT) or magnetic resonance imaging (MRI) scans are used to assess for complications. In addition, a cotton swab may be used to collect a sample from the back of the throat.

MEDICAL TREATMENT

Management of bacterial meningitis requires prompt recognition and treatment with antimicrobial agents. In severe infections, broad-spectrum antimicrobials are used after a CSF specimen is obtained. Changes in therapy may be made when the results of culture and sensitivity tests are reported. Bacterial infections usually respond to antimicrobial therapy, but no specific drugs are effective against most viral infections of the

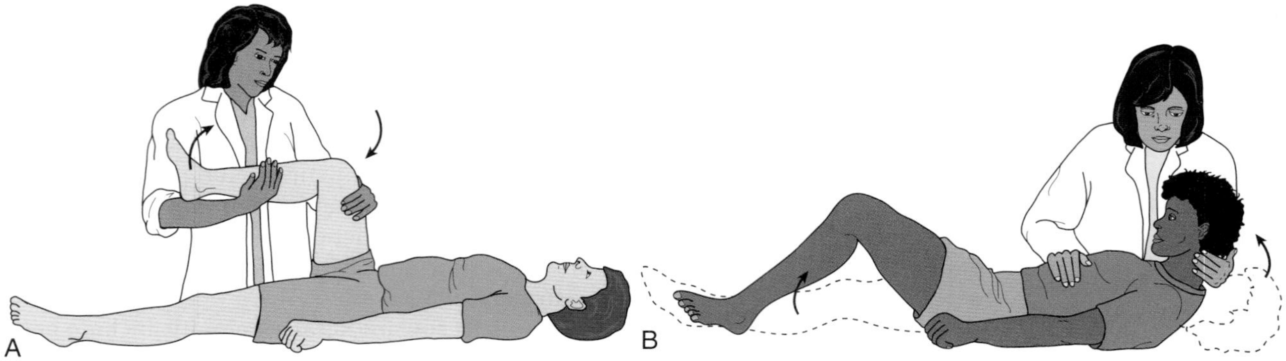

Fig. 22.3 (A) Positive Kernig sign: When the patient's leg is flexed as shown, the patient is unable to completely extend the leg. (B) Brudzinski sign: When the nurse flexes the patient's neck, hip flexion occurs. (From Lewis S, et al.: *Medical-surgical nursing*, ed 7, St. Louis, 2007, Mosby.)

CNS. Treatment for viral meningitis usually includes resting, oral or IV fluids, and medication to treat a fever or headache.

If needed, isolation precautions should be initiated. Organisms responsible for meningococcal meningitis are spread by the respiratory route and appropriate safeguards must be used to protect other patients, family, and staff until the organism is no longer in the nares (see Chapter 25).

Meningococcal vaccines are available for bacterial meningitis to prevent infection. They are recommended for all adolescents, college freshmen living in dormitories, military recruits, and travelers going to areas where meningococcal disease frequently exists (see the Health Promotion Box).

Health Promotion

Meningitis

Preventive measures:

- Vaccination at age 11 or 12 years with a booster at age 16 years
- Vaccinations for people with increased risk for exposure, including travelers to areas of existing epidemics, military recruits, and college freshmen living in dorms

Patients with meningitis and those who interact with them should receive the following interventions as necessary:

- Vaccination to prevent pneumococcal pneumonia and influenza
- Treatment of respiratory and ear infections
- Prophylactic antibiotics for anyone in close contact with bacterial meningitis

NURSING CARE OF THE PATIENT WITH MENINGITIS

FOCUSED ASSESSMENT

The routine neurologic assessment is summarized in Chapter 21, Box 21.2. When a patient has meningitis, assess vital signs and neurologic status frequently to determine further deterioration or the onset of complications.

Patient Problems, Goals, and Outcome Criteria: Meningitis

Patient Problems	Goals and Outcome Criteria
Potential inadequate cerebral tissue perfusion related to increased ICP	Adequate cerebral tissue perfusion: vital signs and level of consciousness consistent with patient norms
Inadequate oxygenation related to depression of the respiratory center	Adequate oxygenation: respiratory rate of 12 to 20 breaths per minute
Acute pain related to irritation of meninges and increased ICP	Pain relief: patient states pain has been relieved, relaxed manner
Potential for injury related to confusion, alterations in mental status, and seizures	Absence of injury: no falls or other trauma
Potential complications of immobility related to bed rest	Absence of complications of immobility: clear breath sounds, intact skin, normal muscle strength and joint mobility, regular bowel movements without straining

INTERVENTIONS

Potential Impaired Cerebral Tissue Perfusion

Elevate the head of the patient's bed as ordered. Instruct the patient to avoid coughing and not to hold their breath during turning because these behaviors increase ICP. Do not use restraints unless they are absolutely necessary to prevent further injury. Monitor for signs of increasing ICP: decreased level of consciousness, headache, nausea, vomiting, abnormal pupillary responses, and respiratory depression. If ICP does increase, administer prescribed treatments (e.g., diuretics, barbiturates, and opioids). Measures to lower the body temperature may be ordered to reduce the metabolic rate.

Inadequate Oxygenation

Monitor the patient's respiratory status and gag and swallowing reflexes. Position the patient to maintain a patent airway (and use suction if necessary). Arterial blood samples should be drawn and analyzed for gas values as ordered. If the respiratory rate is decreasing, the physician should be notified immediately.

Acute Pain

Assess the location and severity of any patient discomfort. Nursing measures to decrease pain include position changes, massage, and a quiet environment. Give analgesics as ordered and document their effect. Chapter 8 provides additional information about the nursing management of pain.

Potential for Injury

Because of the prevailing risk of seizures, take appropriate precautions to ensure patient safety. A subdued environment should be maintained to reduce irritability and contribute to patient comfort. Keep the bed in a low position, with the upper side rails padded and raised. Reorient the patient to the setting as needed and keep the call bell within easy reach. Remind patients who are dizzy not to get up without assistance.

Potential Complications of Immobility

The patient who is confined to bed is at risk for complications of immobility, especially stasis of pulmonary secretions, pressure sores, muscle weakness, joint stiffness, and constipation. Measures to prevent these complications are discussed in detail in Chapter 12.

INFECTIOUS AND INFLAMMATORY CONDITIONS: ENCEPHALITIS

Encephalitis is inflammation of brain tissue that is usually caused by one of several viruses similar to viral meningitis. These viruses may be prevalent during certain times of the year or in a specific geographic area. For example, certain types of mosquitos found in the United States are carriers of a virus commonly associated with encephalitis. In addition, toxic substances or other types of viral infections, such as herpes simplex, may precipitate encephalitis. Complications of encephalitis include changes in level of consciousness, increased ICP, cranial nerve palsies, motor and sensory changes, and speech function. Thus ongoing assessments should monitor for these changes. The complications are not specific to the agent causing the inflammation.

CLINICAL MANIFESTATIONS

The patient with encephalitis has symptoms directly related to the area of the brain that is involved. Fever, nuchal rigidity (stiff neck), headache, confusion, delirium, agitation, and restlessness are commonly seen. However, the patient may also become comatose or exhibit aphasia, hemiparesis, facial weakness, and other alterations in motor activity.

MEDICAL TREATMENT

Care for the patient with encephalitis is focused on enhancing patient comfort and increasing strength. Because seizure activity is a potential problem, you must take appropriate safety precautions.

NURSING CARE OF THE PATIENT WITH ENCEPHALITIS

The nursing plan of care parallels that of the patient with meningitis.

GUILLAIN-BARRÉ SYNDROME

Although its specific cause is unknown, **Guillain-Barré syndrome** (GBS), also known as *acute inflammatory polyneuropathy,* is believed to be an autoimmune response to a viral infection. It is a rapidly progressing disease that affects the motor and sensory component of the peripheral nervous system. Although the spinal nerves are usually affected, the cranial nerves may also be involved.

Patients with GBS often report some recent viral infection or vaccination. This apparently triggers an autoimmune response that destroys the myelin sheath around the peripheral nerves, slowing the conduction of impulses across the involved nerves. The four recognized types of GBS are (1) ascending GBS, (2) descending GBS, (3) Miller Fisher syndrome, and (4) pure motor GBS.

CLINICAL MANIFESTATIONS

GBS has three phases: (1) initial, (2) plateau, and (3) recovery, as described in Table 22.3. The initial phase is characterized by symmetric muscle weakness that typically begins in the lower extremities and ascends to the trunk and upper extremities. The disease process may affect cranial nerves, resulting in visual and hearing disturbances, difficulty chewing, and lack of facial expression. The muscles of respiration may also be affected, resulting in the need for mechanical ventilation.

Table 22.3 Phases of Guillain-Barré Syndrome

PHASE	CHARACTERISTICS	DURATION
Initial	Begins with onset of symptoms	Usually 1 to 3 weeks Ends when disease ceases to progress
Plateau	No further changes; neither deterioration nor improvement	Several days to 2 weeks
Recovery	Gradual improvement	May be as long as 2 years; some residual effects may be permanent

Respiratory dysfunction is the greatest threat to patients with GBS. They require close monitoring for incipient respiratory failure requiring intubation.

Mild paresthesia (abnormal sensations) or anesthesia (numbness) in the feet and hands may be present in a glove or stocking distribution pattern. In addition, some patients experience pain associated with the sensory changes. Despite all the motor and sensory changes, level of consciousness and intellectual functioning remain unchanged.

Effects on the autonomic nervous system may include hypertension, orthostatic hypotension, cardiac dysrhythmias, profuse sweating, paralytic ileus, and urinary retention. Dysautonomia, characterized by the effects just mentioned, occurs most frequently in patients with respiratory involvement and is potentially life-threatening.

In the plateau phase, the patient with GBS remains essentially unchanged. Although no further neurologic deterioration exists, no improvement is seen.

As recovery begins and progresses, remyelination occurs and muscle strength returns in a proximal to distal pattern (head to toes). Because the underlying axon generally remains undamaged, approximately 95% of patients with GBS have a nearly complete recovery. Others have residual numbness, stiffness, or paresis.

MEDICAL DIAGNOSIS

The characteristic onset and pattern of ascending motor involvement provide the basis for the diagnosis of GBS. An elevated protein level in the CSF obtained by lumbar puncture provides additional evidence for the diagnosis. Nerve conduction velocity studies reveal slowed conduction speed in the involved nerves.

MEDICAL TREATMENT

Management during the acute phase of the illness is directed at preserving vital function, particularly respiration. Respiratory status is closely monitored and mechanical ventilation initiated if the vital capacity falls to 15 mL/kg of body weight. In the presence of pharyngeal paresis and difficulty handling secretions, intubation and ventilation can be done earlier.

Massive doses of corticosteroids may be prescribed to suppress the inflammatory process.

Because GBS is believed to be an autoimmune disease, plasmapheresis has emerged as a major treatment. Plasmapheresis is a process in which blood is removed, centrifuged, and returned to the patient. In the process, antibodies that trigger the autoimmune disease are removed from the blood by a machine equipped with a special filtration system. The patient with GBS generally undergoes a series of treatments, ideally delivered within 7 to 14 days after the onset of the disease. Patients who benefit from plasmapheresis often recover faster.

NURSING CARE OF THE PATIENT WITH GUILLAIN-BARRÉ SYNDROME

FOCUSED ASSESSMENT

Assessment of the patient with a neurologic disorder is summarized in Chapter 21, Box 21.2. When GBS is suspected, the health history describes the progression of symptoms. Note the patient's fears, coping strategies, and sources of support. Record information about important social data such as occupation and family roles and responsibilities. The physical examination focuses on cranial nerve, motor, sensory, respiratory, and cardiovascular function.

Patient Problems, Goals, and Outcome Criteria: Guillain-Barré Syndrome

Patient Problems	Goals and Outcome Criteria
Inadequate oxygenation related to neurologic impairment	Adequate oxygenation: normal arterial blood gases and skin color
Inadequate circulation related to labile blood pressure, cardiac dysrhythmias, decreased cardiac output	Normal cardiac output: regular pulse with rate of 60 to 100 beats per minute and blood pressure consistent with patient norms
Potential for complications of immobility related to motor impairment	Absence of complications of immobility: intact skin, no contractures, clear breath sounds, regular bowel movements
Inadequate nutrition related to dysphagia, endotracheal tube	Adequate nutrition: stable body weight
Potential for injury related to loss of sensation in hands and feet, motor impairment, inability to speak	Absence of injury in affected body areas: no falls, bruises, corneal damage, or other injuries
Anxiety related to paralysis, doubts about recovery, loss of verbal communication	Decreased anxiety: patient states anxiety is reduced, calm manner
Lack of knowledge of GBS and its treatment	Knowledge of GBS and its treatment: patient confirms understanding and (if possible) demonstrates self-care

INTERVENTIONS

Inadequate Oxygenation

Some patients with GBS need mechanical ventilation because of neuromuscular failure. Closely monitor the patient for signs of respiratory mechanical failure. Assess the patient's oxygenation status frequently. A respiratory rate greater than 30 breaths per minute, abnormal chest and abdominal movements, and decreasing vital capacity signal increasingly ineffective breathing. Turn the patient at least every 2 hours and suction when indicated by increased pulse or adventitious breath sounds.

Inadequate Circulation

Be alert to rapid or slow cardiac dysrhythmias and administer antidysrhythmic drugs as ordered.

Potential for Complications of Immobility

Immobility is a major issue to address in the patient with GBS. If mobility is severely impaired, the patient is at high risk for disuse syndrome. These patients generally benefit from the use of rotational bed therapy to help promote pulmonary hygiene, peristalsis, and urinary bladder emptying. Careful positioning is crucial, with emphasis on maintaining joint function, muscle tone, and range of motion. Active and passive exercises, splints, and continuous passive motion machines may be used to prevent contractures.

Inadequate Nutrition

Impaired swallowing or the presence of an endotracheal tube mandates an alternative means of feeding. Enteral feedings are usually provided by way of a gastrostomy or nasoduodenal tube. Feedings may be given continuously or intermittently. Elevate the head of the bed 30 degrees during feedings to reduce the risk of aspiration. Aspirate and measure the residual (amount of feeding remaining in the stomach) at intervals to assess emptying of the stomach and prevent overfilling. In some cases, total parenteral nutrition may be used.

Potential for Injury

Progressive weakness makes the patient susceptible to falls. When the patient is in bed, raise the side rails, place the call bell within reach, and put the bed in low position. If the eyes do not close completely, ophthalmic drops or ointments should be applied as ordered. A moisture chamber for the eye is used to prevent eye injury from excessive drying. Carefully inspect the skin, especially areas without sensation, to detect pressure or injury.

Anxiety

Anxiety is understandable with progressive paralysis and increasing dependence on others for basic needs. You must work to develop trust and establish a therapeutic relationship with the patient. If the patient is able to communicate, encourage them to discuss thoughts, fears, and feelings and explore previously used coping strategies. To promote some sense of control, give the patient some choices about aspects of care. Explain equipment and procedures to the patient. Other strategies to reduce anxiety include the use of imagery, music, deep breathing (if possible), and controlling anxiety-producing thoughts. Boredom is a problem that must be considered for the patient with GBS. Orienting devices such as clocks, calendars, and daily schedules are helpful. The patient may enjoy television, radio, CDs, and visits from friends and family (see the Complementary and Alternative Therapies box).

> **Complementary and Alternative Therapies**
>
> Strategies to reduce anxiety include music therapy and massage. The herb *valerian* is used by some people as a sedative; its safety is under study.

One source of anxiety for many patients is impaired communication. While the patient is able to communicate, establish an alternative system of communication, such as blinking (one blink means "yes", two blinks mean "no") or a communication board. If the condition does affect speech or if mechanical ventilation is required, the patient will have a simple, alternative means of expression.

Lack of Knowledge

From admission through rehabilitation, the patient with GBS needs education about the condition and its usual course. Patients can deal with the condition better if they know how the symptoms progress and that reversal and improvement are expected.

Rehabilitation

As function is restored, emphasis is placed on both respiratory and physical rehabilitation. Total recovery of respiratory function determines how quickly physical rehabilitation can begin. Once rehabilitation is initiated, attention must be devoted to maximizing motor function through exercises and occupational therapy. Because complete recovery may take several years, a prolonged rehabilitation period is sometimes necessary. Before the patient is discharged from the hospital, referrals may be made to rehabilitation or home health agencies as appropriate. The patient and family may benefit from a support group for people with long-term or chronic illnesses. The Guillain-Barré Foundation is a source of information (866-224-3301 toll free; www.gbs-cidp.org).

PARKINSON DISEASE

Parkinson disease is a progressive **degenerative** disorder of the basal ganglia that results in an eventual loss of coordination and control of involuntary motor movement. It is generally recognized as a disease of older adults, first appearing in individuals in their 50s, with men affected more often than women. Idiopathic Parkinson disease has no known cause but is related to decreased levels of dopamine in the basal ganglia. A deficiency of dopamine, a neurotransmitter, contributes to the loss of motor function. Other types of **parkinsonism** are caused by atherosclerosis, the long-term use of phenothiazines, and some toxins.

CLINICAL MANIFESTATIONS

Several symptoms are characteristic of Parkinson syndrome. The major triad of symptoms is tremor, rigidity, and bradykinesia. Tremor is a trembling or shaking type of movement most often seen in the upper extremities. Tremors are more pronounced during resting postures and often relieved by movement. Typically, they disappear during sleep. A movement associated with the tremor is pill rolling, in which the tremor repetitively moves the individual's thumb against the fingertips as if rolling a small object. Rigidity is an increased resistance to passive movement or stiffness, and **bradykinesia** refers to extremely slow movements. Other signs and symptoms are loss of dexterity and power in affected limbs, aching, monotone voice, handwriting changes, drooling, lack of facial expression, rhythmic head nodding, reduced blinking, and slumped posture. Those with advanced disease demonstrate cogwheel rigidity (jerky movements with passive muscle stretching) and gait disturbances. The individual may appear to freeze and may have difficulty initiating the action of walking. Fig. 22.4 illustrates the typical facial appearance, posture, and gait of individuals with Parkinson syndrome.

Although Parkinson disease has been traditionally thought of as a motor system disorder, it is now recognized as a complex disorder with diverse clinical features that include neuropsychiatric and nonmotor manifestations:

- Cognitive dysfunction and dementia
- Psychosis and hallucinations
- Mood disorders, including depression, anxiety, and apathy
- Sleep disturbances
- Fatigue
- Autonomic dysfunction
- Olfactory dysfunction
- Gastrointestinal dysfunction
- Pain and sensory disturbances
- Dermatologic findings

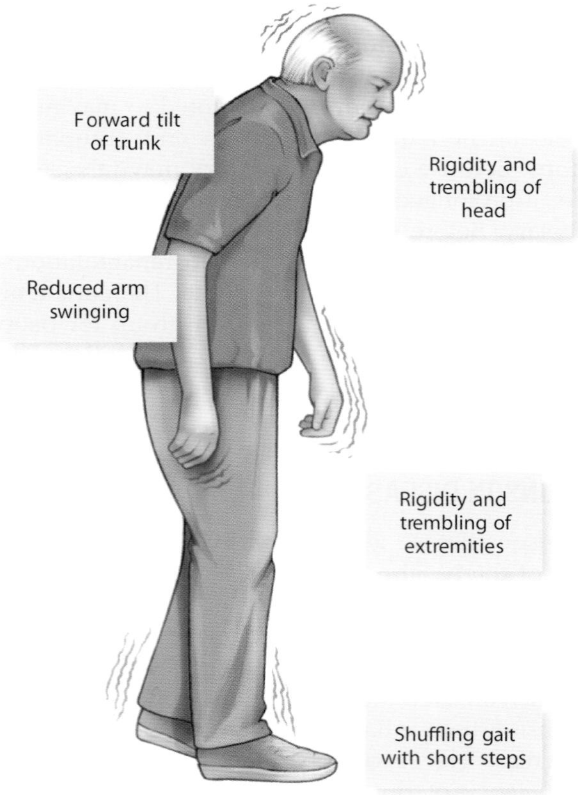

Fig. 22.4 Clinical manifestations of Parkinson syndrome. (From Patton KT, Thibodeau GA: *The human body in health & disease*, ed 7, St Louis, 2018, Elsevier.)

MEDICAL DIAGNOSIS

Parkinson syndrome is diagnosed from the health history and the physical examination results. MRI may be done to rule out other causes of the symptoms.

MEDICAL TREATMENT

Management of the patient with Parkinson syndrome is directed toward controlling the symptoms with physical therapy and drug therapy. The most beneficial physical therapy programs incorporate massage, heat, exercise, and gait retraining. Tai Chi appears to help with balance and stability in mild to moderate disease. Speech therapy has been used with swallowing issues as well as difficulty with speech with variable results.

Drug therapy relieves many of the symptoms of Parkinson syndrome. In the early stage of the disease, dopamine receptor agonists pramipexole (Mirapex) or ropinirole (Requip) are used to maximize the intrinsic dopamine. The cornerstone of therapy is the use of L-dopa (L-dihydroxyphenylalanine). L-dopa can cross the blood-brain barrier and is converted to dopamine in the basal ganglia, thereby supplementing levels of the neurotransmitter and reducing the symptoms of the disease. The conversion of L-dopa to dopamine must occur in the basal ganglia and not in the peripheral tissue. To ensure this, inhibitors are administered to prevent the breakdown of L-dopa by decarboxylase enzymes. The decarboxylase inhibitor most commonly used is carbidopa. It is frequently given in combination as carbidopa/levodopa (Sinemet). When the two drugs are used in combination, therapeutic levels may be achieved with lower doses. Carbidopa/levodopa also comes in orally disintegrating tablets (Parcopa, Carbilev). The enzyme catechol-*O*-methyltransferase (COMT) also breaks down levodopa in the peripheral circulation. Entacapone (Comtan) blocks this breakdown and prolongs the effectiveness of carbidopa/levodopa (Sinemet). Carbidopa/levodopa/entacapone (Stalevo), a combination drug, provides maximum blocking in the peripheral circulation and decreases the number of pills taken at one time. Because the benefits of L-dopa tend to decline after about 2 years, various other drug combinations may be used to control symptoms. Selegiline hydrochloride (Eldepryl), a monoamine oxidase (MAO) inhibitor, is used with Sinemet. MAO is the enzyme that degrades dopamine. Selegiline hydrochloride increases the available dopamine.

Anticholinergic drugs such as trihexyphenidyl (Artane) and benztropine (Cogentin) may be used in patients who have less severe symptoms or who are unresponsive to L-dopa. These are useful in managing tremors. Although the exact mechanism of action is unclear, amantadine (Symmetrel), an antiviral compound, is also used in the management of Parkinson syndrome. Amantadine is thought to release dopamine from storage sites in the neurons. Amantadine is effective for tremor as well as akinesia. It is often used in combination with L-dopa.

Treatment for depression may include antidepressant drug therapy, psychotherapy, and electroconvulsive therapy.

Several surgical procedures, among them thalamotomy, thalamic stimulation, and pallidotomy, may be used to treat Parkinson syndrome, although the benefits are variable. Surgical implantation of fetal dopamine-producing cells continues to be done experimentally. Adrenal medullary transplant entails implantation of the patient's own adrenal cells in the brain. It has produced limited improvement in some patients and is not widely accepted. All these surgical procedures are considered palliative rather than curative.

Put On Your Thinking Cap!

Write a short teaching plan for a home health patient who has started taking selegiline (Eldepryl) for Parkinson syndrome.

NURSING CARE OF THE PATIENT WITH PARKINSON SYNDROME

Nursing management for the patient with Parkinson syndrome is primarily related to maintaining mobility and preventing injury.

FOCUSED ASSESSMENT

The complete neurologic assessment is summarized in Chapter 21, Box 21.2. The health history of a patient with Parkinson syndrome should specifically include assessment for weakness, fatigue, muscle cramps, sweating, **dysphagia**, constipation, difficulty voiding, and unusual movements. Describe the effects of the disease on the patient's life. During the physical examination, be alert for lack of facial expression, eyes fixed in one direction, drooling, slurred speech, tearing, tremors, muscle stiffness, and poor balance and coordination.

As the disease progresses, the patient becomes more immobilized. Additional patient problems are addressed in Chapter 12.

Patient Problems, Goals, and Outcome Criteria: Parkinson Syndrome

Patient Problems	Goals and Outcome Criteria
Decreased mobility related to neuromuscular disease	Maximum possible mobility: patient participates in prescribed exercise program and performs self-care within abilities
Potential for injury related to poor balance and coordination	Absence of injury: no bruises, lacerations, or fractures because of trauma
Inadequate nutrition related to dysphagia, difficulty with self-feeding	Adequate nutritional intake: stable body weight
Inadequate coping related to physical changes and effects of disease on lifestyle	Effective coping with disease effects: patient makes statements confirming ability to deal with condition, adheres to plan of care
Lack of knowledge of disease, management, and self-care	Compliance with the prescribed plan of care: patient correctly describes and adheres to drug therapy, demonstrates exercise routine, uses resources, adapts to continue self-care

INTERVENTIONS

Impaired Mobility

Assess the patient's mobility and ability to perform self-care. Provide assistance as needed, but encourage the patient to remain as independent in self-care as possible. Assistive devices, including walkers and wheelchairs, may enable the patient to be mobile despite some deterioration in coordination and balance. Stress the value of exercise in maintaining strength and mobility. Active and passive range-of-motion exercises may be done. Both the physical and occupational therapists may participate in designing programs to maintain or improve function.

Suggestions to improve mobility with Parkinson syndrome include the following:

- Scoot to the edge of a chair before trying to stand.
- Use satin sheets to make it easier to move in and out of bed.
- March in place before starting to walk.
- Practice lifting the foot as if to step over an object on the floor to initiate walking.

Potential for Injury

The patient with Parkinson syndrome is at special risk for fall-related injuries. Place the call bell within easy reach and instruct the patient to call for assistance when rising. If the patient is ambulatory, remove obstacles on the floor. Recommend firm shoes, which provide better support than soft slippers. Provide assistive devices (e.g., canes, walkers, wheelchairs) as needed. Allow the patient to move at their own speed to decrease the risk of injury. Because this is a chronic condition, the patient's home setting should be evaluated and adapted for safe ambulation.

Inadequate Nutrition

To promote ease of swallowing, position the patient comfortably for meals, with the head elevated and food conveniently arranged. Provide assistance as needed (this may involve simply cutting meat and opening containers or may entail actually feeding the patient). Patients must never be rushed while they are eating. If the patient chokes on liquids, the dietitian should be consulted about the need for semisolids and thick liquids, which are often easier to swallow. Thickening agents can be added to thin fluids to facilitate swallowing. Small, frequent meals may be better tolerated than three large ones. Monitor the patient's weight to assess the adequacy of nutritional intake. Some researchers believe that patients with Parkinson syndrome benefit from a low-protein diet during the day and an evening meal high in protein, but this is still experimental.

Inadequate Coping

Patients with Parkinson syndrome must deal with loss of mobility that may affect their jobs, home and family responsibilities, social relationships, and leisure activities. Voice changes may severely impair verbal communication. Explore how the patient is dealing with these changes. Nurses and other members of the health care team help the patient identify strategies to adapt to changing abilities. These professionals should be alert to expressions of depression and inform the physician of such findings. A referral may be made to a mental health counselor, clinical nurse specialist, or support group. Administer antidepressant drugs as ordered and monitor their effects (see the Complementary and Alternative Therapies box).

Complementary and Alternative Therapies

St. John's wort is used widely as an antidepressant. It is a monoamine oxidase (MAO) inhibitor and can interact with prescribed drugs. Ask the patient to report use of herbal remedies to the physician. Other measures to treat depression are physical exercise, massage, and light therapy.

Caution patients with Parkinson syndrome not to use herbal supplements without physician approval. Kava can worsen symptoms of Parkinson syndrome. Chaste tree fruit interferes with the drug selegiline (Eldepryl). Indian snakeroot interferes with the actions of levodopa and carbidopa.

Lack of Knowledge

Management of this progressive condition requires the patient or a caregiver to understand Parkinson syndrome and how it is treated (see the Patient Teaching box). Supplement verbal information with written material (see the Health Promotion box).

Patient Teaching

Parkinson Disease

- Drugs relieve symptoms but do not cure Parkinson syndrome. You must continue therapy as prescribed to control symptoms.
- Know your drug names, dosages, schedule, and adverse effects that should be reported to your physician.
- Exercise is essential to maintain mobility.
- Resources include the American Parkinson Disease Association (1-800-223-2732; www.apdaparkinson.org), the Parkinson's Foundation (800-457-6676; www.pdf.org), and the National Parkinson Foundation (1-800-473-4636; www.parkinson.org).

Health Promotion

Patients With Parkinson Syndrome

Patients with Parkinson syndrome and those who interact with them should receive the following interventions as necessary:

- Maintain general health and have regular checkups.
- Follow a regular routine of stretching and exercise to maintain mobility and balance.
- Prevent falls through environmental control.

MULTIPLE SCLEROSIS

Multiple sclerosis (MS) is a chronic, progressive degenerative disease that attacks the protective myelin sheath around axons and disrupts the conduction of impulses through the CNS (Fig. 22.5). It may affect motor, sensory, cerebellar, and other pathways. The course of the disease is variable. Several patterns have been identified. The disease may progress steadily (chronic, progressive MS), may be characterized by exacerbations and remissions (exacerbating-remitting MS), may have fewer stable periods than exacerbating-remitting MS (relapsing-progressive MS), or may become stable with no active disease for at least 1 year (stable MS). MS is the second most common neurologic cause of disability. The incidence is highest in persons between 20 and 40 years of age and MS affects women more often than men.

CAUSE

Although the exact cause of MS is unknown, viral infections and autoimmune processes have been implicated. Some studies have implicated a retrovirus in the disease process, but more research is needed to determine whether this is indeed the cause of MS. The myelin sheath surrounding the axons is destroyed, eventually leaving areas of sclerotic tissues (see Fig. 22.5). As the sclerotic tissue develops, the patient may have a period of remission. The involved fibers eventually degenerate, resulting in permanent

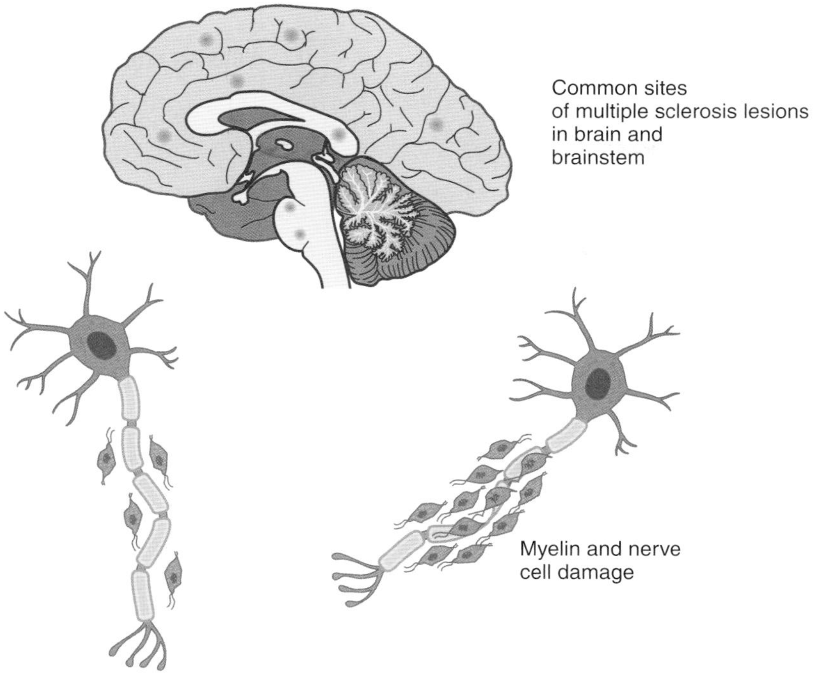

Fig. 22.5 The lesions in multiple sclerosis: location and effects. (From Hopper T: *Mosby's pharmacy technician*, ed 3, St. Louis, 2013, Saunders.)

damage. Nerve impulses then are no longer able to travel down the affected axon.

CLINICAL MANIFESTATIONS

Because the exact pattern of damage varies from patient to patient, the signs and symptoms vary as well. The most common symptoms of MS are fatigue, weakness and tingling in one or more extremities, visual disturbances, problems with coordination, bowel and bladder dysfunction, spasticity, and depression.

For patients who have exacerbating-remitting MS, the progression is variable. As the disease progresses, the periods of remission become shorter and the neurologic deficits present during exacerbations become more severe and permanent.

MEDICAL DIAGNOSIS

The diagnosis of MS is based primarily on the physical examination and history of cyclic remission-exacerbation periods. A familial history of the disease is significant, as is worsening of symptoms when the patient is exposed to warm weather. MRI of the brain and spinal cord may reveal plaques characteristic of MS. Currently, specific MRI requirements support a diagnosis of MS. Slow, absent, or abnormal visual-evoked responses are seen with MS.

MEDICAL TREATMENT

Because of its chronic, progressive nature, the treatment of MS is symptomatic and supportive. Drug therapy during periods of exacerbation may involve administration of adrenocorticotropic hormone (ACTH). Corticosteroids (ACTH, prednisone, methylprednisolone) may be used to control exacerbations, but they do not slow the progression of the disease. Treatment often includes drugs that modulate the immune response and thus the course of the disease. The specific drug will depend on the type of MS. Drugs in this category include interferon beta-1b (Betaseron) and interferon beta-1a (Avonex). Glatiramer acetate (Copaxone) is an immune modulator that is unrelated to interferon. Immunosuppressant drugs such as mitoxantrone (Novantrone) and natalizumab (Tysabri) are also used for exacerbations. When immunosuppressive agents are used, patients must be carefully monitored for bone marrow suppression. Glucocorticosteroids are used for acute exacerbation and relapses. The spasticity experienced by MS patients may respond to treatment with baclofen (Lioresal) or tizanidine (Zanaflex). Carbamazepine (Tegretol) and gabapentin (Neurontin) are used to relieve neuropathic pain. Amantadine (Symmetrel) is used to relieve fatigue associated with the disease. Electrical neuromuscular stimulation is being used to decrease spasticity and improve active movement and function, but studies of its effectiveness have not found consistent evidence of improvement. Urinary retention is treated with cholinergic drugs such as bethanechol (Urecholine) or neostigmine (Prostigmine). Urinary frequency and urgency resulting from spasticity of the bladder can be treated with anticholinergics such as propantheline bromide (Pro-Banthine) or oxybutynin (Ditropan). Tolterodine (Detrol) is a competitive muscarinic receptor antagonist and is more specific for the bladder than oxybutynin. Tamsulosin (Flomax) is also useful for urinary issues related to failure to store and empty urine (see Table 22.4).

Table 22.4 Drug Therapy: Multiple Sclerosis Drugs

DRUG	USE/ACTION	SIDE EFFECTS	NURSING INTERVENTIONS
Corticosteroids			
adrenocorticotropic hormone (ACTH)	Control exacerbations		
prednisone	Intermediate acting glucocorticoid; decreases inflammation by increasing capillary permeability	Thrombophlebitis, embolism, GI hemorrhage, depression, flushing, headache, mood changes; avoid in older adults with high risk of delirium	Evaluate therapeutic response: ease of respirations, decreased inflammation Patient/family teaching: Carry emergency ID that drug is being taken; avoid vaccinations; do not discontinue abruptly, which may result in adrenal crisis; avoid OTC salicylates, cough products with alcohol, cold preparations; report symptoms of infections (fever, sore throat, cough); drug may produce symptoms of Cushing syndrome
methylprednisolone	Intermediate acting glucocorticoid; decreases inflammation	Circulatory collapse, thrombophlebitis, embolism, GI hemorrhage, potassium depletion	Look for signs of potassium depletion: paresthesia, fatigue, nausea and vomiting, depression, polyuria, dysrhythmias, weakness; look for signs of adrenal insufficiency: weight loss, nausea, vomiting, confusion, anxiety, hypotension, weakness Patient/family teaching: Carry emergency ID that drug is being taken; avoid vaccinations; do not discontinue abruptly, which may result in adrenal crisis; avoid OTC salicylates, cough products with alcohol, cold preparations; report symptoms of infections (fever, sore throat, cough); drug may produce symptoms of Cushing syndrome
Dexamethasone (Decadron)	Long-acting glucocorticoid; decreases inflammation	Depression, hypertension, nausea, vomiting, peptic ulcer, hypokalemia, fluid retention	Weigh daily, notify health care provider of weekly gain >5 lb; monitor BP and pulse; notify health care provider of chest pain Patient/family teaching: Carry medical alert ID; take with food or milk; bruising may occur easily; do not discontinue abruptly to avoid adrenal crisis; avoid exposure to chickenpox or measles, persons with infections
Skeletal Muscle Relaxants			
baclofen (Lioresal)	Decreases frequency and severity of muscle spasms; used for spasticity with MS	Dizziness, nausea, weakness, fatigue, drowsiness, disorientation, seizures,	Observe for improvement in spasms and spasticity; look for symptoms of withdrawal such as agitation, tachycardia, insomnia, or increased temperature Patient/family teaching: Avoid hazardous activities because dizziness or blurred vision may occur; avoid OTC medications with alcohol or other CNS depressants; take PO with food or milk; do not discontinue medication quickly but taper off gradually over 1 to 2 weeks.
tizanidine (Zanaflex).	Reduces spasticity; management of muscle tone with MS	Somnolence, dizziness, nervousness, hypotension, dry mouth, constipation, blurred vision, urinary frequency, tremors, rash; avoid drug in older men—may cause urinary retention	Observe for side effects; monitor blood pressure sitting and standing to rule out orthostatic hypotension Patient/family teaching: Patient should rise slowly from lying or sitting to standing position to prevent orthostatic hypotension; avoid drinking alcohol; use chewing gum or lozenges for dry mouth; ask for assistance if dizziness or sedation occur; discontinue medication gradually

Table 22.4 Drug Therapy: Multiple Sclerosis Drugs—cont'd

DRUG	USE/ACTION	SIDE EFFECTS	NURSING INTERVENTIONS
Immune Modulators			
interferon beta-1a (Avonex, Rebif) interferon beta-1b (Betaseron, Extavia)	Immune modifier; antiviral Used for ambulatory patients with relapsing or remitting multiple sclerosis	Headache, fever, pain, chills, mental status changes, depression, suicide attempts, seizures, migraine, palpitations, hypertension, diarrhea, constipation, vomiting, abdominal pain, sweating, injection site reactions, sinusitis	Premedicate with acetaminophen or ibuprofen and give at bedtime to lessen flulike symptoms; rotate injection sites to minimize reactions; do not inject into an area where skin is irritated, reddened, bruised, infected or scarred; check site after 2 hours for redness, edema or tenderness; look for signs of suicidal thoughts Patient/family teaching: Blurred vision, hearing loss, sweating may occur; female patients may experience irregular menses, dysmenorrhea or breast pain; use sunscreen to prevent photosensitivity; notify health care provider of increased temperature, chills, muscle soreness, fatigue, depression
Glatiramer acetate (Copaxone, Glatopa)	May modify immune responses Decreases frequency of relapses in MS	Anxiety, tremor, vertigo, agitation, migraine, palpitations, syncope, tachycardia, dyspnea, blurred vision, ear pain, nausea, vomiting, diarrhea, bruising, rash, pruritis, sweating	Watch for side effects, allergic reactions Patient/family teaching: Take medication as directed; do not stop taking or change schedule; teach self-injection technique
mitoxantrone (Novantrone)	Antineoplastic, antiinfective, immunomodulator; decreases MS relapses	Seizures, cardiac dysrhythmias, blue-green urine, renal failure, nausea, vomiting, diarrhea, anorexia, anemia, sepsis	Rinse mouth 3–4 times a day with water, club soda; brush teeth 2–4 times a day with soft brush or cotton-tipped applicators for stomatitis; use unwaxed dental floss Patient/family teaching: Immediately report bleeding, dyspnea, possible infections, seizure, jaundice, fever, cough, or dyspnea; avoid hot foods or those with citric acid or rough texture; report any bleeding, white spots or ulcerations in mouth; examine mouth daily; avoid crowds or persons with infections; sclera or urine may turn blue; hair loss may occur; notify health care provider if pregnancy is suspected or planned; use effective contraception
natalizumab (Tysabri)	Used for ambulatory patients with relapsing/remitting MS who have not responded to other treatments	Headache, fatigue, depression, abdominal discomfort, rash, arthralgia, lower respiratory tract infection	Observe for side effects, tell patient and family to report side effects that would indicate infection, including sore throat, cough, increased temperature, infusion-site reactions
Cholinergics			
propantheline bromide (Pro-Banthine)	Antispasmodic; used for urinary frequency and urgency resulting from spasticity of the bladder Not recommended for persons over 65 because of highly anticholinergic properties and uncertain effectiveness as an antispasmodic	Palpitations, tachycardia, confusion, dizziness, drowsiness, headache, weakness, insomnia, nervousness, blurred vision, urinary retention, nausea, vomiting, constipation, decreased sweating, anaphylaxis	Be vigilant for side effects, especially in older adults Patient/family teaching: Avoid hazardous activities because dizziness or blurred vision may occur; avoid OTC medications with alcohol or other CNS depressants; avoid hot weather or strenuous activity because drug decreases perspiration

Continued

Table 22.4 Drug Therapy: Multiple Sclerosis Drugs—cont'd

DRUG	USE/ACTION	SIDE EFFECTS	NURSING INTERVENTIONS
oxybutynin (Ditropan, Uromax, Oxytrol).	Relaxes smooth muscle in urinary tract; used for urinary frequency and urgency resulting from spasticity of the bladder	Anxiety, restlessness, dizziness, drowsiness, palpitations, sinus tachycardia, blurred vision, dry eyes or mouth, nausea, vomiting, anorexia, constipation, urinary retention, hyperthermia, anaphylaxis, angioedema	Observe for side effects Patient/family teaching: Avoid hazardous activities because dizziness or blurred vision may occur; avoid OTC medications with alcohol or other CNS depressants; avoid hot weather or strenuous activity because drug decreases perspiration
bethanechol (Urecholine, Duvoid, Myotonachol)	Urinary tract stimulant; used for urinary retention	Nausea, bloody diarrhea, belching, vomiting, cramps, fecal incontinence; orthostatic hypotension, cardiac arrest	Take on an empty stomach; check BP and pulse, monitor intake and output to check for urinary retention; note signs of toxicity: bradycardia, hypotension, headache, dizziness, seizures, respiratory depression (if these occur, discontinue drug) Patient/family teaching: Take drug 1 hour before meals or 2 hours after meals to avoid nausea; make position changes slowly to prevent orthostatic hypotension; avoid hazardous activities until effects are known
Anticonvulsants			
Carbamazepine (Tegretol)	Decreases neuropathic pain and spasticity associated with MS	Drowsiness, dizziness, suicidal thoughts, hypertension, nausea, rash	Take with food or milk; avoid grapefruit juice; avoid use in older adults because drug may cause ataxia, impaired psychomotor function; give hard candy or chewing gum to alleviate dry mouth Patient/family teaching: Avoid hazardous activities, especially if dizziness or drowsiness occurs during first 3 days of treatment; decrease medication gradually; note that urine may turn pink to brown
gabapentin (Neurontin)	Decreases neuropathic pain and spasticity associated with MS	Depression, double vision, dizziness, fatigue	Note location, duration, and characteristics of pain; notify health care provider if mental status changes: mood, sensorium, affect, behavior, suicidal thoughts; avoid use in older adults; do not use within 2 h of antacid
Antiviral			
amantadine (Symmetrel, Osmolex ER, Endantadine)	Prevents penetration virus to host; causes release of dopamine from neurons; used for treatment of fatigue in MS	Headaches, dizziness, anxiety, depression, hallucinations, insomnia, orthostatic hypotension, nausea, vomiting, urinary frequency or retention; may cause increased psychiatric disorders, especially in the elderly	Evaluate therapeutic response: decreased fatigue; change body position slowly to prevent orthostatic hypotension; be alert for side effects of drug
Urinary Tract Innervators			
tolterodine (Detrol)	Relaxes smooth muscle in urinary tract; used for overactive bladder (urinary frequency, urgency), urinary incontinence	Dizziness, headache, nausea, vomiting, anorexia	Avoid in older adults with delirium or at high risk for delirium, monitor for confusion frequently; no liquids before bedtime; observe for signs of infection, skin effects, shortness of breath, urinary retention
tamsulosin (Flomax)	Useful for urinary issues related to failure to store and empty urine.	Dizziness, headache, orthostatic hypotension	Monitor BP sitting and standing; make position changes slowly to prevent orthostatic hypertension; administer medication ½ hour after same meal each day

BP, Blood pressure; *CNS*, central nervous system; *ID*, identification; *MS*, multiple sclerosis; *OTC*, over the counter; *PO*, per os.

NURSING CARE OF THE PATIENT WITH MULTIPLE SCLEROSIS

FOCUSED ASSESSMENT

Complete assessment of the patient with a neurologic disorder is summarized in Chapter 21, Box 21.2. When a patient has MS, the health history specifically includes the onset and progression of symptoms, especially those that affect mobility, vision, eating, and elimination. Explore the effects of the disease on the person's lifestyle (see the Health Promotion box). In addition, identify the patient's usual coping strategies. Important aspects of the physical examination are evaluation of range of motion and strength and observation for gait abnormalities, tremors, and muscle spasms.

Health Promotion

Patients With Multiple Sclerosis

Patients with MS should receive the following interventions as necessary:

- Maintain general health through diet and exercise.
- Avoid or minimize effects of triggers for MS such as infections, trauma, climate changes, and immunizations.
- Seek regular medical checkups for disease prevention.

Patient Problems, Goals, and Outcome Criteria: Multiple Sclerosis

Patient Problems	Goals and Outcome Criteria
Impaired mobility related to weakness or spasticity	Maximal possible mobility: patient continues physical activity within capabilities
Potential for injury related to neurologic impairment	Absence of injury associated with impaired sensation: intact skin without redness related to pressure, no falls
Inability to manage self-care (dressing, bathing, feeding, toileting) related to impaired voluntary movements and poor coordination	Achievement of self-care: ADL completed independently or with assistance as needed
Impaired urinary elimination (functional incontinence, difficulty voiding) related to impaired conduction of bladder nerve impulses	Normal bladder filling and emptying: bladder not palpable, no uncontrolled passage of urine
Potential for infection related to inadequate resistance	Absence of infection: normal body temperature and white blood cell count
Inadequate coping related to chronic illness, uncertain course of disease	Adaptation to changes in physical functioning: behavior and statements reflect intent to maximize abilities
Lack of knowledge of disease, treatment, and self-care	Patient understands disease, treatment, and self-care: patient accurately describes MS, its treatment, and self-care measures to reduce risk of complications

INTERVENTIONS

Impaired Mobility

Encourage the patient to be as independent as possible. Provide assistance with ambulation as needed; a cane or walker may enable the patient to walk safely. If the patient has muscle spasms, administer muscle relaxants as ordered. To prevent contractures, the patient should perform range-of-motion exercise. If the patient cannot do the exercises independently, teach a caregiver how to do the exercises. Physical therapy may be ordered. The patient who is not able to move independently is at risk for disuse syndrome. If the patient becomes disabled to this extent, decisions must be made about home nursing services or care in a long-term facility.

Potential for Injury

If the patient has impaired sensation, give special attention to the skin. Inspect extremities and pressure points for signs of pressure or trauma and encourage the patient to wear shoes when out of bed to prevent injury. Other measures instituted to prevent injury include using caution with sources of heat and cold.

Inability to Manage Self-Care (Bathing, Feeding, Dressing, Toileting)

Encourage patients to do as much as they can for themselves. Provide assistance as needed to carry out ADL. Difficulty with feedings, especially if the patient is dysphagic, may result in inadequate food intake. Alternative means of feeding may be necessary. Discuss with the patient and family their needs for assistance with caregiving. Home nursing care can support the patient who wishes to remain in a home setting.

Impaired Urinary Elimination (Functional Incontinence, Difficulty Voiding)

Palpate the patient's lower abdomen for bladder distention and carry out intermittent catheterization as ordered. If urine retention is a problem, assess the patient for signs and symptoms of urinary tract infection: fever, burning on urination, foul odor, sediment. If the patient has urinary incontinence, take steps to reduce the incontinent episodes as described in Chapter 14. Incontinence briefs may be needed, and meticulous skin care is a must. Loss of bladder control is very distressing, and you must be sensitive in helping the patient to deal with it.

Potential for Infection

The MS patient who is being treated with immunosuppressive drugs has decreased resistance to infection. Take steps to reduce the risk of infection, including protecting the patient from people with infections (e.g., avoiding crowds during seasons with increased respiratory infections). Encourage intake of fluids to maintain adequate hydration and emphasize good hygiene practices. In addition, teach the patient and family the signs of infection that should be reported promptly to the physician.

Inadequate Coping

MS is a chronic, progressive disease. Most patients have increasing disability, which requires considerable adaptation. Because the initial symptoms typically occur in young adults, patients often must learn to balance work, home, and family responsibilities. Provide the patient with opportunities to talk about the illness and its effects. Be accepting of the patient's concerns and guide the patient to identify strengths, abilities, and usual coping strategies (see the Complementary and Alternative Therapies box). With the patient's permission, a referral may be made to the clinical nurse specialist, mental health counselor, or spiritual counselor. Support groups can be helpful to many patients and their families.

> **Complementary and Alternative Therapies**
>
> Guided imagery, breathing exercises, and progressive relaxation can help the MS patient to reduce stress. Various special diets and nutritional supplements (commonly fatty acids, niacin, zinc, magnesium, selenium, beta-carotene, and vitamins C, B_6, and B_{12}) have been proposed, but research has not consistently shown benefits to the MS patient.

Lack of Knowledge

Assess what the patient knows about MS and what they would like to know. The teaching plan is individualized to the patient's needs and may include problems associated with immobility and measures to prevent complications.

AMYOTROPHIC LATERAL SCLEROSIS

CAUSE

Amyotrophic lateral sclerosis (ALS), also known as *Lou Gehrig's disease,* is a degenerative neurologic disease. It affects males two to four times as often as females and most often strikes those between 40 and 70 years of age. The disease generally progresses rapidly, and death occurs approximately 3 years after the onset of symptoms. Although a viral cause has been suspected, the exact cause is unknown.

PATHOPHYSIOLOGY

In ALS, degeneration of the anterior horn cells and the corticospinal tracts occurs, so the patient exhibits both upper and lower motor neuron symptoms. Evidence of upper motor neuron disease includes spasticity and hyperreflexia. Lower motor neuron disease produces weakness, atrophy, cramps, and muscle twitching. Some patients have difficulty swallowing and slurred speech. Despite involvement of the motor nuclei of the brainstem, intellectual ability, sensory perception, vision, and hearing are all unaffected.

CLINICAL MANIFESTATIONS

Initially the patient exhibits weakness of voluntary muscles of the upper extremities, particularly the hands. In addition, some patients may experience difficulty in swallowing and speaking because of progressive weakness of the oropharyngeal muscles. Spasticity of the involved muscle groups may be evident. The disease progresses steadily until the patient is completely incapacitated. Eventually, respirations become shallow and the patient has difficulty clearing the airway of pulmonary secretions. Death results from aspiration, respiratory infection, or respiratory failure.

MEDICAL DIAGNOSIS

The patient's history and physical examination findings lead to the diagnosis of ALS. EMG provides supporting evidence of impaired impulse conduction in the muscles. More sophisticated tests are used to rule out other degenerative motor diseases such as MS or myasthenia gravis.

MEDICAL TREATMENT

Because no known cure or treatment for ALS exists, therapy is supportive, focusing on the prevention of complications and the maintenance of maximum function.

NURSING CARE OF THE PATIENT WITH AMYOTROPHIC LATERAL SCLEROSIS

FOCUSED ASSESSMENT

The complete neurologic assessment is outlined in Chapter 21, Box 21.2. When a patient has ALS, it is important to obtain a patient history to determine the presence of dyspnea, dysphagia, muscle cramps, weakness, twitching, and joint stiffness. Describe the effects of the disease on the patient's lifestyle. During the physical examination, anticipate finding weakness, muscle atrophy, abnormal reflexes and gait, and paralysis.

Patient Problems, Goals, and Outcome Criteria: Amyotrophic Lateral Sclerosis

Patient Problems	Goals and Outcome Criteria
Inadequate oxygenation related to paralysis of respiratory muscles	Patent airway: respiratory rate of 12 to 20 breaths per minute without crackles or wheezes
Decreased mobility related to progressive weakness and atrophy	Maximal possible mobility: patient participates in activities to maintain joint mobility
Inadequate nutrition related to dysphagia	Adequate nutritional intake: stable body weight
Inability to communicate effectively related to oropharyngeal muscle weakness	Effective communication: patient conveys needs without excessive frustration
Potential for disrupted skin tissue integrity related to immobility	Normal skin integrity: intact skin without signs of pressure (redness, blanching)
Anticipatory grief related to progressive, fatal disease	Adaptation to losses: patient verbalizes losses, their importance, and acceptance of losses; makes realistic plans
Altered self-concept related to loss of independence	Stable or improved self-concept: patient makes positive statements about self
Altered family dynamics related to progressive illness of patient	Family adapts to patient condition: positive family communication and interactions; patient's role shifted

INTERVENTIONS

Inadequate Oxygenation

Monitor the patient's respiratory rate and effort, breath sounds, and pulse rate to detect inadequate oxygenation. Provide instructions or assist the immobile patient in turning, coughing, and deep breathing at least every 2 hours. Chest physiotherapy may be ordered to mobilize secretions to prevent atelectasis and pneumonia. If the patient has difficulty removing secretions, gentle suction may be needed. Oxygen therapy is indicated if evidence of hypoxia (restlessness, tachycardia) is noted.

Decreased Mobility

Progressive muscle wasting, spasticity, and paralysis cause increasing immobility. Perform active or passive range-of-motion exercises to prevent contractures and give antispasmodic drugs as ordered. Maintain extremities in functional positions and encourage use of assistive devices (e.g., cane, walker, wheelchair) as needed to maintain mobility as long as possible. Monitor the patient's ability to perform ADL and provide assistance as needed. The patient who is immobile is at high risk for complications of immobility. Nursing care of the immobile patient is discussed in Chapter 12.

Inadequate Nutrition

Muscle weakness and cranial nerve involvement eventually make it difficult for the patient to consume adequate food for good nutrition. Monitor the patient's weight to assess adequacy of the diet. Meals may be supplemented with high-protein snacks. Because constipation is a common problem, recommend high-fiber foods if the patient can eat them. Adequate fluids are needed but may be difficult to swallow. The patient may be able to increase fluid intake by eating semisolids such as ice cream, milkshakes, or gelatin desserts.

The patient with ALS is at risk for aspiration because of impaired swallowing. While the patient is eating, the head of the bed must be elevated or the patient must be seated in a chair. Consult the dietitian about providing a diet of the appropriate texture for the patient, and arrange dietary instruction for any caregivers who might be involved in preparing food for the patient. A speech therapist can recommend techniques to facilitate swallowing. Eventually, oral intake becomes inadequate. The decision to insert a feeding tube should be based on the desires of the patient and family. If a feeding tube is in place, administer feedings and monitor for tube placement and residual. Teach the family or other caregivers how to do the feedings.

Inability to Communicate Effectively

Speech becomes impaired by muscle weakness and dyspnea. Establish alternatives to verbal communication. These might include the use of blinks or gestures or the use of boards with pictures, words, or letters that the patient can select. Use questions that can be answered with "yes" or "no" and give the patient time to respond. Electronic communication devices can prolong the patient's ability to communicate.

Potential for Disrupted Skin Tissue Integrity

Muscle wasting, incontinence, and immobility put these patients at risk for skin breakdown. Reposition them at least every 2 hours and inspect bony prominences for redness. Special beds that alternate or distribute pressure may be used. Promptly change wet or soiled clothing to avoid skin irritation. Meticulous skin care is essential. Once again, if the patient will be cared for at home, caregivers must be able to care for the skin.

Anticipatory Grief

Once the implications of a diagnosis of ALS are understood, patients and their families may begin the grieving process. Encourage patients to talk; listen compassionately and help them to make realistic plans. Remember the stages of grief and be understanding when patients and families show anger, denial, and depression (see the Cultural Considerations box). Referrals to visiting nurse agencies and hospice services can provide needed emotional and physical support at various times in the progress of the disease.

Cultural Considerations

What Does Culture Have to Do With Incurable Illness?

Patients facing progressive, incurable illness may find comfort in religious symbols, charms, incense, candles, and native healers.

Impaired Self-Concept

Explore the patient's thoughts, feelings, and concerns about living with this progressive, terminal disease. Although it is difficult not to offer false reassurance, let the patient cry or otherwise express grief and anger. Stress the patient's strengths, abilities, and contributions and identify and enlist sources of support (e.g., family, friends, support groups, spiritual counselors, therapists). Stress-reducing techniques include imagery, breathing exercises, and progressive relaxation. To preserve the patient's dignity, it is important to provide privacy during personal care and to help the patient attend to grooming and appearance.

Altered Family Dynamics

The disease is painful for both the patient and the family as it steadily takes its toll. Patients with ALS are often middle-aged, with family responsibilities, jobs, and places in the community. The family must plan for transfer of responsibilities and care of the patient when they become disabled. Issues that need to be discussed are patient's feelings about advance directives, insurance, and wills. These topics may be difficult to address but are best handled while the patient can participate. Care of the dying patient is discussed in Chapter 19.

HUNTINGTON DISEASE

Huntington disease is an inherited degenerative neurologic disorder. It usually begins in middle adulthood with abnormal movements, emotional disturbance, and intellectual decline. Symptoms progress steadily, with increasing disability and death in 15 to 20 years. Medical and nursing care are supportive; no cure exists.

MYASTHENIA GRAVIS

Myasthenia gravis is a chronic, progressive disease in which a defect exists at the neuromuscular junction, where electrical impulses are transmitted to muscle tissue.

CAUSE

Evidence indicates that myasthenia gravis has an autoimmune basis. Some patients display an increase in the titer of acetylcholine receptor antibody. The presence of these antibodies interferes with the normal activity at the acetylcholine receptor sites and reduces muscle strength. Some patients have antibodies to muscle-specific receptor tyrosine kinase (MuSK). This polypeptide is found on the muscle side of the myoneural junction.

PATHOPHYSIOLOGY

Normally, as a nerve impulse travels down a peripheral nerve, the neurotransmitter acetylcholine is released at the presynaptic membrane (Fig. 22.6). The impulse is then transmitted across the synaptic junction to postsynaptic receptor sites on the effector muscle. This causes contraction of the involved muscle.

In myasthenia gravis, insufficient receptor sites exist at the junction of the motor nerve with the muscle. With repeated stimulation, the muscle becomes exhausted and is eventually unable to contract at all. If respiratory muscles become involved, death from respiratory insufficiency or arrest is a possibility.

CLINICAL MANIFESTATIONS

Myasthenia gravis is characterized by the following features: weakness of voluntary muscles, particularly those of chewing, swallowing, and speaking; partial improvements of strength with rest; and dramatic improvement with the use of anticholinesterase drugs.

The onset of symptoms is gradual, and early weakness may be so subtle that it goes unnoticed. Muscles responsible for fine movements, such as eye, facial, or hand muscles, are often affected early in the disease process. Ptosis and diplopia are commonly seen. The patient becomes unable to perform any activity that demands sustained muscular contractions, such as brushing the hair, walking upstairs, or holding the

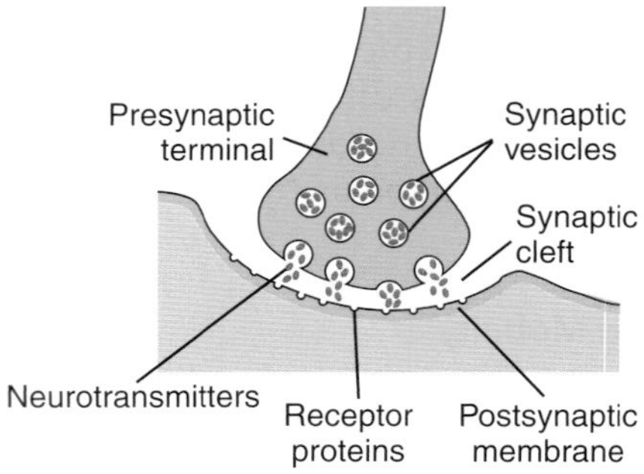

Fig. 22.6 Neurotransmitters (norepinephrine, acetylcholine, dopamine) are released from the axon, travel across the synaptic cleft, and produce some response in the receptors of target cells. (From Black JM, Hawks JH, Keene AM. *Medical-surgical nursing: clinical management for continuity of care*, ed 6, St. Louis, 2001, Saunders.)

hands over the head. The fatigue may abate with rest but rapidly returns when the activity is tried again. If the diaphragm or intercostal muscles are involved, breathing is compromised.

MEDICAL DIAGNOSIS

To make a diagnosis, edrophonium (Tensilon), an anticholinesterase drug, is administered. Edrophonium increases the relative amount of acetylcholine in the neuromuscular junction by destroying acetylcholinesterase. In the patient with myasthenia gravis, muscle tone is markedly improved within 1 minute of injection and this improvement persists for 4 to 5 minutes. The serum is tested for antiacetylcholine receptor antibodies. CT and MRI are performed to screen for thymoma (a tumor of the thymus gland).

MEDICAL TREATMENT

Anticholinesterase Drugs

Therapy is directed primarily toward pharmacologic management with anticholinesterase drugs and corticosteroids. Neostigmine and pyridostigmine (Mestinon) are anticholinesterase drugs that increase the availability of acetylcholine at the neuromuscular junction. Both drugs inhibit the action of cholinesterase, the enzyme that destroys acetylcholine. The availability of acetylcholine is improved, thereby enhancing muscle strength. Dosages are individualized for each patient, based on response and needs rather than a standardized dosing schedule. Stress or sustained levels of activity can alter the need for these agents. The patient must be monitored for pyridostigmine (Mestinon) overdose, which is characterized by gastrointestinal (GI) discomfort, diarrhea, nausea, and vomiting. The adverse events of increased bronchial and oral secretions are particularly risky for patients with dysphagia and respiratory involvement. Other common adverse events are cramping and muscle fasciculation.

Neuromuscular blockers must be used very cautiously in the patient with myasthenia gravis.

Corticosteroids

Corticosteroids may be useful in those patients who do not respond well to the anticholinesterase drugs. ACTH or prednisone is administered concurrently with the anticholinesterase drug to induce remission. During the first 7 to 10 days of therapy, symptoms may worsen, requiring hospitalization to monitor for respiratory depression. With improvement, corticosteroids may be tapered and maintained at the lowest effective dose.

Cytotoxic Therapies

Cytotoxic therapies are useful in patients who are unable to significantly taper corticosteroid drugs. Azathioprine and cyclosporine have been used in these cases.

Thymectomy

Because many patients with myasthenia gravis have hyperplasia of the thymus gland, thymectomy is performed early after the initial diagnosis. Close monitoring is essential postoperatively because a risk of respiratory compromise exists as a result of the possibility of a pneumothorax. About 40% of patients enjoy some degree of remission after thymectomy.

Plasmapheresis

Plasmapheresis is an adjunctive therapy based on the autoimmune theory of myasthenia. It is a process of plasma exchange in which the acetylcholine receptor antibodies are washed from the plasma. A temporary catheter, similar to a renal dialysis access catheter, is used for venous access. Blood is then routed through a pheresis field, where the antibodies are separated from the plasma. The washed blood is then returned to the patient. The procedure takes 3 to 4 hours and is repeated over several days to ensure adequate treatment. Improvement in muscle strength may be noted within 24 to 48 hours after treatment. As progress is made with plasmapheresis, drug doses may be decreased.

Myasthenic and Cholinergic Crises

Emergency respiratory support requiring mechanical ventilation may be necessary in the event of myasthenic or cholinergic crises. Myasthenic crisis is marked by a sudden exacerbation of myasthenic symptoms, including difficulty swallowing and breathing, with possible respiratory arrest. Infection often precipitates the event and symptoms do not decrease even with increased doses of medications.

Cholinergic crisis presents with sudden, extreme weakness and respiratory impairment. It is precipitated by overmedication with anticholinesterase drugs, which literally bombard the receptor sites with excess amounts of acetylcholine. Intubation and mechanical ventilation are required to manage the respiratory compromise.

Because the two crises present similarly, differentiation is critical. Once again, edrophonium is used to distinguish the two entities. Rapid improvement in muscle strength after administration of edrophonium indicates an underlying myasthenic crisis. If no improvement is observed, the patient is experiencing a cholinergic crisis.

Because myasthenia gravis is a chronic neurologic disease, the patient is generally managed at home. However, hospitalization is likely on the initial diagnosis and during periods of crisis and respiratory compromise.

Pharmacology Capsule

Edrophonium (Tensilon) rapidly reverses a myasthenic crisis but has no effect on a cholinergic crisis.

NURSING CARE OF THE PATIENT WITH MYASTHENIA GRAVIS

FOCUSED ASSESSMENT

The complete neurologic assessment is outlined in Chapter 21, Box 21.2. When the patient has myasthenia gravis, a history describes the onset of symptoms, particularly muscle weakness, diplopia, dysphagia, slurred speech, breathing difficulties, and loss of balance. Record the effects of the condition on the patient's lifestyle. In the physical examination, evaluate muscle strength, balance, respiratory effort, and oxygenation status.

Patient Problems, Goals, and Outcome Criteria: Myasthenia Gravis

Patient Problems	Goals and Outcome Criteria
Inadequate oxygenation related to impaired conduction of nerve impulses	Adequate oxygenation: respiratory rate of 12 to 20 breaths per minute without dyspnea
Decreased mobility and inability to manage self-care (bathing, feeding, dressing, toileting) related to muscle weakness, fatigue	Improved mobility and self-care: performance of ADL without excessive fatigue
Inability to communicate effectively related to weakness of the muscles involved in speech	Effective communication: patient makes needs known
Inadequate nutrition and potential for aspiration related to impaired swallowing because of muscle weakness	Adequate intake of fluids and food: stable body weight and absence of respiratory distress associated with aspiration
Lack of knowledge of disease and treatment	Patient understands disease and treatment: patient accurately describes condition and treatment, follows plan of care

INTERVENTIONS

Inadequate Oxygenation

You must monitor the patient for early signs and symptoms of ineffective breathing and hypoxia (tachycardia, restlessness). Progressive symptoms that do not respond to prescribed drug therapy may require mechanical ventilation. Management of the patient on a ventilator is discussed in Chapter 25.

Decreased Mobility and Inability to Manage Self-Care (Bathing, Feeding, Dressing, Toileting)

Because of weakness, the patient may be relatively inactive and unable to provide self-care. Monitor the patient's capabilities and assist as needed (see the Patient Teaching box). Measures to prevent complications, discussed in Chapter 12, include turning and repositioning at least every 2 hours.

Patient Teaching

Myasthenia Gravis

- Myasthenia gravis is a chronic disease that can be treated but not cured.
- Know your drug names, dosages, schedule, side effects, and adverse effects that should be reported to the health care provider. Take the prescribed drugs on time.
- Myasthenic crisis indicates too little acetylcholine.
- Cholinergic crisis occurs when too much acetylcholine is present.
- Difficulty swallowing and breathing are symptoms of both types of crises and each requires immediate medical treatment.
- Adjust your routine based on your symptoms.
- A good source of information is the Myasthenia Gravis Foundation of America (1-800-541-5454; www.myasthenia.org), which may have a local chapter where you live.

Inability to Communicate Effectively

Patients may have weakness of the muscles used in speech, especially when drug effects are wearing off, and after a long conversation. Thus delay questioning when the patient's voice is fading.

Inadequate Nutrition and Potential for Aspiration

Patients may have difficulty chewing and swallowing. Anticholinesterase drugs may be ordered 30 minutes before meals to improve muscle strength. The patient should be seated upright for meals and allowed (or assisted) to eat in an unhurried manner. Teach the patient to lower the chin toward the chest when swallowing to help prevent aspiration. Small, frequent meals may be tolerated better than three large ones. A soft diet is usually ordered so that minimal chewing is required. If swallowing is severely impaired, a feeding tube may be inserted and liquid feedings given as ordered. Adequate fluid intake is important to maintain hydration and prevent constipation.

Inadequate Knowledge

Patient teaching with myasthenia gravis is essential because this chronic condition requires lifelong treatment (see the Health Promotion box).

Health Promotion

Patients With Myasthenia Gravis

Patients with myasthenia gravis should receive the following interventions as necessary:

- Maintain general health through diet.
- Seek regular medical checkups for disease prevention.
- Plan rest periods.
- Tailor activities to conserve energy.

TRIGEMINAL NEURALGIA (TIC DOULOUREUX)

Trigeminal neuralgia is characterized by intense pain along the distribution of one of the three branches of the trigeminal nerve (fifth cranial nerve): (1) ophthalmic, (2) mandibular, or (3) maxillary (Fig. 22.7). The pain has an abrupt onset and is usually unilateral in nature, lasting from seconds to a few minutes. Despite the intense pain, no associated motor or sensory deficit exists. The pain may be crippling, restricting the patient's daily routine. Attacks may be triggered by ingestion of hot or cold liquids, chewing, shaving, or washing the face. Between episodes, the patient may experience a dull ache or be pain free.

CAUSE

Although the exact cause of trigeminal neuralgia is undetermined, various contributing factors can be identified. Trauma or infection may precipitate the characteristic pain, as may compression of the nerve by an aneurysm, artery, or tumor.

MEDICAL DIAGNOSIS

Because no specific test exists, the diagnosis is based on the history. Stimulation of certain trigger points may precipitate the pain.

MEDICAL TREATMENT

Pharmacologic management is the preferable course of therapy. Phenytoin (Dilantin) and carbamazepine (Tegretol) are most commonly used to suppress the pain episodes. During the acute attack, alcohol or phenol may be injected into the affected branch of the trigeminal nerve, with pain relief lasting from 8 to 16 months.

Patients with the most severe, debilitating pain may undergo surgical intervention. Electrocoagulation, a procedure in which heated electrodes are used to destroy the sensory fibers of the nerve, is effective in providing lasting pain relief without compromising motor or tactile function.

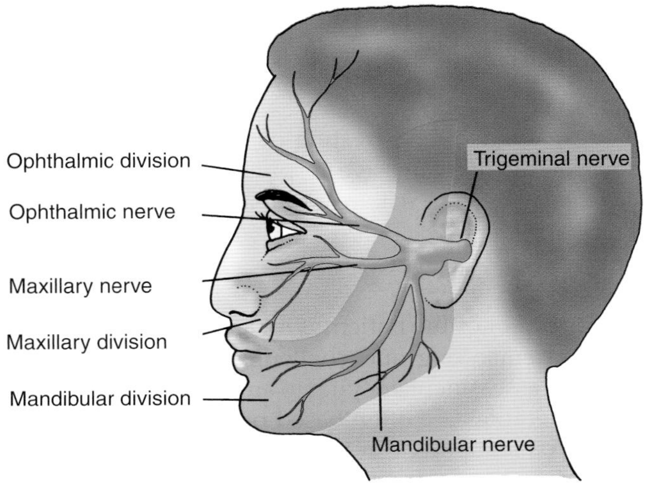

Fig. 22.7 Distribution of the trigeminal nerve and its three divisions: (1) ophthalmic, (2) maxillary, and (3) mandibular. (From Ignatavicius DD, Workman ML: *Medical-surgical nursing: patient-centered collaborative care*, ed 6, St. Louis, 2010, Saunders.)

NURSING CARE OF THE PATIENT WITH TRIGEMINAL NEURALGIA

FOCUSED ASSESSMENT

Assessment of the patient with trigeminal neuralgia focuses on describing the pain, factors that trigger it, and treatments found to be effective or ineffective. Describe the effects of the condition on the patient's life.

Patient Problems, Goals, and Outcome Criteria: Trigeminal Neuralgia

Patient Problems	Goals and Outcome Criteria
Acute pain related to disease process	Reduced frequency and severity of attacks: patient reports fewer attacks and pain is lessened
Inability to manage self-care related to debilitating pain	Self-care activities accomplished: ADL completed independently
Inadequate nutrition related to pain associated with chewing	Adequate nutrition: stable body weight
Fear related to anticipated painful episodes	Lessened fear: patient expresses less fear and increased confidence in ability to manage condition
Lack of knowledge of trigeminal neuralgia and its treatment	Patient understands condition and treatment: patient accurately describes condition, prevention of episodes, and treatment

INTERVENTIONS

The focus of nursing care for the patient with trigeminal neuralgia is pain assessment and management. It may be beneficial to assist the patient in developing alternative strategies for pain relief, such as guided imagery or relaxation therapy. Because of the debilitating nature of the pain, the patient may need encouragement and assistance in performing self-care activities. Nutrition may be affected because chewing may trigger pain. Psychologic effects are also a consideration in management because the fear of engaging in some activity that may trigger pain can lead to social isolation. Chapter 8 provides additional information about care of the patient in pain. Patient teaching emphasizes the nature of the condition and avoidance of factors that trigger episodes.

NEUROFIBROMATOSIS, TYPES 1 AND 2

Neurofibromatosis type 1, also known as *von Recklinghausen disease*, is characterized by multiple subcutaneous nerve tumors. The tumors are benign but may be removed to relieve compression of the nerves or for cosmetic reasons. Neurofibromatosis type 2 is characterized by tumors affecting the inner ear, cranial and peripheral nerves, and brain tissue. The primary treatment is surgical intervention.

BELL'S PALSY

Bell's palsy is acute paralysis of the seventh cranial nerve, which serves the face. The condition usually begins with pain behind the ear or on the face. The patient then has a pulling sensation followed by paralysis of the muscles on the affected side. The affected eyelids do not close, taste is impaired, and eating may be difficult. Most patients recover during a period of weeks or months, but some have residual weakness.

Bell's palsy is treated on an outpatient basis with prednisone and analgesic drugs. Artificial tears are needed if the eyelids do not close and the affected eye should be closed, and an eye shield used on the affected eye at night to prevent drying of the cornea. When function begins to return, the patient can do simple exercises to improve muscle tone: grimacing, opening and closing the eye, whistling, and puffing out the cheeks. Be sensitive to the patient's concerns about the condition and their appearance.

CEREBRAL PALSY

Cerebral palsy is a paralysis associated with a loss of motor coordination caused by cerebral damage. Although the cause is uncertain, the damage is generally believed to occur at birth and to be related to hypoxia, premature birth, or birth trauma.

Individuals with cerebral palsy can be frustrated by people who equate the disorder with mental retardation. Although the staggering gait and unclear speech may resemble a stereotype of a person with mental retardation, the individual with cerebral palsy is fully capable of comprehending their situation and is willing to strive for as much independence as possible.

TYPES OF CEREBRAL PALSY

The three types of cerebral palsy are: (1) spastic paralysis, (2) athetoid, and (3) ataxic. Spastic paralysis is characterized by exaggerated reflexes and muscle spasms. Random, purposeless movement with extreme muscle tone is indicative of the athetoid type, whereas the ataxic variety is characterized by poor balance, an uncoordinated, staggering gait, and speech or vision defects.

MEDICAL TREATMENT

Although no cure exists for cerebral palsy, early muscle training and exercises can be beneficial to prevent complications and promote optimal function. Orthopedic surgery, braces, and casts may be useful in limiting deformities and disabilities.

NURSING CARE OF THE PATIENT WITH CEREBRAL PALSY

Nursing care of the patient with cerebral palsy is covered in depth in pediatric nursing texts because it is typically a lifelong condition diagnosed in infancy. Thus, although many adults have cerebral palsy, it is not discussed in detail here.

POLIOMYELITIS AND POSTPOLIO SYNDROME

Poliomyelitis or "polio" is an acute infectious disease caused by the poliovirus in which motor neurons of the spinal cord and brainstem are damaged. Two types of polio vaccines are used to prevent poliomyelitis: an inactive poliovirus given by injection (developed by Dr. Jonas Salk in 1954) and a weakened poliovirus given by mouth. The World Health Organization recommends that all children be fully vaccinated against polio.

The symptoms of polio mimic those of viral meningitis, including neck stiffness, headache, fever, and vomiting, as well as muscle pain. These symptoms are followed by acute flaccid weakness in one or more muscle groups that can result in quadriplegia and respiratory failure. A diagnosis is made by identifying the virus in the stool, cerebrospinal fluid or throat. Transmission of the disease is through fecal-hand-oral contamination as well as pharyngeal spread. Treatment of poliomyelitis includes pain management, physical therapy, and mechanical ventilation for respiratory failure. Secondary conditions common among polio survivors are new muscle weakness, chronic pain, contractures, depression, fatigue, and sleep problems. No established antiviral therapies exist for poliomyelitis.

Postpolio syndrome (PPS) occurs approximately 35 years after the initial polio episode. About one-third to one-half of poliomyelitis survivors develop PPS. The greater the recovery from the initial disease, the more likely PPS will occur. The cause of postpolio syndrome is unknown. Symptoms include progressive muscle weakness, fatigue and pain in the muscles or joints, and respiratory problems typical of polio infections. Medical and nursing care are primarily supportive, aimed at helping the patient to adapt to the symptoms and maintain maximum possible function. If tolerated, nonfatiguing exercise programs are recommended as well as energy conservation techniques such as spacing of physical activities, avoiding and treating obesity, and using assistive devices. Noninvasive respiratory support may be beneficial for those with respiratory disfunction.

SUMMARY

Management of the patient with a neurologic disorder can be demanding and challenging. Astute observation and assessment are vital to any treatment plan and other therapies are often based on the nursing assessment. As is apparent from this chapter, many patient problems and modes of management are common to almost any patient with a neurologic disorder. Because of the complicated nature of many of these disorders, the management of other body systems must also be considered in a comprehensive care plan.

Get Ready For The NCLEX® Examination!

Key Points

- Seizures are abnormal activity and behavior caused by chaotic electrical impulses in the brain that may be treated with anticonvulsant therapy and, when possible, measures to correct the cause.
- Nursing care of the patient with a seizure disorder addresses potential for injury, inadequate coping, and lack of knowledge.
- Nursing care of the patient with a head injury may focus on inadequate cerebral tissue perfusion, inadequate oxygenation, potential for injury, potential for infection, decreased mobility, altered self-concept, and inability to perform usual roles.
- Meningitis and encephalitis are infections of the nervous system.
- GBS, thought to be an autoimmune response to a viral infection, is characterized by progressive ascending neurologic deficits that, in most cases, eventually resolve.
- Nursing care of the patient with GBS addresses inadequate oxygenation, inadequate circulation, potential for disuse syndrome, inadequate nutrition, potential for injury, anxiety, and lack of knowledge.
- Parkinson syndrome, a progressive disorder that results in loss of coordination and control over involuntary movement, is treated with physical therapy and drugs that increase dopamine levels in the brain.
- The focus of nursing care for the patient with Parkinson syndrome is decreased mobility, potential for injury, inadequate nutrition, inadequate coping, and lack of knowledge.
- MS is a progressive degenerative disease that disrupts the motor pathways of the CNS and may lead to severe neurologic disabilities.
- ALS is a rapidly progressive degenerative disease that usually results in death from respiratory complications within 3 years.
- The patient with ALS has increasing needs for nursing care, eventually becoming completely dependent for all aspects of care.
- Myasthenia gravis is caused by a defect in impulse conduction that is manifested as weakness of voluntary muscles and is treated with anticholinesterase drugs and corticosteroids.
- Trigeminal neuralgia is intense pain along a branch of the trigeminal nerve that may be treated with drug therapy or surgical intervention.
- Cerebral palsy is associated with a loss in motor coordination caused by cerebral damage.

Additional Learning Resources

SG Go to your Study Guide for additional learning activities to help you master this chapter content.

Go to your Evolve website (http://evolve.elsevier.com/Linton/medsurg) for the following learning resources and much more:

- Fluid & Electrolyte Tutorial
- Review Questions for the NCLEX® Examination

Clinical Judgment and Next-Generation NCLEX® Examination-Style Questions

1. **Factors that may trigger migraine headaches include which of the following? (Select all that apply.)**
   1. Alcohol
   2. Menstruation
   3. Exposure to bright light
   4. Changes in environmental temperature
   5. Certain foods

   NCLEX Client Need: Physiological Integrity: Reduction of Risk Potential

2. **Nursing measures when a patient has a generalized seizure include which of the following? (Select all that apply.)**
   1. Apply soft arm restraints to prevent injury.
   2. Insert a tongue blade between the teeth to prevent biting of the tongue.
   3. Turn the patient to one side to maintain a patent airway.
   4. Move objects away from the patient to prevent injury.
   5. Note the time the seizure began.

   NCLEX Client Need: Physiological Integrity: Physiological Adaptation

3. **A postoperative craniotomy patient has an external ventricular drainage system. Proper management of the system includes which of the following instructions? (Select all that apply.)**
   1. Do not clamp the drainage tube under any circumstances.
   2. Use strict aseptic technique to cleanse the insertion site.
   3. Keep the zero point of the drip chamber at the level of the external auditory canal.
   4. Irrigate the tube with sterile normal saline at least every 8 hours.

   NCLEX Client Need: Physiological Integrity: Reduction of Risk Potential

4. **Which one of the following is a nursing measure used to decrease ICP?**
   1. Suction the patient frequently.
   2. Encourage isometric exercises.
   3. Avoid flexing the neck and hips.
   4. Provide continuous stimulation.

   NCLEX Client Need: Physiological Integrity: Reduction of Risk Potential

5. **Parkinson syndrome is associated with a deficit of which neurotransmitter?**

   NCLEX Client Need: Physiological Integrity: Reduction of Risk Potential

6. **Single-Episode Case Test Items: Seizures**

   Question 1: Recognize cues using enhanced hot spot test item type

A 74-year-old male has been residing in a skilled nursing facility for several months because of chronic pain and limited mobility related to osteoarthritis, mild dementia, and inability to manage self-care. He has a history of epilepsy and generalized tonic-clonic seizures for which he receives carbamazepine (Tegretal). He is drowsy and prefers to stay in bed. His urinary output is minimal, although he feels the need to void. His last seizure was about six weeks ago.

Highlight or place a check mark next to the assessment findings that require follow up by the nurse.

- Blood pressure = 170/90 mm Hg
- Pulse = 82 beats per minute
- Respirations = 18 breaths per minute
- T = 100.8º F
- Decreased urinary output
- Drowsy

Cerebrovascular Accident

23

http://evolve.elsevier.com/Linton/medsurg

Objectives

1. Discuss the risk factors for cerebrovascular accident (CVA).
2. Identify the two major types of CVA.
3. Describe the pathophysiology, signs and symptoms, and medical treatment for each type of CVA.
4. Describe the neurologic deficits that may result from CVA.
5. Explain the tests and procedures used to diagnose CVA and nursing responsibilities for patients undergoing those tests and procedures.
6. List drugs, side effects, and nursing interventions used to treat patients with CVA.
7. Discuss criteria used to identify patients eligible for treatment with recombinant tissue plasminogen activator (rt-PA).
8. List data to be included in the nursing assessment of the CVA patient.
9. Assist in developing a nursing care plan for a CVA patient during the acute and rehabilitation phases.
10. Specify criteria used to evaluate the outcomes of nursing care for the CVA patient.
11. Identify resources for the CVA patient and family.

Key Terms

aphasia (ă-FĀ-zhă)
diplopia (dĭ-PLŌ-pē-ă)
dysarthria (dĭs-ĂR-thrē-ă)
dysphagia (dĭs-FĀ-zhă)
dyspraxia (dĭs-PRĂK-sē-ă)
expressive aphasia
global aphasia
hemiplegia (hĕm-ē-PLĒ-zhă)
homonymous hemianopsia (hō-MŎN-ĭ-mŭs hĕm-ē-ă-NŎP-sē-ă)
intracerebral (ĭn-tră-sĕ-RĒ-brăl)
nonfluent aphasia
ptosis (TŌ-sĭs)
receptive aphasia
subarachnoid (sŭb-ă-RĂK-nōyd)
transient ischemic attack (TRĂN-zē-ĕnt ĭs-KĒ-mĭk ă-TĂK)

A *cerebrovascular accident* (CVA) or *stroke* is the fifth leading cause of death and the leading cause of adult disability in the United States. Approximately 795,000 Americans experience strokes each year, resulting in the deaths of approximately 130,000 people annually. Acute care and rehabilitation of stroke patients is a long and expensive process. Advances in care have improved the outlook for many individuals who experience a stroke. More than half of stroke victims acquire independence in activities of daily living (ADL) within 1 year after the stroke. Some 30% of stroke survivors return to work or productive lives within 1 year. These are important figures to remember when caring for the stroke patient.

The signs and symptoms of a stroke come on suddenly. They include numbness or weakness of the face, arm, or leg, especially on one side of the body; confusion, trouble speaking or understanding; trouble seeing in one or both eyes; trouble walking, dizziness, loss of balance or coordination; and severe headache with no known cause. An easy way to remember symptoms of a stroke that is especially helpful for the general public is the acronym "FAST" in which each letter stands for a common symptom of a stroke. Some experts suggest adding the term "BE-FAST" by adding two more symptoms (Box 23.1).

A *transient ischemic attack* (TIA) is a warning sign for stroke. "Ten to 15% of patients have a stroke within 3 months, with half occurring within 48 hours" after a TIA (Easton et al., 2009). Approximately 30% of individuals who experience a TIA have a stroke within 5 years. One tool used to assess the risk of stroke after TIA is the ABCD^2 score. Points are assigned based on age, blood pressure on first evaluation, clinical symptoms, and duration of symptoms and diagnosis of diabetes. The score can range from 0 to 7; the greater the score is, the more increased the risk of stroke is within 2 days. Try out the ABCD^2 score at www.mdcalc.com/abcd2-score-for-tia/.

RISK FACTORS FOR CEREBROVASCULAR ACCIDENT

Stroke experts believe that the majority of strokes could be prevented. Unfortunately, the public has limited knowledge about stroke in relation to signs and symptoms of impending stroke, prevention of stroke, or medical treatment available. Nurses are becoming more involved in community education through outreach programs directed at assisting the public to learn more about stroke, identify risk factors, and teach individuals methods to adopt a healthy lifestyle to reduce their risk of suffering a stroke. The national Know Stroke campaign aims to educate the public to recognize the signs and symptoms of stroke and to take immediate action. To learn more, visit the Know Stroke website at http://stroke.nih.gov/.

Risk factors for stroke are classified as *modifiable* and *nonmodifiable*. Nonmodifiable factors are risk factors that cannot be changed: age, race, gender, heredity, having had a previous TIA or CVA, fibromuscular disease, and patent foramen ovale. CVAs are more common in men, African Americans, Mexican Americans, low income populations, people 51 to 74 years of age, and those with a family history of CVA. Stroke has been considered mostly a disease of older individuals but at least 5% of strokes occur in individuals younger than 45 years of age. Causes of strokes among the young include drug abuse, use of birth control pills in combination with smoking, congenital heart conditions, mitral valve prolapse, atrial fibrillation, infectious endocarditis, sickle cell anemia, rheumatic fever, and leukemia (see the Cultural Considerations box).

Cultural Considerations

What Does Culture Have to Do With Stroke?

For unknown reasons, the southeastern United States, sometimes known as the "stroke belt," has a higher prevalence and mortality rate than the rest of the country.

Box 23.1 Signs of a Stroke Using BE-FAST

- **F**ace: Does the person's face look uneven or droop on one side?
- **A**rm: Does the person have weakness or numbness in one or both arms? Does one arm drift down if the person tries to hold both arms out?
- **S**peech: Is the person having trouble speaking? Does their speech sound strange?
- **T**ime: If you notice any of these stroke signs, call for an ambulance; you need to act FAST. The sooner the treatment begins, the better the chances of recovery. Additional symptoms:
- **B**alance: Is the person having trouble standing or walking
- **E**yes: Is the person having trouble with their vision?

For more information on risk factors, visit: www.stroke.org. Modifiable risk factors are those that can be eliminated or controlled, thereby dramatically reducing the risk for CVA. Modifiable risk factors are listed in Table 23.1 along with the interventions used for each factor. A common denominator of many of the risk factors (hypertension, cardiac disease, diabetes mellitus) is atherosclerosis. Therefore, many interventions include measures to slow the progression of atherosclerosis (see Chapter 34 for more complete coverage).

(For a discussion of the nation's goals for stroke prevention and implications for nurses, see the Health Promotion box.)

Table 23.1 Modifiable Cerebrovascular Accident Risk Factors and Related Interventions

MODIFIABLE RISK FACTOR	INTERVENTIONS TO MODIFY EFFECTS OF RISK FACTOR
Pathologic Disorders	
Hypertension	Antihypertensive drugs, weight control, stress management, smoking cessation, limited alcohol consumption, low-fat diet, reduced sodium intake.
Cardiac disease	Drug therapy to improve blood flow and prevent clots. Treatment of atrial fibrillation. Treatment of hyperlipidemia.
Diabetes mellitus	Balanced program of drug therapy, diet, weight control, exercise. Blood glucose monitoring.
Conditions that increase risk of blood clotting (e.g., sickle cell anemia)	Good hydration. Drug therapy as appropriate.
Lifestyle Factors	
Excessive alcohol consumption	Limit alcohol to 1 ounce of pure alcohol or less (not more than 1 ounce of pure alcohol per day: 2 cans of beer, 2 small glasses of wine, 2 average cocktails). Avoid binge drinking.
Cigarette smoking	Advise patients of risks of tobacco use. Explain that risk falls with smoking cessation. Recommend self-help programs. Refer to physician for drug therapy.
Obesity	Encourage patient to maintain normal body weight. Instruction in proper diet. Weight control programs that help patients modify eating behaviors and establish healthy nutritional practices. Exercise programs as specified by the physician.
High-fat diet	Instruction in meal planning and preparation. Reduce saturated fats in diet.
Drug abuse	Drug abuse treatment programs.
Sedentary lifestyle	Education, structured exercise program.

Health Promotion

HEALTHY PEOPLE 2030: IMPLICATIONS FOR NURSES

Healthy People 2030 presents a comprehensive set of disease prevention and health promotion objectives developed to improve the health of all people in the United States during the third decade of the 21st century. Nurses are in a unique position within the community to promote and participate in this initiative.

Objectives related to stroke include:

- Reduce stroke deaths
- Increase the proportion of adult stroke survivors who participate in rehabilitation service
- Increase the proportion of people with strokes who get mechanical thrombectomy within 16 hours of symptom onset
- Increase the proportion of stroke patients who get intravenous (IV) reperfusion therapy within 3 hours of symptom onset
- Increase aspirin use for secondary prevention of atherosclerotic cardiovascular disease

ROLE OF THE NURSE IN STROKE PREVENTION AND TREATMENT

- Spread the word about risk factors for and warning signs of stroke.
- Assist patients in addressing and lowering their risks for stroke.
- Participate in community education programs for cardiovascular health.
- Get involved in Operation Stroke in your community.
- Participate in stroke and blood pressure screenings.
- Promote evidence-based care and best practices for a healthy lifestyle.
- Engage in and promote physical activity.
- Participate in antismoking campaigns and assist patients to locate such programs.
- Recognize depression after stroke and help patients to obtain adequate treatment.

TRANSIENT ISCHEMIC ATTACK

A **transient ischemic attack** (TIA) is a "transient episode of neurologic dysfunction caused by focal brain, spinal cord, or retinal ischemia, without acute infarction" (Furie, 2020). Blood vessels may be occluded by spasms, fragments of plaque, or blood clots. It is believed that at least 85% of blood flow to an area must be blocked before signs and symptoms of a TIA appear. These episodes of temporary neurologic changes were previously thought to be "benign." It is now known that TIAs are important warning signs for the individual who could potentially experience a full stroke in the future. Previously, TIA was defined as lasting less than 24 hours, but it is now defined as *a temporary onset of stroke symptoms without permanent damage*. It is recommended that a patient experiencing a TIA receive a full medical evaluation within 24 hours. This may be completed in an inpatient or outpatient setting.

CLINICAL MANIFESTATIONS

With TIA, neurologic signs and symptoms resolve with no permanent effects. Some common signs and symptoms of TIA are dizziness, momentary confusion, loss of speech, loss of balance, tinnitus, visual disturbances, ptosis, dysarthria, dysphagia, drooping mouth, weakness, and tingling or numbness on one side of the body. The nature and severity of the symptoms depend on the area of the brain involved and the extent of tissue deprived of adequate oxygen.

MEDICAL DIAGNOSIS

TIA is generally suspected based on the health history and physical examination findings. Confirmation requires brain imaging studies, preferably with magnetic resonance imaging (MRI). In addition, noninvasive imaging of blood vessels, laboratory studies, and cardiac evaluation may be ordered to detect risk factors for TIA and stroke. Noninvasive vascular studies can show narrowing of cervical and cerebral blood vessels. Doppler studies may also be done to assess cerebral blood flow. Ultrasonic duplex scanning is useful in detecting carotid artery disease. Computed tomography (CT) and electroencephalogram (EEG) may be used to rule out intracranial lesions such as tumors, aneurysms, and abscesses. Key features of diagnostic tests are presented in Chapter 21, Table 21.6.

TREATMENT

Treatment of TIA depends on the cause. The common causes of TIA are thought to be carotid artery disease, large or small artery disease from atherosclerosis, and atrial fibrillation. The treatment of atherosclerotic disease depends on the location of the narrowed vessel and the degree of narrowing. Based on research evidence, the American Stroke Association recommends initial treatment with acetylsalicylic acid (aspirin) alone or a combination of acetylsalicylic acid and extended-release dipyridamole (Aggrenox), or a combination of acetylsalicylic and clopidogrel bisulfate (Plavix) to decrease platelet clumping. In atrial fibrillation, microscopic emboli are believed to form, which later are released from the heart and travel to the arteries of the brain to cause TIA or stroke. There are new anticoagulant medications available for the prevention of cardioembolic TIA. The only options used to be warfarin (Coumadin) and heparin for patients exhibiting a cardioembolic TIA. The dosage for warfarin therapy is based on the prothrombin time (PT) and the international normalized ratio (INR). For therapeutic anticoagulation, the PT is usually kept in a therapeutic range of 1.5 to 2.0 times normal and the INR at 2.0 to 3.0. The effect of unfractionated heparin therapy is monitored with the activated partial thromboplastin time (aPTT). Rivaroxaban (Xarelto) and dabigatran (Pradaxa) are also indicated for stroke prevention in nonvalvular atrial fibrillation. The decision for medication should be individualized to the patient based on the medical evaluation of the TIA, possible risk factors, how the patient tolerates the medication, and other health issues (Kernan et al., 2014). If low-molecular-weight heparin (enoxaparin and others) is used, laboratory values for heparin anti-Xa may be monitored. Statin drugs are recommended for patients with elevated lipids or coronary artery disease, or when evidence exists that the TIA is related to atherosclerosis. Treatment of hypertension is recommended as well. Additional information about drug therapy is provided in Table 23.2.

Because of the operative risks and controversy about the value of surgical intervention in terms of stroke prevention, surgery is often reserved for the most serious stenosis. The most common surgical procedures are carotid endarterectomy (Fig. 23.1) and transluminal angioplasty. Carotid endarterectomy is the surgical removal of plaques in the artery to permit improved blood flow. Patients who are at high risk for surgical intervention

Table 23.2 Medications for Cerebrovascular Accident

DRUG	USE/ACTION	SIDE EFFECTS	NURSING INTERVENTIONS
Corticosteroids			
Dexamethasone (Decadron)	Reduces ICP by reducing inflammation in brain after stroke.	Fluid retention, hypertension, hypokalemia, hyperglycemia, suppressed response to infection, fat deposits in cheeks and upper back, gastric ulcers, insomnia, easy bruising, mood swings. Dose usually tapered over 7 to 10 days to prevent acute withdrawal and adrenal insufficiency.	Monitor I&O, BP, blood glucose in people with diabetes. Protect from infection. Report even minor signs of infection. Protect from bumps and other minor injuries.
Hyperosmotic Agents			
Mannitol (Osmitrol) Glycerin (Osmoglyn)	Induces diuresis, which reduces ICP. Mannitol is first-choice drug.	Circulatory overload, heart failure, hypertension, renal failure.	15% to 25% mannitol solutions should be filtered. Monitor infusion site; stop flow and restart if infiltrated to avoid tissue damage. Monitor for signs of fluid volume excess: hypertension, bounding pulse, edema, urine output less than fluid intake.
Anticoagulants			
Unfractionated heparin sodium (Liquaemin sodium)	Prevents formation of new blood clots; does not dissolve existing clots.	Bleeding or hemorrhage resulting from excessive anticoagulation, hyperkalemia, alopecia allergy period.	Effect is monitored by partial thromboplastin time (PTT) or activated partial thromboplastin time (aPTT). Therapeutic goal is 1.5 to 2.0 times the control of 30 to 40 s. If patient's aPTT is greater, withhold drug and contact physician. Assess for bruises, bleeding from GI and urinary tracts, mouth, or nose. Contraindicated with active bleeding. Heparin antidote is protamine sulfate. Caution with venipuncture; apply pressure to site.
Low-molecular-weight heparin: enoxaparin, dalteparin, and others	Prevents formation of new blood clots; does not dissolve existing clots.	Bleeding or hemorrhage, allergic reactions, injection site reactions, increases in liver enzyme tests.	Lab values not routinely followed. If monitored, the anti-Xa assay will be used. Protamine as an antidote will only be partially effective. Assess for bruises, bleeding from GI and urinary tracts, mouth, or nose. Contraindicated with active bleeding.
Warfarin sodium (Coumadin, Panwarfin)	Prevents formation of new blood clots; does not dissolve existing clots.	Bleeding or hemorrhage resulting from excessive anticoagulation.	Effect is monitored by prothrombin time (PT) and international normalized ratio (INR). Therapeutic goal is a PT of 1.5 to 2.0 times control and INR of 2.0 to 3.0. Check PT/INR before initiating medication daily until maintenance dose is reached. Assess for bruising, bleeding from GI and urinary tracts, mouth, or nose. Apply pressure after venipuncture. Antidote for warfarin overdose is vitamin K_1 (AquaMEPHYTON).

Table 23.2 Medications for Cerebrovascular Accident—cont'd

DRUG	USE/ACTION	SIDE EFFECTS	NURSING INTERVENTIONS
Dabigatran (Pradaxa)	A direct thrombin inhibitor indicated to reduce the risk of stroke for patients with nonvalvular atrial fibrillation.	Can cause serious and sometimes fatal bleeding. Promptly evaluate signs and symptoms of blood loss.	Do not break, chew, or empty the contents of the capsule. Discontinuing abruptly may increase risk of new stroke. Antidote not available.
Rivaroxaban (Xarelto)	A direct factor Xa inhibitor indicated to reduce the risk of stroke for patients with nonvalvular atrial fibrillation.	Can cause serious and sometimes fatal bleeding. Promptly evaluate signs and symptoms of blood loss.	Do not break or chew tablet. Take with meal, at the same time each day. Do not stop taking rivaroxaban without consulting your prescribing doctor. Antidote is not available.
Thrombolytics			
Recombinant tissue plasminogen activator (rt-PA) (Altavase)	Emergency drug that initiates dissolution of clots by breaking down fibrin.	Hemorrhage, especially within the first 24 h after administration.	Minimize venipunctures; protect arterial line sites; assess for bleeding; monitor coagulation studies.
Platelet Aggregation Inhibitors			
Aspirin	Reduces risk of stroke in patients with recurrent ischemic attacks. May be given in combination with other antiplatelets.	Excessive bruising, bleeding; bronchoconstriction; nausea, vomiting, gastric bleeding, urticaria, confusion, drowsiness, tinnitus. May be given in combination with other antiplatelets.	Tinnitus and confusion suggest overdosage. Teach patients that aspirin can be harmful if not taken properly.
Dipyridamole (Persantine)	Prevents thromboembolism with heart valve prostheses. Used with Coumarin anticoagulants.	Hypotension, dizziness. Caution with hypotensive patients. MI, dysrhythmias with IV use. Constipation, dry mouth.	Teach patient to manage orthostatic hypotension. Monitor pulse and blood pressure.
Aspirin/extended-release dipyridamole (Aggrenox)	Prolongs bleeding time, decreasing the risk of stroke.	Rash, diarrhea, itching, bruising. Not associated with neutropenic purpura as with Ticlid.	May be given with or without food; assess for bruising.
Clopidogrel (Plavix)	Reduces risk of stroke by inhibition of clotting.	GI bleeding, epistaxis, neutropenia, intracranial hemorrhage, hypertension, dyspnea. Risk of hemorrhage increases if given with aspirin.	Give with food. Advise patients of need for periodic lab studies, including liver function tests with long-term therapy.
Ticagrelor (Brilinta)	Platelet inhibitor; prevention of thromboembolism.	Serious, fatal bleeding; headache, dizziness, fatigue, hypotension.	Observe for bleeding; monitor blood pressure; note chills, fever, bruising; take with or without meals.
Calcium-Channel Blockers			
Nimodipine (Nimotop)	Prevents spasms in cerebral blood vessels after a hemorrhagic stroke.	Headache, fatigue, depression, confusion, dysrhythmias, hypotension, MI, renal failure.	Monitor pulse and blood pressure. Assess for edema. Monitor urine output. Count pulse before each dose; withhold if less than 60 bpm.

BP, Blood pressure; *GI*, gastrointestinal; *I&O*, intake and output; *ICP*, intracranial pressure; *IV*, intravenous; *Lab*, laboratory; *MI*, myocardial infarction.

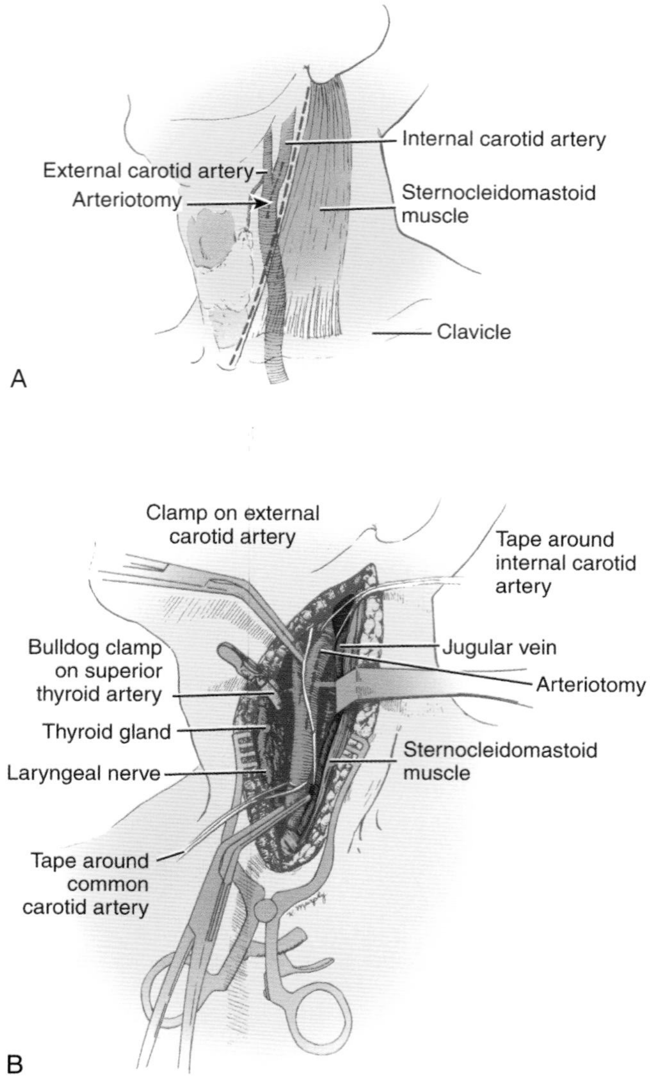

Fig. 23.1 Carotid endarterectomy. Plaques are removed from the artery to improve blood flow. (From Hershey FB, Calman CH: *Atlas of vascular surgery*, ed 3, St. Louis, 1973, Mosby.)

because of other health problems may benefit from angioplasty. A stent may be placed in the artery to keep it open. Transluminal angioplasty improves blood flow by dilating the narrowed artery with a balloon that is inserted into the artery. A patent foramen ovale is sometimes identified in the patient with TIA. Closure of this defect in the heart can be accomplished through an open surgical approach or a transcatheter closure.

Pharmacology Capsule

When patients are taking antiplatelet or anticoagulant medications, take care to prevent injuries and bleeding.

STROKE

A stroke is an abrupt impairment of brain function resulting in a set of neurologic signs and symptoms caused by impaired blood flow to the brain that last more than 24 hours. When symptoms progress over hours or days, the condition is described as *stroke in evolution*. When the neurologic deficits do not change for 2 to 3 days, the stroke is said to be *completed*. Unlike TIA, a completed stroke causes lingering motor, sensory, or cognitive damage with varying disabilities.

PATHOPHYSIOLOGY

The two main classifications of stroke are (1) hemorrhagic and (2) ischemic.

Hemorrhagic Stroke

Hemorrhagic stroke accounts for only about 13% of all strokes. In hemorrhagic stroke, a blood vessel in the brain ruptures and bleeding into the brain occurs. As a result, intracranial pressure (ICP) may increase, disrupting normal cerebral function. Hemorrhagic strokes are further classified by location. An **intracerebral** (within the cerebrum) hemorrhage, 10% of all strokes, is associated with trauma, uncontrolled hypertension, and aneurysms. When a hemorrhage occurs within the spaces of the brain, the terms *subdural, subarachnoid,* or *ventricular* are used to describe the location. Hemorrhagic strokes often are sudden in onset and require emergent, life-sustaining treatment.

A **subarachnoid** hemorrhage, 3% of all strokes, occurs between the arachnoid and pia mater layers of the brain covering. The pia mater is the thin membrane covering the brain. The arachnoid covers the pia mater. Subarachnoid hemorrhage may be caused by congenital malformations of blood vessels in the brain or by rupture of an aneurysm.

Ischemic Stroke

An ischemic stroke is caused by the obstruction of a blood vessel by an atherosclerotic plaque, a blood clot, a combination of the two, or other debris released into the vessel that impedes blood flow to an area of the brain. Brain cells deprived of blood flow become ischemic and die. Ischemic strokes account for 87% of all strokes, including embolic and thrombotic strokes. In an embolic stroke, the clot or plaque fragment is "traveling" through a blood vessel from an area outside of the brain until it lodges in a cerebral artery. Mitral valve stenosis, atrial fibrillation, and myocardial infarction are cardiovascular conditions that may lead to the development of clots that become emboli.

A thrombotic stroke develops when an obstruction forms in a blood vessel of the brain. The atherosclerotic process, which often affects large cerebral arteries, produces most of the thrombotic strokes. Patients may experience stroke in evolution, in which symptoms worsen during approximately 48 hours. As the obstruction progresses, neurologic impairment increases. Fig. 23.2 illustrates each type of stroke. Patients who have thrombotic strokes may have a history of TIAs.

A lacunar stroke results from occlusion of the small penetrating arteries deep within the brain. Lacunar

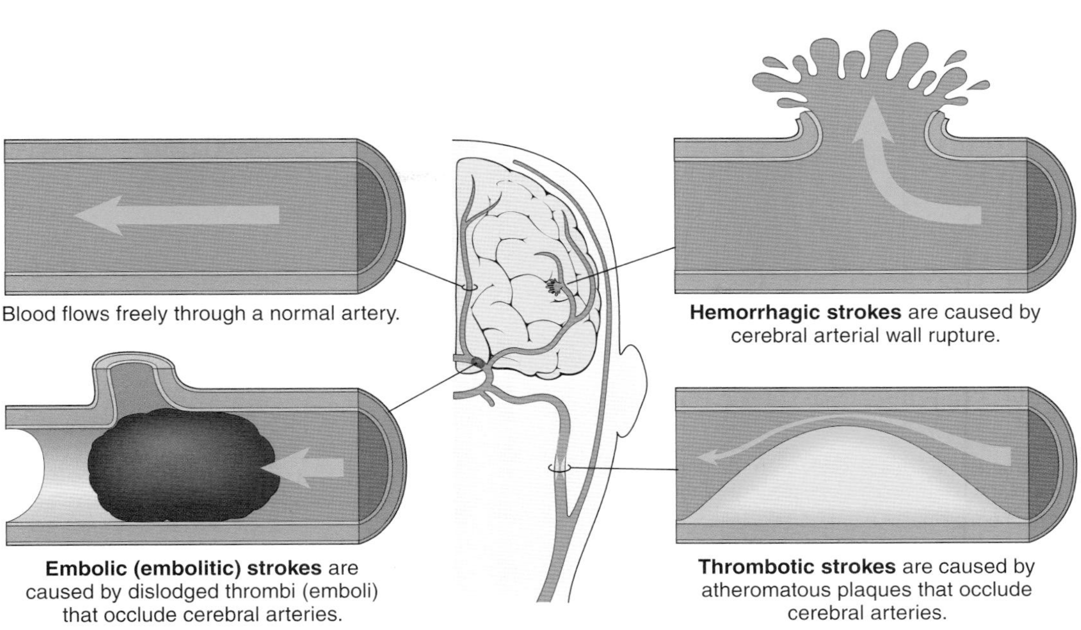

Fig. 23.2 Types of stroke. (From Ignatavicius DD, Workman ML: *Medical-surgical nursing: critical thinking for collaborative care*, ed 4, Philadelphia, 2002, Saunders.)

strokes account for about 25% of all ischemic strokes. A lacuna is defined as an "empty space," the result of tissue death from an occlusive process in the small arteries of the brain. The clinical features associated with lacunar strokes are usually less severe and produce less pronounced neurologic changes. Risk factors for lacunar strokes include advanced age, chronic hypertension, smoking, and diabetes mellitus.

Put On Your Thinking Cap!

Why would patients with atrial fibrillation be treated with anticoagulants?

CLINICAL MANIFESTATIONS

A stroke may produce various signs and symptoms, depending on the type, location, and extent of brain injury. Symptoms of a hemorrhagic stroke generally occur suddenly and may include severe headache that the patient describes as "the worst headache of my life." Other symptoms are stiff neck, loss of consciousness, vomiting, and seizures.

Symptoms of an embolic stroke also often appear without warning. The specific symptoms depend on the area of the brain affected by the lack of blood supply. One or more of the following signs and symptoms may be present: one-sided (unilateral) weakness, numbness, visual problems, confusion and memory lapses, headache, dysphagia (difficulty swallowing), and language problems. Language problems may be in the form of difficulty understanding, difficulty speaking, or both. Reading and writing may also be affected.

The signs and symptoms of a thrombotic stroke may be the same as those of an embolic stroke. However, because the obstruction forms gradually through the atherosclerotic process, the symptoms may develop more gradually. Sudden onset of symptoms may occur with either embolic or thrombotic stroke.

Regardless of the type of stroke, symptoms can be devastating. Whereas some symptoms improve with time and therapy, others may be permanent. Many signs and symptoms are related to the location of the damage and whether the right or the left side of the brain is affected. Fig. 23.3 compares right-sided and left-sided stroke. Long-term effects that merit further discussion include: aphasia, dysarthria, dysphagia, dyspraxia, hemiplegia, sensory impairment, unilateral neglect, homonymous hemianopsia, personality change, emotional lability, impaired cognition, and bladder dysfunction.

Aphasia

The speech center is located in the left hemisphere in more than 90% of all people. In left-handed persons, the speech center is sometimes located in the right hemisphere. If the speech center is damaged, communication is affected. **Aphasia** is a defect in the use of language: speech, reading, writing, or word comprehension. Aphasia is classified as *receptive* or *expressive.* The patient with **receptive aphasia** has difficulty understanding spoken or written words. The patient with **expressive aphasia** has difficulty speaking and writing. Aphasia can also be classified as *fluent* or *nonfluent.* The patient who has fluent aphasia sounds normal but makes little sense, whereas the person with **nonfluent aphasia** has difficulty initiating speech. Although these types of aphasia are distinctly defined, some patients have components of both types. The term **global aphasia** is sometimes used when speech is impaired to the

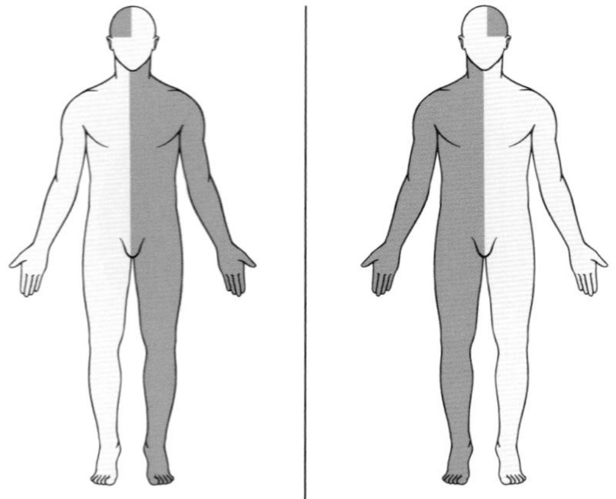

Right-brain damage (stroke on right side of the brain)	Left-brain damage (stroke on left side of the brain)
• Paralyzed left side: hemiplegia • Left-sided neglect • Spatial-perceptual deficits • Tends to deny or minimize problems • Rapid performance, short attention span • Impulsive, safety problems • Impaired judgment • Impaired time concepts	• Paralyzed right side: hemiplegia • Impaired speech/language aphasias • Impaired right/left discrimination • Slow performance, cautious • Aware of deficits: depression, anxiety • Impaired comprehension related to language, math

Fig. 23.3 Comparison of right-sided and left-sided stroke. (From Lewis SM, Dirksen SR, Heitkemper MM, et al.: *Medical-surgical nursing: assessment and management of clinical problems,* ed 9, St. Louis, 2015, Mosby.)

point that the person has almost no ability to communicate. Terms describing communication problems of the stroke patient are defined in Table 23.3.

Dysarthria

Dysarthria is the inability to speak clearly. It is caused by neurologic damage that prevents normal control of muscles used in speech. Dysarthric patients are difficult to understand but they understand what is said and have no difficulty putting together their thoughts.

Dysphagia

Patients with dysarthria are also likely to have **dysphagia** (swallowing difficulty), which may require extensive rehabilitation. This is a very serious problem because of the risk of aspiration and pneumonia and because it can interfere with adequate nutrition. Dysphagia can be especially discouraging for the patient when attempts to eat result in choking, frustration, and fear. A gastrostomy tube may be inserted for long-term feeding purposes. Speech-language pathologists (SLPs) are trained to diagnose and treat patients with dysphagia.

Dyspraxia

Dyspraxia is the partial inability to initiate coordinated voluntary motor acts. Any part of the body with motor function may be affected. For instance, the patient may not be able to walk or transfer to a chair without assistance even though the patient is not paralyzed. Patients with dyspraxia may be able to spontaneously perform a motor act yet be unable to initiate such an act willfully. This contradictory behavior can lead uninformed family, friends, or caretakers to assume that the person is being "difficult." The difficulty initiating motor actions seen in dyspraxia is quite different from the inability to perform motor acts because of hemiplegia. The person who has apraxia can move the affected parts but cannot perform specific purposeful actions such as walking or dressing.

Table 23.3 Types of Communication Disorders After Cerebrovascular Accident

TYPE	LOCATION OF BRAIN LESION	CHARACTERISTICS
Receptive aphasia	Wernicke area	Unable to comprehend spoken or written words
Expressive aphasia	Broca area	Difficulty speaking or writing
Dysarthria	Upper motor neurons	Speaks slowly with great effort; words prolonged, hard to understand

Hemiplegia

Hemiplegia is defined as paralysis of one side of the body. The affected side is opposite (*ipsilateral*) from the side of the brain in which the stroke occurred because nerve fibers in the brain cross over as they pass into the spinal cord. Hemiplegia is characterized at first by flaccidity (decreased muscle tone) and then by spasticity (increased muscle tone). Recovery from hemiplegia is a gradual process and the extent of improvement varies widely.

Sensory Impairment

Impaired sensory function is common after a stroke. The patient may be unable to feel touch, pain, or temperature in affected body parts. Conversely, some hemiplegic individuals with sensory impairment perceive every sensation to the affected area as painful. Patients may feel as if their bodies are limp or flaccid. Altered sensations put the patient at risk for injury from pressure and excess heat or cold. Injuries may be ignored because the patient is not aware of them.

Unilateral Neglect

Patients may experience what is called *unilateral neglect*, in which they do not recognize one side of their body as belonging to them. Unilateral neglect is most common with right hemisphere damage and results in failure to attend to the left side of the body. The condition often resolves after about 3 months.

Homonymous Hemianopsia

Homonymous hemianopsia is a perceptual problem that involves loss of one side of the field of vision. Homonymous hemianopsia translates to a half-blinded field of vision that occurs on the same side in both eyes. At mealtime, the patient may leave half of the plate untouched, the half on the affected side. As another example, the patient may shave his face completely on one side and leave the whiskers untouched on his affected side.

Intellectual and Emotional Effects

Many patients experience emotional changes after a stroke, sometimes to the point of personality change. Emotional lability is a frequent problem after a stroke. The patient may seem quite happy and then suddenly burst into tears for no apparent reason. Angry outbursts, childlike behavior, and inappropriate sexual behavior may occur. Emotional changes such as these are thought to be caused by neurochemical imbalances in the brain or by loss of the brain's ability to inhibit inappropriate behavior. It has also been found that cognitive processes may be slowed after a stroke, even without obvious deficits in thinking and responding.

Elimination Disturbances

In the acute phase of stroke and sometimes into the rehabilitation phase, the patient may experience a neurogenic bladder. A neurogenic bladder is further classified depending on the type of symptoms identified. A flaccid bladder (one without muscle tone) cannot empty completely. In some cases, the coordination to be able to store urine in the bladder or wait once the urge to void is felt is lost (dyssynergia), which also leads to incontinence.

Bowel incontinence may also be a physiologic consequence of stroke. However, confusion, disorientation, and immobility may contribute to incontinent episodes and to chronic constipation.

With both bladder and bowel incontinence, it is important to determine if the cause is physiologic or related to other factors such as infection from a urinary catheter or the inability of the patient to communicate the need to go to the bathroom. Bladder and bowel retraining programs should be implemented as soon as possible.

MEDICAL DIAGNOSIS

When a patient is admitted to a hospital with a tentative diagnosis of a stroke, the following procedures may be ordered: blood studies, electrocardiogram (ECG), CT, MRI, carotid ultrasound studies, cerebral and carotid angiography, EEG, positron emission tomography (PET), and single-photon emission CT.

Blood studies and the ECG are done to identify the presence of risk factors for stroke, such as abnormal clotting, hyperlipidemia, and atrial fibrillation. If subarachnoid hemorrhage is suspected and the CT scan is negative for blood, a lumbar puncture may be performed to obtain cerebrospinal fluid (CSF) for examination. Grossly bloody CSF indicates hemorrhagic rather than ischemic stroke. This finding has important implications for treatment because anticoagulants are contraindicated after hemorrhagic stroke. A lumbar puncture is not done if increased ICP is suspected. In Chapter 21, Table 21.6 summarizes nursing care of patients who have neurologic diagnostic tests and procedures.

COMPLICATIONS

Patients who suffer an acute stroke are at risk for many complications related to impaired neuromuscular function. The patient with severe motor impairment is at risk for constipation, dehydration, contractures, urinary tract infections, thrombophlebitis, pressure injuries, and pneumonia. Sensory losses put the patient at risk for traumatic and thermal injuries. Swallowing difficulties place the patient at risk for pulmonary complications such as choking and aspiration pneumonia. Some patients experience disabling pain, called *central poststroke pain* (CPSP), after stroke.

PROGNOSIS

The prognosis for patients experiencing a TIA or stroke is becoming increasingly hopeful. The critical variables that affect recovery are the patient's condition before the stroke, the length of time between the occurrence of stroke and diagnosis, the treatment and support for the patient in the acute phase (usually the first 48 hours), the severity of the patient's symptoms, and access to rehabilitative therapy. Patients with acute stroke who have access to emergent care and are treated with recombinant tissue plasminogen activator (rt-PA) within 90 minutes of symptom onset have a better cure rate after 3 months than those treated later or not at all (Bahouth and LaMonte, 2005). To accomplish this requires a structured multidisciplinary approach to stroke care. Current national recommendations include medical systems to offer prehospital assessment and transportation, stroke centers, stroke units, and organized stroke teams. Because not all hospitals are equipped to handle the rapid evaluation and treatment of acute stroke, it is important that emergency medical services work closely with recognized stroke centers to transport patients to appropriate locations for this treatment.

The long-term recovery of the stroke patient may well depend on the care received immediately after the stroke. Most recovery from stroke takes place in the first 3 to 6 months but progress often continues long after that.

The nurse's role in providing care to stroke patients is a vital one and has a significant effect on patient outcome.

MEDICAL TREATMENT IN THE ACUTE PHASE

The acute phase of a stroke begins with the onset of signs and symptoms and continues until the patient's vital signs, particularly blood pressure and neurologic condition, stabilize. This phase usually lasts 24 to 48 hours. Patients are often placed in a monitored setting for close observation and treatment during the acute phase. A challenge for the physician is to provide immediate care for acute problems while considering preexisting conditions as well. Management of chronic conditions such as diabetes mellitus, heart disease, arthritis, and gastrointestinal (GI) disturbances must continue during the acute phase of stroke. Many medical management interventions are directed at minimizing complications and deterioration of the patient's condition after a stroke. There are several major focus areas, including (1) hypertension, (2) oxygenation, (3) hyperthermia, (4) hyperglycemia, and (5) arrhythmias. It is very important to monitor patients and report any changes in vital signs, oxygenation, temperature, or glucose levels.

Hypertension

The majority of patients admitted with an acute stroke have high blood pressure during and immediately after a stroke. It is important to be cautious in treating high blood pressure during this phase because sudden reductions in blood pressure have been associated with decreased cerebral perfusion and may lead to worsening of brain tissue damage. Even without treatment, blood pressure naturally begins to decrease within 48 hours and gradually falls for 10 to 14 days. If a patient is to receive thrombolytic therapy, blood pressure control measures will be more aggressive. A small group of patients may present or develop low blood pressure after a stroke. This is often related to dehydration and should be identified and treated right away to avoid a decrease in blood flow to the brain. In patients experiencing a hemorrhagic stroke, blood pressure control will be maintained much tighter and hypertension will be avoided to reduce the risk of more bleeding into the brain.

Oxygenation

Oxygenation is a priority immediately after a stroke, especially if the patient is unconscious, because hypoxemia can extend the area affected and therefore worsen the stroke. Oxygen therapy and monitoring of oxygen saturation will be ordered if the oxygen saturation is less than 94%. For patients who are comatose, intubation and mechanical ventilation may be required to provide adequate ventilation. Respiratory exercises, including incentive spirometry, may be ordered for the alert patient.

Hyperthermia

Fever is common after a stroke. Fever may be related to stress response or to the stroke itself. Hyperthermia of any degree has now been shown to extend the area of damage and potentially worsen the outcome after stroke. Recent studies support keeping the patient's temperature as close to normal as possible. Fever can be adequately managed with medications such as acetaminophen (Tylenol). A device such as a surface cooling system or an indwelling catheter temperature control system is sometimes used.

Hyperglycemia

Individuals experiencing a stroke will often develop hyperglycemia (elevated blood glucose). This often occurs in the absence of having a history of diabetes. Hyperglycemia during the acute phase of a stroke may represent the body's stress response to stroke. It has been shown to contribute to brain damage and worsen the outcome of a patient. Current recommendations require treating hyperglycemia with insulin if the serum glucose is found to be more than 200 mg/dL. In the first 2 days, blood glucose should be measured every 1 to 2 hours in patients who have received thrombolytic therapy and every 6 hours in other patients.

Arrhythmia

Cardiac rhythms may become abnormal after a stroke. Management guidelines recommend continuous cardiac monitoring to identify ischemic heart changes and arrhythmias such as atrial fibrillation.

Drug Therapy

Tissue plasminogen activator (t-PA) (alteplase [Activase, Activase rt-PA]) may be given to dissolve clots in patients with acute ischemic strokes. This is the only medication approved by the U.S. Food and Drug Administration (FDA) to reverse the effects of an ischemic stroke. To be given intravenously, this medication should be initiated within 3 hours from the onset of stroke symptoms. Based on research evidence, the American Stroke Association affirms the value of rt-PA therapy within 3 hours for best outcomes but further recommends that it can be given to selected patients between 3 and 4.5 hours after the onset of symptoms. This narrow window of time has limited the use of rt-PA with acute ischemic stroke. Patient selection criteria are also very strict because this medication is associated with an increased risk of cerebral hemorrhage in patients who have received it. A CT scan or MRI is used to determine whether and where the hemorrhage exists in the brain. The final decision to use or not to use intravenous rt-PA is at the discretion of the treating physician. Once it is determined that the stroke is from an ischemic event and hemorrhage has been ruled out, the patient should be evaluated for treatment with rt-PA.

Intravenous Recombinant Tissue Plasminogen Activator (rt-PA) Administration Screening List

Inclusion Criteria

- Age 18 years or older
- Diagnosis of ischemic stroke causing measurable neurologic deficit
- Clinical diagnosis of stroke, with a National Institutes of Health Stroke Scale (NIHSS) score less than 22
- Time of onset of stroke is known and is 3 hours or less

Exclusion Criteria

- Significant head trauma or prior stroke in previous 3 months
- Symptoms suggest a subarachnoid hemorrhage
- History of previous intracranial hemorrhage
- Intracranial neoplasm, arteriovenous malformation or aneurysm
- Recent intracranial surgery
- Elevated blood pressure: systolic greater than 185 mm Hg, or diastolic greater than 110 mm Hg
- Active internal bleeding
- Blood glucose less than 50 mg/dL or more than 400 mg/dL
- Evidence of hemorrhage on CT scan or MRI

Relative Exclusion Criteria

- Only a minor or rapidly resolving stroke
- Seizure at onset of stroke
- Major surgery or serious trauma within previous 14 days
- Recent gastrointestinal or urinary tract hemorrhage (within previous 21 days)

Criteria for Extending Intravenous rt-PA Treatment 3 to 4.5 Hours From Symptom Onset

- Patient is 80 years of age or older
- Patient does not have a history of both diabetes and stroke
- Patient is not taking warfarin (Coumadin) or any other anticoagulant regardless of INR/coagulation results
- NIHSS is 25 or more
- Written informed consent must be obtained from patient and/or family for intravenous rt-PA within the 3 to 4.5 hours window

Endovascular Interventions. Patients eligible for intravenous rt-PA should receive it first, as they are evaluated for an endovascular intervention and possible mechanical thrombectomy. Endovascular therapy with clot retrievers is the recommended treatment after intravenous rt-PA, if the patient qualifies. These intracranial procedures are conducted by an interventional neuroradiologist under radiologic guidance, in a procedure laboratory where a catheter is inserted into the groin and threaded to the brain at the point of the clot. Once the catheter has reached the clot, an endovascular clot retrieval procedure or mechanical thrombectomy may be implemented. Stroke centers with interventional neuroradiologists can offer clot retrieval procedures. As with rt-PA, the less time from stroke symptom onset to reperfusion with endovascular therapy, the better the outcome for the patient. Reperfusion within 6 hours of stroke onset has shown the best benefit (Powers et al., 2015). With careful evaluation, endovascular therapy is also an option for patients who have a contraindication to intravenous rt-PA

Other Medications. The trauma of a CVA causes edema in the affected tissues and surrounding tissues. Cerebral edema is sometimes treated with osmotic diuretics such as mannitol and with hyperventilation. In severe cases, surgical intervention may be required. Nimodipine (Nimotop), a calcium-channel blocker, may be ordered to prevent spasms in cerebral blood vessels after subarachnoid hemorrhage. Phenytoin (Dilantin) and phenobarbital are anticonvulsants that may be ordered if the patient has seizures. The efficacy and safety of heparin and heparinoid drugs have been challenged in recent years and are no longer routinely used as a first-line treatment with a TIA or an acute ischemic stroke unless a cardioembolic stroke is suspected. Small doses of these medications given subcutaneously are recommended in the prevention of deep vein thrombosis (DVT) associated with acute stroke. When appropriate, heparin is given intravenously followed by oral warfarin. Later the regimen may be changed to aspirin, which decreases the risk of thrombus by preventing platelets from clumping. Newer drugs such as dabigatran (Pradaxa) or rivaroxaban (Xarelto) may also be considered for long-term anticoagulation instead of warfarin.

Medical management is often directed at preventing a subsequent or future stroke. Examples of drugs given to prevent strokes caused by thrombi are acetylsalicylic acid (aspirin), clopidogrel (Plavix), and extended release dipyridamole (Aggrenox). Drugs used to prevent or treat CVA are included in Table 23.2.

Pharmacology Capsule

It is important to remember that recombinant tissue plasminogen activator (rt-PA), which is used to dissolve clots, is most effective when given within 3 hours of the onset of stroke symptoms.

Surgical Intervention

Surgical intervention is an option for some patients with hemorrhagic strokes. Decisions about surgery are based on the patient's age, the ICP, and the location of the hemorrhage.

Fluids and Nutrition

Intravenous fluids are usually administered for the stroke patient in the acute phase. This route provides fluids, electrolytes, and an access for the intravenous administration of drugs. Following an acute stroke, nothing by mouth (NPO) is ordered until a swallowing evaluation is completed by a speech-language pathologist (SLP). The diet is based on the patient's nutritional requirements and ability to eat. Once permitted, food may be regular, soft, or pureed, depending on how well the patient can chew and swallow. Vitamins and electrolyte supplementation may also be given.

Total parenteral nutrition (TPN) may be administered to the malnourished patient. Sometimes a nasogastric tube is inserted for feeding purposes. If long-term enteral feedings are indicated, a gastrostomy tube may be placed.

Urine Elimination

Sometimes an indwelling catheter is used to manage urinary incontinence. Intermittent catheterization is a method of controlling incontinence caused by a flaccid bladder that is less likely to lead to infection. Intermittent catheterization is done every 4 to 6 hours as ordered. The frequency of catheterization is based on the amount of urine obtained each time. Bedside ultrasound bladder scanning may be used by to determine the need for intermittent catheterization.

NURSING CARE IN THE ACUTE PHASE OF STROKE

Once a stroke has occurred, it is important to rapidly identify the type and extent of the stroke so that appropriate treatment can be initiated. The most important aspects of care during the acute phase of a stroke are assessment and stabilization of the patient to prevent further brain injury. This phase is sometimes referred to as *hyperacute.* Management in this phase focuses on identifying the type and extent of the stroke so that appropriate treatment can be initiated, maintenance or improvement of vital physiologic functions, and support of the patient and family (see the Nursing Care Plan).

Nursing Care Plan Patient With a Stroke

FOCUSED ASSESSMENT

Health History

An obese 78-year-old male was admitted with weakness on the right side and slurred speech. His daughter assisted with the history because the patient had some difficulty responding verbally. He has had type 2 diabetes mellitus for 10 years, which he treats with an oral hypoglycemic, and had a myocardial infarction at 75 years of age. He has no recent changes in vision but does wear reading glasses. He has good hearing and no headaches. He is right-handed. He was unable to stand when he awoke this morning. He tried to drink some water but had difficulty swallowing. He has had no loss of bowel or bladder control. He is divorced. An adult daughter and her two teenagers live with him. He is a retired construction worker; his hobbies are carpentry and watching television.

Physical Examination Vital signs: blood pressure 210/104 mm Hg, pulse 96 beats per minute, respiration 22 breaths per minute, temperature 97° F (36° C) measured orally. Height 6′1″, weight 285 lb. Acknowledges he is in the hospital but is uncertain about day or date and time. Uses gestures to respond to some questions when he seems unable to find the right words. Pupils are equal and react to light. Ptosis of right eyelid is noted. Hand grips; voluntary movements; and reflexes of leg, arm, and hand are normal on left side but diminished on right side. Leans toward right side when not supported.

Patient Problems	Goals and Outcome Criteria	Interventions
Fluid volume deficit related to inadequate intake, dysphagia	The patient will maintain adequate hydration, as evidenced by moist mucous membranes, dilute urine, and pulse and blood pressure within usual range.	Record fluid intake and output. Administer intravenous fluid as ordered. After assessment by the speech-language pathologist (SLP), monitor oral fluid intake and assess swallowing. Assist the patient to sit up while eating and drinking. If thin fluids are difficult to swallow, try semisolids such as ice cream, pudding, and popsicles. Have an oral suction device available in case of choking or aspiration. Detect and report signs and symptoms of fluid volume deficit: tachycardia, concentrated urine, and dry mucous membranes.
Inadequate nutrition related to dysphagia, inability to feed self	The patient will maintain adequate nutrition as evidenced by stable weight.	Document food intake. Assist with meals as needed. Use positioning and food consistency guidelines as provided by the SLP. Seat the patient upright for meals. Do not make him feel rushed. Provide alternative means of feeding (nasogastric or gastrostomy tube, total parenteral nutrition [TPN]) as ordered. Weigh weekly to assess adequacy of food intake.

Nursing Care Plan Patient With a Stroke—cont'd

Patient Problems	Goals and Outcome Criteria	Interventions
Inability to communicate effectively related to aphasia	The patient will use nonverbal means to supplement verbal communication and will participate in speech therapy exercises.	Establish a code system of blinks or nods for nonverbal communication; use pictures or cards that the patient can select to express his needs. Encourage verbalization but recognize his frustration and provide words if he cannot retrieve them. Discuss referral to SLP with the physician. Tell the patient that improvement is usually possible with therapy.
Decreased mobility related to weakness, paralysis, poor balance	The patient will maintain intact skin, joint mobility, regular bowel and bladder elimination, good peripheral circulation, and normal breath sounds.	While on bed rest, assist the patient to change positions at least every 2 hours. He should not lie on his right side for more than 30 minutes at a time. Use positioning techniques and devices to reduce pressure points. Inspect the skin for redness and edema associated with pressure. Position the limbs in functional alignment and perform range-of-motion exercises 3 times a day. Do not pull on the affected side. Monitor bowel and bladder function. Administer stool softeners and laxatives as ordered. Encourage fluids and fiber when able to take orally. Palpate the lower abdomen for bladder distention and catheterize as ordered as necessary. Use bladder scanner if available to assess need for urinary catheterization. Report any tenderness, pain, or swelling in calves. Exercise the legs with each position change. Apply graduated compression stockings or sequential compression devices (SCDs) as ordered. Ambulate using gait belt when able. Discuss consults for physical therapy (PT) and occupational therapy (OT) with physician. Encourage coughing and deep breathing with each position change. Auscultate lung fields for breath sounds, wheezes, or rales. Report temperature elevation.
Potential for injury related to paralysis	The patient will have no falls or injuries associated with motor impairment or altered sensory perception.	Keep the bed in low position with the side rails raised according to hospital policy. Put the call bell within reach on nonparalyzed side and instruct the patient to call for help getting out of bed. A bed check device may be implemented when patient has difficulty understanding directions or is in a confused state. Check on him frequently. Monitor the position of affected extremities to prevent trauma that might not be detected because of poor sensation. Use a sling or brace if ordered to support affected limbs. Assess the effects of ptosis on vision. If vision is impaired, approach the patient from the unaffected side and arrange personal articles on that side. When the patient is out of bed, be sure he is seated safely. Use pillows to prevent excessive leaning to one side. When ambulatory, use a gait belt if needed and assist the patient as appropriate.
Anxiety related to loss of function or fear of disability	The patient will have a reduction in anxiety, as evidenced by calm manner and patient statement.	Acknowledge signs of anxiety and attempt to identify sources. Provide information about what is happening, what you are doing, and what the patient can expect. Check on him often. Encourage his family to visit.
Altered family function related to anticipated need of patient for assistance after discharge	The patient and family will plan for altered roles and responsibilities to support the patient during and after discharge.	Give family members an opportunity to ask questions and share their concerns. Provide information and facilitate communication with the physician as needed. Refer them to sources of support and resources, including a social worker and community agencies. Start planning for discharge. Assess family strengths and resources and willingness to help care for the patient after discharge. Identify new responsibilities they might need to assume and discuss how these can be fulfilled.

CRITICAL THINKING QUESTIONS

1. What effect might this patient's stroke have on his daughter and her family?
2. Describe three examples of signs of anxiety that the patient may exhibit.
3. What data in this assessment are consistent with stroke?

Box 23.2 Cincinnati Prehospital Stroke Scale

The patient is asked to show teeth or smile.

- Normal—Both sides of face move equally well.
- Abnormal—One side of face does not move as well as the other side.

The patient is asked to close both eyes and hold both arms straight out, with palms up, for 10 seconds.

- Normal—Both arms move the same, or both arms do not move at all.
- Abnormal—One arm does not move, or one arm drifts down.

The patient is asked to repeat a simple phrase, such as, "You can't teach an old dog new tricks."

- Normal—Patient uses correct words with no slurring.
- Abnormal—Patient slurs words, uses the wrong words, or is unable to speak.

From Kothari RU, Pancioli A, Liu T, et al.: Cincinnati Pre-Hospital Stroke Scale: reproducibility and validity, *Ann Emerg Med* 33(4):373–378, 1999. Copyright 1999, with permission from American College of Emergency Physicians.

FOCUSED ASSESSMENT

The initial nursing assessment is directed at identifying the symptoms that indicate a possible stroke and responding with the appropriate assessments to determine the type and extent of the stroke. During the hyperacute time, information related to the onset of stroke symptoms is very important, such as the time of onset of symptoms and details about the symptoms experienced (e.g., activity). Several tools are available to assess patients experiencing signs of a stroke. The Cincinnati Prehospital Stroke Scale is a quick and easy tool that is often used in the prehospital phase by emergency medical technicians. This is a three-step test, shown in Box 23.2, to assess facial muscles, arm movement, and speech function. Abnormality in any one of these strongly suggests that the patient may be having a stroke. Nursing assessments should also reveal risk factors for CVA and identify nursing care needs of the patient. Details of the neurologic assessment are covered in Chapter 21 and summarized in Box 21.2.

The National Institutes of Health Stroke Scale (NIHSS) (Table 23.4) is a tool used to assess patients who have experienced a stroke. This tool provides a method to guide systematic assessment of neurologic deficits often associated with an acute stroke. The examination addresses motor function, visual fields, ataxia, speech, language, cognition, and motor and sensory abnormalities. A point system is used to rate function; then points are combined to offer a "score." A research neurologist designed it to standardize and document neurologic assessments of stroke patients. To standardize the scale, all clinicians must complete education and maintain a current certificate of examination to conduct the NIHSS assessment and scoring.

Patient Problems, Goals, and Outcome Criteria: Acute Phase of Stroke

Depending on location and extent of brain damage, appropriate patient problems and goals may include the following.

Patient Problems	Goals and Outcome Criteria
Inadequate oxygenation related to impaired cough reflex, altered consciousness, impaired swallowing	Patent airway: breath sounds clear to auscultation
Inadequate oxygenation related to interrupted breathing pattern because of impaired cerebral circulation, increased intracranial pressure (ICP)	Adequate oxygenation: normal respiratory rate and depth, arterial blood gases within normal limits
Potential for injury related to seizure activity, confusion, motor and sensory impairment, increased ICP, hemorrhage after recombinant tissue plasminogen activator (rt-PA) administration	Absence of injury: no bruising, skin breaks, falls, or fractures; stable neurologic status (level of consciousness, pupil equality and reaction to light)
Potential for fluid volume imbalance related to inadequate intake or excessive diuresis	Adequate hydration: balanced fluid intake and output
Potential for fluid volume imbalance related to overhydration	Normal extracellular fluid volume: pulse and blood pressure consistent with patient norms, no edema, breath sounds clear
Inadequate nutrition related to dysphagia, inability to feed self, inability to chew	Adequate intake of nutrients: maintenance of body weight
Elevated body temperature related to effects of neurologic impairment and/or metabolic processes	Effective thermoregulation: temperature within patient's normal range
Potential for impaired cognition related to inadequate cerebral circulation	Improved mental function: patient is oriented to self and environment
Inability to communicate effectively related to aphasia	Effective communication: patient successfully communicates needs
Decreased mobility (bed, transfers, wheelchair, walking) related to weakness, paralysis, spasticity, impaired balance	Absence of complications of immobility: joints have full range of motion, skin intact

Patient Problems, Goals, and Outcome Criteria: Acute Phase of Stroke—cont'd

Patient Problems	Goals and Outcome Criteria
Functional urinary incontinence related to inability to manage toileting process, impaired cognition. Difficulty voiding related to initial effects of stroke	Improved control of urine elimination: episodes of uncontrolled voiding decrease; patient voids voluntarily
Constipation related to immobility, dehydration, drug side effects	Normal bowel elimination: regular passage of soft, formed stool without straining
Loss of bowel control related to impaired conduction of impulses	Controlled bowel elimination: no involuntary bowel evacuation
Inadequate coping related to adapting to neurologic deficits	Effective coping strategies: patient verbalizes acceptance of stroke and strives for maximum recovery
Altered family function related to disruption of family roles and functions	Adaptation of the family to the patient's condition: family demonstrates willingness and ability to adapt to patient's condition

INTERVENTIONS

Inadequate Oxygenation

To ensure adequate oxygenation, maintain the patient's body alignment and elevate the head of the bed 25 to 30 degrees. Closely monitor the patient's respiratory status. Maintaining a patent airway is a priority for patients who have suffered strokes. Neurologic deficits may cause altered breathing patterns and impaired swallowing, gag, and cough reflexes. Increasing ICP may affect the respiratory center in the brain, causing respiratory depression. If the patient exhibits signs of increased ICP (e.g., rising blood pressure, bradycardia, abnormal pupil response, decreasing level of consciousness), elevate the head of the bed 30 degrees and notify the physician.

After a stroke, the patient is at risk for airway obstruction for a number of reasons. If the patient is unconscious, the tongue may fall back and block the airway. A side-lying position helps to prevent such obstruction. An oral or nasal airway is sometimes used to keep the airway open.

Immobility and dehydration cause thick secretions to be retained in the respiratory tract, possibly leading to pneumonia and atelectasis. Good hydration helps to thin respiratory secretions for easier expectoration. Dysphagia may cause the patient to aspirate fluids or food, causing airway obstruction and contributing to the development of pneumonia. Pneumonia is, in fact, the most frequent cause of death after stroke. Feeding the patient with dysphagia is discussed in Chapter 38.

Suctioning and frequent position changes can help to prevent aspiration and promote removal of secretions. Respiratory treatments for the patient, with regular reminders to do deep-breathing exercises, can be helpful. Forceful coughing may be discouraged in the acute phase after a hemorrhagic stroke because it tends to increase ICP. Ask the physician if and when coughing is permitted. Administer oxygen therapy as ordered.

Potential for Injury

Many factors place the stroke patient at risk for injury. Seizures may occur, causing the patient to lose consciousness and to have abnormal motor activity. Therefore it is important to raise bed side rails and pad them according to agency protocol to reduce trauma if the patient strikes the rails. During a seizure, turn the patient to one side and move hard objects away from the patient. Never force anything between the patient's clenched teeth. To do so may injure the teeth and gums. Additional information about seizures is presented in Chapter 22.

Safety precautions are also essential for confused patients and patients with motor impairments. Orient patients to their surroundings and explain why they should not get up unassisted. The staff must respond promptly to the patient's calls for help. Although restraints are needed at times, they should only be used as a last resort because they often agitate the patient and can actually cause injuries. A bed check system may be of more benefit when the patient is having difficulty with understanding directions. Get sufficient help or use mechanical devices to assist the patient in and out of the bed.

Sensory perceptual problems in the stroke patient may include visual disturbances, sensory deprivation or overload, and impaired tactile sensation. Among the visual disturbances are **diplopia** (double vision), loss of the corneal (blink) reflex, **ptosis** (drooping of the upper eyelid), homonymous hemianopsia, and inability to close the eyelids on the affected side. All of these pose threats to safety and self-care. They may also contribute to confusion. The cornea is susceptible to injury when not protected and, in healthy patients, kept moist by the closed eyelid and the blink reflex. Artificial tears may be used to provide moisture in patients with disturbed corneal reflex.

Patients who have homonymous hemianopsia see only half of the field of vision. Some patients have unilateral neglect, a condition in which visual fields are intact but the patient does not attend to certain parts of the fields. Unilateral neglect is most common in patients with right-brain damage. These patients may not attend to one side of the body and may overlook objects on one side of the visual field.

Table 23.4 National Institutes of Health Stroke Scale

1a. Level of consciousness	0 Alert 1 Not alert, but arousable with minimal stimulation 2 Not alert, requires repeated stimulation to attend 3 Coma
1b. Ask patient the month and their age	0 Answers both correctly 1 Answers one correctly 2 Both incorrect
1c. Ask patient to open and close eyes and grip and release hand	0 Obeys both correctly 1 Obeys one correctly 2 Both incorrect
2. Best gaze (only horizontal eye movement)	0 Normal 1 Partial gaze palsy 2 Forced deviation
3. Visual field testing	0 No visual field loss 1 Partial hemianopia 2 Complete hemianopia 3 Bilateral hemianopia (blind including cortical blindness)
4. Facial paresis (ask patient to show teeth or raise eyebrows and close eyes tightly)	0 Normal symmetric movement 1 Minor paralysis (flattened nasolabial fold, asymmetry on smiling) 2 Partial paralysis (total or near total paralysis of lower face) 3 Complete paralysis of one or both sides (absence of facial movement in the upper and lower face)
5. Motor function—arm (right and left) Right arm— Left arm—	0 Normal (extends arms 90 [or 45] degrees for 10 seconds without drift) 1 Drift 2 Some effort against gravity 3 No effort against gravity 4 No movement
6. Motor function—leg (right and left) Right leg— Left leg—	0 Normal (holds leg at 30 degrees for 5 seconds) 1 Drift 2 Some effort against gravity 3 No effort against gravity 4 No movement 9 Untestable (joint fused or limb amputated)
7. Limb ataxia	0 No ataxia 1 Present in one limb 2 Present in two limbs
8. Sensory (use pinprick to test arms, legs, trunk, and face—compare side to side)	0 Normal trunk and face 1 Mild-to-moderate decrease in sensation 2 Severe-to-total sensory loss
9. Best language (describe picture, read items, read sentences)	0 No aphasia 1 Mild-to-moderate aphasia 2 Severe aphasia 3 Mute
10. Dysarthria (read several words)	0 Normal articulation 1 Mild-to-moderate slurring of words 2 Near unintelligible or unable to speak 9 Intubated or other physical barriers
11. Extinction and inattention	0 Normal 1 Inattention or extinction to bilateral simultaneous stimulation in one of the sensory modalities 2 Profound hemi-inattention or extinction to more than one sensory modality (e.g., does not recognize own hand)

It is helpful to encourage patients to scan the affected side. Differences in the nursing approaches during the acute and rehabilitative phases are well contrasted here. In the acute phase, position patients with homonymous hemianopsia so that the staff approaches the unimpaired side to reduce stress to the patients. In rehabilitation, the patient should be positioned so that deliberate scanning by and use of the affected side are required. This is designed to stimulate return of function. Balanced sensory input is essential to reduce the risk of sensory deprivation or overload. The environment should be pleasant but not overly stimulating.

Another type of sensory disturbance after stroke is diminished sensation in affected body parts. The patient who does not feel pressure or pain is susceptible to injury. For example, a paralyzed foot can easily slip between the bed frame and side rails. Catheter tubing under the leg may create pressure that the patient cannot feel. Protect susceptible areas and remind the patient of the need for extra caution. In addition, check positioning of affected extremities to ensure that they are free of pressure and reposition them as needed.

If rt-PA is administered for ischemic stroke, the patient must be monitored closely for hemorrhage for 24 to 36 hours. Intracranial bleeding is the most common location of hemorrhage associated with rt-PA therapy. Signs of intracerebral hemorrhage include change in level of consciousness, elevation in blood pressure, deterioration in motor function, new headache, and nausea and vomiting. Treatment of the bleeding requires administration of factor VIII and platelets. With any change in patient status, the provider should be notified. An urgent CT scan is indicated. Cerebral edema is common after large cerebral infarctions, especially in younger patients. It is most common 3 to 5 days after an ischemic stroke. Early signs of increased ICP include deterioration in level of consciousness and motor function, headache, visual disturbances, change in respiratory pattern, and changes in blood pressure and heart rate. Keep the head of the bed elevated at 30 degrees and maintain the alignment of the head with the rest of the body. Medical interventions include diuretic and barbiturate drugs, hyperventilation, and in some cases surgical intervention.

Potential for Fluid Volume Imbalance

Close monitoring of fluid status is especially important in the acute phase of stroke. Accurate intake and output records are essential. Measure vital signs, compare for trends suggesting excess or deficient fluid volume, and assess the mouth for moisture. In a well-hydrated person, the mucous membranes of the mouth are moist. Evaluate tissue turgor, remembering that it is not a very reliable indicator of fluid status in the older person. Age-related changes in the skin and subcutaneous structures cause a loss of tissue elasticity that may be mistaken for dehydration. Laboratory studies, including urine specific gravity, serum electrolytes, and hematocrit, are also useful indicators of fluid balance.

The patient is at risk for excess fluid volume if excessive intravenous fluids are administered or if the patient's kidneys are unable to eliminate excess fluid rapidly enough. Excess fluid volume may lead to edema and heart failure. Signs of excess fluid volume are fluid intake greater than output, bounding pulse, venous distention, increased blood pressure, crackles in the lungs, and edema. Report evidence of excess fluid to the registered nurse (RN) or physician. The rate of intravenous fluid may be decreased, and diuretics may be ordered. Explain to the patient and family the need to temporarily restrict fluids. If the patient is thirsty, frequently provide small amounts of fluids in small containers and record all intake.

Factors that place the stroke patient at risk for deficient fluid volume include age, dysphagia, drug therapy with diuretics, and immobility. The stroke patient is likely to be older, and older people are less able to conserve water through the kidneys. The patient with dysphagia may be unable to take in adequate oral fluids. If diuretics are given for excess fluid volume or increased ICP, they can precipitate excess loss of water and electrolytes. The patient with motor deficits may not be able to obtain fluids independently.

Deficient fluid volume contributes to constipation, skin dryness, urinary tract infections, and renal calculi (stones). Signs of deficient fluid volume are a thready pulse, tachycardia, low blood pressure, low urine output, concentrated urine, dry mucous membranes, and sometimes confusion. Report evidence of deficient fluid volume to the RN or physician. If intravenous fluids are being administered, the physician may order an increase in the hourly flow rate. Fluids may also be given through enteral feeding tubes.

To reduce the risk of deficient fluid volume, monitor the fluid intake record to ensure that the patient is getting at least eight 8-oz glasses of fluids each day (unless contraindicated). All staff and family members should know to offer fluids and record the amounts taken.

Place fluids within sight and easy reach of the patient and explain the need for adequate hydration. If the patient has hemiplegia, the fluids must be placed on the nonparalyzed side. Spill-proof containers that are easily held with one hand can facilitate independent drinking. If the patient is able to take oral fluids but has difficulty swallowing, it is important to proceed slowly. Have suction equipment on hand in case of aspiration. Thin liquids are more readily aspirated. Jell-O, ice cream, popsicles, and frozen juice may be substituted to provide adequate fluids. Thickening agents can be added to other liquids as needed, as prescribed by the SLP.

Inadequate Nutrition

The patient's nutritional status is of concern throughout stroke treatment. Factors that may lead to inadequate nutrition include dysphagia, paralysis, difficulty chewing, and depression. The patient who is malnourished is at risk for skin breakdown and infection. Obesity hampers mobility and can interfere with rehabilitation.

The patient who has dysphagia may not be able to consume adequate nutrients orally. Sometimes a nasogastric tube is inserted for feeding purposes. The physician may order TPN for the malnourished patient. Aggressive treatment of dysphagia is delayed until the rehabilitative phase. Dysphagia often resolves spontaneously during the first few months of recovery. Feeding the dysphagic patient is discussed in Chapter 38.

If the patient has a nasogastric or nasointestinal feeding tube in place, check its placement and residual according to agency policy. Be certain to provide the correct formula and to ensure that it flows at the prescribed rate. Bolus feedings may be ordered at intervals or pumps may be used to dispense continuous feedings. Keep the head of the patient's bed slightly elevated to reduce the risk of fluid flowing back into the esophagus and being aspirated. The nasogastric tube irritates the naris and the nasal passages. Gently cleanse the naris several times a day. Concentrated formulas may cause diarrhea. If that happens, the physician should be consulted about diluting the formula or changing to another type of formula.

TPN is given through an intravenous line inserted in a large vein (a central line). Unlike enteral feedings, the flow of TPN fluids is always controlled with a mechanical infusion pump. The nurse hangs new bottles of prescribed fluids. The insertion site requires special care to prevent infection so change dressings according to agency protocol, using strict aseptic technique. Patients on TPN may develop hyperglycemia; therefore it is important to monitor blood glucose levels at regular intervals. Care of the patient receiving TPN is explained in Chapter 6.

Elevated Body Temperature

After a stroke, the body's temperature-regulating mechanism may be impaired, causing the temperature to rise. Metabolic processes that are also in play may increase the body temperature. It is important to monitor the patient's temperature and treat elevations promptly. Fever is treated aggressively, most often with antipyretic drugs. Some studies even suggest a decrease in infarction size in those patients aggressively treated for hyperthermia. Always assess the patient for an underlying infection as a potential cause for any temperature elevation.

Potential for Impaired Cognition

After a stroke, patients may suffer functional losses, alterations in sensation and perception, and impaired communication. In addition, they find themselves in the hospital, where they are poked, monitored, and prodded by strangers and where days and nights all seem the same. All of these factors combined can cause the patient to become disoriented or confused. Neglect associated with right-brain strokes may also be manifested as denial. In extreme cases, patients deny that they have even had a stroke.

To orient patients, introduce yourself as often as necessary, remind patients where they are, and tell them what is being done and why. Be sure that eyeglasses and hearing aids are worn if the patient normally uses them. In addition, place clocks and marked calendars in view and tell the patient what time it is and what to expect next. Confused patients require frequent reassurance and reinforcement. Instructions and information should be concise and repeated as needed. Sometimes a familiar person can be helpful with a confused patient. If the visitor is disturbed by the patient's behavior, provide guidance on how to deal with the patient.

Inability to Communicate Effectively

The alert patient who has aphasia is understandably anxious about the inability to speak, to understand words, or both. Use brief, clear statements accompanied by gestures, pictures, and facial expressions. Questions that can be answered with "yes" or "no" may allow the patient to respond more easily. Pause attentively when the patient struggles to respond (excessive chatter can be distressing to the aphasic patient). Explain the communication problem and approaches to the family. Speech therapy may be initiated once the patient's medical condition is stable. Speech rehabilitation is discussed further in the section titled "Nursing Care in the Rehabilitation Phase."

Decreased Mobility (Bed, Transfers, Wheelchair, Walking)

Impaired motor function is common after stroke and places the patient at risk for complications of immobility. Care of the immobilized patient is discussed in detail in Chapter 12 and is summarized here.

Skin Tissue Integrity. The potential for skin breakdown in this patient population is great because of motor impairment, altered consciousness or sensation, poor nutritional status, and incontinence. Measures to maintain skin integrity include cleanliness, pressure relief, and good hydration and nutrition. When skin is dry, as it often is in older patients, it is important to reduce bathing frequency, use soap sparingly, and apply lotions to retain skin moisture.

It is essential to turn and reposition the acute stroke patient at least every 2 hours. Skin breakdown can occur at vulnerable pressure points after just 30 minutes in one position. If reddened pressure areas remain when it is time to turn the patient, shorten the intervals between turnings. Do not allow the patient to lie on the affected side for more than 30 minutes. Because of impaired sensation, the risk of excessive pressure and trauma is much greater on the affected side. Pressure must be alternated on main pressure points such as hips, knees, heels, and lower back. An air floatation mattress or fluidized bed may be used for the high-risk patient. Some of the newer therapeutic beds automatically turn patients. These beds do not stress the usual pressure points of the patient, but regular skin assessments and breathing exercises are still required. As soon as possible, position the patient comfortably in a chair for brief periods. Remember to monitor for a drop in blood pressure when getting the patient out of bed.

Good nursing care is time consuming, so take advantage of this time to stimulate the patient with conversation and explanations of care. This is helpful even if the patient is unresponsive.

Joint Mobility. The immobilized patient is at risk for muscle atrophy and joint contractures. In the stroke patient, the affected side is especially vulnerable when loss of voluntary movement occurs. During the acute phase, be concerned with maintaining joint mobility. This can be done with frequent, gentle range-of-motion exercises and proper positioning. Determine whether the patient had any preexisting limitations of joint mobility. Older patients may have arthritic changes that reduce the range of motion. Never force movement to resistant joints. Once the acute phase has passed, the patient is usually referred for vigorous physical therapy.

Affected extremities must be supported. Never grab or pull the extremities on the patient's affected side. Dislocation or further injury can easily occur because the patient may not be able to accurately perceive the pressure or pain that is normally felt.

Circulation. DVT is a major complication of immobility, especially in this patient population. Regular passive and active range-of-motion exercises encourage venous blood return, thereby reducing the risk of thrombus formation. The physician may order alternating pressure wraps to promote venous return. If the patient received rt-PA, low-dose anticoagulation therapy may be initiated no earlier than 24 hours after the rt-PA infusion is completed, to help prevent thrombus formation. Ambulation is generally encouraged (if the patient is able) as soon as possible after the medical condition stabilizes.

Functional Urinary Incontinence and Difficulty Voiding

It is not unusual for urinary incontinence to occur after stroke. This may be caused by a temporarily flaccid bladder or an inability of the brain to coordinate information to be able to store urine in the bladder or wait once the urge to void is felt. Check the patient hourly for wetness and remove wet clothing and linens promptly. Wash the skin, rinse, and pat dry. A variety of incontinence products are available to minimize the contact of urine with the skin (see Chapter 14). Sometimes an indwelling catheter is ordered to prevent incontinence. The catheter protects the skin and allows for more accurate measurement of output. The disadvantage is that an indwelling catheter is frequently the cause of urinary tract infections. A regular toileting schedule with bladder scanning and intermittent catheterization is a better alternative to indwelling catheterization. External condom catheters are options for male patients. Bladder retraining, discussed in Chapter 14, is actively pursued in the rehabilitation phase.

Constipation and Loss of Bowel Control

As with urinary incontinence, the ability of the brain to coordinate the information to wait once the urge to move the bowels is felt may be damaged. During the acute phase of stroke, it is especially important to monitor bowel elimination, because the patient may develop constipation or incontinence. It is helpful to know the patient's usual patterns of elimination, although they cannot always be determined.

Constipation may develop as a result of immobility, dehydration, and drug therapy. A bowel program, consisting of a mild laxative or stool softener and a high-fiber diet, can help to prompt regular fecal elimination. Explain to patients and family members the importance of sufficient fluids to prevent dry stools. Some older people are laxative dependent. It is unrealistic to try to reverse the effects of years of laxative use during the acute phase of stroke. Inform the health care provider of the pattern and document bowel movements. Laxatives and enemas may be needed to maintain bowel elimination in these patients.

Bowel incontinence may be related to the inability to toilet independently or to confusion and can often be prevented in the alert patient by taking the patient to the toilet at the usual time of defecation. A raised toilet seat with armrests is easier and safer for the patient with hemiplegia. If incontinence occurs, take special care to clean the skin thoroughly. Be careful not to make comments that embarrass the patient. Remember that incontinence, especially with liquid stools, may indicate a fecal impaction. Removal of an impaction usually requires repeated enemas and manual removal of hard stool. Restoration of bowel control receives more attention in the rehabilitation phase and is detailed in Chapter 14.

Inadequate Coping

The effects of stroke may be temporary or permanent. It is difficult to predict how much function will be lost permanently or returned during recovery. Patients typically exhibit responses that reflect the grief process: shock, denial, depression, withdrawal, anger, and bargaining. Determine how the patient is coping and whether the coping strategies are constructive and effective.

An example of unhealthy coping is the patient who denies having problems with vision or balance and refuses to call for help when getting out of bed. Another example is the depressed and withdrawn patient who resists doing therapeutic exercises that would minimize complications. In this type of situation, the nurse can point out the behavior to the patient, explain its consequences, and encourage the patient to take an active role in rehabilitation activities. Depression is a major problem associated with stroke and can occur in up to 70% of stroke patients. The depression seen after a stroke may be the result of a loss of brain chemicals associated with the injury or a reaction to the loss of one's functional abilities. Antidepressant medications may be ordered for patients experiencing depression after a stroke and have been associated with improved outcomes in those patients treated. Sometimes a mental health counselor or support group is beneficial to help the patient learn to deal with the effects of stroke more constructively.

Altered Family Function

In the acute phase of stroke, family members are often frightened and confused. They may fear the patient's death or severe disability. They may also experience emotional and financial strain during the long rehabilitation process. Family members have to assume roles and responsibilities normally carried by the patient. It is important to recognize that the family, as well as the patient, experiences a sense of loss when a loved one has a stroke. Provide support by telling family members what is happening, what is being done, and how they can help the patient. If necessary, a referral may be made to a social worker, mental health specialist, or spiritual counselor.

NURSING CARE IN THE REHABILITATION PHASE

A patient's transition from the acute phase to the rehabilitation phase of stroke is an important one. Early and attentive care for the stroke patient shortens the recovery time and hastens the return of function. The general goals of treatment in the rehabilitation phase are to maximize functional abilities and to teach new ways to compensate for losses. Stabilization of vital signs with no further neurologic deficits indicates that the patient has entered the rehabilitation phase of stroke. At this time, the patient's functional and cognitive problems can vary widely, depending on the location and extent of brain damage. The patient may regain complete independent functioning, partially recover previous abilities, or lose functional abilities completely.

The rehabilitation phase is usually managed by a multidisciplinary team that includes nurses, physicians, physical therapists, occupational therapists, SLPs, social workers, psychologists, recreational therapists, vocational rehabilitation counselors, and dietitians.

During the rehabilitation phase of a stroke, vast changes can occur in the brain. The extent to which collateral blood circulation and alternative neuronal pathways develop affects the ultimate outcome for the patient. The goals of rehabilitation to enhance the ultimate recovery of functional abilities are reached through a program of stimulation and practice.

FOCUSED ASSESSMENT

In the rehabilitation phase, reassess the patient's abilities as well as their expectations, knowledge, motivation, and resources.

Patient Problems, Goals, and Outcome Criteria: Rehabilitation Phase of Stroke

Patient Problems	Goals and Outcome Criteria
Inability to manage self-care (bathing, dressing, feeding, toileting) related to sensory and motor impairments	Self-care needs met: care accomplished with assistance as needed
Potential for injury related to sensory and motor impairments	Absence of injury: no falls, bruises, skin tears, pressure sores
Inadequate coping related to cognitive impairments	Adequate coping: patient uses adaptive strategies to cope with disability
Inability to communicate effectively related to aphasia, dysarthria	Effective communication: meaningful verbalizations or effective use of nonverbal communication to make needs known
Inadequate nutrition related to dysphagia, anorexia	Adequate nutrition: achievement and maintenance of ideal body weight
Impaired mobility (bed, transfers, wheelchair, walking) related to residual motor impairment	Improved physical mobility: increasing independent physical activity
Constipation related to inactivity	Normal bowel elimination: regular, formed stools without straining
Difficulty voiding and/or functional urinary incontinence related to neurologic and motor impairment	Normal urine elimination: voluntary urination, decreasing incontinent episodes

INTERVENTIONS

Inability to Manage Self-Care (Bathing, Dressing, Feeding, Toileting)

The main focus of the rehabilitation phase is to return the stroke patient to the highest level of functioning possible. One of the most frustrating problems after a stroke for many patients and caregivers is the patient's inability to complete ADL. To improve, patients need to use affected parts as much as they are able. It is important for the nurse to demonstrate patience and a supportive attitude. Allow time for patients to try to do things for themselves.

Discouragement is a major factor in unsuccessful rehabilitation and demands prompt attention by the rehabilitation team.

A variety of personal devices and environmental adaptations can foster a return to independence. Prosthetic devices that assist patients with dressing, bathing, and eating are available. Simple measures such as replacing buttons with Velcro fasteners and replacing complicated trousers with elastic-waist pants can make a big difference. Collaboration between the nurse and the occupational therapist will help to identify equipment and environmental adaptations that will support the patient's progress in rehabilitation.

A referral for follow-up at home should be initiated so that the safety and accessibility of the home environment can be assessed before discharge. The trend toward shorter hospital stays means that this must be addressed very early. Many patients are discharged to rehabilitation or skilled nursing facilities until they are ready to return home. A home visit by the patient, home health nurse, physical therapist, and occupational therapist can be made to identify problems and make plans for adaptations. Adaptations should promote access in and out of the home and enable patients to be as independent as possible. The addition of a raised commode seat, bathtub handrails, shower seat, or other devices can facilitate toileting and bathing. Cooking may be assisted by adjusting the height of counters, creating shelves that roll out, and rearranging cabinet contents to improve access. Patients need to practice daily tasks under conditions similar to those at home. Rehabilitation centers usually have activity centers that allow patients to practice self-care skills with their disabilities.

Potential for Injury

Alterations in motor function, sensation, and vision are distressing changes that affect the patient's ability to carry out self-care and pose a threat to safety.

Motor Function. Alterations in motor functioning may leave the patient at risk for injury. Safety precautions are a vital part of nursing care of the patient. Teaching should include calling for assistance as needed, using assistive devices for mobilization, and adaptation of the environment to promote safety (Fig. 23.4). Physical and occupational therapists are invaluable in assisting with providing a safe environment.

Sensation. As noted previously, patients may have altered sensation in the affected body parts after a stroke. This may appear as loss of sensation or as exaggerated response in which every sensation is perceived as painful. The patient may be injured without even knowing it because of impaired sensation. Teach the patient and family to assess the affected area frequently for signs of pressure and to protect it from injury. In addition to teaching the patient how to avoid pressure, advise the patient not to apply heat or cold to that area because of the risk of injury. Remind the patient and family not to pull on the affected side or use that side to move or support the patient in ambulation.

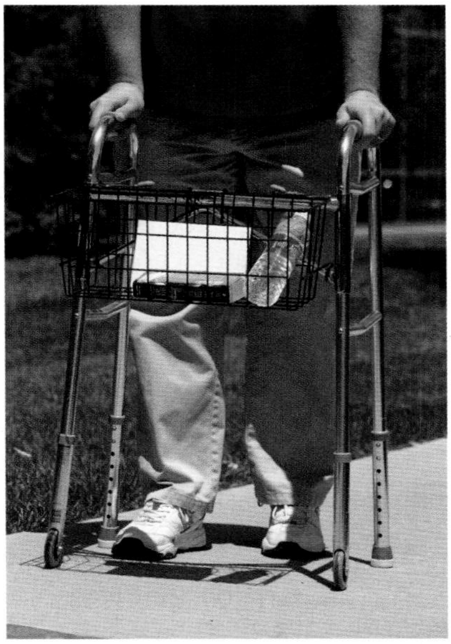

Fig. 23.4 Assistive devices can enable a person with mobility impairment to be active at home and in the community. (From Birchenall J, Streight E: *Mosby's textbook for the home care aide*, ed 3, St. Louis, 2012, Mosby.)

Patients with abnormal pain perception may benefit from regular physical therapy, using a kind of desensitization. During therapy, the patient is reminded and encouraged that the pain is not real and is only misinterpreted by the brain.

Vision. Homonymous hemianopsia, in which half of the field of vision is lost, also presents problems with self-care and safety. In the acute phase, the patient's environment is arranged so that important items are available on the unaffected side. In the rehabilitation phase, the patient is challenged more to promote adaptation to the disability. For example, objects are placed in the field of the visual deficit. Remind the patient to scan the affected visual field, especially when walking, wheeling, and eating. The patient forms new habits of observation through constant practice.

Inadequate Coping

Intellectual and emotional changes after stroke are distressing to patients and their families. Explain these changes and demonstrate how to help patients adapt. Cognitive processes may continue to be slow for quite some time after the stroke. It is important to avoid rushing the patient. The patient may become frustrated and give up trying. Emotional lability is manifested as sudden laughing, crying, or outbursts of anger without apparent reason. Caregivers and families may attribute this emotional unpredictability to depression. It is generally believed that depression is frequently associated with brain trauma of any kind. The patient can often be easily distracted from crying or from anger with simple redirection to the task at hand. This is an indication that the depression, if it exists, may be of a different type than the usual emotional state and requires specific interventions. Treatment of depression, whatever the cause, is an important part of the rehabilitation process. Research clearly demonstrates a positive relationship to outcomes when patients are identified and treated aggressively for depression after a stroke.

Inability to Communicate Effectively

Helping the patient to improve or regain effective communication is an extremely important goal of the rehabilitation phase. Aphasia may affect the ability to understand spoken words or to use words to express oneself. Types of aphasia were explained with the signs and symptoms of stroke (see Table 23.3).

Patients with aphasia need encouragement as they struggle to communicate. Be patient because the aphasic person requires more time to plan and deliver a response. Take time to allow the patient to respond while providing verbal cues or picture boards to avoid frustrating the patient. The physician often refers patients with severe communication impairments to SLPs.

Inadequate Nutrition

The patient with dysphagia must be closely followed and reevaluated at intervals for the ability to swallow. With each evaluation, there should be new recommendations for oral intake based on the new assessment. If the patient is not progressing as expected, a video fluoroscopic test of swallowing may be ordered. This test, conducted by the SLP and the radiologist, traces the route of swallowed fluid to detect swallowing abnormalities.

The patient who has some difficulty swallowing may be placed on a supervised feeding program. SLPs are trained to help patients relearn swallowing but everyday feeding falls to the nursing staff. Through use of radiologic procedures, the SLP will determine the patient's best position to ensure safe swallowing and eating. Often, this will be sitting with the head tilted forward and toward the unaffected side. Fluid intake must still be encouraged for the dysphagic person, despite the increased work for patient and staff. Special utensils can greatly facilitate self-feeding (Fig. 23.5). Acknowledge even small improvements as the patient struggles in rehabilitation.

Nutrition Considerations

1. A major nutritional concern for the stroke patient is dysphagia (difficulty swallowing), which may lead to malnutrition and dehydration because of inadequate intake.
2. Swallowing thin liquids is frequently a problem. Thin liquids can be thickened with dry milk powder, cornstarch, fruit and vegetable flakes, or commercial thickening agents.
3. Very warm or chilled foods stimulate the swallowing reflex better than bland, lukewarm foods.
4. In addition to thickened liquids, foods that are better for chewing and swallowing are soft bread, cooked cereal, ice cream, yogurt, cooked eggs, moist ground beef, canned fruits and vegetables, thick soups, and puddings.

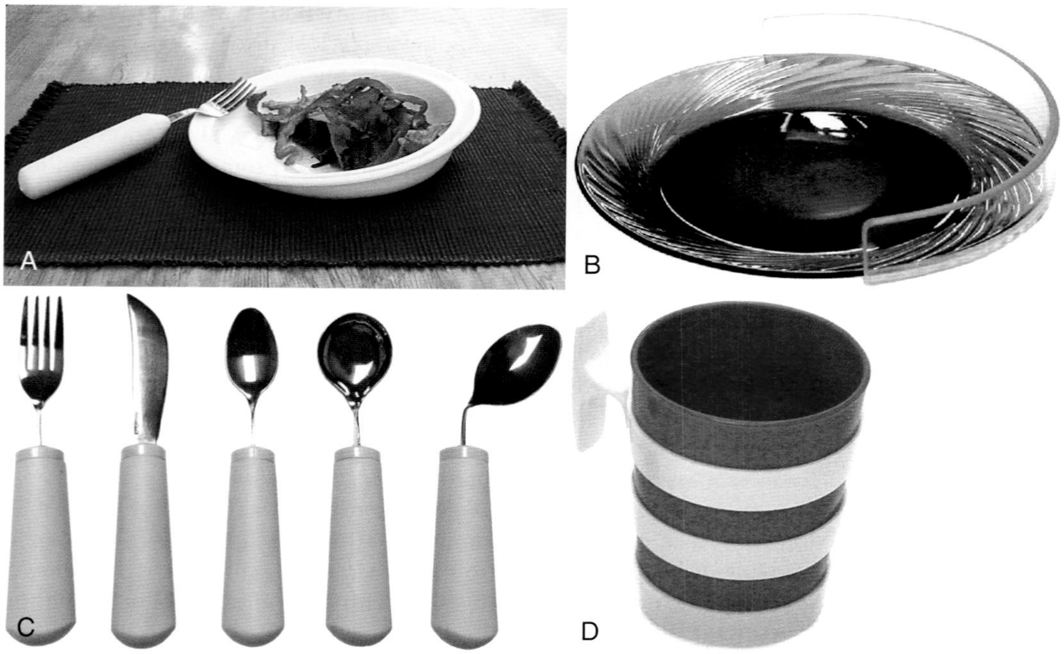

Fig. 23.5 Assistive devices for eating. (A) A scoop plate keeps food from being pushed off the edge. (B) Plate guards keep food on the plate. (C) Utensils adapted to special needs. The rocker blade knife allows a person to cut with only one hand. (D) The special handle is easier to grasp and hold. (Courtesy Kinsman Enterprises Inc.)

Impaired Mobility (Bed, Transfers, Wheelchair, Walking)

Mobility can continue to be a problem for patients in the rehabilitation phase. Hemiplegia, dyspraxia, and visual field disturbances all create unique problems. Hemiplegia is rarely a motor problem alone. It is often accompanied by disturbances in balance and spatial perception (Fig. 23.6).

Regular physical therapy and occupational therapy promote optimal return of motor function. Regular exercise can facilitate a dramatic return of function for some patients. Thus affected arms and legs need to be used to maintain muscular function and circulation if and until neurologic ability is recovered. In the meantime, assistance is needed with motor activities. When the patient is moving, assess gait (if applicable), strength in arms and legs, and balance. Correct body mechanics and transfer techniques are essential when working with the patient. A gait belt helps the patient in transfers and in ambulation and may protect the patient and staff members from injury. This is a fabric belt with a toothed buckle that is applied between the nipple line and the waist and is used to support and assist the patient. Assistive devices such as the quad cane and walkers may improve safety with ambulation (Fig. 23.7).

Patients who have dyspraxia are unable to initiate voluntary motor acts. It is interesting to note that they sometimes exhibit those actions spontaneously. To help the patient remember to initiate voluntary responses, provide verbal cues. Teach family members about dyspraxia and advise them to be patient and to use cues to induce the desired motor performance. Remind the patient who has unilateral neglect to use and support the affected side.

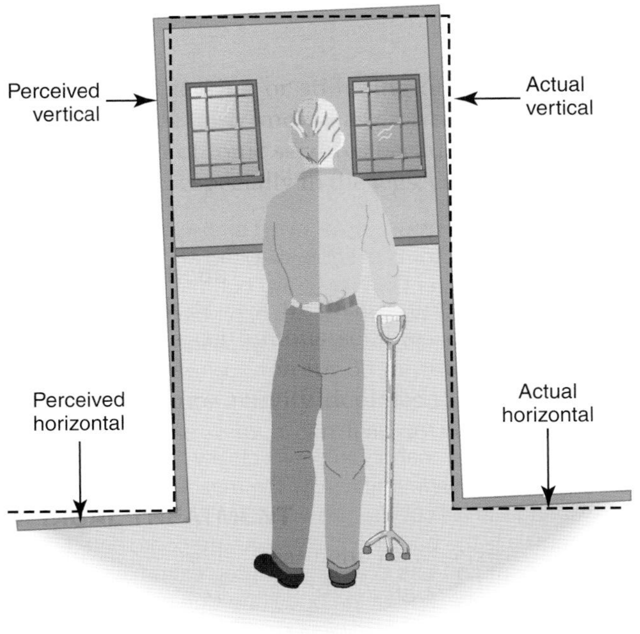

Fig. 23.6 Perceptual disturbances in hemiplegia may affect the patient's ability to maneuver safely in the environment. (From Black JM, Hawks JH: *Medical-surgical nursing: clinical management for positive outcomes*, ed 8, St. Louis, 2009, Saunders.)

> **Put On Your Thinking Cap!**
>
> Use a towel or other material to make an arm sling. Place your dominant arm in the sling while you prepare a meal, eat, and clean up. Immediately after this exercise, write down: (1) what adaptations you had to make, (2) what things you were unable to do unassisted, (3) how you felt during the exercise, and (4) how you behaved during the exercise. Compare responses with your classmates. Discuss implications for patient care.

Constipation

Bowel elimination problems may continue into the rehabilitation phase. Incontinence is not usually a problem for the alert patient except when it is caused by inability to access toileting devices or manage clothing. Document the timing of incidents of bowel incontinence so that a toileting schedule can be developed. Often simply taking the patient to the toilet at the usual time of defecation eliminates bowel incontinence. Additional discussion of bowel incontinence is found in Chapter 14.

Constipation is a common challenge in the rehabilitation phase. A regular bowel program with toileting, orientation, and reminders is needed. Provide sufficient fluids to promote bowel regularity. Many stroke patients do not receive adequate fluid intake because of dysphagia or fear of incontinence. In addition, caregivers may not take the extra time needed to provide fluids for the patient who responds slowly. Stool softeners, laxatives, and suppositories may be used to reestablish regular bowel elimination and then gradually be discontinued. Some patients continue to need stool softeners. As noted earlier, some patients with long-standing laxative dependency

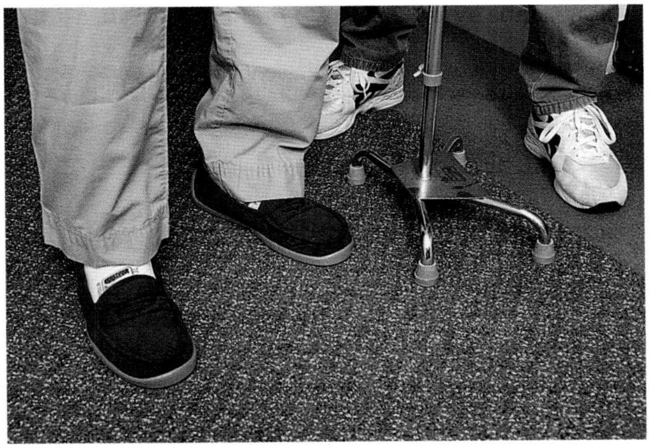

Fig. 23.7 A quad cane provides good support for a patient with hemiplegia. (From Potter PA, Perry AG, Stockert PA, Hall AM. *Fundamentals of nursing*, ed 8, St. Louis, 2013, Mosby.)

may not respond to more conservative measures to promote bowel elimination.

Impaired Urinary Elimination and Functional Urinary Incontinence

If an indwelling catheter was inserted in the acute phase of stroke treatment, it will probably be removed and efforts made to restore bladder control. Immediately after the catheter is removed, the patient may have poor sphincter control or may retain urine. Thus it is important to monitor urine output and check for bladder distention until normal voiding is established. Perineal muscle exercises (see Chapter 14) may be prescribed to improve sphincter control.

Intermittent catheterization may continue to be necessary in the rehabilitation phase. The urine volume obtained is measured and intermittent catheterization is done every 4 to 6 hours, depending on the volume obtained. Bedside ultrasound scanners may be used by the nurse, as ordered and available, to assess the amount of urine in the bladder and to determine the need for intermittent catheterization.

Incontinence of urine is more difficult to correct than bowel incontinence. A bladder program should be initiated promptly. Document the patient's fluid intake and frequency of voiding. Scheduled toileting based on the patient's usual pattern often helps to control incontinence.

Put On Your Thinking Cap!

List all of the factors you can think of that might cause a patient recovering from a stroke to be incontinent of urine besides the physiologic effects of the stroke on the bladder.

DISCHARGE

Patients may be discharged to their homes or may go to specialized rehabilitation centers for continued therapy. Outpatient therapy is an option for some patients. The rehabilitation phase is defined in various ways. In acute rehabilitation settings, patients will be evaluated by all disciplines and goals will be set. Continuous assessments and goal setting occur throughout the rehabilitation process. When able, patients are transitioned back to the home setting. It is essential to include family, friends, and significant others in this process. Medicare defines the rehabilitation phase as 3 months after the stroke. Rehabilitation specialists say that rehabilitation continues indefinitely but progress slows down. A great deal of evidence indicates that rehabilitation helps patients recovering from a stroke to achieve a high level of functioning and improve safety after returning home.

During and after the rehabilitation phase, patients and families need to be made aware of resources to help them deal with continuing disabilities. Patients and families should be referred to the American Heart Association, American Stroke Association, National Stroke Association, and other local agencies within the community. Support groups are available in many communities to offer assistance and generally have a positive effect on the stroke survivor.

Although stroke remains a major health problem, the risk can be reduced. The acute phase of stroke, from diagnosis to stabilization of blood pressure, requires support and careful evaluation of the patient's remaining abilities. In rehabilitation, the patient is respectfully challenged to return to the highest level of function possible.

Get Ready for the NCLEX® Examination!

Key Points

- CVA, commonly called a *stroke*, is an interruption of blood flow to part of the brain.
- The risk factors for CVA are atherosclerosis, atrial fibrillation, hypertension, diabetes mellitus, cardiac disease, excessive alcohol consumption, and, for women, smoking while taking oral contraceptives.
- CVA can be classified as a *TIA, a stroke in evolution,* or a *completed stroke.*
- TIA is an episode of temporary neurologic dysfunction caused by focal brain, spinal cord, or retinal ischemia that occurs without acute infarction.
- TIA, sometimes considered a warning sign of impending stroke, is treated with diet modification, exercise, drug therapy to prevent clot formation, surgery to clear or bypass obstructed blood vessels, or a combination of these therapies.
- A stroke is a set of neurologic signs and symptoms caused by impaired blood flow to the brain that persists for more than 24 hours.
- A hemorrhagic stroke is caused by rupture of a blood vessel in the brain, and an ischemic stroke is caused by obstruction of a blood vessel by an embolus or a thrombus.
- Signs and symptoms of stroke depend on the type, location, and extent of brain injury but may include one-sided weakness, numbness, visual problems, confusion and memory lapses, headache, dysphagia, and speech problems.
- Aphasia is the inability to understand words or respond with appropriate messages.
- Dysarthria is the inability to speak clearly because of neurologic damage that affects the muscles of speech.
- Dysphagia is difficulty swallowing.
- Dyspraxia is the partial inability to initiate coordinated voluntary motor acts in a nonparalyzed extremity.
- Paralysis of one side of the body (the side opposite the brain injury) is called *hemiplegia.*
- Medical treatment of CVA may use oxygen therapy, diuretics, corticosteroids, anticoagulants, thrombolytics, intravenous fluids, dietary modifications, and catheterization, as well as treatment of risk factors.

- After experiencing a stroke, the patient may regain complete independent functioning, partially recover previous abilities, or lose functional abilities completely.
- The goal of rehabilitation after stroke is to enhance the recovery of functional abilities through a program of stimulation and practice.

Additional Learning Resources

SG Go to your Study Guide for additional learning activities to help you master this chapter content.

Go to your Evolve website (http://evolve.elsevier.com/Linton/medsurg) for the following learning resources and much more:

- Fluid & Electrolyte Tutorial
- Review Questions for the NCLEX® Examination

Clinical Judgment and Next-Generation NCLEX® Examination-Style Questions

1. In which part of the brain are the structures that control respirations and heart rate located?

NCLEX Client Need: Physiological Integrity: Physiological Adaptation

2. The licensed vocational nurse/licensed practical nurse (LVN/LPN) recognizes symptoms of a TIA in a homebound patient. Why is it important for the nurse to recognize a TIA?

1. Because TIA is a symptom of a brain tumor
2. Because TIA can cause permanent disability
3. Because TIA is a warning sign of future stroke
4. Because TIA occurs shortly before a hemorrhage

NCLEX Client Need: Physiological Integrity: Physiological Adaptation

3. Which of the following may be present in both TIA and stroke? (Select all that apply.)

1. Visual disturbances
2. Dysphagia
3. Drooping mouth
4. Confusion
5. Weakness

NCLEX Client Need: Physiological Integrity: Physiological Adaptation

4. How are TIAs and strokes different?

1. Weakness and loss of balance are symptoms of TIA but not stroke.
2. Imaging studies show circulatory changes with stroke but not with TIA.
3. Anticoagulants are used with some strokes but not with TIAs.
4. An infarction occurs with stroke but not with TIA.

NCLEX Client Need: Physiological Integrity: Physiological Adaptation

5. A clinic patient who is taking an anticoagulant to reduce the risk of stroke has regular blood tests to measure INR. The LVN/LPN knows that the physician should be notified if the INR exceeds which of the following measurements?

1. 1.5
2. 2.0
3. 2.5
4. 3.0

NCLEX Client Need: Physiological Integrity: Pharmacological Therapies

6. Which of the following is the most common type of stroke?

1. Ischemic
2. Incomplete
3. Hemorrhagic
4. Subarachnoid

NCLEX Client Need: Physiological Integrity: Physiological Adaptation

7. Ms. Y. is recovering from a stroke. She is able to follow directions and communicate nonverbally. However, she struggles to speak, and her words are slurred. When you can understand her, her message is appropriately expressed. What is the correct term to describe this pattern?

NCLEX Client Need: Physiological Integrity: Physiological Adaptation

8. Which of the following are modifiable risk factors for stroke? (Select all that apply.)

1. Age
2. Obesity
3. Gender
4. Hypertension
5. Cigarette smoking

NCLEX Client Need: Physiological Integrity: Reduction of Risk Potential

9. Which of the following are necessary for the most successful use of rt-PA in the stroke patient? (Select all that apply.)

1. Patient not currently taking warfarin (Coumadin)
2. Administration only after an ischemic stroke
3. Intravenous administration within 3 hours of the onset of symptoms
4. Concurrent use with heparin to prevent additional clots from forming
5. Deep intramuscular administration into a large muscle mass

NCLEX Client Need: Physiological Integrity: Pharmacological Therapies

10. A patient with aphasia is admitted to a long-term care facility. The care plan should include which nursing interventions? (Select all that apply.)

1. Insist that patients try to express needs verbally
2. Help them to find the right word if they become frustrated
3. Give praise when patients attempt to verbalize
4. Encourage families to speak for patients rather than expecting patients to speak
5. Establish a system such as blinks for the nonverbal patient to communicate

NCLEX Client Need: Psychosocial Integrity and Physiological Integrity: Physiological Adaptation

11. SLO/Objective: Prioritize nursing care for patients with a cerebral vascular accident (CVA).

NGN Item Type: Cloze

Cognitive Skill: Prioritize Hypotheses

An obese 78-year-old man was admitted with weakness on the right side and slurred speech. He was unable to stand when he awoke this morning. He tried to drink some water but had difficulty swallowing. He was incontinent of urine twice during the night. He uses gestures to respond to some questions when he seems unable to find the right words. Hand grips; voluntary movements; and reflexes of leg, arm, and hand are normal on left side but diminished on right side. Leans toward right side when not supported.

- Blood pressure = 210/104 mm Hg
- Pulse = 96 beats per minute
- Respirations = 22 breaths per minute
- Temperature = 97º F.
- Slurred speech
- Difficulty finding words
- Diminished movement and reflexes on right side
- Urinary incontinence

Choose the *most likely* options for the information missing from the statements below by selecting from the list of options provided.

His right sided weakness is *most likely* the result of (1)____________. The nurse would monitor (2)____________________, (2)____________________, (2)____________________.

OPTIONS FOR 1	OPTIONS FOR 2
Right sided brain damage	Potential for injury
Hypertension	Potential for falls
Expressive aphasia	Blood pressure
Left sided brain damage	Intake and output
Receptive aphasia	Skin tissue integrity
Difficulty swallowing	Ability to communicate

Spinal Cord Injury

24

http://evolve.elsevier.com/Linton/medsurg

Objectives

1. Explain the effects of spinal cord injury.
2. Describe the diagnostic tests used to evaluate spinal cord injuries and related nursing responsibilities.
3. Explain the physical effects of spinal cord injury.
4. Describe the medical and surgical treatment during the acute phase of spinal cord injury.
5. List the data to be included in the nursing assessment of the patient with a spinal cord injury.
6. Identify patient problems, goals, interventions, and outcome criteria for the patient with a spinal cord injury.
7. State the goals of rehabilitation for the patient with spinal cord injury.
8. Describe the nursing care for the patient undergoing a laminectomy.

Key Terms

autonomic dysreflexia (ăw-tō-NŌ-mĭk dĭs-rē-flĕk-sē-ă)
dermatome (DĔR-mă-tōm)
flaccid (FLĂ-sĭd)
myelinated (MĪ-ĕ-lĭ-nā-tĕd)
paraplegia (pār-ă-PLĒ-jă)
spasticity (spas-TĬ-sĭ-tē)
tetraplegia (tĕ-tră-PLĒ-jă)

Few injuries are as physically and emotionally distressing to a person as a permanent spinal cord injury (SCI). The National Spinal Cord Statistical Center (2020) estimates that 17,810 new cases of spinal cord injuries occur each year in the United States, and approximately 294,000 people are living with SCI. Since the 1970s, the average age at injury has increased from 29 years to 42 years. About 78% of new SCI cases are male. The leading causes of spinal cord injuries are motor vehicle crashes, followed by falls, acts of violence (primarily gunshot wounds) and sports/recreational activities. Non-Hispanic White Americans account for more than half of spinal cord injuries followed by about 12.8% of non-Hispanic Black Americans. Re-hospitalizations occur in about 30% of persons with SCI, with genitourinary system disease the leading cause, followed by skin disease. Respiratory, digestive, circulatory, and musculoskeletal disorders also are common contributing factors. Life expectancy decreases after SCI, and the major causes of death are pneumonia and septicemia.

Medical advances and more rapid transport of accident victims to trauma centers have increased the life expectancy of individuals with SCI. However, the effects of the injury may lead to other health problems that require long-term care and potentially affect quality of life. Quality nursing care during the acute and rehabilitative phases of injury can minimize the effect of lifelong problems that plague the person with an SCI. Thus, the potential for rehabilitation and full quality of life can be enhanced.

ANATOMY AND PHYSIOLOGY OF THE SPINAL CORD

To understand the effects of SCI fully, it is important to know the anatomy and physiology of the spinal cord. Normal spinal cord function requires an intact cord with a good blood supply and bony support. Disruption of any one of these components can result in neurologic dysfunction.

VERTEBRAL COLUMN

The bony vertebral column consists of 33 vertebrae: 7 cervical (C1 through C7), 12 thoracic (T1 through T12), 5 lumbar (L1 through L5), 5 sacral (S1 through S5), and 4 coccygeal, which are fused (Fig. 24.1). The individual vertebra consists of a body and an arch, as shown in Fig. 24.2. The body is the round structure that forms the anterior portion of the vertebra. The arch is the posterior portion of the vertebra. The spinal cord passes through an opening in the center of each arch. The structures that form the posterior section of the arch are called *laminae*. Each arch has articulating surfaces against which adjacent vertebrae smoothly glide with movement. In addition, each arch has locations

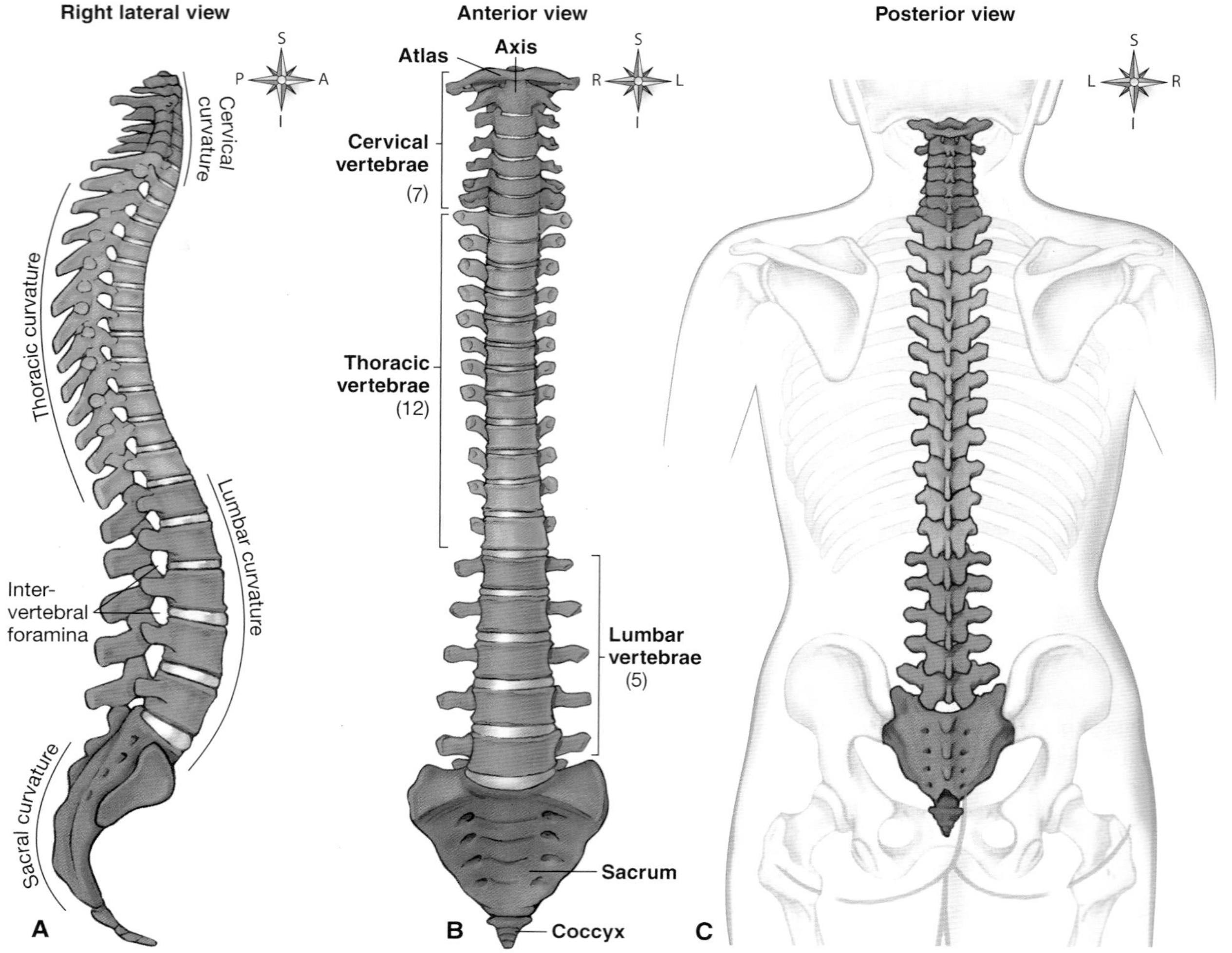

Fig. 24.1 The bony vertebral column consists of 33 vertebrae. (From Patton KT, Thibodeau GA: *The human body in health & disease*, ed 7, St. Louis, 2018, Elsevier.)

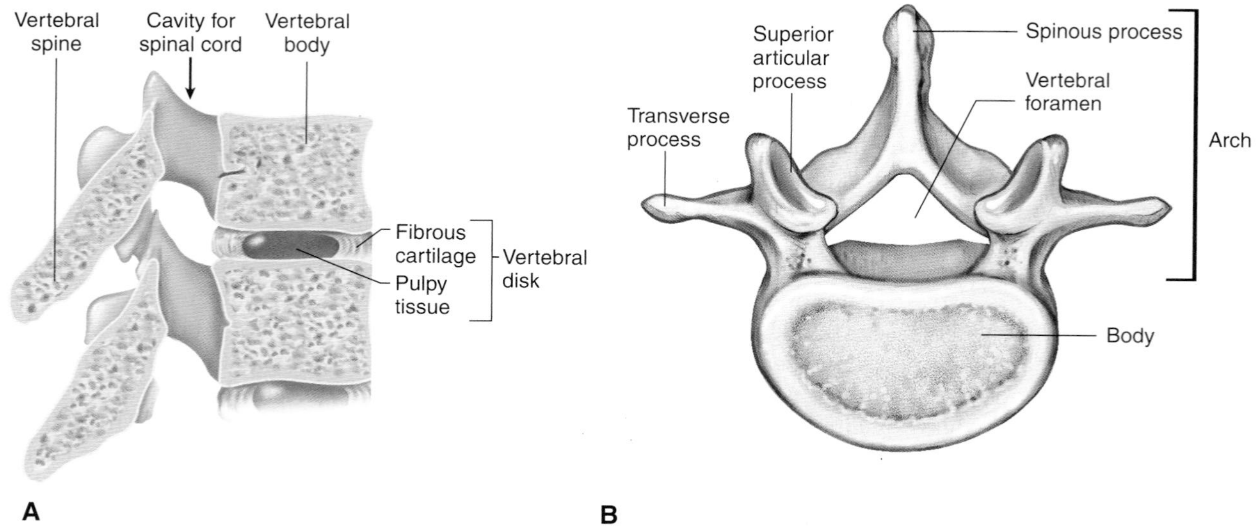

Fig. 24.2 Intervertebral disks separate the vertebrae, each of which consists of a body (A) and an arch (B). (From Patton KT, Thibodeau GA: *The human body in health & disease*, ed 7, St. Louis, 2018, Elsevier.)

for the attachment of ribs and muscles. Muscles and ligaments, which permit mobility and flexibility, support the bony column.

DISKS

Vertebrae are separated by intervertebral disks, which serve as shock absorbers for the vertebral column (see Fig. 24.2). Disks are composed of the annulus fibrosus and the nucleus pulposus. The annulus fibrosus is the fibrous ring of tissue that encircles the nucleus pulposus. The nucleus pulposus is the central sac-like structure with a gelatinous filling that has a high-water content. As a person increases in age, the nucleus pulposus loses a great deal of its water, so it becomes less effective as a shock absorber. Thus older people are at increased risk for back injuries and herniated disks.

SPINAL CORD

The spinal cord extends from the brainstem to the level of L2 in the pelvic cavity (Fig. 24.3). It has a central canal, which is continuous with the fourth ventricle of the brain. Three protective meningeal layers surround the cord: (1) the dura mater, (2) the arachnoid, and (3) the pia mater. The dura mater is the outermost layer.

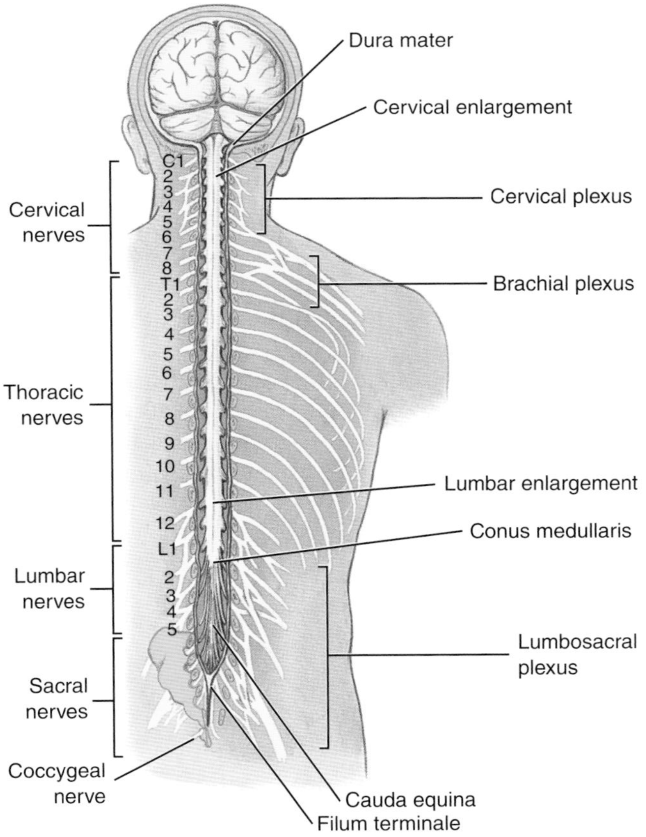

Fig. 24.3 The spinal cord extends from the medulla of the brainstem to the level of the second lumbar vertebra. (From Applegate E: *The anatomy and physiology learning system*, ed 4, St. Louis, 2011, Saunders.)

The arachnoid, the middle layer, is a network of spaces containing cerebrospinal fluid (CSF). The pia mater is the innermost layer that directly covers the spinal cord. The CSF circulates through the brain and spinal column, bathing and protecting the entire central nervous system (CNS).

A cross-section of the spinal cord reveals an inner area of H-shaped gray matter surrounded by white matter. The gray matter consists of the bodies of nerve cells that control motor and sensory activities. The white matter, which is **myelinated** (surrounded by a sheath), consists of bundles of fibers. These fibers, known as *columns* or *tracts*, convey information between the brain and the spinal cord. The tracts may be either ascending or descending. Ascending tracts carry sensory information from the spinal cord to the brain. Descending tracts carry motor information from the brain to the spinal cord (Fig. 24.4).

Blood supply to the spinal cord is vital. Any disruption in blood flow can lead ultimately to neurologic damage. The major arterial supply to the spinal cord consists of the vertebral arteries posteriorly and the anterior spinal artery.

Spinal cord function may be classified as either *reflexive* or *relay* in nature. With reflexive activity, the sensory stimulus is received, and a response is initiated at the level of the spinal cord. The knee jerk is an example of reflexive activity. When the knee is tapped, impulses travel by sensory neurons to the spinal cord, where they are relayed to motor neurons. The impulse travels back to the muscles at the front of the thigh, causing muscle contraction and jerking of the leg. This circuit of impulse transmission is called a *reflex arc*.

With relay activity, the stimulus enters the spinal cord and travels up the ascending tracts to relay sensory signals from the external environment to the brain. Information is processed in the brain and responses are initiated by impulses transmitted to the body by way of descending tracts.

The descending white matter tracts also participate in the relay function of the spinal cord. These tracts relay motor information, with messages being sent from the brain, down the cord, to muscles, which affect various kinds of responses. Four of the most important spinal cord tracts are summarized in Table 24.1.

Information is conveyed by the senses to the brain and spinal cord via the peripheral nervous system. This system consists of 31 pairs of spinal nerves (8 cervical, 12 thoracic, 5 lumbar, 5 sacral, and 1 coccygeal), which branch from the cord and pass between the vertebrae to muscles and visceral organs. Each spinal nerve has a dorsal root, which transmits sensory information, and a ventral root, which transmits motor information. The 12 cranial nerves, arising from the brainstem, are also part of the peripheral nervous system.

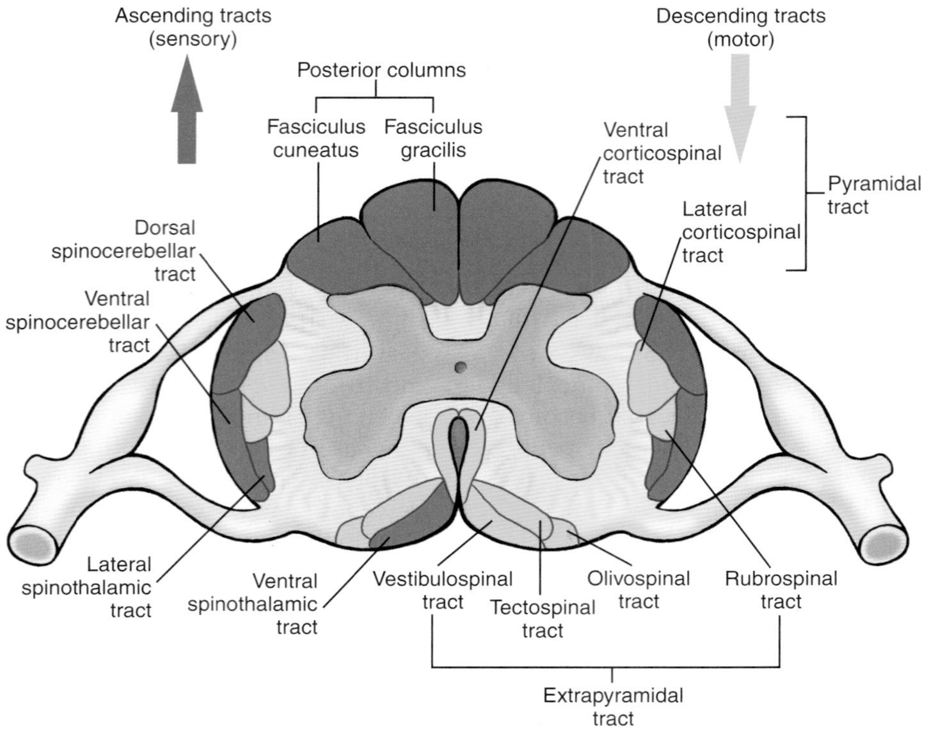

Fig. 24.4 Cross-section of spinal cord. Sensory tracts convey sensory information to the brain; motor tracts convey information from the brain.

Table 24.1 Summary of the Four Major Spinal Cord Tracts

TRACT	TYPE	FEATURES	FUNCTION
Spinothalamic	Ascending (sensory: pain and temperature)	Originates in spinal cord and ascends to thalamus in brain; on entering cord, impulses cross over to opposite side (contralateral)	Carries pain and temperature lateral sensation from opposite side
Corticospinal, lateral	Descending (motor)	Initiates in motor tract of brain, crosses over to opposite side at level of medulla, proceeds down to appropriate spinal cord level	Controls voluntary motor action
Spinocerebellar	Ascending (sensory)	Initiates in spinal cord and terminates in cerebellum	Assists in coordination of muscle contraction
Posterior columns	Ascending (sensory: touch, vibration, position sense)	Made up of several tracts that relay messages from body to brain; initiates in sensory fibers of spinal nerves, crosses over in medulla, and terminates in sensory cortex of opposite hemisphere	Carries touch, deep pressure, vibration, and position sense

PATHOPHYSIOLOGY OF SPINAL CORD INJURY

Traumatic injury creates abnormal forces on the neck and structural components of the spinal cord. The cervical vertebrae support the head and neck and permit movement in various directions. The thoracic vertebrae, on the other hand, permit little movement because of the restrictions of the ribs. Because the thoracic spine has limited flexibility, the neck and cervical spine are extremely vulnerable to injury.

TYPES OF INJURIES

Spinal cord injuries may be classified (1) by location, (2) as open or closed, and (3) by extent of damage to the cord. Injuries classified by location are described as *cervical*, *thoracic*, or *lumbar*, depending on the level of the cord affected.

Closed injuries involve trauma in which the skin and meningeal covering that surrounds the spinal cord remain intact. However, it is important to keep

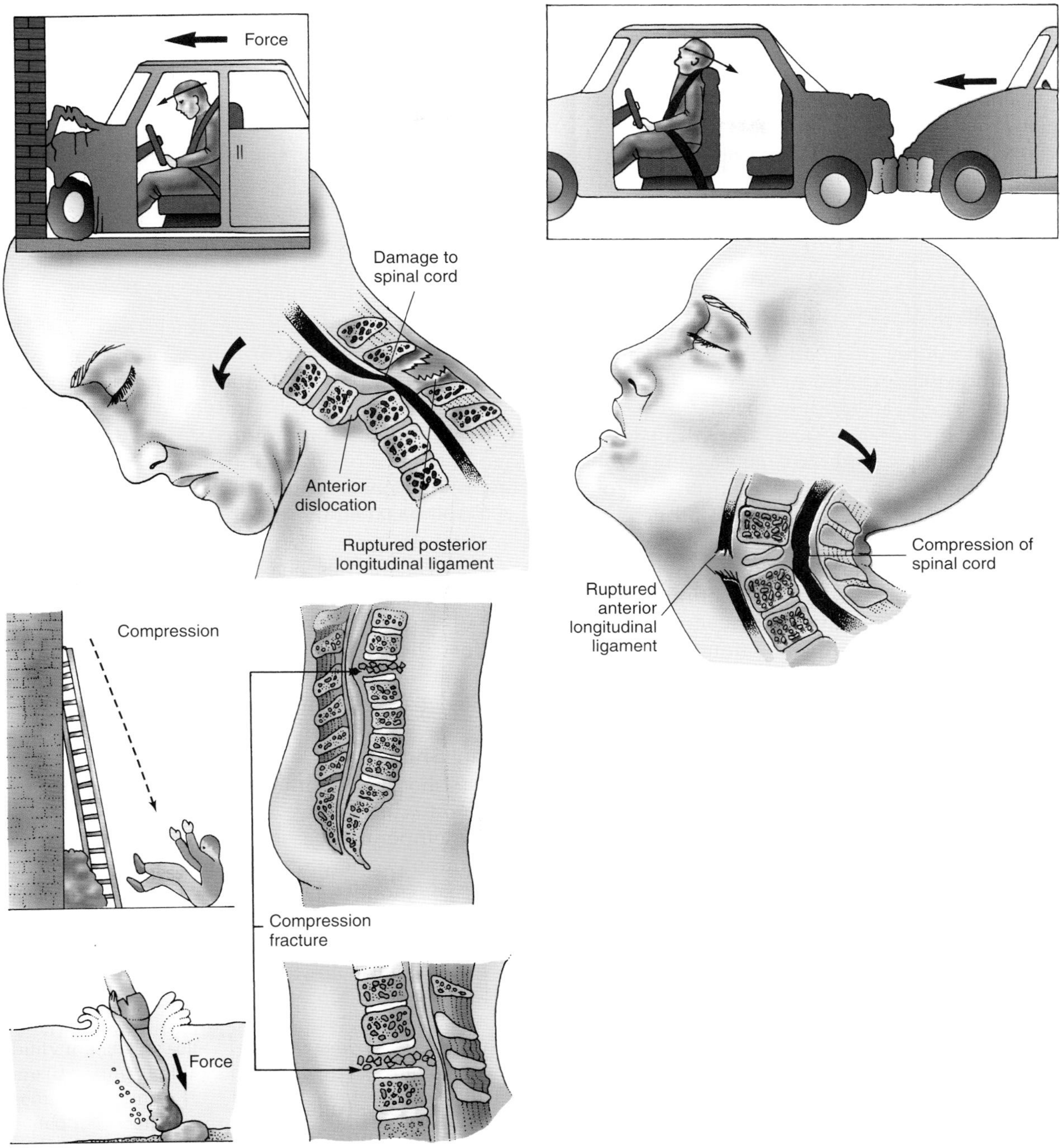

Fig. 24.5 Mechanisms of spinal cord injury. (From Ignatavicius DD, Workman ML: *Medical-surgical nursing: patient-centered collaborative care*, ed 8, St. Louis, 2016, Saunders.)

in mind that stretching or twisting the spinal cord can lead to injury as extensive as partial or complete transection (i.e., cutting all the way through). Common causes of closed injuries include compression, flexion, hyperextension, rotation, and blunt trauma (Fig. 24.5). Degeneration of the vertebrae or intervertebral disks, hematomas, or spinal cord tumors may also compress the cord or one of the spinal nerves. Fractures of the vertebral bodies may cause a subluxation (partial dislocation) of bone fragments, which may further damage the cord. Open injuries with damage to protective skin and meninges are most commonly caused by bullets or stabbing.

The injury may be classified as *complete* or *incomplete*, depending on the extent to which the cord is transected (i.e., cut across). A complete SCI occurs when the cord has been completely severed whereas an incomplete injury results from partial cutting of the cord. Open injuries often result in either complete or partial transection of the cord.

Table 24.2 Incomplete Injuries and Related Neurologic Deficits

INJURY	MECHANISM OF INJURY	ACCOMPANYING DEFICIT
Anterior cord syndrome	Herniation of disk occurring with flexion injury or dislocation of vertebrae	Loss of bilateral pain and temperature perception and motor function below level of lesion without loss of position sense
Central cord syndrome	Hyperextension injury	Motor and sensory loss in upper extremities
Brown-Séquard syndrome	Transverse hemisection of cord	Ipsilateral loss of motor function with contralateral loss of pain and temperature perception

EFFECTS OF SPINAL CORD INJURY

Early recognition of the effects of SCI is vital to maintain maximum possible function. Factors that determine the effects of SCI include the extent of the damage and the level of the injury. Sometimes the extent of injury cannot be fully determined because the symptoms of spinal cord edema may mimic partial or complete transection. A complete injury cuts all descending and ascending tracts. The result is disruption of all voluntary motor and sensory activity below the level of the injury. However, reflex activity continues below the level of injury because it occurs by completing the reflex arc without the transmission of impulses to and from the brain.

Trauma may also produce a variety of incomplete spinal cord injuries. These are injuries in which some function remains below the level of the injury. Specific tracts may be involved, causing certain patterns of neurologic dysfunction. Table 24.2 describes the major types of incomplete injuries and the resulting neurologic losses.

The higher the level of the injury is, the more encompassing is the neurologic dysfunction (because increasingly more of the body is affected). High cervical spine injuries may result in the loss of motor and sensory function in all four extremities. This condition, previously known as *quadriplegia*, is now referred to as **tetraplegia**. Injuries at or below T2 may cause **paraplegia**, which is paralysis of the lower part of the body. Table 24.3 describes the activities that are possible with SCI at various levels.

Respiratory Impairment

The phrenic nerve, which is formed by the nerve roots of C1 to C4, innervates the diaphragm. Thus injuries at or above the level of C5 (called *high cervical injuries*) may result in instant death because the nerves that control respiration are interrupted. Many patients with high cervical injuries die before reaching the hospital. If these patients receive immediate attention and rapid transport to an acute care facility, mechanical ventilation may be possible. However, they remain dependent on ventilators and face challenges for rehabilitation.

Modern technology affords the ventilator-dependent patient a variety of options for pulmonary rehabilitation. A small portable ventilator can be mounted on the back of a mechanized wheelchair, enabling the patient to be mobile. Phrenic nerve stimulators may also be implanted in the patient to help stimulate diaphragmatic movement and enhance respiratory function. Even with a ventilator or phrenic nerve stimulator, pulmonary hygiene is an issue because these patients may have difficulty clearing the airway.

Cervical injuries below the level of C4 spare the diaphragm but can involve impairment of intercostal and abdominal muscles. Patients with these injuries can usually breathe independently but often experience some degree of respiratory compromise related to weakened exhalation and cough.

Spinal Shock

Spinal shock is an immediate, transient response to injury in which reflex activity below the level of the injury temporarily ceases. It may appear as early as 30 to 60 minutes after the injury and may persist for days, weeks, or months. During the period of spinal shock, paralysis is described as **flaccid**, meaning that the involved extremity or muscle group has no tone. The involved neurons in the spinal cord gradually regain their excitability. Resolution of spinal shock is marked by the appearance of spastic, involuntary movements of the extremities.

Autonomic Dysreflexia

One of the most serious and potentially dangerous problems for the patient with SCI is **autonomic dysreflexia**, an exaggerated response of the autonomic nervous system to some noxious (painful) stimuli. It occurs in patients whose injury is at or above the level of T6. As spinal shock begins to subside and reflex activity returns, the risk of autonomic dysreflexia increases. It may occur even in patients with long-standing injuries.

Excessive stimulation of sensory receptors below the level of the injury precipitates autonomic dysreflexia. The sympathetic nervous system is stimulated but an appropriate parasympathetic modulation response cannot be elicited because of the SCI that separates the two divisions of the autonomic nervous system. Arterioles constrict, causing severe hypertension,

Table 24.3 Degree of Loss and Functional Capability With Injury to Each Level of the Spinal Cord

CORD LEVEL	DEGREE OF LOSS	FUNCTIONAL CAPABILITY
C1–C4	Motor and sensory function from neck down Respiratory function Bowel and bladder control	Mechanical ventilation with home care
C5	Motor and sensory function below shoulders Intercostal function in ventilation Bowel and bladder control	Has remaining head control, which facilitates use of "joystick" for writing, typing, and control of mechanical wheelchair
C6	Motor and sensory function below shoulders but increased degree of sensation in arm and thumb Intercostal function in ventilation Bowel and bladder control	Requires some assistive devices for upper extremity use but may be able to help feed and dress self Requires mechanical wheelchair but may be capable of using hand control
C7	Motor control of portion of upper extremities Sensation below clavicle Intercostal function Bowel and bladder control	Remaining intact muscles enhance ability to carry out activities of daily living (ADLs) Increased ability to manage specially equipped wheelchair and automobile
C8	Motor control of portions of upper extremities Sensation below chest Intercostal function Bowel and bladder control	Improved upper extremity mobility enhances hand grasp, independence in ADLs, and use of wheelchair Capable of self-catheterization
T1–T6	Trunk muscles below midchest Sensation from midchest Some intercostal function Bowel and bladder control	Complete control of upper extremities makes independence in wheelchair and ADLs possible Employment possible
T6–T12	Motor control below waist Sensation below waist Bowel and bladder control	Capable of unassisted respiratory function Good upper back and abdominal strength, making increased wheelchair activities and athletics possible
L1–L3	Motor and sensory function to lower extremities Sensation to lower abdomen Bowel and bladder function	Full control of upper extremities allows independence in wheelchair and appropriate athletic activity
L3–L4	Motor and sensory function to distal portions of lower extremities Bowel and bladder control	Control of hip extensors remains, making ambulation possible with leg braces
L4–S5	Variable motor and sensory function to knee, ankle, and foot Sensation to perineum Variable bowel and bladder control	Ambulation with braces possible Considerable independence in ADLs can be expected

which may lead to seizures or a stroke if not corrected. To reduce the excessively increased blood pressure, regulatory mechanisms cause the blood vessels to dilate. The vasodilating response is effective only above the level of the injury, where superficial vasodilation, flushing, and profuse sweating occur. The patient experiences nasal congestion, facial flushing, and a pounding headache.

Increased blood pressure also stimulates the vagus nerve, causing bradycardia. Normally, vagal stimulation would also serve to dilate the constricted vessels. However, because the cord has been severed, these impulses never reach the affected blood vessels below the level of the lesion.

Autonomic dysreflexia is triggered by a variety of stimuli, including a distended bladder, constipation, renal calculi, ejaculation, or uterine contractions, but may also be caused by pressure sores, a skin rash, enemas, or even sudden position changes. In the event of autonomic dysreflexia, indwelling catheters must be inspected for possible occlusions or kinks. If no indwelling catheter exists and the bladder is distended, intermittent catheterization may be done. If constipation is the triggering event, disimpaction may be necessary. Pressure injuries need to be treated with a topical anesthetic to decrease the stimuli, and skin rashes can be treated with appropriate topical ointments to decrease itching.

Autonomic dysreflexia is an emergent situation. It is important to obtain a history related to autonomic dysreflexia on any tetraplegic being cared for in a health care setting. This will allow the provider to be on the alert for symptoms and respond in a timely manner.

Spasticity

Most patients with SCI display some degree of **spasticity** (increased muscle tone) after the resolution of spinal shock. Muscle spasms may prove to be quite incapacitating for these patients, hampering efforts at rehabilitation. In general, after 1 or 2 years, a gradual reduction in spastic episodes occurs.

Muscle tone is evaluated by assessing the amount of resistance to passive movement. The spastic muscle displays a brief period of increased resistance, which is followed by a sudden relaxation. Reflexes are also assessed because hyperactive reflexes accompany spasticity. Passive movement, positioning, or even the slight stimulation of a sheet moving over the lower extremities may cause spastic activity. Medications are available to treat spasticity.

Impaired Sensory and Motor Function

As stated earlier, the higher the level of the lesion, the more extensive the neurologic dysfunction. Any complete cord injury results in the loss of motor and sensory function below the level of the lesion. The effects of incomplete lesions on sensation and motor function are variable. Impaired motor function can significantly affect the patient's mobility and self-care and thus result in complications from immobility. Loss of sensation puts the patient at risk for skin breakdown and other injuries because pressure and pain are not perceived.

Put On Your Thinking Cap!

1. In the community, observe (without being noticed) a person who is using a wheelchair to determine any difficulties they may have with access to public facilities, including buildings, transportation, water fountains, and restrooms.
2. Describe any insights this experience provided that could help you to take care of a patient with SCI who uses a wheelchair.

Impaired Bladder Function

During the period of spinal shock, all bladder and bowel function ceases. An indwelling catheter is inserted to empty the bladder and permit close monitoring of urinary output. As soon as the patient's fluid status is stabilized, the indwelling catheter is often removed and the bladder drained by intermittent catheterization. Once spinal shock resolves, reflex activity returns. The bladder becomes spastic and may spontaneously empty. Bladder retraining protocols can be specifically designed for individual patients.

Medications may be used to aid in the prevention of urinary tract infections. Methenamine mandelate (Mandelamine) is a urinary antiseptic that may be used in the regimen. Because the action of methenamine requires an acidic environment, vitamin C (ascorbic acid) is often prescribed to lower urine pH.

Impaired Bowel Function

The absence of bowel activity in the first day or two after injury may require insertion of a nasogastric tube for decompression. Peristalsis usually returns by the third day postinjury. Most patients with SCI can maintain bowel function because the large bowel musculature has its own neural center that responds to distention by the fecal mass. To assist in evacuation of the bowel, the patient must take advantage of the abdominal muscles as well as have an appropriate diet. Bowel retraining programs are initiated to aid in the regular evacuation of the bowel.

Impaired Temperature Regulations

Depending on the level of the injury, the patient may have difficulty maintaining body temperature within a normal range. If a person becomes too cold, the body normally responds with vasoconstriction and shivering to increase the temperature. If a person becomes too hot, sweating helps to dissipate heat. The patient with SCI may lose these regulatory mechanisms and be unable to adapt to temperature extremes. The tetraplegic person is especially vulnerable to environmental temperature changes because such a large part of the body is affected.

Impaired Sexual Function

Spinal levels S2, S3, and S4 control sexual function, so injury at or above these levels results in sexual dysfunction. The ability of the male patient to achieve erection and ejaculation is variable, depending on the level of injury. In women, menses resumes normally after injury. Women with SCI can have sexual intercourse but lack vaginal sensation. Some women with SCI do experience orgasm, although it is not vaginally triggered. They can also bear children, regardless of the level of the lesion. In the event of pregnancy, vaginal delivery is possible if pelvic proportions are adequate. If the lesion is high, however, the woman will not be aware of labor contractions.

Impaired Skin Integrity

Immobility and loss of sensation put the patient at risk for skin problems. Pressure injuries are common complications in spinal cord injuries. Because the immobile patient is unable to change positions, skin in the sacral area and across the bony prominences may break down. This presents a portal for infection in the patient. In addition, the presence of a pressure sore in the sacral area impedes early rehabilitation efforts because the patient is unable to begin wheelchair training until the ulcer heals.

The complete SCI also interrupts the vasomotor tone of the vascular system. This loss of tone results in vasodilation and pooling of blood in the periphery, impeding perfusion of the skin and encouraging the development of pressure sores.

Disturbed Body Image

The effect of SCI on the patient's self-concept and body image is significant. Depending on the extent of the injury, every aspect of the patient's life (e.g., occupation, family roles and responsibilities, socialization, hobbies) may be affected. Timing of information is essential to prevent overwhelming the patient and family after injury. For some patients, psychologic counseling may be helpful. Psychologic adaptation occurs over time. Because patients are in the acute care setting for shorter periods, they do not have time to fully process the meaning of the injury to their personhood. The sudden nature of SCI precipitates a crisis. As with many crisis situations, it is met with shock, disbelief, and denial. These stages are incompatible with acceptance of the situation.

The patient moves into a period of reaction, which may last a long time. The reaction can include anger, rage, depression, bargaining, inappropriate sexual behavior, verbal abuse, and suicidal ideation. Any mention of suicide should be taken seriously. Appropriate referrals should be made while protecting the patient from harm. As the period of reaction resolves, the patient begins to seek information about the injury and the future. Patient independence and control should be facilitated, at this time.

MEDICAL TREATMENT IN THE ACUTE PHASE

The goals of medical treatment guide the plans for the patient with SCI through all phases of the injury. Three major medical goals exist for the patient with spinal injury: (1) to save the patient's life, (2) to prevent further injury to the cord, and (3) to preserve as much cord function as possible. Each medical goal has specific implications for nursing care and is directed at maximizing the patient's potential for recovery and rehabilitation.

SAVING THE PATIENT'S LIFE

The patient with SCI may have additional life-threatening injuries. As mentioned earlier, patients with high cervical cord injuries (C1 to C4) often die from impaired respiratory function before arriving at the hospital.

The first priority is to establish a patent airway. The conventional head-tilt–chin-lift method of opening the airway is inappropriate in patients with SCI because of the risk of increasing cord damage. The risk of additional damage is especially high with cervical injury. Avoid flexion of the neck, even that caused by a pillow or other support. The jaw-thrust method of opening the airway is preferred for these patients. Once the airway has been opened, 100% oxygen may be administered by mask and manual resuscitator (e.g., an Ambu bag).

An endotracheal or tracheostomy tube may be placed to allow direct access to the airway and to facilitate optimal oxygenation. Any injury that compromises ventilation must be treated immediately.

PREVENTING FURTHER CORD INJURY

Immobilization is essential to prevent further damage to the spinal cord after the initial injury. At the scene of an accident, emergency personnel apply a hard cervical collar, also known as a *Philadelphia* or *Aspen collar*, around the patient's neck to immobilize the spinal column. Various types of devices and traction may be used once the patient arrives at an acute care facility.

Traction

Initially, immobilization with skeletal traction is often used to manage cervical SCI. A variety of skull traction devices may be used, including Gardner-Wells and Crutchfield tongs. Gardner-Wells tongs are secured just above the ears but do not actually penetrate the skull. Crutchfield tongs, which are less commonly used now than in the past, are applied directly to the skull, just behind the hairline. The tongs allow traction to be applied, which separates and aligns the vertebrae to prevent further cord damage and reduces painful muscle spasms (Fig. 24.6). After the tongs are applied, radiographs are ordered to confirm alignment of the spine. Ongoing neurologic assessment is done to monitor for further deficits.

The halo vest is used to immobilize and align the cervical vertebrae and usually is placed at the time of surgery that is done to internally stabilize fractures and relieve the compression of nerve roots (Fig. 24.7). A ring is applied to the skull using four pins and then attached to a fiberglass vest by adjustable rods. The vest allows the paralyzed patient to be moved out of bed and allows the patient who is not paralyzed to be ambulatory. Because good

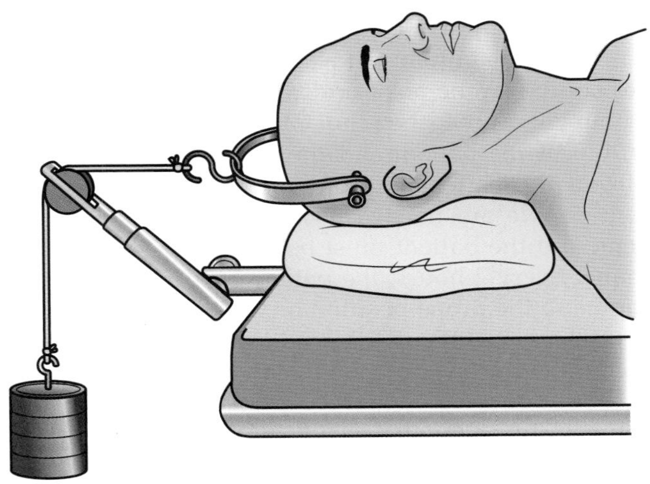

Fig. 24.6 Gardner-Wells tongs are used to immobilize the cervical spine.

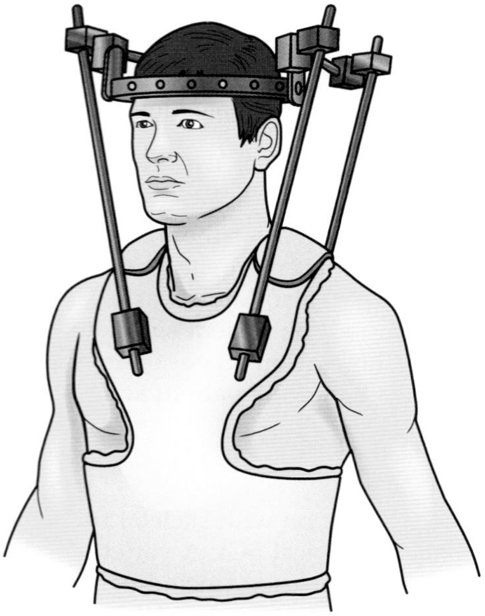

Fig. 24.7 The halo device immobilizes and aligns the cervical vertebrae.

immobilization of the spine is achieved, attention can be turned to other aspects of treatment and rehabilitation can be initiated.

Special Beds and Cushions

Special beds help prevent complications of immobility while maintaining spinal immobilization. A kinetic bed, such as the RotoRest bed, slowly but continually rotates the patient from side to side (Fig. 24.8). This rotation is especially helpful in preventing pulmonary complications by mobilizing secretions. Overlay air mattresses are flotation devices that are placed on standard hospital beds. Air-fluidized and flotation beds may be used after the spine has been stabilized, but they are never used when a patient is in tongs because of the potential damage that could occur if the bed should unexpectedly deflate.

The Stryker wedge frame is a canvas and metal frame bed that may be used to help turn the patient. It is not used as often as it was in the past. The patient lies supine on the posterior frame for approximately 2 hours at a time; then the anterior frame is secured on top of the patient and the device is turned over so that the patient is prone on the anterior frame. Two people are needed each time to turn the patient, and the patient must be tightly secured to the frame. Every 2 hours, the patient is turned from the supine to the prone position or vice versa. Many patients have a difficult time adjusting to such a bed because the prone position leaves the patient feeling as though suspended in midair. Because of this, most patients are managed on a conventional or other specialty bed.

Once the patient has the ability to be up in a chair, cushioning is needed to prevent excessive pressure and pressure injuries. Types of cushions include

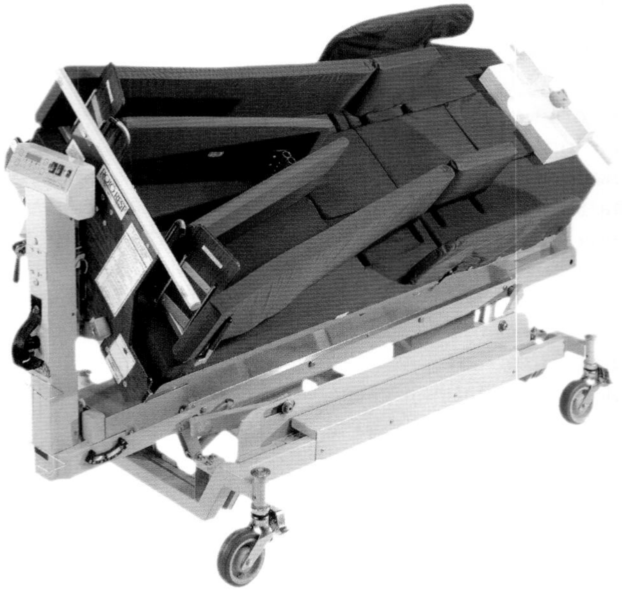

Fig. 24.8 The RotoRest bed slowly turns the patient from side to side. (Courtesy ArjoHuntleigh.)

those inflated with air, flotation devices, and gel pads. Examples of pressure-reducing cushions are the ROHO cushion, Bye Bye Decubiti (BBD) cushion, Jay cushion, AKRO cushion, and VARILITE cushion. The cushion that best meets the needs of the individual patient is selected. The physical therapist is a good resource person to consult for this recommendation.

Drug Therapy

Until the early 1990s, management of the patient with SCI relied almost exclusively on surgical and immobilization techniques. However, the use of methylprednisolone to reduce the damage to the cellular membrane has become standard practice in the acute management of SCI. The optimal time of administration is within the first 8 hours of injury. Completely paralyzed patients have been found to regain about 20% of function whereas those partially paralyzed have regained up to 75% of function. This treatment modality is controversial.

Pharmacology Capsule

The administration of high doses of methylprednisolone sodium succinate during the first 8 hours after spinal cord injury (SCI) may help to limit the neurologic effects of injury.

PRESERVING CORD FUNCTION

Early surgical intervention may be necessary to repair cord damage. Situations in which surgery is required include cord compression by bony fragments, compound vertebral fractures, and gunshot and stab wounds. In these cases, surgery within the first 24 hours is most desirable.

A laminectomy involves removing all or part of the posterior arch of the vertebra to alleviate compression on the cord or spinal nerves. If multiple vertebrae are involved, spinal fusion may also be done to stabilize the area. A spinal fusion entails placing a piece of donor bone, commonly taken from the hip, into the area between the involved vertebrae. After healing, the fusion immobilizes the affected section of the spine. Postoperative immobilization of the area is necessary to allow for adequate healing, permanent fusion, and correct alignment. If the cervical area is involved, a halo jacket will be used. If the thoracic or lumbar area is involved, other brace-like devices may be fitted to the patient. Neither laminectomy nor spinal fusion can be attempted until the patient has been fully stabilized during the acute phase of the injury.

NURSING CARE IN THE ACUTE PHASE

FOCUSED ASSESSMENT

Nursing assessment of the patient with a neurologic disorder is described in Chapter 21.

A complete assessment may be delayed until the patient is stabilized. Until then, monitor the patient's level of consciousness, vital signs, respiratory status, motor and sensory function, and intake and output.

Patient Problems, Goals, and Outcome Criteria: Acute Phase of Spinal Cord Injury

Patient Problems	Goals and Outcome Criteria
Inadequate oxygenation related to neurologic impairment	Adequate oxygenation: normal respiratory rate and measures of oxygenation (blood gases, oximeter)
Potential for injury related to involuntary muscle spasms, lack of motor and sensory function, orthostatic hypotension	Decreased potential for injury: protective measures are taken to prevent injury associated with uncontrollable movement or sensory loss
Potential for injury related to autonomic dysreflexia because of bladder or bowel distention, renal calculi, pressure sores	No signs of autonomic dysreflexia: pulse and blood pressure consistent with patient norms
Potential for complications of immobility related to pathologic or prescribed immobilization (or both)	Absence of complications of immobility: no pressure sores, maximal possible range of motion, clear breath sounds
Loss of bowel control related to impaired conduction of impulses	Controlled bowel elimination: regular bowel movements under controlled circumstances
Difficulty voiding related to sensory and motor impairment	Absence of urinary retention and urinary infection: no bladder distention, urine clear with normal odor
Potential for infection related to skeletal traction pins	Pin sites free of infection: minimal redness and swelling around pins, no purulent drainage
Elevated body temperature related to spinal cord trauma	Maintenance of normal body temperature: temperature within normal range
Impaired performance of ADLs (Feeding, dressing, grooming, toileting) related to neurologic impairment	Adaptation to impaired ADLs: patient participates in self-care as much as possible, accepts help as needed
Altered sexual function related to altered body function	Adaptation to altered sexual function: patient verbalizes sexual capabilities and adaptive techniques
Inadequate coping related to overwhelming losses and limited potential for recovered function	Adequate coping: patient expresses feelings about losses, makes realistic plans for future
Ineffective self-care management related to lack of knowledge, physical impairment, denial, depression	Effective management of self-care within patient's capabilities: follows plan of care, plans realistically, uses resources

Interventions

Inadequate oxygenation. Respiratory problems may result from neurologic damage or may be associated with immobility. The patient with an injury at or above C5 has complete loss of spontaneous respirations and requires mechanical ventilation. When a person has an injury to the lower thoracic cord, abdominal and intercostal muscles are affected, resulting in weakened exhalation and cough. Nursing care is individualized for these patients depending on the extent of respiratory impairment. Ventilator-dependent patients may be taught techniques to allow independent breathing for limited periods of time. The ventilator-dependent patient needs special care, as described in Chapter 25.

A variety of techniques may be used to help patients with spontaneous but impaired breathing to clear the airway more effectively. These include breathing exercises, assisted coughing, and vibration and percussion with postural drainage. For assisted coughing, apply firm pressure to the diaphragm just below the rib cage as the patient exhales or coughs. Because timing is important, it is vital to establish some form of communication with the patient (e.g., a blink) to identify when inspiration is completed. You should be properly trained in this technique before using it.

Turn and reposition the immobile patient as permitted to decrease pooling of secretions in the lungs. If the patient is breathing independently, coach the patient in deep-breathing exercises and use of the incentive spirometer. Adequate hydration helps to thin secretions so that they can be removed more readily.

Potential for injury. Safety is of prime consideration during the period of spastic paralysis. Involuntary muscle spasms can be so violent that the patient may be thrown from the wheelchair or bedside chair. Thus it is imperative that the patient be adequately secured with a protective strap across the chest. Even while in bed, the patient requires protection. It is important to avoid undue stimulation of the spastic extremity or muscle group. Avoid grasping the muscle when performing range-of-motion exercises or positioning the patient. Instead, support the joints above and below the affected muscle groups with the palms of the hands.

Position changes must be done by "logrolling" the patient in cervical traction on a conventional bed. A minimum of three nurses is needed to correctly logroll a patient. Some prior planning must be done so that the movement is coordinated. Identify the desired position and place pillows and equipment in the proper locations before turning the patient. One nurse stands at the head of the bed and stabilizes the traction by placing their hands firmly on the patient's head and neck without flexing the neck. The second nurse prepares to move the patient's shoulders while the third nurse prepares to move the patient's hips and legs. After explaining the procedure to the patient, turn the patient as a unit (logroll) to the desired position while maintaining proper alignment. Then place pillows against the patient's back and shoulders and between the legs (to protect any pressure spots and to promote comfort). The nurse holding the head and neck should not release the patient until all movement has been completed to ensure that traction does not slip out of place.

Venous thromboembolism prevention is essential. Sequential compression devices are important to promote venous return. Use these when the patient is in bed. Pressure stockings can decrease venous stasis and edema.

If injections are necessary, administer them above the level of paralysis for two reasons: (1) decreased drug absorption because of impaired circulation below the level of injury, and (2) increased risk for infection when the skin integrity is broken in affected parts of the body.

Patients with a complete SCI suffer sensory loss and are unable to detect any temperature or pain sensation below the level of the injury. For example, they cannot determine if a painful stimulus, such as a burn, is present. Thus the nurse must provide meticulous skin care and take all necessary measures to protect the patient from harm.

Potential for injury related to autonomic dysreflexia. The focus of nursing management for the patient at risk for autonomic dysreflexia is directed primarily toward the prevention of the triggering stimulus. Teach the patient and family members the causes, signs and symptoms, and management of autonomic dysreflexia.

When autonomic dysreflexia occurs, it is a medical emergency. Once it is recognized, immediate action is required to raise the patient's head to a 45-degree angle or to place the patient in a sitting position to help decrease the pressure. If the cause can be identified, make every effort to eliminate it. Check the indwelling catheter for occlusion. If the bladder is distended and no indwelling catheter is present, straight catheterization may be indicated. Fecal impactions, if present, need to be digitally removed after the application of a local anesthetic as ordered. Monitor the patient with severe hypertension for seizures or signs of a stroke. Immediately notify the physician so that appropriate medications or other interventions can be initiated. Administer antihypertensive drugs as ordered. Features of autonomic dysreflexia are summarized in Box 24.1.

Box 24.1 Autonomic Dysreflexia

CAUSES

- Distended bladder or plugged catheter
- Fecal impaction
- Urinary calculi
- Pressure injury
- Ejaculation
- Uterine contractions

SIGNS AND SYMPTOMS

- Sudden hypertension
- Pounding headache
- Anxiety
- Flushed face
- Diaphoresis
- Nasal congestion
- Bradycardia
- Vasoconstriction below lesion with cold skin and "goose flesh"
- Vasodilation above lesion with warm, moist skin

POTENTIAL EFFECTS

- Seizures
- Stroke

MANAGEMENT

- Assessment to identify cause
- Elevation of head of bed
- Irrigation or replacement of urinary catheter
- Intermittent catheterization
- Application of topical anesthetic and digital disimpaction
- Removal of pressure from irritated skin
- Administration of antihypertensives as ordered

Potential for complications related to immobility. To avoid the development of pressure injuries, turn the patient at least every 2 hours. Massaging the bony prominences may be harmful and is not recommended. As the patient is turned, inspect the back and sacral area for skin breakdown or signs of pressure and provide back care using a gentle lotion or other agent designed specifically to prevent skin breakdown. It is vital to relieve pressure on any reddened or broken areas. When the patient is resting in the lateral supine position, place a pillow between the legs to keep the heels free of pressure and to prevent pressure between the knees. Keep bed linens clean, dry, and free of wrinkles. Teach the patient and caregiver how to inspect the skin and recognize signs of pressure.

Specialty beds and cushions may also be used to help alleviate pressure and enhance circulation. Even if special padding is used, patients in wheelchairs should still be instructed or assisted to reposition at least every 15 minutes. Some wheelchairs designed for tetraplegic patients can be tilted backward to allow shifting of body weight.

Patients with tongs are maintained on strict bed rest. Thus it is imperative that meticulous skin care be provided. With the vertebral column stabilized, the patient may be turned for position changes and skin assessment.

When the patient has spasticity, nursing management is directed toward preventing contractures and muscle atrophy. Pharmacologic agents, such as diazepam (Valium), baclofen (Lioresal), and dantrolene sodium (Dantrium), may be effective muscle relaxants. Electrical stimulators, used with heat and physiotherapy, may also help to relieve spasms. Nursing management of the patient with muscle spasms is summarized in Box 24.2.

During the time of flaccid paralysis, you must diligently perform passive range-of-motion exercises and position and align the patient's extremities to reduce the risk of subluxation or contractures. A more complete discussion of the nursing care of the immobilized person is given in Chapter 12.

Box 24.2 Management of Spasticity in the Patient With Spinal Cord Injury

- Perform passive range-of-motion exercises at least 4 times a day.
- Properly position and splint extremities to prevent contractures.
- Limit tactile stimuli.
- Avoid incidence of noxious stimuli, such as anxiety, pain, bladder or bowel distention, and pressure injuries.
- Turn and reposition at least every 2 hours.
- Properly administer medications to reduce spasms.

Pharmacology Capsule

Muscle relaxants may be ordered to control muscle spasticity.

Loss of bowel control. In the early postinjury period, an ileus may develop, meaning that peristalsis ceases. The abdomen becomes distended and bowel sounds are absent. If this happens, fluids are administered intravenously and nothing is given by mouth. A nasogastric tube may be inserted and connected to suction for decompression. Peristalsis usually returns by the third day postinjury.

Once peristalsis resumes, the patient is given oral fluids and food. Encourage adequate fluids and high-fiber foods to promote soft stools and administer bulk laxatives, stool softeners, suppositories, and lubricants as ordered. It is important to document bowel movements and institute measures to prevent constipation and impaction. Work with the patient to determine the best schedule for bowel elimination and to help the patient carry out the program. A bowel retraining program must be a cooperative effort between the caregiver and the patient. The program can succeed only when the patient is prepared physically and emotionally. Bowel retraining is discussed in detail in Chapter 14.

Difficulty voiding. While the patient has an indwelling catheter, meticulous catheter care is essential. Because catheterization increases the risk of urinary tract infections, monitor the patient's temperature and assess the urine for cloudiness and foul odor. Administer prescribed urinary acidifiers, antiseptics, and antimicrobials as ordered. In addition, encourage the oral intake of fluids, when permitted, to maintain dilute urine. Discourage the ingestion of dairy products because they contain calcium, which may promote formation of urinary calculi.

In the rehabilitation phase, bladder retraining is addressed. As bladder retraining is instituted, work with the patient to carry out the retraining program. To help improve tone and relieve bladder spasms, the catheter may be periodically clamped and then released to increase bladder capacity. When the bladder can hold 300 to 400 mL of urine, the catheter may be removed for a trial period. Details of bladder retraining are provided in Chapter 14.

Put On Your Thinking Cap!

D.J. is a 22-year-old male who has a spinal cord injury (SCI) at T5. His physician has indicated that he no longer is experiencing spinal shock. How would you know that spinal shock has resolved? Why is management of the bowel and bladder very important at this time?

Potential for infection. The risks of pulmonary and urinary infections have already been discussed. If the patient has skeletal traction (Gardner-Wells tongs, halo ring), a risk of infection exists at the pin insertion sites. It is important to provide specific skin care as ordered or per agency policy. Minimize the risk of infection by cleaning the pin site twice daily with sterile saline and keeping it dry. After the initial healing, the area can be cleaned with soap and water. Report increasing redness or purulent drainage at the pin sites to the physician.

Elevated body temperature. Maintain the environmental temperature at a level that avoids chilling or overheating the patient. A room temperature of 70°F (21°C) will keep the tetraplegic's body temperature stable at 95°F. To prevent hypothermia, provide adequate clothing and blankets and promptly change wet clothing and linens.

To prevent excessive warming (hyperthermia), the patient should avoid the outdoors during very hot, humid weather. Some patients carry a water spray bottle when outdoors in the heat or during intense activity. The water can be sprayed on the skin, where it evaporates and cools the body. Fans can also help to cool the patient. An increase in temperature after exercise is normal.

Impaired performance of activities of daily living (feeding, dressing, grooming, toileting). Continually reassess the patient's abilities and need for assistance with self-care activities. The patient may need total care initially. As soon as the patient is able, begin preparing them for self-care consistent with the patient's expected abilities. During rehabilitation, the patient learns to use specialized equipment and strategies to be as independent as possible in self-care.

Altered sexual function. Sexuality and sexual function in the patient with SCI must be addressed when the patient first brings up the subject. Sexual function is controlled by spinal levels S2 to S4. Because sexual gratification is an important aspect of emotional and psychologic well-being, it is an issue that requires thoughtful discussion and counseling. Patients must be apprised of their physical abilities to achieve erection or to bear children. Information about the possibility of pregnancy and about birth control should be provided if the patient expresses a desire to know.

Advise the patient of resources available in the agency and in the community. The expertise of a trained counselor usually is necessary, and the counselor is usually a member of the rehabilitation team. Honest discussion must occur between the patient and the counselor. Both parties must be willing to explore the physical and emotional aspects of the injury. Additional information on management of impaired sexual function is presented in Chapters 52 and 54.

Inadequate coping. Ineffective coping may occur at any phase but is particularly evident during rehabilitation as the patient begins to deal with the realities of their situation. Ineffective coping may present as hopelessness. Hopelessness may manifest as withdrawal, passive behavior, and decreased affect. A person who feels hopeless sees few or no personal choices available and cannot mobilize the energy needed to move forward. Offer opportunities for the patient to discuss feelings about their situation and future. Listen actively and accept the patient's feelings. When the patient is withdrawn, encourage (but do not force) participation in self-care. As the patient begins to acknowledge the injury and assess its effect, encourage them to identify strengths and coping strategies. Refocus attention on things other than the injury and losses. Begin rehabilitation efforts in earnest and give generous praise for effort.

The health care team also works with the patient's significant others to create a supportive atmosphere that conveys hope, acceptance, and confidence. Patients and families often continue to hope for physical improvement that is unlikely. For example, they may interpret the movement associated with spastic paralysis as a return of voluntary motor function. You can avoid this misconception by explaining this phenomenon in advance and emphasizing that it is expected and does not signify improved function.

Inability to manage self-care. During the acute phase of SCI, explain routines and procedures. The health care provider usually informs the patient of the extent of the injury and probable effects. The nurse reinforces that information and helps the patient and family to obtain any additional information requested. An important resource is the National Spinal Cord Injury Association (www.spinalcord.org; 1-800-962-9629), which has a 24-hour service to provide information about rehabilitation, research, organizations, and local contacts. Many communities have local chapters of the Spinal Cord Society, Paralyzed Veterans of America, and National Spinal Cord Injury Association that can provide information and resources.

The following are the essential components of the teaching plan. The details will vary with the level of the injury:

- Effects of SCI
- Types of treatments and their purposes
- Breathing exercises and adaptive techniques
- Range-of-motion exercises and positioning
- Management of orthostatic hypotension
- Skin care and assessment (see the Health Promotion box)
- Management of bowel and bladder elimination
- Recognition of signs and symptoms of infection
- Changes in sexual function and resources for information about adaptation
- Protection of body areas that lack sensation

Box 24.3 Case Study: Spinal Cord Injury

Todd is a 16-year-old teenager who was injured while playing football in the park. His friends called emergency medical services and kept him motionless until their arrival. After his arrival at the hospital, his radiographs revealed a C5 fracture dislocation. The fracture was immobilized using tongs and he received methylprednisolone before admission to the intensive care unit. His condition has stabilized, and he now has a halo brace in place for stabilization of the fracture. He is being transferred to your floor before future admission to rehabilitation.

CRITICAL THINKING QUESTIONS

1. What strategies would you use to ease the patient's transition to your unit?
2. Identify key components of the nursing care plan to consider based on the level of the patient's injury.
3. Does the patient have a potential risk for autonomic dysreflexia? If it occurs, what assessment data would you gather and what would you do during this crisis?

- Adaptive techniques and devices to maximize self-care
- Emotional responses to SCI and coping strategies
- Community resources

See Case Study (Box 24.3).

REHABILITATION

The saying "rehabilitation begins at admission" may sound trite, but for the patient with SCI its truth is astounding. The newly paralyzed person is faced with many sobering physical and psychologic challenges. The acute care staff and the rehabilitation staff strive to ensure that the patient is fully equipped to face the challenge.

Health Promotion

Skin Care: Key Points for the Patient With Spinal Cord Injury

- Avoid excessive pressure, shearing force, and trauma.
- Bathe in tepid water with mild soap; dry thoroughly.
- Soak the feet for 20 minutes once a week; keep toenails trimmed and smooth.
- Keep the skin dry and free of contact with urine or stool.
- Avoid tight clothing with heavy seams.
- Wear cotton undergarments and avoid clothing made of fabrics that do not absorb moisture.
- Eat a balanced diet with adequate vitamins A and C and protein.
- Drink 2000 to 3000 mL of fluid (8–12 8-oz glasses) each day unless directed otherwise.
- In bed, turn at least every 2 hours.
- In a chair, shift your weight at least every 15 minutes.
- Inspect the skin every morning and every evening for redness, bruising, blisters, and dryness and feel for swelling and hardness.
- If redness is present, try to determine the cause. Are you turning or shifting your weight often enough? Are you transferring correctly? Are your cushions in good condition?

Nursing care during the acute phase of the injury focuses on preventing further disability and avoiding complications that could prolong hospitalization and hamper rehabilitation. Rehabilitation is best described as those activities that assist the individual to achieve the highest possible level of self-care and independence.

The rehabilitation process involves a well-organized interdisciplinary team that can address all aspects of function. Members of the team include the physician, nurse, physical therapist, occupational therapist, speech therapist, dietitian, social worker, psychologist, and counselor. Each plays a vital role in helping the patient to achieve the highest level of independence. What once was regarded by the patient as a normal lifestyle or occupation may no longer be possible. Rather, modifications and adjustments must be made. The patient and family must be emotionally and physically prepared to make those adjustments. The team not only helps the patient to accomplish activities of daily living (ADLs) and self-care but also addresses successful adjustment to social integration and gainful employment in the workplace. Although this phase of treatment may take more than a year to accomplish, the patient, family, and rehabilitation team can take pride in the realization that the patient's life can once again be productive and happy.

Put On Your Thinking Cap!

You are assigned to a 19-year-old man who sustained a C8 spinal cord injury (SCI) 2 weeks ago. His condition is stable at this time, and he is alert and oriented. When the nursing assistant brings his breakfast tray, he closes his eyes, says he is not hungry, and asks her to turn off the lights and close the drapes.

1. What phase of adjustment do you think the patient's behavior represents?
2. With adequate support, education, and encouragement, the patient will move into the next phase of adjustment. Describe expected behaviors at that time.

NURSING CARE OF THE LAMINECTOMY PATIENT

Laminectomy is the removal of part of a vertebra. It is usually done to relieve pressure on spinal nerves. In addition to traumatic cord injury, it may be used to treat herniated disks or spinal tumors. See Chapter 17 for general surgical care.

Preoperatively, record the patient's vital signs and neurologic status to establish baselines. Determine the patient's understanding of surgical routines and tell the patient what to expect in the immediate postoperative period.

For the patient who has undergone a laminectomy, postoperative care focuses on ongoing assessment of neurologic status and on promoting healing

Box 24.4 Nursing Care After Laminectomy

NEUROLOGIC ASSESSMENT AND VITAL SIGNS
Frequently assess movement, strength, and range of motion.
Assess the patient's ability to localize sensory stimulus.
Frequently measure vital signs to determine any postoperative complications, such as hemorrhage or infection.

CIRCULATION AND RESPIRATION
Maintain elastic stockings on lower extremities to prevent deep vein thrombosis (DVT).
Encourage range-of-motion exercises 4 times a day.
Encourage deep breathing exercises every 2 hours.
Auscultate breath sounds every 2 to 4 hours.
Have the patient perform incentive spirometry every 2 hours while awake.

PROGRESSIVE AMBULATION AS APPROPRIATE
Help the patient to progress from sitting at the edge of the bed to ambulating with assistance.
Encourage increasing distances and independence while ambulating.
Ensure that the patient uses a back brace or other apparatus as ordered.

BED OR POSITIONING
Maintain the bed flat or only slightly elevated to reduce strain on the operative site.
Maintain a soft collar for cervical laminectomy.
Encourage position changes every 2 hours.

BOWEL AND BLADDER FUNCTION
Measure urinary output.
Assess the patient for urinary distention and complete emptying of the bladder after spontaneous void.
Encourage fluid intake.
Perform intermittent catheterization (as needed) if the patient is unable to void.
Auscultate bowel sounds.
Initiate a bowel program as appropriate.

SURGICAL INCISION
Change the dressing aseptically.
Check the dressing for blood or cerebrospinal fluid (CSF) drainage.

PAIN OR DISCOMFORT
Medicate the patient for pain and spasms as needed.
Encourage ambulation, if possible, to reduce spasms

at the operative site. Specific nursing responsibilities are summarized in Box 24.4.

FOCUSED ASSESSMENT

After a laminectomy, monitor the patient's vital signs, neurologic status, and breath sounds. Frequently assess movement, strength, range of motion, and ability to localize sensory stimulus. Measure fluid intake and output. In addition, auscultate the abdomen for bowel sounds and palpate for bladder distention. Inspect the surgical dressing for bleeding, clear CSF drainage, and foul drainage. If the patient has pain, obtain a complete description of it for the record.

Patient Problems, Goals, and Outcome Criteria: After Laminectomy

Patient Problems	Goals and Outcome Criteria
Potential for injury related to immobility, neurologic trauma, spinal fluid leakage	Freedom from injury: stable or improving neurologic and vital signs, absence of bleeding or cerebrospinal fluid (CSF) drainage, absence of fever, normal white blood cell count
Inadequate circulation related to hypovolemia, obstruction to blood flow	Adequate tissue perfusion: normal pulse, blood pressure, respirations, skin color, and tissue turgor
Acute pain related to tissue trauma, muscle spasms	Pain relief: patient states pain relieved, relaxed expression
Difficulty voiding related to sensory motor impairment, prescribed position restrictions	Normal urine elimination: spontaneous, controlled voiding; no bladder distention; urine output approximately equal to fluid intake
Constipation related to immobility, neurologic trauma, drug therapy	Normal bowel elimination: regular passage of formed stool without discomfort
Decreased mobility related to neuromuscular impairment, weakness, prescribed restrictions	Improved physical mobility: daily increase in walking distance without fatigue
Lack of knowledge of course of recovery, self-care activities, and limitations related to lack of exposure to information	Patient understands routines, self-care, and limitations: patient describes and demonstrates appropriate self-care

Interventions

Potential for injury. Monitor the patient for complications of surgery and notify the physician of any deviations in vital signs, including increased pulse and respirations, hypotension, and fever. In cervical surgeries, difficulty breathing or swallowing may be indicative of impending upper airway obstruction because of edema or hematoma formation; this is a medical emergency. Compare neurologic findings with preoperative assessments and report any decreasing sensory or motor responses to the physician. Assist the patient with measures to prevent complications of immobility (e.g., breathing and leg exercises) within the limitations of postoperative restrictions. Inform the health care provider if clear drainage is observed coming from the incision; this usually indicates a CSF leak. When changing the dressing, use aseptic technique to reduce the risk of wound contamination.

Inadequate circulation. Measures are taken to promote oxygenation and circulation. Apply elastic or pneumatic stockings to the lower extremities as ordered to promote venous return and prevent deep vein thrombosis (DVT). Teach or help the patient to do range-of-motion exercises at least 4 times daily or as ordered. Auscultate breath sounds every 2 to 4 hours and support the patient in deep breathing and coughing to remove pulmonary secretions. The incentive spirometer may be used every 2 hours while the patient is awake. Position the patient in good alignment and teach them to keep the back straight and avoid twisting when turning or getting out of bed.

A soft collar may be ordered after cervical laminectomy. Back braces may be prescribed after lumbar or thoracic spinal fusions. Typically, the braces are worn at all times at first. Use of the device is decreased as muscle strength returns. In some situations, corsets and casts are used to support and stabilize the spine. When supportive devices are worn, inspect the skin carefully to ensure that they are not creating pressure that could result in skin breakdown.

Acute pain. Assess and record the patient's level of discomfort and to keep the bed flat (or with the head slightly elevated) to reduce strain on the operative site. Administer analgesics and muscle relaxants as ordered. Other pain control measures, such as relaxation techniques, cutaneous stimulation, and imagery, are described in detail in Chapter 8. If the prescribed medications and nursing interventions do not provide pain relief, discuss the problem with the health care provider to determine whether other measures can be tried.

Difficulty voiding. Take measures to promote voiding. Intravenous fluids are usually ordered, but fluids can also be given orally as soon as the patient is able to tolerate them. Document voiding and measure urine output and assess the bladder for distention. Promote voiding by providing privacy and positioning the patient as comfortably as allowed. Running water may stimulate voiding. If the patient is unable to void, intermittent catheterization may be ordered.

Constipation. Stool softeners may be ordered to prevent constipation. In addition, ingestion of adequate fluids and fiber is helpful. Ambulation, when permitted, also promotes normal bowel elimination.

Decreased mobility. Patient activity progresses from sitting on the edge of the bed to ambulating with assistance. Encourage the patient to gradually increase distance and independence in ambulating. If the patient is to wear a back brace or other apparatus, ensure that it is applied properly. Physical therapy may be ordered.

Lack of knowledge. Postoperative teaching is directed toward promoting recovery from the surgery and preventing future injuries. Determine activity restrictions and discuss these with the patient.

Get Ready for the NCLEX® Examination!

Key Points

- SCIs most often result from trauma but may also be caused by degenerative conditions and tumors.
- SCIs may be classified by location, as open or closed, and by extent of damage to the cord.
- After SCI, motor and sensory function is monitored by assessing movement, muscle strength, sensation, and reflex activity.
- Effects of SCI may include respiratory impairment, spinal shock, autonomic dysreflexia, spasticity, impaired sensory and motor function, impaired bladder function, impaired bowel function, impaired temperature regulation, impaired sexual function, impaired skin integrity, and altered self-concept and body image.
- Injuries at or above the level of the fifth cervical vertebra may result in instant death because of interruption of the nerves that control respirations.
- Autonomic dysreflexia is an exaggerated sympathetic response to stimuli such as bladder distention, constipation, renal calculi, ejaculation, and uterine contractions that produces severe hypertension with the potential for seizures and stroke.
- Muscle tone is usually flaccid immediately after injury, but spasticity develops when spinal shock resolves.
- Goals of medical care after spinal injury are to sustain life, prevent further cord injury, and repair cord damage.
- Immobilization is essential to prevent further damage to the cord after injury.
- Nursing care after SCI is concerned with inadequate oxygenation, potential for injury, potential for autonomic dysreflexia, potential complications of immobility, bowel incontinence, urinary incontinence, potential for infection, elevated body temperature, decreased body temperature, impaired ADLs (feeding, dressing, grooming, toileting), altered sexual function, inadequate coping, and inability to manage treatment program.
- Rehabilitation assists the patient to achieve the highest possible level of self-care and independence.
- Laminectomy is a surgical procedure that may be done for several reasons, including SCI.

Additional Learning Resources

SG Go to your Study Guide for additional learning activities to help you master this chapter content.

Go to your Evolve website (http://evolve.elsevier.com/Linton/medsurg) for the following learning resources and much more:

- Fluid & Electrolyte Tutorial
- Review Questions for the NCLEX® Examination

Clinical Judgment and Next-Generation NCLEX® Examination-Style Questions

1. **A patient's chart notes that he has had complete transection of the spinal cord at T8. Which of the following should you expect the patient to be?**
   1. Ventilator dependent
   2. Paraplegic
   3. Comatose
   4. Tetraplegic

   NCLEX Client Need: Physiological Adaptation

2. **Various patients on a spinal cord injury unit exhibit all of the findings listed subsequently. Which finding would indicate that spinal shock is resolving?**
   1. Spastic, involuntary movements of the extremities
   2. Blood pressure returns to normal range
   3. No muscle tone in extremities
   4. Patient senses light touch and pressure

   NCLEX Client Need: Physiological Adaptation

3. **A patient with SCI reports a pounding headache. He is flushed, diaphoretic, and extremely anxious. His blood pressure is 210/120 mm Hg. Which complication should be suspected?**

   ____

   NCLEX Client Need: Physiological Adaptation

4. **After spinal shock was resolved, a patient's bladder began to empty spontaneously. What is the most likely explanation for this emptying?**
   1. The spinal cord is beginning to heal.
   2. The patient is regaining normal bladder control.
   3. Intact reflex activity is causing bladder emptying.
   4. The patient is not a candidate for bladder retraining.

   NCLEX Client Need: Physiological Adaptation

5. **Patient teaching for women with spinal cord injuries should include which of the following? (Select all that apply.)**
   1. Pregnancy is still possible.
   2. The menstrual cycle will resume.
   3. Sexual intercourse is discouraged.
   4. If pregnancy occurs, cesarean section will be necessary.
   5. Although vaginal sensations are lacking, some women have orgasms.

   NCLEX Client Need: Physiological Adaptation

6. **Immediate care after a suspected SCI should include which of the following? (Select all that apply.)**
   1. Gently lift the patient's chin and tilt the head
   2. Prop the patient's head to maintain slight flexion
   3. Administer 100% oxygen by mask
   4. Use the jaw-thrust method to open the airway
   5. Maintain alignment and immobilization of the spinal column

   NCLEX Client Need: Reduction of Risk Potential

7. **Which of the following is the purpose of a skeletal traction device after SCI?**
   1. To align and immobilize the vertebrae to prevent further cord damage
   2. To apply tension to the spinal cord to keep it straight
   3. To maintain the neck in the best position to ensure an open airway
   4. To permit healing of the SCI

   NCLEX Client Need: Reduction of Risk Potential

8. **A patient admitted with SCI has an order for methylprednisolone. The nurse knows that the rationale for giving this drug is:**
   1. To prevent allergic reactions to dyes used in diagnostic procedures
   2. To boost the patient's immune system
   3. To reduce damage to the cellular membrane of the spinal cord
   4. To promote regeneration of neurons

   NCLEX Client Need: Physiological Integrity: Pharmacologic Therapies

9. **Nursing care during the acute phase of SCI should include which of the following? (Select all that apply.)**
   1. Avoid grasping the muscles when performing range-of-motion exercises.
   2. Encourage patients in cervical traction to turn themselves every 2 hours to maintain muscle strength.
   3. For the best absorption and to avoid injury, administer injections above the level of paralysis.
   4. Because the patient will require a permanent indwelling catheter, begin teaching catheter care.
   5. After a halo vest is applied, the patient must remain on strict bed rest.

   NCLEX Client Need: Reduction of Risk Potential

10. **Postoperative nursing care for the laminectomy patient should include which of the following? (Select all that apply.)**
    1. Inspect the skin under a back brace for signs of pressure or irritation.
    2. Adjust the bed to keep the patient in a high Fowler position.
    3. Use analgesics and nonpharmacologic measures to manage pain.
    4. Observe for bloody drainage, which is usually CSF.
    5. Compare neurologic check findings with preoperative findings.

11. **SLO/Objective: Apply knowledge of anatomy, physiology, and pathophysiology to determine which assessment data require follow-up by the nurse.**

NGN Item Type: Enhanced Hot Spot

Cognitive Skill: Recognize Cues

A 42-year-old male has been hospitalized for four days after a motorcycle accident in which he sustained a complete spinal cord injury at the level of T6. He is experiencing spastic involuntary movements of the extremities and suddenly has begun having symptoms of pounding headache, anxiety, flushed face, nasal congestion, diaphoresis, hypertension, and bradycardia.

- Blood pressure 200/92 mm Hg
- Pulse 58 beats per minute
- Respirations 18 breaths per minute
- Headache
- Flushed face
- Diaphoresis
- Spastic involuntary movements of the extremities
- Anxiety
- Nasal congestion

Highlight or place a check mark next to the assessment findings that require follow up by the nurse.

12. **SLO Objective: Assist in developing a nursing plan of care for the patient with an SCI.**

NGN Item Type: Cloze

Cognitive Skill: Analyze Cues

A 42-year-old male has been hospitalized for eight days after a motorcycle accident in which he sustained a complete spinal cord injury at the level of T6. He is experiencing spastic involuntary movements of the extremities and suddenly has begun having symptoms of headache, flushed face, diaphoresis, anxiety, and nasal congestion.

- Blood pressure 200/92 mm Hg
- Pulse 58 beats per minute
- Respirations 18 breaths per minute
- Headache
- Flushed face
- Diaphoresis
- Spastic involuntary movements of the extremities
- Anxiety
- Nasal congestion

Choose the most likely options for the information missing from the statements below by selecting from the lists of options provided.

Based on the patient's assessment data, the nurse determines that the patient's vital signs findings are because of (1)____________. These symptoms were precipitated by (2)______ ______, (2)_________, and (2)_________.

OPTIONS FOR 1	OPTIONS FOR 2
Respiratory impairment	Urinary incontinence
Spinal shock	Diarrhea
Respiratory impairment	Nausea and vomiting
Autonomic dysreflexia	Fecal impaction
Cardiogenic shock	Pressure injury
Spinal hemorrhage	Hemorrhage
Bronchospasms	Distended bladder

13. **SLO Objective: Assist in developing a nursing care plan for the patient with an SCI.**

NGN Item Type: Extended multiple response

Cognitive Skill: Prioritize hypotheses

A 42-year-old male has been hospitalized for four days after a motorcycle accident in which he sustained a complete spinal cord injury at the level of T6. He is experiencing spastic involuntary movements of the extremities and suddenly has begun having symptoms of pounding headache, anxiety, flushed face, nasal congestion, diaphoresis, hypertension, and bradycardia.

- Blood pressure 200/92 mm Hg
- Pulse 58 beats per minute
- Respirations 18 breaths per minute
- Headache
- Flushed face
- Diaphoresis
- Spastic involuntary movements of the extremities
- Anxiety
- Nasal congestion

When planning care for this patient, for which **priority** potential complications would the nurse monitor? (Select all that apply.)

Seizure
Bruising
Hemorrhage
Nausea and anorexia
Stroke
Kidney failure
Respiratory failure

14. **SLO Objective: Assist in developing a nursing care plan for the patient with an SCI.**

NGN Item Type: Matrix

Cognitive Skill: Generate solutions

A 42-year-old male has been hospitalized for four days after a motorcycle accident in which he sustained a complete spinal cord injury at the level of T6. He is experiencing spastic involuntary movements of the extremities and suddenly has begun having symptoms of pounding headache, anxiety, flushed face, nasal congestion, diaphoresis, hypertension, and bradycardia.

Use an X for the nursing actions listed below that are *Indicated* (appropriate or necessary), *Contraindicated* (could be harmful), or *Nonessential* (makes no difference or not necessary) for the patient's care at this time.

NURSING ACTION	INDICATED*	CONTRAIN-DICATED	NONESSEN-TIAL
Identify cause			
Put in Tren-delenburg position			
Elevate head of bed			
Irrigate catheter			
Turn on soft music			
Administer anti-hypertensive medication as ordered			

***Note:** This column could be labeled as "Anticipated."

15. **SLO Objective: Discuss content to be included in teaching patients to learn to live with an SCI.**

NGN Item Type: Matrix

Cognitive Skill: Take action

A 42-year-old white male has been hospitalized for four days after a motorcycle accident in which he sustained a complete spinal cord injury at the level of T6. He is experiencing spastic involuntary movements of the extremities and continues to have symptoms of pounding headache, anxiety, flushed face, nasal congestion, diaphoresis, hypertension, and bradycardia.

Use an X for the health teaching below that is *Indicated* (appropriate or necessary), *Contraindicated* (could be harmful), or *Nonessential* (makes no difference or not necessary) before the patient's discharge at this time.

HEALTH TEACHING	INDICATED	CONTRAINDI-CATED	NONESSEN-TIAL
Let the nurse know if you are experiencing a headache			
Stay flat in bed			
Tell the nurse if you are feeling anxious			
Be sure to check your catheter for blockage			
Put on soft music with a darkened room			

16. **SLO Objective: Identify data to be collected in evaluating the outcomes of nursing care.**

NGN Item Type: Matrix

Cognitive Skill: Evaluate outcomes

The fifth day of hospitalization, the patient is assisted to transfer into a chair and feeling more comfortable. He is eating well and has no complaints of nausea or vomiting. He is talking about going to rehab soon.

For each assessment finding, use an X to indicate whether the interventions were *Effective* (helped to meet expected outcomes, *Ineffective* (did not help to meet expected outcomes), or *Unrelated* (not related to the expected outcomes).

ASSESSMENT FINDING	EFFECTIVE	INEFFECTIVE	UNRELATED
Heart rate stabilizes			
No swelling or discoloration of left hand			
Shows signs of urinary retention			
Absence of emergent neurological reactions			
Blood pressure stabilizing			
No dizziness with position changes			
Pulse is 80 beats per minute			
Pupils equal and reactive to light			
Persistent pain in left wrist			

Respiratory System Introduction

25

http://evolve.elsevier.com/Linton/medsurg

Objectives

1. Discuss the anatomy and physiology of the respiratory system.
2. List the components of the nursing assessment of the patient with a respiratory disorder.
3. Describe the diagnostic tests and procedures used to evaluate respiratory function and the nursing responsibilities associated with each.
4. Identify the uses, side effects, and nursing interventions associated with common drug therapies used in patients with respiratory disorders.
5. Identify nursing actions when selected therapeutic measures are ordered for patients with respiratory disorders.

Key Terms

apnea
crackles
cyanosis
dyspnea
epistaxis
hypoxia
orthopnea
rhonchus
wheezes

Respiration is basic to life. The respiratory system provides fuel for bodily activities and energy to sustain life. Respiration is defined as the exchange of oxygen (O_2) and carbon dioxide (CO_2) through the inspiration of air from the atmosphere and the expiration of air from the lungs. The function of the respiratory system is to supply O_2 for the metabolic needs of the cells and to remove CO_2, one of the waste products of cellular metabolism.

ANATOMY AND PHYSIOLOGY OF THE RESPIRATORY SYSTEM

To reach the lungs, air must travel through several passages, including the nose, mouth, pharynx, larynx, trachea, and bronchi (Fig. 25.1). Each passage has an effect on the quality of the air that reaches the lungs.

NOSE

The nose can be divided into internal and external sections. The external nose is made up of bone, cartilage, and mucous membrane. Only the upper one-third of the external nose has a bony skeleton. The remainder is shaped by cartilage.

The internal nose is divided by the nasal septum, a thin wall that creates two passages. The openings on each side of the septum are the nares. The outermost portion of the internal nose, called the *vestibule*, is covered by skin that contains nasal hairs. The rest of the interior is lined with mucous membrane. The internal nose is well supplied with blood by branches of the internal and external carotids.

A layer of mucus covers the membrane. The mucus traps inspired particles and moisturizes dry air. Mucus also protects the airway because it is acidic and contains an enzyme that destroys most bacteria. Cilia sweep particles that are trapped in the mucus toward the throat to be swallowed.

Olfactory cells line the roof of the nasal cavity. These are specialized sensory cells that detect odors and relay information about odors to the brain by way of the first cranial nerve (the olfactory nerve).

The side walls of the internal nose have folds of tissue called *turbinates*. Turbinates are projections, which increase the surface area that inspired air crosses. As air swirls over the turbinates, it is quickly warmed to body temperature. The turbinates also contain openings through which secretions drain from the sinuses.

SINUSES

The sinuses are spaces in the bones of the skull. They are lined with mucous membrane and filled with air. The sinuses produce mucus that drains into the nasal cavity. They also act as sound chambers for the voice and reduce the weight of the skull. The sinuses around the

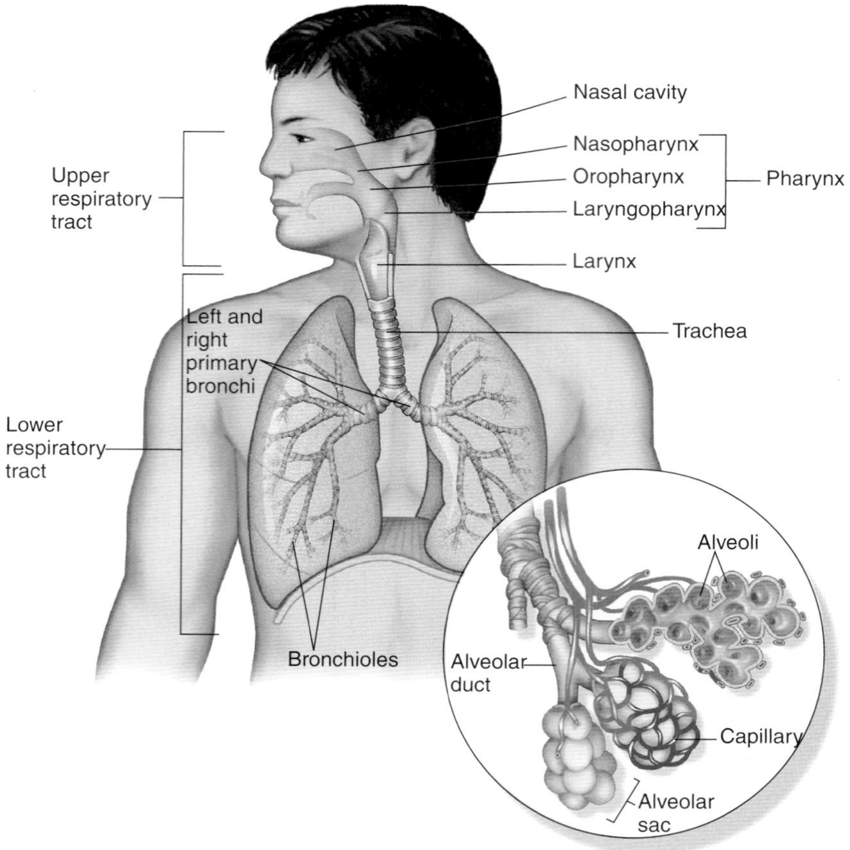

Fig. 25.1 Anatomy of the respiratory system. (From McCance KL, Huether SE: *Understanding pathophysiology,* ed 6, St. Louis, 2013, Mosby.)

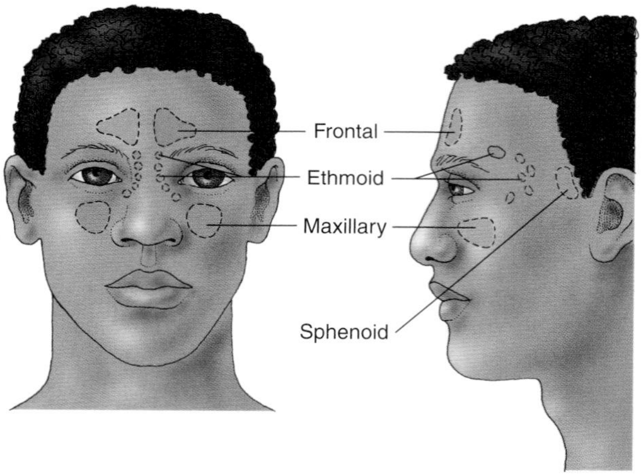

Fig. 25.2 The paranasal sinuses. (From Ignatavicius DD, Workman, ML: *Medical-surgical nursing*, ed 8, St. Louis, 2016, Elsevier.)

nose are called the *paranasal sinuses.* They include the maxillary, frontal, ethmoid, and sphenoid sinuses. Pairs of sinuses are found on either side of the face (Fig. 25.2).

THROAT

The throat, or pharynx, extends from the back of the nasal cavities to the esophagus. It provides passageways from the nose and mouth to the digestive and respiratory tracts. The eustachian tubes that originate in the middle ear open into the nasopharynx. These tubes serve as pressure vents to prevent excessive pressure from building up in the middle ear.

Other important structures in the throat are the tonsils and adenoids. Tonsils and adenoids are masses of lymphatic tissue that guard against bacterial invasion of the respiratory and digestive tracts.

The larynx is the passageway between the throat and the trachea and is commonly referred to as the *voice box.* Two bands of tissue, the vocal cords, stretch across the interior of the larynx. The cords tighten and relax, producing different pitch sounds, as air moves through them. The sounds produced are modified and refined by the oral, nasal, and sinus cavities.

The epiglottis lies on top of the larynx. It is a flap that works like a trapdoor, closing during swallowing to prevent food and fluid from entering the airway.

Trachea

The trachea, or windpipe, is a 4- to 5-inch tube descending from the larynx into the bronchi. It is made up of cartilage, smooth muscle, and connective tissue lined by a layer of mucous membrane. The trachea functions as a passageway for air to reach the lungs.

Bronchi

The bronchi provide a passageway for air going to and from the lungs. Two primary bronchi split to the right and left from the trachea. The right bronchus is shorter and wider and runs straighter up and down than the left bronchus. In addition, the right bronchus branches off before the left bronchus. Because of these factors, foreign bodies from the trachea usually enter the right bronchus.

The larger bronchi divide into smaller, or secondary, bronchi, which then divide again into even smaller tertiary bronchi. The tertiary bronchi divide into smaller units called *bronchioles*, which eventually lead to tiny air sacs called *alveoli* located in the lungs. It is through the walls of the alveoli that the exchange of O_2 and CO_2 takes place.

LUNGS

The lungs are located in the right and left sides of the thoracic cavity within the chest wall. The thoracic cavity is separated from the abdominal cavity by the diaphragm, a large sheet of muscle. The lungs are divided into lobes: three lobes on the right and two on the left. Each lung is covered by a membrane called the *pleura*. The pleura is a sac containing a small amount of fluid that acts as a lubricant for the lungs when they expand and contract.

RESPIRATORY PHYSIOLOGY

Mechanism of Breathing

The process of air entering the lungs is called *inspiration*, and the process of air leaving the lungs is called *expiration*. The terms *inhalation* and *exhalation* are used interchangeably with inspiration and expiration. The movement of the diaphragm and the muscles in the chest accomplish both of these processes. Inspiration involves an active contraction of the muscles and diaphragm and can be noted by an enlargement of the chest cavity. Expiration is a passive process during which the muscles relax, and the chest returns to its normal size (Fig. 25.3).

During normal, quiet breathing, approximately 500 mL of air is inhaled and exhaled. Most of the air movement occurs because of the contraction and relaxation of the diaphragm. A temporary interruption in the normal breathing pattern in which no air movement occurs is called **apnea**. Shortness of breath is called **dyspnea**. Difficulty with breathing in a lying position is called **orthopnea**. Different types of breathing patterns are described in Table 25.1.

Respiratory Center

Breathing is controlled by the respiratory center, which is located in the medulla. The medulla is part of the brainstem immediately above the spinal cord. The respiratory center is stimulated by changing levels of CO_2 and O_2 in arterial blood. Chemoreceptors in the aorta and carotid artery monitor the pH and the amount of CO_2 and O_2 in the bloodstream. Changes in the pH, increased levels of CO_2, or decreased levels of O_2 cause signals to be sent to the phrenic nerves, which in turn, send signals to the respiratory muscles to carry out the major work of breathing. See Box 25.1 for common changes in the respiratory tract in advanced age.

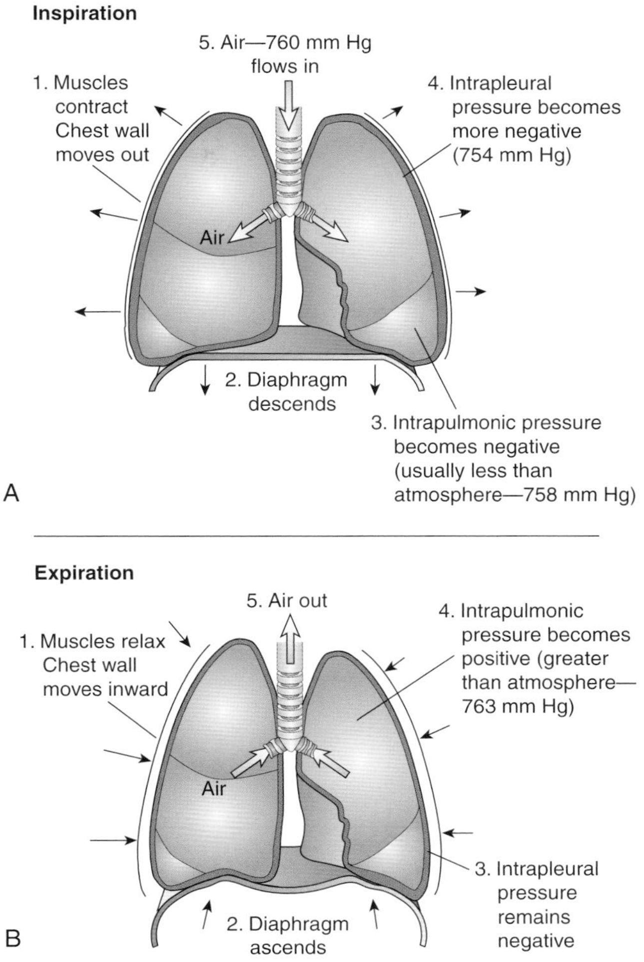

Fig. 25.3 (A) Normal inspiration and (B) normal expiration. Note the visceral pleura, pleural space, and parietal pleura, as well as the changes in pressure in the alveoli and pleural space on inspiration and expiration. (From VanMeter KC, Hubert RJ: *Gould's pathophysiology for the health professions*, ed 5, St. Louis, 2014, Saunders.)

Put On Your Thinking Cap!

Identify three implications of the age-related changes in the respiratory system. For example, a weakened esophageal sphincter may permit reflux of gastric contents into the esophagus.

NURSING ASSESSMENT OF THE RESPIRATORY TRACT

HEALTH HISTORY

Reason for Seeking Care

Patients often seek medical attention for symptoms related to the respiratory system. Among the common

Table 25.1 Types of Breathing Patterns

PATTERN	CHARACTERISTICS	CAUSES
Normal	Pattern: regular Depth: even Rate: 12–20 breaths per minute	Normal respiratory drive
Tachypnea	Pattern: regular Depth: even Rate: faster than 20 breaths per minute	Fever, pain, anxiety
Hyperpnea	Pattern: regular Depth: increased Rate: faster than 20 breaths per minute	Normal during exercise
Bradypnea	Pattern: regular Depth: even Rate: slower than 12 breaths per minute	Sedatives, opioids, and alcohol; brain, metabolic, and respiratory disorders
Apnea	Pattern: respirations cease for several seconds. Persistent cessation is respiratory arrest	
Cheyne-Stokes respirations, apnea	Breaths progressively deeper, then becoming more shallow, followed by period of apnea	Severe brain pathology
Kussmaul respirations (with hyperventilation)	Pattern: regular Depth: deep Rate: faster than 20 breaths per minute	Metabolic acidosis; diabetic ketoacidosis, renal failure
Biot's respirations; apnea	Pattern: abnormally shallow for several breaths, followed by irregular period of apnea	Neurologic disorders

Modified from Kersten LD: *Comprehensive respiratory nursing*, Philadelphia, 1989, Saunders; and Fetzer, S. Vital signs. In: Potter PA, Perry AG, Stockert PA, Hall AH, editors: *Fundamentals of nursing*, ed 9, St. Louis, 2017, Elsevier.

Box 25.1 Age-Related Changes in the Respiratory Tract

- Nose: softening of the nasal cartilage may cause obstruction
- Mucous membranes
- Thinner and more fragile
- Less mucus production
- Increased risk of **epistaxis** (nosebleed)
- Sense of smell declines
- Pharynx and larynx
- Muscles atrophy
- Loss of elasticity of the laryngeal muscles and cartilages; vocal cords slacken
- Esophageal sphincter: weakens
- Trachea: may deviate from midline
- Lungs
- Decreased lung elasticity
- Enlargement of the bronchioles
- Decreased number of functioning alveoli
- Respiratory defense mechanisms: less effective
- Respiratory muscles: atrophy
- Rib cage: more rigid
- Diaphragm: flattens

complaints are "runny nose," sore throat, hoarseness, cough, dyspnea (shortness of breath), and chest pain. You can assist by obtaining a detailed description of the patient's complaints. The data collected by the licensed vocational nurse/licensed practical nurse (LVN/LPN) contribute to a complete nursing assessment. However, if the patient is in respiratory distress, focus on the immediate problem. Detailed assessment, as described later, may be deferred until the patient's respiratory status improves.

Present Health

To describe a cough, include the onset, duration, frequency, type (wet or dry), severity, and related symptoms such as sputum production and pain. Document the frequency of expectoration and the sputum characteristics (i.e., color, consistency, odor, amount). Also record the patient's efforts to self-treat the cough with measures such as medication, vaporizers, and humidifiers, as well as the response to the treatments.

If the patient complains of dyspnea, determine the onset, duration, severity, and precipitating events. Note whether the dyspnea becomes worse with activity or certain positions and whether it is more frequent during certain seasons. Identify associated symptoms, such as fatigue or palpitations. Describe the effectiveness of methods used to manage dyspnea, which might include medications, O_2, and positioning.

When the patient has chest pain, the location, severity, onset, duration, and precipitating events (trauma, coughing, inspiration) should be recorded. Determine whether the pain causes shallow breathing and whether it radiates up to the jaw or down the arms. Record the presence of fever, sweating, or nausea, and document measures that bring relief, such as splinting, heat, analgesics, and antitussive medications.

Past Health History

The patient's past medical history determines previous respiratory disorders, allergies, trauma, and surgery. Conditions that are important to document when a patient has a respiratory disorder include allergies, colds, pneumonia, tuberculosis, chronic bronchitis, emphysema, asthma, cancer of the respiratory tract, cystic fibrosis, sinus infections, streptococcal infections, ear infections, diabetes mellitus, and heart disease. It is especially important to note conditions that suppress the immune response, making the patient more susceptible to infection. Document surgical procedures on the respiratory structures. Record all recent and current medications, including the use of over-the-counter (OTC) drugs, and the dates of the most recent chest radiograph and tuberculin skin test. Inquire about immunizations against pneumonia and influenza.

Family History

Inquire about the respiratory health of close family members. In addition, ask the patient about exposure to smoke or other respiratory irritants in the household. Document a history of tuberculosis in family members.

Review of Systems

The review of systems assesses signs and symptoms that may be directly or indirectly related to the respiratory disorder. Ask about fatigue, weakness, fever, chills, and night sweats. Other data that may be significant are earaches, nasal obstructions, sinus pain, sore throat, hoarseness, edema, dyspnea, and orthopnea.

Functional Assessment

Describe the patient's occupational history, including any exposure to pathogens or to substances that might irritate or harm the respiratory tract. Note exposure to any fumes, toxins, coal dust, silica, or sawdust. Ask the patient to describe a typical day, and to give particular attention to any limitations imposed by the respiratory disorder. Ask about the usual diet and fluid intake. In addition, a smoking history is important; for the cigarette smoker, this is usually reported in pack-years (see the Cultural Considerations box). Pack-years are calculated by multiplying the number of years the patient smoked cigarettes by the number of packs smoked each day. To illustrate, a person who smoked two packs a day for 30 years would have a 60 pack-year smoking history (see the Health Promotion box). The functional assessment also includes the patient's role in the family, sources of stress, and coping strategies.

Cultural Considerations

What Does Culture Have to Do With Smoking?

In the United States, rates of smoking vary by ethnicity: non-Hispanic Native Americans and Alaska natives have the highest rate at 20.9%. Next is non-Hispanic Whites (15.5%), followed by Hispanics (8.8%) and non-Hispanic Asians (7.2%). Most tobacco users start using those products during adolescence.

Health Promotion

How to Calculate Pack-Years

Number of years the patient has smoked × Number of packs smoked each day

Put On Your Thinking Cap!

A patient has smoked one pack of cigarettes each day for 15 years. Calculate the pack-years of the patient's smoking history.

PHYSICAL EXAMINATION

The physical examination begins with observing the patient's general appearance. Note facial expression, posture, alertness, speech pattern, and any obvious signs of distress. Take the vital signs and measure height and weight. Be alert to unusually rapid or slow breathing and to tachycardia, which may be a sign of **hypoxia** (low oxygen level in the blood). The normal respiratory rate for adults is 12 to 20 breaths per minute.

Head and Neck

Examine the head and neck. Inspect the nose for symmetry and deformity and gently palpate for tenderness. The patency of each naris can be assessed by closing one at a time and asking the patient to breathe in through the nose. Note flaring of the nares because it is a common sign of air hunger. Use a nasal speculum to inspect the nasal cavity for swelling, discharge, bleeding, or foreign bodies. The nasal mucosa is normally light red in color. Tilt back the patient's head to inspect for deviation of the nasal septum, the structure that separates the nares. A deviation may be seen as a hump in the nasal cavity. Palpate the sinuses for tenderness by using the thumbs to apply pressure over the frontal and maxillary sinuses.

Inspect the lips, the tip of the nose, the top of the auricles, the gums, and the area under the tongue for **cyanosis**—a bluish color related to inadequate tissue oxygenation. Document the presence of pursed-lip breathing, a common technique for decreasing dyspnea with chronic respiratory disease. Inspect the pharynx for redness and tonsil exudate or enlargement, which are signs of infection.

Inspect the trachea to see if it is midline; if not midline, it is said to be *deviated*. A deviated trachea can be indicative of serious conditions that will be explained in subsequent chapters. Place the thumbs on either side of the trachea just above the clavicles and gently move the trachea from side to side. Compare the spaces between the sternocleidomastoid muscles on either shoulder and the trachea. An experienced examiner palpates for enlargement and tenderness of the lymph glands in the neck.

Thorax

Inspect the chest for deformities and lesions and observe the breathing pattern and effort. The rise and fall of the chest should be regular and symmetric. See Table 25.1 for the different types of breathing patterns. Palpate the thorax for tenderness and lumps. In addition, more sophisticated aspects of the examination that require special training include palpating for symmetric chest expansion and tactile fremitus. The skilled examiner may also percuss (tap) the thorax in a systematic manner to elicit sounds that give clues about the density of underlying tissues.

Using the diaphragm of the stethoscope, auscultate the lungs bilaterally in a systematic manner (Fig. 25.4), usually the posterior, the sides, and then the anterior chest. Listen for the normal movement of air in and out of the lungs and for abnormal breath sounds: **wheezes**, rhonchi, and crackles. A wheeze is a high-pitched sound caused by air passing through narrowed passageways that may be present with asthma or chronic obstructive pulmonary disease (COPD). A **rhonchus** is a dry, rattling sound caused by partial bronchial obstruction. **Crackles** are abnormal sounds associated with many cardiac and pulmonary disorders. Fine crackles are the result of fluid accumulation in the alveoli and do not clear with coughing. To demonstrate the sound of fine crackles, rub a few strands of hair between the thumb and forefinger next to the ear. Coarse crackles are described as sounding like a Velcro fastener opening. Course crackles are caused by secretions accumulating in the larger airways and usually clear with coughing. One other abnormal sound that may be heard on auscultation is a pleural friction rub, which is indicative of pleurisy. A pleural friction rub is a grating, scratchy noise similar to a creaking shoe.

In addition to the examination of the thorax and the auscultation of lung sounds, assess for signs of circulatory disorders that could affect respirations. Inspect the abdomen for distention that might interfere with full expansion of the lungs. Inspect the extremities for color, and palpate for edema. Examine the fingers for clubbing, which is associated with chronic respiratory problems (Fig. 25.5). Deep veins in the legs and pelvis are the source of most pulmonary emboli, so it

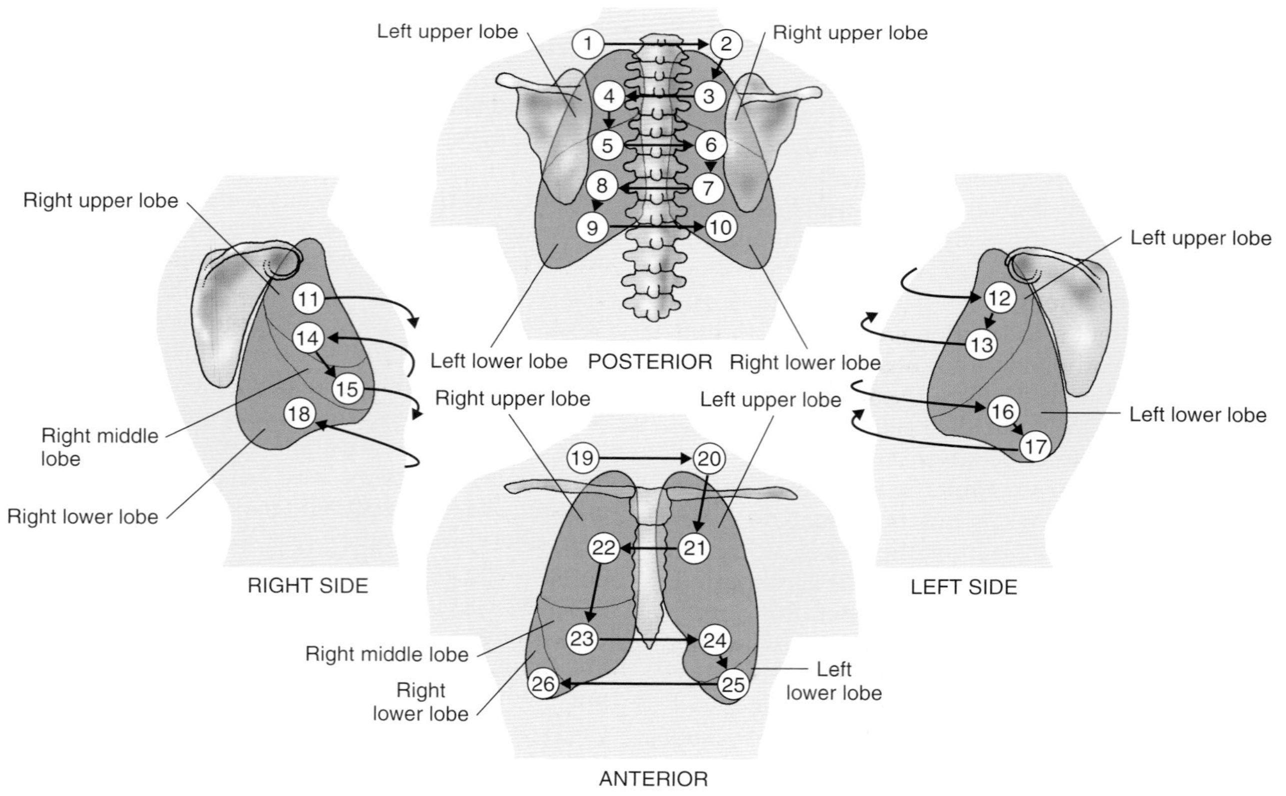

Fig. 25.4 Sequence for percussion and auscultation of the lungs. (From Ignatavicius DD, Workman ML: *Medical-surgical nursing*, ed 8, St. Louis, 2016, Elsevier.)

is important to assess for any circulatory changes in the lower extremities. Assess for unilateral leg or calf swelling, pitting edema confined to one leg, and localized redness and tenderness along the distribution of the deep venous system. Patients with a history of previous pulmonary emboli or deep vein thrombosis, recent surgery or immobilization, or a diagnosis of cancer are at an increased risk for developing a deep vein thrombosis. If a deep vein thrombosis is suspected, it is important to avoid moving the leg vigorously and to immediately notify the health care provider. The nursing assessment of the patient with a respiratory disorder is summarized in Box 25.2.

DIAGNOSTIC TESTS AND PROCEDURES

A variety of tests and procedures may be performed to diagnose disorders of the respiratory system. These tests and procedures are described here. Patient preparation and postprocedure care are presented in Table 25.2.

THROAT CULTURE

Throat cultures are done to isolate and identify infective organisms. A throat culture is usually done when streptococcal sore throat ("strep throat") is suspected. The procedure can also be used to screen for carriers of *Neisseria meningitides*. Carriers harbor the organisms without showing evidence of the disease. If the physician orders the culture and antibiotics at the same time, obtain the culture specimen before starting the antibiotics. The throat should not be swabbed if acute epiglottitis is suspected because the swab could trigger spasms that block the airway. Instead of culture, radiographs of the neck are ordered to confirm epiglottitis.

Kits are available to collect and contain the specimen. The kit consists of a sterile swab or applicator and a tube of culture medium. To obtain the specimen, good lighting is essential. Tilt the patient's head back and depress the tongue with a tongue blade. Firmly, but gently, rotate the swab over the back of the throat, tonsils, and any obvious lesion. The swab should not touch any other area of the mouth. Because patients often gag or cough, stand to one side or wear a mask (Fig. 25.6). Immediately place the swab in the tube of culture medium. Many commercial kits have an ampule of medium that must be broken to release the liquid. Carefully follow the directions on the kit. The results are reported in 24 to 48 hours. For results in a matter of minutes, the rapid antigen detection test (RADT) can be done. The RADT detects the presence of beta-hemolytic streptococcus antigen. Regardless of the results, the culture still should be done for confirmation and to detect other pathogens.

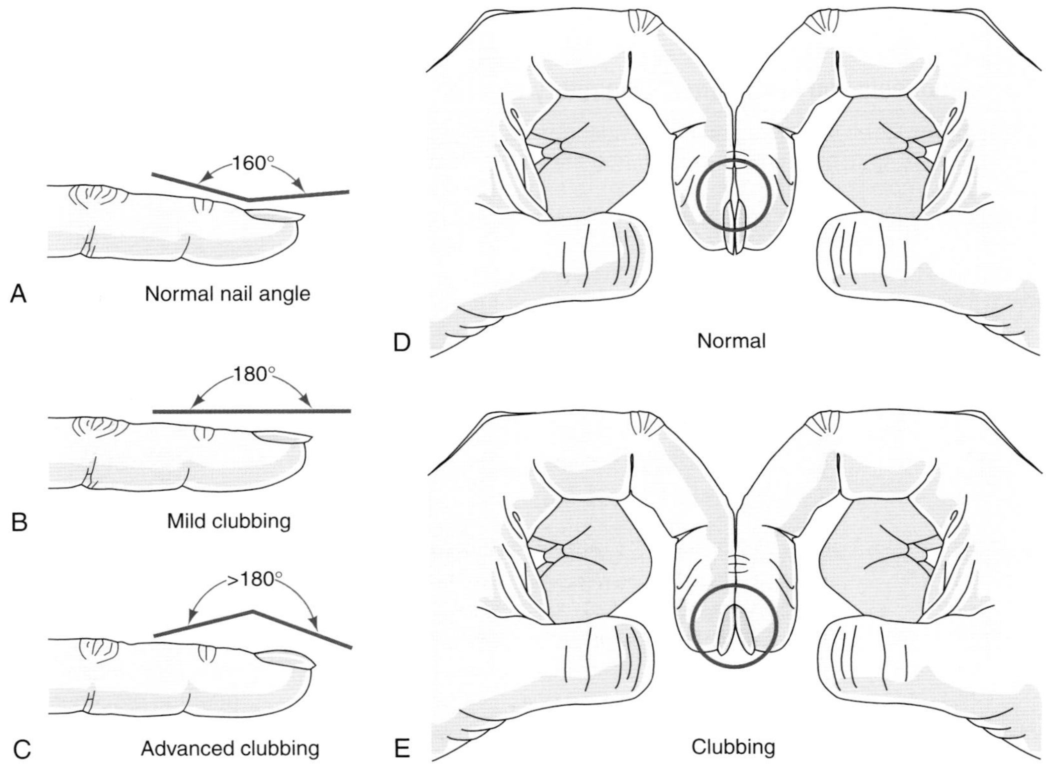

Fig. 25.5 Clubbing is a flattening of the angle between the nail and skin. (A) Normal angle of 160 degrees. (B) Early clubbing: the angle is flattened to 180 degrees. (C) Advanced clubbing: the angle is greater than 180 degrees. (D) The Schamroth technique: the patient puts the nails of the index fingers of each hand together. The examiner then looks at the space between the touching nails. If no clubbing exists, the space is diamond shaped. E. With clubbing, no diamond-shaped space exists. (From Copstead LEC, Banasik JL: *Pathophysiology*, ed 5, St. Louis, 2013, Saunders.)

Box 25.2 Assessment of the Patient With a Respiratory Disorder

HEALTH HISTORY

Reason for Seeking Care

If the patient is in acute respiratory distress, focus on immediate problem. Delay complete assessment until status improves

Present Health

Cough: onset, duration, frequency, severity, type (wet or dry), sputum production and characteristics, pain, self-treatments used and effectiveness

Dyspnea: onset, duration, severity, precipitating events, associated symptoms, self-treatments used and effectiveness

Chest pain: onset, duration, location, severity, precipitating events, radiation, associated symptoms, self-treatments used and effectiveness

Past Health History

Allergies. Previous respiratory disorders: colds, pneumonia, tuberculosis, chronic bronchitis, emphysema, asthma, cancer of the respiratory system, cystic fibrosis, sinus infections, streptococcal infections, ear infections, immune system disorders, surgical procedures and trauma related to respiratory system. Recent and current medications. Dates of last chest radiograph, tuberculin skin test, pneumonia and influenza immunizations

Family History

Major respiratory conditions, smoking history

Review of Systems

Fatigue, weakness, fever, chills, night sweats, earaches, nasal obstruction, sinus pain, sore throat, hoarseness, edema, dyspnea, orthopnea

Functional Assessment

Occupation, exposure to pathogens or irritating substances. Typical day. Limitations imposed by respiratory symptoms. Diet and fluid intake. Smoking history. Role in family, sources of stress, coping strategies

Physical Examination

General Survey: appearance, facial expression, posture, alertness, speech pattern, obvious distress

Height and Weight

Vital Signs

Nose: symmetry, deformity, tenderness, patency of nares, nasal flaring. Nasal cavity: swelling, discharge, bleeding, foreign bodies, septal deviation

Sinuses: tenderness

Lips: color, pursed-lip breathing

Pharynx: redness, tonsil enlargement or exudate

Neck: Tracheal deviation from midline. Palpable, tender lymph nodes

Thorax: deformities, lesions, breathing pattern and effort, symmetry with breathing. Tenderness, lumps, fremitus, percussion. Auscultation: breath sounds, wheezes, rhonchi, crackles, pleural friction rub.

Abdomen: distension

Extremities: skin color, edema, clubbing of fingers, redness and tenderness over veins

Table 25.2 Diagnostic Tests and Procedures: Respiratory System

General nursing actions: Confirm orders and check agency protocol.
Always tell the patient what to expect before, during, and after the procedure.
When a venous blood sample is required, tell the patient to expect a venipuncture.
Following venipuncture, apply pressure and a Band-Aid. Check for oozing.
If patient is taking anticoagulants, the drug may be withheld for a specified period before invasive procedures.
If patient will be sedated for an outpatient procedure, a driver must be available to take the patient home.
If contrast medium (dye) will be used, ask about allergy to iodine or shellfish. Inform radiologist if patient is allergic.

MISCELLANEOUS PROCEDURES

TEST AND PURPOSE	PATIENT PREPARATION	POSTPROCEDURE CARE
Throat culture: done to identify infective organisms.	Tell the patient a swab will be used to collect a specimen from the back of the throat. Analysis of the specimen will reveal the infecting organism, if any.	No special care is required.
Laryngoscopy: permits visualization of the larynx. Video laryngoscopes may be used.	Patient should be NPO for several hours before the procedure. Administer drugs as ordered to decrease secretions and to relax the patient. Note allergies to local anesthetics on the patient's chart and identification band.	Monitor vital signs and respiratory status according to agency protocol. NPO until the gag reflex returns. Then provide lozenges or gargles as ordered for sore throat. Discourage talking, coughing, or clearing the throat for several hours after the procedure.
Pulmonary Function Tests		
Used to evaluate lung function, gas exchanges, pulmonary blood flow, and acid-base balance.	Advise the patient not to smoke or eat a heavy meal for 4 to 6 hours before the test. Patient should void before the tests. Determine whether any medications or treatments should be withheld.	Resume medications. No special care is required.

Table 25.2 Diagnostic Tests and Procedures: Respiratory System—cont'd

MISCELLANEOUS PROCEDURES		
TEST AND PURPOSE	**PATIENT PREPARATION**	**POSTPROCEDURE CARE**
Flexible Bronchoscopy		
Used to visualize abnormalities, take biopsy samples of lesions, or remove foreign bodies. Moderate sedation may be used.	Obtain signed consent. Patient should be NPO for 6 to 8 hours or as specified. Have the patient remove any dentures and provide oral hygiene. Document any loose teeth. Ask the patient not to smoke. Administer sedative and drugs used to dry secretions as ordered.	NPO until gag reflex returns. Semi-Fowler position. Monitor vital signs. Immediately report the following signs of complications: gross hemoptysis, swelling of face and neck, stridor, decreased or asymmetric chest movement, diminished lung sounds, and dyspnea.
Thoracentesis		
Pleural fluid is aspirated with a needle inserted between the ribs. Ultrasound guidance may be used. Fluid is examined for pathogens and other abnormal components. Cells are studied for malignancy.	Obtain signed consent. Stress the importance of not moving or coughing during the procedure. Support the patient during the thoracentesis and monitor their skin color, respiratory rate, and general response. Label any specimens and send them to the laboratory.	Document the amount and color of fluid removed. Monitor the patient's vital signs, lung sounds, and chest movement. Check the dressing for bleeding. Immediately report dyspnea and asymmetric chest movement if present.
Radiographic and Imaging Studies		
General nursing actions: Confirm that signed consent has been obtained, if required. Inform the patient what to expect during the procedure. Inform patient if fasting is required. **Dye precautions:** If contrast dye is to be used, assess for allergy to iodine or shellfish; notify radiologist if patient reports allergy. When dye is given, increased fluids after the procedure are advised to promote dye excretion.		
Chest Radiography		
Used to screen and diagnose some respiratory disorders.	Patient will be asked to remove jewelry on the neck and chest and clothing above waist and to put on hospital gown.	No special care is required.
Fluoroscopy		
Used to provide motion radiographs of lungs.	Preparation is the same as for chest radiography.	No special care is required.
Ventilation-Perfusion Scan (Lung Scan)		
Used to demonstrate lung ventilation and perfusion. Detects pulmonary embolism (PE) and other obstructive conditions.	Assure the patient that the radiation dose is small, that the isotope is quickly eliminated, and that the procedure is painless except for venipuncture. If sedation is needed for agitated patients or small children, the patient is usually maintained NPO for 4 hours. The procedure takes approximately 30 minutes to 1 hour. Monitor the patient for 1 hour after the procedure for anaphylaxis.	Check the venipuncture site. Apply a small dressing and pressure if needed. Radioactive material is excreted in the urine. Tell the patient to wash their hands after voiding. Anyone who handles the patient's urine should wear rubber gloves. Gloves and hands should be washed after urine is discarded.
Computed Tomography		
Used to visualize lesions, tumors, and fractures. Contrast medium may be used.	Inform the patient that the procedure is painless. Stress the importance of remaining still during the scanning. Dye precautions (see above). NPO status may be required.	Assess the patient for side effects of contrast: headache, nausea, vomiting.
Magnetic Resonance Imaging		
Produces images of multiple body planes without radiation. Used to detect abnormalities, lesions, and tumors. Contrast medium may be used.	Obtain signed consent. Inform the patient that they will lie on a stretcher that slides into a tube-like device; mechanical clanging noises are heard as the machine operates. Aneurysm clips, intraocular metal, heart valves made before 1964, and middle-ear prostheses generally contraindicate MRI. MRI may also affect metal implants such as cardiac pacemakers and orthopedic implants, but they are not absolute contraindications. Assess the patient for claustrophobia; if found, report it to the physician. Patients who are anxious or restless may require sedation. Special equipment must be used for oxygen (O_2) therapy or mechanical ventilation. Have the patient remove metal watches and other jewelry.	Use safety precautions if the patient is sedated; otherwise, no special care is needed.

Continued

Table 25.2 Diagnostic Tests and Procedures: Respiratory System—cont'd

MISCELLANEOUS PROCEDURES		
TEST AND PURPOSE	**PATIENT PREPARATION**	**POSTPROCEDURE CARE**
Laboratory Studies		
General nursing actions: Inform the patient that a blood sample or urine sample will be required and whether fasting is necessary. After venipuncture, apply pressure and a Band-Aid; check for oozing.		
Arterial Blood Gas Analysis		
Used to detect alkalosis or acidosis and alterations in oxygenation status.	Tell the patient that a blood sample will be drawn from an artery (usually the radial artery). An Allen test or modified Allen test *must* be done before an arterial puncture to ensure that the arteries to the hand are patent. (Arterial punctures require specialized training.) Rotate sites for repeated punctures.	Apply pressure to the puncture site for 5 to 10 minutes. Note on the laboratory slip the concentration of any O_2 therapy. Transport the blood gas syringe containing the specimen to the laboratory in an ice bath within 15 minutes. Follow agency procedure for handling and transporting specimen to lab.
Sputum Analysis		
Volume, consistency, odor, color provide clues to clinical disorders. Sputum culture and sensitivity (C&S) reveals pathogens and effective antimicrobials. Sputum for cytology detects malignant cells and inflammatory changes.	Collect the specimen early in the morning before breakfast. Provide a sterile container. Instruct the patient to (1) brush the teeth and rinse the mouth, (2) cough deeply and expectorate directly into the container, (3) immediately cap the container, and (4) inform the nurse that the specimen is ready.	For cytology, a special container and solution must be used for specimens. Send the specimen to the laboratory promptly. Refrigerate if it will be more than 1 hour before delivery to the laboratory. Notify the laboratory if an unusual agent is suspected or if the patient is suspected of having a highly contagious disease.
T-SPOT TB Test		
Blood test used to detect tuberculosis. Preferred over skin test for persons who have received BCG vaccine.	No special preparation	No special aftercare
Quantiferon-TB Gold		
Blood test that assists in diagnosis of active or latent tuberculosis. Is an alternative to the tuberculin skin test.	No special preparation	No special aftercare. Follow laboratory instructions for handling specimen very carefully or the results may be invalid. Results in 24 hours.
Tuberculin Skin Test		
Used to determine past or present exposure to tuberculosis. A small amount of a purified protein derivative is injected. A person who has been exposed to TB will have a local reaction in 2 to 3 days.	Inform the patient that the procedure causes brief pain. Cleanse the skin, and inject it intradermally into the lower anterior forearm. Mark and record the site. Tell the patient that a skin reaction may persist for 1 week and not to scratch it. Stress the need to return to the clinic in 48 to 72 hours so that the reaction can be read. A reaction (swelling, redness) of 5 mm or more is positive for tuberculosis exposure. A patient who has ever been vaccinated with BCG may test positive regardless of actual exposure.	Follow-up depends on the response to the test. If it is positive, the patient will be evaluated for active tuberculosis.

BCG, Bacillus Calmette-Guérin; *MRI*, magnetic resonance imaging; *NPO*, nothing by mouth.

LARYNGOSCOPY

Laryngoscopy is the inspection of the larynx to aid in diagnosis of abnormalities or to remove foreign bodies. A laryngoscopy may be either direct or indirect. In the direct procedure, the physician uses a fiberoptic laryngoscope (a flexible lighted tube). The indirect procedure uses mirrors to visualize the larynx. Contrast medium is sometimes instilled to outline the structures in the larynx. A tissue specimen may be taken for examination.

FIBEROPTIC BRONCHOSCOPY

A bronchoscopic examination is performed by inserting a flexible fiberoptic scope through the nose or mouth

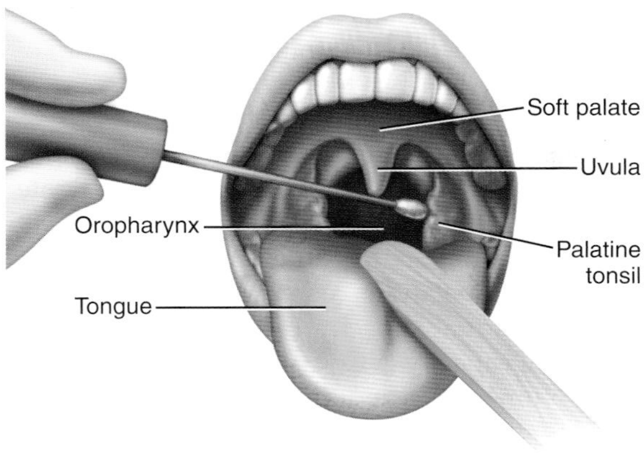

Fig. 25.6 Throat culture technique. (From Harkreader H, Hogan MA, Thobaben M: *Fundamentals of nursing: caring and clinical judgment*, ed 3, St. Louis, 2007, Saunders.)

into the bronchial tree after local anesthesia of the patient's throat. The scope allows for direct visualization of the bronchial tree structures for assessment, diagnosis, or removal of foreign bodies or mucus plugs. Lesions suggestive of malignancy may be located and a biopsy performed as well. Before the procedure, signed consent should be obtained. Have the patient remove dentures. Give sedatives as ordered. Afterward, monitor the patient's respiratory status and level of consciousness. The patient should take nothing by mouth (NPO) until the gag reflex returns. Complications of bronchoscopy include bronchospasm, bacteremia, bronchial perforation, pneumonia, laryngospasm, hemorrhage, and pneumothorax. Alternatives to flexible bronchoscopy include rigid bronchoscopy, virtual bronchoscopy (using imaging technology).

RADIOLOGIC STUDIES

Chest Radiography

Radiographic examination of the chest is one of the most frequently used methods for respiratory screening and diagnosis. It is also used to assess progression of a disease and response to treatment. The radiograph (x-ray) produces a picture in which the bony structures (e.g., ribs, sternum, clavicle), heart shadow, trachea, bronchi, and blood vessels are visible. Bone appears white on the film because it is very dense and does not absorb much energy. In contrast, the lungs appear black because they are filled with air and absorb the x-ray energy. Chest films are usually taken posteroanterior (back to front), anteroposterior (front to back), and lateral (side) to view the chest cavity from different angles.

Fluoroscopy

Fluoroscopy is a radiograph of the chest taken to observe deep structures in motion. It is possible to observe both lungs at the same time during inspiration and expiration. Instead of producing a single, still image, the screen registers a constant image of the chest.

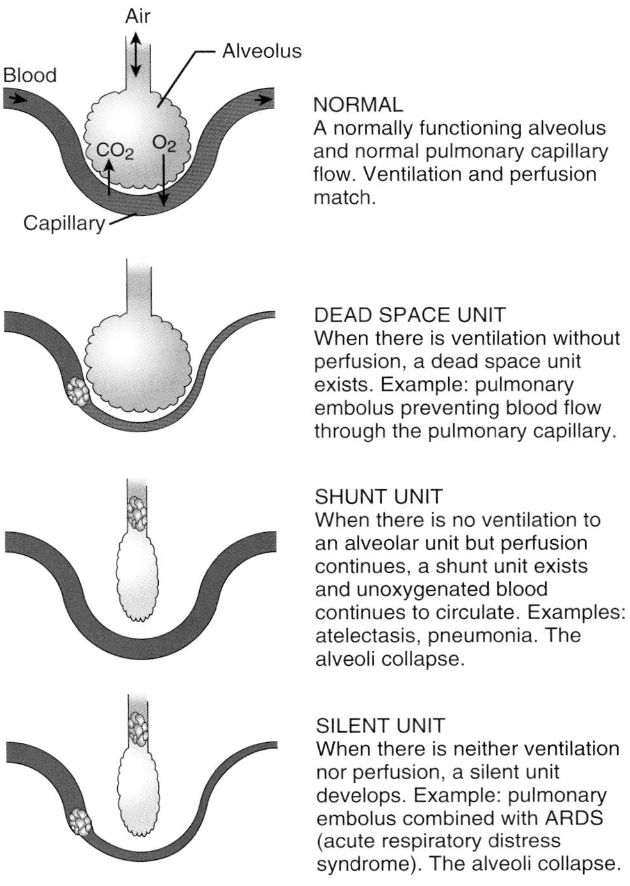

Fig. 25.7 Normal functioning alveolus and pulmonary capillary blood flow. When both are normal, the ventilation and perfusion match. Blockage of the bronchiole or the pulmonary capillary creates a ventilation-perfusion mismatch. CO_2, Carbon dioxide; O_2, oxygen. (From Black JM, Hawks JH: *Medical-surgical nursing: clinical management for positive outcomes*, ed 8, St. Louis, 2009, Saunders.)

The fluoroscopic examination can give information about the speed and degree of lung expansion and structural defects in the bronchial tree.

Ventilation-Perfusion Scan

When the lungs are working efficiently, a balance exists in the ventilation-perfusion ratio, which means that areas receiving ventilation are well perfused with blood and areas perfused with blood are well ventilated. When the alveolus and pulmonary blood flow are normal, ventilation and perfusion are said to match. A mismatch occurs when there is ventilation without perfusion or perfusion without ventilation, as illustrated in Fig. 25.7.

A lung scan or ventilation-perfusion scan is used to assess lung ventilation and lung perfusion. Its chief purpose is to detect pulmonary embolism (PE) or some other obstruction. The patient is given a radioactive substance either by inhalation (to evaluate ventilation) or intravenously (to evaluate perfusion). Ventilation images are compared with the pictures taken during the perfusion scan to determine whether an equal amount of radioactivity exists on both the ventilation and the perfusion pictures. Any areas indicating good ventilation but poor perfusion suggest the presence of a pulmonary embolus or obstruction.

IMAGING PROCEDURES

Computed Tomography

Tomography or tomograms allow visualization of slices or layers of the chest. A computed tomography (CT) scan is a computerized method of tomography in which a camera rotates in a circular pattern around the body to provide a three-dimensional assessment of the thorax. The test is usually used to look for the presence of lesions or tumors.

Radioactive dye containing iodine may be injected intravenously. Each layer of the chest is photographed before and after the injection of the dye. It is extremely important to find out whether the patient is allergic to iodine before the procedure is performed. Make sure to ask the patient about allergies to shellfish, which contain iodine. Failure to determine sensitivity to iodine could result in an allergic reaction, anaphylaxis, and death.

Pharmacology Capsule

Dyes used in computed tomography (CT) contain iodine, which can produce fatal reactions in people with iodine allergies. Patients known to be allergic to iodine can be premedicated with antihistamines and corticosteroids to prevent a reaction, or a nonallergenic contrast medium that does not contain iodine can be used.

Magnetic Resonance Imaging

A magnetic resonance imaging (MRI) scan is similar to a CT scan but without the harmful radiation. The MRI scanner encloses the patient in a donut-shaped magnet and picks up signals from the body to make electronic images. The patient must remain as quiet and as motionless as possible during the procedure. No preparation is necessary, but patients should be warned that no metal may be worn inside the unit (with the exception of dental fillings). Patients with implanted devices, such as pacemakers and orthopedic plates, pins, or screws may be ineligible for MRI scanning.

Positron Emission Tomography

Positron emission tomography (PET) scans of the lungs are used most often to distinguish malignant from benign cells and to evaluate the effectiveness of cancer treatment. PET scans use special radionuclides attached to a natural body compound, usually glucose. This substance is administered to the patient intravenously and the radioactivity localizes in the appropriate areas of the body and is detected by the PET scanner. Cancerous tissue, which uses more glucose than normal tissue does, will accumulate more of the substance and appear brighter than normal tissue on the PET images. The patient must remain quiet, avoiding movement or talking during the test. Because glucose is the substance most often tagged with the radionuclides, it is important to ensure that the patient has not eaten for at least 4 hours before the test.

PULMONARY FUNCTION TESTS

Pulmonary function tests are used to diagnose pulmonary disease, monitor disease progression, evaluate the extent of disability, and assess the effects of medication. The tests measure lung volumes and capacities including total lung capacity, forced expiratory volume (FEV), functional residual capacity (FRC), inspiratory capacity (IC), vital capacity (VC), forced vital capacity (FVC), minute volume (MV), and thoracic gas volume (TGV).

A clip is applied to the nose, and the patient breathes through a mouthpiece as directed while various measurements are taken to assess the mechanics of breathing (flow rates of gas in and out of the lungs) and to measure diffusion (the movement of the gas across the alveolar-capillary membrane).

Spirometry

A spirometer is an instrument that measures the ventilatory function of the lung. It measures the volume of air that the lung can hold, the rate of flow of air in and out of the lung, and the compliance (elasticity) of lung tissue. The test enables the physician to detect impaired pulmonary function, classify the pulmonary impairment, estimate the severity of the impairment, monitor the cause of pulmonary disease, evaluate treatment, give information helpful in planning care, and provide preoperative assessment.

The test involves inserting a mouthpiece; taking as deep a breath as possible; and blowing as hard, as fast, and for as long as possible. Patients should be encouraged to continue blowing out until exhalation is complete.

Spirometry measures FVC and FEV. These and other lung volumes and capacities are defined in Table 25.3.

People who are to undergo spirometry should be taught what to expect during the test and how to prepare. They may be anxious about taking a breathing test if they have respiratory problems because they may fear increased dyspnea or exhaustion. They should be advised not to smoke or use bronchodilator medications for 4 to 6 hours before testing.

Pharmacology Capsule

Bronchodilators should not be given before pulmonary function testing because they can alter the results.

Arterial Blood Gas Analysis

Ventilation and diffusion are also measured by testing for concentrations of O_2 and CO_2 in the arterial blood to determine whether the exchange is adequate across the alveolar membrane. Blood gas analysis is useful in the care of patients with respiratory disorders, problems of circulation and distribution of blood, body fluid imbalances, and acid-base imbalances. Drawing an arterial blood sample requires special training. Samples

Table 25.3 Lung Volumes and Capacities

VOLUME	DEFINITION	SIGNIFICANCE OF INCREASE	SIGNIFICANCE OF DECREASE
Total lung capacity	Total lung volume when fully inflated	Overdistention of lung caused by obstructive lung disease	Restrictive lung disease
Forced expiratory volume (FEV)	Volume of air expired during specified time intervals (0.5, 1.0, 2.0, 3.0 seconds)	Not significant	Restrictive or obstructive lung disease depending on measurements at time intervals
Functional residual capacity (FRC)	Volume of air remaining in the lungs after normal exhalation	Chronic obstructive pulmonary disease (COPD)	Acute respiratory distress syndrome (ARDS)
Inspiratory capacity (IC)	Maximum volume of air that can be inhaled after a normal exhalation	Excessive use of positive end-expiratory pressure	Restrictive lung disease
Vital capacity (VC)	Total volume of air that can be exhaled after maximum inspiration	Not significant; increased or normal VC with normal flow rates: pulmonary edema	Decreased VC with normal or increased flow rates: impaired respiratory effort
Forced vital capacity (FVC)	Total volume of air exhaled rapidly and forcefully after maximum inhalation	Not significant	Obstructive or restrictive lung disease
Minute volume (MV)	Total amount of air breathed in 1 min	Not significant	Restrictive parenchymal lung disease; fatigue
Thoracic gas volume (TGV)	Total volume of air in the lungs, including ventilated and nonventilated areas	Obstructive lung disease with air trapping	Not significant

are often obtained from the radial artery after first performing the Allen test to ensure adequate circulation to the hand from other arteries (Fig. 25.8). After the arterial puncture, pressure must be applied for 5 to 10 minutes to ensure no bleeding. If the radial artery cannot be used, several other options including the brachial artery are available. In the critical care setting, the physician may place an arterial line, commonly called an *ART line*. This line allows for frequent monitoring of arterial blood gases without repeated arterial punctures.

The arterial blood sample is analyzed for pH, $PaCO_2$ (partial pressure of carbon dioxide in arterial blood), PaO_2 (partial pressure of oxygen in arterial blood), HCO_3^- (bicarbonate), and O_2 saturation to detect alkalosis or acidosis and alterations in oxygenation status. Normal values for adults are pH 7.35 to 7.45, $PaCO_2$ 35 to 45 mm Hg, PaO_2 80 to 100 mm Hg (some references give a lower limit of 75 mm Hg), HCO_3^- 22 to 26 mEq/L, and O_2 saturation 96% to 100%.

PULSE OXIMETRY

Pulse oximetry permits the noninvasive measurement of O_2 saturation. A sensor is clipped to an earlobe or fingertip. A beam of light passes through the tissue, and the amount of light absorbed by O_2-saturated hemoglobin is measured. The O_2 saturation is presented as a percentage and registered on a digital readout. Factors that interfere with accurate measurement of the oximeter are hypotension, hypothermia, vasoconstriction, and finger movement. Normal pulse oximetry is 95% or higher. Notify your supervisor or the physician of readings lower than 90%.

SPUTUM ANALYSIS

Sputum is material that originates in the bronchi. Sputum analysis may be performed when respiratory disease is suspected. The mucous membrane lining of the lower respiratory tract responds to acute inflammation by increasing the production of secretions, which may contain bacterial or malignant cells. These cells may be detected by examination of sputum. Sputum specimens are also examined for volume, consistency, color, and odor. Sputum that is thick, foul smelling, and yellow, green, or rust colored may indicate a bacterial infection. Instruct the patient to expectorate the specimen directly into a sterile container after coughing deeply. If the patient is unable to expectorate a specimen, sputum production may be induced with aerosol therapy or obtained by suctioning.

Culture and Sensitivity

Sputum culture and sensitivity tests are ordered to determine the presence of bacteria, identify the specific organisms, and identify appropriate antimicrobials. Collect specimens before antimicrobial therapy begins to ensure that sufficient bacterial growth is present.

Acid-Fast Test

An acid-fast test on a sputum specimen is performed to determine the presence of acid-fast bacilli, which include the bacteria that cause tuberculosis. Specimens are usually collected on 3 consecutive days. Keep each sputum specimen covered and refrigerated or delivered to the laboratory within 1 hour. Use a new sterile container for each collection.

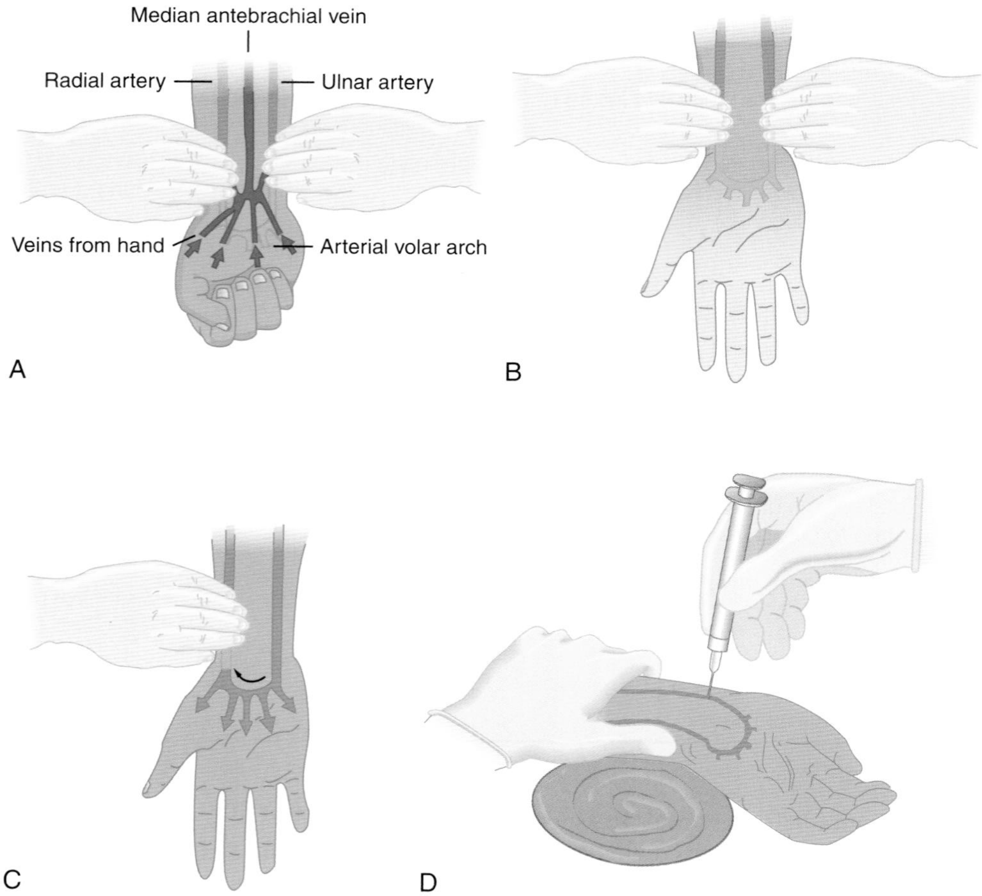

Fig. 25.8 The Allen test should be done before each radial arterial puncture to ensure adequate collateral circulation. Because an arterial puncture may injure the radial artery, the adequacy of blood supply to the area by other arteries must be determined. A puncture is not done on an artery if the other blood supply is not adequate. (A) To perform the Allen test, occlude the radial and ulnar arteries and have the patient make a fist. (B) While maintaining pressure on the arteries, have the patient open the hand. The hand is pale if the arteries are occluded. (C) Release the pressure on the ulnar artery. If collateral circulation is adequate, color will return to the hand. This is a positive Allen test result; the puncture can proceed on the radial artery. If color does not return, the Allen test result is negative, and the radial artery should not be punctured. (D) A blood sample is drawn from the radial artery after a positive Allen test result. (From Black JM, Hawks JH: *Medical-surgical nursing: clinical management for positive outcomes*, ed 8, St. Louis, 2009, Saunders.)

Cytologic Specimens

Sputum specimens are obtained for cytologic examination to determine the presence of lung carcinoma or infectious conditions. Because sputum contains cells from the tracheobronchial tree, malignant cells may be detected in the specimen. A special container with fixative solution may be used for this type of specimen collection. Consult the agency laboratory manual for directions.

Additional details about diagnostic tests and procedures are presented in Table 25.2.

COMMON THERAPEUTIC MEASURES

Classes of drugs used to treat conditions of the respiratory system include adrenergic agents (sympathomimetics), anticholinergics, antihistamines, corticosteroids, antipyretics, analgesics, anesthetics, and antiinfectives. Examples of these drugs, their uses and side effects, and nursing interventions are presented in Table 25.4.

NOSE DROPS

Some drugs are given by the nasal route, primarily to decrease nasal congestion and obstruction. Many OTC nasal decongestants are available. Occasional use is not thought to be harmful, but frequent use is believed to damage the protective mechanisms in the nose. This increases the likelihood of additional obstruction and infection.

To administer nose drops, the patient may be sitting or lying down and the head must be tilted back so that the solution flows into the back of the nose. First ask the patient to blow the nose unless contraindicated. Gently push the tip of the nose upward. Place the dropper at the opening of the nostril, and squeeze to deliver the prescribed amount of medication. The dropper should not touch the nose. The patient should keep their head tilted back for several minutes. The patient may report feeling medication run down the throat. Provide a tissue for any nasal

Table 25.4 Drug Therapy: Drugs Used to Treat Respiratory Disorders

DRUG CLASSES AND EXAMPLES	USE AND ACTION	SIDE EFFECTS	NURSING INTERVENTIONS
Topical Anesthetics			
Lidocaine spray (Xylocaine, Lidoderm)	Applied to nasopharynx and oropharynx before bronchoscopy for anesthetic effect.	Allergy, sensitization, rash, burning, stinging. When sprayed on throat, can decrease gag reflex and cause dysphagia. If absorbed, lidocaine can cause drop in pulse and BP.	Assess gag reflex before giving oral fluids or food. Monitor pulse, BP, and mental status.
Decongestants			
Oral: pseudoephedrine (Sudafed) **Topical:** azelastine (Astepro) **Topical and oral forms:** phenylephrine (e.g., Neo-Synephrine) Numerous other decongestants available.	Constricts blood vessels to reduce swelling of mucous membranes. Used to treat nasal discharge, common cold.	Occasional mild CNS stimulation, especially in older adults. Toxicity can cause dizziness, tachycardia, palpitations, nausea, vomiting, hallucinations, and seizures.	Monitor pulse, BP, and mental and emotional state. Sudafed used with caution in those with severe hypertension and coronary artery disease, as well as those who are breastfeeding. Contraindicated in pregnancy. Tell patients to swallow extended-release tablets whole.
Antitussives			
Opioid antitussives: codeine, hydrocodone **Nonopioid antitussives:** dextromethorphan (Benylin, Robitussin, et al.) diphenhydramine (e.g., Benadryl), benzonatate (Tessalon, Zonatuss)	Suppresses cough reflex. Appropriate to control nonproductive cough or cough that interferes with rest or wound healing. Lack of evidence of value with common cold.	Codeine antitussive is a Schedule V controlled substance. Is an opioid and therefore has abuse potential and can cause sedation. Overdose can cause respiratory depression. Dextromethorphan does not depress respiration; can cause euphoria in high doses.	Encourage fluids unless contraindicated to facilitate expectoration of secretions. Take safety measures with codeine.
Antihistamines			
First-generation sedating: diphenhydramine (Benadryl) **Second-generation nonsedating:** loratadine (Claritin), cetirizine (Zyrtec)	Blocks histamine. Dries respiratory secretions. Antiemetic and sedative effects. Used to treat allergic reactions and prevent motion sickness.	Drowsiness with first-generation drugs. Dry mouth, blurred vision, photophobia, thickening of mucus secretions, decreased sweating, constipation, urinary retention, and increased heart rate. Some patients experience nervousness, stimulation, sleep disturbances.	Take safety precautions if the patient is drowsy and monitor pulse and respiratory status (not recommended for patients with asthma). Encourage fluids if not contraindicated. Monitor elimination. Oral hygiene. Give with food if drug causes gastric distress.
Expectorants			
guaifenesin (e.g., Mucinex, Robitussin)	Increases and thins respiratory secretions for easier expectoration.	Nausea and vomiting with large doses.	Assess the patient's cough productivity. Do not crush sustained-release capsules.
Mucolytics			
acetylcysteine (Acetadote) hypertonic saline	Given by inhalation to reduce viscosity and elasticity of mucus.	Both can trigger bronchospasm. Acetylcysteine has unpleasant odor.	Monitor response for increased dyspnea. Administer bronchodilator as ordered 10 to 15 min before acetylcysteine.

Continued

Table 25.4 Drug Therapy: Drugs Used to Treat Respiratory Disorders—cont'd

DRUG CLASSES AND EXAMPLES	USE AND ACTION	SIDE EFFECTS	NURSING INTERVENTIONS
Bronchodilators			
• Methylxanthines • Adrenergic agonists: nonselective and $beta_2$ selective • Anticholinergics **Note:** The following drugs combine a bronchodilator and a corticosteroid: Symbicort, Advair Diskus, Dulera			
	All relax smooth muscle in the bronchial tree to relieve bronchial constriction.		
Methylxanthines oral theophylline (e.g., Theo-24, Elixophyllin)	Methylxanthines also cause increased heart rate and force of cardiac contraction, CNS stimulation, and increased gastric acid secretion.	Anxiety, restlessness, tachypnea, tachycardia, dysrhythmias, and GI distress. Rapid intravenous administration can cause hypotension and fatal dysrhythmias.	Monitor vital signs, mental state, and serum drug levels. Measure the intake and output. Give drug with milk or food to decrease GI distress. Do not administer the drug before bedtime because it may keep the patient awake.
Nonselective beta-adrenergic agonists: epinephrine, isoproterenol hydrochloride (Isuprel), ephedrine	Nonselective adrenergic drugs also decrease mucus secretion, increase mucociliary clearance, and stabilize mast cells. Significant cardiac stimulation.	Restlessness, anxiety, tachycardia, headache, hypertension, disorientation, nausea, vomiting, and diarrhea.	Do not exceed the prescribed dosage. Teach the patient to use an inhaler and to rinse the mouth after inhalation to decrease dryness and irritation. Avoid excessive caffeine. Monitor the respiratory and cardiovascular status.
Selective $beta_2$-adrenergic agonists: **Inhaled short-acting:** albuterol (Proventil, et al.), levalbuterol (Xopenex, et al.). **Inhaled long-acting:** aclidinium (Tudorza), formoterol (Perforamist), salmeterol (Serevent Discus). **Oral agents:** albuterol (VoSpire ER), terbutaline (generic only)	Relax muscles in bronchi to relieve bronchoconstriction.	Selective $beta_2$ agonists can cause tachycardia, angina, and tremors. Less cardiac stimulation than nonselective adrenergics. Adverse effects vary with route of administration and duration of action.	Monitor respiratory and cardiac status. Teach patient how to use inhaler: wait 1 min between inhalations. Explain whether drug is PRN or to be taken on fixed schedule.
Anticholinergic (muscarinic) bronchodilators **Inhaled muscarinics:** ipratropium bromide (Atrovent HFA), tiotropium (Spiriva), aclidinium (Tudorza Pressair)	Inhaled drugs act directly on the respiratory passages to cause bronchodilation. Not effective for acute asthma attacks.	Dry mouth, irritation of pharynx. Increased intraocular pressure with narrow-angle glaucoma. Rare: hypotension.	Monitor respiratory status. Evaluate the patient for improvement. Tell the patient not to use more than two inhalations at a time and to rinse the mouth after inhaling to reduce dry mouth and throat. Avoid excessive caffeine intake.
Antiinflammatory Drugs			
• Corticosteroids • Mast cell stabilizer: cromolyn • Leukotriene modifiers • IgE Antagonist: omalizumab			

Table 25.4 Drug Therapy: Drugs Used to Treat Respiratory Disorders—cont'd

DRUG CLASSES AND EXAMPLES	USE AND ACTION	SIDE EFFECTS	NURSING INTERVENTIONS
Corticosteroids **Oral:** prednisone (e.g., Novo-prednisone), methylprednisolone (e.g., Singulair), prednisolone (e.g., Orapred) **Inhalation:** beclomethasone (QVAR), budesonide (Pulmicort Flexhaler), circlesonide (Alvesco), et al.	Stabilize mast cells to reduce the release of mediators that cause inflammation and edema. Restore bronchodilator response to sympathomimetics in treating acute bronchial constriction. Administration routes include oral, parenteral, and inhalation.	Systemic therapy: water and sodium retention, potassium loss, abnormal fat distribution, hypertension, and GI distress. Masks signs of infection. Abrupt withdrawal can trigger adrenal insufficiency. Inhaled steroids: hoarseness oral yeast infections; systemic effects are possible with long-term use.	Monitor vital signs, weight, and electrolytes. Assess for subtle signs of infection and encourage the patient to rinse the mouth after inhalation.
Mast Cell Stabilizer			
cromolyn sodium (Intal)	Reduce the production of chemicals by the mast cells that cause bronchial constriction, edema, and inflammation. Help to reduce the frequency and severity of asthma attacks but do not stop asthma attacks. Administration routes include inhalation, nasal.	Wheezing, sneezing, and coughing. Occasional bronchoconstriction is possible. Rare side effects include allergies, headache, nausea, and increased urinary frequency.	Instruct the patient in self-medication and inform that excessive use can actually cause bronchoconstriction. Stress that the drug acts to prevent acute attacks; not treat them. Rinse the mouth after using an inhaler to reduce dry mouth effects. Monitor medication effects.
Leukotriene Inhibitors/Modifiers			
zafirlukast (Accolate)	Inhibit synthesis or receptors of substances that mediate allergic responses.	Headache, nausea, diarrhea, infection.	Take on empty stomach.
zileuton (Zyflo)	Prevent acute asthma attacks.	Elevated liver enzymes, pain, nausea, and headache.	Can be taken with or without food. Monitor the patient's liver function.
montelukast (e.g., Singulair)	Prevent bronchospasm.	Well tolerated and does not seem to cause liver damage.	Phenytoin can lower blood levels.
IgE Antagonists/Monoclonal Antibodies			
omalizumab (Xolair), mepolizumab (Nucala), reslizumab (Cinqair), roflumilast (Daliresp)	Given subcutaneously to relieve allergy-related asthma when preferred drugs (inhaled glucocorticoids) fail.	Risk of anaphylaxis and cancer. Injection site reactions, upper respiratory infection, headache. VERY expensive.	Observe the patient for 2 hours after each of the first three injections. Then, observe for 30 min after subsequent injections. Access to emergency services must be immediately available.
Sublingual Immunotherapy			
Oralair	Treats sneezing, runny nose, itching, and nasal congestion caused by grass allergy. Started 4 months before grass allergy season and continued until the end of the season.	Contains grass pollen extract. Can cause severe allergic reactions including facial and oral edema, esophagitis, anaphylaxis, throat tightness.	Instruct patient to allow tablet to dissolve under the tongue. Monitor patient for 30 min after first dose. If no adverse effects, subsequent doses can be taken at home. Instruct patient in use of epinephrine pen in case allergic reaction occurs.

BP, Blood pressure; *CNS*, central nervous system; *GI*, gastrointestinal; *ICH*, inhaled corticosteroids; *IgE*, immunoglobulin E.

drainage or expectorated solution. Discard any unused solution that remains in the dropper rather than returning it to the bottle.

Put On Your Thinking Cap!

When instilling nose drops, why should the dropper not touch the nose?

Some medications are available as sprays. Many sprays have pumps that administer metered doses. These require that the pump be depressed several times before using to fill the dose chamber. The drug is administered by holding the head upright, inserting the tip into the nostrils, and pumping 2 or 3 times. The patient then should inhale deeply through the nose.

Pharmacology Capsule

Chronic use of nasal decongestant sprays may damage the protective mechanisms of the nose and cause rebound congestion in which nasal blood vessels dilate and congestion recurs.

THORACENTESIS

A thoracentesis is the insertion of a large-bore needle through the chest wall into the pleural space. Usually the physician performs the procedure at the patient's bedside. Thoracentesis is done to remove pleural fluid, blood, or air or to instill medication. Pleural fluid may be removed to reduce respiratory distress caused by fluid accumulation in the pleural space. In addition, fluid obtained in the procedure may be studied to obtain blood cell counts or to measure protein, glucose, lactic dehydrogenase, fibrinogen, or amylase levels. The study of pleural fluids may aid in the diagnosis of infectious diseases and cancer.

The patient sits on the side of the bed and leans the upper torso over the bedside table with the head resting on folded arms or pillows (Fig. 25.9). If the patient is unable to sit up, a side-lying position with the head of the bed elevated 30 degrees may be used. The skin is cleansed thoroughly, and a local anesthetic is injected. The physician inserts a 20-gauge or larger needle between the ribs and through the parietal membrane. Fluid or air is then aspirated, the thoracentesis needle is removed, and a sterile dressing is applied to the puncture site. The patient is positioned on the unaffected side. A chest radiograph may be ordered after the procedure to detect any pulmonary complications caused by accidental injury to the lung. Complications of thoracentesis include air embolism, hemothorax, pneumothorax, and pulmonary edema. Immediately report uneven chest movements, respiratory distress, or hemorrhage to the supervisor and the physician. Details of nursing responsibilities are included in Box 25.2.

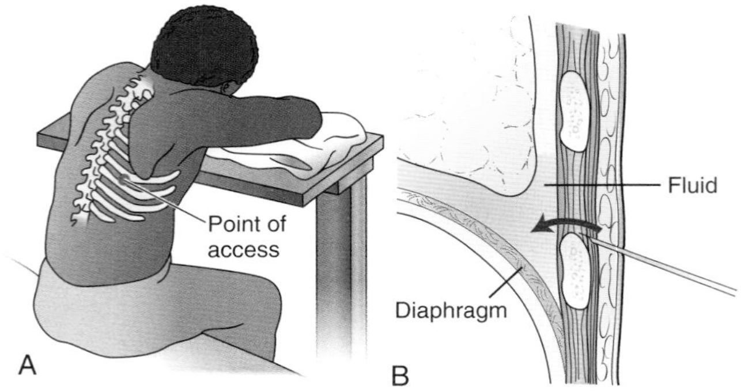

Fig. 25.9 (A) The patient is positioned for a thoracentesis. (B) The needle is inserted into the pleural space, avoiding lung tissue and the diaphragm. The exact location of the puncture varies. (From Buck CJ: *Step-by-step medical coding 2017*, St. Louis, 2017, Elsevier.)

BREATHING EXERCISES

Deep-Breathing and Coughing Exercises

Deep-breathing and coughing exercises are performed to aid in lung expansion and expectoration of respiratory secretions. They are indicated when patients are immobilized or after general anesthesia. Instructions to the patient include the following:

1. Sit in a semi-Fowler position for maximal lung expansion.
2. Place one hand on the abdomen to feel it rise and fall with breathing.
3. Inhale deeply through the nose, pause 1 to 3 seconds, and exhale slowly through the mouth.
4. After 4 to 6 deep breaths, cough deeply from the lungs to aid in the expectoration of sputum.
5. After thoracic or abdominal surgery, splint the incision with a pillow to minimize discomfort and support the incision.

Pursed-Lip Breathing

Another type of breathing exercise is pursed-lip breathing. It is used to inhibit airway collapse and to decrease dyspnea in patients with chronic lung disease. Instruct patients to pucker the lips as if to whistle, blow out a candle, or blow through a straw. They should then inhale through the nose and slowly exhale through pursed lips. Exhalation should last twice as long as inhalation.

Sustained Maximal Inspiration

Sustained maximal inspiration is used to ensure deep inspiration for maximal expansion and aeration of the lungs. An incentive spirometer is an instrument that is frequently used to encourage maximal inspiration. Spirometers basically consist of a cylinder that contains balls or disks and a tube through which the patient inhales. As the patient inhales through the tube, the balls or disks rise (Fig. 25.10). Instruct the patient to inhale deeply and slowly to move the balls or disks in the cylinder upward. For maximum effect, the spirometer is

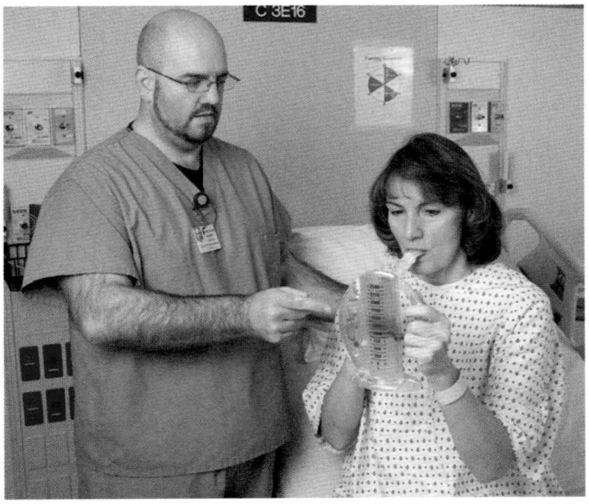

Fig. 25.10 Incentive spirometry encourages deep breathing by providing a visual cue to the patient about the efficiency of deep breathing. (From Potter PA, Perry AG, Stockert P, Hall A, editors: *Fundamentals of nursing*, ed 8, St. Louis, 2013, Mosby-Elsevier.)

kept upright because tilting the device reduces respiratory effort. Some spirometers provide a digital readout of the volume of air displaced. If the patient's maximal inspiration can be measured before surgery, that reading can be used as a target after surgery.

CHEST PHYSIOTHERAPY

Chest physiotherapy consists of percussion, vibration, and postural drainage. These mechanical techniques are used to facilitate the mobilization and expectoration of secretions in patients with large mucus-producing or chronic mucus-retaining respiratory disorders, such as chronic bronchitis and cystic fibrosis. Although this therapy is usually performed in the acute care setting by a respiratory therapist, the nurse often does this in long-term and home-care settings. Therefore you should be familiar with the procedures and be able to evaluate the patient's response. In an outpatient setting, you may also monitor the caregiver's technique in administering the treatment. Chest physiotherapy should be performed before meals to reduce the risk of regurgitation and aspiration of stomach contents. Chest physiotherapy can also cause a decrease in appetite, so the timing of the treatment should allow adequate time for the patient to regain their appetite.

Chest Percussion and Vibration

Chest percussion and vibration are performed to facilitate the movement of respiratory secretions, so that sputum can be expectorated. Percussion is clapping of the cupped palms against the chest wall to dislodge and mobilize respiratory secretions (Fig. 25.11A). The procedure is performed with the hands cupped to create a pocket of air when striking the patient's chest—first with one hand, and then with the other. Percussion is confined to areas protected by the rib cage and is never done over the sternum, kidney, liver, spleen, stomach, or spine. In general, percussion is done for 20 to 30 seconds, followed by vibration.

Vibration is performed by the therapist placing one hand on the top of the other, keeping the arms straight, and pressing the hands flat against the patient's chest (Fig. 25.11B). As the patient exhales, the therapist creates a shaking (vibrating) movement with the palms. The therapist pauses during inhalation. The vibration is repeated during three or four breathing cycles.

Devices designed to loosen and mobilize secretions include various mechanical vibrators, ultra-low-frequency airway oscillation devices, and manual percussor cups. Contraindications to percussion and vibration include lung cancer, bronchospasm, pain in the area being treated, hemorrhage, hemoptysis, increased intracranial pressure, chest trauma, PE, pulmonary edema, gastric reflux, pneumonectomy with open pericardium, extreme agitation or anxiety, and high risk for rib fractures.

Postural Drainage

Postural drainage is the technique of positioning the patient to facilitate gravitational movement of respiratory secretions toward the bronchi and trachea for expectoration. Various positions are used to drain all 18 segments of the lungs. If a patient cannot tolerate a specific position, it should be omitted or modified. Instruct the patient to breathe slowly and deeply throughout the procedure. Drain the upper lobes first and the posterior basal segments of the lower lobes last. The patient should not sit up between position changes. Provide tissues and a disposal receptacle. Maintain each position for 5 to 15 minutes. Perform postural drainage before meals or tube feedings. It may be ordered after respiratory treatments with bronchodilators. The frequency is ordered by the physician. Discontinue the procedure and inform the physician if the patient experiences a heart rate over 120 beats per minute, dysrhythmias, hypertension, hypotension, dizziness, or signs of hypoxemia.

Alternative Airway Clearance Techniques

Although the chest percussion and vibration are time-honored techniques for airway clearance, other techniques that are available are autogenic drainage, active cycle of breathing, and huffing. These are used by cystic fibrosis patients and are described by the Cystic Fibrosis Foundation at https://www.cff.org.

HUMIDIFICATION AND AEROSOL THERAPY

The upper respiratory system is designed to moisturize and warm the air that is inspired through the nose. Humidity is necessary in the respiratory tract to prevent secretions from becoming inspissated (thickened and dried). Inspissated secretions irritate the mucosa, making it more susceptible to bacterial infection.

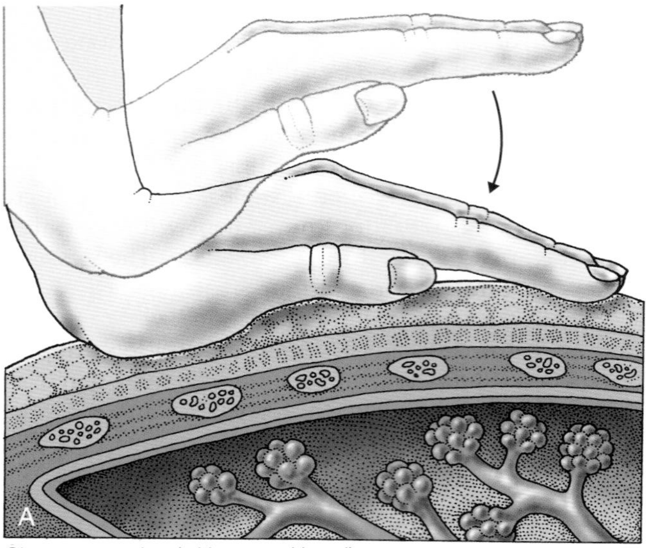

Chest percussion (with cupped hand)

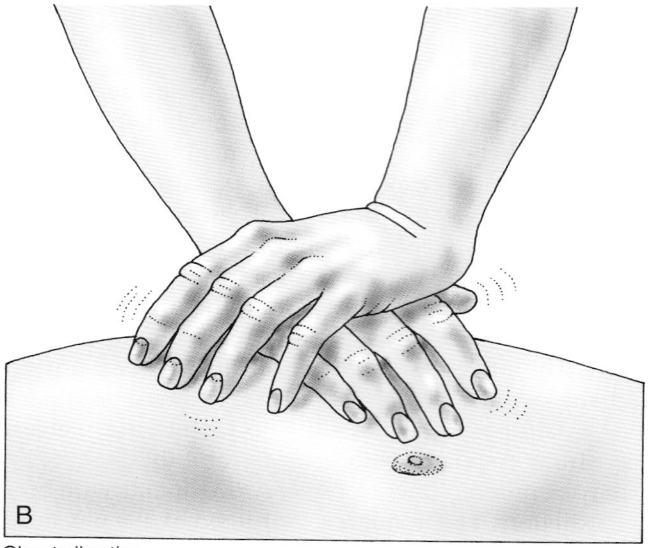

Chest vibration

Fig. 25.11 Chest physiotherapy. (A) Percussion. (B) Vibration. (Modified from Ignatavicius DD, Workman ML: *Medical-surgical nursing: patient-centered collaborative care*, ed 6, St. Louis, 2010, Saunders.)

Humidifiers

Inspiring dry air is uncomfortable, causes loss of body fluid, and can contribute to upper airway infections. Mouth breathing, necessitated by nasal obstruction, bypasses the turbinates that normally moisturize inspired air. A variety of devices are available to increase the humidity of inspired air.

Room humidifiers work in one of two ways: (1) by creating an aerosol or (2) by creating steam. Aerosols dispense tiny droplets of water into the room. Steam humidifiers increase humidity by distributing vaporized water (i.e., steam).

Because steam production requires raising water to the boiling point, steam humidifiers are not likely to become contaminated. Aerosol humidifiers, however, are easily contaminated. Therefore sterile distilled water should be used with aerosol units. Plain distilled water is acceptable with steam units.

With any type of room humidifier, the fluid reservoir should be checked and refilled regularly. Daily cleaning reduces the risk of bacterial contamination. Patients who use humidifiers at home should be shown how to care for the devices. Patients who use tap water in home units can clean them with a solution of 1 cup of white vinegar in 1 gallon of water. Advise them not to inhale aerosol directly from units that do not contain sterile water.

After nasal or sinus surgery, a bedside room humidifier may be ordered. A more effective option is a face tent or aerosol mask. Patients who have a tracheostomy inspire air directly into the trachea. Until the airway adjusts to this situation, humidification is essential to prevent excessive drying of the mucosa and secretions.

Aerosol Therapy

Aerosol therapy is used to liquefy and mobilize respiratory secretions and to deliver medications. Aerosols are suspended liquid particles of bronchodilators or inactive fluids such as water or saline that are delivered by devices called *nebulizers*. Nebulizers deliver a humidified aerosol through large tubing, which may be connected to an O_2 mask or a handheld device. When handheld nebulizers are used, the patient should sit upright and slowly inhale the nebulizer aerosol deeply, hold the breath briefly, and exhale slowly. Once secretions are mobilized, the patient may require deep-breathing and coughing techniques, postural drainage, suctioning, or a combination of these techniques to clear the secretions. Because aerosols can cause bronchospasm, bronchodilators may be ordered before administering some types of aerosol therapy. A risk of fluid retention, infection, and drug toxicity also exists.

Pharmacology Capsule

Oxygen (O_2) should be thought of as a pharmacologic agent with risks of adverse effects.

OXYGEN THERAPY

Air in the atmosphere contains approximately 21% O_2. Usually this is sufficient for oxygenation to maintain the tissue's ability to function normally. In the presence of cardiopulmonary disease or injury, it may be necessary to provide a patient with supplemental O_2, to enrich the atmospheric air with increased concentrations than the patient normally breathes. O_2 should be treated as a pharmacologic agent, as serious side effects (as well as benefits) may occur from its use.

O_2 therapy requires a medical order that should be carried out like any other drug order. If a patient

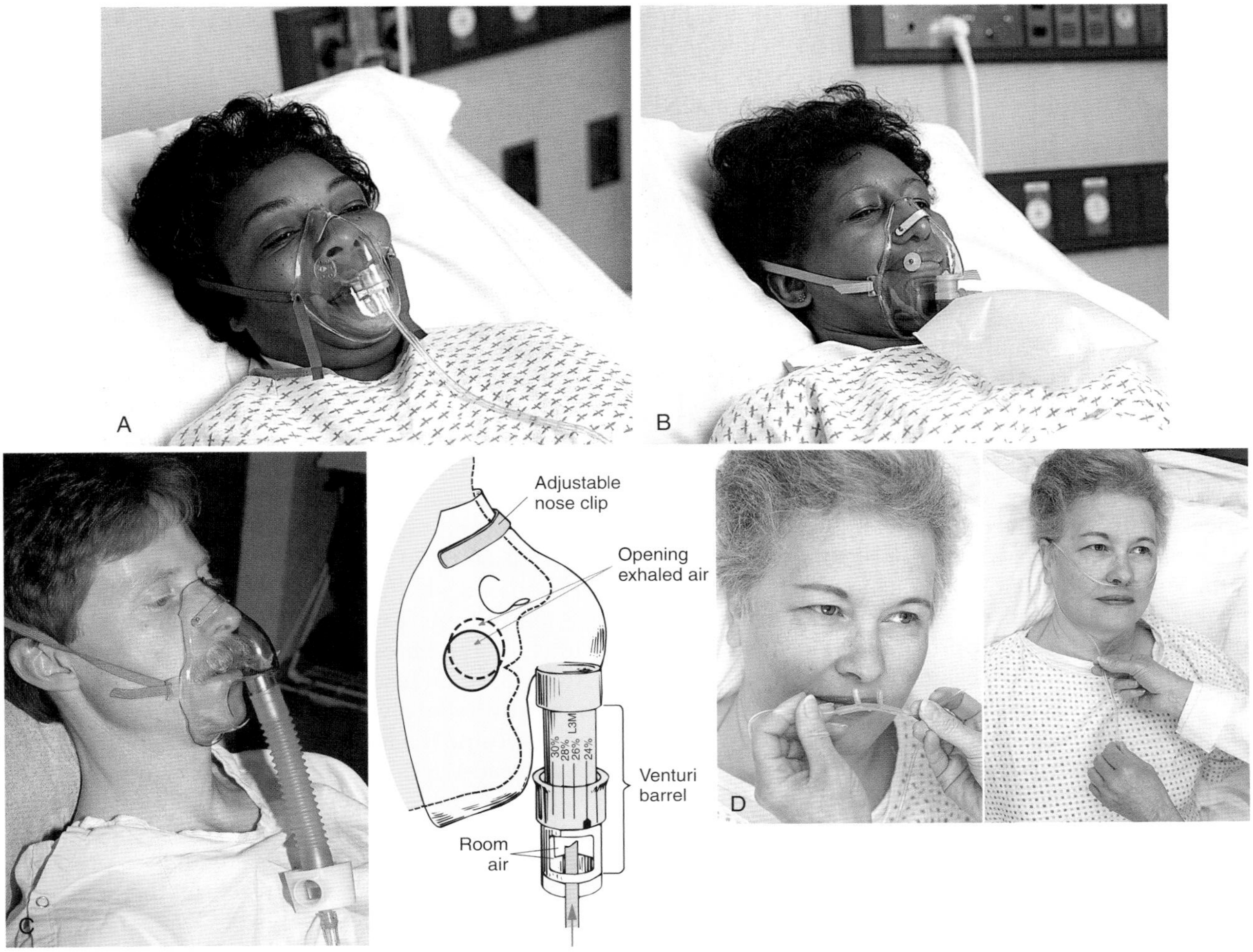

Fig. 25.12 Oxygen (O_2) delivery systems. (A) Standard O_2 mask. (B) Partial rebreathing O_2 mask. (C) Venturi O_2 mask. (D) Nasal cannula. (From Potter PA, Perry AG, Stockert P, Hall A, editors. *Fundamentals of nursing*, 8th ed. St. Louis, Mosby-Elsevier, 2013.)

is observed becoming lethargic or bradypneic (abnormally slow breathing), the nurse should immediately notify a supervisor or physician because these are symptoms of adverse effects of O_2 therapy.

To administer O_2 to the patient, it is necessary to alter the gas from a compressed form such as a bulk O_2 supply or cylinder to a form with a usable, safe flow rate. Modern hospitals have bulk O_2 systems with wall adapters to which flowmeters are attached. When patients with O_2 must be transported, a cylinder on wheels is necessary. A regulator with a flowmeter must be used. After a flowmeter has been attached to the O_2 source, it may be necessary to humidify the gas before delivering it to the patient. Humidification is usually unnecessary when using a low-flow cannula at a flow setting of 2 L (or less) per minute or when using an air entrainment (Venturi mask) O_2 delivery system.

A tube is needed to connect the flowmeter to the specific O_2 delivery device being used. In some devices, the tube is incorporated as an integral component, but in others it is not. It is possible to use extension tubes for some devices, but increasing the length of the tube increases the resistance to gas flow, thus causing pressure to back up in the system so that the patient may not receive the desired O_2 flow.

O_2 therapy is ordered in liters per minute—or fraction of inspired O_2 (FiO_2). This measurement is written, for example, as 0.30 FiO_2, which means 30% O_2 concentration. Various devices can deliver different amounts of O_2 (Fig. 25.12).

The most commonly used device is the nasal cannula, which fits around the face and directly into the nares by way of two prongs. It is designed to deliver a low flow of O_2 from 1 to 6 L/min with an approximate FiO_2 of 0.24 to 0.40 (24%–40% O_2). The nasal catheter is also a low-flow device that is inserted into one naris, and then into the pharyngeal space approximately at the uvula. The FiO_2 and flow rates are the same as those for the cannula. This catheter is rarely used, except during short-term procedures.

Four types of masks are available: (1) the simple oxygen mask, (2) the partial rebreathing mask,

(3) the nonrebreathing mask, and (4) the air entrainment (Venturi) mask. The simple O_2 mask is designed to deliver an FiO_2 ranging from 0.35 to 0.55 (35%–55% O_2). Flow rates from the flowmeter may be adjusted from 6 to 10 L/min. The minimum flow rate of 6 L/min is necessary to prevent any chance of CO_2 buildup from occurring. The partial rebreathing mask includes a reservoir bag to elevate the potential FiO_2. It is unique because the patient actually rebreathes part of the exhaled gas in the system. However, it is designed so that the rebreathed gas contains almost no CO_2 from the patient's lungs—only enriched O_2. The expected FiO_2 range is 0.35 to 0.60 (35%–60%). The flowmeter setting must be from 6 to 10 L/min. The nonrebreathing mask is so named because none of the patient's exhaled gas is rebreathed. Like the previous mask, it also includes a reservoir bag to enhance the FiO_2, but it has a series of valves to direct the flow of O_2 in such a way that the patient receives a fresh supply of gas with each breath. The expected FiO_2 should be near 1.0 (100%). However, experimental research has shown that the highest FiO_2 obtained is approximately 0.7 (70%). The air entrainment mask is designed to provide a specific FiO_2. This device has been called a *Ventimask* or a *Venturi mask* in the past and may still be referred to by these names. The manufacturers of these devices list a specific flowmeter setting for the desired FiO_2. It is also necessary either to adjust a setting on the device or to place a specific attachment on the mask to obtain the desired results. Read the literature accompanying the mask and, if there is confusion, consult a respiratory therapist.

Transtracheal O_2 therapy delivers O_2 through a small, flexible catheter that is inserted into the trachea through a small incision or with a special needle. This approach is used when long-term therapy is indicated.

Occasionally, an O_2 mask must be removed (e.g., for oral care, for eating and drinking). Ask the physician to write an order for the temporary use of a cannula during these times.

Advances in outpatient O_2 therapy have the potential to improve greatly the quality of life for patients with chronic pulmonary or cardiac conditions. Whereas patients used to have to rent large cylinders for home use, they can now rent O_2 concentrators that process room air and deliver air with an increased percentage of O_2. The concentrator is about the size of a canister vacuum cleaner and has a 50-foot tubing connected to a nasal cannula. This allows the patient considerable freedom of mobility in the home setting.

To leave the home, patients can use small tanks of compressed O_2. The tanks weigh approximately 3 lb and can deliver 2 L/min of O_2 for approximately 3 hours. A device that can be used with the canister delivers O_2 only "on demand," when the patient inhales. This conserves the O_2, making the canister last longer. Portable liquid O_2 canisters that can deliver a very high flow of O_2 are also available. These canisters can be refilled from a larger tank that can be kept in the patient's home. A weekend version of the tank fits in the backseat of a car and lasts several days. These devices allow considerable freedom for the patient.

The nurse must recognize the complications of O_2 therapy, including hypoventilation, toxicity, atelectasis, and ocular damage. Patients at the greatest risk for O_2-induced hypoventilation are those with chronic respiratory disorders. Because they may have become insensitive to high CO_2 levels in the blood, low O_2 levels in the blood serve as the stimulus for respirations ("hypoxic drive"). O_2 administration raises the level of O_2 in the blood, and the patient who has hypoxic drive may hypoventilate or even have apnea. The primary goal of supplemental oxygen for the patient with a chronic respiratory disorder is to maintain the pulse oxygen saturation (SpO_2) at 90% to 93% and the PaO_2 at 60 to 70 mm Hg. O_2 toxicity can result from exposure to a high concentration of O_2 for a prolonged period of time. Toxicity progresses from tracheobronchitis to lung fibrosis and atelectasis and may be fatal. Atelectasis can result from the replacement of nitrogen normally in the alveoli with O_2. O_2 is readily absorbed, predisposing the alveoli to collapse. Exposure to 100% O_2 can cause retinal injury and visual impairment.

The following are key points to consider when a patient is receiving O_2 therapy:

1. Monitor the liter flow to be sure it is as prescribed.
2. Assess the patient's response to O_2 therapy; monitor reports of blood gas analyses.
3. Inspect the tubing for kinks, obstructions, and loose connections; listen for a hissing sound in the O_2 mask; feel for adequate O_2 flow.
4. Maintain sterile water in the humidifier reservoir.
5. Clean and replace O_2 therapy equipment according to agency policy.
6. Post a NO SMOKING sign, and advise the patient and visitors that smoking is not allowed because O_2 supports combustion.
7. Monitor for potential skin breakdown around the oxygen delivery device.

INTERMITTENT POSITIVE PRESSURE BREATHING TREATMENTS

Intermittent positive pressure breathing (IPPB) treatments are used to achieve maximal lung expansion. The IPPB equipment delivers humidified gas with positive pressure, which forces air into the lungs with inhalation and allows passive exhalation. This facilitates maximal exchange of O_2 and CO_2 gases in the alveoli and promotes a productive cough. Aerosol medications, including mucolytics (which liquefy secretions) and bronchodilators, can be administered through IPPB treatments with a nebulizer device. Although respiratory therapists administer most IPPB treatments, in some settings, nurses administer them.

In the past, IPPB was used for a wide range of conditions. The American Association for Respiratory Care now recommends it only for specific conditions, including atelectasis, decreased lung compliance with kyphoscoliosis, and cardiogenic pulmonary edema. In addition to its limited usefulness, IPPB is losing favor because it may cause a tension pneumothorax in patients with COPD. It may also cause respiratory alkalosis because of hyperventilation. The desired effects of IPPB can usually be achieved by other, less expensive measures such as incentive spirometry and handheld nebulizers.

ARTIFICIAL AIRWAYS

Artificial airways are sometimes required to maintain a patent airway. Artificial airways include the oral airway, nasal airway, endotracheal tube, and tracheostomy tube.

Oral Airway

The oral airway is a curved tube used to maintain an airway temporarily. The oropharyngeal airway is inserted by tilting the head back, opening the mouth, and inserting the airway into the patient's mouth with the tip pointed toward the roof of the mouth. The tube is turned over while being advanced so that the end of the tube rests on the base of the patient's tongue.

Nasal Airway

A nasopharyngeal airway is a soft rubber tube that is inserted through the nose and extended to the base of the tongue. After ruling out a deviated septum, the nasal airway is coated with a water-soluble lubricant and inserted upward into the nose so that the distal end is located in the pharynx at the level of the base of the tongue. A nasal airway should be changed from one naris to the other every 8 hours.

Endotracheal Tube

An endotracheal tube is a long tube inserted through the mouth or nose into the trachea. These tubes have cuffs—inflatable balloons that seal the trachea to prevent aspiration of foreign material and to facilitate mechanical ventilation. Insertion of an endotracheal tube and care of the patient who is intubated require specialized training.

Tracheostomy Tube

A tracheostomy is a surgically created opening through the neck into the trachea. A variety of tracheostomy tubes exist, and they may be used with or without cuffs. Tracheostomy care and suctioning are discussed later in this chapter.

MECHANICAL VENTILATION

Mechanical ventilation is the process of providing respiratory support by means of a mechanical device called a *ventilator*. Ventilators are required most commonly for patients with acute respiratory failure who are unable to maintain adequate gas exchange in the lungs. This may be evidenced by tachypnea or bradypnea with an elevated or a stable $PaCO_2$, low PaO_2, or low pH. To ventilate a patient mechanically, a cuffed endotracheal or tracheostomy tube must be used to deliver the air. Once the tube is in place, the cuff must be inflated to create a closed system in the patient's airway. Otherwise, air being forced into the lungs could simply flow back out through the trachea.

A volume-limited ventilator is used most commonly for patients with acute respiratory failure. It inflates the lungs with a preset volume of oxygenated air that is delivered under pressure during the inspiratory cycle. The expiratory cycle may be conducted passively or with pressure as indicated.

Three types of positive pressure ventilators exist: (1) volume cycled, (2) pressure cycled, and (3) time cycled. A volume-cycled ventilator, which delivers a constant preset amount of oxygenated air to the patient, is the most commonly used type. A pressure-cycled ventilator, which pushes air into the lungs until a preset pressure is reached, is not widely used for continuous mechanical ventilation. Time-cycled ventilators deliver oxygenated air during a preset length of time. This type is used most frequently in infants and children.

Depending on the patient's needs, ventilators may be programmed to control or assist the rate of ventilation. The most frequently used modes are intermittent mandatory ventilation and synchronized intermittent mandatory ventilation. These modes provide assistance with ventilation by allowing the patient to breathe spontaneously between a preset number of ventilator breaths. Ventilators deliver O_2 ranging in concentration from 21% O_2 (atmospheric air) to 100% O_2. The O_2 concentration, or FiO_2, is adjusted for individual patient needs.

Tidal volume is the preset amount of oxygenated air delivered during each ventilator breath. This is usually 10 to 15 mL/kg of the patient's body weight.

The respiratory rate setting is the total number of breaths delivered per minute. The ventilator alone may govern the respiratory rate, or the ventilator and the patient's spontaneous respirations may determine it.

Positive end-expiratory pressure may be prescribed to keep the pressure in the lungs greater than the atmospheric pressure at the end of expiration. This reduces collapse of small airways and alveoli, thereby increasing the FRC and improving ventilation.

Other mechanical ventilation modalities include options, such as pressure support ventilation, flow-by ventilation, continuous positive airway pressure (CPAP) ventilation, and high-frequency ventilation. These are mentioned only for completeness and not for discussion. If the nurse encounters any of these modalities, specific training is needed that is beyond the scope of this text.

Like much other health care technology, mechanical ventilation can now be managed in the home. With proper training, a family member can manage these devices. Individuals with sleep apnea use a CPAP unit. CPAP maintains positive pressure in the airway during sleep, thereby preventing periods of apnea. CPAP units are small and have a face mask that is worn during sleep.

Nursing care of patients on mechanical ventilation requires special training, but key aspects of care include the following:

1. Monitor settings to ensure that they are set as prescribed.
2. Ensure that high- and low-pressure alarm settings are activated.
3. Have a manual resuscitator and O_2 source readily available.
4. Do not allow water to accumulate in the tubing.
5. Monitor the patient's vital signs and breath sounds; suction as necessary.
6. Establish an alternate method of communication because the patient cannot speak while intubated.

CHEST TUBES

Chest tubes are inserted to drain air or fluid from the pleural space of the lungs. This permits reexpansion of a collapsed lung in the patient with a hemothorax, pneumothorax, or pleural effusion. The physician inserts chest tubes under sterile conditions in the operating room or at the patient's bedside. Multiple tubes may be inserted. A small incision is made to insert one chest tube in the second to fourth intercostal space to remove air. A tube placed in the eighth or ninth intercostal space is for fluid removal. The tubes are sutured in place, and an airtight sterile dressing is applied. The distal ends of the plastic chest tubes are connected to sterile rubber tubing that leads to a pleural drainage device composed of three compartments: (1) the collection chamber, (2) the water seal chamber, and (3) the suction control chamber (Fig. 25.13). Chest fluid and air drain into the collection chamber. Air is diverted to the water seal chamber, where it can be seen bubbling up through the water. Suction pressure is controlled in the suction control chamber. The tubing in the suction chamber is partially submerged in water; the depth of the tube in the water regulates the amount of suction. After the tubes have been inserted, a chest radiograph is obtained to confirm placement.

Monitor the patient's vital signs, breath sounds, and oxygen status frequently. Assess the dressing to ensure that a tight seal is maintained. Tape tubing connections and inspect the connections frequently to detect air leaks. Coil extra tubing on the bed to avoid kinks and keep the drainage system on the floor. Monitor the drainage for blood clots or lung tissue, which may have to be gently kneaded downward to keep the tube patent. Agency and physician preferences dictate whether chest tubes are stripped or milked (Fig. 25.14). Observe the chambers for bubbling. When the system is initially connected to the patient, bubbles are usually seen in the water seal chamber. After a short time, bubbling in this chamber will stop until the lung has reexpanded or the tubing is occluded. If suction is prescribed, you will also see bubbling in the suction control chamber.

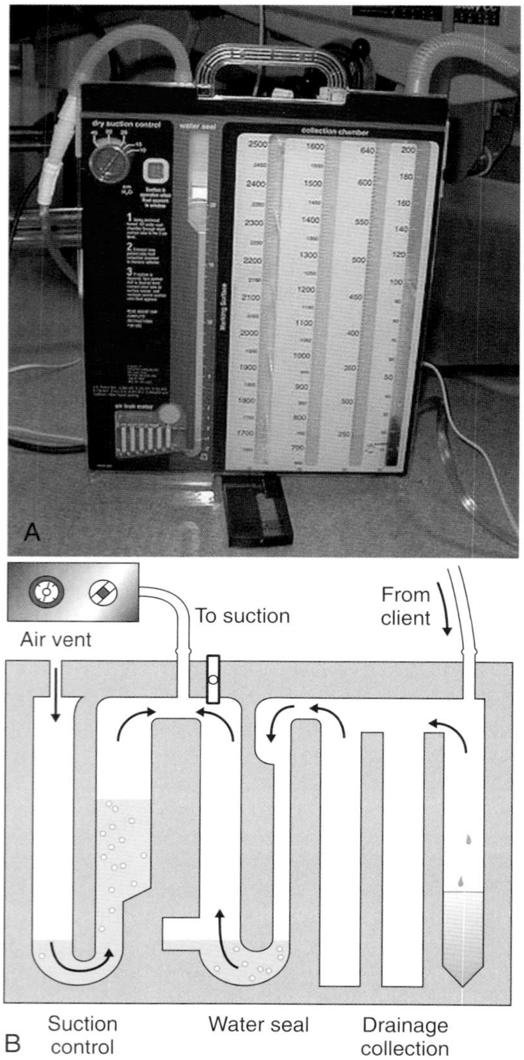

Fig. 25.13 (A) A commonly used disposable chest drainage system. (B) Diagram of chambers of water seal chest drainage. (A, From Vincent JL, Abraham E, Moore FA, et al.: *Textbook of critical care*, ed 7, Philadelphia, 2017, Elsevier. B, From Ignatavicius DD, Workman ML: *Medical-surgical nursing: patient-centered collaborative care*, ed 8, St. Louis, 2016, Elsevier.)

The rate of drainage is monitored by marking the drainage level on the drainage receptacle. The middle water seal chamber is observed for the expected rise in the fluid level with inspiration and the expected fall with expiration. This is called *tidaling*. Continuous

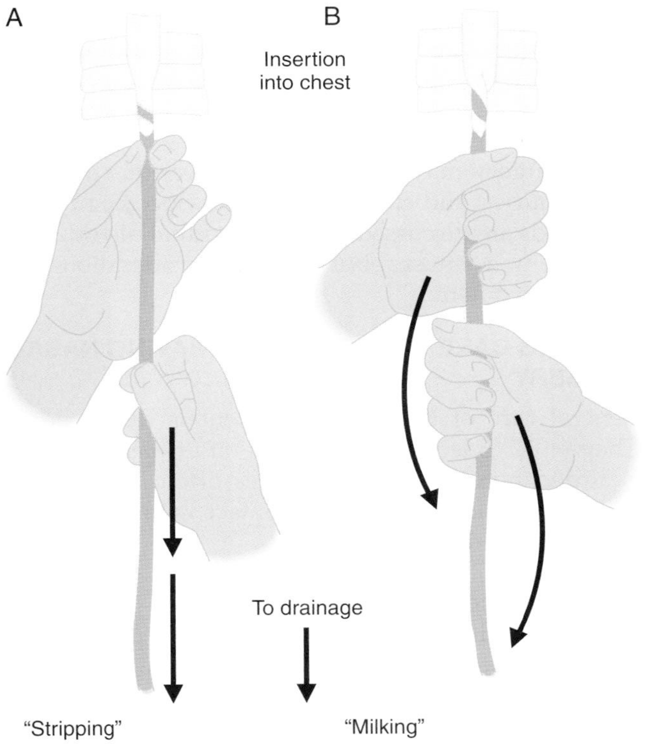

Fig. 25.14 Two techniques for removing blood clots from chest tubes. (A) Stripping. (B) Milking. Both can create excessive negative pressure in the pleural space, but milking is safer than stripping. Follow agency policies and physician orders in relation to these procedures. (From Black JM, Hawks JH, Keene AM: *Medical-surgical nursing: clinical management for continuity of care*, ed 6, Philadelphia, 2001, Saunders.)

bubbling in the water seal chamber suggests an air leak. If an air leak is suspected, agency policy may permit the tubing to be clamped for a maximum of 10 seconds while locating the leak. Wet or dry drainage systems may be used. Wet chambers are regulated by maintaining the water level that is ordered by the physician. Gentle bubbling is expected in the wet suction chamber. Dry chambers are regulated by adjusting the dry suction until the float appears. The drainage receptacle is not usually changed unless the drainage chamber is full. Use sterile technique to change the receptacle. Know the agency policies and procedures for managing chest tubes.

An alternative to the large chest drainage systems is the Heimlich flutter valve. The valve is a disposable unit that is attached to the chest tube and to a sterile drainage receptacle. Air and fluid can flow into the receptacle but cannot flow backward into the chest. The patient who has a flutter valve can assume any position and can ambulate easily. A system with a flutter valve can be attached to chest suction if necessary.

TRACHEOSTOMY SUCTIONING

Suctioning is done to remove secretions from the upper airway. It is especially important for patients who cannot clear their upper airways effectively. Depending on the site of the secretions, you may need to suction the oral cavity, the oropharynx, the nasopharynx, or the trachea.

Suction *only* when evidence indicates that it is necessary. Signs that indicate a need for suctioning include increased heart and respiratory rates, restlessness, and noisy expiration. Patients with tracheostomies also need suctioning when mucus is apparent in the tracheostomy tube. An indication for suctioning when a patient is on a ventilator is increased peak airway pressure.

Suctioning is not done unless indicated because it can cause complications, including hypoxia, tissue trauma, infection, vagal stimulation, and bronchospasm. The following are key points to remember when suctioning a patient's trachea:

1. Use sterile technique. Wear a face shield if secretions may be splashed.
2. Use a water-soluble rather than an oil-based lubricant to avoid getting oil into the respiratory tract.
3. Oxygenate the patient before suctioning:
   A. Instruct the patient to take three deep breaths if able.
   B. Patients who cannot take deep breaths should be ventilated with 100% O_2 for 30 seconds to 3 minutes by manual resuscitator or by O_2 mask.
4. During insertion of the catheter, the vent should be open so that suctioning does not occur.
5. Apply suction intermittently while rotating the catheter back and forth as it is withdrawn. If the catheter adheres to the mucosa, briefly release the suction.
6. Removal of the catheter and suctioning should not take more than 10 to 15 seconds per agency procedure protocol. Holding your breath while suctioning the patient reminds you not to suction for too long.
7. Rinse the catheter by suctioning normal saline through it.
8. Suction the mouth and pharynx, if needed, after suctioning the trachea.
9. Oxygenate the patient again after suctioning.
10. With a cuffed tracheostomy tube, the oropharynx and trachea are suctioned before deflating the cuff.
11. Document respiratory status before and after suctioning.

Put On Your Thinking Cap!

Why should you limit suctioning to 10 to 15 seconds?

TRACHEOSTOMY CARE

In addition to suctioning, the tracheostomy requires care to maintain cleanliness and protect the integrity of the surrounding skin. In the early postoperative phase, you will provide this care for the patient. The patient with a permanent tracheostomy should begin to participate as soon as they are able. Start the teaching process by placing a mirror so that the patient can see and by enlisting the patient's assistance.

A procedure manual should be consulted for details, but the following are key points to remember when doing tracheostomy care:

1. Use Standard Precautions.
2. Suction the tracheostomy before removing the old dressings.
3. Don sterile gloves to remove and clean the inner cannula. Note that the nurse does not remove the outer cannula.
4. Use a sterile solution of normal saline or other solution per agency procedure to clean the inner cannula.
5. Rinse and dry the inner cannula with normal saline or sterile water before reinserting it into the outer cannula.
6. Cleanse the stoma and surrounding skin with normal saline or sterile water and pat dry.
7. Be careful not to get solution into the stoma.
8. Change tracheostomy ties if soiled. If an assistant is not available, leave the old ties in place until the new ties are secure.
9. Replace the tracheostomy dressing with a precut pad or with a gauze pad folded as illustrated in Fig. 25.15. Do not cut a pad, because fibers will get into the stoma.
10. Tie the ties at the side of the neck in a square knot (not a bow).

Document the procedure and observations, including the appearance of the stoma, surrounding skin, and secretions.

NASAL SURGERY

Nasal surgery may be indicated for various obstructions, injuries, and chronic infections. Specific nursing care needs are discussed under individual disorders of the nose and sinuses, but general considerations are summarized here.

❖ NURSING CARE OF THE PATIENT HAVING NASAL SURGERY

General care of the surgical patient is discussed in Chapter 17. Specific nursing care after nasal surgery is added here. These procedures often are done in ambulatory surgery, so your contact with the patient may be limited.

Focused Assessment

After nasal surgery, collect data related to pain, bleeding, anxiety, and dyspnea. Monitor the patient's vital signs to detect signs of excessive blood loss (i.e., tachycardia, restlessness, tachypnea, hypotension). Take the patient's temperature to detect fever associated with infection. The patient with nasal packing will not be able to close the mouth for an oral temperature, so an alternate route will be necessary. Patients often have nasal packing in place with a mustache dressing to absorb drainage. Note the number of dressings saturated

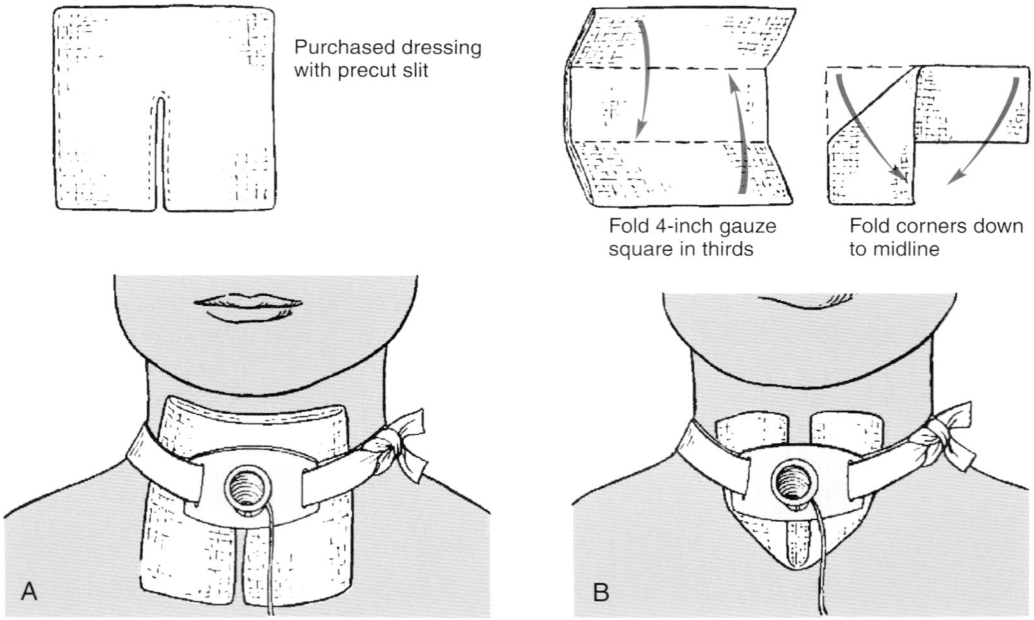

Fig. 25.15 Tracheostomy dressings. (A) Manufactured dressing with a precut slit has no fine threads that could enter the stoma. (B) A 4- × 4-inch gauze pad folded for use as a tracheostomy dressing has no cut edges that could fray and permit fibers to enter the airway. The slit can be placed downward or upward. (From Black JM, Hawks JH, Keene AM: *Medical-surgical nursing: clinical management for positive outcomes*, ed 8, St. Louis, 2009, Saunders.)

and the frequency of changes. Remember that bleeding from the nasal cavity may flow into the throat and be swallowed while the dressing remains dry. Therefore check the back of the throat for bleeding. In addition, be alert for frequent swallowing, which may be a response to bleeding into the throat. Inspect vomitus and stool for signs of blood (i.e., bright-red or "coffee ground" emesis and red, maroon, or black stools).

Patient Problems, Goals, and Outcome Criteria: Nasal Surgery, Postoperative

Patient Problems	Goals and Outcome Criteria
Decreased cardiac output related to blood loss from vascular nasal passageways	Normal cardiac output: pulse and blood pressure (BP) consistent with patient norms
Acute pain related to tissue trauma, edema, or packing	Pain relief: patient states pain reduced, appears relaxed
Inadequate oxygenation related to airway obstruction	Adequate gas exchange: respiratory rate and effort and heart rate consistent with patient norms
Altered body image related to facial bruising	Improved body image: patient accepts temporarily altered appearance; patient acknowledges that facial discoloration is temporary, resumes normal activities

Interventions

Decreased cardiac output. The nasal cavity has an extensive blood supply, so a risk of hemorrhage exists after nasal surgery. To reduce the risk of bleeding, advise the patient not to do anything that increases pressure in the nose. This includes blowing the nose and straining. Laxatives or stool softeners may be ordered to prevent straining because of constipation. The patient should not take any products containing aspirin because aspirin interferes with coagulation.

Notify the physician of indications of excessive bleeding: frequent, steady saturation of dressings with blood; increased pulse and respirations; restlessness; decreased BP; frequent swallowing; hematemesis (i.e., blood in vomitus); and melena (i.e., dark stools associated with blood in stool).

Acute pain. After nasal surgery, some nasal pain is expected because of the trauma and swelling. Semi-Fowler to high Fowler position helps to control swelling. Administer analgesics and apply ice packs as ordered. Cold decreases pain by decreasing swelling. Other sources of discomfort after nasal surgery are dry mouth and sore throat. Frequent mouth care and, when allowed, oral fluids are soothing.

Inadequate oxygenation. Nasal packing is commonly used after nasal or sinus surgery, often with a mustache dressing in place on the upper lip to absorb drainage. Only the physician removes the packing, but nurses can change the mustache dressing as needed.

Nasal packing, especially posterior packing, can interfere with breathing. Position the patient in a semi-Fowler position with the head flat against the bed. When the nasal cavity is packed, the patient breathes through the mouth. A humidifier helps to decrease dryness of the mucous membranes. Frequent oral hygiene is also comforting. Because of the nasal packing, the patient will hear a sucking sound when swallowing. Reassure them that this is normal. It is also common for patients to have poor appetites when the packing is present.

Altered body image. Some types of nasal surgery tend to cause "black eyes." The application of cool compresses to both eyes may reduce or prevent this effect. Reassure the patient that this effect is temporary, but be sensitive to any patient distress about it.

THORACIC SURGERY

A thoracotomy is the surgical opening of the chest wall. Surgical procedures on the lung include pneumonectomy, lobectomy, segmental resection, and wedge resection. Pneumonectomy is the removal of an entire lung, whereas a lobectomy is removal of one lobe of a lung. The extensive dissection and removal of a section of the lung is called a *segmental resection.* A wedge resection is the removal of a small, triangular section of lung tissue. Other procedures that require a thoracotomy are *decortication* and *thoracoplasty.* Decortication is stripping of the membrane that covers the visceral pleura, and thoracoplasty is the removal of ribs. Among the most common purposes for thoracic surgery are evaluation of chest trauma, removal of tumors and cysts, and treatment of empyema.

❖ PREOPERATIVE NURSING CARE OF THE PATIENT WITH A THORACOTOMY

Preoperative nursing care is described in Chapter 17. Before thoracotomy, the nurse should emphasize postoperative breathing exercises. If the insertion of a chest tube is anticipated, the nurse should explain the procedure to the patient.

Focused Assessment

After surgery, the nurse should monitor vital signs, lung sounds, mental status, dressings, and chest tube function and drainage.

Patient Problems, Goals, and Outcome Criteria: Thoracotomy

General postoperative patient problems are presented in Chapter 17. Diagnoses and goals specific to the patient who has had a thoracotomy may also include the following.

Patient Problems	Goals and Outcome Criteria
Inadequate oxygenation related to ventilation-perfusion mismatch	Improved oxygenation: vital signs consistent with patient's norms, arterial blood gases within normal limits
Impaired ventilation related to preexisting respiratory disease or pain	Effective ventilation: regular respirations without cyanosis or dyspnea
Airway obstruction related to dry secretions or ineffective cough	Effective airway clearance: breath sounds clear to auscultation

Interventions

Inadequate oxygenation. After a thoracotomy, the patient is at risk for pneumonia and atelectasis because of the effects of anesthesia (which impairs ciliary motion), drugs that dry secretions, and immobility. To improve gas exchange, position the patient with the head of the bed elevated 20 to 40 degrees. In the immediate postoperative period, the patient is usually placed on the unaffected side. Thereafter, various positions are permitted depending on the specific surgical procedure. Avoid the operative side after wedge resection or segmentectomy to encourage expansion of remaining lung tissue on the affected side. After pneumonectomy, also avoid the complete side-lying position on the affected side because this may encourage mediastinal shift. Administer oxygen as ordered.

Impaired ventilation. Splint the thoracic incision, while assisting the patient to breathe deeply and cough. An incentive spirometer may be used to encourage full expansion of the lungs. Adequate pain control enables the patient to breathe more effectively. Chest physiotherapy and bronchodilators are indicated for some patients. When permitted, assist the patient to sit on the edge of the bed with the feet flat on the floor. An overbed table can be placed in front of the patient, who can lean on it with folded arms. This position fosters movement of the diaphragm and chest expansion.

Airway obstruction. Adequate oral fluid intake reduces the viscosity of mucus; therefore encourage fluids if not contraindicated. If the patient cannot tolerate adequate oral fluids, intravenous fluids may be ordered. For management of chronic respiratory conditions, see Chapter 28.

VIDEO THORACOSCOPY

Many procedures that formerly required thoracic surgery can now be done with video thoracoscopy. Thoracoscopy is performed by inserting an endoscope through a small thoracic incision. Procedures that can be done with this instrument include resection of pulmonary and mediastinal lesions, biopsy, drainage of effusions, sympathectomy, vagotomy, and thymectomy. Potential complications of thoracoscopy include atelectasis, pneumonia, air leaks, and injury to thoracic organs. A chest tube is usually needed to promote full reexpansion of the lung on the operative side. Otherwise, patient care is much less complicated than it is after thoracotomy. Monitor the patient's respiratory status, including lung sounds. Immediately report sudden dyspnea or other signs of respiratory distress to the surgeon. Document the amount and appearance of chest tube drainage. Inspect the closed drainage system for proper functioning. Incentive spirometry may be used to encourage lung expansion. Administer analgesics as ordered. Patients are usually permitted out of bed 4 to 6 hours after surgery and can return to work in 1 week. Before discharge, instruct the patient to notify the physician of dyspnea or a temperature greater than 101°F (38.3°C).

Get Ready for the NCLEX® Examination!

Key Points

- The function of the respiratory system is to supply O_2 for the metabolic needs of the cells and to remove CO_2.
- The functions of the nasal cavity are to warm and moisturize inspired air, trap and remove inspired particles, destroy some bacteria, and convey information about odors to the brain.
- The Eustachian tubes prevent excessive pressure in the middle ear.
- Tonsils and adenoids guard against bacterial invasion of the respiratory and digestive tracts.
- The epiglottis prevents food and fluid from entering the airway during swallowing.
- The actual exchange of O_2 and CO_2 occurs in the alveoli.
- Most air movement in the lungs occurs because of contraction and relaxation of the diaphragm.
- The respiratory center is located in the medulla, which is part of the brainstem above the spinal cord.
- Age-related changes in the respiratory system make the older adult more susceptible to epistaxis, nasal obstruction, esophageal reflux, and lower respiratory infections.

- Dyspnea is shortness of breath; orthopnea is shortness of breath when reclining.
- A smoking history is reported in pack years, which is obtained by multiplying the number of years of smoking times the number of packs smoked per day.
- Cyanosis is a bluish color related to inadequate tissue oxygenation.
- Abnormal breath sounds that may be heard on auscultation are wheezes, rhonchi, pleural friction rubs, and coarse or fine crackles.
- The legs are included in the respiratory assessment because pulmonary emboli often result from thrombi in the deep veins of the legs and pelvis.
- A ventilation-perfusion mismatch occurs when there is ventilation without perfusion or perfusion without ventilation.
- Dyes used in imaging procedures contain iodine, which can produce a fatal reaction in a patient who is allergic to iodine.
- Arterial blood gas analysis measures blood concentrations of O_2 and CO_2, pH, bicarbonate, and O_2 saturation.
- After an arterial puncture, pressure must be applied to the site for 5 to 10 minutes to ensure no bleeding.
- Cheyne-Stokes and Biot's respirations are specific breathing patterns associated with neurologic pathology.
- Kussmaul respirations are typical of metabolic acidosis, diabetic ketoacidosis, and/or renal failure.
- Common therapeutic measures used for upper respiratory conditions include nasal drops, humidification, suctioning, tracheostomy care, nasal surgery, thoracic surgery, and video thoracoscopy.
- Patient problems for the patient having nasal surgery include decreased cardiac output, pain, inadequate oxygenation, and altered body image.
- Patient problems for the patient having thoracic surgery may include inadequate oxygenation, inadequate ventilation, and airway obstruction.

Additional Learning Resources

SG Go to your Study Guide for additional learning activities to help you master this chapter content.

Go to your Evolve website (http://evolve.elsevier.com/Linton/medsurg) for the following learning resources and much more:

- Fluid & Electrolyte Tutorial
- Review Questions for the NCLEX® Examination

Clinical Judgment and Next-Generation NCLEX® Examination-Style Questions

1. **Which of the following is the function of the turbinates in the internal nose?**
   1. To trap inspired particles
   2. To destroy microorganisms
   3. To warm inspired air
   4. To detect odors

   NCLEX Client Need: Health Promotion and Maintenance

2. **A training program for new nurses in a long-term care facility includes common anatomic and physiologic changes in older people. Which of the following changes in the upper respiratory tract should be included? (Select all that apply.)**
   1. Thinning of the mucous membrane
   2. Nasal obstruction more common
   3. Decreased mucus production
   4. Decreased sense of smell
   5. Less risk of epistaxis

   NCLEX Client Need: Health Promotion and Maintenance

3. **Why is it important to limit the time that suction is applied during tracheal suctioning?**
   1. Suctioning removes oxygen that may cause hypoxemia.
   2. Suctioning is traumatic to the lining of the trachea.
   3. Suctioning may induce vomiting.
   4. Suctioning is painful.

   NCLEX Client Need: Physiological Integrity: Reduction of Risk Potential

4. **During the focused assessment, a patient tells the LVN/LPN that he sleeps in a recliner because he cannot breathe well when lying flat in bed. What is the most appropriate term to describe this symptom?**
   1. Dyspnea
   2. Bradypnea
   3. Tachypnea
   4. Orthopnea

   NCLEX Client Need: Physiological Integrity: Basic Care and Comfort

5. **A patient history notes that an 80-year-old patient has a cigarette smoking history of 93 pack-years. Which of the following is the formula for determining pack years?**
   1. Packs smoked per day multiplied by the number of years of smoking
   2. Number of years of smoking added to the patient's age
   3. Packs smoked per year divided by the patient's age
   4. Patient's age subtracted from the number of packs smoked per year

   NCLEX Client Need: Health Promotion and Maintenance: High Risk Behaviors

6. **Wheezes heard during auscultation of a patient's lungs are indicative of which of the following?**
   1. Fluid accumulation in the alveoli
   2. Narrowed airways
   3. Pleural inflammation
   4. Secretions in larger airways

   NCLEX Client Need: Physiological Integrity: Physiological Adaptation

7. **A patient is scheduled for an imaging procedure with radioactive dye. Before the procedure, it is most important to determine whether the patient is allergic to which of the following?**
   1. Eggs
   2. Penicillin
   3. Iodine
   4. Morphine

   NCLEX Client Need: Physiological Integrity: Reduction of Risk Potential

8. **Which of the following pulse oximeter readings should be reported to a supervisor immediately?**
   1. 85%
   2. 90%
   3. 95%
   4. 100%

   NCLEX Client Need: Physiological Integrity: Reduction of Risk Potential

9. **What is the advantage of second-generation antihistamines over first-generation antihistamines?**
   1. Less chance of allergic reaction
   2. Lower dose required
   3. Less drowsiness
   4. More rapid onset of action

   NCLEX Client Need: Physiological Integrity: Pharmacological Therapies

10. **SLO/Objective: Discuss the anatomy and physiology of the respiratory system.**

    NGN Item Type: Enhanced hot spot

    Cognitive skill: Recognize cues

    An 86-year-old woman is brought to the emergency department after an auto accident. She was the driver and was wearing her seatbelt. She is alert and has an anxious expression. A quick assessment reveals no external wounds or bleeding, Moves all extremities without pain. Reports no chronic illnesses except arthritis in her knees and hips for which she takes Motrin. She has a smoking history of 50 pack years but quit 20 years ago. She has frequent respiratory infections. A more detailed assessment yielded these data:
    - Oral temperature 98°F
    - Blood pressure 140/90 mm Hg
    - Heart rate 96 beats per minute, slightly irregular
    - Respirations 24 breaths per minute, shallow
    - O_2 saturation (via oximetry) 88%
    - Breath sounds clear to auscultation
    - Pain in right rib cage (rated 6)
    - Abdomen soft with active bowel sounds

    Highlight or place a check mark next to the assessment findings that require follow-up by the nurse.

    NCLEX Client Need: Physiological Integrity: Physiological Adaptation

Upper Respiratory Disorders

26

http://evolve.elsevier.com/Linton/medsurg

Objectives

1. Explain the pathophysiology, signs and symptoms, complications, and medical or surgical treatment of selected disorders of the nose, sinuses, and throat.
2. Assist in developing nursing care plans for patients with disorders of the nose, sinuses, or throat.

Key Terms

allergen (ĂL-ĕr-jĕn)
antihistamine (ăn-tĭ-HĬS-tă-mēn)
coryza (kŏ-RĪ-ză)
decongestant (dē-kŏn-JĔS-tĕnt)
epistaxis (ĕ-pĭ-STĂK-sĭs)
laryngectomy (lā-rĭn-JĔK-tō-mē)
laryngitis (lā-rĭn-JĪ-tĭs)
polyps (PŎ-lĭps)
rhinitis (rī-NĪ-tĭs)
rhinosinusitis (rī-nō-sī-nə-sī-təs)
sinusitis (sī-nŭ-SĪ-tĭs)
tonsillitis (tŏn-sĭ-LĪ-tĭs)
triad disease

DISORDERS OF THE NOSE AND SINUSES

SINUSITIS AND RHINOSINUSITIS

Sinusitis is inflammation of the sinuses, most often the maxillary and frontal sinuses. It may be caused by bacteria, virus, or, rarely, a fungus. The infection usually spreads from the nasal passages into the sinuses. The term **rhinosinusitis** is used when both the nasal mucosa and the sinuses are inflamed.

Sinusitis can be acute or chronic. Acute sinusitis follows obstruction of the flow of secretions from the sinus. Causes of acute sinusitis include allergic rhinitis, deviated septum, nasal polyps, tumors, airborne pollutants, and inhaled drugs such as cocaine. Chronic sinusitis is a permanent thickening of the mucous membranes in the sinuses after repeated infections.

Clinical Manifestations

Patients with acute sinusitis usually report pain or a feeling of heaviness over the affected sinus. They may report purulent drainage from the nose. When the maxillary sinuses are affected, the pain may seem like a toothache. Headache is common, especially in the morning. Fever may be present and the white blood cell (WBC) count may be elevated.

Symptoms of chronic sinusitis are often nonspecific. Commonly, patients experience facial or dental pain, nasal congestion, and increased drainage. Fever is not usually present.

Complications

Although most patients recover without serious effects, sinus infections can be dangerous. Chronic sinusitis may follow acute sinusitis. Other potential complications are meningitis, brain abscess, osteomyelitis, and orbital cellulitis. The possibility of brain infection exists because of the location of the sinuses in the skull. Suspect neurologic complications if the patient has a high fever, vomiting, chills, seizures, or blurred vision.

Medical Diagnosis and Treatment

Sinusitis is usually suspected based on the history and physical examination. It can be confirmed with computed tomography (CT) or magnetic resonance imaging (MRI). A culture of material obtained by aspiration of the sinus may be done, usually by a specialist. Nasal drainage has so many contaminants that it is not very useful for culture.

Initial treatment may focus on symptom management. Medications may include **decongestants** to promote drainage, intranasal corticosteroids to decrease inflammation, and over the counter analgesics to relieve pain. Warm, moist packs applied to the face can promote drainage and reduce pain. Other measures to promote drainage include twice-daily hot showers, increased fluid intake, and use of a humidifier. After hot showers or use of a humidifier, the patient is encouraged to blow the nose thoroughly. Sleeping with the head of the bed elevated helps promote drainage. Nasal saline sprays or washes are sometimes indicated.

Irrigating solutions can be prepared at home using sterile water (1 quart), pickling/canning salt (1 to 1 1/2 heaped teaspoons), and baking soda (1 teaspoon). Tap water and table salt should NOT be used. Because most cases of sinusitis are caused by viruses, antibiotics are not indicated. However, antibiotic therapy may be prescribed for bacterial infections.

Surgical Treatment

Chronic sinusitis is sometimes treated surgically. Surgery may correct the underlying problem, remove the thickened membrane, or enlarge the opening through which secretions drain. Underlying problems that might be treated surgically include deviated septum, nasal polyps, and hypertrophy of turbinates.

The most common surgery used for sinusitis that does not respond to medical treatment is functional endoscopic sinus surgery (FESS). FESS is an outpatient procedure in which specialized instruments are passed into the sinuses through the nasal cavity. Diseased tissue can be removed and the sinus ostia (i.e., the openings that drain the sinuses) can be enlarged. Nasal packing may be done to control bleeding. The packing is usually removed after a few hours. Complications of FESS can include nasal bleeding and scarring. Although rare, cerebrospinal fluid (CSF) leakage and injury to the optic nerve are possible. Another surgical option is sinus ostial dilation (SOD), which uses a balloon to enlarge the openings in the sinuses to promote drainage. SOD can be done in outpatient settings. Less commonly, external sphenoethmoidectomy is done through a small incision on the side of the nose that permits removal of diseased sphenoidal or ethmoidal sinus mucosa.

◆ NURSING CARE OF THE PATIENT HAVING SINUS SURGERY

Nursing care after sinus surgery is essentially the same as that described in Chapter 25 for nasal surgery. After FESS, the patient is usually able to return to work in 4 to 5 days. Saline nasal sprays may be ordered to prevent crusting and promote healing. After external surgery, the semi-Fowler position is recommended to prevent swelling and promote drainage. Apply cold compresses as ordered during the first 24 hours. Nasal packing is usually left in place until the first postoperative day. Antral packing is left in place for 36 to 72 hours. Caution the patient to avoid blowing the nose or straining, which could cause bleeding and tissue damage. After the procedure (3–5 days), nasal saline sprays may be ordered to moisten the nasal mucosa.

NASAL POLYPS

Nasal **polyps** are swollen masses of sinus or nasal mucosa and connective tissue that extend into the nasal passages. Small polyps are typically asymptomatic. Larger polyps may grow and eventually obstruct the nasal airway. Polyps resemble white grapes in size and shape. The exact cause is unknown, but patients often have a history of allergic rhinitis or infections. Patients who have nasal polyps, asthma, and aspirin allergy are said to have **triad disease**.

The size of the polyps may be reduced by removing allergens or treating the allergic response. Corticosteroids inhaled nasally may be prescribed. However, surgical removal under local anesthesia is often necessary. Unfortunately, nasal polyps tend to recur.

◆ NURSING CARE OF THE PATIENT HAVING NASAL POLYP SURGERY

Nursing care after surgery for nasal polyps is like that described earlier for sinus surgery. This procedure is often done in an outpatient surgical facility, so patient teaching before discharge is especially important. Advise the patient not to take aspirin; it increases the risk of bleeding and some patients are allergic to aspirin.

ALLERGIC RHINITIS

Allergic **rhinitis**, or "hay fever," is a common condition. It is classified as intermittent (seasonal) or persistent (perennial). The condition is considered persistent when symptoms are present for more than 4 days a week for more than 4 weeks per year.

Pathophysiology

Allergic rhinitis follows exposure to a substance that causes an allergic response (**allergen**). An allergic response is a reaction to the release of chemicals, including histamine, that causes vasodilation and increased capillary permeability. Fluid leaks from the capillaries, causing swelling of the nasal mucosa. Occasionally these changes are triggered by overuse of decongestant nose drops or sprays.

Intermittent allergic rhinitis is most often caused by exposure to pollens. It typically lasts several weeks, resolves, and does not return until the offending pollens reappear. The persistent form is more likely because of allergens that are continuously in the environment, such as house dust and animal dander.

Clinical Manifestations

Signs and symptoms of allergic rhinitis include sneezing, watery and itchy eyes, nasal obstruction, clear nasal discharge, and frontal headache. The nasal mucosa is often pale, but it can be red or bluish.

Medical Diagnosis

Diagnosis is made based on a detailed history. With chronic symptoms, the patient may be instructed to keep a diary describing all episodes. This can help to identify possible allergens.

Medical Treatment

The patient may also be referred to an allergist for further evaluation. The allergist applies solutions of common allergens to the skin. The allergens are applied in a specific pattern so that the patient's reaction to them can be assessed individually. Immunotherapy (also called desensitization) may be advised to decrease the patient's reaction to the offending allergens. Patients often call these injections "allergy shots." The injections are composed of dilute solutions of the allergens to which the person reacts. The strength of the solution is gradually increased as the patient's tolerance grows. In a sense, this process causes the body to get used to the allergen so that it no longer reacts with an allergic response. Another outcome of allergy testing is that it identifies substances the patient should avoid.

Numerous prescription and over-the-counter (OTC) drugs are available. The drugs used to treat allergic rhinitis are primarily intranasal corticosteroids and oral or intranasal **antihistamines**. Second-generation antihistamines (e.g., Zyrtec) are preferred over first-generation antihistamines (e.g., Benadryl) because they are less sedating. Decongestants help to relieve symptoms. Many such medications are available without a prescription. In general, these products should be used only on a short-term basis. First-generation antihistamines should be used cautiously in older patients because they are sedating, which could lead to falls. Advise patients to consult with a physician or a pharmacist about the most appropriate over-the-counter drugs.

◆ NURSING CARE OF THE PATIENT WITH ALLERGIC RHINITIS

Patients with allergic rhinitis are usually treated as outpatients. The nurse who works in a clinic or physician's office may need to reinforce teaching about immunotherapy and drug therapy. Patients are usually advised to begin intranasal corticosteroids several weeks before allergy season.

ACUTE VIRAL CORYZA

Acute viral **coryza**, known as the *common cold*, can be caused by any of some 30 viruses. It is contagious and spread by droplet infection.

Clinical Manifestations

Signs and symptoms of the common cold are well known to most people. They usually consist of fever, fatigue, nasal discharge, and sore throat.

Complications

The infection usually runs its course in approximately 1 week. Complications that sometimes develop include otitis media, sinusitis, bronchitis, and pneumonia. Complications are more common in people with weakened resistance.

Medical Treatment

Medical management of the common cold is directed primarily at relief of symptoms. Drug therapy includes antihistamines, decongestants, antitussives, and antipyretics. Combination products are available. However, if a patient has only one symptom, they should choose a single agent to avoid multiple side effects. Patients often expect to receive antibiotics. You can inform them that antibiotics are not effective against infections caused by viruses. Inappropriate use of antibiotics promotes the development of resistant strains of bacteria.

Prevention

Prevention of the common cold is best accomplished by avoidance of people with colds. People with colds are most contagious during the first 2 or 3 days after symptoms appear. The very young, the very old, and those with weakened immune systems especially should be protected from exposure

> **Put On Your Thinking Cap!**
>
> Design a short teaching plan on prevention of colds for first-grade children. Be creative!

◆ NURSING CARE OF THE PATIENT WITH ACUTE VIRAL CORYZA

Nursing intervention related to the common cold is primarily public education about prevention and about drugs prescribed for treatment (see the Complementary and Alternative Therapies box). Encourage patients to rest and to drink plenty of fluids.

> **Complementary and Alternative Therapies**
>
> Despite the common belief that echinacea can prevent and treat colds, research has not found convincing evidence of its effectiveness. However, it is generally considered safe for short-term use of less than 10 days. There is substantial controversy about the effectiveness of vitamin C for treating the common cold. The majority of evidence shows that taking high doses of vitamin C orally may decrease the duration of cold symptoms by a few days.

TUMORS

Clinical Manifestations

Tumors sometimes develop in the nasal passages and sinuses. They can be benign or malignant. Risk factors include smoking, being male, being infected with human papillomavirus, and certain occupations, notably furniture making, carpentry, leather work, and bakery work. This suggests that exposure to certain chemicals or dust may be a factor. The primary symptom is nasal obstruction. Either one or both sides may be affected. Another sign suggestive of a tumor is a bloody discharge from one nasal passage.

Cancers of the nasal cavity and paranasal sinuses are rare, comprising only 3% to 5% of cancer diagnoses each year. Four out of five cases occur in people who are at least 55 years of age.

Medical Diagnosis

A diagnosis is based on biopsy or removal of the entire tumor for examination. When cancer is confirmed or highly suspected, CT, MRI, and positron emission tomography (PET) scans may be done to assess the extent of the disease. The earlier a malignancy is detected and treated, the better the chances of survival. Unfortunately, carcinomas in the nasopharynx tend to metastasize to the neck, liver, and lungs fairly early. These cancers have often spread by the time they are diagnosed. Therefore, a physician should examine any patient with persistent nasal obstruction or bleeding.

Medical Treatment

Treatment of nasal malignancies may include surgery, radiation therapy, chemotherapy, targeted therapy, and/or palliative treatment. The plan of treatment depends on the stage of the cancer and the general health of the patient. Surgical procedures may be extensive and disfiguring, depending on the site and extent of the cancer. Reconstructive surgery or prostheses may be needed.

Benign tumors do not metastasize but are likely to require removal because they still can obstruct the nasal passages.

◆ NURSING CARE OF THE PATIENT WITH NASAL CANCER

The general nursing care of patients having nasal surgery was discussed in Chapter 25 under Common Therapeutic Measures. A diagnosis of cancer has special implications for the nurse. The patient may be especially anxious and fearful of disfigurement or even death. Be supportive and encourage the patient to ask questions and express concerns. Nursing care of the patient with cancer is discussed in detail in Chapter 7.

DEVIATED NASAL SEPTUM

The nose is divided into two passages by a cartilaginous wall called the *septum*. In most adults, the septum is slightly deviated, meaning that it is off center. Minor deviations cause no symptoms and require no treatment. Major deviations, however, can obstruct the nasal passages and block sinus drainage. The patient may complain of headaches, sinusitis, and **epistaxis** (i.e., nosebleeds).

Treatment

Conservative treatment includes management of nasal allergies. Septal deviations can be corrected by a surgical procedure called a *nasal septoplasty*. The procedure is usually done under local anesthesia. The mucosa is repositioned, and the nasal passage is packed with petrolatum gauze. The physician removes the packing after 24 to 48 hours.

The two major complications of septoplasty are tears of the septum and saddle deformity. Saddle deformity is collapse of the bridge of the nose caused by removal of excessive support tissue or by contraction of the surgical scar. Nursing care of the patient having nasal surgery was described in Chapter 25 under Common Therapeutic Measures.

EPISTAXIS

The nose has an abundant blood supply that permits it to bleed easily. The medical term for a nosebleed is *epistaxis*. Causes of nosebleeds include trauma, hypertension, low humidity, allergies, upper respiratory infections, foreign bodies, chemical irritants, overuse of decongestant nasal sprays, nasal surgery, and tumors. Most nosebleeds occur in the anterior portion of the nasal cavity and can be self-treated. Posterior nosebleeds may require medical treatment and often occur secondary to other health problems, like hypertension.

First Aid

When epistaxis occurs, the patient should sit down and lean forward from the waist. Patients should keep their head elevated but not hyperextended. Direct pressure should be applied for 10 to 15 minutes, as illustrated in Chapter 63, Fig. 63.4, unless the patient has had a traumatic injury to the face. Facial trauma suggests a possible nasal fracture and direct pressure may do more harm. An ice pack or a cold compress can be applied to the nose regardless of whether facial trauma has occurred. Once the bleeding stops, advise the patient not to blow the nose for several hours because this may trigger renewed bleeding.

Medical Treatment

If bleeding continues, medical attention is needed. Following the application of a topical anesthetic, the physician may treat anterior bleeding with a topical vasoconstrictor (oxymetazoline nasal prep) or silver nitrate cauterization. If bleeding is not controlled, the next step is direct pressure to the nasal cavity. This can be accomplished with a nasal balloon catheter or nasal packing.

Nasal balloon catheter. The physician may pass a nasal balloon catheter into the nasal cavity. Then the balloon is inflated to apply pressure to the blood vessels. Smaller balloons anchor the catheter in place. Several different types of nasal catheters with single or double cuffs are available, including the Rhino, the Epistat, and the Storz T-3100. Balloons maybe used for both anterior and posterior bleeding.

Nasal packing. The physician may pack the anterior or posterior nasal cavity, or both. Anterior packing uses gauze and an antibacterial ointment. Posterior nasal packing is more complicated and requires close patient monitoring. Packing may be accomplished by using nasal sponges, gauze, or nasal tampons. The packing is inserted into the nares and advanced along the floor of the nasal cavity. The packing expands and applies pressure to stop the bleeding.

Complications. Complications related to packing and balloons include impaired breathing, infection, and blockage of the Eustachian tube. If a gauze pad is applied to a posterior bleeding site, it can depress the soft palate, causing airway obstruction. If the packing should slip out of place, it could block the airway. Packing is usually left in place for 2 to 3 days.

NURSING CARE OF THE PATIENT WITH EPISTAXIS

Focused Assessment

Severe epistaxis is an emergency, so collect only priority data until the patient is stabilized. The priority data when a patient has severe epistaxis are evidence of uncontrolled bleeding and excessive blood loss. Inspect the nose and back of the throat for obvious bleeding and observe for frequent swallowing. Monitor the patient's level of consciousness and vital signs to detect signs of hypovolemia (i.e., restlessness, tachycardia, tachypnea, hypotension). Document allergies and major illnesses.

Once a nasal balloon catheter or nasal packing is in place, monitor for early signs of infection and airway obstruction (i.e., dyspnea, anxiety, tachycardia). In addition, ask the patient about pain in the nose, pharynx, or ears.

Patient Problems, Goals, and Outcome Criteria: Epistaxis

Patient Problems	Goals and Outcome Criteria
Decreased cardiac output related to hypovolemia secondary to hemorrhage	Normal cardiac output: pulse and blood pressure (BP) consistent with patient's norms
Anxiety related to threat of excessive bleeding or unpleasant procedures	Reduced anxiety: patient calm, able to cooperate, states less anxious
Potential for injury related to pressure (of packing, balloon) and possible airway obstruction	Absence of complications of balloon or packing: respiratory rate of 12 to 20 breaths per minute without distress
Potential for infection related to presence of nasal packing	Absence of infection: no fever

Interventions

Decreased cardiac output. Throughout the period of care for epistaxis, monitor for signs of continued and excessive blood loss. Immediately report signs and symptoms of hypovolemia (i.e., increased pulse, restlessness, decreased urine output) to the physician.

Anxiety. When a nasal balloon or packing is used, support the patient and assist the physician during placement of the device. The patient is probably frightened by the visible blood and needs calm reassurance. Because of the discomfort and anxiety associated with posterior nasal packing, a mild sedative may be ordered.

Pharmacology Capsule

Patients who are prone to bleeding are usually advised to avoid aspirin and other nonsteroidal antiinflammatory drugs (NSAIDs) because they inhibit blood clotting.

Potential for injury and potential for infection. Because nasal packing and the epistaxis balloon can depress the soft palate and impair breathing, check the patient's respiratory status frequently. Patients are usually hospitalized when posterior nasal packing is in place for constant monitoring. Frequent mouth care is needed because the patient must breathe through the mouth. Monitor the patient's temperature for elevation, which may indicate infection of the nasopharynx. Inspect the oral cavity. If posterior gauze packing is in place, it should not be visible. If it is visible, the physician should be contacted to adjust the position.

Under normal circumstances, the physician removes the packing. This procedure is uncomfortable; premedicate the patient before the procedure. You can assist by supporting the patient in a sitting position and providing an emesis basin to receive the packing. Drape the patient to protect the clothing. Once the packing is removed, the patient appreciates mouth care.

DISORDERS OF THE THROAT

PHARYNGITIS

Pharyngitis is inflammation of the mucous membranes of the throat or pharynx. Pharyngitis can be a viral, bacterial, or fungal infection. Most cases of pharyngitis are viral. Bacterial infection occurs about 5% to 10% of the time and is usually caused by group A beta-hemolytic streptococci (strep throat). Fungal infections can develop with prolonged antibiotic use or inhaled corticosteroids.

Clinical Manifestations

Signs and symptoms of pharyngitis are dryness, pain, dysphagia (i.e., difficulty swallowing), and fever. The throat appears red and the tonsils may be enlarged. Viral and bacterial pharyngitis differ in several respects. Compared with viral pharyngitis, bacterial pharyngitis has a more abrupt onset and is characterized by fever, enlarged lymph nodes, tonsillar exudate (i.e., drainage), and absence of cough.

Complications

Patients with bacterial pharyngitis are more likely to have serious complications than those with viral pharyngitis. The most important complications are acute glomerulonephritis and rheumatic fever.

Medical Diagnosis

Pharyngitis is diagnosed based on the patient history and physical examination. A more specific diagnosis of viral or bacterial pharyngitis is made after the results of a rapid antigen detection test and/or a throat culture and a complete blood count (CBC) are obtained.

Medical Treatment

Pharyngitis is treated with rest, fluids, analgesics, and throat gargles or irrigations. If the patient's oral intake is low, intravenous fluids may be ordered. A soft or liquid diet may be ordered because of painful swallowing. A cool-mist vaporizer or humidifier may also be ordered to increase moisture in the room air.

Treatment of viral pharyngitis focuses on symptom management. Bacterial pharyngitis is treated with antibiotics. Penicillin is the treatment of choice and is given for 10 days to prevent complications of rheumatic fever. Fungal infections are treated with nystatin.

Prevention

To reduce the risk of pharyngitis, people with weakened resistance should avoid others with upper respiratory infections. Measures that help maintain resistance to throat infections include good nutrition, adequate rest, and avoidance of inhaled irritants. People who have pharyngitis are contagious in the early stages and should avoid contact with susceptible people.

◆ NURSING CARE OF THE PATIENT WITH PHARYNGITIS

Focused Assessment

Mild pharyngitis is usually treated on an outpatient basis, unless the patient is having difficulty breathing. Nursing interventions are limited. Relevant data include the presence of throat pain, dysphagia, muscle and joint pain, nausea and vomiting, and rash. Take the patient's temperature and inspect the throat for redness and enlarged tonsils.

Patient Problems, Goals, and Outcome Criteria

The primary patient problem for the patient with pharyngitis is ineffective self-care management related to lack of understanding of treatment and importance of follow-up care. The goal of nursing care is appropriate self-care by the patient. The criteria for goal achievement are the patient correctly describing self-care measures—including drug therapy and symptoms that should be reported—and making and keeping a follow-up appointment.

Interventions

Reinforce the physician's directions for drug therapy, if ordered. Stress the importance of completing prescribed antibiotics. Encourage patients to take 2000 to 3000 mL of fluids daily unless contraindicated. Fluids must be increased cautiously in older adults because they do not adjust well to sudden changes in blood volume. Advise patients that they are contagious at first and should avoid people with poor resistance.

TONSILLITIS

Tonsillitis is inflammation of the tonsils and other lymphatic tissue in the throat. It is most common in children.

Causes

Tonsillitis is usually caused by a virus but can be caused by bacteria. Tonsillitis is not contagious, but the viruses and bacteria that cause it are contagious. Frequent handwashing will help prevent its spread. A person may have repeated infections that respond to treatment or may have a chronic infection.

Clinical Manifestations

A patient with tonsillitis usually reports a sore throat, difficulty swallowing, fever, bad breath, and sometimes chills. If swollen tissue blocks the Eustachian tubes, pain may also be felt in the ears.

The tonsils are typically enlarged and red. Purulent drainage or yellowish or white patches may be seen on the tonsils. Lymph nodes in the neck may be tender and enlarged.

Medical Diagnosis

The physician will conduct a physical examination and ask about symptoms and medical history. Diagnosis can be made based on a rapid strep test, a throat culture, or both. The culture and sensitivity identify the pathogenic organisms present and what antibiotics are likely to be effective. A chest radiograph may also be ordered to assess for respiratory complications.

Medical Treatment

The medical treatment of tonsillitis depends on the cause. If the cause is a virus, treatment of symptoms is appropriate. If the cause is bacterial, treatment will include antibiotics. Analgesics and lozenges may be prescribed for pain and antipyretics for fever. Remember that children and teenagers should avoid use of aspirin; do not give lozenges to children under the age of 4 years. Warm saline gargles and use of a humidifier may help decrease swelling. Rest and adequate fluids promote comfort and facilitate recovery.

Complications

A peritonsillar abscess may develop with streptococcal tonsillitis. A peritonsillar abscess is an infection of the tissue surrounding the tonsil. The affected side is very painful, and the patient has difficulty swallowing, talking, and opening the mouth. The immediate treatment is drainage of the abscess. Once the acute infection has subsided, tonsillectomy is performed.

Surgical Treatment

When a patient (usually a child) is diagnosed with strep throat 7 or more times in 1 year, the physician may suggest surgery to remove the tonsils (tonsillectomy). Tonsillectomy is also considered when enlarged tonsils cause difficulty breathing, or when they contribute to obstructive sleep apnea (OSA). Tonsillectomy is normally an elective surgery. The decision to remove a child's tonsils must be weighed against the risks of anesthesia and bleeding, as well as the missed school days to recover from the procedure.

◆ NURSING CARE OF THE PATIENT HAVING A TONSILLECTOMY

Preoperative nursing care is discussed in detail in Chapter 17. Postoperative nursing care is as follows (see Nursing Care Plan: Patient Having a Tonsillectomy).

Nursing Care Plan Adult Patient Having a Tonsillectomy

FOCUSED ASSESSMENT

Health History

A 20-year-old college student has had tonsillitis 3 times this year, resulting in absences from school. Her symptoms included sore throat, dysphagia, fever and chills, muscle aches, and headache. She has had no other serious illnesses. She takes no medications except occasional acetaminophen for headache. She was admitted for tonsillectomy, which was performed under local anesthetic this morning. She expressed hope that it will relieve her recurrent illness. She clutches her throat and complains of throat pain.

Physical Examination Vital signs: blood pressure 110/88 mm Hg, pulse 100 beats per minute, respirations 18 breaths per minute, temperature 98°F (36.7°C) measured orally. Height 5′8″, weight 150 lb. Patient is drowsy but responds appropriately. She has a small amount of sanguineous drainage. Respiratory effort and breath sounds are normal. Intravenous fluids are infusing into the antecubital space of the left arm.

Patient Problem	Goals and Outcome Criteria	Interventions
Potential for decreased cardiac output related to excessive bleeding	The patient will maintain normal cardiac output, as evidenced by vital signs consistent with preoperative readings, minimal visible bleeding, and absence of restlessness.	Report signs of excessive bleeding: tachycardia, restlessness, frequent swallowing. Advise the patient not to cough or clear her throat. Inspect drainage for bleeding. Report continued or excessive bleeding to the surgeon. When oral fluids are permitted, have the patient sip from a glass or cup rather than use a straw.
Potential for airway obstruction related to bleeding, edema, effects of anesthesia	The patient will maintain a patent airway, as evidenced by clear breath sounds and respiratory rate of 12 to 20 breaths per minute.	Position the patient on one side until fully alert. Elevate the head of the bed 45 degrees. Monitor for signs and symptoms of inadequate oxygenation: tachycardia, restlessness. Auscultate breath sounds. Have suction equipment in the room.
Acute pain related to tissue trauma	The patient will state that pain is relieved and will appear more relaxed.	Administer analgesics as ordered. Apply an ice collar as ordered. Give cold or frozen liquids when permitted. Provide simple explanations and reassurance.
Inability to perform self-care related to lack of knowledge of postoperative care	The patient will describe postoperative self-care.	Before discharge, teach the following: 1. Consume a soft, high-protein, high-calorie diet for 10 days. Omit rough foods. 2. Drink 8 to 12 8-oz glasses of fluids daily. No citrus juices. 3. Avoid strenuous activity or straining for 2 weeks. 4. Do not take aspirin or other NSAIDs. 5. Earaches are common. 6. White patches naturally form over tonsillectomy sites. 7. Report any bleeding to the physician.

CRITICAL THINKING QUESTIONS

1. What is the significance of frequent swallowing?
2. Why are patients not encouraged to cough after tonsillectomy?
3. Why is it important for tonsillectomy patients to sip from a glass instead of using a straw while drinking liquids?

Focused Assessment

In the immediate postoperative phase, frequently monitor the patient's responsiveness and vital signs. Increased pulse rate and restlessness are early signs of hypovolemia. Cyanosis (i.e., bluish discoloration of the nail beds or lips) is a late sign of inadequate oxygenation. Inspect drainage from the mouth or vomited fluid for blood. Blood-tinged drainage is normal at first but should gradually decrease. Note excessive swallowing, which may indicate bleeding. Monitor respiratory effort and skin color to evaluate oxygenation. Evaluate pain and dysphagia.

Patient Problems, Goals, and Outcome Criteria: Tonsillectomy

Patient Problems	Goals and Outcome Criteria
Potential for decreased cardiac output related to excessive bleeding	Normal cardiac output and decreasing bleeding: pulse and blood pressure (BP) consistent with patient's norms, decreasing bloody drainage
Potential for airway obstruction related to bleeding, edema, or effects of anesthesia	Effective airway clearance and adequate oxygenation: no restlessness, normal skin color, no respiratory distress
Acute pain related to tissue trauma	Pain relief: patient states pain relieved, relaxed manner
Inability to perform self-care related to inadequate knowledge of postoperative care	Performs appropriate self-care: patient describes and carries out self-care as prescribed

Interventions

The two major problems that may develop in the postoperative phase are (1) hemorrhage and (2) respiratory distress.

Potential for decreased cardiac output. To reduce the risk of bleeding, remind the patient not to cough or clear the throat. If suctioning is needed, do so very gently because it may cause further bleeding. Once oral fluids are permitted, the patient should not use a straw. The sucking may dislodge the clots that form at the surgical site.

Potential for airway obstruction. A patient who has had local anesthesia is at less risk for respiratory complications than one who has had general anesthesia. After local anesthesia, position the tonsillectomy patient with the head of the bed elevated at a 45-degree angle. After general anesthesia, the bed should be flat and the patient positioned on the side or semiprone. This promotes drainage of fluid from the mouth that might otherwise be aspirated. Once the patient is fully awake, they may prefer a semi-Fowler position. Increased pulse rate, restlessness, and confusion may be early signs and symptoms of inadequate oxygenation.

Acute pain. Analgesics are ordered for pain. Ice collars may be applied to the neck as ordered to decrease swelling and pain. A clear liquid diet is ordered first. Cold or frozen liquids are especially soothing after tonsillectomy. Red food and drinks are avoided because they could be mistaken for blood in sputum or emesis. Dairy products are commonly excluded because of the belief that they cause mucus to be thicker and more difficult to expectorate.

Inability to perform self-care. Before discharge, advise the patient of measures to promote healing and prevent complications. Teaching points are listed in the Patient Teaching box.

Patient Teaching

Tonsillectomy

- The diet should be soft and high in protein and calories for the next 10 days.
- Avoid strenuous activity and straining for 2 weeks.
- Avoid aspirin and other NSAIDs such as ibuprofen, which interfere with blood clotting.
- Aspirin should be avoided in children and teenagers.
- Avoid smoking, which may disrupt healing.
- Drink 8 to 12 8-oz glasses of fluid daily.
- Avoid citrus juices, which irritate healing tissues.
- Earaches are common and are not cause for alarm.
- White patches normally form over the tonsillectomy sites. This tissue will slough off.
- Report bleeding to the physician.

OBSTRUCTIVE SLEEP APNEA

OSA is a condition marked by airway obstruction during sleep. It is caused by narrowing of the airway with relaxation of muscle tone during sleep and/or the tongue and soft palate falling backward, partially or completely blocking the airway and causing apnea (i.e., cessation of breathing) and hypopnea (i.e., abnormally slow, shallow breathing). The patient's blood oxygen (O_2) level falls and the carbon dioxide (CO_2) level rises. These changes stimulate ventilation and cause the patient to arouse. The patient startles, snorts, and gasps, causing the tongue and soft palate to move forward so the airway is open. These episodes occur repeatedly during sleep, as depicted in Fig. 26.1A–C.

Symptoms of OSA are related to the disrupted sleep pattern. The patient is often irritable and sleepy during the day. The sleeping partner may report loud snoring or episodes of apnea. The symptoms can dramatically affect many aspects of life. Concentration and memory may be impaired. Hypertension and cardiac dysrhythmias may occur. OSA is confirmed

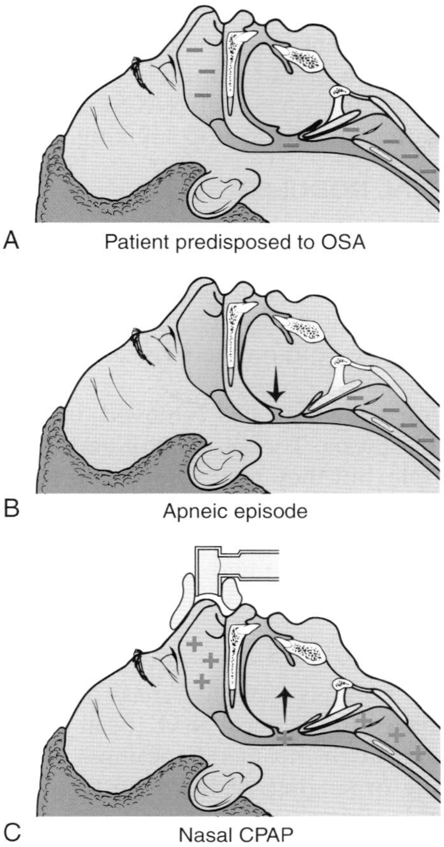

Fig. 26.1 Sleep apnea. (A) The patient predisposed to obstructive sleep apnea (*OSA*) has a small pharyngeal airway. (B) During sleep, the pharyngeal muscles relax, allowing the airway to close. Lack of airflow results in repeated apneic episodes. (C) With nasal continuous positive airway pressure (*CPAP*), positive pressure splints the airway open, preventing airflow obstruction. (From Lewis SM, Dirksen SR, Heitkemper MM, et al.: *Medical-surgical nursing: assessment and management of clinical problems*, ed 8, St. Louis, 2011, Mosby.)

by polysomnography, which may be done in a sleep laboratory or in the patient's home.

There is no single cause of OSA. Risk factors include obesity and smoking. Conservative treatment of OSA includes weight loss if obese and avoidance of sedatives and alcohol for 3 to 4 hours before bedtime. Advise the patient to elevate the head of the bed and sleep on the side rather than the back. An oral appliance that shifts the mandible and tongue forward may be effective. More serious symptoms are treated with nasal continuous positive airway pressure (CPAP). For sleep, the patient wears a mask that is attached to a blower (Fig. 26.2). The device maintains a pressure that prevents airway closure. Some patients have trouble exhaling against the sustained high pressure. Bilevel positive airway pressure (BiPAP) is preferred by some patients because it adjusts to deliver higher pressure during inspiration and lower pressure during expiration. If the patient is unable to tolerate the traditional face mask, several variations are available that might be more acceptable.

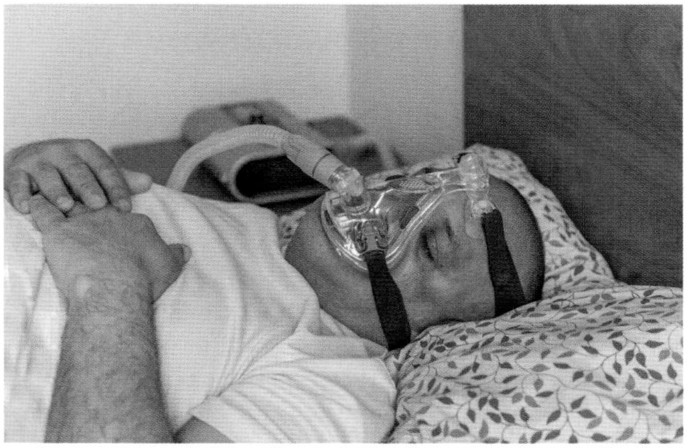

Fig. 26.2 Management of sleep apnea often involves sleeping with a nasal mask in place. The pressure supplied by air coming from the compressor opens the oropharynx and nasopharynx. (Copyright © yelo34/iStock/istock.com.)

Surgical procedures to reduce obstructing tissue are used only when other measures have not been effective. Surgery is not considered a first-line treatment.

DISORDERS OF THE LARYNX

LARYNGITIS

Laryngitis is inflammation of the larynx. It may occur alone, or it may accompany other upper respiratory infections. A number of factors may lead to laryngitis. Upper respiratory infections, voice strain, smoking, alcohol ingestion, gastroesophageal reflux disease (GERD), and inhalation of irritating fumes are all possible factors. Some patients have chronic laryngitis caused by prolonged exposure to irritants.

Clinical Manifestations

Symptoms of laryngitis include hoarseness, cough, and scratchy or painful throat. The patient may report "losing" their voice. This absence of sound production is called *aphonia*, and it occurs in varying degrees. Changes in the voice may be permanent after long periods of chronic inflammation.

Medical Diagnosis

Diagnosis of laryngitis is based primarily on the patient's history and symptoms. The physician may use a laryngeal mirror to examine the larynx for color, edema, and growths such as polyps and tumors. Inflamed vocal cords appear red and swollen. If an upper respiratory infection is suspected, a throat culture may be done to determine the pathogen and best treatment.

Medical Treatment

Treatment of acute laryngitis is aimed primarily at reducing irritation of the larynx. Voice rest is advised, meaning that the patient is to rest the larynx by not talking. An important aspect of treatment for chronic laryngitis is removal of the irritant.

◆ NURSING CARE OF THE PATIENT WITH LARYNGITIS

Patients with laryngitis rarely require hospitalization; however, laryngitis may occur in patients who have been hospitalized for other reasons.

Focused Assessment

For the patient with laryngitis, collection of relevant data begins with a history of the problem. Document the severity and duration of the condition and any factors that seem to aggravate or precipitate it. Information about the patient's occupation and hobbies may provide some clues to the cause of the laryngitis. Take the patient's temperature and describe respiratory status to detect possible infection.

Patient Problems, Goals, and Outcome Criteria: Laryngitis

Patient Problems	Goals and Outcome Criteria
Impaired verbal communication related to aphonia or prescribed voice rest	Effective communication: patient uses nonverbal communication means
Inability to manage self-care related to lack of knowledge	Effective management of therapeutic regimen: patient practices voice rest as ordered, avoids irritants

Interventions

When voice rest is prescribed, explain to the patient that it allows the larynx to heal. Meanwhile, an alternative means of communication must be established. Provide a pad and pencil for written communication. For patients who cannot read or write, hand signals or pictures may be needed. A sign over the bed is needed to advise staff and visitors that the patient should not speak. It is also a good idea to put a notice on the intercom at the nurses' station that the patient cannot (or should not) speak. This alerts staff to go to the patient's room rather than ask what is needed on the intercom.

The teaching plan focuses on comfort and avoiding future episodes of laryngitis. Discourage smoking. Advise the patient to remain in an environment with a constant temperature because sudden changes in temperature tend to aggravate laryngitis. If the air is very dry, a room humidifier reduces the discomfort of a dry nose and throat. Lozenges containing a topical anesthetic may also be ordered to soothe the irritation (see Chapter 25, Table 25.4).

When the patient has chronic laryngitis, the primary goal of treatment is to remove the irritant. Advise the patient who smokes that stopping smoking is likely to improve the symptoms. Changes in the voice may be permanent after long periods of chronic inflammation.

Teach patients that irritants can lead to laryngitis. Patients need to recognize irritants in the home and workplace and know how to protect themselves from harm. If the patient is inclined to stop smoking, provide information about resources in the community. The American Cancer Society (ACS) is a good source of information on how to stop smoking.

LARYNGEAL NODULES

Laryngeal nodules are benign masses of fibrous tissue that result primarily from overuse of the voice, but they can also follow infections. Singers and public speakers are prone to development of nodules because of the strain they put on their voices. The only symptom is hoarseness.

Nodules are surgically removed under local or general anesthesia. The removal of nodules is usually fairly simple, but they may recur if the voice is again misused. After the procedure, the patient is placed on voice rest for several days. Explain voice rest as described in the section titled "Laryngitis" and emphasize the need to avoid strain on the voice.

LARYNGEAL POLYPS

A laryngeal polyp is a swollen mass of mucous membrane attached to the vocal cord. It can cause continuous or intermittent hoarseness. Causes include excessive talking or singing, or irritation (commonly from smoking).

In heavy smokers, flabby masses of tissue may develop on both vocal cords. A procedure called *stripping of the vocal cords* is necessary to treat this condition. Unless the patient continues smoking, the condition usually does not return. Voice rest is prescribed for patients who have polyps removed.

CANCER OF THE LARYNX AND HYPOPHARYNX

The larynx is the "voice box"; it has three anatomical regions: the supraglottis (above the vocal cords), the glottis (which contains the larynx), and the subglottis (below the larynx). The hypopharynx is the part of the throat beside and behind the larynx. Because of their close proximity, laryngeal and hypopharyngeal cancers are considered together. The American Cancer Society (2020) predicted there would be 12,370 new cases of laryngeal and hypopharyngeal cancer in 2020. Approximately 3750 people will die from these cancers in 2020. The rate of new cases of laryngeal cancer is falling by about 2% to 3% a year, most likely because fewer people are smoking.

Factors believed to predispose to laryngeal cancer are exposure to smoke or other noxious fumes, exposure to asbestos, alcohol consumption, poor nutrition, vocal strain, human papilloma virus (HPV) of the throat, and chronic laryngitis. People who smoke and use alcohol are at particularly high risk.

Malignant tumors can develop at various points throughout the larynx: above the glottis, on the vocal cords, or below the vocal cords. For laryngeal cancers, survival rates differ based on which part of the larynx the cancer started in (supraglottis, glottis, or subglottis). Most malignancies of the larynx are squamous cell carcinomas.

The cure rate is highest for patients with tumors that are confined to the vocal cords. Unfortunately, malignancies in the larynx tend to spread fairly early. The most common site of metastasis is the lung. The more widespread the cancer is, the more difficult it is to treat. Lung cancer is the leading cause of cancer death in both men and women.

Clinical Manifestations

Early symptoms of cancer of the true vocal cords include persistent hoarseness or sore throat and ear pain. Subglottic and supraglottic laryngeal tumors can become very large without affecting the voice. Encourage patients to seek medical evaluation if these symptoms last more than 2 weeks. Some patients report throat discomfort or the sensation of a "lump" in the throat. Later signs and symptoms of laryngeal cancer are hemoptysis (i.e., blood in sputum) and difficulty swallowing or breathing. Pain and anorexia leading to weight loss are usually late symptoms of the disease.

Prevention

The most important measures to reduce the risk of cancer of the larynx are for people to stop smoking and drinking alcohol. The public should also be educated to recognize the signs and symptoms of laryngeal cancer and seek prompt medical attention. Early treatment may be able to preserve the voice.

Medical Diagnosis

A diagnosis of cancer of the larynx is confirmed by study of a tissue sample obtained during a laryngoscopy or panendoscopy, which visualizes the larynx, esophagus, and bronchi. Imaging studies (CT and PET scans, MRI) are done to define the extent of the cancer.

Medical Treatment

Treatment involves the use of surgery, radiation, chemotherapy, and/or targeted therapy. The treatment plan depends on the stage of the cancer and the patient's overall health state and ability to cope with the effects of specific treatments. Organ preservation (of the larynx) is a goal, if possible. Depending on the stage of the cancer and the patient's overall health status, various combinations of treatment may be recommended.

Radiation alone can cure some small cancers that have not spread to surrounding tissues. It may also be used in patients who are too weak to have surgery. Brachytherapy is a form of radiotherapy that involves placing thin, hollow needles into and around the tumor. Radioactive seeds are then placed in the needles to emit continuous radiation to the area.

Chemotherapy is often given along with radiation as the main treatment for more advanced cancers of the larynx. Chemotherapy may also be administered as palliative treatment, before surgery to reduce tumor size, or postoperatively to reduce the risk of metastasis. Care of the patient undergoing radiation or chemotherapy is discussed in Chapter 7.

Targeted therapy may be used in combination with chemotherapy and radiation. Targeted therapy is more specific to the cancer cells and less harmful to healthy cells. An example is the EGFR inhibitor cetuximab (Erbitux), which specifically targets epidermal growth factor receptors.

Surgical Treatment

Surgical procedures for cancer of the larynx and hypopharynx range from simple removal of the tumor to extensive procedures such as laryngectomy and modified or radical neck dissection. Laser surgery may be used alone or with radiation therapy for small tumors. A **laryngectomy** can be total or partial. The voice can be preserved with hemilaryngectomy or supraglottic laryngectomy. However, total laryngectomy causes permanent loss of the natural voice. Fig. 26.3 illustrates airflow before and after laryngectomy.

Radical neck dissection is often done at the same time as laryngectomy, especially if lymph nodes are positive for cancer. Radical neck dissection is the excision of the sternocleidomastoid muscle, jugular vein, submaxillary salivary gland, and surrounding soft tissue. The spinal accessory nerve is cut, causing the shoulder to droop on the affected side. Fig. 26.4 illustrates the appearance of the incisions after radical neck dissection. A modified radical neck dissection spares the internal jugular vein; the major cervical lymphatic vessels; and the sympathetic, vagus, and spinal accessory nerves.

◆ NURSING CARE OF THE PATIENT HAVING A TOTAL LARYNGECTOMY

General preoperative nursing care is discussed in Chapter 17. This section addresses the specific needs of the patient facing surgery for laryngeal or hypopharyngeal cancer. Try to find out which procedure will be done so that preoperative teaching can be individualized.

If the patient will lose the ability to speak, information about other means of communication should be available. The physician and speech therapist can advise the patient about appropriate alternatives. The anticipated loss of the voice is very stressful to patients. The full effect may not hit the patient until later, because the first concern is eliminating the cancer. Listen compassionately and accept the patient's expressions of anger or despair. Some patients benefit from meeting a volunteer from an organization for people who have had a laryngectomy. Consult the patient about this before inviting a volunteer.

The patient who will have a laryngectomy and radical neck dissection can expect to be in a monitored unit for several days. This allows close monitoring and maintenance of a patent airway with the new tracheostomy. Advise the patient in advance that this is routine

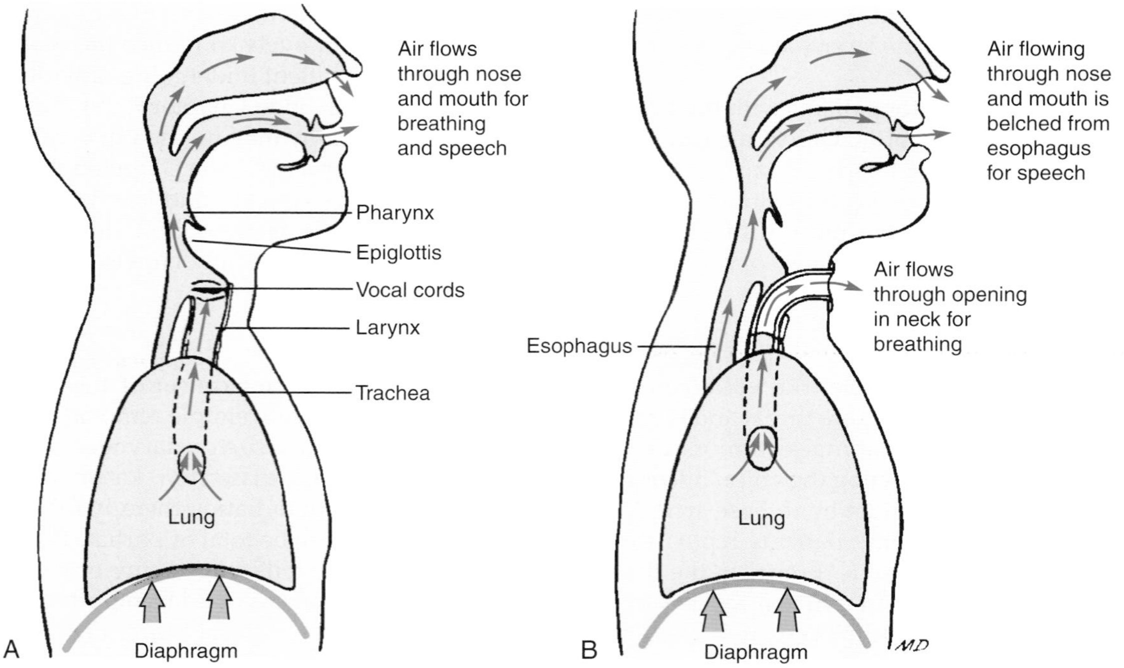

Fig. 26.3 The throat (A) before and (B) after total laryngectomy. *Arrows* indicate the route of airflow. (From Black JM, Hawks JH: *Medical-surgical nursing: clinical management for positive outcomes,* ed 8, St. Louis, 2009, Saunders.)

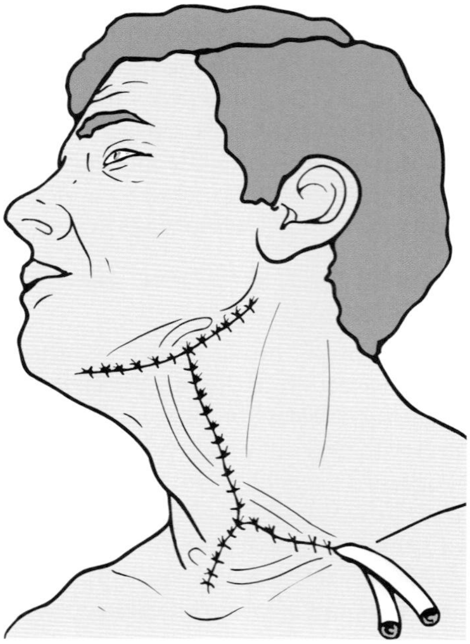

Fig. 26.4 A Radical neck dissection incision with drain tubes in place. (From Lewis SM, Dirksen SR, Heitkemper MM, et al.: *Medical-surgical nursing: assessment and management of clinical problems*, ed 8, St. Louis, 2011, Mosby.)

and does not mean that anything has gone wrong. You can also help prepare the patient to expect intravenous lines, wound drains, a feeding tube, and, perhaps for a short time, a ventilator.

Postoperative care varies with the exact procedure. Procedures include partial laryngectomy, supraglottic laryngectomy, and total laryngectomy. Nursing care of the patient with a total laryngectomy is presented in detail. The unique needs of the patient with a partial or supraglottic laryngectomy are identified.

A total laryngectomy involves removal of the entire larynx, vocal cords, and epiglottis, as well as supportive tissues. The opening of the pharynx to the trachea is closed and the tracheostomy is created by bringing the trachea to the opening in the neck. The upper airway is no longer connected to the lower airway. The patient breathes through the trachea. Fig. 26.3 illustrates the changes with total laryngectomy. A radical or modified radical neck dissection is often done because of the high risk of metastasis to the neck.

Complications

Complications of total laryngectomy with radical neck dissection include salivary fistula, carotid artery rupture (rare), and tracheal stenosis. A salivary fistula is a drainage pathway that forms when saliva leaks through a defect in the suture line in the pharynx. It usually closes spontaneously but sometimes requires surgical closure. Until the fistula closes, the patient must be fed through a nasogastric tube. Otherwise, whatever the patient eats leaks out of the fistula.

Patients at highest risk for carotid artery rupture are those who had radiation therapy before surgery and acquired a salivary fistula after surgery. Although rare, carotid rupture is an emergency that must be corrected surgically.

Tracheal stenosis is narrowing of the trachea that develops weeks or months after surgery. If the airway becomes obstructed, surgical correction is necessary.

The general nursing care of the postoperative patient is discussed in Chapter 17. This section addresses the special needs of the patient with total laryngectomy.

Focused Assessment

In the immediate postoperative period, the assessment focuses on oxygenation, circulation, and comfort. You assist by collecting relevant data. Document the patient's level of consciousness. Ask about pain and observe for signs of discomfort. Measure vital signs at frequent intervals. Continuous electrocardiogram (ECG) monitoring and pulse oximetry may also be used to assess oxygenation and circulation. Record fluid intake and output and describe the characteristics of wound drainage.

Additional aspects of assessment after total laryngectomy are weight changes, ability to swallow, and effectiveness of alternate means of communication. The patient's response to the surgery, coping strategies used, and sources of support are also very important. During the rehabilitation phase, members of the health care team help the patient to anticipate the effects of the surgery on everyday life and the adaptations that need to be made. In addition, collect data that indicate the patient's readiness and ability to participate in self-care.

Patient Problems, Goals, and Outcome Criteria: Total Laryngectomy, Postoperative

Patient Problems	Goals and Outcome Criteria
Potential for airway obstruction related to increased pulmonary secretions or weak cough	Patent airway: respiratory rate 12 to 20 breaths per minute without dyspnea, breath sounds clear
Anxiety related to revised airway, uncertain outcome of cancer surgery, or threat to self-concept	Reduced anxiety: patient calm, states anxiety is reduced
Potential for decreased cardiac output related to excessive blood loss	Adequate cardiac output: pulse and blood pressure (BP) consistent with patient norms, fluid intake and output equal Minimal blood loss: decreasing bleeding, drainage lightens in color
Acute pain related to tissue trauma	Pain relief: patient states pain reduced, relaxed manner
Potential for injury related to excision of muscles in the neck or altered upper airway	Reduced risk for injury: patient demonstrates protection of incision during movement, avoids introduction of harmful substances into trachea
Inadequate nutrition related to dysphagia or diminished sense of smell	Adequate nutrition: stable body weight, maintenance of patient's admission weight if normal
Impaired verbal communication related to surgical excision of larynx	Effective communication: patient uses a means of communication that meets their needs
Inadequate coping related to loss of verbal communication or altered appearance	Effective coping with body changes: patient makes realistic plans to adapt lifestyle to physical and functional changes
Potential for infection related to altered airway or interrupted skin integrity	Absence of infection: normal body temperature and white blood cell (WBC) count, no purulent drainage or secretions
Inability to manage self-care related to lack of knowledge and skills for tracheostomy care	Patient assumes self-care: correctly demonstrates care of tracheostomy

Interventions

Potential for airway obstruction. As previously emphasized, oxygenation status must be monitored frequently. If the patient is on a ventilator, it is usually discontinued within 1 day after surgery. At first, the patient has a laryngectomy tube in the tracheostomy. The laryngectomy tube is shorter and wider than a tracheostomy tube but care of the two tubes is essentially the same.

Because the new tracheostomy bypasses the upper airway, the respiratory tract has to adjust to a dramatic change. The mucous membranes respond to the unexpected trauma and irritation by increasing secretions. Because normal humidification is absent, the secretions tend to be drier than normal, making it more difficult to remove them from the airway.

The trachea and laryngectomy tube must be kept open at all times (or the patient would suffocate). Data that indicate the need for suctioning include increased pulse, restlessness, and audible or visible mucus. Use sterile technique to clear the airway as needed. Tracheostomy suctioning and care are described in Chapter 25. Consult a procedure manual for additional details.

Factors that affect respiratory status are positioning, fluids, and humidification. Semi-Fowler or Fowler position permits maximal lung expansion. Turning, coughing, and deep breathing prevent pooling of secretions in the lungs. Intravenous fluids and enteral feedings maintain hydration and nutrition. Good hydration helps to thin secretions. A tracheostomy collar is used to provide O_2 and humidification of inspired air.

Anxiety. Be sensitive to the patient's anxiety. A calm approach, attentive monitoring, and simple explanations help to reduce anxiety. A tendency exists to treat the patient who cannot speak as if they cannot hear either. Therefore you must also remember to talk to the patient!

Potential for decreased cardiac output. The patient is at risk for excessive bleeding in the early postoperative period. Observe for restlessness and monitor vital signs for increasing pulse and respiratory rates, which may indicate hemorrhage. Inspect secretions for excessive bleeding. Drains are usually in place to remove excess fluid. Note the color and the amount of the drainage. Over the first few postoperative days, the color should change from bright red to pink to clear or straw colored. The amount of drainage should also decrease steadily.

Acute pain. Administer analgesics as ordered after surgery. The patient who has had a radical neck dissection may have less pain than you expect. Because the procedure is so extensive, many nerves are cut, so sensation is impaired. Some areas of numbness are permanent.

Potential for injury. The patient may be fearful of moving their head, especially after radical neck surgery. You can help at first by placing a hand behind the patient's head when they get out of bed. The patient can also learn to roll on one side and support the head while rising from the bed.

The tracheostomy is open to the environment and must be protected from foreign substances. Teach the patient to avoid dusty places and to cover the tracheostomy loosely during shaving or haircuts. The patient cannot submerge the neck or allow bath water to splash into the trachea because the water would go directly into the airway. A plastic collar can be worn for showering.

Inadequate nutrition. Nutrition is often a problem after laryngectomy. The patient's sense of smell is impaired because inspired air no longer goes through the nose. The patient may also have some difficulty swallowing because of tissue trauma around the surgical site. Nasogastric tube feedings are given initially. Oral fluids and foods are reintroduced gradually. After supraglottic laryngectomy, which includes excision of the epiglottis, the patient must learn supraglottic swallowing to prevent aspiration (see the Nutrition Considerations box). The patient's weight should be monitored. Implement nursing interventions for anorexia and for tube feedings, as discussed in Chapters 15 and 38.

Nutrition Considerations

1. Malignancies of the upper airway often lead to inadequate nutritional intake.
2. Patients who have had a supraglottic laryngectomy are at high risk for aspiration while learning to swallow again.
3. Gastrostomy or nasogastric tubes may be placed to maintain nutrition after partial laryngectomy.

Impaired verbal communication. Three types of options exist for restoring some form of oral communication to the patient with laryngectomy. These are esophageal speech, the artificial larynx (electrolarynx), and tracheoesophageal voice restoration. The speech-language pathologist (SLP) and the physician will recommend appropriate methods for the individual patient (Fig. 26.5). It is important that the SLP is trained in rehabilitating people who have had a laryngectomy. The SLP will play a major role in helping the patient learn to communicate.

Some patients are able to learn to use "esophageal speech." Air is swallowed and held in the upper esophagus. The patient then belches. The patient learns to control and use the air to produce sounds. The voice is deep but understandable. Considerable motivation and practice are needed to master esophageal speech. Patients and their families are likely to have periods of discouragement. You can help by acknowledging their feelings and demonstrating patience.

A second option is the use of an artificial larynx or electrolarynx. A variety of such devices are available (Fig 26.5 A and B). One device which looks like a small flashlight is held against the throat and detects vibrations from silently mouthed words, which are then converted into electronic sounds. One of the newer devices (UltraVoice) has a component that is placed inside the mouth. A controller transmits radio waves to the oral unit which creates speech.

One concern is that the "voice" has a mechanical, computerized sound that tends to attract attention. Technological advances continue to improve the quality of the sound. A demonstration of the voice quality with an electrolarynx can be heard on https://UltraVoice.com.

The third option for speech is the tracheoesophageal prosthesis. The surgeon creates a fistula between the trachea and the esophagus. A catheter is placed in the fistula until it heals. When the catheter is removed, a prosthesis is inserted into the fistula. A one-way valve allows air to flow only from the trachea to the esophagus. The patient will need to occlude the stoma with a finger during speech unless a hands-free unit is used that has a special speaking valve. An example is the Blom-Singer speech assistive device. See Fig 26.5C. Use of this device can be seen at https://www.luminaud.com.

Those patients who are unable to use any form of speech must rely on written communication, gestures, or some assistive devices. A word board is a computerized device that enables the patient to select words that are "spoken" by the computer. A personal communicator produces a printed message that the patient enters on a keyboard.

It is especially important to direct the laryngectomy patient to community resources. Organizations such as the Lost Chord Club or New Voice Club are especially useful because the members have had personal experiences with laryngectomies. The ACS can provide information about resources in the local community.

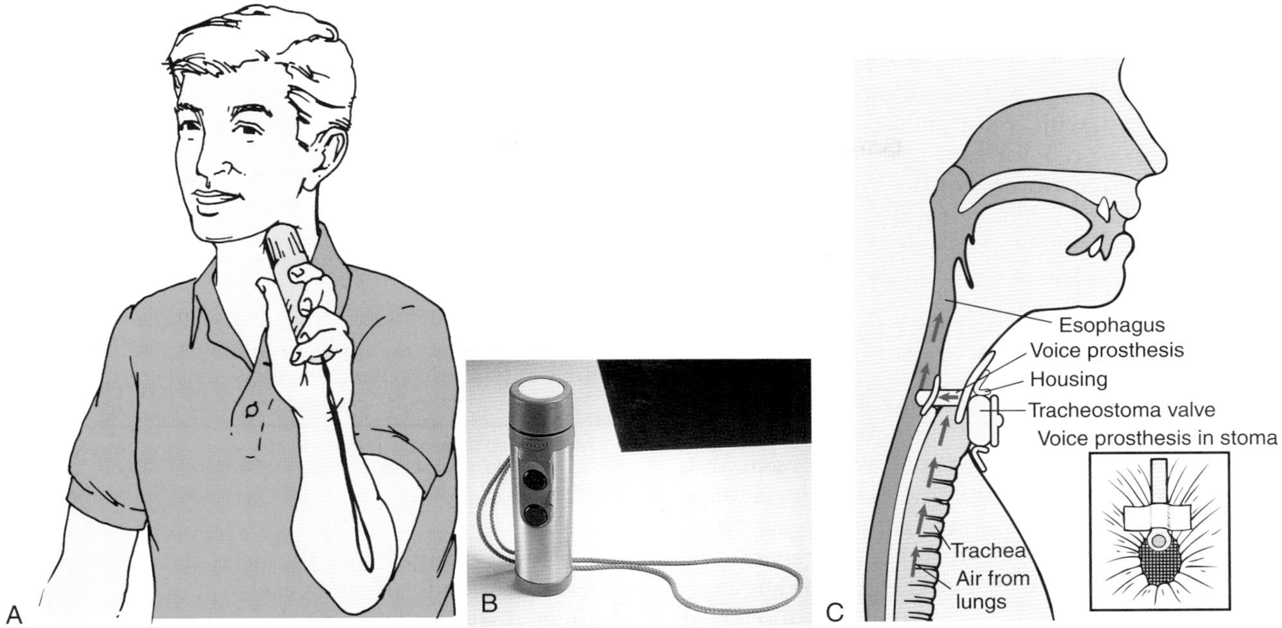

Fig. 26.5 Postlaryngectomy speech aids. (A and B) Patient using the Servox Electrolarynx artificial larynx, which is held against the throat to detect vibrations from silently mouthed words and convert them to electronic sounds. (C) Blom-Singer trapdoor tracheoesophageal prosthesis. (A, From Black JM, Hawks JH: *Medical-surgical nursing: clinical management for positive outcomes*, ed 8, St. Louis, 2009, Saunders.)

Inadequate coping. It has been said that language separates humans from animals. The permanent loss of the ability to communicate verbally is very traumatic. Patients who require laryngectomy usually have some time to prepare for this procedure, but the actual event still evokes a variety of emotional responses. Learning to live with a permanent tracheostomy and loss of the natural voice requires considerable adjustment. The patient may demonstrate behaviors typical of any loss situation: denial, anger, depression, bargaining, and acceptance. Depression may be reflected in withdrawal or refusal to learn about self-care and rehabilitative measures.

Acknowledge the patient's feelings and gently urge participation in self-care and use of alternative means of communication. The patient who learns to care for the tracheostomy and to communicate effectively feels more confident in their ability to cope. Support groups can be especially helpful because the patient sees potential role models of successful adaptation to tracheostomy. The family also requires support, encouragement, and teaching.

Potential for infection. The tracheostomy permits unfiltered air to enter the respiratory tract. The effects are drying of the mucous membranes, increased secretions, and increased risk of infection. Use sterile technique during tracheostomy care. Protect the patient from people who have respiratory infections.

Inability to manage self-care. As soon as the patient is able, encourage participation in self-care. At first, ask the patient simply to hold some supplies. Explain what is being done and why. Gradually, the patient should assume more responsibility for care of the tracheostomy. Even if the patient seems quite competent by discharge, a referral to a home health agency or visiting nurse association is recommended. The home care nurse helps the patient learn to adapt care to the home setting and to deal with various unanticipated problems. A family member or significant other should be taught tracheostomy care as well. Verbal teaching should be accompanied by written information and/or videos for later use. Remember that people recall only a small percentage of what they hear.

◆ NURSING CARE OF THE PATIENT HAVING A SUPRAGLOTTIC LARYNGECTOMY

For patients whose cancer is located above the vocal cords, supraglottic laryngectomy and radical neck dissection are the usual procedures. These patients also have temporary tracheostomies. Cuffed tubes are used at first because of the danger of aspiration. These patients require oral and tracheal suctioning.

Nursing care of the patient having supraglottic laryngectomy is in many ways like that of the patient having total laryngectomy except that the tracheostomy is temporary, the voice is not lost, and swallowing is more problematic. Therefore additional nursing interventions are indicated to maintain good nutrition. Enteral feedings may be needed for a long time, so begin to instruct the patient in self-feeding. Some patients never regain the ability to swallow without aspirating and total laryngectomy is recommended for them. An example of the swallowing techniques taught to these patients is outlined in Box 26.1.

When the patient has a tracheostomy, any aspirated food or fluids may be ejected through the tracheostomy. The patient with a supraglottic laryngectomy is also at increased risk for aspiration pneumonia. Be alert for signs and symptoms of this complication: increased pulse and respiratory rates; dyspnea; cough; crackles and rhonchi; fever; wheezing; and frothy, pink sputum. Keep a suction machine readily available.

◆ NURSING CARE OF THE PATIENT HAVING A PARTIAL LARYNGECTOMY

If a patient has a partial laryngectomy, a temporary tracheostomy for 2 to 5 days can be expected. Intravenous fluids and enteral feedings are usually ordered at first. Like the patient with a supraglottic laryngectomy, these patients have considerable difficulty swallowing when oral nourishment is resumed. In general, the nursing care is similar to that of the patient having a supraglottic laryngectomy. To prevent aspiration, seat the patient upright with the head flexed slightly forward. Semisolids are often easier to manage than thin liquids. A suction machine should be on hand.

Box 26.1 Steps for Performing the Supraglottic Swallow

1. Take a deep breath to aerate the lungs.
2. Perform the Valsalva maneuver to approximate the cords.
3. Place food in the mouth and swallow. Some food will enter the airway and remain on top of the closed vocal cords.
4. Cough to remove the food from the top of the vocal cords.
5. Swallow so that food is moved from the top of vocal cords.
6. Breathe after the cough-swallow sequence to prevent aspiration of food collected on top of the vocal cords.

From Lewis SM, Dirksen SR, Heitkemper MM, et al.: *Medical-surgical nursing: assessment and management of clinical problems*, ed 8, St. Louis, 2011, Mosby.

Get Ready for The NCLEX® Examination!

Key Points

- Sinusitis is an acute or chronic inflammation of the sinuses that can lead to meningitis, brain abscess, osteomyelitis, and orbital cellulitis.
- Rhinosinusitis commonly occurs with sinusitis; the term is used when both the nasal mucosa and the sinuses are inflamed.
- Sinusitis is treated with drug therapy or with surgery to remove obstructions and to improve drainage.
- Nasal polyps are masses of tissue that extend from the sinuses into the nasal passage; they can be surgically excised.
- Allergic rhinitis is an allergic response to a substance that produces sneezing; nasal obstruction; clear nasal discharge; frontal headache; and itchy, watery eyes. It may be treated with antihistamines and decongestants or with desensitizing injections of identified allergens.
- Acute viral coryza, the common cold, is caused by a virus; is contagious; and is treated symptomatically with antihistamines, decongestants, and antipyretics.
- Tumors of the nasal passages typically cause nasal obstruction requiring surgical excision.
- Malignant tumors of the nasal passages and pharynx tend to metastasize early and may be treated with some combination of surgery, chemotherapy, and radiation therapy.
- Carcinomas of the external nose: (1) squamous cell carcinomas grow rapidly and tend to metastasize, and (2) basal cell carcinomas grow more slowly and are less invasive.
- A deviated nasal septum may obstruct the nasal passages and interfere with sinus drainage.
- Septoplasty is a surgical procedure to correct a deviated nasal septum.
- Epistaxis can usually be controlled with external pressure but may require cauterization, a nasal balloon catheter, or packing.
- Tonsillitis is more common in children but is more often severe in adults. It may be treated with drug therapy, irrigations, or surgical excision.
- Nursing care after tonsillectomy focuses on potential for decreased cardiac output, potential for airway obstruction, pain, and inability to perform self-care.
- Cancer of the larynx may be treated with surgery, radiation therapy, chemotherapy, or a combination of these.
- After laryngectomy, the nurse addresses problems of potential for airway obstruction, anxiety, potential for decreased cardiac output, pain, potential for injury, inadequate nutrition, impaired communication, inadequate coping, potential for infection, and inability to perform self-care.

After laryngectomy, speech may be restored with esophageal speech or with assistive devices: the artificial larynx, and the tracheoesophageal prosthesis.

Additional Learning Resources

SG Go to your Study Guide for additional learning activities to help you master this chapter content.

Go to your Evolve website (http://evolve.elsevier.com/Linton/medsurg) for the following learning resources and much more:

- Fluid & Electrolyte Tutorial
- Review Questions for the NCLEX® Examination

Clinical Judgment and Next-Generation NCLEX® Examination-Style Questions

1. **After nasal surgery, a patient has packing in place and a nasal drip ("mustache") dressing on the upper lip. When the mustache dressing has become saturated, which of the following should you do?**
   1. Replace the packing and the mustache dressing.
   2. Remove the mustache dressing.
   3. Reinforce the mustache dressing.
   4. Change the mustache dressing.

   NCLEX Client Need: Physiological Integrity: Reduction of Risk Potential

2. **A patient who had nasal surgery is restless. His pulse rate has increased from 70 to 90 beats per minute, and his respiratory rate is 20 breaths per minute. His nasal dressing has no fresh bleeding. What should you do first?**
   1. Order 1 U of blood.
   2. Take his vital signs again.
   3. Inspect the back of his throat.
   4. Encourage increased fluid intake.

   NCLEX Client Need: Physiological Integrity: Reduction of Risk Potential

3. **The most serious complication of sinusitis is:**
   1. Headache
   2. Pain
   3. Meningitis
   4. Rhinitis

   NCLEX Client Need: Physiological Integrity: Physiological Adaptation

4. **A patient who has triad disease has which of the following? (Select all that apply.)**
   1. Asthma
   2. Nasal polyps
   3. Aspirin allergy
   4. Laryngeal nodules
   5. Sinusitis

   NCLEX Client Need: Physiological Integrity: Physiological Adaptation

5. **A patient rushes into the urgent care clinic holding a bloody towel to her face. She says that her nose started bleeding suddenly, and she cannot control it. Immediate treatment of epistaxis involves having the patient do which of the following?**
   1. Sit up, lean slightly forward, and pinch the nostrils.
   2. Assume a semi-Fowler position with the head tilted back.
   3. Lie supine and apply a cold pack to the nose.
   4. Sit up and lean forward to put the head between the knees.

   NCLEX Client Need: Physiological Integrity: Reduction of Risk Potential

6. **The postoperative nursing care plan for a patient who had a total laryngectomy 24 hours ago includes the subsequent patient problems. Which is the priority patient problem for this patient?**
   1. Anxiety
   2. Pain
   3. Potential airway obstruction
   4. Impaired communication

   NCLEX Client Need: Physiological Integrity: Reduction of Risk Potential

7. **Mr. P. is going to surgery for a supraglottic laryngectomy, and Mr. S. is going to have a total laryngectomy. Which of the following describes the differences in their postoperative needs? (Select all that apply.)**
   1. Mr. S. will be able to swallow more easily than Mr. P.
   2. Mr. S.'s voice will be preserved; Mr. P.'s voice will not be preserved.
   3. Mr. P. will have a temporary tracheostomy; Mr. S.'s tracheostomy will be permanent.
   4. Mr. P. will be at greater risk of aspiration than Mr. S.
   5. Mr. P. is more likely to have a radical neck dissection than Mr. S.

   UNFOLDING CASE TEST ITEMS: Total Laryngectomy

Phase I

Question 1. Recognize cues using enhanced hot spot test item type

A 60-year-old man was diagnosed with cancer of the larynx. After a total laryngectomy and radical neck dissection, he was admitted to intensive care for 3 days. He was moved to a medical-surgical unit today. He has a nasogastric tube in place for enteral feedings, is receiving oxygen via his tracheostomy, and intravenous fluids. A wound drain is in place in the neck incision. The nurse's initial assessment includes the following:

- BP 140/70 mm Hg
- Heart rate 94 beats per minute
- Respirations 24 breaths per minute
- Temperature 98°F
- Weak cough
- Drowsy but responds appropriately
- Oriented to person and place
- Pain level 3 on a 1 to 10 pain scale
- Bright red blood in drain receptacle

Highlight or place a check mark next to the assessment findings that require follow up by the nurse.

Question 2. Analyze cues using Cloze Test Item

A 60-year-old man was diagnosed with cancer of the larynx. After a total laryngectomy and radical neck dissection, he was admitted to intensive care for 3 days. He was moved to a medical-surgical unit today. He has a nasogastric tube in place for enteral feedings, is receiving oxygen via his tracheostomy, and intravenous fluids. A wound drain is in place in the neck incision. The nurse's initial assessment includes the following:

- BP 140/70 mm Hg
- Heart rate 94 beats per minute
- Respirations 24 breaths per minute
- Temperature 98°F
- Weak cough
- Drowsy but responds appropriately
- Oriented to person and place

- Appears anxious
- Pain level 3 on a 1 to 10 pain scale
- Wound drainage is pink
- Pulse oximetry: O_2 saturation at 89%

Choose the most likely options for the information missing from the statements below by selecting from the lists of options provided

The FIRST priority when caring for a patient with a new tracheostomy is (1)________ . The patient's vital signs suggest that the nurse should (2)__________. Factors that are likely contributing to his anxiety include (3)________, (3)_________, and (3)________.

OPTIONS FOR 1	OPTIONS FOR 2	OPTIONS FOR 3
Assessing for hemorrhage	Reposition the patient	Hypoxia
Maintaining oxygenation	Increase his IV fluid rate	Loss of voice
Providing hydration	Suction his tracheostomy	Hunger
Reducing anxiety	Administer pain medication	Loneliness
Providing pain relief	Encourage him to relax	Fear of suffocation

Phase II

Question 3. Prioritize hypotheses using extended multiple response test items

A 60-year-old man was diagnosed with cancer of the larynx. After a total laryngectomy and radical neck dissection, he was admitted to intensive care for 3 days. He was moved to a medical-surgical unit today. He has a nasogastric tube in place for enteral feedings, is receiving oxygen via his tracheostomy, and intravenous fluids. A wound drain is in place in the neck incision.

When planning care for this patient, for which priority potential complications would the nurse monitor? Select all that apply.

a. Salivary fistula
b. Bowel obstruction
c. Urinary tract infection
d. Carotid artery rupture
e. Tracheal stenosis
f. Muscle atrophy

Phase III

Question 4. Take action using matrix test item

A 60-year-old man was diagnosed with cancer of the larynx. After a total laryngectomy and radical neck dissection, he was admitted to intensive care for 3 days. He was moved to a medical-surgical unit today. He has a nasogastric tube in place for enteral feedings, is receiving oxygen via his tracheostomy, and intravenous fluids. A wound drain is in place in the neck incision.

Use an X for the health teaching below that is: *Indicated* (appropriate or necessary), *Contraindicated* (could be harmful), or *Nonessential* (makes no difference or not necessary) before the patient's discharge at this time.

HEALTH TEACHING	INDICATED	CONTRAIN-DICATED	NONES-SENTIAL
"In a few months, the tracheostomy will be closed, so your normal airway will be restored."			
"Many options for communication. The speech therapist will help you select the best one for you."			
"When your feeding tube is removed, you will be able to gradually take liquids and solid foods."			
"Modern devices can restore your natural voice."			
"Cover your tracheostomy when shaving, for haircuts, and when showering."			
"Always use fluoride toothpaste."			

Acute Lower Respiratory Tract Disorders

27

http://evolve.elsevier.com/Linton/medsurg

Objectives

1. For selected acute respiratory disorders, describe the pathophysiology, signs and symptoms, complications, diagnostic measures, and medical treatment.
2. Assist in developing a nursing care plan for the patient who has an acute respiratory disorder.

Key Terms

atelectasis
empyema
hemoptysis
hemothorax
hypercapnia
pleurisy
pneumothorax

ACUTE BRONCHITIS

CAUSE AND RISK FACTORS

Acute **bronchitis** is inflammation of the bronchi in the lower respiratory tract. Most acute bronchial infections are viral in origin, often following a viral infection such as a cold or influenza. Bacterial causes such as *Streptococcus pneumoniae* or *Haemophilus influenzae* and noninfectious inhaled toxins such as cigarette smoke can also cause acute bronchitis. Irritation and inflammation may occur throughout the upper respiratory tract, resulting in an increased production of mucus.

CLINICAL MANIFESTATIONS

Symptoms of acute bronchitis include cough (productive and nonproductive), sputum production, fatigue, dyspnea on exertion, wheezing or rhonchi, fever, chest pain, and other symptoms similar to upper respiratory tract infections such as nasal congestion, runny nose, and sore throat.

MEDICAL DIAGNOSIS

Acute bronchitis is usually diagnosed based on the health history and clinical presentation.

MEDICAL TREATMENT

Medications that may reduce symptoms include antitussive agents such as dextromethorphan or the expectorant guaifenesin. Chest tightness caused by constricted airway can be relieved with beta-2 agonists such as albuterol. Routine antibiotic treatment for uncomplicated acute bronchitis is not recommended. Hospitalization is usually not necessary.

❖ NURSING CARE OF THE PATIENT WITH ACUTE BRONCHITIS

Because acute bronchitis is usually managed in outpatient settings, nursing care focuses on symptom management and patient education. Humidifying the air and eliminating environmental cough triggers may be helpful. If the patient is prescribed antibiotics, teach the patient the importance of taking the full course of their antibiotics to prevent recurrence and antibiotic resistance. Emphasize good handwashing, covering the mouth when coughing, and proper disposal of tissues. The patient should avoid contact with vulnerable individuals while symptomatic.

INFLUENZA

Influenza, commonly called *flu,* is an acute respiratory infection caused by influenza viruses. There are four types of influenza viruses: A, B, C, and D. Human influenza A and B viruses cause seasonal epidemics of disease almost every winter in the United States. Influenza A viruses are divided into subtypes and strains. Current subtypes of influenza A found in people are the "2009" H1N1 (so called after the influenza pandemic of 2009) and H3N2. Influenza A is the most virulent of the flu viruses and can infect both humans and animals. There are over 100 influenza A viruses found in birds (avian flu), pigs (swine flu), horses, seals, and dogs. Influenza type C infections usually cause only mild respiratory illness and are not thought to be responsible for epidemics, whereas influenza D viruses primarily affect cattle and do not infect or cause illness in people. Those most susceptible to the influenza virus are very young children, older adults, pregnant and postpartum women, extremely obese persons, people living in institutional settings, people with chronic illnesses, people on immunosuppressants, Native Americans and Alaska natives, and health care personnel.

COMPLICATIONS

Influenza complications can affect the respiratory, cardiac, and central nervous systems (CNS). The most common complications of influenza are bronchitis, viral or bacterial pneumonia, and sinus or ear infections. Acute respiratory failure secondary to flu is a life-threatening condition that requires immediate medical attention. Multiple organ dysfunction syndrome (MODS) may ensue. Cardiac complications include EKG abnormalities, acute myocardial infarction, myocarditis, and pericarditis. Possible CNS complications are encephalitis, aseptic meningitis, encephalopathy, and Guillain-Barré syndrome.

CLINICAL MANIFESTATIONS

Influenza is similar to the common cold in the way it is spread (i.e., through droplet infection); however, its symptoms differ from those of the common cold. People with colds experience nasal symptoms, sore throat, chest discomfort, and are usually afebrile (without fever) with a gradual onset of symptoms; whereas those with influenza typically experience an abrupt onset of symptoms with a characteristically high fever (102°F–104°F; 38°C–40°C) that lasts 3 to 4 days. Other flu symptoms include headache, general body aches and pains, exhaustion, and fatigue and weakness. These symptoms are commonly accompanied by respiratory tract symptoms, particularly cough and sore throat. However, a wide spectrum of clinical presentations may occur, ranging from a mild, afebrile upper respiratory illness to prostration and severe systemic signs and symptoms. Older adults may have milder symptoms, no fever, but altered mental status.

MEDICAL DIAGNOSIS

A diagnosis of influenza is usually based on the patient's history and clinical symptoms. There are currently a number of flu tests available to detect influenza viruses. The most common tests are called *rapid influenza diagnostic tests (RIDTs)* that can provide results in about 10 to 15 minutes, and *rapid molecular assays* that produce results in about 15 to 20 minutes. However, neither test type is definitive (a person can test negative and still have the flu). There are other, more sensitive and accurate flu tests that are available in specialized laboratories such as those found in hospitals. All of these tests require a nasal, throat, or nasopharyngeal swab.

MEDICAL TREATMENT

Treatment of influenza is similar to the treatment of the common cold: rest, fluids, proper diet, antipyretics, and analgesics. There are currently six prescription influenza antiviral agents available in the United States. These drugs, used to treat or prevent influenza include: oral oseltamivir (Tamiflu) and baloxavir (Xofluza), inhaled zanamivir (Relenza), and intravenous peramivir (Rapivab). Specific agents are identified each year based on the specific viral strain. For the latest information on the use of antivirals to treat influenza, visit www.cdc.gov/flu/professionals/antivirals.

The most effective way to prevent flu is to have a yearly vaccine. The vaccine is recommended for everyone 6 months of age or older. Influenza A (H1N1), A (H3N2), and one or two influenza B viruses (depending on the vaccine) are included in each year's influenza vaccine. Getting a flu vaccine can protect against flu viruses that are the same or related to the viruses in the vaccine. The seasonal flu vaccine does not protect against influenza C viruses. In addition, flu vaccines will not protect against infection and illness caused by other viruses that also cause influenza-like symptoms. There are many nonflu viruses that can result in influenza-like illness (ILI) that spread during flu season. An antiviral drug may be prescribed for people who are at increased risk of acquiring viral infections.

Complementary and Alternative Therapies

Scientific studies have found that echinacea has no effect on the incidence, severity, or duration of colds.

Pharmacology Capsule

Antiviral drugs must be administered ideally within 48 hours after the onset of influenza symptoms to be effective.

❖ NURSING CARE OF THE PATIENT WITH INFLUENZA

Nursing care of the patient with influenza is similar to care of the patient with the common cold. Ongoing monitoring is particularly important with influenza because of the risk of serious complications, especially in older adults. Although routine annual influenza vaccination is now recommended for all persons 6 months of age and older, it is most important for those individuals at high risk: those with serious chronic cardiopulmonary disorders, residents of long-term care facilities, health care providers who have contact with high-risk patients, people older than 65 years of age, and those who have chronic metabolic disorders such as diabetes mellitus.

CORONAVIRUS

CAUSE AND RISK FACTORS

The virus that causes COVID-19 disease is severe acute respiratory syndrome 2 (SARS-CoV-2). Almost anyone can become infected with COVID-19, especially those who spend time in crowded locations. Most people recover, but the elderly and those with underlying health conditions, immune suppression, obesity, and Down syndrome are at greater risk for severe illness (i.e., requiring hospitalization, intensive care, and mechanical ventilation) and death.

COMPLICATIONS

Complications of COVID-19 disease are:

- Respiratory failure: pneumonia, acute respiratory distress syndrome (ARDS), mechanical ventilation required by 12% to 20% of patients
- Cardiac and cardiovascular problems: arrhythmias, acute cardiac injury, shock
- Thromboembolism: pulmonary embolism, acute stroke
- Neurological problems: encephalopathy, movement disorders, motor and sensory deficits, ataxia, seizures, cognitive impairment
- Generalized inflammation: persistent fever, elevated serum inflammatory markers (McIntosh, November 20, 2020)

CLINICAL MANIFESTATIONS

Among the more common symptoms that should alert the health care provider to possible COVID-19 include new onset fever, cough, dyspnea, disturbances in smell and taste, myalgias (muscle aches), and sometimes diarrhea.

MEDICAL DIAGNOSIS

To diagnose COVID-19, a specimen is collected from the upper respiratory tract (usually the nose, nasopharynx, or oropharynx) and submitted for testing. Tests include the NAAT and serologic tests. The NAAT has several variations but is generally considered the most accurate. The antigen test is less sensitive than the NAAT but may be especially useful when supplies for NAAT testing are limited. Serologic tests detect antibodies, therefore, they are most useful 3 to 4 weeks after the onset of symptoms. Serologic tests alone should not be used to detect COVID-19 infection.

MEDICAL TREATMENT

Patients with COVID-19 may be treated at home, seen in ambulatory settings, or in inpatient facilities. Patients who are eligible for home care should have relatively mild symptoms, be able to self-isolate, and reliably report worsening symptoms. If telehealth is available, the health care provider can monitor the patient at home. Criteria for patients who can be managed through a dedicated clinic include those with mild to moderate dyspnea, mild dyspnea with risk factors for severe disease, oxygen saturation between 91% and 94%, and other concerning symptoms. Individuals with severe dyspnea, oxygen saturation of 90% or below, or altered mental status should be evaluated in the emergency department (Cohen & Blau, November 30, 2020).

The optimal treatment of COVID-19 is uncertain at this time. The latest recommendations from the National Institutes of Health (NIH) (October 31, 2021) are listed in Table 27.1. For the most recent information, see COVID-19 Treatment Guidelines at https://www.covid19treatmentguidelines.nih.gov/.

The value of convalescent plasma (which contains antibodies from patients who have recovered from COVID-19) is still being evaluated.

Drugs that have not been shown to have a clear benefit and that have the potential for toxicity are hydroxychloroquine, chloroquine, and/or azithromycin, HIV protease inhibitors, and nitazoxanide.

The care of critically ill patients is beyond the scope of this textbook. Their treatment may also require:

- vasopressors for hypotension
- continuous renal replacement therapy for acute kidney injury
- high-flow nasal cannula oxygen, prone positioning, mechanical ventilation for hypoxemia
- antithrombotic agents for thromboembolic risks

❖ NURSING CARE OF THE PATIENT WITH CORONAVIRUS

Nursing care related to COVID-19 covers a broad spectrum of interventions in various settings. Nurses may provide community education, screening and monitoring in clinics, home health care for mild symptoms, inpatient care for moderately ill persons, and intensive care for critically ill patients. Critical care is beyond the scope of this textbook.

Of special concern with COVID-19 is that it is highly communicable. Caregivers must take isolation precautions to protect themselves and other patients. Individuals with preexisting health conditions are at greater risk than healthy persons and are advised to avoid crowds and contact with others who are risk. As of late 2020, vaccines have been developed and are being distributed.

PNEUMONIA

CAUSE AND RISK FACTORS

The term *pneumonia* describes inflammation of certain parts of the lung such as the alveoli and bronchioles. Pneumonia may be caused by either infectious or noninfectious agents. Examples of infectious agents are bacteria, fungi, and nonspecific viruses.

Noninfectious agents may include irritating fumes, dust, or chemicals that are inhaled or foreign matter that is aspirated.

Hospital-acquired pneumonia (nosocomial pneumonia) is a health care–associated lung infection occurring in a nonintubated patient after 48 hours of hospitalization, and whose infection was not present on admission.

Community-acquired pneumonia is an acute infection occurring in individuals who have not been hospitalized or lived in a community residence in the previous 14 days.

Aspiration pneumonia results from the inhalation into the lungs of some type of foreign matter (liquid or solid).

People who are most likely to contract pneumonia are smokers; those with altered consciousness; those who are immunocompromised; chronically ill people who are malnourished or debilitated; and people on bed rest with prolonged immobility.

Patients at increased risk for aspiration pneumonia are those with impaired swallowing or cough reflexes, decreased gastrointestinal (GI) motility, esophageal abnormalities, tube feedings, tracheostomies, and endotracheal tubes.

PATHOPHYSIOLOGY

Viruses, bacteria, and fungi can all cause pneumonia. Common causes of viral pneumonia are influenza and respiratory syncytial virus (RSV). A common cause of bacterial pneumonia is *Streptococcus pneumoniae* (pneumococcus). Pneumocystis pneumonia (PCP) is caused by a fungus (*Pneumocystis jirovecii*) and can occur in immunocompromised individuals such as those with human immunodeficiency virus/acquired immunodeficiency syndrome (HIV/AIDS). Pneumonia can also result from being on a ventilator, which is known as *ventilator associated pneumonia* (VAP).

The pathophysiology of pneumonia follows a predictable course. When pathogens invade the lungs, the inflammatory process causes fluid to accumulate in the affected alveoli. In a process called *hepatization*, capillaries dilate and neutrophils, red blood cells (RBCs), and fibrin fill the alveoli, causing the lung to appear red and granular. Next, blood flow decreases and leukocytes (white blood cells) and fibrin infiltrate the area and consolidate (solidify). As the infection resolves, the consolidated material dissolves and is ingested and removed by macrophages.

COMPLICATIONS

Although most people recover fully from pneumonia, it remains one of the leading causes of death in the United States, especially in those 65 years of age and older (https://www.cdc.gov.nchs/faststats/leading-causes-of-death.htm). Relatively common pulmonary complications of pneumonia include pleurisy, atelectasis, and pleural effusion. Pleurisy is inflammation of the pleura that causes pain with breathing. Pleural effusion is the accumulation of fluid between the pleura that encases the lungs and the pleura that lines the thoracic cavity. A large amount of fluid can lead to collapse of the lung. **Atelectasis** refers to collapsed alveoli. Other, less common pulmonary complications of pneumonia include lung abscess, bacteremia, pneumothorax, meningitis, acute respiratory failure, sepsis/septic shock, and empyema. **Empyema** is the presence of purulent exudate in the pleural cavity.

CLINICAL MANIFESTATIONS

Usual symptoms of pneumonia are abrupt onset of fever, chills, cough, and side pain. Sputum production, **hemoptysis** (coughing up blood), dyspnea, headache, and fatigue may also occur. Older adults frequently exhibit fewer symptoms, and confusion or delirium may be the initial manifestation. People with bacterial pneumonia may experience an abrupt explosive onset: severe, shaking chills; sharp, stabbing lateral chest pain, especially with coughing and breathing; and intermittent cough with rusty sputum. Viral pneumonia is characterized by burning or searing chest pain in the sternal area; a continuous, hacking, barking cough producing small amounts of sputum; and headache.

MEDICAL DIAGNOSIS

Diagnosis of pneumonia is based on the findings of the history and clinical presentation, sputum culture and Gram stain, chest radiograph, complete blood count, blood culture, and pneumococcal urinary antigen.

MEDICAL TREATMENT

Treatment usually consists of adequate fluid intake to avoid dehydration, limited activity or bed rest, antipyretics and analgesics, and in some cases oxygen (O_2) therapy. Bacterial pneumonias are treated with appropriate antibacterial agents; however, antibacterials are not used with viral pneumonias because they do not kill viruses.

The Centers for Disease Control and Prevention (CDC) publishes a schedule of recommended vaccinations to prevent pneumococcal pneumonia. Whereas there are general recommendations for all healthy people, the schedule may be different for people with certain health problems. To access the latest information, see https://www.cdc.gov.

❖ NURSING CARE OF THE PATIENT WITH PNEUMONIA

FOCUSED ASSESSMENT

Assessment of the patient with a respiratory disorder is summarized in Chapter 25, Box 25.2 (see also Nursing Care Plan: Patient With Pneumonia).

Patient Problems, Goals, and Outcome Criteria: Pneumonia

Patient Problems	Goals and Outcome Criteria
Airway obstruction related to increased sputum production, thick secretions, ineffective cough	Patent airway: clear breath sounds without wheezes or crackles
Inadequate oxygenation related to obstruction of airways by edema and secretions or atelectasis	Adequate oxygenation: normal arterial blood gases, heart rate, and respiratory rate
Fatigue and dyspnea related to obstruction of airways by edema and secretions or atelectasis	Improved tolerance of activity: performance of daily activities without fatigue or dyspnea
Inadequate nutrition related to anorexia, dyspnea, fatigue	Optimal nutritional status: stable body weight
Potential for fluid volume deficit related to inadequate fluid intake, fever, mouth breathing	Normal hydration: fluid intake approximately equal to fluid output, moist mucous membranes, blood pressure consistent with patient norms
Acute pain related to inflammation, cough, muscle aches	Pain relief: patient statement of pain relief, relaxed appearance

Interventions

Airway obstruction. Accumulated secretions in the respiratory tract impair gas exchange and may result in alveolar collapse. Therapeutic measures are taken to decrease the production and promote the expectoration of secretions. Administer antimicrobials, decongestants, and expectorants as ordered. A good cough is essential for removal of secretions, but antitussive medications may be given as ordered if the patient becomes exhausted because of constant coughing. Encourage or assist the patient to change positions at least every 2 hours to help mobilize secretions. Other measures used to mobilize secretions are deep-breathing and coughing exercises, chest physiotherapy, and aerosol therapy. The patient who has a very weak cough may require suctioning. Provide tissues and a receptacle for disposal of secretions. Note the amount, color, and consistency of secretions. Auscultate lung sounds frequently to assess the effects of interventions to clear the airways.

Inadequate oxygenation. The edema and secretions that occur with pneumonia interfere with the exchange of gases in the lungs. The patient may have hypoxemia, meaning that the level of O_2 in the blood is low. At the same time, excess carbon dioxide (CO_2) may accumulate in the blood, a condition called **hypercapnia**. Because normal oxygenation is essential for all body tissues, efforts must be made to improve the patient's gas exchange.

To assess gas exchange, monitor vital signs, lung sounds, and skin color. Be alert for signs of hypoxemia: restlessness, tachycardia, and tachypnea. If arterial blood gases are being measured, report abnormal results to the physician. Hemoglobin may also be measured. Low hemoglobin is significant because it indicates the reduced O_2-carrying capacity of RBCs.

Measures that mobilize secretions, discussed earlier, are important in improving gas exchange. In addition, elevate the head of the bed. Some patients are more comfortable in a reclining chair that permits alterations in position. A semi-Fowler position decreases the pressure of the abdominal organs on the diaphragm so that the patient breathes more easily. Maintain O_2 therapy as ordered.

Fatigue and dyspnea. Activity is usually restricted for the patient with pneumonia and may range from complete bed rest to limited activities. Organize nursing care to prevent overtiring and allow periods of uninterrupted rest. Provide assistance as needed until the patient is able to resume self-care. Keep conversations short and encourage visitors not to tire the patient with long visits. When the patient begins to resume activities of daily living (ADL), evaluate the ability to tolerate daily activities.

Inadequate nutrition. Good nutrition is essential to combat the infection and to promote healing (see the Nutrition Considerations box). Assess the patient's usual dietary habits to provide baseline information so that the diet may be individualized. Monitor weight to determine the adequacy of nutrition. Weigh the patient before breakfast using the same scale each time. Monitor albumin, electrolyte, glucose, and blood urea nitrogen (BUN)/creatinine levels to detect low levels that are common with inadequate nutrition.

A typical diet for the patient with pneumonia is a high-protein, soft diet. Unfortunately, fatigue, dyspnea, and anorexia may interfere with adequate food intake. Provide the diet as ordered, assist the patient with the meal if needed, and document intake. To enhance the appetite, provide oral care before and after

Nutrition Considerations

1. Adequate fluids may help to mobilize pulmonary secretions for expectoration. Nutritional support for patients with respiratory failure should be part of the plan of care on admission to the hospital.
2. A dietary referral for patients with respiratory failure should be obtained.
3. A diet for patients who have been in acute respiratory failure should provide adequate calories to meet or exceed basal energy expenditure.
4. Small, frequent meals with proportionally more fat and protein (e.g., eggs, fish, lean meat, nuts) and fewer carbohydrates are recommended.

Nursing Care Plan Patient With Pneumonia

FOCUSED ASSESSMENT

Health History

A 77-year-old retired teacher comes to the clinic complaining of chills and fever, cough, sore throat, and chest pain. The physician diagnosed viral pneumonia and recommended hospitalization. She states that she had a cold for about 1 week and seemed to get progressively worse. She states that she has "a little" shortness of breath and tires very easily. Her chest pain is aggravated by coughing. She has been taking over-the-counter (OTC) cold remedies. She has a history of hypertension and heart failure (HF), for which she takes an angiotensin-converting enzyme (ACE) inhibitor and a diuretic. She lives alone in a one-story apartment. She has a close friend next door who visits frequently.

Physical Examination

Vital signs: blood pressure 160/94 mm Hg, pulse 92 beats per minute, respiration 24 breaths per minute, temperature 100.6°F (38.1°C) measured orally. Height 5′9″, weight 175 lb. Oxygen saturation 93%. Alert, slightly dyspneic. Skin color pale. Nail beds slightly dusky. Lung sounds clear to auscultation over right lung fields. Wheezes and crackles auscultated in left lung. Frequent cough producing greenish sputum. No retractions or use of accessory muscles of respiration. Abdomen soft.

Patient Problems	Goals and Outcome Criteria	Interventions
Airway obstruction related to increased sputum production and thick secretions	The patient will have a patent airway, as evidenced by clear breath sounds without wheezes or crackles.	Administer decongestants and expectorants as ordered. Administer antitussive medications as ordered if the cough interferes with rest. Suction only if necessary. Have the patient turn, deep breathe, and cough at least every 2 hours. Perform chest physiotherapy and provide aerosol therapy as ordered. Assess response. Monitor lung sounds, respiratory rate, and characteristics of secretions. Dispose of tissues in a sanitary manner.
Inadequate oxygenation related to obstruction of airways by edema and secretions or atelectasis	The patient will have adequate oxygenation, as evidenced by normal arterial blood gases and vital signs, oxygen saturation 95% or higher.	Monitor vital signs, lung sounds, skin color, blood gas reports, and level of consciousness. Be alert for signs of hypoxemia: restlessness, tachycardia, and tachypnea. Report abnormal findings to the physician. Elevate the head of the bed. Administer oxygen (O_2) therapy as ordered. Notify registered nurse or physician if oxygen saturation is below 90%.
Impaired ability to manage self-care related to fatigue or hypoxia	The patient will perform activities of daily living (ADL) as permitted without excessive fatigue or dyspnea.	Instruct the patient in activity restrictions. Plan care to allow periods of uninterrupted rest. Assist the patient with ADL as needed. Gradually encourage increased activity while monitoring for dyspnea and fatigue. Keep interactions short and limit visitors.
Inadequate nutrition: related to anorexia, dyspnea, or fatigue	The patient will maintain optimal nutritional status, as evidenced by stable body weight.	Monitor food intake and weight. If intake is poor, consult with the dietitian about patient preferences. Suggest small, frequent meals. Provide a pleasant environment for meals. Position the patient for comfort. Use an O_2 cannula during meals if permitted. Weigh the patient daily.
Potential for fluid volume deficit related to inadequate fluid intake, fever, or mouth breathing	The patient's hydration will remain normal, as evidenced by fluid intake equal to output, moist mucous membranes, and blood pressure consistent with patient's norms.	Monitor the patient's fluid status for signs of fluid volume deficit: decreased skin turgor, concentrated urine, decreased urine output, dry mucous membranes, and elevated hemoglobin and hematocrit levels. Administer intravenous fluids as ordered. Encourage fluids by mouth up to 3 L/day as permitted. Record intake and output. Monitor the patient's temperature and treat fever as ordered. Keep the patient dry and lightly covered. Administer tepid sponge baths as ordered for fever but do not induce shivering. Use hypothermia blanket as ordered.
Acute pain related to inflammation, cough, or muscle aches	The patient will report pain relief, as measured with a pain scale.	Use a pain scale to assess the patient's pain. Administer analgesics as ordered. Reposition the patient for comfort. Splint painful areas during coughing and deep breathing. Use massage and relaxation techniques. Document the effects of interventions.

CRITICAL THINKING QUESTIONS

1. Identify the factors that make fluid balance a challenge for this patient.
2. What are the risks that occur when patients self-medicate?
3. How is body temperature related to fluid balance?

meals, elevate the head of the bed, and arrange the tray in an attractive and convenient manner. The diet should conform to the patient's preferences as much as possible. If oxygen is needed, a nasal cannula is recommended during meals. If the patient tires quickly, more frequent meals with smaller servings may be better received.

The patient who is malnourished is at increased risk for respiratory infections because of impaired immunity and possible impairment of defense mechanisms.

Potential for fluid volume deficit. The patient with pneumonia may lose excess fluid because of fever and mouth breathing, and fluid intake may be inadequate because of fatigue and dyspnea. Dehydration causes respiratory secretions to be thicker and more difficult to mobilize. Signs and symptoms of deficient fluid volume include decreased skin turgor, concentrated urine, dry mucous membranes, and elevated hematocrit levels. Although there is no specific recommendation for the amount of oral fluids a patient should consume, the patient's hydration status should be continuously assessed. If the patient's oral intake is low, intravenous fluids may be ordered. Intake and output records may be kept (see the Patient Teaching box).

Patient Teaching

Pneumonia

The teaching plan for the patient with pneumonia should include the following points:

- Gradually increase your activities as you recover because fatigue may persist for several weeks.
- Avoid people with colds or other infections.
- You need plenty of rest, good nutrition, and plenty of fluids.
- Complete any prescribed drugs after discharge.

Monitor the patient's temperature every 2 to 4 hours to detect fever. Administer antipyretics as ordered. Keep the patient dry and lightly covered. Keep the room at a comfortable temperature that avoids chilling. Tepid (slightly warm) sponge baths may be given for high fevers as ordered, but do not allow the patient to shiver. A cooling blanket may be needed to reduce very high body temperature.

Acute pain. Treat pain with ordered analgesics. Also use positioning, splinting painful areas during deep breathing and coughing, and massage to promote comfort. Document the effects of comfort measures and notify the physician if the patient's pain is unrelieved or worsens. Other measures to manage pain are detailed in Chapter 8.

PREVENTION OF ASPIRATION PNEUMONIA

Aspiration pneumonia may be prevented by using measures to avoid aspiration or to treat aspiration promptly should it occur. If a patient is at risk for aspiration, keep suction equipment on hand. Position patients with dysphagia (difficulty swallowing) upright with the neck in a neutral position or slightly bent forward during meals. Because semisolids are swallowed more easily than thin liquids, thickening agents may be added to liquids.

If a patient is receiving enteral feedings, elevate the head of the bed while the feeding is being delivered and for 30 minutes afterward. Check tube position per agency policy before each bolus feeding or at specified intervals. Measure residual before each bolus feeding and withhold the feeding according to physician orders or agency policy. Oral hygiene should be performed frequently.

Stop continuous feedings for 20 to 30 minutes before lowering the patient's head. If a patient must be kept flat, the best position is on the right side. Check residual per physician orders and agency policy.

To reduce the risk of aspiration, position the unconscious patient on alternating sides with the head of the bed elevated unless contraindicated. Do not put fluids in the patient's mouth until the presence of a gag reflex has been established.

If aspiration is suspected, use suction to try to remove the foreign material. A side-lying position, if not contraindicated, may promote drainage from the airway. Stop the enteral feeding until it is ruled out as the source of the aspirated material. Monitor the patient closely and notify the physician. Administer O_2 as ordered.

PLEURITIS (PLEURISY)

Pleuritis, commonly called Pleurisy is inflammation of the pleura. The most common causes are pneumonia, tuberculosis, injury to the chest wall, pulmonary embolism, some autoimmune conditions, exposure to some toxins, and cancer. The most characteristic symptom of pleuritis is abrupt and severe pain. The pain almost always occurs on one side of the chest, and patients can usually point to the exact spot where the pain is occurring. Breathing and coughing aggravate the pain.

Treatment of pleuritis is aimed at the underlying condition and at pain relief. Analgesics, antiinflammatory agents, antitussives, antimicrobials, and local heat therapy may be ordered.

❖ NURSING CARE OF THE PATIENT WITH PLEURITIS

FOCUSED ASSESSMENT

Assessment of the patient with a respiratory disorder is summarized in Chapter 25, Box 25.2.

Patient Problems, Goals, and Outcome Criteria: Pleuritis

The primary patient problems when a patient has pleuritis are listed here. Other problems related to the underlying cause of pleuritis are possible.

Patient Problems	Goals and Outcome Criteria
Acute pain related to inflammation	Pain relief: patient statement of pain relief, relaxed expression
Inadequate oxygenation related to splinting, pleural effusion	Adequate oxygenation: vital signs within patient norms, normal breath sounds, oxygen saturation at 95% or higher.

Interventions

Acute pain. When the patient reports pain, obtain a complete description including location, severity, precipitating factors, and alleviating factors. Use analgesics and splinting of the affected side to relieve pain. It is also helpful to splint the rib cage when coughing. If ordered, apply heat to the painful area and give antitussives to decrease painful coughing. If bed rest is prescribed, assist the patient with regular position changes. Administer acetaminophen or nonsteroidal antiinflammatory drugs (NSAIDs) as ordered to reduce pain and inflammation (see the Patient Teaching box). Monitor patients on NSAIDs for GI distress and bleeding.

Patient Teaching

Pleurisy

- Take deep breaths every 1 to 2 hours while awake.
- Sitting upright will make breathing more comfortable.
- If being discharged on nonsteroidal antiinflammatory drugs (NSAIDs), avoid taking aspirin at the same time because it increases the risk of bleeding.
- Take NSAIDs with food, milk, or antacids if gastrointestinal (GI) distress occurs.

Inadequate oxygenation. Monitor the patient's breathing pattern with attention to the symmetry of chest movement. Encourage the patient to turn, take deep breaths and cough, and ambulate if permitted to mobilize secretions and maximize ventilation. Elevate the head of the bed to improve lung expansion. If pleural effusion develops, the patient experiences progressive dyspnea, decreased or absent breath sounds in the affected area, and decreased chest wall movement on the affected side. A thoracentesis may be done to remove the accumulated fluid. If the procedure is done at the bedside, the nurse assists as described in the section titled "Common Therapeutic Measures" in Chapter 25.

CHEST TRAUMA

Traumatic chest injuries fall into two major categories: (1) nonpenetrating injuries and (2) penetrating injuries. Nonpenetrating or blunt injuries most commonly result from automobile accidents, falls, or blast injuries. The extent of the injury depends on the force and effect of the trauma. Common nonpenetrating injuries include rib fractures, pneumothorax, pulmonary contusion, and cardiac contusion. Penetrating injuries most commonly result from gunshot or stab wounds to the chest. Common penetrating injuries include pneumothorax and life-threatening tears of the aorta, vena cava, or other major vessels.

Chest trauma can result in changes in normal pressure relationships between air inside and outside the body, interference with normal breathing patterns and protective mechanisms such as cough, disturbances in blood flow to the lungs, swelling, and pain. Patients are therefore at risk for air entering the pleural space, infection and increased secretions in the tracheobronchial tree, hemorrhage, and abnormal fluid collection in the lung.

CLINICAL MANIFESTATIONS

Signs and symptoms of chest injury may include obvious trauma to the chest wall (e.g., bruising); chest pain; dyspnea; cough; asymmetric movement of the chest wall; marked cyanosis of the mouth, face, nail beds, and mucous membranes; rapid, weak pulse; decreased blood pressure; deviation of the trachea; distended neck veins; and bloodshot or bulging eyes.

MEDICAL TREATMENT

Immediate care of a person with a chest injury is directed at stabilization and prevention of further injury. Remove clothing to assess injury sites and to observe for other injuries such as bleeding. Immediately treat bleeding. Cover any open chest wound with an airtight dressing taped on three sides. This is called a *vented dressing*; it permits air to escape through the chest wound but prevents additional air from entering the chest through the wound. If you were to completely seal an open chest wound, air could continue to leak from the lung into the pleural space. With no exit, the leaking air could accumulate in the pleural space and create a tension pneumothorax (discussed under "Pneumothorax" later).

If an airtight dressing has been applied, be alert for worsening respiratory status (increasing dyspnea, cyanosis, distended neck veins, trachea deviated from midline, decreased breath sounds on the affected side), which requires removal of the airtight dressing. Do not remove impaled objects but stabilize them with bulky dressings. Monitor vital signs and level of consciousness, keeping in mind the potential for shock. Oxygen may be administered by nasal cannula. To facilitate breathing, put the patient in a semi-Fowler position or on the injured side.

PNEUMOTHORAX

Chest injuries often cause **pneumothorax**, which is an accumulation of air in the pleural cavity that results in complete or partial collapse of a lung. Pneumothorax occurs in nearly half of the people who have chest injuries. Air enters the space between the chest wall and the lung, either through a hole in the chest wall or through a tear in the bronchus, bronchioles, or alveoli. A pneumothorax can also occur due to the spontaneous rupture of air sacs in the lungs.

Two types of pneumothorax exist: (1) open and (2) tension. An open pneumothorax results from a chest wound that allows air to move in and out freely with inspiration and expiration. The lung on the affected side collapses. The heart, trachea, esophagus, and great blood vessels may shift back and forth toward

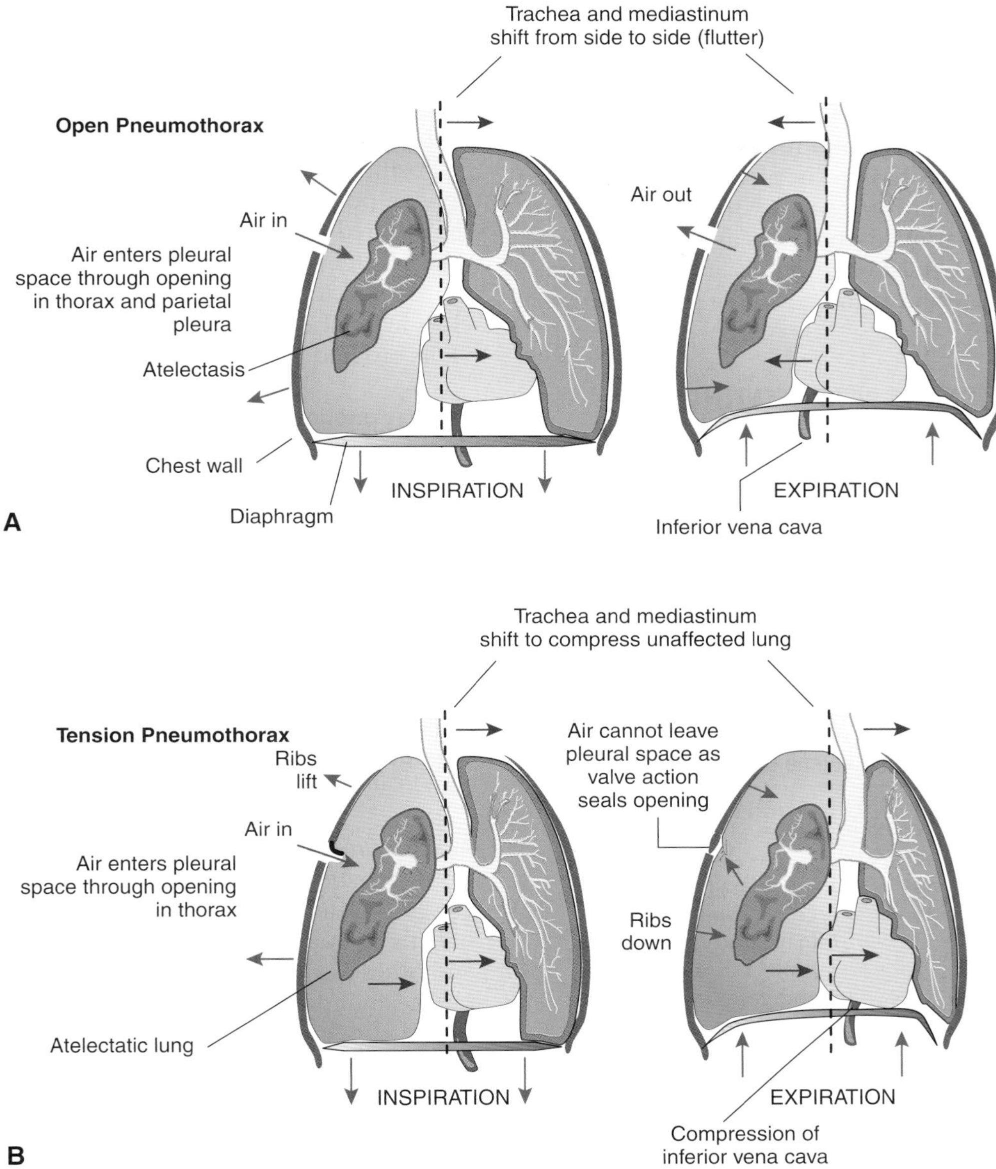

Fig. 27.1 (A) Open pneumothorax. Air movement (*blue arrows*); structural movement (*red and purple arrows*). On inspiration, air is sucked into the pleural space through the open chest wound and the lung on the affected side collapses. The mediastinal contents shift toward the unaffected side. On expiration, air exits through the open wound and the mediastinal contents swing back toward the affected side (mediastinal flutter). (B) Tension pneumothorax may follow an open chest wound that admits air on inspiration, but then closes so that air accumulates in the pleural space. The contents of the mediastinum shift toward the unaffected side and impair circulatory and respiratory function (mediastinal shift). (From VanMeter KC, Hubert RJ: *Gould's pathophysiology for the health professions*, ed 5, St Louis, 2014, Saunders.)

the unaffected side with inspiration, and then toward the affected side with expiration. This condition, called *mediastinal flutter,* is potentially fatal (Fig. 27.1A and B).

With a tension pneumothorax, air repeatedly enters the pleural space with inspiration, causing the pressure to rise. Because air is not escaping from the wound, the accumulating pressure causes the affected lung to collapse. The heart, trachea, esophagus, and great blood vessels shift toward the unaffected side. This is called a *mediastinal shift*, a condition that interferes with blood return to the heart. This is a medical emergency because both the respiratory and the circulatory systems are affected. If not corrected, cardiac output will fall and the patient will die (see Fig. 27.1).

CLINICAL MANIFESTATIONS

Symptoms of pneumothorax are dyspnea, tachypnea, tachycardia, restlessness, pain, anxiety, decreased movement of the involved chest wall, asymmetric chest wall movement, diminished breath sounds on the injured side, and progressive cyanosis. In trauma cases, a chest wound may be present. If air can be heard or felt moving in and out of the wound, it is called a *sucking* chest wound.

MEDICAL TREATMENT

The physician may insert a needle through the chest wall into the pleural space, aspirate accumulated air or fluid, and insert a chest tube. An alternative is to omit the needle aspiration and immediately insert the chest tube. If air is entering the pleural space from a tear in the lung or bronchus, surgery may be needed to repair the tear. A variety of materials are being studied for use in sealing persistent air leaks, including intrapleural tetracycline and autologous (the patient's own) "blood patches."

NURSING CARE OF THE PATIENT WITH PNEUMOTHORAX

FOCUSED ASSESSMENT

The complete assessment of the patient with a respiratory disorder is outlined in Chapter 25, Box 25.2. In addition, if the patient has a chest tube, the nurse should monitor the insertion site as well as the amount and characteristics of any drainage from the tube. Care of patients with chest tubes is covered in the "Chest Tubes" section.

Patient Problems, Goals, and Outcome Criteria: Pneumothorax

Patient Problems	Goals and Outcome Criteria
Inadequate oxygenation related to decreased lung expansion	Adequate oxygenation: regular respirations at a rate of 12 to 20 breaths per minute, normal arterial blood gases, no dyspnea, normal skin color, O_2 saturation 95% to 100%
Fear related to difficulty breathing	Decreased fear: calm demeanor, patient statement that fear is reduced
Inadequate circulation related to mediastinal shift and decreased cardiac output	Adequate circulation: pulse and blood pressure consistent with patient norms
Acute pain related to trauma, altered pressure in chest cavity, chest tube	Pain relief: patient statement that pain is reduced or relieved, relaxed manner
Potential for infection related to traumatic injury, chest tube insertion	Absence of infection: normal body temperature, normal white blood cell count

Interventions

Inadequate oxygenation. Monitor the patient closely for increasing respiratory distress as indicated by tachycardia, dyspnea, cyanosis, restlessness, and anxiety. Inspect the trachea for deviation that may be caused by mediastinal shift. Check arterial blood gas results for hypoxemia (low blood O_2) and hypercapnia (high blood CO_2). Immediately report signs and symptoms of deteriorating respiratory status to the physician. After the chest tube has been inserted, protect the tube and monitor its function.

Position the patient for comfort in a Fowler or semi-Fowler position. Avoid the side-lying position until the affected lung has reexpanded because this position could foster mediastinal shift. Support and encourage the patient to do deep-breathing and coughing exercises at least every 2 hours while awake. Administer O_2 as ordered.

Fear. A pneumothorax is frightening. Patients feel like they are suffocating and may fear that they are dying. Speak to the patient calmly and explain what is happening. Tell the patient that the chest tube will allow the lung to reexpand and relieve the dyspnea. Also tell the patient how to prevent dislodging the tube. Give the patient the opportunity to ask questions and express fears.

Inadequate circulation. Monitor the patient's pulse and blood pressure. If cardiac output decreases because of mediastinal shift, the blood pressure falls and the pulse rate increases. Immediately notify the physician of signs of this potentially life-threatening change.

Acute pain. Be alert for signs of pain and document the characteristics of the patient's pain. Administer analgesics as ordered and document the effects. In addition to drug therapy, use positioning, massage, distraction, and other measures described in Chapter 8. Notify the physician if pain is not relieved.

Potential for infection. Monitor the patient for signs and symptoms of infection: fever, increased pulse and respirations, foul drainage from the tube insertion site, and elevated white blood cell count. Various possible sites of infection must be considered: traumatic wounds, chest tube insertion site, intravenous infusion sites, indwelling catheter, and lungs. Use sterile technique for invasive procedures and dressing changes and administer prescribed antimicrobials. Encourage increased activity when permitted. Monitor hydration status and promote adequate fluid intake. Before discharge, instruct the patient to keep the chest tube insertion site clean and dry and to notify the physician of signs of infection: fever or increasing redness, swelling, or drainage from the insertion site.

HEMOTHORAX

Hemothorax is an accumulation of blood between the chest wall and the lung that is often associated with pneumothorax. Hemothorax results from lacerated or torn blood vessels or lung tissues, lung malignancy, or pulmonary embolus. It may also be a complication of anticoagulant therapy. When air or blood collects in the pleural space, pressure around the lung increases, causing partial or complete collapse. Hemothorax is essentially treated like a pneumothorax, and the nursing care is similar. Surgical intervention may be needed to control the source of bleeding. In addition, the patient is at risk for decreased cardiac output because of hemorrhage.

RIB FRACTURES

Rib fractures are the most common chest injuries. The most common cause is a blunt injury, especially the impact of the steering wheel against the chest in an automobile accident. Ribs 4 through 10 are most frequently fractured because they are least protected by chest muscles. It takes approximately 6 weeks for rib fractures to heal.

CLINICAL MANIFESTATIONS

Signs and symptoms of fractured ribs include pain at the site of injury (especially on inspiration), occasional bruising or surface markings, swelling, visible bone fragments at the site of the injury, and shallow breathing or holding the chest protectively to minimize painful chest movements.

MEDICAL TREATMENT

Depending on the patient's age and overall health status, inpatient treatment is usually recommended if 3 or more ribs are fractured. Treatment is aimed at relief of pain so that the patient can have good chest expansion for adequate breathing. Intercostal nerve blocks with local anesthesia are most frequently used. Analgesics along with mild sedatives may also be given for pain relief. Surgical stabilization is also an option.

NURSING CARE OF THE PATIENT WITH RIB FRACTURES

FOCUSED ASSESSMENT

The nursing assessment of the patient with a respiratory disorder is outlined in Chapter 25, Box 25.2. After rib fractures, the nurse is especially alert for signs of increasing respiratory distress that may indicate a pneumothorax caused by a bone fragment.

PATIENT PROBLEM, GOAL, AND OUTCOME CRITERIA

The primary patient problem for the patient who has fractured ribs is inadequate oxygenation related to pain that occurs with ventilation. The goal of nursing care when a patient has fractured ribs is for the patient to have an adequate oxygenation. Outcome criteria include vital signs within normal range, absence of dyspnea, and breath sounds clear to auscultation.

Interventions

Breathing exercises are necessary to prevent pulmonary complications after rib fractures. Instruct the patient in supporting the fractured ribs while deep breathing and coughing. The patient will perform these exercises better with adequate pain control. Incentive spirometry is often used to promote lung expansion. Assess the patient's pain every 2 hours, asking the patient to rank the pain intensity from 0 (no pain) to 10 (worst pain imaginable). Encourage the patient to report pain and offer reassurance that measures will be taken to provide relief. Because pain typically persists for 5 to 7 days, administer prescribed analgesics. After medications are given, provide a calm environment and encourage the patient to rest. Other nursing measures described in Chapter 8 (i.e., guided imagery, distraction, rhythmic breathing) may be used to manage pain as well. Evaluate the effects of pain management measures and inform the physician if the patient's pain cannot be controlled.

FLAIL CHEST

The term **flail chest** refers to an injury in which two adjacent ribs on the same side of the chest are each broken into two or more segments. The affected section of the rib cage is, in a sense, detached from the rest of the rib cage. This permits it to move independently so that the segment moves "in" with inspiration and "out" with expiration. The pattern of movement is exactly the opposite of the movement of an intact chest wall. Therefore it is called *paradoxical movement.* Ventilation is impaired, and the patient becomes hypoxemic. In addition, contusion (bruising) of underlying lung tissue may cause fluid to accumulate in the alveoli. Fractured ribs may tear the pleura or the lung itself, resulting in a pneumothorax or hemothorax. The loss of chest wall stability and collapse of a lung may permit the mediastinum to flutter, swinging back and forth with respirations. Progressive hypoxemia and hypercapnia may be fatal.

CLINICAL MANIFESTATIONS

Signs and symptoms of flail chest include dyspnea, cyanosis, tachypnea, tachycardia, and paradoxical movement of the chest.

MEDICAL DIAGNOSIS

Diagnosis is based on the history, clinical presentation, and chest radiographs. Arterial blood gases may be measured to assess the adequacy of ventilation.

MEDICAL AND SURGICAL TREATMENT

The treatment of flail chest varies depending on the severity of the condition. If the patient is able to maintain adequate oxygenation, treatment may consist of deep breathing and coughing, incentive spirometry, and pain management. The patient in respiratory distress usually requires intubation and mechanical ventilation. Radiographs and arterial blood gas tests are often repeated at intervals to monitor oxygenation and detect additional pulmonary complications such as pneumonia.

In some circumstances, surgical rib stabilization is needed to maintain oxygenation and to relieve pain that interferes with pulmonary function. Titanium plates are secured to the broken ribs with locking screws. The use of surgical intervention is controversial. However, research comparing medical and surgical treatment has demonstrated fewer complications with surgical intervention. Other studies have found that measures of pain and quality of life are similar with either type of treatment (Sarani, May 12, 2020).

NURSING CARE OF THE PATIENT WITH FLAIL CHEST

FOCUSED ASSESSMENT

The nursing assessment of the patient with a respiratory disorder is outlined in Chapter 25, Box 25.2. When the patient has flail chest, defer the complete assessment until the patient's condition stabilizes. The initial assessment focuses on respiratory status, vital signs, other medical diagnoses, and a drug history.

Patient Problems, Goals, and Outcome Criteria: Flail Chest, Treated Medically

Patient Problems	Goals and Outcome Criteria
Inadequate oxygenation related to loss of rib cage integrity	Adequate oxygenation: normal pulse and respiratory rates, normal arterial blood gases, no dyspnea
Acute pain related to fractures	Pain relief: patient statement of pain relief, patient rates pain at 4 or less
Anxiety related to lack of understanding of injury and treatment	Reduced anxiety: patient statement of reduced anxiety, calm manner

Interventions

Nursing interventions for patients with flail chest are similar to those for the patient with fractured ribs. Because flail chest is more serious and the patient may be acutely ill, anxiety may be very high. To reduce anxiety, respond promptly to the patient's needs, provide simple explanations, and acknowledge the patient's concerns. Anxiety may be especially high if mechanical ventilation is needed. The detailed care of patients who require mechanical ventilation is beyond the scope of this book. A general discussion of mechanical ventilation is included in the section titled "Common Therapeutic Measures" in Chapter 25.

PULMONARY EMBOLUS

An **embolus** is a foreign substance that is carried through the bloodstream. Emboli are usually blood clots but may be fat, air, tumors, bone marrow, amniotic fluid, or clumps of bacteria.

CAUSE AND RISK FACTORS

Risk factors for development of emboli include surgery of the pelvis or lower legs, immobility, obesity, estrogen therapy, and clotting abnormalities. Most pulmonary emboli originate in the deep veins of the thigh or pelvis. A thrombus that develops in the veins can break away and become an embolus. The embolus flows with the blood until it reaches a vessel too narrow to pass through. The embolus lodges and obstructs blood flow so that perfusion to the area is diminished. When a portion of a pulmonary blood vessel is occluded by an embolus, the patient is said to have a pulmonary embolism (PE). The effects depend on the extent of the lung tissue that is deprived of blood. Small emboli usually do not cause dramatic symptoms but disrupt perfusion nevertheless. The alveoli in the affected area are ventilated but without blood flow, gas exchange cannot occur. The result is a ventilation-perfusion mismatch that results in hypoxemia. If a large pulmonary vessel is obstructed, alveoli collapse, cardiac output falls, constriction of the bronchi and the pulmonary artery occurs, and sudden death may ensue.

CLINICAL MANIFESTATIONS

Classic signs and symptoms of PE include dyspnea, chest pain, hemoptysis, cough, orthopnea, and unilateral calf or thigh pain and/or swelling. The onset of dyspnea is often rapid, usually within seconds to minutes. A spontaneous onset of chest wall tenderness without a history of trauma should raise a red flag. The patient may be apprehensive and diaphoretic with a cough and hemoptysis. Wheezing and crackles may be heard on auscultation of the lungs, and the patient may have fever and tachycardia.

MEDICAL DIAGNOSIS

A diagnosis of PE is suggested by the history and clinical presentation and is confirmed by imaging procedures such as computed tomography pulmonary angiography (CTPA) or ventilation-perfusion scanning. Other tests that may done are arterial blood gas analysis, D-dimer blood test, and an electrocardiogram (ECG). Lower extremity ultrasound with Doppler is used to detect venous thromboemboli because veins in the legs are a common source of pulmonary emboli.

MEDICAL AND SURGICAL TREATMENT

Anticoagulation therapy is the cornerstone of treatment for PE. From the day of diagnosis to the tenth day of treatment, the patient is given one of the following:

- low molecular weight heparin
- unfractionated heparin
- a direct acting Xa thrombin inhibitor (e.g., dabigatran)
- a selective factor Xa inhibitor (e.g., fondaparinux).

These and other anticoagulants are discussed in Chapter 33 and summarized in Table 33.9. Heparin prevents the development of new thrombi; it also prevents the extension of existing thrombi but does not dissolve them. Patients on heparin are eventually transitioned to an oral or subcutaneous anticoagulant. The drug is typically continued for 3 to 12 months. Some patients will be prescribed the anticoagulant for an indefinite period of time. A fibrinolytic agent, or tissue plasminogen activator (t-PA), may be given intravenously to dissolve the clots.

Hypoxemia may be managed with O_2 therapy, endotracheal intubation, and mechanical ventilation. Intravenous fluids and drugs to improve cardiac function are indicated to treat hypotension. Intravenous morphine sulfate is commonly used to relieve chest pain and apprehension.

A number of surgical interventions have been used for PE, including embolectomy, vena cava interruption, and venous thrombectomy. Embolectomy, surgical removal of the embolus from the obstructed pulmonary arteries, is reserved for patients who are not candidates for fibrinolytic therapy. Vena cava interruption is most often done by placing a filter in the inferior vena cava to strain clots before they reach the pulmonary circulation (Fig. 27.2).

NURSING CARE OF THE PATIENT WITH A PULMONARY EMBOLUS

FOCUSED ASSESSMENT

Assessment of the patient with a respiratory disorder is outlined in Chapter 25, Box 25.2. When a patient has a PE, the nurse must monitor cardiopulmonary function but must also assess risk factors that may have led to the embolism.

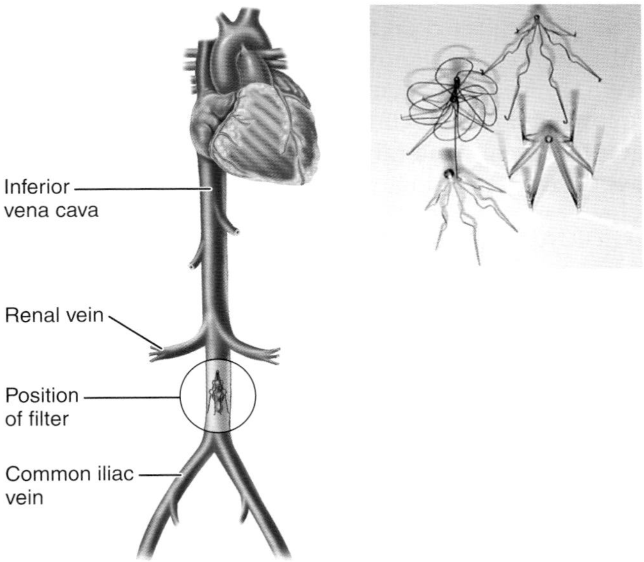

Fig. 27.2 Greenfield and umbrella filters are examples of filters that may be placed in the inferior vena cava to prevent emboli traveling to the lung. (From Black JM, Hawks JH: *Medical-surgical nursing: clinical management for positive outcomes*, ed 8, St. Louis, 2009, Saunders.)

Patient Problems, Goals, and Outcome Criteria: Pulmonary Embolism

Patient Problems	Goals and Outcome Criteria
Inadequate oxygenation related to interruption of blood flow to the alveoli	Sufficient oxygenation: vital signs consistent with patient norms, no dyspnea, normal arterial blood gases
Anxiety related to dyspnea, fear of dying	Reduced anxiety: patient statement of reduced or no anxiety, calm manner
Potential for bleeding related to anticoagulant therapy	Decreased risk of excessive bleeding: anticoagulant blood level within therapeutic range, absence of excessive bruising or bleeding

Put On Your Thinking Cap!

Pulmonary emboli often originate in the veins of the legs and pelvis. Draw the pathway by which the emboli travel from the legs to the lungs.

Interventions

Inadequate oxygenation: Monitor the patient's respiratory rate and effort, breath sounds, skin color, pulse, and blood pressure. Note arterial blood gas results as a measure of tissue perfusion and notify the physician if they are abnormal. Elevate the head of the patient's bed. Administer oxygen as ordered, usually by nasal cannula. Enforce prescribed activity limitations to decrease oxygen demands. After anticoagulants have been started, early ambulation is usually encouraged (Gregory & Hull, May 7, 2020). Administer prescribed intravenous fluids and inotropic drugs. Measure and record fluid intake and output.

Interventions to decrease the risk of further emboli include active and passive range-of-motion exercises for immobilized patients, early ambulation after treatment has begun, and elastic graduated compression stockings (GCS) and pneumatic compression stockings. Although evidence of benefits from GCS are limited, they are widely used and may be helpful in combination with other therapies. Do not place cushions and pillows under the legs where circulation might be impaired.

Anxiety. The patient in respiratory distress and pain is understandably anxious. Remain calm and tell the patient what is being done. Explain equipment and procedures in terms the patient can understand (see the Patient Teaching box). Encourage the patient to express concerns and ask questions. Permit a reassuring family member to remain with the patient.

Patient Teaching

Plumonary Embolism: Anticoagulant Therapy

Patients who have had a pulmonary embolism (PE) must be taught how to manage their anticoagulant therapy because they usually remain on these drugs for at least several months. The following are important points:

- Use a soft toothbrush and electric razor to avoid trauma and bleeding.
- Report red or dark urine, which suggests urinary bleeding.
- Report vomited blood, nosebleed, and red or black stools, which suggest intestinal bleeding.
- Do not take any over-the-counter (OTC) medications without consulting with the physician or pharmacist. Some drugs, especially aspirin, prolong the bleeding time, which could cause excessive bleeding.
- To reduce the risk of a future PE: stand up and walk around every 1 to 2 hours; if you smoke, stop; wear loose, comfortable clothes; shift your position while seated and move your legs and feet often; drink plenty of fluids; wear knee-high compression stockings; avoid alcohol.

Potential for bleeding. Anticoagulant therapy poses a risk of uncontrolled bleeding. While the patient is hospitalized, assess for excessive bruising or bleeding. Symptoms that may be caused by internal bleeding include severe headache and abdominal or back pain. Inspect the urine for hematuria. Apply pressure to venipuncture sites to control bleeding.

To reduce the risk of bleeding in the patient receiving heparin, the patient's activated partial thromboplastin time (aPTT) is monitored every 1 to 2 days until stabilized at 1.5 to 2.5 times the normal rate. Anticoagulant therapy for patients with a PE is usually changed to an oral or subcutaneous drug that can be self-administered at home. Warfarin sodium (Coumadin) was the first oral anticoagulant. The effect of warfarin sodium is monitored by assessing the prothrombin time (PT) which is reported as the international normalized ratio (INR). The therapeutic range for the INR should be 2.0 to 3.0. The dose is adjusted based on the INR. Devices to measure prothrombin time at home are available.

Pharmacology Capsule

Monitor the patient's activated partial thromboplastin time when on heparin. Watch for bleeding. Options for long-term oral anticoagulation therapy include anticoagulant factor Xa inhibitors (rivaroxaban, apixaban, or edoxaban), thrombin inhibitors (dabigatran), and a vitamin K antagonist (warfarin). These drugs do not require frequent blood tests or monitoring. The decision on which agent to use is made based on the risks of bleeding, patient comorbidities, preferences, cost, and convenience.

RESPIRATORY ARREST

See current American Heart Association guidelines for treatment of respiratory arrest.

ACUTE RESPIRATORY DISTRESS SYNDROME

CAUSE AND RISK FACTORS

Acute respiratory distress syndrome (ARDS) is a progressive pulmonary disorder that follows some trauma to the lung. From 6 to 72 hours after the trauma, pulmonary infiltrates develop and lung compliance decreases. Fluid shifts into the interstitial spaces in the lungs and into the alveoli, causing pulmonary edema. Production of pulmonary surfactant decreases, leading to atelectasis. Lung compliance decreases, and the patient rapidly becomes hypoxemic.

Some patients recover and heal completely, while lung fibrosis develops in others. The fibrosis may be mild or severe and sometimes occurs after the patient appears to be recovering. Progressive fibrosis may lead to death. Systemic complications of ARDS include cardiac dysrhythmias, renal failure, stress ulcers, thrombocytopenia, and disseminated intravascular coagulation. In addition, these patients are at risk for O_2 toxicity and sepsis.

CLINICAL MANIFESTATIONS

The first sign of ARDS is usually tachypnea. Auscultation of the lungs may reveal fine crackles. Respiratory distress is usually evident, and the patient may be restless, agitated, and confused. The pulse rate increases, and a cough may be present. These early signs are followed by progressively worsening dyspnea with retractions, cyanosis, and diaphoresis. Diffuse crackles may be heard on auscultation.

MEDICAL DIAGNOSIS

Multiple diagnostic studies are needed to rule out conditions such as heart failure and fluid overload. ARDS is suspected based on the patient's history and physical examination. Findings that support a diagnosis are: (1) respiratory symptoms developed in the week following a known clinical insult; and (2) chest radiographs reveal bilateral opacities; the patient must be hypoxemic at minimal ventilator settings.

MEDICAL TREATMENT

Early detection and treatment are critical factors in treating ARDS successfully. The patient is usually intubated and placed on a mechanical ventilator with positive end-expiratory pressure. Patient anxiety and restlessness may require sedation and short-term neuromuscular blockade. Prone positioning has been shown to improve oxygenation in the majority of patients with ARDS. Specific drug therapy depends on the underlying cause of ARDS. For example, the patient with sepsis is treated with antimicrobials.

NURSING CARE OF THE PATIENT WITH ACUTE RESPIRATORY DISTRESS SYNDROME

The patient with ARDS is critically ill and should be treated in an intensive care setting. Critical care nursing is beyond the scope of this text. However, all nurses must be aware of the risk of ARDS and respond promptly when a patient exhibits progressive respiratory distress. The rapid progression of the condition is frightening to the patient and the family. It is important to recognize their anxiety and fear and offer emotional support and simple explanations.

Get Ready for the NCLEX® Examination!

Key Points

- Influenza is an acute viral respiratory infection that can lead to pneumonia, especially in debilitated people.
- Influenza immunizations do not protect everyone from influenza but do reduce the incidence of the infection and are recommended for people who have poor resistance to infection.
- Symptoms of COVID-19 include new onset fever, cough, dyspnea, disturbances in smell and taste, myalgias (muscle aches), and diarrhea.
- Pathogenic organisms and noninfectious agents such as inhaled irritants, including aspirated gastric contents, may cause pneumonia.
- Patient problems for the patient with pneumonia may include inadequate oxygenation; airway obstruction; fatigue and dyspnea; inadequate nutrition; potential for fluid volume deficit; and acute pain.
- Pleurisy (pleuritis) is inflammation of the pleura that is treated with analgesics, antiinflammatory drugs, antitussives, antimicrobials, and local heat therapy.
- Patient problems for the patient with pleuritis may include pain and inadequate oxygenation.
- Pneumothorax is the accumulation of air in the pleural space, which may cause the lung to collapse.
- The immediate treatment of an open chest wound is coverage with a vented dressing followed by careful monitoring to detect signs of a tension pneumothorax.
- With a tension pneumothorax, air accumulates in the affected side, collapsing the affected lung and causing the heart, trachea, esophagus, and great blood vessels to shift toward the unaffected side (mediastinal shift, a life-threatening condition).
- Patient problems when a patient has pneumothorax may include inadequate oxygenation, fear, inadequate circulation, acute pain, and potential for infection.
- Flail chest is the loss of thoracic integrity caused by fractures of two adjacent ribs into two or more segments on the same side of the chest.
- A pulmonary embolus (PE) is a foreign substance carried through the bloodstream into the lung, where it lodges and blocks blood flow.
- Patient problems for the patient who has a PE may include inadequate oxygenation, anxiety, and potential for bleeding.
- ARDS, a progressive pulmonary disorder that may lead to fibrosis of lung tissue and death, is treated with mechanical ventilation and treatment of the underlying cause.

Additional Learning Resources

SG Go to your Study Guide for additional learning activities to help you master this chapter content.

Go to your Evolve website (http://evolve.elsevier.com/Linton/medsurg) for the following learning resources and much more:

- Fluid & Electrolyte Tutorial
- Review Questions for the NCLEX® Examination

Clinical Judgment and Next-Generation NCLEX® Examination-Style Questions

1. **The nurse completes a functional assessment of a patient who is hospitalized with pneumonia. Which is the best example of the nurse's documentation of the respiratory assessment?**
    1. The patient expectorated a moderate amount of tenacious, green sputum.
    2. The patient reports coughing up a lot of mucus during the current shift.
    3. Physical activity seems to cause the patient to have severe coughing spells.
    4. The patient is coughing up less sputum today than yesterday.

    NCLEX Client Need: Physiological Integrity: Physiological Adaptation

2. **A community education project is designed to encourage older adults to have influenza immunizations. A participant asks about the difference between influenza and the common cold. What is the most appropriate reply?**
    1. Influenza is just a very severe cold.
    2. Bacteria cause colds, whereas a virus causes influenza.
    3. Influenza is more likely to cause fever and chills.
    4. They are equally likely to have serious complications.

    NCLEX Client Need: Physiological Integrity: Physiological Adaptation

3. **A patient who has pneumonia has become restless; vital signs are as follows: temperature 100°F (37.8°C), heart rate 110 beats per minute, respiration 28 breaths per minute, blood pressure 130/72 mm Hg. You should suspect ________________.**

    NCLEX Client Need: Physiological Integrity: Physiological Adaptation

4. **In the emergency care of a patient who has a sucking chest wound, why is a vented dressing preferred instead of a dressing that completely seals the wound?**
   1. The vented dressing permits the drainage of blood from the pleural sac.
   2. Sealing the wound increases the risk of bacterial contamination.
   3. The vented dressing prevents air from escaping from the injured lung.
   4. Sealing the wound could lead to a tension pneumothorax.

   NCLEX Client Need: Physiological Integrity: Reduction of Risk Potential

5. **You witness a serious auto accident in which a driver slammed into the steering wheel. While waiting for emergency medical services (EMS) to arrive, the driver develops respiratory distress. You observe that a part of the rib cage moves inward with inspiration and outward with expiration. Which of the following describes this pattern?**
   1. Paradoxical movement
   2. Tension pneumothorax
   3. Compensatory breathing
   4. Cheyne-Stokes respirations

   NCLEX Client Need: Physiological Integrity: Physiological Adaptation

6. **Measures to prevent PE (pulmonary embolism) in postoperative patients include which of the following? (Select all that apply.)**
   1. Apply compression stockings as ordered.
   2. Assist with range-of-motion exercises.
   3. Enforce bed rest until wound healing is complete.
   4. Support the legs with pillows to promote circulation.
   5. Encourage ambulation as soon as permitted.

   NCLEX Client Need: Physiological Integrity: Reduction of Risk Potential

7. **SLO Objective: Apply knowledge of pathophysiology to recognize signs and symptoms of COVID-19.**

   NGN Item Type: Enhanced Hot Spot

   Cognitive Skill: Recognize Cues

   A 72-year-old woman calls the office of her primary care provider. She is concerned because someone who sat next to her in church last week has tested positive for COVID-19. The nurse interviews her via telephone and collects the following data:
   - No appetite; food is tasteless
   - Oral temperature of 100.5°F
   - Low back pain
   - Dry cough
   - Had influenza vaccine 2 months ago

   Highlight the assessment findings that the nurse should recognize as possible symptoms of COVID-19.

8. **SLO Objective: Plan actions to reduce the risk of pulmonary embolism in patients with limited mobility.**

   NGN Item Type: Matrix

   Cognitive Skill: Generate Solutions

   A 45-year-old woman had an exploratory laparotomy (abdominal surgical procedure) with excision of multiple adhesions yesterday. She has a history of deep vein thrombosis during her last pregnancy. She was assisted out of bed for a brief walk on the evening of her surgery. Today she says she is too exhausted to walk. She reluctantly gets into a bedside chair for 30 minutes then wants to return to bed.

   Use an X for the nursing actions listed below that are *Indicated/Anticipated* (appropriate or necessary), *Contraindicated* (could be harmful), or *Nonessential* (makes no difference or not necessary) for the patient's care at this time.

NURSING ACTION	INDICATED	CONTRAINDICATED	NONESSENTIAL
Apply compression stockings as ordered			
Assist with active range of motion of legs			
Place a pillow under her legs when in bed			
Monitor heparin infusion			
Explain how exercise helps prevent blood clots			
Encourage high fiber foods			

9. **SLO Objective:** Assist in developing a nursing care plan for a patient on anticoagulant therapy.

NGN Item Type: Matrix

Cognitive Skill: Take Action

A patient with a pulmonary embolism is started on anticoagulant therapy. She is being discharged on oral dabigatran (Pradaxa).
Use an X for the health teaching below that is Indicated (appropriate or necessary), Contraindicated (could be harmful), or Nonessential (makes no difference or not necessary before the patient's discharge at this time.

HEALTH TEACHING	INDICATED	CONTRAINDICATED	NONESSENTIAL
Use a soft toothbrush to avoid trauma			
When seated, move your legs and feet often			
For minor pain, use aspirin or ibuprofen			
Take daily multi-vitamins			
Wear loose fitting clothing			
Your dose may be adjusted based on your prothrombin time.			
You can stop taking this medication once you resume an active lifestyle.			

10. **The nurse in a long-term care facility is orienting new Certified Nursing Assistants to elder care. Many residents have some difficulty swallowing. To reduce the risk of aspiration, which measures are appropriate? (Select all that apply.)**

 1. Seat the patient upright with the neck neutral or slightly bent forward for feeding.
 2. If patients are receiving enteral feedings, elevate the head during and 30 minutes after the feeding.
 3. A suction machine should be on hand when feeding patients who choke easily.
 4. Thin liquids are easier to swallow than thick liquids.

28 Chronic Lower Respiratory Tract Disorders

http://evolve.elsevier.com/Linton/medsurg

Objectives

1. Identify examples of chronic inflammatory, obstructive, and restrictive pulmonary diseases.
2. For selected chronic respiratory disorders, describe the pathophysiology, signs and symptoms, complications, diagnostic measures, and medical treatment.
3. Assist in developing a nursing care plan for the patient with a chronic respiratory disorder.
4. Explain the relationship between cigarette smoking and chronic respiratory disorders.

Key Terms

asbestosis (ăs-bĕs-TŌ-sĭs)
asthma (ĂZ-mă)
brachytherapy (brăk-ē-THĔR-ă-pē)
bronchiectasis (brŏn-kē-ĔK-tă-sĭs)
cor pulmonale (kŏr pŭl-mō-NĂ-lē)
emphysema (ĕm-fĭ-SĒ-mă)
exacerbation
granuloma (grăn-yū-LŌ-mă)
pneumoconiosis (nū-mō-kō-nē-Ō-sĭs)
pneumonitis (nū-mō-NĪ-tĭs)

This chapter focuses on chronic disorders of the lower respiratory system. A review of respiratory structure and function, common diagnostic procedures, common therapeutic measures (including drug therapy), and the nursing assessment of respiratory function are covered in Chapter 25.

OBSTRUCTIVE PULMONARY DISORDERS

Obstructive respiratory diseases are characterized by airway obstruction or narrowing that increases resistance to airflow. The most common types are asthma, chronic obstructive pulmonary disease (COPD), cystic fibrosis, and bronchiectasis.

A common diagnostic procedure for obstructive pulmonary disease is the pulmonary function test (PFT). PFTs provide information about airway dynamics, lung volumes, and diffusing capacity. *Airway dynamics* refers to the patient's ability to inhale or exhale by force. Some of the lung volumes measured include vital capacity (VC), inspiratory capacity (IC), expiratory reserve volume (ERV), residual volume (RV), and total lung capacity. The diffusing capacity is a measurement of the ability of gases to diffuse across the alveolar capillary membrane. PFTs are performed under laboratory conditions by trained personnel. These tests are effort dependent, meaning that the patient must be mentally alert, cooperative, and able to follow directions. Additional information about PFTs is presented in Chapter 25.

ASTHMA

Asthma is an obstructive airway disease usually characterized by chronic airway inflammation. . The inflammatory process results in bronchial hyperresponsiveness, bronchial constriction and edema, thickening of bronchial walls, and the production of thick mucus. In relation to asthma, the term *hyperresponsiveness* means that the airway is especially sensitive to stimuli. It is classified as an *obstructive disorder* because of the narrowing of the airways and presence of mucus plugs. Several types of asthma that differ in clinical features and treatment responses are also recognized. Patients with eosinophilic asthma have high eosinophils in their blood and sputum. Elevated eosinophils contribute to airway inflammation, frequent asthma exacerbations, a high degree of airflow limitation, and remodeling. A high eosinophil count is predictive of future exacerbations.

The incidence of asthma has been increasing. It occurs across the lifespan, from the very young to the very old. It is a highly complex condition that can be a mild nuisance or a very serious, life-threatening condition (see the Cultural Considerations box).

Cultural Considerations

WHAT DOES CULTURE HAVE TO DO WITH ASTHMA?

Black Americans and Hispanic Americans have a greater incidence of asthma than do White Americans. The reason for the difference is not clear, but genetics is likely to play a part.

Pathophysiology

Although the cause of asthma is unknown, it appears to be the result of innate (inborn) immunity, genetics, and environmental factors. Variations in the process of development, persistence, and severity of asthma suggest that various types of this condition exist. Asthma was once thought to be simply a condition in which allergies induced episodes of bronchoconstriction. However, researchers now know that it is much more complicated than this and that it has long-term consequences. Patients with asthma periodically have acute **exacerbations** (recurrent symptoms), also called *flare-ups* or *attacks*, of varying intensity. Exacerbations have two distinct phases. The early phase of an acute exacerbation begins when "triggers" (e.g., allergens, irritants, infections, exercise, gastroesophageal reflux, stress) activate the inflammatory process. The airways constrict (bronchoconstriction or bronchospasm) and become edematous. Mucus secretion increases, forming plugs in the airways, and tenacious sputum is produced. Obstruction causes air to be trapped in the alveoli, creating a ventilation-perfusion mismatch. That is, the alveoli are perfused with blood but not ventilated with fresh air. The effect is hypoxemia with compensatory hyperventilation. The early phase usually begins within 30 to 60 minutes after exposure to the trigger and resolves some 30 to 90 minutes later (Fig. 28.1).

The late phase begins 4 to 8 hours after the early-phase response, when airway inflammation is pronounced. Red blood cells (RBCs) and white blood cells (WBCs) infiltrate the swollen tissues of the airways. During this phase, which lasts several hours or days, the airways are hyperresponsive. The patient is at risk for another acute exacerbation until the late phase subsides.

It is important to note that asthma is not an emotional disorder! Stress does not cause asthma, although an emotional response to episodes of difficulty breathing is understandable. It is possible that the patient's emotional state plays some role in acute exacerbations, but this is not fully understood.

Complications

Severe, persistent bronchospasm is called *status asthmaticus.* If not corrected, status asthmaticus can lead to right-sided heart failure, pneumothorax, worsening hypoxemia, acidosis, and respiratory or cardiac arrest. Over time, repeated exacerbations can cause hypertrophy of bronchial smooth muscle, thickening of the tissues in the airways, hypertrophy of mucus glands, air trapping in the alveoli, and hyperinflation of the lungs. These permanent changes are referred to as *airway remodeling*.

Clinical Manifestations

During an asthma exacerbation, the patient may exhibit dyspnea, productive cough, use of accessory muscles of respiration (scalenes and sternocleidomastoids), audible expiratory wheezing, tachycardia, and tachypnea. Air moving through the narrowed airways causes wheezing. Findings that suggest that respiratory arrest is imminent include drowsiness, confusion, absence of wheezing, bradycardia, and retractions above the sternum.

Medical Diagnosis

A diagnosis of bronchial asthma is based on the health history, the physical examination, and spirometry. Typical symptoms reported are wheezing, dyspnea, chest tightness, and cough. In some cases, additional

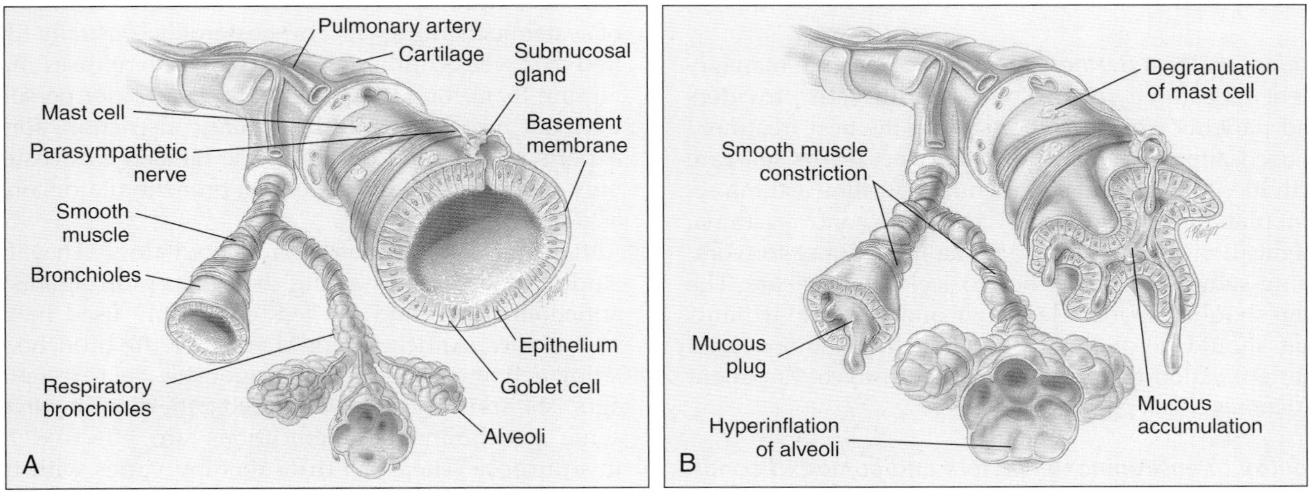

Fig. 28.1 Comparison of bronchioles, respiratory bronchioles, and alveoli (A) in a normal lung and (B) in the lung of a person with bronchial asthma. (From McCance KL, Huether SE. *Understanding pathophysiology*, 5th ed. St. Louis, Mosby, 2013. Modified from Des Jardins T, Burton GG. *Clinical manifestations and assessment of respiratory disease*, 5th ed. St. Louis, Mosby, 2016.)

PFTs may be done. Spirometry typically reveals that the airflow coming from the patient's lungs is significantly less than expected. Arterial blood gas measurements and oximetry may be monitored if the patient has moderate-to-severe symptoms. The eosinophils in blood and sputum may be assessed. The diagnosis may be classified as intermittent, mild persistent, moderate persistent, or severe persistent asthma.

Medical Treatment

The primary goal of medical therapy is to control asthma so that functional limitations and risks (progressive decline in lung function or adverse drugs effects) are reduced. The four key components of asthma care are assessment and monitoring, education, environmental control, and pharmacologic therapy.

Assessing and monitoring asthma severity and control. Medical therapy is selected on the basis of symptom severity and adjusted as needed to achieve and maintain control. Severity and control are determined in relation to current impairment and future risk. The extent of impairment is based on the frequency and intensity of symptoms and the patient's functional limitations. Future risk is estimated by the likelihood of asthma exacerbations, progressive decline in lung function, or risk of adverse drugs effects. In addition to patients' reports of their symptoms, peak flow monitoring is an important tool to determine control. Daily peak flow monitoring is advised for certain persons, such as those with moderate or severe persistent asthma. Periodic spirometry may be done to assess the effectiveness of therapy. Global Initiative for Asthma (GINA) guidelines (2020) recommend follow-up 1 to 3 months after treatment is started, and every 3 to 12 months thereafter, with a review visit within 1 week of an exacerbation. The health care provider should assess asthma control, adherence, and inhaler technique at every visit.

Education for a partnership in care. Effective management of asthma requires that health care providers and patients work together so that the best treatment is used and the patient (or caregiver) learns self-care activities. The patient should have a written asthma action plan that includes daily actions to control asthma, medication adjustments to make in response to worsening symptoms, and when to seek medical care. The plan should also include known allergens and irritants that should be avoided. Research has demonstrated that education for self-management improves patient outcomes.

Control of environmental factors and comorbid conditions that affect asthma. Many irritants and allergens in the environment trigger or aggravate asthma symptoms. The patient's environment should be inspected for common allergens. Skin testing may be done to identify substances to which a patient is sensitive. This informs the patient which triggers to avoid or to remove, if possible. Based on the skin test results, patients may be given subcutaneous injections to desensitize them to the specific allergens. Indoor air-cleaning devices reduce airborne dog and cat allergens, mold spores, and particulate tobacco smoke but they have little effect on cockroach, dust mite, and rodent allergens. Other strategies can be implemented to reduce exposure to these allergens in the home.

Comorbid conditions include all the patient's other diagnoses. Some of the comorbid conditions that can interfere with asthma management are gastroesophageal reflux, obesity, obstructive sleep apnea, rhinitis or sinusitis, stress, and depression. Management of these conditions can improve asthma control. Some patients have features of both asthma and COPD defined by the term *Asthma COPD Overlap Syndrome* (ACOS).

Pharmacology Capsule

Immunotherapy ("allergy shots") should be given in a medical facility where support is available if a life-threatening reaction occurs.

Medications. A variety of medications, including bronchodilators and antiinflammatory drugs, are used to prevent or treat asthma symptoms. Drugs used to treat asthma can be classified as those that provide long-term control ("controllers") and those that relieve acute symptoms ("relievers"). Controllers are antiinflammatory drugs that include inhaled glucocorticoids, leukotriene modifiers, mast cell stabilizers, monoclonal antibodies, long-acting inhaled beta-adrenergic agonists (LABAs) such as salmeterol and formoterol, methylxanthines (oral theophylline), and the inhaled anticholinergics ipratropium, tiotropium, and aclidinium. Systemic corticosteroids may be used for asthma that does not respond to other controllers. The course of systemic therapy with corticosteroids is usually limited to 2 weeks, although especially severe cases may require them for a longer time. Because older persons may not recognize mild bronchial constriction, some experts recommend that they use inhaled corticosteroids on a regular basis instead of bronchodilators only as needed.

Relievers are primarily bronchodilators. They include inhaled short-acting beta$_2$-receptor agonists, anticholinergics, and the less commonly used methylxanthines. Anticholinergics enhance the bronchodilating action of beta$_2$-receptor agonists. Beta$_2$-receptor agonists are the most often used relievers; however, some anticholinergic medications are effective for this purpose. The exact drug therapy varies with the severity of the condition. People with mild asthma may have to use inhaled bronchodilators only when they have symptoms, whereas those with moderate to severe asthma may be advised to use the inhalers

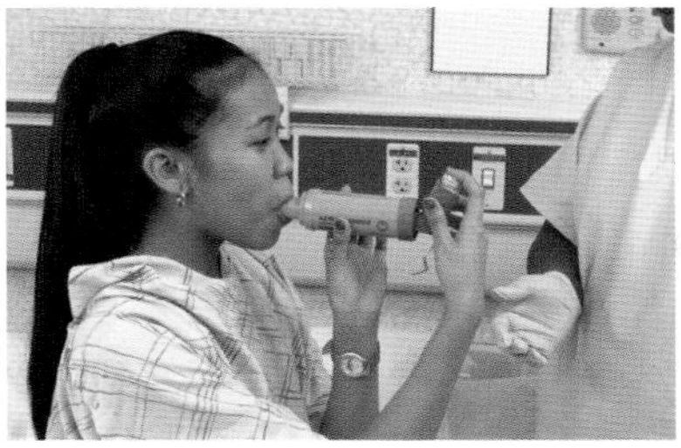

Fig. 28.2 Use of metered-dose inhaler for administration of inhalant medication. (From Lilley LL, Collins SR, Snyder JS. *Pharmacology and the nursing process*, 8th ed. St Louis, Elsevier, 2017.)

daily. Patients with severe asthma may also require other agents, such as aerosol corticosteroids (Fig. 28.2). Some combination preparations are available. Advair contains both a corticosteroid and a bronchodilator, Combivent contains an anticholinergic and a bronchodilator, and Dulera is a combination of mometasone (a synthetic corticosteroid) and formoterol (a bronchodilator).

In 2020 , the *Asthma Management Guidelines* (NHLBI) provided an update of the medications and dosages first published in the classic *Guidelines from the National Asthma Education and Prevention Program Expert Panel Report 3* (2007). Those recommendations are presented as a stepwise approach to asthma management in Fig. 28.3 (see the Complementary and Alternative Therapies box). An option that is sometimes used for patients who do not respond well to medications is bronchial thermoplasty. This treatment requires a series of bronchoscopies in which a heated device is introduced into to the airway. The intended effect is to shrink the muscle tissue in the enlarged airways allowing better air flow. At this time, it is not clear if the outcomes justify the risks of this procedure.

Complementary and Alternative Therapies

Ephedra, marketed as *má huáng*, is a herbal product that can relieve bronchospasm and is sometimes used for weight loss because it is a stimulant. Because of the risk for cardiac and CNS toxicity, the U.S. Food and Drug Administration (FDA) has banned its sale as a dietary supplement.

Status asthmaticus is a severe, life-threatening episode of asthma that does not respond to the patient's usual treatment. It is treated with inhaled and intravenous bronchodilators and oxygen (O_2) therapy. Endotracheal intubation and mechanical ventilation are sometimes necessary. Drugs used to treat respiratory disorders are presented in Chapter 25, Table 25.4.

Pharmacology Capsule

Patients who have severe persistent asthma, nasal polyps, and a history of allergy to aspirin or other nonsteroidal antiinflammatory drugs (NSAIDs) are at risk for life-threatening reactions if they use these drugs.

Put On Your Thinking Cap!

Write a teaching plan (including at least three facts) for an asthma patient who is prescribed an inhaled corticosteroid combined with formoterol.

◆ NURSING CARE OF THE PATIENT WITH ASTHMA

Focused Assessment

The complete assessment of the patient with a respiratory disorder is summarized in Chapter 25, Box 25.2.

Reason for seeking care. When the patient has asthma, it is important to collect essential data (e.g., medications, allergies, known cardiac disease, sleep disruption) and immediately take steps to relieve acute symptoms; then more complete data can be collected.

Health history. Information about the frequency and severity of exacerbations, the factors known to trigger exacerbations, the effect of the condition on the patient's life, the strategies used to manage the condition, the sources of stress and support, and the patient's knowledge of asthma and its treatment should be obtained. In addition, the patient's ability to afford medical care and drug therapy should be explored. If the patient uses an inhaler, have them demonstrate its use. Improper technique may fail to deliver the appropriate amount of the drug to the lungs.

Each time the patient sees a health care provider, the level of asthma symptom control in the past 4 weeks should be assessed by collecting the following data:

- Have you had daytime symptoms more than twice in a week?
- Have you awoken at night because of asthma?
- Have you needed to use a reliever drug more than twice in a week?
- Do you have any activity limitations resulting from asthma?

A person with well-controlled asthma will answer "no" to all of these questions. The patient who answers "yes" to one or two of these questions is considered partly controlled. The patient who answers "yes" to three or four of these questions is considered uncontrolled. This tool enables the prescriber to make decisions about changes in the treatment plan.

Physical examination. Important aspects of the physical examination include measurement of vital signs and auscultation of lung sounds. In addition, note the patient's skin color and respiratory effort. During an acute exacerbation, wheezing on exhalation is common initially. If the episode progresses, wheezes may be heard on both inhalation and exhalation. If breath sounds become severely diminished or absent and the patient is distressed, the situation is life-threatening.

Ages 12+ years: Stepwise approach for management of asthma

	Intermittent asthma	Management of persistent asthma in individuals ages 12+ years				
Treatment	Step 1	Step 2	Step 3	Step 4	Step 5	Step 6■
Preferred	PRN SABA	Daily low-dose ICS and PRN SABA or PRN concomitant ICS and SABA ⅄	Daily and PRN combination low-dose ICS-formoterol ⅄	Daily and PRN combination medium-dose ICS-formoterol ⅄	Daily medium-high dose ICS-LABA + LAMA and PRN SABA ⅄	Daily high-dose ICS-LABA + oral systemic corticosteroids + PRN SABA
Alternative		Daily LTRA* and PRN SABA or Cromolyn,* or nedocromil,* or zileuton,* or theophylline,* and PRN SABA	Daily medium-dose ICS and PRN SABA or Daily low-dose ICS-LABA, or daily low-dose ICS + LAMA,⅄ or daily low-dose ICS + LTRA,* and PRN SABA or Daily low-dose ICS + theophylline* or zileuton, * and PRN SABA	Daily medium-dose ICS-LABA or daily medium-dose ICS + LAMA, and PRN SABA ⅄ or Daily medium-dose ICS + LTRA,* or daily medium-dose ICS + theophylline,* or daily medium-dose ICS + zileuton,* and PRN SABA	Daily medium-high dose ICS-LABA or daily high-dose ICS + LTRA,* and PRN SABA	
		Steps 2–4: Conditionally recommend the use of subcutaneous immunotherapy as an adjunct treatment to standard pharmacotherapy in individuals ≥ 5 years of age whose asthma is controlled at the initiation, build up, and maintenance phases of immunotherapy ⅄			Consider adding asthma biologics (e.g., anti- IgE, anti-IL5, anti-IL5R, anti-IL4/IL13)**	

Assess control

- First check adherence, inhaler technique, environmental factors,⅄ and comorbid conditions.
- **Step up** if needed; reassess in 2–6 weeks
- **Step down** if possible (if asthma is well controlled for at least 3 consecutive months)

Consult with asthma specialist if step 4 or higher is required. Consider consultation at step 3.

Control assessment is a key element of asthma care. This involves both impairment and risk. Use of objective measures, self-reported control, and health care utilization are complementary and should be employed on an ongoing basis, depending on the individual's clinical situation.

Abbreviations: ICS, inhaled corticosteroid; LABA, long-acting beta$_2$-agonist; LAMA, long-acting muscarinic antagonist; LTRA, leukotriene receptor antagonist; SABA, inhaled short-acting beta$_2$-agonist

⅄ Updated based on the 2020 guidelines.

* Cromolyn, nedocromil, LTRAs including zileuton and montelukast, and theophylline were not considered for this update, and/or have limited availability for use in the United States, and/or have an increased risk of adverse consequences and need for monitoring that make their use less desirable. The FDA issued a boxed warning for montelukast in march 2020.

** The AHRQ systematic reviews that informed this report did not include studies that examined the role of asthma biologics (e.g. anti-IgE, anti-IL5, anti-IL5R, anti-IL4/IL13). Thus, this report does not contain specific recommendations for the use of biologics in asthma in steps 5 and 6.

■ Data on the use of LAMA therapy in individuals with severe persistent asthma (step 6) were not included in the AHRQ systematic review and thus no recommendation is made.

December 2020

Fig. 28.3 Ages 12+ Years: Stepwise approach for management of asthma. (From *2020 Focused updates to the asthma management guidelines: A report from the National Asthma Education and Prevention Program Coordinating Committee Expert Panel Working Groups*. National Heart, Lung, and Blood Institute, 2020.)

Patient Problems, Goals, and Outcome Criteria: Asthma

Patient Problems	Goals and Outcome Criteria
Inadequate oxygenation related to air trapping	Adequate oxygenation: regular respirations, 12 to 20 breaths per minute, without dyspnea or wheezing, oxygen saturation of at least 95%
Airway obstruction related to bronchospasm, air trapping, increased secretions	Patent airway and improved airflow: normal skin color, normal pulse and respiratory rates, arterial blood gases within normal limits
Anxiety related to perceived threat of suffocation, hypoxemia	Reduced anxiety: patient statement of lessened anxiety, calm manner

Interventions

Inadequate oxygenation. Monitor the patient's respiratory rate, pattern, and effort, and lung sounds. Support the patient in the Fowler position and give O_2 as ordered. In addition, administer prescribed bronchodilators and monitor for improvement or adverse effects of drug therapy. It is important to remain with the patient during an acute exacerbation. If the patient does not respond to these interventions, immediate medical care is essential because the condition may be life threatening.

Because asthma is a chronic condition, patient teaching is critical. Patients must understand their drugs, how they should be used, and any possible adverse effects that should be reported to the physician. If the patient is unable to afford these drugs, consult a social worker or case manager for assistance. Patients should be taught to use peak expiratory flow rate (PEFR) meters routinely. The patient uses the meter twice daily to establish a baseline (personal best) PEFR and then daily to monitor level of control. When a daily PEFR reading is 80% to 100% of the patient's personal best, the patient should continue current medications. A reading that is 50% to 80% of the personal best indicates that something is triggering the asthma. The patient should have a written asthma management action plan that specifies what to do in this situation. A reading of 50% or less requires prompt action according to the action plan (Table 28.1).

Airway obstruction. Monitor for signs and symptoms of impending respiratory failure: tachypnea, shallow respirations, diaphoresis, reddening skin, tachycardia, cardiac dysrhythmias, initial hypertension, later hypotension, restlessness, drowsiness, or loss of consciousness. Check arterial blood gas values and notify the registered nurse (RN) or physician if the partial pressure of oxygen in arterial blood (PaO_2) decreases, the partial pressure of carbon dioxide in arterial blood ($PaCO_2$) increases, and the pH falls. Administer O_2 as ordered, usually 4 to 6 L/min unless the patient has COPD, in which case O_2 therapy is limited to 3 L/min. A nasal cannula is preferred over a face mask because the mask may increase the patient's feeling of suffocation.

If the patient has tenacious secretions that cannot be expectorated, chest physiotherapy (CPT) and suctioning may be necessary. Because good hydration helps to thin secretions, a daily fluid intake of 2500 to 3000 mL is recommended unless contraindicated. Intravenous fluids may be ordered to improve hydration and provide venous access for administration of emergency drugs.

Anxiety. The feeling of not being able to breathe is very frightening. In addition, with moderate to severe asthma, PaO_2 decreases, which causes a feeling of restlessness and anxiety. Anxiety may serve to aggravate the physical symptoms. While taking steps to improve the patient's oxygenation, try to reduce anxiety by remaining calm, establishing eye contact, providing quiet reassurance, and explaining what is being done. The family may also need information and reassurance to calm their fears so that they can be more supportive of the patient (see the Patient Teaching box).

Patient Teaching

ASTHMA

Management of asthma requires a partnership between the patient and the health care provider so that the patient can learn to manage it. After the acute attack has subsided, initiate patient teaching by providing the following information to the patient:

- Your physician may order long-term control medications daily to prevent symptoms; these drugs will not provide quick relief unless they include a bronchodilator.
- Acute asthma exacerbations can be triggered by allergic reactions to substances in the environment, by exercise, and by infection; stress can aggravate it.
- To reduce environmental triggers, keep pets with fur or hair outdoors or confined to specific rooms, remove carpet and cloth upholstery, never leave food out, have the house treated by pest control, and clean moldy surfaces. During allergy season, stay indoors with the windows closed, especially between midday and afternoon.
- To reduce the occurrence of exacerbations, avoid irritating substances, including tobacco smoke; have infections treated promptly; and learn to manage stressful situations.
- If you need to take your reliever more than 2 days per week, inform your health care provider. An adjustment in your controller may be indicated.
- If you have symptoms during exercise, use your prescribed inhaler as directed 30 minutes before you exercise.
- Drugs for asthma must be taken as prescribed; report adverse effects to your health care provider (see Chapter 25, Table 25.4).
- Seek emergency medical care if your symptoms worsen and do not respond to your medications.
- Drink 10 to 14 8-oz glasses of fluids daily if approved by your physician.
- The Asthma and Allergy Foundation of America is a resource for information about the treatment and management of asthma.
- To deliver drugs effectively, metered-dose inhalers must be used correctly. (Teach correct use and have patients practice, using the manufacturer's directions.)

Table 28.1 Asthma Action Plan

American Lung Association.

My Asthma Action Plan

Name: ____________________ **DOB:** ____ / ____ / ____

Severity Classification: ☐ Intermittent ☐ Mild Persistent ☐ Moderate Persistent ☐ Severe Persistent

Asthma Triggers (list): ____________________

Peak Flow Meter Personal Best: __________

Green Zone: Doing Well

Symptoms: Breathing is good – No cough or wheeze – Can work and play – Sleeps well at night

Peak Flow Meter __________ (more than 80% of personal best)

Flu Vaccine—Date received: ______ **Next flu vaccine due:** ______ **COVID19 vaccine—Date received:** ______

Control Medicine(s)	Medicine	How much to take	When and how often to take it

Physical Activity ☐ Use Albuterol/Levalbuterol ____ puffs, 15 minutes before activity
☐ with all activity ☐ when you feel you need it

Yellow Zone: Caution

Symptoms: Some problems breathing – Cough, wheeze, or tight chest – Problems working or playing – Wake at night

Peak Flow Meter ______ to ______ (between 50% and 79% of personal best)

Quick-relief Medicine(s) ☐ Albuterol/Levalbuterol ____ puffs, every 4 hours as needed

Control Medicine(s) ☐ Continue Green Zone medicines
☐ Add ____________ ☐ Change to ____________

You should feel better within 20–60 minutes of the quick-relief treatment. If you are getting worse or are in the Yellow Zone for more than 24 hours, THEN follow the instructions in the RED ZONE and call the doctor right away!

Red Zone: Get Help Now!

Symptoms: Lots of problems breathing – Cannot work or play – Getting worse instead of better – Medicine is not helping

Peak Flow Meter __________ (less than 50% of personal best)

Take Quick-relief Medicine NOW! ☐ Albuterol/Levalbuterol ____ puffs, ____________ (how frequently)

Call 911 immediately if the following danger signs are present:

- Trouble walking/talking due to shortness of breath
- Lips or fingernails are blue
- Still in the red zone after 15 minutes

Emergency Contact Name ____________________ Phone (____) ____ - ____

Emergency Contact Name ____________________ Phone (____) ____ - ____

Date: ____ / ____ / ____

1-800-LUNGUSA | Lung.org

ALA Asthma AP V1 3 18 2020

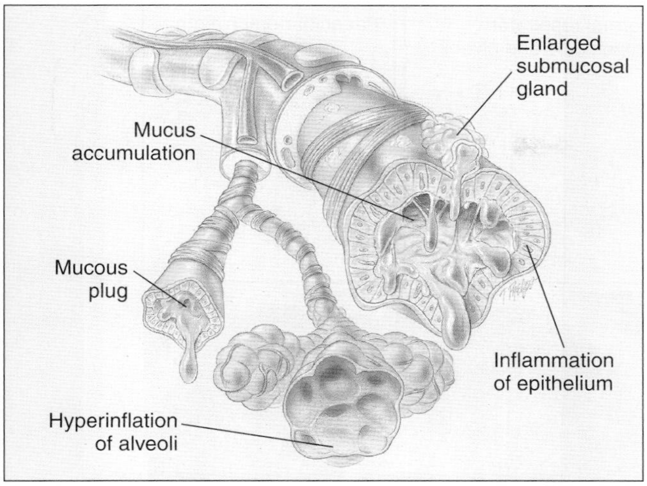

Fig. 28.4 Chronic bronchitis. (From McCance KL, Huether SE. *Understanding pathophysiology*, 5th ed. St. Louis: Mosby; 2013. Modified from Des Jardins T, Burton GG. *Clinical manifestations and assessment of respiratory disease*, 5th ed. St. Louis, Mosby; 2006.)

Health promotion. Vaccination for seasonal influenza is safe and recommended for patients with asthma.

CHRONIC OBSTRUCTIVE PULMONARY DISEASE

The term *chronic obstructive pulmonary disease* (COPD) describes a condition marked by progressive, largely irreversible airflow obstruction that cannot be explained by any other diagnosis such as asthma. Although chronic bronchitis and emphysema can occur independently, patients with COPD often have both. Therefore the two conditions are both discussed in this section. Note that some COPD patients also have asthma.

Pathophysiology

The early stage of COPD is chronic inflammation of the respiratory bronchioles, alveoli, and pulmonary blood vessels (Fig. 28.4). The inflammation is a response to the inhalation of noxious particles and gases with smoking being a frequent source. However, the inflammation is much more destructive than that seen in persons without COPD. Inflammatory cells (neutrophils, macrophages, lymphocytes) attract inflammatory mediators (e.g., leukotrienes, cytokines) leading to structural changes in the lungs. Not only does tissue damage occur, but the normal defense mechanisms and repair processes are disrupted.

Protease is an enzyme that breaks down connective lung tissue. Antiproteases are enzymes that inhibit protease activity. Normally, protease and antiprotease maintain a natural balance, but in COPD protease activity increases and antiprotease activity decreases. This imbalance results in increased mucus secretion and fluid in the lungs. The patient is said to have chronic bronchitis when the increased production of mucus and chronic cough persist for at least 3 months of the year for 2 consecutive years.

Peripheral airways become obstructed, trapping air during expirations. Elastic tissue in the small airways is damaged so that elastic recoil is lost, contributing to air trapping. Trapping leads to expansion of the chest so that it becomes barrel shaped. Over time, the alveolar walls are destroyed. Abnormal enlargement of air spaces beyond the terminal bronchiole is called **emphysema**. The two types of emphysema are centriacinar and panacinar (Fig. 28.5). Centriacinar emphysema, which is associated primarily with cigarette smoking, affects mainly the respiratory bronchioles. The walls of the bronchioles enlarge and break down leaving the alveoli intact. Panacinar emphysema, which affects the respiratory bronchioles and the alveoli, is caused more often by a hereditary deficiency of the enzyme inhibitor alpha 1-antitrypsin. The walls of the alveoli and respiratory bronchioles break down, causing air to be trapped and decreasing the surface area for gas exchange. A patient may have both types of emphysema at the same time. The lungs become hyperinflated, causing the diaphragm to flatten and increasing the reliance on accessory muscles for breathing.

Large air spaces in the lung tissue (bullae) and next to the pleura (blebs) form. With no capillary beds, bullae and blebs contain air but cannot exchange gases. Blebs can rupture causing the affected lung to collapse. A ventilation-perfusion mismatch results in hypoxemia (low level of O_2 in the blood). In severe disease, obstruction of peripheral airways also contributes to the ventilation perfusion mismatch. These factors, along with impairment of respiratory muscles may lead to hypercapnia (high level of CO_2 in the blood).

In the late stage of COPD, pulmonary hypertension may develop because of hypoxic changes in the small pulmonary arteries. As the disease progresses, the right ventricle may become enlarged, a condition called **cor pulmonale**. Right-sided heart failure may ensue. These changes first cause hypoxemia during exercise, and later hypoxemia at rest.

The same chronic inflammation that underlies COPD is a factor in the development of other systemic conditions: cardiovascular disease, skeletal muscle wasting, osteoporosis, diabetes, and metabolic syndrome.

Put On Your Thinking Cap!

Refer to Chapter 6 to figure out why a patient with chronic obstructive pulmonary disease might develop respiratory acidosis.

Put On Your Thinking Cap!

Why is a patient with chronic obstructive pulmonary disease likely to develop failure of the right side of the heart before developing left-sided heart failure?

Complications

The most serious complications of COPD are respiratory failure and heart failure. Respiratory failure is

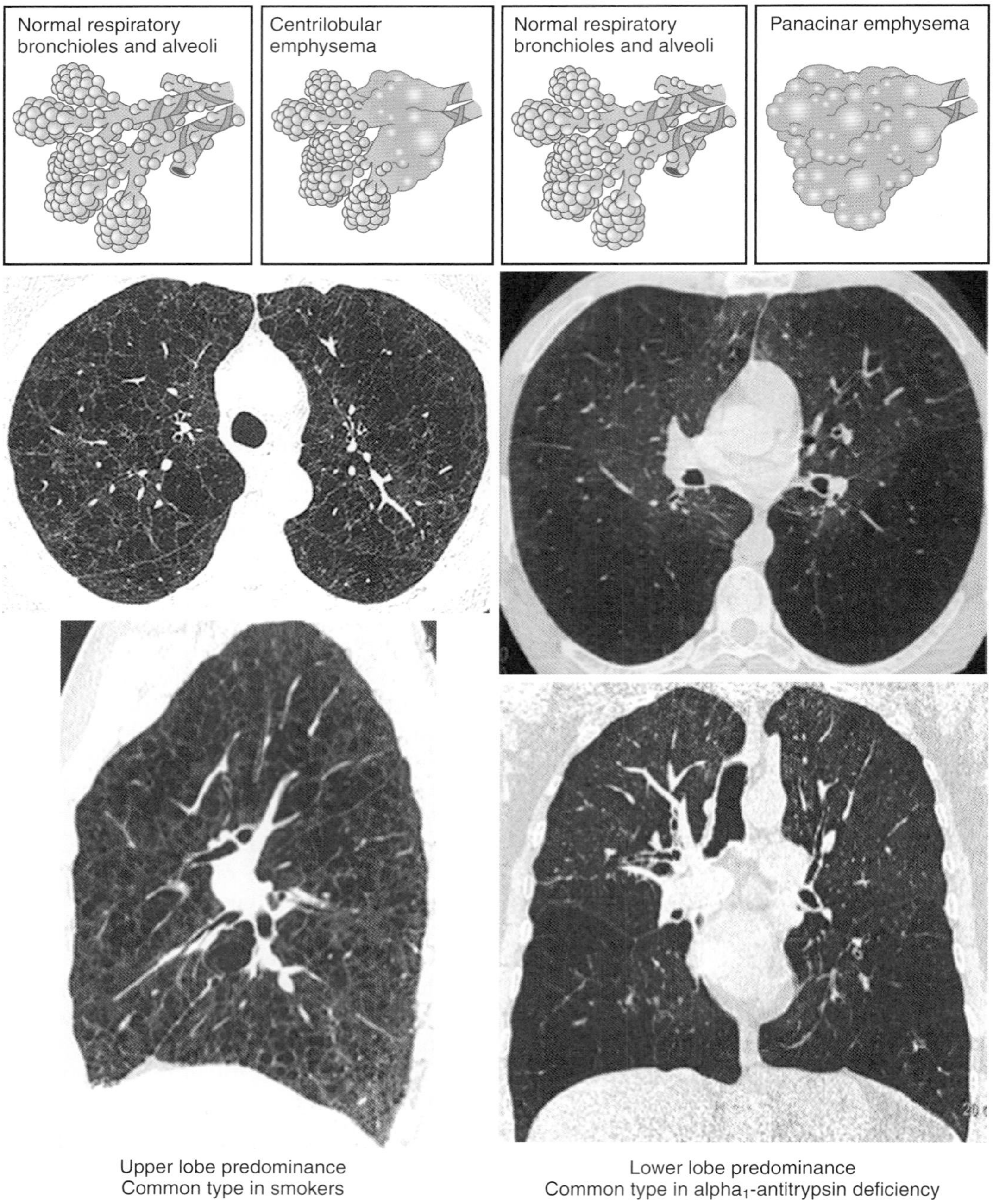

Fig. 28.5 Types of emphysema. (From Spiro SG, Silvestri GA, Agustí A. *Clinical respiratory medicine*, 4th ed. Philadelphia, Saunders, 2012.)

marked by hypoventilation and ventilation-perfusion mismatch with rising $PaCO_2$, declining PaO_2, and respiratory acidosis. Factors that may lead to complications include infection, air pollution, continued smoking, left ventricular failure, myocardial infarction, pulmonary embolism (PE), spontaneous pneumothorax, and adverse effects of drugs.

Clinical Manifestations

The earliest sign of COPD is commonly a chronic cough. The patient may report dyspnea upon exertion and a sense of heaviness in the chest. Wheezing may or may not be heard on auscultation. As the disease progresses, the patient may have dyspnea even at rest. The overinflated lungs cause the diaphragm to flatten. The patient must then use the intercostal and accessory muscles for breathing. Weight loss and fatigue are common. With chronic hypoxemia, the RBC count is typically elevated (polycythemia) to compensate for the inadequate PaO_2. The patient with cor pulmonale may demonstrate signs and symptoms of right heart failure, including increasing dyspnea, cyanosis, and peripheral edema.

Signs and symptoms related to chronic bronchitis include productive cough, exertional dyspnea, and wheezing. The main symptom of emphysema is dyspnea on exertion. As the disease progresses, the patient may also have dyspnea when at rest. Patients are often thin and may be observed using accessory muscles of

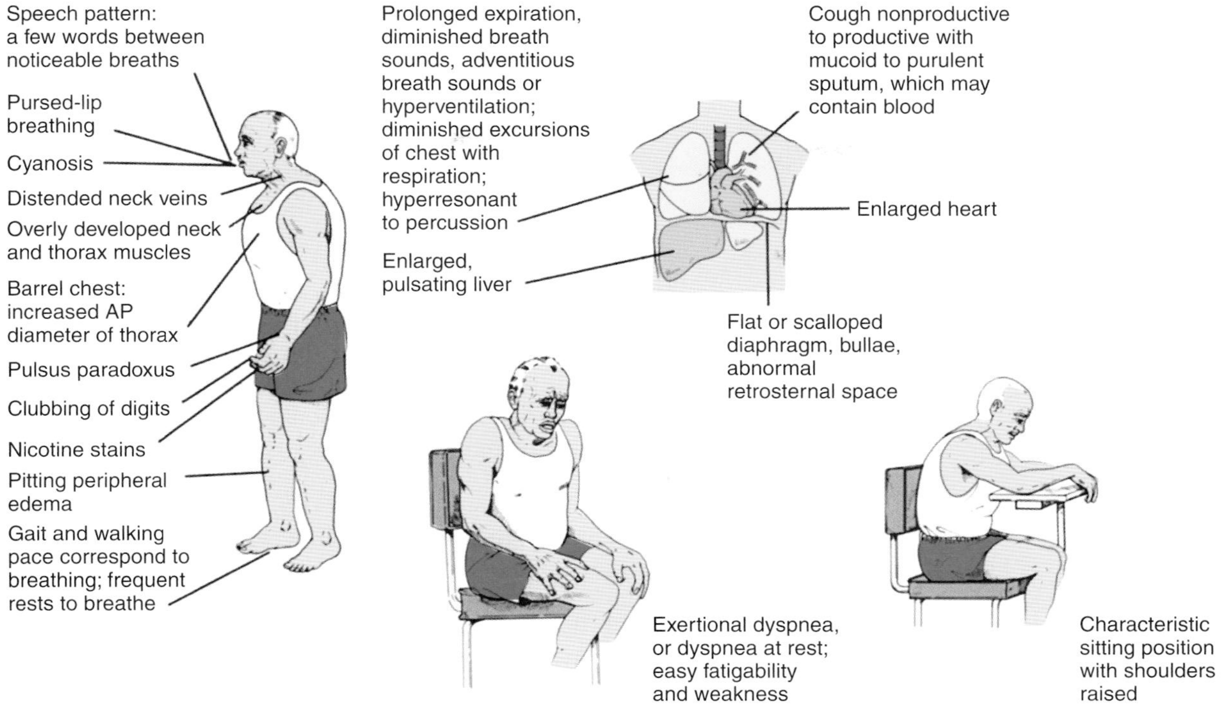

Fig. 28.6 Signs and symptoms of chronic obstructive pulmonary disease. *AP*, Anteroposterior. (From Black JM, Hawks JH. Medical-surgical nursing: clinical management for positive outcomes, 8th ed. St. Louis, Saunders, 2009.)

respiration. Increased anteroposterior diameter of the chest creates what is called a barrel chest (Fig. 28.6). Despite dyspnea, patients who have emphysema without chronic bronchitis often have normal arterial blood gases until the disease is very advanced. Therefore skin color may be normal. Depression and irritability are common in the patient with COPD.

Medical Diagnosis

COPD is suspected on the basis of the patient's health history and physical examination. The most reliable diagnostic tests for COPD are the PFTs, which reveal a decreased forced expiratory volume (FEV) and forced vital capacity (FVC) accompanied by increases in functional residual capacity (FRC) and RV. Total lung capacity (TLC) can be increased or normal. Other diagnostic tests that may be done are spirometry with a bronchodilator, oximetry, a chest radiograph, arterial blood gases, computed tomography (CT) scan, and the 6-minute walk test. The 6-minute walk test measures how far the patient can walk in 6 minutes, allowing for rest periods as needed; pulse oximetry is used during the walk. If a genetic cause is suspected, measurement of serum alpha 1-antitrypsin may be done. People with a severe deficiency of alpha 1-antitrypsin are at increased risk for developing COPD, especially if they smoke cigarettes.

Medical Treatment

The goals of medical treatment are to attain symptom relief, slow disease progression, improve exercise tolerance, prevent or treat complications, and improve overall health. The medical treatment plan begins with education and smoking cessation. Depending on the severity of the disease, additional interventions may include drug therapy, pulmonary rehabilitation, O_2 administration, and surgery. Patients with COPD are encouraged to have influenza and pneumococcal vaccinations.

Drug therapy. Drug therapy plays an important part in treating COPD. Many drugs used to treat asthma are also used to treat COPD (Box 28.1). Bronchodilators, including beta$_2$-adrenergics and anticholinergics, are ordered to decrease airway resistance and the work of breathing. Phosphodiesterase type 4 inhibitors (e.g., roflumilast [Daliresp]) which reduce inflammation, cough, and excessive mucus production, may be used in combination with a bronchodilator or an inhaled glucocorticoid. A person with mild COPD may be prescribed a short-acting inhaled beta-adrenergic agonist (SABA) or a short-acting inhaled anticholinergic drug for use only as needed. For those with moderate or severe COPD, a long-acting bronchodilator may also be prescribed. The preferred route of administration is by inhalation using a metered-dose inhaler. Some evidence indicates that anticholinergic drugs such as ipratropium bromide (Atrovent) or tiotropium (Spiriva) are more effective than beta-adrenergic agents for treating COPD and have fewer side effects.

Oral theophylline is a rather weak bronchodilator, but it may be beneficial if given with inhaled bronchodilators. However, it is not commonly used because of the risk of drug toxicity, particularly cardiac stimulation. If theophylline is used, periodic blood levels must be determined.

Inhaled corticosteroids are commonly used to reduce airway inflammation. These drugs reduce the

Box 28.1 Drugs Used to Treat Asthma

ANTIINFLAMMATORY AGENTS

Glucocorticoids
- beclomethasone (QVAR)
- budesonide (Pulmocort Flexhaler, Pulmicort Respules)
- ciclesonide (Alvesco)
- flunisolide (AeroBid)
- fluticasone propionate (Flovent HFA, Flovent Diskus)
- mometasone furoate (Asmanex Twisthaler)

Monoclonal Antibodies
- omalizumab (Xolair)
- mepolizumab (Nucala)
- reslizumab (Cinqair)

Leukotriene Modifiers
- zileuton
- zafirlukast
- montelukast

BRONCHODILATORS

Beta-2 Adrenergic Agonists
- Inhaled short acting (SABA)
- albuterol (ProAir HFA, Proventil HFA, Ventolin HFA)
- levalbuterol (Xopenex, Xopenex HFA)
- Inhaled long acting (LABA)
- formoterol (Foradil Aerolizer)
- indacaterol (Arcapta Neohaler)
- salmeterol (Serevent Diskus)
- Oral agents:
- albuterol (VoSpire ER, generic)
- terbutaline (generic only)

Methylxanthines
- theophylline (Theo-24, Elixophyllin)

Anticholinergic Agents
- ipratropium (Atrovent HFA)
- tiotropium (Spiriva)
- aclidinium (Tudorza Pressair)

Glucocorticoid-LABA Combinations
- fluticasone/salmeterol (Advair Diskus, Advair HFA)
- budesonide/formoteril (Symbicort)
- mometasone/formoterol (Dulera)

Note: Additional information about asthma drugs is detailed in Chapter 25, Table 25.4

(From Burchum JR, Rosenthal LD. *Lehne's pharmacology for nursing care*, 9th ed, St. Louis, Elsevier, 2016.)

frequency of exacerbations, especially when used in combination with a LABA. However, patients using inhaled corticosteroids are at increased risk for pneumonia. The long-term use of *oral* corticosteroids is not recommended because the benefits do not justify the adverse effects, which include fluid and electrolyte disturbances, increased risk for infection, elevated blood glucose, osteoporosis, and suppression of the adrenal cortex. Antidepressant drugs may be indicated and can improve the quality of life. More detailed information about drugs is presented in Chapter 25, Table 25.4.

Pharmacology Capsule

Bronchodilators are used to relieve symptoms, whereas antiinflammatory agents are used to prevent acute symptoms.

Oxygen therapy. O_2 therapy may be prescribed but must be used cautiously. The goal of O_2 therapy is to maintain the PaO_2 between 50 and 60 mm Hg. The initial liter flow is usually 1 to 3 L/min. The appropriate flow rate can be determined by adjusting the rate by 1 L increments at 15 minute intervals until the O_2 saturation remains above 90% (Niewoehner, 2016).

Periodically, the pulse oximeter should be correlated with actual blood gas laboratory values. High levels of O_2 are not administered because patients with COPD may rely on hypoxic drive to breathe. A comparison of respiratory stimuli in healthy people and people with COPD helps to explain the concept of hypoxic drive. A healthy person's respirations are stimulated by rising $PaCO_2$ levels. The patient with COPD who retains CO_2, however, has adapted to high blood CO_2 and relies on low PaO_2 to stimulate breathing. A high concentration of O_2 may raise the PaO_2 level so that the patient's stimulus to breathe is lost and respiratory depression may result. Not all people with COPD rely on hypoxic drive; retention of CO_2 must be confirmed by blood gas analysis.

For outpatient use, patients can rent O_2 tanks or cylinders, O_2 concentrators, and portable O_2 therapy equipment. O_2 concentrators compress and filter room air and deliver O_2 to the patient through a nasal cannula. Using long tubing, the patient can be mobile in the home setting. Suitcase models can be used for travel. Portable equipment includes liquid O_2 reservoirs that are carried easily on a shoulder strap and compressed-gas units that deliver O_2 only "on demand" so that a small quantity lasts longer than with standard cylinders.

Patients who meet specific criteria may be prescribed long-term oxygen therapy (LTOT), defined as the use of O_2 therapy for a minimum of 18 hours per day. LTOT has been shown to not only prolong survival in people with COPD but also improve exercise capacity, lung function, and mental state.

Chest physiotherapy. Chest physiotherapy (CPT), described in Chapter 25, may be ordered to mobilize secretions in the patient with COPD.

Pulmonary rehabilitation. The patient may be referred to a rehabilitation program that includes exercise reconditioning. Programs are individualized but usually use progressive exercise—either walking or pedaling a stationary cycle. A typical program might have the patient walk 10 to 15 minutes every day or every other day. Every week or two, the exercise time is increased by 5 to 10 minutes. The goal is to enable the patient to exercise comfortably for 45 minutes to 1 hour daily or every other day. Of course, some patients may not improve this much but improvement in walking performance and general well-being has been found in patients who consistently walked as little as 12 minutes every day for 2 months. Unfortunately, benefits tend to fade quickly after the program is completed.

Sometimes bronchodilators are prescribed before exercise.

Nutrition. Nutrition is important for the patient with COPD because malnutrition causes decreased energy and decreased resistance to infection and because obesity increases the work of breathing. No special diet is indicated; however, supplementary feedings may be needed for some patients. Good hydration helps to thin pulmonary secretions (see the Nutrition Considerations box).

Nutrition Considerations

1. Malnutrition and pulmonary disease are strongly related.
2. Starvation and malnutrition often cause impaired pulmonary function and pulmonary disease may result in malnutrition.
3. Pulmonary disease causes an increase in energy expenditure because of increased work of breathing and chronic infection.
4. Reduced dietary intake in lung disease results from fluid restriction, shortness of breath, anorexia, gastrointestinal (GI) distress, and vomiting.
5. Food allergies can be a trigger for asthma attacks.
6. Approximately 70% of patients with chronic obstructive pulmonary disease (COPD) exhibit weight loss.
7. Strategies for increasing intake and weight gain include eating high-calorie and high-fat foods; small, frequent meals; and resting before meals.

Treatment of respiratory failure. On average, COPD patients require hospitalization once each year for exacerbations. Classic signs of exacerbations are changes from the patient's usual dyspnea, cough, and/or sputum. These events may be related to infection, air pollution, heart failure, not taking medications correctly, medication adverse effects, and infection. Measures to treat acute exacerbations include O_2 therapy, aerosol bronchodilators, systemic corticosteroids, antibiotics if indicated, noninvasive positive pressure ventilation (NPPV), and mechanical ventilation (if the patient is becoming exhausted). NPPV has been found to improve survival and decrease the need for intubation. It uses a tightly fitted nasal or full facial mask attached to a positive pressure ventilator.

Surgical Treatment

When medical interventions fail, surgical options are available for selected patients. These procedures include lung volume reduction surgery (LVRS), bullectomy, and lung transplantation. LVRS is most likely to benefit those with poor exercise tolerance whose emphysema is mostly in the upper lung zones. LVRS involves the removal of up to 30% of the hyperinflated lung tissue so that remaining lung tissue can function better. Other surgical procedures that may benefit selected patients are bullectomy (removal of bullae) and lung transplantation.

◆ NURSING CARE OF THE PATIENT WITH CHRONIC OBSTRUCTIVE PULMONARY DISEASE

Focused Assessment

Assessment of the patient with a respiratory disorder is summarized in Chapter 25, Box 25.2. When a patient has COPD, record any presenting symptoms—often dyspnea, cough, chest pain, or a combination of these problems. In addition, a complete medical history is required unless the patient's symptoms make it difficult to participate in a long interview. Sometimes it is necessary to break the interview into smaller portions to avoid exhausting the patient who is dyspneic. A list of current medications and drug allergies is essential. Obtain a functional assessment to explore the effect of the condition on the patient's activities of daily living (ADL) and inquire about exposure to smoke or other respiratory irritants (see the Nursing Care Plan: Patient With Chronic Obstructive Pulmonary Disease box).

During the physical examination, observe the patient's posture, skin color, respiratory effort, and use of accessory muscles of respiration. Measure vital signs and examine the patient for signs of hypoxemia,

Nursing Care Plan Patient With Chronic Obstructive Pulmonary Disease

FOCUSED ASSESSMENT

Health History

A 73-year-old woman is being admitted for increasing dyspnea. She has had chronic bronchitis and emphysema for 3 years. Her past medical history includes frequent upper respiratory infections with two hospitalizations for pneumonia in the past year. She had a myocardial infarction in 2010 and is being treated for hypertension, for which she takes amlodipine. She also uses a tiotropium (Spiriva) inhaler once a day. She is allergic to penicillin. The review of systems notes fatigue, increasing dyspnea with exertion and at rest, orthopnea, and productive cough with yellow sputum. Patient states that she is depressed. She is a retired nurse who volunteers at a local homeless shelter 1 day a week. She lives alone and has no family in the area. She reports that her appetite is poor and that she has lost "a little" weight during the past few weeks. She has smoked one pack of cigarettes daily for 45 years. She states that she knows she should quit and has tried many programs but has never lasted longer than 1 week.

Physical Examination

Vital signs: blood pressure 140/94 mm Hg, pulse 100 beats per minute, respiration 28 breaths per minute, temperature 100.6° F (38.1° C) measured orally. Height 5′6″, weight 102 lb. The patient is seated with her hands on her knees to elevate her shoulders. She appears to be in mild distress. Skin color is normal. Pursed-lip breathing noted. Accessory muscles of respiration are tense. The thorax is barrel shaped. Abdomen is soft. Abdominal muscles are used in respirations. No peripheral edema.

Nursing Care Plan Patient With Chronic Obstructive Pulmonary Disease—cont'd

Patient Problems	Goals and Outcome Criteria	Interventions
Inadequate oxygenation related to alveolar destruction, bronchospasm, air trapping	The patient will have improved oxygenation , as evidenced by pulse, respirations, and arterial blood gases with normal pH, partial pressure of oxygen in arterial blood (PaO_2) a minimum 60 mm Hg, and partial pressure of carbon dioxide in arterial blood ($PaCO_2$) at baseline.	Monitor the patient's vital signs and arterial blood gases for tachycardia, tachypnea, increasing $PaCO_2$, decreasing pH. Administer oxygen (O_2) at 1–3 L/min per nasal cannula as ordered. Assist the patient to a comfortable position: high-Fowler position in bed or supported at bedside. Reinforce pursed-lip and abdominal breathing techniques. Provide a bronchodilator as ordered. Assess the patient's inhaler use technique. Assess the patient's respiratory status before and after use of the bronchodilator (inhaler). Monitor the patient for adverse drug effects: dry mouth, headache, nausea, blurred vision, and palpitations.
Airway obstruction related to increased secretions, weak cough	The patient will maintain a patent airway, as evidenced by absence of crackles on auscultation and expectoration of secretions.	Auscultate breath sounds at least every 4 hours (q4h). Support the patient during coughing and deep breathing. Document the amount and color of sputum. Encourage 2500–3000 mL of fluid daily unless contraindicated. Request chest physiotherapy per the physician's order. Have suction equipment available if the patient cannot expectorate secretions.
Anxiety related to hypoxemia	The patient will verbalize decreased anxiety and will appear calm.	Respond to the patient's needs promptly. Provide comfort measures. Be accepting of irritability. Acknowledge anxiety and try to identify stressors in addition to hypoxemia. Include the patient in planning care.
Inadequate nutrition related to anorexia, dyspnea	The patient will maintain or increase body weight during hospitalization.	Provide a pleasant environment for meals. Schedule respiratory treatments at least 1 hour before meals. Assist the patient with oral hygiene. Offer to arrange smaller, more frequent meals. Consult with the dietitian to consider patient preferences.
Decreased activity tolerance related to inability to meet O_2 needs	The patient will accomplish activities of daily living (ADL) without dyspnea or excessive fatigue.	Allow for periods of uninterrupted rest during the day. Use comfort measures such as backrubs and massage to promote rest. Allow the patient to do what she can for herself but assist when needed to avoid excessive tiring. Include the occupational therapist and social worker to discuss plans for discharge and ways to reduce effort of activities at home. Discuss a pulmonary rehabilitation program with the physician. Encourage ambulation as permitted.
Potential for infection related to stasis of respiratory secretions, effects of continued smoking	The patient will have a normal body temperature, clear or white sputum, no peripheral edema.	Monitor sputum color and body temperature. Administer antimicrobials as ordered. Encourage fluid intake. Protect the patient from people with respiratory infections. Monitor the patient for signs of heart failure, especially peripheral edema.
	The patient will express intent to attempt smoking cessation.	Explore smoking cessation programs the patient has tried. Be nonjudgmental and avoid scolding. Inform her of newer options such as varenicline (Chantix), nicotine patches, gum, lozenges, and nasal spray. Tell her that drug therapy has been helpful for some people and that she may want to ask the physician about this. Provide literature from American Cancer Society and American Lung Association with suggestions to facilitate smoking cessation.
Decreased cardiac output related to right-sided heart failure	The patient will have improved cardiac output, as evidenced by absence of dependent edema or distended neck veins.	Monitor the patient for signs of right-sided heart failure, especially peripheral edema.

Critical Thinking Questions

1. Explain the basis for this patient's symptoms: fatigue, dyspnea, and productive cough.
2. How would you determine whether a patient will be able to use an inhaler properly after discharge?
3. Explain why patients with chronic obstructive pulmonary disease are often irritable.

including restlessness, confusion, and lethargy. Note any pursed-lip breathing. Inspect the neck for distention of veins, inspect the shape of the patient's thorax for the classic barrel chest, and auscultate the lung fields for diminished breath sounds. Examine the patient's nails for clubbing, pallor, or cyanosis and inspect and palpate the feet and ankles for edema. Finally, note any muscle wasting.

Patient Problems, Goals, and Outcome Criteria: Chronic Obstructive Pulmonary Disease

Patient Problems	Goals and Outcome Criteria
Inadequate oxygenation related to damaged alveoli and/or terminal bronchioles, bronchospasm, air trapping	Improved oxygenation: vital signs and arterial blood gases consistent with patient norms
Airway obstruction related to increased secretions, weak cough	Patent airway: breath sounds clear to auscultation
Anxiety related to hypoxemia	Decreased anxiety: calm manner, patient statement of decreased anxiety
Inadequate nutrition related to anorexia, dyspnea	Adequate nutrition: stable body weight
Potential for infection related to decreased ciliary action, increased secretions, weak cough	Absence of infection: normal body temperature, white or clear sputum
Decreased activity tolerance related to inability to meet oxygen (O_2) demands	Improved activity tolerance: completion of activities of daily living (ADL) without excess fatigue
Decreased cardiac output related to right-sided heart failure	Improved cardiac output: absence of dependent edema and distended neck veins

Interventions

Inadequate oxygenation. Monitor the patient's vital signs and arterial blood gases for signs of inadequate oxygenation: tachycardia, tachypnea, increasing $PaCO_2$ level, and decreasing pH level. We have been cautioned to never administer more than 2 to 3 L of O_2 per minute to COPD patients. This was based on the belief that COPD patients became desensitized to a high level of CO_2 and rely on low O_2 in the blood to stimulate respirations. This phenomenon, called *hypoxic drive*, does occur in some COPD patients but not all. To determine the appropriate liter flow for the COPD patient, the health care provider may order 1 L per minute initially. As described earlier, the flow rate may then be increased by 1 L every 15 minutes until the patient's pulse blood oxygen saturation (SpO_2) reaches 90%. When pulse oximetry is not available, maintain the low flow 1 to 3 L per minute until the results can be evaluated. Place the patient in a high-Fowler position or seat the patient on the bedside with the arms folded on the overbed table to promote full expansion of the lungs (Fig. 28.7). Teach pursed-lip breathing by instructing the patient to breathe in through the nose and exhale slowly through the mouth, with the lips almost closed. Pursed-lip breathing reduces the collapse of airways with exhalation and reduces dyspnea.

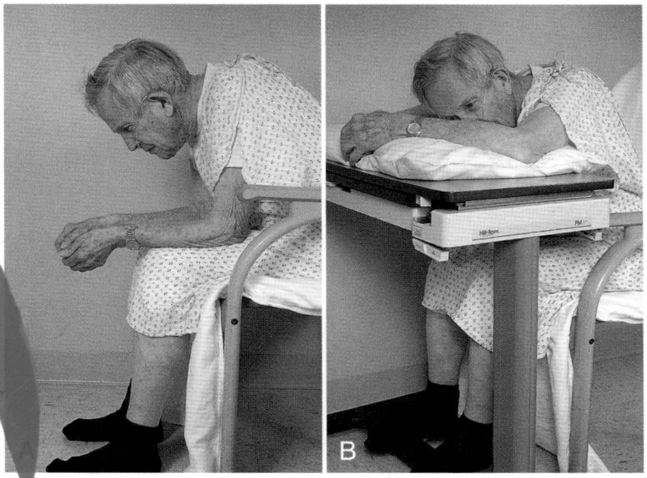

Fig. 28.7 Sitting on the edge of the bed with the arms folded and elevated allows the accessory muscles of respiration to function more effectively. (A) Posture impairs chest. (B) Sitting with the arms folded and elevated improves chest expansion and oxygenation. (From Perry AG, Potter PA, Ostendorf WR. *Nursing interventions & clinical skills*, 6th ed. St. Louis, Elsevier, 2016.)

Administer prescribed bronchodilators and monitor for therapeutic and adverse effects.

Smoking cessation is an important aspect of the management of chronic bronchitis and emphysema as well as of other cardiovascular and respiratory conditions. One-fifth of all deaths in the United States is related to smoking. Health care providers should discourage smoking but must be careful not to be judgmental of the patient. Most patients are aware of the relationship between smoking and respiratory disease, but many find that they are unable to overcome the addiction to nicotine. Ask patients if they have considered quitting smoking and if they would like information about programs that might be helpful.

The physician may order drug therapy or nicotine patches, gum, lozenges, or nasal spray for the patient who wants to try to withdraw from smoking. Some studies have found that the success rate for these products when combined with counseling is only approximately 25% but other types of smoking cessation programs typically have less success, with rates of approximately 10% to 20%. Success is defined as abstinence from smoking for at least 1 year. A recent study reported a 52% success rate among smokers in a program who took varenicline and received 12-month follow-up support (Politis, Ioannidis, Gourgoulianis, Daniil, & Hatzoglou, 2017). The American Cancer Society and the American Lung Association sponsor programs to support people who are trying to quit smoking.

In addition to nicotine, the drugs that have shown the most promise to help people quit smoking are varenicline (Chantix) and bupropion (Zyban, Buproban). Chantix is prescribed for a 12-week course of treatment, followed by a second 12-week course if indicated. It should not be used with nicotine patches because

Box 28.2 Facts About Smoking

- Smoking is the major preventable cause of death in the United States, where more than 480,000 smoking-related deaths occur each year.
- Smoking causes lung cancer, COPD (chronic bronchitis, emphysema) heart disease, stroke, diabetes mellitus, and erectile dysfunction.
- Smoking increases the risk of tuberculosis, osteoporosis, reproductive complications, premature skin wrinkling, cataracts, and fire-related injuries.
- Environmental tobacco smoke is classified as a *carcinogen.* One in five smoking-related deaths is the result of secondhand smoke exposure.
- Smokeless tobacco is not recommended as an alternative to smoking because it has other adverse effects, including oral cancers.

Data from Fast Facts: Smoking and Tobacco Use. Retrieved from https://www.cdc.gov/tobacco/data_statistics/fact_sheets/ December 27, 2020.

the combination may increase the blood pressure. Although 70% of smokers indicate that they would like to quit, the addictive quality of nicotine makes it very difficult to do so. Box 28.2 includes facts about smoking and Box 28.3 provides some helpful information about aids that can be used to encourage smoking cessation in patients.

Pharmacology Capsule

Drugs that have been approved for smoking cessation include nicotine, varenicline (Chantix), and bupropion (Zyban, Buproban).

Put On Your Thinking Cap!

Think of some ways to discourage smoking by deglamorizing it. Make a poster aimed at teenagers to illustrate your strategy.

Box 28.3 Aids to Smoking Cessation

MEDICATION	PATIENT TEACHING
NICOTINE REPLACEMENT	
Gum, lozenge	User controls dosage. Do not eat or drink while in mouth. Lozenge may be easier to use than gum. Gum sticks to dentures.
Transdermal patch	Follow product instructions whether to remove at night or wear around the clock. Use the full-dose patches for 1–3 months; then use the lower-dose patches for 2–4 weeks to taper off of the medication. Alternate sites to avoid skin irritation.
Nasal spray (Nicotrol NS)	Deliver one spray to each nostril every 30–60 minutes. Initial irritation (e.g., nasal burning, sneezing, watery eyes) resolves after 24–48 hours of use.
Inhaler (Nicotrol Inhaler)	The inhaler resembles a plastic cigarette that delivers nicotine flavored with menthol. Most patients use it 6–16 times a day for 3 months and then taper off over 2–3 months.
Bupropion (Zyban, Buproban)	This drug is usually prescribed for 7 days before the patient attempts to quit smoking; then it is continued for 6–12 weeks. Bupropion can be used with a nicotine patch.Do not exceed the prescribed dosage. Overdose can cause seizures.Advise your physician if you have a history of seizures or an eating disorder, both of which are contraindications for bupropion.
Varenicline (Chantix)	Prescribed for a 12-week course of treatment, followed by a second 12-week course if indicated. Do not use this drug with nicotine patches; the combination may increase the blood pressure. Report suicidal thoughts.

Airway obstruction. Monitor the patient for signs and symptoms of airway obstruction, including tachycardia, increasing dyspnea, and abnormal or absent breath sounds. It is helpful to demonstrate effective coughing techniques and assess the patient's efforts in using them. In addition, encourage the patient to drink at least 2500 to 3000 mL of fluid each day unless contraindicated to help liquefy secretions for easier expectoration. Advise the patient to use a humidifier to decrease the drying of secretions. CPT, which includes postural drainage, percussion, and vibration, may be ordered. Mechanical devices that may be used to mobilize secretions include the Flutter, Acapella, and TheraPEP Therapy System. These devices, if available, are quite effective and more efficient than manual CPT. CPT should be performed only by an individual with proper training. The nurse follows up to evaluate the effects. If the patient is unable to expectorate, suctioning may be needed to remove secretions.

Anxiety. The most important intervention for relieving anxiety is helping the patient to breathe more easily. Positioning and O_2 therapy can be instituted promptly. In addition, explain any unfamiliar procedures and equipment to the patient. Remain calm and reassuring until the patient is more comfortable and relaxed. Remember that irritability and anxiety are related to hypoxemia and that the patient is not simply "being difficult." If possible, encourage a family member or friend who has a calming influence on the patient to remain at the bedside. When leaving the patient, place a call bell within reach and instruct the patient in its use. Finally, check on the patient often to provide reassurance that help is nearby if needed.

Inadequate nutrition. The work of breathing is increased with COPD, which in turn increases the patient's caloric requirements. Some patients with COPD have difficulty maintaining adequate nutritional intake. The patient should be weighed daily or weekly, depending on the situation, to monitor fluid and nutritional status. A patient with heart failure may gain weight because of fluid retention. Weight loss may indicate elimination of excess fluid or loss of body weight as a result of inadequate nutrition. Inadequate nutrition may be associated with dyspnea, anorexia, depression, or inability to obtain and prepare food.

The patient who is dyspneic may be given a soft diet with frequent small meals rather than three large meals daily. High-calorie, high-protein supplements may be provided as well. Try to plan care so that the patient is not excessively tired or coughing during meals. To combat anorexia, request a dietary consultation so that meals can be adapted to patient preferences. Assist the patient with oral hygiene before meals and create a pleasant environment by removing soiled tissues and emesis basins. If the agency permits, encourage a family member to eat with the patient to provide a more social atmosphere. If the patient is unable to consume adequate nutrients, tube feeding or total parenteral nutrition (TPN) may be instituted. If the patient is obese, the benefits of weight loss should be discussed.

Potential for infection. Because of pooled secretions and poor nutritional status, the patient with chronic bronchitis and emphysema is at risk for respiratory infections. In addition, because corticosteroids decrease a patient's immune response, a patient on these medications has an increased risk for infection. Monitor for fever and for green or yellow sputum. In addition, promote good hydration and nutrition and administer prophylactic antimicrobials as ordered. Advise patients to take annual influenza immunizations and to avoid people who are ill with infectious respiratory diseases. The physician may prescribe a Pneumovax vaccine if the patient has not already received it to prevent pneumococcal pneumonia.

Decreased activity tolerance. During hospitalization, it is important to attempt to schedule treatments, meals, and exercise so that the patient has time to rest. If the patient becomes excessively dyspneic or experiences tachycardia during activity, pause until the patient recovers. When preparing a patient for discharge, help the patient to plan a daily schedule that spaces out more demanding activities and allows scheduled rest periods (see the Patient Teaching box). Portable O_2 therapy may be ordered to permit increased mobility while receiving supplemental O_2. At home, environmental adaptations may be needed, such as rearrangement of furniture to permit easy access to bathrooms and ramps to replace steps.

Patient Teaching

CHRONIC OBSTRUCTIVE PULMONARY DISEASE

Patients with chronic obstructive pulmonary disease need to know how they can manage the condition. However, instruction is best done in small units to prevent overtiring and overwhelming the patient. Supplement verbal instructions with written material and encourage the patient to do the following:

- Take your prescribed drugs as instructed; report adverse effects to the physician.
- Avoid substances that irritate the airway.
- Cover the nose and mouth when outside in cold weather.
- To reduce risk of infection, avoid infected people.
- Report fever or increased symptoms to your physician promptly.
- Schedule activities to allow adequate rest.
- If oxygen (O_2) therapy is ordered, do not exceed the prescribed liter flow; to do so may depress your breathing.
- Smoking cessation can improve your symptoms. Programs and assistance are provided by the local chapter of the American Lung Association and the American Cancer Society.

If the patient is participating in a rehabilitation program to improve exercise tolerance, monitor their progress and provide encouragement and feedback.

Decreased cardiac output. Patients with COPD are at risk for right-sided heart failure that eventually affects the left side of the heart as well. Therefore it is important to monitor for signs of failure: increasing dyspnea, decreasing urine output, tachycardia, and dependent edema. Management of heart failure (CHF) is discussed in Chapter 34 (see the Coordinated Care box).

Coordinated Care

WORKING WITH THE CERTIFIED NURSING ASSISTANT

- Demonstrate proper positioning of the patient with dyspnea to the certified nursing assistant (CNA).
- Although the CNA can count the patient's respiratory rate, the nurse should collect additional data, including lung sounds.

Coordinated Care

WORKING WITH THE CERTIFIED NURSING ASSISTANT

- Demonstrate proper positioning of the patient with dyspnea to the certified nursing assistant (CNA).
- Although the CNA can count the patient's respiratory rate, the nurse should collect additional data, including lung sounds.

BRONCHIECTASIS

Bronchiectasis is an abnormal permanent dilation and distortion of the bronchi and bronchioles that is usually confined to one lung lobe or segment. It typically follows recurrent inflammatory conditions, infections, or obstructions. Frequent infections may be caused by immunodeficiency or a genetic abnormality in ciliary activity. It may also occur with COPD.

The most prominent signs of bronchiectasis are coughing and the production of large amounts of purulent sputum. The patient may also have fever, hemoptysis, nasal stuffiness, sinus drainage, fatigue, and weakness. The clinical course of the condition varies. Some patients have few or no symptoms, some have daily cough with sputum production, and others have occasional or frequent exacerbations.

The goals of medical treatment are to reduce symptoms, decrease the frequency of exacerbations, improve the quality of life, alter the course of the disease, and to prevent the spread to other areas of the lungs. Maintenance therapy for advanced disease may use antibiotics, antiinflammatory drugs, and airway clearance therapy (CPT, positive expiratory pressure, and various oscillatory devices that mobilize secretions). If the patient has an immune deficiency, replacement therapy is an option. Inhaled bronchodilators (budesonide and formoterol) may be ordered to decrease airway reactivity but their value is still being investigated. Acute exacerbations are treated with antibiotics specific to the infecting organism and CPT. An investigational drug, brensocatib, is showing promise for reducing the frequency of exacerbations. If medical treatment fails and the condition is confined to a limited area, severe bronchiectasis may be treated with surgical excision of the affected portion of the lung. Some patients are eligible for lung transplantation. Nursing care includes administration of prescribed drugs and treatments and documentation of the patient's response. Encourage good hydration and the avoidance of respiratory irritants.

CYSTIC FIBROSIS

Cystic fibrosis is a hereditary disorder that is characterized by dysfunction of the exocrine glands and the production of thick, tenacious mucus. Exocrine glands include those that secrete mucus, sweat, saliva, and digestive enzymes. Cough is the first pulmonary symptom. It eventually becomes productive of thick, purulent sputum that obstructs the airways. Cystic fibrosis also results in obstruction of the pancreatic ducts so that pancreatic enzymes cannot be delivered to the gastrointestinal (GI) tract. Without pancreatic enzymes, patients cannot effectively absorb proteins, fats, and fat-soluble vitamins. Their stools become bulky and foul smelling. Patients may develop diabetes because of damage to the pancreas caused by obstruction of the exocrine ducts. In most men, the vas deferens is absent, rendering them infertile. Women have reduced fertility as well. Patients lose more sodium and chloride in sweat than is normal, putting them at risk for salt depletion, especially in hot environments. Acute exacerbations are characterized by cough, dyspnea, decreased exercise tolerance, fatigue, increased sputum production, and a change in sputum color.

During a period of years, symptoms progress, with increasing dyspnea, decreasing exercise tolerance, and weight loss. Airway obstruction and decreased resistance to infections lead to chronic bacterial infections, emphysema, atelectasis, and respiratory failure.

Treatment

At one time, people with cystic fibrosis were unlikely to survive the early childhood years. However, improved treatment has resulted in more people with cystic fibrosis surviving to adulthood, so they are now more commonly seen in adult care settings. People born between 2014 and 2018 who have cystic fibrosis are expected to live 44 years. Those who live the longest typically are more stable, have milder gene mutations, and a very slow decline in lung function. Treatment consists of pancreatic enzyme replacement, CPT, and aerosol and nebulizer treatments with hypertonic saline or recombinant human deoxyribonuclease (DNase) to reduce mucus viscosity. CFTR modulators are a relatively new type of drug that benefits certain CF patients. Current modulators in use are elexacaftor, tezacaftor, ivacaftor, and lumacaftor. Various combinations of these drugs are used based on the patient's genotype. For eligible patients, CFTR modulators have been shown to significantly improve lung function, weight, and sweat chloride in patients who have specific gene mutations. Supplementary fat-soluble vitamins (A, D, E, and K) are needed because they are poorly absorbed from food sources. Whenever the patient sweats excessively, additional dietary salt is needed. Alternatives to manual CPT include the flutter mucus clearance device, a handheld tool that vibrates to loosen secretions and promotes movement of secretions out of the lungs. An inflatable vest that achieves similar results is also available. Infections are treated with antibiotic therapy, administered orally, by inhalation, parenterally, or via multiple routes. Sometimes antibiotic therapy is continued on a long-term basis. Treatment of infections is complicated by the emergence of bacterial strains that are resistant to commonly used antibiotic medications. Patients with a hyperresponsive airway usually benefit from short courses (5 days) of oral corticosteroids. Inhaled corticosteroids have not been effective. Mechanical ventilation is necessary for ventilatory failure unless the patient has decided against it. It is hoped that gene therapy eventually will provide effective treatment of cystic fibrosis.

NURSING CARE OF THE PATIENT WITH CYSTIC FIBROSIS

The goals of nursing care are to maintain a patent airway, prevention or treatment of infection, adequate nutrition, and effective management of treatment regimen by patients and their families. Measures to clear the airway include administering prescribed medications, maintaining hydration, and performing CPT. Infection prevention focuses on medical asepsis and protecting the patient from others with infections. To maintain adequate nutrition, administer pancreatic enzymes as ordered, allow for rest around mealtimes, and encourage the patient to consume adequate nutrients. In addition, it is important to monitor the patient's stools to assess the adequacy of replacement enzymes (frothy, bulky stools indicate inadequate enzymes). For adult patients with cystic fibrosis, the therapeutic regimen has been a way of life. Allow the patient to maintain as much personal control as possible and try to maintain the patient's usual routines during hospitalization. Finally, identify any teaching needs with the patient and family and design a teaching plan as appropriate.

CHRONIC RESTRICTIVE PULMONARY DISORDERS

In general, restrictive pulmonary disorders are those that result in reduced lung volumes with a normal to elevated ratio of forced expiratory volume in 1 second (FEV_1) to FVC. Examples of restrictive disorders presented here are tuberculosis (TB), interstitial lung diseases including idiopathic pulmonary fibrosis, sarcoidosis, several occupational lung diseases, and lung cancer.

TUBERCULOSIS

TB was a leading cause of death in the United States until effective drugs became available in the 1940s and 1950s. The incidence in 2019 was at the lowest point ever in the United States. The TB rate was 15.5 times greater in foreign-born Americans than in those born in the United States, with the highest numbers among Asian, non-Hispanic Black, and Hispanics/Latino peoples. Among individuals born in the United States, the rates were highest among Native American/Alaska natives and Native Hawaiian/Pacific Islanders. People in California, Texas, New York, and Florida account for approximately one-half of all cases in the United States. Although the incidence has greatly decreased in the United States, it remains a major public health threat in other parts of the world.

Cause and Risk Factors

Mycobacterium tuberculosis, an acid-fast aerobic bacterium, causes TB. The disease is spread through droplets emitted during coughing, laughing, sneezing, and singing. Drug-resistant strains include multidrug-resistant TB (MDR-TB) and extensively drug-resistant TB (XDR-TB).

Anyone may become infected with TB; fortunately, most healthy people are not infected through brief contact. Those at increased risk for TB include older adults, the economically disadvantaged and homeless, those with substance use disorders, children younger than 5 years, people who are immunosuppressed, and some racial and ethnic groups (see the Cultural Considerations box).

> **Cultural Considerations**
>
> **WHAT DOES CULTURE HAVE TO DO WITH TUBERCULOSIS?**
>
> In the United States, the incidence of tuberculosis is increased among non-White Americans and immigrants from Asia and Mexico. These populations should be provided education and screening.

Pathophysiology

A patient's initial TB infection is called the *primary infection*. Most people in whom primary infections develop do not acquire active (symptomatic, progressive) TB. When the TB bacterium invades the lung, a small area becomes inflamed. The body's immune response attempts to destroy the infecting organisms but some may escape and be carried into the lymph nodes or throughout the body. The site of the primary infection may undergo necrotic degeneration. Cavities develop that are filled with cheese-like infectious material that eventually liquefies. This material can drain into the tracheobronchial tree and be coughed up as sputum. The infected site usually heals, creating scar tissue (the lesion is called a *tubercle*) followed by calcification; it sometimes shelters inactive bacteria. In some patients, however, the infectious process progresses and active TB develops. In addition, it is possible for inactive bacteria to be reactivated, causing illness at a later time.

TB is primarily an infection of the lungs, but the organisms may spread and cause infection in the bones, meninges, genitourinary tract, lymph nodes, pleurae, pericardium, abdomen, and endocrine glands. *M. tuberculosis* infection outside the lungs is called *extrapulmonary TB*.

Clinical Manifestations

Signs and symptoms of pulmonary TB may include cough, night sweats, chest pain and tightness, fatigue, anorexia, weight loss, and low-grade fever. The cough is often persistent and productive and may produce bloody sputum (hemoptysis). Older adults may have only vague symptoms and fever of undetermined origin. TB should be considered in patients who have pneumonia that does not respond to usual therapy.

Medical Diagnosis

The patient's history and physical examination may lead the physician to suspect TB, especially if known exposure to high-risk people exists. Tuberculin skin tests are commonly used for screening. People who have been infected mount an immune response that causes a local reaction when tuberculin, a protein fraction of the tubercle bacillus, is injected intradermally. The patient is said to have a *positive reaction* if a hard area (induration) of 5 mm or more develops at the site within 48 to 72 hours. A positive reaction may indicate active or inactive infection (see Chapter 25, Table 25.2). A number of factors may cause inaccurate reactions. For example, a person with poor immune function may not develop induration even though the person does have the infection. A positive screening test does not mean a person has active TB, only that they have antibodies which means they have been exposed to the infection. Follow-up tests must be done to make a diagnosis.

A variety of tests are available, but each has advantages and disadvantages. The gold standard for diagnosing TB is culture on solid media or liquid media followed by drug susceptibility testing. However, this process takes 2 to 6 weeks. Blood tests used to diagnosis TB more quickly are interferon-gamma release assays (IGRAs), which include the QuantiFERON-TB Gold In-Tube test, the QuantiFERON-TB Gold test, and the T-SPOT.TB test. IGRA results are available in 24 hours. IGRA does not distinguish between active and past infections. Another option is the Xpert MTB/RIF test (*Mycobacterium tuberculosis*/resistance to rifampicin), which detects *M. tuberculosis* in respiratory secretions and determines susceptibility to rifampin within 2 hours, however, it is very expensive. Nucleic acid amplification tests (NAATs) include a variety of tests on respiratory specimens. The acid-fast bacilli (AFB) smear uses body fluid (usually sputum) to identify TB; however, it may give false-positive results if a mycobacterial infection other than TB is present. Chest radiographs and CT scanning also aid in making the diagnosis.

Bacillus Calmette-Guérin (BCG) vaccination against TB is given in some countries. However, it is not routinely given in the United States because the risk of TB is considered low, the protection during adulthood is not dependable, and it may cause false-positives in future skin testing. People who have been vaccinated with BCG may have a positive response to the tuberculin test even though they have never had the disease. This would be called a false-positive reaction to the tuberculin test. The Centers for Disease Control and Prevention (CDC) recommends that people who received BCG be tested with one of the TB blood tests instead of skin testing.

Medical Treatment

Patients who have positive results for TB on skin tests and negative results on chest radiographs but who are at increased risk for the disease are usually treated prophylactically to prevent development of active TB. These individuals are said to have latent TB. It is treated with one of three regimens: INH weekly for 3 months, daily rifamycin for 4 months, or daily INH and rifampin for 3 months (cdc.gov, Feb 13, 2020).

For patients with active TB, the CDC recommends combination drug therapy selected from the first-line drugs that include INH, ethambutol, rifampin, and pyrazinamide. An example of an initial regimen for a person with culture-positive pulmonary TB caused by drug-sensitive organisms is as follows: INH, rifampin, pyrazinamide, and ethambutol given daily, twice weekly, or 3 times weekly for 2 months. The patient would then continue therapy with only INH and rifampin daily on a daily, twice weekly, or thrice weekly schedule. Numerous second-line drugs are available for patients who cannot tolerate or do not respond to first-line drugs.

The usual course of therapy for active TB ranges from 6 to 24 months after sputum cultures become negative. Most drugs can be given in daily or twice-weekly doses. Neither MDR-TB nor XDR-TB is destroyed by INH or rifampin; therefore various combinations of other drugs must be used over a 2-year period. The risk of adverse effects with long-term drug therapy is significant, so patient monitoring is essential. Adverse effects are especially common in older adults. Individuals with both TB and human immunodeficiency virus (HIV) infection require unique drug combinations because rifampin decreases the effectiveness of some anti-HIV drugs.

Most people are treated as outpatients and many can continue their usual activities during treatment. However, hospitalization is sometimes indicated when drug therapy is initiated. Because the organism that causes TB readily develops resistance to drugs, it is extremely important that patients take the correct drug doses for the prescribed period of time. Incomplete courses of therapy foster resistant organisms and relapses of the infection. Therefore directly observed therapy (DOT) may be recommended to ensure that patients are taking the drugs as prescribed. DOT is recommended in the case of pulmonary TB with positive sputum smears, treatment failure, disease relapse, drug resistance, HIV infection, psychiatric illness, substance abuse, memory impairment, and history of nonadherence to therapy.

Pharmacology Capsule

Peripheral neuropathy is an adverse effect of isoniazid (INH) that can be prevented or treated with the administration of pyridoxine (vitamin B_6).

Pharmacology Capsule

A common treatment plan for active tuberculosis begins with a 2-month course of isoniazid (INH), rifampin, pyrazinamide, and ethambutol that is followed by 4 months of INH and rifampin alone.

NURSING CARE OF THE PATIENT WITH TUBERCULOSIS

Focused Assessment

Assessment of the patient with a respiratory disorder is outlined in Chapter 25, Box 25.2. When TB is suspected or confirmed, a complete health history and a physical examination are essential because the infection may not be confined to the lung. The nurse may be responsible for reading the reaction to the skin test.

Patient Problems, Goals, and Outcome Criteria: Tuberculosis

Patient Problems	Goals and Outcome Criteria
Inadequate oxygenation related to respiratory secretions, destructive effects of the infectious process	Improved oxygenation: no dyspnea
Social isolation related to medically or self-imposed isolation, fear of contagious disease	Reduced social isolation: less feeling of loneliness or rejection
Potential for injury related to spread of the infection, reactivation of the infection secondary to lowered resistance	Knowledge of measures to decrease disease progression and reactivation of infection: patient demonstrates precautions
Fatigue related to infection, weight loss, coughing	Improved activity tolerance: patient reports decreased fatigue
Inadequate nutrition related to anorexia, fatigue, inadequate financial resources, lack of knowledge	Improved nutritional status: stable body weight; normalization of weight if malnourished
Ineffective management of treatment regimen related to lack of understanding of treatment and risk of reactivation, lack of financial resources	Effective management of prescribed therapy: patient states intention to comply, obtains and takes drugs as prescribed

Interventions

Inadequate oxygenation. Routinely monitor the patient's respiratory status and instruct the patient in effective coughing to expectorate secretions. Encourage ambulation as tolerated, within medically prescribed limits. Although dyspnea is not common except with pleural effusion, it is important to remember to elevate the head of the bed when working with dyspneic patients.

Social isolation. The patient who is thought to have active TB is isolated at first. Nurses must practice good hand washing and wear high-efficiency particulate absorption (HEPA) masks during contacts. Gowns are unnecessary unless gross contamination of clothing occurs. The patient may feel rejected and be fearful that others will avoid contact. It is important to encourage the patient to express feelings about the diagnosis and the isolation. Instruct visitors in measures to reduce the risk of infection and assure the patient that isolation is a temporary measure used to protect others from the infection.

Potential for injury. Once antibiotic therapy has been initiated and the patient's sputum cultures demonstrate low counts of acid-fast bacilli, the patient can usually be discharged. Tell the patient how the infection is transmitted and how to protect others. They should always cover the nose and mouth when sneezing or coughing; disposable tissues should be used and discarded in a sanitary way. Members of the patient's household are tested for active disease. Those who have positive skin tests but are asymptomatic are usually given prophylactic therapy to prevent development of active TB. One problem with the homeless population is that it is often difficult to locate contacts. Finally, emphasize the importance of the patient completing the full course of therapy; if this is not done, the infection may be reactivated.

Fatigue. Fatigue is fairly common with TB. Therefore it is important to adjust the patient's schedule to allow for periods of rest and assure the patient that fatigue diminishes as treatment progresses.

Inadequate nutrition. Anorexia and nausea are common adverse effects of antitubercular drugs. Monitor the patient's weight at regular intervals. Some measures that may reduce the drug's side effects include taking it at bedtime and taking antinausea drugs. Explain the role of nutrition in recovering from an infectious disease and encourage the patient to eat a balanced diet (see the Cultural Considerations box). Five or six small meals may be more acceptable than three large ones to the patient who has a poor appetite. A patient's food preferences should be respected as much as possible. For patients who are homeless or have a low income, ask the social worker to locate services that provide food or prepared meals. Some foods can cause serious reactions if consumed with antitubercular medications. Provide a written list of any foods that the patient should avoid (see the Patient Teaching box).

Cultural Considerations

WHAT DOES CULTURE HAVE TO DO WITH PATIENT TEACHING?

To be effective, the teaching plan for the patient with tuberculosis must consider the patient's native language, vocabulary, lifestyle, and financial resources.

Patient Teaching

TUBERCULOSIS

People with tuberculosis are usually hospitalized for just a short time if at all, so you must implement efficient patient teaching and supplement verbal instructions with written material. Subjects to include in the teaching plan are as follows:

- Tuberculosis is spread by airborne droplets. Protect others by covering your mouth when coughing, laughing, or sneezing. Wash your hands often. Use disposable tissues and discard them in bagged trash.
- Effective treatment requires taking drugs exactly as prescribed for the full course of therapy to prevent reinfection. Notify your physician of adverse effects of your drugs but do not stop taking them unless advised to do so by the physician.
- If you are taking isoniazid (INH), you must avoid foods containing tyramine (e.g., aged cheeses, smoked fish) and histamine (e.g., tuna, sauerkraut). These foods combined with INH can make you very ill.
- Good hygiene, nutrition, and hydration can help you to recover.
- Rifampin causes body fluids to become red-orange and may stain soft contact lenses.

Ineffective management of therapeutic regimen. A major problem with treating TB is failure to complete the lengthy prescribed drug therapy. Nurses must realize that patients do not take drugs as ordered for many reasons, including denial of the illness, lack of understanding, adverse drug effects, and inability to pay for medical care. Intervention should be based on the reason for the patient's nonadherence. Explain the infectious process and its treatment, reinforce the physician's instructions for the drugs, and emphasize that failure to complete the course of therapy could result in the reactivation of an infection that will be more difficult to treat. Tell the patient to report any adverse drug effects so that solutions can be provided to make them more tolerable. If the patient cannot afford the medications, consult a social worker to help the patient obtain financial assistance. For patients who are unable to manage daily self-medication, DOT may be instituted. The drugs are given 2 or 3 times a week in a health care setting, at the patient's worksite, or in their home.

INTERSTITIAL LUNG DISEASES

Interstitial lung diseases include several conditions in which inflammation of the lower respiratory tract and thickening and fibrosis of the alveolar walls, capillaries, acini, bronchioles, and pulmonary parenchyma beyond the gas exchange units render the alveoli nonfunctional. The pleura, lymphatics, and sometimes the lymph nodes may be involved. Although inhaled substances or connective tissue disorders may cause the disease, sometimes no specific cause is identified. Some examples of interstitial lung diseases are idiopathic pulmonary fibrosis, acute interstitial pneumonia, hypersensitivity pneumonitis including occupational lung diseases, neurofibromatosis, and sarcoidosis.

IDIOPATHIC PULMONARY FIBROSIS

Pathophysiology

Idiopathic pulmonary fibrosis is the formation of scar tissue in the lung tissue after inflammation or irritation. It may be related to cigarette smoking, frequent aspiration, or exposure to environmental or occupational substances. Discussion of some specific occupational lung diseases follows.

Complications

Severe fibrosis may lead to pulmonary hypertension (increased pressure in the pulmonary artery caused by obstruction to blood flow in pulmonary vessels), cor pulmonale, and ventilatory failure, in which case the patient is said to have end-stage disease.

Clinical Manifestations

The primary symptom of idiopathic pulmonary fibrosis is progressive dyspnea with exertion. Inspiratory crackles are heard in the lungs on auscultation.

Medical Treatment

The condition is treated with a corticosteroid (prednisone), an immunosuppressant drug (azathioprine [Imuran]), a mucolytic (*N*-acetylcysteine), and O_2 therapy. Corticosteroid treatment reduces inflammation and may prevent additional damage but does not correct existing fibrosis. None of these treatments significantly improves survival or quality of life. The patient should avoid additional exposure to offending substances. Lung transplantation may be recommended for end-stage disease.

◆ NURSING CARE OF THE PATIENT WITH IDIOPATHIC PULMONARY FIBROSIS

Focused Assessment

The complete assessment of the patient with a respiratory disorder is summarized in Chapter 25, Box 25.2.

Patient Problems, Goals, and Outcome Criteria: Idiopathic Pulmonary Fibrosis

Patient Problems	Goals and Outcome Criteria
Inadequate oxygenation related to pulmonary scarring	Improved oxygenation: normal pulse and respirations, no cyanosis, normal blood gases
Decreased activity tolerance related to inadequate oxygenation	Stable activity tolerance: modified activities of daily living, minimal dyspnea on exertion
Potential for infection related to immune suppression by corticosteroids	Reduced risk of infection: patient practices infection control measures

Patient Problems, Goals, and Outcome Criteria: Idiopathic Pulmonary Fibrosis—cont'd

Patient Problems	Goals and Outcome Criteria
Airway obstruction related to increased secretions	Patent airway: clear breath sounds, normal pulse, expectoration of secretions
Anxiety related to dyspnea or possible disabling illness	Decreased anxiety: calm manner, patient statement of lessened anxiety

Interventions

Nursing interventions are similar to those described for the patient with COPD.

SARCOIDOSIS

Pathophysiology

Sarcoidosis is an inflammatory condition that may affect the skin, eyes, lungs, liver, spleen, brain, bones, salivary glands, joints, and heart (see the Cultural Considerations box). An unknown factor triggers a series of immune processes leading to the formation of clusters of cells and debris in affected tissues called **granulomas**. Granulomas in the lungs may resolve or may progress to fibrosis, in which case a restrictive pulmonary condition exists. The course of sarcoidosis is variable. In some patients, it is acute and resolves even without treatment. Others have periods of remission and exacerbations, which may progress to disabling restrictive lung disease.

Cultural Considerations

WHAT DOES CULTURE HAVE TO DO WITH SARCOIDOSIS?

In the United States, sarcoidosis more commonly affects Black Americans than White Americans and is twice as common in Black-American women as in Black-American men.

Clinical Manifestations

Although many patients with sarcoidosis have no symptoms, others experience dry cough, dyspnea, chest pain, hemoptysis, fatigue, weakness, weight loss, and fever.

Medical Diagnosis

A diagnosis of sarcoidosis is based on results of chest radiography and other imaging procedures, PFTs, flexible bronchoscopy with transbronchial lung biopsy, or biopsy of other affected organs.

Medical Treatment

If the patient is asymptomatic, no treatment is indicated. Symptoms usually respond well to a 6- to 12-month course of systemic corticosteroids. In some situations, methotrexate, azathioprine, or hydroxychloroquine is used as an alternative to corticosteroids. Lung transplantation is the only option for patients with end-stage pulmonary disease who do not respond to drug therapy.

◆ NURSING CARE OF THE PATIENT WITH SARCOIDOSIS

Nursing care of the patient with sarcoidosis focuses on monitoring the patient for progressive dysfunction and teaching about drug therapy, if prescribed. Care of the patient with severe pulmonary symptoms is similar to that for patients with COPD.

OCCUPATIONAL LUNG DISEASES

The inhalation of various particles in the work setting can lead to lung conditions classified as occupational lung diseases. Examples of offending substances are dust, ammonia, chlorine, plant and animal proteins, silica, asbestos, and coal dust. The Occupational Safety and Health Administration provides regulations that are intended to protect workers from exposure that could lead to occupational lung diseases.

Categories of occupational lung diseases are described here briefly. The nursing care of patients with occupational lung diseases varies with the severity of symptoms but is similar to that provided to the patient with COPD.

ACUTE RESPIRATORY IRRITATION

The inhalation of gases such as ammonia or chlorine causes acute respiratory irritation. The effects are usually temporary, but if the lower airways are affected, the patient may have pulmonary edema or alveolar damage and airway obstruction. The patient may experience coughing, wheezing, and dyspnea. Symptoms resolve within a few days to several weeks and usually no permanent lung damage exists. The treatment focuses on management of the symptoms and avoidance of future exposure.

OCCUPATIONAL ASTHMA

Inhalation of plant or animal proteins may cause an allergic reaction referred to as *occupational asthma.* Treatment is the same as that for bronchial asthma. Although the initial acute symptoms usually last only a few hours, the patient may continue to have a hyperreactive airway for years. This means that future exposure to irritants may trigger acute asthmatic symptoms. The patient should avoid continued exposure to the offending substance.

HYPERSENSITIVITY PNEUMONITIS

Hypersensitivity **pneumonitis** is an allergic inflammatory response of the alveoli to inhaled organic particles. The reaction may resolve within a few days or the patient may contract pulmonary edema or interstitial fibrosis with permanent restrictive or restrictive-obstructive disease. The condition may be treated with corticosteroids and avoidance of the irritants. Respiratory support may be needed if symptoms are severe.

PNEUMOCONIOSIS

Lung disease caused by inhalation of various dusts is called **pneumoconiosis**. Pneumoconiosis develops in response to repeated exposure to silica, asbestos, or coal dust and is characterized by diffuse pulmonary fibrosis and restrictive lung disease. The effects are usually aggravated by cigarette smoking, so advise patients to avoid the offending dust and cigarette smoke. Otherwise, treatment is symptomatic.

Asbestosis is a pneumoconiosis caused by occupational exposure to asbestos, an insulating material. Symptoms commonly appear decades after exposure. Asbestos exposure has been linked to pleural effusions, pleural fibrosis, and malignant mesotheliomas (cancer of the pleura, peritoneum, or both). The primary symptoms are cough and dyspnea on exertion. The lung disease may progress to the point that transplantation is the only therapeutic option.

LUNG CANCER

Cause and Risk Factors

Lung cancer is the second most common cancer among men and women, and the leading cause of cancer death in the United States. Since 1987 the death rate from lung cancer has exceeded that from breast cancer in women.

Cigarette smoking is the leading cause of lung cancer. The risk is increased even more for smokers who are exposed to other carcinogenic substances, such as arsenic, asbestos, and radioactive materials. Secondhand smoke poses a threat to nonsmokers as well. Air pollution may be an additional risk factor. Genetic susceptibility also appears to play a role in the development of lung cancer.

Pathophysiology

Two major categories of lung cancer exist: (1) small cell ("oat cell") lung carcinoma (SCLC) and (2) nonsmall cell lung carcinoma (NSCLC). NSCLC, the most common type, includes squamous cell carcinomas, adenocarcinomas, and large cell carcinomas. Less common pulmonary tumors include bronchial carcinoid tumors, lymphoma, and others. Small cell and large cell undifferentiated carcinomas grow rapidly; other lung cancers grow slowly. They all can metastasize to other body organs. Enlarging tumors or metastatic lesions may compress the laryngeal and phrenic nerves, the esophagus, and the major blood vessels. SCLCs, which grow rapidly, tend to metastasize early. They can invade the pericardium, causing pericardial effusion (fluid accumulation in the pericardial sac) and possibly triggering dysrhythmias.

Clinical Manifestations

The warning signs of lung cancer are persistent cough, hemoptysis, chest pain, and recurring pneumonia or bronchitis. Patients may also have dyspnea; weight loss; and pain in the shoulder, arm, or hand. Some variation exists with the type of cancer and the location. Other signs and symptoms may be related to metastatic lesions. For example, invasion of the tumor into the ribs produces bone pain and invasion of the pericardium may produce cardiac dysrhythmias. A small percentage of patients develop the syndrome of inappropriate antidiuretic hormone secretion (SIADH), which causes fluid retention and edema. Unfortunately, patients commonly have no symptoms until the disease is advanced.

Medical Diagnosis

Diagnostic tests and procedures for lung cancer include radiographic and imaging procedures (i.e., chest radiography, CT and positron emission tomography [PET], magnetic resonance imaging [MRI]); fiberoptic bronchoscopy; sputum cytology studies; and biopsy of tissue obtained through bronchoscopy, percutaneous transthoracic fine-needle biopsy, thoracotomy, or other methods. Information about specific diagnostic procedures appears in Chapter 25, Table 25.2. Unfortunately, lesions often are not detectable until they are no longer localized. Radionuclide scans of the bones, liver, or brain may be ordered to detect metastatic lesions.

Medical Treatment

Early detection is the key to survival of lung cancer, but this is difficult because metastasis often occurs before the lesion can be seen on radiographs. Treatment decisions are made based on tumor type, lymph node involvement, evidence of metastasis, and the patient's general state of health. The most commonly used options are radiotherapy, chemotherapy, targeted biologic therapies, and surgery.

Radiotherapy. Radiotherapy may be used alone or in combination with other treatment methods. It may be curative in some situations but may also be used to temporarily relieve symptoms by reducing the size of the lesion. Radiotherapy for lung cancer may include external beam irradiation and brachytherapy. **Brachytherapy** is direct irradiation by placement of the radiation source at the site of the tumor. Complications of endobronchial irradiation are pulmonary hemorrhage and radiation bronchitis and stenosis. Other general complications of radiotherapy are discussed in Chapter 7.

Chemotherapy. Chemotherapy may be used alone or with radiation in the treatment of SCLC. Debate exists about the value of chemotherapy in other types of lung cancers, but research continues to explore various treatment combinations of agents. Chemotherapeutic agents are discussed in Chapter 7.

Targeted biologic therapies. An array of targeted biologic therapies that block the activity of growth factor receptors are being studied for their value in cancer treatment. Examples of these agents are cetuximab (Erbitux), bevacizumab (Avastin), gefitinib (Iressa), erlotinib (Tarceva), afatinib, crizotinib, and certinib. Additional information about these drugs is available in Chapter 7.

Surgical Treatment

Surgical intervention is the treatment of choice for early NSCLC. The goal of surgery is to remove the entire tumor while removing as little healthy surrounding

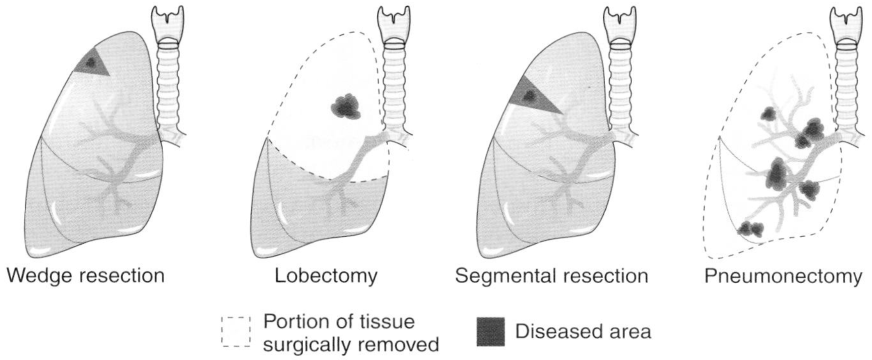

Fig. 28.8 Pulmonary resections. (From Shiland BJ. *Mastering healthcare terminology*, 5th ed. St. Louis, Mosby, 2016.)

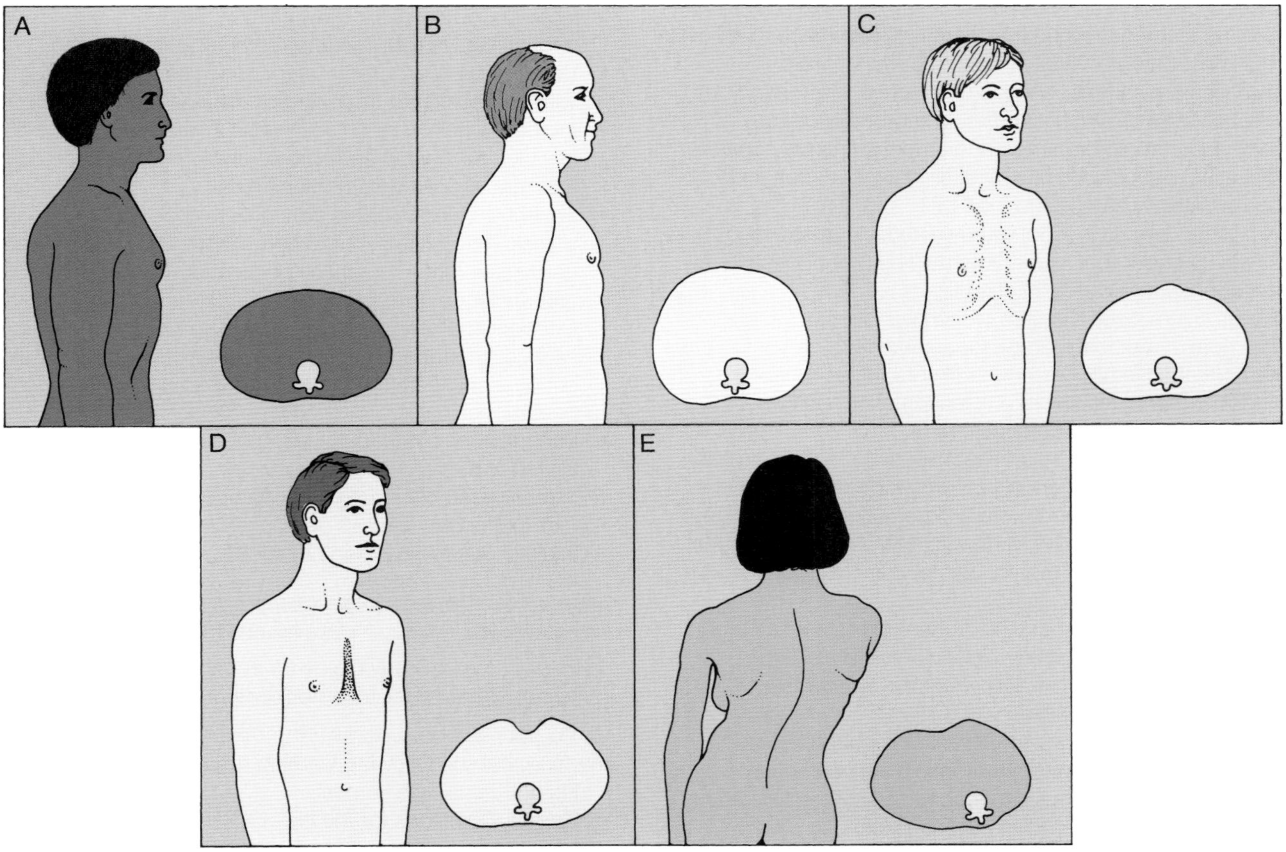

Fig. 28.9 (A) Normal adult chest and (B–E) chest deformities that may affect respiratory function. (B) Increased anteroposterior diameter (barrel chest). (C) Pectus excavatum (funnel chest). (D) Pectus carinatum (pigeon chest). (E) Thoracic kyphoscoliosis. (From Black JM, Hawks JH. *Medical-surgical nursing: clinical management for positive outcomes*, 8th ed. St. Louis, Saunders, 2009.)

tissue as possible. Unfortunately, many patients are not surgical candidates because of poor general health. Removal of a section of tissue is called a *resection*. With lung surgery, the procedure may be a wedge resection, sleeve lobectomy, segmental resection, lobectomy, or pneumonectomy (Fig. 28.8). Tumors that are accessible with a bronchoscope are sometimes treated with laser therapy or photodynamic therapy. Radiotherapy, chemotherapy, or both may be used before or after surgery. Newer therapies use targeted agents.

Despite advances in treatment, the 5-year survival rate for lung cancer remains 15%. Survival improves with early treatment, but American Cancer Society data indicate that only 16% of all lung cancers are detected while still localized. The outlook is best for stages I and II NSCLC treated surgically.

◆ NURSING CARE OF THE PATIENT WITH LUNG CANCER

Nursing care of the patient with cancer is detailed in Chapter 7. Care of the patient who has a thoracotomy is discussed in Chapter 25. In addition, nurses must continue to educate the public about the dangers of cigarette smoking to help eliminate the primary cause of lung cancer.

EXTRAPULMONARY DISORDERS

This chapter and the two preceding chapters describe disorders of the respiratory system. However, many other disorders can also result in significant impairment of respiratory function. For example, chest deformities, as seen in Fig. 28.9, may interfere with lung expansion. Neuromuscular diseases such as myasthenia gravis and amyotrophic lateral sclerosis (ALS) affect the muscles of respiration. Head or spinal cord injuries can disrupt the breathing center in the brain or the neural control of the diaphragm. Heart failure with pulmonary edema fills the lungs with fluid, interfering with the exchange of gases. The specific interventions are covered with each of these conditions in other chapters.

Get Ready for the NCLEX® Examination!

Key Points

- Obstructive respiratory diseases are characterized by airway obstruction or narrowing that increases resistance to airflow.
- The most common types of obstructive respiratory diseases are asthma, chronic obstructive pulmonary disease (COPD), cystic fibrosis, and bronchiectasis.
- Although chronic bronchitis and emphysema are separate diseases, people with COPD often have both conditions; some patients have asthma as well.
- Bronchial asthma is a potentially reversible obstructive airway disorder that is characterized by bronchospasm as a response to a variety of stimuli.
- Status asthmaticus is severe bronchospasm that can be fatal.
- The goal of medical therapy for asthma is to prevent acute asthma attacks using bronchodilators, $beta_2$-receptor agonists, mast cell stabilizers, leukotriene modifiers, anticholinergics, and corticosteroids.
- Patient problems for the patient with asthma may include inadequate oxygenation, airway obstruction, and anxiety.
- Chronic bronchitis is bronchial inflammation characterized by increased production of mucus and chronic cough that persists for at least 3 months of the year for 2 consecutive years.
- Pulmonary emphysema, which often coexists with chronic bronchitis, is a degenerative, nonreversible disease characterized by the breakdown of the alveolar septa distal to the terminal bronchioles.
- Centrilobular pulmonary emphysema is characterized by breakdown of respiratory bronchioles; panlobular pulmonary emphysema is characterized by breakdown of alveolar walls and respiratory bronchioles.
- Patient problems for the patient with chronic bronchitis and emphysema may include inadequate oxygenation, airway obstruction, anxiety, inadequate nutrition, potential for infection, decreased activity tolerance, and decreased cardiac output.
- Smoking cessation is an important aspect of management of COPD and other cardiovascular and respiratory conditions, but success rates for stop-smoking programs are low.
- Bronchiectasis is an abnormal dilation and distortion of the bronchi and bronchioles that causes coughing and the production of large amounts of sputum and is often associated with infection.
- Restrictive pulmonary disorders result in reduced lung volumes.
- Examples of restrictive pulmonary disorders are TB, interstitial lung diseases including idiopathic pulmonary fibrosis, sarcoidosis, several occupational lung diseases, and lung cancer.
- TB is an infectious disease of the lungs and other body tissues that requires long-term drug therapy.
- Patient problems for the patient with TB may include inadequate oxygenation, airway obstruction, social isolation, potential for injury, fatigue, inadequate nutrition, and ineffective management of therapeutic regimen.
- Sarcoidosis is an inflammatory condition that may resolve with corticosteroid treatment or may lead to fibrosis.
- Idiopathic pulmonary fibrosis is an inflammatory condition in which thickening and fibrosis of the alveolar walls occurs that render the alveoli nonfunctional.
- Patient problems for the patient with idiopathic pulmonary fibrosis may include inadequate oxygenation, decreased activity tolerance, potential for infection, airway obstruction, and anxiety.
- Occupational lung diseases are caused by the inhalation of various substances and include acute respiratory irritation, occupational asthma, hypersensitivity pneumonitis, and pneumoconiosis.
- Lung cancer, the leading cause of cancer death in the United States, is usually caused by cigarette smoking and is most treatable if detected while still localized.
- Extrapulmonary causes of respiratory problems may be skeletal, neuromuscular, neurologic, or cardiac.

Additional Learning Resources

SG Go to your Study Guide for additional learning activities to help you master this chapter content.

Go to your Evolve website (http://evolve.elsevier.com/Linton/medsurg) for the following learning resources and much more:

- Fluid & Electrolyte Tutorial
- Review Questions for the NCLEX® Examination

Clinical Judgment and Next-Generation NCLEX® Examination-Style Questions

1. **A patient is being admitted from the emergency department. He has been stabilized after the initial phase of an acute asthma attack. The nurse knows to anticipate the late phase of the asthma attack, which is characterized by:**
   1. Bronchospasm
   2. Increased mucus secretion
   3. Hypoxemia
   4. Hyperresponsive airway

   NCLEX Client Need: Physiological Integrity: Physiological Adaptation

2. **The nurse is preparing a review of asthma drugs for nursing staff. She should inform the audience that appropriate drugs for relieving acute symptoms of asthma include: (Select all that apply.)**
   1. $Beta_2$-receptor agonists
   2. Corticosteroids

3. Anticholinergics
4. Leukotriene modifiers
5. Decongestants

NCLEX Client Need: Physiological Integrity: Pharmacological Therapies

3. **An asthma patient has been advised to measure her peak expiratory flow rate (PEFR) every morning. The nurse should explain that the reason for monitoring PEFR is to:**
   1. Determine whether controller medications are needed that day
   2. Assess the adequacy of asthma control with current drug therapy
   3. Promote deep breathing and effective coughing to clear secretions
   4. Assess what level of activity the patient will be able to tolerate each day

   NCLEX Client Need: Physiological Integrity: Reduction of Risk Potential

4. **A patient's health history includes "reports persistent productive cough for 3 to 4 months each winter for the past 5 years." You recognize these symptoms as typical of which of the following?**
   1. Centriacinar emphysema
   2. Asthma
   3. Chronic bronchitis
   4. TB

   NCLEX Client Need: Physiological Integrity: Physiological Adaptation

5. **What is the nursing implication when a patient with COPD has hypoxic drive?**
   1. The patient needs deep-breathing exercises to improve oxygenation.
   2. The patient's O_2 therapy can depress respirations if the flow rate is too high.
   3. The patient is unable to tolerate any activity and should remain in bed.
   4. The patient is in respiratory acidosis and requires emergency care.

   NCLEX Client Need: Physiological Integrity: Physiological Adaptation

6. **In a long-term care facility, the licensed vocational nurse/licensed practical nurse (LVN/LPN) observes that a patient with COPD has had increased dyspnea since the previous day, a heart rate of 92 beats per minute, and edematous ankles. Which of the following actions should the LVN/LPN take?**
   1. Increase the patient's O_2 flow rate to 5 L/min
   2. Encourage the patient to walk more to promote circulation
   3. Document the findings and check for improvement the next day
   4. Contact the nursing supervisor to report signs of possible heart failure

   NCLEX Client Need: Physiological Integrity: Reduction of Risk Potential

7. **Which of the following is the first priority patient problem for the patient with cystic fibrosis?**
   1. Airway obstruction
   2. Potential for infection
   3. Inadequate nutrition
   4. Potential for fluid volume deficit

   NCLEX Client Need: Physiological Integrity: Physiological Adaptation

8. **Objective: Assist in developing a nursing care plan for the patient with a chronic respiratory disease.**

   NGN Item Type: Matrix

   Cognitive Skill: Take Action

   A 50-year-old woman has been diagnosed with active tuberculosis. She is being treated initially with INH, rifampin, pyrazinamide, and ethambutol three times weekly for 2 months. Then, she will take only INH and rifampin three times weekly.

   Use an X for the health teaching below that is *Indicated* (appropriate or necessary), *Contraindicated* (could be harmful), or *Nonessential* (makes no difference or not necessary) before the patient's discharge at this time.

HEALTH TEACHING	INDICATED	CONTRAINDICATED	NONESSENTIAL
A balanced diet helps your body to recover from an infectious disease.			
You must complete the entire course of therapy to prevent a recurrence of TB.			
Cover your mouth when coughing to prevent spreading the infection.			
As long as you take your medications, you cannot transmit TB to other people.			
Increase your intake of aged foods such as cheese and smoked fish to promote absorption of INH.			
Practice good oral hygiene when being treated for tuberculosis.			
People in your household should be tested for active disease.			
Taking your antitubercular drugs at bedtime may reduce nausea and vomiting.			

9. **What is the primary drug used for the prevention and treatment of TB? ________________**

NCLEX Client Need: Physiological Integrity: Pharmacological Therapies

10. **What is the primary drug used for the prevention and treatment of TB? ________________**

NCLEX Client Need: Physiological Integrity: Pharmacological Therapies

11. **What is the leading cause of lung cancer? ________________**

NCLEX Client Need: Physiological Integrity: Physiological Adaptation

Hematologic System Introduction

29

http://evolve.elsevier.com/Linton/medsurg

Objectives

1. List the components of the hematologic system and describe their role in oxygenation and hemostasis.
2. Identify data to be collected when assessing a patient with a disorder of the hematologic system.
3. Describe tests and procedures used to diagnose disorders of the hematologic system and nursing considerations for each.
4. Describe nursing care for patients undergoing common therapeutic measures for disorders of the hematologic system.

Key Terms

anemia (ă-NĒ-mē-ă)
ecchymosis (ĕk-ĭ-MŌ-sĭs)
hemostasis (hē-mō-STĀ-sĭs)
orthostatic vital sign changes (ŏr-thō-STĂ-tĭk)
oxygenation (ŏk-sĭ-jĕ-NĀ-shŭn)
petechiae (pĕ-TĒ-kē-ă)
purpura (PŬR-pūr-ă)
universal donor
universal recipient

The primary functions of the hematologic system are to transport oxygen and carbon dioxide, control bleeding (**hemostasis**), combat infection, and maintain intravascular volume. Disorders of the hematologic system can be either a primary disease or a complication of another disease. The diagnosis and treatment of these disorders can be very complex. The nurse plays an important role in helping to assess, plan, and manage the care of these patients.

ANATOMY AND PHYSIOLOGY OF THE HEMATOLOGIC SYSTEM

ANATOMIC STRUCTURES AND COMPONENTS OF THE HEMATOLOGIC SYSTEM

Important structures and components of the hematologic system are the bone marrow, the kidneys, the liver, the spleen, the lymph system, and the blood.

Bone Marrow

The bone marrow is the spongy center of the bones where stem cells are manufactured. Stem cells are immature, undifferentiated cells that have the capacity to mature into red blood cells (RBCs), white blood cells, and platelets. The marrow of all bones produces these cells; however, the majority of RBCs and platelets are produced in the vertebrae, ribs, sternum, skull, pelvis, and long bones of the legs.

Kidneys

The kidneys are located in the back of the abdominal cavity to the right and left of the aorta and inferior vena cava. The kidneys perform many functions for different body systems. As part of the hematologic system, the kidneys manufacture hematopoietin, a hormone that is released by the kidneys in response to hypoxia. Hematopoietin stimulates the production of RBCs in the bone marrow.

Liver

The liver is located in the upper right quadrant of the abdomen, under the rib cage and below the diaphragm. The liver performs many functions for different body systems. As part of the hematologic system, the liver manufactures clotting factors. In addition, the liver clears old and damaged RBCs from circulation.

Spleen

The spleen is located in the upper left quadrant of the abdomen. Like the liver, the spleen performs many functions for different body systems. As part of the hematologic system, the spleen removes old RBCs from circulation.

Blood

Blood is a type of connective tissue made up of plasma and blood cells. Plasma is the liquid component of the

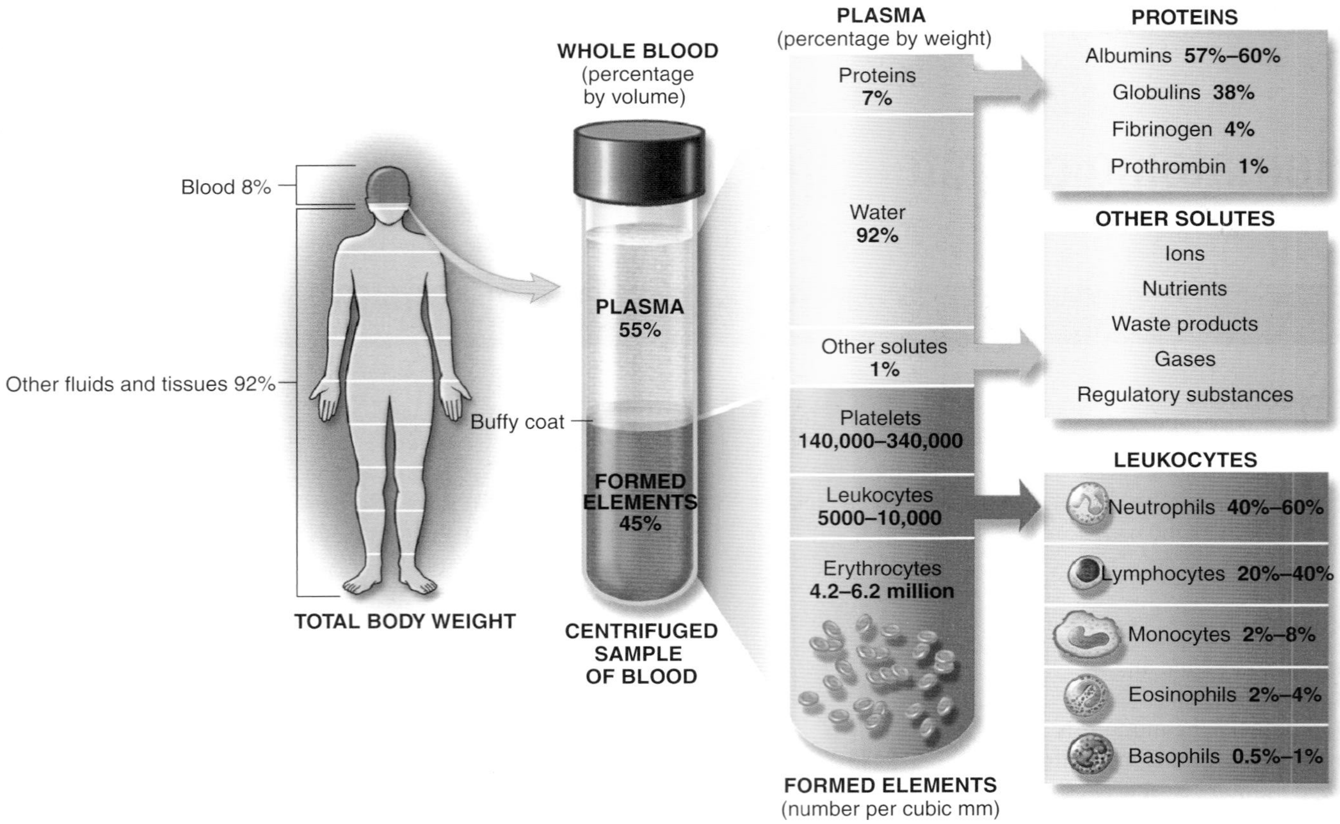

Fig. 29.1 Blood is composed of plasma (~55%) and cellular elements (~45%). Cellular elements include leukocytes (white blood cells), thrombocytes (platelets), and erythrocytes (red blood cells). There are 600 times as many erythrocytes as leukocytes. (From McCance KL, Huether SE: *Understanding pathophysiology*, ed 5, St. Louis, 2013, Mosby.)

blood. The cells in the blood include red blood cells, white blood cells, and platelets (Fig. 29.1). Blood serves many functions but as part of the hematologic system, it carries the cells that transport gases between the lungs and tissues, combat invasion by pathogens, and maintain hemostasis. A healthy adult has about 5 to 6 L of blood circulating through the body.

Red blood cells (or erythrocytes). RBCs, also known as *erythrocytes*, are made in the bone marrow. Once released from the marrow, they circulate in the body, transporting O_2 from the lungs to the tissues and carbon dioxide (CO_2) from the tissues back to the lungs. Hemoglobin (Hgb) in the RBCs makes the transport of O_2 and CO_2 possible. The tough, flexible membrane of the RBCs allows these disk-shaped, biconcave cells to maneuver through the smallest capillaries. After about 120 days, the old RBCs are filtered out of circulation by the liver and spleen. The iron and heme in the old RBCs are recycled to make new RBCs.

RBCs normally have various proteins, called *antigens*, as part of their cell membranes. The two major antigens are named *A* and *B*. Based on the presence or absence of the A and B antigens, a person's blood type is determined. People with type A blood have the A antigen, those with type B blood have the B antigen, those with type AB blood have both the A and B antigens, and those with type O blood have neither the A nor the B antigen. Rhesus (Rh) is another type of RBC antigen that is either present or absent. People with the Rh antigen are designated *Rh positive* (Rh^+) whereas those without the Rh antigen are designated *Rh negative* (Rh^-). Both blood type and Rh factor are genetically determined.

Platelets (thrombocytes). Platelets are also produced in the bone marrow. Platelets activate the blood-clotting system by going to a break in a blood vessel and forming a platelet plug. At the same time, other clotting mechanisms are activated, and the body begins repairing itself. Once released into circulation from the bone marrow, the normal life span of a platelet is 10 days.

Clotting factors. Once platelets activate the blood-clotting system, several clotting factors are activated. The clotting factors are numbered I through XIII and include fibrinogen (factor I) and thrombin (factor II). The clotting factors form a stable fibrin matrix over the wounded area, protecting the injured site while the healing process is completed.

Plasma. Plasma is the clear, straw-colored fluid that carries the red and white blood cells, platelets, and clotting factors through the circulatory system. Plasma is primarily water. In addition to water, plasma contains proteins, electrolytes, gases, nutrients, and waste. The plasma proteins are albumin and globulin.

PHYSIOLOGIC FUNCTIONS OF THE HEMATOLOGIC SYSTEM

Oxygenation

RBCs transport O_2 from the lungs to the tissues and carry CO_2 from the tissues back to the lungs for excretion. The Hgb in the RBCs combines easily with O_2 and CO_2 to accomplish oxygenation.

Hemostasis

Hemostasis means control of bleeding. It is how the body maintains the integrity of the circulatory system. If a blood vessel is injured, three things occur: (1) the blood vessel constricts, reducing the amount of bleeding; (2) platelets adhere to the injured blood vessel, forming an unstable platelet plug; and (3) the coagulation cascade is initiated, forming a stable fibrin matrix, which is commonly recognized as a scab. The *coagulation cascade* is a term used to describe the series of events that occur in the process of blood clotting (Fig. 29.2). See Box 29.1 for age-related changes in the hematologic system.

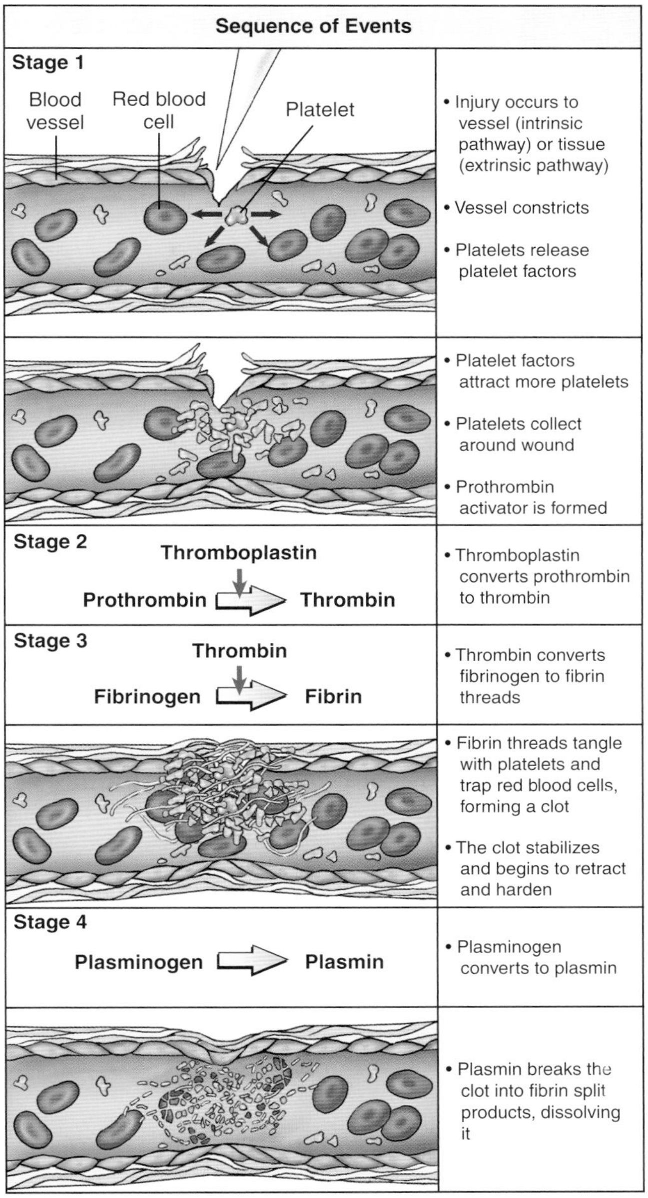

Fig. 29.2 Formation of a blood clot. (From Monahan F, Sands J, Neighbors M, et al.: *Phipps' medical-surgical nursing: health and illness perspectives*, ed 8, St. Louis, 2016, Mosby.)

Box 29.1 Age-Related Changes in the Hematopoietic System

Although bone marrow becomes less productive with age, hematologic function is generally not affected significantly unless a person is unusually stressed with trauma, a chronic illness, or treatment for cancer. Yet even with conditions necessitating increased production of blood cells, the bone marrow can usually respond to the increased demand, given time.

NURSING ASSESSMENT OF THE HEMATOLOGIC SYSTEM

Many subtle findings on the physical examination can suggest changes in the patient's hematologic system that should be documented and reported to a registered nurse (RN) or physician for evaluation. Box 29.2 outlines the nursing assessment of patients with a disorder of the hematologic system. Even though the RN performs the comprehensive assessment, the licensed vocational nurse/licensed practical nurse (LVN/LPN) will assist with data collection and needs to be aware of important findings.

HEALTH HISTORY

Reason for Seeking Care

Pay special attention to the patient who remarks that they bruise easily, bleed for an unusually long time, or are chronically fatigued. These may be the symptoms of an underlying hematologic disorder.

Present Health

Ask the patient to describe the onset of symptoms, severity of symptoms, precipitating events, self-care measures, and effects of those measures.

Past Health History

A patient could have an underlying hematologic problem if they report any of the following: cancer or prior treatment for cancer, human immunodeficiency virus (HIV) infection, liver disease, kidney disease, malabsorption disease, prolonged bleeding or delayed healing with surgery or dental extractions, a history of blood transfusion, placement of prosthetic heart valves, or placement of an indwelling venous access device (indicating that the patient needed long-term venous access). Also note any history of blood transfusions.

Box 29.2 Assessment of Patients With Disorders of the Hematologic System

HEALTH HISTORY

Reason for Seeking Care

Bruising, prolonged bleeding, chronic fatigue

Present Health

Onset of symptoms, severity of symptoms, precipitating events, self-care measures and effects.

Past Health History

Cancer or prior treatment for cancer, human immunodeficiency virus (HIV) infection, anemia, liver disease, kidney disease, malabsorption disorder; prolonged bleeding or delayed healing with surgery or dental extractions; history of having blood transfused; placement of prosthetic heart valves or placement of an indwelling venous access device, indicating that the patient needed long-term venous access; current medications, including over-the-counter (OTC) medications and any recent changes in medication. Use of alcohol or intravenous drugs

Family History

Blood disorders, death of a family member at a young age for reasons other than trauma

Review of Systems

Integumentary: Change in skin color, dryness, pruritus, brittle fingernails or toenails

Neurologic: Dizziness, vertigo, confusion, pain, headache, mental status changes, change in vision

Respiratory: Epistaxis, hemoptysis, dyspnea

Cardiovascular: Palpitations, chest pain, dizziness or fainting with position changes

Gastrointestinal: Change in eating habits, nausea, vomiting, bleeding, abdominal pain, change in bowel habits, blood in stool

Genitourinary: Blood in urine, heavy menses in women

Musculoskeletal: Numbness or pain in bones or joints

Endocrine: Fatigue, cold intolerance

Functional Assessment

Occupation and hobbies, self-concept, activities and exercise, sleep and rest, nutrition, interpersonal relationships, coping and stress, perception of health

Physical Examination

Vital Signs: Tachycardia, tachypnea, hypotension, orthostatic vital sign changes

Height and Weight

General Survey: Responsiveness, mood, expression, posture

Skin: Color, dryness, brittle fingernails and toenails, bruising, petechiae, purpura, ecchymoses

Head and Neck: Bleeding, cracking at the corners of the mouth

Thorax: Respiratory rate, breath sounds, heart rate

Abdomen: Liver enlargement, stool guaiac test, dipstick urine sample for blood

Medications the patient is currently using or a recent change in medication may suggest an underlying hematologic problem. It is important to find out what over-the-counter (OTC) medications the patient uses because many of these contain aspirin or other nonsteroidal antiinflammatory drugs (NSAIDs) that may prolong bleeding.

Family History

Note any family history of blood disorders such as sickle cell disease or hemophilia. Death of a family member at a young age for reasons other than trauma may indicate a genetic hematologic disorder.

Review of Systems

The review of systems is aimed at finding out what symptoms the patient has been experiencing over the past weeks or months that might provide clues as to what specific medical disorder the patient may now have.

In relation to the integumentary system, ask the patient about changes in skin (color, dryness, pruritus [itching]) and brittle fingernails or toenails. Data relevant to the assessment of the neurologic system include dizziness, vertigo, confusion, and pain. Patients with low RBC counts may have headaches. If the patient has had headaches, record the location, duration, and intensity of the pain, as well as what, if anything, relieves the pain. Patients with intracranial bleeding from low platelet counts may report sudden mental status changes or severe headaches. Note changes in vision, which may indicate bleeding behind the eye. While collecting data about the respiratory and cardiovascular systems, ask the patient about epistaxis (nosebleeds), hemoptysis (coughing up blood), dyspnea (shortness of breath), heart palpitations, and chest pain, which may be symptoms of a low RBC count. Heart palpitations accompanied by dizziness may occur with position changes as the heart beats faster to move what little blood exists quickly from the lungs to the body tissues to deliver O_2. Significant data for assessment of the gastrointestinal (GI) system include any changes in eating habits, including changes in appetite or episodes of nausea or vomiting. Inquire about bleeding or pain in the mouth, gums, or tongue. In addition, record the patient's normal bowel function and any recent changes in frequency of bowel movements or consistency of the stool. Also note any report of blood in the stool as well as any report of blood in the urine as an abnormality of the genitourinary system. Ask female patients about unusually heavy menses, which may indicate a bleeding disorder. Any musculoskeletal numbness or pain should also be noted; joint pain can occur if bleeding has taken place in the joint (hemarthrosis). Finally, to collect data about the endocrine system, ask the patient about fatigue or cold intolerance, which may be a symptom of a low RBC count.

Functional Assessment

Patients newly diagnosed with blood disorders may not experience dramatic changes in their functional abilities. However, many blood disorders are chronic conditions that the patient has lived with for many years.

Occupation and hobbies. Knowing a patient's job and hobbies can alert the nurse to unusual chemical exposures. Because the bone marrow and blood can be affected by various chemicals, it is important to document any recent chemical exposure. For example, someone who builds models for a hobby may be exposed to unusual glues or paints, which may affect the blood count.

Self-concept. Assess the patient's self-concept by exploring the patient's feelings about themselves. For many people, their self-concept is related to their job. If the patient is unable to work, their self-concept can be adversely affected. In addition, medical insurance is often contingent on employment. Loss of medical insurance and the need to receive state or federal assistance can further erode a patient's self-concept. Another factor that can adversely affect the patient's self-concept is a change in appearance because of the disease.

Activity and exercise. Describe the patient's current activity level and the effects of the disease and treatment on the patient's usual pattern of activity and exercise. Ask about the layout of the patient's home, specifically the location of bathrooms in relation to living areas and bedrooms. Determine if the patient must climb stairs to enter the home or get to a second floor. Having to climb stairs can quickly tire a patient with a hematologic disorder. Inquire about what the patient does for recreation and whether these activities can still be done during times of decreased energy.

Sleep and rest. Note the number of continuous hours the patient sleeps every night, whether any sleeping aids are used, what interrupts the patient's sleep, and whether the patient naps during the day.

Nutrition. Ask the patient to describe their usual diet and any recent changes in appetite or weight (see the Nutrition Considerations box). Identify factors that might be interfering with eating, such as nausea, vomiting, and taste changes. Depression and loneliness can adversely affect a patient's nutritional status. Limited financial resources can also affect a patient's ability to maintain a nutritious diet.

Nutrition Considerations

A balanced diet should include foods rich in iron, which is required for hemoglobin (Hgb) production. Foods rich in iron include red meats, fish, dried fruits, beans, and dark-green vegetables.

Interpersonal relationships. Explore the patient's view of themselves as a husband or wife, father or mother, son or daughter, friend, and co-worker. Discuss the effects of the disease on these relationships and on the patient's roles in the home. In addition, ask what household chores the patient is responsible for and who does the shopping, cooking, and cleaning. If the patient has children who need to be cared for, note whether the patient is able to perform the usual child care.

Coping and stress. Ask what worries the patient has and how they usually deal with stress. In addition, explore sources of support, which might include family, support groups, and spiritual beliefs and practices.

Perception of health. Ask the patient to discuss feelings about their own health and health practices. This might include measures taken to prevent complications from the disease and keeping regular medical appointments.

PHYSICAL EXAMINATION

Begin the physical examination by measuring the patient's vital signs, height, and weight. Be alert for tachycardia (pulse >100 beats per minute), tachypnea (respiratory rate >20 breaths per minute), and hypotension (systolic blood pressure <90 mm Hg).

Patients with low RBC counts may experience **orthostatic vital sign changes** in pulse and blood pressure when they rise. The body tries to maintain the blood pressure when the patient changes position from lying to standing. If the patient's blood volume is inadequate, the heart rate increases and the blood pressure decreases as the patient stands. This can be why patients complain of feeling dizzy or light-headed when they stand up quickly. Box 29.3 describes how to assess for orthostatic changes in vital signs. Patients

Box 29.3 Assessing for Orthostatic Changes in Vital Signs

1. Have the patient lie down on a bed or in a reclining chair for at least 1 minute.
2. Record the patient's heart rate and blood pressure.
3. Have the patient sit up.
4. After the patient has been sitting for no more than 30 seconds, record the heart rate and blood pressure again.
5. Have the patient stand up. Stay near the patient to ensure the safety of the individual.
6. After the patient has been standing no more than 30 seconds, record the heart rate and blood pressure again.
7. If the blood pressure decreases 10 to 15 points with the change from the lying to the standing position and the heart rate increases 10 to 15 points from lying to standing, the patient is described as having orthostatic or tilt-positive changes.

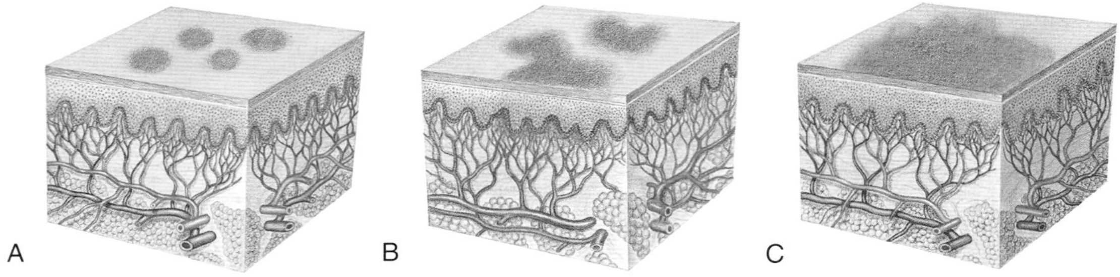

Fig 29.3 Petechiae (A), purpura (B), and ecchymosis (C). (From Harding MM, Kwong J, Roberts D, et al.: *Lewis's medical-surgical nursing: assessment and management of clinical problems*, ed 11, St Louis, 2020, Elsevier.)

who have orthostatic changes in their vital signs usually need some type of hydration. Often the patient is simply dehydrated and needs extra fluids. However, a patient with a low RBC count who needs a blood transfusion can also be orthostatic.

General Survey

Note the patient's responsiveness, mood, expression, and posture. Throughout the examination, carefully inspect and describe any reddened, swollen, or painful areas the patient identifies.

Skin

Note the general color of the skin. A patient with a low RBC count may appear pale. In dark-skinned people, this may be difficult to assess. Look at the conjunctiva of the eyes, the nail beds, and around the mouth to detect any paleness. Patients may also appear jaundiced, or yellow, if many RBCs have been destroyed or if the body is having trouble clearing the blood of old RBCs. Indications of a vitamin deficiency that might cause a blood disorder include dry, itchy skin and scalp or brittle fingernails and toenails (see the Complementary and Alternative Therapies box).

> **Complementary and Alternative Therapies**
>
> Be sure to note any herbal products that the patient uses. Herbs that can affect blood clotting include black cohosh, feverfew, garlic, ginkgo, and ginseng.

Describe any bruising. **Petechiae** are small (1–3 mm), red or reddish-purple pinpoint spots on the skin resulting from blood capillaries breaking and leaking small amounts of blood into the tissues. Petechiae are often confused with a skin rash. Petechiae almost always signal that the patient has a very low platelet count. Severe coughing can cause petechiae on the chest, neck, and face of a patient. A blood pressure cuff pumped up to greater than 250 mm Hg on a patient with a low platelet count can cause petechiae on the arm below the blood pressure cuff as the small capillaries break with the high cuff pressure. This is not dangerous but can be frightening to the patient and the nurse if it happens. Red or reddish-purple spots denote **purpura** and are the result of larger blood vessels breaking. Purpura are larger than petechiae, usually 3 mm or more. Purpura can suggest a low platelet count or a problem with clotting factors in the blood. Ecchymoses are larger purplish areas of skin resulting from a larger amount of blood leaking outside the blood vessels. The common name for **ecchymosis** is a *bruise*. Ecchymoses do not necessarily indicate a bleeding disorder, but if the patient has a number of ecchymotic areas or notes that they bruise easily, it may be a symptom of a blood disorder. Fig 29.3 illustrates common findings in the skin assessment.

Head and Neck

When evaluating the eyes, ears, nose, mouth, and throat, note any signs of bleeding. Look for cracking at the corners of the mouth, which may be a symptom of iron or B vitamin deficiency.

Thorax

Lungs. Count the patient's respiratory rate, note effort, and auscultate breath sounds. Patients with low RBC counts often are dyspneic, or short of breath, because they do not have enough RBCs to carry O_2 to all their tissues, yet the lungs will sound clear to auscultation without wheezing, crackles, or rhonchi. As a result, they are tachypneic, with a respiratory rate greater than 20 breaths per minute, to oxygenate what little blood they have. Any strenuous activity may exacerbate the shortness of breath.

Heart and vascular system. Count the patient's heart rate, take resting blood pressure, and note blood pressure response to position changes. Patients with low RBC counts can be tachycardic, with a heart rate greater than 100 bpm. Again, because not enough RBCs exist to carry O_2 to all the tissues, the heart beats faster to move what little blood exists quickly from the lungs to the body tissues to deliver O_2.

Abdomen

Inspect and palpate the patient's abdomen for distention and tenderness. The examiner with advanced skills may also palpate for organ enlargement. The liver and spleen can become enlarged with blood cell disorders, causing abdominal fullness and tenderness. If a stool specimen is available, a guaiac test may be done to detect microscopic blood. If the patient can provide a urine sample, it can also be tested for blood.

DIAGNOSTIC TESTS AND PROCEDURES

Primarily, blood studies determine the function of the patient's hematologic system. Diagnostic tests and procedures done to diagnose disorders of the hematologic system are described in Tables 29.1 and 29.2. The laboratory performing the test should provide normal values for the various blood tests. Ranges of normal values can be found in various textbooks of laboratory and diagnostic tests.

BLOOD TESTS

The complete blood count (CBC) is a very common test used to help diagnose blood or systemic disorders, and to monitor response to treatments. The RBC count, the Hgb, and the hematocrit (Hct) are the three main blood tests used to monitor RBCs. The RBC count is the total number of RBCs found in a cubic millimeter (mm^3) of blood. The Hgb indicates the O_2-carrying capacity in the blood. The Hct is the percentage of RBCs in whole blood. Normally, the Hct is approximately 3 times the Hgb value. Iron is an essential part of RBCs; therefore serum iron, total iron-binding capacity (TIBC), and ferritin are measured to assess the patient's resources for producing RBCs.

The WBC count and differential measures the total WBCs and the percent of the total contributed by neutrophils, lymphocytes, monocytes, eosinophils, and basophils. Increased WBCs are consistent with infection, inflammation, tissue necrosis, or leukemic neoplasia. A low WBC count reflects reduced bone marrow activity.

Table 29.1 Diagnostic Tests and Procedures: Laboratory Studies

General Interventions: Check your agency procedure manual for diagnostic tests and procedures. Always tell the patient what to expect when tests are ordered. Before a venipuncture, tell the patient to expect a brief sharp pain as the needle goes through the skin. Afterward, apply pressure for 1 minute and elevate the arm. If the patient's blood clotting is impaired, apply pressure for 5–10 minutes. Apply dressing for at least 1 hour.

Different blood tests are collected in different laboratory tubes containing specific reagents or no reagents at all. Usually the tubes have color-coded tops. Be sure to collect the blood in the blood tube specific for the blood test ordered. Usually each institution's laboratory publishes a manual identifying what colored tube to use for each blood test.

COMPONENT	NORMAL VALUES	SIGNIFICANCE OF VALUES
Complete Blood Count		
Red blood cell (RBC) count	Adult male: 4.7–6.1 million/mm^3 Adult female: 4.2–5.4 million/mm^3	Low: anemia, hemorrhage, hemolysis, iron or vitamin B_{12} deficiency, genetic variations, bone marrow failure, renal disease, some drugs High: dehydration, some drugs
Hemoglobin (Hgb)	Adult male: 14–18 g/dL or 8.7–11.2 mmol/L (SI units) Adult female: 12–16 g/dL or 7.4–9.9 mmol/L Older adult: slight decrease	Low: anemia, dilutional overhydration, some blood disorders, some drugs High: dehydration, high altitude, heavy smoking, some drugs
Hematocrit (Hct)	Adult male: 42%–52% or 0.42–0.52 volume fraction Adult female: 37%–47% or 0.37–0.47 volume fraction Older adult: slight decrease	Variations same as RBC count (as mentioned earlier)
RBC Indices	Values for all adults:	Helps to determine type of anemia
• Mean corpuscular volume (MCV)	MCV: 80–95 fL	
• Mean corpuscular Hgb (MCH)	MCH: 27–31 pg	
• Mean corpuscular Hgb concentration (MCHC)	MCHC: 32–36 g/dL (or 32%–36%)	
• Red blood cell distribution width (RDW)	RDW: 11%–14.5%	
White blood cell (WBC) count and differential	All adults: 5000–10,000/mm^3	Low: bone marrow failure High: infection, inflammation, tissue necrosis, leukemia neoplasia
• Neutrophils	55%–70% or 2500–8000 (per mm^3)	High: acute bacterial infection and trauma
• Lymphocytes	20%–40% or 1000–4000	High: chronic bacterial infection, acute viral infection

Continued

Table 29.1 Diagnostic Tests and Procedures: Laboratory Studies—cont'd

COMPONENT	NORMAL VALUES	SIGNIFICANCE OF VALUES
• Monocytes	2%–8% or 100–700	High: monocytic leukemia
• Eosinophils	1%–4% or 50–500	High: allergic reaction, parasitic infection
• Basophils	0.5%–1.0% or 25–100	High: allergic reaction, parasitic infection
Coagulation Measures		
Prothrombin time (PT)	Normal PT: 11.0–12.5 seconds Warfarin therapeutic PT range 1.3–1.5 Normal INR: 1 Warfarin therapeutic INR range; 2–3	Short: diet high in fat or leafy vegetables, some drugs Prolonged: liver disease, oral anticoagulant therapy, biliary obstruction, some drugs
Partial thromboplastin time, activated (aPTT)	aPTT: 30–40 seconds (should not exceed 70 seconds.)	Prolonged: hemophilia, biliary obstruction, liver disease, heparin and some other drugs including salicylates.
Partial thromboplastin time (PTT)	PTT: 60–70 seconds (should not exceed 100 seconds) On anticoagulant therapy: 1.5–2.5 times control value in seconds	
Platelet count	All adults: 150,000–400,000/mm^3	Low: bone marrow failure; hemorrhage; platelet destruction by drugs, infection, antibodies; DIC High: estrogens, oral contraceptives, high altitude

DIC, Disseminated intravascular coagulation; *fL*, femtoliter; *INR*, international normalized ratio.
From Pagana KD, Pagana TJ: *Mosby's manual of diagnostic and laboratory tests*, ed 5, St. Louis, 2014, Elsevier/Mosby. Burchum JR, Rosenthal LD: *Lehne's Pharmacology for nursing care,* ed 10, St. Louis, 2019, Elsevier.

Table 29.2 Diagnostic Tests and Procedures: Bone Marrow Biopsy

TEST/STUDY	PURPOSE AND PROCEDURE	PATIENT PREPARATION	POSTPROCEDURE NURSING CARE
Bone marrow biopsy	A bone marrow biopsy is used to evaluate how well the bone marrow is making white blood cells (WBCs), red blood cells (RBCs), and platelets. The patient is positioned on an examining table according to the location of where the bone marrow biopsy will be collected. The most common site is the posterior iliac spine, requiring the patient to be in the prone position, although the anterior iliac crest, tibia, fibula, rib, or sternum can also be biopsy sites, allowing for alternative positioning. The selected site is prepared and draped as for a minor surgical procedure. A local anesthetic is injected. A special needle is forced into the bone marrow. For a bone marrow aspiration, only fluid and cells are withdrawn for examination. For a biopsy, solid marrow tissue and cells are taken. The needle is removed, and a pressure dressing is applied to the site. A laboratory technician or trained assistant must be present during the procedure to immediately fix and stain the specimens.	Explain the purpose and procedure to the patient. A permit must be signed. No fasting is necessary. Some local discomfort may be experienced as the local anesthetic is injected. The patient usually feels pressure as the Jamshidi needle is inserted into the bone and a momentary sharp pain down the leg as the bone marrow fluid is aspirated. The procedure takes approximately 30 minutes. Sometimes a short acting benzodiazepine such as midazolam (Versed) is given to sedate the patient during the procedure.	If intravenous sedation is used, monitor the patient's pulse, blood pressure, respirations, and pulse oximetry until the patient is fully recovered. Check puncture site for bleeding. The pressure dressing can be removed in 2 hours. Bed rest may be ordered for 10–15 minutes after the procedure. Instruct the patient to report tenderness and/or redness at the puncture site.

From Pagana KD, Pagana TJ: *Mosby's manual of diagnostic and laboratory tests*, ed 5, St. Louis, 2014, Elsevier/Mosby. Zehnder JL: Bone marrow aspiration and biopsy: Indications and techniques. *UpToDate*. January 31, 2020. Retrieved January 7, 2020 from www.uptodate.com.

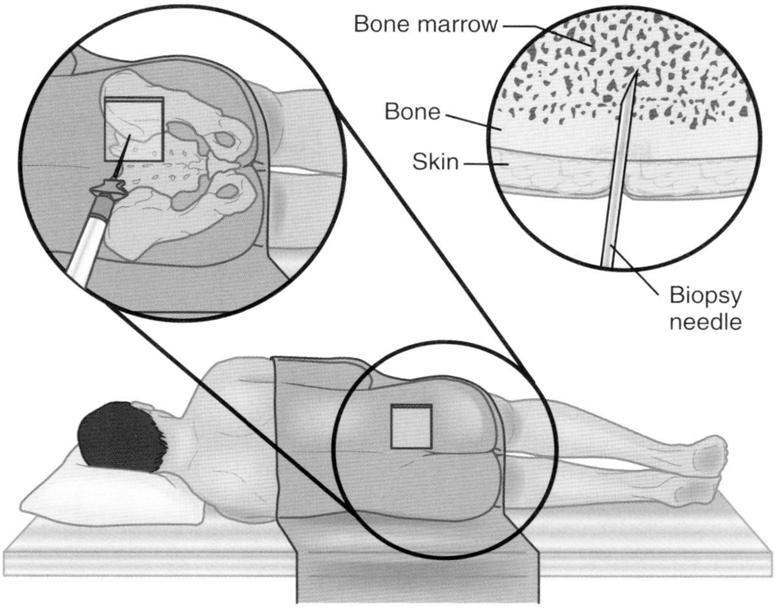

Fig. 29.4 Bone marrow aspiration from the posterior iliac crest. (From Harding MM, Kwong J, Roberts D, et al.: *Lewis's medical-surgical nursing: Assessment and management of clinical problems*, ed 11, St. Louis, 2020, Elsevier.)

The different types of WBCs help to identify the specific type of disorder that is triggering the increase in WBCs. For example, neutrophils increase in the presence of acute bacterial infections or trauma.

Normal platelet counts range from 140,000 to 440,000 platelets/mm^3 of blood. Many times, the platelet count is abbreviated as a multiple of 1000. For example, a platelet count of 200,000 is abbreviated 200K.

The function of the clotting factors is measured with the prothrombin time (PT), the partial thromboplastin time (PTT), and the bleeding time. If the results of these tests are abnormal, other blood tests that may be done to determine the specific abnormality include measurements of fibrinogen; thrombin time (TT); fibrinogen degradation products (FDP), also known as *fibrin split products* (FSP); and D-dimers. If the patient is taking heparin to anticoagulate the blood, the PTT is used to monitor therapy. If the patient is taking warfarin (Coumadin) to anticoagulate the blood, the PT, the international normalized ratio (INR), or both are used to monitor therapy.

BONE MARROW BIOPSY

If blood tests show abnormalities, the physician may perform a bone marrow biopsy to see how well the blood cells are being made in the bone marrow (Fig. 29.4). Table 29.2 describes the bone marrow biopsy procedure.

COMMON THERAPEUTIC MEASURES

Treatment of disorders of the hematologic system is aimed at correcting the underlying problem or replacing deficient components. Blood product transfusions and colony-stimulating factors are used to symptomatically manage the patient.

Box 29.4 Nursing Actions for the Patient at Risk for Injury From Insufficient Oxygenation Related to Low Red Blood Cell Counts (Anemia)

1. Administer oxygen (O_2) as prescribed.
2. Administer blood products as prescribed (see Tables 29.3 and 29.4 and Box 29.5).
3. Administer the hematopoietic growth factor erythropoietin as prescribed (see Table 29.5).
4. Monitor position changes from bed or chair to standing to ensure safety.
5. Allow for rest between periods of activity because the patient with anemia can tire easily.
6. Elevate the patient's head on pillows for shortness of breath.
7. Provide extra blankets if the patient feels too cool.
8. Teach the patient and family about the underlying pathophysiology and how to manage the symptoms of anemia.

From Young-McCaughan S, Jennings BM: Hematologic and immunologic systems. In: Alspach JG, editor: *Core curriculum for critical care nursing*, ed 5, Philadelphia, 1998, Saunders.

NURSING ACTIONS FOR THE PATIENT AT RISK FOR INJURY FROM LOW RED BLOOD CELL COUNTS

Box 29.4 outlines typical nursing actions for the patient at risk for injury from low RBC counts (**anemia**).

NURSING ACTIONS FOR THE PATIENT AT RISK FOR INJURY FROM BLEEDING

Box 29.5 outlines typical nursing actions for the patient at risk for injury from bleeding.

Box 29.5 Nursing Actions for the Patient at Risk for Injury From Bleeding

1. Administer blood product transfusions as prescribed. If a platelet transfusion is to be given in preparation for a procedure, then it is best to give the transfusion immediately before the procedure so that the greatest number of platelets will be available to stop bleeding caused by the procedure (see Table 29.3 and Box 29.6).
2. Minimize the number of invasive procedures done to the patient that might result in prolonged bleeding by taking the following measures:
   a. Draw blood for as much laboratory work as possible with one venipuncture.
   b. Avoid prolonged tourniquet use.
   c. Apply direct pressure for 5 to 10 minutes after all invasive procedures such as venipuncture or bone marrow biopsies.
   d. Avoid intramuscular injections.
3. Avoid damage to the rectal mucosa that might cause bleeding by taking the following measures:
   a. Avoid taking rectal temperatures.
   b. Avoid use of suppositories.
   c. Avoid use of enemas.
   d. Prevent constipation by increasing fiber in the diet or administering stool softeners as ordered.
4. When measuring blood pressure, inflate the cuff only until the pulse is obliterated to prevent petechiae along the arm. Set automated sphygmomanometers to the lowest appropriate pressure.
5. Instruct the patient to use a soft-bristled toothbrush. If oral bleeding occurs, then toothettes or mouth rinses can be used to maintain oral hygiene.
6. Instruct the patient to use an electric razor to shave, not a straight-edged razor.
7. As much as possible and as prescribed by the physician, avoid the use of drugs that interfere with platelet function such as aspirin, aspirin-containing drugs (e.g., Pepto-Bismol, Percodan), and the nonsteroidal antiinflammatory drugs (NSAIDs).
8. Teach the patient and family about the underlying pathophysiology that puts the patient at risk for hemorrhage and precautions to minimize the risk of bleeding.

From Young-McCaughan S, Jennings BM: Hematologic and immunologic systems. In: Alspach JG, editor: *Core curriculum for critical care nursing*, ed 5, Philadelphia, 1998, Saunders.

BLOOD PRODUCT TRANSFUSIONS

Because of the risk for infections, such as with hepatitis or HIV, blood product transfusions are no longer automatically given when the patient's laboratory values fall below a certain value. Instead the patient is evaluated clinically, and a decision is made with the patient whether or not to administer a blood transfusion. Symptoms of a low RBC count that would prompt an RBC transfusion include shortness of breath, tachycardia, decreased blood pressure, chest pain, light-headedness, or extreme fatigue. For each unit of packed red blood cells (PRBCs) transfused, the patient's Hgb should increase approximately 1 g/dL and the Hct approximately 3%. Table 29.3 provides an overview of commonly transfused blood components.

Typing for Transfusions

Before a blood transfusion, a sample of the patient's blood is sent to the blood bank for typing and crossmatching. As discussed previously, depending on which antigens are present in the RBC membrane, a person has either type A, B, AB, or O blood. In addition, depending on the presence or absence of the Rh antigen, a person is either Rh^+ or Rh^-. People with any of these antigens cannot be given blood containing a different antigen. Therefore persons with type O^- blood are considered **universal donors** because their blood does not contain any of the A, B, or Rh antigens and can safely be given to anyone. Those with AB^+ blood are considered **universal recipients** because their blood contains the A, B, and Rh antigens. They can safely receive any type of blood. Unless it is a medical emergency, blood banks exactly match the blood to be transfused with the blood of a patient needing a transfusion.

Transfusions of Packed Red Blood Cells

The physician should counsel and get the signed consent of the patient before any blood transfusion. A blood sample is drawn from the patient and sent to the blood bank for type and crossmatch. One procedure for administering a PRBC transfusion is outlined in Box 29.6. The policies for administering blood products vary from hospital to hospital, so the LVN/LPN must be familiar with their institution's policies.

One way to prevent the risks of infection and reactions with blood transfusions is to collect the patient's own blood before a planned procedure and then transfuse the patient's own blood back into the patient if needed as an autologous RBC transfusion. The patient donates their own blood several times before the planned procedure. The blood is stored by the blood bank and reinfused into the patient if needed intraoperatively or postoperatively. Autologous transfusion (using the patient's own blood) is recommended if significant blood loss is expected during the procedure, especially if the patient has a rare blood type or religious beliefs against receiving donated blood.

Platelet Transfusions

Like RBC transfusions, platelet transfusions are not automatically administered when the patient's platelet count falls below a certain value. However, the lower a patient's platelet count goes, the greater is the chance of bleeding. In general, when the platelet count falls below 20,000 cells/mm^3, platelets are administered.

Table 29.3 Commonly Transfused Blood Products

BLOOD COMPONENT	INDICATIONS	USUAL AMOUNT IN ONE UNIT	RECOMMENDED INFUSION RATE	SPECIAL CONSIDERATIONS
Packed red blood cells (PRBCs)	Symptomatic anemia caused by low hematocrit (Hct) or hemoglobin (Hgb), such as shortness of breath, tachycardia, decreased blood pressure, chest pain, light-headedness, or fatigue	225–350 mL	2–4 h/unit. Start slowly (1–2 ml/min for first 15 mins) and observe for adverse reaction. If tolerated well, increase rate to deliver within 4 hours.	An 18- or 20-gauge needle must be used to prevent damage to RBCs. The transfusion should be started within 30 minutes of leaving the blood bank.
Platelets/apheresis platelets	Bleeding related to thrombocytopenia; patients at serious risk for bleeding	30–60 mL/pack; usually 1 unit of apheresis platelets or 4–6 packs of units derived from whole blood	Run at 2–5 mL/min the first 15 minutes, watching for any transfusion reaction, and then increase rate as patient can tolerate, usually 1–2 hours. Complete within 4 hours.	Platelets should be stored on an agitator before administration to maximize oxygenation of the cells and prolong their effectiveness.
Fresh frozen plasma (FFP) and a variety of other preparations	Clotting deficiencies, TTP (thrombotic thrombocytopenic purpura), hemophilia A and B, rapid reversal of warfarin (Coumadin), massive RBC transfusions	200–250 mL/U Some preparations are 400–600 mL	Run infusion at 2–5 mL/min the first 15 minutes, watching for any transfusion reaction, and then increase rate as patient can tolerate. Complete within 4 hours.	FFP contains all clotting factors except platelets.
Cryoprecipitated AHF, pooled cryo-precipitated AHF	TTP, hemophilia A	10 mL/bag; usually 10 bags are pooled for transfusion	Run infusion slowly the first 15 minutes, watching for any transfusion reaction, and then increase rate as patient can tolerate. Complete within 4 hours.	Cryoprecipitate contains factors I (fibrinogen) and VIII.

Data from American Association of Blood Banks, America's Blood Centers, American Red Cross: Circular of information for the use of human blood and blood components (revised October 2017). http://www.aabb.org/tm/coi/Documents/coi1017.pdf. Silvergleid AJ: Transfusion-associated circulatory overload (TACO). *UpToDate*. February 5, 2020. Retrieved January 7, 2021) from www.uptodate.com.

Box 29.6 Administration of a Red Blood Cell Transfusion

1. After the patient has been counseled and has given signed consent for the transfusion, draw a sample of blood and send it to the blood bank with a request for a type and crossmatch. Start a peripheral intravenous (IV) line of normal saline using an 18- or 20-gauge needle. Blood should not be infused through a cannula smaller than 20 gauge because of the chance of lysing (destroying) the individual blood cells as they go through the cannula. Similarly, normal saline is used in the administration of blood products rather than 5% dextrose solution or lactated Ringer solution to avoid the possibility of agglutination and/or hemolysis of the transfused blood in the IV line.
2. When the blood arrives, two licensed people should check them at the patient's bedside. Be certain to check the expiration date of the blood. Once the blood has arrived from the blood bank, the transfusion should be started within 30 minutes. In many states, licensed vocational nurses/licensed practical nurses (LVNs/LPNs) cannot initiate a blood transfusion. However, the LVN/LPN is responsible for monitoring the patient while the transfusion is in progress. Check the practice laws in your state and your institution's policies.
3. Take and record the patient's vital signs.
4. To administer blood, use a special blood transfusion tubing that has a built-in filter to screen for clots. Piggyback the blood into the normal saline line. Each unit of blood is usually between 250 and 300 mL. In general, blood is infused over 2 to 4 hours.
5. Stay with the patient for 5 to 10 minutes after the blood is started to observe for any immediate untoward reactions that might signal a reaction to the transfusion, such as back pain, fever, chills, or decreased blood pressure.
6. Continue to monitor vital signs during the transfusion per your institution's policy.
7. When the transfusion is complete, document the procedure, the patient's vital signs, and how the patient tolerated the procedure.
8. Subsequent units of blood can be hung immediately as just described. Sometimes the same blood tubing can be used for administering several units of blood.

Box 29.7 Administration of a Platelet Transfusion

1. After the patient has been counseled and has given signed consent for the transfusion, draw a sample of blood and send it to the blood bank with a request for typing and crossmatch. Start an intravenous line of normal saline using at least a 24-gauge needle. Platelets are smaller than red blood cells (RBCs); therefore a smaller intravenous needle can be used to administer the platelets without risk of lysing the cells.
2. When the platelets arrive, two licensed people should check them at the patient's bedside. Once the platelets have arrived from the blood bank, the transfusion should be started immediately. In many states licensed vocational nurses/licensed practical nurses (LVNs/LPNs) cannot initiate a blood product transfusion. However, the LVN/LPN is responsible for monitoring the patient while the transfusion is in progress. Check the practice laws in your state and your institution's policies.
3. Take and record the patient's vital signs.
4. Run the platelets through blood transfusion tubing that has a built-in filter in the system. Piggyback the platelets into the normal saline line. Platelets can be infused as fast as the patient can tolerate them.
5. Stay with the patient for 5 to 10 minutes after the platelets are started to observe for any immediate untoward reactions that might signal a reaction to the transfusion, such as back pain, fever, chills, or decreased blood pressure.
6. Continue to monitor the patient's vital signs during the infusion per your institution's policy.
7. When the transfusion is complete, document the procedure, the patient's vital signs, and how the patient tolerated the procedure.

If the platelet count is greater than 20,000 cells/mm^3, platelets are usually not given unless the patient is actively bleeding. For each multidonor (from multiple donors) pack of platelets, the patient's platelet count should increase by 5000 to 10,000 cells/mm^3.

As with blood transfusions, the physician should counsel and get the signed consent of the patient for the platelet transfusion. A blood sample is drawn from the patient and sent to the blood bank for typing. If the patient has been previously typed and crossmatched for either an RBC transfusion or a platelet transfusion, the blood bank can usually use this information to provide platelets. Platelets are commonly ordered in four-packs or six-packs. Each pack contains approximately 60 mL. One procedure for administering a platelet transfusion is outlined in Box 29.7. Because the policies for administering blood products vary from hospital to hospital, the LVN/LPN must be familiar with their institution's policies.

If platelets are ordered before an invasive procedure that might cause bleeding, such as a lumbar puncture or endoscopy, the platelets should be administered just before the procedure is started. No indication exists to "get the platelets in early" for a procedure scheduled for later in the day. Instead, with the physician, the nurse should plan to administer the platelets just before the procedure begins.

Fresh Frozen Plasma Transfusions

Plasma is separated from whole blood by centrifugation and quickly frozen. Therefore when plasma is to be transfused, usually fresh frozen plasma (FFP) is ordered. FFP contains all of the clotting factors and plasma proteins. Cryoprecipitate, which contains only fibrinogen and factor VIII, can be further separated out from plasma and administered alone if indicated.

Reactions to Blood Transfusions

Four main types of transfusion reactions can occur with transfusions of blood or any of the blood components: (1) hemolytic, (2) anaphylactic, (3) febrile, and (4) circulatory overload. If the patient experiences back or chest pain, fever, chills, a decreased blood pressure, urticaria, wheezing, dyspnea, coughing, or blood in the urine during the transfusion, stop the transfusion immediately and keep the intravenous line open with normal saline. Notify the physician, nursing supervisor, and blood bank immediately; be prepared to administer O_2, epinephrine, Solu-Cortef, furosemide (Lasix), and antipyretics as prescribed by the physician. Save the unused portion of the blood bag for the blood bank. Also be prepared to collect blood and urine samples from the patient for evaluation. Documentation of the event is important; usually each institution has a blood transfusion reaction form that needs to be completed. A delayed hemolytic reaction can also occur 2 to 14 days after the transfusion in patients previously treated with RBC transfusions and alloimmunized so that the patient's own immune system attacks the transfused RBCs. Usually delayed hemolytic reactions do not require treatment. Table 29.4 outlines the types, symptoms, and treatments for the different blood transfusion reactions.

COLONY-STIMULATING FACTORS

Colony-stimulating factors are naturally occurring hormones that stimulate the bone marrow to produce more blood cells. Certain of the colony-stimulating factors have been isolated and are available for therapeutic use. Erythropoietin (Epogen) and darbepoetin (Aranesp) stimulate the bone marrow to produce more RBCs, whereas oprelvekin (Neumega) stimulates the bone marrow to produce more platelets. The effects of these drugs on the Hct and platelet count are not apparent for several days; therefore they are not an option for patients who need to elevate their blood cell counts immediately. These patients need a transfusion of the appropriate blood component. Erythropoietin and darbepoetin are predominantly used by hemodialysis patients who are chronically anemic as a result of dialysis; these medications have also been used to prevent the complications and relieve the symptoms of anemia in patients with cancer or HIV infection. Table 29.5 describes the nursing care of patients receiving these drugs.

Table 29.4 Blood Transfusion Reactions

Standard Response to Transfusion Reaction

1. **Stop the infusion**
2. **Maintain intravenous access with normal saline**
3. **Confirm correct product**
4. **Notify health care provider and blood bank/transfusion service**

REACTION	MECHANISM	SYMPTOMS	OCCURRENCE	TREATMENT
Acute hemolytic transfusion reaction (AHTR)	Antigen-antibody reaction to transfusion of ABO-incompatible blood	Fever, chills, nausea, dyspnea, chest pain, back pain, hypotension, hematuria (blood in urine)	Shortly after starting transfusion	Stop the transfusion. Notify the physician immediately. Be prepared to provide supportive therapy to maintain heart rate and blood pressure.
Anaphylactic transfusion reaction	Type I hypersensitivity reaction to plasma proteins	Urticaria, wheezing, dyspnea, hypotension	Within 30 minutes of starting transfusion	Stop the transfusion. Notify the physician immediately. Be prepared to administer epinephrine and corticosteroids.
Febrile nonhematologic transfusion reaction (FNHTR)	Recipient's antibodies react to donor leukocytes	Fever, chills	Within 30–90 minutes of starting transfusion	Stop the transfusion. Notify the physician immediately.
Transfusion-associated circulatory overload (TACO)	Patient's cardiovascular system is unable to manage the additional fluid load	Cough, frothy sputum, dyspnea, cyanosis, decreased blood pressure	Any time during transfusion and up to 12 hours after completing the transfusion	Stop the transfusion. Call for help. Be prepared to administer oxygen (O_2) and/or furosemide (Lasix). Ventilatory support may be needed.
Transfusion related acute lung injury (TRALI)				
Primary hypotensive reaction	Exact cause unknown. Risk increased in patients on ACE inhibitors. Uncommon	Drop in BP of 30 mm Hg (systolic, diastolic, or both) or more	Within minutes of start of transfusion.	Stop infusion
Delayed hemolytic reactions	Reaction occurs in patients previously treated with red blood cell (RBC) transfusions and alloimmunized so that patient's own immune system attacks transfused RBCs	Unexplained fever, unexplained decrease in hemoglobin (Hgb) and hematocrit (Hct)	2–14 days after transfusion	Most delayed reactions require no treatment.
Primary hypotensive reaction				
Urticarial transfusion reaction (UTR)	Antigen-antibody interaction	Hives		Antihistamine may be given.
Sepsis	Transfusion of contaminated blood	Fever, chills, hypotension		Broad spectrum antibiotics.

Table 29.5 Drug Therapy: Drugs Used to Treat Disorders of the Hematologic System

DRUG	USE AND ACTION	SIDE EFFECTS	NURSING INTERVENTIONS
Erythropoietic Growth Factors			
epoetin alfa (Epogen) darbepoetin alfa (Aranesp)	Stimulates bone marrow to produce red blood cells (RBCs)	Hypertension, headache, arthralgia. Risk of cardiac arrest, heart failure, stroke and MI, especially if given when Hgb approaches 11 g/dL or when Hgb rises too rapidly.	Usually administered by subcutaneous injection; may also be administered intravenously. Patient is usually treated 3 times per week with epoetin alfa or once per week with darbepoetin alfa until the hematocrit (Hct) is 30–33.
Thrombopoietic Growth Factor			
oprelvekin (Neumega)	Stimulates bone marrow to produce platelets. Used to minimize platelet deficiency in patients on certain chemotherapy drugs.	Retention of water and sodium, dysrhythmias, severe allergic reactions, visual disturbances, dizziness, insomnia, dyspnea, oral candidiasis	Given by subcutaneous injection once a day for up to 21 days. Most patients receiving this drug experience side effects. Monitor heart rate and rhythm. Observe for signs of allergic reaction: rash, urticarial, flushing, fever, hypotension, chest pain, wheezing, dyspnea, edema of face and tongue. Do not administer if patient has a history of allergic reactions to oprelvekin.
romiplostim (Nplate) eltrombopag (Promacta)	Increase platelet production in patients with idiopathic thrombocytopenic purpura (ITP) eltrombopag (Promacta),	Arthralgia, dizziness, insomnia, pain in abdomen, shoulders, and extremities. Uncommon but serious: bone marrow fibrosis, hematologic malignancy, thromboembolic events. Eltrombopag: hepatotoxic	Romiplostim: weekly SUBQ injections with dosage based on platelet count. Discontinue if platelets exceed 400 × 10^9/L Eltrombopag: PO, rarely used.
plerixafor (Mozobil)	Increases HSCs before bone marrow ablation in non-Hodgkin lymphoma and multiple myeloma	Injection-site reactions, diarrhea, nausea, dizziness.	SUBQ. Given on specific schedule related to HSC harvest. Dosage reduced in patients with reduced renal function.
Leukopoietic growth factors: filgrastim (Neupogen) pegfilgrastim (Neulasta) sargramostim (Leukine)	Stimulate production of white blood cells to decrease risk of infection in patients on chemotherapy or having bone marrow transplantation	Diarrhea, weakness, rash, malaise, bone pain. Uncommon: pleural and pericardial effusion.	Routes and dosages specific to each drug. Schedule based on chemotherapy or bone marrow transplantation.
Drugs for Deficiency Anemias			
Oral iron preparations: ferrous iron salts (e.g., Feosol, Fer-In-Sol, Fergon, Ferro-Sequels, Aspartate)	Iron replacement	Constipation or diarrhea, black stools, mild nausea, heartburn. Can aggravate peptic ulcers, ulcerative colitis, and regional enteritis. Toxic in large amounts.	Give with food initially; then transition to between meals for best absorption. Give with food only if GI effects are intolerable. If the patient is taking liquid iron, dilute the drug and administer it through a straw to prevent the drug from staining the teeth.

Table 29.5 Drug Therapy: Drugs Used to Treat Disorders of the Hematologic System—cont'd

DRUG	USE AND ACTION	SIDE EFFECTS	NURSING INTERVENTIONS
A variety of parenteral preparations are available. Iron dextran is the only parenteral form approved for iron deficiency of all causes	Iron replacement when oral form is ineffective or infeasible.	Hypersensitivity reactions, brown skin discoloration at the injection site	Test dose the patient before starting treatment. IV preferred. Give intramuscular (IM) injections deeply in a large muscle mass using the Z-track technique. To give an injection using the Z-track technique, firmly pull the skin over the upper, outer quadrant of the buttock laterally. Insert the needle. Slowly inject the medication. Remove the needle and let go of the skin. Use single-dose vial without preservative for IV route: flush line with 10 ml of NS before and after iron dextran. Infuse iron dextran at rate no more than 1 mL (50 mg) per minute. Instruct patient to remain recumbent for 30–60 minutes. Monitor closely. Have epinephrine on hand.
Oral and parenteral: vitamin B_{12} (cyanocobalamin) Intranasal: cyanocobalamin (Nascobal)	Vitamin B_{12} replacement	Diarrhea, hypokalemia; itching, rash at injection site; RARELY heart failure, anaphylaxis	Given PO, intranasal, IM, or deep SUBQ injection. For patients with irreversible anemia, vitamin B_{12} must be given for the rest of the person's life. With intranasal preparation, no hot food for one hour before or after drug administration.
hydroxyurea (Droxia)	Prevention of sickle cell crisis	Nausea, vomiting, severe bone marrow suppression. Harm to a fetus; avoid during pregnancy.	Reinforce to the patient that this drug must be taken regularly to prevent sickle cell crises and that it is of no use once a crisis occurs. Monitor blood cell counts frequently.

GI, Gastrointestinal; *Hgb*, hemoglobin; *HSCs*, hematopoietic stem cells; *IV*, intravenous; *MI*, myocardial infarction, *NS*, normal saline; *PO*, orally; *SUBQ*, subcutaneous.
From Burchum JR, Rosenthal LD: *Lehne's pharmacology for nursing care*, ed 9, St. Louis, 2016, Elsevier.

Get Ready for the NCLEX® Examination!

Key Points

- The hematologic system includes the bone marrow, kidneys, liver, spleen, lymph system, and blood.
- A healthy adult has about 5 to 6 L of blood circulating through the body.
- Components of the blood are plasma, RBCs (erythrocytes), platelets (thrombocytes), clotting factors, and WBCs (leukocytes), proteins, electrolytes, hormones, and enzymes.
- Signs of hematologic abnormalities can include petechiae, purpura, and ecchymoses.
- The four major blood groups are A, B, AB, and O; each group may be Rh^- or Rh^+.
- People with type O^- blood are universal blood donors and people with type AB^+ blood are universal blood recipients.
- For an autologous transfusion, the patient's own blood is collected for administration when significant blood loss is expected during a procedure. This may be done when the patient has a rare blood type or religious objections to donor transfusions.
- Types of reactions that can occur when blood or blood components are transfused include hemolytic, anaphylactic, febrile, and circulatory overload.
- If the patient experiences back or chest pain, fever, chills, a decreased blood pressure, urticaria, wheezing, dyspnea, coughing, or blood in the urine during a blood transfusion, stop the transfusion immediately, keep the intravenous line open with normal saline, and notify the physician, nursing supervisor, and blood bank immediately.
- Depending on the type of reaction, the patient may be treated with oxygen, epinephrine, a corticosteroid, furosemide (Lasix), and/or antipyretics.
- Colony-stimulating factors such as erythropoietin (Epogen) and darbepoetin (Aranesp), stimulate the bone marrow to produce more RBCs, whereas oprelvekin (Neumega) stimulates the bone marrow to produce more platelets.

Additional Learning Resources

SG Go to your Study Guide for additional learning activities to help you master this chapter content.

Go to your Evolve website (http://evolve.elsevier.com/Linton/medsurg) for the following learning resources and much more:
- Fluid & Electrolyte Tutorial
- Review Questions for the NCLEX® Examination

Clinical Judgment and Next-Generation NCLEX® Examination-Style Questions

1. **If a person has no A or B antigens, what is their blood type?** ________________

   NCLEX Client Need: Health Promotion and Maintenance

2. **When inspecting a patient's skin, you notice multiple ecchymoses and petechiae. This should lead you to suspect a deficiency of which blood component?** ________________

   NCLEX Client Need: Physiological Integrity: Physiological Adaptation

3. **A patient says that he is a "universal donor." This means his blood type is ______________?**

   NCLEX Client Need: Health Maintenance and Promotion

4. **While receiving a blood transfusion, a patient complains of chest and back pain and chills. Which of the following should be your *initial* action?**
   1. Notify the blood bank
   2. Take vital signs
   3. Administer acetaminophen
   4. Stop the transfusion

   NCLEX Client Need: Physiological Integrity: Reduction of Risk Potential

5. **During the shift handoff, it is reported that a patient has orthostatic changes in vital signs. Based on this information, which action should the LVN/LPN take?**
   1. Tell the certified nursing assistant (CNA) to take vital signs hourly.
   2. Withhold cardiac drugs and contact the supervisor.
   3. Have the patient remain in bed until seen by the physician.
   4. Instruct the CNA to assist the patient to get up slowly from a lying or sitting position.

   NCLEX Client Need: Physiological Integrity: Reduction of Risk Potential

6. **The LVN/LPN notices that an older patient has small reddish pinpoint spots on her skin. What is the appropriate term for these lesions?**
   1. Ecchymoses
   2. Purpura
   3. Petechiae
   4. Bruises

   NCLEX Client Need: Health Promotion and Maintenance

7. **When a patient is scheduled for a bone marrow biopsy, what points should be included in the teaching plan? (Select all that apply.)**
   1. A local anesthetic will be injected before the biopsy puncture.
   2. Your physician may administer an intravenous sedative before the procedure.
   3. You may feel some pressure as the needle is inserted into the bone.
   4. You should consume no food or fluids for 8 hours before the procedure.
   5. The bone marrow specimen is usually obtained from the femur.

   NCLEX Client Need: Physiological Integrity: Reduction of Risk Potential

8. **A patient with a low platelet count is at risk for:**
   1. Stroke
   2. Bleeding
   3. Infection
   4. Blood clots

   NCLEX Client Need: Physiological Integrity: Reduction of Risk Potential

9. **A teenage boy is receiving chemotherapy that puts him at risk for bleeding. Which information should be included in the teaching plan? (Select all that apply.)**
   1. Shave with an electric razor.
   2. Take aspirin or ibuprofen for mild pain.
   3. Use a soft toothbrush.
   4. Avoid contact sports.
   5. Consume 2 L of liquids each day.

   NCLEX Client Need: Physiological Integrity: Reduction of Risk Potential

10. **Erythropoietin (Epogen) is ordered for a patient on renal dialysis. The purpose of this drug is to do which of the following?**
    1. Increase platelets in the blood.
    2. Decrease toxins in the blood.
    3. Increase RBCs.
    4. Decrease WBCs.

    NCLEX Client Need: Physiological Integrity: Reduction of Risk Potential

11. **What are the LVN/LPNs responsibilities when a patient is receiving a platelet transfusion?**
    1. Stay with the patient for the first 5 to 10 minutes to observe for any adverse reaction.
    2. Stop the infusion if the patient complains of headache.
    3. Assign a CNA to monitor the patient until the transfusion is completed.
    4. Monitor the urine output throughout the transfusion.

    NCLEX Client Need: Physiological Integrity: Reduction of Risk Potential

12. **Objective:** Describe nursing care for patients undergoing common therapeutic measures for disorders of the hematological system.

    NGN Item Type: Enhanced Hot Spot

    Cognitive Skill: Recognize Cues

    A patient who suffered multiple injuries in a motorcycle accident is to receive a unit of packed blood cells. His baseline vital signs are: BP 122/70, P 86 bpm, R 18/min, T 98°F. The nurse remains with him for 15 minutes after the infusion is started. Assessment data in this time period include the following:
    - Drowsy but responsive and oriented
    - Packed cells infusing at 10 mL/min
    - Tight feelings in chest
    - BP 140/110
    - Temperature 97°F
    - Hives and itching
    - Ringing in ears (tinnitus)

    Highlight the data that requires immediate action by the nurse.

Hematologic Disorders

30

http://evolve.elsevier.com/Linton/medsurg

Objectives

1. Describe the pathophysiology, signs and symptoms, medical diagnosis, and medical treatment for selected disorders of the hematologic system.
2. Assist in planning nursing care for a patient with a disorder of the hematologic system.

Key Terms

disseminated intravascular coagulation
hemolytic anemia
hemophilia
pernicious anemia
polycythemia vera
sickle cell anemia
thrombocytopenia

RED BLOOD CELL DISORDERS

Patients with red blood cell (RBC) disorders may have either too many RBCs (i.e., polycythemia vera) or too few RBCs (i.e., anemia). Having too few RBCs is more common. Because the main function of RBCs is oxygenation, anemia results in tissue hypoxia. Anemia can result from a major blood loss over a short period of time, too few RBCs being made, or increased RBC destruction. Acute blood loss, such as with an arterial rupture, dramatically changes the patient's hemodynamic status, requiring emergency intervention. Chronic RBC deficiency, such as with sickle cell disease, allows the body to compensate. Depending on whether the anemia is acute or chronic, the body compensates in three ways: (1) by increasing heart rate and respiratory rate to circulate the existing RBCs as quickly as possible with as much oxygen (O_2) as possible; (2) by redistributing the blood away from the skin, gastrointestinal (GI) tract, and kidneys to the brain and heart; and (3) by increasing the production of erythropoietin, the hormone that stimulates the bone marrow to produce more RBCs. Anemia can be a primary disease or a symptom of another disease. Descriptions of the different types of RBC disorders follow.

PRIMARY POLYCYTHEMIA (POLYCYTHEMIA VERA)

Primary polycythemia is a condition in which too many RBCs, WBCs, and platelets are produced. The increased number of cells makes the blood more viscous, or thicker, so that it does not circulate freely through the body. Symptoms of polycythemia vera include headache, dizziness, ringing in the ears, and blurred vision. Patients with this disorder may have a ruddy (reddish) complexion. They commonly report intense pruritus after a warm bath or shower. Hypertension is common. The liver and spleen may be enlarged. The condition puts the patient at risk for both thrombosis and hemorrhage. Depending on the severity of the condition, complications may include angina, heart failure, peptic ulcers, gout, and stroke. Treatment for polycythemia vera is to have 1 U of blood (250–500 mL) phlebotomized, or taken off, to keep the patient's hematocrit (Hct) normal. This procedure is usually done in the blood bank. A large-bore intravenous needle is inserted in the patient's antecubital vein and 1 U of blood is drawn (taken off). This is the same procedure used when a person goes to the blood bank to donate blood; however, the blood taken from the patient with polycythemia vera cannot be used as donor blood. Additional measures that may be indicated, depending on the severity of the condition and history of complications (thrombosis) include low-dose aspirin, hydroxyurea, and some anticancer drugs that suppress blood cell production.

APLASTIC ANEMIA

Aplastic anemia results from the complete failure of the bone marrow. The term *aplastic anemia* is misleading because patients with this condition have more than an extremely low RBC count; they also have extremely low white blood cell (WBC) counts and low platelet counts because their bone marrow is not making any of these cells. Certain drugs, such as streptomycin and chloramphenicol, as well as exposure to toxic chemicals or radiation, can cause bone marrow failure. Yet in many cases, the cause of a patient's bone marrow failure is never identified.

Signs and symptoms of aplastic anemia can include pallor, extreme fatigue, tachycardia, shortness of breath, hypotension, bruising, unusually prolonged or spontaneous bleeding, and frequent infections that do not resolve. In addition to abnormally low RBC, WBC, and platelet counts on blood tests, patients with aplastic anemia have abnormally low numbers of blood-making cells in their bone marrow.

Medical treatment for aplastic anemia focuses on identifying and treating the cause. Drugs that may cause the condition are discontinued. Transfusions are given to replace RBCs and platelets. Antibiotics or antivirals are given to prevent or treat infections. Immunosuppressant drugs may also be given to prevent the immune system from attacking healthy cells in the bone marrow. If the patient's bone marrow does not recover on its own, a bone marrow transplant may be considered if a donor can be found. The patient with aplastic anemia is critically ill and requires intensive nursing support. Care of the patient who is undergoing a bone marrow transplant is described in Chapter 31.

AUTOIMMUNE HEMOLYTIC ANEMIA

Several types of **hemolytic anemia** exist. The most common type is called warm autoimmune hemolytic anemia because the antibodies that destroy red blood cells are active at body temperature. With autoimmune hemolytic anemia, the bone marrow makes adequate amounts of the blood cells but they are destroyed once they are released into the circulation. Causes of autoimmune hemolytic anemia can include certain infections, drug reactions, and certain cancers. It has also been associated with systemic lupus erythematosus, rheumatoid arthritis, ulcerative colitis, and pregnancy. Hemolytic anemia of the newborn can occur after delivery if the mother has rhesus negative (Rh^-) blood and the baby has rhesus positive (Rh^+) blood. Blood transfusions can cause hemolytic anemia if lymphocytes in the transfused blood make antibodies against the person receiving the blood. Many times, the cause of the hemolytic anemia is never identified. Patients with hemolytic anemia have a positive result on a direct Coombs blood test. Among the complications are thromboembolic events.

Signs and symptoms of hemolytic anemia include pallor, extreme fatigue, tachycardia, shortness of breath, jaundice, and hypotension. Patients with hemolytic anemia usually have high bilirubin levels in their blood from all the RBCs being lysed (broken down).

Medical treatment of this type of anemia focuses on identifying and treating the cause. Blood transfusions may be needed to replace RBCs. Glucocorticoids and rituximab may be administered to the patient. The patient usually recovers in a few days to weeks, however, relapses are not uncommon.

Pharmacology Capsule

Rituximab is a monoclonal antibody that can cause fatal infusion-related reactions, especially with the first dose. Patients are usually premedicated with acetaminophen and an antihistamine and must be monitored closely.

IRON DEFICIENCY ANEMIA

Iron deficiency results from a diet too low in iron, from the body not absorbing enough iron from the GI tract, or from blood loss. Once iron stores are depleted and the body does not have enough iron to make adequate amounts of hemoglobin (Hgb), the result is iron deficiency anemia. Symptoms of this anemia include fatigue, weakness, headache, decreased exercise tolerance, irritability, depression, and pallor. Less common symptoms are pica (specifically ice craving) and restless leg syndrome. In severe cases, patients may have orthostatic changes in their heart rate and blood pressure. In addition to a low RBC count, a low Hgb value, and a low Hct, patients with iron deficiency anemia have a low serum iron level, a low ferritin level, and a high total iron-binding capacity (TIBC). Some older adults suffer from anemia because of poor eating habits and reduced absorption of oral iron. Other risk factors for iron deficiency anemia are gastric bypass surgery, celiac disease, atrophic gastritis, and *H. pylori* infection.

Options to treat iron deficiency anemia include oral iron supplements such as ferrous sulfate or intravenous iron preparations such as iron dextran and low molecular weight iron dextran (LMW ID). Although oral drugs are less expensive and easy to administer, some patients cannot tolerate the side effects. The effects include nausea, metallic taste, flatulence, constipation, diarrhea, epigastric distress, and/or vomiting. Chapter 29, Table 29.5 describes the nursing care of the patient taking iron supplements. Nurses caring for patients with iron deficiency anemia can suggest incorporating foods high in iron in the diet. Foods that are rich in iron include liver, oysters, red meats, fish, dried fruits, dried beans, peas, dark-green vegetables, and iron-enriched whole-grain breads and cereals (see the Nutrition Considerations box).

Nutrition Considerations

1. Inadequate dietary intake of iron or inadequate absorption of dietary iron causes iron deficiency anemia.
2. The lack of intrinsic factor, which is normally manufactured in the stomach, prevents the absorption of vitamin B_{12} and leads to pernicious anemia.

Pharmacology Capsule

Large doses of supplemental iron can be toxic to the gastrointestinal tract and eventually to the brain and liver if not recognized and treated. Caution patients not to exceed recommended dose and to keep the drug out of the reach of children.

PERNICIOUS ANEMIA (VITAMIN B_{12} ANEMIA)

Pernicious anemia occurs when a person does not absorb vitamin B_{12} from the stomach. The person may lack intrinsic factor, a substance made in the stomach that is essential for B_{12} absorption. The individual may have had a gastrectomy, or gastric bypass in which part or all of the stomach was surgically removed, and so cannot make intrinsic factor and therefore cannot absorb vitamin B_{12}. In addition to the fatigue and pallor commonly seen with all anemias, symptoms of pernicious anemia characteristically include weakness, a sore tongue, and numbness of the hands or feet. If severe, the patient may have jaundice, ataxia, and cognitive impairment. Pernicious anemia is treated by prescribing vitamin B_{12}. If the patient has neurologic symptoms, a monthly intramuscular injection of vitamin B_{12} (cyanocobalamin) is needed. Other patients may be prescribed large doses of oral vitamin B_{12}. Table 29.5 in Chapter 29 describes the nursing care of patients receiving vitamin B_{12}.

SICKLE CELL ANEMIA

Sickle cell anemia is a chronic inherited disease characterized by abnormal hemoglobin that alters the shape of RBCs, causing them to become stiff and sickle shaped (Fig. 30.1). These misshapen blood cells are much more fragile than normal RBCs, having a life span of only 10 to 20 days. These abnormally shaped, sickled cells can become stuck in the small capillaries of the body, obstructing blood flow (a vaso-obstructive event). Also, the spleen breaks down the abnormal cells leading to anemia.

Sickle cell anemia occurs almost exclusively in Black Americans. Some 8% of Black Americans carry the genetic trait for sickle cell anemia. Because sickle cell anemia is carried on a recessive gene, a person must inherit the gene from the mother and father to actually have the disease. A person with the trait for sickle cell on only one gene experiences only mild symptoms, or none at all. Newborn screening for sickle cell hemoglobin (HbS) can be done to identify infants with sickle cell disease and to educate parents about the disease and prevention of crises.

Symptoms of sickle cell anemia include persistently low red blood cell (RBC) counts, fatigue, and jaundice. The chronically low RBC counts can cause the heart to enlarge (cardiomegaly) and beat faster to oxygenate the body's tissues. A sickle cell crisis occurs when the sickled cells become stuck in larger blood vessels of the body, obstructing blood flow and causing severe pain.

Clinical Manifestations of Sickle Cell Crisis

Various stressors can trigger a sickle cell crisis. They include dehydration, infection, overexertion, cold weather changes, excessive alcohol consumption, and smoking. Symptoms vary depending on where circulation is blocked by the sickled RBCs. Commonly during a sickle cell crisis, circulation to the chest, abdomen, bones, joints, bone marrow, brain, or penis may be compromised. With circulation obstructed, tissue hypoxia occurs, causing severe pain. Patients in a sickle cell crisis often have a fever, either because infection precipitated the crisis or as part of the inflammatory response to tissue hypoxia.

Medical Diagnosis of Sickle Cell Disease

A variety of blood studies are used to diagnose sickle cell disease and to determine the specific type. Patients with known sickle cell disease who complain of severe pain are suspected of being in crisis. No test exists to determine that a patient is in sickle cell crisis. Rather, physicians use clinical judgment to make the diagnosis. Crises can last anywhere from 1 to 10 days. Some patients experience crises every few weeks, whereas other patients can go months without experiencing painful episodes. Radiographs and scans of the painful area are usually taken to evaluate for bleeding.

Medical Treatment of the Patient With Sickle Cell Disease

The only cure for sickle cell disease is a hematopoietic stem cell transplant which, at this time, is limited to

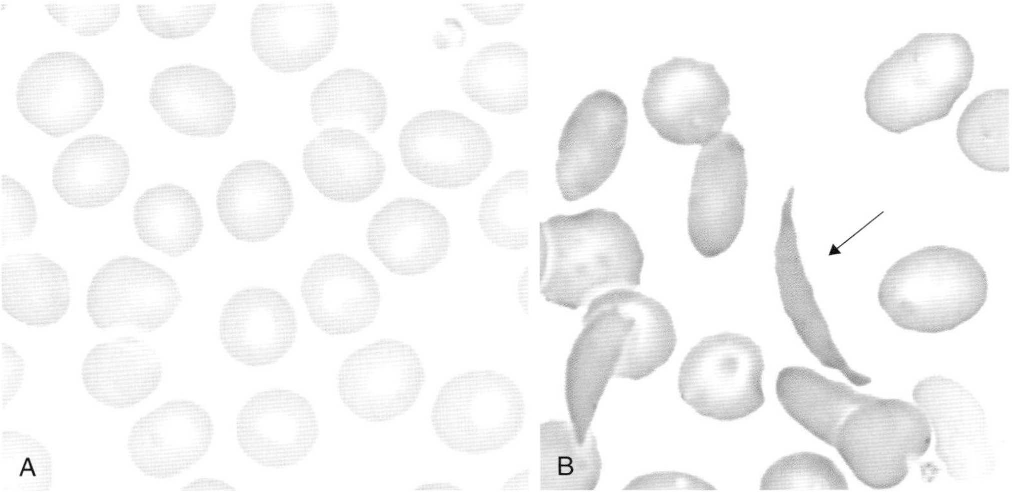

Fig. 30.1 Comparison of (A) normal red blood cells and (B) sickled cells (*arrow*). (From Carr JH, Rodak BF: *Clinical hematology atlas*, ed 3, St. Louis, 2009, Saunders.)

children. Hydroxyurea can be prescribed as a preventive treatment for patients who experience frequent crises. The drug stimulates the production of a certain type of Hgb that is resistant to sickling. Patients with sickle cell disease who regularly take hydroxyurea experience fewer crises. However, once a patient is in crisis, hydroxyurea does not work quickly enough to reduce either the severity or the duration of the crisis. Table 29.5 in Chapter 29 describes the nursing care of patients receiving hydroxyurea.

Medical treatment for patients experiencing a sickle cell crisis is symptomatic. The physician usually prescribes intravenous fluids and pain medication. Aggressive intravenous hydration helps the kidneys to clear the metabolic wastes from ruptured RBCs. The pain can be very severe, and the patient needs adequate pain relief during these episodes, even if they last for several days. Intravenous opioids are commonly prescribed for pain relief. Patients with sickle cell disease can become addicted to opioids. Therefore physicians try to transition the patient quickly from intravenous opioids to oral opioids to nonopioid pain relievers as the crisis resolves. RBC transfusions may be prescribed to correct the anemia and help the body to oxygenate tissues. Although O_2 therapy is often prescribed, it is of little benefit in reversing the crisis.

◆ NURSING CARE OF THE PATIENT IN SICKLE CELL CRISIS

Patients in sickle cell crisis have specialized needs beyond treatment of the simple anemia (see the Nursing Care Plan: Patient in Sickle Cell Crisis box).

Nursing Care Plan Patient in Sickle Cell Crisis

FOCUSED ASSESSMENT

Health History

A 19-year-old Black American woman was diagnosed with sickle cell anemia at age 12 years. She has been in stable health until 3 days ago, when she complained of nausea and began to have diarrhea and vomiting. She has taken only soup and cola beverages since that time. When she began to complain of severe pain in her abdomen, she was brought to the emergency department by her mother, who suspected sickle cell crisis.

Physical Examination

Vital signs: blood pressure 110/56 mm Hg, pulse 106 beats per minute, respiration 24 breaths per minute, temperature 102° F (38.9° C) measured orally. Oral mucosa dry. Skin dry and warm to touch. Breath sounds clear to auscultation. Abdomen soft but tender to light palpation. Bowel sounds hyperactive in all four quadrants. No bladder distention. Mild joint enlargement noted in both knees.

Patient Problems	Goals and Outcome Criteria	Interventions
Acute pain related to sickle cell crisis	The patient states that pain has been relieved or reduced significantly (4 or less on pain scale) and appears relaxed.	Administer analgesics as prescribed. Assess the effects and notify the physician if pain is not relieved. Have the patient rate her pain (0 = no pain, 10 = worst pain) before and after medication administration. Use the distraction technique. Respond to calls quickly. Reassure the patient.
Anxiety related to pain and hospitalization	The patient states that anxiety is reduced and appears calm.	Respond quickly to the patient's needs. Check on her often. Assign a consistent caregiver. Listen and use attention and touch to convey concern.
Potential for injury related to orthostatic hypotension	The patient experiences no injuries or falls caused by dizziness.	Assist the patient to get out of bed when permitted. Have her sit on the side of the bed and exercise her legs before rising. Check the patient's blood pressure in lying, sitting, and standing positions to detect orthostatic hypotension. Advise her to sit and lower her head if she feels dizzy.
Potential for fluid volume deficit related to inadequate intake and excess loss of fluids	The patient is adequately hydrated and has a consistent intake of 4 to 6 L of fluid daily. In addition, she has moist oral tissues and normal urine specific gravity.	Administer intravenous fluids as ordered. Teach the patient the importance of fluid intake. Weigh the patient daily to assess any change in fluid status. Monitor her fluid intake and output and note urine characteristics.
Ineffective self-care management related to lack of knowledge of disease process and self-care	The patient accurately describes the disease process and implications of self-care measures.	Assess what the patient knows about sickle cell disease. Initiate teaching when the crisis has resolved. Make sure she knows to avoid smoking, alcohol, and high altitudes. Emphasize the need to maintain good hydration (4–6 L of fluids each day) and to keep regular medical appointments.

CRITICAL THINKING QUESTIONS

1. Why would genetic counseling be recommended for a young woman with sickle cell disease?
2. Describe the order in which you should implement the listed interventions for this patient.

Focused Assessment

Obtain a complete description of the pain that the patient in sickle cell crisis is experiencing. Note the location, intensity, duration, and precipitating events. Measure vital signs every 4 hours. Be especially alert for a fever, which may indicate an infection that precipitated the crisis. Investigate any symptoms of an infection, such as sore throat, cough, abnormal breath sounds, dysuria, or diarrhea. In addition, monitor the patient for signs and symptoms of dehydration, such as concentrated urine, low blood pressure, or poor skin turgor, which may have precipitated the crisis.

Patient Problems, Goals, and Outcome Criteria: Sickle Cell Crisis

Problems	Goals and Outcome Criteria
Acute pain related to sickle cell crisis	Pain relief: patient states pain has been relieved or reduced to 4 or less on the pain scale, relaxed manner
Anxiety related to pain and hospitalization	Reduced anxiety: patient states anxiety is reduced, calm manner
Potential for injury related to orthostatic hypotension	Absence of injury: no falls caused by dizziness
Potential for fluid volume deficit related to inadequate intake or excess loss of fluids	Adequate hydration: consistent intake of 4 to 6 L of fluid daily
Ineffective self-care related to lack of knowledge of the disease process and management	Effective management of condition: patient accurately describes disease process and implications for self-care measures

Interventions

Acute pain. Give pain medications as prescribed. Usually an intravenous opioid is prescribed. Initially it is not unusual for patients to need large amounts of medication to control their pain. One option for medication delivery is patient-controlled analgesia. Closely monitor the patient's pain level and medication use. Good documentation can contribute to effective pain management. Keeping a flow sheet of patient reports of pain on a 10-point scale can be helpful, especially if different nurses care for the patient throughout the day. A *0* represents no pain and a *10* represents the worst pain that a patient has ever experienced. The patient report of pain, coupled with the amount of pain medication they are receiving, can guide you and the physician in determining the appropriate type and amount of pain medication for the patient. A detailed discussion of pain management strategies is presented in Chapter 8.

Anxiety. Sickle cell crises can be extremely frightening to a patient, especially because of the severe pain that accompanies these crises. Patients fear not obtaining adequate pain relief. The unpredictability of the timing and severity of the crises can be especially frustrating to patients. Provide consistent care to the patient in sickle cell crisis to establish a trusting relationship. In addition, listening closely to the patient can reduce anxiety. Once the patient is discharged from the hospital, they can contact one of the many support groups available for patients with sickle cell disease and their families. Patients should be encouraged to attend meetings of these groups so that they can better cope with this chronic disease.

Potential for injury. The primary treatment for anemia in sickle cell disease is RBC transfusions. Nursing considerations in administering blood transfusions are outlined earlier in the chapter. Nursing actions that should be taken when patients are anemic are outlined in Chapter 29, Box 29.4. Procedures for administering an RBC transfusion are outlined in Chapter 29, Box 29.6.

Potential for fluid volume deficit. Administer intravenous fluids as prescribed and keep records of fluid intake and output management. Measure weight daily to assess gross fluid status and encourage the patient to drink 4 to 6 L of fluids each day to maintain adequate hydration.

Ineffective self-care management. When the patient is not in crisis, they should be taught about the disease (see the Patient Teaching box). Help the patient to identify stressors that bring on a crisis and strategies to avoid these stressors. Encourage the patient not to smoke or drink large amounts of alcoholic beverages, because these are two common stressors that can bring on a crisis. Traveling to high altitudes where less O_2 exists can bring on an attack, so caution the patient about vacationing at high altitudes. Drinking 4 to 6 L of nonalcoholic fluids a day helps to maintain adequate hydration. Regular medical follow-up is extremely important in keeping the patient with sickle cell disease out of a crisis. Genetic counseling can be done with people who have the sickle cell gene to inform them of the risk of passing on the trait or disease to their children. With this information, some people choose not to have their own children and risk passing on this painful, life-threatening disease. Several resources are available for patients, families, and health care providers. An example is the Sickle Cell Disease Association of America (https://www.sicklecelldisease.org). This and other such organizations provide excellent free literature on sickle cell disease and can help to locate groups in specific regions of the country.

Patient Teaching

Sickle Cell Anemia

- To prevent crises, maintain good hydration and avoid smoking, alcoholic beverages, and high altitudes.
- Drink 4 to 6 L of fluid each day to maintain adequate hydration.
- Genetic counseling can help you with decisions about having children by exploring the risk of passing on sickle cell trait or disease.
- You can get additional information from the Sickle Cell Disease Association of America.

Put On Your Thinking Cap!

How would a high fluid intake decrease the risk of sickle cell crisis?

Put On Your Thinking Cap!

Why would immunizations be particularly important for people with sickle cell disease?

COAGULATION DISORDERS

Coagulation disorders can result from a platelet abnormality or from a clotting factor deficiency.

THROMBOCYTOPENIA

Thrombocytopenia is a condition in which a person has too few platelets circulating in the blood. This may be because not enough platelets are being made in the bone marrow or because too many platelets are being destroyed in circulation.

Although thrombocytopenia has many causes, the major cause is treatment of cancer with chemotherapy or radiation therapy. Chemotherapy and radiation therapy kill rapidly dividing cells. Unfortunately, the therapy cannot tell the difference between rapidly dividing cancer cells and rapidly dividing normal cells like those that produce platelets. In patients treated with chemotherapy or radiation therapy, thrombocytopenia can be expected 10 to 14 days after treatment and lasts until the bone marrow is able to make more platelets, which is usually 1 week.

Two examples of thrombocytopenia resulting from too many platelets being either destroyed or consumed are idiopathic thrombocytopenic purpura (ITP) and thrombotic thrombocytopenic purpura (TTP). Both of these disorders are abnormal immunologic processes that result in thrombocytopenia. ITP and TTP are discussed in more detail in Chapter 32.

Symptoms of thrombocytopenia include petechiae and purpura, gingival bleeding, epistaxis (nosebleeds), or any other unusual or prolonged bleeding. The diagnosis is made with blood tests and possibly a bone marrow biopsy. Treatment for thrombocytopenia is to treat or stop the causative factor. If the cause is cancer chemotherapy or radiation therapy, platelet transfusions may be prescribed. Nursing actions for the patient who is at risk for injury from bleeding are outlined in Chapter 29, Box 29.5. Procedures for administration of a platelet transfusion are outlined in Chapter 29, Box 29.7.

ACUTE DISSEMINATED INTRAVASCULAR COAGULATION

Disseminated intravascular coagulation (DIC) is a hypercoagulable state, meaning that blood clotting is abnormally increased. DIC occurs when an imbalance exists between the processes of coagulation and fibrinolysis (breakdown of fibrin). Overstimulation of the normal coagulation cascade results in depletion of clotting factors leading to simultaneous thrombosis and hemorrhage. DIC is always secondary to another pathologic process, such as overwhelming sepsis, shock, major trauma, crush injuries, burns, cancer, acute tumor lysis syndrome, or obstetric complications such as abruptio placentae or fetal demise (death). Coagulation occurs at so many sites in the body that eventually all available platelets and clotting factors are depleted and uncontrolled hemorrhage results.

Blood tests that help to diagnose DIC include the prothrombin time (PT) and activated thromboplastin time (aPTT), fibrinogen degradation products (FDPs), and D-dimers (a product of fibrin breakdown). A patient with DIC has an increased PT/aPTT, FDPs, D-dimers, and decreased fibrinogen.

Medical treatment focuses on correcting the underlying cause, providing hemodynamic and ventilatory support as needed, and aggressive hydration. If bleeding is severe, blood component replacement therapy consisting of red blood cell and platelet transfusions, fresh frozen plasma, and clotting factors may be prescribed. However, the specific treatments vary with the severity of the condition and the individual patient's blood component results. Heparin may be prescribed to interrupt the DIC cycle and allow the body to replenish platelets and clotting factors. However, heparin therapy is controversial because some physicians believe that it only makes the bleeding worse. Nursing actions for the patient who is at risk for injury from bleeding are outlined in Chapter 29, Box 29.5.

Put On Your Thinking Cap!

Explain how heparin could be helpful for a patient with **disseminated intravascular coagulation**.

CHRONIC DISSEMINATED INTRAVASCULAR COAGULATION

Whereas acute DIC is life threatening, a chronic form may occur when the pathologic process progresses to a lesser degree which allows the body to compensate. Most often the precipitating factor is advanced malignancy of the pancreas, stomach, ovaries, or brain.

The patient with chronic DIC is more likely to develop venous or arterial thromboembolic events instead of bleeding. The patient may have no symptoms, normal clotting times, and mild or absent thrombocytopenia. Heparin may be prescribed in selected situations. If the patient is not bleeding, the only treatment may be focused on the underlying condition.

HEMOPHILIA

Hemophilia is a genetic disease in which the affected person lacks some of the blood-clotting factors normally found in plasma. The incidence of hemophilia is 1 case per 5000 to 30,000 persons, depending on the type of hemophilia. In hemophilia A, factor VIII is missing, whereas in hemophilia B, factor IX is missing. Hemophilia A has a much higher incidence than hemophilia B. The disease may be mild, moderate, or severe, depending on the level of clotting factor VIII or IX, bleeding tendency and frequency, and the occurrence of joint bleeding.

Because the trait is carried on the X chromosome, women carry the trait and can pass it on to their sons, who manifest the disease. However, approximately 30% of cases arise from a spontaneous mutation in patients without any family history of hemophilia. Whether the trait is inherited or spontaneous, it is rare for women to have this disease.

Clinical Manifestations

Uncontrollable bleeding is the hallmark of hemophilia. Bleeding generally occurs after some sort of trauma; however, bleeding can also occur spontaneously for no clear reason. Most commonly, bleeding occurs into the joints, causing swelling and severe pain. Bleeding can also occur into the skin; from the mouth, gums, and lips; and from the GI tract. Because any surgical procedure puts the patient at great risk for bleeding, a complete preoperative evaluation must be done. In addition, the availability of replacement factors for transfusion must be confirmed (see the Cultural Considerations box).

Cultural Considerations

What Does Culture Have to Do With Blood Transfusions?

Members of some religious groups do not accept blood transfusions from other people. Autotransfusion may be an acceptable alternative.

Medical Diagnosis

The diagnosis of hemophilia is made by measuring factors VIII and IX in the blood. In addition, the aPTT is prolonged in people with hemophilia.

Medical Treatment

No cure exists for hemophilia. Medical treatment for patients experiencing a bleeding episode is symptomatic. The physician usually prescribes transfusions of fresh-frozen plasma (FFP) or cryoprecipitate, or both. Patients with hemophilia A need factor VIII, which is found in FFP and cryoprecipitate. Patients with hemophilia B need factor IX, which is found in FFP (Tables 30.1 and Tables 30.2). A number of commercial factor VIII and factor IX replacement products are available that can be used on a regular basis to prevent acute bleeding episodes. They also are given on a PRN (as needed) basis to stop ongoing or excessive bleeding. Desmopressin may effectively stop bleeding in

Table 30.1 Selected Products for Patients With Hemophilia A

SELECTED FACTOR VIII PRODUCTS FOR PATIENTS WITH HEMOPHILIA A	
Factor VIII Standard Half-Life Products	**Factor VIII Longer-Lasting Products**
• Advate	• Adynovate
• Hemofil	• Afstyla
• Kogenate FS	• Eloctate
• Koate	• Esperoct
• Kovaltry	• Jivi
• Novoeight	
• Nuwiq	
• Recombinate	
• Xyntha	
Drugs for Patients With Factor VIII Inhibitors[a]	
• Activated Factor VII (Factor VIIa)	
• Anti-Inhibitor Coagulant Complex (AICC)	
• Factor VII Concentrate	
• Porcine Factor VIII	
Pituitary Hormone That Increases Release of Factor VIII	
• Intravenous desmopressin (DDAVP)	
• Intranasal desmopressin (Stimate)	

[a]Patients receiving factor VIII can develop antibodies that render replacement factors ineffective.

From Burchum JR, Rosenthal LD: *Lehne's pharmacology for nursing care*, ed 10, St. Louis, MO, 2019, Elsevier. Hoots WK, Shapiro AD: Hemophilia A and B: routine management including prophylaxis. *UpToDate*, September 23, 2020. Retrieved January 16, 2021 from www.uptodate.com.

Table 30.2 Selected Products for Patients With Hemophilia B

FACTOR IX PRODUCTS FOR PREVENTION AND TREATMENT OF BLEEDING	
Standard Half-Life Products	**Longer-Lasting Products**
• AlphaNine SD	• Alprolix
• BeneFIX	• Idelvion
• Ixinity	• Rebinyn
• Mononine	
• Rixubis	
DRUGS FOR PATIENTS WITH FACTOR IX INHIBITORS[a]	
• Activated Factor VII (Factor VIIa)	
• Anti-Inhibitor Coagulant Complex (AICC)	

[a]Patients receiving factor IX can develop antibodies that render replacement factors ineffective.

From Burchum JR, Rosenthal LD: *Lehne's pharmacology for nursing care*, ed 10, St. Louis, MO, 2019, Elsevier. Hoots WK, Shapiro AD: Hemophilia A and B: routine management including prophylaxis. *UpToDate*, September 23, 2020. Retrieved January 16, 2021 from www.uptodate.com.

persons with mild hemophilia A. Desmopressin works by promoting the release of factor VIII from the vascular epithelium. Unfortunately, some patients develop antibodies against the replacement factors. Drugs are available for hemophilia A patients who have antibodies against the replacement factors, but few options exist for those with hemophilia B. Tables 30.1 and 30.2 list the products used to treat hemophilia. RBC transfusions are frequently used to replace blood lost from the profuse bleeding to which hemophiliacs are prone.

The pain associated with bleeding episodes can be very severe. The patient needs adequate pain relief during these episodes, even if they last several days. Intravenous opioids are commonly prescribed for pain relief. Because patients with hemophilia can become addicted to opioids, pain must be assessed carefully. Usually physicians try to transition the patient quickly from intravenous opioids to oral opioids to nonopioid pain relievers as the crisis resolves.

Coordinated Care

Helping the Certified Nursing Assistant to Care for Patients With Blood Disorders

- Instruct the certified nursing assistant (CNA) to allow periods of rest for patients with anemia (low red blood cell counts).
- Show the CNA how to handle patients with thrombocytopenia (low platelet counts) gently to prevent trauma and bleeding.
- Stress the importance of maintaining accurate records of oral fluid intake of patients in sickle cell crisis.

◆ NURSING CARE OF THE PATIENT WITH HEMOPHILIA

Focused Assessment

Assess the patient for bleeding and pain, noting what measures have stopped the bleeding and relieved the pain in the past. In addition, monitor vital signs and urine output.

Patient Problems, Goals, and Outcome Criteria: Hemophilia

Problems	Goals and Outcome Criteria
Potential for injury related to bleeding	Cessation of bleeding: no visible bleeding, stable vital signs
Acute pain related to bleeding into closed spaces, creating pressure on nerves	Pain relief: patient states pain is relieved, relaxed manner
Ineffective self-care management related to lack of knowledge about the disease process and management	Effective management of condition: patient accurately describes condition and demonstrates self-care measures

Interventions

Potential for injury. The primary treatment to control bleeding in hemophilia is to transfuse FFP, cryoprecipitate, or both (see the Coordinated Care box). Nursing considerations in administering these products are outlined in Chapter 29, Table 29.3. Bleeding precautions that should be taken when patients have hemophilia are similar to bleeding precautions taken when patients are thrombocytopenic (see Chapter 29, Box 29.5).

Acute pain. Administer pain medications as prescribed. If the patient is experiencing a great deal of pain, patient-controlled analgesia may be appropriate. Closely monitor the patient's pain level on a scale of 0 to 10. Keeping a flow sheet of patient reports of pain on a 10-point scale can be helpful, especially if different nurses care for the patient throughout the day. The patient's report of pain, coupled with the amount of pain medication they are receiving, can guide the nurse and physician in selecting the appropriate type and amount of pain medication. A detailed discussion of pain management is presented in Chapter 8.

Ineffective self-care management. People with hemophilia bleed with even the smallest blow or abrasion (see the Patient Teaching box). Patients and their families should be taught to prevent injury and to safeguard their environment against accidents as much as possible. Some patients and families are taught to administer the replacement concentrate at home so that, should an injury occur, prompt treatment can be initiated and blood loss minimized. Genetic counseling can be done with people who have the hemophilia gene to inform them of the risk of passing on the disease to their children. With this information, some people choose not to have their own children and risk passing on this painful, life-threatening disease. The National Hemophilia Foundation; (www.hemophilia.org) provides information and support to patients with hemophilia and their families. Other resources are the Designated Hemophilia Treatment Centers (HTCs). The Centers for Disease Control and Prevention lists these centers on its website. (www.cdc.org)

Patient Teaching

Hemophilia

- Protect yourself from injuries by avoiding activities that could result in trauma.
- Know the emergency treatment of bleeding episodes: first-aid measures (apply pressure, immobilize and elevate affected part if possible), seek medical attention, administer replacement concentrate (if prescribed).

Do not take aspirin or NSAIDs such as ibuprofen as they increase the risk of bleeding.

Get Ready for the NCLEX® Examination!

Key Points

- Anemia is a deficiency of RBCs or Hgb that may be caused by blood loss, an iron-deficient diet, vitamin B_{12} deficiency, bone marrow failure, or genetic abnormalities.
- Pernicious anemia is caused by the inability to absorb adequate vitamin B_{12} owing to a lack of intrinsic factor in the stomach.
- Aplastic anemia is caused by bone marrow failure, resulting in deficient RBCs, WBCs, and platelets.
- Sickle cell anemia is an incurable genetic condition in which RBCs can become abnormally sickle shaped so that they rupture easily and can obstruct capillaries.
- Sickle cell crisis occurs when blood flow is obstructed. Patients in crisis can experience severe pain.
- Patient problems during sickle cell crisis focus on the patient's acute pain, anxiety, potential for injury, potential for fluid volume deficit, and ineffective self-care management.
- Thrombocytopenia is a deficiency of platelets that can lead to excessive or prolonged bleeding.
- Hemophilia is an incurable genetic disease in which some of the factors needed for blood clotting are absent.
- Patient problems for the patient with hemophilia include the patient's potential for injury, acute pain, and ineffective self-care management.

Additional Learning Resources

SG Go to your Study Guide for additional learning activities to help you master this chapter content.

Go to your Evolve website (http://evolve.elsevier.com/Linton/medsurg) for the following learning resources and much more:

- Fluid & Electrolyte Tutorial
- Review Questions for the NCLEX® Examination

Clinical Judgment and Next-Generation NCLEX® Examination-Style Questions

1. **The body compensates for anemia with which of the following mechanisms? (Select all that apply.)**
   1. Increasing blood flow to the brain and heart
   2. Increasing the heart rate
   3. Decreasing the respiratory rate
   4. Suppressing the production of erythropoietin
   5. Reducing blood flow from the skin and intestinal tract

   NCLEX Client Need: Physiological Integrity: Physiological Adaptation

2. **The nurse is inspecting a patient's skin and notices multiple ecchymoses and petechiae. This should lead the nurse to suspect a deficiency of which blood component?**
   1. RBCs
   2. WBCs
   3. Platelets
   4. Proteins

   NCLEX Client Need: Physiological Integrity: Physiological Adaptation

3. **A patient tells the LVN/LPN that he has been diagnosed with pernicious anemia. The patient states he is taking iron tablets rather than going to the clinic for prescribed monthly injections. Which nurse response is most appropriate?**
   1. "The iron tablets should manage your condition very well."
   2. "Ask your care provider whether you can take oral vitamin B_{12}."
   3. "People with pernicious anemia are unable to absorb iron."
   4. "Try taking a multivitamin that includes iron and vitamin B_{12}."

   NCLEX Client Need: Physiological Integrity: Pharmacological Therapies

4. **Which of the following nursing interventions are appropriate for a patient with a low RBC count? (Select all that apply.)**
   1. Avoid taking rectal temperatures and using suppositories
   2. Allow for rest between periods of activity
   3. Encourage increased fluids and dietary fiber
   4. Do not allow fresh flowers in the room
   5. Provide extra blankets as needed to maintain warmth

   NCLEX Client Need: Physiological Integrity: Physiological Adaptation

5. **A patient's laboratory report reflects a deficiency of RBCs, WBCs, and platelets. The nurse recognizes that these findings are characteristic of which condition?**
   1. Aplastic anemia
   2. Hemolytic anemia
   3. Sickle cell anemia
   4. Iron deficiency anemia

   NCLEX Client Need: Physiological Integrity: Physiological Adaptation

6. **The nurse is teaching the parents of a child with sickle cell disease about the condition. Which statement would explain the circumstances that lead to sickle cell crisis?**
   1. Cells lack sufficient Hgb to transport O_2.
   2. Sickled cells are unable to transport adequate O_2.
   3. Sickled cells form clumps that obstruct blood flow.
   4. The bone marrow stops producing RBCs.

   NCLEX Client Need: Physiological Integrity: Physiological Adaptation

7. **Objective: Assist in planning nursing care for a patient with sickle cell disease.**

   NGN Item Type: Enhanced Hot Spot

   Cognitive skill: Recognize Cues

   A patient with sickle cell anemia is seen in the hematology clinic. The nurse collects data to help assess the patient's status. Highlight the data that require follow-up by the nurse.
   - Daily fluid intake approximately 2 L
   - Oral temperature of 100.6°F
   - Walks 2 miles daily
   - Adheres to a vegetarian diet
   - Sleeps 8 to 9 hours per night

- Smokes half a pack of cigarettes each day
- Preparing to go on a ski trip

"Highlight the data that require follow-up by the nurse"

NCLEX Client Need: Physiological Integrity: Physiological Adaptation

8. **A patient is being admitted in the acute phase of a sickle cell crisis. The nurse anticipates that pain management usually requires which of the following?**
   1. Nonsteroidal antiinflammatory drugs
   2. Physical therapy
   3. Nerve blocks
   4. Opioid analgesics

   NCLEX Client Need: Physiological Integrity: Pharmacological Therapies

9. **Overstimulation of the normal blood-clotting process can result in which of the following?**
   1. DIC
   2. ITP
   3. TTP
   4. Hemophilia

   NCLEX Client Need: Physiological Integrity: Physiological Adaptation

10. **Hemophilia A is treated with which factor?**

    ____

    NCLEX Client Need: Physiological Integrity: Pharmacological Therapies

Immunologic System Introduction

31

http://evolve.elsevier.com/Linton/medsurg

Objectives

1. List the components of the immune system and describe their role in innate immunity, acquired immunity, and tolerance.
2. List the data to be collected when a patient has a disorder of the immune system.
3. Describe the tests and procedures used to diagnose disorders of the immune system and nursing considerations for each.
4. Describe the nursing care for patients undergoing common therapeutic measures for disorders of the immune system.
5. For common drugs used to treat immunologic disorders, describe the general actions, side effects, and nursing implications.

Key Terms

allogeneic bone marrow transplant
allograft
autologous bone marrow transplant
cytokines
eicosanoids
graft-versus-host disease
immunoglobulin (ĭ-MŪ-nō-GLŎB-ū-lĭn)
macrophages
syngeneic bone marrow transplantation

The immune system is the body's defense network against infection. It is an inherently complex system that recognizes, isolates, and quickly destroys pathogens and foreign antigens and mutated cells. Disorders of the immune system leave the patient susceptible to overwhelming, life-threatening infections. The nurse plays an important role in helping to assess, plan, and manage the care of patients with these disorders.

ANATOMY AND PHYSIOLOGY OF THE IMMUNE SYSTEM

ANATOMIC STRUCTURES AND COMPONENTS OF THE IMMUNE SYSTEM

Bone Marrow

The bone marrow is the spongy center of the bones where the white blood cells (WBCs) are made. The marrow of all bones produces these cells; however, in adults, the majority of WBCs are produced in the vertebrae, ribs, sternum, skull, pelvis, and iliac crests, the femurs.

Stem Cells

Stem cells are called *progenitor cells*, or *precursor cells*, because they are capable of developing into the various WBCs, red blood cells (RBCs), or platelets (Fig. 31.1). Although the majority of stem cells are located in the bone marrow, some stem cells circulate in the blood.

White Blood Cells (Leukocytes)

The bone marrow produces WBCs. Five major types of WBCs exist: (1) neutrophils, (2) monocytes, (3) eosinophils, (4) basophils, and (5) lymphocytes. Each type of WBC combats certain types of microorganisms. Normally, WBCs identify and destroy foreign antigens or proteins by ingesting them. Because this process destroys the WBCs themselves, the normal life span for a WBC is only a few hours to a few days. Neutrophils may live as little as 6 hours. Other cells called *macrophages* clean up the WBC debris. If the dead WBCs build up faster than the macrophages can clean them up, pus is formed. This is why pus is a classic sign of infection and should be reported to a nurse or a physician immediately and carefully monitored.

Neutrophils. Neutrophils fight bacterial infections. They are the most numerous of the WBCs, comprising approximately 60% of all WBCs. These cells are known by many names, including *polymorphonuclear neutrophils (PMNs, polys)*, *neuts*, *granulocytes (grans)*, or *segmented neutrophils (segs)*. The bone marrow is capable of producing huge numbers of neutrophils to fight infection.

Monocytes and macrophages. Once released from the bone marrow, monocytes circulate in the bloodstream for approximately 1 day before leaving the peripheral circulation and entering tissue. When monocytes enter

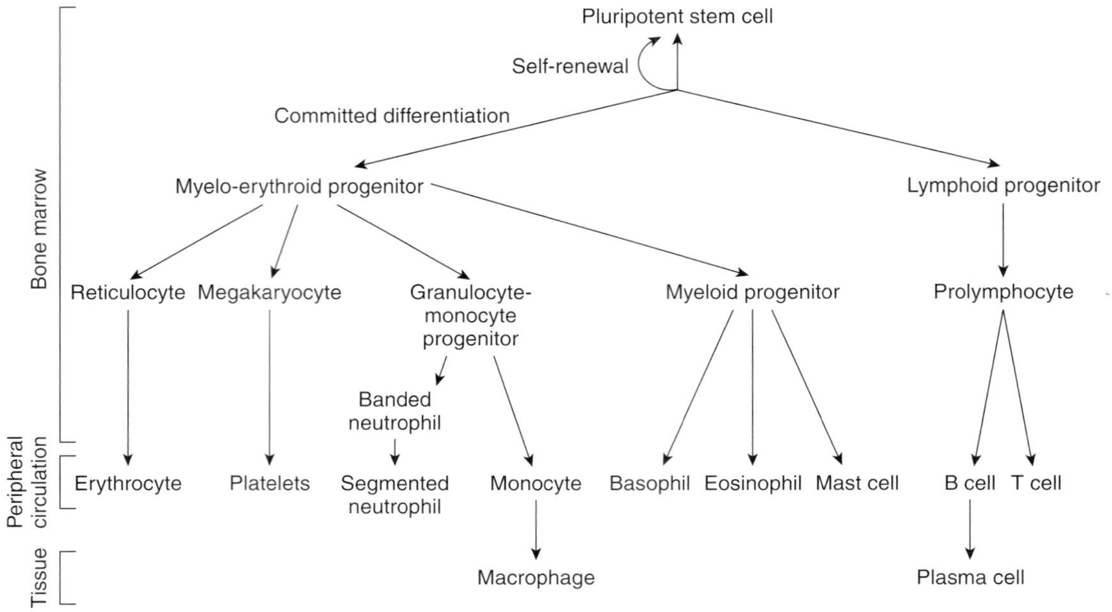

Fig. 31.1 Maturation of cells constituting the hematologic and immune systems. (From Young-McCaughan S, Jennings BM: Hematologic and immunologic systems. In: Alspach JG, editor: *Core curriculum for critical care nursing*, ed 5, Philadelphia, 1998, Saunders.)

tissue, they are called **macrophages**. Some macrophages move throughout the body, whereas others stay in one particular tissue monitoring for microorganisms. Unlike neutrophils, which are destroyed during phagocytosis, macrophages can ingest many foreign antigens and survive months to years.

Eosinophils. Eosinophils combat parasitic infections. They are also associated with allergic reactions and other inflammatory processes.

Basophils. Basophils can initiate a massive inflammatory response that quickly brings other WBCs to the site of infection. Basophils work in conjunction with immunoglobulin E (IgE). When IgE identifies a foreign antigen, it triggers basophils to release histamine from cell vesicles located in the basophils. Histamine is a potent vasodilator that increases blood circulation to the site, quickly bringing other WBCs to the site of infection.

Mast Cells. Like basophils, mast cells also store histamine in cell vesicles that can be released by IgE. Even though mast cells progenitors are made by the bone marrow, they do not become mast cells until they leave the blood and reside in body tissues. The other white blood cells are mature when produced and circulate in the blood.

B Lymphocytes (B cells). B cells manufacture antigen-binding proteins, called **immunoglobulin** (Ig), on their cell membrane. When the B cell Ig binds with a particular antigen, the B cell is stimulated to produce plasma cells and memory B cells. Plasma cells are antibody factories that immediately produce large amounts of Ig. Memory B cells go into a resting state but can be reactivated quickly to produce plasma cells and antibodies if exposed to the same antigen in the future.

Once the Ig is released from the membrane of either the B cell or the plasma cell, it is called an *antibody*. Four major types of antibodies exist. IgM is the first Ig to be secreted during the primary immune response to an antigen. IgG is secreted during the secondary immune response and is more specific to a particular antigen. IgA is present in secretions such as mucus and mother's milk. IgE attaches to the cell membranes of basophils and mast cells, where it triggers the cell to release histamine.

T Lymphocytes (T cells). Two major types of T lymphocytes exist: T helper (T_H) cells and T cytotoxic (T_C) cells. T_H cells are also called *CD4 cells* because of the protein complex CD4 found on their cell membranes. When T_H cells come in contact with foreign antigens, they secrete cytokines that activate other components of the immune system to facilitate the body's immune response. These are the cells that can become infected with the human immunodeficiency virus (HIV). T_C cells are also called *CD8 cells* because of the protein complex CD8 found on their cell membranes. When T_C cells come in contact with foreign antigens, they can directly destroy the invader.

Cytokines

Cytokines are hormones secreted by cells to signal other cells. Examples of cytokines include interferon, interleukin, tumor necrosis factor (TNF), granulocyte-macrophage colony-stimulating factor (GM-CSF), granulocyte colony-stimulating factor (G-CSF), and erythropoietin (EPO).

Eicosanoids

Eicosanoids are a class of fatty acids that regulate blood vessel vasodilation, temperature elevation, WBC

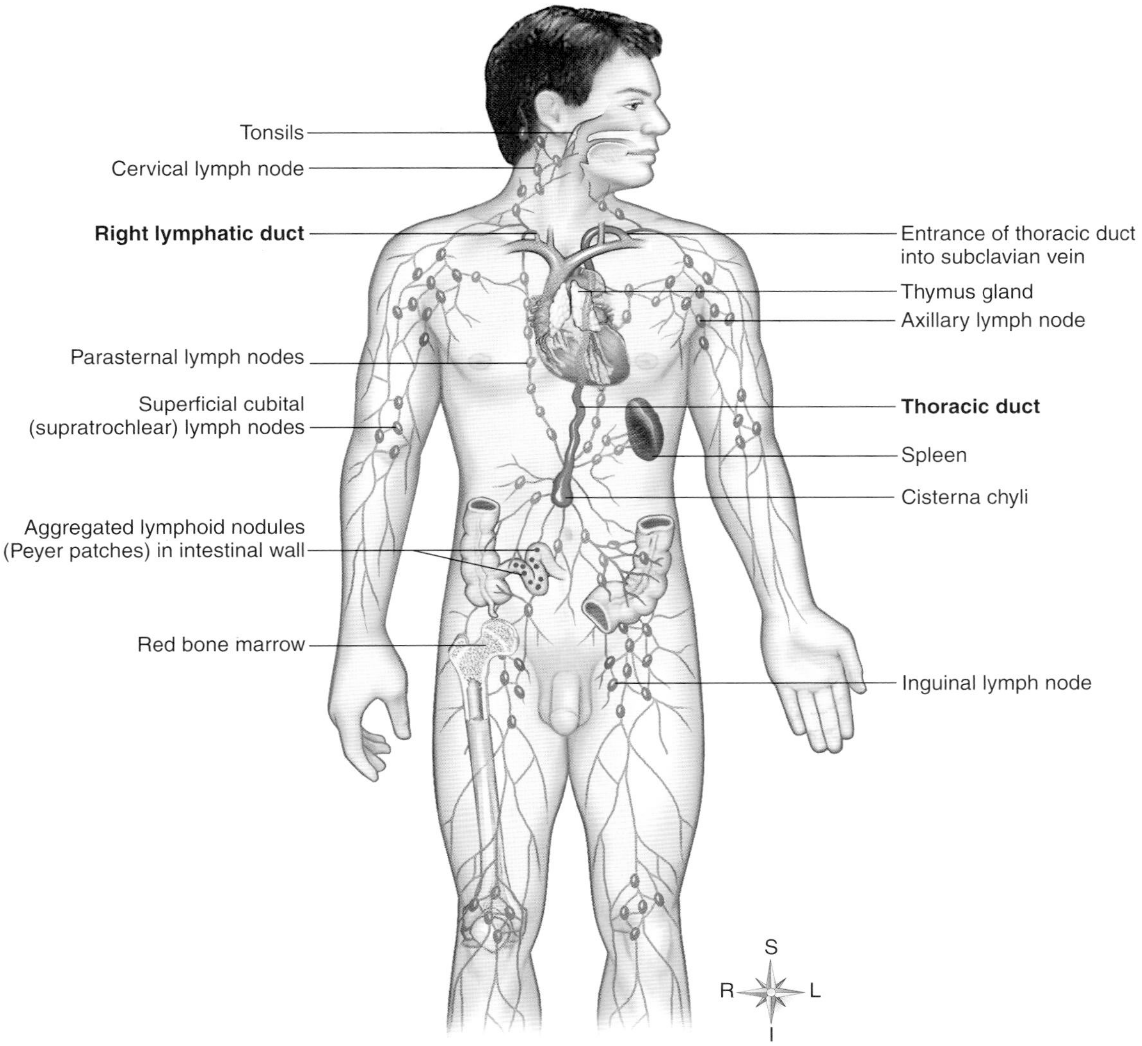

Fig. 31.2 Diagram of the lymphatic system. (From Thibodeau GA, Patton KT: *Anatomy and physiology*, ed 8, St. Louis, 2013, Mosby.)

activation, and other physiologic processes involved in immunity. Many commonly prescribed drugs, such as nonsteroidal antiinflammatory drugs (NSAIDs), disrupt eicosanoid production, thereby affecting a person's ability to mount an immunologic response.

Thymus

The thymus is a lymphoid organ located in the upper chest below the thyroid. Early in life, certain WBCs, called *lymphocytes*, migrate from the bone marrow where they are produced to the thymus where they mature into T lymphocytes, or T cells. Mature T lymphocytes are then released into circulation. After puberty, the T cell population has been maximized. These mature T cells continue to live and function throughout a person's life. At this point, the thymus stops growing and eventually shrinks because it is no longer needed to mature T cells.

Lymph, Lymphatics, and Lymph Nodes

When blood flows through the capillary beds to deliver oxygen (O_2) and pick up carbon dioxide (CO_2), not all of the plasma returns to the veins to be recirculated. The lymphatic system is a network of open-ended tubes—separate from the blood circulation system—that collects the plasma left behind in the tissues and returns it to the venous system. In addition, various WBCs that travel through tissues and organs to monitor for infection reenter the blood circulation via the lymphatic system. This mixture of plasma and cells is known as *lymph fluid.* Lymph fluid is propelled along the lymphatic system by the normal contraction of skeletal muscles. One-way valves located in the lymphatic vessels prevent the lymph fluid from pooling in the periphery. The lymphatic vessels empty into the venous system through the right lymphatic duct of the right subclavian vein and the thoracic duct of the left subclavian vein. Fig. 31.2 shows a diagram of the lymphatic system. The lymphatic vessels can be damaged during surgery or following radiation therapy. As a result, lymph fluid can build up in the tissues distal to the affected area, resulting in lymphedema of the extremity.

Lymph nodes are small patches of lymphatic tissue located along the lymphatic system that filter microorganisms from the lymph fluid before it is returned to the bloodstream. Lymph nodes are located throughout the body, as shown in Fig. 31.2. Individual lymph nodes can become swollen with infection and also with some cancers. During surgery for cancer, the surgeon will usually biopsy nearby lymph nodes and have the pathologist check the specimens to see if the cancer has spread. The nodes closer to the surface of the body in the neck, under the arm, and in the groin can be palpated when they are swollen. Usually, lymph nodes deeper in the body cannot be palpated but can be visualized with computed tomography (CT) if they are larger than 2 cm.

Liver

The liver is located in the upper right quadrant of the abdomen. One of the many functions of the liver is to filter microorganisms from the blood so that macrophages can destroy them.

Spleen

The spleen is located in the upper left quadrant of the abdomen. Like the lymph nodes, the spleen filters microorganisms from the blood. Once trapped in the spleen, microorganisms are destroyed by the WBCs that reside in the spleen.

Under some circumstances, the spleen is surgically removed. Trauma from an accident can rupture the victim's spleen, necessitating removal. Anyone without a spleen is at increased risk for certain kinds of infections such as pneumococcal infections. If possible, patients should receive a Pneumovax vaccine before undergoing splenectomy so that the body can form its own antibodies against pneumococcal bacteria. Vaccinations are not always possible for the individual undergoing an emergency splenectomy.

Peyer Patches

Peyer patches are lymphoid tissue found in the small intestine where it transitions into the large intestine. Macrophages and both B and T lymphocytes found in this lymphoid tissue attach any foreign microorganisms that attempt to enter the bloodstream and could cause infection.

PHYSIOLOGIC FUNCTIONS OF THE IMMUNE SYSTEM

Innate Immunity

Innate immunity is operational at all times, whether or not a pathogen is present. At birth, innate immunologic defense systems are immediately functional. Innate immunologic systems include anatomic and physiologic barriers, inflammatory response, and the ability of certain cells to phagocytose foreign invaders.

Anatomic and physiologic barriers. The skin and mucous membranes are the body's first line of defense, acting as a protective covering and secreting substances that inhibit the growth of pathogens. Sweat glands secrete lysozyme, an antimicrobial enzyme. The skin and the mucosa of the gastrointestinal (GI) and genitourinary systems are acidic, which inhibits the growth of many pathogenic organisms. Secretions from the respiratory and GI tracts contain the antibody IgA, as well as phagocytes. Skin and mucous membrane surfaces are colonized by normal bacterial flora, which prevent pathogens from attaching and gaining access to the body. Normal flora is a mixture of organisms regularly found at any anatomic site. In addition, coughing and sneezing, peristalsis in the GI tract, emptying the bladder, and sloughing of dead skin cells all serve to remove microorganisms from the body, thus preventing their invasion and overgrowth.

Inflammation. The body initially responds to an injury or infection by dilating the capillary bed and increasing the capillary permeability of the affected area. This brings WBCs to the site and allows them to enter the tissue to attack microorganisms. This multistep process is called *inflammation* and is recognized by rubor (redness), tumor (swelling), calor (heat), and dolor (pain) at the site of injury or infection.

Phagocytosis. Phagocytosis is the process of ingesting and digesting invading pathogens, dead cells, and cellular debris. Neutrophils, monocytes, and macrophages are capable of phagocytosis and are sometimes called *phagocytes.*

Acquired Immunity

Whereas innate immunity fights any type of invader and is operational at all times, acquired immunity is specific to a particular pathogen and is activated only when needed. The two types of acquired immunity are antibody mediated and cell mediated.

Antibody-mediated immunity. An antibody-mediated immune response is initiated when the IgM on the surface of B lymphocytes detects a foreign antigen. With the help of T_H cells, the B lymphocytes secrete additional IgM and differentiate to produce antibody-secreting plasma cells and memory B cells. The newly made plasma cells can produce and secrete large amounts of IgM antibody. When antibodies bind to an antigen, they do not actually destroy the pathogen, but they make the antigen readily recognizable to neutrophils, monocytes, and macrophages, which can phagocytose the pathogen. If, in the future, this same pathogen tries to reenter the body, the memory B cells are triggered to immediately produce large amounts of IgG antibody. IgG is similar to IgM except that it is more specific to one particular pathogen, based on previous experience with that same pathogen.

Acquired antibody immunity can be active or passive. Active acquired immunity occurs when a

Box 31.1 Age-Related Changes in the Immunologic System

- Bone marrow: less productive in older persons
- Lymphatic tissue: tissue shrinks; lymph nodes are smaller and fewer
- Despite changes, immunologic function is generally adequate unless a person is unusually stressed by trauma, a chronic infection, or treatment for cancer

person synthesizes their own antibodies in response to a pathogen. A person is exhibiting active acquired immunity when they manufacture antibodies in response to an infection or a vaccination. Active acquired immunity is permanent. Passive acquired immunity occurs when an antibody produced by one person or an animal is transferred to another person. For example, IgA antibodies in mother's milk confer passive immunity to breast-fed babies. Another example of passive acquired immunity is the gamma globulin that may be given to a person exposed to hepatitis. Gamma globulin contains IgG antibodies that help to destroy the hepatitis virus. Passive acquired immunity lasts only 1 to 2 months after the antibodies have been received.

Cell-mediated immunity. Antibody-mediated immune responses are aimed primarily at invading microorganisms such as bacteria. In contrast, cell-mediated immunity is aimed primarily at intracellular defects caused by viruses and cancer. Cell-mediated immunity is also responsible for delayed hypersensitivity reactions and rejection of transplanted tissue. T_C cells are the primary component of cell-mediated immunity. When T_C cells recognize foreign antigens in cells, they secrete cytotoxic substances that destroy the defective cells. Unfortunately, a transplanted tissue graft, such as a kidney transplant or a heart transplant, may be recognized by the organ recipient's immune system as foreign and is attacked by T_C cells in this same way.

Tolerance

As part of initiating an immunologic response, the immune system must be able to recognize its own proteins and not mount an immune response against itself. This process of self-recognition occurs as part of normal neonatal growth and development. Autoimmune diseases occur when a breakdown of tolerance takes place. The immune system inappropriately identifies its own proteins as foreign and mounts a response to destroy these self-proteins. Examples of autoimmune diseases include idiopathic thrombocytopenic purpura (ITP), thrombotic thrombocytopenic purpura (TTP), acute rheumatic fever, type 1 diabetes mellitus, systemic lupus erythematosus (SLE), rheumatoid arthritis, multiple sclerosis, Graves' disease, and Hashimoto thyroiditis (Box 31.1).

Box 31.2 Assessment of a Patient With Disorders of the Immune System

HEALTH HISTORY

Present Health

Frequent or persistent infections, prolonged bleeding, easy bruising, chronic fatigue

Past Health History

Cancer or prior treatment for cancer, human immunodeficiency virus (HIV) infection, history of splenectomy, history of organ transplant, placement of an indwelling venous access device indicating that the patient needed long-term venous access, recent infections, current medications (including over-the-counter [OTC] medications, recent changes in medication, herbal products), recent immunizations

Family History

Cancer, death of a family member at a young age for reasons other than trauma

Review of Systems

Integumentary: Rash, breaks in the skin, ulcers, lesions, or enlarged lymph nodes; red, swollen, or painful areas

Neurologic: Weakness, lethargy, malaise, restlessness, apprehension, headache

Respiratory: Sinus pain, dyspnea, cough

Gastrointestinal: Mouth ulcerations, sore throat, pain with swallowing, pain with defecation, unplanned weight loss or weight gain, diarrhea

Genitourinary: Pain or burning with urination

Musculoskeletal: Pain in bones or joints

Endocrine: Fatigue

Functional Assessment

Occupation and hobbies, changes in ability to do activities of daily living (ADL), roles at home and work, self-concept, activities and exercise, sleep and rest, nutrition, interpersonal relationships, stressors, coping style

Physical Examination

Height and Weight

Vital Signs: Fever, tachycardia, tachypnea, hypotension

General Survey: Responsiveness, mood, expression, posture

Skin: Color

Head and Neck: Enlarged, swollen, or draining areas; enlarged lymph nodes

Thorax: Enlarged lymph nodes, respiratory rate, breath sounds, heart rate

Abdomen: Organ enlargement, enlarged lymph nodes

NURSING ASSESSMENT OF THE PATIENT WITH AN IMMUNOLOGIC DISORDER

Data collected by the licensed vocational nurse/licensed practical nurse (LVN/LPN) contributes to the complete nursing assessment as described here. Many subtle findings in the assessment can suggest changes in the patient's immune system that should be reported to the registered nurse (RN) or the physician for evaluation. Box 31.2 outlines the nursing assessment of patients with disorders of the immune system.

HEALTH HISTORY

Reason for Seeking Care

Pay special attention to the patient who remarks that they have frequent or persistent infections, bleed for a long time when cut, bruise easily, or have chronic fatigue. These symptoms may reflect an underlying immunologic disorder.

Present Health

Document details of the reported symptoms including onset, severity, and precipitating and aggravating factors. Note any treatment measures that have been tried and the effects of those measures. Also ask about recent exposure to infectious conditions.

Past Health History

A patient could have an underlying immunologic problem if they report any of the following: cancer or prior treatment for cancer; HIV infection; history of splenectomy; history of organ transplant; or placement of an indwelling venous access device, indicating that the patient needed long-term venous access. Medications the patient is currently using or a recent change in medication may suggest an underlying immunologic problem. It is important to find out what over-the-counter (OTC) medications (including herbal products) the patient uses, because many of these products contain aspirin or NSAIDs, which may disrupt immunologic function. Ask the patient about any recent changes in medications and any recent immunizations.

Family History

Note any family history of immunologic disorders such as cancer. Death of a family member at a young age for reasons other than trauma may indicate a genetic immunologic disorder.

Review of Systems

The review of systems is aimed at finding out what symptoms the patient has been experiencing over the past weeks or months. These symptoms might provide clues as to what specific medical disorder the patient may now have. The primary symptom of an immunologic disorder is infection. The patient should be carefully questioned about any reddened, swollen, painful, or unusually warm areas that might indicate an infectious process. Ask about fever, chills, or night sweats. Night sweats can occur when the patient's temperature rises at night but the patient does not awaken until the temperature falls, causing sweating. Night sweats can occur normally in women undergoing menopause. However, night sweats can also be a symptom of infection (e.g., tuberculosis, malaria), leukemia (cancer of the WBCs), or lymphoma (cancer of the lymph nodes).

Begin the review of systems with the integument. Ask about any red, swollen, or painful areas (which could be sites of infection) and any breaks in the skin, ulcers, lesions, or enlarged lymph nodes (which could indicate a site of infection). Relevant data about the neurologic system include weakness, lethargy, malaise, restlessness, apprehension, or headache, which could indicate a central nervous system (CNS) infection. In relation to the respiratory system, ask about sinus pain, dyspnea, or cough, which could indicate an infection. If the cough is productive, ask the patient to describe the sputum. When assessing the GI system, ask about sore throat, any pain with swallowing, and any pain with defecation. Ask about any unplanned weight loss or weight gain and characteristics and consistency of bowel movements. When reviewing the genitourinary system, ask about any pain or burning with urination, any change in the frequency of urination, and any blood in or discoloration of the urine. Finally, when assessing the endocrine system, ask about any unusual fatigue.

Functional Assessment

Patients newly diagnosed with an immunologic disorder may not experience dramatic changes in their functional abilities. However, many immunologic disorders are chronic conditions that the patient has lived with—and been treated for—for many years.

Occupation and hobbies. Knowing a patient's job and hobbies can alert the nurse to unusual chemical exposures. Because various chemicals can affect the bone marrow and blood, note any recent chemical exposure. For example, someone who builds models for a hobby may be exposed to unusual glues or paints that may affect the blood count.

Self-concept. The patient's self-concept can be assessed by exploring the patient's feeling about themselves. For many people, one's self-concept depends on one's job. If the patient is unable to work because of an immunologic disorder, their self-concept can be adversely affected. In addition, medical insurance is often contingent on employment. Loss of medical insurance and the need to go on state or federal assistance can diminish a patient's self-concept. Another factor that can adversely affect the patient's self-concept is a change in appearance because of the disease or the treatment.

Activity and exercise. Document the current activity level as well as the effects of the disease and treatment on the patient's usual pattern of activity and exercise. Ask about the layout of the patient's home, specifically the location of bathrooms in relation to living areas and bedrooms. Ask if the patient must climb stairs to enter the home or get to a second floor; stair climbing can quickly tire a patient with an immunologic disorder. Also ask what the patient does for recreation and whether these activities can still be done during times of decreased energy.

Sleep and rest. Note the number of continuous hours the patient sleeps every night as well as whether any sleeping aids are used, what interrupts the patient's sleep, and whether the patient naps during the day.

Nutrition. Ask the patient to describe their usual diet and any recent changes in appetite or weight. Identify factors that might be interfering with eating, such as nausea, vomiting, and taste changes (see the Nutrition Considerations box). Depression and loneliness can adversely affect a patient's nutritional status. Limited financial resources can also limit a patient's ability to maintain a nutritious diet.

Nutrition Considerations

1. Because food contains microorganisms, patients with low white blood cell (WBC) counts are often discouraged from eating raw fruits and vegetables and from drinking milk. However, it is not clear that this actually reduces infection in these patients.
2. Patients with human immunodeficiency virus (HIV) require high calorie and nutrient intake to combat wasting.

Interpersonal relationships. Explore the patient's view of themselves as a husband or wife, partner, father or mother, son or daughter, friend, and co-worker. Discuss the effects of the disease on these relationships and the patient's roles in the home. Ask what household chores the patient is responsible for doing as well as who does the shopping, cooking, and cleaning. If the patient has children who need care, ask whether the patient is able to perform the usual child care activities.

Coping and stress. Ask what worries the patient has and how they usually deal with stress. Explore sources of support, which might include family, support groups, and spiritual beliefs and practices.

Perception of health. Discuss the patient's view of their own health and health practices. This might include measures taken to prevent complications from disease and keeping regular medical appointments.

PHYSICAL EXAMINATION

The physical examination begins with measurement of vital signs and height and weight. Be alert for fever, tachycardia, tachypnea, and hypotension.

General Survey

Note the patient's responsiveness, mood, expression, and posture. Throughout the examination, carefully inspect and describe any reddened, swollen, or painful areas the patient identifies.

Skin

Inspect the patient's skin from head to toe, noting the general color, texture, turgor, temperature, and integrity. Also palpate for any swollen or painful areas.

Head and Neck

When examining the eyes, ears, nose, mouth, and throat, it is important to note any enlarged, swollen, or draining areas that might indicate an infection. Examples might be swollen, draining sinuses; a canker sore in the mouth; or enlarged tonsils with exudate. The examiner with advanced skills may palpate the neck for enlarged lymph nodes.

Thorax

The examiner with advanced skills may palpate the axilla for enlarged lymph nodes.

Lungs. Document the patient's respiratory rate and effort and auscultate for wheezing, crackles, or rhonchi. Patients with a respiratory tract infection may have abnormal breath sounds or a cough.

Heart and vascular system. Record the patient's heart rate and blood pressure. Patients with a severe infection may be tachycardic or hypotensive.

Abdomen

The examiner with advanced skills may palpate the abdomen for tenderness. The liver and spleen can become enlarged with blood cell disorders, causing abdominal fullness and tenderness. The advanced practice examiner may palpate the patient's groin for enlarged lymph nodes.

DIAGNOSTIC TESTS AND PROCEDURES

Various blood studies are used to screen the function of the patient's immunologic system. Blood studies, as well as other tests and procedures done to diagnose disorders of the immune system, are described in Tables 31.1 and 31.2. The laboratory performing the test should provide normal values for the various blood tests. Ranges of normal values can be found in various textbooks of laboratory and diagnostic tests.

BLOOD TESTS

The complete blood count (CBC) is a common blood test done in most laboratories; it reports the total number of WBCs as well as what percentage of the total number of WBCs are neutrophils, monocytes, eosinophils, basophils, and lymphocytes. Both the total number of WBCs in the body and the differential, or percentage of each of the specific types of WBCs in the body, are evaluated. Normal WBC counts range between 5000 and 10,000 WBCs per cubic millimeter (mm^3) of blood. The majority of the WBCs (60%) are neutrophils. See Table 29.1 for additional details. Physicians and nurses are interested primarily in the number of neutrophils because these are the cells that fight bacterial infections. To calculate the absolute neutrophil count (ANC), one multiplies the percentage of

Table 31.1 Diagnostic Tests and Procedures: Laboratory Studies to Evaluate the Immune System

General Interventions: Check your agency procedure manual for diagnostic tests and procedures. Always tell the patient what to expect when tests are ordered and whether fasting is necessary. Wear gloves for exposure to body fluids. Before a venipuncture, tell the patient to expect a brief sharp pain as the needle goes through the skin. Afterward, have the patient apply pressure for 1 minute; elevate the arm and maintain pressure for 5–10 minutes if the patient's blood clotting is impaired. Apply dressing for at least 1 hour.

Different blood tests are collected in different laboratory tubes containing specific reagents or no reagents at all. Usually the tubes have color-coded tops. Be sure to collect the blood in the blood tube specific for the blood test ordered. Usually each institution's laboratory publishes a manual identifying what colored tube to use for each blood test.

TEST/STUDY	PURPOSE AND PROCEDURE	PATIENT PREPARATION	POSTPROCEDURE NURSING CARE
Blood tests (CBC, ANA, LE prep)	Used to measure various blood components.	Choose the correct blood tube in which to collect the blood.	Standard venipuncture care.
HIV serologic and virologic tests	Serologic tests, virologic tests, immunoassays, and urine tests can detect antigens and antibodies associated with HIV infection. Initial testing is followed by confirmatory testing. Home testing kits are available.	Nonfasting. Recognize patient's concerns about test results. Written patient consent may be required.	In addition to standard care, follow-up is critical. Patient confidentiality must be maintained. A positive HIV test is frightening, and the patient will need support and education.
Blood cultures	Used to detect and identify microorganisms in the blood. Specimen should be drawn by a trained person.	If possible, the sample should be collected before starting antibiotics or shortly before the next dose. Inform laboratory if patient is on antibiotics. Vacuum blood culture containers with culture media must be used; one for aerobic and another for anaerobic cultures. Cleanse the vein site with an antiseptic solution (alcoholic chlorhexidine) and allow to dry. Also prepare the tops of the blood culture bottles with 70% isopropyl alcohol and allow to dry for 30 to 60 seconds. Do not touch the draw site except with sterile gloves. Draw at least 10 mL of blood for each culture container. Draw a second specimen from a different site. Send the specimens to the laboratory immediately.	Standard venipuncture care. Preliminary results may be available in 24 hours; final results take 48 to 72 hours. Anaerobic organisms may take longer. Tell the patient that results may take up to 4 days.
Sputum cultures	Used to detect and identify microorganisms in the sputum.	Collect specimen before starting antibiotics. Inform laboratory if patient is already on antibiotics. Have the patient rinse mouth and collect sputum in a sterile cup the next time they cough, at least 1 hour after eating. Caution the patient not to collect saliva. Sputum comes from the lungs with coughing. A minimum of 1 tsp is needed. Send the specimen to the laboratory immediately.	No special care required. Inform patient that final results usually take 48 hours. However, cultures for fungus take 6 to 8 weeks.
Urine cultures	Used to detect and identify microorganisms in the urine. Midstream ("clean catch") specimen is preferred. Other options are aspiration from port of indwelling catheter, and catheterization.	Give the patient wipes and a sterile container. Explain how to obtain a clean catch specimen. Assist as needed. If catheterization is necessary, follow procedure described in Chapter 41. If the patient has an indwelling catheter, obtain the sample via the catheter port per agency policy. Send the specimen to the laboratory immediately.	No special care is required after the procedure. If catheterization is used, advise patient that a burning sensation may occur with urination following procedure.
Stool cultures	Used to detect and identify microorganisms in the stool.	Wear gloves and use a sterile tongue blade to collect a specimen from a clean bedpan. Transfer the specimen, including mucus and blood streaks, to a sterile container. Send the specimen to the laboratory immediately.	No special care is required after the procedure.

ANA, Antinuclear antibody; *CBC*, complete blood count; *HIV*, human immunodeficiency virus; *IFA*, immunofluorescence assay; *LE prep*, lupus erythematosus preparation, *tsp*, tea spoon.
From Pagana KD, Pagana TJ: *Mosby's manual of diagnostic and laboratory tests*, ed 5, St. Louis, 2014, Elsevier.

Table 31.2 Diagnostic Tests and Procedures: Special Procedures to Evaluate the Immune System

General Interventions: Check your agency procedure manual for diagnostic tests and procedures. Always tell the patient what to expect when tests are ordered and whether fasting is required. Before nuclear scans, report allergies to any radionuclides (technetium-99m, gallium, thallium, iodine). Record the patient's age and weight. Following procedures with radionuclides, special precautions are indicated for 12 hours. Patients should wash their hands after elimination. The toilet should be flushed several times after using. Soiled clothing should be washed separately from other items.

TEST/STUDY	PURPOSE AND PROCEDURE	PATIENT PREPARATION	POSTPROCEDURE NURSING CARE
Lymphangiography (LAG). Contrast enhanced study.	LAG demonstrates the anatomy of the lymphatic vessels and nodes, and detects the site of chyle leak. In diagnostic radiology, a 1- to 2-inch incision is made on the dorsum of each foot or hand. The lymphatic vessels are cannulated and dye is injected. Radiographs are taken as the dye moves up the extremities. Additional scans are done after 12 to 24 hours.	Explain the purpose and procedure to the patient and obtain signed consent. Ask the patient about any allergies to contrast media. Nonfasting. A local anesthetic will be injected to numb the top of the feet or hands. Incisions may stain blue from the dye. The procedure takes approximately 3 hours. Additional scans are made 12 to 24 hours later.	Check vital signs every 4 hours (q4h) for 48 hours. Keep the incisions clean and dry after the procedure. Elevation of the legs or arms may be ordered. Sutures may be in left place for 5 to 7 days.
Computed tomography (CT) of the spleen. Various types of CT exist for various purposes.	The CT can reveal splenic trauma, tumors, hematomas, and cysts. It is a radiographic procedure that may include enhanced imaging with a radioactive dye injected into a vein. The amount of dye taken up by the spleen is measured.	Report any allergies to dye (contrast media), iodine, shellfish. Nonfasting. An IV line is used to inject the dye. The procedure takes less than 30 minutes.	Encourage fluids to promote excretion of contrast media. Watch for delayed reaction to the dye 2 to 6 hours after procedure: dyspnea, rash, tachycardia, and hives; treated with steroids and antihistamines.
Positron Emission Tomography (PET scan)	Can reveal lymphoma. An IV radionuclide is given followed by scanning.	No fluids or food for 4 hours before test. Avoid caffeine, alcohol, and tobacco for 24 hours before PET scan. The scan takes 40 to 90 minutes. Empty the bladder before the test begins.	Drink fluids to remove the radioactive chemicals. Change from lying to standing position slowly to avoid postural hypotension.
Skin tests	Skin testing is done to detect sensitivity to allergens (e.g., pollen), to determine sensitivity to pathogens (e.g., tuberculin), and to assess cell-mediated immune functions. After cleaning the inner side of the patient's forearm, the test material is injected intradermally using a 26- or 27-gauge needle and tuberculin syringe.	Tell the patient that they will feel a needlestick as the needle goes through the skin.	No special care is required after the procedure. Tell the patient to return in 2 to 3 days to determine the results of the testing. Swelling at the site of injection indicates that the body's cell-mediated immune system is functioning. Instruct patient not to take any antihistamine or other allergy medicine unless instructed by physician as these can interfere with test results.

IV, Intravenous.
From Pagana KD, Pagana TJ: *Mosby's manual of diagnostic and laboratory tests*, ed 5, St. Louis, 2014, Elsevier. Sax PE. Acute and early HIV infection: Clinical manifestations. *UpToDate*. November 11, 2020. Retrieved January 20, 2021 from www.uptodate.com.

neutrophils indicated on the differential of the CBC by the total number of WBCs. See Box 31.3 for a sample calculation.

Other blood tests are specific to the diagnosis of a particular disease. The antinuclear antibody (ANA) test detects antibodies in the blood that may be indicative of SLE or other autoimmune disorders. A lupus erythematosus preparation (LE prep) is a blood test more specific to SLE.

HIV Testing

A number of blood tests are available to diagnose HIV infection. The CDC classifies these as *nucleic acid tests* (NATS), *antigen/antibody tests*, and *antibody tests*. NATS is very expensive and not commonly used for screening. Antigen/antibody tests detect both antigens and antibodies, and antibody tests (enzyme-linked immunoassay [ELISA]) detect only antibodies against HIV. Most home tests and rapid tests are antibody tests. The virus is undetectable immediately after infection, so it is a challenge to detect the infection as soon as possible. Less common are tests of urine and oral mucosal transudate. Repeat testing is done to confirm screening results. Note that positive antibody tests do not mean the patient will develop acquired immunodeficiency syndrome (AIDS).

HIV Viral Load

HIV viral load is not a screening test. However, the amount of HIV present in the blood of an infected patient provides information about the progression of the disease and the response to therapy. Viral load, along with CD4 counts, provides a basis for decisions about initiating or changing drug therapy. A falling viral load suggests a positive response to therapy. If the CD4 count falls below 200/mm^3, the patient is at risk for AIDS and other HIV complications.

Cell Surface Immunophenotyping

CD4 (t helper cells) and CD8 (t-cytotoxic cells) counts are predictive of the course of the HIV disease and the prognosis. An increase in CD4 counts is seen with successful HIV therapy. The ratio of CD4 to CD8 T lymphocytes is another important measure of the body's response to HIV infection.

CULTURES OF BLOOD, URINE, SPUTUM, AND STOOL

Cultures are done to detect infections in the blood, sputum, urine, or stool. When a patient has a fever without an obvious source of infection, all of these specimens are obtained to look for the source of the infection.

SKIN TESTS

Skin tests can serve as a barometer of immune system functioning, pointing out either hyposensitivities or hypersensitivities to a particular antigen. Examples of allergens used in skin testing include dust, pollen, animal dander, purified protein derivative, tuberculin bacillus, and *Candida albicans*.

Box 31.3 Calculating Absolute Neutrophil Count From Complete Blood Count

COMPLETE BLOOD COUNT REPORT

White blood cells (WBCs) × 10^3	6.5
Red blood cells (RBCs) × 10^6	4.51
Hemoglobin (Hgb) in g/dL	14.0
Hematocrit (Hct) %	40.8
Mean corpuscular volume (MCV) in fL	90.5
Mean corpuscular hemoglobin (MCH) in pg	30.9
Mean cell hemoglobin concentration (MCHC) in g/dL	34.2
Platelet count (PLT) × 10^3	333

AUTOMATED DIFFERENTIAL

Lymphocytes %	35.0
Monocytes %	10.3
Neutrophils %	46.3
Eosinophils %	7.3
Basophiles %	1.0

MANUAL DIFFERENTIAL

Segmented neutrophils %	49.0
Banded neutrophils %	1.0
Lymphocytes %	32.0
Monocytes %	8.0
Eosinophils %	9.0
Basophils %	1.0

To calculate the absolute neutrophil count (ANC), use the manual differential because it is more accurate. Multiply the percentage of segmented neutrophils (49% in this example) plus the percentage of banded neutrophils (1% in this example) by the total number of WBCs (6500 in this example). Banded neutrophils are included in the calculations of the ANC because they are developmentally nearly mature neutrophils and can function as mature neutrophils (see Fig. 31.1). If a manual differential has not been done, the automated differential can be used; however, if the total WBC count is >10,000/mL or <3000/mL, a manual differential should be requested.

GENERIC CALCULATION

ANC = (% neutrophils +% banded neutrophils) × WBCs

CALCULATIONS FOR THIS EXAMPLE

(0.49 + 0.01) × 6500.00 = 3250.00

COMMON THERAPEUTIC MEASURES

DRUG THERAPY

A variety of drugs are used to treat disorders of the immune system. This chapter will address those drugs only in relation to immunologic disorders, although you will see most of them included in other chapters because of their range of applications. Table 31.3 presents only examples of these drugs. They are powerful drugs with many adverse effects, so when you have a patient receiving any of them, use your drug handbook for more complete information. Also, various combinations of drugs are commonly used when treating immunologic disorders. You will see that these drugs suppress the immune system, so you can anticipate a risk of anemia, thrombocytopenia, and leukopenia. This leaves the patient at risk for fatigue, bleeding, and infection. Most of these drugs are used for more than one disease. However, the drugs used to treat HIV are mostly specific to that infection. You will find those drugs with the HIV content in Chapter 32.

Patient Teaching

Patients Taking Corticosteroids

- Take this drug before 9 AM each morning to reduce the risk of adrenal complications.
- This drug reduces your resistance to infection. Avoid people with contagious diseases. Wash your hands often. Inform prescriber of any signs of infection: sore throat, fever.
- You may have fluid retention. Report swollen ankles and weight gain to prescriber.
- Your potassium level may fall. Notify your prescriber if you have an irregular heartbeat, muscle weakness, or muscle cramps. Eat potassium-rich foods such as bananas and citrus fruits.
- You are at risk for peptic ulcers. Do not take NSAIDs (ibuprofen, aspirin, etc.). Report upper abdominal pain or black, "tarry" stools.
- You may experience mood changes such as anxiety or irritability. Inform your prescriber of severe disturbances.
- Always keep extra doses with you.
- Wear a medical alert tag or bracelet stating that you are taking corticosteroids. If you have an emergency, this is critical information for the health care provider.

ORGAN TRANSPLANTATION

Organ and tissue transplantation has become increasingly common as antirejection drugs have been developed. Specific types of transplant are discussed in the chapters where those organ/tissues are covered. When patients undergo kidney, heart, liver, or other organ or tissue transplantation, their own healthy immune systems may recognize the **allograft** (transplanted organ or tissue) as foreign and try to destroy it. Rejection can be classified as active antibody-mediated rejection (ABMR), chronic active ABMR, or C4D staining without evidence of rejection. Rejection that occurs within 24 hours after transplantation requires removal of the transplanted organ. It is caused by preexisting antibodies against the transplanted organ, which destroy blood vessels. Acute rejection usually occurs within 6 months after transplantation and can usually be reversed with immunosuppressant drugs. It is the result of an immune response that is activated against the donated organ or the formation of antibodies by the patient. Chronic rejection occurs months or years after transplantation. Large numbers of T and B cells infiltrate the transplanted tissue causing fibrosis and scarring. In this way, the allograft is slowly rejected over months to years. Treatment is supportive as there is no clearly established treatment for chronic rejection.

Tissue matching of donor to recipient minimizes the chance of the recipient's immune system attacking the allograft after transplantation. Various combinations of drugs are given to suppress the recipient's immune system and minimize the immune response to the allograft. However, these drugs also suppress the patient's ability to fight bacteria, viruses, fungi, and parasites, putting the patient at increased risk for infection. Combinations of steroid drugs, methotrexate, cyclosporine, tacrolimus, azathioprine, and mycophenolate are commonly used to chronically suppress the immune system after an organ transplant. Table 31.3 describes these drugs and related nursing interventions. In addition, several newer drugs target the T cells while preserving B cell function and thus more of the patient's immune function. Patients who have undergone organ or tissue transplantation may have to take immunosuppressive therapy for the rest of their lives to preserve the allograft (see the Complementary and Alternative Therapies box). The following section describes stem cell transplantation and provides an example of pre- and postprocedure care.

Complementary and Alternative Therapies

Patients with immunologic disorders should consult with their physicians before using complementary and/or alternative therapies, because they have adverse effects and can interact with some medications.

Put On Your Thinking Cap!

Explain what would happen if transplant recipients did not take immunosuppressant drugs to prevent organ rejection.

HEMATOPOIETIC STEM CELL TRANSPLANTATION

Hematopoietic stem cell transplantation (HSCT or HCT) can be a life-saving treatment for patients with a variety of types of cancer (e.g., certain leukemias and lymphomas) and nonmalignant conditions such as aplastic anemia. The goal of this procedure is to repopulate the bone marrow with blood-producing cells, thereby restoring the patient's hematologic and immunologic systems. The earliest procedure used harvesting of bone marrow, so it was called *bone marrow transplantation*. Stem cells can now be obtained from peripheral circulating blood or from umbilical cord blood, so the term *HSCT* is more often used.

Allogeneic bone marrow transplantation requires a donor whose human leukocyte antigens (HLAs) match those of the patient. When a perfect match cannot be found, partially matched relatives or cord blood may be used. High doses of chemotherapy and radiation therapy are given to the patient to destroy all of the cancerous bone marrow. It is administered to the patient just like a blood transfusion through an intravenous line. The infused stem cells seek out the patient's bone marrow, where they start growing and producing healthy WBCs, RBCs, and platelets.

HLA typing is similar to blood typing but is much more specific. Because these HLAs are genetically determined, brothers and sisters of the patient are initially tested to determine whether they can be bone

Table 31.3 Drugs Used to Treat Immunologic Disorders

DRUG	USE AND ACTION	SIDE EFFECTS	NURSING INTERVENTIONS
The following drugs are hazardous to the nurse and require special handling: calcineurin inhibitors, mTOR inhibitors, cytotoxic agents, methotrexate			
Immunosuppressants			
Corticosteroids • prednisone, numerous other preparations for oral, parenteral, intranasal, inhalation, and topical use. Can also be injected into joints and lesions.	Suppresses immune response via multiple mechanisms. Used to prevent rejection of grafted tissue, and to treat rheumatoid arthritis, systemic lupus erythematosus, multiple sclerosis, and other conditions.	Adrenal insufficiency, osteoporosis, increased risk of infection, muscle wasting, thin skin, fluid and electrolyte imbalances, glucose intolerance, psychologic disturbances, peptic ulcer disease.	Doses must be tapered off when discontinued to prevent acute adrenal insufficiency. Protect patient from sources of infection. Protect fragile skin from trauma. See the Patient Teaching box for patients taking corticosteroids.
Calcineurin inhibitors (CI) • cyclosporine (e.g., Sandimmune Gengraf, Neoral) • tacrolimus (e.g., Prograf, Astagraf XL, Envarus XR)	Used to prevent rejection of transplanted tissue by reducing proliferation of B cells and cytotoxic T cells.	Nephrotoxicity, infection, hepatotoxicity, lymphoma, hypertension, rarely anaphylaxis with IV route.	Consult handbook for specific drug information. Be aware of multiple drug interactions. Grapefruit juice inhibits metabolism, raising CI blood level. Oral solutions can be mixed with milk or apple or orange juice. See package directions for pipette used to draw up cyclosporine. Monitor for signs of infection. Advise patient of importance of regular kidney and liver tests.
mTOR (mammalian target of rapamycin) inhibitors • sirolimus (Rapamune) • everolimus (Zortress)	Suppresses activation of B cells and T cells. Used to prevent rejection of transplanted organs. . Everolimus also used for liver transplant recipients.	Risk of infection; elevated serum lipids; rash, acne, photosensitivity anemia, thrombocytopenia, joint pain, diarrhea, hypokalemia; severe complications in liver and lung recipients. Thrombosis in transplanted kidney. Everolimus can also cause new-onset diabetes.	Be aware of numerous drug and food interactions. Grapefruit juice raises serum drug levels. Drugs should be taken consistently with or without food. Patient should avoid sun exposure. Use sunscreen.
Cytotoxic agents* • cyclophosphamide • azathioprine • mycophenylate mofetil (CellCept)	Prevents rejection of transplanted tissue by killing B and T lymphocytes. Also used to treat severe rheumatoid arthritis, systemic lupus erythematosus, and other autoimmune disorders.	Bone marrow suppression: neutropenia, thrombocytopenia. Infection, GI disturbances, hair loss, reduced fertility. Increased risk of malignancy.	Stress importance of regular blood studies. Protect patient from sources of infection. Teach good handwashing.

Table 31.3 Drugs Used to Treat Immunologic Disorders—cont'd

DRUG	USE AND ACTION	SIDE EFFECTS	NURSING INTERVENTIONS
Folate Antagonist/Antimetabolite			
methotrexate (Rheumatrex, Trexall)	Suppresses B and T lymphocyte production by interfering with folate metabolism. Used to treat psoriasis, arthritis, various types of cancer, acute lymphoblastic leukemia. CNS prophylaxis with leukemia therapy, prevention of graft-versus-host-disease after transplant.	Antirejection dose is lower than dose used for cancer, so it does not suppress bone marrow but may cause liver damage. Dosage for cancer treatment can cause nausea, vomiting, rash, diarrhea, leukopenia, anemia, thrombocytopenia, headache, confusion, hair loss.	Hazardous drug that requires special handling to protect the nurse. Protect patient from infection. Stress need for regular blood tests. Inspect skin for serious rash. Tell patient to report sore throat, fever, bleeding. If hair loss is a concern, refer to American Cancer Society for strategies.
Pyrimidine Analog			
cytarabine	Affects the biosynthesis of DNA and RNA. Used to treat AML, ALL, non-Hodgkin lymphoma.	Neutropenia, anemia, thrombocytopenia, nausea and vomiting, fever, stomatitis, liver damage, headache, conjunctivitis, pulmonary edema, cerebellar toxicity.	Monitor for excessive bruising, prolonged bleeding. Avoid exposure to infections. Teach good hygiene.
Anthracyclines			
daunorubicin (Cerubidine, DaunoXome) idarubicin (Isamycin)	Destroys target cells by inhibiting DNA and preventing DNA repair. Used to treat AML in adults. Unlabeled uses: non-Hodgkin lymphomas, AML and ALL, and some other cancers.	Neutropenia, anemia, thrombocytopenia, cardiotoxicity, nausea and vomiting, reversible hair loss, stomatitis, liver and kidney toxicity, anorexia, conjunctivitis.	Inform patient that the drug will turn urine and sweat red and that extremities may become pigmented. IV route only.
Monoclonal Antibodies			
belimumab (Benlysta) rituximab (Rituxan) basiliximab (Simulect) lymphocyte immune globulin (Atgam) Muromonab-CD3 (Orthoclone OKT3)	Belimumab treats systemic lupus erythromatosis. Basiliximab used only to prevent rejection of kidney allograft. Lymphocyte immune globulin for renal transplants and aplastic anemia. Others used to treat non-Hodgkin lymphoma, systemic lupus erythematosus, some leukemias (ALL).	First dose can cause chills, fever, chest pain, nausea, vomiting. Resolves quickly. Anaphylaxis (rarely). Immune globulin: mild immune reactions (chills, fever, leukopenia, skin reactions; anaphylaxis possible). Does not increase risk for infection.	Be prepared for possible anaphylaxis with epinephrine and facilities for respiratory support.
Tyrosine Kinase Inhibitors			
imatinib (Gleevec) nilotinib (Tasigna) dasatinib (Sprycel)	Inhibits proliferation and promotes death of cancer cells. Treats chronic myelogenous leukemia, some GI tumors.	Neutropenia, anemia, thrombocytopenia. Nausea, diarrhea or constipation, myalgia, rash, edema, liver injury, fluid retention, pulmonary edema, cardiac dysrhythmias.	Monitor respiratory status. Report dyspnea, edema, bleeding. Inspect skin for serious rash. Stress to patient importance of regular blood tests. Assess peripheral and apical pulses for irregularity. Take with food or liquids, same time each day. See drug handbook for directions specific to each drug.

ALL, Acute lymphocytic leukemia; *AML*, acute myeloid leukemia; *CNS*, central nervous system; *DNA*, deoxyribonucleic acid; *GI*, gastrointestinal; *IV*, intravenous; *RNA*, ribonucleic acid.

marrow donors for their sibling. A 25% chance exists that a sibling will be an HLA match to a patient needing a bone marrow transplant. If the patient has an identical twin, the twin will be a perfect HLA match. In this situation, the procedure is called a **syngeneic bone marrow transplantation**. A possibility exists that someone in the general population might be HLA matched to the patient, but the chances of finding a matched unrelated donor (MUD) are very small. For many patients, an allogeneic bone marrow or peripheral stem cell transplant is not possible because a matched donor cannot be found.

Another type of transplant harvests the patient's own bone marrow or peripheral stem cells before chemotherapy and radiation therapy. After therapy, the patient's own bone marrow or stem cells are returned to the patient. This type of transplant, called an **autologous bone marrow transplant** or *autologous HSCT*, is the best option for patients with a solid tumor that has not metastasized to the bone marrow (i.e., patients with lymphoma). An autologous transplant is generally not an option for patients with leukemia or those who have a cancer that has metastasized to the bone marrow, because healthy bone marrow must be reinfused in the patient after chemotherapy and radiation therapy to prevent cancer recurrence.

A third type of transplant is a *peripheral blood stem cell transplant*. For this type of transplant, colony-stimulating factors are administered to the patient to stimulate the bone marrow to produce large numbers of WBCs. Then apheresis is performed to collect the patient's peripheral stem cells. Apheresis is a procedure similar to hemodialysis. A large-bore apheresis catheter is placed into the subclavian vein that allows simultaneous blood withdrawal and blood reinfusion. The patient's blood is first drawn off into the apheresis machine. The apheresis machine centrifuges, or spins, the blood, separating it into WBCs, RBCs, and plasma. The stem cells in the WBC layer are removed and stored and the rest of the WBCs, RBCs, and plasma are returned to the patient. When enough of these peripheral blood stem cells are harvested and stored, the patient is treated with chemotherapy and radiation therapy. The specific treatment varies with the patient diagnosis and general condition. Some regimens are more toxic than others. After treatment, the peripheral blood stem cells are returned to the patient. Stem cells re-engraft more quickly than bone marrow, reducing the duration of neutropenia and therefore the risk of infection. Often peripheral blood stem cell transplants are administered concurrently with autologous bone marrow transplants. Peripheral blood stem cell transplants have been so successful that they have become the most common type of transplant.

Major complications of bone marrow transplantation and peripheral blood stem cell transplantation include infection, thrombocytopenia, renal insufficiency, hepatic venoocclusive disease, and graft-versus-host disease. Infection is a constant concern in the care of patients undergoing bone marrow or stem cell transplantation. For approximately 2 weeks after transplantation, when the new bone marrow is engrafting, patients are severely neutropenic and at very high risk for infection. Even when WBCs and neutrophil counts approach normal levels, the patient's cell-mediated immune function can be compromised for more than 1 year.

Thrombocytopenia can be profound and prolonged in the patient undergoing bone marrow transplantation or peripheral blood stem cell transplantation because of the high doses of chemotherapy and radiation therapy.

Renal insufficiency can occur if the kidneys are damaged with high doses of nephrotoxic drugs such as cisplatin chemotherapy or the antibiotic gentamicin. Kidney function can be further compromised if blood flow to and through the kidneys is not maintained.

Hepatic venoocclusive disease can occur if the liver is damaged with high doses of chemotherapy and radiation therapy. Blood flow into and out of the liver can be obstructed, resulting in ischemia, ascites, and increasing serum bilirubin.

Graft-versus-host disease is a complication of allogeneic bone marrow transplants in which T lymphocytes in the transplanted bone marrow identify the patient's tissue as foreign and try to destroy the patient's tissues. The transplanted T lymphocytes attack primarily epithelial cells of the skin, GI tract, biliary ducts, and lymphoid system, resulting in a skin rash; large amounts of green, watery, heme-negative diarrhea; and elevated liver enzyme levels.

Patients undergoing bone marrow transplantation or peripheral blood stem cell transplantation as treatment for a hematologic or immune system disorder are frequently hospitalized in a specialized transplant unit and need intensive nursing care and long-term follow-up to ensure that their new immune system is functioning and that the underlying disease does not recur.

Put On Your Thinking Cap!

Compare and contrast the three types of bone marrow transplants in relation to the following: patient preparation, source of cells, advantages, disadvantages, and complications.

NURSING ACTIONS FOR THE PATIENT AT RISK FOR INJURY FROM INFECTION

The lower a patient's WBC count is (in particular, the lower their neutrophil count), the greater is the patient's risk of infection. Box 31.4 outlines compromised host precautions for the patient at risk for infection.

Box 31.4 Nursing Actions for the Patient at Risk for Infection: Compromised Host Precautions

1. The patient should have a private room. It does not have to be an isolation room. The door may be left open. A *Compromised Host Precaution* sign should be posted on the door.
2'. All persons entering the patient's room must wash their hands before touching the patient for any reason. This is the most important way to prevent infection. The patient and family should be encouraged to remind all staff and visitors to wash their hands before touching the patient.
3. Monitor the patient's vital signs every 2 to 4 hours. Notify the physician immediately of a temperature >101° F to consider the need for an infectious fever workup and initiation or changing of antibiotics. An infectious fever workup usually includes two sets of blood cultures, a chest radiograph, sputum culture, urine culture, wound culture, and cultures of other sites suggestive of infection. Patients with a central line or permanent, indwelling venous access device usually have one set of specimens for culture drawn from the line and one set drawn from a peripheral site. Mark the culture bottles clearly regarding where the specimen was obtained to assist with localization of the infection. Blood cultures are more likely to yield the "offending organism" if the blood is drawn as the patient's temperature is rising instead of after the patient's temperature has peaked.
4. Invasive procedures should be kept to a minimum. Invasive devices such as catheters and tubes should be removed as soon as the patient's medical condition permits.
5. Careful attention to aseptic technique must be observed, especially when performing phlebotomy, handling intravenous lines, or performing other invasive procedures.
6. Designate a particular stethoscope and thermometer to be used exclusively in caring for the patient.
7. Masks are not required; in fact, they are discouraged. Staff with upper respiratory tract or other infections should not care for the patient.
8. Clean table tops, equipment, and the floor frequently with hospital-approved disinfectant, clean cloths, and clean mops.
9. The patient should be taught to wash their hands before and after eating, using the toilet, and doing any self-care procedure. If possible, the patient should shower every day. Liquid soap instead of bar soap should be used.
10. Encourage the patient to cough and deep breathe every 4 hours. Mobility should be encouraged. Smoking should be discouraged.
11. Only canned or cooked foods may be served. Raw fruits, raw vegetables, and milk products may not be served because of the risk of *Escherichia coli*, *Pseudomonas aeruginosa*, and *Klebsiella* spp. bacteria on or in these food items. The patient should be encouraged to choose appropriate foods from the menu. The diet roster should be annotated *compromised host precautions* so that the nutrition care staff can verify that appropriate choices are being made.
12. Tests, scans, and appointments away from the patient's room should be coordinated in advance to eliminate or minimize waiting time in common waiting areas.
13. The patient should wear a clean mask when outside the room, especially in heavily traveled public areas such as corridors, elevators, and waiting rooms. The mask may be removed when the patient is in less public areas. A new mask should be used for each trip out of the room.
14. Some hospitals allow flowers and plants in the patient's room; however, they should not be handled by the patient because of the possibility of *E. coli* contamination of the water and soil.
15. No humidifiers with standing water should be used in the patient's room. If a wall humidifier is needed, the water should be changed every day.
16. Teach the patient and family about the underlying pathophysiology that puts the patient at risk for infection and about precautions to minimize the risk for infection.

Get Ready for the NCLEX® Examination!

Key Points

- The immune system is the body's defense network against infection; it provides the body with resistance to invading organisms and enables it to fight off invaders once they have gained access.
- Body organs that are part of a functioning immune system include the bone marrow, lymph nodes, spleen, and thymus.
- Stem cells are called progenitor cells, or precursor cells, because they are capable of developing into WBCs, RBCs, or platelets.
- Antigens are foreign substances that stimulate a response from the immune system, whereas antibodies are proteins that are produced by the immune system to help eradicate antigens.
- Innate immunity is present in the body at birth, whereas acquired immunity develops after birth as a result of the body's immune response to specific antigens.
- Many types of leukocytes (WBCs) act as nature's cleanup mechanism by migrating to infected or inflamed areas and engulfing and destroying antigens through a process known as phagocytosis.
- The two types of acquired immunity are antibody mediated and cell mediated.
- Acquired immunity depends on the proper development and functioning of specific WBCs called B and T lymphocytes.
- Immunodeficiency occurs when the body is unable to launch an adequate immune response, resulting in an increased risk for infection.

- Autoimmune diseases occur when the immune system inappropriately identifies its own proteins as foreign and mounts a response to destroy these self-proteins.
- Frequent or persistent infections, prolonged bleeding when cut, easy bruising, and chronic fatigue may reflect an underlying immunologic disorder.
- The primary symptom of an immunologic disorder is infection.
- Because the bone marrow becomes less responsive with age, the older person's immune response may be inadequate under stressful situations.
- The patient with a low WBC count is at risk for infection.
- Tests to diagnose HIV infection include NATS, antigen/antibody tests, and antibody tests.
- Following a positive HIV screening test, a second confirmatory test should be done.
- Patients who are treated with immunosuppressant drugs are at risk for anemia, leukocytopenia, and thrombocytopenia.
- When patients undergo organ or tissue transplantation, their own healthy immune system may recognize the allograft (transplanted organ or tissue) as foreign and try to destroy it.
- Rejection that occurs within 24 hours after transplantation requires removal of the transplanted organ.
- Acute rejection, which usually occurs within 6 months after transplantation, results from an immune response against the donated organ or the formation of antibodies by the recipient and is treated with immunosuppressant drugs.
- Chronic rejection occurs months or years after transplantation and results in tissue fibrosis and scarring; treatment is supportive.
- Tissue matching of donor to recipient minimizes the chance of the recipient's immune system attacking the allograft after transplantation.
- Stem cells can be obtained from the bone marrow or from peripheral blood.
- Hematopoietic stem cell transplantation is a procedure that reconstitutes the hematologic and immunologic systems after certain cancer therapies.
- Major complications of bone marrow transplantation and peripheral blood stem cell transplantation include infection, thrombocytopenia, renal insufficiency, hepatic venocclusive disease, and graft-versus-host disease.

Additional Learning Resources

SG Go to your Study Guide for additional learning activities to help you master this chapter content.

Go to your Evolve website (http://evolve.elsevier.com/Linton/medsurg) for the following learning resources and much more:
- Fluid & Electrolyte Tutorial
- Review Questions for the NCLEX® Examination

Clinical Judgment and Next-Generation NCLEX® Examination-Style Questions

1. **A patient has a neutrophil count that is 70% of his total WBC count. You should suspect infection caused by ____________________.**

   NCLEX Client Need: Physiological Integrity: Physiological Adaptation

2. **Mr. B. had chickenpox as a child. When he was exposed to chickenpox years later, he did not become infected. His resistance was most likely the result of which type of acquired immunity? ____________________**

   NCLEX Client Need: Physiological Integrity: Physiological Adaptation

3. **Which of the following correctly describe(s) the effects of age-related changes in the immune system? (Select all that apply.)**
   1. The bone marrow becomes less productive with advancing age.
   2. The immune system functions well under normal circumstances.
   3. Lymphatic tissue shrinks so that fewer and smaller lymph nodes exist.
   4. Older people have better immune function than most young adults.
   5. The bone marrow can usually respond to increased demand, given more time.

   NCLEX Client Need: Health Promotion and Maintenance

4. **Following hematopoietic stem marrow transplantation, patients are at greatest risk for infection during which time frame?**
   1. 24 hours
   2. 2 weeks
   3. 1 month
   4. 6 months

   NCLEX Client Need: Physiological Integrity: Reduction of Risk Potential

5. **When the nurse is collecting data about the patient with an immunologic disorder, which of the following is the priority?**
   1. Signs and symptoms of infection
   2. Unexplained changes in weight
   3. Increased blood pressure
   4. Characteristics of urine

   NCLEX Client Need: Physiological Integrity: Physiological Adaptation

6. **During a report, it is noted that your patient's WBC is 20,000. What is the best interpretation of this laboratory finding?**
   1. Your patient could have a mild infection.
   2. Your patient's infection is resolving.
   3. Your patient could have a severe infection.
   4. Your patient is producing excess neutrophils, artificially raising the WBC.

   NCLEX Client Need: Physiological Integrity: Physiological Adaptation

7. **When the nurse is assigned to a patient who is on compromised host precautions, which of the following precautions are required? (Select all that apply.)**
   1. Visitors and staff should wash their hands before patient contact.
   2. The patient can have no fresh, raw fruits and vegetables.
   3. Staff should always wear masks when in the patient's room.
   4. Vital signs should be monitored at least every 8 hours.
   5. The patient will be placed in an isolation room.

   NCLEX Client Need: Physiological Integrity: Reduction of Risk Potential

8. **A patient with severe allergies cannot tolerate cigarette smoke. The smoke is an example of a/an:**
   1. phagocyte
   2. antigen
   3. antibody
   4. pathogen

   NCLEX Client Need: Physiological Integrity: Physiological Adaptation

9. **A patient is scheduled for an autologous hematopoietic stem cell transplant. Which of the following statements by the patient indicate that he correctly understands the procedure? (Select all that apply.)**
   1. A donor with tissue similar to mine is being sought.
   2. Donor bone marrow will be injected into my hip bone.
   3. I will be given healthy stem cells to prevent cancer recurrence.
   4. I will be given chemotherapy and radiation.
   5. I can return home the day after the procedure.

   NCLEX Client Need: Physiological Integrity: Reduction of Risk Potential

10. **What is the correct name of the stem cell transplantation procedure in which a patient's stem cells are harvested and returned after chemotherapy or radiation?**
    1. allogeneic
    2. autologous
    3. syngeneic
    4. myelogenous

    NCLEX Client Need: Physiological Integrity: Reduction of Risk Potential

11. **Objective: Describe the tests and procedure used to diagnose and treat disorders of the immune system and nursing considerations for each.**

    NGN Item Type: Cloze

    Cognitive skill: Prioritize Hypotheses

    A patient who has cancer is scheduled for a *peripheral blood stem cell transplant.* For this type of transplant, colony-stimulating factors are administered to the patient to stimulate ________ to produce large numbers of ________. Then ________ is performed to collect the patient's peripheral stem cells. The patient's blood is withdrawn and centrifuged to separate cells from plasma. Stem cells are removed and _______; the other blood components are returned to the patient. Then the patient is usually treated with ___________ and _________. After treatment, the peripheral blood stem cells are returned to the patient. The cells migrate to the ___________ where they engraft and begin to produce healthy blood cells.

    Use the options below to fill in the blanks. Options may be used more than once.

OPTIONS
Chemotherapy
Apheresis
Bone marrow
Red blood cells
Radiation
White blood cells
Platelets
Stored
Hemodialysis
Discarded
Radiated

12. **Objective: List the data to be collected when assessing a patient with a disorder of the immune system.**

    NGN Item Type: Enhanced Hot Spot

    Cognitive skill: Recognize Cues

    One week after a peripheral stem cell transplant, the nurse's assessment data are listed below.

    Highlight **those** findings that may indicate complications.
    - Oral temperature 101°F
    - Multiple bruises on both arms and legs
    - Lab report: increased neutrophils
    - Fluid intake 2200 mL; urine output 1100 mL last 24 hours
    - Heart rate 80 bpm
    - Lab report: increased bilirubin

32 Immunologic Disorders

http://evolve.elsevier.com/Linton/medsurg

Objectives

1. Describe the pathophysiology, signs and symptoms, medical diagnosis, and medical treatment for selected disorders of the immune system.
2. Explain measures to reduce the risk of transmission of human immunodeficiency virus (HIV).
3. Explain the difference between HIV and acquired immunodeficiency syndrome (AIDS).
4. Name the major classes of HIV drugs, side effects, and nursing considerations.
5. List key points to include in the teaching plan for patients with an immunologic disorder.
6. Assist in developing a nursing care plan for a patient with a disorder of the immune system.

Key Terms

acquired immunodeficiency syndrome (AIDS) (ĬM-myū-nō-dē-FĬ-shĕn-sē)
antiretroviral therapy (ART) (ĂN-tē-rĕ-trō-vī-rŭl)
autoimmune disorder
human immunodeficiency virus (HIV)
immunotherapy
neutropenia

WHITE BLOOD CELL DISORDERS OF THE IMMUNE SYSTEM

The main function of the white blood cells (WBCs) is to protect the body against pathogens. Patients are at great risk for infection when the WBCs are inadequate or not functioning properly.

NEUTROPENIA

Neutropenia occurs when the total number of neutrophils is abnormally low (an absolute neutrophil count [ANC] of <1500 cells/μL), putting the patient at increased risk of infection. Decreased bone marrow production (e.g., because of infiltration with malignant cells), chemotherapy, radiation therapy, certain drugs (e.g., zidovudine, clozapine), or an autoimmune reaction (e.g., systemic lupus erythematosus [SLE], rheumatoid arthritis) can cause neutropenia. The longer the patient is neutropenic, the greater is the chance of infection. Because these patients do not have adequate numbers of WBCs to mount an immunologic response, classic signs of infection (e.g., redness, swelling, pain) may be absent. Fever may be the only sign of infection.

The most common sites of infection in neutropenic patients are the lung (pneumonia), blood (septicemia), skin, urinary tract, and gastrointestinal (GI) tract (mucositis, esophagitis, perirectal lesions). Most infections in neutropenic patients are caused by bacteria; however, fungi and viruses can also infect these patients. The goal of antibiotic therapy is to support the patient until the patient's own WBCs are available to fight the infection. In addition to administering prescribed antibiotics, it is important to minimize the patient's exposure to infectious agents by instituting compromised host precautions, described in Chapter 31, Box 31.4.

NON-HODGKIN LYMPHOMAS

Non-Hodgkin lymphomas (NHLs) are a group of cancers of the lymph system that can spread to other organs. Although the various types have differing courses and survival rates, cure is possible for most patients. The American Cancer Society estimated that 81,560 new cases of NHL would be diagnosed in 2021, and that it would account for 20,720 deaths. Although NHL is more common in older people, individuals of any age and gender may get the disease. NHLs are staged as low grade, intermediate grade, or high grade. The higher the grade of lymphoma, the more aggressive the cancer. The terms *indolent* and *aggressive* are also used to differentiate lymphomas based on their progressions. Medical treatment of NHL can include **immunotherapy**, targeted therapy, radiation therapy, and chemotherapy in various combinations depending on the stage of the disease and specific histologic type. High-dose chemotherapy with hematopoietic stem cell transplantation (HSCT) is an option for some patients who suffer recurrent disease after standard treatment. In some cases, patients with nonsymptomatic, early-stage, lower-grade lymphomas may be monitored and treatment deferred until the disease progresses. Survival rates vary widely depending on the grade of the disease at diagnosis. The overall 5-year survival rate for patients with NHL is 73%.

HODGKIN LYMPHOMA

Hodgkin lymphoma is characterized by Reed Sternberg cells in the lymph nodes. According to the American Cancer Society, more than 8,830 new cases of Hodgkin lymphoma would be diagnosed in 2021 and 960 people would die from the disease. The incidence of the disease is highest for people in their 20s and their 50s. Men are more likely than women to have the disease. Medical treatment of Hodgkin lymphoma may include radiation therapy, chemotherapy, and/or immunotherapy depending on the stage of the disease. Chemotherapy typically uses multiple drug combinations. High-dose chemotherapy and radiation therapy with HSCT is an option for patients who do not respond to standard treatment or who suffer recurrent disease after standard treatment. A variety of immunotherapeutic agents such as monoclonal antibodies are available.

Patients sometimes have late effects of therapy that occur months or years after Hodgkin treatment. Among these late effects may be various cancers, infections, infertility, and hypogonadism. Survival rates vary widely depending on the stage of the disease at diagnosis. The overall 5-year survival rate for patients with Hodgkin lymphoma is 87%.

LEUKEMIA

Leukemia is a cancer of the WBCs in which the bone marrow produces too many immature WBCs. These nonfunctioning, immature WBCs leave the patient unprotected against microorganisms and at great risk for life-threatening infections. The American Cancer Society estimated that 61,090 cases of leukemia would be diagnosed in 2021, and 23,660 would die. Although for most cases no cause is identified, factors that may be associated with the development of leukemia are exposure to large doses of ionizing radiation or exposure to certain chemicals such as benzene, a compound found in gasoline. Persons with Down syndrome and certain other genetic abnormalities are at increased risk for developing leukemia.

Two main types of leukemia exist: (1) myelogenous and (2) lymphocytic. Each type of leukemia can be either chronic or acute. The chronic leukemias—chronic myelogenous leukemia (CML) and chronic lymphocytic leukemia (CLL)—occur most often in adults. In both types of chronic leukemias, the WBC count slowly increases over months or years. The disease can usually be controlled with oral chemotherapy for many years. Patients being treated for chronic leukemia generally feel healthy. They do not lose their hair and usually do not experience nausea. Most of these patients can continue to work. A drug for patients with CML, imatinib mesylate (Gleevec), has revolutionized the treatment of this particular leukemia. Gleevec is a protein tyrosine kinase inhibitor that targets the leukemic cells while sparing normal cells. It is an oral medication taken once a day. Only minimal side effects have been reported. Research continues to determine the optimal length of treatment and follow-up needed for these patients. The average life expectancy after diagnosis for a patient with CML ranges from 3 to 8 years, depending on the stage of the disease at diagnosis. It is anticipated that life expectancy will increase with Gleevec treatment. The life expectancy for a patient with CLL ranges from 2 to 10 years, again depending on the stage of the disease when diagnosed. After this time, the chronic leukemias often transform into an acute leukemia that is very difficult to treat. Patients generally die shortly after they enter this accelerated phase.

Each of the chronic forms of leukemia—lymphocytic and myelogenous—also has an acute form. Acute lymphocytic leukemia (ALL) occurs most often in children between the ages of 2 and 6 years. Acute myelogenous leukemia (AML), also called *acute nonlymphocytic leukemia (ANLL),* occurs more often in adults. The acute leukemias appear very suddenly. The patient's WBC count can skyrocket in days, crowding out the normal red blood cells (RBCs) and platelets and leaving the patient at severe risk for infection and bleeding. Treatment with chemotherapy must be started as soon as possible. Approximately 38% of adults diagnosed with ALL will be alive in 5 years. Only 26% of adults diagnosed with AML will be alive in 5 years. For CLL and CML, the 5-year survival rates are 86% and 70% respectively.

Clinical Manifestations of Acute Leukemia

Patients with leukemia commonly have infections because their bone marrow is producing huge numbers of immature WBCs that cannot effectively fight infection; fevers and night sweats are in response to the infection. Because the leukemic WBCs crowd out the normal cells in the bone marrow, patients may have symptoms related to low RBC counts, such as fatigue, paleness, tachycardia, and tachypnea. Concurrently, patients may have symptoms related to low platelet counts, such as petechiae or purpura, epistaxis (nose bleeds), gingival bleeding (from the gums), melena (blood in the stool), or menorrhagia (heavy menstrual bleeding). Some patients have bone pain because of the crowding created by rapidly dividing leukemic cells in the bone marrow. Patients may report weight loss and swollen lymph nodes.

Medical Diagnosis of Acute Leukemia

A complete blood count (CBC) with an extremely high WBC count indicates that leukemia might be present. A bone marrow biopsy enables diagnosis of the specific type of leukemia. Chapter 29, Tables 29.1 and 29.2 describe these diagnostic procedures.

Medical Treatment of the Patient With Acute Leukemia

Among the treatment options for acute leukemias are chemotherapy (Table 32.1), targeted therapy, immunotherapy, and hematopoietic stem cell transplant (HSCT). The HSCT process and nursing care are described in Chapter 31. Examples of drugs commonly used to treat leukemia are listed in Table 32.1.

NURSING CARE OF THE PATIENT WITH ACUTE LEUKEMIA

Patients with acute leukemia require intensive nursing care. Patients undergoing HSCT are normally hospitalized for only 2 to 3 weeks and are critically ill most of that time. Once a patient's vital signs stabilize and the patient has no signs or symptoms of infection, they can be discharged from the hospital and followed as an outpatient until normal bone marrow function returns and adequate numbers of WBCs, RBCs, and platelets are being made. The physical and psychologic nursing care of these patients is intensive.

Focused Assessment

Infection is the leading cause of death in patients with leukemia. Therefore, patients are frequently assessed for any signs or symptoms of infection. The most common sites of infection are the lungs, blood, skin, urinary tract, and GI tract. Take complete vital signs every 4 hours. Fever is the hallmark of infection. Other vital sign changes caused by sepsis or widespread infection include tachycardia, tachypnea, and hypotension. Auscultate the patient's breath sounds every shift and note changes. A cough, especially a productive cough, may indicate an early pulmonary infection. If sputum is produced, note the amount and color. The physician may want the sputum cultured. Each day, carefully inspect the patient's skin for any reddened, swollen, painful, or draining areas. This is most easily done when helping the patient with personal hygiene. Because patients with leukemia do not have normal WBCs, pus may not be seen even though an infection may be present. Redness, swelling, pain, or a combination of these may be the only symptoms of a serious infection. Inspect the patient's mouth and pharynx, looking for any reddened, swollen, painful, or draining areas. In addition, ask the patient about any pain or burning on urination, indicating a possible bladder infection.

While monitoring for infection, also look for any evidence of bleeding. The lower the platelet count is, the greater is the patient's risk for bleeding. A platelet count below 50,000 cells/mm^3 is cause for concern. Note any petechiae, purpura, or ecchymoses. Patients may report epistaxis, gingival bleeding, melena, or menorrhagia. Perform a guaiac test to assess for blood on all bowel movements as directed.

In addition, note any side effects from the chemotherapy, such as nausea and vomiting or stomatitis, so that the appropriate interventions can be taken. Remember that most patients lose their hair from chemotherapy for acute leukemia beginning 1 to 2 weeks after treatment. While doing a physical examination, also assess how much the patient knows about the disease and their treatment, as well as how the patient is coping with this life-threatening disease and the side effects of treatment.

Table 32.1 Treatment of Leukemia

Acute Lymphocytic Leukemia (ALL)	Chronic Lymphocytic Leukemia (CLL)
Drug Therapy • vincristine • prednisone • l-asparaginase • daunorubicin • methotrexate • cyclophosphamide • cytarabinemethotrexate • 6-mercaptopurine • cytarabine • blinatumomab Other Therapies • cranial radiation therapies • intrathecal methotrexate or cytarabine • allogenic HSCT • CAR-T cell therapy	Drug Therapy • fludarabine • cyclophosphamide • bendamustine • rituximab • obinutuzumab • alemtuzumab Other Therapies • radiation • splenectomy • colony-stimulating factors • allogeneic HSCT
Acute Myelogenous Leukemia (AML)	**Chronic Myelogenous Leukemia (CML)**
Drug Therapy • anthracycline • cytarabine • idarubicin • daunorubicin • inotuzumab ozogamicin Other Therapies • allogenic HSCT	Drug Therapy • imatinib • nilotinib • dasatinib • ponatinib • bosutinib • omacetaxinhydroxyurea • cytarabine • decitabine • busulfan • 6-mercaptopurine Other Therapies • Radiation • HSCT • alpha-interferon • leukapheresis

HSCT, Hematopoietic stem cell transplant.

Patient Problems, Goals, and Outcome Criteria: Acute Leukemia

Patient Problems	Goals and Outcome Criteria
Potential for injury related to infection, thrombocytopenia, and anemia	Absence of injury from infection, bleeding, and inadequate oxygenation: normal body temperature, no bruising or frank bleeding, pulse and respiratory rates within patient's norms

Patient Problems, Goals, and Outcome Criteria: Acute Leukemia—cont'd

Patient Problems	Goals and Outcome Criteria
Fatigue related to the disease process and treatment	Reduction in fatigue: patient reports tolerance of activity has improved
Impaired oral tissue integrity related to stomatitis	Intact oral mucous membranes: oral tissues normal in color without lesions
Inadequate nutrition related to nausea and vomiting	Adequate intake of nutrients: stable body weight
Anxiety related to the disease, treatment, and uncertain outcome	Reduced anxiety: patient reports anxiety is reduced, calm manner
Ineffective management of treatment regimen related to lack of knowledge about the disease process and treatment	Patient manages side effects of treatment effectively: patient resumes self-care; verbalizes disease process, treatment, and implications

Interventions

Potential for injury

Infection. Infection presents the greatest risk to patients with leukemia. Most hospitals institute compromised host precautions when a patient's ANC (absolute neutrophil count) falls below 1000 cells/mm^3. Thorough hand washing is of extreme importance in caring for these patients. Hospital personnel who do not diligently wash their hands risk transmitting microorganisms to compromised patients. Encourage patients to shower every day to remove bacteria from the skin and perianal area. Because patients with low WBC counts often become infected with their own microorganisms through their GI tract, consider discouraging patients from eating fresh fruits or vegetables and from drinking milk products. Uncooked foods naturally contain the bacteria *Escherichia coli*, *Pseudomonas aeruginosa*, and *Klebsiella*. A normal immune system can destroy the bacteria in uncooked foods. However, patients undergoing treatment for leukemia are at high risk for infection after being exposed to even small amounts of these bacteria. Chapter 31, Box 31.4. outlines typical compromised host precautions for patients with low WBC counts. Once the patient's ANC climbs above 1000 cells/mm^3, compromised host precautions can be discontinued and a regular diet resumed without restrictions.

Thrombocytopenia. In addition to infection, patients with leukemia are at great risk for bleeding related to thrombocytopenia (a low platelet count). The primary treatment for thrombocytopenia is a platelet transfusion. However, physicians try not to prescribe platelet transfusions for patients unless they are actively bleeding or their platelet count is below 20,000 cells/mm^3 because of the risks associated with blood product administration. Nursing considerations in administering platelet transfusions and care of patients who are thrombocytopenic are discussed in Chapters 29 and 30, respectively.

Anemia. Anemia, or hematocrit (Hct) below 30% and hemoglobin (Hgb) below 10 gm/dL, is a common finding in patients with leukemia. Expect anemia along with neutropenia and thrombocytopenia. As with neutropenia and thrombocytopenia, the leukemic cells crowding out the healthy red cells in the bone marrow may cause anemia, or it may be the result of chemotherapy. The primary treatment for anemia is an RBC transfusion. Nursing considerations in administering blood transfusions are covered in Chapter 29. Other precautions for patients with anemia are outlined in Box 29.4.

Fatigue. Almost all patients with acute leukemia experience fatigue, which has been described as an overwhelming tiredness or exhaustion. Causes of fatigue in these patients can include a low RBC count (anemia) from both the disease and the treatment, the buildup of metabolic wastes as the leukemic cells are being destroyed and cleared from the body, disrupted sleep, and the psychologic stress of the disease and treatment. A discussion of fatigue is presented in the Nursing Care of the Patient With Cancer section in Chapter 7.

Impaired oral tissue integrity. Stomatitis, an inflammation of the mucous membranes, is also a common side effect of chemotherapy. Discussion of the nursing management of stomatitis is presented in Chapters 7 and 38.

Inadequate nutrition. Nausea, with or without vomiting, is a common side effect of chemotherapy. Persistent nausea and vomiting can adversely affect a patient's nutritional status and psychologic state. The licensed vocational nurse/licensed practical nurse (LVN/LPN) can play an important role in managing this most distressing side effect. A discussion of the nursing management of nausea and vomiting related to chemotherapy is presented in Chapter 7.

Anxiety. A diagnosis of leukemia is likely to be alarming to patients and their families. Patients must deal not only with the disease and treatment but also with the feelings and emotions of facing a life-threatening illness. Encourage patients to ask questions and talk about their feelings. Often a patient's fears are caused by a lack of knowledge about the disease and treatment. The oncology clinical nurse specialist or other specially trained oncology nurse can answer many of the patient's and family's questions. Often information is what the patient and family need to deal with their anxieties. However, a referral to a social worker, chaplain, or mental health counselor may be indicated if the patient and family are having continued anxiety and difficulty in coping. It is important to know what the patient understands about the disease, the treatment, and the prognosis so that correct information can be reinforced.

Ineffective management of therapeutic regimen. The patient must receive accurate, consistent information from all members of the health care team. An oncology clinical nurse specialist or other specially trained oncology nurse can usually provide comprehensive information about the disease and its treatment to the patient and family and answer questions as they arise during hospitalization. All nurses reinforce this teaching. The Leukemia & Lymphoma Society (www.lls.org; telephone: 1-800-955-4572) provides excellent, free literature on the different types of leukemia. The National Cancer Institute, through the Cancer Information Service, also provides excellent, free literature on chemotherapy for people receiving treatment. It can be reached by calling 1-800-4-CANCER or on the internet at www.nci.nih.gov. The American Cancer Society (www.cancer.org; telephone: 1-800-227-2345) offers various local support services for people with all forms of cancer, including leukemia. Many resources provide answers to questions online, using email, and via live chat sessions with experts.

OTHER IMMUNE SYSTEM DISORDERS

HYPERSENSITIVITY REACTIONS

Hypersensitivity reactions, or allergies, are exaggerated immune responses that can be uncomfortable and potentially harmful to the patient. The four types of hypersensitivity reactions are classified according to the time between exposure and reaction, the immune mechanism involved, and the site of reaction.

Type I immediate hypersensitivity reactions are mediated by immunoglobulin (Ig) E reacting to common allergens such as dust, pollen, animal dander, insect stings, or various drugs. Type I reactions can be either local (resulting in local swelling and discomfort) or systemic (resulting in anaphylaxis and possible death if not recognized and treated promptly). Type I anaphylactic (systemic) hypersensitivity reactions occur in the following way. After a first, sensitizing exposure to a specific allergen, subsequent exposures to the same allergen trigger an exaggerated antibody reaction. For example, in a person with a hypersensitivity reaction to insect stings, one insect sting results in the production of abnormally large amounts of IgE antibodies. When this person is stung again by the same type of insect, the circulating IgE immediately triggers the release of histamine and other cytokines from mast cells, causing bronchial constriction, peripheral vasodilation, and increased capillary permeability. These individuals can experience airway obstruction, pulmonary congestion, peripheral edema, hypotension, shock, and circulatory collapse. Prompt diagnosis and treatment of anaphylaxis with epinephrine, antihistamines, corticosteroids, and hemodynamic support are of paramount importance.

Type II immediate hypersensitivity reactions are mediated by antibody reactions. Type II hypersensitivity reactions can occur with a mismatched blood transfusion or as a response to various drugs.

Type III immediate hypersensitivity reactions result in tissue damage resulting from precipitation of antigen-antibody immune complexes. Type III hypersensitivity reactions can occur with autoimmune reactions, with some occupational diseases, or as a response to various drugs.

Type IV delayed hypersensitivity reactions result from immune cells migrating to the site of exposure days after the exposure to the antigen. Type IV hypersensitivity reactions can occur with contact dermatitis, measles rash, tuberculin skin testing, or various drugs. Transplanted graft rejection occurs because of a type IV hypersensitivity reaction. Hypersensitivity reactions to drugs, or drug allergies, are one of many possible adverse drug reactions. Drug-induced hypersensitivity reactions can be any of the four types of hypersensitivity.

AUTOIMMUNE DISEASES

As mentioned earlier in the description of tolerance and how the body learns to recognize itself, autoimmune diseases occur when a breakdown of tolerance occurs. The immune system inappropriately identifies its own proteins as foreign and mounts a response to destroy these self-proteins. Examples of autoimmune diseases are idiopathic thrombocytopenic purpura (ITP), thrombotic thrombocytopenic purpura (TTP), acute rheumatic fever, type 1 diabetes mellitus, SLE, multiple sclerosis, rheumatoid arthritis, Graves disease, and Hashimoto thyroiditis.

IDIOPATHIC (IMMUNE) THROMBOCYTOPENIC PURPURA

ITP is an antibody-mediated **autoimmune disorder** in which IgG mistakenly helps to destroy the patient's own platelets. Drugs known to induce ITP include beta lactams (penicillin cephalosporins), thiazide diuretics, chlorpropamide, heparin, vancomycin, and rifampin. Patients with human immunodeficiency virus (HIV) infection are at increased risk for developing ITP. The condition sometimes resolves without treatment, but it may become chronic and require medical intervention.

Treatment for ITP can include platelet infusions and glucocorticoids or intravenous immune globulin (IVIG). For patients who do not respond to initial therapy, second line treatments include splenectomy, rituximab, and thrombopoietin receptor agonists (TPO-Ras). Adult patients with ITP commonly sequester (store) platelets in the spleen and so splenectomy may be done to remove this storehouse, thereby increasing the circulating blood levels of platelets. Immunosuppressive therapy with cytotoxic drugs such as cyclophosphamide or azathioprine can be used in patients who do not respond to splenectomy. The monoclonal antibody rituximab is being used off label with dexamethasone and is showing promising results. Drugs that boost platelet production include the thrombopoietin receptor agonists romiplostim (Nplate) and eltrombopag (Promacta). Nursing actions for the patient who is at risk for injury from bleeding from ITP are outlined in Box 29.5.

Pharmacology Capsule

Advise patients taking glucocorticoids to take them early in the day because these drugs can disrupt sleep.

THROMBOTIC THROMBOCYTOPENIC PURPURA

TTP is characterized by extensive blood clot formation and decreased blood flow to affected tissues. These patients become critically ill, developing fever, thrombocytopenia, hemolytic anemia, renal impairment, and neurologic symptoms. TTP may be inherited or acquired. The acquired condition is caused by antibodies that block the activity of an enzyme that is involved in blood clotting. Factors that may trigger TTP include some conditions (e.g., pregnancy, HIV, lupus), medical procedures (e.g., surgery, stem cell transplant), some drugs (e.g., ticlopidine, clopidogrel, chemotherapy, hormone therapy), and quinine.

The main treatment for TTP is plasma exchange (PEX), also called plasmapheresis, which aims to remove the immunologic agent that triggered the TTP from the plasma. The patient's blood is centrifuged in an apheresis machine that separates the blood components so that the plasma can be selectively removed. Critically ill patients can become hemodynamically unstable during this procedure and need close monitoring and timely interventions to maintain cardiac output and blood pressure. Other treatments include drug therapy with corticosteroids and rituximab. Caplaxizumab (Cablivi) is ordered for selected patients. Platelet transfusions are usually contraindicated because they may contribute to the abnormal clotting process. Nursing actions for the patient who is at risk for injury from bleeding are outlined in Box 29.5.

SYSTEMIC LUPUS ERYTHEMATOSUS

SLE is an autoimmune disease in which the person's immune system loses its ability to recognize itself and mounts an immune response against its own proteins. Damage results from antibodies and immune complexes directed against organ systems that may include the skin, joints, kidneys, central nervous system (CNS), cardiovascular system, membranes lining body cavities, and hematologic and immune systems. The four types of SLE are systemic, cutaneous, drug-induced, and neonatal. Approximately 1.5 million people in the United States have the disease.

The cause of SLE is unknown; however, genetics, environmental triggers, and altered immune function all appear to play a role in the occurrence of the disease. Ninety percent of cases occur in women, usually of childbearing age. The disease is much more common in Black, Latino, and Asian Americans than in White Americans (see the Cultural Considerations) box. Damage to affected organs is progressive in this disease. The most common causes of death in these patients are infection and diseases of the cardiovascular system, renal system, pulmonary system, and CNS. Factors associated with a poor outcome include increased creatinine, hypertension, large amounts of protein excreted in the urine, anemia, and low socioeconomic status.

Cultural Considerations

What Does Culture Have to Do With Lupus?

Although the cause of systemic lupus erythematosus (SLE) is unknown, a genetic predisposition is thought to exist. The disease is more common in women and is 3 times more common in Black American women than in White American women.

Clinical Manifestations

Patients with SLE can experience long periods of remission alternating with periods of symptom exacerbation ("flares"). Individual patients present with various combinations of symptoms depending on which organs are affected. The most common symptoms, experienced by 95% of patients at some time during the course of their disease, are fatigue, malaise, fever, anorexia, nausea, and weight loss. Musculoskeletal symptoms, also experienced by 95% of patients at some time during the course of their disease, include arthralgias (joint pain) and myalgias (muscle pain). Joints are often swollen, tender, stiff, and painful with movement. Cutaneous symptoms can include a rash and photosensitivity. The classic skin lesion is a butterfly-shaped rash across the bridge of the nose and the cheeks. This rash can extend to the neck, upper trunk, and arms. Life- and organ-threatening symptoms can include inflammation of the kidneys, heart, and lungs resulting in organ failure. Inflammation of the retina of the eye can result in sudden-onset blindness.

Medical Diagnosis

No single test confirms the diagnosis of SLE. Blood work may detect antinuclear antibodies (ANAs), but a positive ANA assay is not specific for SLE. A negative ANA assay makes the diagnosis of SLE unlikely but not impossible. A variety of other blood tests for specific antibodies may be done to assist in the diagnostic process. Blood test results, along with clinical manifestations, are used to make a diagnosis of definite SLE, probable SLE, or possible SLE. The more manifestations the patient has, the more likely SLE is present. Because symptoms come and go, the diagnosis of SLE can be very difficult to make and can take a long time. One set of criteria has been established by The American College of Rheumatology (ACR). Using the ACR criteria, a diagnosis of SLE can be made if a patient experiences any four of the following:

- Characteristic "butterfly" rash
- Discoid rash (red, scaly patches that cause scarring)
- Photosensitivity with exposure to sunlight
- Oral ulcers
- Arthritis (i.e., peripheral joint tenderness, swelling, or effusion in absence of erosion)
- Serositis: pleuritis or pericarditis (i.e., inflammation of the lining of the lungs or heart)
- Renal disorder (e.g., proteinuria or cellular casts)
- Neurologic disorder (e.g., seizures, psychosis)
- Hematologic disorder (e.g., anemia, leukopenia, thrombocytopenia)
- Immunologic disorder (as evidenced by detection of abnormal antibodies in the blood)
- Positive ANA test

Medical Treatment

No cure for SLE exists. The medical treatment of SLE is symptomatic and aimed at minimizing symptoms, preventing organ damage, and maintaining quality of life. Care is individualized because some patients have relatively mild symptoms, whereas others are severely affected. Fever, arthralgias, myalgias, and rash are managed with acetaminophen, nonsteroidal antiinflammatory drugs (NSAIDs), corticosteroids, and the antimalarial drug hydroxychloroquine. Some topical alternatives to corticosteroids for skin rash are tacrolimus and pimecrolimus. If symptoms are not controlled with these drugs or if organ function is threatened, immunosuppressive agents (e.g., voclosporin [Lupkynis], azathioprine [Imuran], mycophenylate mofetil [CellCept], cyclophosphamide [Cytoxan], methotrexate [Rheumatrex]) can be used to suppress the abnormal immune response. Voclosporin and the monoclonal antibody belimumab (Benlysta) are being used to treat lupus nephritis.

◆ NURSING CARE OF THE PATIENT WITH SYSTEMIC LUPUS ERYTHEMATOSUS

The nursing care of the patient with SLE varies depending on the severity of the symptoms the patient may be experiencing. Patients are treated primarily as outpatients. Because patients with SLE are frequent consumers of medical care, they often become very knowledgeable about their disease and want to be fully informed about all treatments they are receiving as well as the possible side effects of the treatments. The goal of care is quality of life.

Focused Assessment

The complexity of SLE requires a thorough health history and physical examination. Data collected by the LVN/LPN helps to determine the effects of the symptoms on the patient's activities of daily living (ADL) and quality of life.

Patient Problems, Goals, and Outcome Criteria: Systemic Lupus Erythematosus

Nursing goals and diagnoses for the patient with SLE are extremely individualized but may include the following.

Patient Problems	Goals and Outcome Criteria
Fatigue related to the disease process and treatment	Decreased fatigue: patient manages daily routines without excessive tiring
Pain related to acute and/or chronic inflammation of joints and muscles	Pain relief: patient states pain is relieved, appears relaxed
Altered body image related to skin rash, joint deformity	Improved body image: patient makes positive statements about self, takes measures to improve appearance
Inadequate coping related to stress of chronic illness	Effective coping: patient uses positive coping skills to reduce stress
Ineffective management of therapeutic regimen related to lack of knowledge about disease process and treatment	Patient resumes self-care: patient accurately describes disease process, treatments, and side effects of treatment

Interventions

Fatigue. Almost all patients with SLE report experiencing fatigue. Causes of fatigue in these patients can include a low RBC count from both the disease and the treatment, chronic pain, disrupted sleep, and the psychologic stress of the disease and treatment. The nursing management of fatigue is discussed in Chapter 7.

Pain. Inflammation of muscles and joints, as well as inflammation of various organs, can cause pain. Closely monitor the patient's pain level and medication use. Keeping a flow sheet of patient reports of pain on a 10-point scale can be helpful, especially as different nurses care for the patient throughout the day. A *0* represents no pain while a *10* represents the worst pain a patient has ever experienced. The patient's report of pain coupled with the amount of pain medication they are receiving can guide the nurse and physician as to the appropriate type and amount of pain medication. Pharmacologic and nonpharmacologic pain management strategies are presented in Chapter 8.

Altered body image. Encourage the patient to avoid prolonged exposure to the sun and to use sunscreen with a sun protection factor (SPF) rating of at least 30 to prevent the skin rash and exacerbation of symptoms.

Inadequate coping. A diagnosis of SLE is often a shock to patients and their families. Patients must deal not only with the disease and treatment but also with the emotions of facing a chronic illness. Encourage patients to ask questions and to talk about their feelings. A referral to a social worker, chaplain, or mental health counselor may be indicated if the patient and family are having difficulty coping.

Ineffective management of therapeutic regimen. The patient must receive accurate, consistent information from all members of the health care team. A clinical nurse specialist or other specially trained nurse can usually provide comprehensive information about the disease and its treatment to the patient and family and answer questions as they arise. It is important to know what the patient has been told about the disease, the treatment, and the prognosis so that correct information can be reinforced (see the Patient Teaching box). The patient's interpretation and understanding of the information is essential. The Lupus Foundation of America (www.lupus.org; telephone: 1-800-558-0121) provides excellent, free literature on SLE and can help to locate support groups in specific regions of the country.

Patient Teaching

Systemic Lupus Erythematosus

- Know the names, dosages, schedule, and side effects of your drugs.
- Avoid prolonged exposure to the sun and use sunscreen with a sun protection factor (SPF) rating of at least 30.
- You can get additional information from the Lupus Foundation of America and The National Resource Center on Lupus (https://www.lupus.org/resources).

HUMAN IMMUNODEFICIENCY VIRUS

Few viruses have descended on human beings as swiftly and wreaked as much devastation as **human immunodeficiency virus (HIV)**. The disease it causes, **acquired immunodeficiency syndrome (AIDS)**, has been seen in every country on the globe and claims victims without regard to age, race, class, gender, or sexual orientation. Despite advances, a cure has not been found; however, reason for hope exists. In the developed world, the disease has come to be viewed less as a fatal illness and more as a manageable chronic condition. However, in the developing world, where access to health care and medications is often difficult, the picture is less optimistic. Worldwide, only about 1 in 5 people at risk of becoming infected with HIV has access to prevention services.

HISTORY

The virus may have appeared as early as the 1940s, but it was not recognized as a new pathogen until the early 1980s. Young men generally have normally functioning immune systems, so epidemiologists (physicians who study patterns of illness) began to take note when immune deficiency conditions such as oral candidal infection (thrush); herpes; *Pneumocystis jirovecii* pneumonia; and Kaposi sarcoma (KS), a rare type of cancer, began to show up in the United States, primarily among urban populations of men who have sex with men (MSM). In 1986 two types of the HIV (HIV-1 and HIV-2) were isolated as the viruses that cause AIDS. HIV-1 is the predominant type around the world, whereas HIV-2 is mostly confined to West Africa. Within these types are multiple groups and subtypes. Some differences exist between the types, with HIV-1 being more easily transmissible and more likely to be progressive than HIV-2. When references are made to HIV without specifying a type, it can be assumed to be HIV-1 because it is so much more common.

MSM were just the first population to be recognized. Infection was soon seen in other populations, including the following:

- Individuals with hemophilia who must use blood products to treat the blood clotting disorder
- Patients who received a transfusion with HIV-infected blood or blood products
- Newborns and breast-fed infants of HIV-infected mothers (perinatal transmission)
- Injection drug users
- Partners, including heterosexuals, who had unprotected sex with those infected with the virus
- In some developing countries, such as those in sub-Saharan Africa, HIV infects more heterosexuals than homosexuals (see the Cultural Considerations box). It is transmitted by exposure to body fluids (e.g., blood, semen, breast milk, vaginal secretions) that contain the virus, not by lifestyle or sexual orientation.

DEMOGRAPHICS

According to the Centers for Disease Control and Prevention (CDC, 2020), the estimated number of persons in the United States living with diagnosed HIV infection is over 1.2 million. Six out of seven infected persons know they have the virus, meaning that a significant number of infected persons are unaware of their status. From 2014 to 2018, the number of new diagnoses declined by 7%. According to the CDC, 37,968 new cases were diagnosed in 2018.

Although HIV can infect anyone, infection rates are often reported by demographics, such as age, race, and gender.

- Age group. In 2018 the highest rate of new diagnoses was among persons aged 25 to 34 years. An estimated 10% of new diagnoses are among people aged 55 years or older.
- Gay or bisexual males accounted for most new cases (69%) (CDC, 2020).

- Race and ethnicity. The highest rate and the largest percentage are among Black Americans, followed by Hispanic/Latino Americans, White Americans, persons of multiple races/ethnicities, and Asian Americans. Native Hawaiians, other Pacific Islanders, Native Americans, and Alaska Natives had the lowest rates.
- Gender. In 2018 males accounted for the greatest percentage of all diagnoses of HIV infection among adults and adolescents (CDC, 2020).
- Drug Use. Some 7% of newly diagnosed HIV cases were persons who injected drugs.
- Another way of reporting HIV rates and AIDS diagnoses is by mode of transmission. The CDC has established five primary transmission categories:
  1. Male-to-male sexual contact
  2. Injection drug use
  3. Heterosexual (male-to-female) contact
  4. Mother-to-child (perinatal) transmission
  5. Other (which includes blood transfusions and unknown causes)

HIV is transmitted by blood and body fluids (i.e., breast milk, semen, and vaginal fluids). The virus has been found in low concentrations in the saliva, tears, and urine of infected individuals, but no recorded cases of transmission from these fluids exist. The risk of HIV transmission by various behaviors can be seen on a continuum from low risk to high risk. The levels of risk of HIV transmission via various behaviors can be found at https://www.cdc.gov/hiv/risk/estimates/riskbehaviors.html.

Cultural Considerations

Because HIV is disproportionately represented in some cultural groups, prevention programs need to be culturally sensitive to reach target audiences.

PATHOPHYSIOLOGY

Infection with HIV causes destruction of immune cells. HIV falls into a category of viruses called *retroviruses.* In these viruses, transcription of genetic material is reversed. Ribonucleic acid (RNA) is made into deoxyribonucleic acid (DNA) rather than the normal pattern of DNA to RNA. Reverse transcriptase is an enzyme that catalyzes the transcription of RNA into DNA.

Life Cycle of Human Immunodeficiency Virus

HIV first penetrates the body through blood and body fluids. HIV is spherical in shape and has two protein markers that protrude from the virus. These markers are like keys that attach themselves to protein markers found on macrophages and T4 helper cells or CD4 cells. Macrophages and T4 helper cells are distributed throughout the body, especially in mucous membranes and body orifices. Once HIV attaches to the macrophages and T4 helper cells, it infuses its genetic material into the host cell. The reverse transcriptase enzyme then transcribes HIV RNA into HIV DNA and inserts the HIV DNA into the host's DNA. Once the HIV DNA is incorporated into the host cell's DNA, billions of copies of HIV are made. Over time, the HIV destroys CD4+ T cells faster than the body can replace them. When the patient's immune response is severely impaired, opportunistic infections can gain access. A diagnosis of AIDS is made when the CDC criteria are met.

Body's Response to Human Immunodeficiency Virus Infection

Once infected with HIV, the body mounts a defense with antibodies and T cells. *Viral load* is a term used to describe how much virus is found in the blood. Especially high levels of viral load have been documented in the early phases of HIV infection. Approximately 12 weeks after infection, the body produces enough antibodies to be detected by standard HIV testing. Once sufficient antibodies are produced, the HIV viral load begins to drop, indicating partial effectiveness of the body to rid itself of HIV. Throughout the course of HIV infection, the body maintains high levels of HIV antibodies. However, CD8 cells and CD4 cells continue to decline throughout the course of the illness.

Health Promotion

The Centers for Disease Control and Prevention recommends HIV screening of all persons between the ages of 13 and 64 years so that cases can be detected early and treatment initiated. Men who have sex with men should be screened at least once each year. More frequent screenings may be advised for others at high risk (CDC, August 11, 2017, 2017).

STAGES OF HUMAN IMMUNODEFICIENCY VIRUS INFECTION

The initial stage of HIV infection lasts 4 to 8 weeks from the time of exposure. High levels of the virus are in the blood. About 50% of people who become infected with HIV experience generalized flu-like symptoms; the other 50% have no symptoms of infection. The virus then enters a latent stage during which it is inactive in the infected resting CD4 host cells. When the resting CD4 host cells are activated for an immune response, the virus begins to replicate. Levels of virus are high in the lymph nodes where CD4 cells reside but are low in the blood. The latent stage can last 2 to 12 years, during which time the patient is asymptomatic although the number of CD4 cells declines. During the third stage of HIV infection, the patient begins to experience opportunistic infections. These infections are called *opportunistic infections* because one can say that these microbes take advantage of the opportunity to infect the person who is HIV positive when their T cells are low. Levels of CD4 cells are usually less than 500 cells/mm^3 and declining while levels of virus in the blood are increasing. This stage can last 2 to 3 years. When the CD4 cell level falls below 200 cells/mm^3, the patient is considered to have AIDS. Virus levels in the blood are high.

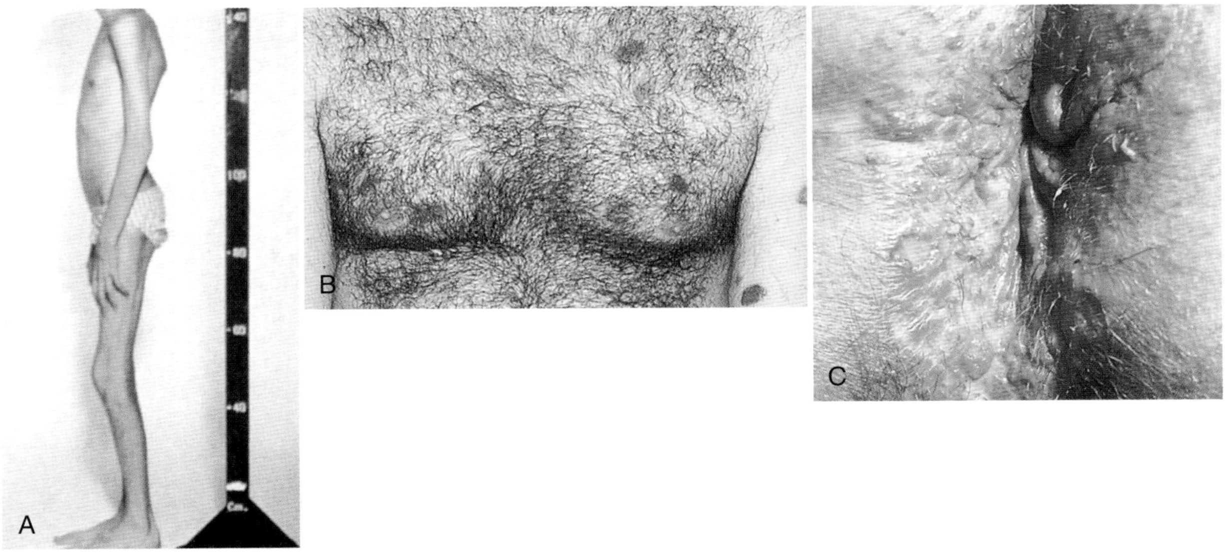

Fig. 32.1 Clinical Symptoms of Acquired Immunodeficiency Syndrome. (A) Severe weight loss and anorexia. (B) Biopsy-proven Kaposi sarcoma (KS) lesions. (C) Perianal vesicular and ulcerative lesions of herpes simplex infection. (A, from Taylor PK: *Diagnostic picture tests in sexually transmitted disease*, London, 1995, Mosby. B and C, From Morse SA, Ballard BC, Holmes KK, et al., editors: *Atlas of sexually transmitted diseases and AIDS*, ed 3, London, 2003, Mosby.)

With the initiation of triple antiretroviral drug therapy in the 1990s, HIV-related deaths dropped by two-thirds in developed countries. Antiretroviral drug regimens are abbreviated to ART and are also referred to as highly active **antiretroviral therapy** (HAART). With multidrug regimens and improved treatment of HIV complications, 80% of those diagnosed with HIV have now survived 10 years after being diagnosed. In July 2017, the CDC announced that 49% of people with HIV in the United States had the virus under control through HIV treatment. HIV/AIDS is increasingly becoming a chronic, managed disease rather than a terminal illness.

CLINICAL MANIFESTATIONS

Patients in the initial stage of HIV infection may experience only generalized flu-like symptoms such as malaise, nausea, and vomiting, decreased appetite, rash, and diarrhea. Because the symptoms are vague, HIV infection is not often diagnosed in the early stage. During the second, latent stage of the disease, patients may not experience any symptoms. Eventually they begin to experience frequent and persistent infections. Patients may present for medical care complaining of fever, night sweats, swollen lymph nodes, or other symptoms specific to the site of infection, such as headache, skin lesions that do not heal, sore throat, dyspnea, burning with urination, or diarrhea. Patients may also report extreme fatigue and weight loss. Any of these symptoms coupled with a history of unprotected sexual contact with persons possibly infected with HIV, a history of intravenous drug use with shared needles, or a history of a blood transfusion before 1989 warrants consideration of a diagnosis of HIV infection.

COMPLICATIONS

The major complications of HIV infection are opportunistic infections, wasting, secondary cancers, and dementia. Patients with AIDS are at very high risk for opportunistic fungal, parasitic, and viral infections. Infections that these patients commonly experience include oral candidiasis, *P. jirovecii* (formerly *P. carinii*) pneumonia, herpes simplex, cytomegalovirus retinitis, *Cryptosporidium* enteritis, *Cryptococcus neoformans* meningitis, and toxoplasmosis (Fig. 32.1). Almost all patients with HIV infection experience a wasting syndrome characterized by weight loss and malnutrition. Reduced food intake, malabsorption of nutrients, and altered metabolic pathways all contribute to this wasting syndrome. Cancers such as KS, NHL, anal cancer, and cervical cancer occur in 40% of patients with HIV infection. Presumably this increased incidence of cancer is caused by the inability of the patient's crippled immune system to identify and destroy cells that undergo malignant changes. The virus can affect the CNS, causing encephalopathy, cognitive impairment, and dementia.

Fig. 32.2 shows tissues that may be affected by HIV infection.

Opportunistic Infections

Once the body's CD4 cells, CD8 cells, or HIV antibodies (or a combination of these) fall below normal levels, infections and cancers that the body normally could resist take advantage of this opportunity and cause infection or cancer in the body. That is why these infections are called *opportunistic infections.* Parasites, fungi, bacteria, and viruses can cause opportunistic infections. Table 32.2 provides details of these diseases.

Parasitic Infections

Opportunistic parasitic infections include cryptosporidiosis, cystoisosporiasis, and toxoplasmosis. They are treated with antiprotozoal and other antiinfective drugs.

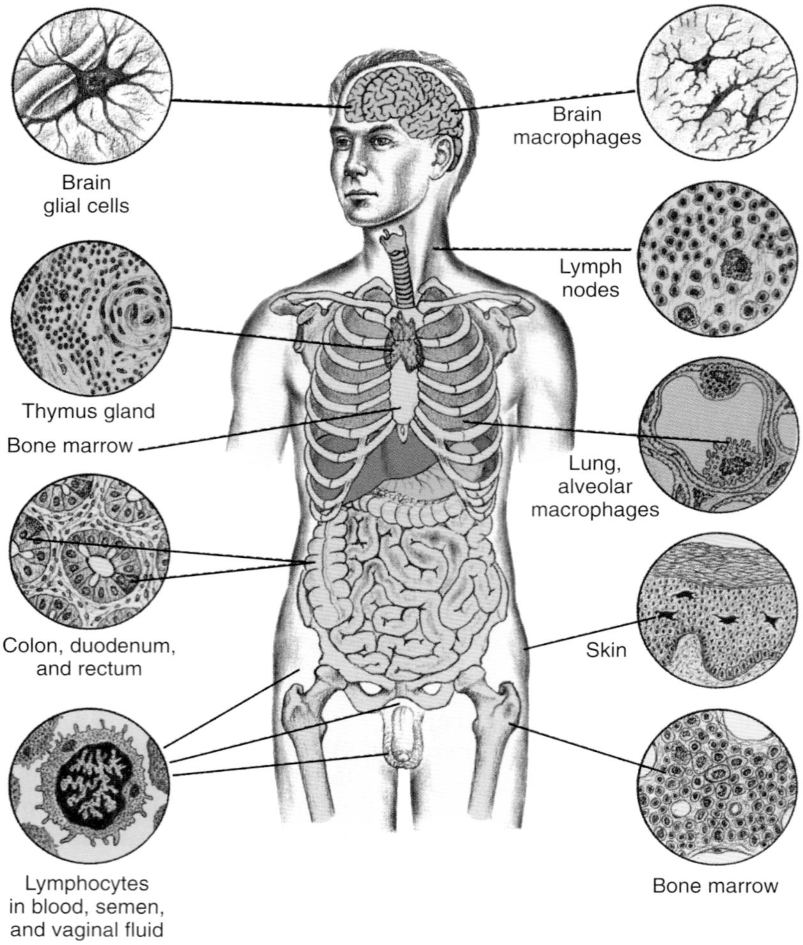

Fig. 32.2 Distribution of tissues that can be infected by human immunodeficiency virus. Infection is closely linked to the presence of CD4 receptors on host tissue, with the possible exceptions of glial cells in the brain and chromaffin cells in the colon, duodenum, and rectum. (From Monahan F, Sands J, Neighbors M, et al.: *Phipps' medical-surgical nursing: health and illness perspectives*, ed 8, St. Louis, 2006, Mosby.)

Fungal Infections

Opportunistic fungal infections include microsporidiosis, *P. jirovecii* pneumonia, aspergillosis, candidiasis, coccidioidomycosis, cryptococcosis, and histoplasmosis. These infections may be treated with various antifungal drugs, such as amphotericin B (Amphotec), itraconazole, nystatin, clotrimazole, fluconazole, ketoconazole, and flucytosine. Some antimalarial, antiinflammatory, antiprotozoal, and antiinfective drugs may be used for specific fungal infections.

Pharmacology Capsule

Amphotericin B, which is administered intravenously, causes fever, rigors, and headache. Pretreatment with diphenhydramine (Benadryl) and acetaminophen (Tylenol) as ordered will minimize this reaction. Rigors may be treated with meperidine (Demerol) or dantrolene (Dantrium). Amphotericin B can also cause electrolyte disturbances and is toxic to the kidneys.

Viral Infections

Opportunistic viral infections include various types of cytomegalovirus (CMV) infections, herpes simplex, herpes zoster, oral hairy leukoplakia (OHL), and progressive multifocal leukoencephalopathy (PML). Antiviral drugs are limited in number and work primarily by suppressing viral replication rather than killing the virus. Some of the antiviral drugs used are ganciclovir, famciclovir, valacyclovir, foscarnet, and acyclovir. Various combinations of these drugs may be used. See the Patient Teaching box.

Patient Teaching

Herpes Simplex Virus or Herpes Zoster Virus

When a patient has open sores on the skin, they should be instructed to do the following:

- Maintain good hygiene without drying out the skin.
- Avoid deodorant astringent soap.
- Use tepid water; pat the skin dry and do not rub it.
- Apply lotion after bathing and at bedtime.
- Do not scratch.
- Use a separate cloth for affected areas.
- Remember that some wounds need special care.
- Avoid contact with people who have never had chickenpox.

Bacterial Infections

Opportunistic bacterial infections include bacillary angiomatosis (BA), *Mycobacterium avium* complex (MAC), and tuberculosis. Treatments use various antibacterial drugs depending on the infecting organism. Patients need to understand the importance of taking antibacterials exactly as prescribed and completing the prescribed course of therapy. In persons with HIV infection, antiinfective drugs sometimes are ordered prophylactically when the CD4 cell count falls below certain levels.

Table 32.2 provides additional information about these infections.

Oncologic Conditions

Oncologic conditions that occur most often in persons with HIV infection include KS and lymphoma. Other cancer sites are the rectum and the vagina.

Table 32.2 Opportunistic Infections

INFECTION	MANIFESTATIONS	MODE OF TRANSMISSION	PREVENTION
Parasitic			
Cryptosporidiosis and cystoisosporiasis	Watery diarrhea, often severe	Contaminated water	Good hygiene. Clean water source
Toxoplasmosis	CNS (most common site in immunosuppressed people): dull, constant headache, weakness, seizures, altered level of consciousness, hemiparesis, cerebellar tremor, and visual field defects. Pulmonary: dyspnea, nonproductive cough Eyes: loss of visual acuity, photophobia	Cats, mammals, and birds harbor the parasite. Spread by ingestion of contaminated food or contact with animal feces.	Good hygiene Avoid undercooked and raw meats. Wear gloves and wash their hands after changing cat litter box (CDC, 2017).
Fungal			
Pneumocystis jirovecii pneumonia	Lungs: pneumonia* with dyspnea on exertion, fever, nonproductive cough *previously known as *Pneumocystis* pneumonia (PCP).	Inhalation	Prophylactic treatment with trimethoprim-sulfamethoxazole
Aspergillosis	Fever, cough, dyspnea, chest pain, and hemoptysis. High mortality rate among immunocompromised patients.	Inhalation of *Aspergillus* spores found in soil, water, and air; e.g., potted plants, marijuana, wicker, household dust	Avoid wet, cool places.
Candidiasis	Mouth: "thrush," white plaques that can be scraped off, inflamed tongue and mucosa Esophagus: dysphagia, ulceration Vagina: vaginitis, thick, cheesy white or yellow discharge; intense itching; redness and swelling of labia and vulva Anus: inflammation Retinal and systemic involvement possible	Normally present in mouth, GI tract, and vagina. Also found in most foods, soil, and inanimate objects	Prophylactic drug therapy for immunosuppressed patients
Coccidiomycosis	Pulmonary: fever, weight loss, fatigue, dry cough, pleuritic chest pain Systemic effects: skin lesions, joint pain (knees, back), meningitis	Inhalation; endemic in the southwestern United States and northern Mexico	Avoid exposure to disturbed soils in endemic areas.
Cryptococcosis	CNS: altered mental status, stiff neck, visual disturbances, severe headache, malaise, nausea and vomiting Pulmonary: fever, cough, dyspnea; possible acute respiratory insufficiency in immunocompromised patients	Inhalation Found in soil and bird droppings	Prophylactic antifungal therapy for HIV-infected patients with low CD4 counts

Continued

Table 32.2 Opportunistic Infections—cont'd

INFECTION	MANIFESTATIONS	MODE OF TRANSMISSION	PREVENTION
Histoplasmosis	Pulmonary: fever, night sweats, weight loss, dyspnea Systemic: hypotension, liver and spleen enlargement, skin and mucous membranes lesions, decreased blood cell counts, acute respiratory failure	Inhalation. Found in soil and bird droppings, especially in the central and southern parts of the United States	Avoid disturbed soil, bird droppings, caves, contact with bird cages
Viral			
Cytomegalovirus (CMV) infection	Eye: inflammation (retinitis) Spinal cord: inflammation, paraplegia, disturbances in urinary and rectal sphincter control Nerve roots: inflammation (polyradiculitis): initial perineal and leg pain; then progressive paralysis, loss of reflexes, urinary retention and rectal incontinence CNS: subacute encephalitis with headache, impaired cognition and sensorium, apathy, social withdrawal Lungs: pneumonia GI tract: inflammation (colitis): diarrhea, weight loss, fever	Acquired throughout life. Present in semen, cervical secretions, saliva, urine, blood, and organs. Transmitted mainly by blood and body fluids through unprotected sex.	Avoid exposure to body fluids with safe sex practices
Herpes simplex virus (HSV) and herpes zoster virus (HZV) infections	Initial or reactivated HSV infection: Skin: lesions, perineal ulcerations Mouth: ulcerations, "cold sores" Esophagus: inflammation (esophagitis) Colon: inflammation (colitis) Lung: inflammation (pneumonitis) Male genitalia: penile lesions Female genitalia: lesions of vulva, vagina, cervix Virus is transmissible even when no signs are present HZV reactivation: shingles	In patients who are HIV positive, infection is usually caused by reactivation of the dormant virus from an earlier infection. Fever, stress, ultraviolet light also can reactivate HSV.	Prophylactic antiviral drugs may suppress activity, but are not curative. Condoms for sexual activity whether lesions are present or not. See the *Patient Teaching* Box for HSV
Oral hairy leukoplakia	Epstein-Barr virus causes firm plaques on the sides of the tongue; lesions eventually resolve	Usually acquired in childhood or adolescence via saliva. Resides in B lymphocytes. Sheds at intervals without symptoms.	No specific preventive measures except to suppress virus with HAART
Progressive multifocal leukoencephalopathy (PML)	Jamestown Canyon (JC) virus rarely causes PML unless patient is immunosuppressed. Initial signs: weakness, speech and language abnormalities, behavioral and cognitive disturbances. In some patients: gait disturbances, sensory loss, visual impairment, seizures, problems with balance. Prognosis has improved greatly with HAART	Transmitted by mosquito and tick bites	Protect against insect bites

Table 32.2 Opportunistic Infections—cont'd

INFECTION	MANIFESTATIONS	MODE OF TRANSMISSION	PREVENTION
Bacterial			
Bacillary angiomatosis (BA)	Causative bacteria: *Bartonella henselae* and *B. quintana* Primarily manifests in skin lesions: papules and plaques anywhere on the skin. Can affect other organs.	Usually transmitted by cats and their fleas. Most patients with BA have been bitten or scratched by a cat.	Warn patients with HIV about the risk of being around cats; the patient should avoid rough play with cats and ensure that cats are treated for fleas
Mycobacterium avium complex (MAC)	Causative bacteria: *Mycobacterium avium* May affect any organ of the body, causing fever, fatigue, weight loss, night sweats, abdominal pain, and diarrhea.	Found everywhere in most food, animal, and soil sources. Not contagious.	Prophylactic treatment should be considered when CD4 cell counts drop below 50 cells/mm^3
Tuberculosis	Causative bacterium *Mycobacterium tuberculosis.* Primarily affects the lungs but may involve other organs, especially in patients with HIV. Tuberculosis is discussed in Chapter 28.	Inhalation or ingestion of infected droplets. Patients with HIV infection are much more likely than healthy persons to develop tuberculosis if exposed and if CD4 cell counts drop below 200 cells/mm^3	Protection from infected persons. Good handwashing.

CNS, Central nervous system; *CDC*, Centers for Disease Control and Prevention; *GI*, gastrointestinal; *HAART*, highly active antiretroviral therapy; *HIV*, human immunodeficiency virus.

Kaposi sarcoma. KS is a common type of neoplasm that develops in people with AIDS. It is caused by KS-associated herpes virus that is transmitted by exchange of saliva. KS affects the skin first, appearing as a macular, painless, nonpruritic lesion. KS can vary in color—pink, red, purple, and brown. As the disease advances, the lesions may become swollen, ulcerated, and painful. Other symptoms develop when tumors spread to the GI system, oral palate, and lungs. Sometimes when KS shows on the skin, it has already affected the body internally. When KS affects the GI system, bleeding may result, causing anemia. When KS affects the respiratory system, hypoxia may occur. Less often, the liver, bones, and soft tissue are affected. KS is diagnosed by clinical appearance, but the most definitive method of diagnosis is a biopsy.

No cure exists for KS, and the goal of treatment is long-term remission. Among the usual treatment options are antiretroviral drugs, chemotherapy, doxorubicin, daunorubicin, and paclitaxel. Surgical intervention, cryotherapy, and radiotherapy are used less often. To help patients with self-care, see the Patient Teaching box.

Patient Teaching

Patient With Kaposi Sarcoma

- Tumor growth varies from patient to patient.
- Regardless of therapy, KS tends to recur.
- Various therapies are available; each has risks and benefits.
- For patients with cutaneous KS: report blood in stool or abdominal pain.

Lymphoma. Lymphoma is cancer that originates in lymphoid tissue—bone marrow, spleen, or thymus gland. Immunodeficient patients have a much greater risk than the general population of getting one of eight distinct lymphomas. The two types of lymphoma are (1) Hodgkin and (2) non-Hodgkin. NHL is the second most common malignancy found in patients with AIDS.

The prognosis with NHL is poor because the disease has spread widely by the time it is discovered. With chemotherapy, survival rates are as follows:

- 24 months with CD4 cell counts above 100 cells/mm^3
- 4.5 months with CD4 cell counts less than 100 cells/mm^3
- 2 months if the CNS is affected

Symptoms are typically vague, vary according to the site involved, and include chills, fever, night sweats, and weight loss. Having a fever for more than 2 weeks strongly suggests lymphoma. The diagnosis, treatment, and nursing care of patients with lymphoma are covered earlier in this chapter.

MEDICAL DIAGNOSIS

Fourth-generation diagnostic tests for HIV test for both HIV antibodies and the p24 antigen. The p24 antigen is an HIV protein that is elevated in the first few weeks after a person becomes infected. This allows for diagnosis earlier than older tests, because antibodies may not be measurable for as long as 12 weeks. The CDC recommends repeat testing to confirm initial positive results.

The CDC (2013) criteria for a diagnosis of AIDS include the following:

- CD4 cell count of less than 200 cells/mm^3, asymptomatic
- CD4 cell count of less than 200 cells/mm^3, with category B symptoms (which include BA; candidiasis; oropharyngeal, vaginal, and cervical dysplasias; herpes zoster [shingles]; ITP; listeriosis; OHL; pelvic inflammatory disease [PID]; and peripheral neuropathy)
- Category C symptoms, regardless of CD4 cell count (these include candidiasis of bronchi, trachea, or lungs; esophageal or cervical cancer; coccidioidomycosis; cryptococcosis; cryptosporidiosis; CMV; encephalopathy; herpes simplex virus [HSV]; chronic ulcers of longer than 1 month's duration or bronchitis, pneumonitis, or esophagitis; histoplasmosis; isopsoriasis; KS; lymphoma; *M. avium, M. tuberculosis,* or *P. jirovecii* pneumonia; pneumonia—recurrent; progressive multifocal leukoencephalopathy; salmonella; septicemia—recurrent; toxoplasmosis; and wasting because of HIV infection)

Several diagnostic products are available for home testing. The Home Access HIV-1 Test System requires the patient to prick a finger for a small blood sample, apply the sample to a special card, and mail the card to a laboratory for analysis. The results can be available by telephone in as little as one day. OraQuick ADVANCE is a home-testing kit that detects HIV-1 and HIV-2 antibodies in 20 minutes using a cheek swab. False negative results occur in about 8% of infected persons using OraQuick. That means those persons have the infection even though the test indicates they do not. With both of these tests, retesting should be done to confirm initial results.

Home testing is controversial because of the risks of incorrect results as well as the lack of professional counseling about the results. For example, a person in the early stage of infection who tests negative because not enough antibodies exist to be detected might assume that they are free of infection and fail to protect a sexual partner.

MEDICAL TREATMENT

No cure for HIV infection exists. The medical treatment of HIV infection is aimed at reducing the viral load, preventing and treating infections, and treating malignancies. Patients are also encouraged to maintain a balanced diet, exercise regularly, maintain good dental hygiene, avoid smoking and using illicit drugs, limit alcohol intake, minimize stress, and practice safe sexual habits. The Health Promotion box addresses reducing the risk of perinatal transmission of HIV infection. Table 32.3 lists the classes of drugs used to treat HIV infection.

Health Promotion

WOMEN AND HUMAN IMMUNODEFICIENCY VIRUS

Women with human immunodeficiency virus (HIV) infection should be treated with antiretroviral drugs during pregnancy and delivery. As well, the newborn should be treated for the first 6 weeks of life to decrease the risk of transmission of the virus to the baby.

OLDER ADULTS AND HUMAN IMMUNODEFICIENCY VIRUS

Nearly half of people living with HIV in the United States are over 50 years of age, and approximately 40% of those with AIDS are 50 years of age or older. Older adults are at increasing risk for HIV infection, AIDS, and other sexually transmitted infections (STIs). Many factors contribute to the increasing risk of infection in this age group. See the Health Promotion box below.

Health Promotion

Factors That Contribute to Human Immunodeficiency Virus Among Older Adults

- Older people may lack awareness of HIV risk factors.
- Health care providers may not assess HIV risk or perform screening tests in older patients.
- Older patients may be less likely to approach the health care provider about sex and drug use.
- Little HIV prevention education is directed at older people.
- Many older people believe that HIV is a young person's disease.
- Older patients may fail to get "safe sex" education.
- Newly single older persons may have ignored HIV prevention methods when they had a partner.
- Older adults often mistake the symptoms of HIV/AIDS for the aches and pains of normal aging, so they are less likely to be tested for HIV infection.

Pharmacology

Patients with HIV infection are commonly started on a medication regimen when the HIV viral load reaches a certain level. The regimen typically comprises various combinations of protease inhibitors, nucleoside reverse transcriptase inhibitors (NRTIs), and nonnucleoside reverse transcriptase inhibitors (NNRTI). Other categories are fusion inhibitors, chemokine coreceptor antagonists, and integrase inhibitors. Examples of each class of antiretroviral drugs are presented in Table 32.3.

Before the patient with HIV infection is started on a medication regimen, the prescriber must assess the patient's ability and willingness to comply with the therapy. Once a medication regimen is started, the patient with HIV infection should not miss doses. When a dose is missed, the serum drug level falls, which allows the virus to mutate and build resistance to the HIV medications. Resistance is a very serious problem with antiretroviral drugs. If resistance to enough of the HIV medications builds up, the patient will have no medication options, which will ultimately end in their death. Therefore if the

Table 32.3 Medications Used to Treat Patients With Human Immunodeficiency Virus Infection

DRUG	USE AND ACTION	SIDE EFFECTS	NURSING INTERVENTIONS
Drugs that Inhibit HIV Enzymes			
Nucleoside/Nucleotide Reverse Transcriptase Inhibitors (NRTIs)			
abacavir (Ziagen) didanosine (Videx) emtricitabine (Emtriva) lamivudine (Epivir) stavudine (Zerit) tenofovir (Viread) zidovudine (Retrovir) **Note:** Numerous combination drugs are available (e.g., Epzicom, Truvada, Combivir, et al.)	Used to slow the progression of HIV infection by suppressing synthesis of viral DNA. The drug Truvada is a combination of tenofovir and emtricitabine that is used preexposure to prevent HIV transmission.	Anemia, neutropenia, headache, confusion, nausea, diarrhea, fatigue, muscle damage, skin rash, lactic acidosis with enlarged liver and fatty liver, pancreatitis, peripheral neuropathy, and lipodystrophy. *See a drug handbook for effects specific to each drug.*	Some of these drugs should be taken on an empty stomach while others can be taken with or without food; check manufacturer's direction. Neutrophil counts and hemoglobin must be monitored as directed, usually every 2–4 weeks. Liver function will also be monitored. Multiple drug interactions are possible between NRTIs and other drugs; therefore the prescriber must review the patient's complete medication record before beginning these drugs or adding other drugs to the patient's regimen.
Protease Inhibitors (PIs)			
atazanavir (Reyataz) darunavir (Prezista) fosamprenavir (Lexiva) indinavir (Crixivan) lopinavir and ritonavir (Kaletra) nelfinavir (Viracept) ritonavir (Norvir) saquinavir (Invirase) tipranavir (Aptivus)	Used to slow the replication and progression of HIV by blocking protease enzymes so that infected cells cannot produce HIV proteins.	Diarrhea, nausea and vomiting, kidney stones, jaundice, abdominal pain, headache, skin rash, numbness and tingling around the mouth, drooling, dizziness, sleepiness, sore throat, sweating, altered taste, and lipodystrophy.	Advise patient whether specific PIs should be taken on an empty stomach or with food. Multiple drug interactions are possible between PIs and other drugs; therefore the patient's complete medication record must be reviewed before beginning these drugs and before adding other drugs to the patient's regimen after they are started on a protease inhibitor.
Nonnucleoside Reverse Transcriptase Inhibitors (NNRTIs)			
delavirdine (Rescriptor) efavirenz (Sustiva) etravirine (Intelence) nevirapine (Viramune) rilpivirine (Edurant)	Used to slow the progression of HIV by directly interfering with replication inside the T helper/CD4 cell.	Mild to severe skin rash, headache, dizziness[a], drowsiness[a], nightmares[a], nausea, diarrhea, liver damage, and fatigue. Patients with history of mental illness or drug abuse at greater risk. Teratogenic.	Can be taken with or without food. Multiple drug interactions are possible between NNRTIs and other drugs. Inform patients that some of these drugs decrease the effectiveness of hormonal contraceptives. Therefore, the patient's complete medication record must be reviewed before beginning these drugs and before adding other drugs to the patient's regimen after they are started on an NNRTI.
Integrase Strand Transfer Inhibitor (INSTI)R			
raltegravir (Isentress) dolutegravir (Tivicay)	Used to treat HIV infection. Considered a first-choice HIV drug. Inhibits the insertion of HIV into DNA of CD4 cells.	Insomnia and headache. Rhabdomyolysis (muscle destruction releases myoglobin that damages kidneys). Rare: hypersensitivity, liver failure.	Immediately report signs of hypersensitivity: rash, blisters, fever, malaise, fatigue, oral lesions, facial edema, muscle and joint aches. Drug must be discontinued if signs of rhabdomyolysis occur: muscle pain, dark urine, increased CPK.

Continued

Table 32.3 Medications Used to Treat Patients With Human Immunodeficiency Virus Infection—cont'd

DRUG	USE AND ACTION	SIDE EFFECTS	NURSING INTERVENTIONS
Drugs that Block HIV Entry Into Cells			
Fusion Inhibitor			
enfuvirtide (Fuzeon)	Fuzeon is used in combination with other antiretroviral drugs in treatment experienced patients who have increasing HIV levels. This drug prevents the HIV from entering CD4 T cells.	Irritation at injection site, pneumonia, hypersensitivity, neutropenia, fatigue, nausea, and insomnia.	Reconstitute and store as directed. Inject subcutaneously as ordered (usually twice daily) and rotate sites.
Chemokine Receptor 5 (CCR5) Antagonist			
maraviroc (Selzentry)	Blocks the entry of HIV into CD4 cells used in combination with other antiretroviral agents.	Cough, dizziness, fever, rash, abdominal pain, musculoskeletal symptoms, URIs, liver damage. Uncommon: MI.	

[a]Usually resolve within a month.
DNA, Deoxyribonucleic acid; *HIV*, human immunodeficiency virus; *MI*, myocardial infarction; *URIs*, upper respiratory infections.
Modified from Burchum JR, Rosenthal LD: *Lehne's pharmacology for nursing care*, ed 10, St Louis, 2019, Elsevier. Skidmore-Roth L: *Mosby's 2021 nursing drug reference*, ed 34, St. Louis, MO, 2021, Elsevier.)

patient will not comply with the HIV medication regimen, it would be better to not start it. Some common side effects of antiretroviral therapy are as follows:

- Lipodystrophy
- Hepatitis
- Diabetes
- Increased cholesterol
- Increased low-density lipoproteins (LDLs)
- Increased triglycerides
- Pancreatitis
- Hemolytic anemia
- Peripheral neuropathy
- Nephrolithiasis and nephrotoxicity
- Stevens-Johnson syndrome
- Myopathy
- Hypersensitivity reaction
- Hepatotoxicity
- Nightmares
- Nausea, vomiting, and diarrhea

GI upset is a very common side effect of antiretroviral drug therapy and is one of the major reasons for noncompliance. The nurse should make the patient with HIV infection aware that many of the side effects of the regimen are transitory and will subside within a few weeks.

Health Promotion

Prevention of Human Immunodeficiency Virus Transmission

- Sexual abstinence
- Sex only in a mutually monogamous relationship with a person who is HIV negative
- Consistent and correct condom use
- Abstinence from injection drug use
- Consistent use of sterile equipment if unable to cease using injected drugs
- Preexposure prophylaxis (PrEP) with emtricitabine/tenofovir (Truvada) can reduce the risk of HIV transmission by as much as 90%.

PREVENTION

The most effective way to avoid HIV infection is to avoid exposure (see the Health Promotion box). However, exposure may occur for a variety of reasons. When that happens, the person who has been exposed should seek medical care immediately. For preventive drug therapy to be effective, it must be started within 72 hours of the exposure. The health care provider will test the individual for HIV to make sure the person does not already have the infection. Once a negative HIV test is obtained, a 28-day drug regimen of antiretroviral drugs, called postexposure prophylaxis (PEP) will be prescribed. Meanwhile, the person must continue to use condoms with sex partners and avoid sharing needles and drug preparation equipment ("works") with others. Although PEP is highly recommended, it cannot guarantee that the patient will not develop the infection. The health care provider will monitor the patient for up to 6 months to be certain the patient remains HIV-negative.

Preexposure prophylaxis (PrEP) taken daily can reduce the risk of HIV transmission by more than 90% (Mayer & Krakower, 2020). The drug Truvada is a combination of tenofovir disoproxil fumarate and emtricitabine that is highly effective if used as prescribed. The CDC (2018) recommends PrEP as one prevention option for the following:

- Sexually active adult MSM at substantial risk of HIV acquisition
- Adult heterosexually active men and women who are at substantial risk of HIV acquisition
- Adult persons who inject drugs and are at substantial risk of HIV acquisition

The use of PrEP should be explored with heterosexually active women whose partners are known to have HIV infection as one of several options to protect the uninfected partner during conception and pregnancy. An informed decision must be made considering the risks and benefits of PrEP to the mother and the fetus.

Pharmacology Capsule

Truvada must be taken daily to prevent human immunodeficiency virus infection. Truvada may cause nausea initially, but that side effect usually subsides over time.

NURSING CARE OF THE PATIENT WITH HUMAN IMMUNODEFICIENCY VIRUS INFECTION

Care of the patient with HIV infection varies depending on the stage of infection the patient is experiencing (see the Nursing Care Plan). During the early stages of the disease, patients are treated primarily as outpatients. Because patients with HIV infection are frequent consumers of medical care, they often become very knowledgeable about their disease and treatment options and want to be actively involved in all treatment decisions. In the later stages of HIV infection, nursing care is much more intensive as the patient becomes more debilitated. Throughout the course of this disease, the goal of all treatments is good quality of life.

FOCUSED ASSESSMENT

Infection is the leading cause of death in patients with HIV infection. Therefore, it is important to assess the patient frequently for any signs or symptoms of infection. The most common sites of infection are the lungs, mouth, GI tract, skin, blood, and CNS. Any change in the physical examination findings or any change in function should be reported to a registered nurse (RN) or physician. While collecting data about the patient's physical status, determine how much the patient knows about the disease and treatment as well as how the patient is coping with this life-threatening disease. The complete assessment, as done by the RN, is outlined here. The LPN/LVN may collect some of these data.

Health History

A complete health and social history should be obtained from each patient with HIV infection. The history should include the following:

- History of sexually transmitted infections (STIs)
- Surgical history
- Medication history: all current drugs, compliance, allergies, response to HIV drugs
- Immunization history
- Family history
- Sexual history—number of partners the patient has had in the past year
- Needle and blood exposure history—exposure to hepatitis B and C
- History of screening for hepatitis B and C
- Tobacco and alcohol use
- Illegal drug use history—use of intravenous drugs or unsafe behavior while using drugs
- Travel history—travel outside United States to locations where possible exposure to pathogens may have occurred
- Pet history—exposure to cats, birds, or exotic pets
- Occupational history—exposure to pathogens in the workplace
- Nutritional history—usual food and fluid intake
- Gynecologic history—number of pregnancies, knowledge of contraceptives

Physical Examination

A complete physical examination should be performed (review the Nursing Care Plan). The examination should include the following:

- General examination—measurement of height, weight, vital signs
- Skin examination—signs of infections, lesions
- Head, ears, eyes, nose, and throat examination
- Lymphatic system—enlarged lymph glands
- Respiratory system—auscultation for quality of breath sounds
- Cardiovascular examination
- Abdominal examination
- Musculoskeletal examination
- Neurologic examination—orientation, alertness, sensory and cognitive functioning
- Genitourinary examination

Patient Problems, Goals, and Outcome Criteria: Human Immunodeficiency Virus Infection

Patient Problems	Goals and Outcome Criteria
Ineffective management of therapeutic regimen related to lack of knowledge about disease process and treatment, denial, fear	Effective self-care management: patient correctly describes and demonstrates self-care measures
Anxiety related to the disease and treatment	Reduced anxiety: patient reports anxiety is lessened, more relaxed manner
Potential for infection (lung, mouth, gastrointestinal [GI] tract, skin, blood, central nervous system [CNS], eye) related to decreased immunity	Patient remains free of infection: no fever, signs of inflammation, lesions
Impaired oral tissue integrity related to the disease and oral infections	Intact oral mucous membranes: normal color of mouth tissues, no lesions

Continued

Nursing Care Plan Patient With Human Immunodeficiency Virus Infection

FOCUSED ASSESSMENT

Health History

A 25-year-old divorced mother of two children works as a freelance accountant and lives with her parents, who provide financial and emotional support. She was diagnosed with human immunodeficiency virus (HIV) infection during the pregnancy with her daughter, who is now 2 years old and has shown no signs of HIV infection. The patient and her husband have been divorced since her infection was diagnosed. His HIV status is not known. She reports tiring easily but most days is able to work about 6 hours and care for her children. She is seen monthly by a nurse practitioner (NP) at a neighborhood clinic. Her medications are dolutegravir (Tivicay), tenofivir (Viread), and emtricitabine (Emtriva). She reports bouts of depression and anxiety about her own and her children's future. Her most recent blood studies show a decline in the number of T helper (CD4) cells. The CD4 cell count today is 480 cells/mm^3. She has been treated twice this fall for upper respiratory tract infections. She does not sleep well. She has experienced a 10-lb weight loss in the past 3 months and reports poor appetite and frequent diarrhea.

Physical Examination

Healthy-looking young woman. Alert. Converses easily. Vital signs within normal limits (WNL). No fever. Skin intact; no lesions. Lungs clear on auscultation. No lymphadenopathy. Abdomen soft. Bowel sounds present in all four quadrants. Normal reflexes. Full range of motion in all joints.

Patient Problem	Goals and Outcome Criteria	Interventions
Ineffective management of therapeutic regimen related to lack of knowledge about disease process and treatment, denial, and fear	Patient will effectively manage self-care, as evidenced by correctly taking prescribed medications and following medical advice for rest and protection from infection.	Provide written and verbal instructions for any prescribed drugs. Advise her of the kinds of side and adverse effects she might experience. Explain the importance of continuing the drugs under medical supervision. Discuss ways to conserve energy and to promote restful sleep at night. Explore options to obtain assistance with child care.
Anxiety related to disease and treatments	Patient will verbalize decreased anxiety and will appear more relaxed.	Encourage her to ask questions and talk about her feelings. Be accepting of feelings she may express (fear, anger, and depression are common). Provide information or refer her to a social worker, support groups, chaplain, or mental health counselor if needed.
Potential for infection related to impaired resistance	Patient will remain free of infection, as evidenced by absence of fever, lesions, or signs of inflammation.	Encourage her to report any signs of infection immediately. If antibiotics are ordered, encourage her to take them as prescribed. Explain the need to avoid people with infections and crowded public places during seasons when upper respiratory tract infections are common.
Impaired oral tissue integrity related to human immunodeficiency virus (HIV) infection and oral opportunistic infections	Patient will have intact oral mucous membranes with normal color and no lesions.	Teach the importance of regular dental care. Advise her to use a soft toothbrush and to avoid traumatizing oral tissues. Explain how maintaining good fluid intake keeps mucous membranes moist and reduces oral complications.
Inadequate nutrition and fluid volume deficit related to HIV infection, diarrhea, and gastrointestinal (GI) infections	Patient's intake of food and fluids will be adequate, as evidenced by stable body weight, moist mucous membranes, and normal blood pressure and pulse.	Suggest the addition of Carnation Instant Breakfast to her daily diet to increase calorie intake. Weigh her weekly. Talk to the nurse practitioner (NP) about prescribing antinausea medication, an appetite stimulant, and an antidiarrheal drug.

CRITICAL THINKING QUESTIONS

1. How would you explain to the patient the importance of taking the prescribed drugs as ordered?
2. What other suggestions could you give this patient to help her increase her intake of food and liquids throughout the day?

Patient Problems, Goals, and Outcome Criteria: Human Immunodeficiency Virus Infection—cont'd

Patient Problems	Goals and Outcome Criteria
Inadequate nutrition and fluid volume deficit related to the disease, diarrhea, and GI infections	Adequate intake of nutrients and fluids: stable weight, intake and output approximately equal, moist mucous membranes
Confusion related to disease-induced dementia	Resolved confusion: patient's consciousness, attention, cognition, and perception improve to baseline Patient safety: absence of injuries associated with irreversible confusion
Pain related to actual or potential tissue damage	Pain relief: patient states pain is relieved, appears relaxed
Inadequate coping related to perceived lack of support, fear, anxiety	Effective coping: patient demonstrates strategies to cope with feelings about diagnosis in a positive way.

INTERVENTIONS

Ineffective Management of Therapeutic Regimen

It is vital that the patient receives accurate, consistent information from all members of the health care team. A clinical nurse specialist or other specially trained nurse can usually provide comprehensive information about the disease and its treatment to the patient and family and answer questions as they arise during hospitalization. You can reinforce this teaching. Excellent sources of current information about HIV and AIDS for patients, families, and health care providers are available on the internet (e.g., www.thebody.com, www.cdc.gov, www.nih.gov).

Anxiety

A diagnosis of HIV infection is always a shock to patients and their families. Patients must deal not only with the disease and treatment but also with the emotions of facing a life-threatening illness. Encourage patients to ask questions and to talk about their feelings. Often a patient's fears result from lack of knowledge about the disease and treatment. The clinical nurse specialist or other specially trained nurse can answer many of the patient's and family's questions. Often information will help the patient and family to deal with their anxiety. A referral to a social worker, chaplain, or mental health counselor may be indicated if the patient and family are experiencing continued anxiety and difficulty in coping. It is important for the nurse to know what the patient has been told about the disease, the treatment, and the prognosis so that correct information can be reinforced. The patient's interpretation and understanding of the information are essential.

Potential for Infection

As emphasized earlier, patients with HIV infection are at high risk for opportunistic infections. Early detection and prompt treatment of infections are vital. Many patients take antiinfective drugs (e.g., trimethoprim-sulfamethoxazole, pentamidine) prophylactically to prevent infections. Educate the patient about the importance of taking drugs exactly as prescribed. Stopping antibiotic therapy early can result in incomplete treatment and the development of resistant organisms. Many of the antibiotics must be administered intravenously and require nursing coordination for intravenous access and either clinic or home administration.

Impaired Oral Tissue Integrity

Patients with HIV infection can experience altered oral mucous membrane integrity because of the disease and oral infections. Encourage patients to clean their teeth and mouth regularly with dental floss and a soft toothbrush. Debilitated patients may need assistance with mouth care. Encourage noncaffeinated fluids to maintain hydration and keep oral mucous membranes moist. Topical anesthetics to control pain can be applied before eating. Prescribed topical anti-infectives should be reapplied after eating and routine mouth care. Regular dental evaluations can help to prevent and manage oral disease and infections in these patients.

Inadequate Nutrition

Many factors can alter the nutritional needs of the patient with HIV infection. A referral to a dietitian for nutrition education and counseling should be made as soon as the patient is diagnosed with HIV infection. The exact nutritional needs are specific to the individual based on a thorough assessment. When HIV is well controlled, the patient should follow the same principles of healthy eating and fluid intake as other individuals. If appropriate, strategies to maximize calorie and nutrient intake can be discussed. Oral supplements such as Carnation Instant Breakfast, Boost, Ensure, Sustacal, or Resource may be added as indicated. Medications may be prescribed to improve appetite (e.g., megestrol, dronabinol), relieve nausea, and control diarrhea. Deficiencies of vitamin A, zinc, and selenium are common with infectious conditions. However, micronutrient supplementation should be based on documented deficiencies. Caloric needs should be based on individual assessments. Because the resistance to pathogens may be impaired, advise the patient to avoid food that might contain pathogens (e.g., undercooked meat, raw eggs, unpasteurized milk) (see the Nutrition Considerations box).

Nutrition Considerations

Acquired immunodeficiency syndrome (AIDS) wasting is common among patients with AIDS. Factors thought to contribute to wasting include inadequate nutritional intake, the inability of the body to absorb nutrients, and increased metabolic rates from viral replication or disease complications. Among the many reasons for inadequate intake are problems chewing or swallowing, altered gastrointestinal motility, neurologic diseases that affect perceived hunger or ability to eat, psychosocial and economic factors, and anorexia caused by medications. Every patient with human immunodeficiency virus (HIV) infection should be seen by a nutritionist who can help to determine the basis for the inadequate intake and recommend interventions.

- Helpful nutrition teaching for the patient with HIV infection includes the following to reduce the risk of acquiring infections from foods:
- Do not buy expired foods.
- Do not buy cracked eggs.
- Thoroughly cook meats and poultry.
- Wash hands thoroughly before preparing foods.
- Wash all fruits and vegetables before eating them.
- Thaw frozen foods in the refrigerator, not at room temperature.
- Avoid eating leftovers.
- If the CD4 cell counts drop below 100 cells/mm^3, boil water for 1 minute or use sterile water products.
- Remember that many HIV drugs cause hyperlipidemia. If your serum lipids are high, you should eat small, frequent meals that are low in fat and lactose and high in caloric intake.
- Abstain from alcohol and caffeine.
- Eat healthy meals with five to six servings of fruits and vegetables per day.
- Weigh yourself daily and report patterns of weight loss or weight gain to your physician.

Fluid Volume Deficit

Because many HIV patients develop infections or cancers related to the GI tract, they often experience diarrhea, nausea and/or vomiting, or a poor appetite. This will often lead to fluid and electrolyte imbalances. It is very important for the nurse to monitor the patient's intake and output, daily weights, electrolytes, protein and albumin levels; and inform the provider of abnormal levels. HIV patients should be educated about the importance of maintaining a healthy, well-balanced diet, drinking 4 to 6 (8 oz) glasses of water daily, and taking a daily multivitamin if not contraindicated.

Patients who are nauseated or who are vomiting may be prescribed an antiemetic. Patients who have a poor appetite may be prescribed appetite stimulants. It is vital that the nurse assesses the patient frequently for fluid volume and electrolyte and nutritional status.

Confusion

Patients with HIV-induced encephalopathy may experience cognitive and motor impairment. Patients may withdraw from social activities because of embarrassment. They may become depressed, angry, and hostile with the onset of yet another disability. The primary treatment is an antiretroviral drug. Because the patient is likely already on antiretrovirals, the physician may add additional ones. In the hospital and at home, patient safety needs to be reevaluated constantly based on the patient's mental and physical capabilities.

Pain

Pain has been an underrecognized problem for patients with HIV infection. Pain can be caused by opportunistic infections, viral invasion into the nerves and muscles, malignant tumors, and diagnostic procedures. Closely monitor the patient's pain level and medication use. Keeping a flow sheet of patient reports of pain on a 10-point scale can be helpful, especially as different nurses care for the patient throughout the day. A *0* represents no pain while a *10* represents the worst pain a patient has ever experienced. The patient's report of pain, coupled with the amount of pain medication they are receiving, can guide the nurse and physician as to the appropriate type and amount of pain medication. Pharmacologic and nonpharmacologic pain management strategies are presented in Chapter 8.

Inadequate Coping

A diagnosis of HIV/AIDS, with its life-threatening consequences, can overwhelm the patient's ability to cope. Patients and their significant others may experience many emotions, such as fear, anxiety, anger, shame, grief, depression, and loss of self-esteem. Fearing social stigma, patients may be reluctant to share the diagnosis with others. Other than sexual partners and health care providers, the patient is not obligated to inform other persons.

Nurses must be aware of their own feelings, and even fears, about caring for people with HIV infection. Education about self-protection and measures to take in the event of body fluid exposure can relieve some of the nurse's concerns. Sensitivity and touch can be very comforting to patients. When changes in a patient's emotional state are noted, encourage the patient to talk about their feelings. Provide information about support groups and mental health care as needed.

Get Ready for the NCLEX® Examination!

Key Points

- Immunodeficiency occurs when the body is unable to launch an adequate immune response, resulting in an increased risk for infection.
- Neutropenia is an abnormally low neutrophil count.
- The patient with a low WBC count is at risk for infection.
- Lymphomas are cancers of the lymph system that are treated with surgery, radiation, chemotherapy, and hematopoietic stem cell transplant (HSCT).
- Leukemia is a cancer of the WBCs in which the bone marrow produces too many immature WBCs.
- The two main types of leukemia are (1) myelogenous and (2) lymphocytic; there are acute and chronic forms of each type.
- Patients with leukemia may have low RBCs and platelets as well as low WBCs.
- Infection is the leading cause of death in patients with leukemia.
- Allergy or hypersensitivity occurs when a normally inoffensive foreign substance stimulates an atypical or exaggerated immune response.
- An anaphylactic reaction is a life-threatening hypersensitivity event characterized by bronchial constriction, peripheral vasodilation, hypotension, and shock.
- Anaphylaxis is treated with epinephrine, antihistamines, corticosteroids, and respiratory support.
- SLE is an autoimmune disorder that can affect multiple body systems.
- Patient problems for the SLE patient may include: fatigue, pain, altered body image, inadequate coping, and ineffective management of therapeutic regimen.
- A person with ITP is at risk for uncontrolled bleeding.
- HIV is transmitted by body fluid exposure, including intrauterine exposure. HIV infection occurs in heterosexual and homosexual people of all races.
- The drug emtricitabine/tenofovir (Truvada) reduces the risk of HIV infection by approximately 90%.
- Behaviors by which HIV may be transmitted include needle sharing, unprotected sex, and blood transfusions.
- HIV is a retrovirus that enters the body through blood, semen, vaginal fluids, or breast milk.
- If drug therapy fails, HIV infection eventually exhausts the immune response to pathogens.
- CD8 cell count drops drastically in the late stage of HIV infection; CD4 cell count slowly declines throughout the course of the infection.
- A patient is considered to have AIDS when the CD4 cell count drops below 200 cells/mm^3.
- Initial symptoms of HIV infection are usually flulike symptoms.
- During the latent stage, which can last 2 to 12 years, patients may have no symptoms.
- During the later stages of HIV, patients may have fever, night sweats, swollen lymph glands, skin lesions, dyspnea, burning with urination, diarrhea, and other symptoms.
- The major complications of HIV infection are opportunistic infections, wasting, secondary cancers, and dementia.
- Parasites, viruses, bacteria, and fungi can cause opportunistic infections.
- The most common types of cancer associated with HIV infection are KS and lymphoma.
- The most accurate HIV blood tests are those that detect both HIV antigens and HIV antibodies.
- Infections are the leading cause of death in patients with HIV infection.
- Among the classes of drugs used to treat HIV infection are NRTIs, protease inhibitors, NNRTIs, fusion inhibitors, and integrase strand transfer inhibitors.
- Failure to take HIV drugs as scheduled can encourage resistant strains of HIV.
- Patient problems for the patient with HIV infection may include ineffective management of therapeutic regimen, anxiety, potential for infection, impaired oral mucous membrane integrity, inadequate nutrition, fluid volume deficit, confusion, pain, and inadequate coping.
- Inadequate nutritional intake or the inability of the body to absorb and use nutrients causes wasting.

Additional Learning Resources

SG Go to your Study Guide for additional learning activities to help you master this chapter content.

Go to your Evolve website (http://evolve.elsevier.com/Linton/medsurg) for the following learning resources and much more:

- Fluid & Electrolyte Tutorial
- Review Questions for the NCLEX® Examination

Clinical Judgment and Next-Generation NCLEX® Examination-Style Questions

1. **Which of the following is the priority when caring for a patient with neutropenia?**
   a. protection from trauma
   b. education about drug therapy
   c. prevention of infection
   d. promotion of adequate rest

   NCLEX Client Need: Safe and Effective Care Environment: Safety and Infection Control

2. **Which of the following conditions are classified as *autoimmune disorders*? (Select all that apply.)**
   1. Type 1 diabetes mellitus
   2. Hodgkin lymphoma
   3. Rheumatoid arthritis
   4. SLE
   5. Multiple sclerosis

   NCLEX Client Need: Physiological Integrity: Physiological Adaptation

3. **A patient who has an immune disorder has a low platelet count. Which data are most important for the nurse to collect in this situation?**
   1. Take the patient's temperature every 4 hours
   2. Inspect the skin for bruising and bleeding
   3. Measure urine output hourly
   4. Auscultate the breath sounds each shift

   NCLEX Client Need: Physiological Integrity: Physiological Adaptation

4. **An LVN/LPN is giving flu shots in a community clinic. Which emergency medication should be available in case of anaphylactic hypersensitivity?**
   1. epinephrine
   2. isoproterenol
   3. nitroglycerin
   4. norepinephrine

   NCLEX Client Need: Physiological Integrity: Pharmacological Therapies

5. **The nurse collects all of the data listed subsequently for a patient with leukemia who is undergoing chemotherapy. Which data should be reported immediately?**
   1. The patient states that he feels tired all the time.
   2. The patient's skin is pale and dry.
   3. The patient's oral temperature is 101°F.
   4. The patient eats only half of the food served at lunch.

   NCLEX Client Need: Physiological Integrity: Physiological Adaptation

6. **While on a hike, a woman was stung by an insect. Within minutes the site was painful, red, and swollen. This is an example of which type of hypersensitivity reaction?**
   1. Type I immediate hypersensitivity reaction
   2. Type II immediate hypersensitivity reaction
   3. Type III immediate hypersensitivity reaction
   4. Type IV delayed hypersensitivity reaction

   NCLEX Client Need: Physiological Integrity: Physiological Adaptation

7. **During the latent stage of HIV infection, which of the following cells host the HIV?**
   1. CD4 cells
   2. CD8 cells
   3. Antibodies
   4. Natural killer cells

   NCLEX Client Need: Physiological Integrity: Physiological Adaptation

8. **Through which of the following does HIV enter the body?**
   1. Inhaled particles
   2. Body fluids
   3. Contaminated food
   4. Skin contact

   NCLEX Client Need: Physiological Integrity: Physiological Adaptation

9. **What is the leading cause of death in persons with AIDS?**
   1. Cancer
   2. Infection
   3. Heart disease
   4. Renal failure

   NCLEX Client Need: Physiological Integrity: Physiological Adaptation

10. **Most antiretroviral drugs work by which mechanism?**
    1. Direct destruction of the HIV
    2. Stimulation of WBC production
    3. Enhanced production of antiviral phagocytes
    4. Suppression of HIV replication

    NCLEX Client Need: Physiological Integrity: Pharmacological Therapies

11. **A patient with HIV infection has recently become confused. Which of the following explanations should you provide to the patient's partner?**
    1. "Confusion with HIV is rare but irreversible."
    2. "The patient's confusion is probably caused by something other than HIV."
    3. "The patient's mental status may improve with drug therapy."
    4. "Confusion is usually the effect of drug toxicity."

    NCLEX Client Need: Physiological Integrity: Physiological Adaptation

12. **A 52-year-old person with AIDS is seen by the home health nurse. The nurse's assessment data are listed below.**
    - Painless purple lesions on the chest
    - Fever for last 2 days
    - Dyspnea on exertion
    - Recent onset of intermittent confusion
    - Painful perianal lesions
    - Weight gain of 3 kg since previous visit one week ago
    - Six diarrhea stools in 24 hours

    Highlight the assessment findings that should be reported promptly to the primary care provider.

Cardiovascular System Introduction

33

http://evolve.elsevier.com/Linton/medsurg

Objectives

1. Identify specific anatomic and physiologic factors that affect the cardiovascular system.
2. Describe age-related changes in the cardiovascular system.
3. Discuss the nursing assessment of patients with cardiovascular disorders.
4. Explain nursing care related to tests and procedures used to diagnose cardiovascular disorders.
5. Identify common therapeutic measures for cardiovascular disorders.

Key Terms

afterload
atrium/atria
atrioventricular valves
aneurysm (ĂN-yŭr-ĭzm)
blood viscosity (vĭs-KŎ-sĭ-tē)
bradycardia (bră-dĕ-KĂR-dē-ă)
contractility
diastole
dysrhythmia (dĭs-RĬTH-mē-ă)
hypertension
murmur (MŬR-mĕr)
preload
Purkinje fibers
semilunar valves
syncope (SĬN-kă-pē)
systole
tachycardia (tă-kĕ-KĂR-dē-ă)
ventricle

The cardiovascular system carries oxygenated blood and nutrients to the cells and transports carbon dioxide (CO_2) and wastes from the cells. Adequate functioning requires a reservoir for blood coming from the tissues, pumping action to send blood to the lungs and the body, and an intact vascular system to transport the blood. A malfunction in any of these components may affect other body systems and may threaten life or compromise overall health status.

ANATOMY AND PHYSIOLOGY OF THE CARDIOVASCULAR SYSTEM

HEART

The heart, located in the mediastinum, is covered and protected by the sternum and ribs anteriorly and flanked by the lungs laterally. The esophagus, the descending aorta, and the fifth through eighth thoracic vertebrae are directly behind the heart. The heart rests on the diaphragm, with two-thirds of it positioned to the left of the sternum. The right side of the heart is located under the sternum (Fig. 33.1).

The heart is a hollow muscular pump approximately the size of a person's fist. It weighs 10 to 14 oz in an adult and is covered by pericardial membranes called the *visceral* and *parietal pericardium*. The space between the pericardial membranes contains fluid that lubricates the membranes and decreases friction.

Chambers

The heart is divided into four chambers: two upper atria (right and left) and two lower **ventricles** (right and left). The four chambers are separated by septa (walls), with two chambers on the right (atrium and ventricle) and two chambers on the left (atrium and ventricle). Valves separate the atria from the ventricles.

The right and left sides of the heart receive blood from and send blood to different parts of the body. The right atrium (RA) is a thin-walled reservoir receiving blood from the inferior and superior vena cava and from the coronary sinuses. The right ventricle (RV) has thicker walls than the RA and receives blood from the RA through the tricuspid valve. Blood moves rather passively from the RA to the RV. When the RV contracts

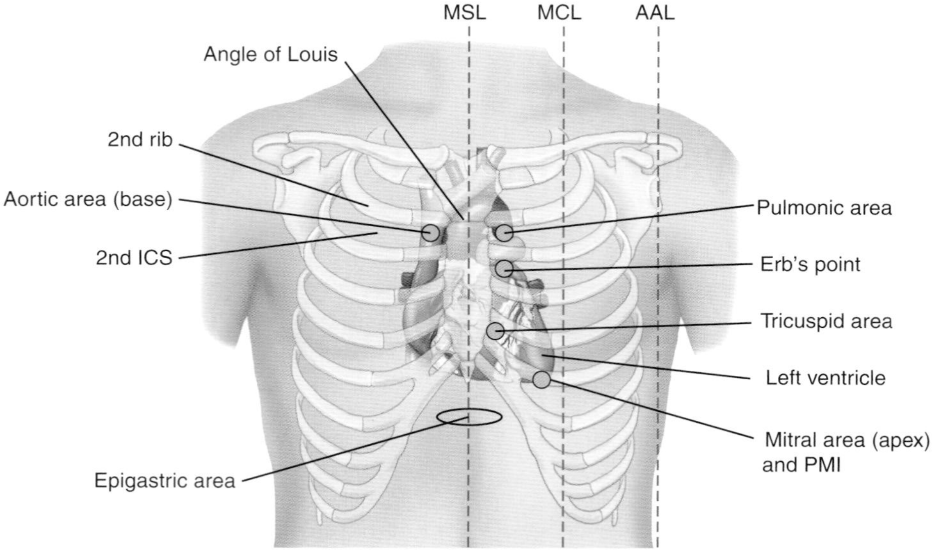

Fig. 33.1 Anatomic location of the heart. *AAL*, Anterior axillary line; *ICS*, intercostal space; *MCL*, midclavicular line; *MSL*, midsternal line; *PMI*, point of maximal impulse. (From Lewis SL, Dirksen SR, Heitkemper MM, et al.: *Medical-surgical nursing: assessment and management of clinical problems*, ed 9, St. Louis, 2015, Mosby.)

(**systole**), blood is ejected through the pulmonic valve into the pulmonary artery. The pulmonary artery carries the blood to the lungs, where it releases CO_2 as waste and picks up oxygen (O_2) to be taken to the tissues. Pulmonary veins carry the blood from the lungs to the left atrium (LA).

The blood passes from the LA through the mitral valve into the left ventricle (LV), the chamber with the thickest, strongest muscle. The LV is cone shaped and contains the apex of the heart located at the midclavicular line at the fourth or fifth intercostal space. An apical pulse is taken by auscultating the heartbeat at this location.

When the LV contracts (systole), blood is ejected through the aortic valve into the aorta and the systemic circulation. The systemic circulation carries O_2 and nutrients to all active cells and transports wastes to the kidneys, liver, and skin for excretion (Fig. 33.2).

The pressures in the RA and RV are very low compared with the pressures in the LA and LV. This is because the LV pumps blood out into the systemic circulation. The pressure in the LV is the highest of all the chambers.

Muscle Layers

Three layers of cardiac muscle tissue exist: (1) the endocardium, (2) the myocardium, and (3) the epicardium. The endocardium is the inner layer that lines the heart chambers. The middle layer, the myocardium, is made of muscle fibers and is responsible for the pumping action of the heart. The thickness of the myocardium varies with each chamber. The outer layer, the epicardium, is also the visceral pericardium. The coronary arteries are embedded in the epicardium.

Valves

Four valves exist in the heart: (1) the mitral, (2) the tricuspid, (3) the aortic, and (4) the pulmonic. Their purpose is to retain blood in one chamber until the next chamber is ready to receive the blood. The valves keep blood flowing in one direction by opening and closing passively, in response to changes in pressure and volume. A valve opens when the pressure behind it is greater than the pressure that is ahead. A valve closes when the pressure ahead of it is greater than the pressure that is behind.

Atrioventricular valves. The mitral and tricuspid valves are called **atrioventricular (AV) valves** because they separate the atria from the ventricles. The tricuspid valve separates the right atrium from the right ventricle. The mitral valve is between the left atrium and the left ventricle. Cusps, or leaflets, are attached by chordae tendineae to the papillary muscles that line the floor of the ventricles. These valves are closed during systole and open during diastole.

Semilunar valves. The **semilunar valves**, called *aortic* and *pulmonic*, separate the ventricles from the aorta and the pulmonary artery, respectively. These valves are open during systole and closed during diastole. The semilunar valves have three cusps (cup-shaped structures) each.

Heart sounds. Closure of the valves produces the heart sounds auscultated over the heart. The first heart sound (S_1), referred to as *lub*, occurs when the ventricles contract during systole and when the mitral and tricuspid valves close. The second heart sound (S_2), called *dub*, occurs during ventricular relaxation or diastole and is caused by the closing of the aortic and pulmonic valves.

CORONARY BLOOD FLOW

The coronary arteries are the first branches of the systemic circulation. These arteries supply blood to the

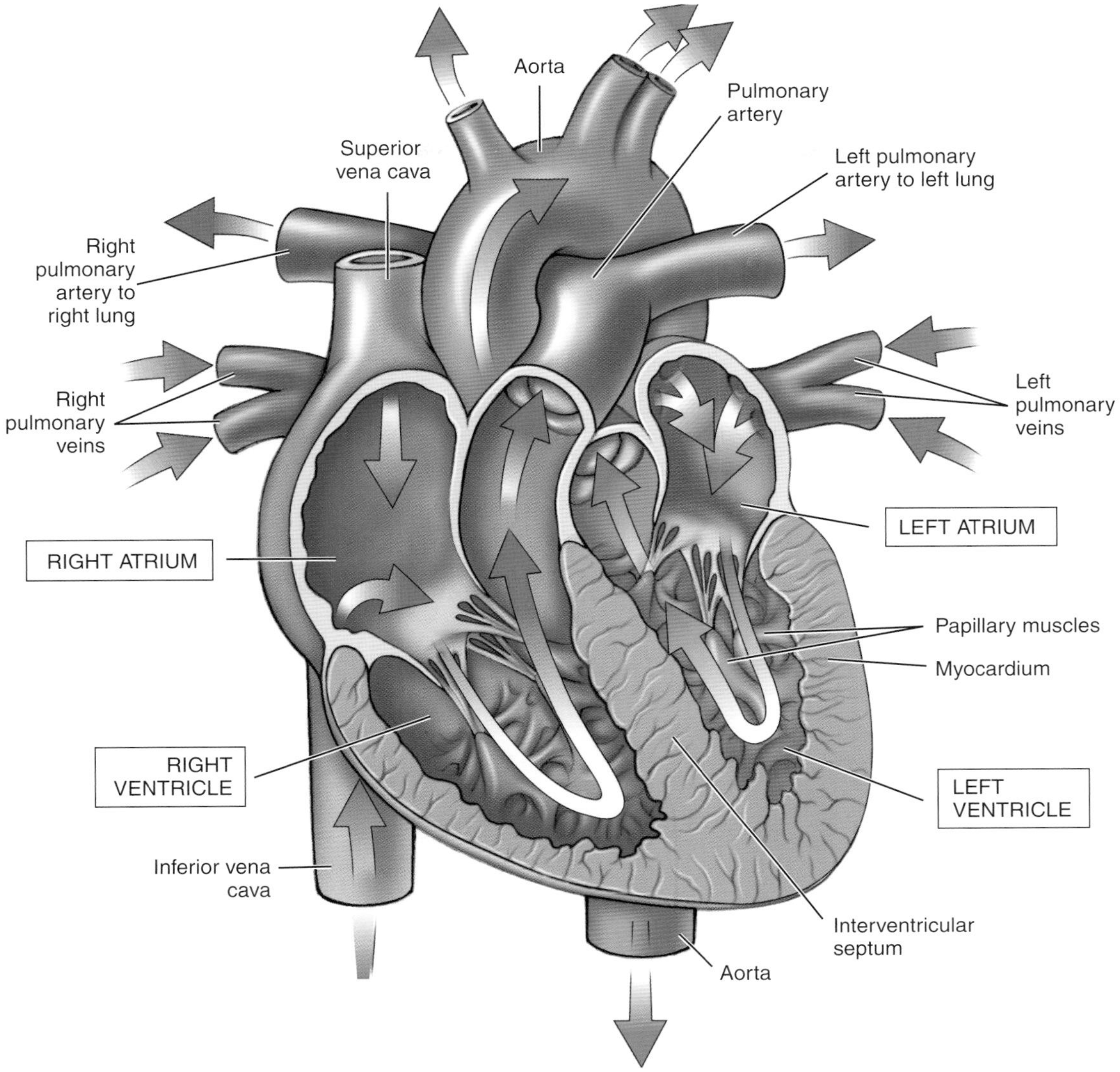

Fig. 33.2 Normal circulation through the heart. (From Herlihy B: *The human body in health and illness*, ed 4, St. Louis, 2011, Saunders.)

myocardium and the conductive tissue of the heart. The two major coronary arteries, the left coronary artery and the right coronary artery, arise from the aorta just beyond the aortic valve. Blood flow through the coronary arteries occurs during diastole. The left coronary artery, which branches into the left anterior descending and circumflex arteries, supplies blood to the LA, most of the LV, and most of the septum between the two ventricles (interventricular septum). The right coronary artery branches to supply the sinoatrial (SA) and the AV nodes, the RA and RV, and the inferior part of the LV. Variations in the pattern of arterial branching are common.

Collateral arteries are connections between two branches of arteries. They are more common in certain areas of the heart. It is thought that collateral circulation protects the heart, and that coronary collaterals develop over time as a result of gradual coronary occlusion.

In general, the venous system parallels the arterial system: the great cardiac vein follows the left anterior descending artery, and the small cardiac vein follows the right coronary artery. The veins meet to form the coronary sinus (the largest coronary vein), which returns deoxygenated blood from the myocardium to the right atrium (Fig. 33.3).

CONDUCTION SYSTEM

For the heart to pump blood through the chambers, nerves must stimulate muscle contractions in an orderly fashion. The conduction pattern follows a particular route. The SA node, also called the *pacemaker*, initiates the impulse. The impulse is carried throughout the atria to the AV node, located on the floor of the right atrium. The impulse is delayed in the AV node, and then transmitted to the ventricles through the bundle of His. The bundle is made up of Purkinje cells and is located where the atrial and ventricular septa meet. The bundle of His divides into the left and right bundle branches. The terminal ends of the right and left branches are called the **Purkinje fibers**. When the

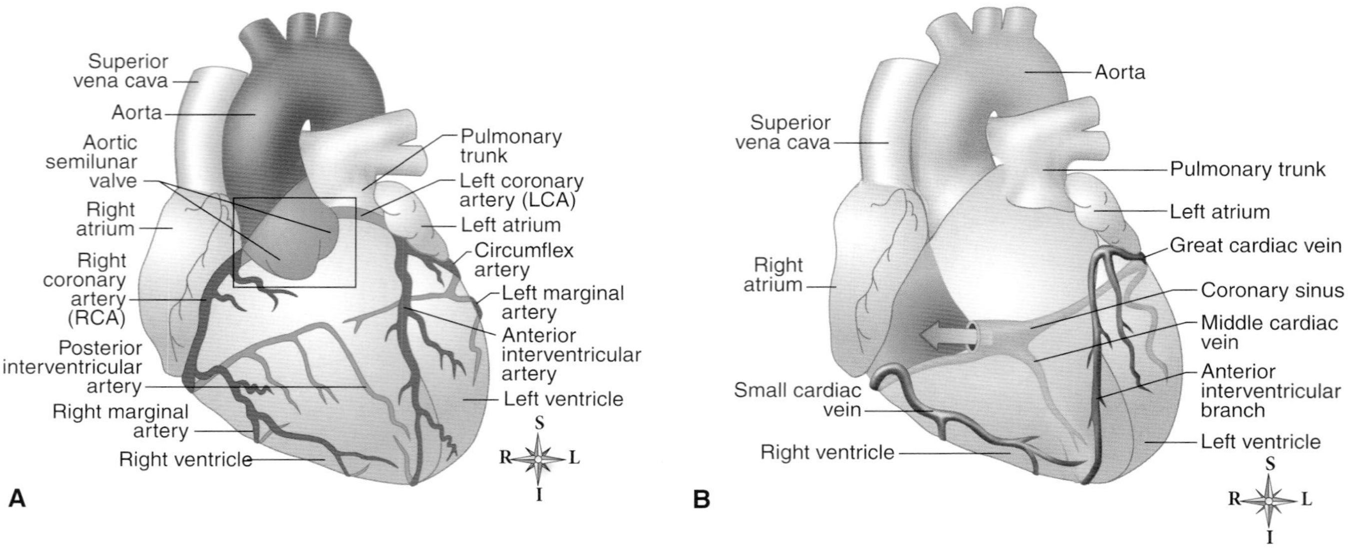

Fig. 33.3 Coronary arteries (A) and veins (B). (From Patton KT, Thibodeau GA: *The human body in health & disease*, ed 7, St. Louis, 2018, Elsevier.)

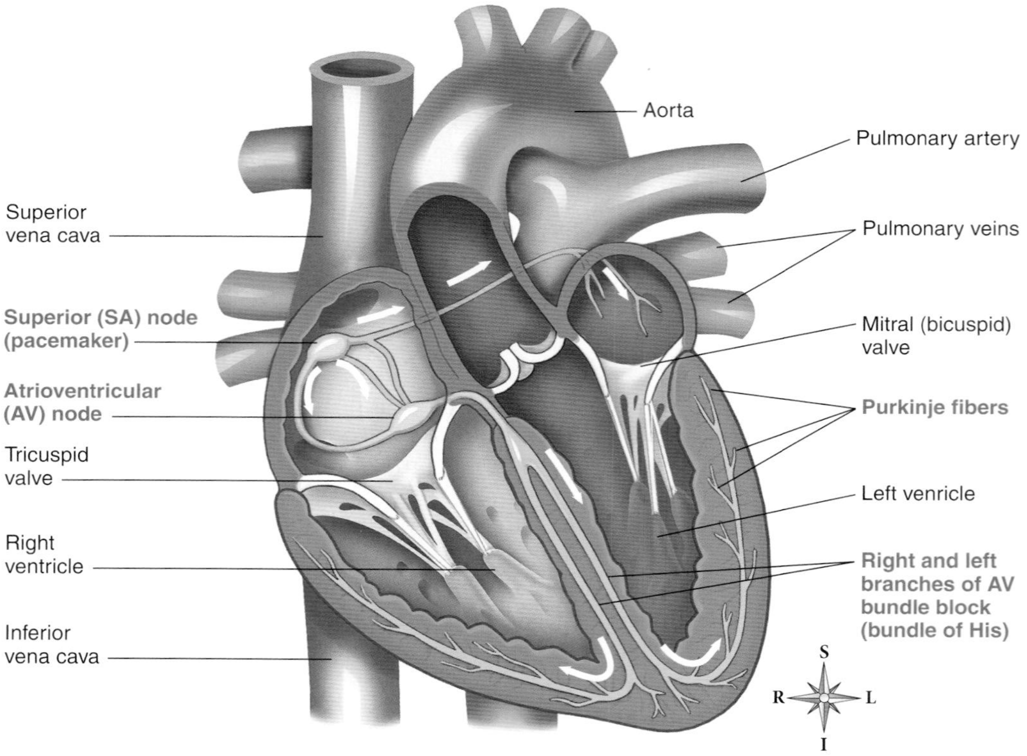

Fig. 33.4 The conduction system of the heart. (From Patton KT, Thibodeau GA: *The human body in health & disease*, ed 6, St. Louis, 2014, Elsevier.)

impulse reaches the Purkinje fibers, the ventricles contract (Fig. 33.4).

The impulse produces a change in the movement of electrically charged ions across the membrane of cardiac cells. Cardiac cells at rest are electrically polarized, with the inside of the cell negatively charged and the outside of the cell positively charged. When stimulated, cardiac cells lose their internal negativity by a process called *depolarization*. Depolarization moves from cell to cell, producing a wave of electrical activity that is transmitted throughout the heart. Once depolarization is complete, the resting state (i.e., the inside of the cell is more negative than the outside) is restored through a process called *repolarization*.

The SA node normally generates these impulses at a rate between 60 and 100 beats per minute. The AV node is also capable of generating an impulse if the SA node should fail. The AV node rate is 40 to 60 beats per minute.

Table 33.1 Intrinsic Heart Rates

INITIATION OF IMPULSE	RATE
Sinoatrial (SA) node	60–100 beats per minute
Atrioventricular (AV) node	40–60 beats per minute
Ventricle	15–40 beats per minute

The Purkinje network can also generate an impulse, but it does so at less than 40 beats per minute, which could prevent cessation of heart function for a short time (Table 33.1).

Cardiac Innervation

Sympathetic and parasympathetic fibers of the autonomic nervous system innervate the heart. Sympathetic fibers are distributed throughout the heart. Sympathetic stimulation results in increased heart rate, increased speed of conduction through the AV node, and more forceful contractions. Parasympathetic fibers, which are part of the vagus nerve, are found primarily in the SA and AV nodes and the atrial tissue. Parasympathetic stimulation results in slowing of the heart rate, slowing of conduction through the AV node, and decreased strength of contraction.

CARDIAC FUNCTION

The primary function of the heart is to pump blood through the pulmonary and systemic circulations. This is accomplished by a continually repeating pattern of contraction and relaxation.

Cardiac Cycle

Contraction and relaxation of the heart make up one heartbeat and are called the *cardiac cycle.* When the ventricles are at rest (relaxation phase), they are filling up with blood coming from the atria. This is called **diastole**. At the end of diastole, the atria contract to eject more blood into the ventricles (called the *atrial kick*). Once the ventricles have filled with blood and the electrical impulse has reached the terminal fibers of the conduction system, the ventricles contract and eject blood into the pulmonary artery from the RV and into the aorta from the LV. This is called *systole.* A person with a heart rate of 60 beats per minute would have 60 cardiac cycles per minute.

Cardiac Output

The amount of blood ejected by the heart each minute is determined by stroke volume and heart rate. Stroke volume is the amount of blood ejected with each ventricular contraction. The normal stroke volume is 60 to 100 mL. Cardiac output (CO) is the amount of blood (in liters) ejected by the heart per minute. It is calculated by multiplying the heart rate (HR) by the stroke volume (SV):

$$CO = HR \times SV$$

The normal cardiac output is 4 to 8 L/min. In the normal heart, cardiac output responds to the increased demands for O_2 and nutrients that occur with exercise, infection, or stress.

Three factors affect stroke volume: (1) preload, (2) contractility, and (3) afterload.

Preload. **Preload** is the amount of blood remaining in a ventricle at the end of diastole or the pressure generated at the end of diastole. Increased preload results in increased stroke volume, and thus increased cardiac output. Factors that increase preload include increased venous return to the heart and overhydration. Factors that decrease preload include dehydration, hemorrhage, and venous vasodilation.

Contractility. **Contractility** is the ability of cardiac muscle fibers to shorten and produce a muscle contraction. *Inotropy* is a term used to refer to the contractile state of the cell. Factors that increase contractility are said to have a positive inotropic effect, and factors that decrease contractility create a negative inotropic effect.

Afterload. **Afterload** is the amount of pressure the ventricles must overcome to eject the blood volume. Afterload is determined primarily by pressure in the arterial system. Afterload is decreased by vasodilation and increased by vasoconstriction.

Myocardial Oxygen Consumption

Myocardial tissue routinely needs 70% to 75% of the O_2 delivered to it by the coronary arteries. Skeletal muscles, by contrast, need 35% at rest and up to 75% during exercise. The only ways to increase O_2 supply to the myocardium are to (1) increase the coronary blood flow by coronary artery vasodilation or (2) increase the O_2 in the blood by administering supplemental O_2.

VASCULAR SYSTEM

The peripheral vascular system comprises arteries, capillaries, veins, and the lymph vessels (Fig. 33.5). The function of this system is to maintain blood flow to supply adequate O_2 and nutrients to all tissues. Any interruption of the blood flow results in tissue hypoxia, which can lead to tissue necrosis (death) if untreated.

Arteries

Arteries are the vessels that carry the blood away from the heart toward the tissues. These vessels are normally elastic and have greater tensile strength than the veins. The aorta, which is the largest artery in the body, transports oxygenated blood from the LV of the heart. Arteries that branch from the aortic arch supply the head and arms. The thoracic branch of the descending aorta supplies intercostal muscles, the esophagus, and some respiratory passages. The abdominal branch of the descending aorta supplies the gastrointestinal (GI) organs, the kidneys, the gonads, the lumbar area of the

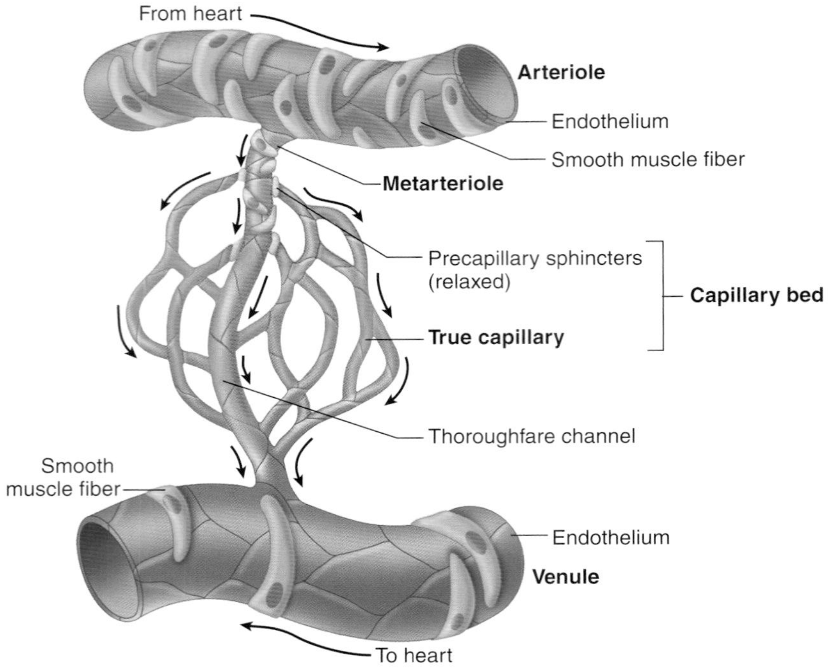

Fig. 33.5 Capillary bed. Foods, nutrients, and oxygen (O_2) are delivered to tissues through the capillaries and wastes are collected from the capillaries for recycling or excretion. Precapillary sphincters help to regulate the flow. (From Patton KT, Thibodeau GA: *Anatomy and physiology*, ed 8, St. Louis, 2014, Mosby.)

back, and the legs. Arteries branch into progressively smaller vessels as they travel away from the aorta. The smallest branches of the arteries are called *arterioles.*

Arteries and arterioles are thick-walled structures with three layers: (1) the intima, (2) the media, and (3) the adventitia (Fig. 33.6). The intima is composed of endothelial cells that form the smooth inner surface of the arteries, allowing the blood to flow with little resistance. The middle layer is the *media*, the primary structure of the artery. The media is composed of smooth muscle, elastic fibers, and connective tissue fibers.

Smooth muscles encircle and control the diameter of arteries and arterioles. Contraction of the muscles constricts the vessels, whereas relaxation of the muscles results in vessel dilation. The autonomic nervous system and other chemical and hormonal factors govern smooth muscle contraction and relaxation.

The outer layer of the arteries and arterioles is the *adventitia*. This layer, which is composed mostly of connective tissue, secures the artery or arteriole to the surrounding structures.

Capillaries

Arterioles branch into progressively smaller and smaller vessels, until they form the capillaries. Capillaries consist of a single layer of endothelial cells that allow the efficient delivery of nutrients and O_2 into the tissues and the removal of metabolic wastes from the tissues. Transfer of O_2 and nutrients between the blood and the tissue cells occurs in the capillaries. Red blood cells (RBCs) must conform to the size of the capillaries by changing their shape to fit through the small diameter.

The tiny vessels that receive blood from the capillaries are venules, which are the smallest veins. The metabolic activity occurring in the tissue determines the distribution of capillaries. Tissues such as skeletal muscles and digestive tract lining have a rich capillary network, whereas tissues such as bone and cartilage have a scanty capillary network.

The amount of blood in the capillary is controlled by sphincters on the arteriolar side of the capillary because capillaries have less smooth muscle than the arteries. Other factors such as chemical stimulation and hormonal changes also influence blood flow and fluid shifts in the capillaries. For example, histamine causes the capillary permeability to increase, allowing more fluid to shift into the tissues.

Veins

The blood is returned to the heart by way of the venules and veins. These vessels are formed as the capillaries organize into larger and larger vessels. The venous system is less sturdy and more passive than the arterial system. The walls of veins and venules are composed of the same three layers as the walls of the arteries and arterioles, but the layers are less defined. Because the walls of the veins and venules are thinner and less muscular, they can stretch more than those of the arterial system. Therefore the venous system can store a large volume of blood under relatively low pressure. As much as 75% of the body's total blood volume is housed in the venous system.

Valves. The venous system is equipped with valves that are composed of endothelial leaflets (Fig. 33.7).

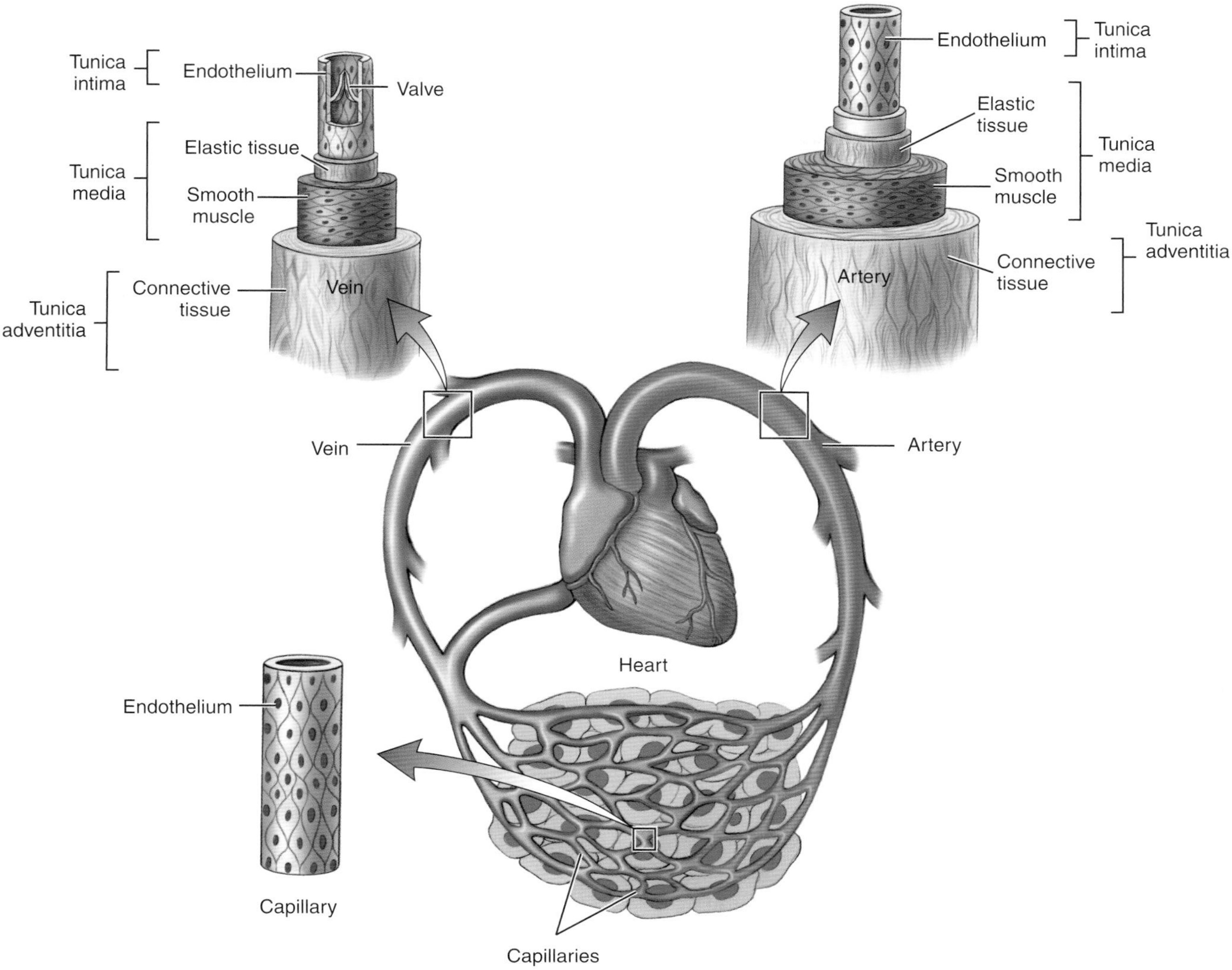

Fig. 33.6 Tissue layers of veins and arteries. (From Herlihy B: *The human body in health and illness*, ed 4, St. Louis, 2011, Saunders.)

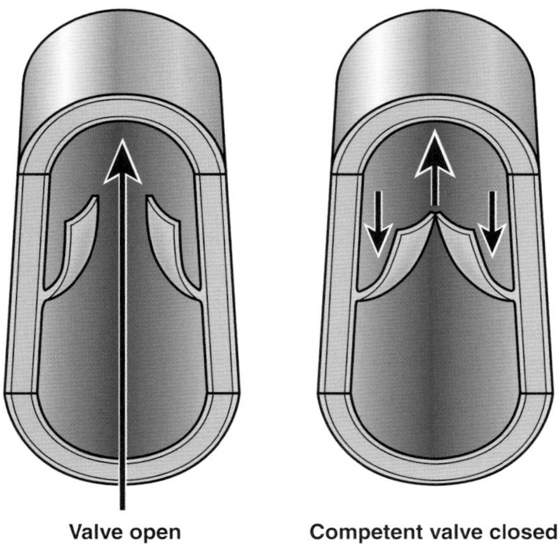

Fig. 33.7 Veins contain bicuspid valves that open in the direction of blood flow but prevent regurgitation of flow when pockets become filled and distended.

Valves allow the blood to move in only one direction and prevent backflow of the blood in the extremities. Skeletal muscle contractions compress the veins, forcing blood back toward the heart. This action reduces venous pooling and increases the circulating blood volume. As deoxygenated blood moves toward the heart, CO_2 and other metabolic wastes are carried to the lungs and kidneys for elimination.

Innervation. The sympathetic nervous system innervates the venous system, acting on the musculature of the veins to stimulate venoconstriction. Blocking of sympathetic nerve stimulation permits venodilation.

Lymph Vessels

The lymph system is an organization of small, thin-walled vessels that resemble the capillaries. These vessels accommodate the collection of lymph fluid from the peripheral tissues and the transportation of the fluid to the venous circulatory system. Because the lymph system interacts with the venous system, it is classified as part of the cardiovascular system. The lymph system comprises two main trunks: (1) the thoracic duct and (2) the right lymphatic duct. Each of these trunks is responsible for collecting and draining fluid from specific areas of the body. (See Chapter 29 for additional information.)

Lymph fluid is composed of plasma-like fluid, large protein molecules, and foreign substances. Because these protein molecules are too large to enter the capillaries or the venules, the lymph fluid carries them to the lymphatic ducts, where they are emptied into the subclavian and internal jugular veins. The movement of lymph fluid is accomplished by the contraction of muscles that encircle the lymphatic walls and surrounding tissues.

Factors That Affect Blood Flow

The body has multiple homeostatic mechanisms to control the systemic and local blood volume. These mechanisms work by changing resistance within the vessels or by changing the blood viscosity.

Resistance. Resistance within the vascular system is controlled by the diameter of the vessels. When vascular diameter increases (dilation), peripheral resistance falls, and blood flow increases. When vascular diameter decreases (constriction), however, peripheral resistance increases, thereby reducing blood flow. As previously noted, the diameter of blood vessels is controlled by the central nervous system, hormones, some ions, and blood pH.

The sympathetic nervous system plays a major role in adjusting vascular resistance. The vasomotor center located in the brain medulla and pons regulates the diameter of peripheral blood vessels. Stimulation of the sympathetic nervous system by either physiologic or psychologic stressors also triggers the adrenal glands to release norepinephrine and epinephrine, which cause vasoconstriction.

Other substances that cause changes in vascular resistance are angiotensin, serotonin, histamine, the kinins, and the prostaglandins. Angiotensin II is a potent chemical released by the kidneys that causes intense vasoconstriction and retention of salt and water by the kidneys. The kinins, histamine, and prostaglandins cause vasodilation, which decreases peripheral resistance. Serotonin, a chemical that is liberated from platelets when vessel walls are damaged, can cause vasoconstriction or vasodilation, depending on tissue conditions.

Blood viscosity. In addition to changes in peripheral resistance, modification of **blood viscosity** helps to regulate blood flow to peripheral tissues. Viscosity describes the thickness of the blood. The blood viscosity is usually constant but can be affected by changes in the proportions of the solid or liquid components. An increase in RBCs or a decrease in body water produces hemoconcentration, which increases blood viscosity. When blood is concentrated, the kidneys usually begin to retain water and the movement of fluid out of the capillaries is restricted.

An important factor that affects blood viscosity is capillary permeability. Hydrostatic and osmotic pressures normally maintain balanced movement of fluids in and out of the capillaries. Any mechanism that alters capillary permeability changes the amount and direction of fluid movement, resulting in a change in blood viscosity. Factors that increase capillary permeability include histamine, bradykinin, leukotrienes, and prostaglandins. Certain muscle metabolites, hypoxemia, malnutrition, and pH imbalances can also increase capillary permeability. When the proportion of serum to solid components in the blood is greater than normal, blood is less viscous and the kidneys excrete excess fluid.

Hypertension

Hypertension, or high blood pressure (HBP), is defined as a persistent systolic blood pressure (SBP) greater than or equal to 140 mm Hg and diastolic blood pressure (DBP) greater than or equal to 90 mm Hg. Approximately 65 million American adults, or nearly 1 in 3, have HBP. The prevalence of hypertension among citizens in the United States and Canada is 32% and 22%, respectively.

HBP is usually detected in people aged between 30 and 50 years; however, it is being found with increasing frequency in children. The development of hypertension in children and adolescents is caused in part by the increasing prevalence of childhood obesity as well as to the growing awareness of this disease. Primary or essential hypertension is more common in adolescents and has multiple risk factors, including obesity and a family history of hypertension. Secondary hypertension is more common in preadolescent children, with most cases caused by renal disease.

Hypertension is a known risk factor for coronary heart disease (CHD) in adults, and the presence of childhood hypertension may contribute to the early development of CHD.

HBP is called "the silent killer" because it often has no symptoms and is not discovered until a serious complication develops. It is estimated that 30% of those with hypertension do not know they have it. Among individuals in the United States with hypertension, 59% are being treated, but only 34% are considered to be in control of their condition. This is unfortunate because it is believed that hypertension can be controlled in most people.

Hypertension and its management among various racial and ethnic groups in the United States demand special attention from health care providers. Black Americans, as compared with other ethnic groups, have the highest prevalence of hypertension in the world. Black Americans develop hypertension at a younger age than White Americans. Black American women have a higher incidence of hypertension than Black American men (see the Cultural Considerations box).

Cultural Considerations

Cultural and Ethnic Health Disparities for Hypertension

- Black Americans, as compared with other ethnic groups, have the highest prevalence of hypertension in the world.
- Black Americans develop hypertension at a younger age than White Americans.
- Black American women have a higher incidence of hypertension than Black American men.
- Hypertension is more aggressive in Black Americans and results in more severe end-organ damage.
- Black Americans have a higher mortality rate related to hypertension than White Americans.
- Black Americans and White Americans living in the southeastern United States have a higher incidence of hypertension than similar ethnic groups living in other parts of the United States.
- Mexican Americans are less likely to receive treatment for hypertension than White Americans and Black Americans.
- Mexican Americans and Native Americans have lower rates of adequate blood pressure control than White Americans and Black Americans.

From Lewis SM, Dirksen S, Heitkemper MM, et al: *Medical-surgical nursing: assessment and management of clinical problems*, ed 8, St. Louis, 2010, Mosby.)

Complications of hypertension, including damage to the heart, blood vessels, kidneys, brain, and eyes, increase after 50 years of age. As BP rises, so does the risk of heart attack, heart failure (HF), stroke, kidney disease, and blindness. Men, especially Black American men, suffer serious complications more often than women. Cardiac disease is the leading cause of death in people with hypertension. Improved management of hypertension has significantly reduced the death rate from stroke in women aged 50 years and older.

AGE-RELATED CHANGES IN THE CARDIOVASCULAR SYSTEM

It is difficult to separate the normal age-related changes in the heart and blood vessels from the changes caused by disease. In general, age-related changes progress slowly, whereas pathogenic changes are more likely to be sudden. Age-related changes are listed in Box 33.1.

Box 33.1 Age-Related Changes in the Cardiovascular System

- Heart muscle density increases and elasticity decreases
- Cardiac contractility declines
- Valves thicken, stiffen, and may not close properly
- Cardiac output decreases
- Pacemaker cells in the sinoatrial node decrease in number
- Nerve fibers in the ventricles decrease in number
- Heart takes longer to respond to stress or exercise and return to normal
- Connective tissue and elastic fibers in arteries become stiffer, increasing peripheral resistance and impairing blood flow
- After 60 years of age, peripheral vascular resistance increases by approximately 1% per year; systolic pressure rises in response to increased peripheral vascular resistance
- Arterial pulse pressure increases
- Veins stretch and dilate, leading to venous stasis and impaired venous return
- Cardiovascular system adapts more slowly to changes in position, frequently resulting in postural hypotension

NURSING ASSESSMENT OF CARDIOVASCULAR FUNCTION

A complete assessment is important for the cardiovascular patient. However, if the patient is having acute symptoms, a detailed assessment must be deferred until the patient is stable.

The nursing assessment of a patient who may have a cardiovascular disorder requires a thorough assessment by a registered nurse (RN), as described in Chapters 34, 35, and 36. The licensed vocational nurse/licensed practical nurse (LVN/LPN) may assist by collecting relevant data.

HEALTH HISTORY

Reason for Seeking Care

Determine the patient's reason for seeking medical care. Common symptoms that may be related to cardiovascular disorders include fatigue, edema, palpitations, dyspnea, and pain. Note when symptoms occur, what aggravates them, and what relieves them.

Present Health

Ask whether the patient has specific conditions that may be related to cardiovascular disease. These include hypertension, kidney disease, pulmonary disease, peripheral vascular disease diabetes mellitus, stroke, rheumatic fever, streptococcal sore throat, anemia, smoking, and alcoholism. List recent and current medications, recording any allergies in the appropriate records. Question whether the patient is taking any vitamins, herbs, or homeopathic remedies. It may be easier to ask something such as "What are you doing to stay healthy or to help you feel better?"

Past Health History

Note previous cardiovascular disorders, illnesses, and hospitalizations.

Family History

Because cardiovascular problems are often familial or hereditary, ask whether immediate relatives have had hypertension, CHD, other cardiac disorders, peripheral vascular disease, or diabetes mellitus.

Review of Systems

Ask whether the patient has experienced the following specific symptoms: weight gain, fatigue, dyspnea (shortness of breath), cough, orthopnea (difficulty breathing in a supine position), paroxysmal nocturnal dyspnea (sudden dyspnea during sleep), palpitations, chest pain, **syncope** (fainting), concentrated urine, or leg edema. If the patient has had dyspnea or orthopnea, it is important to determine when it occurred and whether the onset was gradual or sudden. A person with hypertension may be asymptomatic unless the condition is severe.

Pain. Pain also requires detailed descriptions. Cardiac pain may radiate or be referred to other areas. The pain may radiate down either arm, to the jaw, or to just below the sternum. The severity may range from mild, intermittent discomfort to severe, crushing chest pain. Ask the patient to rate the severity of the pain on a scale of 1 (mildest) to 10 (worst possible). Chest pain may be experienced differently in women, patients with diabetes, and older adults and may be described as *indigestion, a feeling of anxiety, nausea,* or *a feeling of fatigue.* Document the exact description, location, and severity of the pain, as well as whether the pain is radiating, what events cause it, and what relieves the pain.

To determine the nature of pain in the peripheral vascular system, ask the patient to describe any pain or discomfort in the calf, thigh, hip, or buttock areas. Describe the pain (e.g., sharp, throbbing, continuous, intermittent), the location and duration of the pain, the precipitating factors (e.g., exercise, lying down in bed), and any alleviating factors (whatever brings relief).

Intermittent claudication. Intermittent claudication is chronic pain associated with decreased perfusion that is aggravated by exercise and relieved by rest. Intermittent claudication can affect any major muscle group distal to (beyond) the point of arterial occlusion. The pain is described as a feeling of tightness, burning, fatigue, aching, or cramping. Exercise causes the muscle group to become ischemic because blood flow is inadequate to supply nutrients and O_2 and to remove wastes. This results in the development of pain. When the exercise is stopped, the metabolic demands of the muscle tissue decrease, wastes are removed from the tissues, and the pain is relieved.

Rest pain. Rest pain indicates severe arterial occlusion (obstruction). By impeding blood flow, the occlusion causes tissue ischemia in the extremity. For example, a person with arterial occlusion in the lower extremities may experience severe, burning pain in the legs and feet after lying flat for a period of time. The pain is relieved when the extremity is dangled in a dependent position that promotes blood flow by gravity. Frequently, the patient sleeps best in a chair or with the feet in a dependent position.

Box 33.2 Assessment of Patients With Cardiovascular Disorders

HEALTH HISTORY

Reason for Seeking Care

Fatigue, palpitations, dyspnea, syncope, pain, edema

Present Health

Symptom onset, duration, type, location and severity; aggravating and relieving factors; apparent distress

Past Health History

Hypertension, kidney disease, pulmonary disease, diabetes mellitus, stroke, rheumatic fever, streptococcal sore throat, scarlet fever, previous cardiac diseases or conditions, previous hospitalizations, recent and current medications, allergies

Family History

Hypertension, coronary heart disease (CHD) or other cardiac conditions, diabetes mellitus, peripheral vascular disease

Review of Systems

Weight gain, fatigue, dyspnea (shortness of breath), cough, orthopnea (difficulty breathing in a supine position), paroxysmal nocturnal dyspnea (sudden dyspnea during sleep), palpitations, chest pain, syncope (fainting), concentrated urine, or leg edema

Functional Assessment

Effects of illness on usual activities, activity and rest pattern, lifestyle, sources of stress, coping strategies; social support

Physical Examination

Height and weight

Vital Signs: Blood pressure in both arms and while supine, sitting, standing; apical heart rate and rhythm; peripheral pulses: rate, rhythm, quality, equality; respiratory effort and rate

Skin: Color, hair distribution, capillary refill, temperature

Thorax: Heart sounds, heart murmurs, rubs; breath sounds, crackles, wheezes; cough; presence and appearance of sputum

Extremities: Pulses, color, warmth, edema, hair distribution; nails

Functional Assessment

The functional assessment determines the effect of the disease process on the patient's life and the ability to carry out usual activities independently such as walking, bathing, dressing, cooking, and housekeeping. The pain associated with cardiovascular disease can interfere with work and recreation. Inactivity can reduce the patient's stamina.

Describe activity, rest patterns, and social support. Determine whether the patient receives assistance with activities of daily living (ADLs). Ask the patient about sources of stress and coping strategies.

Other aspects of the functional assessment that are relevant to cardiovascular disease are smoking and diet. Smoking causes vasoconstriction and a high fat intake can contribute to arteriosclerosis. Be sure to record salt and fat intake (Box 33.2).

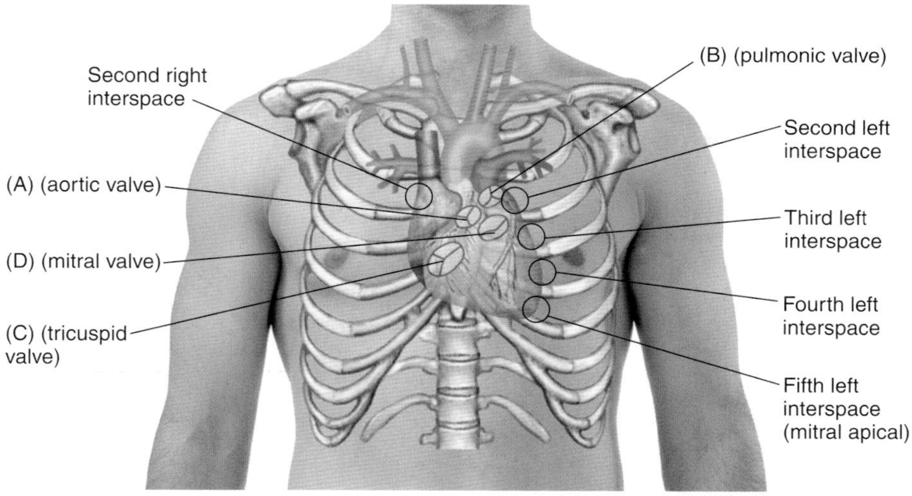

Fig. 33.8 Auscultation of the heart. (A) Aortic valve at the second intercostal space to the right of the sternum. (B) Pulmonic valve at the second intercostal space to the left of the sternum. (C) Tricuspid valve at the fifth intercostal space to the left of the sternum. (D) Mitral valve at the fifth intercostal space in the midclavicular line. (From Seidel HM, Ball JW, Dains JE, et al: *Mosby's guide to physical examination*, ed 7, St. Louis, 2011, Mosby.)

PHYSICAL EXAMINATION

Begin the physical examination with measurement of height and weight and recording of vital signs.

Vital Signs

Blood pressure. The correct size of BP cuff must be used. Position the patient's arm at the heart level, and check the BP in both arms. It is important to note the pulse pressure (difference between the systolic and diastolic pressures) because this is a noninvasive measure of cardiac output. Next, measure BP and pulse rates in the lying, sitting, and standing positions. A BP decrease of 20 mm Hg or more with a position change indicates decreased blood volume or an autonomic response. As BP decreases, the pulse should increase as a compensatory mechanism.

Pulses. Palpate the radial pulses for rate, rhythm, quality, and equality and auscultate the apical pulse for rate and rhythm. Apical and radial pulses may be taken simultaneously to detect a pulse deficit. The normal heart rate is 60 to 100 beats per minute. **Bradycardia** is considered a rate of 60 beats per minute or less. **Tachycardia** is characterized by a heart rate in excess of 100 beats per minute. The rhythm is described as *regular*, *irregular*, or *regularly irregular*. The quality of a palpated pulse is graded on a 4-point scale: *0*, absent pulse (not palpable); *1*, weak or thready pulse (pulse easily obliterated by slight finger pressure, returning as pressure is released); *2*, normal pulse (easily palpable); and *3*, bounding pulse (forceful, not easily obliterated by finger pressure). With a stethoscope, listen at the fifth intercostal space at the midclavicular line to assess the apical pulse. In addition to the radial pulse, assess the carotid, brachial, femoral, popliteal, posterior tibial, and dorsalis pedis pulses at appropriate times during the physical examination.

Respirations. Observe the patient's respiratory effort and skin color; count the respiratory rate; and auscultate the breath sounds for crackles and wheezes. If the patient produces sputum, describe the color, amount, and appearance.

Skin

Inspect the skin for color, hair distribution, and capillary refill, and palpate for temperature. Skin color and temperature should be relatively the same over the entire body.

Heart Sounds

The heart sounds are systole (lub) and diastole (dub). To auscultate heart sounds, place the diaphragm of the stethoscope firmly on the bare anterior chest (not through clothing). Fig. 33.8 shows where the heart sounds, made by closing of the valves, may be heard best. With practice, you can learn to distinguish these. The following pattern of auscultation is recommended:

1. Listen to the aortic area first, and then to the pulmonic. As the aortic and pulmonic valves close, the dub should be louder than the lub in the aortic and pulmonic areas.
2. Listen to the tricuspid and mitral valves in the areas indicated. In these areas, the lub should be louder than the dub.
3. After listening to each area with the diaphragm, repeat the pattern with the bell of the stethoscope. Note additional sounds of S_3 and S_4. The S_3 and S_4 sounds are heard best with the bell of the stethoscope placed at the apex when the patient is positioned on the left side. S_3, also called a *ventricular gallop*, occurs early in diastole. S_3 is normal in children and young adults and may be pathologic after 30 years of age. S_4, also called an *atrial gallop*, occurs late in diastole. S_4 is an abnormal heart sound.

Table 33.2 Grading of Heart Murmurs

GRADE	DESCRIPTION
I	Very faint
II	Faint, but recognizable
III	Loud, but moderate in intensity
IV	Loud and accompanied by a palpable thrill
V	Very loud, accompanied by a palpable thrill, and audible with the stethoscope partially off the client's chest
VI	Extremely loud; may be heard with the stethoscope slightly above the client's chest

From Ignatavicius DD, Workman ML: *Medical-surgical nursing: patient-centered collaborative care*, ed 7, Philadelphia, 2013, Saunders.

Heart murmurs. A heart **murmur** is the sound produced by turbulent blood flow across the valves. Murmurs are recorded as having high, low, or medium pitch, and they are located using the anatomic landmarks where they are heard best. The timing of a murmur relates to when it is heard in the cardiac cycle: systole or diastole. Murmurs are graded according to intensity or loudness (Table 33.2).

A rub is heard when the pericardium is inflamed. A scratchy or muffled sound may be heard best by having the patient sit upright and lean forward. This position brings the pericardium closer to the chest wall. A pericardial friction rub is best heard along the left sternal border throughout the cardiac cycle. It may help to ask patients to hold their breath briefly. If a rub is heard during this brief time, it is a pericardial rub rather than a pleural rub.

Extremities

Examination of the peripheral vascular system helps to determine whether the disease process is arterial or venous in nature. In general, arterial complications involve multiple areas, whereas venous complications remain more localized, usually in the lower extremities. Inspect the skin for color and lesions. Pallor suggests peripheral vasoconstriction or inadequate arterial blood flow. A reddish-brown discoloration called *rubor* in a dependent lower extremity suggests the presence of arterial occlusive disease. In venous disorders, the affected areas of the skin may have a brownish discoloration and be cyanotic when the extremity is dependent.

It is important to be alert for open ulcers and for scars around the ankles that may be associated with either arterial or venous disease. Note the presence of stasis dermatitis, a brown pigmentation with flaky skin over the edematous areas of the ankles. It may take on a bluish cast when the leg is in a dependent position. Arterial stasis dermatitis begins as ulcerations in the toes. The ulcers are painful, pale, crusty, and located over bony prominences. Venous stasis dermatitis begins as ulcers in the ankle area. The ulcers develop very slowly, are usually painless, and are difficult to heal.

Determine capillary refill time in the nail beds to determine the adequacy of peripheral perfusion. To do this, press the nail bed until it blanches (turns pale). Then release the pressure and note the number of seconds it takes for the color to return. Capillary refill time greater than 3 seconds denotes a reduction in peripheral perfusion.

Palpate the affected areas to evaluate the temperature, detect edema, and assess peripheral pulses. Skin temperature should be palpated bilaterally, moving proximally to distally (toward the feet), to detect any ischemic areas. A cool limb suggests an arterial problem and a warm limb suggests a venous problem. A pulsating mass detected on abdominal palpation may be an **aneurysm**.

Dependent edema develops as a result of systemic disorders, lymphatic dysfunction, deep vein thrombosis (DVT), or chronic venous insufficiency. To determine the severity of edema, the examiner presses the thumb into the edematous area for approximately 5 seconds. If the depression of the thumb remains in the edematous area, the edema is said to be *pitting*. The severity of pitting edema is graded from 1+ to 4+. A slight indentation with no apparent leg swelling is graded 1+. Moderate pitting that subsides rapidly is graded as 2+. A deep indentation that remains briefly, with swelling of the leg is graded 3+. Deep pitting that lasts a long time accompanied by gross leg swelling is graded 4+. The same area on both extremities should be compared.

Another aspect of the examination is the evaluation of peripheral pulses (Fig. 33.9). Palpate pulses for presence, symmetry, volume, and rhythm. The peripheral pulses to be palpated in the upper extremities include the brachial, ulnar, and radial arteries. The peripheral pulses appraised in the lower extremities are the femoral, popliteal, dorsalis pedis, and posterior tibial arteries. Pulses should be compared bilaterally, and any absent or asymmetric pulses documented. The palpation of the arteries provides valuable information concerning the condition of the vessels. A sclerotic vessel feels stiff and cordlike, whereas a normal vessel can be palpated as soft and springy.

Homans sign traditionally has been checked to evaluate for peripheral vascular disease (PVD). The assumption was that pain elicited by sharply dorsiflexing the patient's foot (positive Homans sign) indicated the presence of DVT in that leg. However, this test is not reliable and should not be included.

A test that can be beneficial in the assessment of the peripheral vascular system is the Allen test. The Allen test is used to determine the adequacy of arterial circulation to the hand. The patient is asked to tightly clench the fist, while the nurse occludes the radial and ulnar arteries. The patient is then instructed to open the fist, and the nurse releases pressure on the ulnar artery. If

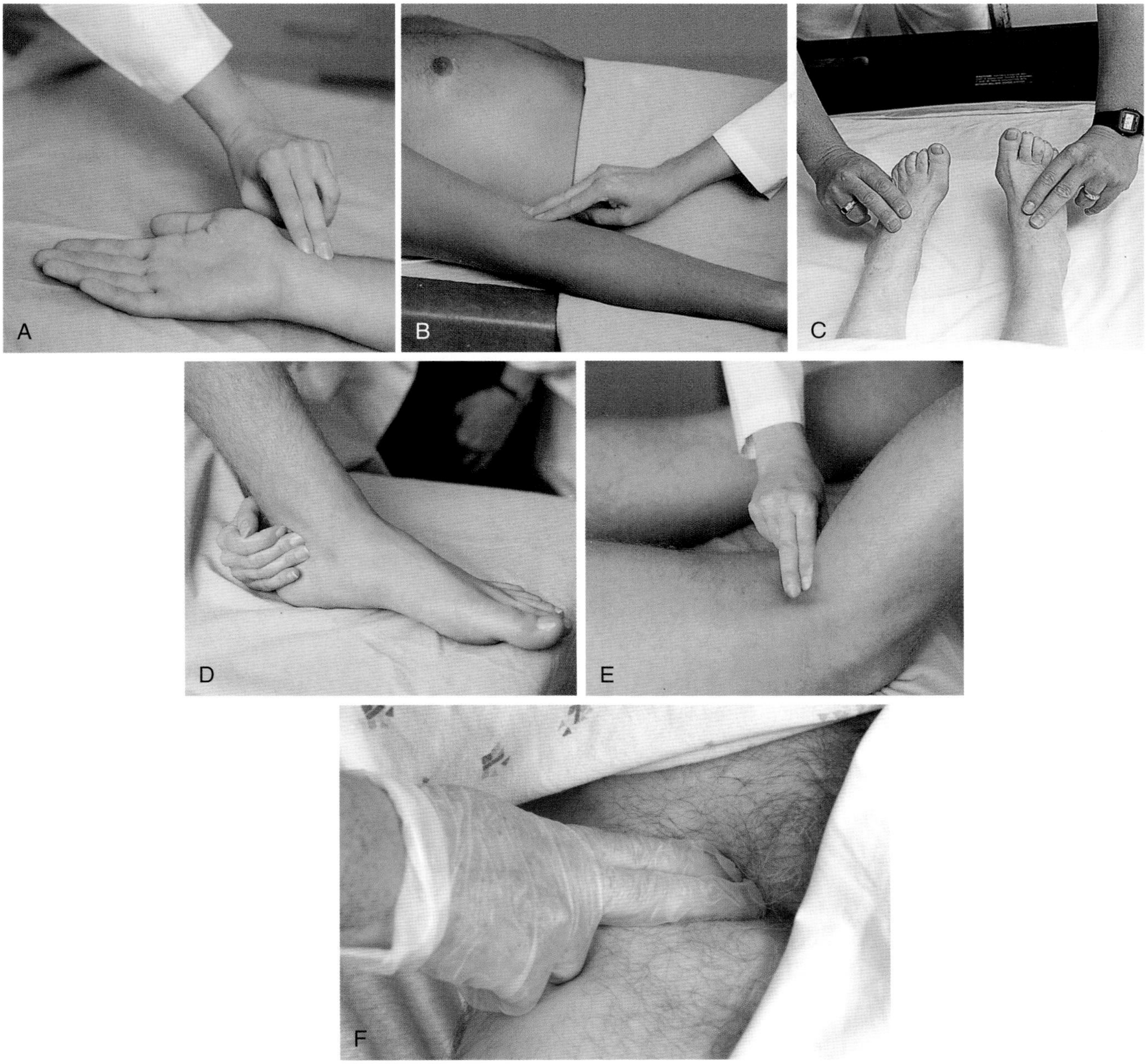

Fig. 33.9 Palpating peripheral pulses. (A) Radial, (B) brachial, (C) dorsalis pedis, (D) posterior tibial, (E) popliteal, (F) femoral. (From Perry AG, Potter PA, Ostendorf W: *Clinical nursing skills and techniques*, ed 9, St. Louis, 2017, Elsevier.)

the ulnar artery is patent, the palm should promptly return to a normal color. A persistence of pallor in the palm area indicates an occlusion of the ulnar artery. The test can be repeated with the ulnar artery being occluded instead of the radial artery to detect occlusion within the radial artery (see Chapter 25, Fig. 25.8).

The nurse with advanced education can further evaluate peripheral vascular function by auscultating the sounds of blood flow through the arteries. Bruits sound like turbulent, fast-moving fluid. The presence of bruits can signal the presence of an aneurysm or the development of chronic arterial occlusive disease long before other signs appear.

DIAGNOSTIC TESTS AND PROCEDURES

A number of tests or procedures may be used to assess cardiovascular structure and function. More common tests are described here. Patient preparation and post-procedure care are detailed in Table 33.3.

PULSE OXIMETRY

Pulse oximetry noninvasively measures arterial O_2 saturation. Light is passed through a pulsating artery and interpreted mechanically to determine the O_2 saturation. The transdermal clip or patch may be applied to a digit (finger or toe), the ear, or the nose (Fig. 33.10).

Table 33.3 Diagnostic Tests and Procedures: Cardiovascular Conditions

TEST	PURPOSE AND PROCEDURE	PATIENT PREPARATION	POSTPROCEDURE NURSING CARE
Electrocardiogram (ECG)	Electrodes are placed on the skin to detect electrical activity of the heart. Detects abnormalities in conduction of impulses, including changes caused by heart damage.	Tell the patient what to expect and that the procedure is painless. No special preparation is needed.	Remove the gel and electrode pads from the patient's skin. No special care is needed.
Holter monitor	Provides continuous ECG monitoring for 24 to 48 hours. Detects occasional dysrhythmias that may be correlated with specific activities noted in the patient's diary.	Tell the patient to wear loose clothing, take only a sponge bath, avoid magnets and metal detectors, and monitor placement of electrodes. Emphasize keeping an accurate diary of activities and to push "event button" if symptoms occur.	Return at the scheduled time. ECG recording will be retrieved for inspection.
Implantable loop	Provides ECG monitoring for longer periods, and saves the information on a memory loop for analysis. Detects dysrhythmias causing syncopal episodes.	Tell the patient, family member, or significant other to activate the recorder when symptoms occur and to keep a written record of events.	Return at the scheduled time. ECG recording will be retrieved for inspection.
Echocardiogram	Uses ultrasound to create images of the heart. Gel is placed on the patient's skin, and a transducer is moved over the area. Detects valve abnormalities, left ventricular hypertrophy, and hypertrophic cardiomyopathy (CMP).	Tell the patient what to expect and that the procedure is painless. No special preparation is needed.	Remove the gel from the patient's skin. No special care is needed.
Transesophageal echocardiogram (TEE)	Used when a conventional echocardiogram is not diagnostic. Probe is inserted through the esophagus into stomach (behind the heart). Has the same purpose as an echocardiogram.	Tell the patient what to expect: throat will be anesthetized, may have intravenous (IV) line installed. Signed consent is needed.	Monitor the patient's vital signs and gag reflex; if sedated, monitor the level of consciousness.
Stress test (exercise tolerance test [ETT])	Assesses the presence and severity of coronary heart disease (CHD) by having the patient exercise during ECG monitoring. Blood pressure is monitored. The test is stopped if symptoms of CHD occur.	Tell the patient what to expect. Nothing by mouth (NPO) for 2 hours before the test. Have the patient wear loose clothing and comfortable shoes. Give a beta-blocker if prescribed. Signed consent is needed.	No special care is needed.
Magnetic resonance imaging (MRI)	Creates images of body structures without radiation. The patient lies on a firm pad that rolls into a circular device. "Open MRI" is better tolerated by claustrophobic patients because the machine does not surround the patient. Clanging sounds are heard as the machine works.	Tell the patient what to expect. All metal must be removed. Sedation may be ordered if the patient is very anxious or unable to be still.	No special care is needed. Safety precautions should be taken if a sedative has been given.
Multiple-gated acquisition (MUGA) scanning	Radioactive material is injected intravenously, and the heart is scanned to evaluate function. May be done at rest or during exercise.	Tell the patient what to expect. NPO for 2 hours before the procedure. Start IV infusion as ordered. Signed consent is needed.	No special care is needed.

Table 33.3 Diagnostic Tests and Procedures: Cardiovascular Conditions—cont'd

TEST	PURPOSE AND PROCEDURE	PATIENT PREPARATION	POSTPROCEDURE NURSING CARE
Myocardial perfusion imaging: • Positron emission tomography (PET) scan • Single photon emission computed tomography (SPECT)	Radioisotope(s) administered by IV route to assess perfusion of the heart. May be done with stress/exercise.	Tell the patient that one or two IVs may be inserted and that they may be asked to use an exercise bike or treadmill during scanning. The patient may be NPO for 4 to 6 hours before the test and should abstain from caffeine, alcohol, and tobacco for 24 hours before the test.	Encourage the patient to change positions slowly to avoid postural hypotension and to drink fluids, if not contraindicated, to help with excretion of the radioisotopes.
Ultrafast computed tomography (CT); also known as *electron beam tomography (EBT)*	Imaging technology that provides images used to assess myocardial perfusion and right and left ventricular muscle mass and function, and to measure calcium deposits in the coronary circulation.	Tell the patient what to expect (e.g., lie on the table, hold very still, you may be asked to hold breath for a few seconds at a time). No special preparation is needed.	No special care is needed.
Cardiac catheterization	A catheter is passed through a vein or artery, and dye is injected. Radiographs are taken to visualize heart structures and blood vessels. The procedure is done in a special room. Blood pressure, pulse, and ECG are monitored throughout test.	Tell the patient what to expect. Assess for allergies to seafood or iodine, and inform the radiologist if they are present. NPO for specified time before procedure. Tell the patient to expect a flushing sensation when the dye is injected. Give a sedative if ordered. Signed consent is needed.	Check the puncture site; maintain pressure per protocol if a vascular sealing device is not used. Monitor vital signs and peripheral pulses on the affected extremity. Enforce bed rest as ordered.
Electrophysiology study (EPS)	A catheter with multiple electrodes is passed into the right side of the heart through the femoral vein. The electrodes record electrical activity of the conduction system and may be used to stimulate the patient's dysrhythmia.	Tell the patient what to expect. NPO for 6 hours before the procedure. Premedicate the patient with prescribed sedatives. Signed consent is needed.	Similar to cardiac catheterization (described previously).
Duplex ultrasound: combines compression ultrasound with Doppler	Uses sound waves to facilitate diagnosis of PVD	Tell the patient the test is painless and has no risks. Patient may be asked to change the position of the extremity being evaluated and perform breathing exercises.	No special care is required.
Plethysmography	Used to detect DVT, to screen patients who are at risk for PVD, and to investigate the possibility of pulmonary emboli	Tell the patient the procedure is safe, painless, and takes about 30 to 45 minutes. Patient's leg will be elevated, and a pressure cuff will be placed on the thigh. Electrodes record information about blood flow in the veins.	No special care is required.
Pressure measurement	Types include segmental limb pressures and pulse volume measurements	Tell the patient blood pressures will be measured in multiple sites over the extremities to assess the blood vessels. Pressures are measured during activity and while at rest. Test is noninvasive, painless, and safe.	No special care is required.

Continued

Table 33.3 Diagnostic Tests and Procedures: Cardiovascular Conditions—cont'd

TEST	PURPOSE AND PROCEDURE	PATIENT PREPARATION	POSTPROCEDURE NURSING CARE
Exercise (treadmill) test	Evaluates the functional abilities of patients with PVD by measuring pulse volumes before, during, and after exercise	Tell the patient the test is noninvasive. Patient will be asked to walk for approximately 5 minutes on a treadmill. The test will be stopped if the patient has pain or dyspnea.	Carefully monitor the patient for any complications that may develop as a result of the test.
Angiography (venography: contrast, CT, MRI; arteriography, and radiographs)	Identifies vascular obstruction, aneurysm, and atherosclerotic plaques	Tell the patient dye will be injected and radiographs taken. Patient may briefly feel a burning sensation when the dye is injected. Signed consent is required. Patient should be NPO for 4 hours before the test. Inform the radiologist if the patient is allergic to iodine or seafood. Risks include hemorrhage at insertion site, dye-induced allergic reaction, thrombosis/embolism, renal insufficiency, and pseudoaneurysm.	Bed rest is required for several hours. Monitor the patient's vital signs and pulses hourly for 6 hours. Assess the injection site for bleeding, hematoma, and pulsating mass (pseudoaneurysm). Neurovascular checks (pulses, sensation, movement, color, warmth) should be conducted.

DVT, Deep vein thrombosis; *PVD*, peripheral vascular disease.

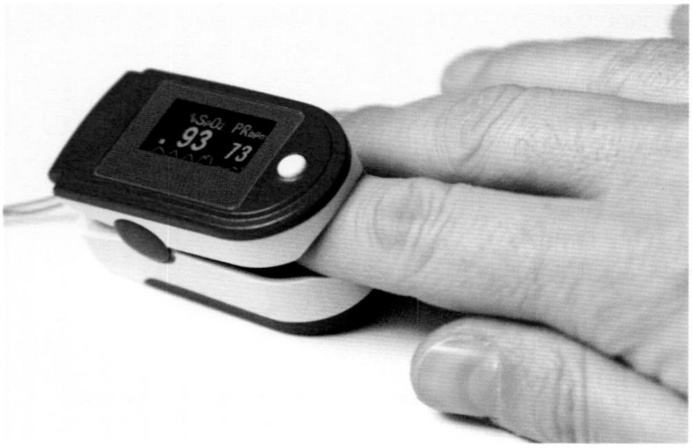

Fig. 33.10 Pulse oximeter. (Copyright © juanrvelasco/iStock/iStock.com.)

ELECTROCARDIOGRAM

The electrocardiogram (ECG) allows study of the electrical activity (conduction system) through the heart muscle. An electrical impulse causes a series of contractions as it passes through the heart muscle. Electrodes placed on the surface of the skin pick up the electrical impulses of the heart. The standard ECG records the electrical activity using 12 leads. Interpreting the 12-lead ECG allows detection of conduction disturbances, ischemia and infarction, electrolyte imbalances, and structural changes.

The ECG is graphed on standardized paper or viewed on an oscilloscope. Each cardiac cycle is represented by a series of P, Q, R, S, and T waves. The activity represented by each wave is explained in the section titled "Interpretation of Electrocardiograms." The ECG is interpreted to detect abnormalities in rate, rhythm, or impulse conduction. The normal finding is called a *normal sinus rhythm*, which is characterized by the following:

1. Rate of 60 to 100 beats per minute
2. Regular rhythm
3. P wave preceding each QRS complex
4. PR interval that is within 0.12 to 0.20 seconds
5. QRS complex that is less than 0.12 seconds

Nurses who work in critical care areas are responsible for monitoring and interpreting ECGs. Patients are usually monitored continuously at the bedside and have intermittent monitoring through a 12-lead ECG.

12-Lead Electrocardiogram

A 12-lead ECG looks at the heart from 12 directions or perspectives. This permits more precise evaluation of the heart's electrical activity. Three leads are placed on the limbs (leads I, II, and III); three leads are augmented (aVR, aVL, and aVF); and six chest, or precordial, leads exist (V_1 to V_6). Electricity flows from the negative to the positive lead. If the depolarization wave flows toward the positive pole (electrode), the deflection is upright. If the wave flows away from the positive pole, the deflection is negative.

Continuous Monitoring

Most units that perform continuous monitoring use the five-lead system, with four limb electrodes and a chest electrode (which is placed at one of the V lead sites). The electrodes are held in place by adhesive

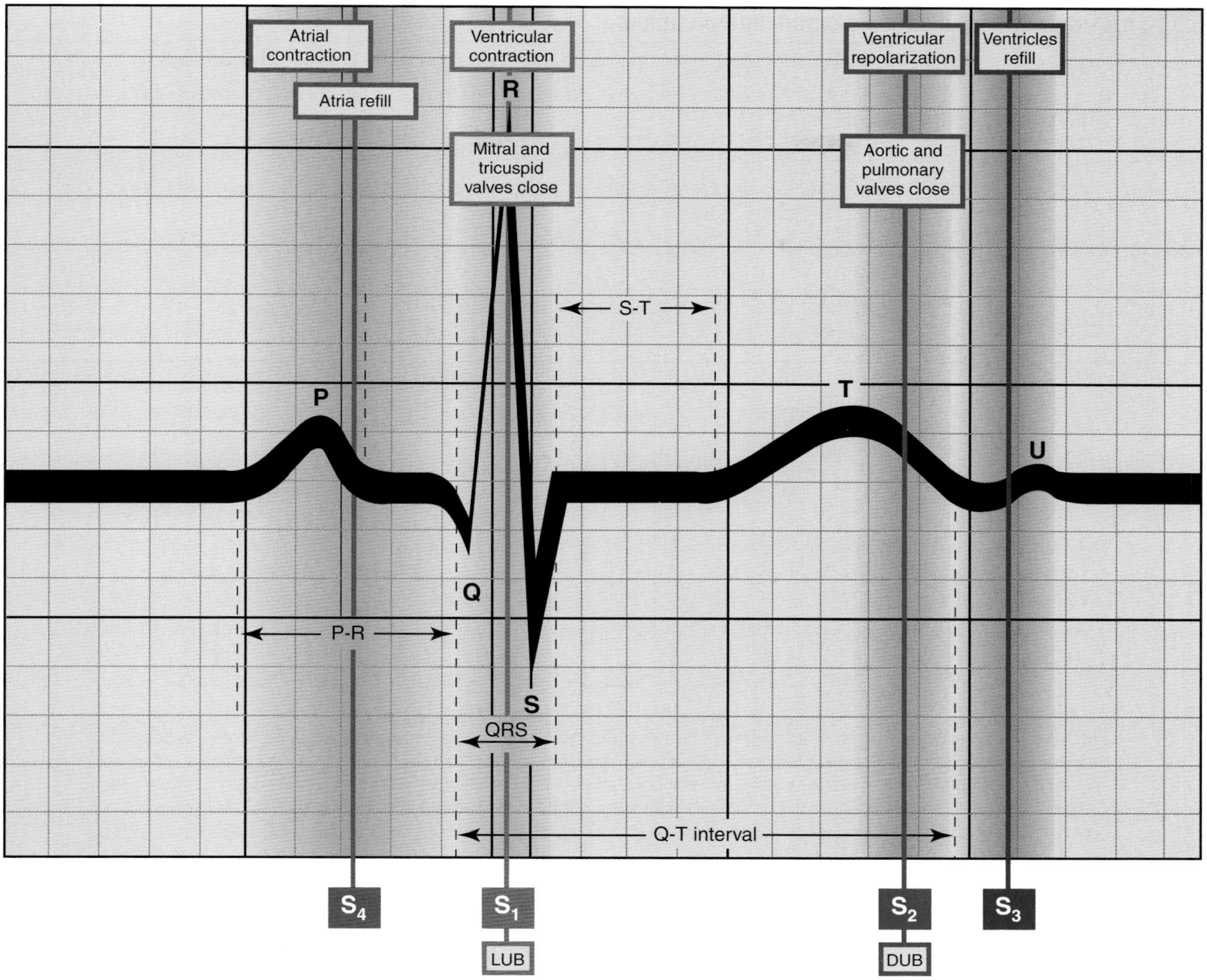

Fig. 33.11 Relationship between the cardiac cycle and the heart sounds. (From Monahan FD, Drake DT, Neighbors M, editors: *Medical-surgical nursing: foundations for clinical practice*, ed 2, Philadelphia, 1998, Saunders.)

pads. Thoroughly clean the electrode sites before applying the pads, and change the pads according to agency policy. In addition, monitor the patient's skin for irritation or breakdown. The lead monitored depends on the purpose of the monitoring (e.g., to detect dysrhythmias, to detect ischemia).

Interpretation of Electrocardiograms

To interpret an ECG strip, refer to Fig. 33.11. The graph paper consists of horizontal and vertical, small and large squares. The horizontal axis measures time; the vertical axis measures voltage. Each small square represents 0.04 second on the horizontal axis and 1 mm on the vertical axis. Each large square, bounded by heavy lines, is made up of five small squares and represents 0.20 second and 5 mm. The electrical activity of the heart is represented by deflections, positive and negative, from the baseline. A deflection is an upward or downward movement from the baseline. The baseline is called the *isoelectric line.* The first positive deflection (upward movement) is the small, rounded P wave that represents atrial depolarization. The second positive deflection is the peaked QRS complex that represents ventricular depolarization. The Q is the first negative deflection, meaning that the line moves below the isoelectric line. The R wave corresponds to the patient's pulse. Atrial repolarization occurs during ventricular depolarization and is obscured by the QRS complex. The third deflection is the rounded T wave, which represents ventricular repolarization. The fourth deflection, if present, is the U wave. It is small, rounded, and usually indicates electrolyte imbalance (hypokalemia).

The PR interval represents the time it takes the impulse to travel from the atria through the AV node to the ventricles. The PR interval is measured from the beginning of the P wave to the Q wave. The normal PR interval is 0.12 to 0.20 second. The QRS complex is measured from the point at which the Q leaves the isoelectric line to the point at which the S returns to the isoelectric line. The normal QRS complex is 0.12 second or less. The ST segment represents the time from ventricular depolarization

Table 33.4 Criteria for Electrocardiogram Interpretation

Rate	Are the atrial and ventricular rates the same as measured by the P-P and R-R intervals?
Rhythm	Is the rate regular or irregular? If irregular, does a pattern exist? Are these ectopic beats? Where do they occur?
P waves	Is there a P wave before every QRS complex? Does each P wave have the same size and shape?
PR interval	Are all the PR intervals the same length? If not, does a pattern exist to the irregularity? Are the PR intervals within normal range?
QRS complexes	Do all QRS complexes look alike? Are all QRS complexes within the normal range (0.06–0.10 seconds)?
ST segment	Is the ST segment isoelectric, depressed, or elevated?
T waves	Do all T waves look alike? Are the T waves upright or inverted?

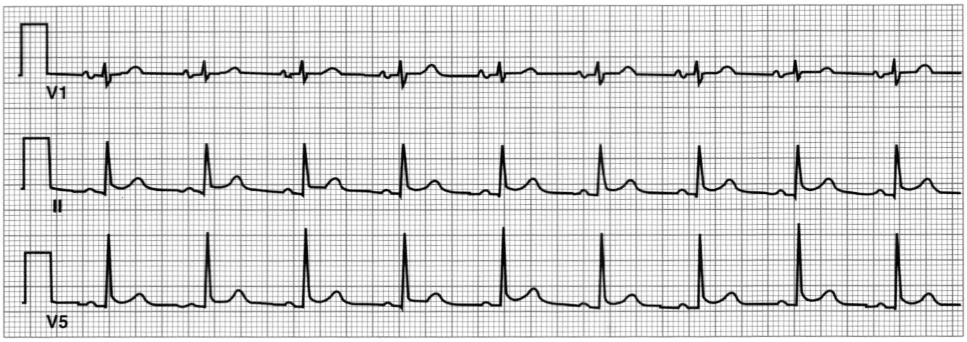

Fig. 33.12 Normal sinus rhythm. Each segment between the dark lines (above the monitor strip) represents 3 seconds, when the monitor is set at a speed of 25 mm/s. Characteristics: rate—60 to 100 beats per minute; regularity—essentially regular (P-to-P and R-to-R intervals are regular with only minor variation); P wave, PR interval—a P occurs before every QRS (each P wave is the same size and shape; PR interval is between 0.12 and 0.20 second); QRS—falls between 0.06 and 0.10 second; T wave—rounded, all the same shape. Interpretation: normal sinus rhythm. (From Aehlert B. *ECGs made easy*, 5th ed. St Louis, Mosby, 2013.)

to ventricular repolarization. The ST segment should be along the isoelectric line.

Criteria for Interpreting Electrocardiograms

Criteria have been established for interpreting an ECG strip. The ECG is evaluated for rate, regularity, P waves, PR interval, and QRS complexes (Table 33.4).

Rate calculation. Most ECG strips have tic marks indicating 3-second time periods. Heart rate can be calculated from the ECG strip in several ways. The most common method is to count the number of P waves (for atrial rate) or R waves (for ventricular rate) in a 6-second strip (between three tic marks or 30 large squares) and multiply by 10 for the estimate of the number of beats per minute. For example, if six R waves are seen in a 6-second strip, the heart rate is 60 beats per minute.

Rhythm. The consecutive P-P intervals for the atria and the consecutive R-R intervals for the ventricles are measured for consistency. Using calipers or a blank piece of paper, the distance between P waves and R waves is noted. If the distances do not vary more than one small square, the rhythm is considered regular. If the distances are greater than one small square, the rhythm is irregular.

P waves. The next evaluation is of P waves. Is a P wave noted before each QRS complex? If so, the rhythm originates in the SA node. Do all P waves appear to be the same size and shape? If so, the impulse originates in the SA node.

PR interval. Does the PR interval fall within the normal range of 0.12 to 0.20 second? If so, no interference occurs in conduction from the SA node to the AV node.

QRS complex. Does the QRS complex fall within the range of 0.06 to 0.12 second? If the QRS is prolonged (>0.12 second), a delay occurs in conduction through the ventricles.

ST segment. Next, the ST segment is examined. Is it isoelectric, depressed, or elevated?

T waves. Are the T waves rounded and the same size and shape? Do the T waves follow the QRS complexes?

Normal Sinus Rhythm

The most common cardiac rhythm is sinus in origin because the impulse originates in the SA node, is conducted normally, and meets all of the criteria established earlier. Normal sinus rhythm is shown in Fig. 33.12.

Common Dysrhythmias

A **dysrhythmia** is a disturbance of the rhythm of the heart caused by a problem in the conduction system. Dysrhythmias are categorized according to the site of origin of the impulse formation. Dysrhythmias originating in the atria are called *atrial dysrhythmias.* Dysrhythmias originating in the AV node are called *junctional* or *escape rhythms.* Dysrhythmias originating below the AV node are called *ventricular.* Blocks are interruptions in impulse conduction and can occur at the AV node (first-degree, second-degree type I, second-degree type II, or third-degree blocks) or in the right or left bundle of His (right or left bundle branch blocks). Dysrhythmias and blocks have unique characteristics that are seen on the ECG and interpreted by specially trained health care providers. See Figs. 33.13–33.19 for examples. Only more common dysrhythmias and lethal dysrhythmias are included in this text. For more in-depth information on ECG interpretation, many resources are available (textbooks, websites, formal classes). Antidysrhythmic drugs are used to treat dysrhythmias and restore normal sinus rhythm.

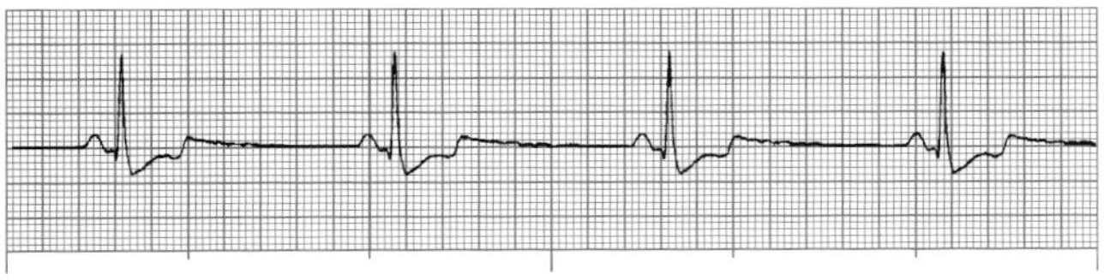

Fig. 33.13 Sinus bradycardia. Characteristics: rate—less than 60 beats per minute; regularity—normal; P wave, PR interval—normal; QRS—normal; T wave—normal. Interpretation: All characteristics are within normal ranges except for the rate, which is slow. Causes: drugs, including digitalis and beta-blockers; vagal stimulation (Valsalva maneuver); severe pain; hyperkalemia; infection; and myocardial infarction. Frequently seen in athletes as a result of conditioning. Symptoms: dizziness, syncope, chest pain, hypotension, sweating, nausea, dyspnea, and disorientation; sometimes no symptoms. Treatment: not treated unless the patient is symptomatic. The underlying cause is treated. Atropine may be given to increase the heart rate. Isoproterenol is used with extreme caution. A pacemaker may be needed. (From Aehlert B: *ECGs made easy*, ed 5, St. Louis, 2013, Mosby.)

HEMODYNAMIC MONITORING

In addition to noninvasive cardiac assessment and ECG monitoring, more sophisticated measures may be needed to determine what is going on within the heart or vascular system. Nurses who work in intensive care areas frequently work with patients who have central venous catheters, pulmonary artery catheters, or arterial lines.

The central venous catheter is placed through the skin, into a venous access (brachial, femoral, subclavian, or jugular sites), and threaded into the RA. The catheter may have one to three lumens. With this catheter, the pressure in the RA (called *right atrial pressure* or *central venous pressure*) can be measured. This catheter may also be used to infuse fluids, blood and blood products, and medications and to withdraw blood for analysis. The pulmonary artery catheter, frequently called a *Swan-Ganz catheter*, is longer than the central venous catheter. The purpose of a pulmonary artery catheter is to measure right-sided heart pressures and pulmonary artery pressures and to assess left-sided heart function. With a pulmonary artery catheter in place, cardiac output can be measured continuously. The normal cardiac output is 4 to 8 L/min. Stress increases the cardiac output. Cardiac output may decrease with myocardial infarction (MI), HF, bradycardia, tachycardia, and some drugs.

An arterial line may be inserted (most often in the radial artery) to provide a direct measurement of SBP and DPB. Once the line is inserted, it is connected to a pressurized solution to keep the catheter patent and to a transducer to assess pressure. The mean arterial pressure (MAP) is an indication of tissue perfusion. This pressure is elevated with sympathetic stimulation and increased heart rate. For more in-depth information on hemodynamic monitoring, many resources are available (textbooks, websites, formal classes).

AMBULATORY ELECTROCARDIOGRAM (HOLTER MONITOR)

An ambulatory ECG uses a portable ECG machine with a memory to provide continuous cardiac monitoring for

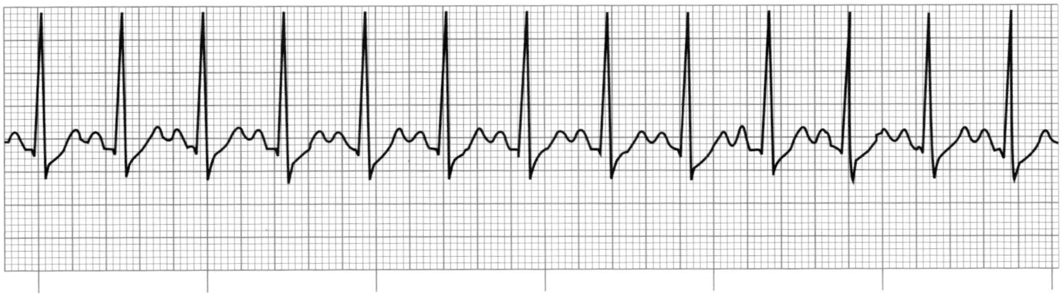

Fig. 33.14 Sinus tachycardia. Characteristics: rate—greater than 100 beats per minute, usually less than 150 beats per minute; regularity—regular; P wave, PR interval—P waves may be buried in T wave of preceding beat with very rapid rates, more than 140 beats per minute; QRS—normal; T wave—normal. Interpretation: All characteristics are within normal range except for the rate, which is excessive. Causes: fever, dehydration, hypovolemia, increased sympathetic nervous system stimulation, stress, exercise, and acute myocardial infarction. Symptoms: palpitations most common. Angina and decreased cardiac output from the decreased ventricular filling time also may occur. Treatment: correction of underlying cause; elimination of caffeine, nicotine, and alcohol; vagal stimulation may decrease the rate but does not treat the cause; beta-blockers. (From Aehlert B: *ECGs made easy*, ed 5, St. Louis, 2013, Mosby.)

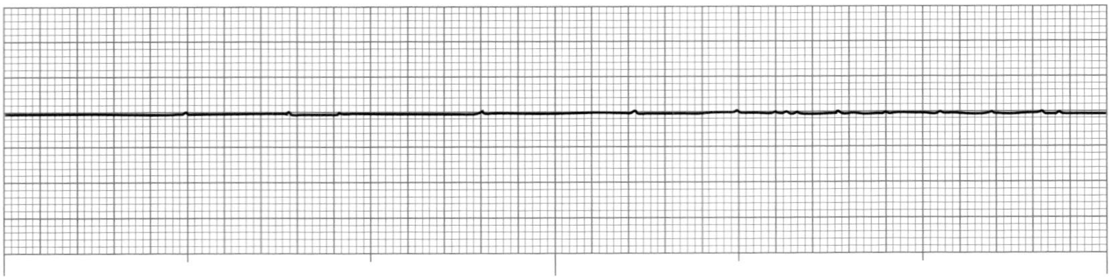

Fig. 33.15 Asystole. Characteristics: rate—none; regularity—none; P wave, PR interval—there may be P waves, but none is conducted, the PR interval is not measurable; QRS—absent; T wave—absent. Interpretation: straight or only slightly wavy baseline. Causes: severe metabolic deficit, acute respiratory failure, and myocardial damage. Symptoms: loss of consciousness, no pulse. Treatment: immediate response with cardiopulmonary resuscitation and advanced cardiac life support; epinephrine, atropine; transcutaneous pacemaker. (From Aehlert B: *ECGs made easy*, ed 5, St. Louis, 2013, Mosby.)

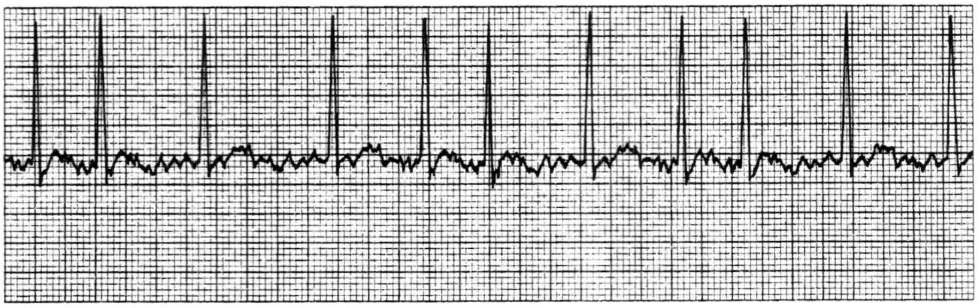

Atrial fibrillation

Fig. 33.16 Atrial fibrillation. Characteristics: rate—atrial rate is greater than 400 beats per minute, if it can be determined at all, ventricular rate is 100 to 150 beats per minute; regularity—very irregular; P wave, PR interval—no P waves, PR interval unmeasurable; QRS—normal; T wave—undeterminable. Interpretation: the baseline between QRS complexes is wavy. Causes: rheumatic fever, mitral valve stenosis, coronary heart disease, hypertension, cardiomyopathy, myocardial infarction, hyperthyroidism, chronic obstructive pulmonary disease, and heart failure. It is frequently seen in older adults after the administration of anesthetic. Symptoms: may have palpitations, angina, and decreased cardiac output. The concerns are development of an atrial thrombus and loss of atrial kick from ineffective atrial function. Treatment: calcium channel blockers or beta-blockers to reduce a rapid ventricular response; anticoagulants to prevent embolization; synchronized cardioversion or drug therapy (amiodarone or ibutilide) to restore a normal rhythm. (From Ignatavicius DD, Workman ML: *Medical-surgical nursing: patient-centered collaborative care*, ed 6, St. Louis, 2010, Saunders.)

24 to 48 hours. A complete record of the heart rhythm is stored and analyzed later. This type of monitoring is used to detect dysrhythmias that occur infrequently, to determine if symptoms correlate with any underlying cardiac disease, to assess the effects of medications, and for research purposes. The patient records in a diary all activity that occurs during the monitoring, such as walking, stair climbing, sleeping, and engaging in sexual activity. The monitor strip is computer scanned, and then interpreted by a physician.

Even more sophisticated monitoring is accomplished by transtelephonic means. An audio signal is sent over telephone lines to a station operated by personnel trained to recognize potentially dangerous dysrhythmias.

IMPLANTABLE LOOP RECORDER

For longer monitoring periods, to record a patient's ECG during syncopal episodes, an implantable loop recorder (ILR) may be used. This device, implanted just under the patient's skin in the chest area, continually monitors the ECG activity of the patient in a memory loop. The patient, family member, or significant other is taught to activate the recorder when symptoms are felt. The ECG can then be analyzed and appropriate treatment implemented.

ECHOCARDIOGRAM

The echocardiogram visualizes and records the size, shape, position, and behavior of the heart's internal structures, especially wall motion and valve function. This painless test may be performed at the bedside or in a laboratory. Gel is applied to the skin and a special device called a *transducer* is moved over the precordium. The transducer picks up sound waves and converts them to electrical impulses that are recorded as waveforms on an oscilloscope, a videotape, or a strip chart. Common echocardiogram types include motion mode (M-mode) and two-dimensional mode (2D mode). Echocardiograms can also be enhanced using Doppler technology (Doppler echocardiogram) and color-flow imaging.

TRANSESOPHAGEAL ECHOCARDIOGRAM

At times, the echocardiogram is not diagnostic and a transesophageal echocardiogram (TEE) is used. A

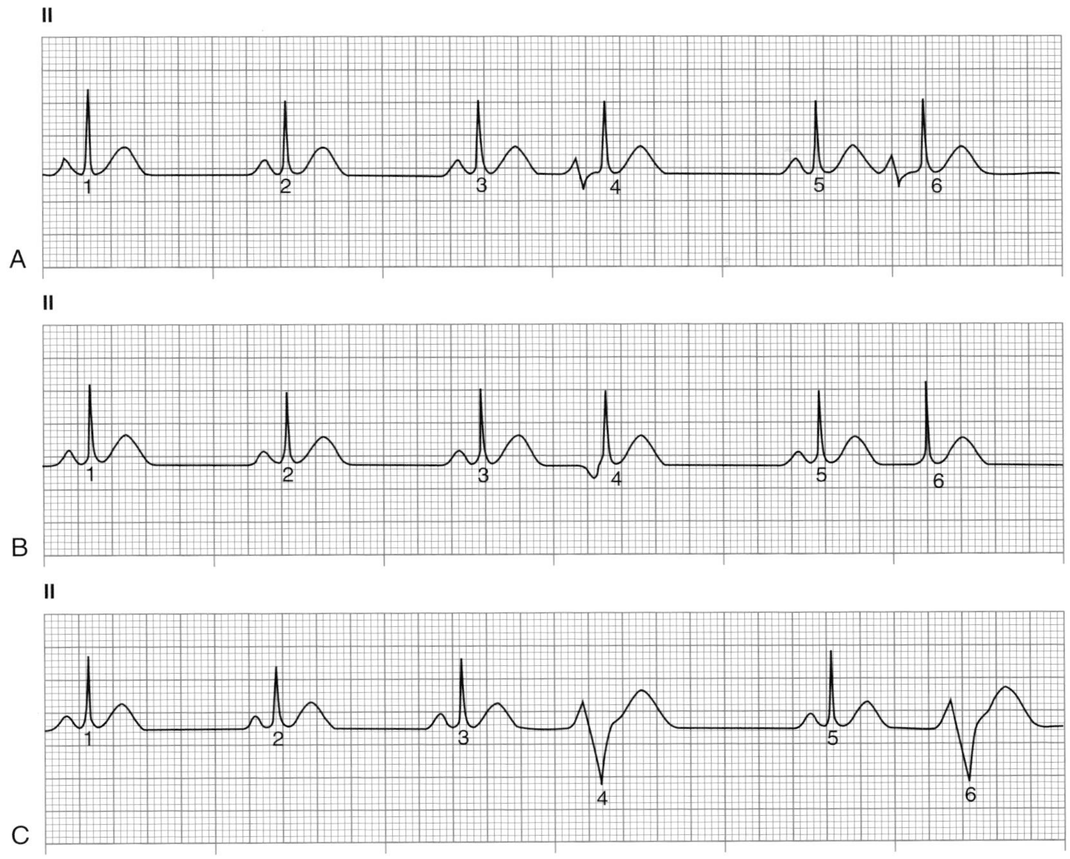

Fig. 33.17 Premature ventricular contractions (PVCs). Characteristics: rate—normal; regularity—irregular because of PVCs; P wave, PR interval—no P wave with the PVC, inverted P wave may follow a PVC, no PR interval occurs with the PVC; QRS—wide and bizarre in the PVC; T wave—opposite deflection to the PVC. Interpretations: wide QRS. Unifocal PVCs originate from one site. Multifocal PVCs arise from different ventricular sites and have a poorer prognosis. Causes: digoxin toxicity, hypokalemia, hypercalcemia, sympathetic nervous system stimulation (stress, caffeine, nicotine), and excess catecholamine release. Symptoms: the patient may or may not note a "skipped" beat. The PVCs are not palpable at peripheral pulse sites, but a pause may be observed. Cardiac output diminishes with frequent PVCs. Treatment: no treatment necessary for infrequent PVCs, which probably occur undetected in most people; treat the cause and administer antidysrhythmic agents for symptomatic or frequent PVCs. (From Grauer K: *A practical guide to ECG interpretation*, ed 2, St. Louis, 1998, Mosby.)

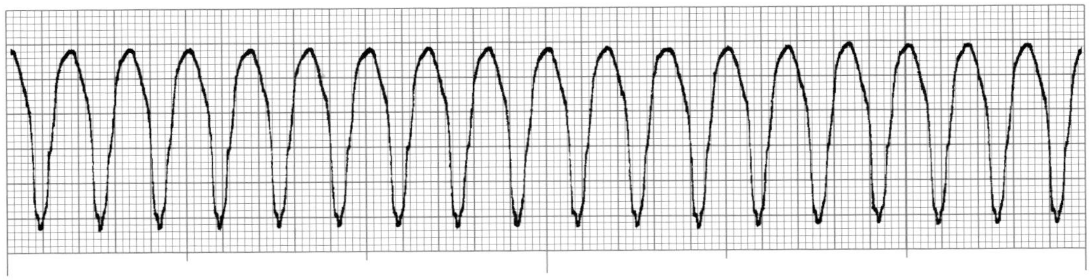

Fig. 33.18 Ventricular tachycardia. Characteristics: rate—100 to 250 beats per minute, no relationship exists between the atrial and ventricular contractions; Regularity—ventricular rhythm usually regular; P wave, PR interval—absent; QRS—wide, bizarre, greater than 0.12 second, may look like PVCs; T wave—opposite deflection to QRS. Interpretation: this is a life-threatening dysrhythmia that often precedes ventricular fibrillation. Causes: myocardial irritation, myocardial infarction, coronary heart disease, rheumatic heart disease, hypokalemia, and digoxin toxicity. Symptoms: initially, palpitations, dizziness, and chest pain, progressing to decreased cardiac output and loss of consciousness. Treatment: assess for pulse, signs, and symptoms. If ventricular tachycardia without pulse: defibrillate and follow advanced cardiac life support algorithm. With pulse, but unstable: synchronized cardioversion. If stable, with pulse: amiodarone, then synchronized cardioversion. (From Grauer K: *A practical guide to ECG interpretation*, ed 2, St. Louis, 1998, Mosby.)

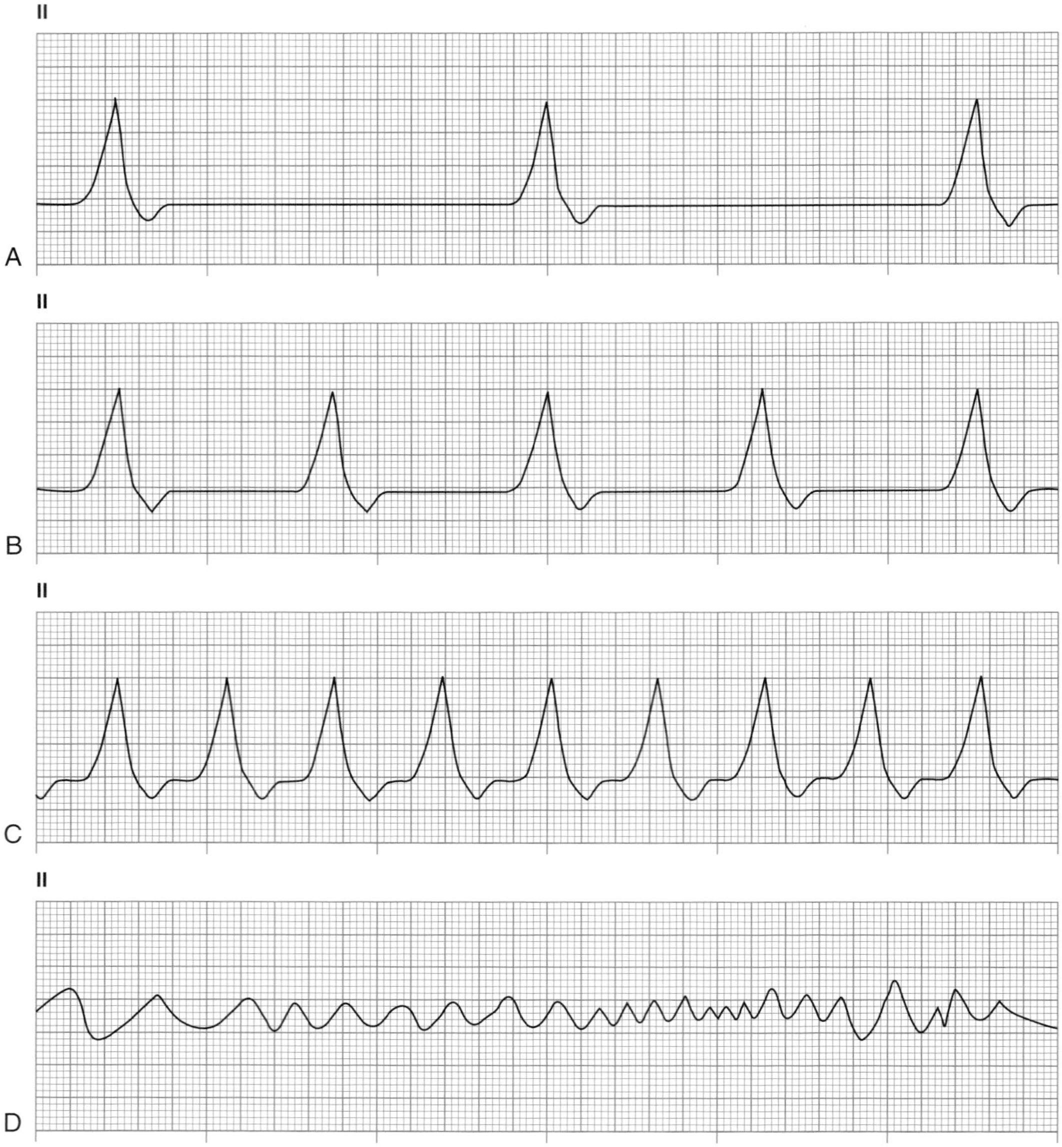

Fig. 33.19 Ventricular fibrillation. Characteristics: (A) rate—undeterminable; regularity—chaotic, wavy baseline; (B) P wave, PR interval—undeterminable; (C) QRS—undeterminable; (D) T wave—undeterminable. Interpretation: this life-threatening dysrhythmia must be terminated quickly if the patient is to resume useful function. Causes: coronary heart disease, acute myocardial infarction, untreated ventricular tachycardia, electrolyte and acid-base imbalances, electric shock, and hypothermia. Symptoms: loss of consciousness, cessation of heartbeat and respirations, dilation of pupils. Treatment: cardiopulmonary resuscitation, defibrillation, and advanced cardiac life support measures. (From Aehlert B: *ECGs made easy*, ed 5, St. Louis, 2013, Mosby.)

flexible endoscopic probe with an ultrasound transducer is passed down the back of the throat into the esophagus. A local anesthetic to the throat decreases the gag reflex. Occasionally, an intravenous (IV) sedative is needed to reduce patient anxiety. Images are obtained from behind the heart as the probe moves down into the stomach. The probe is down for approximately 15 to 20 minutes. The TEE provides information that is useful in the evaluation of ventricular wall motion and function and possible heart valve disorders.

STRESS TEST (EXERCISE TOLERANCE TEST)

The stress test is a noninvasive method of assessing the presence and severity of coronary heart disease by recording a person's cardiovascular response to exercise. It is also used to measure functional capacity for work, sport, or participation in a rehabilitation program. The stress test is not flawless, and false-positive and false-negative results are common. A negative test result does not absolutely exclude CHD. However, the stress test is the best noninvasive screening procedure available. The alternative is the much more invasive cardiac catheterization.

For the stress test, a continuous ECG is monitored while the patient uses a treadmill or a stationary bicycle. Every 2 to 3 minutes the speed and incline angle of the treadmill are increased (or pedal resistance is increased with a bicycle) until (1) the patient cannot continue for whatever reason, (2) the patient's maximum heart rate is achieved (220 − patient's age = maximum heart rate), (3) symptoms intervene, or (4) significant changes are detected on the ECG. The target heart rate is 85% of the predicted maximum heart rate for the patient's age and sex. When patients are unable to exercise, a pharmacologic stress test can be performed using medications that dilate the coronary arteries (e.g., dobutamine, adenoscan).

Significant CHD limits blood flow to the myocardium. The increased demands of exercise may cause the patient to have symptoms of CHD, which are angina, dizziness, dyspnea, dysrhythmias, a falling BP, and certain ECG findings. If these symptoms occur, the test must be stopped immediately.

Contraindications for the test include acute systemic illness, severe aortic stenosis, uncontrolled HF, severe hypertension, angina at rest, and significant dysrhythmia. Although the mortality rate for test participants is very low, cardiopulmonary resuscitation (CPR) equipment must be available.

MAGNETIC RESONANCE IMAGING

A magnetic resonance imaging (MRI) scan provides high-resolution, three-dimensional images of body structures. Cardiac tissue is imaged without lung or bone interference. The patient is enclosed in a chamber for approximately 30 to 90 minutes for an MRI scan of the heart. No loose metallic objects are permitted in the chamber during the procedure. Patients with intracranial aneurysm clips, intraocular metal foreign bodies, and some middle ear prostheses should not have MRI scans because the devices may be affected by the magnetic field or may interfere with the MRI. Other implanted devices that contraindicate MRI include pacemakers, automatic implantable cardioverter defibrillators (AICDs), and implanted infusion pumps. For patients who are claustrophobic, an open MRI may be available.

ELECTROPHYSIOLOGY STUDY

The electrophysiology study (EPS) is used to record the heart's electrical activity from within the heart using catheters with multiple electrodes inserted through the femoral vein into the right side of the heart. The electrodes record the electrical activity of the heart's conduction system. In addition, the electrodes can be used to stimulate dysrhythmias that will help to locate the source of the patient's dysrhythmia.

MULTIPLE-GATED ACQUISITION SCAN

In a multiple-gated acquisition (MUGA) scan, the patient is injected with a radioactive tracer. The heart is then scanned to assess LV structure and function, to evaluate myocardial wall motion, to assess valvular disease, and to identify location and size of an MI. Assessment of ventricular function can be done while the patient is resting or exercising. Sublingual nitroglycerin may be administered to assess its effect on ventricular function.

MYOCARDIAL PERFUSION IMAGING

Myocardial perfusion imaging (MPI) is a noninvasive study that shows how well blood is perfusing the heart. Areas that are not receiving enough blood flow will be evident. There are two types of MPI: the positron emission tomography (PET) scan and the single photon emission computed tomography (SPECT) or radionuclide ventriculography (SPECT/RVG). These scans are noninvasive and use a radioactive tracer and a gamma camera to assess the coronary arteries and how well blood is flowing to the cardiac muscle. The scans show healthy and damaged cardiac muscle. Both scans are often used in conjunction with stress testing (exercise or drug induced).

ULTRAFAST COMPUTED TOMOGRAPHY

Ultrafast computed tomography (CT), also known as *electron beam tomography (EBT)*, is a fast form of imaging technology that allows for high-quality images that are not affected by the movement of the heart as it contracts and relaxes. The images obtained are used to assess myocardial perfusion, along with RV and LV muscle mass and function. In addition, ultrafast CT can measure calcium deposits in the coronary arteries, and a coronary calcium score can be derived. The greater the amount of coronary calcium is, the higher the score, and hence the risk of coronary occlusive disease.

CARDIAC CATHETERIZATION (CARDIAC ANGIOGRAPHY, CORONARY ARTERIOGRAPHY)

Cardiac catheterization is a procedure in which a catheter is inserted into a vein or artery and is threaded into the heart chambers, coronary arteries, or both under fluoroscopy (Fig. 33.20). A contrast dye is injected through the catheter, and films are made of the visualized heart structures. Vital signs and ECG are monitored during the procedure.

In a catheterization of the right side of the heart, the catheter is inserted into a vein and threaded into the vena cava, RA, RV, and pulmonary artery. Pressures in the RA, RV, and pulmonary artery may be determined. The function of the pulmonic and tricuspid valves may be assessed.

In a catheterization of the left side of the heart, the catheter is inserted into an artery and threaded against the flow of blood into the coronary arteries or the LV. The function of the coronary arteries and the aortic and mitral valves may be assessed. Blood samples may be drawn, and pressures in the various structures are measured. The femoral vein and artery are the preferred insertion sites for cardiac catheterization.

Complications of cardiac catheterization include bleeding, hematoma formation, infection, and embolus or thrombus formation. Nursing care before and after the procedure is very important.

Angiography may also be used to confirm the diagnosis of PVD, to distinguish clot formation from

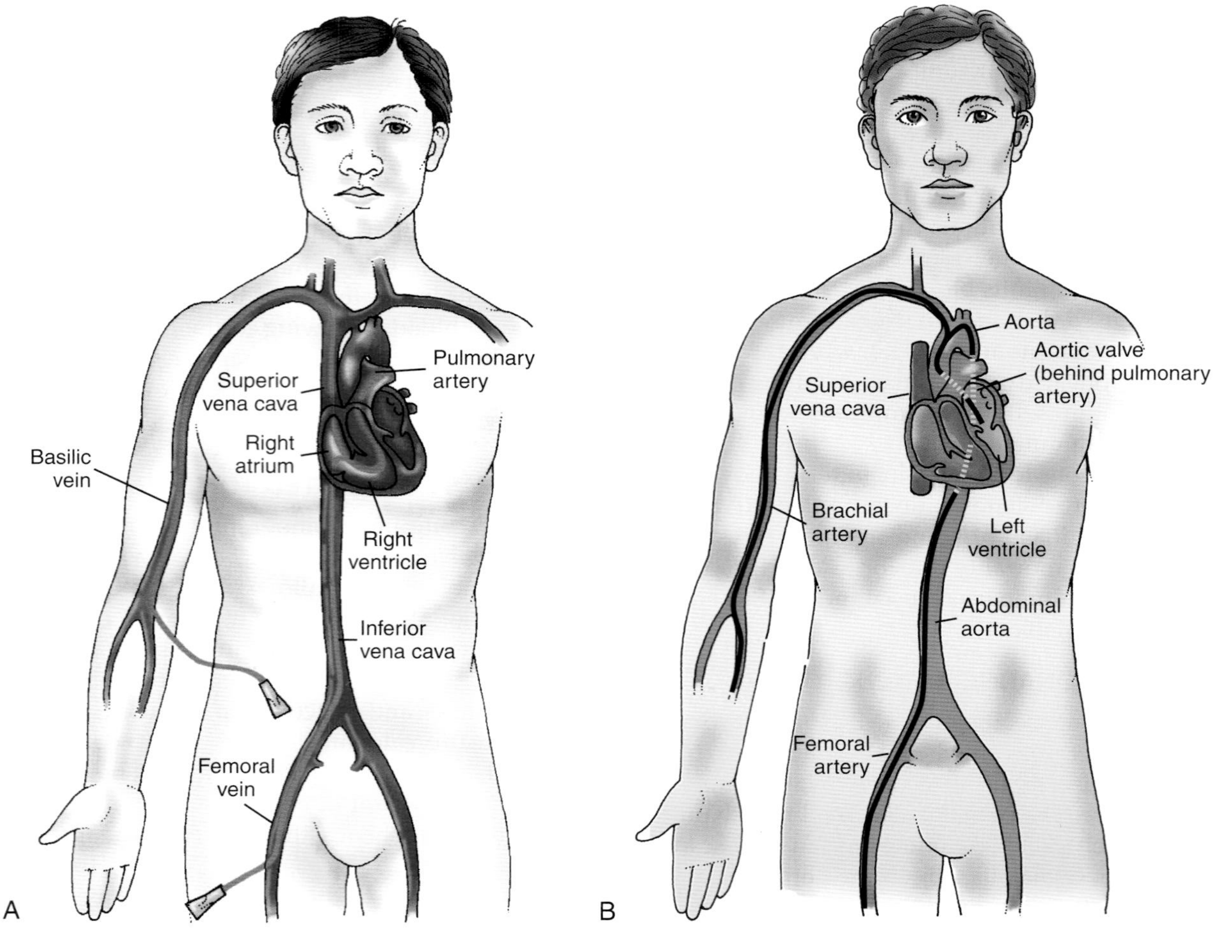

Fig. 33.20 Right-sided (A) and left-sided (B) heart catheterization.

venous obstruction, and to locate a suitable vessel for grafting. Angiography is an invasive procedure that requires the injection of dye into the vascular system, which makes the vessels visible on radiographs. The two types of angiography are (1) arteriography, which examines arteries, and (2) venography, which examines veins. Abnormalities can be visualized and assessed during the procedure. The risks associated with these tests are hemorrhage at the IV insertion site, dye-induced allergic reactions, thrombosis at the insertion site, and emboli. The patient is exposed to relatively high doses of radiation.

PRESSURE MEASUREMENTS

Plethysmography is a noninvasive study used to measure blood flow in the extremities. Multiple BP cuffs are applied to different parts of the extremities. Variations in pressure from one site to another can reveal vascular occlusions or obstructions. Although plethysmography is less accurate than arteriography and venography, it is very safe and can be used to assess patients who are too ill to undergo arteriography.

LABORATORY TESTS

A number of laboratory tests may be used to assess cardiovascular structure and function. More common tests are described here. Patient preparation and post-procedure care are detailed in Table 33.5.

Arterial Blood Gases

Arterial blood gases (ABGs) are analyzed to determine the body's ability to maintain the acid-base balance. Acidity or alkalinity is determined by pH. If the serum pH is less than 7.35, the blood is acidic; pH greater than 7.45 indicates alkalinity. Carbonic acid breaks down into CO_2 and water. The lungs regulate CO_2. A partial pressure of carbon dioxide in arterial blood ($PaCO_2$) greater than 45 with an acidic pH is respiratory acidosis and indicates that the body is unable to excrete the excess CO_2 through the lungs. With a pH in excess of 7.45 and a $PaCO_2$ of less than 35, respiratory alkalosis is present.

The kidneys regulate bicarbonate (HCO_3^-) through excretion and retention. The HCO_3^- (or base excess, a combination of all serum bases) is assessed to determine metabolic causes of imbalance. If the pH is less

Table 33.5 Laboratory Tests for Cardiovascular Conditions

TEST	PURPOSE AND PROCEDURE		
Arterial blood gases (ABGs)	Assesses acid-base balance by measuring pH, partial pressure of carbon dioxide in arterial blood ($PaCO_2$), partial pressure of oxygen in arterial blood (PaO_2), bicarbonate (HCO_3^-), and base excess.	Tell the patient about arterial puncture. Prepare a heparinized syringe, and obtain a blood sample.	Remove air bubbles from the sample. Place the tube on ice, and send it out for immediate analysis. Apply pressure to the puncture site for 5 minutes. Report any results.
Troponin	Measures protein released after myocardial injury: cardiac troponin T (cTnT) and cardiac troponin I (cTnI).	Tell the patient a blood sample will be drawn. No special preparation is needed.	Check the venipuncture site. Apply pressure if it is oozing.
Cardiac enzymes (creatine kinase [CK], creatine kinase-MB fraction [CK-MB], lactate dehydrogenase [LDH])	Measures enzymes that rise in a predictable pattern with myocardial damage.	Tell the patient a blood sample will be drawn. No special preparation is needed. To detect acute myocardial infarction (MI), draw a specimen before other invasive procedures.	Check the venipuncture site. Apply pressure if it is oozing.
Myoglobin	Measures myoglobin levels in the blood. Rises soon after myocardial injury. Also elevated by strenuous exercise, renal failure, and some other conditions.	Tell the patient a blood sample will be drawn. No special preparation is needed.	Check the venipuncture site. Apply pressure if it is oozing.
Complete blood count (CBC)	Counts white blood cells (WBCs) and red blood cells (RBCs), hemoglobin (Hgb) and hematocrit (Hct), RBC indices, and sometimes platelets. (Normal values are listed in Table 33.8.)	Tell the patient a blood sample will be drawn. No special preparation is needed.	Check the venipuncture site. Apply pressure if it is oozing.
Lipid profile	Measures common serum lipids (cholesterol, triglycerides, lipoproteins). Used to evaluate risk of coronary heart disease (CHD).	Tell the patient to expect venipuncture. Nothing by mouth (NPO) for 12 hours before the sample is drawn. Remind patient to eat usual diet for 2 weeks before the test.	Check the venipuncture site. Apply pressure if it is oozing.
B-type natriuretic peptide (BNP)	Measures naturally occurring BNP levels that are elevated in heart failure (HF) and cardiomyopathy (CMP). Helps to differentiate dyspnea related to cardiac problems from noncardiac-related dyspnea.	Tell the patient a blood sample will be drawn. No special preparation is needed.	Check the venipuncture site. Apply pressure if it is oozing.
C-reactive protein (CRP)	Acute phase protein that is elevated in system inflammation. Elevated levels seen with acute coronary syndrome.	Tell the patient a blood sample will be drawn. No special preparation is needed.	Check the venipuncture site. Apply pressure if it is oozing.

than 7.35 and the HCO_3^- is less than 22, the body is in metabolic acidosis. With a pH greater than 7.45 and an HCO_3^- greater than 26, the interpretation is metabolic alkalosis (Table 33.6).

Cardiac Markers

Cardiac markers are released when heart cells die as a result of damage. These markers (enzymes and other proteins) are measured in the serum, and their values rise as indicators of damage to the heart cells. Table 33.7 lists normal cardiac marker levels.

Troponin. Troponin is a protein involved in the contraction of muscles. Two subtypes, cardiac troponin T and cardiac troponin I, are specific to cardiac muscle and are released into the circulation with any myocardial injury. Troponin levels, generally not detectable in healthy individuals, will elevate significantly after an MI. Troponin levels rise in 3 to 6 hours from onset of symptoms, peak in 12 hours, and remain in the circulation for up to 10 to 14 days. This test is done in the emergency department because even very low levels of troponin are treated quickly and aggressively.

Table 33.6 Interpreting Arterial Blood Gases

CONDITION	pH	$PaCO_2$	HCO_3^-
Normal range	7.35–7.45	35–45	22–26
Respiratory acidosis	↓	↑	Normal
Respiratory alkalosis	↑	↓	Normal
Metabolic acidosis	↓	Normal	↓
Metabolic alkalosis	↑	Normal	↑

↑, Elevated; ↓, decreased; HCO_3^-, bicarbonate; $PaCO_2$, partial pressure of carbon dioxide in arterial blood.
If the arrows are in the same direction, a metabolic problem exists. If arrows are in opposite directions, a respiratory problem exists.

Table 33.7 Cardiac Biomarkers and Enzymes

TEST[a]	NORMAL VALUES
Creatine kinase (CK)	Male subject: 55–170 U/L Female subject: 30–135 U/L
CK isoenzymes	MM fraction: 100% MB fraction: 0% BB fraction: 0%
Cardiac troponin T (cTnT)	<0.1 ng/mL
Cardiac troponin I (cTnI)	<0.03 ng/mL
Myoglobin	<90 mcg/mL

[a]Values may vary according to the laboratory equipment used.

Table 33.8 Complete Blood Count

TEST[a]	NORMAL VALUES
White blood cells (WBCs)	5000–10,000/mm^3
Differential	
Neutrophils	60.0%–70.0%
Eosinophils	1.0%–4.0%
Basophils	0.5%–1.0%
Lymphocytes	20.0%–40.0%
Monocytes	2.0%–6.0%
Red blood cells (RBCs)	
Male subject	4,200,000–5,400,000/mm^3
Female subject	3,600,000–5,000,000/mm^3
Hematocrit (Hct)	
Male subject	40.0%–54.0%
Female subject	37.0%–47.0%
Hemoglobin (Hgb)	
Male subject	13.5–17.5 g/dL
Female subject	12.0–16.0 g/dL
Platelets	150,000–350,000/mm^3

[a]Values may vary according to the laboratory equipment used.

Complete Blood Count

The complete blood count (CBC) is a basic screening test. Included in this test are the white blood cell (WBC) count, the RBC count, the hemoglobin (Hgb) and hematocrit (Hct) measurements, the RBC indices, and (in some laboratories) the platelet count. Components of the CBC are presented in Table 33.8.

White blood cell count. The WBC count indicates the body's ability to defend itself against infection and inflammation. The WBC level is usually elevated with inflammatory processes such as MI and bacterial infections, but it may be below normal with viral infections and bone marrow depression.

Red blood cell count. The RBC count is assessed to determine the ability of the blood to carry O_2 from the lungs to the tissues and CO_2 from the tissues to the lungs. The RBC level may be below normal with anemia and malignancies and may be elevated in dehydration.

Hematocrit. The Hct is the percentage of packed red blood cells (PRBCs) in the total sample of whole blood. With severe dehydration, the plasma portion of the blood decreases and the Hct is elevated. In anemia and hemorrhage, the Hct is below normal. In general, the Hct is 3 times the Hgb measurement.

Hemoglobin. Hgb is the main component of the RBCs. Its function is to transport O_2 to the cells. The Hgb measurement may be below normal in anemia and hemorrhage. It is elevated in dehydration, chronic obstructive pulmonary disease (COPD), and CHF. A Hgb of less than 5 g/dL leads to HF and death if not corrected.

Platelet (thrombocyte) count. The platelets (thrombocytes) are the smallest of the formed elements in the blood. They are necessary for coagulation. The platelet count is below normal with anemia, bone marrow depression, and bleeding. The count may be increased in acute infections and some heart diseases. A count of less than 20,000 may result in spontaneous bleeding.

Lipid Profile

A lipid profile is a battery of tests that measure the most common serum lipids: cholesterol, triglycerides, and lipoproteins.

Cholesterol is a blood lipid produced by the liver. It is used to form bile salts for the digestion of fat and the production of adrenal, ovarian, and testicular hormones. The normal adult serum cholesterol level is less than 200 mg/dL. Elevated cholesterol levels (hypercholesterolemia) are associated with increased risk of CHD, hypertension, and MI. The cholesterol accumulates in the arterial lumen and, in time, results in decreased blood flow and occlusion.

Several forms of cholesterol are identified; however, the high-density lipoproteins (HDLs) and low-density lipoproteins (LDLs) are the two that most closely correlate with CHD. The HDLs are desirable because they promote the excretion of cholesterol; therefore higher levels of HDLs are encouraged. Conversely, elevated LDL levels are associated with a higher risk of CHD; thus, lower LDL levels are encouraged. A good way to remember the difference is that HDLs are healthy and LDLs are lethal. Currently, the recommendations are for HDL levels greater than 45 mg/dL (for men) or greater than 55 mg/dL (for women) and for LDL levels less than 130 mg/dL (Pagana et al., 2017). See the Health Promotion box for advice on increasing HDL levels.

Health Promotion

LOW HIGH-DENSITY LIPOPROTEIN LEVELS

Raising low levels of high-density lipoprotein (HDL) can be accomplished by being physically active at least 30 minutes every day, by not smoking, and by losing weight (or maintaining a healthy weight).

Triglycerides are a major contributor to coronary heart disease. They are produced in the liver. Triglyceride levels increase when LDL levels increase. The normal triglyceride level is 40 to 160 mg/dL in men and 35 to 135 mg/dL in women (Pagana et al., 2017)

B-Type Natriuretic Peptide

B-type natriuretic peptide (BNP) is a cardiac hormone released when ventricular dilation and stretch (such as occurs in HF) occur. Less than 100 pg/mL is considered a normal BNP level, and elevated levels relate closely to the severity of HF (e.g., the higher the levels, the more severe the failure). In addition, BNP levels can be monitored to assess the effectiveness of treatment.

C-Reactive Protein

C-reactive protein (CRP) is an acute-phase protein and a marker for systemic inflammation. Elevated levels of CRP are present in patients with acute coronary syndrome. CRP can be used to predict an individual's risk for cardiovascular disease or events.

COMMON THERAPEUTIC MEASURES

DRUG THERAPY

Commonly used cardiovascular drugs are cardiac glycosides, antianginals, antidysrhythmics, anticoagulants, vasodilators, diuretics, and lipid-lowering agents. Information about these medications is presented in Table 33.9.

Cardiac Glycosides

Cardiac glycosides, such as digoxin (Lanoxin) have several important pharmacologic actions on the heart. They slow the heart rate (negative chronotropic effect) and increase the force of myocardial contraction (positive inotropic effect), causing increased stroke volume and cardiac output. Cardiac glycosides are widely used in the treatment of HF. They are also used to treat some cardiac dysrhythmias.

When rapid effects are needed, a patient can be given a loading dose (called a *digitalizing dose*) of cardiac glycosides. Once therapeutic blood levels are obtained, a maintenance dose is prescribed to maintain the therapeutic effects. These drugs have high potential for toxicity and require close monitoring. Common practice is to count the apical pulse before giving each dose. If the rate is less than 60 beats per minute in adults, withhold the dose and contact the health care provider. Because patients are often on cardiac glycosides for long-term therapy, they must be taught to monitor their own pulse and to report symptoms of toxicity (anorexia, nausea, visual disturbances).

Antianginals

Drugs used to treat angina (chest pain related to myocardial ischemia) include nitrates, beta-adrenergic blockers, and calcium channel blockers. Nitrates are used to treat actual anginal episodes and to prevent angina. Beta-adrenergic blockers and calcium channel blockers are used in the long-term management of angina.

Antidysrhythmics

Drugs used to treat abnormal cardiac rhythms are called *antidysrhythmics* or *antiarrhythmics*. Four main classes of antidysrhythmics exist, each with various actions. In general, they work by slowing the rate of impulse conduction, depressing automaticity, or increasing resistance to premature stimulation. All antidysrhythmics have the potential to cause additional dysrhythmias.

Examples of these drugs, their actions, and adverse effects, as well as associated nursing considerations, are provided in Table 33.9.

Angiotensin-Converting Enzyme Inhibitors

Angiotensin-converting enzyme (ACE) inhibitors work against the renin-angiotensin-aldosterone (RAA) system to dilate arteries and decrease resistance to blood flow in the arteries (reduced afterload). In addition, less fluid is retained because aldosterone release is blocked. ACE inhibitors are prescribed for patients with HF, in some cases of hypertension, and in some cases after MI. Examples of these medications are captopril (Capoten), enalapril (Vasotec), and quinapril (Accupril). Some patients do not tolerate the ACE inhibitors. In these cases, angiotensin receptor blockers (ARBs) may be prescribed. Examples of ARBs are

Table 33.9 Selected Medications for Cardiovascular Disorders

DRUG	USE AND ACTION	SELECTED NURSING INTERVENTIONS
Cardiac Glycosides		
digoxin (Lanoxin)	Delays impulse conduction through the AV node to slow the heart rate (negative chronotropic effect). Increases strength or force of myocardial contraction (positive inotropic effect). Increases stroke volume and CO. Used for HF, atrial fibrillation and flutter, and paroxysmal atrial tachycardia.	Obtain baseline vital signs, ECG, and electrolytes before administering the first dose. Assess apical pulse for 1 minute; hold the drug, and notify the health care provider if the patient's pulse is <60 beats per minute. Monitor potassium (K^+) levels because low potassium increases the risk of digoxin toxicity. Decreased renal function may delay excretion and lead to toxicity. Toxicity may be indicated by dysrhythmias, pulse <60 beats per minute, anorexia, nausea, syncope, visual disturbances, and abdominal pain. Therapeutic level: 0.8–2.0 ng/mL; toxic level: >2.0 ng/mL. Teach the patient the following: • Take your radial pulse for 1 minute at the same time each day.
Antianginal Agents		
nitroglycerin (available as sublingual tablets, ointment, transdermal patch, buccal tablets, mist, sustained-release oral tablets, and injectable [IV])	Acts as a vasodilator (arteries and veins). Relaxes all smooth muscles, especially vascular smooth muscle. Decreases preload, afterload, BP, CO, and systemic vascular resistance. Used to prevent and treat angina.	Assess the patient's BP and pulse before administration. Teach the patient the following: • Sit or lie down at onset of chest pain. • Place the tablet under the tongue; the tablet causes tingling sensation if effective (older adults may not detect this). • Repeat every 5 minutes for a total of three doses; if chest pain is not relieved, call 911. Note: some sources advise to seek medical care if pain is not relieved by one tablet. • Keep the tablets in the containers in which they are supplied; the drug decomposes on exposure to light and air. • Headache decreases with tolerance. • Drug may be taken before activities likely to cause angina (e.g., exercise, sex).
isosorbide dinitrate (Isordil)	Acts as a vasodilator that works by relaxing smooth muscles. Decreases preload, afterload, left ventricular end-diastolic pressure, and myocardial oxygen (O_2) consumption. Used for acute angina and maintenance of chronic angina.	Assess vital signs before administration. Teach the patient: • Take the drug 1 to 2 hours before meals and at bedtime. • Sit when taking the sublingual or chewable medications. • Change positions slowly to avoid orthostatic hypotension. • Headache decreases over time. • Alcohol potentiates hypotension.

Table 33.9 Selected Medications for Cardiovascular Disorders—cont'd

DRUG	USE AND ACTION	SELECTED NURSING INTERVENTIONS
atenolol (Tenormin) and metoprolol tartrate (Lopressor)	Acts as a cardioselective beta-adrenergic blocker used to treat angina and hypertension. Reduces HR, BP, CO, and myocardial O_2 consumption.	Monitor vital signs. Provide continuous ECG monitoring with IV administration of metoprolol tartrate. Take apical pulse before each dose. Teach the patient: • Take the drug with or after meals. • Do not discontinue abruptly. • Take your pulse, and report to the health care provider if it is <60 beats per minute. • Avoid alcohol and smoking. • Avoid OTC cold medication.
diltiazem hydrochloride (Cardizem)	Acts as a calcium channel blocker. Dilates coronary arteries; increases the availability of O_2 to the myocardium. Decreases total vascular resistance, afterload, and systolic BP. Slightly decreases myocardial contractility. Prolongs AV node refractory period. Used in chronic stable angina, coronary artery spasm, atrial fibrillation, and hypertension.	Dose may need to be reduced in older adult patients. Teach the patient: • Take your radial pulse for 1 minute. • Grapefruit juice can increase the serum concentration of diltiazem. • Change positions with caution to prevent postural hypotension. • Take the drug before meals and at bedtime.
nifedipine (Procardia)	Acts as a calcium channel blocker. Decreases myocardial O_2 consumption. Dilates coronary arteries. Decreases vascular resistance. Increases CO. Used for angina, mild to moderate hypertension, vascular headaches, and coronary artery spasms.	Monitor BP during titration (i.e., during dose adjustment). Teach the patient: • Smoking is contraindicated (nicotine constricts coronary arteries). • Do not discontinue this drug abruptly. • Limit caffeine intake.
Antidysrhythmic Agents		
amiodarone hydrochloride (Cordarone)	Acts as an antidysrhythmic. Increases action potential duration and effective refractory period. Increases CO. Decreases PVR, coronary artery resistance, and HR. Used for severe tachycardia and supraventricular tachycardias.	Observe ECG, as bradycardia can occur. Assess vitals, as hypotension can also occur. Observe for liver toxicity by monitoring liver enzymes. Observe for pulmonary complications, as pulmonary toxicity can occur. Teach the patient the following: • Take your radial pulse daily. • Photosensitivity and photophobia may occur. • Pharmacologic action may have a delayed onset of 5 days to 3 months. • Skin discolorations fade with time.
disopyramide phosphate (Norpace)	Reduces the rate of spontaneous diastolic depolarization in pacemaker cells. Increases SVR. Decreases myocardial conductivity. Suppresses ectopic focal activity. Used to suppress and prevent recurrent PVCs and ventricular tachycardia.	Assess apical pulse before administration. Hold the drug if the pulse is <60 or >120 beats per minute, and notify physician. Monitor BP. Monitor intake and output. Urinary retention and constipation may occur. Teach the patient: • Take your radial pulse daily. • Weigh yourself daily; observe for edema. • Change position slowly. • Do not drink alcohol (severely decreases BP). • Relieve dry mouth with sugarless gum or dry candy. • Avoid sunlight (photosensitivity).

Continued

Table 33.9 Selected Medications for Cardiovascular Disorders—cont'd

DRUG	USE AND ACTION	SELECTED NURSING INTERVENTIONS
flecainide acetate (Tambocor)	Acts as an antidysrhythmic. Used to treat PVCs, atrial tachycardia, and other dysrhythmias not responsive to other antidysrhythmics.	Monitor ECG.
lidocaine (Xylocaine)	Increases the electrical stimulation threshold of the ventricular conduction system. Used for rapid control of ventricular dysrhythmias during MI, cardiac surgery, cardiac catheterization, and digitalis intoxication.	Administer the drug with an infusion pump. Monitor BP and ECG. May precipitate malignant hyperthermia (tachycardia, tachypnea, elevated temperature). Assess breath sounds for crackles.
mexiletine hydrochloride (Mexitil)	Acts as an antidysrhythmic for the management of life-threatening ventricular arrhythmias.	Administer the drug with food or antacids. Monitor ECG.
verapamil (Calan) diltiazem (Cardizem)	Calcium channel blockers used for atrial fibrillation and atrial flutter.	Monitor heart rate and BP. Teach the patient to change positions slowly, as orthostatic hypotension can occur. Teach the patient to report signs of HF that can occur with these drugs: shortness of breath, swelling, or distended neck veins.
Anticoagulant Agents		
Noac (Novel Oral Anticoagulant)		
dabigatran (Pradaxa) Others that are the same here: rivaroxaban (Xarelto) apixaban (Eliquis) edoxaban (Savaysa)	Prevents blood clot formation. Used to prevent the risk of stroke and serious blood clots in patients with atrial fibrillation.	Monitor for bleeding. Be aware that a reversal agent for dabigatran exists: idarucizumab (Praxbind) Teach the patient: • Take with or without food. • Do not stop the medication suddenly without the direction of the health care provider. • Check with your health care provider before beginning any OTC medications.
Antiplatelet Agents		
clopidogrel (Plavix)	Decreases platelet aggregation. Prolongs bleeding time. Used to prevent thromboembolic disorders, such as stroke and MI.	Monitor bleeding time, CBC with differential, and platelet count. Avoid OTC medications with aspirin or NSAIDs unless prescribed by the health care provider. Teach the patient: • Report bleeding. • Keep appointments for blood work.
ticlopidine (Ticlid)	Same as Plavix.	Monitor liver function studies, CBC, and prothrombin time (PT). Teach the patient: • Report bleeding. • Take the drug with food. • Keep appointments for blood work.
abciximab (ReoPro)	Inhibits platelet aggregation. Given IV to reduce ischemic complications with angioplasty or atherectomy.	Used only in the hospital. Monitor vital signs, ECG, and level of consciousness. Assess hemoglobin (Hgb), hematocrit (Hct), platelet count, and clotting factors frequently. Watch for bleeding. Protect from trauma.

Table 33.9 Selected Medications for Cardiovascular Disorders—cont'd

DRUG	USE AND ACTION	SELECTED NURSING INTERVENTIONS
Lipid-Lowering Agents		
cholestyramine (Questran)	Prescribed when diet, exercise, and weight loss fail to bring cholesterol levels under control. Lowers LDL cholesterol. Increases HDL cholesterol.	Interferes with absorption of some other drugs, so check drug-drug interactions before giving this medication. To get the best effect, teach patients to: • Continue diet and exercise. • Increase fluid intake to counter constipating effects.
gemfibrozil (Lopid), nicotinic acid (niacin)	Decreases synthesis and secretion of VLDL by liver. Decreases triglyceride levels.	For best effect, teach the patient: • Continue diet and exercise. • Take the drug with meals.
pravastatin (Pravachol), simvastatin (Zocor), lovastatin (Mevacor), atorvastatin (Lipitor)	Increases rate of removal of LDL from plasma. Decreases synthesis of LDL.	Monitor liver function tests. For best effect, teach the patient: • Continue diet and exercise. • Report muscle tenderness. • Take as single dose in the evening. • Have routine eye examinations.
ezitimibe (Zetia)	Inhibits absorption of cholesterol through the small intestine.	Monitor liver function tests. Notify the health care provider if you have muscle pain or weakness. Take at the same time each day.
Miscellaneous and Emergency Agents		
atropine sulfate	Acts as a vagal blocker. Increases HR and CO in heart blocks and severe bradycardia. Used in symptomatic bradycardia and bradydysrhythmias.	Assess HR, rhythm, and BP.
calcium chloride	Necessary for cardiac rhythm, tone, and contraction. Increases muscle tone and force of contraction. Used in cardiac resuscitation and in cardiac irregularities associated with hyperkalemia.	Monitor ECG, BP, and arterial blood gases (ABGs). Avoid extravasation; causes necrosis. Alkalosis decreases the absorption of calcium. Acidosis increases the absorption of calcium.
dobutamine (Dobutrex)	Acts as beta-adrenergic agonist and inotrope. Increases CO with less increase in HR and BP than other catecholamines. Used in CHF and after cardiac surgery to increase myocardial contractility, stroke volume, and CO.	Continuous monitoring of ECG, cardiac parameters, and urinary output; titrate to HR and BP. Urinary output should increase with improved CO and renal function. Often used with nitroprusside or dopamine for additive effects. Causes less increase in HR, PVR, and dysrhythmias than dopamine.
dopamine hydrochloride (Intropin)	Acts as a neurotransmitter (a precursor to norepinephrine). Increases CO and BP. Improves renal blood flow and urine output with lower doses. Used for hemodynamic support in shock.	Avoid extravasation; causes necrosis. Monitor vital signs, ECG, urine output, and extremity color. Titrate to target BP; use an infusion pump. Peripheral vasoconstriction is noted with cold upper and lower extremities.
epinephrine hydrochloride (Adrenalin chloride)	Acts as a catecholamine. Strengthens myocardial contraction; increases BP, HR, and CO. Dilates bronchial tree. Used in anaphylactic shock and to restore cardiac rhythm in cardiac arrest.	Monitor vital signs and ECG continuously. Avoid extravasation; causes sloughing. Titrate to cardiac response. *Caution:* Drug is available in several concentrations, be sure to check for the prescribed solution. May be administered by endotracheal tube because drug is rapidly absorbed from the lungs.

Continued

Table 33.9 Selected Medications for Cardiovascular Disorders—cont'd

DRUG	USE AND ACTION		SELECTED NURSING INTERVENTIONS
sodium nitroprusside (Nipride)	Acts as a vasodilator. Decreases preload and afterload. Used in hypertensive crises.		Nipride is light-sensitive and should be protected from light. The drug must be diluted and infused with a pump. Titrate to maintain CO. Continuously monitor BP. Discard the solution 4 hours after preparation. Monitor for signs of cyanide toxicity (bradycardia, confusion, convulsions).
norepinephrine (Levophed)	Acts as a catecholamine (vasoconstrictor and cardiac stimulant). Produces increased BP, myocardial O_2, and coronary artery blood flow. Used in acute hypotensive states, MI, and cardiac arrest.		The drug must be diluted and administered as a continuous infusion via pump. Continuously monitor and titrate the drug to the desired BP. Monitor peripheral blood flow. Avoid extravasation.
sodium bicarbonate	Acts as a systemic alkalinizer. Used to correct metabolic acidosis in cardiac arrest.		Do not infuse the drug with calcium. Monitor ABGs. Avoid extravasation; causes severe tissue damage.
milrinone (Primacor)	Acts as an inotropic agent. Increases myocardial contractility and CO. Vasodilation decreases preload and afterload. Used to treat HF that does not respond to usual therapy.		Monitor vital signs, intake and output, and daily weight during therapy. Monitor ECG continuously.
Anticoagulant Agents: Most Effective Against Venous Thrombosis			
unfractionated heparin	Interferes with blood clotting; prevents formation of new clots; does not affect existing clots. Rapid effect. Used to treat pulmonary embolism, evolving stroke, and massive DVT. Prevents clotting during open heart surgery and renal dialysis. May be used *with* a thrombolytic agent for AMI. Low-dose heparin may be used to prevent postoperative venous thrombosis.	Thrombocytopenia (reduced platelets and increased clotting), hemorrhage, nausea and vomiting, and local irritation at injection site. Allergic response: chills, fever, and hives. Osteoporosis with long-term, high-dose use.	Regular blood testing must be done to monitor effect on clotting. Check aPTT before each dose (not necessary with low-dose therapy). Goal is aPTT 1.5–2.0 times normal (60–80 seconds). Monitor the patient for bleeding. Monitor platelet counts. Avoid trauma. Heparin should be given via IV or deep SC route. Draw up with 20- to 22-gauge needle, but use a 25-gauge needle for an SC injection. After an SC injection, apply pressure 1–2 minutes; do not massage. Rotate injection sites. Move heparin locks every 2–3 days. Protamine sulfate should be available as an antidote.
LMWH: enoxaparin (Lovenox), dalteparin (Fragmin), tinzaparin (Innohep)	Prevents formation of fibrin and thrombin. First-line therapy to prevent and treat thromboembolism. Approved to prevent DVT after some surgeries (e.g., hip or knee replacement), to treat DVT, and to prevent complications of specific cardiac conditions. Used off-label to prevent DVT after general surgery and in patients with multiple trauma or acute spinal injury.	Bleeding, thrombocytopenia, anemia, edema, nausea, fever, confusion, cardiac toxicity, and bruising. Severe neurologic injury in patients having spinal puncture.	Remember that this drug is given deep SC only! Do not aspirate. Rotate sites. Leave a bubble in the syringe when administering the drug. Administer the drug at the same time each day. Do not give the drug IM. Teach the patient to report any bleeding, to use a soft toothbrush and electric razor, and to not take aspirin. Monitoring of aPTT is not necessary. Overdose is treated with protamine sulfate.
warfarin sodium (Coumadin)	Interferes with blood clotting; may prevent extension of existing clots and formation of new clots. Can be used long term to prevent thrombosis in patients with prosthetic heart valves and atrial fibrillation.	Bruising, hemorrhage, nausea, and anorexia. Long-term use may weaken bones.	May be required to report PT and INR to physician before each dose. Dose may be individualized based on PT and INR. Monitor the patient for bleeding. Teach the patient not to take aspirin with warfarin.

Table 33.9 Selected Medications for Cardiovascular Disorders—cont'd

DRUG	USE AND ACTION		SELECTED NURSING INTERVENTIONS
Direct thrombin inhibitor: dabigatran etexilate (Pradaxa, Pradax)	Inhibits thrombin. Used to prevent stroke with atrial fibrillation and, in Canada, to prevent VTE after knee or hip replacement surgery.	Safer than warfarin but can still cause serious bleeding and GI disturbances (nausea and vomiting, abdominal pain, GERD, gastritis, ulcer). No specific antidote exists.	Take with food to reduce GI distress. Swallow capsules intact. Drug is unstable when exposed to moisture, so keep in original container. Use within 60 days of opening.
Direct factor Xa inhibitor: rivaroxaban (Xarelto)	Inhibits production of thrombin. Used to prevent DVT and pulmonary embolism after knee and hip surgery and to prevent stroke related to atrial fibrillation.	Bleeding. Hematoma after spinal or epidural puncture. No specific antidote exists.	Compared with warfarin, has rapid onset, fixed dosage, lower bleeding risk, few drug interactions, and no need to monitor INR.
Platelet Aggregation Inhibitors and Antiplatelet Agents: Primarily Used to Prevent Arterial Thrombosis			
Cyclooxygenase inhibitor: aspirin	Inhibits platelet aggregation, decreases inflammation and fever, and reduces pain.	GI irritation, tinnitus, pruritus, headache, and bleeding.	Assess the patient for bruising and bleeding. Give the drug with milk or food if GI irritation occurs.
cilostazol (Pletal)	Inhibits platelet aggregation. Pletal is used to treat intermittent claudication.	Cardiac dysrhythmias, headache, dizziness, and diarrhea.	Monitor the patient for bleeding and signs of HF. Blood work must be done during therapy. May take up to 12 weeks for effects.
Glycoprotein IIb/IIIa receptor antagonist: abciximab (ReoPro), eptifibatide (Integrilin), tirofiban (Aggrastat)	Intended for short-term use to prevent ischemia with acute coronary syndromes and to prevent reocclusion after certain angioplasty and atherectomy procedures. Usually given with low-dose heparin and aspirin.	Risk of major bleeding.	Immediately report GI, urinary, or puncture site bleeding. Infusion should be stopped if major bleeding occurs. Route of administration is IV.
Adenosine diphosphate receptor antagonist: clopidogrel (Plavix), ticlopidine (Ticlid)	Inhibits platelet aggregation. Plavix used to prevent blockage of coronary artery stents and to reduce thrombotic events in various cardiac conditions. Ticlid used to prevent thrombotic stroke.	Both can cause GI disturbances, rash, and TTP. A lower risk of bleeding exists with clopidogrel than with ticlopidine. Ticlopidine can also cause various blood dyscrasias.	Explain to the patient the importance of having regular blood tests and reporting any bleeding, bruising, or rash. Taking the drug with food decreases GI symptoms.
Thrombolytic Agents ("Clot Busters"): Used to Treat Existing Thrombi			
streptokinase (Streptase), urokinase (Abbokinase), alteplase (tissue plasminogen activator [t-PA]) (Activase), tenecteplase (TNKase), reteplase (Retavase)	Dissolves existing clots. Used to treat acute coronary thrombosis, DVT, and massive pulmonary embolism. Alteplase can be used for ischemic stroke. Urokinase is approved to clear IV catheters.	Minor to major bleeding; transient thrombocytopenia and alopecia, hypersensitivity and hypotension with streptokinase; and cardiac dysrhythmias with restored blood flow.	Monitor tests of clotting activity. Monitor ECG and vital signs. Assess the patient for bleeding, and protect from trauma. Educate the patient that chest pain or other symptoms of MI should be evaluated immediately. Early thrombolytic therapy (within 4–6 hours) may reduce myocardial damage. To reduce the risk of bleeding, handle the patient gently, and avoid IM and SC injections and invasive procedures.
Vasodilators			
Calcium Channel Blockers			
nifedipine (Procardia), amlodipine (Norvasc), diltiazem (Cardizem)	Dilates peripheral and coronary arteries. Used to treat hypertension, angina pectoris, and cardiac dysrhythmias.	Drowsiness, dizziness, cardiac dysrhythmias, CHF, MI, hypotension, and polyuria.	Monitor the patient's BP and pulse. Check for edema. Tell the patient to limit caffeine, avoid alcohol, and swallow extended-release tablets and capsules whole. Teach the patient how to manage postural hypotension.

Continued

Table 33.9 **Selected Medications for Cardiovascular Disorders—cont'd**

DRUG	USE AND ACTION		SELECTED NURSING INTERVENTIONS
Alpha-Adrenergic Blockers			
prazosin (Minipress), terazosin (Hytrin)	Decreases vascular resistance and lowers BP. Used to treat hypertension, Raynaud disease, urinary symptoms associated with BPH.	Dizziness, headache, drowsiness, nausea, orthostatic hypotension, edema, and palpitations.	Teach the patient to manage orthostatic hypotension, to take safety precautions if dizzy, and to monitor their weight daily. Take first dose or any increased dose at bedtime because of potential hypotension. Monitor BP and pulse.
Hemorheologic Agent			
pentoxifylline (Trental)	Decreases blood viscosity, fibrinogen, and platelet aggregation; increases flexibility of RBCs to allow passage through small vessels; used to treat intermittent claudication.	Dyspepsia, epistaxis, dizziness, nausea, vomiting, angina, tachycardia, cardiac dysrhythmias, leukopenia, headache, tremors, and rash.	Assess the patient's vital signs. Administer the drug with meals to decrease GI upset. Take safety precautions if the patient is dizzy. Tell the patient to report a rapid or irregular pulse. Explain how to manage epistaxis if it occurs. Monitor the patient's WBC count.

AMI, Acute myocardial infarction; *aPTT*, activated partial thromboplastin time; *AV*, atrioventricular; *BP*, blood pressure; *BPH*, benign prostatic hypertrophy; *CBC*, complete blood count; *CHF*, congestive heart failure; *CO*, cardiac output; *DVT*, deep vein thrombosis; *ECG*, electrocardiogram; *GERD*, gastroesophageal reflux disease; *GI*, gastrointestinal; *HDL*, high-density lipoprotein; *HF*, heart failure; *HR*, heart rate; *IM*, intramuscular; *INR*, international normalized ratio; *IV*, intravenous; *LDL*, low-density lipoprotein; *LMWH*, low-molecular-weight heparin; *MAP*, mean arterial pressure; *MI*, myocardial infarction; *NSAIDs*, nonsteroidal antiinflammatory drugs; *OTC*, over-the-counter; *PT*, prothrombin time; *PVC*, premature ventricular contraction; *PVR*, peripheral vascular resistance; *RBC*, red blood cell; *SC*, subcutaneous; *SVR*, systemic vascular resistance; *TTP*, thrombotic thrombocytopenic purpura; *VLDL*, very-low-density lipoprotein; *VTE*, venous thromboembolism; *WBC*, white blood cell.

valsartan (Diovan), losartan (Cozaar), and telmisartan (Micardis).

Vasodilators

Vasodilators are used to relax the vascular smooth muscle, which reduces resistance in the vessels and results in increased blood flow. Commonly used vasodilators are calcium channel blockers and alpha-adrenergic inhibitors.

Diuretics

Diuretics are often prescribed for cardiovascular conditions. Many patients with heart problems, hypertension, and PVD have fluid retention that is treated with diuretic drugs. The most frequently used diuretics are loop diuretics, such as furosemide (Lasix), thiazide diuretics, such as hydrochlorothiazide (Microzide), and potassium-sparing diuretics, such as spironolactone (Aldactone). Information about these and other diuretics is presented in Chapter 41, Table 41.3.

Anticoagulants

Anticoagulant therapy is used to prolong the clotting time, hinder the extension of a thrombus, and inhibit the formation of a thrombus during the postoperative period. The primary anticoagulant medications used are heparin, low-molecular-weight heparin (LMWH), and warfarin sodium (Coumadin) derivatives. A newer group of oral anticoagulants known as direct oral anticoagulants (DOACs) are used to prevent blood clots as well as treat existing blood clots. Examples include dabigatran (Pradaxa), rivaroxaban (Xarelto), apixaban (Eliquis), and edoxaban (Savayasa).

Heparin is given intravenously for immediate response and subcutaneously for maintenance or prophylaxis. LMWH is given only subcutaneously and warfarin is given orally. The clinical indications for anticoagulant treatment are venous thrombosis, pulmonary embolism, and risk for embolism.

When anticoagulant therapy is used, regular coagulation tests are done to assess the effectiveness of the treatment regimen. The effective range for the activated partial thromboplastin time (aPTT) during heparin treatment is 1.5 to 2.5 times the control. Warfarin dosage is based on the patient's prothrombin time (PT) and international normalized ratio (INR). The target PT and INR depend on the condition being treated. LMWH has advantages over heparin because a fixed dose can be administered, laboratory monitoring is not necessary, and one or two doses daily are sufficient. Direct oral anticoagulants do not require frequent monitoring of laboratory results or frequent visits to the health care provider. However, these medications are not recommended for patients with heart valve replacements, and patients on these medications still need to be monitored closely for signs of bleeding.

Pharmacology Capsule

Heparin dose is adjusted based on the patient's activated partial thromboplastin time (aPTT). Warfarin dose is adjusted based on the patient's prothrombin time (PT) and international normalized ratio (INR).

The fundamental complication of anticoagulant therapy is spontaneous bleeding that can occur anywhere in the body and may be evident in the urine, stool, emesis, or integument. Because of the risk of bleeding, the antidotes for each type of anticoagulant should be accessible. The antidote for heparin and LMWH is protamine sulfate; for warfarin sodium, it is vitamin K. Medications such as some antibiotics, mineral oil, nonsteroidal antiinflammatory drugs (NSAIDs), aspirin, and tolbutamide can intensify the anticoagulant effects of warfarin sodium. Some drugs that decrease the effectiveness of warfarin are antacids, barbiturates, oral contraceptives, and adrenal corticosteroids.

All patients on anticoagulants must be monitored closely for any signs of bleeding. In addition, patients should be taught how to reduce the risk of bleeding (see the Patient Teaching box).

Pharmacology Capsule

Patients taking anticoagulant drugs must be monitored for bleeding.

Patient Teaching

Anticoagulant Therapy

- Anticoagulants help to prevent blood clots from forming. Take your medications exactly as prescribed.
- Anticoagulant drugs can interfere with normal blood clotting; notify your physician of excessive bruising, bleeding gums, or blood in stools or urine.
- Consult your physician before taking any additional medications, because some drugs affect the action of your anticoagulant.
- Keep appointments for regular blood tests to monitor the serum level of your drugs when taking heparin sodium or warfarin. Test results are used to ensure that your dosage is safe and effective.
- Wear a medical alert bracelet noting anticoagulant therapy.

Antiplatelet Agents

Antiplatelet therapy is often used after an MI to prevent additional MIs and strokes. The dose of aspirin as an antiplatelet agent in MI and stroke prevention continues to be studied extensively in various groups (e.g., women, men, older adults, diabetics). Aspirin should be used under the direction of a health care provider so that each patient's unique situation can be taken into consideration. Clopidogrel (Plavix) also exhibits antiplatelet effects and may be prescribed for patients who are unable to tolerate aspirin.

Glycoprotein (GP) IIb/IIIa inhibitors block the platelet receptor sites that bind with fibrinogen and lead to platelet aggregation. GP IIb/IIIa inhibitors, such as abciximab (ReoPro) and eptifibatide (Integrilin) are used in combination with heparin and aspirin as part of the medical treatment for unstable angina and MI. They are also being used after MI in conjunction with fibrinolytic therapy, percutaneous coronary interventions (PCIs), or both. Pentoxifylline is used to treat PVD by improving the passage of RBCs through small vessels.

In addition to drugs that prevent clot formation, patients may also be taking medications such as hypoglycemic agents for diabetes and antihypertensives for HBP because those conditions contribute to the development of heart conditions and PVD.

Fibrinolytic Agents

Whereas anticoagulants and antiplatelet agents prevent the continued formation of clots, the fibrinolytic agents (also called *thrombolytic agents*) act to destroy clots that have already formed. These medications are often referred to as *clot busters.* Examples of thrombolytic medications are streptokinase (Streptase), urokinase (Abbokinase), alteplase (tissue plasminogen activator [t-PA]) (Activase), reteplase (Retavase), and tenecteplase (TNKase). Thrombolytic therapy is used to treat acute myocardial infarction (AMI), pulmonary embolism, DVT, and arterial thrombosis or embolism. They are best used as soon as evidence of clot formation is seen. They are administered intravenously when certain criteria have been met. Administration is continued until evidence of reperfusion is noted or until the maximum dose has been given. Uncontrolled bleeding can result from thrombolytics; thus, the patient must be monitored continuously during the treatment regimen.

Pharmacology Capsule

Anticoagulants prevent the formation of blood clots; thrombolytics dissolve existing blood clots.

Lipid-Lowering Agents

Lipid-lowering drugs are frequently part of the overall treatment plan, along with diet and exercise, for many patients with cardiovascular disease. The goal of therapy is for the patient to have decreased serum triglyceride and LDL levels and an improved HDL level. Patients taking these medications need to be encouraged to adhere to diet restrictions, exercise, and quitting smoking (see the Complementary and Alternative Therapies box). Serial laboratory tests (lipid profile and liver function) are closely monitored.

Complementary and Alternative Therapies

Many herbal remedies interact with conventional drugs. Feverfew, garlic, ginger root, and ginkgo enhance the effects of antiplatelet drugs. St. John's wort can decrease the effectiveness of warfarin. Caution patients against using herbal remedies while on prescribed anticoagulants.

Pharmacology Capsule

Monitor patients for hypotension when taking vasodilators. Teach them how to manage orthostatic hypotension.

COMMON THERAPEUTIC MEASURES FOR CARDIAC CONDITIONS

Diet Therapy

Reduction of body weight lessens the workload on the heart. A low-fat, high-fiber diet is usually recommended for patients with cardiac disorders. Patients are encouraged to eat a well-balanced diet that includes an emphasis on fruits, vegetables, grains, and proteins low in fat (fish, legumes, poultry, and lean meats). Cholesterol intake should be limited to 200 mg/day for individuals with heart disease or at high risk for heart disease. Saturated fats should be limited to no more than 5% to 6% of total caloric intake. An exercise program may help the patient to achieve optimal weight.

Sodium. If fluid retention accompanies the cardiac problem, the health care provider may order a sodium restriction diet containing less than 1500 mg/day. More severe restrictions of sodium intake are difficult to achieve, and patients find it difficult to comply with the dietary regimen. Salt substitutes are available.

Potassium. Patients taking potassium-wasting diuretics (e.g., furosemide, hydrochlorothiazide) need to include adequate potassium in the diet to counteract the depletion. Patients taking large doses of potassium-wasting diuretics need to have potassium supplements prescribed.

Pharmacology Capsule

Potassium-wasting diuretics such as furosemide and hydrochlorothiazide may cause hypokalemia, which can lead to dangerous dysrhythmias.

Priority Care for Chest Pain

Chest pain is often a presenting sign of CHD. Nitroglycerin is used to produce vasodilation. The vasodilation often decreases the pain. If the pain does not decrease, then IV nitroglycerin is used, and morphine may be administered. Morphine relieves pain, reduces anxiety, and can produce vasodilation in the coronary arteries, which can also decrease chest pain.

Oxygen Therapy

The myocardium needs an adequate blood supply to function properly. Any patient complaining of chest pain unrelieved by nitroglycerin should have supplemental O_2 administered. A nasal cannula or facemask should be applied and set to deliver the prescribed liter flow; the patient's response to this therapy should be monitored.

Cardiopulmonary Resuscitation

CPR is the restoration of heart and lung function after cardiac arrest. The procedure is used in basic cardiac life support and advanced cardiac life support. The reader is referred to materials prepared by the American Heart Association for current, in-depth coverage of the procedure. Advanced cardiac life support (ACLS) incorporates CPR with defibrillation, advanced airway management, and cardiac dysrhythmia care. The ability to perform ACLS requires additional training and certification by the American Heart Association.

Defibrillation. Defibrillation is the delivery of an electrical shock to the heart to restore normal cardiac conduction and contraction in the patient experiencing ventricular fibrillation or pulseless ventricular tachycardia. Defibrillation needs to be used as soon as possible when one of these abnormal rhythms is detected. There are standard defibrillators (usually biphasic) available in acute care facilities and portable, automated defibrillators known as *automated external defibrillators (AEDs)* available in most locations where people gather (airports, malls, schools, etc.). The use of a standard defibrillator is taught in ACLS, and the use of an AED is part of the CPR and ACLS courses.

Cardioversion. Cardioversion is the delivery of a synchronized shock to terminate atrial or ventricular tachydysrhythmias (rapid abnormal heart rhythms). Cardioversion may be done as an emergency or elective procedure. The shock is synchronized with the R wave of the QRS complex on the ECG to avoid shocking during the vulnerable period of the T wave. A shock delivered during ventricular relaxation can initiate ventricular fibrillation.

If the patient is receiving digoxin, the drug is withheld for 24 hours before the procedure. Emergency drugs are made available, and the patient has a patent IV line in place before the procedure. Explain the procedure and obtain informed consent. A short-acting sedative is usually given. The cardioverter is set to the synchronized mode, and two electrodes are placed on the chest. One electrode is placed to the right of the sternum just below the clavicle, and the other is placed at the apex of the heart. The initial impulse varies from 50 to 100 J, depending on the type of dysrhythmia. If the initial impulse does not convert the dysrhythmia to normal sinus rhythm, the impulse energy is increased and the procedure is repeated.

After cardioversion, the patient usually recovers very quickly from the sedation and does not remember the event. Inspect the skin under the electrodes for irritation, and monitor the patient's heart rate and rhythm, vital signs, and neurologic status. Transient dysrhythmias and a drop in BP are common. Be especially alert for atrial fibrillation, which can contribute to the formation of atrial wall thrombus and emboli.

Automatic implantable cardioverter defibrillator. The AICD is used to treat patients who have survived life-threatening recurrent ventricular tachycardia or fibrillation or who are at high risk for development of either of these. The device senses heart rate, identifies rhythm changes, and treats ventricular dysrhythmias. The AICD generator is implanted in the subcutaneous tissue over the pectoral muscle. The lead system is placed via a subclavian vein into the endocardium. The cardioverter recognizes ventricular fibrillation and ventricular tachycardia and uses the shocks to convert the dysrhythmia to normal sinus rhythm. When the AICD senses these lethal dysrhythmias, it delivers a shock of up to 25 J to defibrillate. If the heart rhythm does not return to normal, the device can continue to deliver shocks. The patient is instructed to sit or lie down when experiencing a shock and to keep a record of the number of shocks delivered. Patients report that the shocks feel like a blow to the chest. In addition to defibrillation, AICDs can also function as antitachycardia and antibradycardia pacemakers.

Complications. Complications associated with the AICD are inappropriate shocks, broken or displaced leads, and failure to deliver shocks as a result of battery failure or failure to recognize a dysrhythmia.

NURSING CARE OF THE PATIENT WITH AN AUTOMATIC IMPLANTABLE CARDIOVERTER DEFIBRILLATOR

Postinsertion care is similar to that for pacemaker insertion. In addition to postprocedure care, nurses can promote psychosocial adaptation in patients with AICDs. The patient may be concerned with body image change or develop a fear of shocks. Addressing anxiety about being shocked is important. Some patients become very dependent on the device. People who touch the patient during a shock will feel a tingling sensation, which is not harmful. An established support group for the patient and family is very helpful. The family must be instructed in CPR. An identification bracelet and a card with instructions about the AICD setting are carried at all times. Patients and families should be instructed about what to do if the AICD fires. For example, the patient should sit or lie down if the device fires and if the device shocks more than one time or the patient is not feeling well. Call emergency medical services (EMSs). Advise patients to avoid strong magnetic fields (e.g., metal detectors, power plants, MRI). The device should be checked for correct function at appropriate intervals determined by the health care provider.

Pacemakers

A pacemaker is a device used to restore regular rhythm and to improve cardiac output and tissue perfusion. Pacemakers may be temporary or permanent. Methods for temporary pacing are transcutaneous, transvenous, or epicardial. Transcutaneous pacemakers deliver impulses through the skin from externally placed electrode pads. A transvenous pacemaker has a pacing electrode that is threaded through a vein into the right side of the heart. Epicardial pacing wires are placed into the epicardial wall of the heart during cardiac surgery, and the wires are brought through the chest wall. Temporary pacemakers all require an external pulse generator to provide the electrical energy needed to stimulate depolarization. A permanent pacemaker is a small device that is surgically placed subcutaneously in the wall of the chest, with the electrical leads placed into the heart through a vein. Impulses are conducted from the power source (external pulse generator or implanted pacemaker) to the heart to stimulate contraction of the myocardium.

Pacemakers can be used to stimulate the atrium or ventricle (called *single-chamber pacing*), or they can be used to stimulate both chambers (called *dual-chamber pacing*). Dual-chamber pacing produces conduction and contraction that is near normal. Pacemakers have multiple settings related to pacing and sensing.

Temporary pacemakers. Temporary pacemakers can be used electively or for emergency situations. Elective uses include gaining control of very rapid supraventricular tachycardic rhythms, assessing the need for permanent pacing in patients with bradycardias, and after cardiac surgery.

Permanent pacemakers. Permanent pacemakers are indicated in a number of patient situations in which conduction defects or dysrhythmias compromise the normal function of the heart. Several clinical conditions indicate the need for permanent pacing. A few of these conditions are heart blocks, sinus node dysfunction, and symptomatic tachycardia. A permanent implantable pacemaker is inserted under local anesthesia. The batteries, usually lithium, have an 8- to 10-year expected life. Permanent pacemakers are inserted in the operating room, catheterization laboratory, or special procedures area. The pacing lead(s) are positioned (through the subclavian or cephalic vein) in the RA, RV, LV, or a combination of these (depending on the patient's problem). The generator is placed in a subcutaneous pocket, usually under the clavicle or in the abdomen.

Nursing Care of the Patient With a Pacemaker

Patients with inserted pacemakers recover on a telemetry unit. Monitor the patient for proper pacemaker functioning by observing for the pacemaker "spike." The pacemaker spike is a mark observed on the ECG tracing that represents the impulse generated by the pacemaker. Assess vital signs, and inspect the incision frequently for bleeding. Once stable, most patients may be up and active but should limit movement of the arm and shoulder on the implanted side. The health care provider may order immobilization of the arm. Limited arm and shoulder movement reduces the risk of lead dislodgement. Prophylactic antibiotics may be administered before and after insertion of a pacemaker. Monitor the patient for elevated temperature, signs of infection at the site, and an elevated WBC count.

After insertion of a temporary pacemaker, microshock precautions should be followed. Monitor the patient's ECG monitor and transport the patient with a portable cardiac monitor and a nurse in attendance. Assess the pacemaker for misfiring, and plan a gradual increase in activities.

Three major problems can occur with pacing: (1) failure to pace, (2) failure to capture, and (3) failure to sense. Failure to pace means that a pacemaker does not initiate an electrical stimulus when it is supposed to fire. Frequently caused by battery failure or lead wire displacement, it is recognized by the lack of a pacer spike on the ECG tracing. Failure to capture means that electrical stimulus from the pacemaker is not followed by electrical activity in the patient's heart. Failure to capture is often caused by dislodgement of the lead or the pacemaker output setting set too low and is recognized by noting the presence of a pacer spike without ECG activity after the spike. Failure to sense means that the pacemaker does not sense the patient's cardiac rhythm and initiates an electrical impulse when it is not needed. Failure to sense is most often caused by displacement of the electrode and can be recognized by pacer spikes that fall too close to the patient's rhythm.

When a permanent pacemaker has been inserted, teach the patient how to count the pulse for 1 full minute daily and keep a record to share with the health care provider. Explain wound care and the healing process, and advise the patient to notify the physician of symptoms of decreased cardiac output: dyspnea, dizziness, syncope, weakness, fatigue, and chest pain. In addition, instruct the patient to carry an identification card describing the type of pacemaker implanted.

THERAPEUTIC MEASURES FOR PERIPHERAL VASCULAR DISEASE

The primary goals for the patient with PVD are to increase the arterial blood supply to the extremities, reduce venous congestion, dilate blood vessels to increase arterial blood flow, prevent vascular compression, provide relief from pain, attain or maintain tissue integrity, and encourage adherence to the treatment plan.

Exercise programs, stress management, pain management, smoking cessation, elastic stockings, intermittent pneumatic compression units, body positioning, drug therapy, surgical interventions, and patient education are used in the management of the disease process.

Exercise

The simple act of walking stimulates the movement of blood from the dependent areas of the extremities toward the heart. Walking causes the muscles of the lower extremities to contract, pushing venous blood upward toward the heart and promoting the development of collateral circulation. For patients with vascular disease, the physician must prescribe an exercise program. Patients who have leg ulcers, gangrene, or acute thrombotic occlusion may be restricted to bed rest until the condition improves.

A specific type of exercise program that is effective in the management of PVD is the use of Buerger-Allen exercises or active postural exercises (Fig. 33.21) (see the Patient Teaching box).

Patient Teaching

Buerger-Allen Exercises

These exercises allow gravity to fill and empty the blood vessels.

- Lie flat on your back and raise your legs above the level of your heart for 2 minutes or until they become very pale.
- Lower the legs to a dependent position, and flex and extend your feet for 3 minutes or until color returns to your legs.
- Keep your legs flat for 5 minutes.
- Go through the entire process 6 times in each session if you can tolerate it. Three to four sessions a day provide the best results.
- Stop the exercises immediately if you have pain or severe skin color changes.

Stress Management

Emotional stress causes peripheral vasoconstriction, which is detrimental to a patient whose circulation is already compromised. Resistance to blood flow is increased, which reduces blood flow to the tissues. Emotional stress cannot be avoided entirely but can be reduced with a stress management plan, which may include lifestyle changes, massage, relaxation, or other stress-reducing activities.

Pain Management

The patient with PVD often limits ambulation because of pain. However, immobility tends to worsen circulatory problems. Thus pain management is an important aspect of care. Pain can be managed by promoting circulation to the affected area, by administering prescribed analgesics, or both. When intermittent claudication occurs, the patient should stop the exercise. Rest decreases circulatory demands and alleviates the pain. Once the pain is relieved, the activity may be resumed. Advise the patient to avoid constrictive garments such as girdles, garters, belts, and tight pantyhose that can cause pain by obstructing blood flow.

Smoking Cessation

Smoking cessation is critical to effective management of PVD because smoking causes vasoconstriction (constriction of the blood vessels). Vasoconstriction can be documented for up to 1 hour after a cigarette has been smoked. In addition, the nicotine in tobacco causes

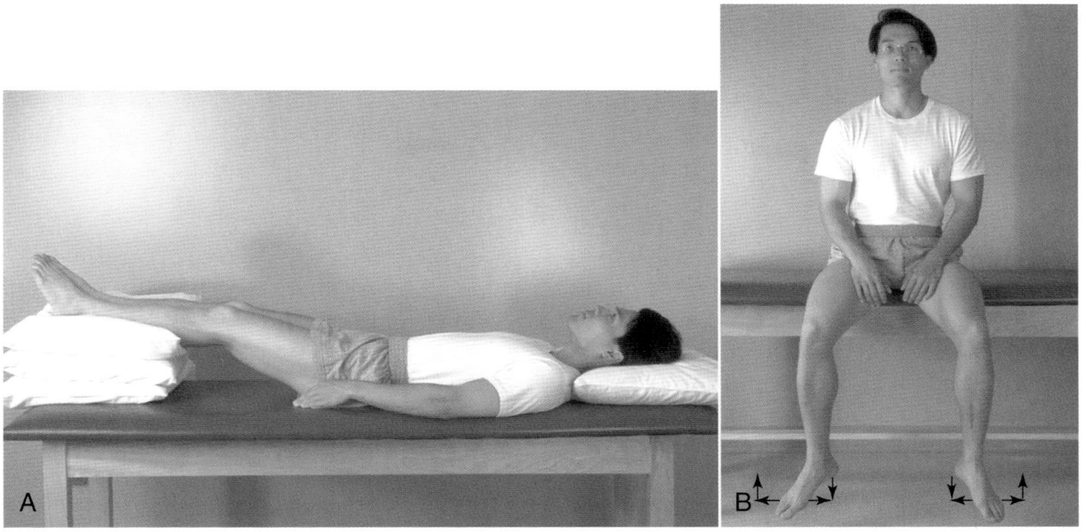

Fig. 33.21 Buerger-Allen exercises for peripheral vascular disease. (A) Elevate and support the legs at a 45- to 90-degree angle for 2 to 3 minutes, or until the skin blanches. (B) Sit with feet in a dependent position so that the skin turns red. Support the legs in this position for 5 to 10 minutes, then flex, extend, pronate, and supinate each foot three times. Finally, lie flat in a supine position for 10 minutes. (From Monahan FD, Drake DT, Neighbors M, editors: *Medical-surgical nursing: foundations for clinical practice*, ed 2, Philadelphia, 1998, Saunders.)

vasospasms, which drastically restrict the peripheral circulation. Measures to help the patient include encouragement; reinforcement; teaching about the nature of tobacco addiction, the harm of smoking, and the benefits of stopping; self-help materials or "Quit Kits" that are available from various agencies; and pharmacotherapy. Nicotine (patches, spray, gum, inhalers), varenicline (Chantix), and bupropion (Zyban) enhance the chances of success. Even though the best smoking cessation programs have about a 25% to 30% success rate, that rate is significant when one realizes that 45 million Americans smoke cigarettes, and that smoking is responsible for about 430,700 preventable deaths in the United States annually.

Pharmacology Capsule

Drugs that help some people who are trying to quit smoking are nicotine, varenicline, and bupropion.

Elastic Stockings

Another therapy that is useful in the management of PVD is the use of elastic stockings or antiembolism hose. These stockings provide sustained, evenly distributed pressure over the entire surface of the calves and thighs. The correct placement of elastic stockings compresses superficial veins, resulting in improved blood flow to the deeper veins. It is important to take care when applying these stockings because they can become tourniquets if applied incorrectly. The proper size of elastic stockings must be determined for each patient by using the instruction sheet provided by the manufacturer. Elastic stockings are best applied in the morning before rising from bed, because swelling is usually at its lowest level at this time of the day. With the stocking inside out, begin by pulling the stocking onto the foot with firm, even support (Fig. 33.22). Once the elastic stocking is positioned over the heel, pull from the sides so that it distributes evenly over the entire length of the leg. The stockings should be smooth when the application process is completed. If the top is allowed to roll or turn down, circulatory stasis occurs. The stockings should be removed for 10 to 20 minutes twice a day, during which time, it is best for the patient to be resting in bed or with the extremities in a nondependent position. When the elastic stockings are removed, it is also important to inspect the skin for any signs of irritation, pressure, or tenderness, which could reflect developing complications. Document the inspection and findings.

Intermittent Pneumatic Compression

Intermittent pneumatic compression or a pulsatile antiembolism system may be used for patients who are confined to bed after surgery or a traumatic injury. The primary function of these devices is to prevent DVT. With intermittent pneumatic compression, elastic stockings are applied that are sequentially inflated from the ankles, calves, and thighs, and then deflated. This expansion and contraction mimics the muscle pumping of the lower extremities, prevents venous pooling, and stimulates the circulation.

Positioning

Body positions play an important part in the management of PVD. Frequently, patients are restricted to bed during the acute phases of the disease process. It is important to use different positions to mobilize the blood volume that has become stagnant in the dependent areas. Lowering the extremities below the level of the heart enhances arterial blood supply. Elevating the

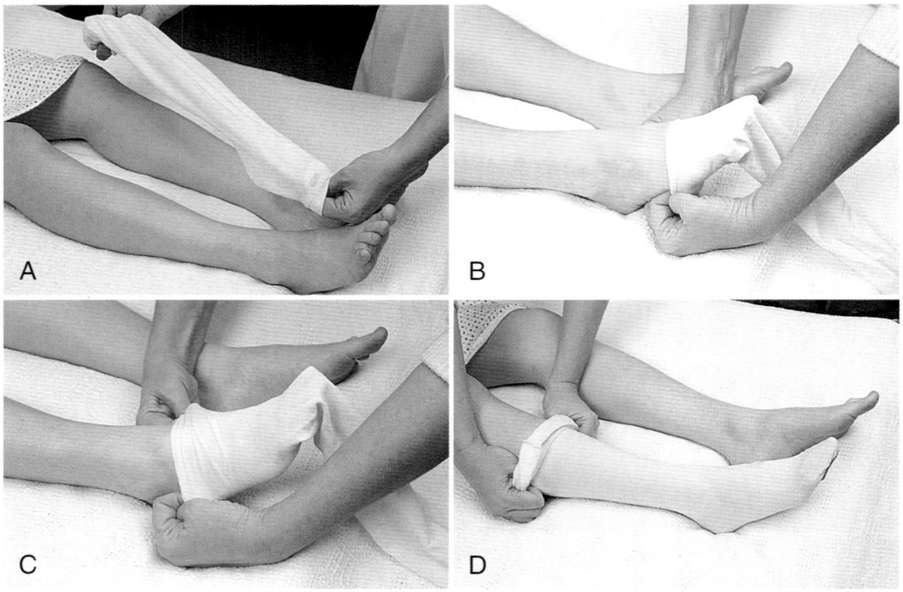

Fig. 33.22 Elastic stockings provide sustained, consistently distributed pressure over the entire surface of the calves and thighs to promote venous return. (From Elkin MK, Perry AG, & Potter PA: *Nursing interventions and clinical skills*, ed 4, St. Louis, 2007, Mosby.)

lower extremities above the level of the heart promotes venous return and reduces venous stasis. For patients who are not restricted to bed, prolonged standing puts strain on the venous system. Instruct the patient to sit down and elevate the extremity to a nondependent position whenever possible.

Thermotherapy

Thermotherapy (either warm or cold) can be used for its effects on the circulatory system. Heat, whether dry or moist, works as a vasodilator that promotes arterial flow to the peripheral tissues. Heat should be used cautiously, however, because patients with PVD may suffer burns because they have impaired sensation as a result of tissue ischemia. Blood vessels constrict in response to cold. Clothing can be used effectively to promote warmth and to prevent chilling and vasoconstriction.

Protection

Affected extremities must be protected from trauma because the healing process is usually impaired with PVD. To prevent injury to poorly perfused tissues, the patient must avoid scratching and vigorous rubbing. Caution the patient to wear properly fitting shoes and clean socks or hose, to keep fingernails and toenails trimmed and smooth, and not to walk about barefoot. Inform the physician of ingrown toenails, blisters, or skin injuries so that prompt treatment can be initiated.

Patient Teaching

Patient education is important in the management of PVD. The patient must understand the disease process and the prescribed therapies. The teaching plan should include cleanliness, warmth, safety, comfort measures, prevention of constricting blood flow, exercise, signs and symptoms that should be reported to the health care provider, drug therapy, and the importance of smoking cessation.

Dietary Interventions

The dietary interventions used with PVD are like those recommended for cardiovascular health. Atherosclerotic plaques create rough vessel walls and contribute to peripheral vascular complications. Low-fat diets reduce serum cholesterol levels, thereby reducing the risk of atherosclerotic plaque formation. A weight reduction diet may be prescribed if the patient is obese, because obesity causes a strain on the heart, increases venous congestion, and reduces peripheral circulation. Adequate vitamin B, vitamin C, and protein are needed to promote healing and improve tissue integrity. (See the Nutrition Considerations box.)

CARDIOVASCULAR SURGERY

Nursing care needs vary considerably depending on the type of surgical procedure. Care specific to particular conditions is discussed in Chapters 35 and 36. In addition, see Chapter 17 for thorough coverage of care of the surgical patient. This section addresses needs common to many patients having cardiovascular surgery.

The most common surgical procedures involving the heart are pacemaker or AICD insertion, heart surgery to repair or replace valves, and coronary artery bypass surgery. Coronary artery bypass surgery is described as a surgical treatment for MI under "Cardiac Disorders."

For some of the surgical procedures on the heart, the heart muscle must be at rest during the procedure. This requires placing the patient on a bypass machine to direct the blood away from the heart and lungs and to maintain appropriate O_2 and CO_2 levels. The heart's rhythm is interrupted by an electrolyte solution and may be restarted after the surgery by electrical stimulation.

During this type of surgery, the patient's core temperature is usually reduced to decrease the O_2 needs of the entire body, especially the brain.

Common vascular surgeries include embolectomy, percutaneous transluminal angioplasty (PTA), endarterectomy, sympathectomy, vein ligation and stripping, sclerotherapy, and laser or light therapy. These procedures are discussed more specifically in Chapter 36, Vascular Disorders.

PREOPERATIVE NURSING CARE OF THE CARDIOVASCULAR SURGERY PATIENT

The patient with severe cardiovascular disease may have activity restrictions to reduce the demands on the circulatory system until the surgical procedure is done.

Assessment

When a patient is facing cardiovascular surgery, the nurse must also assess the patient's fears and anxiety (see the Patient Teaching box). Patients are usually very concerned when surgery is recommended. It is important to determine what patients know about the surgery and what more they would like to know.

Patient Teaching

Cardiovascular Surgery, Preoperative

The specifics of the teaching plan depend on the exact procedure and agency procedures. General content of the teaching plan includes the following:

- Preoperative routines: nothing by mouth (NPO), monitoring, diagnostic tests, any special preparation.
- Postoperative care setting: the room and the equipment.
- Postoperative routines: how to turn, cough, deep breathe, and exercise the leg muscles; monitoring; procedures.
- Postoperative pain: amount of pain to expect; relief measures, such as splinting, positioning, medication.
- Communication: means of communication established before surgery (because many patients are intubated for 4 to 8 hours after more extensive cardiac surgery).

Patient Problems, Goals, and Outcome Criteria: Preoperative Cardiovascular Surgery

Patient Problems	Goals and Outcome Criteria
Stress related to perceived threat of death or unfamiliarity with setting and procedures	Reduced stress: patient states being less fearful, demonstrates relaxed manner
Anxiety related to threat to health status or uncertain outcome	Reduced anxiety: patient states being less anxious, calmer

Interventions

Stress and anxiety. Encourage the patient to identify feelings, and then explore the basis of those feelings. Do not assume that you know how the patient feels. Accept the patient's feelings and avoid trite reassurance (e.g., "Don't worry; everything will be fine."). Accurate information about what to expect helps to reduce fear of the unknown. Physical comfort measures, such as a massage or back rub may also be soothing. If the patient's anxiety level remains high, notify the health care provider.

Good patient teaching is essential to address fear and anxiety. The health care provider reviews necessary diagnostic tests, the surgical procedure itself, and what to expect after surgery. Nevertheless, the nurse must be able to clarify and further explain what the patient will experience. If the surgery is done on an emergency basis, little time is available for preoperative teaching. However, planned cardiovascular surgery allows time for the patient to accept the need for surgery and to explore why the procedure is necessary. Include the family in the preoperative teaching to decrease their anxiety, and allow them to participate in the patient's recovery. The patient teaching plan must be individualized for the type of surgical procedure.

Put On Your Thinking Cap!

A patient who has a low degree of health literacy is scheduled for cardiovascular surgery and requests more education about the surgery. What information should the nurse include and what strategies could be used to educate the patient?

◆ POSTOPERATIVE NURSING CARE OF THE CARDIOVASCULAR SURGERY PATIENT

Assessment

After surgery, be especially alert to changes in the patient's vital signs, breath sounds, urine output, mental alertness, and color. In the intensive care unit, monitor cardiac rhythm, ABGs, and hemodynamic pressures. It is also important to assess chest tube function and frequently inspect all dressings for type and amount of drainage. Examine the patient's surgical wound site and the insertion sites of tubes and cannulas for increasing redness, swelling, and purulent drainage. In addition, assess urine amount, appearance, and odor.

Patient Problems, Goals, and Outcome Criteria: Postoperative Cardiac Surgery

Patient Problems	Goals and Outcome Criteria
Inadequate pulmonary oxygenation related to mechanical ventilation, general anesthesia, pain, or restrictive surgical dressings	Adequate oxygenation: arterial blood gases (ABGs) within normal limits for the patient
Acute pain related to tissue trauma	Pain relief: patient states pain reduced or relieved, relaxed manner

Continued

Patient Problems, Goals, and Outcome Criteria: Postoperative Cardiac Surgery—cont'd

Patient Problems	Goals and Outcome Criteria
Decreased body temperature related to cooling during surgery	Normal body temperature: temperature of at least 36.7°C (98°F) orally
Decreased cardiac output related to fluid loss or decreased fluid intake	Normal cardiac output: fluid intake equal to output
Potential for infection related to altered skin integrity	Absence of infection: no fever; decreasing drainage, redness, and swelling of wound
Anxiety related to unfamiliar routines and stressful experience	Reduced anxiety: patient states anxiety is reduced

Interventions

Inadequate pulmonary oxygenation. Patients with open heart or bypass surgery may be unresponsive on arrival in the intensive care unit. Ventilatory assistance is of primary importance until the patient is awake and extubated. Reassess breath sounds and ABGs frequently, and connect chest tubes to water seal drainage. (See Chapter 25 for the care of chest tubes.) Reposition the patient often to promote removal of pulmonary secretions and improve respiratory excursion.

When the patient is extubated, use an O_2 mask or nasal cannula as ordered to provide supplemental O_2. Also assist the patient to cough and deep breathe frequently. A pillow or a blanket in a pillowcase can be used as an incisional splint during coughing. An incentive spirometer is usually ordered; monitor its use, and remind the patient to use it. Assist the patient with early ambulation, as ordered, to reduce the risk of pulmonary complications.

Pain. Effective pain relief makes it easier for the patient to turn, cough, and deep breathe. Assess the patient's pain: location, severity, aggravating factors, and relieving factors. Administer analgesics as ordered; IV morphine in small doses is prescribed most frequently. You may also use independent measures, including position changes, back rubs, relaxation techniques, and imagery. Assess the effectiveness of the interventions in managing pain, and provide for periods of rest and sleep after pain relief efforts.

Decreased body temperature. Warming blankets may be used to assist with rewarming. Monitor the patient's body temperature continuously until the patient is stable.

Inadequate cardiac output. While in the intensive care unit, the patient's cardiac pressures are monitored continuously until they stabilize. Prescribed medications are adjusted based on vital signs, hemodynamic pressures, and cardiac rhythms. Pacing wires are connected to a temporary pacemaker. It is important to monitor fluid and blood administration and assess urinary and other drainage outputs. Volume expanders (i.e., albumin) and vasoactive drugs may be necessary to maintain BP. Oral fluids are ordered shortly after extubation.

Potential for infection. The patient is at risk for incisional, respiratory tract, and urinary tract infections. In addition, the presence of multiple tubes and cannulas provides additional sites for potential nosocomial infection. To reduce the risk of infection, it is vital to practice good hand-washing technique and use aseptic technique when handling dressings and invasive equipment. Provide wound care as ordered (or per agency policy), and administer antibiotics as ordered. Before discharge, begin teaching the patient how to care for the surgical wounds. Emphasize signs or symptoms that should be reported to the physician (e.g., fever, increasing or purulent wound drainage, increasing redness or swelling, separation of wound margins).

Anxiety. Explain to the patient and family what is being done and how the patient is responding. Remember to talk to the patient and offer reassurance. When the patient is on a ventilator, use the previously established nonverbal means of communication. It is often necessary to repeat instructions because of the effects of pain, medications, and anxiety (see the Complementary and Alternative Therapies box). As the patient improves, explain the importance of follow-up care and rehabilitation.

Complementary and Alternative Therapies

For pain relief, many complementary therapies are used with analgesics. Examples are massage, relaxation techniques, and imagery.

Get Ready for the NCLEX® Examination!

Key Points

- The peripheral vascular system comprises arteries, capillaries, veins, and lymph vessels, each of which plays a critical role in the oxygenation and nourishment of body tissues.
- Risk factors for PVD include older age, heredity, smoking, obesity, physical inactivity, hypertension, and diabetes mellitus.
- Common age-related changes in the vascular system include arteriosclerosis (stiffening of blood vessel walls), decreased Hgb, slower heart rate, and decreased cardiac output.
- Six *P*s characteristic of PVD are (1) pain, (2) pulselessness, (3) poikilothermy, (4) pallor, (5) paresthesia, and (6) paralysis.
- Intermittent claudication is pain in any major muscle group that is precipitated by exercise and relieved by rest.
- Poikilothermy describes an area of the body that is cooler than the rest of the body because of local ischemia.
- Tests and procedures used to diagnose PVD include Doppler ultrasound, duplex ultrasonography, pressure measurement, exercise testing, and angiography.
- Common therapeutic measures used in the management of PVD are exercise programs, drug therapy, stress management training, pain management, smoking cessation, elastic stockings or intermittent pneumatic compression devices, positioning, thermotherapy, protection, and patient teaching.
- Common surgical interventions for PVD include PTA, stenting, endarterectomy, embolectomy, sclerotherapy, laser therapy, light therapy, and vein ligation and stripping.
- Blood flow may be improved with drug therapy using anticoagulants, thrombolytics, platelet aggregation inhibitors, and vasodilators. NSAIDs and other analgesics may be needed for pain and inflammation.
- Persons with vascular disorders usually are prescribed a low-fat diet, and a weight reduction program may be advised if appropriate.

Additional Learning Resources

SG Go to your Study Guide for additional learning activities to help you master this chapter content.

Go to your Evolve website (http://evolve.elsevier.com/Linton/medsurg) for the following learning resources and much more:

- Fluid & Electrolyte Tutorial
- Review Questions for the NCLEX® Examination

Clinical Judgment and Next-Generation NCLEX® Examination-Style Questions

1. **Which individuals are at greatest risk for severe complications of hypertension?**
   1. White American men
   2. White American women
   3. Black American men
   4. Black American women

   NCLEX Client Need: Physiological Integrity: Physiological Adaptation

2. **At which of the following levels does the exchange of O_2 and nutrients occur?**
   1. Arteriole
   2. Capillary
   3. Venule
   4. Lymphatic

   NCLEX Client Need: Physiological Integrity: Physiological Adaptation

3. **Nursing students in a gerontology course learn that the intima layer of blood vessels thicken and harden with age. The students recognize that such changes put the older adult at risk for which of the following?**
   1. Anemia
   2. Bradycardia
   3. Emboli
   4. Hypotension

   NCLEX Client Need: Physiological Integrity: Physiological Adaptation

4. **A patient complains of pain and cramping in the legs that occurs when walking and is relieved by rest. What term is used to describe this complaint? ________________**

   NCLEX Client Need: Physiological Integrity: Physiological Adaptation

5. **When inspecting a patient's legs, you press your thumb into an edematous area around each ankle. Each time you remove your thumb, a moderate indentation appears that soon subsides. Which of the following should you document?**
   1. 1+ edema noted
   2. Pitting edema, both ankles
   3. Mild edema, both ankles
   4. 2+ edema, both ankles

   NCLEX Client Need: Physiological Integrity: Physiological Adaptation

6. **Which of the following is an invasive diagnostic procedure used to assess the vascular system?**
   1. Ultrasound
   2. Plethysmography
   3. Angiography
   4. Exercise test

   NCLEX Client Need: Physiological Integrity: Reduction of Risk Potential

7. **Measures used to improve venous return in the patient with PVD include which of the following? (Select all that apply.)**
   1. Exercise
   2. Elastic stockings
   3. Thermotherapy
   4. Elevation of extremities
   5. Smoking cessation therapy

   NCLEX Client Need: Physiological Integrity: Reduction of Risk Potential

8. **Mr. J. has been on warfarin (Coumadin) to prevent a stroke related to atrial fibrillation. Mr. J.'s doctor is changing him from warfarin to dabigatran (Pradaxa). When Mr. J. asks the home health nurse why he should change medications, what should he be told? (Select all that apply.)**
   1. Dabigatran does not require regular blood testing.
   2. He will be able to take the same dose every day.
   3. Dabigatran is not affected by food or other drugs.
   4. Bleeding is less likely with dabigatran than with warfarin.
   5. An overdose of dabigatran can be readily reversed.

   NCLEX Client Need: Physiological Integrity: Pharmacological Therapies

9. **Which of the following is included in discharge teaching for the patient with peripheral arterial disease affecting both legs?**
   1. Elevate your feet when sitting
   2. Exercise is contraindicated
   3. Promptly report any injury to the feet or legs
   4. Take prescribed vasoconstrictors as ordered

   NCLEX Client Need: Physiological Integrity: Physiological Adaptation

10. **Which statement correctly describes one of the three factors that affect stroke volume?**
    1. Contractility is the ability of cardiac muscle fibers to shorten and produce a muscle contraction.
    2. Preload is the amount of blood remaining in the atria at the end of diastole.
    3. Cardiac output is the amount of blood ejected by the heart with each ventricular contraction.
    4. Afterload is the amount of blood remaining in the ventricles at the end of systole.

    NCLEX Client Need: Physiological Integrity: Physiological Adaptation

11. **The nurse hears a murmur when auscultating the heart sounds of an 80-year-old patient. The nurse recalls that age-related changes in the circulatory system that can cause heart murmurs include which of the following? (Select all that apply.)**
    1. Decreased elasticity of connective tissue in the heart muscle
    2. Arterial stiffening caused by changes in connective tissue and elastic fibers
    3. Heart valves that are stiff do not close properly
    4. Stretching and dilation of veins result in impaired venous return
    5. The aging heart responds more slowly to increased demands

    NCLEX Client Need: Physiological Integrity: Physiological Adaptation

12. **Before administering digoxin, the nurse counts a patient's apical heart rate and finds that it is 62 beats per minute. The patient's usual rate ranges from 65 to 75 beats per minute. Should the nurse administer the digoxin?**

    NCLEX Client Need: Physiological Integrity: Physiological Adaptation

13. **The licensed vocational nurse/licensed practical nurse (LVN/LPN) is administering medications to patients in long-term care. Three of the patients are taking various antidysrhythmic drugs. Which of the following is a potential adverse effect common to all antidysrhythmic drugs?**
    1. Fluid and electrolyte imbalance
    2. Drowsiness
    3. Diarrhea
    4. Additional dysrhythmias

    NCLEX Client Need: Physiological Integrity: Pharmacological Therapies

14. **When cardiac output falls, compensatory mechanisms include which of the following? (Select all that apply.)**
    1. Elimination of excess fluid by the kidneys
    2. Constriction of blood vessels in the extremities
    3. Stimulation of the parasympathetic nervous system
    4. Enlargement of the ventricular myocardium
    5. Increased heart rate

15. **Take Action Using Matrix Test Item**

    The nurse is preparing a teaching plan for a cardiac patient who lives at home. The plan should include which of the following dietary recommendations?
    Use an X for the health teaching below that is *Indicated* (appropriate or necessary), *Contraindicated* (could be harmful), or *Nonessential* (makes no difference or not necessary) before the patient's discharge at this time.

HEALTH TEACHING	INDICATED	CONTRAIN-DICATED	NONES-SENTIAL
"Restrict sodium intake to 1 g/day."			
"Avoid raw fruits and vegetables that are difficult to digest."			
"Use unsaturated fats, such as vegetable oil instead of butter."			
"Limit saturated fats by eating no more than 12 oz of meat per day."			
"Include foods that contain omega-3 fatty acids."			
"Avoid starchy vegetables."			
"Raw vegetables are more nutritious that cooked vegetables."			

Hypertension

34

http://evolve.elsevier.com/Linton/medsurg

Objectives

1. Define hypertension.
2. Explain the physiology of blood pressure regulation.
3. Discuss the risk factors, signs and symptoms, diagnosis, treatment, and complications of hypertension.
4. Identify the nursing considerations when administering selected antihypertensive drugs.
5. List the data to be collected during the nursing assessment of a person with known or suspected hypertension.
6. Describe the nursing interventions for the patient with hypertension.
7. Identify the patient problems, goals, and outcome criteria for the patient with hypertension.
8. Discuss new methodologies and trends for management of hypertension.

Key Terms

dyslipidemia (dĭs-lĭp-ĭ-DĒ-mē-ă)
epistaxis (ĕp-ĭ-STĂK-sĭs)
hypertension (hī-pĕr-TĔN-shŭn)
hypertrophy (hī-PĔR-trō-fē)
orthostatic hypotension (ŏr-thō-STĂ-tĭk hī-pō-TĔN-shŭn)
syncope (SĬN-kō-pē)

INTRODUCTION

Hypertension (HTN) or elevated blood pressure (BP) is the leading cause of death globally, accounting for 10.4 million deaths per year. The *International Society of Hypertension* (ISH) has created initiatives to reduce the global burden of elevated BP. New developments include redefining hypertension, initiating treatment with single pill combination therapy, advising out-of-office blood pressure measurement, and lower BP targets (Unger T, 2020). The ISH, upon extensive review of guidelines and standards of care, has developed worldwide practice guidelines for the management of hypertension.

DEFINITIONS

In the United States, the most widely used classification of blood pressure for adults aged 18 or over is from the 2003 *Seventh Report of the Joint National Committee on Prevention, Detection, Evaluation, and Treatment of High Blood Pressure (JNC 7)*, which defines normal blood pressure (BP) as systolic pressure of less than 120 mm Hg and diastolic pressure of less than 80 mm Hg. In 2017, the American College of Cardiology and the American Heart Association (ACC/AHA) updated these guidelines, recommending 130 mm Hg, but generally, the JNC 7 guidelines endure (Table 34.1).

Although still controversial, the current ISH global classification system is listed here:

- Optimal: systolic lower than 120 mm Hg and diastolic lower than 80 mm Hg
- Normal: Systolic 120 to 129 mm Hg and/or diastolic lower than 85 mm Hg
- High normal: Systolic 130 to 139 mm Hg and/or diastolic 85 to 89 mm Hg
- Grade 1: Systolic 140 to 159 mm Hg and/or diastolic 90 to 99 mm Hg
- Grade 2: Systolic 160 to 179 mm Hg or greater and/or diastolic 100 to 109 mm Hg
- Grade 3: Systolic 180 mm Hg or greater and/or diastolic 110 mm Hg or greater
- Isolated systolic: 140 mm Hg or greater and diastolic lower than 90 mm Hg

The Systolic Blood Pressure Intervention Trial (SPRINT) demonstrated a 25% decrease in cardiovascular events or death with targeting a systolic BP of less than 120 mm Hg versus 140 mm Hg in patients at increased cardiovascular risk. Future guidelines will likely incorporate the results of the SPRINT trial into target BP recommendations.

The *Eighth Report of the Joint National Committee on Prevention, Detection, Evaluation, and Treatment of High Blood Pressure (JNC 8)* summarizes key points for practice:

- Pharmacologic treatment should be initiated when BP is 150/90 mm Hg in adults 60 years and older, or 140/90 mm Hg in adults younger than 60 years.

Table 34.1 Guidelines for Diagnosis of Hypertension in Persons 18 Years of Age and Older[a]

CATEGORY	SYSTOLIC BLOOD PRESSURE (mm Hg)		DIASTOLIC BLOOD PRESSURE (mm Hg)
Normal[b]	<120	and	<80
Prehypertension	120–139	or	80–89
Hypertension[c]			
Stage 1	140–159	or	90–99
Stage 2	≥160	or	≥100

[a]Not taking antihypertensive drugs, and not acutely ill.
[b]Optimal blood pressure (BP) with respect to cardiovascular risk is below 120/80 mm Hg. However, unusually low readings should be evaluated for clinical significance.
[c]Based on the average of two or more readings taken at each of two or more visits after an initial screening.
From The Joint National Committee on Prevention, Detection, Evaluation, and Treatment of High Blood Pressure: *The seventh report of The Joint National Committee on Prevention, Detection, Evaluation, and Treatment of High Blood Pressure*, Bethesda, MD, 2003, Department of Health and Human Services, National Institutes of Health, National Heart, Lung, and Blood Institute.

- In patients with hypertension and diabetes, pharmacologic treatment should be initiated when BP is 140/90 mm Hg or higher, regardless of age.
- Initial antihypertensive treatment should include a thiazide diuretic, calcium channel blocker (CCB), angiotensive converting enzyme inhibitor (ACE), or angiotensin II receptor blocker (ARB) in the general non-Black population or a thiazide diuretic or a CCB in the general Black population.
- If the target BP is not reached in 1 month after initiating therapy, the dosage of the initial medication should be increased, or a second medication should be added.

Readings classified as *stage 1* and *stage 2* **hypertension** (HTN) are outlined in Table 34.1. If the systolic and diastolic pressures fall into different stages, the higher measurement is used to classify the stage of HTN. Complications and death increase directly with the stage of HTN.

In addition to staging, patients with HTN are classified as being in risk group A, B, or C. Individuals in risk group A have no major risk factors, no target organ damage, and no clinical cardiovascular disease. Individuals in risk group B have one or more risk factors, not including diabetes; no target organ damage; and no clinical cardiovascular disease. Individuals in risk group C have target organ damage and clinical cardiovascular disease, diabetes, or all of these conditions, with or without other risk factors.

Some people have only occasional elevations in BP and normal readings at other times. These findings are called *isolated pressure elevations.* Isolated systolic blood pressure (SBP) elevations of 160 mm Hg or more frequently occur in older adults. The elevations are usually caused by atherosclerosis (narrowing of arteries caused by plaques of fatty material on the inner walls).

ANATOMY AND PHYSIOLOGY OF BLOOD PRESSURE REGULATION

Two factors determine BP: cardiac output (CO) and peripheral vascular resistance (PVR):

$$BP = CO \times PVR$$

CO is the volume of blood pumped by the heart in a specific period of time (usually 1 minute).

PVR is the force in the blood vessels that the left ventricle (LV) must overcome to eject blood from the heart. Resistance to blood flow is determined primarily by the diameter of the blood vessels and blood viscosity (thickness). Increased PVR results from a narrowing of the arteries and arterioles or an increased fluid volume in the blood vessels that results from sodium and water retention. Increased PVR is the most prominent characteristic of HTN.

The diameter of blood vessels is regulated largely by the vasomotor center. The vasomotor center is located in the medulla of the brain. Sympathetic nervous system tracts from the medulla extend down the spinal cord to the thoracic and abdominal regions. Stimulation of the sympathetic nervous system causes release of the hormones norepinephrine and epinephrine. These hormones, called *catecholamines*, are vasoconstrictors, meaning that they cause the blood vessels to constrict, making their diameters smaller. By constricting blood vessels, norepinephrine increases PVR and raises BP. Epinephrine constricts blood vessels and increases the force of cardiac contraction, causing BP to rise.

Vasoconstriction decreases blood flow to the kidneys, which then release renin. Renin leads to the formation of angiotensin, another potent vasoconstrictor. Angiotensin stimulates the adrenal cortex to secrete aldosterone, a hormone that promotes sodium and water retention. This results in an increased blood volume. Vasoconstriction, cardiac stimulation, and retention of fluid all contribute to HTN. Fig. 34.1 illustrates how various factors raise BP.

TYPES OF HYPERTENSION

HTN is classified as *primary* (essential) or *secondary.* Primary HTN accounts for 90% to 95% of all cases of HTN. Even though the cause for primary HTN is unknown, several contributing factors, including increased sodium intake, greater than ideal body weight, diabetes mellitus, and excessive alcohol consumption, have been identified.

Secondary HTN is caused by underlying factors such as kidney disease, certain arterial conditions, some drugs, and occasionally pregnancy.

PRIMARY (ESSENTIAL) HYPERTENSION

Risk Factors

The most significant risk factors for primary (essential) HTN are **dyslipidemia** (abnormally elevated

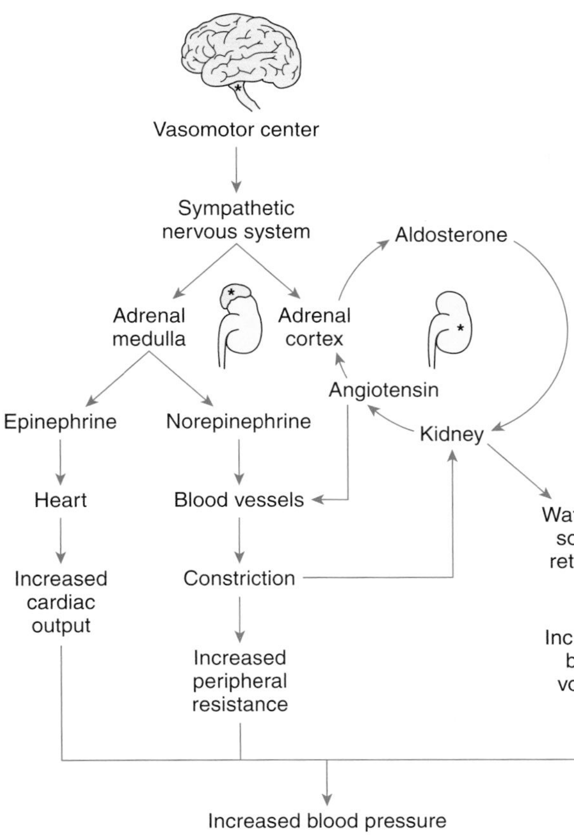

Fig. 34.1 Factors that increase blood pressure.

cholesterol or lipids in the blood), atherosclerosis, diabetes mellitus, tobacco use, age over 55 years for men or over 65 years for women, family history (i.e., father or brother diagnosed with heart disease before 55 years of age; mother or sister diagnosed with heart disease before 65 years of age), and sedentary lifestyle. Obesity, defined as weight 20% over ideal body weight, is also a risk factor. The additional weight and fat cause increases in the number of blood vessels, circulating blood volume, and cardiac workload. Atherosclerosis decreases the elasticity of the arteries and arterioles, causing increased PVR. The inhalation of nicotine in cigarettes or e-cigarettes constricts blood vessels and stimulates the release of epinephrine and norepinephrine. As mentioned, these hormones also constrict blood vessels and raise heart rate and BP. Lack of physical activity leads to pooling of blood in the extremities and increases the workload of the cardiovascular system.

Other risk factors include stress; overstimulation; and a family history of obesity, HTN, or dyslipidemia. Stress caused by such factors as a high-pressure job, financial worries, or family problems increases secretion of catecholamine (hormones that cause vasoconstriction). Stimulants that may contribute to or aggravate HTN include caffeine, nicotine, and amphetamines. Caffeine is found in tea, coffee, and chocolate. Nicotine is consumed by smoking or chewing tobacco products.

Clinical Manifestations

Many people with HTN have no symptoms. Symptoms that may accompany HTN include occipital headaches that are more severe on arising, lightheadedness, and **epistaxis** (nosebleed). If HTN has damaged blood vessels in the heart, kidneys, eyes, or brain, the patient may have symptoms of impaired function of those organs.

Complications

The most serious consequences of HTN are heart attack, heart failure (HF), stroke, kidney disease, and blindness. Complications occur because the long-term effect of prolonged HTN is replacement of elastic arteriolar tissue with stiffer, fibrous collagen tissue. Thickening of the arteriolar wall decreases its ability to distend, resulting in increased PVR and decreased blood flow to various organs. The organs that are most sensitive to these changes are the heart, kidneys, brain, and eyes. Patients with HTN must be assessed frequently for damage to these sensitive ("target") organs (Fig. 34.2).

Heart. Coronary heart disease (CHD) develops in patients with HTN 2 to 3 times more frequently than in people with normal BP. CHD reduces blood supply to the myocardium, which can result in angina, myocardial infarction (MI), and congestive heart failure (CHF). MI, commonly called a *heart attack*, results when the blood supply to the heart muscle is inadequate and the myocardium is deprived of oxygen (O_2).

Sustained HTN requires the LV to work harder to overcome increased peripheral resistance. The increased workload may cause the LV to **hypertrophy** (enlarge), and it may eventually fail.

Kidneys. Narrowing of the renal arteries may decrease renal function and lead to chronic renal failure. Initial indicators of renal failure are nocturia (need to urinate during the night) and azotemia (accumulation of nitrogen waste products in the blood). In addition, urinalysis may reveal protein (proteinuria), blood (hematuria), or both in the urine.

Brain. Prolonged HTN constricts and damages cerebral arteries, putting the patient at risk for transient ischemic attacks (TIAs) and cerebrovascular accidents (CVAs). A TIA, sometimes called a *little stroke*, is a temporary neurologic dysfunction caused by cerebral ischemia.

A CVA, or *stroke*, results from interrupted blood flow in the brain caused by a thrombus (clot) that occludes the vessel or by a rupture of a blood vessel. People with HTN have a sevenfold increased incidence of CVAs compared with those with normal BP.

Eyes. Damage to the eyes may include narrowing of the retinal arterioles, retinal hemorrhages, and papilledema (edema of the optic nerve). These changes may lead to blindness.

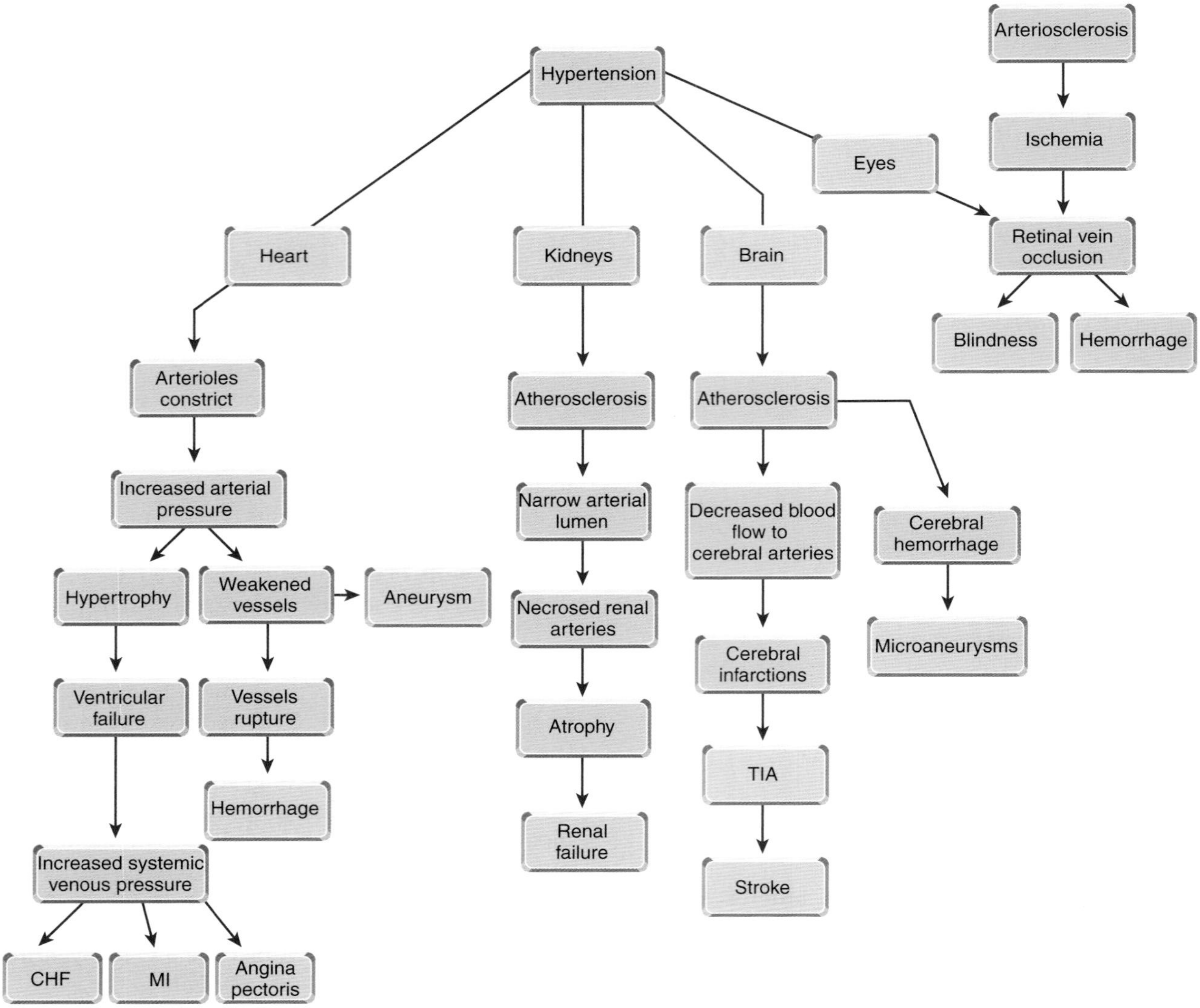

Fig. 34.2 How hypertension affects major target organs. *CHF*, Congestive heart failure; *MI*, myocardial infarction; *TIA*, transient ischemic attack. From Monahan FD, Drake DT, Neighbors M, editors: *Medical-surgical nursing: foundations for clinical practice*, ed 2, Philadelphia, 1998, Saunders.

Diagnostic Tests and Procedures

Diagnosis of HTN is based on direct and indirect data. HTN is confirmed by repeated findings of average pressures of 140/90 mm Hg or higher. When elevations are found in clinics or in screenings, the physician might have patients monitor their own BPs at home for comparison.

Ambulatory BP monitors (ABPMs), that can be programmed to record readings every 15 to 30 minutes for 24 hours, typically provide readings lower than clinic readings. These readings provide a better foundation for the diagnosis of HTN than a few isolated readings. The process is not cost effective for all patients but is appropriate in selected situations. The ABPM report provides clear, concise, measurable information to patients and providers. ABPM diagnoses "white coat" hypertension, described as BP over 140/90 mm Hg in the office (based upon several readings) but normal outside the office. These reports, when reviewed with the patients, seem to allay fears and educate patients about their chronic illness. ABPM is increasingly used in research to provide unbiased BP information (Ford, 1997).

On finding an elevated BP, a health care provider collects data about the patient's lifestyle, other cardiovascular risk factors, and other medical diagnoses, such as diabetes. The patient is examined for effects of HTN on the heart, eyes, kidneys, and brain. An electrocardiogram (ECG) and blood and urine studies should be ordered. Blood studies include glucose, hematocrit, potassium, calcium, creatinine, and a lipid profile. If kidney damage exists, the serum creatinine level is elevated. Abnormal serum lipids and lipoproteins may indicate atherosclerosis. A chest radiograph may show enlargement of the heart or pulmonary blood vessels.

Health care providers disagree about the need to try to determine the cause of HTN. If no evidence suggests an underlying disease process, the consensus is to limit diagnostic tests to those that are most significant, thus reducing patient care costs.

Table 34.2 Principles of Lifestyle Modification

- Encourage healthy lifestyles for all individuals.
- Prescribe lifestyle modifications for all patients with prehypertension and hypertension.
- Components of lifestyle modifications include weight reduction, DASH (Dietary Approaches to Stop Hypertension) eating plan, dietary sodium reduction, aerobic physical activity, and moderation of alcohol consumption.

Lifestyle Modification Recommendations

MODIFICATION	RECOMMENDATION	AVERAGE SYSTOLIC REDUCTION RANGE[a]
Weight reduction	Maintain normal body weight (body mass index [BMI] 18.5–24.9 kg/m^2).	5–20 mm Hg/10 kg
DASH eating plan	Adopt a diet rich in fruits, vegetables, and low-fat dairy products with reduced content of saturated and total fat.	8–14 mm Hg
Dietary sodium reduction	Reduce dietary sodium intake to ≤100 mmol/day (2.4 g sodium or 6 g sodium chloride).[b]	2–8 mm Hg
Aerobic physical activity	Engage in regular aerobic physical activity (e.g., brisk walking) at least 30 minutes/day, most days of the week.	4–9 mm Hg
Moderation of alcohol consumption	Men should be limited to ≤2 drinks[c] per day. Women and lighter-weight persons should be limited to ≤1 drink[c] per day.	2–4 mm Hg

[a]Effects are dose and time dependent.
[b]National Research Council recommends daily sodium intake of 1500 mg with upper limit of 2300 mg per day.
[c]1 drink = ½ oz or 15 mL ethanol (e.g., 12-oz beer, 5-oz wine, 1.5-oz 80-proof whiskey).
From The Joint National Committee on Prevention, Detection, Evaluation, and Treatment of High Blood Pressure: *The seventh report of The Joint National Committee on Prevention, Detection, Evaluation, and Treatment of High Blood Pressure*, Bethesda, MD, 2003, Department of Health and Human Services, National Institutes of Health, National Heart, Lung, and Blood Institute.

Medical Treatment

In 2017, the American College of Physicians (ACP) recommended treatment initiation in patients aged 60 or older who have persistent systolic blood pressure (SBP) above 150 mm Hg to reduce the risk of stroke, cardiac events, and death. Treatment should be intensified if patients over 60 are at higher risk because of diabetes, chronic kidney disease, or other cardiovascular disease.

The goal of therapy for HTN is to gradually reduce peripheral vascular resistance (PVR) and BP. Lowering BP to less than 140/90 mm Hg significantly decreases cardiovascular risks. For patients who have diabetes or renal disease, the medical goal is less than 130/80 mm Hg. Optimal BP is usually defined as a diastolic pressure of less than 80 mm Hg and a systolic pressure less than 120 mm Hg. Treatment of underlying conditions may lower the BP in people with secondary HTN.

For treatment of primary HTN, a conservative, nonpharmacologic method is usually tried first. Drug treatment may be added if needed.

Lifestyle modifications. A nonpharmacologic approach includes weight reduction, smoking cessation, sodium and alcohol restriction, exercise, and relaxation techniques. Reduction of weight can reduce BP by reducing the cardiac workload. Stopping smoking eliminates vasoconstriction caused by nicotine. Reduction of sodium in the body reduces water retention and decreases the blood volume. A planned program of exercise improves cardiac efficiency by increasing CO and decreasing PVR. Exercise also decreases the patient's blood glucose and cholesterol levels and promotes a sense of well-being. Isotonic (muscular contraction) exercises, such as walking, bicycling, and swimming help to reduce weight and promote relaxation.

Additional information for successful lifestyle modifications.

- Smoking cessation: Likely need a combination of behavioral interventions plus pharmacotherapy. E-cigarettes/vaping are not recommended.
- Weight loss: Best goal is ideal body weight, but aim for at least 1-kg (2.2 lbs.) reduction.
- Healthy diet: DASH (Dietary Approaches to Stop Hypertension) is a diet rich in fruits and vegetables, whole grains, low-fat dairy products. (DASHdiet.org)
- Reduced sodium: Optimal goal is under 1500 mg/day. Check food labels.
- Enhanced intake of dietary potassium: Aim for 3500 to 5000 mg/day by consuming fruits, vegetables, and other potassium-rich foods.
- Physical activity: Goal is 90 to 150 minutes per week of aerobic exercise.
- Moderation in alcohol intake: Men less than two drinks daily, women less than one drink daily. One standard drink contains 14 g alcohol (12 oz beer, 5 oz wine, and 1.5 oz distilled spirits).
- Reduce stress: Meditation, biofeedback, and behavior modification are techniques to lower stress.

Lifestyle modifications are recommended for individuals with all stages of HTN regardless of the risk group (Table 34.2). However, according to Dr. Raymond Townsend, director of Hypertension Program at the Perelman School of Medicine, University of Pennsylvania, "the biggest hurdle is fostering adherence to lifestyle and medications. Years of research showing weight loss and salt restriction and exercise help. But getting people to be adherent [to management of hypertension] is still a challenge."

Pharmacologic therapy. Drug therapy is indicated if the BP is very high initially (systolic ≥ 160 mm Hg, diastolic ≥ 100 mm Hg) or if conservative therapies for less severe HTN are not effective within 3 to 6 months. Drug therapy must be individualized for each patient and may be recommended at earlier stages. The goal of drug therapy is to normalize BP using the smallest number of the safest drugs at the lowest effective dosages. A single agent is preferred if good control can be achieved, because patients are more likely to take one drug as prescribed than multiple agents. However, most patients require two or more drugs to achieve control. There are many combination drugs on the market at this time, improving adherence.

Specific antihypertensive drugs. First-line antihypertensive drugs recommended by *JNC 8* include thiazide diuretics, ACE inhibitors, angiotensin II receptor (ARB) blockers, and calcium channel blockers. Other categories that may be used are alpha$_1$-adrenergic blockers, beta-blockers, central alpha$_2$ agonists and other centrally acting drugs, and direct vasodilators. A number of combination drugs are available, and these reduce the number of tablets the patient must take. Each medication class lowers the blood pressure in a different way. Most diuretics offer a generic choice, making these drugs more affordable (Table 34.3).

Diuretics. Diuretics increase urination which reduces sodium and fluid in the body. That can help lower blood pressure because it lowers blood volume. Mild hypertension can sometimes be treated using diuretics alone. They are often used in combination with other blood pressure medications.

Thiazide diuretics. The most common thiazide diuretics are hydrochlorothiazide (HCTZ) and chlorthalidone. Thiazide-type diuretics decrease the reabsorption of sodium and water in the distal convoluted tubule, which lowers BP by reducing blood volume. These diuretics are especially effective in treating Black American patients with HTN.

Patients taking diuretics must be monitored for fluid and electrolyte imbalances, especially hypovolemia (decreased blood volume) and potassium imbalances. Older patients are especially susceptible to hypokalemia. Hypokalemia (low potassium) is a potentially serious problem except with potassium-sparing diuretics. The nurse should monitor for signs of hypokalemia: confusion, irritability, muscle weakness, cardiac dysrhythmias, and anorexia. Severe hypokalemia can lead to respiratory arrest and disruptions in cardiac rhythm. To prevent hypokalemia, it is important to encourage the patient to consume additional dietary potassium. Sources of potassium include bananas and orange juice. After blood levels are drawn to determine the need for potassium supplementation, some patients require supplementary potassium as ordered.

Loop diuretics. Loop diuretics prevent the reabsorption of sodium and potassium (in the thick ascending loop of Henle) into the blood stream as urine moves through the kidney, thus increasing the excretion of sodium and potassium in the urine. The most common loop diuretics are furosemide and torsemide. Loop diuretics are potent drugs. Potassium is needed for proper muscular movement and a deficiency can result in weakness, fatigue, and even heart problems. These patients usually need a potassium supplement.

Potassium-sparing diuretics. These diuretics work in the distal renal tubule to increase the excretion of sodium, but not potassium. The most common potassium-sparing diuretics are spironolactone, amiloride, and triamterene.

Combination diuretics. These medications include both a traditional diuretic and a potassium-sparing agent. Most common are amiloride/HCTZ, spironolactone/HCTZ, and triamterene/HCTZ.

Pharmacology Capsule

When patients are taking diuretics, monitor for signs and symptoms of hypokalemia: cardiac dysrhythmias, muscle weakness, and diminished bowel sounds.

Beta-adrenergic receptor blockers. Beta-adrenergic receptor blockers, commonly called *beta-blockers*, reduce BP by blocking the beta effects of catecholamine (stress hormone that raises BP). Examples of beta-blockers used to treat HTN are atenolol (Tenormin), metoprolol (Lopressor), and propranolol (Inderal). When beta receptors are stimulated, they stimulate the heart and relax bronchial smooth muscle. Beta-blockers prevent this stimulation, resulting in decreased heart rate, decreased strength of cardiac contraction, and bronchial constriction. A number of beta-blockers have slightly different effects. Some affect cardiac function more; others have an increased effect on the bronchi. Beta blockers should not be used when the lungs are compromised, (e.g., in asthma, chronic obstructive pulmonary disease [COPD]). Except for labetalol (Normodyne) and carvedilol (Coreg)—both combination alpha/beta blockers—beta-blockers are less effective than other types of antihypertensive drugs in Black American patients (see the Cultural Considerations box).

Cultural Considerations

What Does Culture Have to Do With Antihypertensive Drugs?

Genes affect the way people metabolize drugs. Therefore, ethnicity and race explain some variations in effects of antihypertensive drugs. For example, Asian Americans respond better to beta-blockers than do White Americans. Black Americans are best treated with thiazide diuretics and/or calcium channel blockers.

Table 34.3 Drug Therapy: Antihypertensive Drugs and Nursing Interventions

General Considerations

1. Monitor blood pressure (BP) regularly with patient in supine, sitting, and standing positions.
2. Encourage patients to take medications and keep follow-up appointments even when they are feeling well.
3. Teach patients with orthostatic hypotension to rise slowly, avoid prolonged standing, and avoid hot baths and showers.
4. Advise patients to consult physician or pharmacist about safety of over-the-counter (OTC) drugs.
5. Do not stop drugs abruptly because rebound hypertension may occur.

DRUG CLASSES AND EXAMPLES	USE AND ACTION	SIDE EFFECTS	NURSING INTERVENTIONS
Centrally Acting Agents (Alpha$_2$-Agonists)			
clonidine (Catapres), methyldopa (Aldomet)	Acts on the central nervous system (CNS) to block vasoconstriction, which lowers BP; also reduces anxiety.	Drowsiness, dry mouth, weakness, depression, and retention of sodium and water. Orthostatic hypotension occurs with some drugs.	Monitor the patient's BP. Take safety precautions and encourage good oral hygiene. Assess the patient for edema. Teach the patient to manage orthostatic hypotension.
Alpha-Adrenergic Receptor Blockers (Antagonist)			
doxazosin (Cardura), prazosin (Minipress), terazosin (Hytrin)	Blocks the effects of norepinephrine, causing vasodilation.	Reflex tachycardia, palpitations, headache, dizziness, drowsiness, and nausea. Potentially severe orthostatic hypotension can occur with first or increased dose of prazosin.	Monitor the patient's pulse and BP. Advise the patient that most side effects diminish over time. Give the first or increased dose of prazosin at bedtime. Advise the patient of possible orthostatic hypotension. Change positions slowly.
Beta-Adrenergic Receptor Blockers			
propranolol (Inderal), atenolol (Tenormin)	Decreases cardiac stimulation.	Bradycardia, fatigue, drowsiness, depression, hypoglycemia, and bronchial constriction.	Monitor the patient's pulse, BP, and respiration. Assess the patient's emotional status. Monitor patients with asthma for dyspnea and patients with diabetes for low blood glucose.
Direct Vasodilators			
hydralazine (Apresoline)	Relaxes vascular smooth muscle, causing vasodilation.	Reflex tachycardia, headache, dizziness, nausea and vomiting, anorexia, and hypotension.	Monitor the patient's pulse and BP.
Calcium Channel Blockers			
verapamil (Calan), diltiazem (Cardizem), amlodipine (Norvasc), amlodipine and atorvastatin (Caduet), nifedipine (Procardia)	Decreases the force of cardiac contraction and dilates the peripheral blood vessels.	Bradycardia, flushing, dizziness, headache, edema, and palpitations.	Monitor the patient's pulse. Elevate the legs when sitting to reduce edema.
Angiotensin-Converting Enzyme Inhibitors			
captopril (Capoten), enalapril (Vasotec), lisinopril (Zestril, Prinivil)	Reduces aldosterone secretion and prevents the formation of angiotensin II, thus decreasing peripheral resistance and fluid volume.	Skin rash, headache, dizziness, neutropenia, and cough. Renal failure can occur in patients with renal artery stenosis.	Monitor the patient's blood cell counts. Report any changes in urine output to the physician.

Continued

Table 34.3 Drug Therapy: Antihypertensive Drugs and Nursing Interventions—cont'd

DRUG CLASSES AND EXAMPLES	USE AND ACTION	SIDE EFFECTS	NURSING INTERVENTIONS
Diuretics			
hydrochlorothiazide (HCTZ), furosemide (Lasix)	Reduces fluid volume; may cause vasodilation; sodium loss may reduce vasoconstriction.	Fluid volume deficit, hyponatremia, and hypokalemia (except with potassium-sparing diuretics).	Monitor the patient's fluid balance: hydration, urine output, mental status, and muscle tone. Recommend foods high in potassium (e.g., bananas, orange juice) unless potassium-sparing diuretics are being given.
Angiotensin II Receptor Antagonists			
losartan (Cozaar), valsartan (Diovan)	Blocks the action of angiotensin II; causes vasodilation; increases renal excretion of sodium and water.	Dizziness.	Take safety precautions to prevent injury to the patient who may experience dizziness.

Common side effects of beta-blockers include bradycardia (heart rate <60 beats per minute) and hypotension, hypoglycemia, and increased low-density lipoprotein (LDL) in the blood. Beta-blockers are usually not recommended in patients with asthma, COPD, or heart block. When a patient is taking a beta-blocker, the nurse should monitor for bradycardia and hypotension. People with diabetes should be watched carefully for hypoglycemia because beta-blockers lower blood glucose and suppress the usual signs of hypoglycemia. Diaphoresis (excessive perspiration) may be the only sign of hypoglycemia when people with diabetes are taking beta-blockers. Older adult patients are at increased risk compared with young patients for hypotension and bradycardia associated with beta-blockers. Therefore, they should be started on low doses that are increased cautiously if needed.

Pharmacology Capsule

Monitor people with diabetes for low blood glucose if they are taking beta-blockers.

Calcium antagonists. Calcium antagonists are called *calcium channel blockers* because they block the movement of calcium into cardiac and vascular smooth muscle cells. This action reduces the heart rate, decreases the force of cardiac contraction, and dilates peripheral blood vessels. Because dilated vessels present less resistance to blood flow, BP is reduced. Diltiazem (Cardizem), isradipine (DynaCirc), nicardipine (Cardene), nifedipine (Procardia), amlodipine (Norvasc), amlodipine and atorvastatin (Caduet), and verapamil (Calan) are examples of calcium channel blockers used for HTN.

Common side effects of calcium channel blockers are flushing, dizziness, and headache. The nurse should also monitor for hypotension, bradycardia, and edema.

Angiotensin-converting enzyme inhibitors. ACE inhibitors prevent the conversion of angiotensin I to angiotensin II, a potent vasoconstrictor. Blocking the production of angiotensin II decreases peripheral resistance. ACE inhibitors also decrease fluid retention by decreasing the production of aldosterone. Potassium is preserved. Examples of ACE inhibitors are captopril (Capoten), lisinopril (Zestril, Prinivil), Ramipril (Altace), and enalapril (Vasotec). ACE inhibitors with diuretics are often effective for Black American patients. Adverse effects can include a chronic cough, dizziness, headache, fatigue, angioedema, hyperkalemia, and hypotension. Combination pills with HCTZ increase effectiveness and lessen the side effects of hypokalemia. ACE inhibitors are recommended as first-line treatment for diabetic patients because of their potential for prevention and control of chronic kidney disease.

Angiotensin II receptor antagonists. Angiotensin II receptor antagonists prevent vasoconstriction in response to angiotensin. They also prevent the release of aldosterone, which increases excretion of salt and water, thereby reducing blood volume. Potassium is preserved. Examples of angiotensin II receptor antagonists are losartan (Cozaar), olmesartan (Benicar), and valsartan (Diovan). Unlike the ACE inhibitors, the only significant adverse effect of these drugs has been dizziness in some patients. These drugs are often given in combination (losartan/HCTZ—Hyzaar). ARBs are also used as first-line drugs for diabetic patients because of the potential antiinflammatory qualities. They are used for prevention and control of chronic kidney disease (CKD).

Central adrenergic blockers. Central adrenergic blockers inhibit impulses from the vasomotor center in the brain that maintain the muscle tone in blood vessels. The effects of this type of drug are to reduce peripheral resistance and lower BP. Examples of centrally acting adrenergic blockers are clonidine (Catapres), guanfacine (Tenex), and methyldopa (Aldomet).

Alpha-adrenergic receptor blockers. Stimulation of alpha receptors produces constriction of arterioles.

Table 34.4 JNC 8 2014 Hypertension Management Guidelines for Individuals Aged 18 and Older

AGE	BP GOAL	DRUG THERAPY	LIFESTYLE MODIFICATIONS
≤60 years	SBP <150 mm Hg DBP <90 mm Hg	Thiazide diuretic or ACE inhibitor or ARB or CCB, alone or in combination	Yes
<60 years	SBP <140 mm Hg DBP <90 mm Hg	Non-Black American: Thiazide diuretic or ACE inhibitor or ARB or CCB, alone or in combination Black American: Thiazide diuretic or CCB, alone or in combination	Yes
All ages with DM; no CKD	SBP <140 mm Hg DBP <90 mm Hg	Non-Black American: Thiazide diuretic or ACE inhibitor or ARB or CCB, alone or in combination Black American: Thiazide diuretic or CCB, alone or in combination	Yes
All ages with CKD; with or without DM	SBP <140 mm Hg DBP <90 mm Hg	ACE inhibitor or ARB, alone or in combination with another drug class	Yes

ACE, Angiotensin-converting enzyme; *ARB,* angiotensin-receptor blocker; *BP,* blood pressure; *CCB,* calcium channel blocker; *CKD,* chronic kidney disease; *DBP,* diastolic blood pressure; *DM,* diabetes mellitus; *SBP,* systolic blood pressure.
From 2014 Evidence-based guideline for the management of high blood pressure in adults: report for the panel members appointed to the Eighth Joint National Committee (JNC 8), *JAMA,* 311(5): 507–520, 2014.

Drugs such as doxazosin (Cardura), terazosin (Hytrin), and prazosin (Minipress) block alpha receptor stimulation and lower BP by reducing peripheral resistance. The most important adverse effect is orthostatic hypotension, which is most severe with initial or increased dosages. Patients should lie down for 2 hours after taking a first or increased dose of this drug. Thus, it is best given at bedtime. Alpha-blockers can also cause dizziness, headache, and drowsiness.

Direct vasodilators. Direct vasodilators lower BP by relaxing arteriolar smooth muscle. Examples of direct vasodilators are fenoldopam (Corlopam), minoxidil (Loniten), hydralazine (Apresoline), diazoxide (Hyperstat IV), and sodium nitroprusside (Nipride). Fenoldopam, nitroglycerin, sodium nitroprusside, hydralazine, and diazoxide are used to treat hypertensive crisis. Most emergency vasodilators are diluted in intravenous fluids and administered at the rate needed for the desired results. Diazoxide is given by direct intravenous injection (IV push), usually in small, repeated doses until the BP reaches the target reading. These drugs are used in severe hypertension and emergent situations.

Pharmacology Capsule

Studies have shown that blood pressure medicine taken at bedtime works better that medication taken in the morning. People have better overnight blood pressure control, while maintaining control in the daytime. In addition, there are fewer adverse drug reactions and better kidney function.

Nursing implications. The nurse must be familiar with the drugs commonly prescribed for HTN. Nursing responsibilities include administering the drugs to inpatients, monitoring for therapeutic and adverse effects, and teaching patients about their drugs. Additional information about antihypertensive drugs and nursing interventions is presented in Table 34.3.

Older adults respond differently to drug therapy. Older patients are at increased risk for adverse effects of medications because of reduced liver and kidney function. They are especially susceptible to orthostatic hypotension because their blood vessels respond more slowly to position changes. This creates increased risk for falls.

Older people may respond differently to beta-blockers and to diuretics. The effectiveness of beta-blockers may be reduced because beta receptor activity is lessened in older adults. In addition, diuretics may produce a more profound decrease in blood volume in these patients. Older patients are often taking medications for other conditions. Drug interactions can alter therapeutic effects or enhance side effects. Dosages for antihypertensive medications may need to be reduced or adjusted depending on what conditions the patient has.

JNC 8 Recommendations for Treatment of Hypertension. The management guidelines for HTN recommended by the *JNC 8* are listed in Table 34.4. If lifestyle modifications have not achieved the BP goal, initial drug choices are made on the basis of individual factors. Different recommendations are made depending on whether the patient has stage 1 or stage 2 HTN. Stage 1 HTN is defined as an SBP of 140 to 159 mm Hg or a diastolic blood pressure (DBP) of 90 to 99 mm Hg; Stage 2 HTN is defined as a SBP of 160 mm Hg or more or a DBP of 100 mm Hg or more. Some patients have "compelling indications for individual drug classes." Specific classes of drugs are recommended for patients with HF, diabetes, and chronic kidney disease, as well as for patients who have had an MI, are at high risk for cardiovascular disease, or are being treated to prevent a recurrent stroke.

Put On Your Thinking Cap!

You have been asked to give a talk on hypertension to members of a senior center. The members are low income and have minimal education. Some speak limited English.

1. How might you explain the effects of hypertension on the body?
2. Select one lifestyle modification, and explain how it reduces the risk of hypertension.

SECONDARY HYPERTENSION

Secondary HTN, which has a specific known cause, is less common than primary HTN. Causes include renal disease, excess secretion of adrenal hormones, narrowing of the aorta, increased intracranial pressure, and some drugs such as vasoconstrictors.

◆ NURSING CARE OF THE PATIENT WITH HYPERTENSION

Focused Assessment

Early detection, education, and promotion of adherence to treatment are the keys to controlling BP. Periodic BP checks detect new or unknown people with HTN and provide data to evaluate the effect of therapy in known people with HTN.

The nursing assessment of the person with known or possible HTN begins with a complete history and physical examination by the registered nurse (RN). The licensed vocational nurse/licensed practical nurse (LVN/LPN) may be involved in initial BP screenings and monitoring and provides important data to evaluate treatment effectiveness.

Reason for seeking care. The patient's reason for seeking care should be noted. Because HTN often has no symptoms, the visit may be related to some other problem.

Past health history. It is important to explore the patient's past health to determine whether they have ever had HTN or renal, cardiac, or endocrine disorders. Note the date and readings of the last BP measurement. Ask the female patient about pregnancy and about hormone replacement therapy, if appropriate. List current medications, including over-the-counter (OTC) drugs. In the family health history, inquire about HTN, MI, or CVAs among relatives.

Review of systems. Review the body systems for significant signs and symptoms, particularly headaches, epistaxis, dizziness, visual disturbances, dyspnea, angina, or nocturia. Information about the patient's usual functioning may detect some potential risk factors for HTN. This includes occupation, exercise and activity, sleep and rest, nutrition, interpersonal relationships, and stressors.

Physical examination. While taking the health history and beginning the physical examination, observe the patient's general appearance, noting any obvious distress. Measure height, weight, and vital signs. The nurse may be the first to detect elevated pressure, so accurate measurement of BP is very important. The patient should be seated comfortably in a chair with their feet on the floor. Position the arm on a surface at the level of the heart. The proper cuff size is essential; the bladder of the cuff should encircle at least 80% of the circumference of the patient's arm. A cuff that is too small may give a false high reading, whereas a cuff that is too large may give a false low reading. For a more accurate reading, determine the systolic pressure first by palpation. To do this, palpate the radial or brachial pulse while inflating the cuff. The pressure when the last pulse is felt is the palpated systolic pressure. Then deflate the cuff, and take the pressure by auscultation, being careful to reinflate the cuff above the palpated systolic pressure.

For the initial assessment, usually done by an RN or physician, multiple readings should be taken. The BP should be assessed in both arms first with the patient in the supine position, then with the patient sitting, and finally, standing. It is normal for the SBP to fall approximately 10 mm Hg and the DBP to rise approximately 5 mm Hg between the supine and standing readings. In general, BP readings obtained in the home are more valid measures because patients are more relaxed there than in a clinic or office.

In addition to BP and pulses, assess respiratory rate and effort and inspect extremities for edema and color. Note any abnormalities in neurologic or muscular function.

Nursing assessment of the patient with known or possible HTN is summarized in Chapter 33, Box 33.2.

◆ NURSING ASSESSMENT OF CARDIOVASCULAR CONDITIONS

When screening persons for HTN, if the BP is elevated initially, reassess it after 1 to 5 minutes. If the pressure remains elevated, refer the patient for medical evaluation. Remember that a single elevated reading does not mean that the patient has HTN. If the BP is severely elevated (diastolic pressure of ≥115 mm Hg), the patient is in imminent danger of a stroke and immediate medical care is needed.

Patient Problems, Goals, and Outcome Criteria: Hypertension

Patient Problems	Goals and Outcome Criteria
Ineffective self-care management related to lack of knowledge about management of hypertension, drug side effects, difficulty maintaining lifestyle changes	Effective self-care management of prescribed treatment: patient correctly explains hypertension and its treatment. Patient adheres to prescribed treatment plan: lowered blood pressure (BP), evidence of positive lifestyle changes (weight loss, cessation of smoking)
Potential for injury related to orthostatic hypotension secondary to antihypertensive drug therapy, sedation	Absence of injury: no falls or other incidents associated with orthostatic hypotension or sedation
Inadequate coping related to depression secondary to drug side effects	Effective coping: patient reports positive emotional state
Altered sexual function related to drug side effects	Satisfactory sexual function: patient's statement of ability to manage effects of drug therapy on sexual function

Interventions

Ineffective self-care management. Adherence to therapy requires commitment and active participation on the part of the patient. Lifestyle changes may be required, and pharmacologic side effects may be unpleasant. Failure to follow the prescribed regimen is often referred to as *noncompliance.* Some people prefer the term *nonadherence* as being less judgmental. In counseling the patient, it must be stressed that HTN is a chronic disease that requires long-term management. Sometimes patients discontinue drug therapy inappropriately because they have no symptoms and current BP readings (while on medications!) are normal.

Patient education is critical for effective management of HTN. Education begins as soon as the condition is diagnosed and continues throughout life. As with any patient teaching, begin by finding out what the person already knows and is most interested in learning. Addressing the patient's immediate concerns first builds trust that should facilitate further teaching. It is important to present measures to manage HTN as health practices that are beneficial to everyone, rather than as a long list of what the patient should or should not do. Include members of the patient's household, especially a spouse, in the teaching. Their understanding and cooperation can be very supportive to the patient.

Teaching patients about their medications can promote adherence. Information in writing and a chart with times for medication administration may be helpful. Patients who do not take their medications as prescribed often cite the adverse side effects as reasons for noncompliance. It is important to teach patients to report unpleasant drug side effects to the physician promptly. A change in dosage or in the medication itself may reduce undesirable effects, but the patient should not make changes unless advised to do so by the physician. Common side effects of antihypertensive drugs that may affect adherence are orthostatic hypotension (sudden drop in BP when standing up), sedation, sexual dysfunction, and depression.

Diet therapy. The nurse and the dietitian should cooperate in teaching patients about their prescribed dietary alterations. If someone other than the patient prepares the food at home, that person should be included in the dietary teaching (see the Cultural Considerations box). If the patient is taking a potassium-wasting diuretic, dietary potassium intake may need to be increased or potassium supplements may be recommended.

Cultural Considerations

What Does Culture Have to Do With Diet?

Cultural dietary practices affect the types of foods eaten and how they are prepared. These practices must be considered and incorporated when teaching patients about healthier dietary practices.

The DASH eating plan helps to lower BP in people with HTN, and it decreases the risk of developing HTN in those who currently have BP in the healthy range. It is a good plan for the whole family (Table 34.5).

The Nutrition Considerations box discusses diet and HTN.

Nutrition Considerations

1. Diet and lifestyle changes, including weight reduction, exercise, and stress management, are important in the treatment of hypertension.
2. Weight loss in obese people lowers blood pressure (BP) at a rate of 1 mm Hg/kg (2.2 lb) of body weight.
3. Sodium-restricted diets help to lower BP in many people with hypertension.
4. A high potassium intake may help to lower BP and replace potassium lost with potassium-wasting diuretics. Foods particularly high in potassium are fresh fruits and vegetables.
5. An adequate calcium intake may help in preventing and treating hypertension. Two to three cups of milk or yogurt per day, 4 oz of low-sodium cheese, or calcium supplements (calcium carbonate, 1 to 2 g/day) can provide adequate calcium intake.

Table 34.5 Dietary Approaches to Stop Hypertension Eating Plan

The DASH (Dietary Approaches to Stop Hypertension) eating plan is based on 2000 calories a day. The number of daily servings in a food group may vary from those listed, depending on an individual's caloric needs.

FOOD GROUP	DAILY SERVINGS (EXCEPT AS NOTED)	SERVING SIZES
Grains and grain products	7–8	1 slice of bread 1 cup of ready-to-eat cereal[a] ½ cup of cooked rice, pasta, or cereal
Vegetables	4–5	1 cup of raw, leafy vegetable ½ cup of cooked vegetable 6 oz of vegetable juice
Fruits	4–5	1 medium fruit ¼ cup of dried fruit ½ cup of fresh, frozen, or canned fruit 6 oz of fruit juice
Low-fat or fat-free dairy foods	2–3	8 oz of milk 1 cup of yogurt 1½ oz of cheese
Lean meats, poultry, and fish	2 or fewer	3 oz of cooked lean meat, skinless poultry, or fish
Nuts, seeds, and dry beans	4–5 per week	⅓ cup or 1½ oz of nuts 1 tablespoon or ½ oz of seeds ½ cup of cooked dry beans
Fats and oils[b]	2–3	1 teaspoon of soft margarine 1 tablespoon of low-fat mayonnaise 2 tablespoons of light salad dressing 1 teaspoon of vegetable oil
Sweets	5 per week	1 tablespoon of sugar 1 tablespoon of jelly or jam ½ oz of jelly beans 8 oz of lemonade

[a]Serving sizes vary between ½ cup and 1¼ cup. Check the product's nutrition label.
[b]Fat content changes serving counts for fats and oils. For example, 1 tablespoon of regular salad dressing equals 1 serving, 1 tablespoon of low-fat salad dressing equals ½ serving, and 1 tablespoon of fat-free salad dressing equals 0 servings.
From Mayo Clinic Staff, 2019.

Exercise. Nutrition and exercise go hand in hand. It is very difficult to maintain or lose weight without engaging in some form of exercise. Walking is highly recommended as an exercise that increases cardiovascular functioning, burns calories, relieves stress, and promotes a sense of well-being. Thirty minutes of physical exercise on most days of the week can make a difference. An exercise program can benefit people of all ages, even older adults. Advise patients to ask their physicians before beginning new exercise programs, and instruct them to increase their activities gradually over a period of time.

A program of good nutrition and exercise may allow a patient to eliminate or reduce medications used to control HTN. This information may be motivating to some people.

Stress management. Patients need to understand that stress can raise BP. Help patients to identify stressors in their lives and explore ways to reduce them. Referrals to professional counselors may be positive for patients with complicated or multiple stressors. Some agencies or community centers offer classes in stress management, meditation, or relaxation techniques. There are many new phone and computer apps to help!

Drug therapy. Patients need to be well informed about their medications. Review with the patient the name, dosage, purpose, and side effects of any prescribed medications. Advise patients to never discontinue their drugs or change the dosage without consulting with the physician, even if they feel well. BP can be very high with no symptoms. Suddenly stopping antihypertensive drugs may produce adverse effects, including rebound HTN (sudden return of elevated BP), MI, and CVA. In addition, explain that many OTC drugs, such as cold remedies, contain vasoconstrictors that can counteract BP medications (see the Patient Teaching box).

Box 34.1 Action Items to Help Lower Blood Pressure

- Lose extra pounds, especially waistline, where too much weight increases risk of high BP.
- Exercise regularly.
- Eat a healthy diet.
- Reduce sodium in diet.
- Limit the amount of alcohol: 1 drink a day for women, 2 for men, can actually lower BP, but more can increase BP.
- Quit smoking.
- Cut back on caffeine.
- Reduce your stress: focus on controllable issues, avoid stress triggers like rush-hour traffic, make time for activities you enjoy, and practice gratitude.
- Monitor your BP at home, especially a week before medical appointment.
- Get support: family, friends, and support groups can add an emotional boost.
- If you need drugs to help lower your BP, you still must follow the lifestyle changes just mentioned.
- Use notes and other reminders to help you remember to take your drugs. Ask your family to help you with reminder phone calls and messages.

From U.S. Department of Health and Human Services, National Institutes of Health, National Heart, Lung, and Blood Institute: *Your guide to lowering blood pressure*, Bethesda, MD, 2003, National Institutes of Health.

Patient Teaching

Hypertension

- Good control of hypertension reduces the risk of heart attack and stroke.
- A diet low in saturated fats and sodium may help to lower BP.
- Regular exercise as advised by your physician helps with weight control and reduction of BP.
- Smoking aggravates hypertension; the American Heart Association has programs to help you quit smoking. Smoking cessation aids (prescription medication such as Zyban and patches) can be beneficial.
- Relaxation techniques lower BP.
- Do not stop taking your medications unless instructed to do so by your physician. Suddenly stopping these drugs may cause BP to rise rapidly.
- Keep appointments for follow-up care; feeling better does not necessarily mean that your hypertension is under control.

Box 34.1 summarizes a variety of actions patients may take to help lower their BP.

Potential for Injury

The patient who is taking antihypertensive medications may be at risk for injury because of drug side effects. The effects that pose the greatest potential for injury are orthostatic hypotension and sedation.

Orthostatic hypotension. **Orthostatic** or postural **hypotension** is a sudden drop in SBP, usually 20 mm Hg, when going from a lying or sitting position to a standing position. Monitor for light-headedness, dizziness, and **syncope** (fainting) in patients who are at risk for orthostatic hypotension. In addition, instruct patients who are prone to orthostatic hypotension to exercise their legs, and then to rise slowly from a lying or sitting position. They should avoid activities that cause BP to fall, such as prolonged standing in one place and taking very hot baths or showers.

Sedation. Sedation may be dealt with by taking medications at bedtime to promote sleep. If drowsiness from a medication is unavoidable during the day, the patient should not engage in activities that require alertness during times of peak drug effect.

Inadequate Coping

If depression occurs as a side effect of an antihypertensive drug, the patient should consult the physician so that another drug may be substituted. This side effect should be taken very seriously. Refer patients with severe depression to a mental health professional.

Altered Sexual Function

A common side effect of many antihypertensive medications is sexual dysfunction. Dysfunctions may take the form of decreased libido, inability to achieve an erection, or delayed ejaculation. Many patients consider sexual function to be a very personal subject, so it must be handled in a sensitive manner. Some patients volunteer information about sexual changes; others may fail to relate the problem to their medications and not report it to the nurse or the physician. You can introduce the subject by saying, "Some people who take this medication have changes in sexual function. Has this been a problem for you?" If it is a problem for the patient, advise the physician so that an alternative medication or other intervention can be considered.

Pharmacology Capsule

Advise patients not to discontinue antihypertensive therapy simply because they feel well. Blood pressure can be very high with no symptoms.

Older Patients

Planning nursing care for older patients with HTN requires additional considerations. Response to drug therapy is more difficult to predict, and side effects are more common. Orthostatic hypotension and sedation are especially problematic for the older person, who is prone to fall and suffer serious injuries. Depression must also be taken very seriously because it lowers motivation, impairs quality of life, and can lead to suicide.

Health care providers tend to assume that older adults are not sexually active. Therefore, they often fail to assess sexual function or dysfunction in older people. This is a real disservice to the older person whose sexual functioning is impaired as a result of antihypertensive drugs. The older patient should be treated just like a younger patient in the assessment and management of distressing drug effects.

HYPERTENSIVE CRISIS

Hypertensive crisis is a life-threatening medical emergency. The patient has severe headache, blurred vision, nausea, restlessness, and confusion. Along with a very elevated DBP (130 mm Hg or more), the heart and respiratory rates are increased. This episode may occur because the patient has decided to stop taking antihypertensive drugs or because the patient may have existing malignant HTN, hypertensive encephalopathy, eclampsia, pheochromocytoma (adrenal tumor), or a CVA. Malignant HTN is a specific type of hypertensive crisis in which the diastolic pressure exceeds 140 mm Hg. It has a sudden onset and is seen most often in Black American men 30 to 40 years of age.

Without appropriate treatment, the patient in hypertensive crisis may incur cardiac and renal damage. Death may ensue as a result of a CVA, renal failure, or cardiac failure.

Put On Your Thinking Cap!

Albert Smith, a 34-year-old Black American man, arrives at the emergency department complaining of severe headache and blurred vision. His blood pressure (BP) is 220/146 mm Hg. The physician diagnoses malignant hypertension (HTN). Mr. Smith is anxious and says that his father died of a stroke at 39 years of age. Mr. Smith is a carpenter who reports no history of serious illness except thyroid deficiency. What is his primary risk factor for malignant HTN?

MEDICAL DIAGNOSIS

Assessment in the emergency department reveals elevated BP, pulse, and respiratory rate. Retinal hemorrhage, papilledema, or both can be observed in the fundus (back, interior portion) of the eye.

The health care provider may order blood drawn for arterial blood gases (ABGs), complete blood count (CBC), electrolytes, blood urea nitrogen (BUN), creatinine, and cardiac enzymes. A chest radiograph may be requested. Direct BP monitoring through an arterial catheter is preferred.

MEDICAL TREATMENT

The goal of drug therapy is to rapidly reduce BP to a non–life-threatening level, and then to bring it slowly within normal range. Diuretics and potent vasodilators may be administered, specifically fenoldopam, nitroglycerin, diazoxide, hydralazine, phentolamine, labetalol, and nitroprusside. An intravenous line is usually established because many drugs are given by that route. Oral options for the management of hypertensive crisis include captopril, clonidine, and nifedipine. Drugs used to treat hypertensive crisis are listed in Box 34.2.

Box 34.2 Emergency Antihypertensive Drugs

VASODILATORS
sodium nitroprusside (Nipride)
nitroglycerin
diazoxide (Hyperstat)

CALCIUM CHANNEL BLOCKERS
nicardipine (Cardene)
Clevidipine (Cleviprex)

ADRENERGIC BLOCKERS
labetalol (Normodyne)

DOPAMINE-1 AGONIST
Fenoldopam (Corlopam)

ANGIOTENSIN-CONVERTING ENZYME INHIBITORS
enalaprilat (Vasotec)
captopril (Capoten)

OTHER AGENTS
Hydralazine
Phentolomine

Elliott WJ: Chapter 8 hypertensiive crises. In Kaplan NM, Victor RG, editors: *Kaplan's clinical hypertension*, ed 11, 2010, Wolters Kluwer, p. 263.

◆ NURSING CARE OF THE PATIENT IN HYPERTENSIVE CRISIS

Focused Assessment

The patient in hypertensive crisis must be monitored closely. Frequently check the patient's BP, pulse, respiration, and level of consciousness. Some drugs are given in intravenous fluids, requiring continuous monitoring and adjustment. Maintain a careful record of fluid intake and output. Nausea and vomiting may indicate an impending seizure or coma.

Interventions. The nurse's role in caring for the patient in hypertensive crisis includes administering prescribed drugs, monitoring vital signs before and after each drug dose, monitoring cardiac and renal function, starting and maintaining intravenous therapy and O_2 as ordered, and comforting the patient.

Take appropriate safety measures if the patient shows signs of seizure activity or a decreasing level of consciousness. Bedside rails should be raised and padded if necessary, according to agency policy. Elevate the head of the bed to facilitate breathing and place an oral airway and suction equipment at the bedside. Offer brief explanations or words of encouragement to allay some of the patient's anxiety. Once the patient's condition improves, it is important to explain how to manage HTN and prevent future crises from developing.

TECHNOLOGY AND HYPERTENSION

Telehealth refers to a means of transmission with wired or wireless devices (mobile phones, computers, or wearable sensors) to communicate with a health care provider. Analyses of various telehealth interventions have demonstrated greater SBP and DBP reductions than in those who received usual care without telehealth. However, telehealth has not been effective as a standalone strategy for improving blood pressure control.

Examples of telehealth strategies and technologies to promote effective hypertension management:

- Automated BP data capture and transmission of patient's self-measured BP
- Self-management support, including education, reminders, and feedback
- Medication titration and follow-up monitoring
- Prescription refill reminders
- Integration of behavior change techniques, including e-counseling
- Medication adherence assessment

Commonly used telehealth technologies include wireless smartphones, wired landline phones, website-accessed computers, text messaging, email messaging, social networking, wireless BP measurement devices, and electronic pill dispenser/counters. According to Dr. Raymond R. Townsend, director of Hypertension Program, University of Pennsylvania School of Medicine, telehealth "is getting to be the preferred method nowadays, and Penn is again pressing faculty to discourage in-center visits favoring telemedicine."

Special note: Telehealth technologies have rapidly increased during the COVID-19 pandemic. Will they continue at the forefront of hypertension management? What about reimbursement? Will health care dollars be saved by telehealth? Will outcomes prove more or less positive?

Get Ready for the NCLEX® Examination!

Key Points

- HTN is called "the silent killer" because it often has no symptoms and is not discovered until a serious complication develops, such as damage to the blood vessels in the kidneys, eyes, heart, or brain.
- HTN is defined as a persistent elevation of arterial BP of 140/90 mm Hg or greater.
- Primary (essential) HTN has no known cause, whereas secondary HTN is caused by an underlying factor, such as kidney disease.
- Two factors that determine BP are CO and PVR.
- Primary risk factors for primary HTN are dyslipidemia, obesity, atherosclerosis, use of tobacco, diabetes, sedentary lifestyle, age, and family history of early heart disease.
- BP tends to rise as people age, but age is not a barrier to aggressive treatment of HTN.
- HTN often has no symptoms, but some people experience occipital headaches, lightheadedness, and epistaxis.
- Diagnosis of HTN is usually based on multiple readings and is accompanied by tests to rule out possible correctable causes.
- Conservative measures to treat HTN include weight reduction, smoking cessation, sodium restriction, exercise, relaxation techniques, and modified alcohol intake.
- Pharmacologic treatment is based on the stage of HTN and presence of other factors such as kidney disease and heart failure.
- Types of drugs used to treat HTN include diuretics, beta-adrenergic receptor blockers, calcium channel blockers, ACE inhibitors, angiotensin II receptor antagonists, central adrenergic blockers, alpha-adrenergic receptor blockers, and direct vasodilators.
- Ethnicity affects response to many antihypertensive drugs.
- Nursing care of the person with HTN addresses inability to manage treatment program, potential for injury, inadequate coping, and impaired sexual function.
- Hypertensive crisis, defined as a DBP of 130 mm Hg or more, is a life-threatening medical emergency that is usually treated with diuretics and potent vasodilators.
- Complications of hypertensive crisis include stroke, heart failure, and kidney failure.

Additional Learning Resources

SG Go to your Study Guide for additional learning activities to help you master this chapter content.

Go to your Evolve website (http://evolve.elsevier.com/Linton/medsurg) for the following learning resources and much more:

- Fluid & Electrolyte Tutorial
- Review Questions for the NCLEX® Examination

Clinical Judgment and Next-Generation NCLEX® Examination-Style Questions

1. Which of the following is a persistent BP of 144/99 mm Hg considered to be?

1. Normal
2. High normal
3. Stage 1 HTN
4. Stage 2 HTN

NCLEX Client Need: Physiological Integrity: Reduction of Risk Potential

2. What is the cause of primary (essential) HTN? ______________ ______________

NCLEX Client Need: Physiological Integrity: Physiological Adaptation

3. Complications associated with prolonged HTN include which of the following? (Select all that apply.)

1. Glaucoma
2. Damage to heart valves
3. Renal failure
4. Heart attack
5. Blindness

NCLEX Client Need: Physiological Integrity: Reduction of Risk Potential

4. **To detect hypokalemia in a patient who is taking hydrochlorothiazide, the nurse should monitor for which of the following? (Select all that apply.)**
   1. Edema
   2. Confusion
   3. Irritability
   4. Irregular pulse
   5. Muscle weakness

   NCLEX Client Need: Physiological Integrity: Reduction of Risk Potential

5. **Beta-adrenergic blockers lower BP by which of the following?**
   1. Eliminating excess body fluid
   2. Inhibiting cardiac stimulation
   3. Blocking the movement of calcium into myocardial cells
   4. Preventing the formation of angiotensin II

   NCLEX Client Need: Physiological Integrity: Pharmacological Therapies

6. **The routine measurement of BP should include which of the following?**
   1. Determine the systolic pressure first by auscultation, and then by palpation
   2. Select a cuff with a bladder that encircles 50% of the circumference of the arm
   3. Position the patient's arm above the level of the heart
   4. Have the patient seated with the feet on the floor

   NCLEX Client Need: Physiological Integrity: Reduction of Risk Potential

7. **A patient who takes antihypertensive drugs complains of feeling dizzy when first rising from a supine position. What should you advise the patient to do when this occurs?**
   1. "Change positions slowly, and exercise the legs before standing."
   2. "Discontinue all antihypertensive drugs immediately."
   3. "Go back to bed, and call the physician."
   4. "Increase salt intake to bring BP up to normal."

   NCLEX Client Need: Physiological Integrity: Pharmacological Therapies

8. **An 80-year-old patient who has been diagnosed with HTN is not taking her prescribed medications. She says, "Wouldn't you expect my BP to be up a bit at my age?" Which of the following is the nurse's most appropriate reply?**
   1. "BP tends to increase with age, but treatment reduces the risk of complications regardless of your age."
   2. "As long as you are feeling well, it will not hurt for you to skip your medication."
   3. "High BP medications probably offer little benefit to someone your age."
   4. "Your physician is going to be pretty upset if you don't follow medical orders."

   NCLEX Client Need: Physiological Integrity: Reduction of Risk Potential

9. **The DASH diet plan is low in which of the following? (Select all that apply.)**
   1. Fat
   2. Poultry
   3. Potassium
   4. Red meat
   5. Dairy products

10. **Take Action Using Matrix Test Item**

    A 58-year-old male had an appointment with his primary care provider for blood pressure monitoring and treatment. He had been diagnosed with HTN for the past 3 years. The nurse made an initial assessment of his vital signs that were reported by the patient:
    - BP 140/90 mm Hg, sitting, 160/95 mm Hg, standing
    - Pulse 86 beats per minute

    The patient also was asked about his diet, tobacco use, and exercise, as well as his medication regimen.

    Use an X for the health teaching below that is *Indicated* (appropriate or necessary), *Contraindicated* (could be harmful), or *Nonessential* (makes no difference or not necessary) before the patient's discharge at this time.

HEALTH TEACHING	INDICATED	CONTRAINDICATED	NONESSENTIAL
"Take your medications as prescribed, and contact your health care provider if any problems arise."			
"Cut down on your tobacco use."			
"Try to rest. Don't overexert yourself so that your BP will remain under control."			
"Drink at least 8 glasses of water per day."			
"The DASH eating plan will help you to maintain your normal weight."			
"Adding carbohydrates to your diet will give you added energy."			
"Be aware of stressors in your life; here are a couple of relaxation techniques that you can use."			

Cardiac Disorders

35

http://evolve.elsevier.com/Linton/medsurg

Objectives

1. Explain the pathophysiology, risk factors, signs and symptoms, complications, medical treatment, and nursing care for selected cardiac disorders.
2. List the data to be obtained in assessing the patient with a cardiac disorder.
3. Contribute to the development of nursing plan of care for patients with cardiac disorders.

Key Terms

arteriosclerosis (ăr-tē-rē-ō-sklĕ-RŌ-sĭs)
atherosclerosis (ăth-ĕr-ō-sklĕ-RŌ-sĭs)
myocardial infarction (mī-ō-KĂR-dē-ăl ĭn-FĂRK-shŭn)
regurgitation (rē-gŭr-jĭ-TĀ-shŭn)
thromboembolism (thrŏm-bō-ĔM-bō-lĭzm)

Heart disease is the leading cause of death in the United States, and approximately one in every four deaths or about 655,000 people occur each year. Coronary artery disease is the most common type of heart disease, killing about 366,000 people a year.

CORONARY ARTERY DISEASE

Coronary artery disease (CAD), also referred to as *coronary heart disease (CHD)*, *arteriosclerotic heart disease*, and *ischemic heart disease*, occurs when the major coronary arteries supplying the myocardium are partially or completely blocked. Blockage of the arteries is caused by coronary artery spasm, arteriosclerosis, or atherosclerosis and may result in ischemia or infarction of myocardial tissue. Atherosclerosis is the major cause of CAD.

ATHEROSCLEROSIS

Atherosclerosis begins with soft fat deposits in the arteries that gradually harden with age. Injury to the endothelial cells, which line the wall of the arteries, leads to inflammation and lipid deposits within the intima. Major causes of injury to the epithelium include tobacco use, hypertension, hyperlipidemia, toxins, diabetes, and infection. When these deposits accumulate, they progress to the lesions associated with atherosclerosis: fatty streaks, fibrous or stable plaque, and unstable plaque.

Progression of Lesions

Fatty streak. The fatty streak is the earliest lesion to develop in atherosclerosis. Yellow-colored lipids fill smooth muscle cells, producing streaks. Fatty streaks may begin as early as infancy and continue to develop through childhood. They do not cause obstruction to the affected vessel, and no symptoms are associated with these lesions.

Fibrous plaque. The fibrous plaque is the characteristic lesion of progressing atherosclerosis that develops over time. Smooth muscle cells, chronically stimulated by low-density lipoproteins (LDL) and platelet-activated growth factors, proliferate, produce collagen, and migrate over the fatty streak. This process forms a fibrous plaque that protrudes from the wall of the artery into the lumen. Other substances such as white blood cells (WBCs), platelets, lipids, and calcium adhere to and collect within the plaque. The fibrous plaque is whitish or grayish in appearance, may develop in one portion of the artery or circle the entire lumen, and may have smooth or rough edges. Fibrous plaque, often referred to as *stable plaque*, contributes to the loss of arterial elasticity and impairs the vessel's ability to dilate to meet increased O_2 needs.

Unstable plaque. The outer layer of the fibrous plaque often thins out, making the plaque unstable and increasing the risk of ulceration and rupture. When the plaque ruptures, platelets are activated and trigger the development of a thrombus that partially or completely occludes the artery (Fig. 35.1).

Collateral Circulation

If plaque formation occurs slowly, collateral circulation may develop. Collateral blood vessels are new branches that grow from existing arteries to provide increased blood flow (Fig. 35.2).

Risk Factors

Factors that increase the risk of atherosclerosis include increased serum cholesterol, high blood pressure, tobacco

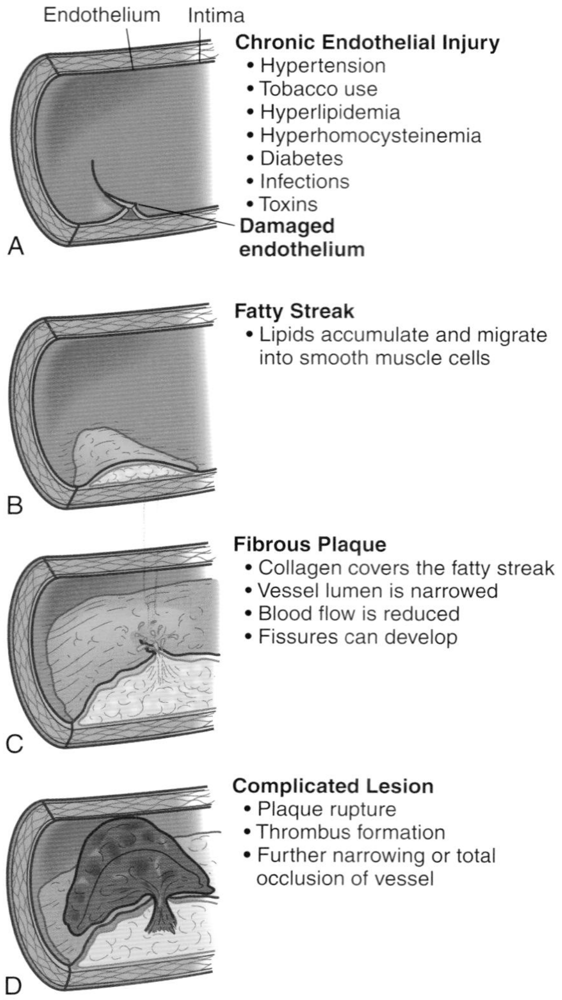

Fig. 35.1 Pathogenesis of atherosclerosis. (A) Damaged endothelium. (B) Fatty streak and lipid core formation. (C) Fibrous plaque. Raised plaques are visible: some are yellow, others are white. (D) Complicated lesion: thrombus is red, collagen is blue. Plaque is complicated by red thrombus deposition. (From Lewis SL, Bucher L, Heitkemper MM, Harding MM: *Medical-surgical nursing: assessment and management of clinical problems*, ed 10, Amsterdam, 2017, Elsevier.)

smoke, diabetes mellitus, obesity, physical inactivity, age, gender, and heredity. These risk factors are divided into two categories: (1) risk factors that cannot be modified and (2) risk factors that can be modified (Table 35.1).

The focus of patient education is on reducing the risk factors that can be modified. See the Health Promotion box.

> **Health Promotion**
>
> **Risk Factor Modification**
>
> Risk factor modification will help to reduce an individual's chances for developing coronary artery disease (CAD), angina, and acute coronary syndrome. Controlling hypertension; reducing serum cholesterol and low-density lipoproteins (LDLs); quitting smoking; participating in regular, moderate exercise; obtaining and maintaining ideal body weight; and learning to handle stress are recommended lifestyle changes that can help to decrease risk (Table 35.2).

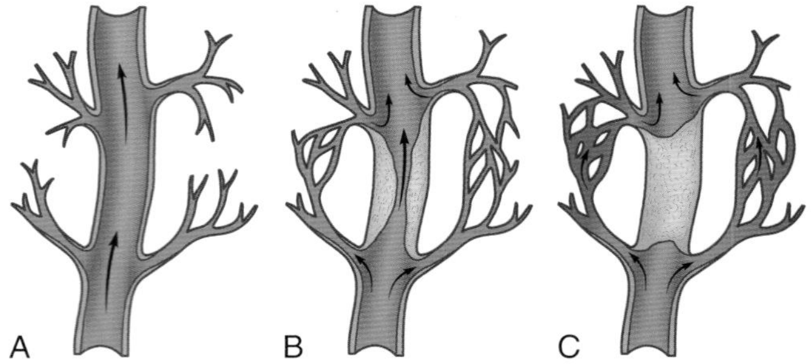

Fig. 35.2 Vessel occlusion with collateral circulation. (A) Open, functioning coronary artery. (B) Partial coronary artery closure with collateral circulation being established. (C) Total coronary occlusion with collateral circulation bypassing the occlusion to supply blood to the myocardium. (From Lewis SL, Bucher L, Heitkemper MM, Harding MM: *Medical-surgical nursing: assessment and management of clinical problems*, ed 10, Amsterdam, 2017, Elsevier.)

Healthy People 2030 set several goals related to heart disease in the third decade of the 21st century (see Box 35.1).

> **Cultural Considerations**
>
> **What Does Culture Have to Do With Heart Disease?**
>
> Native Americans and Black Americans develop coronary heart disease (CHD) at an earlier age than other Americans. The incidence of CHD is highest among middle-aged White men. Latino Americans have lower death rates from CHD than non-Latino Americans. Nurses can educate high-risk patients about risk factors that can be modified: obesity, hypertension, and stress. Role models from the target population are especially influential.

CLINICAL MANIFESTATIONS

CAD is usually asymptomatic until the tissue's blood supply is reduced by at least 50%. Then the clinical manifestations of CAD include chronic stable angina, acute coronary syndrome, unstable angina, myocardial infarction (MI), and sudden cardiac death.

Angina

Angina or chest pain, the most common symptom of CAD, occurs when the demand for O_2 by the myocardial cells exceeds the supply of O_2 delivered. Three different types of angina exist: (1) *chronic stable angina*, (2) *unstable angina*, and (3) *Prinzmetal angina (variant)*. Chronic stable angina takes place intermittently over a long period of time and has a predictable onset. The pain may be triggered by physical exertion, stress, or strong emotions. Other precipitating factors are temperature extremes, heavy meals, tobacco use, sexual activity, and stimulants. The chest pain is usually substernal and described by the patient as vise-like, burning, squeezing, or smothering. The pain may radiate to each arm, the shoulder, the jaw, the neck, or the epigastrium. The pain is rarely described as sharp or stabbing and does not change with position or

Table 35.1 Risk Factors for Coronary Artery Disease

NONMODIFIABLE RISK FACTORS	MODIFIABLE RISK FACTORS

• Increasing age
• Gender (more common in men than in women until 75 years of age)
• Ethnicity (more common in White men than in Black Americans)
• Genetic predisposition and family history of heart disease
	Major
	• Serum lipids:
	  • Total cholesterol >200 mg/dL
	  • Triglycerides ≥150 mg/dL[a]
	  • LDL cholesterol >160 mg/dL
	  • HDL cholesterol <40 mg/dL in men or <50 mg/dL in women[a]
	• BP ≥140/90 mm Hg[a]
	• Diabetes
	• Tobacco use
	• Physical inactivity
	• Obesity: Waist circumference ≥102 cm (≥40 in) in men and ≥88 cm (≥35 in) in women[a]
	Contributing
	• Fasting blood glucose ≥100 mg/dL[a]
	• Psychosocial risk factors (e.g., depression, hostility, anger, stress)
	• Elevated homocysteine levels

[a]Three or more of these risk factors meet the criteria for metabolic syndrome.
From Lewis SL, Bucher L, Heitkemper MM, Harding MM: *Medical-surgical nursing: assessment and management of clinical problems*, ed 10, Amsterdam, 2017, Elsevier.)

breathing. Accompanying symptoms such as diaphoresis and dyspnea may occur. Chronic stable angina lasts only 2 to 5 minutes and is relieved by rest or with nitroglycerin.

Anginal pain that lasts longer or is not relieved by nitroglycerin is called *unstable angina*.

Unstable angina is categorized and treated as acute coronary syndrome. The pain of unstable angina is more severe, occurs at rest or with minimal exertion, is not always relieved by nitroglycerin or requires more frequent nitroglycerin administration, and is not predictable. Associated symptoms that generally accompany unstable angina include dyspnea, diaphoresis, nausea, and vomiting. Unstable angina may occur in a patient with a history of stable angina; the patient may describe a change in the pain pattern or in the severity of the pain. However, unstable angina could also present as the first clinical manifestation of CAD that a patient experiences. In either case, unstable angina is considered more serious than stable angina and is treated differently. Patients with unstable angina are at higher risk for MI and frequently are hospitalized for diagnostic workup and treatment.

Prinzmetal angina, also known as variant angina, is caused by coronary artery spasm and is usually not associated with CAD. This type of angina is unpredictable and often occurs at rest. When the coronary spasm occurs, the patient experiences pain, and, if the patient is being monitored, transient ST segment elevation may be seen. When the spasm subsides, the pain ceases, and the ST segment returns to normal. Prinzmetal angina generally is treated with the administration of calcium channel blockers to prevent the spasms from recurring (Fig. 35.3).

DIAGNOSTIC TESTS

Tests used for diagnosis of cardiac disease are electrocardiogram (ECG), Holter monitor, implantable loop recorder (ILR), echocardiogram, transesophageal echocardiogram (TEE), stress test (exercise tolerance test [ETT]), magnetic resonance imaging (MRI), multiple-gated acquisition (MUGA) scanning, myocardial perfusion imaging, ultrafast computed tomography (CT), cardiac catheterization, and electrophysiology study (EPS). Blood tests include arterial blood gases (ABGs), troponin, cardiac enzymes, myoglobin, complete blood count (CBC), lipid profile, B-type natriuretic peptide (BNP), and C-reactive protein (CRP). Diagnostic tests and nursing interventions for heart conditions are described in Chapter 33, Table 33.3.

MEDICAL TREATMENT

Treatment of CAD includes diet therapy, drug therapy, and reduction of modifiable risk factors (e.g., smoking, obesity, high blood pressure). The American College of Cardiology (ACC) and the American Heart Association (AHA) provide guidelines for the medical management of stable and unstable angina.

There are three classes of drugs that are commonly used in the treatment of chronic stable angina: (1) nitrates, (2) beta-blockers, and (3) calcium channel blockers. The objective is to reduce angina symptoms by decreasing oxygen demand and/or increasing oxygen supply. The goal is to lower the risk of MI and death. Nitrates such as nitroglycerin are used to treat actual episodes and to prevent the occurrence of angina. Various forms of nitroglycerin are prescribed.

Table 35.2 Reducing Risk Factors for Coronary Artery Disease

Include the following instructions when teaching risk reduction for coronary artery disease.

RISK FACTOR	HEALTH-PROMOTING BEHAVIORS
Hypertension	• Monitor home-based BP and obtain regular checkups. • Take prescribed drugs for BP control. • Reduce salt intake. • Stop tobacco use. Avoid exposure to environmental tobacco (secondhand) smoke. • Control or reduce weight. • Perform physical activity daily.
Elevated serum lipids	• Reduce total fat intake. • Reduce animal (saturated) fat intake. • Take prescribed drugs for lipid reduction. • Adjust total caloric intake to achieve and maintain ideal body weight. • Engage in daily physical activity. • Increase amount of complex carbohydrates, fiber, and vegetable proteins in diet.
Tobacco use	• Begin a tobacco cessation program. • Change daily routines associated with tobacco use to reduce desire to smoke. • Substitute other activities for smoking. • Ask caregivers to support efforts to stop smoking. • Avoid exposure to environmental tobacco smoke.
Physical inactivity	• Develop and maintain at least 30 min of moderate physical activity daily (minimum 5 days a week). • Increase activities to a fitness level.
Psychologic state	• Increase awareness of behaviors that are harmful to health. • Alter patterns that add to stress (e.g., get up 30 min earlier so that breakfast is not eaten on way to work). • Set realistic goals for self. • Reassess priorities in light of identified risk factors. • Learn effective stress management strategies (see Chapter 4). • Seek professional help if feeling depressed, angry, anxious, etc. • Plan time for adequate rest and sleep (see Chapter 4).
Obesity	• Change eating patterns and habits. • Reduce caloric intake to achieve body mass index of 18.5–24.9 kg/m^2. • Increase physical activity to increase caloric expenditure. • Avoid fad and crash diets, which are not effective over time. • Avoid large, heavy meals. Consider smaller, more frequent meals.
Diabetes	• Follow the recommended diet. • Control or reduce weight. • Take prescribed drugs for diabetes. • Monitor blood glucose levels regularly.

From Lewis SL, Bucher L, Heitkemper MM, Harding MM: *Medical-surgical nursing: assessment and management of clinical problems*, ed 10, Amsterdam, 2017, Elsevier.

These are administered sublingually or buccally at the onset of pain. They are quickly absorbed and usually effective. Oral, topical, spray, and transdermal nitrates may be ordered to prevent angina attacks.

For some patients, a combination of these drugs is required to control anginal symptoms. In addition, all patients with angina, in the absence of contraindication, should take low-dose aspirin daily, which can inhibit platelet aggregation and reduce the overall risk for MI. If the patient cannot tolerate aspirin, another antiplatelet medication (e.g., Plavix) is prescribed. Beta-adrenergic blockers and calcium channel blockers are prescribed in the long-term management of angina. For patients who have not had an adequate response with standard angina treatment, a newer antianginal agent, ranolazine (Ranexa), may be used. Angiotensin-converting enzyme (ACE) inhibitors also may be prescribed to patients with stable angina to reduce the risk of MI. In addition, some patients may be recommended for further treatment with percutaneous coronary intervention (PCI) such as angioplasty, stent placement, or atherectomy.

After the initial relief and control of the anginal pain, the focus of therapy is on risk reduction, including blood pressure control; smoking cessation; lipid control (diet alone or diet plus lipid-lowering medications), healthy diet; tight glucose control for diabetic patients; increasing physical activity; patient education (non., medication therapy, risk reduction, and what to do if symptoms of an MI occur); and yearly flu vaccine.

Additional information about various drug therapies is presented in Chapter 33, Table 33.9.

Unstable angina may be treated conservatively or more aggressively, depending on the situation. Because unstable angina may be a warning of more serious events, it has been classified as *acute coronary syndrome*. Patients who present with unstable angina should be managed as though they are having an MI until the cause of chest pain is determined. Initial management includes nitrates, beta-blockers, statin therapy, and anticoagulation. Most patients presenting with unstable angina should undergo a cardiac catheterization to assess the scope of disease and determine the proper approach for management.

SURGICAL INTERVENTION

Surgical procedures to treat CAD are discussed in Chapter 33.

Box 35.1 Healthy People 2030 Goals for Heart Health

- Improve cardiovascular health in adults
- Reduce coronary heart disease deaths
- Increase the proportion of adult heart attack survivors who are referred to a rehabilitation program
- Reduce heart failure hospitalizations in adults
- Increase the proportion of heart attack patients who get timely fibrinolytic therapy
- Increase the proportion of heart attack patients who get timely percutaneous intervention
- Reduce the proportion of adults with high blood pressure
- Reduce cholesterol in adults
- Increase cholesterol treatment in adults
- Increase aspirin use for secondary prevention of atherosclerotic cardiovascular disease
- Increase the proportion of adults whose risk for atherosclerotic cardiovascular disease is assessed
- Increase control of high blood pressure in adults

MYOCARDIAL INFARCTION

A **myocardial infarction** (MI) is the death of myocardial tissue caused by prolonged lack of blood and O_2 supply. Approximately 1.5 million cases of MI and about 151,000 deaths occur annually in the United States. There is a 30% mortality rate with MI, and about 50% of the deaths occur before arrival at the hospital. In addition, 5% to 10% of survivors die within the first year after an MI, and about one-half of patients are rehospitalized within one year of their first occurrence.

The death rate for people experiencing an acute MI is approximately three times higher in men than in women. For those under age 75, the death rate is higher in Black Americans than White Americans; however, it equalizes over age 75 years. Latino Americans have a lower mortality rate than either Black Americans or White Americans.

PATHOPHYSIOLOGY

An MI begins with the occlusion of a coronary artery caused by a thrombus that has developed from an aggregation of platelets. An abrupt blockage of blood flow results in irreversible necrosis (cell death) in the heart muscle beyond the blockage. The process takes a period of 4 to 6 hours for the entire thickness of the heart to become necrosed. Deprived of blood and O_2, the affected tissue becomes soft and loses its normal color. With continued ischemia (decreased blood supply), an *infarction*, or death of myocardial tissue, occurs. Ischemia lasting 20 minutes or more is sufficient to produce irreversible tissue damage. The majority of MIs occur in the left ventricle (LV), and the location of the ischemia is related to the site of the blocked artery.

Within 24 hours after an infarction, the healing process begins. By the third day, necrotic tissue has been broken down by enzymes and removed by macrophages. Collateral circulation develops to supply the injured area, and scar tissue begins to form. About 10 to 14 days after the MI, the myocardium is

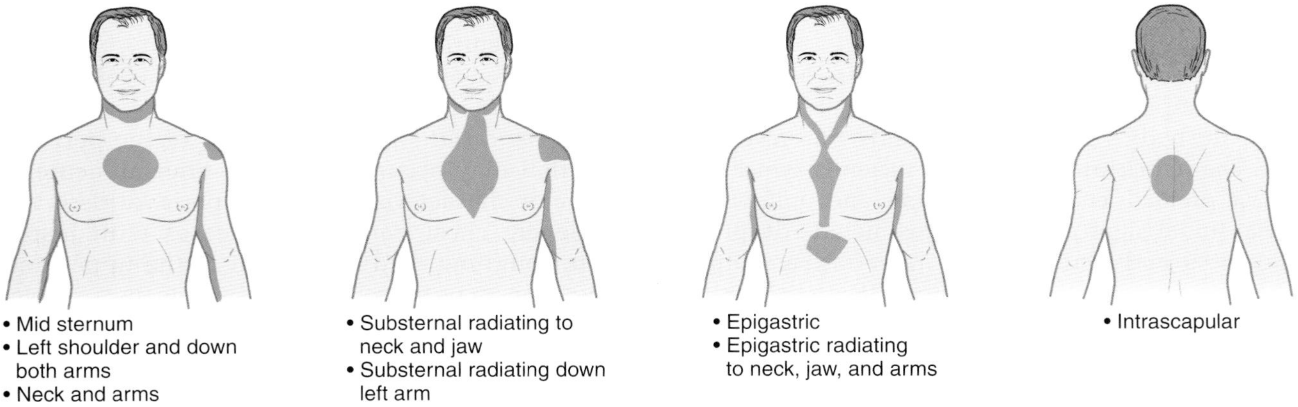

Fig. 35.3 Common locations and patterns of pain during angina or myocardial infarction. (From Lewis SL, Bucher L, Heitkemper MM, Harding MM: Medical-surgical nursing: assessment and management of clinical problems, ed 10, Amsterdam, 2017, Elsevier.)

especially vulnerable to stress because of the weakness of the healing tissue. Complete healing takes about 6 weeks.

CLINICAL MANIFESTATIONS OF MYOCARDIAL INFARCTION

Pain is the classic symptom of an MI. It is typically a heavy or constrictive pain located below or behind the sternum, as described with angina. It may radiate to the arms, back, neck, or jaw. The pain may begin with or without exertion and lasts for more than 20 minutes. The pain is described as more severe than the pain of angina. The patient becomes diaphoretic and lightheaded and may experience nausea, vomiting, and dyspnea. The skin is frequently cold and clammy. The patient experiences great anxiety and often a feeling of impending doom. However, not all patients experience the more classic signs and symptoms. Women, older adults, and diabetic patients frequently have atypical symptoms. Women may report fatigue, shortness of breath, and atypical chest pain. Older adults and diabetic patients may not experience chest pain but will report other symptoms such as shortness of breath, dizziness, and nausea.

COMPLICATIONS

The major complications of MI are dysrhythmias, heart failure (HF), cardiogenic shock, sudden cardiac death, ventricular aneurysm and rupture, and pericarditis.

Dysrhythmias

Dysrhythmias are disturbances in heart rhythm, including excessively rapid, slow, or irregular heartbeats. They occur in approximately 90% of all patients with MI. Because some dysrhythmias are life threatening, continuous cardiac monitoring is essential. This permits early detection and prompt treatment of dysrhythmias. The most frequently observed dysrhythmias are premature ventricular contractions, ventricular tachycardia, and ventricular fibrillation. Recognition and treatment of specific dysrhythmias are addressed in Chapter 33.

Heart Failure

An injured ventricle caused by an MI can lead to decreased pumping action of the heart so that it is unable to meet the body's circulatory demands, thus resulting in HF. The ventricle fails to empty efficiently, which can increase preload leading to systemic and pulmonary edema. Initial signs and symptoms include dyspnea, restlessness, and increased heart rate. Cardiac output and blood pressure fall. Untreated HF progresses to cardiogenic shock and death. HF may become a chronic condition.

Cardiogenic Shock

Cardiogenic shock is the most frequent cause of death after an MI. Cardiogenic shock is usually related to extensive injury to the LV and is more common when the patient has had a previous infarction. Cardiogenic shock is marked by hypotension; cool, moist skin; oliguria; and decreasing alertness.

Sudden Cardiac Death

Sudden cardiac death occurs when heart activity and respirations cease abruptly. CAD is the most common underlying reason for sudden cardiac death. The event usually occurs during ordinary activity and frequently is preceded by ventricular tachycardia or ventricular fibrillation, and occasionally by severe bradydysrhythmias (slow, abnormal cardiac rhythms). Major causes include MI, left ventricular dysfunction, cardiomyopathy (CMP), electrolyte imbalance, electrocution, and pulmonary embolism.

Those who survive an episode of sudden cardiac death need to undergo extensive testing to determine the nature and cause of the episode. Many patients need treatment with medical therapy, PCI, or coronary artery bypass graft (CABG). Most have a potentially lethal dysrhythmia that requires intervention. Diagnostic tests include 24-hour Holter monitoring, stress testing, and an EPS. During the EPS, pacing electrodes are placed in the heart and electrical stimuli are used to elicit the dysrhythmia. This helps the health care provider to determine appropriate medical therapy. In some patients, the dysrhythmia may be treated during the EPS with catheter ablation. The ablation (removal or "burning") of abnormal conduction pathways or irritable sites in the heart can prevent the dysrhythmia from recurring. Still other patients are treated effectively with antidysrhythmic agents such as amiodarone (Cordarone). Preventing the reoccurrence of sudden cardiac death is currently accomplished with the use of automatic implantable cardiac defibrillators (AICDs).

Ventricular Aneurysm and Rupture

Weakened areas of the ventricular wall may bulge during contractions. If scar tissue is inadequate to strengthen the wall, an aneurysm may develop and rupture. Ventricular rupture is fatal.

Pericarditis

Acute pericarditis is inflammation of the pericardium that may occur 2 to 3 days after an acute MI. A major characteristic of acute pericarditis is mild to severe chest pain that increases with inspiration, coughing, and movement of the upper body. The pain may be relieved by sitting in a forward position.

MEDICAL DIAGNOSIS

The diagnosis of MI is based on the patient's history, physical signs and symptoms as well as laboratory evidence and ECG changes.

Cardiac Markers

Troponin. Cardiac troponin T and cardiac troponin I are proteins released from cardiac muscle when the muscle is damaged. Troponin levels elevate in 3 hours after myocardial injury, peak in 12 hours, and remain in the circulation for up to 10 to 14 days. Troponin levels are drawn in the emergency department as even low levels of troponin are treated aggressively to preserve cardiac muscle.

Electrocardiogram

Changes in the normal waveform can be seen on an ECG after an MI. For purposes of diagnosis and treatment, health care providers divide myocardial infarction into two types: (1) Non-ST-elevation MI (NSTEMI) and (2) ST-elevation-MI (STEMI). The ST segment of an ECG is usually flat or isoelectric (see interpretation of ECGs in Chapter 33). With ischemia, the ST segment is depressed and the T wave is inverted. If prolonged total occlusion of a coronary artery has occurred, the ECG will show ST segment elevation (STEMI). If transient or partial occlusion of the artery has occurred, the ECG may not show ST segment elevation (NSTEMI). After infarction, another change often seen on the ECG waveforms is a significant Q wave. A significant Q wave is one that is greater than one-third the height of the R wave (Fig. 35.4).

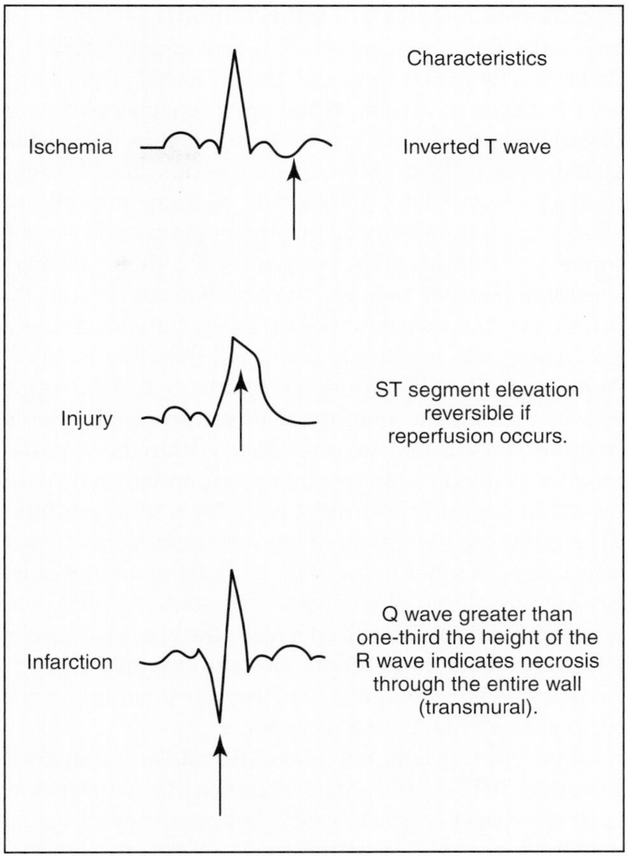

Fig. 35.4 Electrocardiographic changes with myocardial infarction.

Medical Treatment

The goals of medical therapy after an MI are to limit the amount of cardiac muscle injury, to relieve symptoms, and to prevent or minimize complications.

Drug Therapy

Sublingual or intravenous (IV) nitroglycerin is administered to dilate coronary arteries and increase blood flow to the damaged area. Morphine sulfate is also used for chest pain and has many effects in addition to analgesia. Morphine causes peripheral pooling of blood, which decreases the blood returning to the heart and lungs. Morphine also diminishes anxiety, decreases tachypnea, and relaxes bronchial smooth muscles, thereby improving gas exchange.

O_2 should be administered if the patient's O_2 saturation is 90% or below to assist in oxygenating myocardial cells. If the patient is not already on aspirin (or other antiplatelet medication), aspirin is administered.

Thrombolytic (fibrinolytic) therapy is recommended for patients with ST-Elevation-MI (STEMI) when PCI is not available within 120 minutes of first medical contact. Thrombolytics such as streptokinase and tissue plasminogen activator (t-PA) are administered intravenously to dissolve the thrombus. This treatment is most effective when initiated early (within 30 minutes of arrival to hospital) but may be administered up to 12 hours from the onset of chest pain. The patient must meet strict criteria (non., no recent surgery or active bleeding, no history of a stroke, no bleeding disorders) and provide informed consent before the administration of thrombolytic agents. After administration of the thrombolytic agents, heparin is administered to prevent further clot formation. To monitor the effectiveness of this therapy, the nurse should assess for relief of chest pain and the return of the ST segment to baseline. Bleeding is the greatest risk associated with thrombolytic therapy and the nurse should assess for signs of major bleeding:

- Changes in level of consciousness from intracerebral bleeding
- Decrease in hemoglobin (Hgb) and hematocrit (Hct)
- Sudden decrease in blood pressure and increase in heart rate
- Blood in stool, urine, or both

Beta-adrenergic blockers should be administered as soon as the patient can tolerate them and if not contraindicated. Beta-adrenergic blockers improve survival rates by decreasing the heart rate, reducing the work of the heart, and lessening the O_2 demand of the myocardium. ACE inhibitors may be prescribed for some patients to minimize the abnormal shaping or ventricular remodeling that can occur in the damaged ventricular muscle. As the myocardium receives blood and O_2, reperfusion dysrhythmias that require treatment may be noted.

Dysrhythmias often occur as a result of either the MI or medication therapy; they should be treated if they are causing the patient symptoms.

Percutaneous Coronary Intervention

Emergency PCI is the first choice for treatment of an MI, if available. The goal is to reopen the occluded artery within 90 minutes of arrival to the emergency department. Several PCI procedures can be performed in the cardiac catheterization laboratory: percutaneous transluminal coronary angioplasty (PTCA), or balloon angioplasty; intracoronary stent placement; atherectomy, and laser angioplasty. PTCA involves passage of a catheter through a peripheral artery (usually the femoral artery) into the occluded coronary artery. The tip of the catheter contains a balloon that is inflated to compress the atherosclerotic plaque and dilate the artery. The majority of PTCA procedures include the placement of intracoronary stents. Stents are devices that are positioned within the blockage through a balloon-tipped catheter, expanded into place, and left to support the arterial wall. Over time, endothelial cells line the inner wall of the stent completely to produce a smooth inner lining (Fig. 35.5). After an intracoronary stent is placed, the patient is prescribed antiplatelet agents or anticoagulants to decrease the chance of occlusion in the stent. Some stents are coated with a medication that prevents overgrowth of the new inner lining and reduces the incidence of a recurrence.

When appropriate, percutaneous transluminal coronary artery (PTCA) and/or intracoronary stent placement is preferred over coronary artery bypass surgery because it can be done under local anesthetic, is less invasive, and the recovery time is faster. The procedure is safer than bypass surgery but is not without risks. Complications of PTCA and intracoronary stents include coronary artery dissection, dysrhythmias, coronary spasm, hematoma or bleeding at the catheter site, re-stenosis, and death.

Coronary atherectomy is a procedure that widens the coronary artery by removing the atherosclerotic plaque using a device that shaves the plaque off the vessel walls. The laser angioplasty uses a catheter with a laser on its tip. The laser is used to widen the lumen of the artery by destroying atherosclerotic plaque.

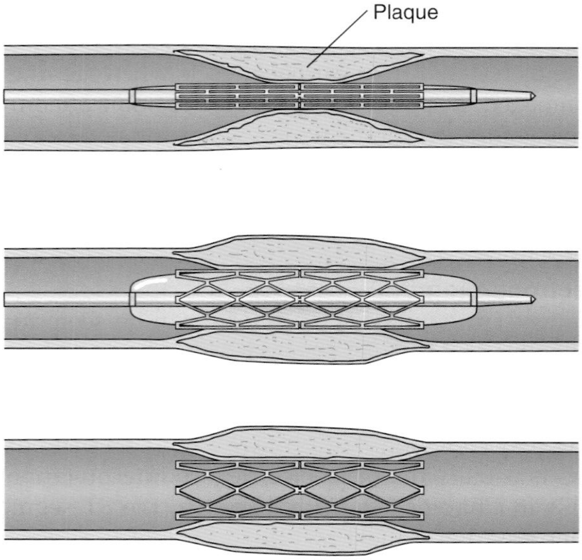

Fig. 35.5 Intracoronary stent. (From Lewis SM, Bucher L, Heitkemper MM: *Medical-surgical nursing: assessment and management of clinical problems*, ed 10, St. Louis, 2017, Elsevier.)

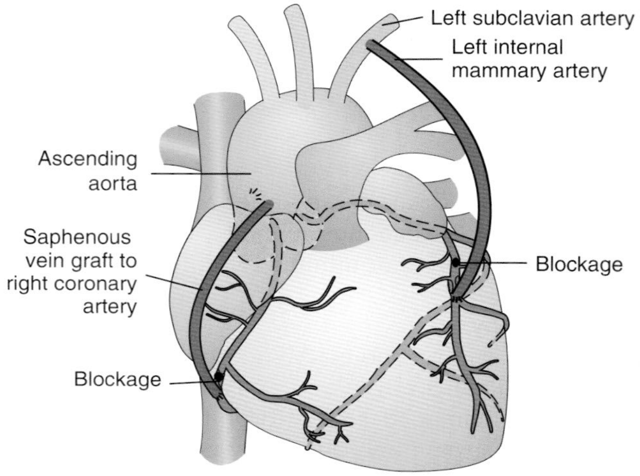

Fig. 35.6 Coronary artery bypass graft surgery. (From Lewis SL, Bucher L, Heitkemper MM: *Medical-surgical nursing: assessment and management of clinical problems*, ed 10, St. Louis, 2017, Elsevier.)

Coronary Artery Bypass Graft Surgery

CABG surgery (also known as *coronary revascularization surgery*) may be performed to improve the blood supply to the myocardium. Arterial bypass surgery uses the patient's own vasculature as a bypass for occluded coronary arteries. Multiple occluded sections may be bypassed during a single surgical procedure. The saphenous veins and the internal mammary artery are most commonly used. The saphenous veins are removed from one or both legs, inspected for patency, and reversed so that the valves do not inhibit blood flow. The bypass vessels are attached to the aorta and below the occlusions in the coronary arteries and serve as new conduits for oxygenated blood to the myocardium (Fig. 35.6). The internal mammary artery is left attached to the subclavian artery (point of origin), dissected from surrounding tissue, and attached to the coronary artery below the occlusion. This is major surgery that requires the heartbeat to be stopped and the patient to be placed on a cardiopulmonary bypass (CPB) machine during the surgery. Use of CPB supports the body's tissue needs during the surgery but several complications are associated with CPB. These include postoperative bleeding, hypothermia, dysrhythmias, unstable hemodynamics, and pulmonary dysfunction. The survival rate is higher in patients who are in stable condition.

Another approach to surgical revascularization is being used on patients who require surgery on the arteries of the anterior heart. This procedure is called *minimally invasive direct coronary artery bypass grafting* (MIDCAB) and is performed through a small anterior thoracotomy incision. The patient's left internal mammary artery is used to bypass the stenosed vessel and the bypass is accomplished on a beating heart. The patient does not have to be placed

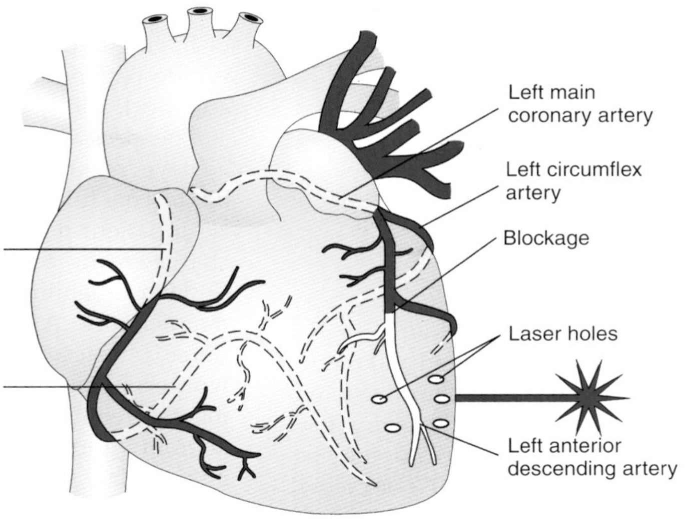

Fig. 35.7 Transmyocardial laser revascularization (TMR). (From Ballard JC, Wood LL, Lansing AM: Transmyocardial revascularization: criteria for selecting patients, treatment, and nursing care. *Crit Care Nurs* 17(1):42–49, 1997. Reprinted with permission.)

on CPB. Postoperative care is similar to that of other cardiac surgery, although patients do not require as lengthy ventilatory support and total hospital stay is shorter.

A third option, off-pump coronary artery bypass (OPCAB), usually uses a full sternotomy incision (as with traditional CABG) to provide the surgeon access to all coronary vessels (anterior and posterior). The OPCAB surgery is then accomplished on a beating heart without the use of CPB. The surgeon uses specially developed vacuum-assisted stabilizers to stabilize the heart and graft site.

A newer approach to CABG, called *totally endoscopic coronary artery bypass* (TECAB), has been used by making three tiny incisions on the patient's chest between ribs and a small camera and two robotic arms are inserted (using the da Vinci surgical system). The surgeon sits at a console to view the surgical area and manipulates the robotic arms with their hands and wrists. The surgery is done on a beating heart, is less traumatic to the patient because of the small incisions and has an easier recovery. However, the time of the procedure is much longer than a traditional bypass, and further research is warranted to determine the role for this approach.

Another method of revascularization, used for patients with diffuse coronary vessel disease who are not candidates for CABG, is transmyocardial laser revascularization (TMR). Tiny holes (between 10 and 50) are drilled in the myocardium using a laser, which helps to provide collateral circulation to the ischemic myocardial muscle (Fig. 35.7).

NURSING CARE OF THE PATIENT WITH ACUTE MYOCARDIAL INFARCTION

FOCUSED ASSESSMENT

General assessment of the cardiac patient is summarized in Chapter 33. When a patient has an MI, be especially concerned with assessment of pain. When chest pain is present, early evaluation and treatment are paramount. Ask the patient to describe the pain, including type, location, duration, and severity. It is recommended that chest pain be assessed using the mnemonic PQRST, as follows:

P Precipitating factors, palliative: What was the patient doing when the pain began? Did anything make the pain better? Worse?

Q Quality: Have the patient describe what the pain feels like (in their own words).

R Region, radiation: Where is the pain located? Does it hurt anywhere else?

S Severity, symptoms: Have the patient rate the pain. Use the 0 to 10 pain scale. Note other symptoms (e.g., nausea, diaphoresis).

T Time: When did the pain start? How long did it last?

Record what the patient was doing when the pain started, what action was taken, and the effects of any actions or treatments. In addition, inspect the patient's skin for color and palpate for temperature and moisture. Frequently assess vital signs and document the patient's mental status and level of anxiety. When cardiac monitoring is initiated, evaluate the rate and rhythm.

Patient Problems, Goals, and Outcome Criteria: Acute Myocardial Infarction

Patient Problems	Goals and Outcome Criteria
Acute pain related to lack of oxygen (O_2) to the myocardium	Pain relief: patient statement of relieved pain, relaxed manner
Inadequate myocardial tissue perfusion related to dysrhythmia and abnormal heart rate	Normal myocardial tissue perfusion: normal pulse, blood pressure, and cardiac rhythm

Continued

Patient Problems, Goals, and Outcome Criteria: Acute Myocardial Infarction—cont'd

Patient Problems	Goals and Outcome Criteria
Anxiety-related to feeling of impending doom, lack of understanding of routines	Reduced anxiety: patient statement of lessened anxiety, calm manner, and self-care

Interventions

Acute pain. Administer analgesics as ordered and monitor for relief of pain. Morphine is usually administered in small amounts (2–4 mg) intravenously every few minutes until pain relief is evident. Aspirin also may be given as ordered. If the O_2 saturation is 90% or below, provide supplemental O_2 as ordered through nasal cannula at 2 to 4 L/min to provide adequate O_2 to the heart muscle. The head of the bed is usually elevated at least 30 degrees. Inform the health care provider if the patient has an increasing respiratory rate or dyspnea.

Inadequate myocardial tissue perfusion. Monitor the patient's vital signs hourly or more frequently until they are stable. Watch the ECG for changes from the normal waveform and for dysrhythmias. Notify the health care provider of changes in the rhythm such as an inverted T wave, ST segment elevation, and/or Q wave. In an intensive care unit, standing orders prescribe drug therapy for specific dysrhythmias. An IV line is established so that emergency drugs can be administered quickly and directly. Prompt treatment of dysrhythmias may prevent fatal alterations in rhythm. Monitor the patient for fluid volume excess (crackles, cough, jugular vein distention) and report any such evidence to the health care provider.

Interventions to decrease demands on the heart include assisting the patient to rest; spacing activities and providing rest periods; providing adequate ventilation and oxygenation; relieving pain; and maintaining a calm, quiet environment.

Anxiety. Provide as calm an environment as possible and explain procedures and equipment to the patient and family, using simple terms. Keep family members informed of the patient's progress. They can be helpful in calming the patient during the acute episode.

During the acute phase of MI, provide simple explanations of the procedures and routines. Reinforce information given by the physician about the diagnosis and treatment. Patient teaching is especially important in the rehabilitation phase.

Cardiac rehabilitation. As soon as the patient is stable, begin rehabilitation by teaching the patient and family about exercise, medications, and diet. If surgical intervention has been proposed, you may also teach the patient about that procedure.

The purpose of rehabilitation is to minimize the risk of having another MI. The goal of rehabilitation is to enable patients to attain the highest level of wellness and work ability.

The program is individualized for the patient to achieve maximal success (see the Patient Teaching box). The four phases of cardiac rehabilitation are (1) inpatient management; (2) immediately after discharge, using telemetry monitoring during exercise; (3) later rehabilitation, which is unmonitored; and (4) maintenance. A team of health care providers (e.g., nurse, physician, physical therapist, nutritionist, social worker) plans the individual program. Education during the rehabilitation process should include normal anatomy and physiology of the heart; pathophysiology of CHD, angina, and MI; risk factor modification; activity and exercise; medications; diet; and when to seek medical advice. See the Nutrition Considerations box for a discussion of dietary considerations for patients with heart disease.

Patient Teaching

Myocardial Infarction

After myocardial infarction (MI), the following are some key points in the discharge teaching plan:

- It is very important to take your medications as prescribed and to contact your health care provider if you have any problems. (Provide written information about drug names, dosages, purpose, interactions with other medications and foods, and adverse effects that should be reported.)
- Your health care provider may prescribe a low-fat, low-sodium diet to decrease weight and to reduce the workload on your heart.
- Participation in cardiac rehabilitation will help you to become active again in a safe manner.
- Stop smoking. Smoking stimulates the heart rate and causes blood vessels to constrict, which makes the heart work harder.
- Maintain normal weight (or lose weight if obese) to decrease the work of the heart.
- The local chapter of the American Heart Association is a helpful resource for information and guidance on diet, smoking cessation, and exercise.

Nutrition Considerations

1. A major part of treatment for people with heart disease is reduction of fat and cholesterol in the diet.
2. When fats are used in cooking or eating, unsaturated fats (vegetable oil such as corn oil, canola oil, or olive oil) should be substituted for saturated fats (animal fat such as butter or lard).
3. Fats and oils used in cooking or eating should be limited to five to eight servings daily in normal adults.
4. Saturated fat can be limited by eating only 5 to 7 oz. of meat daily.
5. Foods that contain omega-3 fatty acids (certain fish, walnuts, and soybeans) lower serum triglycerides and decrease the number of deaths resulting from heart disease.

Put On Your Thinking Cap!

A new patient is being seen in the health care provider's office. Basic information and health history data include the following: 58-year-old White man, blood pressure 152/84 mm Hg, pulse 82 beats per minute, respiration 14 breaths per minute, temperature 98°F (36.7°C) measured orally, height 5'9", weight 190 lb.

PRESENT HEALTH

Real estate salesman (describes himself as "pretty successful" and able to maintain a good quality of life). Plays tennis 3 times a week; walks 2 miles, 4 times a week. Divorced father of three adult children; one son, who recently was admitted to rehabilitation for substance abuse, has no insurance. Patient has conflict with ex-wife related to son's situation. Enjoys a "few beers" in the evening. Has eggs, bacon, biscuits, coffee for breakfast; has lunch (sandwich, fries) at a fast-food restaurant; and cooks dinner (usually "meat and potatoes"). Sleeps 7 to 8 hours; usually rested on arising. Some recent trouble sleeping because of son's problems. No current significant other.

PAST HEALTH

Hypertension for 5 years treated with daily antihypertensive drug; chronic sinusitis; arthritis in left knee related to sports injury.

FAMILY HISTORY

Mother, 78 years of age, living and in moderately good health. Had mild stroke last year without permanent effects. Has diabetes. Father died suddenly at 66 years of age of myocardial infarction (MI). Two living brothers, 52 and 49 years of age. Both are hypertensive.

ANALYSIS

1. Based on the data available, identify modifiable and unmodifiable risk factors for coronary heart disease (CHD).
2. Identify one strategy to address each modifiable factor.
3. Identify current factors that reduce the patient's risk of CHD.

HEART FAILURE

HF is the inability of the heart to meet the metabolic demands of the body because the pumping ability of the heart is ineffective.

CAUSE AND RISK FACTORS

Recently, "heart failure" has replaced the term "congestive heart failure." Congestive heart failure (CHF) is an historic term used for HF because it describes the symptoms seen when the heart fails to pump effectively, causing the blood to "back up" into the vasculature of the lungs, producing congestion. The two terms (HF and CHF) may be seen and used interchangeably in the clinical setting. Causes of HF are primarily of two types: (1) disorders that increase the workload of the heart and (2) disorders that interfere with the pumping ability of the heart. Conditions that may precipitate HF include CAD, MI, cardiomyopathy, hypertension, chronic obstructive pulmonary disorder (COPD), pulmonary hypertension, anemia, disease of the heart valves, and fluid volume overload. Other conditions that increase metabolic needs, such as fever and pregnancy, may also precipitate HF. Approximately 6.5 million Americans have HF, and the number is expected to increase by 46% by 2030.

PATHOPHYSIOLOGY

HF results when the LV, RV, or both ventricles fail to pump blood adequately. The left side of the heart usually fails first. In time, the right side fails as a result of the left-sided failure. HF can be classified as *systolic HF* resulting from ineffective *pumping* of the ventricles or as *diastolic HF* resulting from impaired *filling* of the ventricles. With either classification, cardiac output is decreased. HF can occur acutely, with onset over several hours or days, or it can be chronic, with onset over months to years.

Compensation

Compensation is a term used to describe the cardiac and circulatory adjustments that maintain or restore cardiac output to normal or near normal. Major mechanisms by which compensation occurs are sympathetic nervous system stimulation, regulation of blood volume by the kidneys, and enlargement of the ventricular myocardium.

Sympathetic compensation. The sympathetic nervous system responds to reduced cardiac output and decreased blood pressure. Catecholamines are released that increase heart rate, stroke volume, cardiac output, and venous tone. Increased venous tone promotes systemic vascular resistance, venous return, and ventricular filling.

Renal compensation. The second mechanism that responds to decreased cardiac output is renal compensation. When cardiac output falls, so does renal perfusion, which initiates the renin-angiotensin-aldosterone (RAA) mechanism. Renin, secreted by the kidneys, activates angiotensinogen to convert to angiotensin I. Angiotensin I is converted to angiotensin II, which causes vasoconstriction and triggers release of aldosterone. Vasoconstriction raises the blood pressure by increasing peripheral resistance to blood flow. Aldosterone causes the kidneys to retain sodium and water, which increases blood volume.

Ventricular hypertrophy. The final mechanism is enlargement of the ventricular myocardium, called *ventricular hypertrophy*, in which increased blood volume raises the pressure in the ventricles causing the ventricles to dilate. Eventually the ventricle changes in size and shape, resulting in impaired pumping effectiveness. This process is called *ventricular remodeling*.

With time, the compensatory mechanisms are no longer able to meet the increased demands. When compensatory mechanisms are overwhelmed, acute HF syndrome occurs. Contractility decreases because the heart muscle can stretch only so far before becoming inefficient. The force of contraction of the LV decreases. Stroke volume and cardiac output decrease as pumping action fails. Afterload increases with left-sided HF. Blood backs up in the left atrium (LA) and then in the pulmonary veins. Because of the high pressure in the pulmonary veins (pulmonary hypertension), fluid leaks from the capillaries into the interstitial space and alveoli, causing pulmonary edema. Pulmonary hypertension eventually causes the right side of the heart to fail as well. Then blood returning to the right side of the heart from the body meets resistance from the pulmonary hypertension, which causes blood to back up into the venous system and organs. This results in peripheral edema and enlargement of the liver and spleen. If HF is not corrected, death eventually ensues.

With left-sided HF, the patient has increased LV end-diastolic pressure, increased LA pressure, increased pulmonary pressure, and resulting pulmonary edema as the excess fluid leaks into the lung tissues. In right-sided HF, right ventricle (RV) pressure increases, right atrial (RA) pressure increases, and fluid accumulates in the systemic vasculature.

Natriuretic peptides. Natriuretic peptides are neurohormonal substances released with HF. Atrial natriuretic peptide (ANP) is released in response to increased volume and stretch in the cardiac atria. BNP is released when the cardiac ventricles stretch, usually from increased blood volume. The natriuretic peptides are thought to counter the vasoconstrictive and volume-increasing effects of the sympathetic nervous system and the RAA system. BNP levels can be measured in the blood and can be used as a diagnostic tool for HF.

Put On Your Thinking Cap!

1. Explain why a patient with heart failure (HF) might (1) feel anxious and (2) gain weight.
2. A patient with HF is advised to try to lose 30 lb. What nursing strategies would help the patient to achieve this goal?
3. You suspect that a patient with HF and hypertension is not taking prescribed blood pressure medication regularly. What strategies might improve the patient's compliance?

CLINICAL MANIFESTATIONS

The patient with left-sided HF is typically anxious, pale, weak, and tachycardic. Consecutive blood pressure readings may show a downward trend. Auscultation of the lung fields may reveal crackles, wheezes, dyspnea, and cough. When assessing heart sounds, S_3 and S_4 may be heard as a result of the backup of fluid and the heart's inability to handle the excess fluid. The exchange of O_2 and CO_2 in the lungs is impaired and patients are often restless and confused.

With right-sided HF, the patient has increased central venous pressure, jugular venous distention, abdominal engorgement, and dependent edema. Anorexia, nausea, and vomiting may result from the abdominal engorgement. Patients commonly report fatigue, weight gain, and decreased urinary output.

MEDICAL DIAGNOSIS

The diagnosis of HF is made on the basis of the history, physical examination, radiographs, and laboratory test results. A chest radiograph may reveal hazy lung fields, distended vasculature, and cardiomegaly. An echocardiogram may reveal heart enlargement and ineffective ventricular contraction. Laboratory tests indicative of HF are decreased serum sodium and Hct, resulting from hemodilution and decreased saturated arterial oxygenation from poor pulmonary perfusion. The blood urea nitrogen (BUN) and creatinine are elevated with decreased renal function. BNP levels are elevated in HF, and the higher the levels, the more severe the failure. Liver function test results are elevated with hepatomegaly (liver enlargement). The patient who is critically ill with HF may require more intensive monitoring of hemodynamic parameters.

MEDICAL TREATMENT

Medical treatment of HF includes management of the underlying cause, drug therapy to improve cardiac output and eliminate excess fluid, conservative measures to decrease demands on the heart, and possibly cardiac resynchronization therapy (CRT). Sodium restriction is prescribed for most patients with HF.

Treatment of the underlying problem may involve interventions such as correction of dysrhythmias, management of hypertension, and valve replacement or repair.

Drug Therapy

Drugs used to treat HF include ACE inhibitors, diuretics, beta-adrenergic blockers, inotropic agents, cardiac glycosides, and nitrates. Patients who are worsening or having breathing problems may benefit from BNP (Natrecor). ACE inhibitors decrease preload and afterload by blocking the RAA system, resulting in vasodilation, decreased blood volume, and lower blood pressure. In addition, ACE inhibitors are thought to limit the progression of ventricular remodeling. Diuretics are prescribed to decrease circulating fluid volume and decrease preload. Loop diuretics such as furosemide (Lasix) are usually used in HF. Beta-adrenergic blockers improve survival rates by decreasing the heart rate, reducing the work of the heart, and lessening the O_2 demand of the myocardium. Inotropic agents such as dopamine may be prescribed initially for short-term management to improve cardiac contractility, improve renal perfusion, and decrease fluid retention. Digoxin, a cardiac glycoside with inotropic effects, is often prescribed and used long term to improve pump function by increasing contractility and decreasing heart rate. Nitrates, such as nitroglycerin, are vasodilators that reduce preload for patients with HF. This helps to reduce the workload on the heart. Morphine may be used to decrease anxiety, dilate the vasculature, and reduce myocardial O_2 consumption in the acute stage. Chapter 33 Table 33.9 provides additional information on drugs used to treat HF.

Other Therapies

Other therapies are available to decrease cardiac workload and increase myocardial oxygenation. The intraaortic balloon pump (IABP), ventricular assist devices (VADs), and CRT, also called *biventricular pacing*, may be used. The IABP is a temporary device used in the intensive care unit to increase cardiac output and coronary artery perfusion. VADs can partially or completely support a patient's failing heart. In some patients with HF, a VAD is a temporary intervention, used as a "bridge" to transplantation. Other patients may have long-term therapy, known as *destination therapy*, with a VAD instead of transplantation. CRT is useful in patients with HF who have conduction delays in the right or left bundle branch. The conduction delays lead to the depolarization of the ventricles and out of synchrony contractions, thus decreasing cardiac output and worsening of HF. In CRT, leads are placed in both ventricles and stimulated at the same time. Cardiac contraction occurs in both ventricles at the same time and cardiac output is improved.

Surgery

CABG surgery may be considered in patients with HF who experience angina. Valve repair or replacement is recommended when valve dysfunction contributes to the HF. Partial left ventriculectomy may be useful in some patients. Cardiac transplantation is often the last option for patients with end-stage HF whose symptoms are not responding to conventional therapy.

COMPLICATIONS

Common complications of treatment are dysrhythmias, pulmonary edema, renal failure, and cardiogenic shock.

❖ NURSING CARE OF THE PATIENT WITH HEART FAILURE

FOCUSED ASSESSMENT

Complete assessment of the cardiac patient is outlined in Chapter 33, Box 33.2 (see also the Nursing Care Plan: Patient With Heart Failure). Be sure to assess heart sounds, rate, and rhythm. The point of maximum impulse (PMI) should be noted and the apical and radial pulses assessed frequently. The nurse should inspect for jugular vein distention. A baseline respiratory assessment of rate, rhythm, and breath sounds is vital. In addition, the patient's weight and blood pressure should be measured accurately and the skin inspected and palpated for turgor and edema. Intake and output records and daily weights should be done to evaluate fluid retention or loss. If ordered, central venous pressure and hemodynamic readings should be assessed. The nurse should observe for dysrhythmias with cardiac monitoring. Nurses who work in intensive care units routinely interpret ECGs. Interpretation is discussed under "Electrocardiogram Monitoring" in Chapter 33.

Patient Problems, Goals, and Outcome Criteria: Heart Failure

Patient Problems	Goals and Outcome Criteria
Inadequate cardiac circulation related to mechanical failure	Improved cardiac circulation: normal heart rate and rhythm, fluid intake and output equal
Inadequate pulmonary oxygenation related to decreased pulmonary perfusion	Adequate pulmonary oxygenation: clear breath sounds, respiratory rate 12–20 breaths per minute without dyspnea
Increased extracellular fluid volume related to ineffective cardiac pumping	Normal fluid volume: no edema or dyspnea, blood pressure consistent with patient norms
Decreased mobility related to inability to meet oxygen (O_2) demands	Increase mobility: performance of activities of daily living (ADL) without fatigue
Anxiety related to difficulty breathing	Reduced anxiety: patient statement of reduced anxiety, calm manner

Interventions

Inadequate cardiac circulation. Give medications as ordered and monitor the patient for therapeutic and adverse effects. Older adult patients are more susceptible to adverse drug effects because they may metabolize and excrete drugs more slowly. This is especially true when the older patient is taking digoxin. Advise the patient to report early signs of digoxin toxicity: anorexia, nausea, and visual disturbances. Bed rest and stress reduction decrease the cardiac workload. When the patient is acutely ill, eliminate all unnecessary activity. Give partial baths rather than complete bed baths and assist the patient to change positions at least every 2 hours so that the skin can be inspected for signs of pressure. Visitors may be permitted but advise them to sit quietly with the patient for short periods.

Pharmacology Capsule

Before each dose of digoxin, the apical pulse is counted for 1 full minute. If the heart rate is less than 60 beats per minute, the drug is withheld and the health care professional is notified.

Pharmacology Capsule

The most common adverse effects of diuretic therapy are fluid and electrolyte imbalances.

Inadequate pulmonary oxygenation. Hypoxia is a common finding with left-sided HF because of pulmonary edema. This also occurs with right-sided HF because of decreased blood flow to the lungs. The patient with HF usually breathes easier in a semi-Fowler or high-Fowler position. Elevation of the upper body facilitates breathing by reducing pressure of the abdominal organs on the diaphragm. Supplemental O_2 is used for patients who are hypoxemic (with O_2 saturations of ≤90%) (Colucci, 2017). The O_2 flow rate is based on O_2 saturation and arterial blood gas values and may be reduced to 2 L/min for patients with chronic hypoxia. Assess the patient's respiratory status and blood gases frequently.

Prescribed bed rest can lead to other pulmonary complications related to immobility (i.e., pneumonia, pulmonary emboli, venous thromboembolism). Teach the patient to cough and deep breathe at least every 2 hours to promote respiratory excursion and to mobilize secretions. Other interventions to prevent complications of immobility are detailed in Chapter 12.

On discharge, the health care provider may order portable O_2 for use at home. The nurse or respiratory therapist instructs the patient in the use of the equipment and the safety precautions to take when using O_2 (see Chapter 25).

Increased extracellular fluid volume. Fluid retention is a response to HF (i.e., an attempt to maintain normal cardiac output). Unfortunately, it compounds the problem by increasing the workload on the heart. Thus measures are taken to reduce the fluid volume to normal while improving the function of the heart. Administer diuretics as ordered and monitor the patient for adverse effects. The most common adverse effects of diuretic therapy are fluid and electrolyte disturbances. Signs and symptoms that may indicate fluid or electrolyte disturbances include cardiac dysrhythmias, muscle weakness or twitching, cramps, changes in mental status, and abdominal distention. Frequent serum electrolyte measurements are usually ordered. Note the results and inform the health care provider of any abnormal findings. If hourly urine output is being measured, report an output of less than 30 mL/h to the health care provider as well. The patient should be weighed daily.

An IV catheter is usually placed to provide a route for drug and fluid administration. If IV fluids are administered, monitor the rate of administration very carefully. Fluid overload can occur very quickly in patients that are already experiencing symptoms of HF. If fluid retention is not relieved by other means, fluid restriction may be instituted. All staff should know the exact amount of fluid allowed and must record all intake. Fluid restriction can be very uncomfortable for the patient. Even with fluid volume excess, the patient may feel thirsty because of electrolyte imbalances. Present oral fluids in small containers and offer them at reasonable intervals. Provide frequent mouth care. The patient and family must understand why fluids are restricted so that the patient does not exceed the prescribed intake.

The most common therapeutic dietary measure for chronic HF is sodium restriction (see the Patient Teaching box). The patient may be limited to 1.5 g of sodium per day. Reduced sodium intake decreases fluid retention, thereby reducing the cardiac workload. In addition, reduced sodium intake is associated with better overall health outcomes, including fewer symptoms and hospitalizations and lower health care costs. For a 1.5 g sodium diet, advise the patient to avoid foods high in sodium (a list should be provided), not to add salt before or after cooking, and to use no more than two cups of milk products daily. Patients often have difficulty changing their use of seasonings. Acknowledge the difficulty and explain how sodium limitation contributes to improvement of cardiac function.

Patient Teaching

Chronic Heart Failure

- Reducing sodium in your diet will help to control swelling and reduce the workload on your heart.
- Excess weight makes your heart work harder. Your health care provider may prescribe a weight loss diet for you.
- Take your medications as prescribed to improve your heart function. (Provide written information about drug names, actions, dose, schedule, side and adverse effects, special aspects of administration, and interactions with other medications and food.)
- Gradually increase your activity. Avoid activity that causes shortness of breath or severe fatigue.
- Weigh yourself each morning, before breakfast, on the same scale and wearing the same amount of clothing.
- Contact your health care provider if you gain 3–5 lb in 1 week, develop a persistent cough, or have shortness of breath or chest pain.
- Resources: The American Heart Association provides information about diet and exercise. The Visiting Nurses Association or a home health agency can monitor your condition and help you in your home.

Identifying the type of diet prescribed on discharge as early as possible allows time for a dietary consultation to be arranged. The nurse and dietician often work collaboratively to teach the patient and family measures to adhere to the new diet. The person who prepares the patient's meals at home must be included in the teaching sessions.

Decreased mobility. Frequent rest periods, pacing of activities, and relaxation techniques help the patient to conserve energy. As the fluid volume is decreased and the cardiac output is increased, the patient can expect to be less fatigued.

The patient may be referred to a rehabilitation facility for rehabilitation. In general, the patient is advised to plan rest periods before and after tiring activities. Activity should be increased gradually, with rest periods taken when fatigue or dyspnea occurs. The health care provider may prescribe vasodilators for patients who experience chest pain with some activities. If monitoring is indicated after discharge, contact social services and request a referral to a home nursing agency.

Instruct the patient to notify the health care provider if the following problems develop; increasing dyspnea or edema; excessive fatigue; or pain that is not relieved by rest or prescribed medications. Early recognition of signs and symptoms that the patient's condition is deteriorating is crucial to prevent rehospitalization (see the Health Promotion box). In addition, advise the patient to avoid smoking and smoky environments and refrain from wearing constrictive clothing on the lower extremities.

Health Promotion

Heart Failure: Discharge Instructions

A major goal for patients with heart failure (HF) is to prevent rehospitalization. A critical factor in reaching this goal is for the patient and family members to recognize early signs and symptoms of worsening failure and to contact the health care provider. Examples of symptoms that require action are difficulty breathing (especially with activity); dry, hacking cough; weakness and increased fatigue; foot and ankle swelling; dizziness; and weight gain of 3–5 lb in 1 week or less.

Anxiety. Factors that may cause the patient to become anxious are dyspnea, unfamiliar setting and routines, and uncertainty about what is happening. Acknowledge the patient's anxiety and attempt to identify its basis. While taking immediate measures to relieve dyspnea, calmly explain what is being done. It may be helpful to tell the patient how specific measures help to relieve symptoms. The presence of family members may have a calming effect if the relatives understand that they, too, must remain calm.

Pharmacology Capsule

Older adults are more susceptible to adverse drug effects because they metabolize and excrete drugs more slowly.

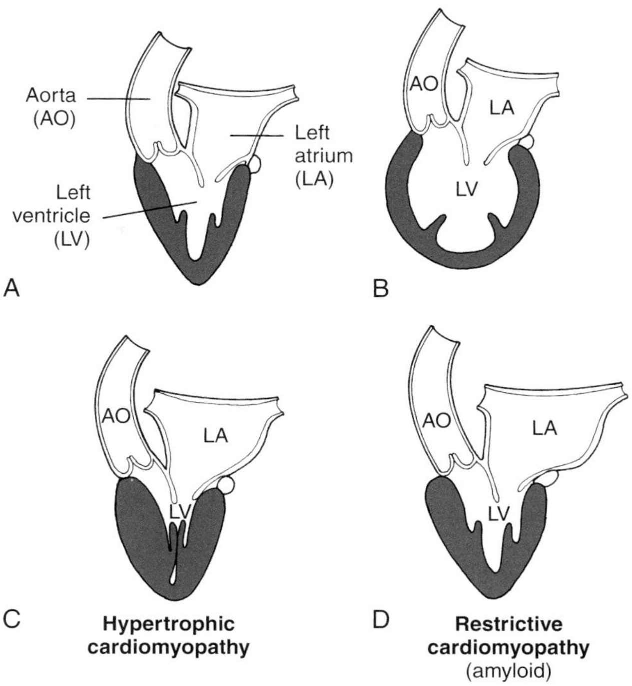

Fig. 35.8 Cardiomyopathy (CMP). (A) Normal heart. (B) Dilated CMP. (C) Hypertrophic CMP. (D) Restrictive CMP. (From McCance KL, Huether SE. *Understanding pathophysiology*, 5th ed. St. Louis, Mosby, 2013.)

Pharmacology Capsule

Patients who are taking immunosuppressive drugs to prevent rejection of transplanted tissue have reduced resistance to infection.

CARDIOMYOPATHY

CAUSE AND RISK FACTORS

Cardiomyopathy (CMP) is disease of the heart muscle. CMP may be secondary to another disease process or may be unknown. The disease usually leads to HF. Three major types of CMP are recognized: (1) dilated, (2) hypertrophic, and (3) restrictive (Fig. 35.8). Dilated CMP is the most common type. Many possible causes of dilated CMP exist, such as ischemia, hypertension, alcohol or drug abuse, infections, chemotherapy, pregnancy, and genetics.

Hypertrophic cardiomyopathy (HCM) is the most common inherited heart defect. In the United States, approximately 500,000 people have HCM, yet most are unaware that they have it. HCM is more common in younger individuals; many young athletes who die suddenly are found to have HCM. HCM can result from valvular heart disease or hypertension.

Restrictive CMP is the least common type of CMP. Amyloidosis, sarcoidosis, and other immunosuppressive disorders may predispose individuals to restrictive CMP.

PATHOPHYSIOLOGY

With dilated CMP, the patient has dilation of the ventricular chamber with severely impaired systolic function, resulting in decreased contractility, decreased ejection fraction and stroke volume, and increased LV end-diastolic pressure. Pressure backup results in dilation of all four chambers and is most pronounced in the ventricles. Excessive back pressure causes LV failure and consequent HF (see Fig. 35.8B).

In HCM, the LV hypertrophies and the ventricular septum thickens. The LV capacity diminishes, and the outflow track of the LV decreases in size. The size of the LA increases as a result of the back pressure. The exterior heart size may appear to be normal. Ventricular dysrhythmias are common (see Fig. 35.8C).

In restrictive CMP, the myocardium becomes rigid and noncompliant. This reduces ventricular filling and cardiac output, resulting in pulmonary and systemic congestion (see Fig. 35.8D).

CLINICAL MANIFESTATIONS

Dilated CMP is a progressive, chronic disease. The onset is gradual, with dyspnea, fatigue, left-sided HF, and moderate to severe cardiomegaly. Mitral valve regurgitation and S_3 and S_4 sounds are evident.

With hypertrophic CMP, the progression of symptoms is slow. Dyspnea, orthopnea, angina, fatigue, syncope, palpitations, ankle edema, and S_4 sounds are found.

With restrictive CMP, the primary symptom is exercise intolerance. Dyspnea, fatigue, right-sided HF, S_3 and S_4 sounds, and mitral valve regurgitation are also noted.

MEDICAL DIAGNOSIS

Diagnosis of dilated CMP is made primarily on the basis of an echocardiogram; cardiac enlargement may be noted on chest radiography. The echocardiogram and chest radiograph are also used to diagnose hypertrophic CMP. An enlarged LV may be accompanied by LA enlargement. The diagnosis of restrictive CMP is demonstrated by decreased cardiac output and HF and must be differentiated from pericarditis. An echocardiogram may show impaired diastolic function and decreased ventricular size.

MEDICAL TREATMENT

Supportive measures are used for dilated CMP. Inotropic drugs to improve cardiac contractility and cardiac output; diuretics to decrease preload; and ACE inhibitors and vasodilators to decrease afterload provide this type of therapy. Anticoagulants may be used to prevent thrombi. If all other measures fail, the patient will need a heart transplant. Medical treatment for hypertrophic CMP includes antidysrhythmic agents, antibiotics, anticoagulants, calcium channel blockers, and beta-blockers. Surgical incision of the hypertrophied septal muscle and resection of some of the hypertrophied muscle may be considered for hypertrophic CMP. A nonsurgical alternative for reduction of the hypertrophied septum is the use of alcohol ablation (cutting) that can be done percutaneously in the cardiac catheterization laboratory. Treatment of restrictive CMP is similar to that of HF therapy. Heart transplantation may be considered. Complications observed with all types of CMP are dysrhythmias, HF, and death.

NURSING CARE OF THE PATIENT WITH CARDIOMYOPATHY

FOCUSED ASSESSMENT

Patients are primarily assessed for HF. Be alert for dyspnea, cough, edema, dysrhythmias, and decreased cardiac output.

Patient Problems, Goals, and Outcome Criteria: Cardiomyopathy

Patient Problems	Goals and Outcome Criteria
Inadequate cardiac circulation related to ventricular failure	Improved cardiac circulation: normal pulse and blood pressure
Decreased mobility related to poor tissue perfusion	Increased mobility: performance of daily activities without excessive fatigue
Anxiety related to a new cardiac diagnosis	More positive outlook: patient's expression of feelings about condition and hopeful statements

INTERVENTIONS

The care of these patients is similar to that of patients with HF. In addition, a hopeful atmosphere and a careful explanation of care requirements are necessary. Encourage the family to support the patient. The teaching plan guides the patient to make lifestyle changes. Increasing knowledge about the disease is often empowering and can encourage the patient to make decisions and choices in living with a chronic illness.

CARDIAC TRANSPLANTATION

Transplantation is considered for end-stage HF that is not responding to therapy, CMP, and severe inoperable CHD. More than 5000 heart transplants occur around the world each year; however, almost 50,000 people are candidates for transplantation. Because of the critical shortage of organs, criteria for heart transplantation have been established to ensure

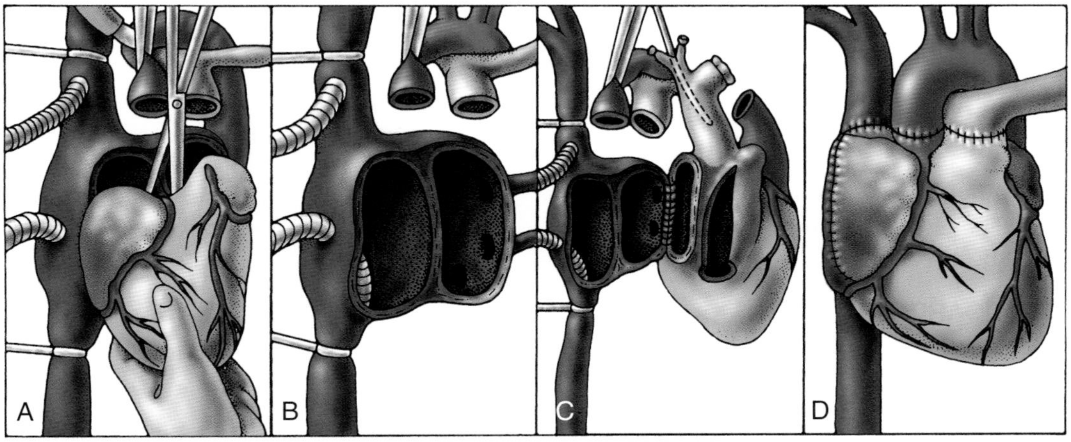

Fig. 35.9 Heart transplantation. (A) After the recipient is placed on cardiopulmonary bypass (CPB), the heart is removed. (B) The posterior walls of the recipient's left and right atria are left intact. (C) The left atrium (LA) of the donor heart is anastomosed to the recipient's residual posterior atrial walls and the other atrial walls, the atrial septum, and the great vessels are joined. (D) Postoperative result.

the best potential outcomes. The United Network for Organ Sharing (UNOS) has a system to fairly distribute available organs for transplantation. A number of factors exclude patients from heart transplantation:

- Systemic illness with a life expectancy less than two years despite heart transplantation
- Irreversible pulmonary hypertension
- Clinically severe symptomatic cerebrovascular disease
- Active substance abuse (drug, tobacco, or alcohol)
- Multiple demonstrations of inability to comply with drug therapy.

Other possible conditions that may be considered include neoplasms, irreversible renal dysfunction, COVID-19, infections, obesity, inadequate social support or a cognitive-behavioral disability, frailty and tuberculosis.

Just as the recipient must meet specific criteria, the donor must as well to ensure the best possible outcomes. The criteria include brain death according to established criteria, no malignancies outside the central nervous system (CNS), free of infection, and not have experienced severe chest trauma. Prolonged advanced life support measures are avoided. The donor and recipient organs are carefully matched with consideration to physical size and needs of the recipient as well as the proximity of the donor to the recipient. The donor heart may be preserved for 4 to 6 hours before transplantation making proximity a critical element in organ allocation.

The recipient is prepared for surgery as with any open-heart procedure. CPB is initiated, and the recipient's heart is removed except for the posterior portions of the atria (Fig. 35.9). The donor heart is trimmed and anastomosed to the remaining native heart. The patient is removed from bypass, the heart is restarted, and the chest is closed.

Aftercare of the patient with a heart transplant is similar to that of the patient after coronary artery bypass surgery. Hemodynamic monitoring, mechanical ventilation, cardiac assessment, care of chest tubes, and accurate intake and output measurements are vital. Immediately after surgery, the patient is placed in a private room in the intensive care unit. Gowns, masks, and careful and frequent hand washing are used to protect the patient from infection. Invasive lines and tubes (e.g., endotracheal tube, pulmonary artery catheter, Foley catheter, chest tubes) are removed as rapidly as possible to decrease the chance of infection. The prevention of postoperative infection is the primary goal. Pulmonary infections are most frequently found after heart transplantations. Moving the patient from the intensive care unit to a private room and then to home as soon as possible decreases the incidence of nosocomial infections. Patients and families are taught the signs and symptoms of infection and to avoid crowds and others with infections.

In addition, the patient with a transplant receives immunosuppressive medications. Lifelong immunosuppression is administered to prevent the body from rejecting the donated heart, which it recognizes as foreign tissue. Initially, large doses of corticosteroids are administered, and the dose is decreased over time. At the first indication of rejection (increased temperature, infection, dyspnea, malaise, fatigue, dysrhythmia), the steroid dose is usually increased. Many other drugs can be used to prevent and treat rejection. Examples include azathioprine (Imuran) and cyclosporine (Neoral). Protocols using several immunosuppressive agents are considered most effective. Reduced dosages of each drug provide for a lower incidence of toxicity.

Rejection is monitored through endomyocardial biopsies. These are performed frequently in the period immediately after transplantation and less frequently over time. Patients are taught to monitor their own progress and to report problems promptly. The transplant team monitors patients closely and observes them for infection, rejection, quality of life, and complications. Common complications noted after heart transplantation, other than rejection and infection, are hypertension, elevated cholesterol, obesity, and malignancies.

INFLAMMATORY DISORDERS

Inflammation of the heart most often results from systemic infections. The endocardium, myocardium, and pericardium may be affected.

INFECTIVE ENDOCARDITIS

Microbial infections of the endocardium primarily affect the valves. Organisms present in the blood easily colonize valves damaged by rheumatic heart disease, congenital defects or a mitral valve that is prolapsed.

Although the incidence of infective endocarditis (IE) has decreased with the use of antibiotic drugs, the problem has increased in IV drug users. The more frequent use of invasive intravascular catheters for severely compromised patients has also contributed to the frequency of IE.

Patients with known valvular disease are also at risk for IE. They should be treated with prophylactic antibiotics before dental or invasive procedures. Immunosuppression or any source of bacterial contamination (lacerations, pneumonia, invasive procedures, IV drug use with contaminated needles) places patients at risk.

Pathophysiology

Pathogens, usually bacteria, enter the bloodstream by any of the previously mentioned means. The pathogen accumulates on the heart valves, the endocardium, or both and forms vegetation. The mitral valve is the most common site for vegetation. The turbulence of the blood flow through the heart weakens the vegetation and causes pieces to break off; these emboli can then obstruct circulation and impair tissue perfusion in the lungs, brain, kidneys, and heart.

Complications

Complications of IE include HF and embolization. HF is the most frequent cause of death with IE.

Clinical Manifestations

Patients usually have fever, chills, malaise, fatigue, and weight loss. The fever may be low grade (99°F–102°F/37.2°C–38.9°C) or higher (102°F–105°F/38.9°C–40.6°C). The fever is accompanied by chills and night sweats. Chest or abdominal pain may be reported, possibly indicating embolization. Vegetative fragments and microembolization can produce petechiae inside the mouth and on the ankles, feet, and antecubital areas. Pea-sized, tender, red to purple lesions known as *Osler nodes* may be on the patient's fingertips or toes. Janeway lesions (flat, red, painless spots) may be noted on palms and soles. A new or changing heart murmur is noted in most patients (usually mitral or aortic).

Medical Diagnosis

The diagnosis of IE is based on the history, physical examination, and results of laboratory studies. A history of recent dental or surgical procedures may precede IE. Auscultation may reveal a heart murmur. Echocardiography helps to visualize vegetation and valvular regurgitation. Right-sided or left-sided HF may be evident. Serial blood cultures may give clues to the causative organism or organisms. The WBC count may be elevated.

Medical Treatment

Antimicrobial drugs, rest, and limitation of activities are the primary therapeutic measures for IE. Antimicrobials are given intravenously for 2 to 6 weeks, depending on the organism. The patient is hospitalized initially and then receives home IV therapy. Prophylactic anticoagulants may be necessary. Surgery may be necessary to replace an infected valve. Historically, prophylactic antibiotics were given before dental, genitourinary, and respiratory procedures for patients with any type of heart murmur. Evidence suggests this does not affect the rate of IE and prophylactic antibiotics are only recommended for a few very high-risk patients before certain dental and procedures.

❖ NURSING CARE OF THE PATIENT WITH INFECTIVE ENDOCARDITIS

Focused Assessment

Complete assessment of the cardiac patient is summarized in Chapter 33, Box 33.2. With IE, review the patient's history for risk factors, recent invasive procedures, known pathologic cardiac conditions, and onset of symptoms. Also assess for temperature elevation, heart murmur, evidence of HF (cough, peripheral edema), and embolization.

Patient Problems, Goals, and Outcome Criteria: Infective Endocarditis

Patient Problems	Goals and Outcome Criteria
Inadequate cardiac circulation related to impaired valve function	Normal cardiac output: normal pulse and blood pressure
Decreased mobility related to fatigue and prolonged intravenous therapy	Resumption of usual physical activities without symptoms: performance of activities of daily living (ADL) without fatigue
Potential for inadequate cardiac tissue perfusion related to embolization	Normal tissue perfusion: absence of dyspnea or signs of circulatory obstruction

Interventions

Administer antibiotics as prescribed. Throughout the course of the illness, it is important to continue to assess cardiac output and monitor for complications. Teach the patient about the medications prescribed and any restrictions imposed. Encourage the patient to get adequate rest, which is necessary during the healing process. Range-of-motion exercises may be necessary during the acute stage and until the patient is ambulatory.

MYOCARDITIS

Myocarditis is an inflammatory disease of the cardiac muscle caused primarily by viruses; however, other pathogens including bacteria, fungi, protozoa, and helminths also may be responsible. Infections such as acute rheumatic fever and autoimmune disorders such as systemic lupus erythematosus are frequently associated with myocarditis. In addition, drug reactions, including cocaine abuse, may be precipitating factors.

Clinical Manifestations

Symptoms may vary according to the type and cause of the condition. Symptoms include HF (tiredness, decreased exercise tolerance, edema of the feet and legs, difficulty breathing); chest pain; arrhythmias, and sudden cardiac death.

Medical Diagnosis

Diagnostic tests include blood tests to measure enzyme levels; ECG; MRI; chest radiograph to observe for pulmonary edema or enlarged heart; and echocardiogram or "echo" to measure the walls and chambers of the heart as well as pumping ability and valve functioning. Cardiac catheterization measures pressures inside the heart and blood vessels. During a cardiac catheterization, coronary angiography may be done that shows blockage or narrowing of cardiac arteries. In addition, a biopsy also may be done during a cardiac catherization.

Medical Treatment

Treatment of myocarditis is similar to that of various types of heart disease, particularly HF, arrythmias, systemic embolus or ventricular thrombus. Specific drugs are used to treat each condition, such as anticoagulation for atrial fibrillation or thrombi, antiarrhythmias for ventricular arrythmias, and diuretics and ACE inhibitors or beta-blockers for HF. Immunosuppressive therapy is suggested for specific types of myocarditis. Nonsteroidal antiinflammatory drugs should be avoided, especially with HF. In addition, heavy alcohol consumption should be discouraged. Physical activity should be restricted to reduce the work of the heart.

NURSING CARE OF THE PATIENT WITH MYOCARDITIS

Nursing care is focused on managing the signs and symptoms of HF. Patients should be kept in a semi-Fowler's position to decrease cardiac workload. Rest is encouraged by providing a quiet environment with spacing of activity and rest periods. Administer medications as ordered. If a patient has anxiety because of the myocarditis diagnosis, take measures to help decrease anxiety such as guided imagery, meditation, and emotional support.

PERICARDITIS

Pericarditis is an inflammation of the pericardial sac (*pericardium*) and can be a primary disease or associated with another inflammatory process. The disease may be acute or chronic. Viruses, bacteria, fungi, trauma, or MI can cause acute pericarditis. Tuberculosis, radiation, or metastases cause chronic pericarditis.

Pathophysiology

In acute pericarditis, the inflammatory process causes an increase in the amount of pericardial fluid and inflammation of the pericardial membranes. In chronic pericarditis (also called *constrictive pericarditis*), scarring of the pericardium fuses the visceral and parietal pericardia together. Loss of elasticity results from the scarring. This constrictive process prevents adequate ventricular filling.

Complications

The major complication of pericarditis is *pericardial effusion* or accumulation of fluid in the pericardial space. This may lead to *cardiac tamponade* (pericardial tamponade) in which fluid in the pericardium builds up, resulting in compression of the heart. The onset may be rapid or gradual. Symptoms typically include those of cardiogenic shock including shortness of breath, weakness, lightheadedness, and cough. Diagnostic signs include hypotension, jugular venous distension and quiet heart sounds (together known as Beck's triad), and peripheral edema. A pericardial rub may be present because of inflammation. Diagnostic tests include ECG, chest radiograph, or cardiac ultrasound. If fluid increases slowly the pericardial sac can expand to contain more than 2 L; however, if the increase is rapid, as little as 200 mL can result in tamponade. When sufficient fluid accumulation decreases ventricular filling, the resulting drop in cardiac output is an emergency. Treatment for pericardial effusion is by pericardiocentesis to drain the accumulated fluid.

Clinical Manifestations

Chest pain is the hallmark symptom of pericarditis. The pain is most severe on inspiration and is most often sharp and stabbing but may be described as *dull* or *burning*. The pain may be relieved by sitting up and leaning forward. Dyspnea, chills, and fever accompany pericarditis. ST segment elevation may be noted on the ECG. A pericardial rub may be present.

Medical Diagnosis

The diagnostic challenge is to differentiate pericarditis from MI. Serial ECGs show that the ST segment elevation resolves in several weeks. QRS complex measurements may decrease because of the accumulated fluid in the pericardial space. An echocardiogram may show pericardial thickening and effusion. Atrial fibrillation may occur because of the irritation. The troponin may be elevated. Blood cultures may identify the causative organism or organisms. One differentiating feature to consider is that position change does not relieve ischemic chest pain or angina whereas the chest pain that accompanies pericarditis is often relieved by a change in position.

Medical Treatment

The patient is treated with analgesics, antipyretics, antiinflammatory agents, and antibiotics. With constrictive pericarditis, the patient would be treated as for HF. As noted earlier, pericardiocentesis to remove the accumulated fluid would be performed with cardiac tamponade. Surgical creation of a pericardial window (removal of a segment of parietal pericardium to allow continuous drainage of pericardial fluid) may be necessary to treat chronic pericarditis with effusion.

❖ NURSING CARE OF THE PATIENT WITH PERICARDITIS

Focused Assessment

General nursing assessment of the cardiac patient is summarized in Chapter 33, Box 33.2. With pericarditis, assessment of heart sounds is especially important.

Patient Problems, Goals, and Outcome Criteria: Pericarditis

Patient Problems	Goals and Outcome Criteria
Pain related to pericardial inflammation	Pain relief: patient statement that pain is reduced, relaxed manner
Impaired cardiac circulation related to pericardial constriction	Improved cardiac output: normal pulse and blood pressure
Anxiety related to illness	Decreased anxiety: patient statement that anxiety is reduced, calm manner

Interventions

Rest and reduction of activity decrease the workload of the heart. Administer medications and teach the patient about them. Emotional support from the nursing staff and significant others is vital. The patient can be instructed in relaxation techniques. Monitor vital signs and auscultate for a pericardial friction rub. The rub is heard during inspiration with the diaphragm of the stethoscope placed between the second and fourth intercostal spaces at the left sternal border. The rub is heard when no fluid accumulation is present. Distant heart sounds may be heard when fluid accumulation exists. Be sure to note pain characteristics and response to analgesics and antiinflammatory agents. Also monitor the ECG for dysrhythmias.

VALVULAR DISEASE

The purpose of the heart valves is to maintain blood flow in one direction. If the valves are damaged through a congenital defect or acquired disease, their function is compromised. Stenosis and insufficiency are the two major valve problems. Stenosis is narrowing of the valvular opening. A stenotic valve limits the amount of blood ejected from one chamber to the next. Regurgitation (also called *insufficiency*) is the inability of the valve to close completely allowing the blood to flow backward when a valve does not close. The left side of the heart is affected most often, and the mitral valve is the most frequently affected of all the valves. The pulmonic valve in the right side of the heart is infrequently affected. Only left-sided valvular disease is discussed here.

Antibiotics have decreased the incidence of valvular disease from rheumatic fever but the incidence of nonrheumatic valvular disease has increased. Longer life span and IV drug use are the primary causes of the increasing incidence of nonrheumatic valvular disease.

MITRAL STENOSIS

Mitral stenosis is a narrowing of the opening in the mitral valve that impedes blood flow from the LA to the LV. The mitral valve leaflets become thickened and fibrotic. Rheumatic heart disease is the leading cause of mitral stenosis. Congenital malformations of the mitral valve occur but are not common. Other causes are calcium accumulation on valve leaflets and atrial myxomas (tumors).

Pathophysiology

The thickening of the valve structures reduces the outflow of blood from the LA to LV. The LA dilates to accommodate the amount of blood not ejected and LA pressure increases. As LA pressure increases, the blood volume backs up into the pulmonary system, increasing pulmonary pressures. This increases the workload on the right side of the heart, leading to RV hypertrophy. Eventually, the RV fails and cardiac output decreases because less blood is delivered to the LV.

Clinical Manifestations

Symptoms may begin soon after the disease process or may be delayed for many years. Dyspnea, fatigue, cough, chest pain, and activity intolerance are the most frequent symptoms. Exertional dyspnea and pulmonary edema occur as blood backs up in the pulmonary system and serous fluid leaks into the pulmonary tissues. Because stenosis causes turbulent blood flow through the valve, a murmur is

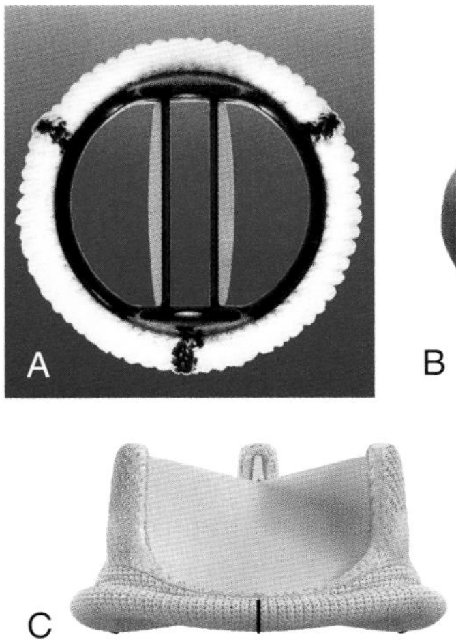

Fig. 35.10 Types of prosthetic and tissue valves. (A) St. Jude Medical Masters HP Series Mechanical Heart Valve. (B) Freestyle Valve. (C) Carpentier-Edwards PERIMOUNT Magna Ease aortic heart valve. (A, St. Jude Medical is a trademark of St. Jude Medical, Inc. or its related companies. Reprinted with permission of St. Jude Medical, Copyright 2014. All rights reserved. B, FreeStyle™ Bioprosthesis valve ©Medtronic 2018. C, Used with permission from Edwards Lifesciences LLC, Irvine, CA. Edwards, Edwards Lifesciences, the stylized E logo, Carpentier-Edwards, Carpentier-Edwards Classic, Magna, Magna Ease, Magna Mitral Ease are trademarks of Edwards Lifesciences Corporation.)

present during diastole (best heard at the apex of the heart).

Medical Diagnosis

Diagnosis is made on the basis of the patient history, physical examination, and results of diagnostic procedures. The chest radiograph shows LA, RV, and pulmonary vascular enlargement. Echocardiography, often TEE, is used to visualize the mitral valve. Cardiac catheterization is used to confirm the diagnosis and determine the extent of the disease process.

Medical Treatment

When symptomatic, the patient with mitral stenosis is treated as for HF with drug therapy, sodium and fluid restrictions, and activity restriction. Digoxin, diuretics, beta-blockers, and antidysrhythmic agents may be prescribed. If the patient has atrial fibrillation, anticoagulant agents may also be prescribed.

Surgical Treatment

Surgical treatment includes commissurotomy, mitral valve replacement, and balloon valvuloplasty. Commissurotomy is excision of parts of the leaflets to enlarge the opening. The mitral valve may be replaced with a biologic or mechanical valve (Fig. 35.10). The choice between biological and mechanical replacement valves is influenced by age, other systemic diseases and personal choice. Mechanical valves most often are implanted in younger patients (age <65 years) and can last between 20 and 30 years. Blood clots may form on mechanical valves, so anticoagulants may be necessary. Biological valves, also known as bioprosthetic valves, primarily come from cows or pigs. Biological valves typically last between 10 and 15 years, so patients may require additional replacement surgery at some point. Anticoagulants are not required because there is a lower risk of blood clots. Biological valves are best for people over age 65, those with kidney disease, who are pregnant, cannot take Coumadin or have a high risk for bleeding. Both commissurotomy and mitral valve replacement require major surgery with CPB.

Balloon valvuloplasty, a procedure done in the cardiac catheterization laboratory, has been very successful in dilating stenosed heart valves. This procedure is less invasive than valve replacement or commissurotomy. To dilate the mitral valve, a balloon catheter (similar to the one used for PTCA) is threaded from the femoral artery to the mitral valve. The balloon is positioned in the valve and inflated until the valve opens sufficiently. After the procedure, the patient is observed closely for dysrhythmias and complications. Complications include valve regurgitation, restenosis, perforation of the myocardium, and, rarely, systemic embolization.

❖ NURSING CARE OF THE PATIENT WITH MITRAL STENOSIS

Focused Assessment

Obtain a complete history as summarized in Chapter 33, Box 33.2 and a record of signs and symptoms being experienced. Take the patient's vital signs and auscultate for heart murmurs. The murmur of mitral stenosis is described as *rumbling* and *low pitched* and is heard best at the apex of the heart. The ECG may show a notched P wave, indicating LA enlargement. Atrial fibrillation, tachycardia, and tachypnea are common signs. The pulse pressure may decrease, indicating low cardiac output. Jugular venous distention and crackles are found with pulmonary congestion.

Patient Problems, Goals, and Outcome Criteria: Mitral Stenosis

The patient problems and goals for mitral stenosis are the same as those for congestive heart failure (CHF) and for all valvular diseases.

Patient Problems	Goals and Outcome Criteria
Inadequate cardiac circulation related to narrowing or insufficiency of the valve	Increased cardiac output: normal pulse and blood pressure
Inadequate pulmonary oxygenation related to pulmonary congestion	Improved pulmonary oxygenation: clear breath sounds, normal arterial blood gases (ABGs)

Continued

Patient Problems, Goals, and Outcome Criteria: Mitral Stenosis—cont'd

Patient Problems	Goals and Outcome Criteria
Decreased mobility related to imbalance between oxygen (O_2) supply and demand	Improved mobility: performance of daily activities without excessive fatigue
Increased extracellular fluid volume related to decreased glomerular filtration rate, increased aldosterone, sodium and water retention, and increased antidiuretic hormone (ADH) release	Normal fluid balance: no edema, clear breath sounds, fluid output equal to or exceeds fluid intake

Interventions

See the section titled "Nursing Care of the Patient With Heart Failure" for the remainder of the nursing process.

MITRAL REGURGITATION

Mitral **regurgitation** (insufficiency) allows blood to flow back into the LA during diastole. The valve does not close completely because one or both of the valve leaflets becomes rigid and shortens.

The LA and LV hypertrophy as a result of the backflow of blood against the incompetent valve. The LV hypertrophies in an attempt to maintain cardiac output. Eventually, the left side of the heart fails, and symptoms are then the same as with mitral stenosis.

The murmur of mitral regurgitation is high pitched and blowing and occurs during systole. This murmur is best heard at the apex and may radiate to the axilla. With severe disease, S_3 and S_4 sounds may be auscultated. Atrial fibrillation occurs as the LA enlarges.

Mitral regurgitation is treated with vasodilators to decrease the afterload and therefore the regurgitation. Other medical treatment includes activity restriction, dietary sodium limitation, diuretics, and digoxin. Surgical treatment includes annuloplasty and mitral valve replacement. Annuloplasty is reconstruction of the leaflets and the aortic annulus, a fibrous ring at the aortic opening to the front and right of the atrioventricular aortic valve.

MITRAL VALVE PROLAPSE

The mitral valve prolapses when one or both leaflets enlarge and protrude into the LA during systole. It has a tendency to run in families and may be caused by heart infections, rheumatic fever, or a wide variety of congenital anomalies. The disease is usually benign but may progress to mitral insufficiency.

In most patients, symptoms do not occur or may occur with stress. Symptoms include chest pain, palpitations, dizziness, and syncope. Some patients exhibit dysrhythmias. The ECG usually shows normal findings. Evidence of mitral valve prolapse may be found on echocardiography. The problem is often controlled with stress reduction techniques. Beta-blockers may be prescribed to decrease syncope, palpitations, and severe chest pain. Therapeutic management is matched to the degree of symptoms.

AORTIC STENOSIS

Cause and Risk Factors

Stenosis of the aortic valve occurs when the valve cusps become fibrotic and calcify. Aortic stenosis may be caused by a congenital malformation or result from rheumatic fever, syphilis, or the aging process (atherosclerosis and calcification). When seen in younger patients, it is most often caused by a congenital malformation. The aortic valve is most commonly diseased in the aging population.

Pathophysiology. The valve opening decreases to one-third its normal size before symptoms occur. As flow becomes impeded through the narrowed valve, the LV hypertrophies to compensate for the extra pressure needed to eject blood. The LA also compensates by delivering a strong atrial kick. These compensatory mechanisms allow normal function until atrial fibrillation disrupts the atrial kick or until the LV hypertrophies to the point of dysfunction, with decreased cardiac output and myocardial ischemia. With LV dysfunction, blood backs up into the LA and the pulmonary system. If uncorrected, eventually the right side of the heart fails.

Clinical Manifestations

The patient reports dyspnea on exertion, angina, and syncope. Fatigue, orthopnea, and paroxysmal nocturnal dyspnea are late symptoms and indicate HF. A systolic murmur may occur.

Medical Diagnosis

The chest radiograph shows atrial and ventricular enlargement, which are late signs. The murmur of aortic stenosis is heard best in the aortic area, the second intercostal space to the right of the sternum. The echocardiogram shows LV wall thickening. An ETT may be ordered to evaluate heart function.

Medical Treatment

HF is treated with digoxin, diuretics, a low-sodium diet, and activity restriction. Surgical treatment includes balloon valvuloplasty and aortic valve replacement.

❖ NURSING CARE OF THE PATIENT WITH AORTIC STENOSIS

The nurse should monitor for a bounding arterial pulse and widened pulse pressure. The nursing process is the same as for HF (see the Nursing Care Plan: Patient With Heart Failure box).

Nursing Care Plan Patient With Heart Failure

FOCUSED ASSESSMENT

Health History

A 73-year-old Chinese-American woman is admitted through the emergency department. She is a retired business owner who lives alone and has no immediate family in the area. She began having dyspnea and orthopnea that has become progressively worse over the past 3 days. Her past medical history includes a myocardial infarction 1 year ago and a 10-year history of hypertension treated with diet and a beta-blocker daily. In addition to the beta-blocker, she takes only an occasional laxative. She reports fatigue, restlessness, nervousness, irritability, insomnia, anorexia, and a productive cough with pink sputum.

Physical Examination Vital signs: blood pressure 168/96 mm Hg, pulse 104 beats per minute with slight irregularity, respiration 24 breaths per minute, temperature 98°F (36.7°C) measured orally. Height 5′2″, weight 152 lb (a 7-lb increase in 1 week). Her oxygen (O_2)saturation is 87. She is alert but appears anxious. Her skin is pale and diaphoretic. An S_3 is present. Jugular vein distention is noted. Auscultation of the lungs reveals crackles in the lower lobes of both lungs. The abdomen is distended. Bowel sounds are present in all four quadrants and 3+ pitting edema exists in both feet and ankles.

She is being admitted to the telemetry unit for treatment, where she will have continuous electrocardiogram (ECG) and be placed on O_2.

Patient Problems	Goals and Outcome Criteria	Interventions
Inadequate cardiac circulation related to decreased myocardial contractility	The patient's cardiac circulation will improve, as evidenced by normal heart rate and rhythm, normal blood pressure, normal hemodynamic measures, and breath sounds clear to auscultation.	Monitor the patient's vital signs, heart and lung sounds, level of consciousness, and electrocardiography. Enforce bed rest, with the head of the bed elevated. Schedule activities to allow rest. Request small, frequent meals. Administer vasodilators and angiotensin-converting enzyme (ACE) inhibitors as ordered.
Inadequate pulmonary oxygenation related to pulmonary congestion	The patient's pulmonary oxygenation will be evidenced by pulse oximetry >95%, normal skin color, absence of dyspnea, and clear lung sounds.	Assess lung sounds and respiratory status every 4 hours. Monitor her O_2 saturation. Elevate the head of the bed. Administer O_2 as ordered. Assist to cough and deep breathe every 2 hours. Administer diuretics as ordered.
Fluid volume excess related to decreased glomerular filtration rate, increased aldosterone, sodium and water retention, and increased antidiuretic hormone (ADH) release	The patient will have normal fluid balance as evidenced by weight of 145 lb, absence of edema, absence of crackles and wheezes in lungs, and ability to participate in activities of daily living (ADL) without dyspnea.	Monitor for jugular venous distention and peripheral edema. Auscultate heart and lung sounds every 4 hours. Measure weight daily and record her intake and output accurately. Maintain intravenous lines and correct fluid infusion rate. Administer diuretics as ordered. Teach the patient about sodium restriction and the rationale behind it. Protect any edematous extremities from pressure or injury.
Decreased mobility related to imbalance between O_2 supply and demand	The patient's mobility will improve, as evidenced by performance of ADL without excessive fatigue or dyspnea.	Assess response to activity when permitted. Monitor her for dyspnea and changes in vital signs. Limit fatiguing activities. Gradually increase activity as her tolerance improves.
Anxiety related to hypoxia, life-threatening situation	The patient's anxiety will be reduced, as evidenced by calm demeanor and statement that she feels less anxious.	Explain the procedures and equipment used. Tell her about heart failure (HF) and how it is being treated. Point out signs of improvement. Visit often and respond to the call bell promptly. Offer to engage the help of a spiritual counselor if desired.
Lack of knowledge of condition, treatment, self-care, and resources related to lack of exposure to information.	The patient will verbalize information about her condition, treatment, self-care measures, and resources.	Provide a simple explanation of heart failure (HF), its effects, and its treatment. As discharge nears, discuss diet, exercise, and drug therapy. Explain signs and symptoms that should be reported to her physician. Advise the patient of services offered by the American Heart Association. Explore sources of support and the need for a visiting nurse or home health services.

Critical Thinking Questions

1. What is the rationale behind sodium restriction in patients with HF?
2. Describe three signs of improvement in a patient with HF.

AORTIC REGURGITATION

Aortic regurgitation (also called *insufficiency*) occurs when fibrosis and thickening of the aortic cusps cause the valve to no longer maintain unidirectional blood flow. Aortic regurgitation is caused primarily by rheumatic fever. Other causes include IE, blunt chest trauma, calcification of the valve, and chronic hypertension.

Regurgitation of blood into the LV during diastole increases the amount of blood in the LV. The LV dilates and hypertrophies. Myocardial ischemia and LV failure occur. Blood backs up into the pulmonary system and eventually RV failure occurs.

The murmur of aortic regurgitation is high pitched and blowing and occurs in diastole. It is auscultated best at the aortic area. The point of maximal impulse may be shifted to the left and down. Tachycardia and palpitations are compensatory mechanisms. Later signs of HF such as fatigue, dyspnea, and ascites develop. A widened pulse pressure (increased difference between systolic and diastolic pressures) results from a low diastolic pressure. S_3 and S_4 sounds are often auscultated.

LA and LV dilation are noted on chest radiography. The echocardiogram shows left ventricular dilation. Cardiac catheterization is used to determine the extent of incompetence.

Digoxin and diuretics are prescribed for LV hypertrophy. Aortic valve replacement provides long-term correction.

Get Ready for the NCLEX® Examination!

Key Points

- Risk factors for atherosclerosis are age, gender, heredity, diabetes mellitus, serum cholesterol, tobacco smoking, hypertension, overweight and obesity, and physical inactivity.
- Stable angina is the pain that results from temporary myocardial ischemia and is treated with vasodilators and rest.
- Procedures used to improve myocardial blood flow include percutaneous coronary balloon angioplasty, stent placement, laser angioplasty, atherectomy, coronary artery bypass graft (CABG), and transmyocardial laser revascularization (TMR).
- Myocardial infarction (MI), caused by partial or complete occlusion of a coronary artery, can lead to dysrhythmias, heart failure (HR), cardiogenic shock, thromboembolism, sudden cardiac death, and ventricular aneurysm and rupture.
- Nursing care of the patient with MI addresses anxiety, pain, and inadequate circulation.
- Patients with acute cardiac conditions often have continuous cardiac monitoring to detect potentially fatal dysrhythmias for prompt treatment.
- Cardiac rehabilitation begins with a cardiac incident, lasts throughout life, and includes the patient and family in teaching about exercise, diet, and medications.
- HF, the inability of the heart to meet the metabolic demands of the body, may be caused by disorders that increase the heart's workload or interfere with its pumping action.
- Treatment of HF may include correction of underlying causes, drug therapy to improve cardiac function and eliminate excess fluid, and measures to decrease demands on the heart.
- Complications of HF are dysrhythmias, pulmonary edema, and cardiogenic shock.
- Nursing care of the patient with HF focuses on increased fluid volume, inadequate oxygenation, anxiety, inadequate circulation, and inability to tolerate activity.
- CMP is a disease of the heart muscle that is treated with supportive measures but may lead to HF that eventually requires cardiac transplantation.
- Patients who have received heart transplants require immunosuppressive drugs for the remainder of their lives to prevent rejection of the foreign tissue.
- Signs and symptoms of cardiac transplant rejection are fever, dyspnea, fatigue, and dysrhythmias.
- Cardiac inflammatory conditions (endocarditis and pericarditis) are treated with drug therapy and rest.
- The primary disorders of the heart valves are stenosis, which interferes with blood movement from one chamber to the next, and regurgitation, which allows blood to flow backward.
- Valve disease may be treated with drug therapy to improve cardiac function, with balloon valvuloplasty to dilate stenosed valves, with commissurotomy to enlarge the opening, and with valve replacement using a biologic or synthetic valve.
- General measures to maintain perfusion of vital organs are O_2, IV fluids, and drugs to maintain or restore blood pressure.
- A dysrhythmia (also called an *arrhythmia*) is a disturbance of the heart rhythm caused by a problem in the conduction system.

Additional Learning Resources

SG Go to your Study Guide for additional learning activities to help you master this chapter content.

Go to your Evolve website (http://evolve.elsevier.com/Linton/medsurg) for the following learning resources and much more:

- Fluid and Electrolyte Tutorial
- Review Questions for the NCLEX® Examination

Clinical Judgment and Next-Generation NCLEX® Examination-Style Questions

1. **Nurses in a retirement community are preparing a program to educate residents about risk factors for atherosclerosis that can be modified. Which of the following risk factors should be addressed? (Select all that apply.)**
   1. Increased serum lipids
   2. Hypertension
   3. Heredity
   4. Physical inactivity
   5. Stress

   NCLEX Client Need: Physiological Integrity: Basic Care and Comfort

2. **Your neighbor was mowing his lawn when he began to have chest pain that radiated to his left shoulder. What is this type of pain called?** ____________________

   NCLEX Client Need: Physiological Integrity: Reduction of Risk Potential

3. **Which of the following drugs may be administered after MI to dissolve thrombi?**
   1. Heparin
   2. t-PA
   3. Aspirin
   4. Lidocaine

   NCLEX Client Need: Physiological Integrity: Physiological Adaptation

4. **Discharge teaching for a patient with HF should include which of the following instructions?**
   1. Immediately begin a vigorous program of exercise.
   2. Inform the physician if you gain more than 3 to 5 lb in 1 week.
   3. Weigh yourself before going to bed each night.
   4. Expect to continue having shortness of breath, chest pain, and cough.

   NCLEX Client Need: Physiological Integrity: Physiological Adaptation

5. **A patient who has had heart transplantation comes to the health care provider's office complaining of fever, fatigue, shortness of breath, and an irregular heartbeat. What problem should the nurse suspect?** ____________________

   NCLEX Client Need: Physiological Integrity: Reduction of Risk Potential

6. **Which of the following findings would the nurse expect in a patient with mitral stenosis?**
   1. Increased LA pressure
   2. Decreased pulmonary pressure
   3. Increased cardiac output
   4. Decreased RV pressure

   NCLEX Client Need: Physiological Integrity: Physiological Adaptation

7. **Take Action Using Matrix Test Item**

   A 76-year-old woman was admitted to the hospital complaining of shortness of breath, dizziness, nausea and mid back pain. Based on her symptoms and ECG findings, the patient was diagnosed and treated for an MI. She has a history of hypertension, diabetes, osteoarthritis, and obesity. The patient has become stable and is ready for discharge.

   Use an X for the health teaching below that is *Indicated* (appropriate or necessary), *Contraindicated* (could be harmful), or *Nonessential* (makes no difference or not necessary) before the patient's discharge at this time.

HEALTH TEACHING	INDICATED	CONTRAINDICATED	NONESSENTIAL
Take your medications as prescribed and contact your health care provider if any problems arise.			
Stop smoking.			
Stay in the house on bedrest" so that your heart can rest.			
Drink at least 8 glasses of water per day.			
Your BMI is in the obesity range, so you should lose weight to reduce the workload of your heart.			
Participate in a cardiac rehab program to become active again.			
Maintain a low sodium, low fat diet.			

36 Vascular Disorders

http://evolve.elsevier.com/Linton/medsurg

Objectives

1. Indicate data to collect for assessment of a patient with selected vascular disorders
2. Describe the pathophysiology, signs and symptoms, complications, and medical or surgical treatments of selected vascular disorders.
3. Assist in developing a plan of nursing care for patients with selected vascular disorders.

Key Terms

aneurysm (ĂN-yŭr-ĭzm)
embolism (ĔM-bō-lĭzm)
ischemia (ĭs-KĒ-mē-ă)
phlebitis (flĕ-BĪ-tĭs)
thrombosis (thrŏm-BŌ-sĭs)
vasoconstriction (vā-zō-kŏn-STRĬK-shŭn)

The delivery of oxygen (O_2) and nutrients to the tissues depends on adequate *perfusion* (blood flow to an organ or tissue), which requires a functionally intact cardiovascular system. When the cardiovascular system is compromised by vascular disease, the homeostasis of the body is affected. Risk factors for vascular disease include advanced age, heredity, smoking, obesity, physical inactivity, hypertension, hyperlipidemia (elevated cholesterol), and diabetes mellitus. Vascular diseases can affect the arterial and venous components of the circulation, resulting in pain, impaired function, and even death.

Atherosclerosis is discussed in Chapter 36. Other peripheral vascular disorders, as well as aortic aneurysm and aortic dissection, are presented here.

PERIPHERAL ARTERIAL DISEASE OF LOWER EXTREMITIES

PATHOPHYSIOLOGY

Lower extremity peripheral artery disease (PAD) affects 12% to 20% of Americans aged over 60 years and nearly 50% in those 85 years and older. The most significant risk factors are hyperlipidemia (high cholesterol), hypertension, diabetes, chronic kidney disease, and smoking (Firnhaber, 2019).

PAD is characterized by pathologic changes in the arteries, typically plaque formations that arise where the arteries branch, veer, arch, or narrow (Fig. 36.1). The most common sites for arterial occlusion are the distal superficial femoral and the popliteal arteries. Occlusions prevent the delivery of O_2 and nutrients to the tissues. Hypoxia affects all tissues distal to the occlusion. Peripheral nerves and muscles are more susceptible to harm from hypoxia than the skin and subcutaneous tissues. Severe O_2 deprivation may lead to **ischemia** and then to necrosis (tissue death).

Because PAD develops gradually, compensatory mechanisms attempt to maintain circulation. These compensatory mechanisms include the development of collateral blood vessels, vasodilation, and anaerobic metabolism. Collateral blood vessels are small new vessels that branch out to supply blood to poorly perfused tissues. The extent of collateral circulation determines the severity of symptoms.

CLINICAL MANIFESTATIONS

The clinical manifestations of PAD develop gradually. A classic sign of PAD is *intermittent claudication*. Symptoms such as aching, cramping, tiredness, and weakness in the legs commonly occur with walking and are relieved by rest; however, *persistent* and *aching* pain that occurs during rest may be present. Complaints of tingling or numbness (or both) in the toes are common. The affected extremity is cold and numb because of the reduction in the flow of blood to the area. Muscle atrophy may be evident. The skin of the affected area is pale because of reduced blood flow. When the extremity is in a dependent position, the color becomes red. Reduced blood supply to toenails can cause the nails to thicken. Other signs of arterial occlusion are shiny, scaly skin; subcutaneous tissue loss; hairlessness on the affected extremity; and ulcers with a pale gray or yellowish hue, especially at the ankles. If one extremity is affected more than the other, size differences between the extremities may be apparent.

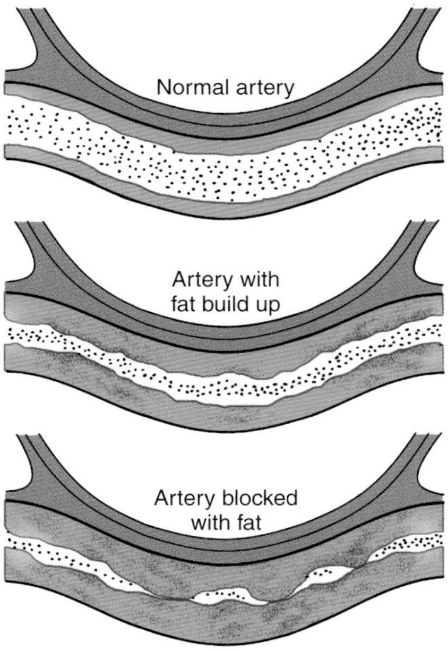

Fig. 36.1 Development of atherosclerosis. (From Ignatavicius DD, Workman ML: *Medical-surgical nursing: patient-centered collaborative care*, ed 7, St. Louis, 2013, Saunders.)

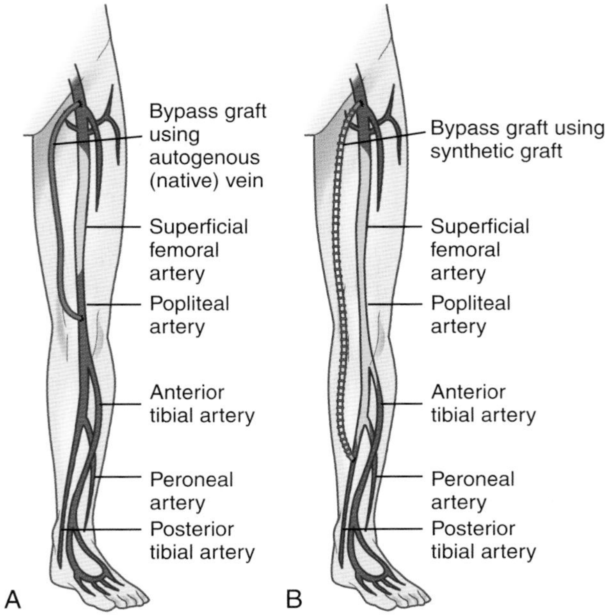

Fig. 36.2 (A) Femoral-popliteal bypass graft around an occluded superficial femoral artery. (B) Femoral-posterior tibial bypass graft around occluded superficial femoral, popliteal, and proximal tibial arteries. (From Lewis LL, et al.: *Medical-surgical nursing*, ed 10, 2017, Elsevier.)

MEDICAL DIAGNOSIS

The ankle-brachial index (ABI) is an inexpensive and reproducible method for assessing lower extremity hemodynamics. The ABI index test compares the blood pressure at the ankle with the blood pressure measurement at your arm. The ABI test can easily be done in the office setting by experienced staff. If results are less than 0.9, the risk of major cardiovascular events and overall mortality nearly doubles. Additional diagnostic tests used to confirm a diagnosis of PAD are duplex imaging, and, if surgery is contemplated, angiography (see Chapter 33, Table 33.3).

MEDICAL AND SURGICAL TREATMENT

The first step in managing PAD is to encourage the patient to make lifestyle changes, including smoking cessation, exercise, and weight management. Smoking cessation is a high priority. The use of e-cigarettes (also known as vaping) is not recommended as a tool to stop smoking tobacco. e-cigarettes introduce nicotine into the body plus noxious substances into the lungs. Success may be enhanced with varenicline (Chantix), nicotine replacement therapy, or bupropion (Zyban). Exercise programs found to be most successful with PAD include at least three sessions of 30 to 60 minutes of exercise each week. Training programs typically use a treadmill that allows gradual increases in speed and grade (incline). The benefits are sustained only as long as the patient continues regular exercise. Treatment should be initiated for hypertension, hyperlipidemia, and diabetes, if present. Angiotensin receptor blockers and angiotensin-converting enzyme (ACE) inhibitors ramipril (Altace) and telmisartan (Micardis) improve outcome.

Among the drugs used to treat claudication are cilostazol (Pletal) and pentoxifylline (Trental), which dilate blood vessels and prevent platelets from clumping. Aspirin or clopidogrel (Plavix) is used for antiplatelet activity. Several new types of drugs under study include recombinant growth factor, immune modulators, and carnitine. Scientists hope that gene therapy will stimulate growth of new blood vessels. See Chapter 33, Table 33.9 for a complete list of medications prescribed for cardiovascular conditions.

Surgical interventions include stenting (to keep the vessel lumen open), endarterectomy, grafting, and catheter-based interventional radiology procedures. Endarterectomy is the surgical removal of the obstruction. Grafting is the surgical replacement of a diseased segment of an artery with a graft of some type, either synthetic or from another blood vessel (Fig. 36.2).

Interventional radiology is done in the catheterization laboratory, is highly successful, and requires a recovery period of only 24 to 48 hours. Percutaneous angioplasty (PTA) is one interventional radiology procedure. By inserting a catheter containing a balloon at the tip into the femoral artery, PTA enlarges the interior diameter of the blood vessel. A stent is placed immediately within the artery to keep it open. Possible complications of PTA are hematoma formation, embolus, arterial dissection, and allergic reaction. Nursing care for the procedure is the same as for a diagnostic angiography (see Table 33.3).

Asymptomatic patients with PAD generally are not candidates for revascularization. However, patients with claudication who have not responded to treatment and supervised exercise therapy should be referred to a vascular surgeon.

◆ NURSING CARE OF THE PATIENT WITH PERIPHERAL ARTERIAL DISEASE

Focused Assessment

Assessment of the patient with PAD is summarized in Chapter 33, Box 33.2. When the patient has had surgical intervention, it is especially important to monitor the pulses distal to the surgical site and compare them with the same pulses in the unaffected extremity. Cessation of a pulse suggests possible arterial occlusion, and the surgeon must be notified immediately. Other important aspects of the postoperative assessment are vital signs, color and temperature of the affected extremity, fluid intake and output, central venous pressure, and mental status. If the patient has pain, document the location, severity, and nature of the pain.

Patient Problems, Goals, and Outcome Criteria: Peripheral Arterial Disease

Patient Problems	Goals and Outcome Criteria
Decreased activity tolerance related to decreased blood flow to extremities	Improved activity tolerance: patient states is increasingly able to perform activities without pain
Chronic pain related to ischemia	Reduced pain: patient states pain is reduced, relaxed manner
Disrupted tissue integrity related to inadequate circulation	Healthy skin: skin intact with normal color and warmth
Altered body image related to muscle atrophy, stasis ulcers, and skin discoloration	Positive body image: positive patient statements about self, patient makes effort to maintain good physical appearance
Inadequate peripheral tissue perfusion related to vascular occlusion	Adequate peripheral tissue perfusion: palpable peripheral pulses, extremity warm with normal skin color
Ineffective self-care management related to lack of knowledge of disease process, treatment, and self-care	Patient carries out proper self-care measures: patient describes and demonstrates self-care

If surgical intervention is performed, additional diagnoses and goals may include the following.

Patient Problems	Goals and Outcome Criteria
Potential for infection related to surgical incision, graft placement	Absence of infection: normal body temperature, decreasing wound redness and drainage

Patient Problems, Goals, and Outcome Criteria: Peripheral Arterial Disease—cont'd

Patient Problems	Goals and Outcome Criteria
Decreased cardiac output related to hemorrhage, diuresis, fluid shifts	Normal cardiac output: pulse and blood pressure consistent with patient norms
Inadequate peripheral circulation related to graft thrombosis	Patent graft: operative extremity warm, with improved color and palpable pulses
Acute pain related to surgical incision	Pain relief: patient relaxed, states that pain is relieved
Decreased mobility related to weakness, fear, surgical procedure	Increased physical mobility: increasing activity without pain

Interventions

Decreased activity tolerance. To monitor the patient's activity tolerance, assess the patient before, during, and after planned activities; then monitor progress as treatment progresses. When planning an exercise regimen, use the following guidelines:

1. Work with the patient to plan the activity schedule and goals.
2. Gradually increase the exercise time as tolerance increases.
3. Discontinue activity if the patient has chest pain, bradycardia, dyspnea, or intermittent claudication. After rest relieves the pain of intermittent claudication, the patient may resume activity.
4. Reduce the intensity of the activity if the pulse takes longer than 3 to 4 minutes to return to the baseline rate or if the patient has severe dyspnea.
5. For patients confined to bed, start exercises with range-of-motion exercises performed twice daily.
6. Patients should not exercise when they have leg ulcers, cellulitis, deep vein thrombosis (DVT), or gangrene.

Chronic pain. The chronic pain associated with ischemia is exhausting and greatly reduces the patient's quality of life. Therefore, pain management must be a priority. The most direct interventions are those that increase circulation or decrease metabolic demands of ischemic tissues. Resting the extremities in a dependent position may help to relieve the pain of arterial occlusive disease. Administer analgesics as prescribed, along with other comfort measures. Nonpharmacologic pain relief measures include relaxation techniques, warm baths, breathing exercises, and back rubs (see the Complementary and Alternative Therapies box). See Chapter 8 for a detailed discussion of pain management.

Complementary and Alternative Therapies

Relaxation, warm baths, breathing exercises, and back rubs can help the patient with chronic pain.

Disrupted tissue integrity. The nursing interventions for maintaining skin integrity focus on improving circulation and avoiding tissue trauma. If the patient has an ulcerated area, keep it clean and free of pressure. Various wound care products may be prescribed to protect the wound and prevent infection. However, unless circulation is improved, healing is unlikely. The physician will prescribe any activity limitations.

The feet are especially susceptible to injury and require special care. Advise the patient not to go barefoot, to wear only shoes that fit properly, to inspect the feet daily for signs of pressure or lesions, and to keep the toenails neatly trimmed. Because of the risk of ingrown nails, nails should not be trimmed too short. Toenails should always be cut straight across rather than in a curved shape. The patient should see a peripheral vascular specialist promptly if any foot problems develop.

Altered body image. Encourage the patient to express any feelings that result from problems associated with PAD, such as activity intolerance, stasis ulcers, discoloration of the extremities, and, for some, amputations. It is important to be supportive and help the patient to identify coping strategies to deal with the feelings.

Inadequate peripheral circulation. Administer vasodilators and other drugs that improve blood flow as ordered. Encourage exercise according to the individualized exercise plan. Maintain adequate warmth and discourage smoking. Elevation of the extremities is not usually recommended with arterial disease.

Additional interventions are indicated for the postoperative patient.

Inability to manage self-care. To cope with PAD, the patient must understand the disease process and treatment. Include the family in patient teaching because their fears and concerns can have an enormous effect on the patient's perception of the situation. The patient teaching plan is the same as for the patient with arterial embolism. Adaptation to lifestyle changes is essential to good management of PAD. Additional interventions are indicated for the postoperative patient.

Potential for infection. After surgery, patients are at risk for infection of the surgical incision and the grafts (especially synthetic grafts) that are used to replace the diseased blood vessel. An infected synthetic graft is very serious because it necessitates removal of the graft and often amputation. Monitor the patient's temperature and report fever to the surgeon. It is vital to inspect the incision for increasing redness, edema, and drainage that suggest infection. Antimicrobials are usually ordered before surgery and may be continued after surgery.

Decreased cardiac output. Monitor for signs and symptoms of deficient fluid volume: tachycardia, restlessness, decreased urine output, pallor, and hypotension. Provide intravenous and oral fluids as ordered and maintain records of fluid intake and output. Monitor daily weights and inspect the surgical dressing for bleeding, which must be reported immediately to the surgeon.

Inadequate peripheral circulation. Thrombus formation can occur in the graft, causing occlusion and impaired blood flow. Monitor the pulses, warmth, and color of the operative extremity and promptly inform the surgeon of diminishing pulses, coolness, and pallor or cyanosis. Some patients are given anticoagulants or thrombolytics to decrease the risk of graft occlusion. Edema for 4 to 8 weeks is common after bypass surgery. The leg is usually wrapped in a light dressing or vascular boot and kept flat initially. Elastic stockings are not used immediately after a vein graft.

Acute pain. Postoperative pain is treated with analgesics, positioning, and relaxation techniques as described in Chapters 17 and 33.

Decreased physical mobility. After surgery, the patient's activities are increased gradually. A specific program of exercises may be prescribed. Assist the patient and assess muscle strength and tolerance of activity.

ARTERIAL EMBOLISM

PATHOPHYSIOLOGY

The development of an arterial **embolism** is a potentially life-threatening event. An arterial embolus usually forms from a thrombus in the heart. Heart conditions that may cause a thrombus include infective endocarditis, mitral valve disease, atrial fibrillation, cardiomyopathy, and prosthetic heart valves. In any artery, roughened atheromatous plaque as well as traumatic injury can lead to thrombus formation. If a thrombus breaks loose, it becomes an embolus traveling through the circulatory system until it lodges in a vessel, blocking blood flow distal to the occlusion. Thrombi from the right side of the heart lodge in the lungs, causing a pulmonary embolism (addressed later), whereas thrombi from the left side usually affect a leg. The effects of arterial occlusion depend on the size of the embolus formed, the organs involved, and the extent to which collateral circulation can maintain sufficient blood supply to affected tissues.

PREVENTION

Increased risks for clots are:

- Smoking
- Minimal exercise
- High blood pressure
- Elevated cholesterol levels
- Diabetes
- Overweight
- Stress

CLINICAL MANIFESTATIONS

Whereas some patients with arterial obstruction have no pain, others experience severe pain and other symptoms of tissue ischemia. When the collateral circulation cannot compensate for the compromised blood flow, the patient has distinct symptoms of reduced blood flow to the tissues. Signs and symptoms of inadequate blood supply in the lower extremities include:

- Severe, acute pain
- Weakness and gradual loss of sensory and motor function in the affected areas
- Pain aggravated by movement or pressure
- Absent distal pulses
- Muscle pain or spasm in the affected area
- Pallor (pale color) and mottling (irregular discoloration)
- A sharp line of color and temperature demarcation (tissue beyond the obstruction is pale and cool)

DIAGNOSIS

An arterial embolism may result in a decreased or absent pulse, absent blood pressure and possible signs of tissue death (darkened skin) in the extremities distal to the obstruction. Specific tests include angiography, Doppler ultrasound, and MRI of the affected extremity. If embolism is suspected in the lung, plethysmography can measure the air volume or if embolism of the brain is suspected, transcranial Doppler examines the arteries of the brain.

MEDICAL AND SURGICAL TREATMENT

Arterial embolism requires prompt treatment at a hospital. The goals of treatment are to control symptoms and to improve the interrupted blood flow to the affected area of the body. Arterial embolism is managed with intravenous anticoagulants and thrombolytics. Anticoagulants (such as warfarin and heparin) and antiplatelet medicines such as aspirin and clopidogrel (oral blood thinner) can prevent new clots from forming. Thrombolytics (called "clot busters") such as streptokinase can dissolve clots. These medications cannot be used with active internal bleeding, cardiovascular accident, recent major surgery, uncontrolled hypertension, and pregnancy. See Chapter 33, Table 33.9 for a complete list of medications and nursing implications for cardiovascular disease. Patients who cannot be treated with medications may be prepared for thrombectomy (surgical removal of the embolus). Failure to restore perfusion results in tissue death and requires amputation of the affected part. Patients at risk for future arterial emboli are often treated long term with oral anticoagulants.

◆ NURSING CARE OF THE PATIENT WITH ARTERIAL EMBOLISM

Focused Assessment

The assessment of the patient with peripheral vascular disease (PVD) is outlined in Chapter 33, Box 33.2, Assessment of Patients With Cardiovascular Disorders.

Patient Problems, Goals, and Outcome Criteria: Arterial Embolism

Patient Problems	Goals and Outcome Criteria
Inadequate peripheral tissue perfusion related to compromised circulation	Improved tissue perfusion: normal skin color, palpable pulses, capillary refill time less than 3 seconds in affected extremity
Stress related to fear of treatments, environment, and risk of limb loss	Reduced stress: patient is calm, states fear is reduced or relieved
Immobility related to the surgical procedure and compromised circulation	Improved mobility: patient increases activity without discomfort
Disrupted tissue integrity related to ischemic changes from the impairment of peripheral circulation	Healthy skin in affected areas: skin intact
Inability to manage self-care related to lack of knowledge of self-care, including drug therapy	Patient knows and practices prescribed self-care measures: patient correctly describes and demonstrates self-care measures and self-medication

Interventions

Nursing interventions are designed to improve circulation and prevent further damage to the affected tissue.

Inadequate tissue perfusion. To promote circulation, maintain the affected extremities at or slightly below the horizontal position. Administer prescribed medications and perform range-of-motion exercises as ordered.

Stress. To decrease fear, orient the patient to the environment and the expected therapies using simple statements to explain the disease process and procedures. Encourage the patient to express feelings of helplessness and anxiety and to identify coping mechanisms that have worked in other situations.

Immobility. Until the thrombus is removed, the affected limb may be immobilized. The physician will order the appropriate level of activity. Improved physical mobility requires instruction in range-of-motion exercises and the development of a progressive exercise plan. This exercise plan usually is limited to 15 minutes, 3 times a day, in the initial days after surgery or treatment. The progression of exercise is determined by the individual patient's response.

Disrupted tissue integrity. With arterial embolism, the affected tissue is highly susceptible to injury. Protect the limb from pressure, trauma, and extreme heat or cold. Edematous tissue is equally susceptible to injury and must be protected.

Inability to manage self-care. Patient teaching enables the patient to participate in the plan of care during and after hospitalization. For information on teaching interventions for patients, see the Patient Teaching box.

Patient Teaching

Arterial Embolism

- Protect affected limbs from pressure, trauma, and temperature extremes.
- Exercise to improve blood flow; gradually increase activity as you are able to tolerate it.
- Report pain, numbness, coolness, and pale or bluish skin color to your health care provider.

CHRONIC VENOUS INSUFFICIENCY

PATHOPHYSIOLOGY

Venous insufficiency is a condition in which the veins have difficulty sending blood from the extremities back to the heart. For example, valves in leg veins normally keep blood moving forward toward the heart. With chronic venous insufficiency, the walls and valves inside the veins are weakened. This causes the veins to stay filled with blood, especially when standing.

Elevated venous pressure causes edema, primarily around the ankles. Red blood cells (RBCs) seep into the tissues and combine with metabolic wastes to impart a brownish color, called *stasis dermatitis*, around the ankles. Ulcers may form because of the pressure exerted by edema or as a result of trauma. The ulcers develop most often on the medial malleolus (the prominent bone on the inner aspect of the ankle). Because of the poor circulation, the ulcers are very resistant to healing and susceptible to infection. Some ulcers eventually necessitate amputation (Fig. 36.3).

RISK FACTORS

Risk factors for venous insufficiency include age, family history, female gender, history of deep vein DVT in the legs, obesity, pregnancy, sitting or standing for long periods, and tall height.

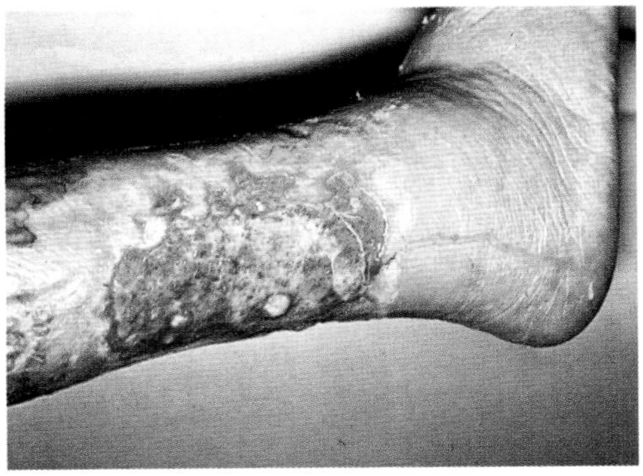

Fig. 36.3 Venous leg ulcer. (From Kamal A, Brockelhurst JC: *Colour atlas of geriatric medicine*, ed 2, Europe, 2017, Mosby-Year Book.)

CLINICAL MANIFESTATIONS

Signs and symptoms of chronic venous insufficiency include edema around the lower legs, pain, leg cramps, brownish skin discoloration (stasis dermatitis), and stasis ulcerations. Patients often describe pain as heaviness or dull ache in the calf or thigh. Discomfort becomes worse when standing and is relieved when the legs are raised. The skin temperature is cool, and nails are normal. Peripheral pulses are present but may be difficult to palpate because of the edema. The feet and ankles often are cyanotic when in a dependent position.

MEDICAL DIAGNOSIS

The physical examination provides evidence of chronic venous insufficiency. The diagnosis usually is made based on the appearance of the leg and leg veins when standing. Noninvasive screening called duplex ultrasound may be done to check how the blood flows in the veins and to confirm the diagnosis of chronic venous insufficiency or to assess its severity. A culture may be ordered to determine the infectious agent if a stasis ulcer has formed and is draining.

MEDICAL AND SURGICAL TREATMENT

Self-care steps to help manage venous insufficiency include avoiding standing or sitting for long periods, losing weight if overweight, and exercising regularly.

The medical management of stasis ulcerations is constantly changing; however, compression, which promotes venous return, remains the key to healing existing ulcers and preventing new ones. Among the many options are elastic or compression stockings and pneumatic compression devices. However, high-pressure compression is contraindicated if the patient's arterial blood flow is poor.

Endovenous laser ablation and radiofrequency ablation are both minimally invasive procedures that can be done in an office or clinic. A tube (catheter) puts heat directly into an affected vein. This closes the vein so less blood pools in the leg. Overall blood flow is improved.

If the patient has an ulcer, treatment typically includes special dressings along with compression. Topical debriding agents may be used to prepare a clean wound bed. Dressings that maintain a moist environment are believed to be superior to dry dressings. However, evidence supporting one type of dressing over another is limited. A wound, ostomy, continence nurse (WOC nurse) can advise on the most current effective treatment for a specific situation. Infected ulcers are treated with systemic antibiotics, which are more effective than topical ointments. Skin grafting or surgical closure of the ulcer along with removal of the associated varicose veins is sometimes done. Hyperbaric O_2 therapy may be prescribed to promote healing of the ulcer by reducing capillary pressure and hyperoxygenating the blood. The overall goal for medical management of ulcerations is to preserve the extremity by stimulating granulation tissue in the ulcer.

NURSING CARE OF THE PATIENT WITH CHRONIC VENOUS INSUFFICIENCY

Focused Assessment

The general assessment of peripheral vascular status is summarized in Chapter 33, Box 33.2. When the patient has chronic venous insufficiency, inspect the lower extremities for rubor and stasis dermatitis, palpate skin temperature, evaluate edema, and determine the presence of pain in the affected extremity (see Nursing Care Plan: Patient With a Venous Stasis Ulcer).

Patient Problems, Goals, and Outcome Criteria: Chronic Venous Insufficiency

Patient Problems	Goals and Outcome Criteria
Inadequate peripheral tissue perfusion related to reduced vascular circulation	Improved peripheral circulation and venous return: absence of edema and lesions, improved skin color
Altered self-concept related to chronic, open stasis ulcerations	Patient adapts to changes in appearance: patient expresses concerns about changes, makes effort to maintain or improve appearance
Potential for infection related to compromised circulation and impaired skin integrity	Decreased risk for infection: healed ulcer, intact skin. Absence of infection: normal body temperature, absence of local redness or drainage
Disrupted skin tissue integrity related to stasis dermatitis and ulcerations	Restored skin integrity: skin intact in affected areas

Interventions

Inadequate peripheral tissue perfusion. To improve circulation in areas of compromised vascular function, the patient should elevate the legs when sitting and wear compression stockings. Stocking size is determined by patient leg measurements. The patient should put on the stockings before rising. The toe opening should be under the toes and the heel section in place. The thigh gusset should be on the inner thigh. The stocking must be smooth and not allowed to roll down at the top. The stocking should be removed for 10 to 20 minutes for bathing and skin care. Stockings should be replaced every 4 to 6 months. The patient should avoid standing still, crossing the legs, and wearing restrictive clothing, especially socks or hose with tight, narrow bands. When sitting, encourage the patient to exercise the feet, ankles, and knees to promote venous return.

Altered self-concept. Encourage the patient to share feelings about body image changes and be accepting and supportive. Encourage the patient to pay attention to grooming; they may prefer clothing that conceals stockings or dressings.

Potential for infection. Carefully monitor for signs of infection such as elevated temperature; chills; general malaise; and localized redness, pain, and purulent drainage. Teach the patient thorough hand washing, good hygiene, and appropriate wound care. The fragile edematous tissue must also be protected from trauma to avoid creating portals for pathogens.

Disrupted skin tissue integrity. Inspect for dermatitis and ulcerations, especially in the ankle area. Apply a moisturizer to dry, intact skin. Patient education is critical because these ulcerations are frequently treated on an outpatient basis. Instruct the patient and family in the management of the ulcerations while in the home setting. A referral for home health care and wound care may be appropriate.

Prognosis. Chronic venous insufficiency tends to get worse over time. It can be managed if treatment is started in the early stages. By taking self-care steps, the condition can be stabilized and most likely prevented from getting worse. If there is an increase in swelling, fever, redness or leg sores, a vascular surgeon should be consulted.

VENOUS THROMBOSIS

PATHOPHYSIOLOGY

A variety of terms are used to describe inflammation and thrombus formation in the veins. **Phlebitis** is inflammation of a superficial vein. When a thrombus forms in the presence of phlebitis, the condition is called *venous* **thrombosis**. Depending on the depth of the affected veins, venous thrombosis is labeled *superficial vein thrombosis* (SVT) or DVT. The superficial vein that is most often the site of thrombus formation is the saphenous vein. The deep veins commonly involved are the femoral, popliteal, and small calf veins. *Venous thromboembolism* (VTE) is a clot that moves. VTE includes both SVT and DVT. Research has identified three factors (called *Virchow's triad*) that contribute to venous thrombus formation: (1) stasis of the blood, (2) damage to the vessel walls, and (3) hypercoagulability (increased tendency of blood to clot). A grave complication of DVT is a pulmonary embolism.

RISK FACTORS

Some of the factors that place a person at risk for the development of thrombi are:

- Recent hospitalization and/or surgery
- Prescribed bed rest or extended travel
- Older age
- Leg trauma resulting in immobilization from casts or traction
- Family history of VTE
- Previous venous insufficiency
- Obesity
- Use of oral contraceptives or hormone replacement therapy
- Recent or recurring cancer
- During and just after pregnancy

CLINICAL MANIFESTATIONS

The signs and symptoms of venous thrombosis vary with the size and location of the thrombus, the amount of obstruction, the collateral circulation, and the existence of other medical problems. SVT is characterized by a vein that feels firm and cordlike when palpated. The area around the vein may be warm, red, and tender. When obstruction occurs in a deep vein, the affected extremity may be edematous and painful with warmth and tenderness at the area of compromise. The patient may have a mild elevation in systemic temperature.

Table 36.1 compares features of arterial and venous disease.

MEDICAL DIAGNOSIS

The primary diagnostic examinations used in the detection of venous thrombi are venography, Doppler ultrasonography, duplex ultrasonography, and MRI. A D-dimer blood test measures a substance in the blood that is released when a clot breaks up. These tests are instrumental in the confirmation of the disease process and determination of the treatment plan. A ventilation-perfusion lung scan, pulmonary angiogram, spiral CT scan or MRI may be done if pulmonary embolism is suspected. See Chapter 33, Table 33.3.

MEDICAL AND SURGICAL TREATMENT

The goals of treatment are to prevent thrombus extension and pulmonary emboli, to reduce the risk of further thrombus formation, and to reduce discomfort. Anticoagulant or thrombolytic therapy (or both) is begun promptly after diagnosis. When anticoagulants cannot be used, a filter can be inserted inside the vena cava to trap the embolus before it reaches the lungs. A treatment plan typically includes patient teaching about the disease; ongoing assessment for pulmonary emboli; bed rest; elevation of the extremity; warm, moist soaks to the affected area; and compression stockings. Ambulation is initiated after the acute phase. Surgery to remove the clot may be considered when the patient cannot receive anticoagulants or thrombolytic therapy or when the possibility of a pulmonary embolus is high.

NURSING CARE

Focused Assessment

Assessment of the patient with PVD is summarized in Chapter 33, Box 33.2.

Patient Problems, Goals, and Outcome Criteria: Venous Thrombosis

Patient Problems	Goals and Outcome Criteria
Disrupted skin integrity related to venous stasis	Intact skin: absence of redness, rash, pallor, lesions
Pain related to impaired circulation and tissue ischemia	Pain relief: patient verbalizes pain relief, relaxed manner
Anxiety related to hospitalization and uncertainty of disease process	Reduced anxiety: patient states that anxiety is reduced, calm manner
Activity intolerance related to leg pain or swelling	Improved ability to tolerate activity: increasing activity without pain
Inadequate peripheral tissue perfusion related to impaired peripheral circulation	Adequate tissue perfusion: pulses present and symmetric, normal skin color and warmth
Inadequate pulmonary oxygenation related to pulmonary embolus	Normal oxygenation: respiratory rate consistent with patient norms, no dyspnea or chest pain
Ineffective self-care management related to the developing disease process, treatment, self-care	Patient adheres to prescribed plan of care: correctly describes and demonstrates self-medication, exercises, and precautions

Pain. The patient's pain must be reduced before activity tolerance can improve. Administer analgesics as prescribed and implement other prescribed comfort measures such as warm, moist soaks, and elevation of the extremity. Massage is contraindicated because it may dislodge a thrombus resulting in an embolus that can obstruct blood flow.

Anxiety. Anxiety may be related to lack of knowledge about the disease and its treatment as well as concerns about the effects of the condition on employment, activities of daily living (ADLs), and quality of life. Patients worry about when and if another blood clot could form and they feel a lack of control. Blood clots are life-changing and traumatic. The patient may even restrict activities out of fear. Many patients say that time is the most critical factor in emotional healing. It is important to talk to people who understand.

Table 36.1 Comparison of Arterial and Venous Disease in the Legs

CHARACTERISTIC	PERIPHERAL ARTERY DISEASE	VENOUS DISEASE
Peripheral pulses	Decreased or absent	Present; may be difficult to palpate with edema
Capillary refill	>3 seconds	<3 seconds
Edema	Absent unless leg constantly in dependent position	Lower leg edema
Hair	Loss of hair on legs, feet, toes	Hair may be present or absent
Skin color	Dark reddish color when in dependent position; pale when elevated	Bronze-brown pigmentation; varicose veins may be visible
Skin texture	Thin, shiny, taut	Thick, hardened, indurated
Skin temperature	Cool, temperature gradient down the leg	Warm, no temperature gradient
Pain	Intermittent claudication or rest pain in foot; ulcer may or may not be painful	Dull ache, heaviness in calf or thigh; ulcer often painful
Ulcers	Location: tips of toes, foot, lateral malleolus Margins: round, smooth Drainage: minimal Color: black or pale pink	Location: near medial malleolus Margins: irregular Drainage: moderate to large amount Color: yellow or dark red
Dermatitis and pruritus	Rare	Frequent

Modified from Lewis SM, Bucher L, Heitkemper MM: Medical-surgical nursing: assessment and management of clinical problems, ed 10, St. Louis, 2017, Elsevier-Mosby.

There are private Facebook groups online. The relief of anxiety can help the patient to move toward an acceptable level of activity and improved quality of life. Understanding the symptoms that need attention immediately (such as shortness of breath, unable to lie flat, and leg pain that inhibits walking) is important to allay fears of unrelated symptoms. Journaling is a helpful tool to clarify timing and severity of symptoms at doctor visits.

Patient Teaching

Venous Thrombosis

- Protect your legs from pressure and trauma.
- Elevate your legs when sitting to improve circulation.
- Do not massage or rub affected areas.
- Gradually increase your activity; slow down or stop if you have pain during activity.
- Avoid prolonged standing and crossing your legs.
- Notify your physician if you have any chest pain or shortness of breath.

Inadequate peripheral tissue perfusion. Improved peripheral circulation aids in tissue perfusion, which decreases pain, improves skin integrity, reduces anxiety, and increases physical activity. Administer prescribed anticoagulants or platelet aggregation inhibitors to prevent new clots or administer thrombolytics to dissolve existing clots and reestablish blood flow to the affected area. Check blood test results before giving anticoagulants and take action according to agency policy. Apply warm, moist packs to the affected area as ordered to improve circulation and assist the patient in the placement of antiembolism hose, if prescribed, to prevent stasis and improve circulation. Explain to the patient how stress reduction and smoking cessation can improve tissue perfusion by reducing vasoconstriction.

Inadequate pulmonary oxygenation. The possibility of a pulmonary embolus developing during the treatment of venous thrombosis is ever present. When an embolus lodges in the lung, the affected blood vessels can no longer exchange gases. Pressure builds in vessels behind the embolus. Symptoms of pulmonary embolism depend on the amount of tissue affected. Small emboli may produce no symptoms. Larger emboli can cause dyspnea, chest pain, tachycardia, cough, fever, anxiety, and a change in mental status. A massive embolus can cause heart failure and shock. Sixty percent of people do not survive massive emboli.

To improve oxygenation when a patient has a pulmonary embolism, elevate the head of the bed to a 45-degree angle and administer O_2 as ordered. It is also vital to monitor and document any changes in the patient's respiratory pattern, address anxiety, teach the patient deep-breathing and coughing techniques, and assist with position changes every 2 hours. Administer drugs as ordered to dissolve existing clots and prevent future clots. Surgical removal of the clot, called *pulmonary embolectomy*, is sometimes indicated. Additional discussion of pulmonary embolism is found in Chapter 27.

Inadequate self-care. To follow the long-term plan of care, the patient must understand the condition and how it can best be managed. Once the acute process has resolved, discharge planning must include patient teaching as outlined. In addition, for more on the care of a patient with venous thrombosis, see the Patient Teaching box.

VARICOSE VEIN DISEASE

PATHOPHYSIOLOGY

Varicose veins are referred to as *varicosities*. Varicosities are dilated, tortuous, superficial veins—often the saphenous veins in the lower extremities. The dilation of the vessels results from incompetent valves in the veins; that is, the valves cannot prevent backflow of blood. Vein incompetence is a result of hereditary weakness made worse by aging, pregnancy, obesity, occupations requiring prolonged standing, or a combination of these. Restrictive clothing aggravates the condition. Varicose veins are classified as *primary* (only superficial veins are affected) and *secondary* (characterized by deep vein obstruction). In addition to peripheral veins, varicosities can occur in other areas such as the esophageal and hemorrhoidal veins. Incompetent valves cannot be repaired.

CLINICAL MANIFESTATIONS

The onset of varicose vein disease is gradual, but the condition is progressive. When only the superficial veins are involved, the signs and symptoms are minimal except for the cosmetic changes that occur. The dilated veins are seen as oversized, discolored (purplish), and tortuous. Symptoms typically include dull aching sensations when standing or walking; a feeling of heaviness in the affected legs; muscle cramps, especially at night; increased muscular fatigue in the affected area; and ankle edema. Over time, some people develop postphlebitic syndrome, which is evidenced by persistent edema, brownish skin discoloration, and ulcers most commonly on the inner aspect of the ankle (Fig. 36.4).

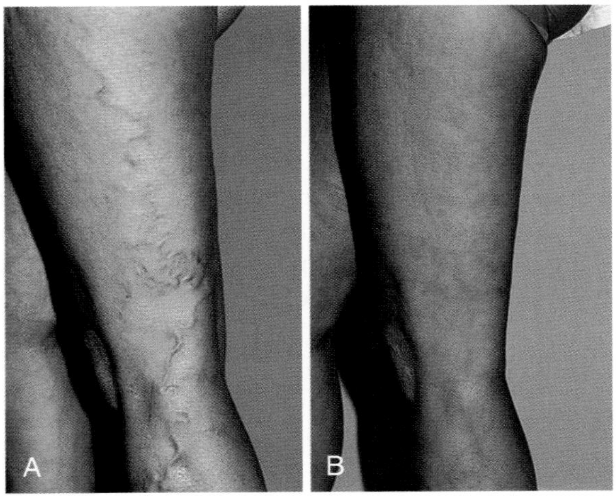

Fig. 36.4 (A) Lateral aspect of varicose veins before treatment. (B) Lateral aspect of varicose veins 2 years after initial treatment with sclerotherapy. (From Goldman MP, Guex JJ, Weiss RA: *Sclerotherapy treatment of varicose and telangiectatic leg veins*, ed 5, Philadelphia, 2011, Mosby.)

MEDICAL AND SURGICAL TREATMENT

Conservative treatments of varicosities are used whenever possible. Advise the patient to avoid restrictive garments, prolonged standing or sitting, crossing the legs or knees, and injury to the compromised areas. If the patient is obese, explain that weight reduction usually reduces pressure on the lower extremities. Support stockings are often ordered, although research on the benefits of this therapy has not consistently shown value. If the physician recommends support stockings, help the patient to learn how to put them on correctly. Compression stockings squeeze the legs, helping veins and muscles move the blood toward the heart more efficiently. (see the Complementary and Alternative Therapies box).

Complementary and Alternative Therapies

Horse chestnut can improve the tone of the veins, making them less permeable and less fragile. Blood flow is increased, and edema is reduced. Feelings of pain, tiredness and heaviness also may be alleviated.

Sclerotherapy (injection of a foam into the vein causing closure of the vein), or laser therapy (sending strong bursts of light into the vein, causing the vein to slowly disappear) may be effective in the treatment of superficial varicosities. Surgery may be recommended for cosmetic reasons or if stasis ulcers develop. The surgical procedure that removes large, dilated veins is called *ligation and stripping*. It requires several incisions along the course of the affected vein. For some patients, a simpler procedure is possible in which the saphenous vein is ligated (tied shut) at the groin, requiring only one incision. Endovenous ablation uses a catheter that is threaded into the vein. The catheter emits energy that causes the vein to collapse. The vein is removed through a small incision.

◆ NURSING CARE OF THE PATIENT WITH VARICOSE VEIN DISEASE

Focused Assessment

When a patient has varicose veins, the health history determines the presence of pain, edema, cramps, and muscle fatigue. Note a family history of varicose veins and document the patient's occupation and usual activities. When taking a pain and discomfort history, determine what measures the patient has used for pain control. The physical examination focuses on inspection of the legs for color, edema, turgor, and capillary refill. Palpate the legs for tenderness. Postoperative assessment is especially concerned with monitoring peripheral circulation and tissue perfusion.

Patient Problems, Goals, and Outcome Criteria: Varicose Veins

Patient Problems	Goals and Outcome Criteria
Chronic pain related to engorgement of the veins	Reduced pain: patient states that pain with activity has decreased
Activity intolerance related to feelings of heaviness and fatigue	Improved ability to tolerate activity: patient reports gradual increase in activity with less discomfort
Inability to manage self-care related to management of the varicosities	Patient carries out appropriate self-care: patient correctly verbalizes and demonstrates self-care

Interventions

The primary nursing role in the care of the patient with varicose veins is teaching self-care. Interventions to improve activity tolerance and to manage pain are outlined in the Patient Teaching box. In general, measures that improve venous return also decrease pain.

For the surgical patient, patient teaching is also of paramount importance because the procedure is usually done as a same-day surgical procedure. While the patient is still in the surgical suite, pressure bandages are placed on the extremities. The surgeon orders specific aspects of postoperative care, such as when the pressure bandages should be removed, what types of stockings are recommended afterward, and how long they should be worn. Activity restrictions and positioning of the legs (usually 15–30 degrees for the first 24 hours) are also ordered at this time. Serious complications are rare; however, bleeding is most likely to occur in the groin area, so the dressing in that area should be monitored. After sclerotherapy or laser therapy, both of which are outpatient procedures, the patient is advised to wear compression stockings for as long as 6 weeks.

Patient Teaching

Varicose Veins

- Exercise regularly to promote circulation.
- Avoid prolonged standing, sitting, and crossing your legs.
- Avoid restrictive clothing.
- Elevate extremities whenever possible.
- Obesity contributes to the development of varicose veins. People who are overweight usually see improvement with weight loss.
- Nonprescription analgesics and frequent position changes usually control pain.
- Wear support hose if recommended by your physician.

THROMBOANGIITIS OBLITERANS

Thromboangiitis obliterans (TO), also called *Buerger disease,* is an inflammatory thrombotic disorder rather than an atherosclerotic process. The exact cause is unknown, but it occurs only in smokers (see the Cultural Considerations box). Small blood vessels become inflamed and swollen. The blood vessels then narrow and are blocked by blood clots (thrombosis). Blood vessels of hands and feet are affected. Arteries are more affected than veins. Average age when symptoms begin is around 35. Young men who smoke heavily or chew tobacco are most often affected. Many people who are afflicted by this condition have poor dental health. Bacteria may be a contributing factor. Signs and symptoms may include intermittent claudication, rest pain, fingers and toes appear pale, red, or bluish and feel cold to the touch, cold sensitivity, severe pain often described as burning or tingling, abnormal sensation, ulceration, and gangrene. Diagnosis is based on a history of young age at onset, physical findings, and arteriography. There are no blood tests that diagnose TO.

Cultural Considerations

What Does Culture Have to Do With Buerger Disease?

Buerger disease affects more people in the Middle East, Asia, the Mediterranean, and Eastern Europe. It is relatively uncommon in the United States. When assessing patients, especially those of Indian, Korean, or Japanese heritage, be alert for related signs and symptoms.

There is no cure for TO. The most important aspect of treatment is smoking cessation. Palliative treatments include sympathectomy (surgery to cut the nerves to the area to control pain), spinal cord stimulation, analgesics for pain, vasodilators, and antibiotics if infected. The prostaglandin iloprost (Ventavist) has shown some benefit in European studies. Gene therapy is under study. Ulcers may respond to treatment with vascular endothelial growth factor. If gangrene develops (most commonly below the knee), amputation is the only treatment option. Forty percent of patients who continue tobacco use eventually require amputations. Nursing care is similar to that of patients with PAD. Emphasis is on smoking cessation measures (see Chapter 28) and protection of the affected extremities.

RAYNAUD DISEASE

PATHOPHYSIOLOGY

Primary and secondary Raynaud phenomena are forms of an intermittent constriction of arterioles that affects the hands primarily, although it can affect the toes and tip of the nose. Increased or unusual sensations of coldness, pain, and pallor reflect temporary constriction of the arterioles.

The first step toward understanding Raynaud disease is determining whether it is primary or secondary. Primary Raynaud phenomenon has no known cause, but is more common in women, especially during winter months. The condition generally is not as severe as secondary Raynaud phenomenon, but it can be very frustrating.

Secondary Raynaud phenomenon occurs from an underlying cause such as connective tissue disease that affects blood flow to tissues and organs. The most common diseases causing secondary Raynaud phenomenon include lupus, Sjogren syndrome (dryness of the eyes and mouth), scleroderma (hardening of skin and tissues) and rheumatoid arthritis. Blood pressure, migraine, cancer medications and birth control pills can also be the cause. Sometimes, people who work with vibrating tools or are around certain chemicals are at risk of acquiring this disorder. Additionally, smokers have an increased risk of Raynaud disease. Gangrene is not common but can develop in the skin on the tips of the digits. The term *primary Raynaud phenomenon* is synonymous with Raynaud disease; secondary Raynaud phenomenon is called simply *Raynaud phenomenon*.

CLINICAL MANIFESTATIONS

The cardinal signs and symptoms of Raynaud disease are chronically cold hands, numbness, tingling, and pallor. Finger involvement is not symmetric and the thumb is not usually affected. During an arterial spasm, the skin color changes from pallor to cyanosis to redness. Pallor is the result of sudden **vasoconstriction**. Cyanosis reflects inadequate oxygenation. As the spasm resolves, vasodilation allows blood flow to return, which produces a red color (Fig. 36.5).

MEDICAL DIAGNOSIS

The diagnosis of Raynaud disease is usually based on the signs and symptoms and on the absence of evidence of occlusive vascular disease. There is no specific blood test to identify Raynaud disease, but a health care provider may order other tests to rule out connective tissue diseases as mentioned above.

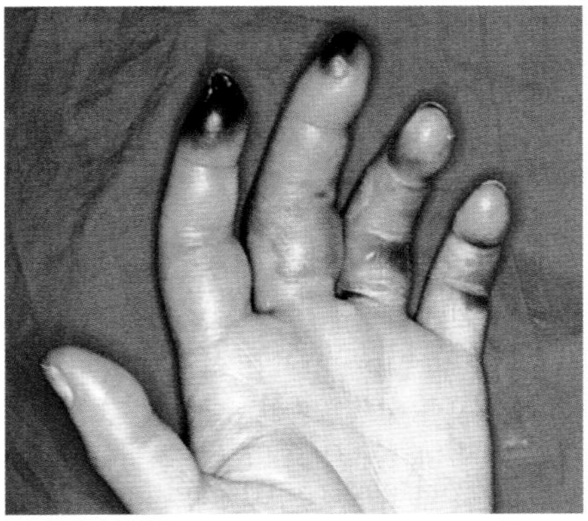

Fig. 36.5 Raynaud phenomenon. (From Kamal A, Brockelhurst JC: *Colour atlas of geriatric medicine*, ed 2, Europe, 2017, Mosby-Year Book.)

MEDICAL AND SURGICAL TREATMENT

The goals of the medical treatment plan for Raynaud disease are to prevent pain and to promote vasodilation in the extremities (see the Complementary and Alternative Therapies box). The most commonly used drugs are calcium-channel blockers or alpha-adrenergic blockers. Other drugs that have been used include transdermal nitroglycerin, an endothelin receptor antagonist (bosentan), phosphodiesterase inhibitors (e.g., sildenafil), and intravenous prostaglandins (e.g., iloprost, alprostadil). In severe cases, the physician may resort to sympathectomy to interrupt the sympathetic nerves. This surgical procedure aids some patients but tends to have temporary effects and is not used routinely.

Complementary and Alternative Therapies

Biofeedback is sometimes helpful in controlling vasospastic episodes with Raynaud disease.

◆ NURSING CARE OF THE PATIENT WITH RAYNAUD DISEASE

Focused Assessment

Assessment of the patient with PVD is summarized in Chapter 33, Box 33.1. With Raynaud disease, assessment of the hands is the priority.

Patient Problems, Goals, and Outcome Criteria: Raynaud Disease

Patient Problems	Goals and Outcome Criteria
Chronic pain related to the ischemia that develops from vasoconstriction	Reduced pain: patient states that pain has decreased, appears relaxed
Inadequate peripheral tissue perfusion related to vasoconstriction	Improved perfusion of peripheral tissue: improved warmth and color of affected areas
Stress related to fear of potential loss of work, difficulty performing activities of daily living (ADL)	Relief from stress: patient states stress is reduced, appears more relaxed

Interventions

Chronic pain and inadequate peripheral tissue perfusion. Nursing interventions to reduce pain and improve tissue perfusion focus on teaching the patient to avoid the stimuli that cause the vasoconstriction: exposure to cold, smoking, and excessive stress. Encourage the patient to take part in a smoking cessation program and to dress warmly when going outside in cold weather. Wear thick socks and gloves or mittens (mittens are better than gloves for maintaining warmth). Sometimes the patient can interrupt an acute attack by placing the affected parts in warm water or by using a hair dryer or hand- and foot-warming devices. In addition to alcohol and caffeine, many over-the-counter (OTC) cold remedies contain vasoconstrictors that can aggravate Raynaud phenomenon. Patients should wear medical alert identification and inform all new health care providers of their diagnosis so that inappropriate medications will not be prescribed.

Pain can be managed by carefully warming the area when vasoconstriction occurs. However, the affected areas must be protected from trauma. Hot water should not be used to warm affected tissue, because the lack of sensation during the period of vasoconstriction could result in serious burns.

Stress. Stress can be addressed in much the same manner as anxiety. Attempt to determine the actual cause of fear, which might be loss of work, loss of limb, or pain. Accept and explore the patient's feelings, provide factual information, encourage problem solving, and help the patient to learn to live with the condition and to manage the prescribed therapy.

ANEURYSMS

PATHOPHYSIOLOGY

An **aneurysm** is a balloon-like bulge in an artery. Aortic aneurysms occur in the aorta, the main artery carrying oxygen-rich blood to the body. There are two types of aneurysms that affect the aorta: abdominal aortic aneurysm (AAA) and thoracic aortic aneurysms (TAA). Aneurysms can be congenital or acquired. Conditions associated with congenital aneurysms are Marfan syndrome and Ehlers-Danlos syndrome. Those affected with Marfan Syndrome are tall and thin with long arms, legs, fingers, and toes. Serious complications involve the heart and aorta. Ehlers-Danlos syndrome, another genetic condition, affects the joints (overly flexible), the skin (stretchy), and the capillaries. These genetic conditions cause abdominal aneurysms and often run in families. Thoracic aneurysms are less common because the wall of the aorta in the thoracic (upper) wall is thicker, muscular, and stronger.

Acquired aneurysms can be caused by atherosclerosis, trauma, or infection. The most common cause is atherosclerosis. Hypertension and high cholesterol are contributing factors. Atherosclerosis weakens elastic fibers in the media, which allows a segment of the vessel to balloon outward. Infections, including syphilis, can also damage the media and result in the formation of aneurysms. The abdominal aorta is the most common site of aneurysm formation.

RISK FACTORS

Risk factors include age (most common in adults aged over 65 years), family history, genes, lifestyle habits (smoking, using cocaine, or weightlifting), medical conditions (chronic obstructive pulmonary disease and other heart related conditions), and male gender.

CLINICAL MANIFESTATIONS

Generally, symptoms that occur before a rupture depend upon location of the aneurysm and whether it has become large enough to affect other parts of the body. People with TAA usually have no symptoms, although some report deep, diffuse chest pain. If the aneurysm puts pressure on the recurrent laryngeal nerve, the patient may complain of hoarseness. Pressure on the coronary arteries can cause angina and pressure on the esophagus may cause dysphagia (difficulty swallowing). If the superior vena cava is compressed, the patient may have edema of the head and arms. Signs of airway obstruction may be present if the aneurysm presses against pulmonary structures.

AAA is usually detected during routine physical examinations or diagnostic procedures. The aneurysm may be palpated as a pulsating mass in the area slightly to the left of the umbilicus. Although most abdominal aneurysms are asymptomatic, pressure on abdominal organs and nerves may cause back pain, epigastric pain, or constipation.

COMPLICATIONS

Complications of aneurysms include rupture, thrombus formation that obstructs blood flow, emboli, and pressure on surrounding structures.

MEDICAL DIAGNOSIS

Certain groups of people should be screened for aneurysm, especially those 65 to 75 years old with a history of smoking and those who have a family member who has had an aneurysm. An aneurysm can develop and grow without any symptoms until it ruptures or dissects—both life-threatening events. If the aneurysm is found early, treatment or surgery may slow its growth and prevent rupture or dissection.

Diagnosis is made on the basis of physical findings and radiologic studies. Studies performed to obtain better visualization of the aneurysm include echocardiography, ultrasonography, computed tomography (CT), MRI, and aortography (see Chapter 33, Table 33.3).

MEDICAL AND SURGICAL TREATMENT

Repair of aneurysms may be done by replacing the dilated segment of the artery with a synthetic graft or, in some cases, by suturing or patching the defective area. For TAA, TEVAR (thoracic endovascular aneurysm repair) has largely supplanted open repair because it lowers morbidity and mortality. For the patient with AAA, endovascular aneurysm repair (EVAR) may be an option. EVAR places an aortic stent graft in the aneurysm through a femoral artery incision. This minimally invasive procedure is less risky than open surgical repair. However, not all patients are candidates for EVAR.

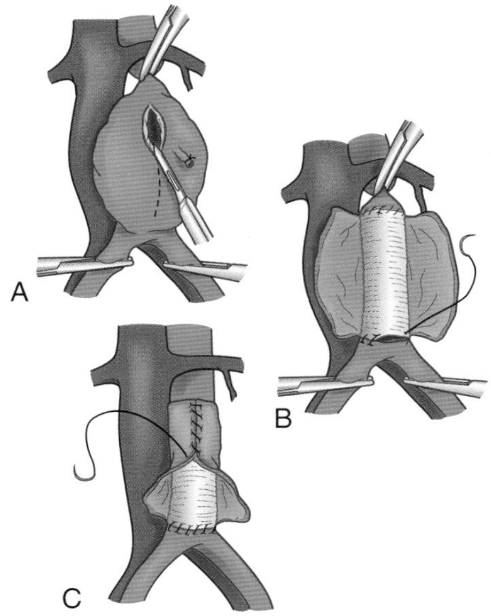

Fig. 36.6 Surgical repair of an abdominal aortic aneurysm. (A) Incising the aneurysmal sac. (B) Insertion of synthetic graft. (C) Suturing native aortic wall over synthetic graft. (From Lewis LL, et al.: *Medical-surgical nursing*, ed 10, 2017, Elsevier.)

Repair is usually done as soon as possible but may be delayed until the patient is evaluated for other problems that increase surgical risk (Fig. 36.6).

Decisions to attempt repair of aneurysms are based on the size of the defect and the patient's general status. For example, an AAA smaller than 5 cm is usually monitored with periodic ultrasound studies. If it begins to enlarge, surgical repair may be recommended.

Complications of AAA surgery vary with the location of the defect. Complications of AAA surgery include myocardial infarction, sexual dysfunction, renal failure, emboli, spinal cord ischemia with paralysis, bowel and bladder incontinence, and impaired sensation. Although EVAR is generally safer, complications can include graft leakage, stent migration, aneurysm rupture, bleeding, and infection.

Because surgical repair of aneurysms is high risk for the patient, research is taking place to better understand AAA pathogenesis and also to lead the development of medical therapies, such as drug-based and cell-based strategies. Aneurysms are caused in part by inflammation. Currently, no drug therapy is available for AAA. A clinical need exists to develop medical therapies that limit or prevent the progressive expansion and rupturing of the aneurysm.

PREOPERATIVE AND POSTOPERATIVE NURSING CARE OF THE PATIENT WITH AN ANEURYSM

When surgical repair of an aneurysm is planned, the patient should be prepared physically and emotionally as described in Chapter 17. Preoperative and postoperative nursing care specifically for cardiovascular patients is described in Chapter 33.

Patient Problems, Goals, and Outcome Criteria: Aortic Aneurysm Repair

In addition to the routine problems of the postoperative patient (see Chapter 17), patient problems for the patient who has had an aortic aneurysm repair may include the following.

Patient Problems	Goals and Outcome Criteria
Impaired urinary elimination related to interrupted blood flow	Normal urinary function: urine output approximately equal to fluid intake
Potential for injury related to ileus	Absence of injury related to ileus: wound margins intact, no abdominal distention, bowel sounds present
Inadequate pulmonary oxygenation because of poor breathing pattern related to abdominal incision or splinting	Adequate breathing pattern and oxygenation: regular respirations, 12 to 20 breaths per minute; clear breath sounds
Decreased cardiac output related to myocardial infarction, occlusion of blood vessels, graft leakage	Adequate cardiac output: pulse and blood pressure consistent with patient norms
Inadequate peripheral circulation related to vascular occlusion	Normal peripheral circulation: warm extremities with palpable pulses

Interventions

Complications of both types of aortic aneurysm repair can occur, and they may be life-threatening. Bleeding and blood loss are the most urgent complications and may need additional surgery or blood transfusions to correct and/or stabilize.

Impaired urinary elimination. During repair of an abdominal aneurysm, the aorta is clamped for a period of time. This poses a risk of renal damage and subsequent renal failure. Thus fluid intake and urine output are measured hourly at first, then less often if output is satisfactory. Declining urine output must be reported promptly to the physician. In addition to daily weights, blood urea nitrogen (BUN), creatinine, and electrolyte levels are usually measured daily to detect increases associated with renal failure. Because fluid retention or circulatory obstruction may cause edema, its presence should be noted. Intravenous fluids should be administered as ordered.

Potential for injury. After abdominal surgery, peristalsis ceases temporarily. A nasogastric tube may be inserted and attached to suction to prevent gaseous distention of the bowel, which is uncomfortable and places stress on the abdominal incision. Ensure that the suction is working properly and monitor for distention and the return of bowel sounds.

Inadequate pulmonary oxygenation. Whether the patient has an abdominal or a thoracic incision, a risk of poor lung expansion exists. After thoracic surgery, patients are at especially high risk for atelectasis and pneumonia. Mechanical ventilation in the immediate postoperative period maintains adequate ventilation until the patient is able to breathe effectively. Thereafter assist the patient to turn, deep breathe, and cough frequently. An incentive spirometer may be used to encourage lung expansion. It is important to support the patient's incision during the breathing exercises. Pain control measures include patient-controlled analgesia (PCA), an epidural catheter, as needed (PRN) parenteral analgesics, and other measures as appropriate. The patient can breathe more effectively if good pain relief is achieved. Monitor lung sounds frequently to assess for abnormalities.

Decreased cardiac output. Cardiac output may fall as a result of myocardial infarction, cardiac dysrhythmias, heart failure, or hemorrhage. Hemorrhage may occur in the incision or by separation of the graft. Closely monitor the patient's vital signs and hemodynamics. In addition, inspect wound dressing and drains for increasing bleeding. Early signs of circulatory failure are restlessness and tachycardia. Later signs are hypotension, cyanosis, and decreased alertness. Immediately notify the physician if evidence of decreasing cardiac output is seen.

Inadequate peripheral circulation. A risk of impaired blood flow below the level of the repaired aneurysm exists. Monitor peripheral pulses and the color and warmth of the extremities. This assessment is especially important when a patient has had a femoral or popliteal aneurysm repair. Signs and symptoms of occlusion include pain, pallor or cyanosis, and coldness distal to the repair. If these manifestations occur, they must be reported to the physician at once.

AORTIC DISSECTION

Aortic dissection is different from an aneurysm. The aorta wall is three layers thick. When the inner layer (called the intima) tears, blood can move between the middle and inner layer of the artery wall and dissect (separate). Blood accumulates between the layers, possibly causing the media to split lengthwise. The split may extend up and down the aorta, where it can occlude major arteries. Fig. 36.7 compares the various types of aortic aneurysms with an aortic dissection.

People at highest risk of an aortic dissection are males and individuals 60 to 70 years old. Precipitating factors include aortic disease, atherosclerosis, trauma,

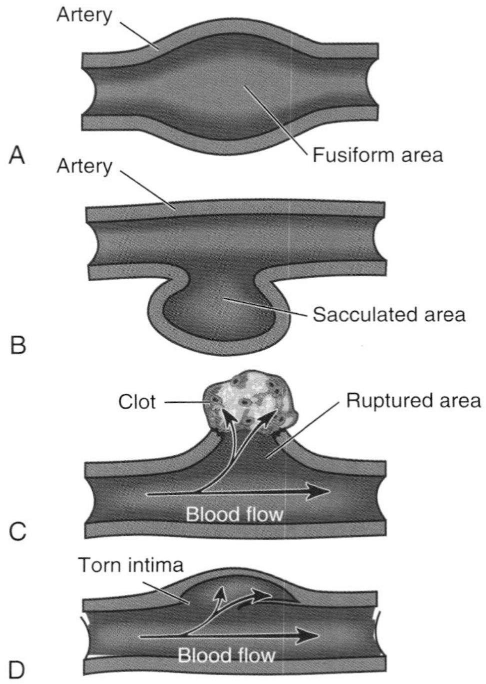

Fig. 36.7 (A) True fusiform abdominal aortic aneurysm. (B) True saccular aortic aneurysm. (C) False aneurysm or pseudoaneurysm. (D) Aortic dissection. (From Lewis LL, et al.: *Medical-surgical nursing*, ed 10, 2017, Elsevier.)

tobacco, cocaine or methamphetamine use, congenital heart disease, connective tissue disorders, family history, history of heart surgery, pregnancy, and poorly controlled hypertension.

Aortic dissections are classified in two ways:

- Type A: The most common and the most dangerous dissection occurs as the aorta descends from the heart.
- Type B: This type of dissection occurs in the lower part of the aorta toward the abdomen

Most patients with Type A aortic dissection experience an abrupt onset of excruciating anterior chest pain, whereas patients with Type B usually experience pain in the back, abdomen or legs. The location of the pain in both types may overlap, and the pain is often characterized as "sharp," "tearing," "ripping," or "stabbing." Older people are less likely to have an abrupt onset of chest or back pain, and instead may have hypotension and vague symptoms.

The risk of life-threatening complications (e.g., rupture, stroke) is much greater when the ascending aorta is involved than when only the descending aorta is affected. If no complications occur, the patient may be managed with antihypertensive agents and drugs that decrease the strength of cardiac contraction. Surgery is generally recommended for an acute Type A dissection, and it is considered a surgical emergency. The affected area containing the intimal tear is replaced with a synthetic graft. The death rate and incidence of neurological complications are high. Preoperatively, the patient should be kept in a semi-Fowler's position in a quiet environment to maintain their blood pressure and heart rate at the lowest safe level possible. Opioids and sedatives should be given as ordered to minimize pain and anxiety. Monitor vital signs frequently and look for changes in peripheral pulses as well as signs of increasing pain, restlessness and anxiety. A key aspect of postoperative care is keeping the blood pressure at the lowest possible level. In other respects, the care is similar to that of a patient who has had an aortic aneurysm repair.

LYMPHANGITIS

PATHOPHYSIOLOGY

Lymphangitis is acute inflammation of the lymphatic channels. The inflammation is the result of an infectious process. Lymphangitis commonly develops after microorganisms gain entry into the lymphatic vessels through a skin wound.

CLINICAL MANIFESTATIONS

The primary characteristic of lymphangitis is enlargement of the lymph nodes along the lymphatic channel. Each node can be palpated along the course of the channel. The patient complains of node tenderness, a wound that is not healing, and feeling sick or weak. A red streak from the infected wound extends up the extremity along the path of the lymphatics, as each node drains into the lymphatic system and the cardiovascular system. These nodes are located in the groin, the axilla, and the cervical regions. The infectious material can localize into an abscess with necrotic, purulent discharge from the area. Lymphangitis can spread to the blood if left untreated. This life-threatening infection is called sepsis, fever and inflammation throughout the body causing a cascade of changes that damage multiple organ systems and sometimes result in death. With prompt medical treatment, recovery is usually rapid, and treatment is highly effective.

MEDICAL DIAGNOSIS

The classic signs and symptoms, supported by wound culture results, are usually adequate to confirm lymphangitis. Lymphangiography, which uses a contrast medium for the radiologic visualization of the lymphatic system, will also provide evidence of lymphangitis.

MEDICAL AND SURGICAL TREATMENT

Antimicrobials (usually delivered intravenously) often are used before culture results to treat lymphangitis. When an abscess develops, the area is incised to drain the purulent material. Other supportive measures that may be ordered are rest and elevation of the limb; warm, wet dressings; and elastic support hose.

NURSING CARE OF THE PATIENT WITH LYMPHANGITIS

Focused Assessment

Care of the patient with lymphangitis includes inspection of the skin for open wounds, signs of inflammation (redness, warmth, edema), and presence of red streaks along the paths of lymphatic channels (see the Nutrition Considerations box). Palpate the lymph nodes in the groin and underarm areas for any enlargements. Report fever or chills.

Nutrition Considerations

1. Edema is frequently treated with a low-sodium diet; sodium-restricted diets vary from 4 g (least restrictive) to 250 mg (severe sodium restriction) daily.
2. Foods high in sodium include salt, monosodium glutamate, smoked or processed meats (ham, bacon, frankfurters, cold cuts), salted foods (potato chips, pretzels, salted nuts, popcorn), prepackaged frozen foods, and canned foods.
3. Older adults who take diuretics are generally not encouraged to restrict sodium intake because they are at risk for the adverse effects of low sodium.
4. Salt substitutes are a source of potassium, which is desirable in patients who are receiving potassium-wasting diuretics; however, a health care provider should approve salt substitutes before they are used.

Patient Problems, Goals, and Outcome Criteria: Lymphangitis

Patient Problems	Goals and Outcome Criteria
Pain related to the inflammatory process in the lymphatic system	Pain relief: patient verbalizes less pain, appears relaxed
Activity intolerance related to pain with movement	Improved activity tolerance: patient increases activity without increased pain
Potential for injury related to infection	Decreased risk for injury: protection of affected tissue Resolution of infection: absence of fever, normal white blood cell count, decreasing swelling and pain

Interventions

Nursing care of the patient with lymphangitis is essentially the same as that for chronic venous insufficiency.

Interventions to relieve pain include administration of the prescribed analgesics and antimicrobials and elevation of the extremity to reduce lymphedema. Nonpharmacologic measures should be used in addition to analgesics. The application of warm, moist soaks to the infected areas as prescribed improves the circulation to the area. As the circulation is improved, white blood cells (WBCs), nutrients, and O_2 are delivered, which aids in the recovery of the healthy tissue. Elastic support hose is used for several months after an acute attack of lymphangitis to prevent the formation of lymphedema.

Nursing Care Plan Patient With a Venous Stasis Ulcer

FOCUSED ASSESSMENT

Health History

A 75-year-old man is being seen in the community clinic for an ulcer on the medial malleolus of the right ankle. The ulcer is shallow and measures 1.5 cm × 2.5 cm. He describes a "heavy" burning sensation in the lower legs. He worked for many years as a tollbooth attendant and has had chronic venous insufficiency for 5 years. He reports having had hypertension in the past but is taking no medication for it. Otherwise he has been in good health and remains active. He is the caregiver for his wife, who has been disabled for 3 years because of a stroke. He has a daughter who helps with her care and who has been dressing his leg ulcer.

Physical Examination

Vital signs: blood pressure 194/102 mm Hg, pulse 64 beats per minute, respiration 16 breaths per minute, temperature 97°F (36.1°C) measured orally. Height 5′9″, weight 170 lb. Alert and oriented. Walks with slight limp. 2+ edema, both ankles. Varicosities noted in both legs. Stasis dermatitis in ankles and calves. Ulcer is 1.5 cm × 2.5 cm and shallow. Ulcer is slightly moist, pink, with no drainage or odor. Ankles and feet are cooler than calves. Pedal pulses faint but palpable, slightly stronger in left foot.

Patient Problem	Goals and Outcome Criteria	Interventions
Inadequate peripheral tissue perfusion related to compromised circulation	Perfusion of blood and oxygen will improve, as evidenced by reduced pain, redness, and edema; skin will be warm to the touch.	Instruct the patient in measures to improve circulation: exercise moderately each day, elevate the legs above the level of the heart when resting, avoid smoking, apply dressings and compression stockings as ordered, avoid prolonged periods of walking or standing still. Teach wound care as ordered. At each visit, assess the condition of his ulcer, peripheral pulses, skin color and warmth, pain, and edema.
Potential for infection related to open wound	The patient will remain free of signs and symptoms of infection: fever, increasing redness, and purulent drainage.	Teach hygienic techniques of hand washing and wound care. Encourage him to choose a diet with adequate protein and vitamins. Teach the signs and symptoms of infection that should be reported to the physician. Instruct him in antimicrobial therapy if prescribed.
Pain related to circulatory impairment	The patient will report pain relief.	Encourage the patient to increase movement and maintain warmth to improve circulation. Teach pain relief measures including relaxation, deep-breathing techniques, cutaneous stimulation, and behavior modification. Explain the use of prescribed analgesics. Assess the effectiveness of pain control measures.
Disrupted skin tissue integrity related to circulatory impairment	The patient's wound will heal completely.	Assess and document the condition of the ulcer during each clinic visit. Advise the patient to use gentle soap for bathing, to avoid trauma, and not to rub the ulcer. Encourage good nutrition and adequate fluid intake. Discuss wound care with the physician or wound, ostomy, continence (WOC) nurse (specialist in wound care).
Ineffective self-care management related to lack of knowledge of chronic venous insufficiency and treatment of stasis ulcer	The patient will correctly explain chronic venous insufficiency and demonstrate correct care of the ulcer.	Assess the patient's understanding of his condition and self-care. Advise him to avoid restrictive clothing, smoking, and weight gain. Explore sources of stress and coping strategies.
Ineffective self-care management related to lack of knowledge of importance of treating hypertension	The patient will verbalize understanding of the need to have his blood pressure evaluated and will make an appointment for evaluation.	Explain the importance of detecting and treating hypertension. Refer the patient to the physician or blood pressure clinic for evaluation.

CRITICAL THINKING QUESTIONS

1. What data will contribute to the assessment of the effectiveness of pain and infection control techniques?
2. What role does nutrition play in the therapeutic treatment of venous stasis ulcers?
3. What data should you collect related to the condition of the ulcer?

Get Ready for the NCLEX® Examination!

Key Points

- The most dangerous complication of venous thrombosis is pulmonary embolism.
- An arterial embolus, an unattached clot or other material in an artery, can lodge in an artery and obstruct blood.
- Nursing care of the patient with an arterial embolus focuses on inadequate peripheral circulation, stress, skin breakdown, immobility, and inability to manage treatment program.
- PAD impairs blood flow and may be treated surgically.
- Nursing care of the patient with PAD focuses on inability to tolerate activity, pain, skin breakdown, altered self-concept, inadequate peripheral circulation, and inability to manage treatment program.
- Thromboangiitis obliterans (Buerger disease) is an inflammatory thrombotic disorder of arteries and veins in upper and lower extremities of smokers; atherosclerosis is not a factor.
- Primary and secondary Raynaud phenomena are characterized by intermittent arteriolar vasoconstriction that is usually treated with vasodilators.
- An aneurysm is a dilated segment of an artery, most often the aorta, which can rupture, serve as a site for thrombus formation, and compress surrounding tissues.
- Aortic dissection results from a tear in the intima that allows blood to escape into the space between the intima and the media, which causes the media to split lengthwise.
- Varicose veins are dilated, tortuous, superficial veins that result from incompetent venous valves; they may lead to chronic venous insufficiency and are treated with conservative measures to improve venous return and sometimes with surgical intervention or laser therapy.
- Phlebitis is inflammation of a vein wall.
- Thrombosis is clot formation and DVT indicates that the clot is located in deep veins, a condition that poses a high risk for pulmonary emboli.
- Risk factors for thrombus formation are bed rest, surgery in people older than 40 years of age, leg trauma and immobilization, previous venous insufficiency, obesity, oral contraceptives, and malignancy.
- Nursing care of the patient with venous thrombosis addresses skin breakdown, pain, anxiety, inability to tolerate activity, inadequate peripheral circulation, inadequate oxygenation, and inability to manage treatment program.
- Chronic venous insufficiency causes edema and stasis dermatitis around the ankles.
- Lymphangitis is an inflammation of the lymphatic channels that is treated with antimicrobials, analgesics, heat therapy, and rest.

Additional Learning Resources

SG Go to your Study Guide for additional learning activities to help you master this chapter content.

Go to your Evolve website (http://evolve.elsevier.com/Linton/medsurg) for the following learning resources and much more:

- Fluid and Electrolyte Tutorial
- Review Questions for the NCLEX® Examination

Review Questions for the NCLEX® Examination

1. Mrs. P. has had an open abdominal aneurysm repair. Her nurse knows that it is especially important to monitor:

1. Reflexes in the lower extremities
2. Intake and output
3. Mental status
4. Electrocardiogram

NCLEX Client Need: Physiological Integrity: Physiological Adaptation

2. Which of the following is the most serious complication of venous thrombosis?

1. Pulmonary embolism
2. Stasis dermatitis
3. Ankle ulceration
4. Pitting edema

NCLEX Client Need: Physiological Integrity: Physiological Adaptation

3. Signs and symptoms of an arterial embolism in the lower extremities are (select all that apply):

1. Severe, acute pain
2. Hypotension
3. Excessive bleeding
4. Absent distal pulses

NCLEX Client Need: Physiological Integrity: Physiological Adaptation

4. Because the patient with an acute aortic embolism is usually immobilized, which actions should be taken by the nurse? Select all that apply.

1. Perform range of motion exercises
2. Protect the affected limb from extreme heat or cold
3. Raise the affected limb above the level of the heart
4. Keep flat in bed

NCLEX Client Need: Physiological Integrity: Basic Care and Comfort

5. For a patient with peripheral arterial disease, the nurse would carry out which of the following actions to help to relieve pain?

1. Elevate foot of bed
2. Administer opioids as prescribed
3. Use relaxation techniques
4. Keep immobilized

NCLEX Client Need: Physiological Integrity: Basic Care and Comfort

6. Raynaud disease is characterized by which of the following signs or symptoms?

1. Cold hands
2. Vasodilation
3. Swollen thumb
4. Symmetrical finger involvement

NCLEX Client Need: Physiological Integrity: Physiological Adaptation

7. **Which is the most common cause of an acquired aneurysm?**
   1. Hypertension
   2. Atherosclerosis
   3. Trauma
   4. Infection

   NCLEX Client Need: Physiological Integrity: Reduction of Risk Potential

8. **A 60-year-old male has been diagnosed with a venous thrombosis in his right lower leg. What signs and symptoms would be expected distal to the obstruction? (Select all that apply)**
   1. Absence of peripheral pulses
   2. Ankle edema
   3. Yellow or dark ulceration
   4. Thick hardened skin

   NCLEX Client Need: Physiological Integrity: Reduction of Risk Potential

9. **Which of the following is the primary nursing role in the care of the patient with varicose veins?**
   1. Teaching self-care
   2. Providing a warm environment
   3. Encouraging fluids
   4. Keeping patient immobilized

   NCLEX Client Need: Physiological Integrity: Basic Care and Comfort

10. **Teaching a patient with a venous thrombosis should include: (Select all that apply)**
    1 Protect legs from pressure and trauma
    2. Elevate legs when sitting
    3. Avoid prolonged standing and crossing your legs
    4. Massage affected area to alleviate pain

    NCLEX Client Need: Health Promotion and Maintenance

11. **SLO/Objective:** Determine appropriate nursing actions for patients experiencing postoperative complications.

    NGN Item Type: Extended Drag and Drop

    Cognitive Skill: Take Action

    A 68-year-old man was admitted to the ICU from the PACU after having a repair of an aortic aneurism. He has a history of hypertension and prostatitis and total knee replacement in his right knee.

    Indicate which nursing action listed in the far left column is appropriate for the potential postoperative complications. Note that not all nursing actions will be used.

NURSING ACTION	POTENTIAL POSTOPERATIVE COMPLICATION	APPROPRIATE NURSING ACTION FOR POSTOPERATIVE COMPLICATION
1. Assess peripheral pulses	Renal failure	
2. Encourage the patient to use an incentive spirometer	Hemorrhage	
3. Measure intake and output	Pneumonia	
4. Monitor patient's vital signs	Heart failure	
5. Inspect wound for bleeding	Vascular occlusion	
6. Elevate feet above heart		
7. Keep patient immobilized		

Digestive System Introduction

37

http://evolve.elsevier.com/Linton/medsurg

Objectives

1. Identify the nursing responsibilities in the care of patients who are undergoing diagnostic tests and procedures for disorders of the digestive tract and the accessory organs.
2. List the data to be included in the nursing assessment of the patient with digestive tract disorders.
3. For each class of drugs used to treat digestive tract disorders, identify related nursing interventions.
4. Describe nursing responsibilities for patients having common therapeutic measures for digestive tract disorders.

Key Terms

ascites
aspiration
cathartic
chime
endoscope
gluconeogenesis
glycogenesis
glycogenolysis
hepatic
hepatomegaly
jaundice
scleral icterus
striae

To remain healthy, the human body must have a steady supply of nutrients and fluids. The primary role of the digestive tract is to extract the molecules essential for cellular function from food and fluids. Disorders of the digestive tract can threaten the patient's nutritional status, leading to disorders in the structure and functioning of other body systems.

ANATOMY AND PHYSIOLOGY OF THE DIGESTIVE TRACT

The digestive tract is also called the *gastrointestinal* (GI) *tract* and the *alimentary tract* (Fig. 37.1). It is a muscular tube about 30 feet long. The main parts of the digestive tract are the mouth, pharynx, esophagus, stomach, small intestine, large intestine, and anus. Other organs that are outside the digestive tract but considered part of the digestive system are called *accessory organs*. Accessory organs include the salivary glands, liver, gallbladder, and pancreas. Each of these organs secretes fluid containing specialized enzymes into the digestive tract. These enzymes play a part in the breakdown or metabolism of foodstuffs. A two-layer membrane, the peritoneum, lines the abdominal cavity and covers the surfaces of the abdominal organs. Lubricating fluid between the two layers permits the organs to move without friction during breathing and digestive movements.

The functions of the digestive tract are ingestion, digestion, absorption of nutrients, and elimination of wastes. Ingestion refers to the intake of nutrients. Digestion is the breakdown of food into simple nutrient molecules that can be used by the cells. The process of digestion requires (1) the adequate intake of food and fluids, (2) the mechanical and chemical breakdown of food, and (3) the movement of food through the digestive tract.

MOUTH

Food is ingested into the mouth, where the teeth, tongue, and salivary glands begin the process of food digestion. As the teeth cut and grind the food, the salivary glands secrete saliva—a watery solution that contains amylase (ptyalin). Amylase is an enzyme that initiates the breakdown of carbohydrates. The tongue helps by mixing saliva with the food and pressing it against the teeth. When the bolus is swallowed, the tongue forces the food into the pharynx.

PHARYNX

The pharynx is a muscular structure that is shared by the digestive and respiratory tracts. It joins the mouth

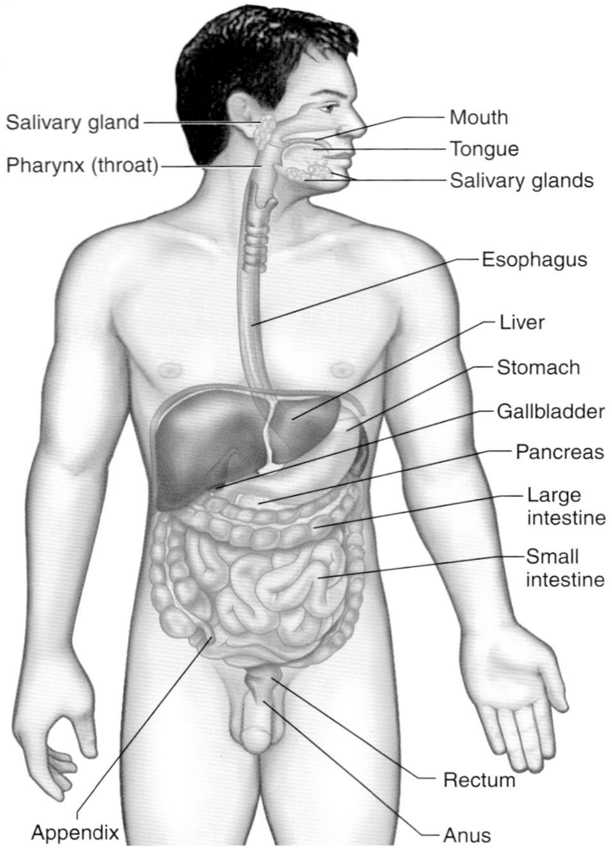

Fig. 37.1 The digestive tract and associated structures. (From Thibodeau GA, Patton KT: *The human body in health and disease*, 6th ed 6, St. Louis, 2014, Mosby.)

and nasal passages to the esophagus. During swallowing, the epiglottis covers the airway like a trapdoor to prevent food from entering the respiratory tract.

ESOPHAGUS

Food moves from the pharynx into the esophagus, a long muscular tube that passes through the diaphragm into the stomach. Gravity helps but is not essential for the movement of food through the esophagus. Circular, wavelike contractions of the muscles of the digestive tract propel food down the tract. This movement is called *peristalsis*.

STOMACH

The stomach is the widest section of the digestive tract. The stomach is not very large when empty, but it expands considerably when food is present. It consists of three sections: (1) the fundus, (2) the body, and (3) the pylorus. A unique arrangement of muscle layers allows the stomach to churn the food, mixing it with gastric secretions until it becomes a semiliquid mass called **chyme**. Gastric secretions include rennin, pepsin, hydrochloric acid, and lipase. Rennin starts to break down milk proteins, lipase breaks down fats, and pepsin and hydrochloric acid partially digest proteins. The pyloric sphincter between the stomach and the small intestine keeps food in the stomach until it is properly mixed.

SMALL INTESTINE

Chyme leaves the stomach and enters the small intestine, where chemical digestion and absorption of nutrients take place. The small intestine is approximately 20 feet long and consists of three sections: (1) the duodenum, (2) the jejunum, and (3) the ileum.

Liver and pancreatic secretions enter the digestive tract in the duodenum. Bile, produced in the liver and stored in the gallbladder, breaks down large fat globules. Pancreatic enzymes further reduce the fat to glycerol and fatty acids, which can be absorbed easily. The functions of the liver, gallbladder, and pancreas are discussed in more detail in Chapter 40 and 50.

Three layers of tissue make up the walls of the small intestine. The mucous membrane layer secretes the digestive enzymes sucrase, lactase, maltase, carboxypeptidase, aminopeptidase, dipeptidase, nucleosidase, lipase, and enterokinase. The inner layer is lined with thousands of microscopic projections called *villi*. Digested food molecules are absorbed through the villi into the bloodstream. Muscle layers contract to continue mixing the chyme, moving it toward the large intestine.

LARGE INTESTINE AND ANUS

Chyme enters the large intestine through the ileocecal valve. The first section of the large intestine is the cecum, where the appendix is located. The large intestine goes up the right side of the abdomen (the ascending colon), across the abdomen just below the waist (the transverse colon), and down the left side of the abdomen (the descending colon). The part of the descending colon between the iliac crest and the rectum is called *the sigmoid colon*. The last 6 to 8 inches of the large intestine is the rectum, which ends at the anus, where wastes leave the body. The presence of sphincters in the anus allows wastes to be stored until voluntary elimination occurs.

Unlike the small intestine, the large intestine has no villi and secretes no digestive enzymes. Its function is to absorb water from the chyme and to eliminate the remaining solid wastes in the form of feces.

See Fig. 37.2 for an illustration of the time required for food and other substances to move through the digestive tract.

ACCESSORY ORGANS

The salivary glands, liver, pancreas, and gallbladder are not actually part of the digestive tract. However, they play such an important part in digestion that they are called *accessory organs*. Dysfunction of any of these structures can have important consequences for the digestive process and the patient's general health.

ANATOMY AND PHYSIOLOGY OF THE LIVER

The liver is the largest internal organ in the body. It is located under the diaphragm in the right upper quadrant of the abdomen (Fig. 37.3). The term **hepatic** refers to the liver.

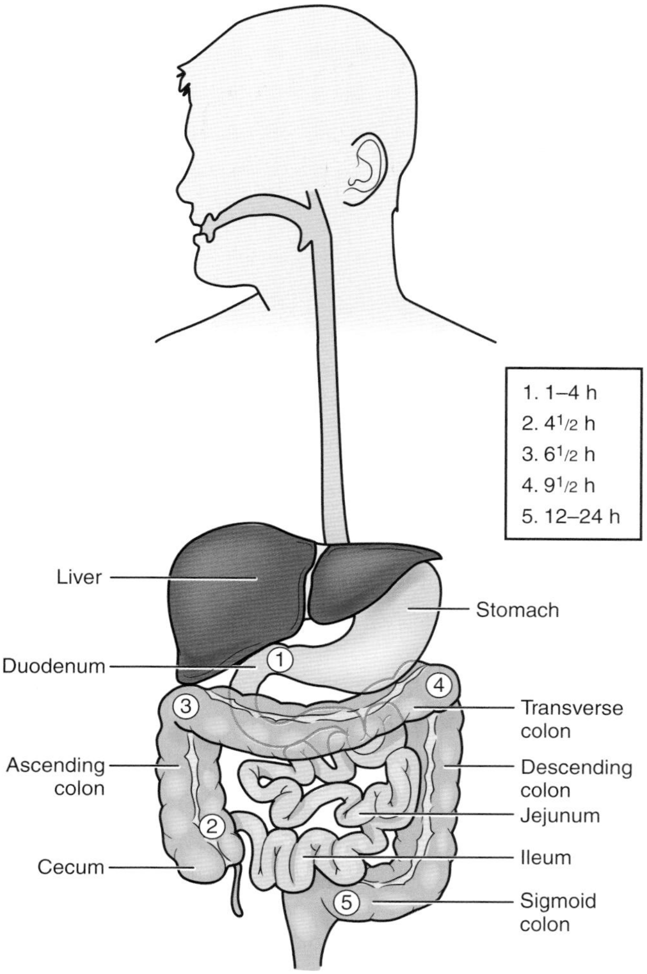

Fig. 37.2 Time required for the passage of substances through the digestive tract.

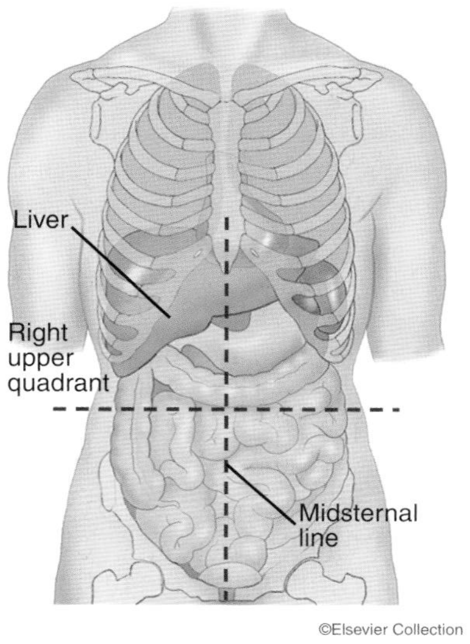

Fig. 37.3 The liver is located under the diaphragm in the right upper quadrant of the abdomen. Anatomic landmarks are noted. (Copyright © Elsevier Collection.)

The liver can be divided into four lobes that are made up of many lobules (Fig. 37.4). Blood from the aorta is delivered to the liver via the hepatic artery. The portal vein delivers blood from the intestines to the liver. Portal blood circulates through the liver and is transported to the inferior vena cava by the hepatic veins. Fig. 37.5 illustrates hepatic circulation.

Specialized hepatic cells allow the liver to carry out many critical functions. Reticuloendothelial cells, called *Kupffer cells*, ingest old red blood cells (RBCs) and bacteria. Parenchymal cells carry out various metabolic functions, including metabolism of carbohydrates, fats, proteins, and steroids and detoxification of potentially harmful substances.

Bile Production and Excretion

Bilirubin is a product of the normal breakdown of old RBCs in the liver. The initial breakdown product is unconjugated or indirect bilirubin. The liver then converts unconjugated bilirubin into conjugated bilirubin and secretes it into the bile. Bile produced in the liver passes through the cystic duct into the gallbladder for storage.

When fats pass into the duodenum, the gallbladder and the liver respond by delivering bile through the common bile duct into the small intestine. Bile emulsifies fat, meaning that it breaks it into small particles that can be absorbed easily. It also neutralizes the acidic chyme as it leaves the stomach. Bile plays a role in the absorption of fat-soluble vitamins and the removal of some toxins.

Bile travels through the intestines with the chyme. In the large intestine, it is converted to urobilinogen and then to stercobilin. This final breakdown product of bilirubin gives stool its characteristic brown color.

Metabolism

Glucose metabolism. The liver helps to maintain the blood glucose within a certain range. After a meal, excess glucose molecules are taken up by the liver, combined, and then stored as glycogen. This process is called **glycogenesis**. When the glucose level in the blood falls, the process is reversed by **glycogenolysis** and the glucose molecules are returned to the blood. **Gluconeogenesis** is the third process by which the liver maintains blood glucose. Fats and protein are broken down in response to low blood glucose levels and the molecules are used to make new glucose.

Protein metabolism. Some nonessential amino acids, plasma proteins (albumin and globulin), and clotting factors are synthesized in the liver. Another important liver function in relation to protein metabolism is the conversion of ammonia to urea. Ammonia is a by-product of the metabolism of amino acids. If ammonia accumulates in the blood, it has toxic effects on brain tissue.

Lipid metabolism. The liver synthesizes lipids from glucose, pyruvic acid, acetic acid, and amino acids. It

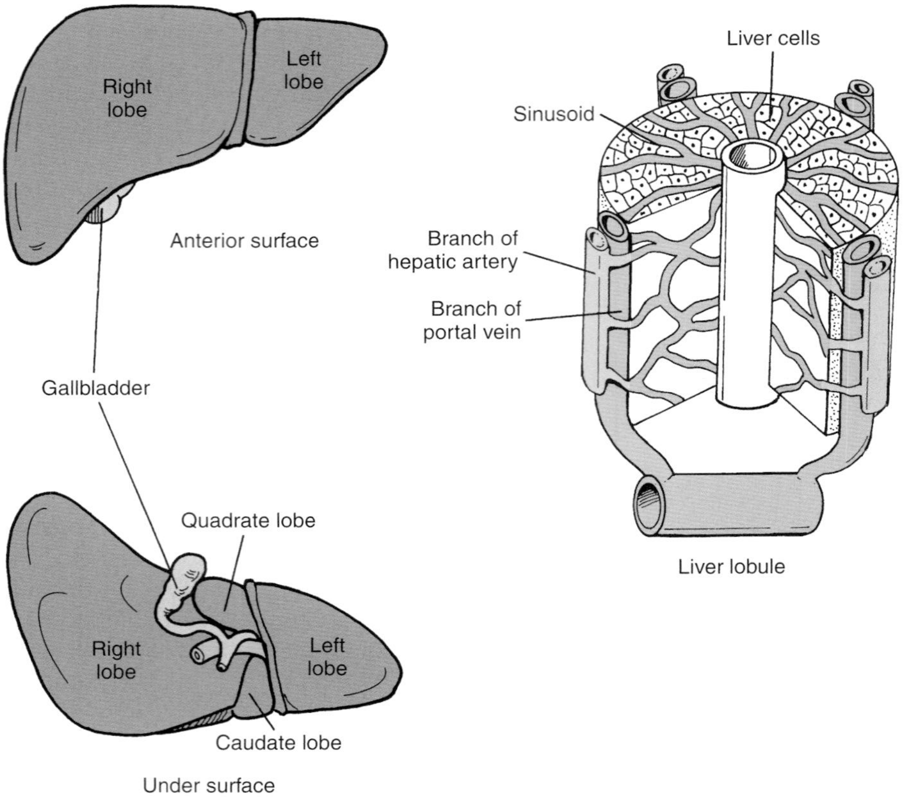

Fig. 37.4 The liver has four lobes, each made up of many lobules.

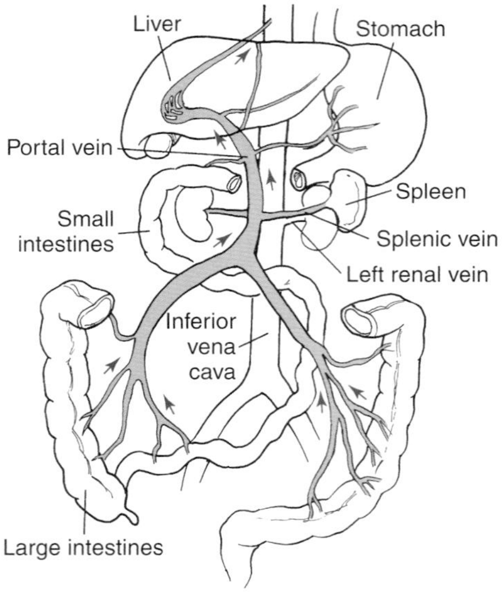

Fig. 37.5 Hepatic circulation. Venous blood from the digestive tract and spleen passes through the liver via the portal vein and is delivered through the hepatic veins to the inferior vena cava.

also synthesizes fatty acids, breaks down triglycerides, and synthesizes and breaks down cholesterol.

Blood Coagulation

Normal blood coagulation (clotting) is a complex process. Two essential elements for coagulation, prothrombin and fibrinogen, are synthesized by the liver.

Detoxification

The liver filters the blood and inactivates many chemicals, including most medications. Therefore, medications are prescribed very cautiously for patients with poor liver function. Patients with liver disease are at increased risk for toxic effects of drugs (see the Complementary and Alternative Therapies box). With age, some decrease in liver function occurs, so lower drug dosages may be adequate. Especially with long-term therapy, the older person should be monitored closely for signs of toxicity.

> **Complementary and Alternative Therapies**
>
> Inform patients that the following herbs can harm the liver: comfrey, borage, coltsfoot, chaparral, and germander.

Immunity

An important protective mechanism is the development of antibodies to resist pathogens. Antibodies and other substances that help to resist infection are produced in the liver.

Hormone Metabolism

The liver plays an important role in the metabolism of adrenocortical hormones, estrogen, testosterone, and aldosterone. If these hormones are not metabolized, they accumulate, causing an exaggerated effect on target organs.

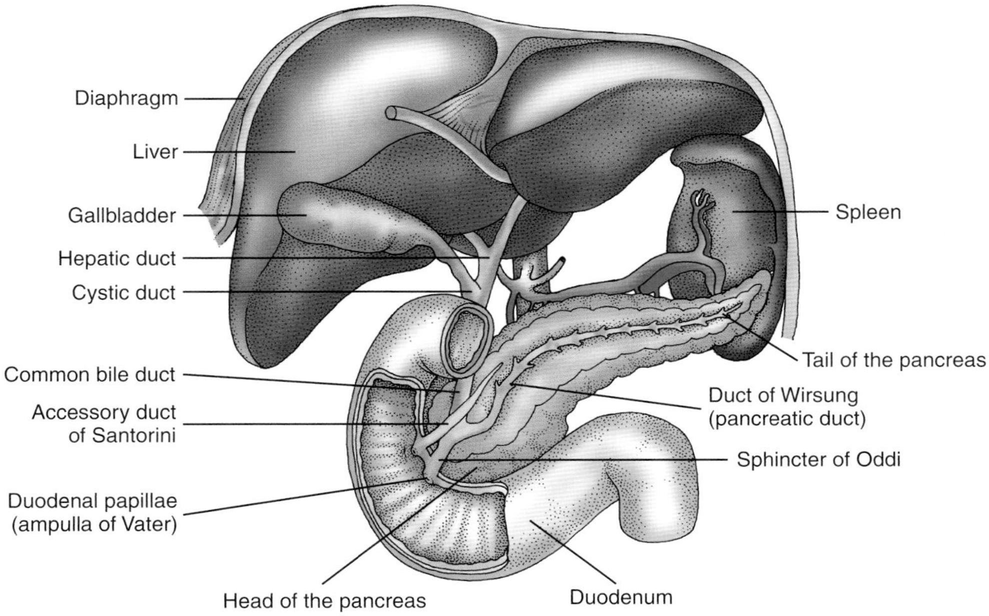

Fig. 37.6 Anatomy of the liver, gallbladder, and pancreas. (From Ignatavicius DD, Workman ML: *Medical-surgical nursing: patient-centered collaborative care*, ed 8, St. Louis, 2016, Elsevier.)

Pharmacology Capsule

Because many drugs are metabolized in the liver, patients with liver disease are at increased risk for toxic effects of drugs.

ANATOMY AND PHYSIOLOGY OF THE BILIARY TRACT

Bile is a yellow-green liquid that has several important functions. It contains bile salts, which are essential for the emulsification and digestion of fats. It also provides a medium for the excretion of bilirubin from the liver.

The biliary tract is made up of the gallbladder and the bile ducts. The function of the biliary tract is to deliver bile from the liver to the duodenum. Bile is produced in the liver and channeled into the common hepatic duct. The common hepatic duct joins the cystic duct to form the common bile duct. The cystic duct leads to the gallbladder, a saclike organ beneath the liver. Bile flows from the liver to the gallbladder, where it is stored and concentrated (Fig. 37.6).

When fats enter the duodenum, the gallbladder contracts and delivers bile to the intestine through the common bile duct.

ANATOMY AND PHYSIOLOGY OF THE PANCREAS

The pancreas is a fish-shaped organ located in the left upper quadrant of the abdomen behind the stomach. The head of the pancreas lies against the duodenum and the tail lies next to the spleen. The pancreatic ducts connect the pancreas to the duodenum. One duct goes directly to the duodenum and the other merges with the common bile duct.

Exocrine Function

The exocrine function of the pancreas is carried out by acinar tissue. Acinar tissue is composed of tiny grapelike clusters of cells that produce pancreatic fluid. Pancreatic fluid contains enzymes needed for the digestion of proteins, fats, and carbohydrates. It is secreted into the duodenum through the pancreatic duct.

The pancreatic enzymes trypsin, amylase, and lipase act on partially digested foods in the small intestine. Trypsin plays a role in the digestion of protein by breaking proteases and peptones into small polypeptides. Normally, trypsin is not activated until it enters the duodenum. Otherwise, it would digest the protein tissue of the pancreas itself. Amylase acts with intestinal enzymes to reduce starch, sucrose, and fructose to glucose, fructose, and galactose. Lipase acts on emulsified fats to yield fatty acids, glycerides, and glycerol.

Endocrine Function

The endocrine function of the pancreas is carried out by clusters of specialized cells scattered throughout the pancreas. These cells are called *islets of Langerhans*. The islets contain alpha, beta, delta, and PP cells. Alpha cells produce and secrete glucagon. Beta cells produce and secrete insulin. Delta cells produce somatostatin, which inhibits the release of glucagon and insulin. PP cells secrete pancreatic polypeptides, a family of peptides known chiefly for their inhibitory functions.

Glucagon is secreted when the blood glucose level falls. It stimulates the liver to convert glycogen into glucose. Insulin is secreted when the blood glucose rises, as after a meal. It stimulates the use of glucose by the cells so that a normal blood glucose level is maintained. The endocrine function of the pancreas is discussed more thoroughly in Chapter 50.

AGE-RELATED CHANGES

Normal aging generally does not significantly impair ingestion, digestion, absorption, or elimination. However, when acute or chronic illnesses occur, the older person is at increased risk for problems with digestion and elimination. Common changes are as follows:

- Teeth: mechanically worn down; appear darker and somewhat transparent.
- Gingiva: tendency to recede
- Tooth loss: common although not a normal effect of aging.
- Jaw: osteoarthritis
- Taste buds: significant loss; may be able to detect sweet better than other tastes.
- Saliva: xerostomia (dry mouth)
- Esophagus and stomach: walls thinner, secretions lessen
- Lower esophageal sphincter: more relaxed
- Hydrochloric acid and digestive enzymes: production decreases
- Gastric motor activity: slows
- Small intestine: no significant changes
- Absorption of vitamins and minerals: absorption of vitamin A may increase; absorption of vitamin D, calcium, and zinc may be reduced.
- Pancreatic secretions decrease in volume but usually remain adequate for normal function.
- Liver changes include reduced blood flow, delayed healing after injury, and delayed clearance of some drugs.
- The risk of gallstones in the gall bladder increases with age.
- Large intestine: atrophy of muscle layer and mucosa; decreased smooth muscle tone and blood flow; increased connective tissue; slower transit time
- Anal sphincter: decreased tone and strength

Constipation is a frequent complaint among older adults, and they use laxatives more often than do young people. Many experts believe that constipation is not a normal age-related change but rather is caused by such factors as low fluid intake, lack of dietary fiber, inactivity, drugs, depression, and hypothyroidism.

NURSING ASSESSMENT OF THE DIGESTIVE TRACT

HEALTH HISTORY

Although the registered nurse (RN) should perform the complete assessment, the licensed vocational nurse/licensed practical nurse (LVN/LPN) contributes to the database.

Reason for Seeking Care

The health history begins with a detailed description of the current complaints or symptoms. These symptoms or complaints may include weight changes, problems with food ingestion, descriptions of digestive disturbances such as vomiting or heartburn, pain, or changes in bowel elimination. Note factors that seem to bring on or relieve the symptoms. The relationship between symptoms and meals may be significant.

Past Health History

Past medical history may disclose recent surgery, trauma, burns, or infections. Note serious illnesses such as diabetes, hepatitis, anemia, peptic ulcers, gallbladder disease, Crohn disease, ulcerative colitis, liver dysfunction, and cancer. Note surgical procedures and blood transfusions. Identify any alternative methods of feeding or fecal diversion such as ileostomy or colostomy. Document any food allergy or intolerance with a description of the reaction. List current medications. The use of estrogen or oral contraceptives is significant in biliary tract disease. The use of thiazide diuretics, furosemide, oral contraceptives, corticosteroids, sulfonamides, and nonsteroidal antiinflammatory drugs (NSAIDs) may be relevant to biliary tract disorders.

> **Pharmacology Capsule**
>
> Many drugs affect gastrointestinal (GI) function, causing anorexia, nausea, vomiting, and diarrhea or constipation.

Functional Assessment

The functional assessment focuses on nutrition, activity, and stressors. Information about general dietary habits should include the daily pattern of food intake (mealtimes, food eaten in a typical day, food likes and dislikes, and use of food supplements), attitudes and beliefs about food, and changes in dietary habits related to health problems. Describe the effects of the chief complaint on usual functioning and note whether the patient is able to obtain and prepare food and eat without difficulty. Because liver disease may be associated with exposure to toxins, ask about exposure to chemicals, potentially toxic drugs, such as acetaminophen, and alcohol use. Some people are reluctant to discuss alcohol use, so handle the subject tactfully and without judgment. People tend to understate the amount of alcohol they typically consume. Note use of street drugs, especially those taken intravenously.

PHYSICAL EXAMINATION

Begin the physical examination with the measurement of the patient's height, weight, and vital signs. Observe the patient's general appearance, noting skin color, texture, moisture, and turgor; posture; motor activity; and responses to instructions. Skin color is especially important in relation to the liver. **Jaundice** is a golden-yellow skin color associated with liver dysfunction or bile obstruction. It is relatively easy to recognize in fair-skinned people.

Head and Neck

Inspection of the mouth determines the condition of the lips, teeth, gums, tongue, and mucous membranes. Describe caries, moisture, color, and lesions and note any unpleasant or unusual odors of the mouth. If the patient has dentures, examine the mouth with and without the dentures in place. Inspect the sclera of the eyes. Like the skin, the sclera may turn yellow with liver disease, a condition called **scleral icterus**. This sign is especially useful when jaundice cannot be seen elsewhere in dark-skinned people.

Chest and Abdomen

Observe for enlargement of breast tissue in men. Such enlargement is called *gynecomastia*. When inspecting the chest, also look for spider angiomas. Spider angiomas are small, visible vessels shaped like spiders.

For the abdominal examination, the patient should be supine, with the head raised slightly and the knees slightly flexed. The areas of the abdomen are commonly described as quadrants. An imaginary line is drawn horizontally across the abdomen at the level of the umbilicus. A second imaginary line extends from the sternum to the pubic bone. This creates the four quadrants: (1) the right upper quadrant, (2) the left upper quadrant, (3) the right lower quadrant, and (4) the left lower quadrant. Findings can then be documented by anatomic location (Fig. 37.7).

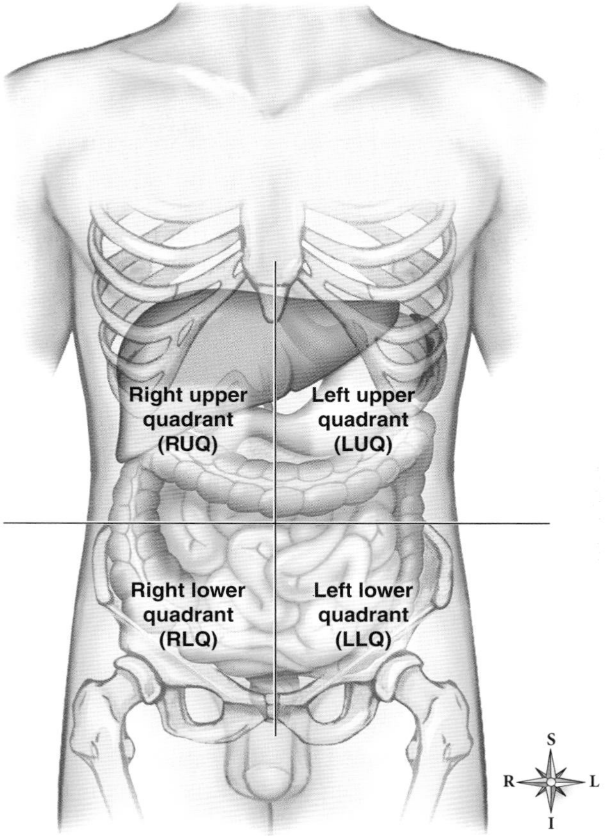

Fig. 37.7 The abdomen is divided into four quadrants. (From Patton KT, Thibodeau GA: *Human body in health & disease*, ed 7, St. Louis, 2018, Elsevier.)

Inspection. Inspect the skin of the abdomen for color, texture, scars, **striae** ("stretch marks"), rashes, lesions, and dilated blood vessels. Describe the general contour of the abdomen as flat, convex (rounded), concave (sunken), protuberant, or distended. Note the location and contour of the umbilicus. Aortic pulsations and peristalsis are sometimes observed, especially in thin people. The examination of the abdomen is especially important in detecting liver disease. Inspect the shape of the abdomen. Note the presence of prominent veins. If significant **ascites** (fluid accumulation in the peritoneal cavity) is present, the abdomen appears distended. Measure the abdomen at the largest circumference to permit comparative measurements later (Fig. 37.8).

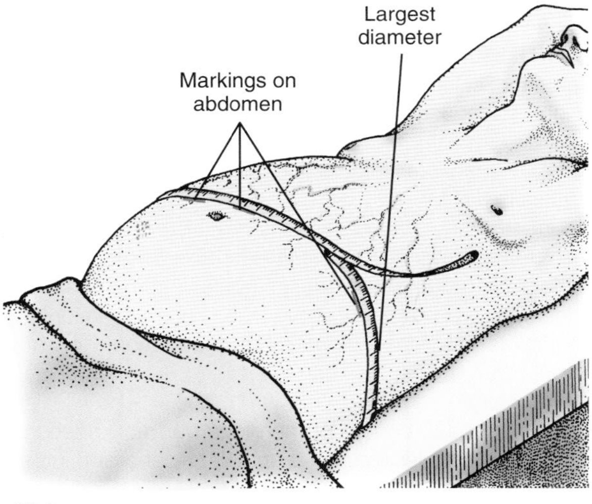

Fig. 37.8 How to measure abdominal girth. Marks are made on the abdominal midline and on both sides so that subsequent measurements can always be made at the same place.

Auscultation. After inspecting the abdomen, auscultate the abdomen to assess bowel sounds. Auscultate before palpating because palpation can alter normal bowel sounds. Warm the diaphragm of the stethoscope and then use it to listen to each quadrant. Normal bowel sounds include clicks and gurgles that occur 5 to 30 times per minute. Listen to each quadrant for at least 2 minutes. If no sounds are heard, it is important to listen for a full 5 minutes before recording bowel sounds as absent. Bowel sounds may be described as present, absent, increased, decreased, high-pitched, gurgling, tinkling, or gushing. Loud gurgling sounds are called *borborygmi*. Note any facial grimacing during auscultation. Record the presence or absence of bowel sounds in each quadrant.

Percussion. Nurses with advanced training in physical examination use percussion and palpation to collect additional data. Percussion is tapping on the skin to detect the presence of air, fluid, or masses in the underlying tissues. It can also be used to locate the margins of internal organs. Percussion over an air-filled organ produces a high-pitched, hollow sound called *tympany*. Tympany is similar to the sound made by a kettle drum. Percussion over a solid or fluid-filled structure sounds dull and flat. Normally, tympany is heard more often than dullness. All four quadrants of the abdomen should be percussed.

Palpation. Palpation is done to detect tenderness, sensitivity, masses, swelling, and muscular resistance. The examiner holds their fingers together and depresses the abdomen gently in all four quadrants. Light palpation depresses the abdominal wall only about 1 cm. Deep palpation uses more pressure. To assess for rebound tenderness, the abdomen is depressed and then quickly released. Grimacing or expressions of discomfort should be noted. Deep palpation and tests for rebound tenderness should be done only by people who are trained in these techniques. Palpate the abdomen for distention and tenderness. Experienced examiners may be able to palpate the liver but, unless it is enlarged, it is difficult to locate under the right rib cage. An enlarged, diseased liver may be felt well below the rib margin. Liver enlargement is called **hepatomegaly**.

Rectum and Anus

Gloves are worn when examining the anus and perianal area. Inspect the perianal skin for color, rashes, and lesions and note the presence of any external hemorrhoids. The rectal examination is performed by a trained examiner. The LVN/LPN may help to position, drape, and comfort the patient. The examiner inserts a gloved, lubricated finger into the rectum and points it toward the umbilicus. The patient is instructed to bear down as if to have a bowel movement. This relaxes the anal sphincter. The examiner palpates for lumps and tenderness in the rectum.

Assessment of the digestive tract is summarized in Box 37.1.

DIAGNOSTIC TESTS AND PROCEDURES

Diagnostic tests and procedures for the digestive tract and accessory organs include endoscopic examinations, imaging and radiologic studies, biopsies, and laboratory studies.

ENDOSCOPIC EXAMINATION

Traditional endoscopic examinations permit direct inspection of hollow, interior organs through a lighted tube called an **endoscope**. Endoscopes may be rigid tubes or flexible fiberscopes. Endoscopic examinations of the gastrointestinal tract include esophagoscopy, gastroscopy, gastroduodenoscopy, esophagogastroduodenoscopy, endoscopic retrograde cholangiography, and colonoscopy.

Box 37.1 Assessment of the Patient With a Disorder of the Digestive Tract or Accessory Organs

HEALTH HISTORY

Reason for Seeking Care

Weight changes, weakness, fatigue, problems with food ingestion, symptoms of digestive disturbances, changes in bowel elimination, skin changes, pregnancy.

Past Health History

Recent surgery, trauma, infections, history of pancreatic disease including diabetes mellitus, liver disease, anemia, peptic ulcer, gallbladder disease, cancer. Alternative methods of feeding: type, amount, schedule. Fecal diversion: type. Allergies: food, drugs. Hepatitis B immunization. Recent and current medications.

Family History

Diabetes mellitus, cancer of the digestive tract, peptic ulcer disease, gallbladder disease, hepatitis, alcoholism, intestinal polyps, obesity.

Review of Systems

General health state: Change in weight
Skin: Change in color, pruritus
Oral cavity: Pain, abnormal tastes or odors, difficulty chewing
Appetite change
Dysphagia
Digestive disturbances: Nausea, vomiting, dyspepsia, heartburn, flatulence (gas), fat intolerance, change in stool frequency or characteristics (amount, color, consistency, abnormal contents including blood and undigested food)
Pain: Location, onset, intensity, duration, aggravating and relieving factors, relation to meals
Urinary symptoms: Change in urine color
Respiratory symptoms: Dyspnea
Extremities: Numbness or tingling

FUNCTIONAL ASSESSMENT

Dietary pattern, alcohol intake, occupation, exposure to toxins, attitudes and beliefs about food, activity, stressors, coping strategies, interpersonal relationships

Physical Examination

General Appearance: Diaphoresis, grimacing, restlessness
Height and Weight: Change
Vital Signs: Tachycardia, tachypnea, fever, hypotension, hypertension
Skin: Dryness, jaundice, spider angiomas, scratches, bruises
Head and Neck: Condition of teeth, gums, tongue, mucous membranes, odors, scleral icterus
Thorax: Gynecomastia
Abdomen: Distention, prominent veins, girth, liver enlargement, bowel sounds

Signed consent is required before endoscopic examinations. Patients usually are not permitted food or fluids for 4 to 8 hours before the examination. However, regular medications may be allowed with a small amount of water. A sedative may be ordered before the procedure to reduce anxiety. The most serious complication of endoscopy is perforation (puncture) of the digestive tract.

An innovation in endoscopy uses a wireless disposable video camera capsule that is about the size of a large vitamin tablet. Several types of capsules are available for specific purposes. The patient swallows the capsule. Leads are applied to the abdomen and connected to a recording device worn on a belt. Images are transmitted as the capsule moves through the digestive tract. The patient can go about usual activities while the capsule is in transit. It is especially useful for visualizing the small intestine, which is not accessible with traditional endoscopy. Patients fast overnight before swallowing the capsule. Bowel preparation may or may not be required, depending on institutional practice.

RADIOLOGIC STUDIES

Radiologic studies include the upper gastrointestinal (UGI or GI) series (barium swallow), small bowel series, and barium enema examination. Radiographs of the gallbladder are obtained as well. These studies allow the radiologist to study the structure and function of the digestive tract. A contrast medium is used in some studies. This is a substance, such as barium sulfate, that can be given orally or by enema. Sometimes air is introduced into the bowel for radiographic studies. This is called an *air contrast procedure*. When radiographs are taken, the contrast medium outlines the hollow organs of the digestive tract (Fig. 37.9).

Most hospitals and clinics have a specific protocol to follow before the examination to ensure that the GI tract is cleansed. If the patient is not properly prepared for the procedure, it may have to be repeated. Fluid restriction and bowel cleansing can be difficult for older or debilitated patients. If they become exhausted or if their vital signs change, the preparation should be stopped and the RN or physician notified. After the procedure, a laxative is usually ordered to clear the barium from the GI tract. Until all barium has been eliminated, the stools are white or gray in color.

In the liver, radiologic studies are used primarily to visualize the hepatic circulatory and biliary structures. They include computed tomography (CT), magnetic resonance imaging (MRI), hepatobiliary scintigraphy (HIDA), and abdominal ultrasound. CT and MRI are noninvasive, painless procedures used to obtain scans of internal organs, including the liver. HIDA is a nuclear imaging scan that uses a radioactive substance. After being injected into a vein, the substance accumulates in the liver. Radiographs are then taken to reveal the size, shape, and position of the liver, as well as tumors, cirrhosis, and abscesses. Ultrasonography uses sound waves to create an image of the liver, spleen, pancreas, gallbladder, and biliary system. It is a noninvasive, painless procedure.

Tests and procedures used to diagnose biliary tract disorders are ultrasonography, oral cholecystography, intravenous cholangiography, T-tube cholangiography, endoscopic retrograde cholangiopancreatography (ERCP), and percutaneous transhepatic cholangiography. Table 37.1 describes common diagnostic tests and nursing implications.

LIVER BIOPSY

A liver biopsy involves removal of a small specimen of liver tissue for examination. The specimen can be obtained by needle biopsy which uses a special type of needle inserted through the abdominal wall. Alternative approaches to the needle biopsy include the open biopsy and the transjugular approach. The open biopsy requires an incision under general anesthesia. The transjugular approach accesses the liver by way of the superior vena cava and hepatic vein. It is preferred for patients with coagulation disorders because the liver capsule is not punctured.

Before either procedure, baseline vital signs should be obtained and blood coagulation studies done. The patient's blood should be typed and crossmatched because of the risk of bleeding. Signed consent is required. Tell the patient what to expect during the procedure. For a needle biopsy, position the patient supine with the right arm behind the head. Place a pad under the right chest. The physician instructs the patient to take a deep breath and hold it during the actual puncture. A sample of liver tissue is aspirated for study.

Afterward, a pressure dressing is placed over the puncture. It should be checked for bleeding every 15 minutes for the first hour, every 30 minutes for the next hour, and then hourly or according to agency protocol. Monitor vital signs at the same time for signs of blood loss (tachycardia, restlessness, hypotension) or pneumothorax (restlessness, tachypnea). The physician usually orders the patient kept on the right side for at least 2 hours to maintain pressure on the puncture site. After being allowed to change positions, the patient may still be kept flat for up to 14 hours.

The primary complications of liver biopsy are hemorrhage and pneumothorax. Bleeding is a possibility because of the liver's rich blood supply and the potential for impaired coagulation in the patient with liver disease. Pneumothorax occurs if the lung is accidentally punctured during the biopsy. Air escapes into the pleural cavity and the lung on the affected side collapses. An alternative to the liver biopsy for some patients is a blood test called FibroSure. It provides an estimate of the extent of fibrosis in a noninvasive manner.

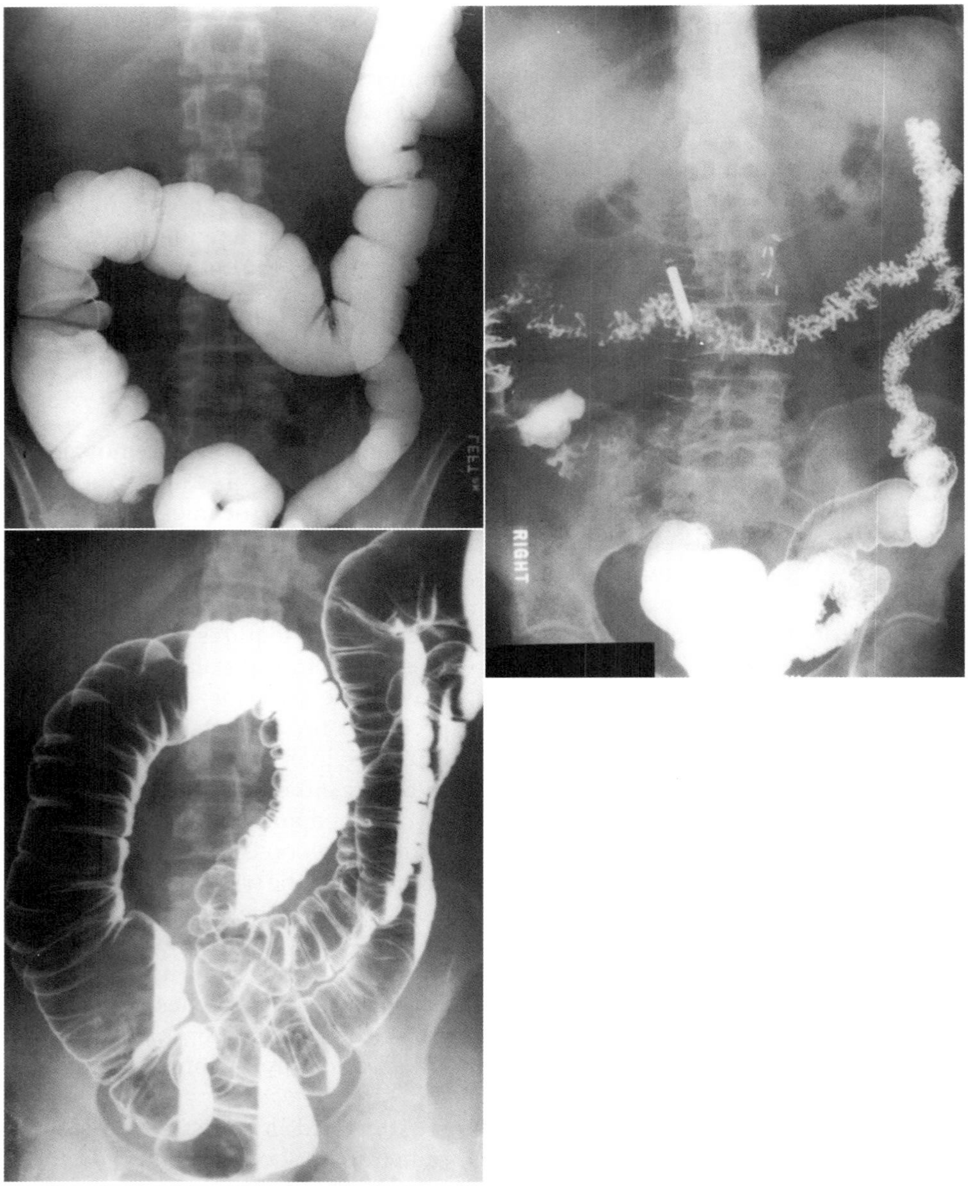

Fig. 37.9 Contrast medium outlines the hollow organs of the digestive tract. (From Laufer I, Levine MC: *Double contrast gastrointestinal radiology*, ed 2, Philadelphia, 1992, Saunders.)

LABORATORY STUDIES

The most common laboratory studies related to the digestive tract and accessory organs are performed on blood and urine. Tests to detect *Helicobacter pylori* include analysis of the breath, urine, serum, stool, and gastric biopsy tissue. Studies that may be done to assess nutritional status include serum albumin, total lymphocyte count, urine creatinine/height index, mean corpuscular volume (MCV), and transferrin saturation. See Chapter 15 for details of the nutritional assessment.

Liver function tests provide basic information about normal activity. When liver disease is suspected, laboratory studies may also be done to measure bilirubin, urinary and fecal urobilinogen, serum proteins, ammonia, vitamin K production, prothrombin time (PT), international normalized ratio (INR), and serum enzymes. Table 37.1 explains the significance of these laboratory tests. Laboratory studies related to the biliary tract include liver function tests, serum and urine bilirubin measurements, alkaline phosphatase (ALP), aminotransferase, and complete blood count (CBC).

Specific blood studies used to assess pancreatic function include measurements of serum amylase, lipase, glucose, calcium, and triglycerides. Urine amylase and renal amylase clearance tests may also be ordered. Stool specimens may be analyzed for fat content.

The secretin stimulation test measures the volume and bicarbonate concentration of pancreatic fluid after secretin is given intravenously to stimulate the production of pancreatic fluid.

Table 37.1 Diagnostic Tests and Procedures for the Digestive Tract and Accessory Organs

TEST AND PURPOSE	PATIENT PREPARATION	POSTPROCEDURE NURSING CARE
General interventions: Check your agency procedure manual for diagnostic tests and procedures. Always tell the patient what to expect when tests are ordered. Explain if fasting (NPO) is necessary. Document the care provided and relevant assessment data. If venipuncture is done, apply a dressing and check the site for oozing. Apply pressure and elevate arm for 1 minute if patient's blood clotting is impaired. **When contrast dye is used:** Before a procedure, assess patient allergy to dye, iodine, or (if agency requires) shellfish. If patient reports allergy, notify radiology. Tell patient that injection of contrast dye can create a feeling of warmth, a salty taste, and nausea. Inform the physician if the patient exhibits any signs of allergic response to the contrast dye. Administer antihistamines as ordered for allergy.		
Radiographic Tests and Other Imaging Procedures		
Upper gastrointestinal (UGI) or gastrointestinal (GI) series: Barium swallow detects abnormalities of esophagus and stomach. Modified barium swallow uses video fluoroscopy.	Inform the patient that they will need to drink a solution containing contrast medium. Radiographs will be taken initially and repeated 6 hours later to see how much barium has passed through the stomach. NPO 6–8 hours before the procedure or per agency protocol.	Monitor stools for at least 2 days for passage of white stools that show that barium is being eliminated (normal stool color returns in 3 days). Laxatives may be ordered to promote elimination. Provide food, extra fluids, and rest.
Small bowel series detects abnormalities of the small intestine.	After the patient drinks a contrast solution, films are taken at 20- to 30-minute intervals as the solution passes through the small intestine. The patient will be asked to assume various positions for the radiographs. The procedure may take several hours. Preparation is the same as for the UGI series.	Care is the same as for the UGI series.
Barium enema detects abnormalities of the large intestine. Largely replaced by endoscopy and CT scanning.	A contrast solution is administered by enema and radiographs are taken with the patient in a variety of positions. The test may take as long as 1¼ hours. The day before the procedure, the patient may be restricted to clear liquids and given a laxative and enemas. NPO after midnight. On the morning of the procedure, enemas are given until the return fluid is clear.	Care is the same as for the UGI series.
Computed tomography (CT) reveals abnormalities of liver and other organs. Contrast dye may be used.	May be NPO. Usually can take medications. Tell the patient they will lie still on a stretcher while a donut-shaped machine moves around them. The procedure is painless. [a]Contrast dye may be injected intravenously (IV). Sedation may be ordered if patient cannot lie still. Dye precautions	Dye precautions
Cholangiography: T-tube, IV, percutaneous transhepatic, surgical, magnetic resonance cholangiopancreatography. All provide images of hepatic and biliary ducts to detect abnormalities. A contrast agent may be injected.	Dye precautions. Food and fluids should be withheld as ordered. The patient is usually NPO after midnight before the study. A laxative may also be ordered the night before. The test takes 4–6 hours.	Dye precautions. A fatty meal helps to eliminate dye, if used. After percutaneous transhepatic cholangiography, watch for signs of bleeding and respiratory distress.
Portal venography and hepatic arteriography use IV contrast dye followed by radiographs to study blood vessels in liver.	Dye precautions	Dye precautions. Care is the same as for T-tube cholangiography.

Continued

Table 37.1 Diagnostic Tests and Procedures for the Digestive Tract and Accessory Organs—cont'd

TEST AND PURPOSE	PATIENT PREPARATION	POSTPROCEDURE NURSING CARE
Liver scan and liver-spleen scan use a radioactive substance that collects in the liver when given IV. Radiographs are taken with the patient in various positions. A scanner maps uptake of radiation, revealing liver tumors and abscesses.	Fasting is not usually required. Assure patient that the small dose of radiation is harmless.	The patient must wash their hands thoroughly after voiding for 24 hours. Report any allergic symptoms.
Gallbladder scan, hepatobiliary scintigraphy, hepatobiliary imaging, biliary tract radionuclide scan, cholescintigraphy After a radionuclide is injected, images are taken of the biliary tract to assess patency and to detect cholecystitis. Patient may be given a fatty meal followed by scans to evaluate emptying of the gallbladder.	A 2–4 hour fast may be required. No morphine or meperidine for specified period before the scan. Tell patient the scan takes about 90 minutes. Repeat imaging may be needed up to 4 hours later.	Encourage the patient to drink fluids to promote elimination of radionuclide, to wash hands after voiding, and to flush immediately. Caregivers should wear gloves to handle urine. Wash gloved hands before removing gloves; wash hands after removing gloves. Dispose of gloves as you would other nuclear waste.
Ultrasonography uses high-frequency sound waves to create an image of the gallbladder, liver, spleen, pancreas, and biliary system to identify abnormalities.	Nonfasting. The patient lies on a table. A technician applies gel to the abdomen and moves an instrument transducer over the abdomen. Images are projected onto a screen. It is not painful.	No special care required
Magnetic resonance imaging (MRI) cholangiopancreatography (MRCP). Noninvasive imaging of biliary tree, gallbladder, pancreas, and pancreatic duct to identify abnormalities. MRI of the liver uses contrast material to reveal liver and biliary tumors.	Fasting may be ordered for some abdominal procedures. Tell patient that MRI is a painless, noninvasive procedure, but the machine is noisy. The patient must remain still on a narrow surface. All metal must be removed before the MRI, including patches with foil backing. Older MRI devices are circular and surround the body like a tunnel. Closing the eyes reduces claustrophobia. Medication can be given for claustrophobia. Open MRI, if available, eliminates claustrophobia.	No special care required unless a sedative was given, then patient needs to be driven home.
Endoscopic Tests		
Upper Digestive Tract and Accessory Organs		
Esophagoscopy visualizes the esophagus. Gastroscopy visualizes the stomach. Gastroduodenoscopy visualizes the stomach and duodenum. Esophagogastroduodenoscopy visualizes the esophagus, stomach, and duodenum. Endoscopic retrograde cholangiography visualizes the bile ducts and gallbladder. Endoscopic retrograde cholangiopancreatography (ERCP) visualizes pancreatic, hepatic and common bile ducts and ampulla of Vater.	NPO for 6–8 hours or per agency protocol. If ordered, give the patient a sedative shortly before the examination. Dentures and eyewear will need to be removed. Inform the patient that the scope will not interfere with breathing. ERCP requires dye so implement general dye precautions: ask if patient is allergic to dye, iodine, or seafood. If yes, inform radiology in advance.	The patient should be NPO until the gag reflex returns. Monitor for signs of trauma: bleeding from the throat or rectum. Monitor for signs of perforation: fever, abdominal distention, cramping pain, and vague discomfort. The patient may have belching or flatulence. Tell the patient that sore throat can be treated with warm gargles or an ice pack to the neck. The patient should contact the physician in the event of severe pain, fever, dyspnea, or hematemesis.

Table 37.1 Diagnostic Tests and Procedures for the Digestive Tract and Accessory Organs—cont'd

TEST AND PURPOSE	PATIENT PREPARATION	POSTPROCEDURE NURSING CARE
Lower Digestive Tract		
Colonoscopy visualizes the anus, rectum, and entire colon. Fiberoptic colonoscopy often visualizes part of the terminal ileum as well. Proctoscopy visualizes the rectum.	NPO for 6–8 hours before the examination. The patient may be restricted to only liquids on the previous day or evening. Bowel cleansing may be done with cathartics, suppositories, and enemas.	Tell patient to report blood in stools (bleeding suggests perforation of colon). Monitor BP and heart rate. Inspect abdomen for distention. Encourage fluids when fully alert to replace loss during preparation.
Sigmoidoscopy visualizes the rectum and sigmoid colon.	Cathartics and suppositories are usually given on the evening before the test. Enemas may be ordered on the morning of the test until the fluid return is clear.	Same as colonoscopy
Capsule Endoscopy		
Capsule endoscopy transmits video images of the entire digestive tract to a recorder worn on a waistband. It is especially useful for the study of the small intestine and may detect obscure GI bleeding, inflammatory bowel disease (IBD), small bowel tumors, malabsorption disorders, and inflammation caused by nonsteroidal antiinflammatory drugs (NSAIDs) or radiotherapy.	A 10-hour overnight fast is required for the small bowel study. Bowel preparation, if any, varies with the agency and health care provider. Study of the esophagus requires a 2-hour fast. Simethicone may be given when the capsule is swallowed to reduce bubbles and improve visualization.	The capsule is normally eliminated painlessly in the stool. No special care is required. If the small intestine is obstructed, the capsule can become lodged at the site, requiring surgical removal. The patient returns to the office in 6–10 hours to turn in the recorder.
Virtual colonoscopy uses a CT scanner and computer software to examine the colon after inflation via a small rubber tube. Fusion CT/positron emission tomography (PET) scan can also determine if an abnormality is malignant.	Cleansing bowel preparation is required as described earlier. No sedation is required.	Because the patient is not sedated, they can leave immediately afterwards and resume regular activities.
Laboratory Tests		
Blood Tests		
Serum electrolytes measure electrolytes in the blood to detect imbalances.	Medications that affect results may be held until blood is drawn.	Resume medications after blood is drawn.
Serum protein electrophoresis measures serum protein, which may be decreased with peptic ulcers, acute cholecystitis, and malabsorption.	Medications that can alter test results (aspirin, isoniazid, neomycin, bicarbonate, sulfonamides) may be withheld until the blood sample is drawn.	Resume medications after blood is drawn.
Carcinoembryonic antigen (CEA) measures a protein in the blood that may indicate GI malignancy, although the test is not specific. This test is also used to monitor the patient's response to cancer therapy.	No special preparation is required. Note whether the patient smokes; if yes, they will most likely test positive for CEA.	General interventions only.
Serum bilirubin. Elevated with cirrhosis, gallstones, bile obstruction.	NPO may be required.	Monitor venipuncture site. Apply pressure. Patients with liver disease may have prolonged clotting time.
Alkaline phosphatase (ALP). Elevated with liver or bone disease.	Overnight fast preferred but not required. Recent meal raises ALP.	Monitor venipuncture site. Apply pressure. Patients with liver disease may have prolonged clotting time.
Serum enzymes. Elevated by tissue damage. Useful in diagnosing hepatic and pancreatic disease. Only ALT is specific to liver disease.	Fasting recommendations vary. See laboratory manual.	Monitor venipuncture site. Apply pressure. Patients with liver disease may have prolonged clotting time.

Continued

Table 37.1 Diagnostic Tests and Procedures for the Digestive Tract and Accessory Organs—cont'd

TEST AND PURPOSE	PATIENT PREPARATION	POSTPROCEDURE NURSING CARE
Serum triglycerides. Elevated in many conditions including pancreatic disorders.	Fasting 12–14 hours or per agency policy. No alcohol for 24 hours before test. Fatty meals increase triglycerides.	General interventions only.
Prothrombin time (PT) and international normalized ratio (INR). Measures clotting ability. Prolonged with liver disease, vitamin K deficiency, anticoagulant therapy.	Nonfasting. If patient is on warfarin, obtain specimen before daily dose. Dose may be adjusted pending test results.	Monitor venipuncture site. Apply pressure. Patients with liver disease may have prolonged clotting time. Check results: nurses should know these values: PT 11.0–14 seconds INR 0.8–1.1 seconds Immediately report PT >46 seconds or INR ≥5
Serum protein. With advanced cirrhosis, albumin is decreased and gamma globulin increased. Results vary with renal disease and chronic inflammation.	Note on laboratory request if patient has had any vaccinations in the past 6 months. Some drugs that affect results may be withheld.	Monitor venipuncture site. Apply pressure. Patients with liver disease may have prolonged clotting time.
Serum amylase. Elevated in pancreatitis, cholecystitis, parotitis.	No special preparation.	General interventions only.
FibroSure/FibroTest: provides a measure of the level of fibrosis in the liver.	Check agency laboratory manual.	General interventions only.
Urine Studies		
Urine amylase. Increased with pancreatitis and some other conditions.	No special preparation. Nonfasting. Record actual time of specimen collection.	No special care required.
Esophageal Function Tests		
Esophageal pH monitoring is used to detect acid reflux. Manometry measures lower esophageal sphincter (LES) pressure and assesses esophageal swallowing waves. For the Bernstein test, hydrochloric acid and normal saline are alternately instilled in the esophagus to see if the patient experiences pain with the acid.	NPO for 8 hours before the test. The procedure takes about 30 minutes. Tell the patient that it will be necessary to swallow several small tubes that will measure the pressure in the esophagus and record esophageal waves during swallowing. In some situations, the pH sensor is left in place for 24 hours.	No special aftercare is required. The patient may have a mild sore throat.
Stool Analysis		
Stool occult blood detects GI bleeding when blood is not readily seen.	Advise the patient of the need to obtain a stool specimen. If the test is done at home, explain the procedure.	No special care is required.
Stool ova and parasites detect parasitic infections.	Preparations are the same as for the stool occult blood test.	No special care is required.
Fecal fat tests for increased fat in stools that occurs with Crohn disease, malabsorption, and pancreatic disease.	Instruct the patient on how to observe a 60-g fat diet for 3–6 days, followed by collection of a stool specimen. No laxatives, enemas, or suppositories may be used for 3 days before the test.	Tell the patient to resume a normal diet.
Multitarget stool DNA testing (e.g., Cologard). Detects DNA shed in stool by colorectal malignancies.	A stool collection kit is delivered by mail. The patient collects a stool sample in the provided container and returns the container by mail so it will be received within 72 hours. No drug or dietary restrictions.	No special care. If positive results, the physician will follow up with additional diagnostic tests.

Table 37.1 Diagnostic Tests and Procedures for the Digestive Tract and Accessory Organs—cont'd

TEST AND PURPOSE	PATIENT PREPARATION	POSTPROCEDURE NURSING CARE
Tests for *Helicobacter pylori*		
Stool antigen assay	Proton pump inhibitors are stopped 1–2 weeks before test. Wait 4 weeks after bismuth/antibiotic therapy.	
Gastric biopsy	Tissue sample taken during endoscopy	
Urea breath test	Patient is given a labeled carbon dioxide isotope PO. *H. pylori* frees labeled carbon dioxide can be detected in the breath. Proton pump inhibitors may be withheld.	
Tests for Pancreatic Function		
Secretin stimulation test measures pancreatic juice secreted in response to IV secretin. Assesses bicarbonate and pancreatic enzymes.	Explain that a tube will be passed through the nose and into the intestinal tract. An IV medication will be given and fluids withdrawn through the tube.	No special care is required.
Fecal elastase-1 test provides a measure of pancreatic function.	Patients taking pancreatic enzymes may be asked not to take them for a specified time before the specimen collection. Urine-free stool specimen must be collected in a clean, dry, leak-proof container. Use cold pack to transport.	No special care required.

If cancer is suspected, blood levels of cancer antigen (CA) 19-9 and carcinoembryonic antigen (CEA), which are considered "markers" for cancer, may be measured. Unfortunately, levels of these antigens are elevated with many types of cancer, so their presence does not specifically indicate pancreatic cancer.

Additional information about diagnostic tests and procedures for the pancreas is provided in Table 37.1.

Occult Blood Test

Occult blood is blood that is not visible with the naked eye. Stool specimens are often tested for occult blood because patients with digestive tract or liver disease sometimes bleed into the tract. To test for occult blood, a small sample of the stool is placed on a special type of paper that is then treated with a chemical. If blood is present, specific color changes are observed on the paper.

Stool Examination

Stool specimens may be examined for blood, bile, pathogenic organisms, parasite ova (eggs), fecal fat, and the white blood cell (WBC) count. Key points when stool examinations are ordered include the following:

- Collect the specimen in a clean, dry container. Urine should not be in the container because it destroys parasites. Do not discard bathroom tissue in the container because the paper contains bismuth, which interferes with some tests.
- Deliver stool specimens to the laboratory immediately. If temporary storage is necessary, specimens for ova and parasites must be kept warm. Specimens for pathogens should be refrigerated.
- Depending on the specific test used, the patient may be instructed not to eat red meat for 2 to 3 days before the specimen is collected. Red meat interferes with the results of some tests.
- Drugs that may interfere with results are salicylates, ascorbic acid, anticoagulants, and steroids.
- If visible blood or mucus is present in the stool, include it in the specimen sent to the laboratory.

COMMON THERAPEUTIC MEASURES

GASTROINTESTINAL INTUBATION

Tubes are inserted most often into the stomach or intestines to deliver feedings or to keep the digestive tract empty (decompression). Tubes that are passed through the nose are called *nasogastric*, *nasoduodenal*, or *nasoenteric tubes*, depending on whether the end is located in the stomach or the small intestine.

A variety of tubes exist for special purposes (Fig. 37.10). Nasogastric tubes such as the Levin and Salem sump tubes may be used for decompression. Nasoenteric tubes used for decompression of the small intestine include the Miller-Abbott, Cantor, and Harris tubes.

The Sengstaken-Blakemore esophageal-gastric balloon tube is a special tube used to control bleeding in the esophagus. It is generally used in patients with severe complications of liver disease stet, restore as written.

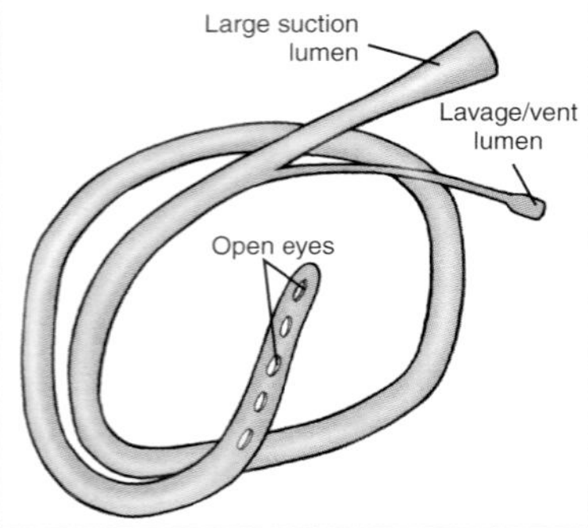

Lavacuator tube
An orogastric tube with a large suction lumen and a smaller lavage/vent lumen that provides continuous suction because irrigating solution enters the lavage lumen while stomach contents are removed through the suction lumen. Used to remove toxic substances from the stomach.

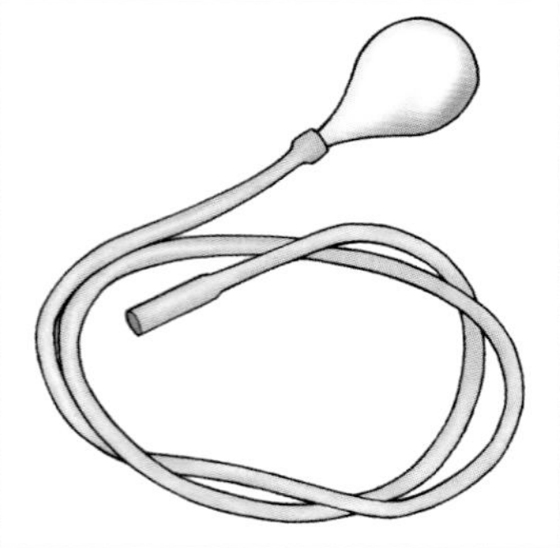

Cantor tube
A single-lumen long tube with a small inflatable bag at the distal end. About 5 to 10 mL of mercury is injected with a needle (gauge 21 or smaller or balloon may leak) and syringe into the bag before insertion of the tube.

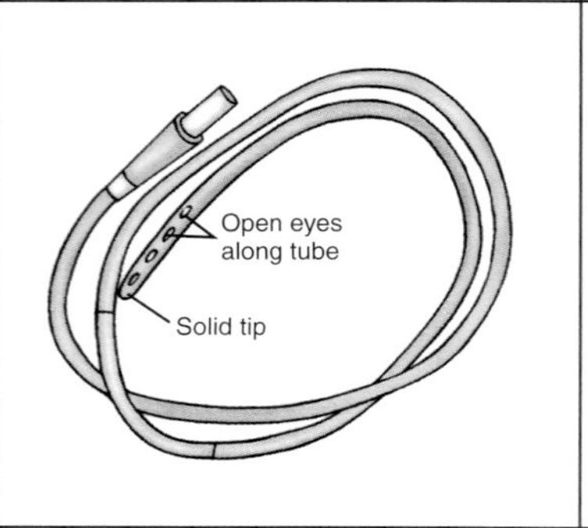

Levin tube
A plastic or rubber single-lumen tube with a solid tip that may be inserted into the stomach via the nose or mouth. Used to drain fluid and gas from the stomach. Single lumen must be used for irrigation and drainage, so continuous irrigation is not possible.

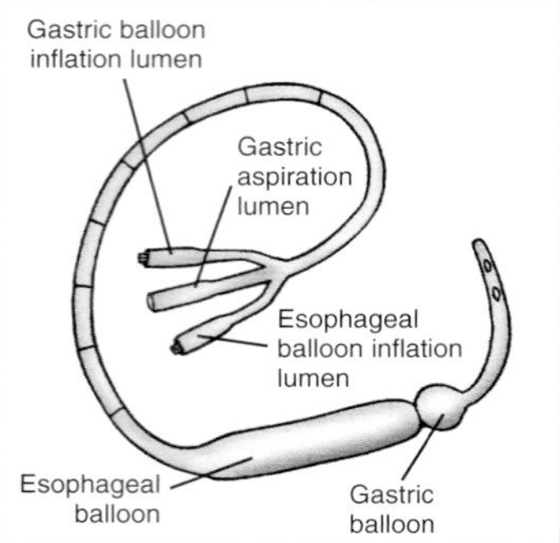

Sengstaken-Blakemore tube
A three-lumen tube. Two ports inflate an esophageal and a gastric balloon for tamponade, and the third is used for nasogastric suction. This tube does not provide esophageal suction, but a nasogastric tube may be inserted in the opposite naris or the mouth and allowed to rest on top of the esophageal balloon. Esophageal suction is then possible, reducing the risk of aspiration.

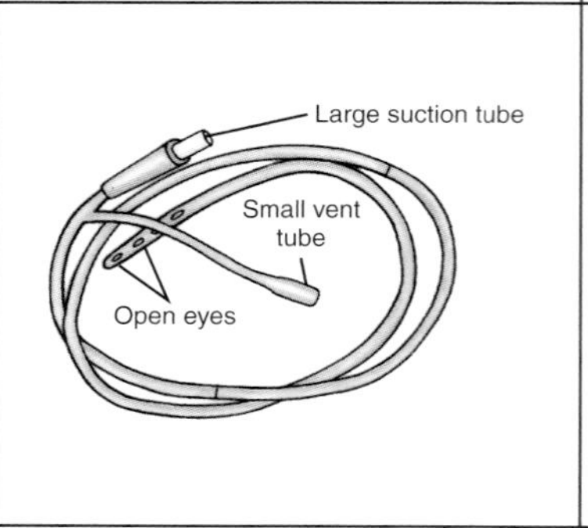

Salem sump tube
A short double-lumen tube. The small vent tube within the large suction tube prevents mucosal suction damage by maintaining the pressure in open eyes at the distal end of the tube at less than 25 mm Hg.

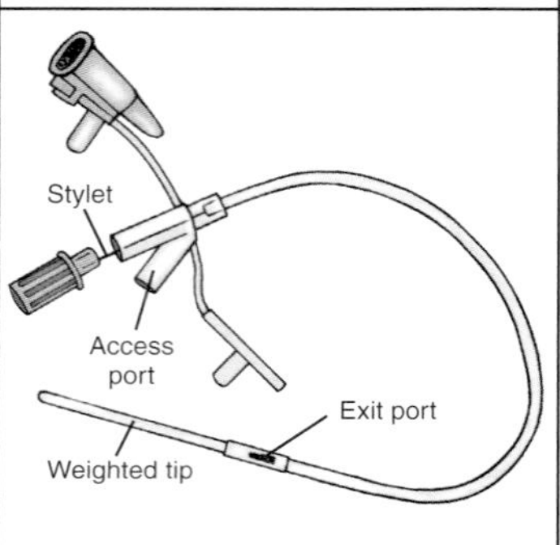

Weighted flexible feeding tube with stylet
Access port with irrigation adapter allows maintenance of the tube without disconnecting the feeding set.

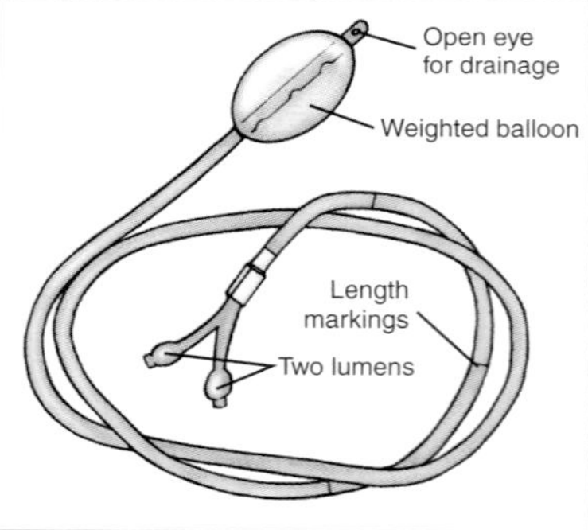

Miller-Abbott tube
A long double-lumen tube used to drain and decompress the small intestine. One lumen leads to a weighted balloon that is filled once it is in the stomach; the second is for irrigation and drainage.

Fig. 37.10 Examples of tubes used in the digestive tract. (From Monahan FD, Drake DT, Neighbors M, editors: *Medical-surgical nursing: foundations for clinical practice*, ed 2, Philadelphia, 1998, Saunders.)

Gastrostomy (PEG) tubes, used for feedings, are placed in the stomach through an opening (stoma) in the abdominal wall (Fig. 37.11). Levin and Dobhoff tubes are used for enteral feedings. The Dobhoff is a small nasoduodenal tube that is weighted so it passes through the stomach into the duodenum.

Enteral Tube Feedings

Enteral feedings were introduced in Chapter 15. This section summarizes key nursing actions when patients are receiving feedings in this manner. The health care provider writes specific feeding orders. Feedings may be delivered by gravity flow or by infusion pump. Without a pump, a syringe barrel or a packaged delivery set is used to put the feeding into the tube. Regardless of the method used, several key points must be remembered about this procedure:

- It is critical to confirm by radiograph that the tube is in the stomach or the duodenum before administering feedings to avoid introducing feedings into the airway. Radiographic confirmation is the most reliable method but is not practical for every feeding. At the bedside, observation of aspirated material is thought to provide the most reliable evidence

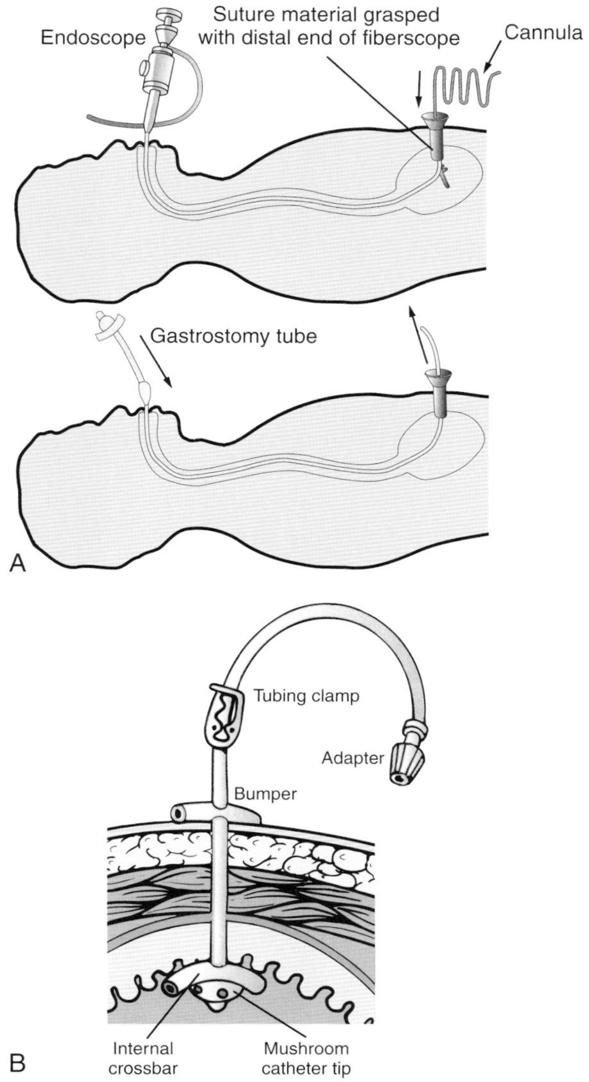

Fig. 37.11 Percutaneous endoscopic gastrostomy (PEG). (A) Placement of PEG tube. Using endoscopy, a gastrostomy tube is inserted through the esophagus into the stomach. A cannula is inserted through the abdominal wall into the stomach. The fiberscope grasps the cannula and the cannula and tube are pulled out through the abdominal wall. (B) A retention disk and bumper keep the tube in place. (From Lewis SM, Heitkemper MM, Dirksen SR, et al.: *Medical-surgical nursing: assessment and management of clinical problems*, ed 9, St. Louis, 2015, Mosby.)

of location. Stomach contents are grassy green, clear and colorless, or brown. The measurement of pH may not be accurate because patient medications may alter the pH of gastric fluid which is normally 5 or less (Hodin and Bordeianou, March 17, 2020). The intestinal pH is normally 6 or higher. Methods that lack scientific support are listening over the stomach area with a stethoscope while injecting air through the tube, placing the end of the tube in water to see if bubbles appear, testing the patient's ability to speak, and observing for respiratory symptoms. When a patient has continuous feedings, placement is usually checked at least once each shift.

- Elevate the patient's head and chest 30 to 45 degrees during and 30 to 60 minutes after the feeding to reduce the chance of **aspiration** (regurgitation and passage of fluids into the respiratory tract).
- Depending on agency policy, residual (formula remaining in the stomach from the previous feeding) may be measured in an effort to prevent overfilling of the stomach. Follow agency procedure to clear the tubing and aspirate contents. Agency policy dictates what action should be taken based on the amount of residual formula. The residual formula should be returned through the tube to prevent loss of electrolytes. Some resources question the value of monitoring residual (Seres, February 4, 2019).
- Be sure to give the right formula (there are many), in the right amount, at the right dilution, on the right schedule, and to the right patient.
- When tube feedings are first started, they are often delivered at a slower rate. If the patient tolerates the formula well, the rate is gradually increased.
- Stop the feeding and notify the health care provider if the patient has nausea or pain.
- Rinse the tube by flushing it with at least 30 mL of water after each bolus feeding.
- If diarrhea occurs, contact the health care provider regarding action to take which might include decreasing the concentration or the rate of delivery, or both, of the formula.
- Dumping syndrome may occur with rapid feedings of concentrated formula. Signs and symptoms are cold sweat, abdominal distention, dizziness, weakness, rapid pulse rate, nausea, and diarrhea.
- If using a syringe to give the feeding, do the following:
  - Remove the plunger from the barrel of the syringe.
  - Attach the barrel to the feeding tube.
  - Pinch or kink the tube while the syringe barrel is filled with formula to reduce the amount of air being forced into the stomach.
  - Hold the barrel no more than 18 inches above the insertion site and allow the fluid to flow by gravity.
  - Flush tubing with water per agency protocol.
- If an infusion pump is used to deliver the feeding, fill the tubing with formula before connecting it to the feeding tube to reduce the amount of air forced into the digestive tract. Continuous feedings are initially given at a rate of 10 to 20 mL/h and increased by 10 to 20 mL every 8 to 12 hours or as ordered to a target rate.
- Bolus feedings are given at specified intervals. The initial feeding is usually 2.5 to 5 mL/kg delivered over 20 to 30 minutes. The amount is then advanced as ordered to the desired amount.
- Oral drugs can usually be given through a nasogastric tube but some drugs should not be crushed. Before administering any medication, consult a drug reference.
- Change administration set tubing and bag every 24 hours.

Gastrointestinal Decompression

GI decompression is used to relieve or prevent distention. A tube is passed through a nostril and into the stomach or intestines (or both) and attached to suction. The suction removes fluid and gases that accumulate when GI motility is impaired or when a patient is intubated for respiratory failure. Conditions that slow motility include peritonitis, obstruction, and any type of surgery performed while the patient is under general anesthesia. Handling of the bowel during abdominal surgery often causes a temporary loss of peristalsis. Decompression may be ordered until bowel activity returns, usually in 3 to 5 days. The following are key points to remember when caring for the patient with GI suction:

- Attach the tube to a suction apparatus as ordered.
- Monitor the patency of the tube. Observe for the movement of fluids through the tubing into the suction container. If the tube does not seem to be draining, change the patient's position. Gently rotate the tube or pull it out very slightly. (Exception: do not reposition tubes after gastric surgery.) Notify the health care provider if drainage does not resume.
- Irrigations should not be done routinely, but they may be ordered occasionally as needed. Frequent irrigations cause acid-base disturbances. For adults, irrigations are usually done with 20 to 30 mL of normal saline. Check the health care provider's order or the agency's procedure manual.
- Monitor the suction output. Record the amount, color, and characteristics every shift. Monitor the patient for successful decompression. If distention is not being relieved effectively, the patient may have nausea and vomiting, shortness of breath, a feeling of fullness, and enlargement of the abdomen.
- Assess for the return of peristalsis, indicated by the presence of bowel sounds and passage of flatus (gas) and stool through the rectum.
- Provide comfort measures. The nasopharynx and throat are often very tender. Because the patient is placed on NPO (nothing by mouth) status, mouth dryness is another source of discomfort. Handle the tubing gently to avoid trauma. Cleanse the nostrils and apply a water-soluble lubricant to reduce drying and irritation. Provide mouth care frequently. Moisturize the lips. Offer oral spray or lozenges as ordered to provide temporary relief of sore throat.
- Once the tube is in place, tape it securely to the nose or upper lip and cheek to prevent it from being pulled out (Fig. 37.12). Do not tape the tubing to the forehead because this puts excessive pressure on the nasal tissues. Wrap the tube with a piece of tape that is pinned to the patient's gown to prevent accidental traction on the tube.

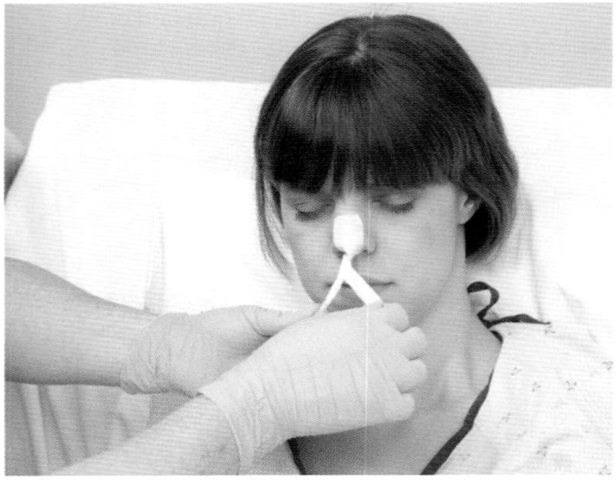

Fig. 37.12 This method of taping a nasogastric tube anchors it securely while avoiding trauma to the nose. (From Potter PA, Perry AG, editors: *Fundamentals of nursing*, ed 8, St. Louis, 2013, Mosby.)

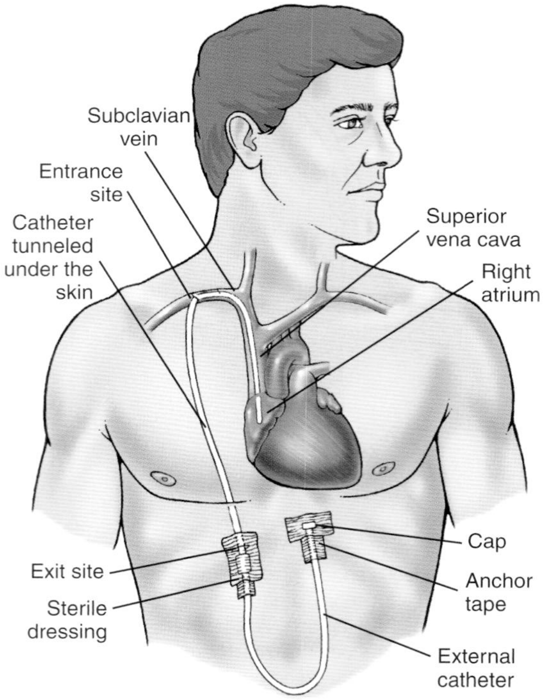

Fig. 37.13 A catheter inserted into the right subclavian vein for total parenteral nutrition. A transparent waterproof dressing allows vapor to escape while maintaining sterility. (From Monahan FD, Drake DT, Neighbors M, editors: *Medical-surgical nursing: foundations for clinical practice*, ed 2, Philadelphia, 1998, Saunders.)

TOTAL PARENTERAL NUTRITION

Sometimes the digestive tract cannot be used for feedings. Total parenteral nutrition (TPN) bypasses the digestive tract by delivering nutrients directly to the bloodstream. A catheter such as a central venous catheter (Fig. 37.13) or peripherally inserted central catheter (PICC) is inserted into a large vein and is used for the feedings. The feeding passes directly into the superior vena cava and the right atrium (RA). This placement allows for rapid dilution of the concentrated feeding. The solution is never administered into a smaller vein because it would cause thrombophlebitis (inflammation of the vein).

When the catheter is inserted, it is sutured to the skin and the insertion site is covered with a sterile dressing. A radiograph is ordered to check placement before the catheter is used for feedings.

Regular intravenous feedings can provide only water, glucose, electrolytes, minerals, and vitamins. This is adequate for short-term problems but does not provide all of the nutrients necessary to maintain health or promote healing.

Two types of solutions are used for TPN therapy. The first is a concentrated solution of glucose, amino acids, vitamins, and minerals. It is administered using a special filter. A lipid solution can also be given through a peripheral vein. The lipids are not mixed with the TPN solution.

Important points to remember when caring for the patient receiving TPN include the following:

- Take great care to prevent infection at the insertion site. Always use sterile technique for site care. The exact procedure should be ordered or written in the agency's procedure manual. With each dressing change, inspect the site for signs of infection (redness, swelling, foul odor, or purulent drainage). Monitor the patient's temperature for elevation.
- Monitor the flow rate. If the solution is given too rapidly, the patient may have circulatory overload, changes in blood glucose, or excessive diuresis (urine output). If the feeding falls behind schedule, do not speed up the rate to catch up.
- Monitor the patient for signs and symptoms of blood glucose changes. The concentrated glucose solution can raise the blood glucose excessively (hyperglycemia). Elevated glucose stimulates the pancreas to produce more insulin, which may then cause a drop in blood glucose (hypoglycemia).
- Label TPN lines and never use the TPN catheter to administer drugs.
- Be sure that all staff who give medications differentiate TPN lines from small-bore enteral feeding tubes. Patient deaths have occurred as a result of oral medications being administered through a TPN line.

> **Pharmacology Capsule**
>
> Never use a total parenteral nutrition (TPN) line to administer drugs.

DRUG THERAPY

Drugs that are commonly used for their effects on the digestive tract include antacids, antiulcer drugs, laxatives, antidiarrheal drugs, antiemetics, antibacterial and antifungal drugs, and antiinflammatory drugs. Other classes that patients with digestive disorders may require include vitamins and minerals, albumin, diuretics, hormones, antihypertensive agents, antispasmodics, pancreatic enzymes, and insulin. These drugs are identified with the conditions for which they are prescribed. In addition, Table 37.2 summarizes the drugs, their actions, and nursing interventions. Weight loss drugs are discussed in Chapter 15 because their use is unique to obesity.

DIGESTIVE TRACT SURGERY

Conditions of the digestive tract that may require surgery include cancer, peptic ulcer disease, diverticulosis, appendicitis, polyps, obstruction, and ulcerative colitis. General care of the surgical patient is discussed in Chapter 17. The following section provides an overview of nursing care when a patient has surgery on the digestive tract. Details specific to certain procedures are included in subsequent chapters.

PREOPERATIVE NURSING CARE OF THE PATIENT HAVING GASTROINTESTINAL SURGERY

Radiographic examinations of the digestive tract are often done before surgery. These may be done on an outpatient basis or after admission to the hospital. The digestive tract is usually cleansed before GI surgery. The extent of the cleansing depends on the exact site of the surgery. Oral preparations such as magnesium citrate or large-volume **cathartic** (intense, rapid-acting laxative) solutions may be prescribed. Use of enemas until the returning fluid is clear may also be ordered. This process is tiring and may exhaust the very ill or older patient. The nurse should offer assistance with toileting and hygiene. Changes in vital signs (abnormal heart rate or rhythm, hypotension) or mental state during the bowel cleansing process should be reported to the health care provider.

Diet is usually limited to liquids for 24 hours before the surgery. The patient should have nothing to eat or drink for a specified period before surgery. Intravenous fluids may be ordered, especially if GI suction is being used. Oral antibiotics may be given to reduce the bacterial flora in the bowel, thereby decreasing the risk of contamination of the peritoneal cavity during surgery.

General anesthesia and abdominal surgery cause a temporary loss of peristalsis. Therefore before or during surgery, a nasogastric tube may be inserted and attached to suction. This prevents the accumulation of fluid and gas in the digestive tract until peristalsis returns.

POSTOPERATIVE NURSING CARE OF THE PATIENT WHO HAS HAD GASTROINTESTINAL SURGERY

Usual postoperative care, discussed in Chapter 17, includes measures to relieve pain; detect complications (hemorrhage, infection); and prevent adverse effects of immobility, anesthesia, and drug therapy. Immediately after surgery on the digestive tract, be especially concerned with preventing gastric or abdominal distention, replacing lost fluids, and maintaining urine elimination. The patient usually has a nasogastric tube in place for decompression. The intermittent removal of fluids and gas decreases the stimulation of the digestive tract and reduces pressure on the internal

Table 37.2 Drug Therapy: Disorders of the Digestive Tract

DRUG	USE AND ACTION	SIDE EFFECTS	NURSING INTERVENTIONS
Drugs Used to Treat Peptic Ulcer Disease			
Antacids			
magnesium hydroxide, aluminum hydroxide, calcium carbonate, sodium bicarbonate.	Reduces pain of peptic ulcers by neutralizing acid in the stomach, decreasing irritation of the stomach lining, and inhibiting production of pepsin. Reduces pain of pancreatitis by indirectly decreasing pancreatic secretions.	Calcium and aluminum salts: constipation. Magnesium salts: diarrhea. Combinations may be used to neutralize these effects.	Teach patients that antacids are nonprescription drugs but still have side effects, interact with other drugs, and can be abused. Shake liquids before pouring. Follow the dose with water or milk to deliver antacid to the stomach. Antacids interfere with absorption of oral drugs if given within 1–2 hours of each other. Tablets should be chewed before swallowing.
H2-Receptor Blockers			
cimetidine (Tagamet), famotidine (Pepcid), nizatidine (Axid)	Reduces secretion of gastric acid and promote healing of ulcers. Decreases HCl so that pancreatic enzymes cannot be activated.	Diarrhea, muscle pain, rash, confusion, and drowsiness. Cimetidine can cause impotence and gynecomastia and impairs the metabolism of many common drugs; confusion in older adults. Other drugs have fewer side effects (and do not cause impotence or gynecomastia).	Give with or after meals. Do not give ranitidine at the same time as antacids. Advise older patients of the risk of confusion and drug interactions with cimetidine.
Proton-Pump Inhibitors			
omeprazole (Prilosec), esomeprazole (Nexium), lansoprazole (Prevacid), pantoprazole (Protonix), rabeprazole (Aciphex)	Inhibits gastric acid secretion in the treatment of peptic ulcer disease, GERD, and Zollinger-Ellison syndrome.	Nausea, diarrhea, and headache	Advise the patient to swallow the capsule whole. For patients who cannot swallow capsules, Prevacid capsules can be opened and the contents mixed in applesauce. A liquid preparation is also available.
Mucosal Barriers			
sucralfate (Carafate)	Permits healing of an ulcer by interacting with acid to form a protective gel that coats the ulcer surface. Adsorbs pepsin.	Constipation, dry mouth, drowsiness, rash, and itching.	Give the drug on an empty stomach 1 hour before meals and antacids. The medication interferes with absorption of some other drugs.
Synthetic Prostaglandins			
misoprostol (Cytotec)	Decreases gastric acid secretion and protects the gastric mucosa. Often used to prevent gastric ulcers caused by NSAIDs.	Contraindicated during pregnancy. Diarrhea, abdominal pain, miscarriage, headache, flatulence, and nausea and vomiting.	Usually given with meals and at bedtime. Explain the importance of avoiding pregnancy during prostaglandin therapy because it can cause spontaneous abortion.

Table 37.2 Drug Therapy: Disorders of the Digestive Tract—cont'd

DRUG	USE AND ACTION	SIDE EFFECTS	NURSING INTERVENTIONS
Anticholinergic Agents			
atropine, pirenzepine (Gastrozepin)	Decreases salivary and gastric secretions by blocking action of acetylcholine. Reduces pain by reducing smooth muscle tone in GI tract.	Dry mouth, constipation, visual disturbance, and urine retention. Pirenzepine side effects much milder than atropine. Older adults may become confused, agitated, or drowsy.	Contraindicated with narrow-angle glaucoma, renal disease, prostatic hypertrophy, or intestinal obstruction. Best given ½ to 1 hour before meals and at bedtime. Assist with oral hygiene and monitor stools and urine output. Report changes in behavior.
scopolamine (Transderm Scōp)	Used to suppress the vomiting center. Often used to prevent motion sickness.	Confusion, delusions and hallucinations, tachycardia, dry mouth, blurred vision, and urinary retention.	Transderm Scōp is a medicated adhesive disk that is placed behind the ear. Contraindicated with narrow-angle glaucoma and urinary tract obstruction.
Laxatives			
Bowel Stimulant			
bisacodyl (Dulcolax) tablets and suppositories senna (Senokot) cascara sagrada	Facilitates bowel elimination. Stimulates the GI tract by irritating the mucosa. Tends to produce diarrhea-like stools. Intended for temporary relief.	Contraindicated with undiagnosed abdominal pain and inflammatory conditions of GI tract. Bisacodyl suppositories: anal irritation. Cascara and senna: pink or brownish urine.	Monitor stools. Encourage adequate fluids and fiber to reduce the need for laxatives. Advise older adults to discuss most appropriate drugs to manage constipation with their health care provider.
Bulk-Forming Laxatives			
psyllium (Metamucil), methylcellulose (Citrucel)	Prevents constipation by retaining water in the stool to increase bulk and fluid, which stimulates peristalsis and the passage of the formed soft stool.	One of safest laxatives for long-term therapy and during pregnancy. Obstruction can occur if it is not taken with adequate fluids or if passage through the intestine is arrested.	The patient must take adequate fluids or the mass can harden. It may take up to 3 days before the effect is evident, so it is used primarily for prevention of constipation.
Saline (Osmotic) Laxatives			
magnesium citrate, magnesium hydroxide (milk of magnesia), sodium phosphate (Fleet Phospho-soda), polyethylene glycol (MiraLAX)	Draws water into bowel to distend and stimulate evacuation. Intended for short-term use only.	Risk of dehydration with frequent or prolonged use. Most of these laxatives are contraindicated with kidney disease, heart failure, hypertension, and edema.	Educate patients about appropriate use. Monitor effects.
Lubricants			
mineral oil	Lubricates feces for easier passage.	Caution: there is a risk of lipid pneumonia if the product is aspirated.	Because mineral oil impairs absorption of fat-soluble drugs and nutrients, it should be given on an empty stomach. Discourage use by older adults.
Fecal Wetting Agents			
docusate calcium (Surfak), docusate sodium (Colace)	Prevents constipation by softening fecal mass. Takes up to 3 days before effects are evident.	Nausea, anorexia, cramps, diarrhea, rash, and throat irritation.	Liquid forms can be given in milk or juice to mask taste.

Continued

Table 37.2 Drug Therapy: Disorders of the Digestive Tract—cont'd

DRUG	USE AND ACTION	SIDE EFFECTS	NURSING INTERVENTIONS
Other Laxative Agents			
lactulose (Cephulac)	Increases fecal water content to stimulate bowel evacuation. Treats hepatic encephalopathy by promoting passage of ammonia through the rectum. Available for oral or rectal administration.	Cramps, flatulence, diarrhea, and hyperglycemia with diabetes.	Can be mixed with full glass of water, milk, or juice to disguise the taste. It is more effective on empty stomach. Report diarrhea because dosage needs to be reduced. For a retention enema, administer the agent with a rectal balloon catheter.
polyethylene glycol-electrolyte solution (GoLYTELY, HalfLytely, MoviPrep, MiraLAX)	GoLYTELY, HalfLytely, and MoviPrep are used to cleanse the bowel before diagnostic procedures. HalfLytely and MoviPrep include other drugs that stimulate the bowel and require less fluid volume than GoLYTELY. MiraLAX is used to treat occasional constipation and as a stool softener.	Nausea, bloating, abdominal discomfort.	GoLYTELY can be used with renal and cardiac disease because it does not disturb the patient's electrolyte balance. When prepared for administration, GoLYTELY comprises 4 L. The patient must drink the solution over a prescribed period of time. The patient should have immediate access to a toilet as the laxative begins to take effect within an hour.
Antidiarrheal Agents			
Opiates			
morphine, diphenoxylate HCl, (Lomotil), loperamide HCl (Imodium)	Decreases intestinal motility so that the liquid portion of feces is reabsorbed. Dosage is less than that used for analgesia.	CNS depression, drowsiness, dizziness, constipation, nausea, and dry mouth.	Do not exceed the maximum dosage. Use safety precautions and encourage good oral hygiene.
Adsorbents			
kaolin, aluminum hydroxide	Binds to substances that may cause diarrhea.		Shake the suspension before pouring. Do not administer it with other oral drugs because adsorbents will interfere with absorption.
Probiotics			
Lactobacillus and *Bifidobacterium* products	Used to replace normal bacterial flora of the bowel.	Flatulence and bloating	May require refrigeration.
Antiemetics			
Serotonin Antagonists			
ondansetron (Zofran), granisetron (Kytril), palonosetron (Aloxi) dolasetron (Anzemet)	Used to prevent nausea and vomiting caused by chemotherapy. Aloxi has a very long half-life (40 hours), so a single dose usually controls initial and delayed chemotherapy side effects.	Medication is usually tolerated well. Most common side effects include the following: headache, constipation, diarrhea, abdominal pain, musculoskeletal pain, shivering, fever, hypoxia, and urinary retention.	After diluting the agent according to directions, it is given IV 30 minutes before a chemotherapy dose as ordered. Advise the patient that drowsiness may occur. Ask about constipation and difficulty voiding. Encourage fluids, fiber, and activity as appropriate. Stool softeners may be needed.

Table 37.2 Drug Therapy: Disorders of the Digestive Tract—cont'd

DRUG	USE AND ACTION	SIDE EFFECTS	NURSING INTERVENTIONS
Substance P/Neurokinin$_1$ Antagonists			
aprepitant (Emend), netupitant/palanosetron (Akynzeo), rolapitant (Varubi)	Used to prevent nausea and vomiting caused by chemotherapy. Used in combination with other antiemetics.	Common side effects include headache, dizziness, diarrhea, constipation, and nausea. Most serious side effects include thrombocytopenia and neutropenia.	Administer the agent as ordered: a 3-day course with the first dose 1 hour before therapy.
Antihistamines			
promethazine HCl Phenergan), dimenhydrinate HCl (Dramamine)	Used to prevent and treat nausea. Decreases the sensitivity of the vestibular apparatus of the inner ear. Suppresses the vomiting center.	Drowsiness and confusion, especially if given with other CNS depressants.	Use these medications cautiously with asthma, glaucoma, and prostatic hypertrophy.
Cannabinoids			
dronabinol (Marinol), nabilone (Cesamet)	Used for chemo-therapy-induced nausea and vomiting for patients who do not respond to preferred agents. Dronabinol stimulates appetite in patients with AIDS.	Tachycardia, hypotension, and drowsiness, subjective effects similar to marijuana create potential for abuse.	Advise patient not to take with alcohol or sedatives. Inform of potential for abuse.
Sedatives			
hydroxyzine (Atarax)	Used to prevent perioperative nausea and vomiting; antianxiety effects.	Drowsiness, confusion, hypotension, dry mouth, nausea, diarrhea, and urinary retention.	Monitor alertness, BP, urine output. Assist with ambulation. Bed in low position, Call bell in reach. Oral care.
Prokinetic Agents			
metoclopramide (Reglan)	Used to speed up gastric emptying into the small intestine.	CNS depression, GI upset, and Parkinson-like symptoms.	Contraindications include the following: GI perforation, obstruction, hemorrhage, and epilepsy.
Antimicrobials **Antibacterials**			
ciprofloxacin (Cipro), erythromycin (E-Mycin), metronidazole (Flagyl), clarithromycin, amoxicillin, metronidazole, bismuth subsalicylate	Used to treat diarrhea caused by pathogens. Cipro: *Escherichia coli, Campylobacter jejuni, Shigella* spp. E-Mycin: *Entamoeba histolytica* Flagyl: *Clostridium difficile;* treatment of Crohn disease. Clarithromycin, amoxicillin, metronidazole, bismuth subsalicylate: *H. pylori*.	Side effects vary with the specific drug.	Advise the patient to complete the entire course of therapy and to report worsening symptoms. Nursing care varies with specific agent.
amoxicillin (Amoxil)	Used to treat *H. pylori* when combined with omeprazole, prostaglandins, or bismuth subsalicylate (or a combination of these medications).	Rash, diarrhea, anaphylaxis, and superinfections (colitis).	Instruct the patient to take the full course of treatment.

Continued

Table 37.2 Drug Therapy: Disorders of the Digestive Tract—cont'd

DRUG	USE AND ACTION	SIDE EFFECTS	NURSING INTERVENTIONS
rifaximin (Xifaxan)	Used alone or with lactulose to prevent/treat hepatic encephalopathy. Reduces ammonia by decreasing GI bacterial flora.	Superinfection, constipation, flatulence, headache, exfoliative dermatitis.	Instruct patient to report diarrhea, especially with bloody stools.
Antifungals			
nystatin (Mycostatin)	Used as an effective treatment against *Candida albicans* (yeast) infections.	Nausea, vomiting, and diarrhea with nystatin.	Instruct the patient to dissolve lozenges in the mouth. Shake suspensions well. Swish in the mouth before swallowing.
clotrimazole (Mycelex)	Used to treat *C. albicans* (yeast) infections.	Nausea, vomiting, and itching.	Vaginal preparations are available.
Antiviral Drugs			
sofosbuvir/ledipasvir (Harvoni) sofosbuvir/velpatasvir (Epclusa) sofosbuvir/velpatasvir/voxilaprevir (Vosevi) flecaprevir/pibrentasvir (Mavyret)	Used to treat adults with chronic hepatitis C	Headache, fatigue, nausea, chills, rash, diarrhea, and neutropenia. Possible reactivation of hepatitis B.	Pregnancy should be ruled out before starting therapy. Tell patient not to stop drug abruptly.
Diuretics			
Potassium-sparing diuretics: spironolactone (Aldactone), amiloride (Midamor), triamterene (Dyrenium) Loop diuretic: furosemide (Lasix) Thiazide diuretic: chlorothiazide (Diuril)	Used to promote excretion of excess fluid in edema and ascites.	Fluid and electrolyte imbalances, including fluid volume deficit, hyperkalemia, and hyponatremia. Most diuretics can cause hypokalemia. Potassium-sparing diuretics (e.g., spironolactone) can cause hyperkalemia.	Monitor the patient's intake, output, and abdominal girth. Check laboratory values for electrolyte imbalances.
Antiinflammatory Drugs			
5-aminosalicylates: sulfasalazine (Azulfidine) mesalamine (e.g., Apriso) olsalazine (Dipentum) Balsalazide (Colazal)	Reduces inflammation in mild to moderate UC. Maintenance therapy with IBD. Crohn disease.	Nausea, fever, rash, arthralgia, crystaluria, blood disorders (anemia, agranulocytosis), headache, abdominal pain, and diarrhea.	Monitor response. Encourage patient to have periodic blood studies as ordered and to report any signs of infection (sore throat, fever). Encourage increased fluid intake to prevent crystal formation.
Glucocorticoids: dexamethasone, budesonide	Primarily used to induce remission in UC and Crohn disease. Reduces inflammation in acute pancreatitis. Antiinflammatory action.	With long-term use: adrenal suppression, osteoporosis, increased susceptibility to infection, fluid retention, and fat redistribution.	Advise patient to avoid people with infections, practice good hygiene.
Immunosuppressants: Cytotoxic drugs: azathioprine, methotrexate, mycophenolate, mercaptopurine, Calcineurin inhibitors (CNIs): tacrolimus, cyclosporine mTOR inhibitors: sirolimus, everolimus	Long-term therapy for UC and Crohn disease when other drugs fail. Prevent rejection of transplanted organs.	Cytotoxic drugs: neutropenia, thrombocytopenia. CNIs: renal and hepatic toxicity hypertension mTOR inhibitors: increased serum lipids, edema, hypertension, and anemia.	

Table 37.2 Drug Therapy: Disorders of the Digestive Tract—cont'd

DRUG	USE AND ACTION	SIDE EFFECTS	NURSING INTERVENTIONS
Immunomodulators: infliximab (Remicade)	Moderate to severe UC and Crohn disease, rheumatoid arthritis, and psoriasis.	Increased susceptibility to infection, infusion reactions, chest pain, dyspnea, and BP changes.	
Miscellaneous Drugs Used to Treat Cirrhosis			
Beta-adrenergic blocker: propranolol (Inderal)	Used to reduce pressure in the portal veins to reduce the risk of bleeding. Target heart rate is 50–55 beats per minute.	Bradycardia, hypotension, and bronchoconstriction. The drug masks signs of hypoglycemia.	Monitor the patient's pulse and notify the physician if it is below the target rate. Monitor blood glucose in patients with diabetes.
Hormones: Octreotide (sandostatin) vasopressin (VP)	Unlabeled use: to reduce pressure in the portal veins to treat bleeding esophageal varices.	Headache, flushing, chest pain, myocardial infarction, nausea, and vomiting. Water intoxication: disorientation, neuro-muscular excitability.	Monitor heart rate, BP, ECG, fluid status, mental status, and lethargy. Safety measures if drowsy and/or dizzy.
Vitamin K: phytonadione (AquaMEPHYTON)	Used to treat serious bleeding disorders caused by deficiency of prothrombin (given cautiously to patients with severe liver disease).	Gastric upset (oral route only), rash, urticaria, flushing, hemolytic anemia, pain and swelling at the injection site.	Check laboratory results for prothrombin time (PT). Report any abnormalities to the physician. Monitor complete blood count (CBC). Assess for bleeding. Apply pressure to needle puncture sites for 5 minutes.
Blood derivative: albumin	Off-label use: Prevents renal dysfunction caused by spontaneous bacterial peritonitis.	Fluid volume excess: elevated BP, distended neck veins, dyspnea, and headache.	Monitor vital signs. Must be reconstituted to prepare for IV administration.
Pancreatic Enzymes			
pancrelipase (Creon, Viokase, Pancreaze, Pertzye, Ultressa, Zenpep)	Supplements normal enzyme secretion. Aids in digestion of fats, carbohydrates, and proteins. Goal is less frequent stools with lower fat content.	Diarrhea, nausea, stomach cramps, abdominal pain hyperuricuria, hypoglycemia or hyperglycemia.	Give with every meal or snack. Capsule should not be chewed or crushed. Do NOT sprinkle capsule contents on alkaline food. Notify health care provider if blood in urine. Monitor stools.

BP, Blood pressure; *CNS*, central nervous system; *GERD*, gastroesophageal reflux disease; *GI*, gastrointestinal; *HCl*, hydrochloric acid; *IV*, intravenously; *NSAIDs*, nonsteroidal antiinflammatory drugs; *RN*, registered nurse; *UC*, ulcerative colitis; *IBD*, inflammatory bowel disease.

incisions. It is important to monitor GI suction to be sure it is functioning. Inspect, describe, and measure the drainage. Inspect and auscultate the abdomen for distention and bowel sounds. Follow the health care provider's orders regarding irrigation. After gastric surgery, do not irrigate or reposition the tube because of the possibility of traumatizing healing tissue. Notify the RN or health care provider if the tube is not draining properly or if the abdomen becomes distended.

Intravenous fluids are given until GI suction is discontinued and oral intake is adequate. Maintain strict intake and output records. The patient is at risk for fluid and electrolyte imbalances when GI suction is used. Because patients often have difficulty voiding after abdominal surgery, an indwelling catheter is usually inserted during the procedure. If no catheter is present, nursing measures may be needed to promote voiding. These measures are discussed in Chapter 41.

Get Ready for the NCLEX® Examination!

Key Points

- Any disorder of the digestive tract can cause nutritional deficiencies by disrupting one or more of its three functions: (1) digestion, (2) absorption, and (3) elimination.
- Accessory organs of the digestive tract are the salivary glands, liver, gallbladder, and pancreas.
- Chemical digestion and absorption of nutrients occurs through villi in the small intestine.
- Liver functions include metabolism of carbohydrates, fats, proteins, steroids, detoxification of potentially harmful substances, and ingestion of old red blood cells and bacteria.
- The liver regulates blood glucose by storing glucose as glycogen (glycogenesis), converting it back to glucose when needed (glycogenolysis), and making new glucose by breaking down fats and protein (gluconeogenesis).
- Patients with liver disease are at increased risk for toxic effects of drugs.
- The pancreas participates in metabolism (exocrine function) and plays a critical role in regulation of blood glucose (endocrine function).
- Numerous changes in the digestive tract can affect the older adult's nutritional status.
- Tooth loss with age is not normal but is common.
- Jaundice is a golden-yellow skin color associated with liver dysfunction or bile obstruction; when the sclera are affected, it is called *scleral icterus.*
- Ascites is fluid accumulation in the peritoneal cavity that causes the abdomen to be distended.
- The correct sequence of the abdominal examination is inspection, auscultation, percussion, and palpation.
- The most serious complication of GI endoscopy is perforation.
- Signs of hemorrhage, which may occur after a liver biopsy, include tachycardia, restlessness, and hypotension.
- Dyspnea after a liver biopsy may indicate a pneumothorax.
- Various tubes may be inserted into the stomach or small intestine to provide feedings or keep the digestive tract empty (decompression).
- When an enteral feeding tube is inserted, placement must be confirmed by radiograph before the first feeding.
- The most accurate way to assess tube placement before each feeding is to aspirate and examine stomach contents.
- Stomach contents are green, clear, or brown and have a pH of 5 or less.
- To prevent aspiration with tube feedings, elevate the patient's head 30 to 45 degrees during and 30 to 60 minutes after the feeding. Follow agency policy for checking residual.
- Clearly label TPN feeding tubes and never use the tube to administer drugs.
- Do not irrigate or reposition a nasogastric tube after gastric surgery because it may traumatize healing tissue.

Additional Learning Resources

SG Go to your Study Guide for additional learning activities to help you master this chapter content.

Go to your Evolve website (http://evolve.elsevier.com/Linton/medsurg) for the following learning resources and much more:

- Fluid & Electrolyte Tutorial
- Review Questions for the NCLEX® Examination

Review Questions for the NCLEX® Examination

1. The nurse is caring for patients with various disorders of the digestive tract. Which of these patients is at the greatest risk for malnutrition?

1. A 60-year-old man with chronic gastritis
2. A 19-year-old woman who had part of her small intestine removed after an abdominal injury
3. A 45-year-old woman who has had a colectomy because of a high risk of cancer
4. A 52-year-old man who has had a partial colectomy because of rectal cancer

NCLEX Client Need: Physiological Integrity: Physiological Adaptation

2. Inspection of the mouth of an older adult reveals all of the data listed subsequently. Which findings should the nurse recognize as normal? (Select all that apply.)

1. Worn chewing surfaces on the teeth
2. Recession of the gingiva (gums)
3. Loss of most of the natural teeth
4. Teeth appear dark and transparent
5. Whitish patches on the border of the tongue

NCLEX Client Need: Health Promotion and Maintenance

3. Other than a radiograph, the most reliable way to assess placement of a nasogastric tube is to do which of the following?

1. Auscultate the epigastrium while injecting air into the tube
2. Examine aspirated stomach contents
3. Place the end of the tube in water and observe for bubbling
4. Listen for air movement at the end of the tube

NCLEX Client Need: Safe and Effective Care Environment: Safety and Infection Control

4. A patient who has had oral surgery complains of dry mouth. Your most appropriate action is to do which of the following?

1. Tell the patient this is normal after oral surgery
2. Provide a commercial mouthwash for rinsing the mouth
3. Check the health care provider's orders for mouth care
4. Suction the mouth after giving the patient sips of water

NCLEX Client Need: Reduction of Risk Potential

5. **Which of the following types of antiulcer drugs work by inhibiting the secretion of gastric acid? (Select all that apply.)**
   1. Antacids
   2. H2-receptor blockers
   3. Mucosal barriers
   4. Proton-pump inhibitors
   5. Synthetic prostaglandins

   NCLEX Client Need: Physiological Integrity: Pharmacological Therapies

6. **Sequence the assessment techniques below in the order they should be performed.**
   1. Palpation
   2. Auscultation
   3. Inspection
   4. Percussion

   NCLEX Client Need: Health Promotion and Maintenance

7. **A patient with liver disease asks why his abdomen is swollen. When explaining the pathophysiology of liver disease, which statement correctly describes the function of the portal vein?**
   1. The portal vein delivers blood from the aorta to the liver.
   2. The portal vein delivers blood from the intestines to the liver.
   3. The portal vein delivers blood from the liver to the inferior vena cava.
   4. The portal vein delivers blood from the aorta to the inferior vena cava.

   NCLEX Client Need: Physiological Integrity: Basic Care and Comfort

8. **Which of the following factors are thought to contribute to constipation in older adults? (Select all that apply.)**
   1. Low fluid intake
   2. Lack of dietary fiber
   3. Inactivity
   4. Drugs
   5. Hyperthyroidism

   NCLEX Client Need: Physiological Integrity: Physiological Adaptation and Health Promotion and Maintenance

9. **SLO Objective: Apply knowledge of anatomy and physiology to determine which assessment data require follow up by the nurse.**

   NGN Item Type: Enhanced Hot Spot

   Cognitive Skill: Recognize Cues

   Shortly after a percutaneous liver biopsy, the nurse performs a focused assessment that yields the following data:
   - Temperature 98°F
   - Heart rate104 beats per minute
   - Respirations 28 per minute
   - Blood pressure 130/60 mm Hg
   - Skin pale and dry
   - Patient on right side
   - Dressing intact and dry
   - Patient states she feels "nervous" and cannot catch her breath

   Highlight or place a check mark next to the assessment findings that require follow up by the nurse.

   NCLEX Client Need: Physiological Integrity: Reduction of Risk Potential

10. **The nurse has inserted a feeding tube and started the first feeding using a pump. After 20 minutes the patient complains of nausea and dizziness. She is sweating, and her pulse is rapid. The nurse should recognize that these are symptoms of which of the following?**
    1. Gastric perforation
    2. Dumping syndrome
    3. Hyperglycemia
    4. Allergic reaction

    NCLEX Client Need: Physiological Integrity: Reduction of Risk Potential

38 Upper Digestive Tract Disorders

http://evolve.elsevier.com/Linton/medsurg

Objectives

1. Describe the pathophysiology, clinical manifestations, complications, and treatment for selected disorders of the upper digestive tract.
2. Assist in developing nursing care plans for patients with disorders of the upper digestive tract.

Key Terms

anorexia
emesis
gingivitis
peritonitis
regurgitation
stomatitis

Disorders of the upper digestive tract can have a profound effect on nutrition, overall health, and quality of life. This chapter will examine problems affecting ingestion, digestion, and absorption caused by pathogens, inflammation, structural changes, and cancer.

DISORDERS AFFECTING INGESTION

Anything that interferes with the ability to eat a balanced diet can cause nutritional deficiencies. Problems can be as basic as anorexia, inability to feed oneself, or dysphagia or they may occur secondary to other problems such as oral infection and inflammation, dental problems, oral cancer, and parotitis (inflammation of the parotid glands, as in mumps).

ANOREXIA

The intake of food depends largely on having an appetite. Lack of appetite is called **anorexia**.

Causes

Anorexia can occur with many physical and emotional disturbances. Nausea, a decreased sense of taste or smell, mouth disorders, and medications are some physical factors that may decrease one's appetite. Emotional problems such as anxiety, depression, or disturbing thoughts may also cause anorexia. Older people often report decreased appetite. This may be attributed to diminished senses of taste and smell, drug effects, decreased activity, and social isolation.

Medical Diagnosis

The physician, nurse practitioner, or dietitian assesses the patient for evidence of malnutrition. Weight may be monitored over several weeks. A complete history and physical examination are done to detect underlying problems and the effects of inadequate intake. Initial diagnostic tests that are likely to be ordered include measurements of serum hemoglobin (Hgb), iron, total iron-binding capacity (TIBC), transferrin, calcium, folate, vitamin B_{12}, and zinc. Tests of thyroid function may be ordered to detect metabolic disorders, and skin tests may be ordered to evaluate allergic responses. A stool specimen may be tested for occult blood. If indicated, the health care provider may perform additional procedures to detect possible cancers of the digestive system, lungs, and breasts.

Medical Treatment

Correctable causes of anorexia are treated but sometimes no physical cause is found. Nutritional supplements may be ordered. The oral route is preferred but enteral feedings or total parenteral nutrition (TPN) may be indicated in extreme cases. Some patients benefit from appetite stimulants such as megestrol (Megace).

◆ NURSING CARE OF THE PATIENT WITH ANOREXIA

Focused Assessment

The general assessment of the patient with digestive disturbances is summarized in Chapter 37, Box 37.1. When a patient has anorexia, try to determine contributing factors such as discomfort, nausea, dental or other oral problems, and emotional state. Sometimes a therapeutic diet is unappealing or different from the patient's customary and cultural dietary preferences. Note the patient's height and weight for recent changes and trends. Engage the registered dietitian for a complete nutrition assessment and recommendations.

Patient Problem, Goal, and Outcome Criteria: Anorexia

Patient Problem	Goal and Outcome Criteria
Inadequate nutrition related to anorexia	Improved appetite and adequate food intake: patient states appetite is better, increased intake of food, stable or increased body weight

Interventions

It is helpful to identify factors that contribute to the patient's anorexia. If the patient has a dry mouth or bad taste in the mouth, assist with oral hygiene before and after meals. If the teeth or gums are in poor condition, teach proper oral hygiene and refer the patient for dental care. Poorly fitting dentures need to be readjusted or relined for a tighter fit or replaced.

When a patient is nauseated, institute measures to relieve the nausea before presenting a meal tray. Nausea and anorexia can be related to unpleasant stimuli in the environment.

Many people enjoy meals more when they are in the company of others. Socialization during mealtime can greatly improve a person's appetite. In long-term care facilities, group dining is usually an option. Also, cultural preferences should be considered when meals are chosen and provided to patients.

Before food is brought in by family or friends, advise them of any dietary restrictions. Small servings are more acceptable than large ones to the anorexic person. Additional nutrients can be provided by between-meal snacks.

FEEDING PROBLEMS

Patients may require assistance with meals because of temporary impairments or long-term disabilities. Patients with paralysis, arthritis, neuromuscular disorders, confusion, weakness, or visual impairment are likely to need assistance. Individualized interventions are needed to ensure adequate nutrition despite disability.

Medical Diagnosis and Treatment

The medical diagnosis is directed at identifying the basic problems and prescribing treatment as appropriate. Patients are often referred to physical therapy and occupational therapy to help them regain basic self-care skills.

NURSING CARE OF THE PATIENT WITH FEEDING PROBLEMS

Focused Assessment

Determine the patient's ability to feed themselves independently. Consider the nature of the patient's difficulty and identify remaining abilities. Some patients are temporarily impaired because they are immobilized or confined to restricted positions as part of their medical treatment. Important aspects of the physical examination are visual acuity, range of motion and muscle strength in both arms, and range of motion and grip strength in both hands. Also evaluate the patient's ability to follow instructions and to chew and swallow without choking or gagging.

Patient Problems, Goals, and Outcome Criteria: Feeding Problems

Patient Problems	Goals and Outcome Criteria
Inability to perform ADLs (feeding) related to paralysis, weakness, poor coordination, confusion, visual impairment, or any other condition or situation	Improved self-feeding: patient participates in feeding within their capabilities
Inadequate nutrition related to inability to feed self	Adequate food intake: stable body weight or attainment of ideal body weight

Interventions

Encourage patients to be as independent as possible in feeding. For some, proper positioning and arrangement of the meal tray are all that is needed. Assistive devices designed for paralyzed and arthritic patients are available. These can be obtained through the physical therapy or occupational therapy department. Simple adaptations such as padding the handles of utensils may enable the patient with limited grasping ability to feed themselves. Thickening liquids may also be used to reduce the risk of choking.

Teach CNAs and caregivers the following points when feeding a patient:

- Check the diet and the patient's name for accuracy.
- Seat the patient upright, with the head tilted slightly forward for easiest swallowing.
- Tuck in a napkin or towel under the patient's chin to catch spills.
- If the patient can communicate, ask in what order the food should be offered. The practice of mixing all food together to ensure that the patient gets a little of everything is unappetizing and not recommended.
- Some patients do not open their mouths voluntarily. Touch the lips with the spoon or gently press just below the lower lip with a finger to encourage them to do so.
- Pacing is important, so observe that the patient has swallowed before offering more food.
- In stroke patients, food may accumulate in the affected side of the mouth. Check the mouth at intervals for accumulated food.
- Offer fluids periodically.
- At the completion of the meal, provide mouth care and record the amount of food taken.

Put On Your Thinking Cap!

Practice feeding a classmate a simple meal. Then reverse roles and permit the classmate to feed you. Assume that the person being fed is unable to speak clearly but understands what is said. Immediately afterward, write down (1) the steps you went through when feeding another person, (2) how you felt while being fed, and (3) what you learned from the experience that you could apply in patient care.

ORAL INFLAMMATION AND INFECTIONS OF THE ORAL CAVITY: STOMATITIS

Stomatitis is a general term for inflammation of the oral mucosa that may affect the gums, cheeks, lips, tongue, and roof of the mouth. It may result from the mechanical trauma of poorly fitting dentures, the irritation of excessive tobacco or alcohol use, poor oral hygiene, inadequate nutrition, pathogenic organisms, radiation therapy, or drug therapy. Disorders of the kidney, liver, or blood can also cause stomatitis. Emotional tension and excessive fatigue seem to make people more susceptible to some types of stomatitis. Medical treatment is directed toward determining the cause and eliminating it. If specific pathogenic organisms are identified, appropriate antibiotics (usually topical), antifungal agents, or antivirals may be prescribed. Table 38.1 summarizes some common types of stomatitis.

❖ NURSING CARE OF THE PATIENT WITH ORAL INFLAMMATION OR INFECTION

Patients with only oral inflammation or infections are usually treated as outpatients, so the nurse's role is limited to reinforcing medical instructions. However, these conditions may develop in long-term care residents and patients who are hospitalized for other reasons. The nurse then has a more active role in treating the condition and teaching patients.

Focused Assessment

The history includes a thorough description of the patient's symptoms. Describe pain location, onset, and precipitating factors and note measures that have helped to relieve pain. Record any known illnesses and treatments, including drugs and radiation therapy. Also describe the patient's habits, including diet, oral care practices, alcohol intake, and tobacco use. Inspect the lips and oral cavity for redness, swelling, and lesions. Inquire about recent or current stresses.

Patient Problems, Goals, and Outcome Criteria: Stomatitis

Patient Problems	Goals and Outcome Criteria
Acute pain related to tissue trauma, irritation, infection	Pain relief: relaxed appearance, patient statement that pain is reduced or relieved
Disrupted oral tissue integrity related to trauma, ineffective oral hygiene, infection, adverse drug effects	Healthy oral mucous membranes: membranes intact, without redness or lesions
Inadequate nutrition related to inflamed or infected oral tissue	Adequate nutrition: usual food intake, stable body weight

Pharmacology Capsule

When drugs are given for candidiasis, the directions may be to "swish and swallow" the medication or to allow tablets to dissolve in the mouth. Be sure to instruct patients appropriately and evaluate their understanding of directions.

Interventions

When acute inflammation is present, gentle oral hygiene and the use of prescribed mouthwashes are soothing. The diet may be modified to exclude rough and spicy food. The teeth and tongue can be cleansed with a soft-bristled toothbrush, sponge, or cotton-tipped applicator. Administer medications as ordered. If poor oral hygiene is a contributing factor, teach the patient proper techniques for brushing and flossing the teeth. Emphasize the importance of daily oral hygiene and good nutrition in preventing recurrences.

DISORDERS OF THE GUMS: PERIODONTAL DISEASE

Periodontal disease begins with **gingivitis** (inflammation of the gums) and progresses to involve other structures that support the teeth. Inflamed gums are typically red, swollen, painful, and bleed easily. If untreated, abscesses develop around tooth roots,

Table 38.1 Common Types of Stomatitis

TYPE	CAUSE	TREATMENT	COMMENTS
Aphthous "canker sore"	Possible virus or immune response	Topical or systemic corticosteroids	Start treatment when earliest symptoms appear
Herpes simplex type 1 "cold sores"	Virus	Oral antiviral drugs: acyclovir, valacyclovir, famciclovir	Triggers: stress, excessive sun exposure, upper respiratory infection
Candidiasis "thrush"	*Candida albicans*—yeast	Antifungal drugs (e.g., nystatin suspension)	Overgrowth of normal flora often triggered by steroid therapy or antibiotics

causing them to loosen and possibly require extraction. Gingivitis results primarily from poor oral hygiene but may occur secondary to some systemic disorders. Growing evidence shows a relationship between gingivitis and cardiovascular disease. Patients should be referred to a dentist for evaluation and treatment of periodontal disease. Treatment may involve teeth cleaning, plaque removal, smoothing root surfaces, and surgical removal of diseased gum tissue. Good oral hygiene and regular dental care can reduce the risk of recurrence.

NURSING CARE OF THE PATIENT WITH A GUM DISORDER

Focused Assessment

Inquire about oral pain or soreness in the health history. Note the usual diet, frequency of dental examinations, and mouth-care practices. When examining the mouth, observe the condition of the teeth and gums and note any missing or broken teeth, caries, redness or lesions of the gums, and gum recession. It is especially important for nurses in long-term care to assess patients' mouths at frequent intervals. Oral problems are often overlooked until they are quite advanced.

Patient Problems, Goals, and Outcome Criteria: Disorders of the Teeth and Gums

Patient Problems	Goals and Outcome Criteria
Acute pain related to dental caries, tissue inflammation	Pain relief: relaxed appearance; patient statement that pain is reduced or relieved
Inadequate nutrition related to oral pain, tooth loss	Adequate nutrition: stable body weight

Interventions

Most dental and gum disorders are treated in dentists' offices. However, sometimes dental problems develop when the patient is receiving nursing care for other reasons. In that case, interventions aim to minimize pain until a dentist can correct the problem. The physician or dentist may order an analgesic for pain. Gentle mouth care should be performed several times each day. In long-term care or home settings, the nurse may be the first to recognize oral problems that require attention.

The nurse should provide oral care for patients who cannot do it themselves. Certified nursing assistants and attendants need to understand the importance of regular mouth care and know how to provide it. It is important to include this care in the daily duties of the certified nursing assistant (CNA).

ORAL CANCER

The most life-threatening disorder affecting the mouth is cancer. Two types of malignant tumors develop in the mouth: (1) squamous cell carcinoma and (2) basal cell carcinoma. Squamous cell carcinomas occur on the lips, buccal mucosa, gums, floor of the mouth, tonsils, and tongue. The most common site for basal cell carcinoma is the lip.

Patient Teaching

Disorders of Gums

Nurses are able to teach patients how to prevent dental caries and gingivitis. Include the following instructions:

- Seek periodic dental examinations so that problems can be detected early and expert instruction in mouth care can be obtained.
- Brush teeth at least twice daily and floss every day.
- Eat a balanced diet with limited sugar intake.

Risk Factors

Cancer of the lip is related to prolonged exposure to irritants, including sun, wind, and pipe smoking. Factors that increase the risk of cancers inside the mouth include tobacco (including smokeless products) and alcohol use (especially in combination), infection with the Epstein-Barr or human papillomavirus, poor nutritional status, and chronic irritation.

Clinical Manifestations

Symptoms of oral cancer include tongue irritation and pain in the tongue or ear. Malignant lesions may appear as ulcerations, thickened or rough areas, or sore spots. The presence of hard, white patches in the mouth is called *leukoplakia*. Leukoplakia is considered a premalignant condition.

Medical Diagnosis and Treatment

A biopsy of suspicious lesions is done to make a medical diagnosis. When a malignancy is confirmed, the health care provider often orders endoscopic examinations and radiographs of the upper digestive and respiratory tracts to see whether evidence of metastases exists. Depending on the extent of the cancer, treatment may include surgery, radiation, or chemotherapy (or a combination of these treatments). One type of surgical procedure is illustrated in Fig. 38.1. Grafts are sometimes needed to close large defects caused by the surgical procedures. The donor site is usually the patient's anterior thigh.

◆ NURSING CARE OF THE PATIENT WITH ORAL CANCER

Focused Assessment

Assessment of the patient with a disorder of the digestive tract is summarized in Chapter 37, Box 37.1. When a patient is being evaluated for possible oral cancer, note a history of prolonged sun exposure, tobacco use, or alcohol consumption. Ask whether the patient or immediate family members have a history of cancer. Significant signs and symptoms to record include difficulty swallowing or chewing, decreased appetite,

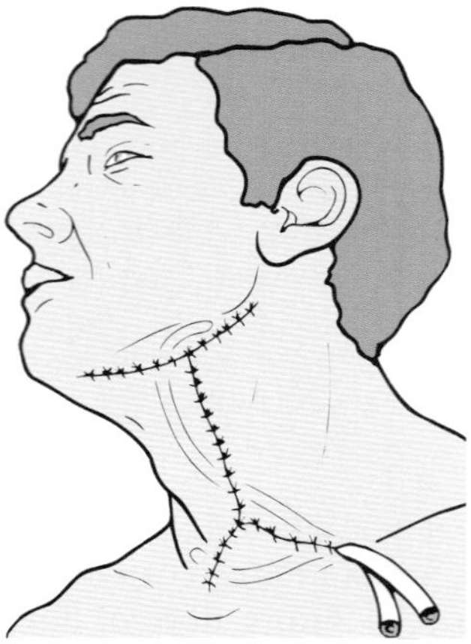

Fig. 38.1 One approach to surgery of the oral cavity for cancer: radical neck dissection for advanced oral and pharyngeal cancers. (From Lewis SL, Dirksen SR, Heitkemper MM, et al.: *Medical-surgical nursing: assessment and management of clinical problems*, ed 8, St. Louis, 2010, Mosby.)

weight loss, change in fit of dentures, and hemoptysis. The physical examination should focus on examination of the mouth for lesions. In addition, assess the neck for limitation of movement and enlarged lymph nodes.

Patient Problems, Goals, and Outcome Criteria: Oral Cancer

Patient Problems	Goals and Outcome Criteria
Disrupted oral tissue integrity related to tumor, edema, secretions	Healthy oral mucosa: membranes intact without lesions, healed surgical incisions
Airway obstruction related to tumor, tissue trauma	Patent airway: normal respiratory rate and effort
Acute pain related to tissue trauma	Pain relief: relaxed appearance, patient statement that pain is reduced or relieved
Inadequate nutrition related to pain, edema, medical restrictions on oral intake	Adequate nutrition: caloric intake sufficient to maintain body weight
Impaired verbal communication related to edema secondary to tissue trauma	Effective communication: patient communicates needs verbally or nonverbally
Altered body image related to effects of surgical or radiation treatment	Adjustment to altered appearance or function: patient statement of acceptance of changes, positive statements about self
Potential for infection related to broken skin, traumatized tissue	Absence of infection: no fever, normal white blood cell (WBC) count, incision free of excessive swelling and redness, no purulent drainage
Inadequate peripheral tissue perfusion of graft related to inadequate blood flow	Adequately perfused graft: warm tissue with normal color

Interventions

Disrupted oral tissue integrity. Mouth care varies with the type of lesion and the treatment performed. Surgical incisions can be extensive, with considerable tissue trauma. Dry mouth is often a problem after radiation of the mouth. Consult with the physician before doing any mouth care for the patient who has had oral surgery or radiation. Temperatures are usually taken by routes other than the mouth after oral surgery. The physician may order specific solutions for rinsing the mouth. One solution that soothes and cleans is half hydrogen peroxide and half normal saline. Another is made by mixing ½ teaspoon of baking soda in 8 oz of water. Good hydration keeps the oral mucosa moist and thins secretions. Other products such as Biotene® come in the form of a mouthwash, lozenges, or gel, which is a saliva substitute used to treat dry mouth. It should not be swallowed but can be used several times during the day as needed.

Airway obstruction. Edema, secretions, and an enlarging tumor can cause obstruction of the airway. Monitor the patient's respiratory status frequently and report signs of inadequate oxygenation (dyspnea, restlessness, tachycardia). If edema or bleeding is present, elevate the head of the bed. Steroids may be ordered to decrease inflammation and production of secretions. Oral suction may be ordered to remove secretions that might be aspirated. A tracheostomy may be performed to prevent or treat airway obstruction. Care of the patient with a tracheostomy is discussed in Chapter 25.

Pain. Patients with oral cancer may have acute pain as a result of the lesion, surgical trauma, or the effects of radiation. Patients who have had grafts often report more pain in the donor site than in the grafted site. Administer analgesics as ordered to manage pain. Inform the registered nurse (RN) or health care provider if the medication is not controlling the patient's pain. In addition to drug therapy, relaxation, mental imagery, and other strategies can be used, as described in Chapter 8.

Inadequate nutrition. If the patient can swallow, a soft or liquid diet may be prescribed. Mouth care before and after meals may improve appetite and keeps the mouth free of food particles. If the patient cannot or should not take oral nutrition, a feeding tube (nasogastric or gastrostomy) will probably be needed. Another option is TPN. Monitor intake and output records and daily weights to assess adequate intake. With large tumors that cannot be completely removed, or after extensive oral surgery, the feeding tube may be needed indefinitely. See Chapter 37 for care of the patient with a feeding tube. When the patient is able to take oral fluids, assess swallowing and monitor the amount of food taken. Therapy may be needed to help the patient learn to swallow again. Speech-language pathologists are experts in evaluating and managing swallowing disorders.

Impaired verbal communication. A large tumor, or one that interferes with movement of the tongue, is likely to affect speech. In addition, surgical procedures can damage structures involved in normal speech. Assess the patient's ability to read and write and devise a system to enable the patient to communicate with others. Keep a white board, electronic messaging device, or pen and pad within the patient's reach; the call bell must also be within reach at all times.

Altered body image. Patients with oral cancer may have body image disturbances as a result of impaired speech, inability to eat, and altered physical appearance. Demonstrate acceptance through attentive care, patience, and listening. Assure the patient that edema related to surgery will resolve. However, some disfigurement may be permanent. Encourage the patient to resume grooming and explore ways to improve their appearance. Professional counseling may be needed to help the patient learn to cope with body image changes.

Potential for infection. Patients with open lesions or surgical incisions are at risk for infection. If tissue has been grafted, the patient's donor site is also a potential site for infection. Be alert for signs and symptoms of infection (e.g., fever, redness, swelling, purulent drainage) and advise the RN or physician if these are present. Prophylactic antibiotics may be ordered. Provide care of external incisions according to the medical orders and agency policy (see the Patient Teaching box).

Patient Teaching

ORAL CANCER PREVENTION

- Avoid known risk factors: tobacco and alcohol use, excessive sun exposure.
- Report any dental problem or pain in the mouth to a dentist or health care provider for early evaluation.
- Good nutrition and mouth care are essential for oral health and wound healing.
- Consider human papillomavirus vaccination of children aged 11 to 12 years.

SELF-CARE

- If the patient is discharged with a feeding tube or tracheostomy, begin teaching self-care as soon as the patient is well enough to participate. If the patient and family need assistance, a referral to a home health agency should be sought.

Inadequate peripheral tissue perfusion of graft. Sometimes tissue is grafted to cover a large defect. The primary concern with the graft is maintaining adequate blood supply so that the tissue remains alive. Monitor graft color and warmth and protect the graft from pressure. Immediately inform the RN or surgeon of any coolness or darkness of the graft.

PAROTITIS

Parotitis is inflammation of the parotid glands. This condition causes painful swelling of the salivary glands below the ear next to the lower jaw. Pain increases during eating. Parotitis may develop in patients who are unable to take oral liquids for a long time, especially if their oral hygiene is poor. Patients who are very weak and have little resistance to infection are also at risk for parotitis.

The condition is treated with antibiotics, mouthwashes, and warm compresses. If chronic inflammation develops, surgical drainage or removal may be necessary. Otherwise, the infected gland can rupture, spreading infection into surrounding tissues. Parotitis might be prevented in susceptible patients by providing chewing gum or citrus-flavored hard candy (if allowed) to stimulate saliva production. Monitor the patient's temperature and comfort level. Report increased swelling of the infected gland. Provide antibiotics and mouth care as ordered.

ACHALASIA

Achalasia is characterized by progressively worsening dysphagia (difficulty swallowing). It is caused by failure of the lower esophageal muscles and sphincter to relax during swallowing. The reason for this failure is unknown but it is thought to be a neuromuscular defect affecting the esophageal muscles. Conservative care includes avoidance of restrictive clothing, identification of the position that works best for eating, elimination of specific foods that seem especially difficult to swallow, and gastric acid suppressants.

Treatment includes drug therapy, esophageal dilation, and surgical measures. Correction of achalasia requires mechanical or balloon dilation or surgical cutting of the lower esophageal sphincter (LES). Esophageal dilation is done on an outpatient basis and brings about improvement in most patients. Its effects are best in people older than 40 years. The main complication of dilation is perforation of the esophagus. Symptoms of perforation are chest and shoulder pain, fever, and subcutaneous emphysema. After dilation, monitor for signs of perforation and bleeding. The patient is usually kept nothing by mouth (NPO) for 1 hour and then allowed only liquids for 24 hours. Instruct the patient to expectorate rather than swallow secretions so that any bleeding can be detected.

ESOPHAGEAL CANCER

Pathophysiology

Cancer of the esophagus is not common but, when it does occur, it has a very poor prognosis. Most esophageal cancers are located in the middle or lower portion of the esophagus. No known cause exists but predisposing factors are cigarette smoking, excessive alcohol intake, chronic trauma, poor oral hygiene, and eating spicy foods (see the Cultural Considerations box).

Cultural Considerations

What Does Culture Have to Do With Esophageal Cancer?

In the United States, the incidence of esophageal cancer is greater among Black American men than among White American men and is related to tobacco use and dietary factors. The incidence is increased in areas of the world where food and soil contamination and nutritional deficiencies are common.

Cancer of the esophagus often has begun to metastasize by the time it is diagnosed. The liver and lung are common sites of metastasis. The lesion can also extend to the aorta, causing erosion and hemorrhage. Other complications are esophageal obstruction and perforation.

Clinical Manifestations

Progressive dysphagia (difficulty swallowing) is the primary symptom of esophageal cancer. The patient has difficulty with meat first, then with soft foods, and eventually with liquids. Pain associated with swallowing may be substernal, epigastric, or located in the back and radiate to the neck, jaws, ear, or shoulder. Some patients report a sore throat and choking. Obstruction is a late sign of esophageal cancer. Weight loss may be dramatic.

Medical Diagnosis

Radiologic studies used to diagnose cancer of the esophagus include radiographs, computed tomography (CT), magnetic resonance imaging scans (MRI), and positron emission tomography scans (PET). Additional information about common diagnostic tests and procedures is summarized in Chapter 37, Table 37.1.

Medical and Surgical Treatment

Esophageal cancer may be treated with surgery, radiation, chemotherapy, or various combinations of these treatments. Neither chemotherapy nor radiation alone can cure esophageal cancer. Surgical procedures used to treat this type of cancer include the following (Fig. 38.2):

- Esophagectomy—removal of all or part of the esophagus and replacement of the resected part with a Dacron graft
- Esophagogastrostomy—resection of the diseased part of the esophagus and attachment of the remaining esophagus to the stomach
- Esophagogastrectomy—resection of the lower part of the esophagus and the upper part of the stomach (the remaining portions of the esophagus and the stomach are reattached)
- Colon interposition (esophagoenterostomy)—replacement of the diseased part of the esophagus with a segment of colon

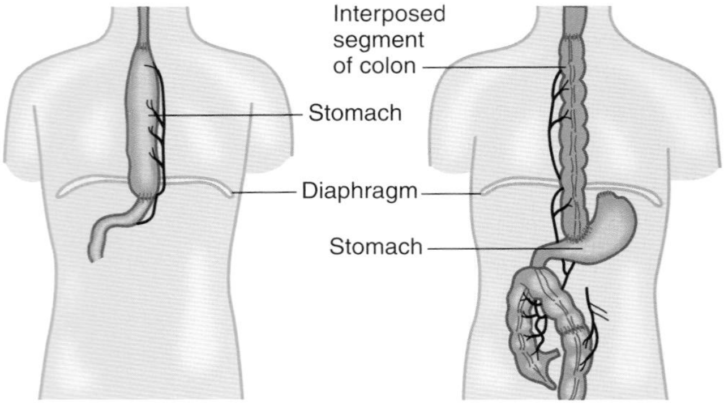

Fig. 38.2 Surgical approaches to the treatment of esophageal cancer.

If the diseased segment cannot be removed, an expandable metal stent may be put in place to keep the esophagus patent. Because maintaining good nutrition is a major challenge, the health care provider may insert a feeding tube, often a gastrostomy tube, to provide adequate nourishment. TPN may be used on a short-term basis preoperatively to improve the patient's nutritional status.

◆ NURSING CARE OF THE PATIENT WITH ESOPHAGEAL CANCER

Focused Assessment

Assessment of the patient with a digestive tract disorder is summarized in Chapter 37, Box 37.1. The nursing assessment of dysphagia includes the patient's description of the problem and observations of the patient while eating. It is important to note the conditions under which the patient has dysphagia as well as the temperature and texture of foods that cause problems. Assess for the presence of hoarseness, cough, anorexia, weight loss, and regurgitation. The functional assessment documents the use of alcohol and tobacco and dietary practices.

General physical appearance and height and weight are important aspects of the physical examination. It is helpful to observe the patient eating. Note body position, size of bites, chewing efforts, and speed of eating.

Patient Problems, Goals, and Outcome Criteria: Esophageal Cancer

Patient Problems	Goals and Outcome Criteria
Acute pain related to esophageal lesion, effect of radiation therapy, trauma of surgical incision	Pain relief: relaxed manner, patient statement of pain reduction or relief

Patient Problems, Goals, and Outcome Criteria: Esophageal Cancer—cont'd

Patient Problems	Goals and Outcome Criteria
Inadequate nutrition related to dysphagia	Adequate nutritional intake: stable or increased body weight
Anxiety related to diagnosis, therapy, uncertain outcome	Decreased anxiety: calm manner, patient statement of lessened anxiety
Potential for injury related to leakage at anastomosis sites	Reduced risk for injury: healed incisions; no signs of complications such as tarry stools, abdominal pain, or distention
Inadequate oxygenation related to incisional pain, splinting, shallow breathing	Adequate oxygenation: normal respiratory effort and rate, clear breath sounds
Inability to manage self-care related to lack of knowledge of wound care, maintenance of nutrition.	Adequate self-care: patient cares for wounds properly and uses measures to maintain nutrition

Interventions

Acute pain. Administer analgesics as ordered. Independent measures to reduce or relieve pain are discussed in Chapter 8.

Inadequate nutrition. Nutrition is a major problem for the patient with esophageal cancer. Daily weights, intake and output measurements, and calorie counts are monitored to assess adequacy of intake. A high-calorie, high-protein diet is recommended. The texture of food (e.g., soft, semisolid) and meal size are adjusted as needed depending on the patient's ability to swallow.

Some general interventions may be helpful in managing dysphagia. A quiet, relaxed environment helps the patient to concentrate on effective swallowing. An erect position is preferred. The head should be tilted slightly forward. Some patients think that they can swallow better with the head thrown back. That position makes swallowing more difficult and increases the risk of aspiration. If dysphagia prevents adequate nutritional intake, an alternative feeding method must be used. Options include nasogastric and gastrostomy feedings and TPN.

Pharmacology Capsule

The patient with dysphagia may be able to take liquid medications more easily than capsules or tablets.

Anxiety. During the diagnostic period, determine the patient's understanding of tests and procedures and offer explanations as needed. Help the patient to select foods that are swallowed comfortably. A diagnosis of cancer evokes many questions and fears. Find out what the patient has been told about the treatment and prognosis so that correct information can be reinforced. Encourage the patient to ask questions and talk about their fears. Be accepting of the patient's feelings and avoid using trite phrases and giving false reassurance. A referral to a spiritual or mental health counselor may be indicated (see the Complementary and Alternative Therapies box).

Complementary and Alternative Therapies

Yoga, Tai Chi, music therapy, massage, meditation, and mental imagery all have been found to be effective in reducing stress and anxiety.

Potential for injury. Depending on the surgical procedure, the patient may have multiple incisions and wound drains. Assist the patient in supporting the incisions during coughing and position changes. Like any surgical patient, the patient who has undergone surgery for esophageal cancer must be monitored for signs and symptoms of hemorrhage (i.e., restlessness, tachycardia, hypotension) and infection (i.e., fever, increased white blood cell [WBC] count, erythema, purulent wound drainage). In addition to the risk of infection, the patient is at risk for leakage at anastomosis sites. If the anastomosis is not secure, digestive fluids leak into the thoracic or abdominal cavity. The risk of leakage is greatest 5 to 7 days after surgery. Signs and symptoms of leakage are fever, tachycardia, tachypnea, and fluid accumulation. The health care provider should be notified immediately if leakage is suspected.

Inadequate oxygenation. Immediately after surgery, the patient may be artificially ventilated to maintain adequate oxygenation. Chest tubes are needed to remove fluid from the thoracic cavity. When the ventilator is discontinued, encourage and support the patient in turning, coughing, and deep breathing. Chest physiotherapy or incentive spirometry may be ordered. Elevate the patient's head to ease chest expansion and to reduce the risk of reflux of gastric contents into the esophagus.

Patients who have stents placed in the esophagus should be told how to reduce the risk of regurgitation of stomach contents. Instruct them to eat only small meals, to remain upright for several hours after meals, and to avoid lying flat at any time. The head of the bed should be elevated at least 30 degrees at all times.

Inability to manage self-care. Postoperatively, it is important to prepare the patient for discharge. Encourage the patient to continue breathing exercises and to gradually increase activity. Discourage bed rest. Point out the characteristics of the healing incisions and teach the patient the signs of wound complications that should be reported. Stress the importance of small, high-calorie, high-protein meals. If nasogastric or other enteral feedings are continued, instruct the patient and family in management of the feedings. Because esophageal cancer often recurs, the patient should know to report increased pain or dysphagia. A referral to a home health agency may be made for assistance after discharge.

DISORDERS AFFECTING DIGESTION AND ABSORPTION

NAUSEA AND VOMITING

Nausea is a feeling of discomfort sometimes referred to as *queasiness*. It may or may not be accompanied by abdominal pain, pallor, perspiration, and cold, clammy skin. Causes of nausea include odors, irritating foods, infectious diseases, radiation, drugs and other chemicals, hormonal changes and imbalances, and distention of the digestive tract. It is common after surgery and in patients with motion sickness, inner ear disorders, and pregnancy.

Nausea and vomiting often occur together. Vomiting **emesis** is the forceful expulsion of stomach contents through the mouth. It occurs when the vomiting reflex in the brain is stimulated. Very forceful ejection of stomach contents is called *projectile vomiting*. **Regurgitation** is the gentle ejection of food or fluid without nausea or retching. Just before vomiting occurs, a person usually senses what is about to happen. Tachycardia and increased salivation are common just before vomiting.

Complications

Prolonged or severe vomiting can lead to significant loss of fluids and electrolytes. In addition to dehydration, metabolic alkalosis may develop because of loss of stomach acids. Patients who are very weak or unable to move are at risk for aspirating the vomited stomach contents. Therefore, nausea and vomiting must be treated to relieve patient discomfort and to prevent complications.

Medical Treatment

Drugs that prevent or treat nausea and vomiting are classified as *antiemetics*. Most antiemetic drugs have multiple uses. They may have local effects (adsorbents), they may act on the central nervous system (CNS), or they may act in more than one way. Centrally acting antiemetics include anticholinergics, antihistamines, dopamine antagonists, glucocorticoids, and cannabinoids. Antiemetics classified as *serotonin antagonists* affect the small intestine as well as the peripheral nervous system and CNS. Examples of these drugs are listed in Table 37.2. A common side effect of most centrally acting antiemetics is drowsiness. They may also cause tachycardia, hypotension, constipation, urinary retention, and dry mouth. Many antiemetics are contraindicated in patients with glaucoma, myocardial infarction, bowel or urinary obstruction, and pregnancy.

Intravenous fluids may be ordered to prevent dehydration. Oral fluids may be limited to clear liquids or withheld completely until the nausea and vomiting stop. At times, a nasogastric tube is inserted and attached to suction to keep the stomach empty. Severe or prolonged vomiting may necessitate TPN to meet the patient's metabolic needs.

Pharmacology Capsule

A common side effect of most antiemetics is drowsiness, so take necessary safety precautions.

◆ NURSING CARE OF THE PATIENT WITH NAUSEA AND VOMITING

Focused Assessment

The nursing assessment plays an important part in the management of nausea and vomiting. The health history should elicit a description of the onset, frequency, and duration of the present illness. Note the conditions under which nausea and vomiting occur. For example, is it before or after meals, at a certain time of day, or after taking a certain medication? If vomiting occurs, record the amount, color, odor, and contents of the vomitus. Contents might include undigested food or medications. Vomitus containing bile has a characteristic green color. A bright-red color suggests recent bleeding in the esophagus or stomach, although it could be the result of recently ingested red food or liquid. When blood has been in the stomach long enough to be acted on by stomach secretions, it turns dark brown and resembles wet coffee grounds.

Patient Problems, Goals, and Outcome Criteria: Nausea and Vomiting

Patient Problems	Goals and Outcome Criteria
Inadequate nutrition related to inability to consume or retain food	Adequate nutrition: stable body weight, retention of food and fluids
Fluid volume deficit related to loss of fluids by vomiting	Normal hydration: pulse and blood pressure consistent with patient norms, urine output approximately equal to fluid intake, moist mucous membranes
Potential for aspiration related to decreased level of consciousness, impaired swallowing, depressed gag reflex, vomiting	Absence of aspiration: respiratory rate 12 to 20 breaths per minute without dyspnea, clear breath sounds

Interventions

Inadequate nutrition and fluid volume deficit. When a patient complains of nausea, assist them in assuming a still, comfortable position. Maintain a cool room temperature and remove any unpleasant stimuli. Provide an emesis receptacle and apply a cool, damp cloth to the face and neck for comfort. Advise the patient that taking deep breaths and swallowing may be effective in suppressing the vomiting reflex. Unless the episode passes promptly, administer an antiemetic drug as ordered. In situations in which nausea can be anticipated, antiemetics are best given before nausea occurs. It is easier to prevent nausea than to treat it.

If the patient vomits, remain close by and offer reassurance. Severe or prolonged vomiting puts the patient at risk for fluid volume deficit. Infants and older adults are especially susceptible to fluid volume deficit because their kidneys are less efficient in conserving body fluids. Monitor intake and output, vital signs, and other measures of hydration. Signs of fluid volume deficit include tachycardia, hypotension, oliguria, confusion, and poor tissue turgor.

When the patient is ready to resume oral intake, they are usually started on clear liquids. Tea, broth, flat carbonated liquids, and gelatin are generally tolerated best. Other liquids may be added if nausea and vomiting do not recur. If permitted, offer dry toast or crackers to help relieve nausea and advise the patient to eat slowly (see the Complementary and Alternative Therapies box).

Complementary and Alternative Therapies

Ginger root is effective in calming upset stomach, reducing flatulence, and preventing motion sickness. However, be aware that it enhances the action of anticoagulants and antiplatelet agents.

Potential for aspiration. The patient who is unconscious or who has impaired swallowing or a depressed gag reflex is at risk for aspiration. This risk is greatly increased when the patient is vomiting. Therefore, position the patient on their side so that vomitus can drain from the mouth. Keep the suction apparatus at the bedside and use it as needed to clear the mouth and upper airway. Monitor the patient's respiratory rate and effort and breath sounds. Notify the health care provider of increasing respiratory rate, dyspnea, and abnormal breath sounds.

HIATAL HERNIA

Pathophysiology

The esophageal hiatus is the opening in the diaphragm through which the esophagus passes. A hiatal hernia is the protrusion of the lower esophagus and stomach upward through the diaphragm and into the chest. Fig. 38.3 illustrates the two types of hiatal hernias: (1) the sliding hernia and (2) the paraesophageal (rolling) hernia. In a sliding hernia, the gastroesophageal junction is above the hiatus. The stomach slides into the thoracic cavity when the patient reclines. It slides back into place when the patient stands or sits up. Sliding hernias are commonly associated with gastroesophageal reflux disease (GERD). Weakness of the esophageal sphincter permits gastric fluids to flow backward into the esophagus. Acidic gastric fluids can cause inflammation of the esophagus. However, not all patients with hiatal hernias have GERD and not all patients with GERD have hiatal hernias. GERD is discussed later.

In a rolling hernia, the gastroesophageal junction remains in place but a portion of the stomach herniates up through the diaphragm through a secondary opening.

Complications of hiatal hernia include ulcerations, bleeding, and aspiration of regurgitated stomach contents. The paraesophageal hernia can also result in strangulation of the hernia, a situation in which the herniated tissue becomes trapped and deprived of blood flow.

Causes

Hiatal hernia may be caused by weakness of the muscles of the diaphragm in the area where the esophagus and the stomach join (the lower esophageal sphincter or LES); however, the exact cause is not known. Factors that contribute to development of hiatal hernia include excessive intraabdominal pressure, trauma, and long-term bed rest in a reclining position. Intraabdominal pressure is increased by obesity, pregnancy, abdominal tumors, ascites, and repeated heavy lifting or strain. Hiatal hernia develops in about half of all people older than 60 years of age.

Clinical Manifestations

Many patients with hiatal hernias have no symptoms at all. Others report feelings of fullness, dysphagia, eructation (belching), regurgitation, and heartburn. Heartburn is a feeling of burning and tightness rising from the lower sternum to the throat. It is triggered by foods and drugs that decrease LES pressure and by lying down or bending over.

Medical Diagnosis

When hiatal hernia is suspected, several tests and procedures may be ordered. A barium swallow examination with fluoroscopy outlines the esophagus and demonstrates esophageal peristalsis. A CT scan or MRI helps to visualize the abnormality. In the patient with hiatal hernia, the reflux of gastric contents is evident. Structural abnormalities and tissue inflammation may be detected with esophagoscopy. Tissue specimens can be taken for biopsy during endoscopy.

Esophageal manometry measures the pressures in the stomach and the esophagus. With the patient sitting up, a small tube is inserted through the nose into the stomach. The patient is then placed in a supine position. Small amounts of water or gelatin are given to the patient to

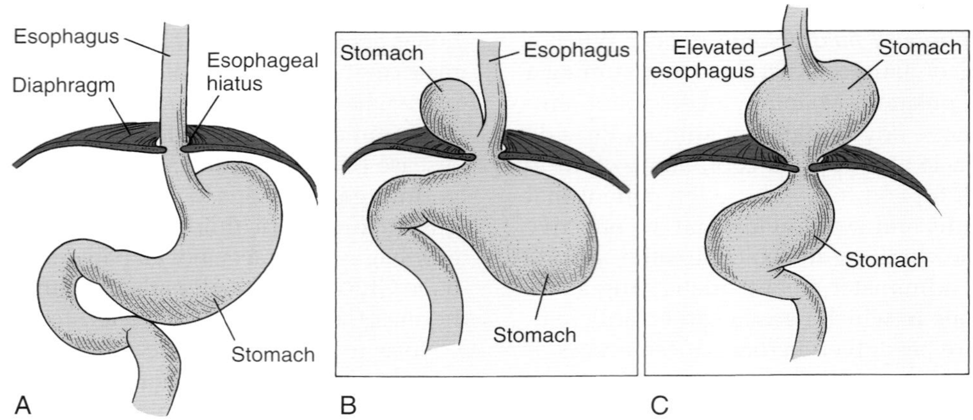

Fig. 38.3 Hiatal hernia. (A) Normal anatomy. (B) Paraesophageal (rolling) hiatal hernia. (C) Sliding hiatal hernia. (From Schlenker ED, Long S: *William's essentials of nutrition & diet therapy*, ed 9, St. Louis, 2007, Mosby.)

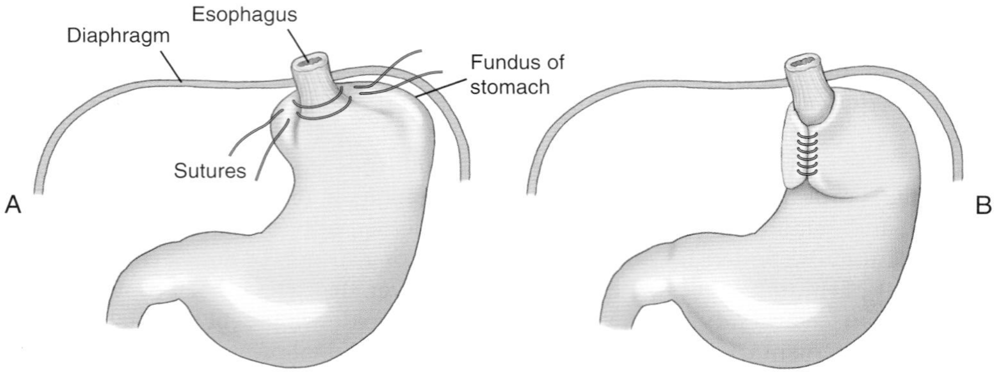

Fig. 38.4 Nissen fundoplication for hiatal hernia repair. (From Lewis SL, Dirksen SR, Heitkemper MM, et al.: *Medical-surgical nursing: assessment and management of clinical problems*, ed 9, St. Louis, 2015, Mosby.)

swallow. Pressure measurements are taken in the stomach and esophagus. For acid reflux testing, a second probe that is sensitive to acid is inserted through the nose into the esophagus. The detection of acid in the esophagus is consistent with esophageal reflux.

Medical Treatment

In many cases, hiatal hernia can be managed with drug therapy, diet, and measures to avoid increased intraabdominal pressure. Drug therapy includes use of antacids that include aluminum hydroxide (Maalox) or calcium carbonate (TUMS); sometimes drugs such as H2-receptor blockers (e.g., cimetidine [Tagamet], famotidine [Pepcid], and Nizatidine [Axid]) or proton pump inhibitors (e.g., omeprazole [Prilosec]) are used to reduce gastric acid secretion.

Surgery may be necessary if severe bleeding or narrowing of the esophagus occurs. Surgical options to treat hiatal hernia include several types of fundoplication such as the Nissen, Toupet, and LINX procedures. Fundoplication (Fig. 38.4) is a minimally invasive form of surgery that strengthens the LES by suturing the fundus of the stomach around the esophagus and anchoring it below the diaphragm. Procedures that can be done laparoscopically are preferred. When laparoscopy is not appropriate, incisions may be made in either the abdomen or the chest. Either way, risk of postoperative respiratory complications exists.

◆ NURSING CARE OF THE PATIENT WITH HIATAL HERNIA

Focused Assessment

Assessment of the patient with a digestive tract disorder is summarized in Chapter 37, Box 37.1. When a patient has hiatal hernia, document the symptoms (e.g., pain, dysphagia, eructation) and record factors that trigger them as well as measures that aggravate or relieve them. Note any abdominal trauma in the past medical history. In addition, describe the patient's dietary habits, use of alcohol and tobacco, and medication history. Also inquire about activities requiring lifting or intense physical exertion.

Patient Problems, Goals, and Outcome Criteria: Hiatal Hernia

Patient Problems	Goals and Outcome Criteria
Acute or chronic pain related to esophageal inflammation	Pain relief: patient statement of less or no pain, relaxed manner

Patient Problems, Goals, and Outcome Criteria: Hiatal Hernia—cont'd

Patient Problems	Goals and Outcome Criteria
Potential for aspiration related to regurgitation of gastric contents	Absence of aspiration: respiratory rate 12 to 20 breaths per minute without dyspnea, clear breath sounds
Inadequate nutrition related to inadequate food intake as a result of dysphagia	Adequate nutrition: stable body weight

Interventions

Acute or chronic pain. The patient may have chronic pain caused by the reflux of acid into the inflamed esophagus. Therefore pain can be reduced by increasing LES pressure, which prevents gastric contents from passing into the esophagus. Administer prescribed drugs that neutralize acid and reduce acid secretion. Evaluate and document the effects of drug therapy. Dietary alterations, position changes, and medications are helpful in reducing the symptoms of hiatal hernia.

Potential for aspiration. Gastric contents that are regurgitated into the esophagus may be aspirated into the respiratory tract, causing aspiration pneumonia. To reduce the risk of aspiration, food and fluids should not be taken for 2 to 3 hours before bedtime. This reduces reflux of stomach contents during sleep. Patients with hiatal hernia should sleep with their heads elevated 6 to 12 inches. Wooden blocks can be placed under the legs of the head of the bed if a mechanical or electrical bed is not available. This sleeping position requires a period of adjustment but is very important to prevent nighttime reflux.

Inadequate nutrition. Monitor weight changes and note excessive weight loss. Advise the patient to eat small, frequent meals because large meals increase pressure in the stomach and delay gastric emptying. Encourage the patient to avoid foods that are known to decrease LES pressure: fatty foods, coffee, tea, cola, chocolate, and alcohol. In addition, acidic and spicy foods may be irritating when the esophagus is inflamed. Counsel the obese patient about the relationship between obesity and increased intraabdominal pressure (see the Patient Teaching box).

Patient Teaching

Hiatal Hernia

- Know the drugs you take, their dosages, schedule, and adverse effects.
- Eat small, frequent meals. Avoid foods and beverages that aggravate the condition (e.g., fatty foods, caffeinated drinks, alcohol).
- Maintain normal weight to decrease intraabdominal pressure.
- Elevate the head of your bed to discourage reflux.
- Avoid smoking.
- Learn stress management techniques.
- To prevent increased intraabdominal pressure, avoid bending forward, lifting, or straining and avoid clothing that is tight around the waist or abdomen.

POSTOPERATIVE NURSING CARE OF THE PATIENT WITH HIATAL HERNIA REPAIR

When the patient has had an abdominal or thoracic approach for hiatal hernia repair, care is similar to that after any major surgery. Turning, coughing, and deep breathing are particularly important for these patients. The patient will probably have a nasogastric tube in place and be connected to suction for 1 or 2 days after surgery. Until bowel function returns, the patient is given only intravenous fluids. Tell the patient to expect mild dysphagia for several weeks.

Following laparoscopic procedures, patients typically require overnight hospitalization before discharge. A liquid diet is recommended for several weeks, then gradually advanced to soft and regular food. The patient should chew food thoroughly and pause between bites. Regular walks are encouraged, and heavy lifting is discouraged. Stool softeners may be recommended to prevent constipation and straining.

GASTROESOPHAGEAL REFLUX DISEASE

GERD is the backward flow of gastric contents from the stomach into the esophagus. A key finding is inappropriate relaxation of the LES. GERD is often associated with a sliding hernia, although the two are not always found together. The term *nonerosive reflux disease* (NERD) is used when a patient has heartburn but no tissue destruction in the esophagus.

Pathophysiology

Factors that contribute to the development of GERD include abnormalities around the LES, gastric or duodenal ulcer, gastric or esophageal surgery, prolonged vomiting, and prolonged gastric intubation. The acidic stomach contents flow backward into the esophagus and eventually cause esophagitis (inflammation of the esophagus). Complications can include esophageal stricture (narrowing) and adenocarcinoma.

Clinical Manifestations

The onset of GERD symptoms may be sudden or gradual. Patients typically report a painful burning sensation that moves up and down, commonly occurs after meals, and is relieved by antacids. If severe, the pain may radiate to the back, neck, or jaw. Acid regurgitation, intermittent dysphagia, and belching are common. Symptoms are likely to occur after activities that increase intraabdominal pressure, such as lifting, straining, and lying supine, or ingestion of specific foods.

Medical Diagnosis

A diagnosis of GERD is suggested by the signs and symptoms. The health care provider may order a trial course of a proton pump inhibitor. If the symptoms cease while on the drug but return after the drug is discontinued, they are assumed to be caused by reflux rather than cardiac disease. Various diagnostic procedures may be done to confirm the diagnosis, assess the severity, and detect complications. These might include radiographic studies, endoscopy, biopsy, gastric analysis, esophageal manometry, 24-hour monitoring of esophageal pH, and acid perfusion tests.

Medical Treatment and Nursing Care

Medical treatment and nursing care are similar to those described earlier for hiatal hernia. In brief, drug therapy may include the following:

- Prokinetic agents (e.g., metoclopramide [Reglan])
- Proton pump inhibitors (e.g., omeprazole [Prilosec])

If medical care is unsuccessful, surgical fundoplication may be done.

Put On Your Thinking Cap!

Draw pictures or create a model to illustrate what a sliding hiatal hernia is and how it causes heartburn.

GASTRITIS

Pathophysiology

Gastritis is an inflammation of the lining of the stomach. The area of the inflammation and the depth of stomach tissue affected vary with different types of gastritis. Despite a variety of causes, the pathophysiology is common to all. The mucosal barrier that normally protects the stomach from autodigestion breaks down. Hydrochloric acid, histamine, and pepsin cause tissue edema, increased capillary permeability, and possible hemorrhage.

Among the many causes of gastritis, *Helicobacter pylori* is thought to be the prime culprit. Gastritis induced by *H. pylori* affects primarily the superficial tissues of the stomach lining. The type of gastritis associated with nonsteroidal antiinflammatory drugs (NSAIDs), stress, and alcohol tends to affect deeper tissue and is more prone to hemorrhage. The role of diet in gastritis is not completely understood. Some foods, such as red and black pepper, can cause superficial erosions in the gastric mucosa. It is interesting to note that chili pepper in small amounts stimulates mucus production but in large amounts can damage the mucosa. Other related factors are reflux of bile salts from the duodenum, prolonged vomiting, intense stress, and CNS lesions.

Chronic gastritis type A is probably induced by immune mechanisms. The changes in the stomach lining with chronic atrophic gastritis result in decreased production of acid and intrinsic factor. Intrinsic factor is needed for the absorption of vitamin B_{12}, which is essential for the maturation of red blood cells (RBCs). Without intrinsic factor, a serious condition called *pernicious anemia* develops. The management of pernicious anemia is discussed in Chapter 30.

Pharmacology Capsule

Although the parenteral form of vitamin B_{12} is traditionally used to treat pernicious anemia, research has shown that it can be treated with high-dose oral vitamin B_{12}.

Clinical Manifestations

Symptoms of acute gastritis usually include nausea, vomiting, anorexia, a feeling of fullness, and pain in the stomach area. Symptoms of chronic gastritis may be the same as acute gastritis. However, some patients have only mild indigestion or no symptoms at all unless they develop pernicious anemia.

Medical Diagnosis

The best means of diagnosing gastritis is endoscopy. The health care provider is able to visualize the interior of the stomach and biopsy any suspicious areas. Laboratory studies may be done to detect occult blood in the feces, low blood Hgb and hematocrit (Hct), and low serum gastrin levels. The presence of *H. pylori* can be confirmed by breath, urine, stool, or serum tests or by gastric tissue biopsy. Because *H. pylori* has been associated with gastric and duodenal ulcers and with gastric cancer, cytologic examination of a tissue specimen is commonly done.

Medical Treatment

Medical management of acute gastritis is concerned with treatment of symptoms and fluid replacement. If hospitalization is considered necessary, oral fluids and foods are usually withheld until the acute symptoms subside. Intravenous fluids can be ordered to prevent or treat dehydration. Medications to reduce gastric acidity (i.e., antacids, H2-receptor blockers, proton pump inhibitors) and to relieve nausea may be given. Analgesics may be ordered for pain relief and antibiotics for *H. pylori*. When nausea and vomiting stop, oral fluids are gradually increased. Typically, the patient progresses from clear liquids to full liquids and then to a soft, bland diet.

Medical management of chronic gastritis focuses on elimination of the cause (e.g., *H. pylori*, alcohol, NSAIDs, or other drugs) and treatment of pernicious anemia. Treatment of *H. pylori* usually requires a combination of omeprazole (Prilosec), which reduces gastric acid secretion, and one or two antibiotics (amoxicillin, clarithromycin, or both). Prepackaged combinations are available. Corticosteroids may also be used to reduce inflammation. Vitamin B_{12} supplements must be given regularly to prevent long-term complications. A bland diet given in six small feedings per day is usually prescribed, with antacids ordered after meals when reflux is most common.

Surgical intervention may be needed if conservative measures fail to correct or control gastritis or if the patient is hemorrhaging. Specific procedures and nursing implications are the same as for peptic ulcer disease, which is discussed later.

NURSING CARE OF THE PATIENT WITH GASTRITIS

Focused Assessment

In taking the health history, first describe the patient's present illness. Patients often complain of pain, indigestion, nausea, and vomiting. Document the onset, duration, and location of pain and note factors that trigger or relieve the symptoms. Document chronic illnesses as well as current and recent medications (see the Patient Teaching box).

Patient Teaching

Gastritis

- Adjust diet as recommended, which may include soft, bland, small meals; avoid irritants.
- Know the name, dosage, schedule, and adverse effects of your medications.
- Some stress reduction techniques that may be helpful are exercise, soft music, and regular leisure activities.
- Notify your primary health care provider if bloody vomitus or dark, tarry stools are present.
- It is vital to avoid using alcohol and tobacco, both of which stimulate acid secretion.
- Do not take aspirin or nonsteroidal antiinflammatory drugs (NSAIDs) because they aggravate gastritis and increase the risk of hemorrhage.

Patient Problems, Goals, and Outcome Criteria: Gastritis

Patient Problems	Goals and Outcome Criteria
Acute pain related to inflammation of the gastric mucosa	Pain relief: patient states less or no pain, relaxed manner
Inadequate nutrition related to anorexia, pain, nausea and vomiting that interfere with food intake	Adequate nutrition: stable weight
Fluid volume deficit related to vomiting, bleeding	Normal hydration: pulse and blood pressure within patient norms, moist mucous membranes, urine output equal to fluid intake Absence of bleeding: normal stool color, no blood in emesis
Inadequate coping related to chronic illness	Effective coping strategies: patient uses stress management techniques and resources

Interventions

Acute pain. Give medications as ordered, including antacids, H2-receptor blockers, proton pump inhibitors, other antiulcer medications, analgesics, and antibiotics. Assess drug effectiveness and inform the health care provider if pain is not relieved. Nonpharmacologic methods of pain control, as described in Chapter 8, may be used as well.

Inadequate nutrition. The most appropriate diet for the patient with gastritis is controversial. In general, patients are encouraged to avoid caffeine and alcohol as well as any other foods that seem to aggravate the symptoms. Many sources recommend a soft, bland diet taken in small meals; however, this pattern may actually increase the total amount of acid secreted. Most sources agree that the patient should avoid large meals before retiring. Note the patient's dietary intake and try to accommodate the patient's dietary choices as well as to reduce pain. Periodic weights may be appropriate to determine whether the patient is receiving adequate nourishment.

Fluid volume deficit. Deficit fluid volume may result from dehydration or hemorrhage. The patient may become dehydrated because of poor oral intake or severe vomiting. Be alert for signs of deficient fluid volume (i.e., oliguria, tachycardia, dry skin and mucous membranes, poor tissue turgor, hypotension). Record intake and output. Inspect vomited fluids for bright-red blood or dark-brown particles that indicate bleeding in the stomach. Examine stools for the maroon or tarry-black appearance characteristic of bleeding from the stomach. Administer intravenous fluids as ordered, monitoring the rate of infusion.

Inadequate coping. Chronic illness drains the patient physically and emotionally. Explore how the patient is dealing with gastritis and what additional supports are needed. Professional counseling may be needed to help the patient learn relaxation and stress management techniques (see the Complementary and Alternative Therapies box).

Complementary and Alternative Therapies

Alternative therapies for stress reduction include acupuncture, therapeutic massage, guided imagery, progressive relaxation, meditation, yoga, and aromatherapy with chamomile, lavender, citronella, and mandarin.

PEPTIC ULCER

Pathophysiology

A peptic ulcer is a loss of tissue from the lining of the digestive tract. Normally, a mucous barrier protects the lining from the digestive fluids. When that barrier fails, pepsin and hydrochloric acid injure the unprotected tissue.

Peptic ulcers may be acute or chronic, depending on the layers of tissue affected. Acute ulcers affect only the superficial layers of the digestive lining, whereas chronic ulcers extend into the muscle layer. Acute ulcers are sometimes called *acute gastric lesions*.

Peptic ulcers are classified as *gastric* or *duodenal*, depending on their location. Gastric and duodenal ulcers differ in depth of injury, amount of gastric secretions, incidence, and signs and symptoms. These differences are presented in Table 38.2.

Eighty percent of peptic ulcers occur in the duodenum. Duodenal ulcers are more common in younger men and in people with type O blood. Duodenal ulcers are found among people in all occupations and income levels.

Causes

Factors that contribute to the development of ulcers are thought to include drugs, infection, and stress. Drugs that are associated with ulcer disease include aspirin and NSAIDs such as ibuprofen. However, most ulcers are caused by the microorganism *H. pylori*. In addition, extremely stressful events such as shock, burns, and trauma are thought to cause a temporary decrease in blood flow to the gastric mucosa. Inadequate blood flow interferes with the mucosal barrier, permitting breakdown of the stomach lining. Ulcers attributed to this process are called *stress ulcers*. Spicy foods often have been blamed for ulcers, but this link has not been proven. With gastric ulcers, gastric acid production is usually normal or decreased. However, an increase in gastric acid is common with duodenal ulcers.

Clinical Manifestations

Gastric ulcers typically produce burning pain in the epigastric area 1 to 2 hours after meals. Nausea, anorexia, and weight loss are sometimes present. Some patients have no pain at all until serious complications develop. Although some patients with duodenal ulcers have no pain, others experience a burning or cramping pain 2 to 4 hours after meals. The pain is located in the area just beneath the xiphoid process. It is often relieved by antacids or food. The patient commonly reports pain that lasts for several weeks or months, disappears, and then returns.

> **Pharmacology Capsule**
>
> Antacids such as Maalox, Pepto-Bismol, and TUMS are drugs and can have adverse effects if taken in excess.

Complications

Peptic ulcers can lead to serious, even life-threatening complications. *Intractability* is the term used to describe symptomatic peptic ulcer disease that does not respond to treatment. Hemorrhage is more common in older adults and in people with gastric ulcers. If the hemorrhage is not brought under control, the patient can bleed to death.

A perforation is a break in the wall of the stomach or the duodenum that permits digestive fluids to leak into the peritoneal cavity, causing inflammation of the peritoneum (**peritonitis**).

The pylorus is the opening between the stomach and the duodenum. With peptic ulcer disease, pyloric obstruction may develop as a result of edema and scarring. Pyloric obstruction causes persistent vomiting that can lead to severe fluid and electrolyte imbalances.

Medical Diagnosis

Tests and procedures used to detect peptic ulcers include barium swallow examination and endoscopy. These studies, including patient preparation and aftercare, are described in Chapter 37, Table 37.1. Several laboratory tests are available to detect *H. pylori* in a specimen obtained from a biopsy of the gastric mucosa. *H. pylori* can also be detected by antibodies in the blood or stool and by a breath test.

Medical Treatment

The goals in treating peptic ulcers are to relieve symptoms, promote healing, prevent or detect complications, and prevent recurrence. Interventions include drug therapy, diet, and stress management.

Drug therapy. Drug therapy is intended to relieve symptoms, heal the ulcer, cure *H. pylori* infections,

Table 38.2 Comparison of Gastric and Duodenal Ulcers

CHARACTERISTIC	GASTRIC ULCER	DUODENAL ULCER
Incidence	More common in older men, working class, those with type A blood, substance abusers, and people under severe stress	More common in younger men, all social classes, those with type O blood, people with chronic illnesses
Ulcer depth	Shallow	Deep
Gastric secretions	Unchanged or decreased	Increased
Signs and symptoms	Burning and pressure in upper left abdomen below rib cage and in back; pain 1 to 2 hours after meals; relieved by food or fluids	Burning and pressure in upper middle abdomen and back; pain 2 to 4 hours after meals; relieved by antacids or foods
Complications	Hemorrhage, perforation, obstruction	Hemorrhage, perforation, obstruction

Table 38.3 Complications of Peptic Ulcer Disease

COMPLICATION	SIGNS AND SYMPTOMS	TREATMENT	NURSING CARE
Hemorrhage	Thready pulse, restlessness, diaphoresis, chills, oliguria, hematemesis, tarry stools, hypotension	Saline lavage, vasopressin, arterial embolization	Assist with procedure; monitor effects of treatment; monitor for water intoxication: headache, coma, tremor, sweating, anxiety; monitor vital signs, intake and output; maintain patent NG tube; give IV fluids as ordered
Perforation	Sudden, sharp mid-epigastric pain that spreads over entire abdomen; rigid abdomen; absence of bowel sounds; shock	NG suction, IV fluids, antibiotics, surgical repair	Monitor vital signs, intake and output; enforce NPO order; give fluids and blood as ordered; keep NG tube patent
Obstruction	Feeling of fullness, nausea after eating, persistent vomiting	NG suction	Monitor vital signs, intake and output; keep NG tube patent

IV, Intravenous; *NG*, nasogastric; *NPO*, nothing by mouth.

and prevent recurrence. Antisecretory drugs decrease gastric acid secretion, which relieves symptoms and allows the ulcer to begin healing. Proton pump inhibitors, H2-receptor blockers, and prostaglandins are examples of antisecretory drugs. Proton pump inhibitors are the most commonly used initial drugs. Examples are omeprazole (Prilosec), esomeprazole (Nexium), and lansoprazole (Prevacid). H2-receptor blockers include cimetidine (Tagamet), famotidine (Pepcid), and nizatidine (Axid). If *H. pylori* infection is confirmed, it is treated with various combinations of drugs such as clarithromycin, amoxicillin, bismuth, metronidazole, and tetracycline. Multiple antibiotics are needed to prevent the development of resistant strains.

Antacids are not used to treat peptic ulcer disease but may be used to relieve occasional heartburn. If used, they are typically given 1 and 3 hours after meals and at bedtime. Because antacids are available without a prescription, patients may think they can do no harm. In fact, they can have serious side effects. They also impair the absorption of many other drugs if taken at the same time. The patient should be cautioned to take the exact amount prescribed and not to adjust dosage on their own.

Some other drugs may be prescribed to treat ulcers. Metoclopramide (Reglan) is a prokinetic agent that causes the stomach to empty more quickly, removing food and drugs that stimulate acid production. Sucralfate (Carafate) is a mucosal barrier. It clings to the surface of the ulcer and protects it so that healing can take place. It is used less often now than in the past.

In some cases, antisecretory therapy may be continued as a preventive measure after the ulcer has healed. The proton pump inhibitor omeprazole (Prilosec) may be used to prevent ulcers in patients who take NSAIDs.

Diet therapy. No evidence exists to support dietary restrictions for ulcer patients. The current approach is to permit the patient almost any foods that do not produce discomfort. Frequent small feedings throughout the day may be recommended. The ulcer patient should be advised not to skip meals.

Managing complications. Complications may be treated medically or surgically. If hemorrhage is suspected, a nasogastric tube is inserted and attached to suction to remove and measure blood in the stomach.

Perforation is treated initially with gastric decompression and intravenous fluids and antibiotics. A small perforation may close spontaneously. Otherwise, surgical repair is needed.

Complications of peptic ulcer disease, signs and symptoms, related treatments, and nursing care are summarized in Table 38.3.

Surgical intervention is indicated to reduce acid secretion or for treatment of complications that do not respond to conservative treatment. Procedures that decrease acid secretion include vagotomy, pyloroplasty, gastroenterostomy, antrectomy, and subtotal gastrectomy. In extreme cases, total gastrectomy is necessary. Some of these procedures are described in Table 38.4.

◆ NURSING CARE OF THE PATIENT WITH PEPTIC ULCER

Nursing care of the patient with peptic ulcer disease can be quite complicated, depending on the severity of the condition and the medical or surgical treatment. Therefore, nursing care of the medical patient and the surgical patient are discussed separately (see Nursing Care Plan: Patient With a Peptic Ulcer).

◆ NURSING CARE OF THE PATIENT WITH PEPTIC ULCER DISEASE MANAGED MEDICALLY

Focused Assessment

Complete assessment of the patient with a disorder of the digestive tract is summarized in Chapter 37, Box 37.1. When the patient has peptic ulcer disease, focus on pain (location, severity, duration, precipitating factors, relieving factors, self-treatment, recent stressors). Ask about nausea and vomiting and whether blood

Table 38.4 Surgical Treatment of Peptic Ulcer Disease

OPERATION	PROCEDURE	PURPOSE	ADVERSE EFFECTS
Truncal vagotomy	Vagus nerve that supplies the stomach is severed.	Decreases stimulation of gastric acid secretion.	Patient may experience delayed gastric emptying. Patient also may have a feeling of fullness, dumping syndrome, and diarrhea.
Selective or super-selective vagotomy	Severs the part of the vagus nerve that stimulates acid production. Spares the nerve supply to the pyloric sphincter.	Decreases stimulation of gastric acid secretion.	Patient may experience delayed gastric emptying.
Pyloroplasty	Widens the pylorus.	Improves the passage of stomach contents into the duodenum. Procedure is usually done with a vagotomy to prevent gastric stasis.	Patient may experience dumping syndrome because of the rapid emptying of the stomach into the duodenum.
Simple gastroenterostomy	Creates a passage between the body of the stomach and the jejunum.	Permits passage of alkaline intestinal secretions into the stomach to neutralize gastric acid.	Patient may experience increased gastric acid secretion.
Antrectomy	Removal of the antrum of the stomach.	Reduces gastric acid by removing the source of acid secretion.	Patient may experience diarrhea, a feeling of fullness after eating, dumping syndrome, malabsorption, and anemia.
Subtotal Gastrectomy			
Gastroduodenoscopy (Billroth I)	Part of the distal portion of the stomach, including the antrum, is removed. Remaining stomach is anastomosed to the duodenum.	Reduces acid by removing the source of acid secretion.	Patient may experience dumping syndrome (less often than with other procedures), anemia, malabsorption, weight loss, and bile reflux.
Gastrojejunostomy (Billroth II)	Part of the distal portion of the stomach, including the antrum, is removed. Remaining stomach is anastomosed to the jejunum.	Removes the source of acid secretion.	Patient may experience dumping syndrome, weight loss, malabsorption, duodenal infection, pernicious anemia, and afferent loop syndrome (obstruction of the duodenal loop).
Total gastrectomy	Removal of the entire stomach. Esophagus anastomosed to the duodenum.	Removes the source of gastric acid secretion.	Patient can consume only small, frequent meals of semisolid foods. Patient may experience pernicious anemia and dumping syndrome.

has been noted in the emesis or stools. Describe pain location, onset, and severity.

Patient Problems, Goals, and Outcome Criteria: Peptic Ulcer Disease

Patient Problems	Goals and Outcome Criteria
Acute pain related to ulceration of stomach or duodenum	Pain relief: patient states pain is reduced or relieved, relaxed manner
Inadequate nutrition related to nausea, vomiting, anorexia, nothing by mouth (NPO) status	Adequate nutrition: stable body weight
Potential for injury related to hemorrhage, perforation, obstruction	Absence of complications: vital signs within patient norms; no vomiting, hematemesis, or tarry stools

Nursing Care Plan Patient With a Peptic Ulcer

FOCUSED ASSESSMENT

Health History

A 47-year-old clinic patient has recently been diagnosed as having duodenal ulcers. He has a history of burning pain 2 to 3 hours after meals. The pain is located in the upper middle abdomen and back and is relieved by antacid agents. Symptoms are sometimes accompanied by nausea but not vomiting. He noticed that his stools have been darker than usual this week. He describes his health as good but is being treated for hypertension.

He states that he rarely drinks alcoholic beverages but smokes 1½ packs of cigarettes daily. He is a truck driver who usually eats only two meals each day, at irregular hours.

Physical Examination Blood pressure, 136/82 mm Hg; pulse, 76 beats per minute; respiration, 16 breaths per minute; temperature, 97.6°F (36.4°C) measured orally. Height, 5′10″; weight, 210 lb. Alert and oriented. Abdomen soft. Bowel sounds present in all four quadrants.

Patient Problem	Goals and Outcome Criteria	Interventions
Acute pain related to ulceration of gastric mucosa	Patient will verbalize pain relief and appear relaxed.	Teach patient about ordered drugs that reduce symptoms by decreasing acid secretion, neutralizing acid, or coating ulcer surfaces. Explore stressors and activities that patient finds restful. Explain the importance of rest and teach relaxation techniques.
Inadequate nutrition related to nausea, vomiting, anorexia, self-imposed dietary restrictions	Patient will maintain adequate nutrition, as evidenced by stable body weight.	Inform patient that he can consume any foods that do not cause discomfort. He may find that small, frequent meals are tolerated better than 2 to 3 large meals. If antiemetic agents for nausea and vomiting are ordered, explain how they should be taken. Monitor the patient's weight at each visit. Consult a dietitian if the patient is losing weight.
Potential for injury related to hemorrhage, perforation, and obstruction	Patient will remain free of complications, as evidenced by normal vital signs and no vomiting, hematemesis, or tarry stools.	Advise the patient to immediately notify the physician of bright red blood in stools; maroon, tarry stools; bloody emesis; or sudden, severe pain.
Inadequate coping related to prescribed alterations in lifestyle	Patient will express intent to implement lifestyle alterations.	Identify behaviors that aggravate peptic ulcer disease. Explain the benefits of altering those behaviors on the disease. Offer information about resources that provide services to help patients give up tobacco.
Inability to manage self-care related to lack of knowledge	Patient will correctly describe self-care measures to promote healing of duodenal ulcers and prevent recurrence.	Advise the patient to avoid alcohol and tobacco because they stimulate the release of gastrin. Stress the importance of taking drugs as prescribed. Explain the side effects and adverse effects and their management. Inform him that NSAIDs should be avoided. Supplement verbal instruction with written information. Encourage follow-up care.

CRITICAL THINKING QUESTIONS

1. What signs and symptoms would alert you to possible hemorrhage?
2. How would you explain to the patient the need to avoid alcohol and tobacco?
3. How might the patient's occupation make it difficult for him to adhere to the plan of care?

Patient Problems, Goals, and Outcome Criteria: Peptic Ulcer Disease—cont'd

Patient Problems	Goals and Outcome Criteria
Inadequate coping related to prescribed alterations in lifestyle	Effective coping: adjustment to prescribed changes in lifestyle, adherence to treatment regimen

Interventions

Acute pain. The most important means of reducing pain associated with peptic ulcer disease are drug therapy, rest, and diet. Drugs reduce pain by neutralizing acid, decreasing acid secretion, or coating the ulcer surface. The environment should be as restful as possible. Encourage relaxation techniques and stress management strategies as described in Chapter 8.

Inadequate nutrition. The patient is advised to avoid any foods that have caused gastric distress in the past.

When nausea and vomiting are present, oral fluids may be restricted to clear liquids or the patient may be placed on NPO status. Administer antiemetics as ordered.

Potential for injury. Monitor the patient for signs and symptoms of complications. Signs of bleeding are hematemesis (vomiting blood) and the presence of blood in the feces. Blood that has passed through the digestive tract is maroon to black and causes the stool to have a sticky or tarry quality. Stools and vomited fluid may be tested for occult blood. When blood loss is significant, the patient may go into shock. Early signs of shock are weakness, tachycardia, and pallor. Hypotension is a relatively late sign.

If hemorrhage occurs, it is vital to notify the RN or health care provider immediately while continuing to monitor the patient's vital signs. Anticipate insertion of a nasogastric tube and saline lavage. Keep the patient quiet and give the patient nothing to eat or drink (NPO status). Maintain intravenous lines and record fluid intake and output. The patient may have to be prepared for transfer to intensive care or surgery.

Perforation is characterized by sudden, sharp pain starting in the mid-epigastric region and spreading across the entire abdomen. Digestive fluids in the abdomen cause peritonitis (inflammation of the peritoneum). With peritonitis, the abdomen is rigid and tender. The patient tends to draw the knees up toward the chest. When perforation is suspected, nursing care is much like that provided for hemorrhage.

Inadequate coping. Explore what the patient thinks about prescribed treatments and how they will affect their lifestyle (see the Patient Teaching box). Resources are available to help patients who have difficulty giving up alcohol or tobacco.

Patient Teaching

Peptic Ulcer

- It is important to know the name, dosage, schedule, and adverse effects of each drug taken.
- Avoid nonsteroidal antiinflammatory drugs (NSAIDs), including aspirin, alcohol, and smoking because they aggravate peptic ulcer disease.
- The only dietary restrictions are to avoid foods that cause discomfort.
- Follow-up care is important to ensure that the ulcer is healing or has not recurred.
- Resources for stress management techniques and alcohol abuse (if appropriate) are available.

◆ NURSING CARE OF THE PATIENT WITH PEPTIC ULCER MANAGED SURGICALLY

Preoperative nursing care is like the care outlined in Chapter 17 for any patient having major surgery. This section emphasizes the special postoperative needs of the patient who has undergone gastric surgery for peptic ulcer disease.

Focused Assessment

Postoperatively, the patient should be assessed for pain, nausea, and vomiting. Measure vital signs at frequent intervals until the patient is stable. In addition, document the amount and type of intravenous fluids. If a nasogastric tube is present, document patency of the tube as well as the color and amount of drainage. Inspect the skin around the nostril where the tube is located for irritation, auscultate breath sounds, and inspect the wound dressing for bleeding. Once the dressing is removed, examine the incision for increased redness, swelling, drainage, and incomplete closure. Describe any drainage from the wound or from drains. Inspect the abdomen for distention and auscultate for bowel sounds. Finally, monitor urine output and palpate for bladder distention.

Patient Problems, Goals, and Outcome Criteria: Gastric Surgery

Patient Problems	Goals and Outcome Criteria
Potential for injury related to gastric dilation, obstruction, perforation	Absence of complications: vital signs within patient norms, minimal vomiting
Inadequate nutrition related to decreased capacity for intake of nutrients	Adequate nutrition: maintains or attains ideal body weight
Decreased cardiac output related to hypovolemia secondary to dumping syndrome	Normal cardiac output: no decrease in blood pressure after meals

Interventions

Potential for injury. Potential complications of gastric surgery include gastric dilation, obstruction, and perforation. Gastric dilation results from accumulation of fluid in the stomach. Tachycardia, hypotension, and hiccups may develop. Obstruction can result from edema at the surgical site, causing pain and vomiting.

A nasogastric tube is usually inserted preoperatively and remains in place after surgery. Specific orders for suction will be written. It is very important to maintain suction and drainage as ordered.

After gastric surgery, do not irrigate or reposition the tube. Doing so may cause the suture line in the stomach to tear. Nasogastric drainage is usually bright red immediately after surgery. The color darkens over the first 24 hours and then turns yellow or green. The tube is removed when peristalsis returns, usually on the third to fifth postoperative day. Document the presence of bowel sounds and the passage of flatus through the rectum.

Inadequate nutrition. After the tube is removed, the diet is gradually advanced from water or ice chips to clear liquids, full liquids, and then solid foods. Special dietary needs depend on the type of surgery (see the Patient Teaching box).

Patient Teaching

Peptic Ulcer, Postoperative

- Know the name, dosage, schedule, and adverse effects of each medication taken.
- After subtotal gastrectomy, eat small, frequent meals until stomach capacity expands. After total gastrectomy, the need to eat small, frequent meals probably will be a requirement for life.
- Promptly inform the physician if nausea, vomiting, abdominal pain, or dark, tarry stools are present.
- Reduce the risk of recurrence by avoiding alcohol, aspirin, and nonsteroidal antiinflammatory drugs (NSAIDs).
- If stressed, try stress management techniques such as relaxation exercises or seek personal counseling.

Gastric surgery can have serious effects on the patient's nutritional status. The absorption of vitamin B_{12}, folic acid, iron, calcium, and vitamin D may be impaired, so supplements will be needed. Without vitamin B_{12}, the patient develops pernicious anemia. Pernicious anemia is more common after a total gastrectomy but can follow a subtotal gastrectomy. As discussed earlier, the parietal cells in the stomach produce intrinsic factor, a substance that is needed to absorb vitamin B_{12}. Vitamin B_{12} is essential for the production of RBCs. When all or part of the stomach is removed, the patient develops a vitamin B_{12} deficiency and, eventually, severe anemia. The condition is easily treated with vitamin B_{12}.

Decreased cardiac output. Some patients experience dumping syndrome after gastric surgery. The symptoms of dumping syndrome may occur in stages. In the first stage, the patient experiences abdominal fullness and nausea within 10 to 20 minutes of eating. These symptoms are thought to be caused by distention of the small intestine by the consumed food and fluids and the shift of a modest amount of fluid from the circulation into the intestines. The patient feels flushed and faint, the heart rate races, and the patient breaks into a sweat as a result of pooling of blood in the abdominal organs. In the intermediate stage, the patient has abdominal bloating, flatulence, cramps, and diarrhea that occur 20 to 60 minutes after eating. These symptoms are probably related to the malabsorption of carbohydrates and other foodstuffs because of a deficiency of digestive enzymes. One to 3 hours later, the late stage may occur. The patient may perspire, feel weak, anxious, shaky, or hungry. These symptoms are blamed on hypoglycemia caused by an exaggerated rise in insulin secretion in response to the rapid delivery of carbohydrates into the intestine.

Dumping syndrome usually disappears within a few months. Meanwhile, the following directions for the patient will help:

1. Consume a diet low in carbohydrates and refined sugar, moderate in fat, and moderate to high in protein.
2. Smaller, more frequent meals may be better tolerated than three large meals.
3. Drink fluids between meals, not with them.
4. Lie down for about 30 minutes after meals.

STOMACH CANCER

Pathophysiology

Cancer of the stomach is expected to be diagnosed in more than 26,000 people in the United States in 2021. The incidence is highest among men, people older than 70 years of age, Asians and Pacific Islanders, Black Americans, Native Americans, and Latinos. (see the Cultural Considerations box).

Stomach carcinoma begins in the mucous membranes, invades the gastric wall, and spreads to the regional lymphatics, liver, pancreas, and colon. Distant metastases are found in the lungs and bones. Unfortunately, no specific signs or symptoms are seen in the early stages. Late signs and symptoms are vomiting, ascites, liver enlargement, and an abdominal mass. By the time late signs appear, the cancer is advanced and the patient's chance of 5-year survival is poor.

Cultural Considerations

What Does Culture Have to Do With Stomach Cancer?

The incidence of stomach cancer is greater in non-White persons than in White persons. In addition, culturally based dietary patterns (high intake of starch, salt, pickled foods, salted meats, and nitrates) increase the risk of stomach cancer.

Risk Factors

No specific cause of gastric cancer is known; however, various factors are known to increase a person's risk for this cancer. Risk factors include *H. pylori* infection, pernicious anemia, chronic atrophic gastritis, achlorhydria (lack of hydrochloric acid), type A blood, and a family history of stomach cancer. Some personal habits that seem to be related to stomach cancer are tobacco use, alcohol consumption, and a diet high in starch, salt, pickled foods, salted meats, and nitrates. Patients who have had the Billroth II procedure (gastrojejunostomy) also have increased incidence of stomach cancer (see the Health Promotion box).

Medical Diagnosis

Endoscopy is used to examine the interior of the stomach and to take specimens for microscopic study. Other procedures that might be used to establish the diagnosis and extent of the cancer are endoscopic ultrasound, upper gastrointestinal (GI) series, CT scan, bone scan, positron emission tomography (PET) scan, magnetic resonance imaging (MRI), and laparoscopy. Laboratory studies may include Hgb and Hct, serum albumin, liver function tests, and carcinoembryonic antigen (CEA). Stool specimens may be tested for occult blood.

Health Promotion

Breaking The Link Between Diet And Digestive Tract Cancers

- People who have a poor diet, do not have enough physical activity, or are overweight may be at increased risk of several types of cancer. Overweight and obese individuals are twice as likely as people of healthy weight to develop a type of esophageal cancer called esophageal adenocarcinoma. A smaller increase in risk has been found for a specific type of stomach cancer that begins in the area of the stomach next to the esophagus.
- Having a healthy diet, being physically active, and maintaining a healthy weight may help to reduce cancer risk. The National Institutes of Health (NIH) recommends the following:
- Eat well: A healthy diet includes plenty of foods that are high in fiber, vitamins, and minerals. This includes whole-grain breads and cereals and five to nine servings of fruits and vegetables every day. In addition, it is important to limit foods high in fat (e.g., butter, whole milk, fried foods, red meat).
- Be active and maintain a healthy weight: Physical activity can help to control weight and reduce body fat. Most scientists agree that it is a good idea for an adult to engage in moderate physical activity (e.g., brisk walking) for at least 30 minutes on 5 or more days each week.

Data from National Cancer Institute: Cancer Trends Progress Report. https://progressreport.cancer.gov/.

Medical Treatment

Stomach cancer may be treated with surgery, chemotherapy, radiation therapy, or various combinations of two or three of these. If the cancer is detected early, surgical options include subtotal gastrectomy with lymph node dissection and total gastrectomy. Sometimes part of the esophagus or duodenum is resected. In more advanced cancer, the surgeon may remove as much of the tumor as possible to relieve or prevent obstruction without removing the entire stomach. In some cases, chemotherapy is given before and after surgery. Gene therapy and immune-based therapy are in early phases of study and may prove useful someday.

◆ POSTOPERATIVE NURSING CARE OF THE PATIENT WITH STOMACH CANCER

General preoperative and postoperative nursing care is discussed in Chapter 17. Chapter 7 discusses general care of the patient who has cancer. The special needs of patients having surgery for gastric cancer are discussed here.

Focused Assessment

Data related to comfort, appetite, and nausea and vomiting are especially important after surgery for stomach cancer. Monitor the patient for weight changes and determine dietary preferences. Identify the patient's support system and coping strategies.

Patient Problems, Goals, and Outcome Criteria: Stomach Cancer: Postoperative Care

Patient Problems	Goals and Outcome Criteria
Acute pain related to tumor, surgical trauma, or both	Pain relief: patient states less or no pain, relaxed manner
Inadequate nutrition related to anorexia, pain, nausea and vomiting	Adequate nutrition: maintains or attains ideal body weight
Inadequate coping related to diagnosis of cancer, poor prognosis	Effective coping: patient verbalizes concerns, seeks and uses resources as needed, makes realistic plans

Interventions

Acute pain. Administer analgesics as ordered in addition to using nonpharmacologic measures to manage pain. Massage, relaxation techniques, and mental imagery are examples of complementary measures to help manage pain.

Inadequate nutrition. Nutritional needs are much like those of the patient who has undergone surgery for peptic ulcer disease.

Inadequate coping. The patient and family may need help in coping with this life-threatening illness. Encourage them to talk and to be accepting of the thoughts and feelings the patient expresses. Help the patient to think about changes in daily routines that may be necessary after discharge (see the Patient Teaching box). If chemotherapy or radiation therapy is planned, the patient needs to know what to expect. Provide the patient with information about community resources such as home health agencies or the American Cancer Society (www.cancer.org).

Patient Teaching

Stomach Cancer: Postoperative Care

- Know the name, dosage, schedule, and adverse effects of each medication.
- Eat six small meals a day and drink fluids between meals rather than with meals.
- Notify the health care provider if the wound shows increasing redness, swelling, pain, or drainage.

If the patient is scheduled for chemotherapy or radiation therapy, explain what the patient can expect.

Get Ready for the NCLEX® Examination!

Key Points

- Any disorder of the digestive tract can cause nutritional deficiencies by disrupting one or more of its three functions: (1) digestion, (2) absorption, and (3) elimination.
- Anorexia, or lack of appetite, may be caused by illness, drugs, or emotional factors.
- Oral inflammations and infections can be caused by irritants, bacteria, viruses, and fungi and can interfere with food intake and enjoyment.
- Cancers inside the oral cavity are usually squamous cell carcinomas related to poor nutrition, chronic irritation, or combined tobacco and alcohol use.
- Cancers of the lip are usually basal cell carcinomas attributed to prolonged exposure to irritants, including sun, wind, and pipe smoking.
- Nursing care of patients being treated for oral cancers focuses on impaired oral tissue integrity, inadequate oxygenation, acute pain, impaired verbal communication, inadequate nutrition, altered body image, potential for infection, and inadequate peripheral tissue perfusion.
- Cancer of the esophagus may be treated with surgery, radiotherapy, chemotherapy, or a combination of these or by palliative measures to maintain a patent esophagus.
- Vomiting, which can result in fluid and electrolyte imbalances, aspiration, and nutritional deficiencies, is treated with antiemetics, fluid and electrolyte replacement, and sometimes GI decompression.
- Treatment of hiatal hernia, the protrusion of the lower esophagus and stomach upward through the diaphragm, may include drug therapy, diet, measures to avoid increased intraabdominal pressure, or surgery.
- Gastritis is inflammation of the stomach lining usually caused by *H. pylori* and aggravated by alcohol, caffeine, and other irritants.
- Peptic ulcer is loss of tissue from the lining of the stomach or duodenum that can lead to hemorrhage, perforation, and obstruction.
- Nursing care of patients with peptic ulcer focuses on acute pain; inadequate nutrition, potential for injury, and inadequate coping.
- Dumping syndrome may occur after gastric surgery, causing weakness, dizziness, diaphoresis, and palpitations.
- Measures to control dumping syndrome include small, frequent meals; reduced intake of carbohydrates and refined sugars; avoiding fluids with meals; and reclining for 30 minutes after meals.
- Nursing care of the patient with stomach cancer, which is often advanced when diagnosed, focuses on acute pain, inadequate nutrition, and inadequate coping.

Additional Learning Resources

SG Go to your Study Guide for additional learning activities to help you master this chapter content.

Go to your Evolve website (http://evolve.elsevier.com/Linton/medsurg) for the following learning resources and much more:

- Fluid & Electrolyte Tutorial
- Review Questions for the NCLEX® Examination

Clinical Judgment and Next-Generation NCLEX® Examination-Style Questions

1. **SLO/Objective: Assist in developing nursing care plans for patients with disorders of the upper digestive tract.**

   NGN Item Type: Matrix

   Cognitive Skill: Generate Solutions

   The nurse is reviewing the admission papers for a new resident of a long-term care facility. The patient was admitted after falling several times in her home. She has diagnoses of mild dementia, achalasia, and type 2 diabetes mellitus.

   Use an X for the nursing actions listed below that are *Indicated* (appropriate or necessary), *Contraindicated* (could be harmful), or *Nonessential* (makes no difference or not necessary) for the patient's care at this time.

NURSING ACTION	INDICATED	CONTRAINDICATED	NONESSENTIAL
Elevate head of bed 30 degrees for meals			
Assess breath sounds daily			
Help patient to select loose clothing			
Maintain intake and output record			
Monitor weight daily			
Assign a CNA to feed patient			
Encourage a nap after noon meal			

   NCLEX Client Need: Physiological Integrity: Reduction of Risk Potential

2. **Which of the following types of antiulcer drugs work by inhibiting the secretion of gastric acid? (Select all that apply.)**
   1. Antacids
   2. H2-receptor blockers
   3. Mucosal barriers
   4. Proton pump inhibitors
   5. Synthetic prostaglandins

   NCLEX Client Need: Physiological Integrity: Pharmacological Therapies

3. **The nurse has been assigned to care for a patient who was recently diagnosed with a hiatal hernia. The patient is experiencing chronic heartburn when eating a meal. The nurse would teach the patient to avoid which of the following situations?**
   1. Lying flat after eating a meal
   2. Ingesting small, frequent meals
   3. Raising the head of the bed on 6- to 8-inch blocks
   4. Taking acetaminophen for minor pain.

   NCLEX Client Need: Physiological Integrity: Basic Care and Comfort

4. **The nurse is providing instructions to a patient who recently had a gastrectomy. The focus is on prevention of dumping syndrome. Which instruction would the nurse include?**
   1. Take a vigorous walk after eating
   2. Eat high-carbohydrate meals
   3. Limit fluids taken with meals
   4. Have an alcoholic beverage with meals

   NCLEX Client Need: Physiological Integrity: Basic Care and Comfort

5. **A patient with a diagnosis of chronic gastritis is at risk for which vitamin deficiency?**
   1. Vitamin A
   2. Vitamin B_{12}
   3. Vitamin C
   4. Vitamin E

   NCLEX Client Need: Physiological Integrity: Reduction of Risk Potential

6. **SLO/Objective:** Apply knowledge of anatomy and physiology and pathophysiology to determine which assessment data require follow-up by the nurse.

   NGN Item Type: Enhanced Hot Spot

   Cognitive Skill: Recognize Cues

   The home health nurse visits a 90-year-old male patient one week after discharge following a prostatectomy for benign hypertrophy. He has a history of hypertension, osteoarthritis, and chronic gastritis. The nurse's focused assessment provides the following data:

   - Oral temperature 97°F
   - Heart rate 96 beats per minute, slightly irregular
   - Respirations 20 breaths per minute
   - BP 130/66 mm Hg
   - Breath sounds clear
   - Skin and mucous membranes pale
   - Tires easily
   - Voiding without difficulty
   - Urine clear

   Highlight or place a check mark next to the assessment findings that require follow up by the nurse.

   NCLEX Client Need: Physiological Integrity: Basic Care and Comfort

Lower Digestive Tract Disorders

39

http://evolve.elsevier.com/Linton/medsurg

Objectives

1. Describe the surgical options for the bariatric surgery patient.
2. Assist in developing a plan of nursing care for the bariatric surgery patient.
3. Describe the pathophysiology, signs and symptoms, complications, and treatment of selected lower digestive tract disorders.
4. Assist in developing nursing care plans for patients who are receiving treatment for lower digestive tract disorders.

Key Terms

flatus (FLĀ-tŭs)
helminths (HĔL-mĭnthz)
steatorrhea (stē-ĂT-ō-rē-ă)
volvulus (VŌL-vyū-lŭs)

Lower digestive tract disorders are those that affect the colon, rectum, and anus.

OBESITY

The term *obesity* is used when a person's body mass index (BMI) is 30 kg/m^2 or more. Obesity is introduced in Chapter 15 where the causes, complications, and medical treatment of obesity were discussed in the context of nutrition. The term *bariatric* refers to the medical specialty that treats for obesity. This chapter will address surgical options because the nursing care is similar to patients with other digestive tract surgery and because the treatments affect the ingestion and absorption of food.

SURGICAL INTERVENTION FOR OBESITY

When extreme obesity (sometimes called *morbid obesity*) persists over a period of years despite conservative treatment, bariatric surgical intervention may be recommended. Bariatric surgical procedures are either malabsorptive or restrictive. Malabsorptive procedures bypass a portion of the small intestine, which reduces food absorption. Restrictive surgery reduces the size of the stomach so that the patient feels full after eating only a small amount of food and takes in fewer calories. These procedures include Roux-en-Y gastric bypass (RNYGBP), sleeve gastrectomy (also called *sleeve gastroplasty*), duodenal switch with biliopancreatic diversion, and laparoscopic adjustable gastric banding (Fig. 39.1).

RNYGBP is a common type of bariatric surgery. A small pouch that allows very small amounts of food and fluid to enter is created at the top of the stomach. The small intestine is then diverted from the main stomach below and connected to the pouch. Remember that the main part of the stomach remains and continues to make digestive juices. The portion of small intestine still attached to the main stomach is then reattached farther down to allow the digestive juices to flow into the small intestines.

Sleeve gastrectomy does not affect the absorption of calories and nutrients in the same way as RNYGBP. Part of the stomach is removed. The smaller stomach cannot hold as much food, which lessens the production of the hormone called *ghrelin*. Less ghrelin may lessen the desire to eat, which in turn helps to decrease food intake.

Duodenal switch with biliopancreatic diversion, like sleeve gastrectomy, entails removal of a large part of the stomach. The distal end of the duodenum is attached to the large intestine so that food bypasses most of the small intestine, thereby reducing the absorption of calories and nutrients. The separated part of the small intestine is reattached to the duodenum to deliver bile and pancreatic digestive juices.

Lastly, laparoscopic adjustable gastric banding involves a band housing an inflatable balloon that is placed around the upper part of the stomach and is then held in place. This position creates a small stomach-like pouch above the band with a narrow opening into the rest of the stomach. The balloon can be deflated or inflated using a port placed under the skin of the abdomen. This procedure restricts the amount of food consumed but does not affect absorption.

VAGAL NERVE BLOCKING THERAPY

An alternative to the surgical procedures just described is the vBLOC Maestro System. This system consists of electrodes that are implanted via laparoscopy above the junction of the esophagus and stomach. A regulator is implanted just underneath the skin. It can be turned on/off, recharged, programmed by an external device.

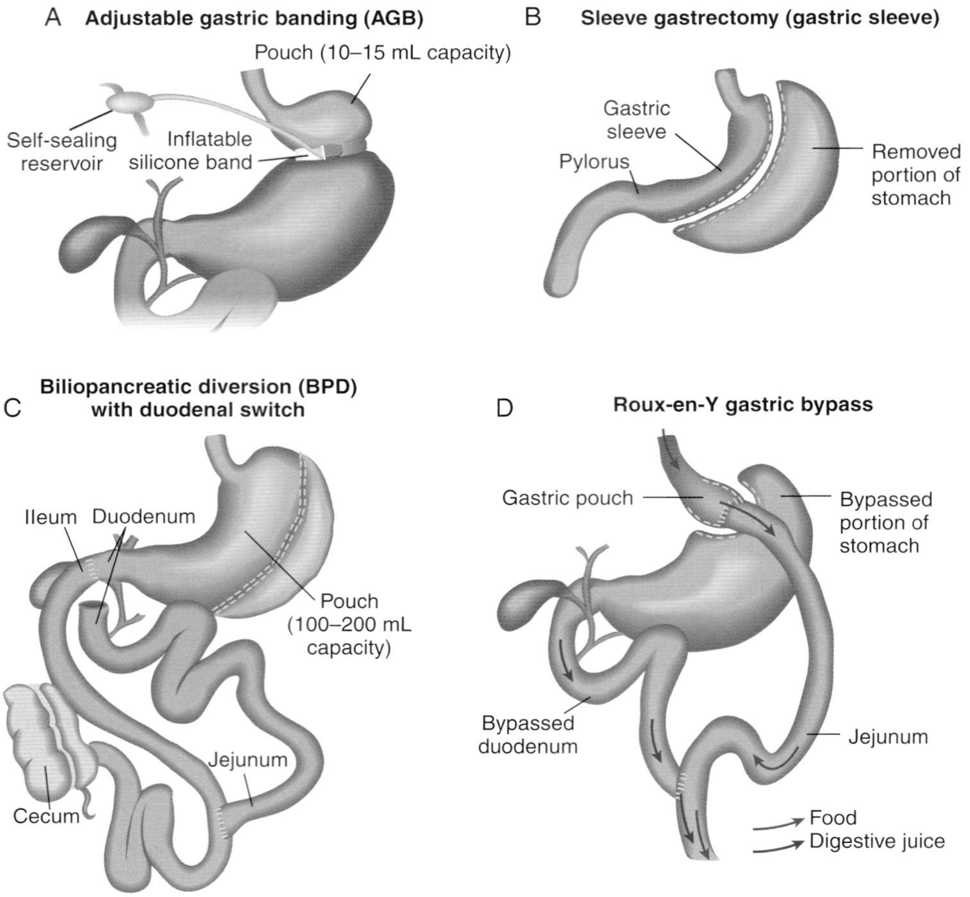

Fig. 39.1 Bariatric surgical procedures: (A) adjustable gastric banding (*AGB*) uses a band to create a gastric pouch. (B) Sleeve gastrectomy involves creating a sleeve-shaped stomach by removing about 75% of the stomach. (C) Biliopancreatic diversion (*BPD*) with duodenal switch procedure creates an anastomosis between the stomach and intestine. (D) Roux-en-Y gastric bypass procedure involves constructing a gastric pouch whose outlet is a Y-shaped limb of small intestine. (From Lewis SL, Bucher L, Heitkemper MM, Harding MM, editors: *Medical surgical nursing: assessment and management of clinical problems*, ed 10, St. Louis, 2017, Elsevier.)

The electrode blocks signals from the vagal nerve which is responsible for informing the brain when the stomach feels empty or full. By blocking feelings of hunger, the patient is assumed to eat less and therefore lose weight (Fig. 39.2). Caution should be taken with use of the vBLOC Maestro System with patients diagnosed with cirrhosis of the liver, dilated veins in the esophagus, hiatal hernia, and patients experiencing increased pressure in hepatic veins.

◆ NURSING CARE OF THE OBESE SURGICAL PATIENT

Focused Assessment

By the time a patient is approved for weight loss surgery, the assessment focuses on the current state of health and factors that might be relevant to surgical success over the long term. Ask about the patient's expectations for the surgery as well as any fears and concerns they may have. Document pertinent chronic illnesses such as cardiac, respiratory, and orthopedic problems, and diabetes mellitus. Ask about a typical day and whether the patient is able to manage self-care, home management, and family needs independently. Inquire about interpersonal relationships, stresses, coping strategies, and sources of support.

Some aspects of the physical examination are more difficult when the patient is obese. For example, it may be difficult to auscultate heart, lung, and bowel sounds. Having the patient lean forward or lie on the left side may make it easier to hear heart sounds. Accurate measurement of blood pressure requires a large cuff. Scales must accommodate heavier patients. Also specialized beds may need to be used to accommodate the obese patient who is admitted for inpatient care.

When collecting these data, it is essential to convey an attitude of respect and concern. Be aware of your personal feelings about obesity and consider how these feelings affect the nurse-patient relationship.

Acknowledge and compliment good grooming and attention to appearance and attributes other than physical size.

INTERVENTIONS AFTER BARIATRIC SURGERY

After bariatric surgery, patients need the same care as any postoperative patient, as discussed in Chapter 17. However, the needs of the obese surgical patient that

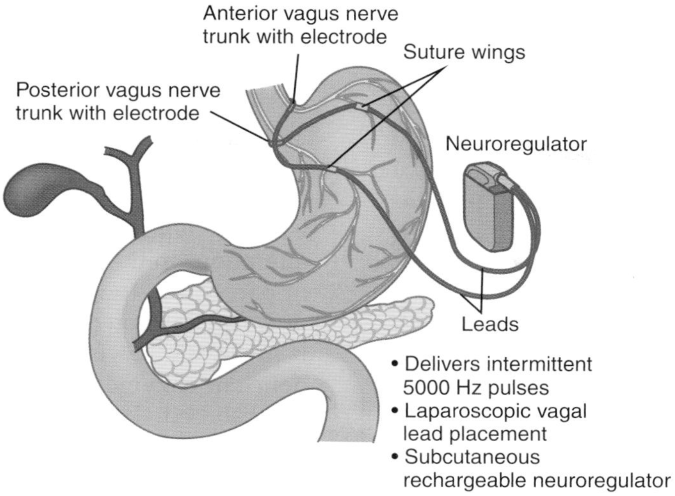

Fig. 39.2 The Maestro Rechargeable System is an electrical stimulator that is surgically implanted into the abdomen. It decreases hunger by sending electrical pulses to the vagus nerve to trigger a feeling that the stomach is full. (From Lewis SL, Bucher L, Heitkemper MM, Harding MM, editors: *Medical surgical nursing: assessment and management of clinical problems*, ed 10, St. Louis, 2017, Elsevier.)

require special attention are covered here. The postoperative assessment focuses on oxygenation, skin integrity, nutrition, prevention of DVTs, and lifestyle changes.

Patient Problems, Goals, and Outcome Criteria: Postoperative Bariatric Surgery

Patient Problems	Goals and Outcome Criteria
Inadequate oxygenation related to weight of fatty tissue on chest.	Adequate oxygenation: vital signs and oxygen (O_2) saturation within normal limits; breath sounds clear
Potential for disrupted tissue integrity related to poor blood supply to adipose tissue, pressure and moisture of body tissue folds.	Skin warm, dry, intact, free of excess pressure: no redness, blanching, or breaks in skin; wound margins closed
Inadequate nutrition related to surgically reduced food ingestion and/or absorption.	Adequate nutrition: patient adheres to prescribed nutrient and supplement intake and loses weight at prescribed rate
Potential for inadequate peripheral circulation (venous thromboembolism) related to limited mobility.	Normal venous circulation: absence of tenderness and swelling in legs
Inability to manage treatment regimen related to lifestyle changes required by weight loss surgery.	Adoption of new eating behaviors with minimal difficulties: patient reports adhering to dietary guidelines and having few episodes of vomiting, diarrhea, or dumping syndrome caused by inappropriate food choices or amounts of food.

Inadequate oxygenation. Some obese people cannot expand the lungs fully because of the weight of fatty tissue on the chest. This increases the risk of postoperative atelectasis and pneumonia and makes breathing exercises and spirometry especially important. Elevating the head of the bed 30 to 45 degrees decreases pressure on the diaphragm and reduces strain on the surgical incisions. Also anesthesia has an affinity for adipose tissue. As the drug is gradually released from the tissue, it can prolong the sedative effects of the drug. If the patient's respirations are depressed, be sure they are positioned to maintain a patent airway. Unless there are complications, they are usually discharged within a few days. If the patient normally uses continuous positive airway pressure (CPAP) or bilevel positive airway pressure (BiPAP) equipment for sleep apnea, it will be needed during hospitalization as well.

Potential for disrupted tissue integrity (skin breakdown). Skin and wound care is especially important for several reasons. The blood supply to adipose tissue is relatively poor, so healing is slow and pressure injuries develop more readily. In addition, tissue folds tend to stay moist, so the patient may develop candidiasis. Therefore, keep the skin clean and dry. Inspect the wound for intact margins. Instruct the patient to avoid strain on incision. Support the abdomen with pillow for coughing and deep breathing. Avoid use of talcum powder and cornstarch; instead, place soft fabric between tissue layers to absorb moisture. Moisture barriers may be needed in the perineal area.

Potential for inadequate circulation (venous thromboembolism). The obese patient is at increased risk for deep vein thrombosis (DVT) and pulmonary emboli when immobilized. Early ambulation is usually ordered and the patient may be treated with low-molecular-weight heparin (LMWH). Position changes, deep breathing, and leg exercises reduce the risk of cardiopulmonary complications. Compression devices for the legs may be ordered. For the obese patient, the foot device may fit better than the long-leg device. Patients are usually assisted out of bed the evening or morning after the surgery and encouraged to walk 3 to 4 times each day. Be sure to have adequate help when assisting the patient out of bed. Facilities that specialize in bariatric surgery are usually equipped and designed for safe movement of obese persons. Monitor the patient's tolerance of physical activity. Tachycardia and dyspnea suggest that the patient's tolerance has been exceeded.

Inadequate nutrition. Before the patient can be fed, imaging studies may be done to ensure that no leaks exist in the surgical sites in the digestive tract. The patient is advanced from water to clear liquids and then to full liquids. Initially the stomach or pouch will hold only 15 to 30 mL. Once solid food is permitted, the typical diet is 800 to 1200 calories per day in four to six small meals. The meals are high in protein and low in fat and carbohydrates. Multivitamin, calcium, and vitamin B_{12} supplementation may be needed. A registered dietitian should develop a nutritional plan and provide patient teaching. However, the nurse can reinforce what the patient has been taught.

Dumping syndrome, described in Chapter 38, is a common problem. The patient can learn to avoid it by selecting appropriate foods in the proper amount.

Inability to manage self care. Adapting to weight loss surgery can be difficult, but the decision to seek the surgery is a huge commitment. Patients are usually excited when they first begin to lose weight but may become discouraged at the long process required to reach the goal weight. Sometimes they feel bad that they were not able to lose weight without surgery. Help them avoid such negative thinking by focusing on their accomplishments. For persons with a history of overeating, learning to eat small meals and avoiding favorite snack food can be especially stressful. Most bariatric centers have counselors to help patients with the emotional adjustment to weight loss surgery. Patient teaching points are listed subsequently.

Patient Teaching

Postbariatric Surgery

- Your diet should be high in protein and low in fat, carbohydrates, and roughage.
- Divide your food intake into 4 to 6 meals per day.
- Do not drink liquids with your meals.
- Food high in sugar or fat may cause you to have acute diarrhea.
- Take dietary supplements as ordered.
- Weight loss is rapid in the first 6 to 12 months.
- You must follow the prescribed diet to sustain and maintain that weight loss.
- Your health care provider may recommend a sleep study to ascertain if CPAP and other forms of respiratory aids are required.

DISORDERS AFFECTING ABSORPTION AND ELIMINATION

MALABSORPTION

Malabsorption is a term used to describe a condition in which one or more nutrients are not digested or absorbed. Among the many causes of malabsorption are bacteria, deficiencies of bile salts or digestive enzymes, alterations in the intestinal mucosa, and absence of all or part of the stomach or intestines. The specific effects of malabsorption depend on the type of deficiency that is present. Likewise, treatment is directed at replacing deficient enzymes or avoiding substances that cannot be absorbed. Two examples of malabsorption are (1) sprue and (2) lactase deficiency.

Two types of sprue exist: (1) celiac (nontropical) and (2) tropical. Celiac disease is caused by a genetic abnormality. It is characterized by severe changes in the intestinal mucosa and impaired absorption of most nutrients. Tropical sprue is caused by an infectious agent and results in malabsorption of fats, folic acid, and vitamin B_{12}.

People with lactase deficiency do not have adequate lactase to metabolize lactose. These people are said to have lactose intolerance. Lactase deficiency may be inherited or acquired. Causes of acquired lactase deficiency include inflammatory bowel disease (IBD), gastroenteritis, and sprue syndrome (see the Cultural Considerations box).

Cultural Considerations

What Does Culture Have to Do With Malabsorption?

Inherited lactase deficiency is most prevalent among Black Americans, Asian Americans, and South Americans. The dietitian should be contacted to help the patient design a culturally appropriate diet.

Clinical Manifestations

A common sign of malabsorption is **steatorrhea**, the presence of excessive fat in the stool. Stools are large, bulky, foamy, and foul smelling. Patients may also have weight loss, fatigue, decreased libido, easy bruising, edema, anemia, and bone pain. Bloating, cramping, abdominal cramps, and diarrhea are symptoms of lactase deficiency that commonly occur within several hours of consuming milk products.

Medical Diagnosis

The diagnosis of celiac disease is based on laboratory studies and endoscopy with small bowel biopsy. Lactase deficiency is diagnosed on the basis of the health history, the lactose tolerance test, a breath test for abnormal hydrogen levels, and, if necessary, biopsy of the intestinal mucosa.

Medical Treatment

Nontropical celiac disease is treated by avoiding products that contain gluten (i.e., wheat, barley, oats, rye).

Tropical sprue is treated with antibiotics, oral folate, and vitamin B_{12} injections.

Lactase deficiency can be treated by eliminating milk and milk products from the diet, although many adults can tolerate small amounts of lactose without symptoms. Lactase enzyme can be mixed with milk or taken before drinking milk to avoid symptoms. Some milk and milk products that have been treated with lactase are also available. If milk products are limited, the diet must be assessed for adequacy of calcium, vitamin D, and riboflavin. Supplements may be advised.

NURSING CARE OF THE PATIENT WITH MALABSORPTION

Document the patient's symptoms and note stool characteristics. In the case of celiac sprue, it is helpful to teach the patient how to eliminate gluten from the diet. Today there are many products that are free of gluten and can be purchased from specialty food stores and supermarkets. Administer antibiotics as ordered for tropical sprue. If folic acid therapy is to be continued, instruct the patient in self-medication. The effect of therapy is evaluated by the return of normal stool consistency. Advise the patient with lactase deficiency of dietary restrictions and alternative products.

DIARRHEA

Diarrhea is defined as the passage of loose, liquid stools with increased frequency. The patient may also have cramps, abdominal pain, and a feeling of urgency before bowel movements.

Causes

Many factors can cause diarrhea. They include spoiled foods, allergies, infections, diverticulosis, malabsorption, cancer, stress, fecal impactions, and tube feedings. Diarrhea is an adverse effect of some medications. A stool sample may be cultured to assess for pathogens.

Complications

Diarrhea is usually temporary and causes no serious problems. However, it does pose an increased threat to the very old, the very young, and those in poor health. These individuals are more likely to become dehydrated and experience electrolyte imbalances and metabolic acidosis. Chronic diarrhea interferes with absorption of nutrients and can lead to malnutrition and anemia.

Medical Treatment

Acute diarrhea is usually treated by resting the digestive tract and focusing on restoration of fluids and electrolytes. Antidiarrheal drugs such as loperamide may be used in the absence of fever and bloody stools. Antibiotics are appropriate in some situations. In the outpatient setting, the patient is advised to consume only clear liquids (see the Complementary and Alternative Therapies box). A variety of liquids, such as broth, gelatin, oral rehydrating solutions, and clear fruit juices, provide water, electrolytes, and some calories. Hospitalized patients may be placed on nothing by mouth (NPO) status and given intravenous fluids. Severe, persistent diarrhea may require total parenteral nutrition (TPN). When diarrhea begins to improve, the diet is gradually expanded to include full liquids, bland solids, and then all other food.

Complementary and Alternative Therapies

Natural substances that can help to control diarrhea include rice water (made by boiling rice and straining the water), potatoes, and unpeeled apples. An herbal remedy is goldenseal, which is effective for diarrhea caused by some bacteria. However, high doses of this herb can cause dangerous central nervous system (CNS) stimulation and uterine contractions, which contraindicate its use during pregnancy.

◆ NURSING CARE OF THE PATIENT WITH DIARRHEA

Focused Assessment

Nursing assessment of the patient with diarrhea can help to determine possible causes, the severity and progress of the condition, the complications, and the effect of treatment. Data that the nurse collects are very important. The history should record the presence of diarrhea and detail the onset, severity, precipitating factors, and measures that bring relief. Describe the pain that accompanies diarrhea and ask the patient about stool characteristics, including amount, color, odor, and unusual contents such as blood, mucus, or undigested food. The functional assessment focuses on usual diet, dietary changes, recent and current medications, and recent travel to a foreign country. It is also important to assess the patient's ability to get to the toilet independently or to call for assistance with toileting.

Important aspects of the physical examination include vital signs, weight, and tissue turgor. Tissue turgor is often assessed by gently pinching the tissue on the forearm. If the pinched tissue flattens as soon as it is released, tissue turgor is generally considered good. This test is not a good indicator of hydration in older adults because their tissue is less elastic, regardless of hydration. Palpate the abdomen for distention or tenderness and inspect the perianal area for irritation. A rectal examination should be performed as agency policy permits if the nurse believes that the patient may have fecal impaction.

Problems that may be experienced by the patient with diarrhea are listed in the following box.

Patient Problems, Goals, and Outcome Criteria: Diarrhea

Patient Problems	Goals and Outcome Criteria
Fluid volume deficit related to fluid loss from diarrhea	Adequate hydration: pulse and blood pressure within patient norms, moist mucous membranes, urine output equal to fluid intake

Continued

Patient Problems, Goals, and Outcome Criteria: Diarrhea—cont'd

Patient Problems	Goals and Outcome Criteria
Inadequate nutrition related to failure to absorb nutrients	Adequate nutrition: patient attains and maintains normal body weight
Acute pain related to abdominal cramping and rectal irritation	Pain relief: patient states less or no pain, relaxed manner
Potential for disrupted tissue integrity related to irritation of diarrhea stool	Intact skin: no perianal redness, lesions
Inability to use perform ADLs (toileting) independently related to weakness or decreased level of consciousness	Improved performance of ADLs: patient uses toilet independently and without injury

Interventions

Fluid volume deficit and inadequate nutrition. The prevention of serious fluid and electrolyte imbalances requires careful monitoring and replacement of fluid losses. When patients have severe diarrhea, keep intake and output records. Whenever possible, measure liquid stools. Stool characteristics are also important and should be recorded. Signs and symptoms that suggest possible fluid imbalances include unequal fluid intake and output; decreased blood pressure; changes in pulse rate or rhythm; changes in respiratory rate or depth; confusion; muscle weakness, tingling, or twitching; dry mucous membranes; and poor tissue turgor. These changes may indicate serious imbalances in water and electrolytes. They should be recorded and reported promptly.

The daily fluid intake should be 2000 to 3000 mL of various fluids. Carefully monitor the flow rates of intravenous fluids. Excessive or rapid fluid replacement can cause heart failure, especially in older adults.

Acute pain. Abdominal cramping associated with diarrhea is often relieved by antidiarrheal drugs that reduce intestinal activity. Record the severity, duration, and location of the pain as well as the effects of drug therapy.

Potential for disrupted tissue integrity. Liquid stool is very irritating to the anal and perianal areas. With frequent bowel movements, skin breakdown may occur. If necessary, assist the patient with perianal care after each stool. Wash the area thoroughly and gently with warm water and mild soap, rinse, and then pat dry with a soft towel. Protective creams, sprays, or lotions can be applied.

Inability to perform activities of daily living (toileting) independently. Older persons or those who are acutely ill may have difficulty with toileting during diarrhea episodes. If possible, they should be placed in rooms close to the nurses' station. Staff should be aware of the need to respond promptly to call bells. A bedside commode is recommended if the toilet is too far from the bed. Patients who are unable to call for help must be checked frequently for the passage of diarrhea stools (see the Coordinated Care box).

Coordinated Care

Helping Certified Nursing Assistants Assist With Toileting

Because certified nursing assistants (CNAs) usually assist patients with personal care, they are most likely to assist with toileting. The CNAs should inform the nurse if the patient has difficulty with defecation or has abnormal stools such as diarrhea or stools containing blood, mucus, or undigested food.

CONSTIPATION

The frequency of defecation varies among healthy people. Bowel movements may occur as often as 2 or 3 times daily or as seldom as once a week. If the stool is soft and is passed without difficulty, the patient is not constipated. Constipation is a condition in which a person has hard, dry, infrequent stools that are passed with difficulty.

Pharmacology Capsule

Laxatives, cathartics, enemas, and suppositories usually relieve constipation promptly but the effects of stool softeners are not seen for several days.

Causes

Many factors can contribute to constipation. When stool is present in the rectum, the urge to defecate occurs. If the urge is ignored, stool remains in the rectum longer than usual and becomes dry. It is then more difficult, and sometimes painful, to have a bowel movement. People who frequently ignore the urge to defecate may become chronically constipated. The frequent use of laxatives or enemas may also contribute to chronic constipation. These agents keep the lower digestive tract empty and eventually interfere with the normal pattern of elimination.

Because physical activity promotes normal bowel elimination, people who are inactive are at risk for constipation. Inadequate water intake can lead to constipation because more water will be reabsorbed from the stool in the large intestine. Diet significantly affects the stool. A diet that is low in fiber and high in foods such as cheese, lean meat, and pasta promotes constipation.

Drugs that slow intestinal motility or increase urine output also contribute to constipation. Examples of these drugs are those used for anesthesia, pain relief, and cold symptoms. Medical conditions that may be related to constipation include diseases of the colon or rectum as well as brain or spinal cord injury.

Abdominal surgery causes a loss of intestinal activity, but it should be temporary.

Many people believe that constipation is normal for older people. Normal age-related changes in the large intestine do not explain the frequent complaints of constipation by older adults. More likely, when constipation does occur, it is related to inactivity, drug therapy, long-term laxative or enema abuse, or some medical condition.

Complications

When people are constipated, they may feel the need to strain to have bowel movements. Straining occurs when a person attempts to exhale with the glottis closed, causing increased pressure in the chest and abdominal cavities. This is called the *Valsalva maneuver*. The pressure slows the flow of circulating blood back into the chest, causing a brief drop in pulse and blood pressure. Relaxation allows a rush of blood back into the chest, with a resulting rise in pulse and blood pressure. The rapid changes in blood flow can be fatal to a patient with heart disease. Therefore, prevention of constipation and straining is very important in the care of cardiac patients.

Chronic constipation also contributes to the development of hemorrhoids. Another complication of constipation is fecal impaction, which is discussed subsequently.

Medical Treatment

Treatment of constipation is directed toward immediate relief of the problem and prevention of future episodes. Laxatives, suppositories, enemas, or a combination is ordered to get prompt results. The health care provider may prescribe stool softeners as well. Stool softeners, as the name suggests, promote normal elimination by allowing more water to be held in the stool so that it is softer and more easily passed. It takes several days for the effects of stool softeners to be seen, so they are not used for acute constipation. They are relatively safe drugs that are often prescribed over a long period of time. The trade names of some stool softeners are Colace, Surfak, and Metamucil.

Metamucil is an example of a bulk-forming stool softener. In the intestinal tract, it absorbs water to produce a gel-like mass to aid in the passage of a soft stool. If the patient does not take adequate fluids, the mass can harden and cause obstruction in the intestine. Table 37.2 provides additional information about drugs used to treat constipation.

NURSING CARE OF THE PATIENT WITH CONSTIPATION

Focused Assessment

The assessment of bowel elimination may detect constipation or risk factors that may cause it. Data that contribute to the assessment include the patient's usual pattern of bowel elimination, including frequency, amount, color, unusual contents (blood, mucus, undigested food), and pain associated with defecation. Note recent changes in any of these factors. Information about diet, exercise, and drug therapy is helpful in revealing potential risk factors for constipation. If any aids to elimination (laxatives, stool softeners, enemas, suppositories) are used, record the type and frequency of use.

Examine the abdomen for distention or visible peristalsis and auscultate for bowel sounds in all four quadrants. When severe constipation is accompanied by mild diarrhea, a rectal examination should be done to detect a fecal impaction if agency policy permits.

Patient Problem, Goal, and Outcome Criterion: Constipation

Patient Problem	Goal and Outcome Criterion
Constipation related to drug therapy, diet, inadequate fluid intake, inactivity, neuromuscular disorder	Establishment of normal bowel elimination: regular passage of formed stools without straining

Interventions

Constipation. The first action is directed at relieving the patient's constipation. Sometimes the health care provider will write an order for a laxative or an enema as needed. An enema or suppository is preferred if the patient is very uncomfortable because it usually acts within 1 hour. A laxative may take as long as 8 to 10 hours.

When a laxative is truly needed, it should be given. However, laxatives are often abused. Laxatives can also produce diarrhea, which may lead to excessive loss of fluids and electrolytes (see the Complementary and Alternative Therapies box). When an enema is indicated for a person aged 70 years or older, a warm water solution is preferred. Phosphate/biphosphate enemas can cause serious electrolyte imbalances in this population (Rao, May 20, 2020).

Complementary and Alternative Therapies

Herbs that have a laxative effect include aloe, cascara sagrada, and senna. Other complementary therapies include abdominal massage in a circular pattern with essential oil of rose, marjoram, fennel, or rosemary.

Nurses are often responsible for managing the bowel elimination of severely disabled people. This is especially true in long-term care facilities. It is critical to record and describe all stools so that problems can be found and treated early. Teach certified nursing assistant (CNAs) the importance of keeping accurate records. If detected early, constipation may be treated easily with a mild laxative or suppository. Severe constipation may require repeated enemas and laxatives for relief (see the Patient Teaching box).

Patient Teaching

Constipation

- Include high-fiber foods such as fruits, raw vegetables, greens, and whole grains in the diet.
- Drink six to eight 8-oz glasses of water each day unless the health care provider has restricted fluid intake for some reason.
- Exercise daily. It need not be strenuous; walking is excellent exercise.
- Go to the bathroom promptly in response to the urge to have a bowel movement.
- Contrary to popular opinion, it is not necessary to have a bowel movement every day. A bowel movement every 2 or 3 days without pain or straining is normal for some people.
- Use a toilet that is comfortable. Feet should touch the floor, causing the hips to bend slightly. Use a footstool if necessary. This helps use of the abdominal muscles.
- Laxatives can be used safely for occasional constipation. Consult the health care provider for a recommended laxative.

In many cases, bowel elimination can be maintained with diet, fluids, exercise, and regular toilet habits. Occasional use of elimination aids is not harmful. However, some patients require nursing interventions to promote elimination over a long period.

Megacolon. Megacolon is a condition in which the large intestine loses the ability to contract effectively enough to propel the fecal mass toward the rectum. These patients usually need regular enemas for bowel cleansing. Other measures are generally not adequate. Patients who have special problems with constipation are those with neurologic conditions such as spinal cord injuries and cerebrovascular accident (CVA). The management of bowel elimination in these patients and the process of bowel retraining are discussed in Chapters 23 and 24.

Fecal impaction. All nursing staff should understand the possibility of fecal impaction in the physically or mentally impaired person. Fecal impaction refers to the retention of a large mass of stool in the rectum that the patient is unable to pass. Some liquid stool trickles around the impaction and may be mistaken for diarrhea.

Consider possible impaction when a patient who has not had a bowel movement for several days has repeated episodes of mild diarrhea. If agency policy permits, assess for impaction by inserting a gloved, lubricated finger into the rectum. The fecal mass is usually easily felt. It may be very hard or soft.

The impaction should be removed following agency protocol or the health care provider's specific orders. This process may require administration of a mineral oil enema to soften hard stool, followed by a soapsuds enema. It may be necessary to break up and remove the mass manually. This procedure is painful and embarrassing for the patient. With good nursing care, manual extraction should rarely be necessary.

INTESTINAL OBSTRUCTION

Causes

Intestinal obstruction can be caused by many factors, including strangulated hernia, tumor, paralytic ileus, stricture, **volvulus** (twisting of the bowel), intussusception (telescoping of the bowel into itself), and postoperative adhesions. When the bowel is obstructed, digestive contents cannot progress. Volvulus and intussusception are illustrated in Fig. 39.3.

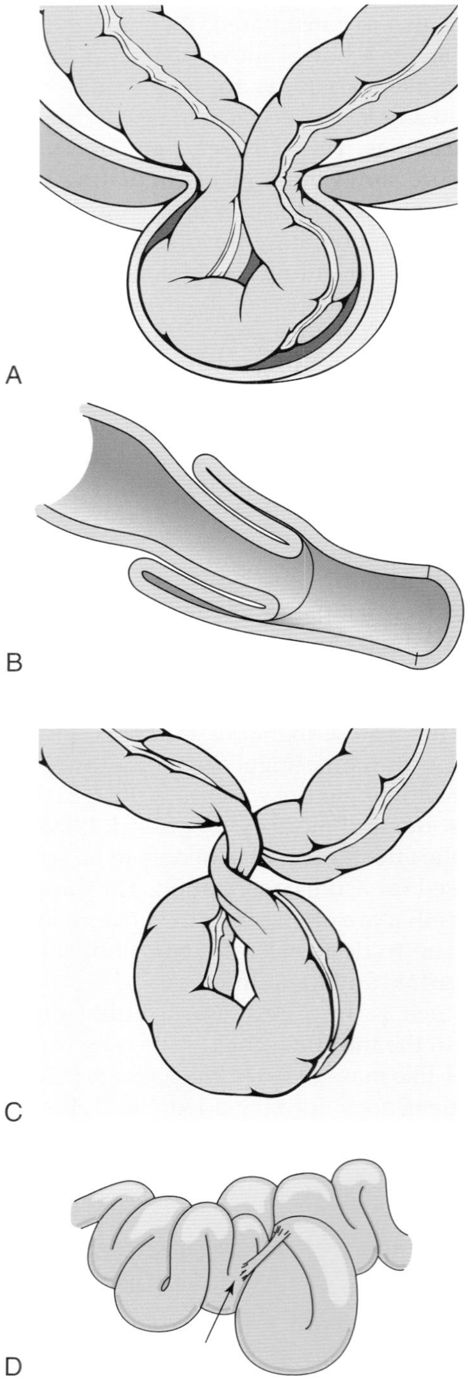

Fig. 39.3 Causes of mechanical bowel obstruction. (A) Incarcerated hernia. (B) Intussusception. (C) Volvulus. (D) Adhesions. (From McCance KL, Huether SE: *Understanding pathophysiology*, ed 5, St. Louis, 2013, Mosby.)

Signs and Symptoms

Symptoms are most acute when an obstruction is located in the proximal portion of the small intestine. Early symptoms of obstruction are vomiting (possibly projectile), abdominal pain, and constipation. Gastric contents are vomited first, followed by bile and then fecal matter. Blood or purulent drainage may be passed rectally. Abdominal distention may develop, especially with colon obstruction.

Complications

If blood supply to the intestine is impaired, gangrene and perforation of the bowel may occur. Untreated obstruction can result in shock and death.

Medical Diagnosis

Intestinal obstruction is suspected based on the patient's history, physical examination, and laboratory studies. It is confirmed by radiologic studies.

Medical Treatment

The initial treatment of obstruction is gastrointestinal (GI) decompression. A nasogastric tube is passed and connected to suction. Intravenous fluids are provided. Depending on the cause of the obstruction, surgical intervention may be necessary.

NURSING CARE OF THE PATIENT WITH INTESTINAL OBSTRUCTION

Focused Assessment

Ask about the patient's symptoms, including pain and nausea, and describe the onset and progression of those symptoms. The past medical history should include potentially related conditions, such as hernia, cancer of the digestive tract, and abdominal surgeries. Ask when the patient's last bowel movement was and if the characteristics were normal.

Take vital signs to detect signs of infection (e.g., fever, tachycardia) and impending shock (e.g., tachycardia, hypotension). Assess skin moisture and tissue turgor along with moisture of the mucous membranes. Inspect the patient's abdomen for distention and visible peristalsis. Auscultate for rapid, high-pitched tinkling bowel sounds and gently palpate for tenderness and guarding. Note any rectal bleeding or drainage.

Patient Problems, Goals, and Outcome Criteria: Intestinal Obstruction

Patient Problems	Goals and Outcome Criteria
Acute pain related to distention	Pain relief: patient states less or no pain, relaxed manner
Fluid volume deficit related to vomiting, intestinal suction	Normal hydration: pulse and blood pressure within patient norms, moist mucous membranes, equal fluid intake and output

Patient Problems, Goals, and Outcome Criteria: Intestinal Obstruction—cont'd

Patient Problems	Goals and Outcome Criteria
Potential for infection related to complications of obstruction	Absence of infection: no fever, normal white blood cell (WBC) count
Inadequate ventilation related to abdominal distention, shallow respirations resulting from abdominal distention	Adequate ventilation: respiratory rate of 12 to 20 breaths per minute without dyspnea, heart rate consistent with patient's usual, O_2 saturation of 95% to 100%
Anxiety related to pain, anticipated surgery	Decreased anxiety: patient states less or no anxiety, calm manner

Interventions

Acute pain. Give analgesics as ordered and assess effectiveness. Use nonpharmacologic interventions such as massage and relaxation.

Fluid volume deficit. Promote fluid balance by providing intravenous fluids as ordered. Monitor the patient's vital signs, intake, and output. If a nasogastric tube is ordered, place it per protocol, monitor output, and ensure drainage at all times.

Potential for infection. Monitor the patient's temperature. Signs of intestinal rupture (i.e., increasing tenderness, sudden sharp pain, abdominal rigidity) must be reported to the health care provider immediately.

Inadequate ventilation. Elevate the patient's head to relieve pressure on the diaphragm. Encourage deep breathing and coughing and administer oxygen as ordered. When surgery is planned, carry out preoperative orders, which may include giving an enema and intravenous fluids.

Anxiety. Give simple explanations of what is being done and what the patient should expect postoperatively if surgery is scheduled. Stress the importance of deep breathing, turning, coughing, and leg exercises.

◆ POSTOPERATIVE NURSING CARE OF THE PATIENT WITH INTESTINAL OBSTRUCTION

Postoperative care depends on the surgical procedure performed.

APPENDICITIS

Pathophysiology

The appendix is a blind pouch in the cecum. Appendicitis is an inflammation of the appendix. Inflammation occurs when the opening of the appendix to the large intestine is blocked by feces, tumors, **helminths** (a worm classified as a parasite), or indigestible substances such as seeds. The tissue becomes infected by bacteria in the digestive tract. Pus accumulates, the blood supply is impaired, and the appendix may rupture. A ruptured appendix allows digestive contents to enter the abdominal cavity, causing peritonitis—a life-threatening surgical emergency. Early detection of appendicitis may permit treatment before the appendix ruptures.

Signs and Symptoms

The initial symptom of appendicitis is usually pain in the epigastric region or around the umbilicus, which then shifts to the right lower quadrant. The classic symptom of appendicitis is pain at McBurney point, which is located midway between the umbilicus and the iliac crest (Fig. 39.4). The patient may have temperature elevation and nausea and vomiting. Because of the pain, the patient may assume a position of hip flexion. The right leg cannot be straightened without pain. An elevated white blood cell (WBC) count indicates the presence of infection.

Signs and symptoms of peritonitis are absence of bowel sounds, severe abdominal distention, increased pulse and temperature, nausea, and vomiting. The abdomen may be rigid, although this sign is often absent with peritonitis in older patients. Consider possible shock if the patient begins to lose consciousness and is cool and pale.

Medical Diagnosis

A diagnosis of appendicitis is based on classic signs and symptoms and a WBC count of 10,000 to 15,000/mm^3.

Medical Treatment

When appendicitis is suspected, the patient is placed on NPO status. Laxatives and heat applications should never be used for undiagnosed abdominal pain. If the appendix is inflamed, heat or laxatives may cause it to rupture.

If rupture has not occurred, immediate surgical treatment is indicated. With a ruptured appendix, surgery may be delayed 6 to 8 hours while antibiotics and intravenous fluids are given. An appendectomy may be performed by laparoscopy or through an open incision. In most situations, the laparoscopic route is used.

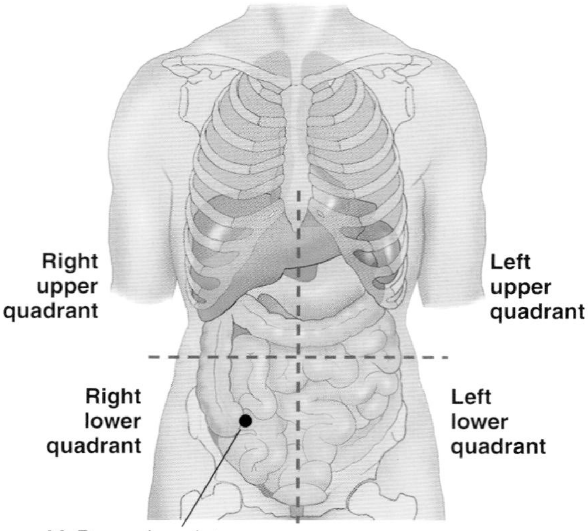

Fig. 39.4 McBurney point is located in the right lower quadrant, midway between the anterior iliac crest and the umbilicus. Localized tenderness here is typical of appendicitis. (From Shiland BJ: *Medical terminology & anatomy for coding*, ed 3, St. Louis, 2018, Elsevier.)

◆ NURSING CARE OF THE PATIENT WITH APPENDICITIS

Focused Assessment

The patient's chief complaint is usually pain. Describe the location, severity, onset, duration, precipitating factors, and alleviating measures in relation to the pain. In the past medical history, note previous abdominal distress, chronic illnesses, and surgeries. Record allergies and any medications the patient may be taking. Review of systems assesses the presence of nausea and vomiting. Significant data in the physical examination are temperature; abdominal pain, distention, and tenderness; and the presence and characteristics of bowel sounds.

Patient Problems, Goals, and Outcome Criteria: Appendicitis

Patient Problems	Goals and Outcome Criteria
Potential for infection (peritonitis) related to appendix rupture	Absence of infection: normal body temperature and vital signs, bowel sounds present, abdomen soft
Fluid volume deficit related to nausea, vomiting, medical restriction of fluid intake	Normal fluid balance: pulse and blood pressure within patient norms, moist mucous membranes, serum electrolytes within normal limits, fluid intake equal to output
Acute pain related to inflammation of appendix or surgical tissue trauma	Pain relief: patient states less or no pain, relaxed manner
Inadequate ventilation related to shallow respirations, incisional pain, or anesthesia	Adequate ventilation: respiratory rate of 12 to 20 breaths per minute, clear breath sounds, O_2 saturation of 95% to 100%
Fear related to sudden emergency status, minimal preoperative teaching	Reduced fear: patient states less or no fear, calm manner

Preoperative Interventions

Before surgery, the patient will probably be most comfortable in a semi-Fowler or side-lying position with the hips flexed. Because the pain location and pattern help the health care provider to make a diagnosis, analgesics may be withheld initially. This should be explained to the patient. If rupture is suspected, elevate the patient's head to localize the infection.

Postoperative Interventions

Postoperatively, the patient receives intravenous fluids. If the appendix had ruptured, antibiotics are likely to be prescribed to treat/prevent peritonitis and GI decompression may be used. Assist the patient in turning, splinting the surgical site when coughing, and deep breathing to promote expansion of the lungs. Incentive spirometry can also be useful. Early ambulation is usually ordered to reduce the risk of postoperative complications. Inspect the abdominal wound for redness, swelling, and foul drainage and provide wound care as ordered or according to agency policy.

After a laparoscopic procedure for uncomplicated appendicitis, the patient may be discharged the same day or next. If the appendix has ruptured, the hospitalization is longer and includes antibiotic therapy. Initially, lifting objects is usually limited to 5 to 10 pounds. Normal activities can be resumed in 2 to 3 weeks.

PERITONITIS

Pathophysiology

Peritonitis is inflammation of the peritoneum (the serous membrane lining the cavity of the abdomen) caused by chemical or bacterial contamination of the peritoneal cavity. Chemical contamination may follow rupture of a digestive tract structure, including the appendix. Bacterial contamination may be caused by rupture of a digestive tract structure or fallopian tube or from nonsterile, traumatic wounds.

When a chemical or bacterial contaminant is present, the body's defenses attempt to wall off the area to contain the injury. Fluid shifts out of the bloodstream into the peritoneal cavity. Peristalsis slows or stops. If defenses are adequate, the offending fluid remains localized and is eventually eliminated. Complications of peritonitis include abscesses, adhesions, septicemia, hypovolemic shock, paralytic ileus, and possible organ failure.

Signs and Symptoms

Signs and symptoms of peritonitis include pain over the affected area, rebound tenderness, abdominal rigidity and distention, fever, tachycardia, tachypnea, nausea, and vomiting. The older patient may have more subtle symptoms with less pain and the absence of abdominal rigidity.

Medical Diagnosis

A diagnosis of peritonitis is suspected on the basis of the patient's history and physical examination. Diagnostic tests and procedures done to confirm the inflammation include a complete blood count (CBC), serum electrolyte measurements, abdominal radiography, computed tomography (CT), and ultrasound. Paracentesis may be done to obtain a specimen of fluid for culture.

Medical Treatment

A nasogastric tube is inserted for GI decompression. Intravenous fluids, antibiotics, and analgesics are ordered. Surgery may be done to close a ruptured structure and to remove foreign material and fluid from the peritoneal cavity.

◆ NURSING CARE OF THE PATIENT WITH PERITONITIS

Focused Assessment

Begin by asking about the patient's present illness. Because pain is the prominent symptom, record the onset, location, and severity of the pain and any related symptoms. When peritonitis is suspected, record a history of abdominal trauma, including surgery. It is also important to take and record vital signs, inspect the abdomen for distention, and auscultate for the presence of bowel sounds. Evaluate fluid status, including tissue turgor, moisture of mucous membranes, and intake and output.

Patient Problems, Goals, and Outcome Criteria: Peritonitis

Patient Problems	Goals and Outcome Criteria
Acute pain related to inflammation	Pain relief: patient states pain is reduced or relieved, has relaxed manner
Decreased cardiac output related to decreased blood volume	Normal cardiac output: pulse and blood pressure within patient norms, skin warm and dry, fluid output equal to intake
Inadequate nutrition related to nausea, vomiting, nothing by mouth (NPO) status	Adequate nutrition: stable body weight
Anxiety related to threat of serious illness and invasive treatment	Decreased anxiety: patient states anxiety is reduced or relieved, calm manner

Interventions

Acute pain. Administer opioid analgesics as ordered for pain. Position the patient with the head elevated and offer comfort measures, such as massage and relaxation techniques. Notify the health care provider if pain relief is not achieved.

Decreased cardiac output. The shift of fluid from the blood into the peritoneal cavity may be so great that the patient develops deficient intravascular fluid volume. Cardiac output falls and perfusion of vital organs is reduced. Administer intravenous fluids as ordered and monitor fluid intake and output. Monitor vital signs and immediately report increasing pulse, restlessness, pallor, and decreasing blood pressure. In addition to deficient fluid volume, the patient may go into shock because of septicemia (the presence of bacteria in the blood). This patient requires intense monitoring and probably will be placed in the intensive care unit. Report findings immediately to the health care provider.

Inadequate nutrition. GI decompression usually eliminates nausea and vomiting but antiemetics may be ordered as needed. Check to ensure that the nasogastric tube is draining at all times.

Anxiety. The patient is likely to be anxious because of pain and uncertainty about what is happening. Even when a sense of urgency exists in caring for the patient, give simple explanations for procedures and tell the patient what to expect. Encourage the patient to ask questions. If surgery is planned, essential preoperative teaching may have to be done quickly. Explain to the patient the importance of breathing and leg exercises after abdominal surgery. The health care provider may order sedatives to calm the patient.

◆ POSTOPERATIVE NURSING CARE OF THE PATIENT WITH PERITONITIS

Postoperative care is like that for any major surgery and is described in Chapter 17. Care specific to surgery on the digestive tract is addressed in Chapter 37 under "Common Therapeutic Measures."

ABDOMINAL HERNIA

Pathophysiology

Muscles play an important role in keeping the abdominal organs in place. Weakness in those muscles may allow a portion of the large intestine to push through the abdominal wall. The bulging portion of intestine through the weak muscle is called a *hernia*. Hernias occur most often in areas where the abdominal wall is already weak. Weak locations include the umbilicus and the lower inguinal areas of the abdomen (Fig. 39.5). Hernias may also develop at the site of a surgical incision.

Hernias are classified as reducible or irreducible. A reducible hernia slips back into the abdominal cavity with gentle pressure or when the patient lies on their back. When the hernia cannot be manipulated back into place, it is said to be irreducible, or incarcerated. An irreducible hernia may impair blood flow to the trapped loop of intestine, causing it to become gangrenous. A hernia that is trapped and deprived of blood is said to be strangulated. This is treated as a medical emergency.

Signs and Symptoms

Hernias are usually diagnosed when a patient reports a smooth lump on the abdomen. The lump may disappear when the patient is lying down or at rest but returns when standing or straining. Heavy lifting or coughing usually causes the hernia to appear.

Hernias are usually not painful unless they become incarcerated. With incarceration, the patient has severe abdominal pain and distention, vomiting, and cramps.

Medical Diagnosis

Hernias are diagnosed on the basis of the health history and physical examination.

Medical Treatment

Surgical repair of hernias is usually recommended even if they are reducible (manually pushing the hernia back into its original compartment or place). Repair prevents the possibility of incarceration. Two surgical procedures are used to repair hernias. Herniorrhaphy is the repair of the muscle defect by suturing. If additional measures are needed to strengthen the abdominal wall, a hernioplasty is done. Strong materials are used to cover and reinforce the defect.

Some patients cannot tolerate the stress of surgical hernia repair. For them, a hernia belt or truss may be advised, although trusses are not used as widely as in the past (see the Patient Teaching box). A truss consists of a pad that is placed over the hernia and a belt that holds it in place. Both devices provide support by applying pressure over the hernia defect.

Patient Teaching

Hernia Belt or Truss

- Put the belt/truss on before rising each morning.
- Check under the pad and belt several times daily for skin irritation.
- The belt/truss does not cure a hernia, so the patient should avoid straining.

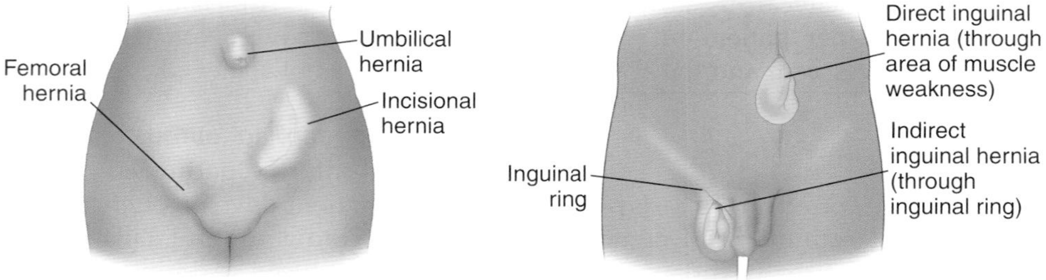

Fig. 39.5 Abdominal hernias. (From Leonard PC: *Building a medical vocabulary with Spanish translations*, ed 10, St. Louis, 2018, Elsevier.)

NURSING CARE OF THE PATIENT WITH ABDOMINAL HERNIA

Focused Assessment

Begin the assessment with the patient's chief complaint, usually a smooth lump in the abdomen that appears and disappears with various activities and positions. Ask about pain and vomiting, which may be present if the hernia is strangulated. Have the patient explain their work and home responsibilities to identify the type of physical exertion required. The most relevant aspect of the physical examination is the assessment of the abdomen. Inspect for abnormalities and listen for bowel sounds in all four quadrants. If the patient wears a belt or truss, examine the skin underneath it for signs of irritation.

Patient Problems, Goals, and Outcome Criteria: Abdominal Hernia

Patient Problems	Goals and Outcome Criteria
Potential for injury related to hernia strangulation or distention	Absence of injury (strangulation): normal pulse and temperature without abdominal pain
Disrupted skin tissue integrity related to pressure created by the belt or truss	Absence of complications caused by truss: intact skin without redness under truss

Preoperative Interventions

Potential for injury. Monitor the patient for signs and symptoms of strangulation (i.e., nausea, vomiting, pain, abdominal distention, fever, tachycardia). If these symptoms develop, it is vital to notify the health care provider immediately. It is important for the nonsurgical patient to know that these symptoms should be reported.

Determine what restrictions the patient has in relation to physical exertion and provide verbal and written instructions to the patient.

Disrupted skin tissue integrity. Teach patients who use a truss what measures to take to avoid injury to the skin.

1. Step into the hernia belt or truss and pull it up over the hips. If a belt is provided, wrap the belt around the abdomen surrounding the area of the hernia.
2. Insert the hernia pad or pads into the truss (if the truss does not already have pads attached). If there are hernias on both sides of the abdomen, insert a second pad.
3. Gently press the pads to push the hernia or hernias back into the abdominal cavity. Secure straps or tighten the belt to hold the pads in place and maintain compression on the hernia or hernias.

Remember, a belt or truss should be worn only for a short period of time. It must be properly fitted and worn to be effective. Wearing a belt or truss is not an alternative form of treatment. Patients should be advised to follow the guidelines and recommendations of their health care provider. Surgical intervention is the usual course of action taken to repair hernias.

Patient Problems, Goals, and Outcome Criteria: Abdominal Hernia Repair

Patient Problems	Goals and Outcome Criteria
Urinary retention related to abdominal surgery, anesthesia	Normal urinary function: urine output approximately equal to fluid intake, no bladder distention
Constipation related to immobility, effects of anesthesia, and abdominal surgery	Normal bowel elimination: formed stools at regular intervals without pain or straining
Acute pain related to scrotal swelling	Pain relief: patient states there is less or no pain, relaxed manner
Potential for injury (wound dehiscence) related to stress on wound margins	Well-healed wound: margins intact, decreasing redness and swelling

Postoperative Interventions

The general postoperative care of patients who have undergone surgery is discussed in Chapter 17. In addition to the routine postoperative assessments, after hernia repair, the nurse should be especially concerned with assessing bowel and bladder elimination, wound healing, and the patient's knowledge about ways to avoid placing stress on the healing surgical wound.

Urinary retention. Many patients have temporary problems with urination after hernia repair surgery. Keep intake and output records, document voiding, and palpate for bladder distention.

Constipation. Bowel activity may also cease temporarily in response to the anesthesia and manipulation of the bowel during surgery. It is important to monitor bowel sounds and note the passage of **flatus**. Like any other patients having major surgery, patients undergoing hernia repair need to keep their lungs clear to prevent complications. Encourage them to turn and deep breathe, but they should not cough or sneeze. Coughing and sneezing put tension on the surgical incision and repaired tissues.

Acute pain. Scrotal swelling is common after inguinal hernia repair. A scrotal support and a cold pack can greatly reduce the painful swelling.

Potential for injury. Activities are usually restricted for 2 to 6 weeks. Reinforce the health care provider's instructions about refraining from exertion and lifting.

Advise the patient to report fever or wound drainage to the health care provider.

INFLAMMATORY BOWEL DISEASE

Pathophysiology

IBD refers to ulcerative colitis and Crohn disease. Crohn disease is also known as *regional enteritis*. In both conditions, inflammation and ulceration of the lining of the intestinal tract occurs. With ulcerative colitis, the inflammation typically begins in the rectum and gradually extends up the bowel toward the cecum. The progression of Crohn disease is different in that it can affect any area of the GI tract. Although the terminal ileum is most often affected, there may be multiple sites interspersed with healthy segments of bowel.

The two conditions have similar symptoms and are treated in much the same way medically. However, surgical options are different.

A patient with IBD may have a few isolated attacks or may have a chronic condition. With chronic IBD, attacks may last for days or even months, followed by periods of remission lasting several weeks to several years.

Causes

The exact cause of IBD is unknown. Possible causes that are being studied include infectious agents, autoimmune reactions, allergies, heredity, and foreign substances (see the Cultural Considerations box). In the past, it was thought that IBD might be caused by stress. However, current thinking suggests that stress is a result of IBD rather than its cause.

Cultural Considerations

What Does Culture Have to Do With Inflammatory Bowel Disease?

Inflammatory bowel disease (IBD) is more common among White Americans and people of Middle-Eastern origin than among Black Americans and Asian Americans.

Signs and Symptoms

The symptoms of IBD vary with the extent of the disease. When ulcerative colitis affects only the rectum, the patient may be constipated. More commonly, however, patients have diarrhea with frequent bloody stools and abdominal cramping. In severe cases, the patient may also have fever and weight loss.

Symptoms of Crohn disease are even more variable, depending on the areas affected. If the stomach and duodenum are involved, symptoms include nausea, vomiting, and epigastric pain. Involvement of the small intestine produces pain, abdominal tenderness, and cramping. An inflamed colon typically causes abdominal pain, cramping, rectal bleeding, and diarrhea. Systemic signs and symptoms include fever, night sweats, malaise, and joint pain.

Complications

The local complications of IBD include hemorrhage, obstruction, perforation (rupture), abscesses in the anus or rectum, fistulas, and megacolon. Patients who have had ulcerative colitis for 10 years have a greatly increased risk of cancer of the large intestine. Patients with Crohn disease are also thought to have an increased risk of colon cancer, although the relationship is less clear.

Systemic complications may also be found with ulcerative colitis. These are conditions outside the intestine but related to the colitis. They include inflammation of the joints and eyes, skin lesions, urinary stones, and liver disease. Of course, severe or prolonged diarrhea can result in malnutrition, anemia, and fluid and electrolyte imbalances.

Medical Diagnosis

IBD is suspected on the basis of the history and physical examination. Abdominal radiography may be done to rule out obstruction before additional tests are done. To confirm the diagnosis, the health care provider may order a colonoscopy with biopsy, a barium enema examination with air contrast, ultrasonography, CT, and cell studies. The video capsule that is swallowed by the patient provides a view of the small intestine that is not accessible by endoscopy.

Medical Treatment

Treatment of IBD addresses the local and the systemic effects of the disorders. Intestinal inflammation is treated with drug therapy, diet, and rest. Some drugs are useful for both ulcerative colitis and Crohn disease; others are specific to one or the other diagnosis. The following drugs may be used alone or in combination, depending on the specific situation:

- Corticosteroids: to decrease inflammation in mild to moderately severe episodes (not for maintenance therapy)
- Immunosuppressant agents: to inhibit the immune response: azathioprine (Imuran), mercaptopurine (Purixan), cyclosporine (Sandimmune et al.), methotrexate
- Antidiarrheal agents: to control diarrhea (except in severe colitis)
- Anticholinergics: to reduce pain and GI motility and secretions
- Antibiotics: to treat mild to moderately severe attacks of Crohn disease: metronidazole, ciprofloxacin; antibiotics are not very useful for ulcerative colitis.
- Aminosalicylates: to reduce symptoms: 5-ASA (mesalamine oral, suppository, or enema; or sulfasalazine); now considered to have limited benefits
- Iron supplements and vitamin B_{12}: to treat anemia
- Immunomodulators: to block the inflammatory process in Crohn disease for patients who do not respond well to azathioprine (may be given in

combination with azathioprine). Examples are infliximab (Remicade), vedolizumab (Entyvio), and ustekinumab (Stelara)

- Tricyclic antidepressants: sometimes helpful

Research is ongoing to develop other drugs for acute and chronic management. Based on the low incidence of IBD among smokers, therapy with nicotine transdermal patches or gum is also being studied.

A low-roughage diet without milk products is prescribed for mild to moderate IBD. Intravenous fluids or TPN may be needed to provide fluid, electrolytes, and nutrients when symptoms are severe.

Although most patients respond to medical treatment, some require surgery. Removal of the colon (colectomy) is curative for ulcerative colitis. When the colon is removed, an artificial opening from the small intestine through the abdominal wall is needed to allow elimination of digestive wastes. The opening is called an *ileostomy*. Although good health is usually restored after this surgery, an ileostomy is permanent and requires special care. Surgery is not usually done unless all other measures have failed. Care of the patient with an ostomy is covered in Chapter 18.

Surgical treatment of Crohn disease is more likely to involve removal of the diseased portion of the intestine. Recurrence is so common that surgery is not usually done unless necessitated by serious complications. Postoperatively the disease typically reappears at the site of anastomosis within 1 year. Newly affected areas may also appear in other sections of the intestine.

Pharmacology Capsule

Corticosteroids suppress the immune and inflammatory responses, so the patient is more susceptible to infection.

NURSING CARE OF THE PATIENT WITH INFLAMMATORY BOWEL DISEASE

The nursing care of a patient during an acute attack of IBD is concerned with ongoing assessment, comfort measures, skin care, emotional support, and administering drugs and monitoring the effects. The nursing needs of the patient with IBD who undergoes surgery are like those of other patients who have undergone GI surgery, as discussed under "Common Therapeutic Measures" in Chapter 37.

Focused Assessment

Assessment of the patient with IBD should identify the symptoms that caused the patient to seek care—usually pain and diarrhea. Record the onset, location, severity, and duration of pain. Note factors that contribute to the onset of pain, such as specific foods or stressors, as well as the onset and duration of diarrhea and the presence of blood. Explore the effect of the illness on the patient's life and coping mechanisms of the patient.

Important aspects of the physical examination are vital signs, height and weight, and measures of hydration (tissue turgor, mucous membrane moisture). Inspect the perianal area for irritation or ulceration. Maintain accurate intake and output records, measuring and counting diarrhea stools as output if possible.

Patient Problems, Goals, and Outcome Criteria: Inflammatory Bowel Disease

Patient Problems	Goals and Outcome Criteria
Chronic pain related to abdominal cramping, perianal irritation	Pain relief: patient states pain is reduced or relieved, manner is relaxed
Diarrhea related to intestinal inflammation	Cessation of diarrhea: stools formed, less frequent
Fluid volume deficit related to diarrhea	Adequate hydration: pulse and blood pressure within patient norms, moist mucous membranes
Inadequate nutrition related to malabsorption	Adequate nutrition: stable body weight
Inadequate coping related to chronic illness	Adequate coping: patient reports strategies to deal with inflammatory bowel disease (IBD), patient sees disease as manageable
Potential for injury related to drug side effects and adverse effects	Absence of adverse drug effects: normal urine output, electrolyte and blood glucose levels within normal limits, no bruising

Interventions

Chronic pain. Perianal pain is treated with gentle cleansing, sitz baths, and skin protectants. Measures to relieve abdominal pain include administration of analgesics and antispasmodics and application of heat to the abdomen as ordered. Positioning, massage, relaxation, imagery, and other strategies, as described in Chapter 8, may also be used.

Put On Your Thinking Cap!

Compare and contrast ulcerative colitis and Crohn disease. How are they similar and how are they different?

Diarrhea. Easy access to a toilet and prompt response to calls for help reduce the chance of episodes of bowel incontinence. After each stool, gently clean and inspect the perianal area. If bedpans or bedside commodes are used, remove and clean them immediately and use room deodorizers to eliminate odors.

Prescribed drugs for diarrhea usually include antidiarrheals, antispasmodics, anticholinergics, antibiotics, and corticosteroids. The patient may be placed on NPO status or may be given only clear liquids when diarrhea is severe. Bed rest may be prescribed, or the patient may be encouraged simply to rest (see the Patient Teaching box).

Patient Teaching

Inflammatory Bowel Disease

Topics for patient teaching include the following:

- Stress reduction measures are recommended to help control your symptoms.
- Because people with inflammatory bowel disease (IBD) have increased risk of cancer, you should have regular colon screening.
- You can facilitate digestion by taking small bites, eating slowly, and chewing well.
- Avoid caffeine and other irritating fluids and foods; consume a high-calorie, low-residue diet.
- You need to know the names, dosages, and schedules of your prescribed drugs and know what effects should be reported to the health care provider.
- Resources: Crohn's and Colitis Foundation: http://www.crohnscolitisfoundation.org/

Fluid volume deficit. Severe diarrhea can quickly deplete the patient's fluid volume. Assess fluid status on an ongoing basis. Signs of fluid volume deficit are dry mucous membranes, hypotension, tachycardia, and decreased urine output. Intravenous fluids and TPN should be administered as ordered.

Inadequate nutrition. The patient with ulcerative colitis needs to avoid only foods that worsen symptoms. For the patient with Crohn disease, TPN and elemental enteral diets (e.g., Ensure) may be prescribed. The patient who is able to take solid food is usually placed on a low-residue diet without caffeine, pepper, or alcohol. Foods that are not allowed include whole grains, nuts, and raw fruits and vegetables. Consult a dietitian to teach the patient about the prescribed diet. Monitor the patient's weight on a routine basis.

Inadequate coping. IBD is painful and stressful and can interfere with the patient's everyday life. Try to establish a trusting relationship with the patient. Encourage independence, participation in care and decision making, and realistic goal setting. People who have IBD may benefit from therapy that assists them with stress management. With the patient's approval, initiate a referral to a mental health professional or spiritual counselor. Report sadness and discouragement to the registered nurse (RN) or health care provider.

Potential for injury. Nursing responsibilities in relation to drug therapy for IBD include administering the drugs, monitoring their effects, and teaching the patient about long-term drug therapy. Depending on the type and severity of IBD and the patient's age, various drugs may be used to treat acute attacks. Sulfasalazine is the antibiotic most often prescribed for patients with ulcerative colitis. It is useful in treating acute attacks and preventing future attacks. After an acute attack has subsided, maintenance therapy may be initiated. A maintenance dose typically is given for 6 to 12 months although some patients are treated longer. The patient is monitored to assess the effects of the drug as well as to detect adverse drug effects. Teach the patient that discontinuing the drug early may result in another acute attack.

If sulfasalazine is used, inform the patient that it can cause crystals to form in the urine (crystalluria), which can damage the kidneys. Patients taking this drug should take enough fluids to maintain a urine output of 1500 mL/day. A high urine output reduces the risk of crystalluria.

Corticosteroids are used in IBD for their ability to reduce inflammation. Unfortunately, this action also decreases the ability of the body to resist infection. Patients on steroids must be monitored for any signs and symptoms of infections. Instruct these patients to avoid unnecessary exposure to others with infectious conditions.

Long-term steroid therapy can have many other serious side effects. These include fluid and electrolyte imbalances, ulcers, increased blood glucose, weight gain, elevated blood pressure, acne, capillary fragility, and hirsutism (abnormal growth of hair).

DIVERTICULOSIS

Pathophysiology

Diverticulosis is a condition characterized by small, sac-like pouches in the intestinal wall called *diverticula*. Diverticula occur when weak areas of the intestinal wall allow segments of the mucous membrane to herniate outward (Fig. 39.6). Most diverticula are found in the sigmoid colon and usually more than one exists.

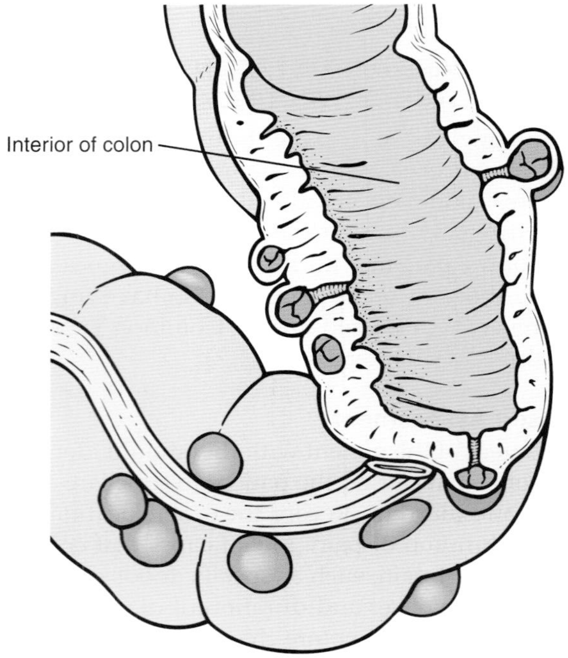

Fig. 39.6 Diverticula in the sigmoid colon. (From Lewis SM, Heitkemper MM, Dirksen SR, et al: *Medical-surgical nursing: assessment and management of clinical problems*, ed 9, St. Louis, 2015, Mosby.)

Risk Factors

Because diverticulosis is most common in Western and industrialized countries, it is thought that lack of dietary fiber is a contributing factor. Other related factors are high intake of red meat, lack of physical activity, obesity, and smoking.

Signs and Symptoms

Diverticulosis is often asymptomatic, but many people report changes in bowel habits. The change may be constipation, diarrhea, or periodic bouts of each. Other symptoms might include rectal bleeding, pain in the left lower abdomen, nausea and vomiting, and urinary problems.

Complications

Intestinal contents can lodge in diverticula, causing inflammation or infection. The patient is then said to have *diverticulitis*. Diverticulitis may be related to irritating foods, alcohol, chronic constipation, and persistent coughing. Contrary to popular opinion, the consumption of nuts, seeds, and popcorn does not cause diverticulitis (Pemberton, December 16, 2019). Symptoms of pain and bleeding are more severe with diverticulitis. The patient may also have a fever.

Possible complications of diverticulitis are severe bleeding, obstruction, perforation (rupture), peritonitis, abscess formation, and fistula formation. A fistula is an abnormal opening. In this case, it is most likely to develop between the colon and the bladder or vagina. The fistula permits bowel contents to pass into these other structures.

Medical Diagnosis

Diverticulosis is often found in patients with no symptoms during a routine colonoscopy. Abdominal CT with contrast is ordered for patients who present with symptoms suggestive of diverticulosis. In addition to the CT scan, the stool is tested for occult blood.

Medical Treatment

Diverticulosis is currently treated with a high-fiber diet with limited red meat. Stool softeners or bulk-forming laxatives are used to treat constipation. If pain is severe, it may be treated with analgesics. Broad-spectrum antibiotics are often prescribed. Anticholinergics may be given to decrease spasms in the colon.

During periods of acute inflammation, the patient is placed on bed rest and clear liquids or NPO status. Intravenous fluids are ordered. GI decompression may also be instituted.

If a diverticulum ruptures, the patient is at risk for peritonitis. The body attempts to "wall off" the area which can result in an abscess. An option is to drain the abscess through an abdominal puncture site. If symptoms persist and complications occur, surgical intervention may be necessary. The affected portion of the colon is removed. A temporary colostomy may be created to rest the colon while the surgical incisions heal. Sometimes elective surgery is recommended because the risk of surgical complications is much lower than it is with emergency surgery.

◆ NURSING CARE OF THE PATIENT WITH DIVERTICULOSIS

Focused Assessment

Monitor the patient's comfort and stool characteristics. Note any nausea and vomiting, monitor the patient's temperature, and examine the abdomen for distention and tenderness.

Patient Problems, Goals, and Outcome Criteria: Diverticulitis

Patient Problems	Goals and Outcome Criteria
Fluid volume deficit related to diarrhea and vomiting	Adequate hydration: pulse and blood pressure within patient norms, urine output approximately equal to fluid intake, moist mucous membranes
Acute pain related to inflammation	Pain relief: patient states pain is decreased or relieved, has relaxed manner
Potential for infection related to perforation	Absence of infection: no fever, normal white blood cell (WBC) count, abdomen soft and not tender

Interventions

Provide fluids as permitted and monitor the patient's intake and output. Give antiemetics as ordered for nausea. Analgesics and anticholinergics may be given as ordered for pain. Be alert for signs of perforation (i.e., fever, abdominal distention, rigidity). Teach the patient about diverticulosis, including the pathophysiology, treatment, and symptoms of inflammation.

If surgery is performed, the nursing care is similar to that described for any major abdominal surgery. General surgical care is discussed in Chapter 17 and care of the patient with an ostomy is discussed in Chapter 18.

COLORECTAL CANCER

Pathophysiology

Colorectal cancer, or cancer of the large intestine, is the third most common cancer in the U.S. People at greater risk for colorectal cancer are those with histories of IBD or family histories of colorectal cancer or multiple intestinal polyps. Some evidence indicates that a high-fat, low-fiber diet and inadequate intake of fruits and vegetables may also contribute to the development of this type of cancer.

Colorectal cancer can develop anywhere in the large intestine. Three-fourths of all colorectal cancers are located in the rectum or lower sigmoid colon.

Signs and Symptoms

Signs and symptoms of colorectal cancer depend on the location of the disease. In the early stages, symptoms are usually mild. If the cancer is located on the right side of the abdomen, the patient may have only vague cramping until the disease is advanced. Unexplained anemia, weakness, and fatigue related to blood loss may be the only early symptoms of right-sided colon cancer.

Cancers on the left side or in the rectum cause more obvious changes in bowel function. Patients may develop diarrhea or constipation and may notice blood in the stool. Stools may become very narrow, causing them to be described as pencil-like because of pressure on the bowel from the growing tumor, which causes a narrowed lumen. The patient may report a feeling of fullness or pressure in the abdomen or rectum. If left untreated, obstruction of the bowel eventually occurs regardless of the tumor site.

Medical and Surgical Treatment

Colorectal cancers are usually treated surgically. The exact surgical procedure depends on the location and extent of the cancer. For cancers above the rectum, the diseased portion of the intestine can often be removed. The healthy ends of the remaining intestine are then anastomosed (connected).

Rectal cancers often require more extensive surgery, with incisions in the abdomen and the perineum (abdominoperineal resection). With removal of the rectum, a permanent colostomy may be created for fecal elimination. However, relatively new procedures may be used to attach the rectal stump to the anus in patients with certain rectal cancers. When this is possible, normal bowel elimination can be maintained and a colostomy can be avoided.

Combination chemotherapy may be recommended postoperatively if the tumor extends through the bowel wall or if lymph nodes are involved. Rectal cancer is sometimes treated with radiation as well as surgery.

◆ NURSING CARE OF THE PATIENT WITH COLORECTAL CANCER

Because the primary treatment for colon cancer is surgery, nursing care focuses on the surgical patient. Preoperative care includes bowel preparation, hydration, emotional support, and teaching postoperative routines to prevent surgical complications. Care of the patient with an ostomy is discussed in Chapter 18 and care of patients who are receiving radiation or chemotherapy is discussed in Chapter 7.

Focused Assessment

In the postoperative period, assess vital signs, intake and output, breath sounds, bowel sounds, and pain. Describe the appearance of wounds and wound drainage. If the patient has a colostomy, measure and describe the fecal drainage. Assess the patient's reactions to the surgical procedure and any other anticipated therapies.

Patient Problems, Goals, and Outcome Criteria: Colorectal Cancer

Patient Problems	Goals and Outcome Criteria
Potential for injury related to extensive surgical trauma, open wounds	Wound healing without infection: no fever, intact wound margins without excessive redness
Inadequate peripheral tissue perfusion circulation related to effects of anesthesia, immobility	Adequate peripheral tissue perfusion: vital signs consistent with patient baseline norms, no edema or tenderness in legs
Acute pain related to tissue trauma	Pain relief: patient states less or no pain, relaxed manner
Sexual dysfunction related to perineal surgery	Patient understands potential for sexual dysfunction: patient describes possible problems and corrective measures
Inadequate coping related to life-threatening illness	Adequate coping: patient uses strategies that promote adaptation to illness

Interventions

Potential for injury. The nursing care of a patient after an abdominoperineal resection is very demanding. The patient has three incisions: one on the abdomen, a second for the colostomy, and a third on the perineum. Check all three incisions for bleeding or drainage. The perineal wound normally drains a large amount of serosanguinous fluid. Serosanguinous fluid is made up of serum and blood. It is a pinkish color and thin in consistency. The wound may be open and packed, partly closed with Penrose drains, or closed and drained with a suction device. An example of a suction drainage system is the Jackson-Pratt drain and fluid collection device. Dressings should initially be reinforced when saturated. Disposable waterproof pads under the patient's hips protect bedding and can be changed easily. A T-binder holds the perineal dressing securely in place.

With so many wounds, especially open ones, these patients are at great risk for infection. Any handling of wound dressings should be done wearing sterile gloves. Always assess the wound for signs of infection (i.e., unusual odor, excessive redness or swelling around the wound, purulent drainage).

If packing has been placed in a wound, it will be removed gradually. Once the packing has been removed completely, the health care provider may order the wound to be irrigated on a regular schedule. Gentle irrigations promote healing by keeping the wound clean. It is important to use strict sterile technique during wound irrigation.

Inadequate peripheral tissue perfusion. Because the abdominoperineal resection requires several incisions and is a lengthy procedure, the patient is at risk for respiratory and circulatory complications. Coughing, deep breathing, and incentive spirometry help to prevent fluid accumulation in the lungs. Encourage and help the patient to change positions at least every 2 hours. Leg exercises are important because the pressure on abdominal blood vessels during the long surgery may contribute to the formation of blood clots in the legs.

Acute Pain. Pain is severe for several postoperative days. Give opioid analgesics as ordered. Inform the health care provider if the drugs do not provide relief. In addition to drug therapy, implement comfort measures such as position changes and back rubs. At first, the patient will probably be most comfortable in a side-lying position. Later, they will be able to tolerate being supine as well.

When the patient is allowed to be up, sitz baths may be ordered several times a day. The warm water cleans, soothes, and increases circulation to the perineum. Supervise the patient in the sitz bath the first few times in case of dizziness or faintness.

Sexual dysfunction. Extensive perineal surgery can cause various types of sexual dysfunction. Be open and sensitive to questions that the patient may bring up about sexual function. Refer questions about the specific effects of particular surgical procedures on sexual function to the health care provider. The nurse should not dismiss or ignore patient concerns about sexuality, but the information given must be accurate. Once the correct answers are known, the nurse can reinforce them.

Inadequate coping. Patients with colorectal cancer and their families often face a difficult period of adjustment. For many people, the thought of having cancer brings up fears of pain, suffering, and a lingering death. These fears may not surface until after the patient recovers from the acute postoperative period. The nurse can help by encouraging the patient to express fears and ask questions and by being a kind listener. Referral to mental health or spiritual counselors or to support groups can be helpful (see the Patient Teaching box).

Patient Teaching

Colorectal Cancer

As the patient improves, the nurse needs to consider long-term needs. The teaching plan should include the following:

- Wound care
- Colostomy care (see Chapter 18)
- Information about resources for treatment of sexual dysfunction (if appropriate)
- Diet (Your diet should be high in fiber. Avoid irritating foods and alcohol.)
- Medications (For each of your medications, know the drug names, dosages, schedule, and adverse effects.)
- Symptoms of inflammation (Notify the health care provider if these symptoms of inflammation occur: bleeding, fever, and increased pain.)
- Resources: Wound Care and Ostomy Nurse (WOCN) (a nurse who is expert in the care of patients with wounds and ostomies); United Ostomy Association of American (www.ostomy.org).

While learning to deal with changes in body image and the threat of a potentially deadly disease, the patient may be faced with receiving chemotherapy and/or radiotherapy as well. Most patients have heard about the side effects of the powerful drugs used in chemotherapy and they may be justifiably fearful of the treatments. The nursing care of patients who are receiving chemotherapy and radiotherapy is discussed in detail in Chapter 7.

POLYPS

Polyps are growths in the intestine. Most are benign, but they can become malignant. Two inherited syndromes, familial polyposis and Gardner syndrome, are characterized by multiple colorectal polyps and almost always lead to cancer. Polyps are usually asymptomatic and are found on routine examination. Potential complications are bleeding and obstruction. Polyps are diagnosed by a barium enema examination or an endoscopic examination. Some of the growths can be removed during the endoscopic examination. Colectomy may be advised for patients with familial polyposis or Gardner syndrome because of the high risk of malignancy.

Patients who are at risk for cancer should be encouraged to seek medical attention. If the patient has surgery, the postoperative care is similar to that of the patient with cancer of the colon. If a colostomy is created, the patient needs special support and teaching, as described in Chapter 18.

HEMORRHOIDS

Hemorrhoids are dilated veins in the rectum. They may be above the sphincter muscles of the anus (internal hemorrhoids) or below these muscles (external hemorrhoids) (Fig. 39.7). If blood clots form in external hemorrhoids, they become inflamed and very painful. Hemorrhoids containing clotted blood are said to be thrombosed.

Risk Factors

A key factor in the development of hemorrhoids is increased pressure in the rectal blood vessels. Pressure is increased by constipation, pregnancy, and prolonged sitting or standing.

Signs and Symptoms

The most common symptoms of hemorrhoids are rectal pain and itching. Bleeding may occur with defecation, especially if the hemorrhoids are internal. External hemorrhoids are easy to see and appear red or bluish.

Medical Diagnosis and Treatment

Hemorrhoids are diagnosed on visual inspection. Nonsurgical treatment of hemorrhoids attempts to relieve pain, swelling, and pressure. Topical medications such as creams, lotions, or suppositories may be ordered to soothe and shrink inflamed tissue (see the Complementary and Alternative Therapies box). Sitz

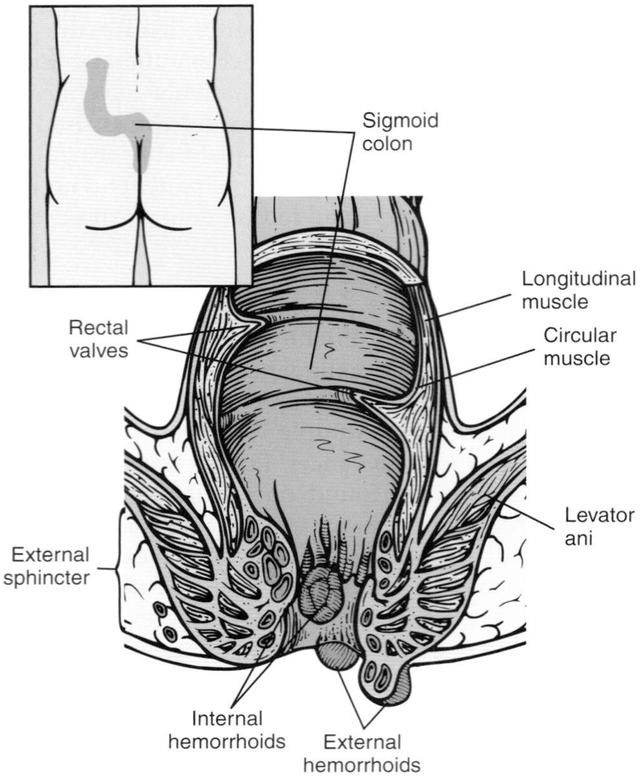

Fig. 39.7 Internal and external hemorrhoids. (From Monahan F, Sands J, Neighbors M, et al.: *Phipps' medical-surgical nursing: health and illness perspectives*, ed 8, St. Louis, 2007, Mosby.)

baths are often comforting. The health care provider may order heat or cold applications. Sometimes, especially with thrombosed hemorrhoids, ice packs may be applied for a few hours, followed by warm packs.

Complementary and Alternative Therapies

Witch hazel compresses applied to the anus after each bowel movement are soothing.

A hemorrhoidectomy is the surgical excision (removal) of hemorrhoids. It is necessary when symptoms are very severe. After the hemorrhoids are removed, the wound may be closed with sutures or packed and left open to heal.

Outpatient procedures for removing hemorrhoids include the following:

- Ligation: tying off with rubber bands. The bands cut off the blood supply so that the vessels shrink and die. Dead tissue eventually breaks off and is eliminated.
- Sclerotherapy: the injection of an agent into the tissue around the hemorrhoids that causes them to shrink. Results often are temporary.
- Thermocoagulation and electrocoagulation: use of different types of devices to remove the hemorrhoid.
- Laser surgery: effective but more expensive and risky.

◆ NURSING CARE OF THE PATIENT WITH HEMORRHOIDS

Medical management of hemorrhoids usually does not require hospitalization. Therefore, this section emphasizes the care of the surgical patient. Preoperative care may include an enema before the procedure. Patient teaching focuses on postoperative measures to manage pain, prevent constipation, and to promote healing.

Focused Assessment

After hemorrhoidectomy, monitor vital signs, intake and output, and breath sounds. Inspect the perianal area for bleeding and drainage.

Patient Problems, Goals, and Outcome Criteria: Posthemorrhoidectomy

Patient Problems	Goals and Outcome Criteria
Acute pain related to tissue trauma	Pain relief: patient states less or no pain, relaxed manner
Disrupted skin tissue integrity related to surgical procedure	Healthy wound healing: surgical incision healed, no signs of infection (excessive redness, purulent drainage, continued pain)
Constipation related to patient fear of pain with defecation	Normal defecation: patient passes stool with minimal pain

Interventions

Acute pain. Hemorrhoidectomy patients have severe postoperative pain that may require opioid analgesics if nonopioid drugs do not bring relief. Sitz baths in warm water are soothing. Because the patient may become lightheaded during the treatment, stay with them initially. Imagery and relaxation techniques also may help to control pain.

Disrupted skin tissue integrity. If wound packing is present, the health care provider removes it a day or two after surgery. After the packing is removed, it is important to assess for rectal bleeding. Sitz baths may then be ordered to soothe and clean the area and to promote circulation. Provide a soft pad or cushion for more comfortable sitting. "Donut" (circular) pads should not be used because they can impair circulation to the operative area.

Constipation. It is especially important to assess and record any stools passed after rectal surgery. The patient will probably dread the first bowel movement, expecting severe pain. Stool softeners or bulk forming agents will probably be ordered to reduce the trauma of defecation. Pain medication can be given as ordered before the patient tries to defecate (see the Patient Teaching box). Someone should stay close by in case the patient feels weak or faint.

Patient Teaching

Hemorrhoids, Postoperative Care

- Notify your surgeon if you have fever or bleeding.
- To prevent recurrence, avoid constipation, prolonged sitting or standing, and straining to have a bowel movement.
- Ingest a high-fiber diet with plenty of fluids to promote regular, soft stools.
- Use stool softeners or bulk-forming agents if prescribed.
- Follow a regular pattern of bowel elimination and do not delay defecation when the urge occurs.
- Follow the activity limitations prescribed by your health care provider.

ANORECTAL ABSCESS

An anorectal abscess is an infection in the tissue around the rectum. Signs and symptoms are rectal pain, swelling, redness, and tenderness. The patient often reports a history of diarrhea. If the abscess becomes chronic, it causes bleeding, itching, and discharge.

Anorectal abscess is treated with antibiotics followed by incision and drainage. The procedure may be done under local or general anesthesia, depending on how extensive the abscess is. Preoperatively, pain is treated with ice packs, sitz baths, and topical agents as ordered. Postoperatively, the nursing care is similar to that after hemorrhoidectomy. Pain is treated with opioid analgesics. Patient teaching emphasizes the importance of thorough cleansing after each bowel movement. Advise the patient to consume adequate fluids and a high-fiber diet to promote soft stools.

ANAL FISSURE

An anal fissure is a laceration between the anal canal and the perianal skin. Fissures may be related to constipation, diarrhea, Crohn disease, tuberculosis, leukemia, trauma, or childbirth. Sometimes a cause is not apparent. Signs and symptoms include pain before and after defecation and bleeding on the stool or tissue. If the fissure becomes chronic, the patient may experience pruritus, urinary frequency or retention, and dysuria. Fissures usually heal spontaneously but they can become chronic. Conservative treatment of anal fissures uses sitz baths, stool softeners, and analgesics. Surgical excision may be necessary. Postoperatively, instruct the patient to cleanse the perianal area after defecation. Pain relief measures and stool softeners are continued.

ANAL FISTULA

An anal fistula is an abnormal opening between the anal canal and the perianal skin. Fistulas can develop from anorectal abscesses or may be related to IBD or tuberculosis. The patient typically complains of pruritus and discharge. Sitz baths provide some comfort. The surgical treatment is excision of the fistula and surrounding tissue. Sometimes a temporary colostomy is done to allow the surgical site to heal. Postoperative care includes analgesics and sitz baths for pain.

PILONIDAL CYST

A pilonidal cyst is located in the sacrococcygeal area. It appears to result from an infolding of skin causing a sinus that is easily infected because of its closeness to the anus. Once infected, it is painful and swollen and may form an abscess. Surgical excision is usually recommended. Care is similar to that for the patient having a hemorrhoidectomy.

PATIENT EDUCATION TO PROMOTE NORMAL BOWEL FUNCTION

Nurses often have the opportunity to teach patients how to promote normal bowel function and detect problems early (see the Nutrition Considerations box later). Acute GI disorders can be caused by irritants or infectious agents. It is helpful for patients to identify and avoid foods that create distress.

Good hand washing and proper food handling reduce the ingestion of infectious agents. Food poisoning can be acquired from food that has been improperly stored, poorly cooked, or exposed to contaminated containers or utensils.

Food poisoning is often a problem for frail older adults who live at home. Poor vision and smell can make food management difficult. It is a good idea for the home health nurse to check the patient's refrigerator and food cabinets to identify potential problems.

People who recognize that stress affects their GI function may benefit from relaxation techniques and stress management training.

Signs and symptoms of possibly serious digestive problems should be reported for prompt diagnosis and treatment if indicated. GI symptoms that could indicate gastric cancer include persistent gastric distress, anorexia, and weight loss. Rectal bleeding, a change in bowel habits, or both often occur with intestinal cancer. As part of the annual physical examination for people older than 40 years, many health care providers do a rectal examination and test the stool for occult blood. For men and women, the American Cancer Society recommends periodic colonoscopy and fecal occult blood tests at intervals (see Chapter 7).

Teaching patients what is normal, how to promote normal bowel function, and how to detect problems can help to avoid serious GI dysfunction (see the Nutrition Considerations box).

Nutrition Considerations

1. Diarrhea is caused by pathogenic organisms, diet, intestinal lesions, or irritations associated with various diseases or conditions.
2. Replacement of lost fluids is the goal of nutritional therapy for diarrhea.
3. Constipation is caused by insufficient fiber intake, insufficient fluid intake, lack of exercise, some drugs, and the habitual use of laxatives.
4. The dietary treatment of constipation consists of increasing fluid (8–10 glasses of water a day) and fiber intake.
5. A hot drink such as coffee or tea enhances peristalsis and promotes defecation.

Get Ready for the NCLEX® Examination!

Key Points

- When conservative efforts at weight loss fail, the obese person may be recommended for bariatric surgery.
- Most weight loss surgical procedures limit the stomach capacity.
- The obese surgical patient is at increased risk for postoperative complications.
- Various types of malabsorption (a condition in which one or more nutrients are not digested or absorbed) exist.
- Diarrhea is the frequent passage of loose or liquid stools. It can lead to fluid and electrolyte imbalances, metabolic acidosis, and malnutrition.
- Constipation is the difficult passage of hard, dry stools. It may be related to inactivity, dehydration, a low-fiber diet, some drugs, and a variety of medical conditions.
- Fecal impaction is the retention of a large mass of stool in the rectum that the patient cannot pass and that may require removal with enemas and manual extraction.
- Factors that can cause intestinal obstruction include strangulated hernia, tumor, paralytic ileus, stricture, volvulus, intussusception, and postoperative adhesions.
- Appendicitis is inflammation of the appendix that requires surgical treatment to prevent rupture and peritonitis.
- A hernia is a portion of intestine that bulges through a weak area in the muscles of the abdominal wall and can become incarcerated (trapped) and obstructed.
- IBD, characterized by inflammation and ulceration of the lining of the intestines, includes ulcerative colitis and Crohn disease.
- Nursing care of the patient with IBD focuses on pain, diarrhea, fluid volume deficit, inadequate nutrition, inadequate coping, and potential for injury.
- Diverticulosis is characterized by small, saclike pouches in the intestinal wall that can become inflamed, causing obstruction, perforation, peritonitis, and fistula formation.
- Nursing care of the patient with colorectal cancer, which is usually treated surgically, focuses on potential for injury, inadequate peripheral tissue circulation, pain, sexual dysfunction, and inadequate coping.
- Polyps are small growths in the intestine that are usually benign but may be removed because they may bleed, cause obstructions, or become malignant.
- Hemorrhoids are dilated rectal veins that can become inflamed and thrombosed; they are treated with topical medications, sitz baths, heat or cold, sclerotherapy, or surgical excision.
- Anal disorders include abscesses, fissures, and fistulas, all of which may be treated surgically.

Additional Learning Resources

SG Go to your Study Guide for additional learning activities to help you master this chapter content.

Go to your Evolve website (http://evolve.elsevier.com/Linton/medsurg) for the following learning resources and much more:
- Fluid & Electrolyte Tutorial
- Review Questions for the NCLEX® Examination

Clinical Judgment and Next-Generation NCLEX® Examination-Style Questions

1. A patient who was admitted with severe abdominal pain is being evaluated for possible appendicitis. The physician should be notified immediately if the nurse's assessment reveals which of the following?

1. The patient's WBC count is 15,000/mm^3.
2. Palpation at McBurney point causes pain.
3. The patient keeps both hips flexed.
4. The patient's abdomen is rigid.

NCLEX Client Need: Physiological Integrity: Physiological Adaptation

2. A patient asks if surgery would cure her Crohn disease. She states that her friend's ulcerative colitis was cured with surgery. The nurse would explain that surgery is used to treat Crohn disease less often than to treat ulcerative colitis for what reason? Crohn disease:

1. usually returns near the site of the anastomosis.
2. typically involves the entire small and large intestines.
3. can usually be cured with combination drug therapy.
4. is associated with an increased risk of surgical complications.

NCLEX Client Need: Physiological Integrity: Reduction of Risk Potential

3. The nurse is asked to speak at a support group for people with ulcerative colitis. Which content should be included in the presentation? (Select all that apply.)

1. Stress management may help to control symptoms.
2. Ulcerative colitis is caused by a bacterial infection.
3. Avoid caffeine and any food that causes symptoms.
4. Have regular colon screening examinations.
5. Medications are needed only when acute symptoms occur.

NCLEX Client Need: Physiological Integrity: Reduction of Risk Potential

4. SLO/Objective: Apply knowledge of anatomy and physiology and pathophysiology to determine which assessment data require follow-up by the nurse.

NGN Item Type: Enhanced Hot Spot

Cognitive Skill: Recognize Cues

A 16-year-old female presents to the camp clinic with abdominal pain. The nurse's focused assessment provides the following data.

- Temperature: 100°F (oral)
- Heart rate: 98 beats per minute
- Respiratory rate: 22 breaths per minute
- Blood pressure: 138/70 mm Hg
- Pain rated 8 on a 10-point scale
- Pain upon palpation of right lower quadrant
- Bowel sounds present all four quadrants

Highlight or place a check mark next to the assessment findings that require follow-up by the nurse.

NCLEX Client Need: Physiologic Integrity

NCLEX Client Need: Health Promotion and Maintenance

5. **The nurse is reviewing the record of a female client with Crohn disease. Which stool characteristics would the nurse expect to find in the patient's history?**
   1. Diarrhea
   2. Chronic constipation
   3. Constipation alternating with diarrhea
   4. Stools constantly oozing from the rectum

   NCLEX Client Need: Safe and Effective Care Environment

6. **The nurse recognizes the need for additional teaching when a patient with celiac disease states:**
   1. "I should suggest that my sister be screened for celiac disease."
   2. Following a gluten-free diet will not cure celiac disease, but will improve symptoms.
   3. "I really don't need to restrict my diet of gluten-containing foods, unless I am having diarrhea."
   4. "It will be difficult to find gluten-free foods, as gluten is part of so many types of food."

   NCLEX Client Need: Safe and Effective Care Environment

7. **As the nurse, you teach your patient with diverticulosis to: (Select all that apply.)**
   1. Use prescribed anticholinergic medications to prevent bowel spasm
   2. Get an annual colonoscopy to detect any possible changes that may be cancerous
   3. Consume a high-fiber diet and take bulk laxatives to increase fecal volume
   4. Avoid whole-grain breads and cereals to prevent further irritation of the bowel

   NCLEX Client Need: Safe and Effective Care Environment

8. **A patient in the clinic is prescribed an immunosuppressant drug for treatment of IBD. Which patient teaching point related to this drug is appropriate?**
   1. Always take your medication with food or milk
   2. Avoid people with active infections
   3. Stop the medication if you have diarrhea
   4. Take this medication only when you have symptoms

   NCLEX Client Need: Physiological Integrity: Pharmacological Therapies

9. **Residents of an assisted living facility have asked how they can reduce the risk of colon cancer. The nurse should recommend a high intake of which of the following? (Select all that apply.)**
   1. Vegetables
   2. Fruits
   3. Fat
   4. Fiber
   5. Proteins

   NCLEX Client Need: Physiological Integrity: Reduction of Risk Potential

40 Liver, Gallbladder, and Pancreatic Disorders

http://evolve.elsevier.com/Linton/medsurg

Objectives

1. Explain the pathology, signs and symptoms, diagnosis, complications, and medical treatment of selected disorders of the liver, gallbladder, and pancreas.
2. Assist in developing a nursing care plan for the patient with liver, gallbladder, or pancreatic dysfunction.

Key Terms

cholecystectomy (kō-lĕ-sĭs-TĔK-tō-mē)
cholecystitis (kō-lĕ-sĭs-TĪ-tĭs)
choledocholithiasis (kō-lĕd-ō-kō-lĭ-THĪ-ă-sĭs)
cholelithiasis (kō-lĕ-lĭ-THĪ-ă-sĭs)
cirrhosis (sĭr-RŌ-sĭs)
eructation (ĕ-rŭk-TĀ-shŭn)
hepatic (hĕ-PĂ-tĭc)
hepatitis (hĕ-pă-TĪ-tĭs)

DISORDERS OF THE LIVER

When referring to the liver, the term **hepatic** is commonly used, as in hepatic circulation, hepatic enlargement, or hepatic pathology.

HEPATITIS

Hepatitis is inflammation of the liver. Globally, the incidence of acute viral hepatitis is decreasing because of improved hygiene and effective vaccines. In the United States, an estimated 71,900 new cases of hepatitis B and C occurred in 2018. However, it is believed that as many as 5.3 million Americans are living with chronic hepatitis B or C. Although many patients have an uneventful recovery, others develop chronic conditions that eventually can lead to liver failure and death.

Pathophysiology

Hepatitis has local and systemic effects. Locally, the inflammatory process causes the liver to swell. If swelling is severe, two important effects occur. First, the bile channels are compressed, damaging the cells that produce bile. This results in an elevation in serum bilirubin and jaundice. Second, blood flow through the liver is impaired, causing pressure to rise in the portal circulation (see Chapter 37, Fig. 37.5).

Systemic effects are related to altered metabolic functions normally performed by the liver and to the infectious response in viral hepatitis. Systemic signs and symptoms of hepatitis include rash, angioedema, arthritis, fever, and malaise.

Types of Hepatitis

Hepatitis can be classified as *infectious* or *noninfectious*. Viruses known to cause infectious hepatitis are classified as types A, B, C, D, and E. Hepatitis G virus and hepatitis GB virus type C have been identified, but their precise role in human liver disease is not well understood. Other viruses that may cause acute inflammatory liver disease include human cytomegalovirus, Epstein-Barr virus, and herpes simplex virus. It is likely that some yet-to-be-identified viruses are also involved. Noninfectious hepatitis is caused by exposure to toxic chemicals, including drugs. Key features of each type of hepatitis are summarized in Table 40.1.

Hepatitis A. Hepatitis A has been called *infectious hepatitis* and *epidemic hepatitis*. It is caused by the hepatitis A virus (HAV), which is transmitted from one person to another by way of water, food, or medical equipment that has been contaminated with infected fecal matter. Hepatitis A is the most common type of viral hepatitis. Fortunately, it is rarely fatal and infected persons do not become asymptomatic carriers.

Hepatitis B. Hepatitis B is caused by the hepatitis B virus (HBV). Because HBV is found in all body fluids of infected persons, modes of transmission include intimate contact with carriers as well as contact with contaminated blood or medical equipment. IV drug users who share needles are also at risk for contracting the virus. Among medical personnel, infection may occur following an injury with sharp items that are contaminated with the body fluids of infected patients. Current screening procedures make it highly unlikely that hepatitis will be transmitted in a blood transfusion. Hepatitis B can be transmitted from an infected mother

Table 40.1 Key Features of Each Type of Viral Hepatitis

TYPE	CAUSE	TRANSMISSION ROUTE	PREVENTION	TREATMENT
Hepatitis A	Hepatitis A virus (HAV)	Fecal-oral route (often via contaminated water or food). Infected food handler, poor sanitation. Incubation period: 15 to 50 days	Wash hands after toileting. Use clean water and food supplies. Use gloves to handle stool specimens and soiled articles. A vaccine is recommended for all children and for adults who wish to be protected. After exposure: HAV vaccine should be given to adults within 2 weeks after exposure.	No curative treatment is available. Usually resolves spontaneously.
Hepatitis B	Hepatitis B virus (HBV)	Contaminated blood introduced through the skin or mucous membranes (often via contaminated needles or other medical or dental equipment). Sexual contact. Newborns may be infected before, during, or after birth. Incubation period: 45 to 180 days	Use disposable needles. Avoid contaminated articles. Screen blood donors. Use caution with body fluids. A vaccine is recommended for infants and others, including nurses, who are at risk for exposure. Hepatitis B immune globulin (HBIG) is given after exposure.	*Acute* hepatitis B: no drugs are available. Treated with rest, good nutrition and hydration, and avoidance of alcohol. *Chronic* hepatitis B: may be treated with interferon alfa-2b, peginterferon alfa-2a, and antiviral such as lamivudine.
Hepatitis C	Hepatitis C virus (HCV)	Contaminated blood introduced through the skin or mucous membranes (often via contaminated needles or other medical or dental equipment). Although rare, it can be transmitted via sexual intercourse. Unborn babies may be infected by their mothers. Incubation period: 14 to 180 days	Use disposable needles. Avoid contaminated articles. Screen blood donors. Avoid risky sexual practices with people who may have hepatitis C. Do not share personal items such as razors. Use caution with body fluids. No vaccine is available.	Treated with peginterferon, ribavirin, and either boceprevir or telaprevir. Side effects of interferon include flulike symptoms, hair loss, low blood count, depression, and thinking difficulties. Success varies with the genotype of HCV.
Hepatitis D	"Delta agent" hepatitis D virus (HDV)	Contaminated blood or equipment or sexual contact. Can cause infection only when HBV is present. Incubation period: 2 to 26 weeks	The hepatitis B vaccine is given. Hepatitis D cannot infect unless hepatitis B is present.	Treated with pegylated interferon.
Hepatitis E	Hepatitis E virus (HEV)	Fecal-oral route (often via contaminated water or food). Incubation period: 15 to 64 days	Wash hands after toileting. Use clean water and food supplies. Use gloves to handle stool specimens and soiled articles. A vaccine has been developed but is not yet available for general use. For prevention, IG can be given before or within 48 hours after exposure.	Usually resolves in several weeks to months without treatment.

to her baby. Adult infections spontaneously resolve in most cases. Individuals who do not clear the infection develop chronic hepatitis and become carriers, meaning that they can transmit the infection to others. Globally, an estimated 257 million people are HBV carriers. Chronic hepatitis B also increases the risk of cirrhosis, liver failure, and liver cancer. Vaccination of children and high-risk groups, including health care workers, has dramatically decreased the incidence of hepatitis B.

Hepatitis C. Hepatitis C (HCV) is transmitted by contact with contaminated blood or medical equipment or by contact with infected body fluids. Like hepatitis B, it can be transmitted from an infected mother to her baby during birth; however, that is rare. HCV infection is commonly asymptomatic and undiagnosed. Although some individuals recover completely from acute hepatitis C, a significant proportion of people with hepatitis C develop chronic infections and become carriers. Many of these people will develop cirrhosis or cancer of the liver. In the United States, 19,000 deaths per year are attributed to HCV infection.

Hepatitis D. Hepatitis D is caused by a virus known as the *delta agent*, which is a defective ribonucleic acid (RNA) virus that can survive only in the company of HBV. Hepatitis D is transmitted percutaneously (through the skin or mucous membranes) with or following HBV infection. The presence of hepatitis D greatly increases the risk that the patient will progress to chronic hepatitis and possible liver failure.

Hepatitis E. Hepatitis E is similar to hepatitis A and is most commonly transmitted via water or food contaminated with infected fecal matter. Hepatitis E infection is rare in the United States, except among people who have traveled in developing countries where the virus is more common. No long-term, chronic form of hepatitis E infection exists.

Noninfectious hepatitis. Although the cause is not always identifiable, noninfectious hepatitis can be the result of exposure to toxins such as mercury and arsenic and drugs such as alcohol and acetaminophen.

Clinical Manifestations

Regardless of the cause, the signs and symptoms of hepatitis are similar. Differences occur in the number and severity of the symptoms from one person to the next. Many patients have no symptoms at all. For those who are symptomatic, the course of the disease is fairly predictable.

Acute hepatitis. Common findings in the acute phase include malaise, severe headache, right upper quadrant abdominal pain, anorexia, nausea, vomiting, fever, arthralgia (joint pain), rash, enlarged lymph nodes, urticaria, and enlargement and tenderness of the liver. The patient may or may not have yellowish skin discoloration called jaundice, light- or clay-colored stools, and dark urine typical of impaired bile production and secretion. Hepatitis patients who do not develop jaundice are said to have *anicteric hepatitis*. The accumulation of bile salts under the skin may cause pruritus. The acute phase usually lasts from 1 to 6 months and is the period when the patient is most infectious.

Convalescence. In the convalescent phase, jaundice fades but fatigue, malaise, and liver enlargement persist for weeks to months. Most patients with hepatitis A and B recover completely although some have relapses where symptoms recur. Some patients with HBV and most patients with HCV progress to chronic hepatitis.

Complications of acute hepatitis include chronic hepatitis, fulminant hepatitis, cirrhosis of the liver, and liver cancer. Some patients with hepatitis B or C become carriers. About one-fourth of those who become carriers will have chronic active hepatitis, which can lead to cirrhosis. Carriers are also at increased risk for liver cancer. People who have had hepatitis cannot donate blood because of the risk of transmitting the disease to a recipient.

Chronic hepatitis. Chronic hepatitis is characterized by a prolonged recovery with continuing fatigue and liver enlargement. Signs and symptoms persist for more than 6 months. Liver damage continues and may lead to cirrhosis. If necrosis of damaged cells occurs without regeneration, fulminant hepatitis results. Severe liver failure may follow and is often fatal unless a liver transplant is done.

Medical Diagnosis

A diagnosis of hepatitis is based on the presence of viral antigens and antibodies and RNA tests specific to each type of hepatitis. If the hepatitis virus is confirmed, viral genotyping may be done to identify the treatment most likely to be successful. The effects of the infection on the liver may cause liver function tests to be abnormal. Typical findings consistent with hepatitis include elevated levels of serum enzymes (aspartate aminotransferase [AST], alanine aminotransferase [ALT], gamma-glutamyl transpeptidase [GGT]), serum and urinary bilirubin, and urinary urobilinogen. The prothrombin time (PT) may be prolonged. Albumin and gamma globulin may be normal or low. A number of other blood studies may be ordered as well. A liver biopsy may be done to evaluate harm caused by chronic hepatitis B or C; however, new tests are noninvasive and safer. They include ultrasound elastography and FibroSure (a blood test) that determine the degree of liver fibrosis.

Medical Treatment

Acute hepatitis A usually requires no treatment as it typically resolves spontaneously and does not become chronic. Most patients with acute hepatitis B spontaneously clear the virus without drug therapy. Chronic hepatitis B can usually be controlled with nucleoside and nucleotide analog antiviral drugs (e.g., lamivudine, tenofovir, entecavir) sometimes in combination with an immune modulator such as pegylated interferon. Acute hepatitis C is treated with direct acting antiviral agent. The goal is to prevent the infection from becoming chronic. The biggest breakthrough in hepatitis treatment has been the development of drugs that are effective against chronic hepatitis C. Combinations of sofosbuvir and various other antiviral drugs have effected a cure in a high proportion of patients with

Box 40.1 Examples of Drugs Used to Treat Chronic Viral Hepatitis B and C

- Immune modulator: pegylated interferon
- Nucleoside and nucleotide analogs
  lamivudine
  telbivudine
  tenofovir
- Direct acting antiviral drugs for HCV
  simeprevir
  declatasvir
  sofosbuvir
- Combination therapies
  elbasvir + grazoprevir (Zepatier)
  ledipasvir + sofosbuvir (Harvoni)

specific strains 1 and 6 of hepatitis C. Two of the combination drugs are marketed as Harvoni and Vosevi. Mavyret, a different combination of drugs, is effective against six strains of the virus (see Box 40.1).

Other drugs may be prescribed to treat symptoms of hepatitis such as fever and nausea. The selection of drugs is important because hepatotoxic drugs (those that are toxic to the liver) should not be given.

Patients with viral hepatitis should consume a well-balanced diet. In some cases, various supplements may be advised based on the patient's nutritional status. Recommended activity depends on the patient's signs and symptoms and liver function tests. Bed rest may be ordered during the acute phase but practices vary.

Pharmacology Capsule

Hepatotoxic drugs are contraindicated for the patient with hepatitis because they can cause further damage to liver cells.

Prevention

As with any infection, the risk of acquiring viral hepatitis can be reduced by good hygiene and avoidance of possible contaminated sources. Individuals with known hepatitis B can protect intimate partners by using condoms during intercourse. Household members should be encouraged to be vaccinated. The infected person should not share personal items such as razors and toothbrushes. Contact with blood should be avoided.

All care providers can reduce their risk of exposure by strict adherence to Standard Precautions. The Centers for Disease Control and Prevention (CDC) recommends that adults up to 40 years of age who are exposed to hepatitis A be given the HAV vaccine within 2 weeks of exposure to prevent infection. In adults over 40 years of age, immunoglobulin (Ig) may be given rather than the HAV vaccine. Active disease may be averted in patients who have been exposed to HBV by administering the HBV vaccine and hepatitis B immune globulin (HBIG), preferably within 24 hours after exposure.

Vaccines are available to immunize people against hepatitis A and B. At this time, no vaccine is available to prevent type C. A hepatitis E vaccine has been developed but its efficacy is still under study. Because hepatitis D can exist only in the presence of the B virus, the vaccine for hepatitis B also protects against type D.

Health Promotion Box

The CDC (April 2020) recommends that all people ages 18 and older have a one-time screening test for HCV. Detection of unrecognized infection permits treatment to avoid future complications.

◆ NURSING CARE OF THE PATIENT WITH HEPATITIS

Focused Assessment

Nursing assessment of the patient with a digestive disease is outlined in Chapter 37, Box 37.1. When taking a health history of the person with hepatitis, essential data include information about general health state; drug and alcohol use; chemical exposure; dietary habits; blood transfusions; recent travel; GI disturbances; and changes in skin, urine, or stools. The physical examination includes vital signs, inspection of skin, weight changes, and mental status.

Patient Problems, Goals, and Outcome Criteria: Hepatitis

Patient Problems	Goals and Outcome Criteria
Decreased activity tolerance related to fatigue and prescribed bed rest	Improved activity tolerance: patient reports less fatigue and improved activity tolerance
Potential for complications of immobility related to fatigue, prescribed bed rest	Absence of complications of immobility: skin intact, breath sounds clear, no calf tenderness
Inadequate nutrition related to anorexia, nausea, and vomiting	Adequate dietary intake: stable body weight
Fluid volume deficit related to inadequate intake, vomiting	Normal hydration status: fluid output equal to intake, vital signs consistent with patient norms, moist mucous membranes
Potential for disrupted skin tissue integrity related to pruritus and scratching	Intact skin: no abrasions
Altered body image related to jaundice	Improved body image: patient expresses acceptance of skin discoloration
Anxiety related to hospitalization, unfamiliar procedures, serious illness	Decreased anxiety: patient states that anxiety is decreased or absent, calm manner
Inability to manage stet self-care related to lack of knowledge	Manages treatment plan: patient describes and adheres to plan of care

Interventions

Decreased activity tolerance and potential for complications of immobility. Most patients with acute viral hepatitis are treated at home, so instructions about activity limitations are needed. The extent of activity limitation depends on the severity of symptoms. Although the patient is asymptomatic, various levels of rest and activity may be advised. Explain that rest allows the liver to heal by regenerating new cells to replace those damaged by hepatitis. Help the patient to plan care activities to permit undisturbed times. Suggest diversions such as reading, television, and "visits" on Zoom or FaceTime to combat boredom. If the patient is being treated at home, explain the importance of rest. Some household tasks may need to be redistributed.

Unless the patient has severe complications, complete bed rest is usually not necessary. If complete bed rest is ordered, the patient is at risk for complications of immobility. Inspect the skin for early signs of pressure (redness, especially over bony prominences). If the patient is unable to turn independently, assist with turning at least every 2 hours. Moisturizing lotions protect the skin and can help to relieve itching associated with jaundice. Teach the patient to cough and deep breathe every 2 hours to reduce the risk of pneumonia. Gentle exercise of the legs promotes circulation and discourages the formation of thrombi. Discourage crossing of the legs. Inactivity tends to lead to constipation and may cause urinary stasis. Record bowel movements and urine output and describe any abnormal characteristics of stool and urine. Care of the immobilized patient is discussed in detail in Chapter 12.

Inadequate nutrition. Good nutrition is essential to decrease demands on the liver (see the Nutrition Considerations box). Specific dietary orders depend on the extent of liver dysfunction. With uncomplicated hepatitis, protein requirements are the same or slightly higher than that for healthy adults. Fat intake may be restricted. Provide written information about dietary needs to the home caregiver.

Unfortunately, anorexia is a common symptom of hepatitis. Measures to manage anorexia include small, frequent meals, a pleasant eating environment, frequent oral hygiene, and explanations of the need for a balanced diet. Occasionally, supplemental feedings are required to increase nutritional intake.

Nausea and vomiting can also contribute to nutritional deficits and fluid and electrolyte imbalances. Best results are usually obtained by administering an antiemetic as soon as nausea is reported. A cool, damp cloth applied to the face and neck is sometimes helpful. When the patient vomits, note the amount and contents of vomitus (emesis) as well as any visible blood. Measure emesis and record the volume as output. Remove soiled clothing, linens, and basins promptly and handle them according to agency infection control guidelines.

Fluid volume deficit. The patient with hepatitis needs to maintain a fluid intake of 2500 to 3000 mL/day unless contraindicated. If the patient is hospitalized, maintain intake and output records. If the patient's fluid intake is low or if vomiting is present, also monitor for dehydration. Signs of dehydration include dry mucous membranes, tachycardia, concentrated urine, and confusion. Patients who are at risk for dehydration may receive intravenous (IV) fluids as prescribed. Patients with liver disease are also at risk for fluid volume excess. Signs of fluid retention include edema, increasing abdominal girth, and rising blood pressure (BP).

Potential for disrupted skin tissue integrity. Pruritus, or itching, is a distressing symptom. Patients naturally respond by scratching, which may cause breaks in the skin. Nursing measures are designed to reduce dryness and irritation. The patient should bathe in tepid water and pat dry. Mild soap may be used unless it seems to increase symptoms. Lubricating lotions or topical antipruritics may be applied. You can suggest that the patient gently pat the skin instead of scratching to reduce the itching sensation. If a patient is confused, trim the fingernails as agency policy permits. Mittens may be needed to prevent skin injury. If conservative measures are not effective, consult the health care provider about ordering an antihistamine.

Altered body image. The patient with jaundice may be self-conscious about their appearance. Demonstrate acceptance of the patient and explain that the skin color usually returns to normal in 2 to 4 weeks.

Anxiety. Diagnostic tests and procedures and possible hospitalization can provoke anxiety in the patient with hepatitis. The patient may also be fearful about the expected course of the disease and the risk of complications. Encourage questions and find out what the patient wants to know. Explain what to expect to reduce the fear of the unknown. Explore how patients usually deal with stress and help them to identify coping strategies. If the patient has a history of drug or alcohol abuse, provide information about support groups such as Alcoholics Anonymous and Narcotics Anonymous.

Inability to manage treatment plan. The patient with chronic hepatitis who does not respond to treatment must learn how to live with the disease (see the Patient Teaching box). Good nutrition, exercise, adequate sleep, and avoidance of illicit drugs and alcohol can slow the progression of the disease. Explain any prescribed treatment and the importance of taking medications as prescribed. If the patient is a sexually active female, explain that many drugs used to treat hepatitis can cause birth defects. Oral contraceptives may be ineffective, so condoms, spermicidal jelly or foam, or a diaphragm should also be used.

Patient Teaching

Hepatitis

Take precautions to avoid exposing others to the virus. Precautions vary with the type of hepatitis, but the following guidelines are helpful:

- People who have had close contact with you should see a physician immediately. A vaccine or immunoglobulin (Ig) may be available to protect them from infection.
- Do not share personal items or utensils with others.
- Wash your hands thoroughly after toileting.
- If you have hepatitis B, use condoms for sexual intercourse; your partner should be vaccinated against the hepatitis B virus (HBV).
- Do not expose others to your blood.

Staff protection. When patients are hospitalized, Standard Precautions are implemented. Nurses are at risk for exposure to hepatitis because they often handle body fluids. The Occupational Safety and Health Administration (OSHA) requires hepatitis B vaccination for nurses and other health care providers. The vaccine is given in a series of three injections and confers long-term immunity on most people. Follow-up testing may be done to assess the titer level, which is a measure of immunity. If the antibody titer is inadequate, up to three booster doses may be given. Vaccination has significantly decreased hepatitis B among health care providers; however, no vaccine exists for hepatitis C.

Table 40.1 summarizes precautions to be used to prevent transmission of hepatitis.

ALCOHOL-ASSOCIATED LIVER DISEASE

Pathophysiology

The three kinds of liver disease related to alcohol consumption are (1) alcohol-associated steatosis (fatty liver), (2) alcoholic hepatitis, and (3) alcohol-associated cirrhosis.

Alcohol-associated steatosis (fatty liver). Most people who drink alcohol in excess develop fatty liver characterized by a buildup of fat cells in the liver. Patients may experience discomfort in the upper abdomen caused by liver enlargement, but many people have no symptoms. Fatty liver is reversible if alcohol intake ceases. The accumulation of fat in the liver not associated with alcohol, hepatitis, or autoimmune disease is called *nonalcoholic fatty liver disease* (NAFLD).

Alcoholic hepatitis. Inflammation of the liver is fairly common with heavy alcohol consumption. It may be acute or chronic. In some cases, life-threatening complications develop. Clinical manifestations may include fever, anorexia, nausea and vomiting, abdominal pain and tenderness, and jaundice.

Alcohol-associated cirrhosis. Individuals who ingest excessive amounts of alcohol are at risk for developing alcoholic cirrhosis, a condition in which normal liver cells are replaced by scar tissue. The risk is increased for individuals who have alcohol-induced liver disease and another chronic liver disease such as hepatitis C. Although cirrhosis is not exclusively related to alcohol use, alcohol is the most common contributing factor. Cirrhosis is discussed next.

CIRRHOSIS

Pathophysiology

Cirrhosis is a chronic, progressive disease of the liver. It is characterized by degeneration and destruction of liver cells. Fibrotic bands of connective tissue impair the flow of blood and lymph and distort the normal liver structure.

As cirrhosis progresses, significant disruption of many physiologic processes occurs. The effects of liver disease include metabolic disturbances, blood abnormalities, fluid and electrolyte imbalances, decreased resistance to infection, accumulation of drugs and toxins, and obstruction of blood vessels and bile ducts in the liver.

Cirrhosis is described as *compensated* or *decompensated*. Both types are characterized by fibrosis and nodules, but the presence of ascites, bleeding varices, encephalopathy, or jaundice defines decompensated cirrhosis.

Incidence

The highest incidence of cirrhosis is in people between the ages of 40 and 60 years. It is the twelfth leading cause of death in the United States (see the Cultural Considerations box). It is more common in men than in women. The pathology is most often related to alcohol-associated liver disease (as described previously), chronic hepatitis C, or nonalcoholic liver disease. However many other factors can lead to cirrhosis.

Cultural Considerations

What Does Culture Have to Do With Cirrhosis?

Native Americans and Alaska Natives have the highest rate of deaths from liver disease in the United States.

Types of Cirrhosis

Four major types of cirrhosis are classified based on cause: (1) alcohol-associated cirrhosis, (2) postnecrotic cirrhosis, (3) biliary cirrhosis, and (4) cardiac cirrhosis. Several other types occur infrequently.

- Alcohol-associated cirrhosis. This type of cirrhosis is caused by exposure to alcohol. The liver enlarges, becomes "knobby," and then shrinks. Alcoholic cirrhosis is not reversible.
- Postnecrotic cirrhosis. Postnecrotic cirrhosis can be a complication of hepatitis in which massive liver

cell necrosis occurs. It may also be related to exposure to liver toxins including some drugs.
- Biliary cirrhosis. Biliary cirrhosis develops as a result of obstruction to bile flow.
- Cardiac cirrhosis. Cardiac cirrhosis follows severe right-sided heart failure. Venous congestion and hypoxia lead to necrosis of liver cells.

Clinical Manifestations

In the early stage, signs and symptoms of cirrhosis are usually subtle. The patient may report slight weight loss, unexplained fever, fatigue, and dull heaviness in the right upper quadrant of the abdomen. These symptoms are probably the result of inflammation and enlargement of the liver. The liver may be palpable below the right rib margin.

As the disease progresses, impaired metabolism of carbohydrates, fats, and proteins causes GI disturbances such as anorexia, nausea, vomiting, diarrhea or constipation, flatulence, and dyspepsia (heartburn). Resistance to blood flow from the intestines to the liver causes circulation to become congested in the intestines, stomach, and esophagus. Elevated pressure in veins in the GI tract causes them to dilate and bulge. Dilated veins in the esophagus are called *esophageal varices* and those in the rectum are called *hemorrhoids*. Prominent veins may be visible on the abdomen.

Anemia, leukocytopenia, thrombocytopenia, and prothrombin deficiency are hematologic disorders associated with cirrhosis. As a result, patients tend to tire quickly and are more susceptible to infections. They bruise easily and may bleed excessively from minor trauma. Epistaxis (nosebleed) is common.

Later signs and symptoms of cirrhosis reflect the liver's inability to perform normal functions. Jaundice develops because of elevated serum bilirubin levels. Two factors contribute to jaundice in the patient with cirrhosis. First, diseased liver cells may be unable to conjugate and excrete bilirubin. Second, structural changes in the liver prevent the normal flow of bile out of the liver. Another effect of impaired bilirubin excretion, as previously mentioned, is the deposition of bile salts under the skin that can cause intense pruritus.

The diseased liver is unable to metabolize estrogen, testosterone, aldosterone, and adrenocortical hormones. Therefore the patient exhibits signs and symptoms of hormone excesses. Testicular atrophy, impotence, and gynecomastia may be noted in men and amenorrhea may be noted in women. Palmar erythema (redness) and spider angiomas are also attributed to hormone excess. Excess aldosterone contributes to sodium and water retention. The failing liver is also unable to metabolize ammonia, a product of protein metabolism. Excess ammonia affects the central nervous system (CNS), leading to confusion and decreasing consciousness.

Cirrhosis impairs the liver's ability to manufacture albumin. Albumin plays a critical role in creating the colloid osmotic pressure that retains water in the vascular compartment. With low serum albumin levels, water leaks from the capillaries, causing decreased blood volume and edema. Ascites is the accumulation of fluid in the peritoneal cavity.

Peripheral neuropathy, characterized by tingling or numbness in the extremities, is common with cirrhosis. This is thought to be caused by dietary deficiencies of vitamin B_{12}, thiamine, and folic acid.

Fig. 40.1 illustrates the clinical picture of the patient with liver disease.

Complications

The patient with cirrhosis is at risk for many complications related to portal hypertension and liver insufficiency. They include esophageal varices, ascites, hepatic encephalopathy, hepatorenal syndrome (HRS), and spontaneous bacterial peritonitis.

Portal hypertension. The portal vein delivers blood from the intestines to the liver. Changes in the liver with cirrhosis obstruct the flow of incoming blood, causing blood to back up in the portal system. High portal pressure, or portal hypertension, causes collateral vessels to develop. Collateral vessels commonly form in the esophagus, the anterior abdominal wall, and the rectum.

Esophageal varices. Distended, engorged vessels in the esophagus are called *esophageal varices*. They are fragile and bleed easily, with the potential for fatal hemorrhage. Circumstances that may trigger bleeding include irritation and increased intraabdominal pressure. Sources of irritation are alcohol, coarse foods, and stomach acid. Intraabdominal pressure is increased by vomiting, coughing, heavy lifting, and straining to defecate.

Ascites. Ascites is an accumulation of fluid in the peritoneal cavity. Factors that contribute to the development of ascites with cirrhosis include portal hypertension, leaking of lymph fluid and albumin-rich fluid from the diseased liver, low serum albumin levels, increased aldosterone levels, and water retention.

Hepatic encephalopathy. The failing liver is unable to detoxify ammonia, a breakdown product of protein metabolism. Excessive ammonia in the blood causes neurologic symptoms, including cognitive disturbances, declining level of consciousness, and changes in neuromuscular function. If the condition is not reversed, the patient lapses into unconsciousness, referred to as hepatic *coma*.

Factors that may precipitate hepatic encephalopathy are infection, fluid and potassium depletion, GI bleeding, constipation, and some drugs.

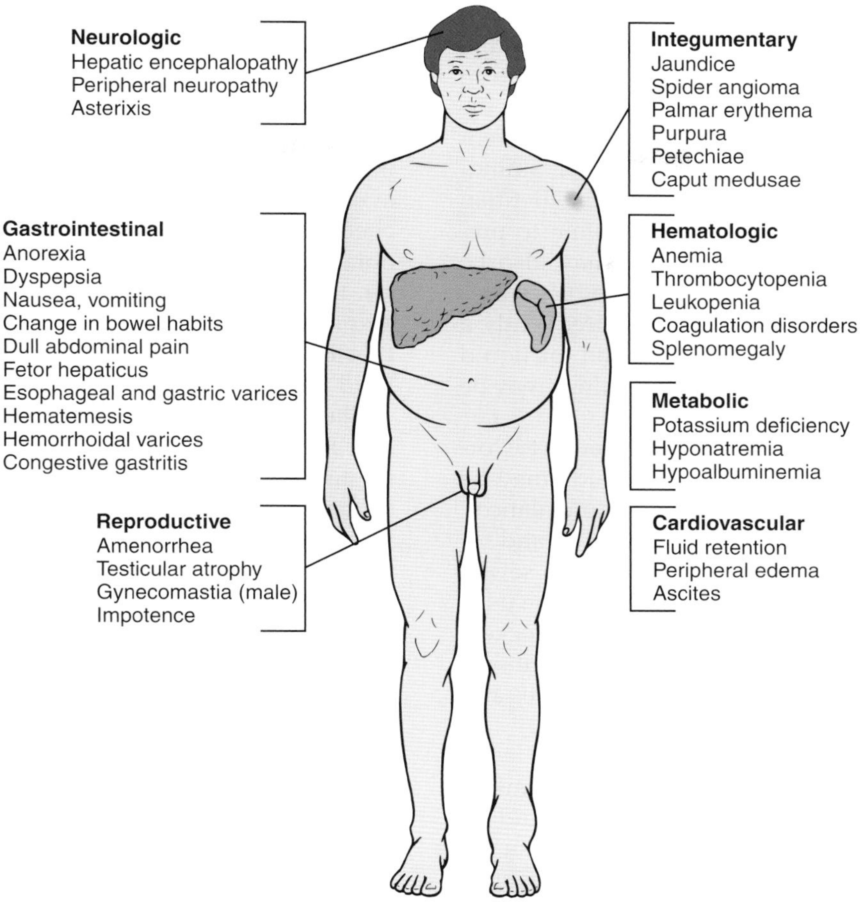

Fig. 40.1 Findings associated with liver disease. (From Lewis SM, Heitkemper MM, Dirksen SR: *Medical-surgical nursing: assessment and management of clinical problems*, ed 5, St. Louis, 2000, Mosby.)

Hepatorenal syndrome. Hepatorenal syndrome (HRS) is renal failure in the patient with cirrhosis that often follows excessive diuresis, paracentesis without albumin infusion, or GI hemorrhage. Vasodilation associated with portal hypertension triggers a physiologic response that constricts renal blood vessels.

Spontaneous bacterial peritonitis. This infection is fairly common among patients with cirrhosis. Although some patients have no symptoms, others have fever, jaundice, and abdominal pain.

Medical Diagnosis

When the patient's history and physical examination suggest cirrhosis, blood and urine tests, imaging procedures, and liver biopsy may be done to confirm or rule out the disease. Results of laboratory tests that are consistent with cirrhosis include elevated serum and urine bilirubin, elevated serum enzymes, decreased total serum protein, decreased cholesterol, and prolonged PT. The complete blood count (CBC) may reveal deficiencies of red blood cells (RBCs), white blood cells (WBCs), and platelets. The liver biopsy is performed to obtain a tissue specimen for microscopic study. Typical cellular changes occur with cirrhosis. Imaging procedures outline the liver features. Transient elastography is a study that uses ultrasound technology to measure liver stiffness. Chapter 37, Table 37.1 summarizes tests and procedures used to diagnose liver disorders.

Liver biopsy. A biopsy removes a small specimen of liver tissue for examination. Most commonly, a local anesthetic is injected, and the specimen is obtained by inserting a 14- or 18-gauge needle into the liver through the abdominal wall. This is the percutaneous route. The procedure takes about 15 minutes. The patient may experience mild discomfort. Nursing care is detailed in Chapter 37.

Medical Treatment

The goals of medical treatment for cirrhosis are to limit deterioration of liver function and to prevent complications, but no specific medical treatment exists. The approach is to promote rest so that the liver can regenerate. The earlier the condition is diagnosed, and measures are taken to promote healing, the better is the chance of recovery. Compensated cirrhosis is managed with treatment of any underlying disease (e.g., antiviral treatment of hepatitis B or C), avoidance of liver toxins, and monitoring for varices and liver cancer.

If the patient is in liver failure, bed rest is usually ordered. Malnutrition is common, and the specific diet depends on individual patient factors. A diet high in calories, carbohydrates, and vitamins is typically ordered. In the past, protein was restricted to prevent encephalopathy caused by accumulation of ammonia. In general, that is no longer the case. The dietitian may recommend normal or increased protein to prevent malnutrition. Supplementary iron may also be ordered. The amount of fat allowed in the diet varies with the patient's condition. Anorexia is frequently a problem with cirrhosis, so small, semisolid, or liquid meals may be better received. Enteral feedings may be needed to provide adequate nutrients.

Other medical treatments may be ordered to correct the complications of cirrhosis. IV fluids may be needed to correct fluid and electrolyte imbalances. Anemia may require blood transfusions. Water and sodium are likely to be restricted in patients with severe fluid retention. Cathartics and antibiotics may be used for hepatic encephalopathy. Beta-adrenergic blockers such as propranolol may be prescribed to reduce portal pressure, thereby decreasing the risk of varices and hemorrhage.

Ascites. The medical management of ascites aims to promote reabsorption and elimination of the fluid by means of sodium restriction and diuretics, usually spironolactone, furosemide, or both. Combinations of various types of diuretics may yield better results than one alone. Albumin may be given intravenously to help maintain blood volume and to increase urinary output. Albumin raises the serum colloid osmotic pressure, causing water to be drawn back into the bloodstream. Chapter 37, Table 37.2 lists drugs used to treat the patient with ascites.

If ascites does not respond to conservative treatment, fluid can be removed with a needle, a procedure called *paracentesis*. Alternatives include the placement of a peritoneal-venous shunt or a transjugular intrahepatic portosystemic shunt (TIPS) (discussed later).

Paracentesis. Paracentesis is the removal of ascitic fluid from the peritoneal cavity. A special instrument called a *trocar* is inserted through the abdominal wall and a catheter is placed to allow the fluid to drain. It is not used frequently because it removes essential protein and electrolytes. In addition, it provides a potential portal of entry for pathogens.

If paracentesis is done to remove ascites, your role is to prepare the patient, assist and support the patient during the procedure, and provide aftercare. The physician should explain what will be done and obtain patient consent. Reinforce explanations and obtain the written consent as agency policy permits. Obtain baseline vital signs, weight, and abdominal girth. Instruct the patient to void.

The procedure is often done at the bedside with the patient in a supine position. During paracentesis, you should support and encourage the patient. The physician may request monitoring of vital signs during the process. Fluid is removed slowly because rapid removal of ascitic fluid could result in circulatory collapse. After paracentesis, a sterile dressing is applied to the puncture site. Monitor vital signs every 15 minutes until the patient is stable and check the dressing for bleeding. Measure the fluid obtained and send a specimen for laboratory analysis. Document the procedure, including the amount and color of the fluid. Monitor for blood in the urine. IV albumin may be ordered based on the amount of fluid removed.

Shunts. Shunts provide a mechanism to collect ascitic fluid and return it to the circulation. Advantages to shunting ascitic fluid rather than removing it are (1) protein-rich serum is retained and returned to the vascular compartment; and (2) urine output increases, which eliminates excess sodium and water. Several types of shunts exist. The TIPS is often the preferred treatment. A catheter is threaded through the jugular vein and the inferior vena cava to the hepatic vein. The hepatic vein is punctured and connected to the portal vein with a stent. This nonsurgical procedure reduces pressure in the portal system and reduces pressure in the varices. One problem with TIPS is that toxins in the blood bypass the liver and may cause encephalopathy. Also not all patients are candidates for this procedure. Two other types of shunts are the portacaval and distal splenorenal shunt; both require surgical procedures. The portacaval shunt involves anastomosing (joining) the portal vein to the inferior vena cava to divert blood from the portal vein to the systemic circulation. The patient with a portacaval shunt is at risk for hepatic encephalopathy because ammonia accumulates in the blood. The distal splenorenal shunt anastomoses the splenic vein to the renal vein. The rerouting of blood flow to the low-pressure renal vein reduces pressure in the varices (Fig. 40.2). The incidence of hepatic encephalopathy is lower with distal splenorenal shunts.

Bleeding esophageal varices. Several techniques can be used to control bleeding esophageal varices. These include drug therapy, sclerotherapy, and endoscopic ligation. Ligation uses rubber rings to "tie off" varices. Although now uncommon, placement of esophageal-gastric balloon tubes may still be useful to control severe hemorrhage.

Acute bleeding episodes may be treated with IV octreotide, which constricts blood vessels and lowers pressure in the hepatic circulation. In addition to blood transfusions, vitamin K and proton pump inhibitors (PPIs) such as pantoprazole (Protonix) may be ordered. Lactulose may be administered to prevent the breakdown of blood in the intestines that would release ammonia, contributing to hepatic encephalopathy. Antibiotics are given (usually IV ceftriaxone

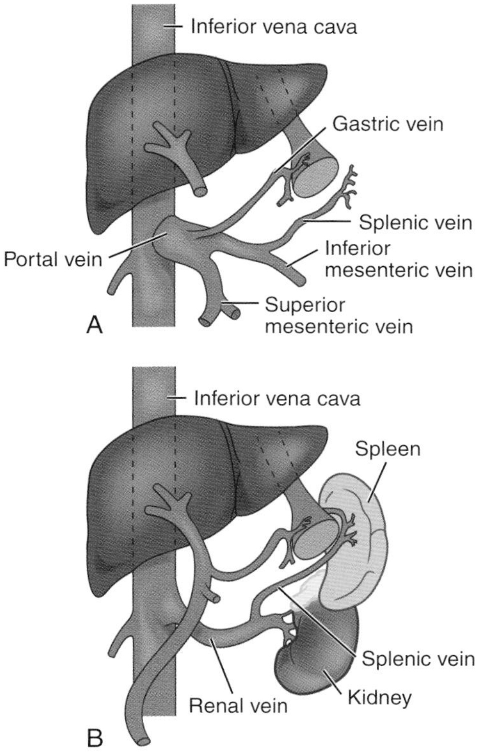

Fig. 40.2 Portosystemic shunts. (A) Portacaval shunt. The portal vein is anastomosed to the inferior vena cava, diverting blood from the portal vein to the systemic circulation. (B) Distal splenorenal shunt. The splenic vein is anastomosed to the renal vein. The portal venous flow remains intact while esophageal varices are selectively decompressed. (The short gastric veins are decompressed.) The spleen conducts blood from the high pressure of the esophageal and gastric varices to the low-pressure renal vein.

or oral ciproflaxin) to prevent bacterial infection and to decrease rebleeding. Beta-adrenergic blockers may be used to reduce BP in the long-term management of patients after acute bleeding episodes.

Surgical treatment of bleeding varices. In an emergency situation, the patient can then be stabilized with endoscopic ligation before a more extensive corrective procedure. Corrective procedures surgically shunt blood from engorged varices to other veins. Shunting the blood, as described earlier, reduces pressure in the portal venous system and the esophageal varices.

Sclerotherapy. Sclerotherapy is a procedure in which a solution is injected into the varices or into the veins that supply them, causing the varices to harden and close (Fig. 40.3). The procedure can be done through an endoscope or through a small surgical incision. Sclerotherapy can be done to prevent or to treat bleeding.

After sclerotherapy, patients often report chest discomfort for several days. The physician usually orders a mild analgesic. If it does not relieve the pain, the physician should be notified, because persistent pain may indicate perforation of the esophagus. Once a patient has had sclerotherapy, extra care must be taken in the insertion of nasogastric tubes.

Hepatic encephalopathy. Hepatic encephalopathy is a deterioration in neurologic function associated with excess ammonia in the body. Ammonia is a product of protein metabolism that is normally broken down by the liver. Manifestations include hand tremor,

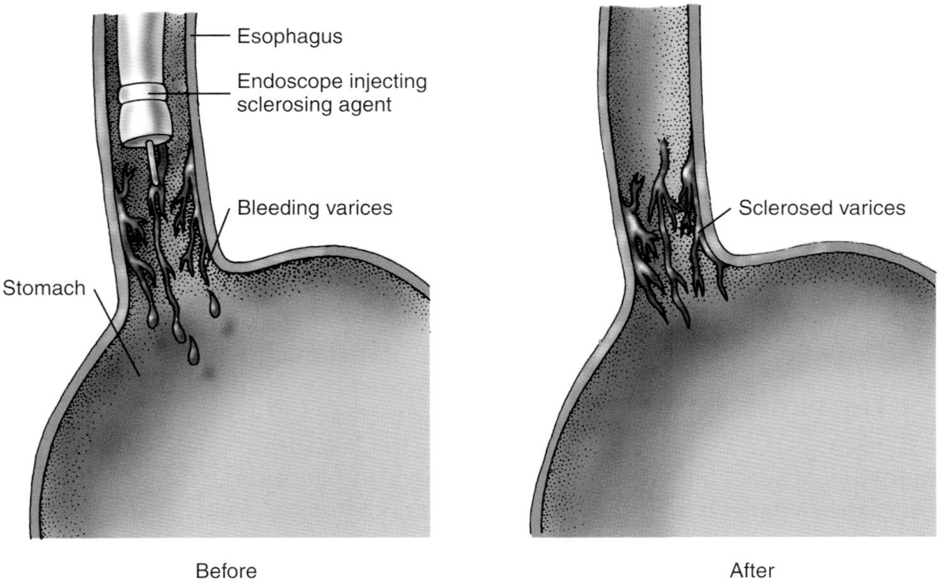

Fig. 40.3 Injection sclerotherapy. (From Monahan FD, Drake DT, Neighbors M, editors: *Medical-surgical nursing: foundations for clinical practice*, ed 2, Philadelphia, 1998, Saunders.)

personality changes, hyperventilation, and lethargy progressing to coma. Many factors can precipitate hepatic encephalopathy, including constipation, GI bleeding, hypokalemia, infection, opioids, dehydration, and renal failure. Treatment is aimed at correcting the cause and reducing the amount of ammonia being produced in the digestive tract. This reduction may be achieved with lactulose. Lactulose is a cathartic that promotes elimination of ammonia from the colon and discourages bacterial growth by making the intestinal contents more acidic. Other drugs used are polyethylene glycol 3350 electrolyte solution and antibiotics such as rifaximin or neomycin. Albumin dialysis is another option to improve neurologic function by removing toxins.

If the patient has been bleeding into the GI tract, laxatives and enemas may be ordered to remove old blood and protein. Patients with recurring hepatic encephalopathy may be candidates for liver transplantation.

Hepatorenal syndrome. HRS is renal failure accompanying cirrhosis. Precipitating factors include paracentesis, diuresis, and GI hemorrhage. It may be treated with a vasoconstrictor (octreotide with midodrine), albumin, a TIPS, or extracorporeal albumin dialysis. Patients should not receive nephrotoxic drugs such as nonsteroidal antiinflammatory drugs (NSAIDs). Medical management is used primarily to support the patient until liver transplantation is available.

Spontaneous bacterial peritonitis. Spontaneous bacterial peritonitis is treated with antibiotics. IV albumin is given to prevent renal dysfunction associated with this infection. Long-term prophylactic antibiotic therapy is reserved for a few circumstances because it leads to antibiotic resistance.

Drug therapy. A variety of drugs may be used to treat the effects of cirrhosis. These drugs and nursing implications are summarized in Chapter 37, Table 37.2. Because most drugs are metabolized by the liver and many drugs are hepatotoxic, the physician is cautious in the selection of drugs.

Pharmacology Capsule

Acetaminophen can cause liver failure if taken in excess. Advise patients not to exceed the maximum recommended daily dose.

◆ NURSING CARE OF THE PATIENT WITH CIRRHOSIS

Focused Assessment

Ongoing assessment of the cirrhosis patient should include daily measurements of weight, intake and output, and abdominal girth. Patients are monitored for signs and symptoms of complications—bleeding, ascites, encephalopathy, and renal failure.

Patient Problems, Goals, and Outcome Criteria: Cirrhosis

Patient Problems	Goals and Outcome Criteria
Inadequate nutrition related to anorexia, metabolic imbalances	Adequate nutrition: stable body weight, consumes meals
Decreased activity tolerance related to fatigue	Improved activity tolerance: performs activities of daily living (ADL) without excessive fatigue
Potential for disrupted skin tissue integrity related to edema, immobility, pruritus, hypoproteinemia	Intact skin: no redness or breaks in skin, no scratching
Inadequate ventilation related to shallow breathing, ascites	Adequate ventilation: respiratory rate of 12 to 20 breaths per minute without dyspnea, heart rate consistent with patient norms
Potential for injury (hemorrhage) related to impaired coagulation	Absence of bleeding: no blood in emesis or stool, vital signs consistent with patient norms
Acute confusion related to elevated blood ammonia	Normal cognitive function: mentally alert, oriented
Fluid volume deficit (hypovolemia) or fluid volume excess (in third space) related to hypoproteinemia, increased aldosterone	Normal fluid distribution in body fluid compartments: balanced fluid intake and output without edema or ascites; pulse and blood pressure (BP) consistent with patient norms
Potential for infection related to liver dysfunction, impaired response to infection, malnutrition	Absence of infection: oral temperature less than 100°F (37.8°C)
Fear related to dyspnea, life-threatening illness	Reduced fear: patient states no or less fear, calm manner

Interventions

Inadequate nutrition. Good nutrition is essential for regeneration of liver tissue. However, it is a challenge for the patient with cirrhosis, who often has anorexia, indigestion, nausea, and vomiting. Furthermore, the diet may be made less palatable by protein or salt restriction.

Explain the need for adequate food intake to the patient and encourage the patient to eat even when they are not hungry. Small, frequent meals may be more acceptable to the anorexic patient. Arrange a dietary consult for the patient to report likes and dislikes.

Make mealtimes as pleasant as possible. Put bedpans, emesis basins, and drainage collection devices out of sight. Ventilate the room to reduce odors. Do not schedule tiring activities immediately before meals. Record daily weights as ordered to monitor both nutritional and fluid status.

Reduced activity tolerance. Some activity limitations are usually imposed, depending on the patient's overall status. Schedule nursing care to allow some periods of undisturbed rest. The patient can generally assume any position that is comfortable.

If the patient spends all or most of the day in bed, there is a risk of complications related to immobility. Assist the patient to change positions, deep breathe, and exercise extremities regularly.

Potential for disrupted skin tissue integrity. The patient with cirrhosis is at risk for skin breakdown for several reasons. Bile salts that are normally processed by the liver may be deposited under the skin, causing intense pruritus. Loss of muscle and fat tissue with advanced disease reduces the padding that normally protects the skin from pressure. Also many patients have edema, which makes tissue more fragile and impairs healing.

Nursing measures to relieve the itching of pruritus include gentle bathing with mild soap and tepid water, thorough rinsing, and application of moisturizing lotions. The patient's nails should be kept short to reduce trauma from scratching. If scratching persists, put soft cotton mittens or gloves on the patient's hands. If itching is severe, consult the physician about ordering a medication to relieve the discomfort. Cholestyramine (Questran) may be ordered to increase the excretion of bile salts.

Inadequate ventilation. Ascitic fluid can cause the abdomen to become greatly distended. While in bed, the patient breathes easier with the head of the bed elevated. Sitting in a chair with the feet elevated, if allowed, may be even more comfortable.

Potential for injury. The patient with cirrhosis is at great risk for injury or hemorrhage because of impaired coagulation and fragile varices. Handle the patient gently to avoid trauma. Use a soft toothbrush or swab for mouth care. Apply firm pressure to injection sites to minimize oozing. Pad side rails if the patient is restless.

An uncommon but effective treatment for bleeding esophageal varices is an esophageal-gastric balloon tube placement. The patient with this type of tube is usually in an intensive care unit because close monitoring is necessary. If you should encounter this procedure, consult your agency procedure manual and manufacturer's instructions to provide appropriate care.

Acute Confusion. Cognitive changes in the patient with cirrhosis are usually caused by hepatic encephalopathy. Nursing care of the patient with hepatic encephalopathy includes monitoring mental and neurologic status. Inform the registered nurse (RN) or physician of changes in status. The patient who is confused or unconscious requires close attention to prevent injury or complications of immobility. Talk to the patient to provide basic information and reassurance. The family may also need an explanation of the patient's behavior. Administer prescribed drugs that decrease ammonia-producing bacteria in the intestines (e.g., lactulose). Be alert for adverse effects of drug therapy, which may include diarrhea or vitamin K deficiency.

Fluid volume deficit or fluid volume excess. Fluid needs vary with the patient's condition. Sodium and water are likely to be restricted if marked edema or ascites exist. Despite the excess in total body water, the patient's blood volume may be dangerously low. Adequate water is present but is not distributed appropriately. Without adequate albumin in the serum, colloid osmotic pressure falls, and water shifts out of the capillaries into the tissues. Administer IV fluids and albumin 25% as ordered. In addition to monitoring vital signs, evaluate fluid intake and output.

Potential for infection. The patient with cirrhosis is at risk for infection for several reasons. The liver is no longer able to filter bacteria from the blood as it comes from the intestines. The function of the spleen is also impaired, which lowers resistance to infection. In addition, these patients tend to be malnourished, so they lack the building materials necessary for tissue repair. Monitor for fever and malaise, which suggest infection. Protect the patient from others with infections. Practice good hand washing and use aseptic technique for invasive procedures.

Fear. Patients with cirrhosis can experience frightening complications, including confusion, dyspnea, and hemorrhage. With advanced cirrhosis, the prognosis is poor, and patients often have repeated emergency admissions. Treatments and diagnostic procedures may be painful and anxiety producing. The nurse can help by recognizing the patient's fear and acknowledging it.

To provide emotional support to cirrhosis patients, you must be aware of your personal reaction to these patients. There is a stigma attached to cirrhosis because it is often associated with alcohol abuse. Health care providers must treat patients in a nonjudgmental manner. Nurses must realize that alcoholism is a complex chronic disease that is not easily controlled and that cirrhosis can be caused by factors other than alcohol (see the Complementary and Alternative Therapies box).

Complementary and Alternative Therapies

Some patients have found acupuncture helpful for the treatment of alcoholism.

Put On Your Thinking Cap!

Identify three functions of the healthy liver. Describe how cirrhosis affects those functions. State one nursing implication related to the change with cirrhosis in each function.

Information can help to reduce fear. When the patient is acutely ill, give simple explanations and answer questions. When the patient improves, explore what they know about cirrhosis and determine what additional information is needed. General teaching points are noted in the following Patient Teaching box.

Patient Teaching

Cirrhosis

- A balanced diet will help prevent additional injury to the liver and reduce risk of complications.
- Avoid specific food as advised by the physician and the dietitian.
- Notify your physician if you have increasing fluid retention, black tarry stools, bloody vomitus, increasing fatigue, or confusion.
- Alcohol is discouraged because of the toxic effects on the liver. Community resources you can use for information and assistance include Alcoholics Anonymous (if appropriate), the American Liver Foundation, and home health nursing services.
- Do not take medications except as approved by your physician. Many drugs, including acetaminophen, can be toxic to the liver.

LIVER FAILURE

Liver failure can be acute or chronic. Acute liver failure, commonly called *fulminant liver failure*, may result from acute hepatitis, drug toxicity (e.g., acetaminophen, isoniazid), or obstruction of the hepatic vein. Complications of acute failure include cerebral edema resulting in brainstem herniation, worsening encephalopathy, coagulation abnormalities, and renal failure. With appropriate management, some patients do recover from acute failure. If recovery is judged to be unlikely, the patient may be transferred to a transplant center because liver transplantation offers the best hope of survival. Chronic liver disease such as cirrhosis can also lead to liver failure. Late-stage cirrhosis is generally considered irreversible; however, some patients respond to therapy and show improvement (Goldberg and Chopra, November 6, 2019).

One advancement in the care of patients with liver failure is albumin dialysis. Using principles of renal dialysis, the patient's blood is filtered through a system that removes toxins and returns the blood to the body. Albumin is used because many toxic molecules including bilirubin bind with it. This technology can support patients while the liver recovers or serve as a temporary treatment while awaiting liver transplantation. Some of the systems currently in use are MARS, the Prometheus system, and single-pass albumin dialysis. ADVOS is a newer system that reports significant reductions in bilirubin, creatinine, and serum blood urea nitrogen (BUN) using a process that rapidly regenerates albumin.

CANCER OF THE LIVER

Cancer rarely begins in the liver, but the liver is a frequent site of metastasis. Cirrhosis is a predisposing factor for liver cancer. Signs and symptoms of liver cancer include liver enlargement, weight loss, anorexia, nausea, vomiting, and dull pain in the right upper quadrant of the abdomen. As the disease progresses, the signs and symptoms are essentially the same as those of cirrhosis. Because the early signs and symptoms of liver cancer are vague, the condition is often not diagnosed until it is advanced.

Tests and procedures used to diagnose liver cancer are liver scan, CT or MRI, biopsy, hepatic angiography, endoscopy, and measurement of alpha-fetoprotein levels. If the cancer is confined to one area, a lobectomy may be done; otherwise, chemotherapy is the primary treatment. Chemotherapy is generally considered to be palliative, meaning that it may slow the progress of the cancer and increase patient comfort but is unlikely to be curative. Transarterial chemoembolization is a procedure in which the chemotherapy drug and a drug that obstructs the blood vessels are injected into the blood vessels that supply the tumor. Other options are liver transplantation and ablation (destruction) of the tumor using heat, cold, alcohol, or acetic acid. Transplantation is an option unless the cancer is widespread.

During the course of the illness, the patient's needs are much like those of the patient with cirrhosis (discussed previously). Additional aspects of nursing care of the patient with cancer are discussed in Chapter 7.

LIVER TRANSPLANTATION

The only possible cure for end-stage liver disease is liver transplantation. Transplantation is also appropriate for patients with cancer that is confined to the liver and for patients with certain congenital disorders. Most livers are obtained from deceased donors, although a suitable living donor is sometimes an option. When a living donor is available, a lobe is transplanted. Patients who are recommended for transplantation are ranked by standard criteria and entered in a national computer network. When a liver becomes available by donation, the best recipient can then be identified. Patients awaiting transplantation must be on standby status in the event that a donor is located. This is a time of alternating hope and fear for patients and families. In the United States, a deficiency of donors means that some eligible patients will die while awaiting transplant.

Patients with hepatitis C are given antiviral drugs preoperatively and postoperatively. After liver transplantation, the patient is cared for in a specialized unit. A transplant patient often has a T-tube, wound drainage devices, a nasogastric tube, and a central line for total parenteral nutrition (TPN). Mechanical ventilation is also used initially.

Nursing assessments focus on neurologic status, vital signs, central venous pressure, respiratory status, and indicators of bleeding. If stable, the patient is moved out of the specialized unit after 3 or 4 days. Continue to monitor vital signs, intake and output, and neurologic status. Provide usual postoperative care, including assistance with turning, coughing and deep breathing, and progressive activity. Lifelong immunosuppressive therapy will be required to prevent rejection of the donor liver. Initially, it is common to prescribe a combination of 3 drugs. They may include a glucocorticoid (e.g., prednisone), a calcineurin inhibitor (e.g., tacrolimus or cyclosporine), and a mycophenolate (e.g., mofetil). If the patient is free of rejection after 6 months, they may be maintained on a single agent, often a calcineurin inhibitor.

Pharmacology Capsule

Rifampin, phenobarbital, ketoconazole, and St. John's wort enhance metabolism of immunosuppressants, making them less effective and increasing the risk of graft rejection.

The transplant recipient must be monitored for signs of rejection. These signs include fever, anorexia, depression, vague abdominal pain, muscle aches, and joint pain. Fever is sometimes the only sign of rejection. In addition to rejection, the patient is at risk for numerous drug adverse effects as well as hepatic complications (see Box 40.2). If rejection occurs and does not respond to treatment, retransplantation may be needed.

Before discharge, the patient should know the signs and symptoms of transplant rejection and infection, wound care, dietary restrictions (usually sodium restriction), and self-medication.

Pharmacology Capsule

Drugs that suppress rejection of transplanted organs reduce the patient's ability to resist infection.

DISORDERS OF THE GALLBLADDER

Gallbladder disease is one of the most common health problems in the United States. The two most common gallbladder disorders are (1) cholecystitis and (2) cholelithiasis. Carcinoma of the gallbladder occurs but is uncommon.

Risk factors for gallbladder disease include obesity, familial tendency, a sedentary lifestyle, and the use of estrogen or oral contraceptives. Women are at greater risk than men, especially women who have had multiple pregnancies. The "five Fs" are sometimes used to describe those at greatest risk for gallbladder disease: (1) female, (2) fat, (3) fair, (4) forty, and (5) fertile.

Box 40.2 Complications Related to Liver Transplantation and Immunosuppression

- Infection
- Metabolic syndrome
  Hypertension
  Diabetes mellitus
  Obesity
  Elevated serum lipids
- Kidney disease
- Cancer
- Skin
  Infections
  Lesions
  Cancer
- Bone loss
- Neurological problems
- Elevated uric acid
- Liver
  Rejection
  Leaks or strictures in biliary tract
  Recurrence of primary liver disease

CHOLECYSTITIS AND CHOLELITHIASIS

Cholecystitis is inflammation of the gallbladder. It is caused most often by the presence of gallstones but can be the result of bacteria, toxic chemicals, tumors, anesthesia, starvation, and opioids. The inflamed gallbladder and cystic duct become swollen and congested with blood. The cystic duct may actually become occluded.

When gallstones are present, the patient is said to have **cholelithiasis**. Most gallstones are composed of cholesterol mixed with bile salts, bilirubin, calcium, and protein. It is not known exactly why gallstones form, but the process is associated with high concentrations of cholesterol. The concentration of cholesterol rises when stasis of bile exists (as occurs with pregnancy, immobility, and inflammation of the biliary tract). Many patients with gallstones have no symptoms; the condition is often diagnosed incidentally during imaging procedures for unrelated complaints.

Cultural Considerations

What Does Culture Have to Do With Gallbladder Disease?

The highest prevalence of gallstones in the United States is among Mexican American women, followed by White American women and Black American women.

Gallstones may be found anywhere in the biliary tract: the gallbladder, the cystic duct, or the common bile duct (Fig. 40.4). The stones may move through the biliary tract with bile flow. If a stone cannot pass through the tract, it lodges and causes an obstruction. Ducts respond to obstruction with spasms to move the stone. This is responsible for an intense, spasmodic pain, called *biliary colic*.

If the cystic duct is obstructed, bile cannot leave the gallbladder and inflammation develops. Cystic duct

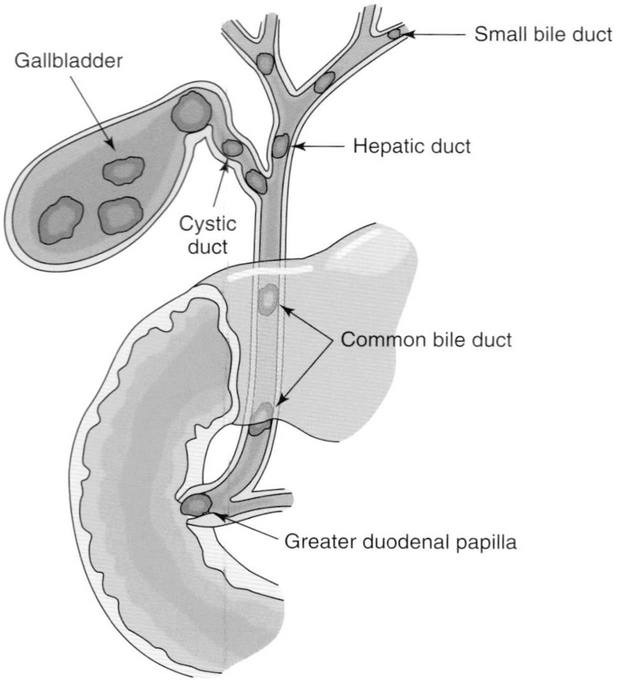

Fig. 40.4 Gallstones within the gallbladder that could obstruct the common bile duct and the cystic duct. (From Monahan F, Sands J, Neighbors M, et al., editors: *Phipps' medical-surgical nursing: health and illness perspectives*, ed 8, St. Louis, 2007, Mosby.)

obstruction does not prevent the flow of bile into the duodenum from the liver. However, if the common bile duct is obstructed (**choledocholithiasis**), bile is unable to flow into the duodenum.

Signs and Symptoms

Signs and symptoms of cholecystitis vary from one patient to the next. Some have only mild indigestion whereas others have severe pain, fever, and jaundice. Other symptoms are nausea, **eructation** (belching), fever, chills, and right upper quadrant pain that radiates to the shoulder or back. Symptoms typically occur about 3 hours after a meal, especially if the food had high fat content.

When bile flow is obstructed, bile production in the liver decreases and the serum bilirubin rises, leading to obstructive jaundice. Some excess bilirubin is excreted in the urine, creating a dark-amber color. Digestion of fats is impaired, causing intolerance of fatty foods and steatorrhea (i.e., excess fat in feces). The absence of urobilinogen in the stool causes it to be a characteristic clay color. The patient is unable to absorb fat-soluble vitamins and may show signs of vitamin deficiencies. Vitamin K deficiency interferes with normal blood clotting, and thus the patient bleeds and bruises easily.

Complications

The most serious complications of cholecystitis and cholelithiasis are pancreatitis, abscesses, cholangitis (i.e., inflammation of the biliary ducts), and rupture of the gallbladder.

Medical Diagnosis

Transabdominal ultrasonography usually confirms a tentative diagnosis of cholelithiasis based on patient history and physical examination findings. Other diagnostic imaging procedures may be used in some circumstances. A technetium-labeled hepatobiliary iminodiacetic acid (HIDA) scan is a specific test for acute cholecystitis.

Blood and urine studies provide additional information. With inflammation or infection, the WBC count is elevated. If bile flow is obstructed, levels of serum and urinary bilirubin and serum enzymes may be elevated. Nursing considerations associated with specific diagnostic tests and procedures are summarized in Table 37.1.

Medical Treatment

Conservative treatment of acute cholecystitis includes analgesics and anticholinergic agents to relieve pain and muscle spasms. Antibiotics are given to treat infection. IV fluids are selected to maintain fluid balance, especially if the patient has been vomiting. A nasogastric tube may be inserted and attached to suction to rest the bowel. This relieves nausea and vomiting and reduces the stimulation of the gallbladder by intestinal contents.

Among the options available for the treatment of cholelithiasis or choledocholithiasis are drug therapy, shock wave lithotripsy, endoscopic sphincterotomy (Fig. 40.5), and cholecystectomy. Nonsurgical options are rarely used now because laparoscopic cholecystectomy is safe and effective. Patients with asymptomatic gallstones usually require no treatment except in special circumstances. Some experts recommend cholecystectomy in patients having bariatric weight loss surgery even if they have no gallstones because 30% will require cholecystectomy within one year after surgery.

Drugs used to treat conditions of the biliary tract are described in Chapter 37, Table 37.2 except those used only to dissolve gallstones which are described in Table 40.2.

Cholecystectomy. **Cholecystectomy** is the standard of care for cholelithiasis. The two procedures that may be used are via laparoscopy (which accounts for 90% of cholecystectomies) or through a right subcostal incision. For laparoscopic cholecystectomy, the surgeon inserts a laparoscope with a camera through a small abdominal incision. Using the camera, the surgeon guides forceps and a laser toward the gallbladder through other small abdominal incisions. The gallbladder is grasped with the forceps, cut free with the laser, and pulled out through one of the small incisions. Stones remaining in the common bile duct can be removed endoscopically. The most serious complication, although rare, is injury to the bile duct, which requires endoscopic repair. Patients are usually discharged the

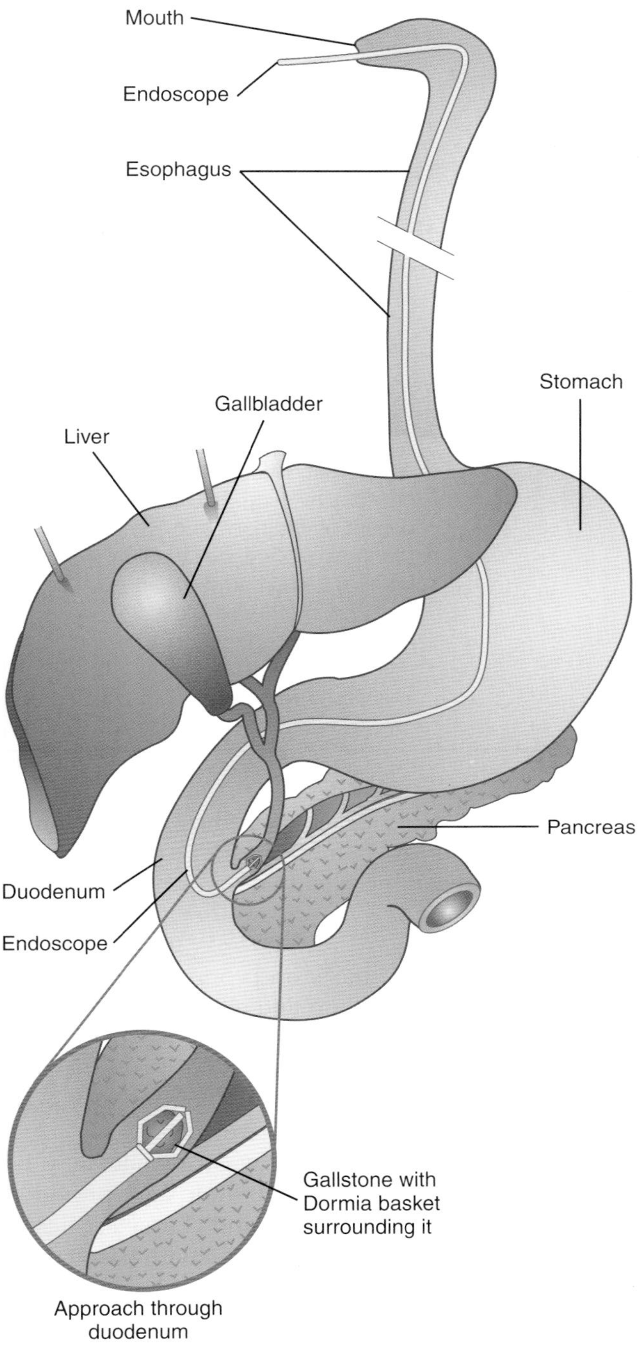

Fig. 40.5 Choledochoscopic removal of gallstones. (From Black JM, Hawks JH: *Medical-surgical nursing: clinical management for positive outcomes*, ed 8, St. Louis, 2009, Saunders.)

same day or on the day after surgery and resume regular activities within a week.

In the classic procedure, an incision is made below the right rib margin. The gallbladder is removed, and the common bile duct is explored for stones. A T-tube may be placed in the common bile duct to maintain bile flow until swelling in the duct subsides (Fig. 40.6). One part of the tubing is brought through the patient's skin and connected to a closed-gravity drainage receptacle. Wound drains may also be present.

When the patient first returns from surgery, the drainage from the T-tube may be bloody but it should soon become greenish brown. Drainage should gradually decrease as edema subsides in the common bile duct. Measure and record the amount of drainage and notify the physician if it exceeds 1000 mL in 24 hours.

Place the patient in a low Fowler position with the tube arranged to drain freely. Protect the tube during movement to prevent dislodging it. The physician specifies the level of the drainage bag and when it should be clamped. If the patient experiences pain, fever, chills, nausea, or distention, the tube should be unclamped. The physician removes the T-tube when the patient tolerates clamping for a prolonged period of time. Cleanse the area around wound drains using aseptic technique and dress per agency protocol.

If the patient is discharged with the T-tube in place, you must teach the patient to care for the tube, including emptying the receptacle, caring for the insertion site, and recognizing when to clamp and unclamp it.

◆ NURSING CARE OF THE PATIENT WITH A GALLBLADDER DISORDER

Focused Assessment

General assessment of patients with problems of the digestive tract is outlined in Chapter 37, Box 37.1. When gallbladder disease is diagnosed or suspected, it is especially important to document pain: location, onset, intensity, duration, and relationship to meals. Ask about indigestion, dyspepsia, nausea, and vomiting. Note whether the patient has pruritus, dark urine, or light-colored stools. Observe the color and moisture of the skin and gently palpate the abdomen for distention and guarding.

Patient Problems, Goals, and Outcome Criteria: Cholelithiasis

Patient Problems	Goals and Outcome Criteria
Acute pain related to biliary colic	Reduced pain: patient states pain is reduced or relieved, rates pain lower on pain scale
Fluid volume deficit related to vomiting, inadequate intake	Adequate hydration: balanced fluid intake and output, vital signs consistent with patient norms
Potential for disrupted skin tissue integrity related to pruritus	Decreased itching: no scratching, patient states less or no itching
Anxiety related to disease, anticipation of invasive procedures	Reduced anxiety: patient states anxiety relieved or reduced, relaxed manner
Potential for injury (bleeding) related to vitamin K deficiency	Absence of bleeding: no abnormal bruising or bleeding

Table 40.2 Drugs Used to Dissolve Gallstones

General Nursing Implications

1. Drugs are effective only against small cholesterol stones.
2. Drug therapy is successful in only about one-third to one-half of patients treated.

Drug	Side Effects	Nursing Interventions
Oral Bile Salts		
chenodeoxycholic acid (Chenix), ursodeoxycholic acid (UDCA) (Actigall)	Diarrhea; cramps; nausea; vomiting; elevated levels of serum enzymes, low-density lipoproteins (LDLs), and cholesterol. UDCA has milder side effects but is very expensive. Contraindications include biliary tract infection, pancreatitis, and pregnancy.	If the patient is a woman, advise her not to become pregnant while taking this drug. Stress the importance of periodic blood tests to determine liver enzyme and serum cholesterol levels.
Dissolution Agents		
methyl tertiary-butyl ether (MTBE)	Abdominal pain and nausea during treatment.	Oral contrast dye is given the previous evening. Position the patient on the right side after the procedure to reduce bleeding. Monitor for hemorrhage, shock, and pneumothorax. Measure the patient's vital signs every 15 minutes until stable; then 3 times at 4-hour intervals. The patient should be kept on bed rest for 24 hours.

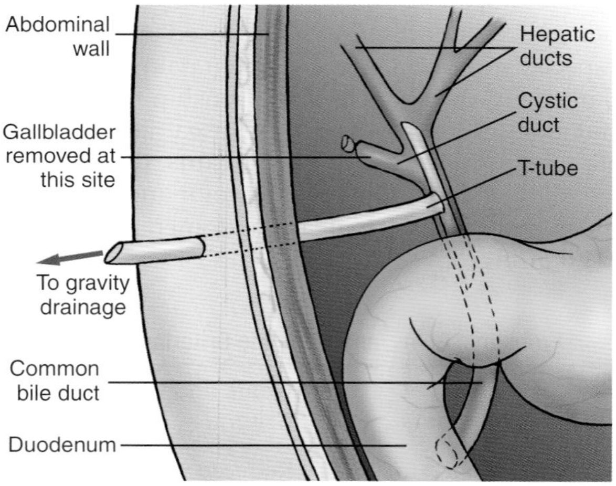

Fig. 40.6 A T-tube in the common bile duct. (From Monahan FD, Drake DT, Neighbors M, editors: *Medical-surgical nursing: foundations for clinical practice*, ed 2, Philadelphia, 1998, Saunders.)

Interventions

Acute pain. The degree of pain with cholecystitis varies, but many patients experience severe pain. Appropriate analgesics include NSAIDs (e.g., ketorolac) and opioids. Evaluate comfort often and medicate the patient as soon as pain is reported instead of waiting for it to become severe. When opioid analgesics are given, take safety precautions because the drugs cause drowsiness. In addition to medications, use position changes, smooth linens, back rubs, and mouth care to promote comfort.

Attacks of biliary colic are caused by stimulation of the gallbladder, most often by fats in the duodenum. A low-fat diet is recommended to decrease the incidence of acute symptoms.

Fluid volume deficit. If nausea and vomiting are present, the patient is at risk for fluid and electrolyte imbalances. Administer antiemetics as ordered. Keep intake and output records. Monitor for signs of fluid volume deficit (hypovolemia): tachycardia, hypotension, dry skin, concentrated urine, decreased urine output.

If vomiting is severe, a nasogastric tube may be inserted and attached to suction. Fluids are provided intravenously. Note the amount and characteristics of aspirated fluid. A problem associated with nasogastric decompression is the continuous removal of gastric secretions. When the fluid is continuously drained, the patient loses significant water, electrolytes, and acid. This puts the patient at risk for fluid volume deficit, potassium deficit, sodium excess, and metabolic alkalosis. Serum electrolytes are monitored and specific IV fluids are ordered to maintain or restore balance.

Potential for disrupted skin tissue integrity. Patients who have obstructive jaundice caused by blockage of the bile ducts often have pruritus caused by accumulated bile salts under the skin. Measures to promote comfort include tepid baths with baking soda or oily lotions, use of soft linens, and maintaining a comfortable room temperature. Patients should be advised not to scratch, but that can be difficult. Short fingernails or even cotton gloves may be suggested to avoid skin injury from scratching. The physician may order a drug such as cholestyramine (Questran) to reduce the discomfort.

Anxiety. Acute pain and unexpected hospitalization can be anxiety provoking for patients and their families. Provide clear explanations about what is being done and what they can expect. Acknowledge their anxiety and take time to answer questions and offer reassurance.

Potential for injury. A patient who has obstructed bile flow may have a deficiency of vitamin K because absorption of this vitamin in the digestive tract requires bile salts. Vitamin K is needed for the production of prothrombin, an essential element for clotting. Indications of vitamin K deficiency include bleeding gums and oozing of blood at injection sites. Minimize trauma by using a soft toothbrush or swab for mouth care and by applying gentle pressure to injection sites (see the Patient Teaching: Cholelithiasis box).

Pharmacology Capsule

Caution patients that supplementary bile salts interfere with the effectiveness of oral contraceptives.

Patient Teaching

Cholelithiasis

- You need to have a low-fat diet with supplementary fat-soluble vitamins (or as ordered by the physician). The dietitian will explain the details of the diet to you.
- Notify your physician of signs of bile duct obstruction: light stools, dark urine, jaundice, and itching.
- If you are taking bile salts, report gastric upset.
- Keep medical appointments to have blood drawn to monitor liver function.
- Do not rely on oral contraceptives; bile salts interfere with their effectiveness.

NURSING CARE OF THE PATIENT AFTER SURGERY FOR CHOLELITHIASIS

Common nursing interventions for the patient who has undergone incisional surgery for cholelithiasis are presented here. Detailed assessment and care of the surgical patient are discussed in Chapter 17. Nursing care after laparoscopic cholecystectomy is much simpler because patients usually recover quickly and are discharged on the same day or within 24 hours. They usually do not need postoperative nasogastric intubation or T-tubes.

Focused Assessment

Postoperatively, take the patient's vital signs until they are stable. Observe chest expansion and auscultate breath sounds. Inspect the dressing for bleeding. If a T-tube is present, note the color and amount of drainage. Examine passive drains to ensure that they are functioning properly. Inspect the skin around the incision or the drain for redness or breakdown. If a nasogastric tube is in place, observe the characteristics and amount of the drainage and ensure that the suction is operational. Inspect the patient's nares for irritation or pressure from the tube.

Patient Problems, Goals, and Outcome Criteria: Incisional Cholecystectomy

Patient Problems	Goals and Outcome Criteria
Acute pain related to surgical incision, nasogastric tube	Pain relief: patient states pain relieved or reduced, relaxed manner
Inadequate ventilation related to shallow respirations because of splinting of the surgical incision	Adequate ventilation: breath sounds clear on auscultation, respiratory rate of 12 to 20 breaths per minute, O_2 saturation of at least 95%
Disrupted skin tissue integrity related to surgical incision	Wound healing without skin breakdown: clean wound margins without excessive redness
Potential for injury related to irritation by wound drainage	
Fluid volume deficit related to gastrointestinal (GI) suction	Normal fluid and electrolyte status: electrolytes within normal limits, balanced fluid intake and output
Potential for infection related to surgical incision, invasive procedure	Absence of infection: normal temperature and white blood cell (WBC) count

Interventions

Acute pain. When the patient undergoes a procedure that requires a surgical incision, pain is expected. In addition to administering ordered analgesics, reposition the patient for comfort and check to ensure that any drainage tubes are functioning. Show the patient how to support the incision with the hands or a pillow during coughing and deep breathing. Other pain relief measures are described in Chapter 8. If pain continues despite these measures, notify the physician.

The patient who has a nasogastric tube in place has an additional source of discomfort. The nose and throat may become very sore. Secure the tube to the patient's upper lip or nose so that it is not moved or tugged easily. Gently cleanse the nares and provide frequent mouth care.

Inadequate ventilation. Potentially ineffective breathing patterns are most likely to be a problem when the patient has a subcostal incision. The incision is located close to the diaphragm, so full lung expansion is painful. The patient tends to guard the surgical area by not breathing deeply. Explain the importance of deep breathing and coughing to prevent atelectasis and pneumonia. Also demonstrate how splinting the area makes breathing and coughing more comfortable. Adequate pain management enables the patient to breathe more effectively. Monitor respiratory rate and breath sounds.

Disrupted skin tissue integrity. Patients who have subcostal incisions often have wound drains in place. These drains allow for removal of fluids that collect at the surgical site. A Penrose drain diverts fluids directly onto the wound dressings. This requires frequent dressing changes to prevent skin irritation. It is especially important if bile is present in the drainage because bile contains digestive enzymes, which are even more irritating. A pouch collection device like those used for stomas can be applied if needed to protect the skin. A passive drain such as the Jackson-Pratt drain has a fluid collection device that keeps fluid away from the skin.

Fluid volume deficit. Postoperatively, measure fluid intake and output. Until oral fluids are permitted, administer IV fluids as ordered. Blood studies may be ordered to assess serum electrolytes. If nasogastric suction is ordered, check frequently to ensure that it is working properly. Otherwise, the patient may have distention that causes vomiting and further loss of fluids and electrolytes.

Potential for infection. The patient who has undergone gallbladder surgery is at risk for infection of the surgical wound. Draining wounds provide a moist environment for bacterial growth. Meticulous wound care can reduce that risk.

A complication of endoscopic sphincterotomy is pancreatitis caused by accidental injury to the pancreatic duct. Early signs of pancreatitis are pain and fever (see the Patient Teaching: Laparoscopic Cholecystectomy box).

Patient Teaching

Laparoscopic Cholecystectomy

After laparoscopic cholecystectomy, usual instructions include the following:

- Avoid fatty foods for several weeks.
- Remove the dressings and bathe or shower normally the next day.
- Notify the physician if redness, drainage, or pus from the incision is noted.
- Report any signs of peritonitis: severe abdominal pain, chills and fever, and vomiting.
- A low-fat diet may be recommended for 4 to 6 weeks.
- In general, avoid heavy lifting for 4 to 6 weeks or as prescribed. Other activities, including sexual intercourse, can usually be resumed when you feel well enough.

CANCER OF THE GALLBLADDER

Cancer of the gallbladder is rare and is thought to be related to chronic cholecystitis and cholelithiasis. The diagnosis is often delayed because early signs and symptoms are essentially the same as those of cholecystitis and cholelithiasis. This explains the 5-year survival rate of less than 10%.

Treatment options include cholecystectomy, chemotherapy, targeted therapy, and immunotherapy; however, the prognosis is generally poor. Often only supportive, symptomatic care is given. Nursing care is similar to that for other patients with gallbladder disease. You also need to focus on the needs of the patient with cancer, as discussed in Chapter 7.

DISORDERS OF THE PANCREAS

◆ NURSING ASSESSMENT OF THE PATIENT WITH A DISORDER OF THE PANCREAS

Assessment of the patient with a disorder of the digestive tract is outlined in Box 37.1. When the patient has a pancreatic disorder, data collection focuses on both digestive and metabolic functions. Ask the patient about digestive disturbances and pain. Significant data in the health history would be biliary disorders and diabetes mellitus. Relevant drugs to note are thiazides, furosemide, estrogens, corticosteroids, sulfonamides, opiates, oral contraceptives, and NSAIDs. The functional assessment includes data about the patient's dietary habits and use of alcohol.

Inquire if the patient has pruritus and inspect the skin for jaundice, dryness, and scratches. Inspect and palpate the abdomen for distention, discoloration, and tenderness. Auscultate bowel sounds.

DIAGNOSTIC TESTS AND PROCEDURES

Tests and procedures used to diagnose pancreatic disorders include laboratory analyses of blood, urine, stool, and pancreatic fluid as well as imaging studies (chest and abdominal radiographs, CT scan, endoscopic ultrasonography, MRI, positron emission tomography [PET] and endoscopic retrograde cholangiopancreatography [ERCP]).

Specific blood studies used to assess pancreatic function include measurements of serum amylase, lipase, glucose, calcium, and triglycerides. Urine amylase and renal amylase clearance tests may also be ordered. Stool specimens may be analyzed for fat content.

The secretin stimulation test measures the volume and bicarbonate concentration of pancreatic fluid after secretin is given intravenously to stimulate the production of pancreatic fluid.

If cancer is suspected, blood levels of cancer antigen (CA) 19-9 and carcinoembryonic antigen (CEA), which are considered "markers" for cancer, may be measured. Unfortunately, levels of these antigens are elevated with many types of cancer, so their presence does not specifically indicate pancreatic cancer.

Additional information about diagnostic tests and procedures for the pancreas is provided in Table 37.1.

PANCREATITIS

Pancreatitis is inflammation of the pancreas. It may be acute or chronic. Pancreatitis is most often associated with alcoholism or obstruction of the pancreatic duct by a gallstone. Other causes include viral infections; peptic ulcer disease; cysts; metabolic disorders (i.e., renal failure, hyperparathyroidism); and trauma from external injury, surgery, or endoscopic procedures. A high-fat diet and cigarette smoking may play a role as well. Chronic pancreatitis, which is often associated with alcohol abuse, may follow the acute condition but often develops independently. In addition, chronic pancreatitis is sometimes associated with cancer of the duodenum or pancreas.

Normally, pancreatic enzymes are activated in the small intestine. With pancreatitis, digestive enzymes (trypsin, elastase, and phospholipase A) are activated by some mechanism that is not well understood and begin to digest pancreatic tissue (a process called *autodigestion*), fat, and elastic tissue in blood vessels. Pancreatic fluid may leak into the surrounding tissues. The effect of this escaped fluid has been compared with an internal chemical burn and it can be devastating.

Put On Your Thinking Cap!

The term *autodigestion* is used to describe the effects of pancreatitis. Explain what this means.

Signs and Symptoms

Abdominal pain is the most prominent symptom of pancreatitis. The pain is typically severe with a sudden onset, is centered in the left upper quadrant or the epigastric region and radiates to the back. Severe vomiting, flushing, cyanosis, and dyspnea often accompany the pain. Other signs and symptoms are low-grade fever, tachypnea, tachycardia, and hypotension.

The abdomen may be tender and distended. Bowel sounds may be absent, suggesting an ileus. Trypsin may damage blood vessels, causing pancreatic hemorrhage and discoloration of the abdomen. Cyanosis or greenish discoloration of the abdominal wall, the flanks, and the area around the umbilicus may be present. Enzymes released into the abdominal cavity increase capillary permeability, permitting protein-rich serum to leak from blood vessels. Bleeding and shifting of fluid reduce blood volume and may lead to shock. Early signs and symptoms of shock are restlessness and tachycardia. Hypotension is a late sign.

Symptoms of chronic pancreatitis are similar to those of the acute disease but usually appear as periodic attacks that become more and more frequent. In addition, patients with chronic pancreatitis may develop diabetes mellitus and malabsorption with steatorrhea.

Complications

Complications of pancreatitis include pseudocyst; abscess; hypocalcemia; and pulmonary, cardiac, and renal complications.

A pseudocyst is a fluid-filled pouch attached to the pancreas. It contains products of tissue destruction and pancreatic enzymes. The fluid can leak into the digestive tract or the abdominal cavity. Symptoms of pseudocyst include abdominal pain, nausea, vomiting, and anorexia. Sometimes a mass can be palpated in the epigastric area. Necrosis within the pancreas can lead to pancreatic abscess, a fluid-filled cavity in the pancreas. Symptoms are similar to those of pseudocyst. Patients usually run a high fever.

Hypocalcemia (low serum calcium) is caused by the action of fatty acids on calcium and increased loss of calcium in the urine. The pulmonary complications of pancreatitis are pneumonia and atelectasis. Pancreatitis can be fatal. In the early stage of acute pancreatitis, cause of death is usually cardiovascular, renal, or pulmonary failure. Later, sepsis and abscesses are the leading causes of death.

A person may recover completely from an attack of acute pancreatitis, have repeated acute episodes, or develop chronic pancreatitis.

Medical Diagnosis

The most important diagnostic findings in acute pancreatitis are elevated serum amylase, serum lipase, and urinary amylase levels. When the kidneys clear amylase more rapidly than they clear creatinine, acute pancreatitis is strongly suspected. Other findings with acute pancreatitis are elevated WBC count, elevated serum lipid and glucose levels, and decreased serum calcium level. Ultrasonography and ERCP may reveal the presence of gallstones, cysts, or abscesses and help to rule out other disorders that might be causing the patient's symptoms.

Tests for chronic pancreatitis include the secretin stimulation test and fecal studies in addition to the tests used for acute pancreatitis. Findings consistent with chronic pancreatitis are decreased volume and bicarbonate concentration of pancreatic fluid, low serum trypsinogen, and high fecal fat content. Imaging procedures reveal the structure of the pancreas and the pancreatic duct.

Medical Treatment

Specific medical interventions vary depending on the severity of the condition. IV fluids are ordered to restore and maintain fluid balance. Urine output is monitored and should be at least 40 mL per hour. Once food is permitted, the patient is usually started on a low residue, low fat, soft diet. If the patient cannot tolerate the oral route, a nasojejunal feeding tube or TPN may be needed to provide adequate nutrients. Because the inflamed pancreas is susceptible to infection, some physicians order prophylactic antibiotics. Fluid that accumulates around the pancreas usually resolves without intervention. However, the fluid is sometimes drained using endoscopy or the percutaneous route.

Drug therapy. Drug therapy for pancreatitis commonly includes analgesics, antispasmodic agents, anticholinergic agents, and gastric acid inhibitors. Pain control is a major problem with pancreatitis. Opioids (e.g., morphine, fentanyl) are the preferred analgesics for acute pancreatitis. Anticholinergic agents decrease secretions, which can reduce spasms and pain. Reducing the secretion of gastric acid decreases the stimulus for pancreatic secretions.

With chronic pancreatitis, pain may be managed with tricyclic antidepressants (amitriptyline), NSAIDs, and opioids (morphine or fentanyl patches). Other options are endoscopic nerve block and dilation of ductal strictures, and various surgical procedures described below. The patient with chronic pancreatitis is likely to need to take pancreatic enzymes to digest food. The enzymes can be taken with meals or snacks. The effect of the enzymes can be determined by examining the stools. Steatorrhea (i.e., bulky, frothy stools with a high fat content) results from inadequate enzymes. If diabetes mellitus develops, insulin or oral hypoglycemic drugs are needed and the patient requires diabetes education.

Other drugs that may be needed are antacids, anticholinergic agents, and histamine blockers to decrease hydrochloric acid in the stomach. Bile salts may also be needed to enhance absorption of fat-soluble vitamins. Drugs used to treat pancreatitis are described in Chapter 37, Table 37.2.

Health Promotion

Nonpharmacologic measures that can improve symptoms of chronic pancreatitis include cessation of alcohol intake and smoking.

Surgical intervention. Various surgical procedures may be indicated. For example, if gallstones are present, endoscopic sphincterotomy followed by cholecystectomy may be done. If an abscess, pseudocyst, or severe peritonitis develops, surgical intervention is indicated. Debridement involves resection of necrotic tissue and irrigation of the cavity to remove harmful fluid. The procedure may need to be repeated more than once. After surgical debridement, multiple sumps may be placed in the abdomen for continuous postoperative irrigation. Each sump tube is connected to a separate suction apparatus. Irrigations may be alternated as ordered. Endoscopic or percutaneous debridement may be used in patients who are poor surgical risks.

◆ NURSING CARE OF THE PATIENT WITH PANCREATITIS

Focused Assessment

General nursing assessment of the patient with a disorder of the digestive tract is outlined in Box 37.1. When a patient has acute pancreatitis, it is especially important to report signs of hypovolemic shock: restlessness, tachycardia, tachypnea, hypotension, and decreased urinary output. The abdomen should be inspected for discoloration, distention, tenderness, and diminished bowel sounds. The flanks should also be examined for discoloration. In addition, the patient's mental status should be monitored. Altered mental status may be the result of metabolic imbalances. Confusion and agitation may occur in the patient who abuses alcohol because of withdrawal (see the Nursing Care Plan).

If the patient has surgery, general postoperative assessment should include the data covered in Chapter 17.

Patient Problems, Goals, and Outcome Criteria: Pancreatitis

Patient Problems	Goals and Outcome Criteria
Acute pain related to inflammation, infection, biliary obstruction, autodigestion	Pain relief: patient states pain is reduced or relieved, relaxed manner
Fluid volume deficit related to vomiting, bleeding, fluid shift from the blood to the abdominal cavity	Normal fluid balance: balanced fluid intake and output, pulse and blood pressure (BP) consistent with patient norms
Potential for infection related to tissue necrosis	Absence of infection: normal body temperature and white blood cell (WBC) count
Potential for inadequate oxygenation related to pain, pulmonary complications	Adequate oxygenation: breath sounds clear to auscultation, respiratory rate 12 to 20 breaths per minute, O_2 saturation of 95% or higher
Inadequate nutrition related to anorexia, vomiting, digestive disturbance	Adequate nutrition: stable body weight
Anxiety related to unfamiliar setting and procedures, acute illness	Reduced anxiety: patient states anxiety is lessened, calm manner
Inability to manage self-care related to lack of knowledge of therapy and measures to reduce risk of recurrence related to lack of exposure to information, acute illness	States self-care needed to manage symptoms: patient states understanding of self-care to prevent recurrence

Nursing Care Plan Patient With Pancreatitis

FOCUSED ASSESSMENT

Health History

Mrs. Sanchez is a 57-year-old Latina admitted with repeated attacks of severe pain in the left upper quadrant that radiates to her back. She reports having vomited repeatedly over the past 24 hours. When the pain is severe, she reports feeling flushed, faint, and short of breath. She has no other related symptoms. Mrs. Sanchez reports having had a gallbladder attack several months ago that resolved without surgery. She is a high school teacher who lives with her husband.

Physical Examination Vital signs: blood pressure 144/84 mm Hg, pulse 92 beats per minute, height 5′2″, weight 150 lb, respiration 24 breaths per minute, temperature 100.2°F (37.9°C), measured orally. The patient appears to be in acute distress but is alert and oriented. Abdomen is tender and distended, with hypoactive bowel sounds in all four quadrants.

Patient Problems	Goals and Outcome Criteria	Interventions
Acute pain related to inflammation, biliary obstruction, autodigestion	The patient will report decreased pain and will appear more relaxed.	Document painful episodes. Treat the patient promptly with analgesics and antispasmodic drugs as ordered. Use distraction, imagery, and relaxation techniques to enhance drug therapy. Advise the physician if pain is unrelieved.
Fluid volume deficit related to vomiting, bleeding, fluid shift from bloodstream to abdominal cavity	The patient's fluid status will stabilize, as evidenced by stable blood pressure (BP) and pulse, normal skin color, and urine output equal to fluid intake.	Insert a nasogastric tube and connect it to low suction as ordered. Initiate intravenous fluid therapy and administer medications as ordered. Monitor the patient's vital signs, intake and output, weight, and electrolyte studies. Report any signs of fluid volume deficit (i.e., tachycardia, hypotension, dry skin, concentrated urine) to the physician.
Potential for infection related to tissue necrosis	The patient will be free of signs and symptoms of infection: fever, tachycardia, and increased white blood cell (WBC) count.	Monitor the patient's vital signs and blood cell counts. Report any signs of infection. Administer antimicrobials as ordered. Use Standard Precautions for invasive procedures.
Potential for inadequate oxygenation related to pain, pulmonary complications	The patient will remain free of pulmonary complications, as evidenced by absence of dyspnea, tachypnea, and abnormal breath sounds.	Assess the patient's respirations and breath sounds. Assist her to change positions, to cough, and to deep breathe at least every 2 hours. Use a semi-Fowler position to promote lung expansion.
Inadequate nutrition related to anorexia, vomiting, digestive disturbances	The patient's body weight will remain stable.	Administer total parenteral nutrition (TPN) if ordered. Monitor the patient for hyperglycemia and administer insulin as ordered. Take daily weights. When oral intake is permitted, monitor the patient's tolerance. Discourage spicy foods, caffeine, and alcohol.
Anxiety related to acute symptoms	The patient will report decreased anxiety and will be calm.	Check on the patient often. Respond to her needs promptly. Ask what questions she has and provide explanations of the condition and the treatment she is receiving.

CRITICAL THINKING QUESTIONS

1. Explain why the patient with pancreatitis has severe pain.
2. Explain why it is necessary to monitor respiratory status in the patient with pancreatitis.

Interventions

Acute pain. Describe the patient's pain and provide ordered analgesics promptly. Reposition the patient for comfort. Other nursing measures for pain are described in Chapter 8 and include distraction, imagery, and cutaneous stimulation (see the Complementary and Alternative Therapies box). Evaluate and record the effectiveness of pain control measures. The physician should be informed if pain is not relieved.

Complementary and Alternative Therapies

Distraction, imagery, relaxation, and cutaneous stimulation can enhance the effects of analgesics to promote pain relief.

Fluid volume deficit. Administer prescribed IV fluids. Monitor the patient's fluid status by measuring vital signs, intake and output, and weight. Signs of fluid volume deficit include tachycardia, hypotension, dry skin, concentrated urine, and decreased urine output. The physician should be informed if the urine output falls below 40 mL/h. Depletion of blood volume causes hypovolemic shock and leads to death if not corrected. Other potential fluid imbalances are metabolic alkalosis from severe vomiting, hypokalemia, hyponatremia, hypocalcemia, and hypochloremia.

Potential for infection. Necrosis of the pancreas and surrounding tissue provides a site for infection. If a surgical procedure is done, there is also a risk for wound infection. Inform the physician of fever, purulent drainage, or separation of wound margins—all signs of infection. Take special care to maintain asepsis during wound care. Administer antibiotics as ordered.

Inadequate oxygenation. Fluid accumulation in the peritoneal cavity puts upward pressure on the diaphragm, thereby limiting lung expansion. Because the acutely ill patient is inactive, secretions may pool in the lungs. Poor lung expansion and inactivity combine to invite pneumonia and atelectasis. Monitor for tachypnea, dyspnea, and abnormal breath sounds.

Measures to prevent pulmonary complications in the patient with pancreatitis include frequent turning, coughing, and deep breathing. The semi-Fowler position promotes lung expansion.

Inadequate nutrition. Initially, the patient may be NPO because food and fluids stimulate pancreatic fluid secretion. When oral intake is resumed, small feedings of a low residue, low-fat soft diet are provided. Spicy foods, caffeine, and alcohol should be avoided (see the Patient Teaching box). TPN (see Chapter 15) is usually needed only with severe malnourishment. Daily weights are used to evaluate the adequacy of the nutrition plan.

The patient with chronic pancreatitis commonly requires pancreatic enzyme replacement taken with meals and supplemental vitamins. Specific dietary recommendations are based on the nutritional assessment. If the pancreas is severely damaged, insulin secretion will be deficient. The patient will have to be managed like a person with diabetes mellitus (see Chapter 50).

Anxiety. Attempt to determine the reasons for the patient's anxiety. Some concerns can be alleviated by telling the patient what is happening and what to expect. Respond promptly to the patient's needs and offer comforting reassurance by checking on the patient frequently. Anxiety can be related to pain or hypoxia as well as to emotional distress, so assess for comfort and oxygenation status and take appropriate corrective actions. During acute attacks, answer questions and give simple explanations. As the patient improves, implement your teaching plan.

Inability to manage self-care. The patient with acute pancreatitis is too ill for systematic teaching. Explain simply what you are doing and why. Answer any questions the patient may ask. As the patient improves, the teaching plan should address the importance of avoiding alcohol and tobacco to prevent recurrences. Explain the rationale for the prescribed diet.

Patient Teaching

Pancreatitis

- Your prescribed diet (usually low residue, low fat) will avoid stimulating your pancreas and will promote healing.
- At first, you may tolerate small, frequent meals better than large meals.
- Abstaining from alcohol and tobacco decreases your risk of recurrence.
- Community resources such as Alcoholics Anonymous can assist if it is hard for you to abstain from drinking alcohol (www.aa.org; telephone: 1-212-686-1100).

CANCER OF THE PANCREAS

Cancer of the pancreas is extremely serious as it quickly spreads to the duodenum, stomach, spleen, and left adrenal gland. It most commonly originates in exocrine tissue. A rare form is pancreatic neuroendocrine tumor (NET). About 60,000 new cases were expected to be diagnosed and 48,220 deaths were predicted in 2021 in the United States. The five year survival rate overall is 10%, but varies greatly with the stage at diagnosis: localized = 39%, regional = 13%, distant = 3% (see the Cultural Considerations box). The risk factors for pancreatic cancer include chronic pancreatitis and smoking. Other probable risk factors are obesity, diabetes mellitus, a high-fat diet, and exposure to certain toxic chemicals. Tumors may develop in the head, body, or tail of the pancreas.

Cultural Considerations

What Does Culture Have to Do With Pancreatic Cancer?

A family history of pancreatic ductal carcinoma and a high-fat diet are two risk factors for pancreatic cancer.

Signs and Symptoms

Signs and symptoms of pancreatic cancer vary with the stage and location but often include pain, jaundice with or without liver enlargement, weight loss, and glucose intolerance. When located in the head of the pancreas, tumors typically obstruct the common bile duct, causing jaundice. In the early stage of the disease, jaundice may be the only sign present. If the patient seeks medical care early, the chance of survival is somewhat better. Other signs and symptoms may be weight loss, upper abdominal pain, anorexia, vomiting, weakness, and diarrhea.

When the tumor is in the body or the tail of the pancreas, the patient may not have any symptoms until the disease is advanced. Then the liver, gallbladder, and spleen may be enlarged. Pressure on the portal veins may cause esophageal and gastric varices (dilated veins) that bleed easily into the GI tract. Pressure on nerves may cause back pain.

Medical Diagnosis

The most useful diagnostic tests and procedures when pancreatic cancer is suspected are CT, MRI, ERCP, magnetic resonance cholangiopancreatography (MRCP), and endoscopic ultrasonography. Blood studies and other imaging procedures can be helpful as well. Blood values associated with pancreatic cancer include elevated serum amylase, lipase, bilirubin, and enzyme levels. The tumor marker CA 19-9 is usually elevated with pancreatic cancer. Percutaneous transhepatic cholangiography and ERCP allow the physician to detect obstructed pancreatic ducts and to take samples of pancreatic fluid and tissue.

Medical and Surgical Treatment

Treatment depends on the location and extent of the malignant tissue. If the tumor is confined to the head of the pancreas, surgery may be an option. A variety of procedures may be used for pancreatic cancer. The most common are side-to-side pancreaticojejunostomy, caudal pancreaticojejunostomy, and radical pancreaticoduodenectomy (Whipple procedure), as illustrated in Fig. 40.7. Potential complications of the Whipple procedure are listed in Table 40.3.

Sometimes surgical procedures are done primarily to relieve obstruction and improve patient comfort. Opioid analgesics are ordered for pain management. At times, a jejunostomy tube is placed below the obstruction so that the patient can be given tube feedings.

Research is continuing to seek the best strategy for this challenging cancer. Radiation therapy and chemotherapy may be advised either preoperatively or postoperatively. Radiation does not appear to improve survival but may reduce pain. For patients who are candidates for surgery, the addition of a 6-month course of 5 fluorouracil (5-FU) or gemcitabine after surgery reduces mortality by about one-third. Some physicians believe that a combination of surgery, radiation, and chemotherapy may be the best approach. These therapies are discussed in detail in Chapter 7.

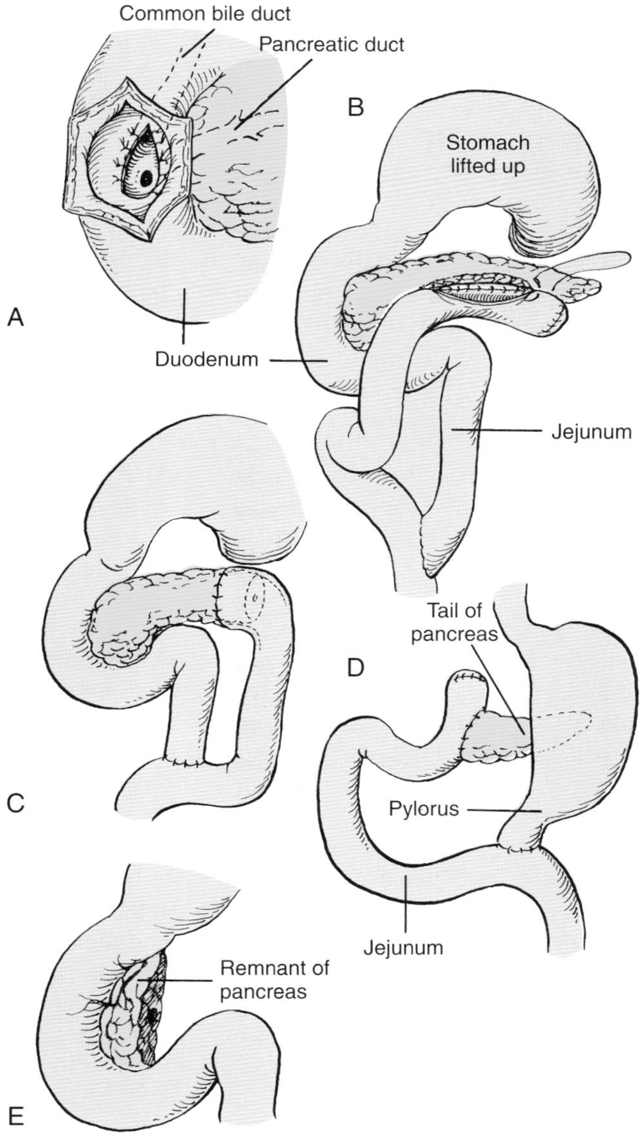

A. **Sphincteroplasty (ampullary)**
Indicated for stenosis of the sphincter of Oddi with dilation of the pancreatic duct. This procedure has limited application in pancreatitis and its use is decreasing.

B. **Side-to-side pancreaticojejunostomy (ductal drainage)**
Indicated when gross dilation of the pancreatic ducts is associated with septa and calculi. The most successful procedure, with rates of 60% to 90%.

C. **Caudal pancreaticojejunostomy (ductal drainage)**
Indicated for the uncommon cases of isolated proximal pancreatic ductal stenosis not involving the ampulla.

D. **Radical pancreaticoduodenectomy (ablative) (with preservation of pylorus) (Whipple procedure)**
Indicated when major changes are confined to the head of the pancreas. Preservation of the pylorus avoids the usual sequelae of gastric resection.

E. **Subtotal pancreatectomy (ablative)**
Indicated when other operations fail and when ducts are unsuitable for decompression. Because metabolic sequelae are significant, this procedure is declining in popularity.

Fig. 40.7 Surgical procedures for pancreatic cancer. (From Black JM, Hawks JH, Keene AM: *Medical-surgical nursing: clinical management for continuity of care*, ed 6, Philadelphia, 2001, Saunders.)

Table 40.3 Potential Complications of the Whipple Procedure

COMPLICATION	NURSING INTERVENTIONS
Hemorrhage	Monitor vital signs for tachycardia and falling blood pressure (BP). Assess for restlessness. Check dressings and drains for excess bleeding.
Fluid and electrolyte imbalances	Assess for cardiac dysrhythmias, muscle weakness or twitching, and changes in mental status. Monitor intake and output as well as tissue turgor. Check laboratory reports and notify the physician of abnormalities.
Respiratory failure	Monitor respiratory rate and effort, skin color, and breath sounds.
Circulatory failure	Monitor for dysrhythmias, tachycardia, and falling BP.
Renal failure	Measure intake and urine output. Report output of less than 30 mL/h. Assess for edema. Maintain prescribed fluid intake.
Hepatic failure	Assess for jaundice, fatigue, confusion, and digestive disturbances.
Wound infection, dehiscence, and fistulas	Assess dressing and drains for excess bleeding, foul odor, and purulent drainage. Check the patient's temperature for fever. Note any elevation in the white blood cell (WBC) count.
Hyperglycemia	Monitor blood glucose as ordered. Note drowsiness, thirst, polyphagia, and polyuria.

◆ NURSING CARE OF THE PATIENT WITH PANCREATIC CANCER

Focused Assessment

General assessment of the patient with a digestive disorder is outlined in Chapter 37, Box 37.1. With pancreatic cancer, pay particular attention to GI function, pain, and emotional state. If surgery is planned, determine the patient's knowledge about preoperative and postoperative care.

Patient Problems, Goals, and Outcome Criteria: Cancer of the Pancreas

Patient Problems	Goals and Outcome Criteria
Acute pain related to obstruction, extensive malignancy	Pain relief: patient states pain is reduced or relieved, more relaxed
Fear and grieving related to diagnosis or poor prognosis	Reduced fear: patient states being less fearful, makes realistic plans; receives family support
Inadequate nutrition related to anorexia, nausea, vomiting	Adequate nutrition: stable body weight
Potential for disrupted skin tissue integrity related to pruritus, inactivity, nutritional deficiencies	Healthy skin: skin intact without reddened area or abrasions
Altered body image related to jaundice, weight loss	Adjustment to physical changes: patient makes effort to improve appearance, attends to grooming and dress
Inability to manage self-care related to lack of knowledge of symptom management and sources of support	Adequate knowledge to manage self-care: patient and family demonstrate understanding of patient care and resources

Interventions

In many ways, the care of the patient with pancreatic cancer is like that discussed under "Nursing Care of the Patient With Pancreatitis." Chapter 7 also provides details of caring for the patient with cancer. Areas that require special attention with pancreatic cancer are discussed here.

Acute pain. Assess and record pain severity, nature, and location. Opioid analgesics are usually needed for severe pain management; however, nonopioids may be effective for mild to moderate pain. Radiation therapy and chemotherapy can reduce pain by shrinking the tumor. A celiac plexus nerve block can be done during surgery or percutaneously and provides excellent pain control for several months. Other options for intolerable pain are patient-controlled analgesia (PCA) and epidural opioids. The effectiveness of drug therapy may be enhanced by distraction, imagery, and cutaneous stimulation, as discussed in Chapter 8.

Fear and grieving. You can help the patient by recognizing and acknowledging their fear, showing compassion, teaching, and providing attentive care. A referral to a mental health professional or spiritual counselor can be made with the patient's consent.

Inadequate nutrition. Monitor the patient's dietary intake and weight. If intake is poor, consult the dietitian. Small, frequent meals may be ordered. Pancrelipase tablets are needed if the patient has malabsorption. Sometimes a jejunostomy tube is placed and feeding is delivered by pump. Feedings are usually started with dilute formula given at a slow rate. Both the concentration and the rate are gradually increased. Inform the physician if the patient develops diarrhea. Some patients require TPN for adequate nourishment (see the Nutrition Considerations box).

Potential for disrupted skin tissue integrity. If pruritus is a problem, special skin care and protection are needed. Eliminate bath soaps and apply emollient lotions. Keep the fingernails short to reduce trauma from scratching. Supply mittens if the patient is unable to avoid scratching. The physician may order diphenhydramine (Benadryl) to reduce pruritus. If a patient has drains or fistulas, irritating digestive fluids may come in contact with the skin. Carefully cleanse the exposed skin. Skin barriers and pouches may be effective in protecting the skin. An enterostomal therapist may be consulted for advice on skin care.

Altered body image. Weight loss and jaundice alter the patient's appearance and may be distressing. Assist patients with grooming and encourage them to look their best.

Inability to manage self-care. People under stress retain only part of what they hear, so information must often be repeated and reinforced. Provide written material in addition to verbal instruction. The patient's family may also need information and support when dealing with a diagnosis of pancreatic cancer. Refer questions about medical decisions and prognosis to the physician. The specific teaching plan will depend on the diagnostic and therapeutic measures prescribed. You should advise the patient of community resources, including the American Cancer Society and home health nursing services.

Surgical Complications and Postoperative Nursing Care

In general, the postoperative care of the patient with pancreatic cancer is like that of any patient undergoing major abdominal surgery. If the Whipple procedure is performed, the patient is at risk for many complications. These include hemorrhage; fluid and electrolyte imbalances; respiratory, circulatory, renal, and hepatic failure; wound infection and dehiscence; fistulas; and hyperglycemia. Therefore ongoing nursing assessments are critical. Closely monitor vital signs, intake and output, and blood glucose values. Assess the wound for bleeding, infection, and separation of margins. Evaluate mental status to detect changes associated with electrolyte imbalances, poor circulation, and hepatic or renal failure.

Nutrition Considerations

1. People with gallbladder disease should follow a low-fat diet because fat intake usually causes pain.
2. For a person with hepatitis, the diet should be high in calories and vitamins with moderate to high protein and moderate to low fat.
3. When the liver is damaged by cirrhosis, protein may be restricted to lower blood ammonia.
4. In hepatitis and cirrhosis, carbohydrates should provide most of the calories.
5. A soft, low residue, low-fat diet is recommended for pancreatitis.
6. Pancreatitis patients must avoid alcohol and foods that stimulate the pancreas.

Get Ready for the NCLEX® Examination!

Key Points

- Signs of liver dysfunction include jaundice (a golden-yellow skin color) and scleral icterus (yellowing of the sclera of the eyes).
- Hepatitis is liver inflammation caused by a viral infection or exposure to toxic substances; it can lead to hepatic failure.
- Nursing care of the patient with hepatitis addresses reduced activity tolerance, potential for complications of immobility, inadequate nutrition, acute pain, potential for disrupted skin tissue integrity, fluid volume deficit, altered body image, and anxiety.
- Health care providers should be vaccinated against hepatitis B because it can be spread through contact with body fluids.
- Cirrhosis is chronic, progressive liver failure that disrupts metabolism and causes blood abnormalities, fluid and electrolyte imbalances, decreased resistance to infection, accumulation of drugs and toxins, and obstruction of blood vessels and bile ducts in the liver.
- Cirrhosis may be caused by nutritional deficiencies, toxins (including alcohol), hepatitis, biliary obstruction, and heart failure.
- Complications of cirrhosis include portal hypertension, esophageal varices, ascites, spontaneous bacterial peritonitis, hepatic encephalopathy, and hepatorenal syndrome.
- Nursing care of the patient with cirrhosis addresses inadequate nutrition, reduced activity tolerance, potential for disrupted skin tissue integrity, pain, inadequate ventilation, potential for injury, acute confusion, fluid volume deficit, fluid volume excess, potential for infection, and fear.
- The only cure for end-stage liver disease is liver transplantation, which requires lifelong treatment with antirejection drugs that suppress the immune system and put the patient at risk for infection.
- Signs and symptoms of transplanted organ rejection are fever, anorexia, depression, vague abdominal pain, muscle aches, and joint pain.
- Bile is produced in the liver, stored in the gallbladder, and delivered to the intestine, where it is essential for emulsification and digestion of fats.
- Cholecystitis is inflammation of the gallbladder, usually caused by gallstones; the gallstones may obstruct bile flow, causing symptoms from mild indigestion to nausea, chills and fever, and right upper quadrant pain that radiates to the shoulder.

- Symptomatic cholelithiasis (stones in the bile) are usually treated with laparoscopic cholecystectomy.
- Nursing care of the patient with cholecystitis and cholelithiasis focuses on acute pain, fluid volume deficit, potential for disrupted skin tissue integrity, anxiety, potential for injury, and, for surgical patients, inadequate ventilation and risk for infection.
- The pancreas has an endocrine function (insulin and glucagon secretion) and an exocrine function (secretion of digestive enzymes).
- Pancreatitis is inflammation of the pancreas; it can lead to pseudocyst; abscess; hypocalcemia; and pulmonary, cardiac, and renal complications.
- Nursing care of the patient with pancreatitis addresses pain, fluid volume deficit, potential for infection, potential for inadequate oxygenation, inadequate nutrition, anxiety, and inability to manage self-care.
- The overall five year survival rate for patients with pancreatic cancer is 10% unless it is detected while still localized in which case the five year survival rate is 39%.
- Nursing care of the patient with pancreatic cancer usually focuses on acute pain, fear, grieving, inadequate nutrition, potential for disrupted skin tissue integrity, altered body image, and inability to manage self-care.

Additional Learning Resources

SG Go to your Study Guide for additional learning activities to help you master this chapter content.

Go to your Evolve website (http://evolve.elsevier.com/Linton/medsurg) for the following learning resources and much more:

- Fluid & Electrolyte Tutorial
- Review Questions for the NCLEX® Examination

Clinical Judgment and Next-Generation NCLEX® Examination-Style Questions

1. **Your focused assessment of a patient with hepatitis reveals jaundice, light-colored stools, and dark urine. These findings are typical of which phase of hepatitis? __________________**

   NCLEX Client Need: Physiological Integrity: Physiological Adaptation

2. **A patient who has hepatitis reports that she is itching and cannot resist scratching. Which measures should help to control the itching? (Select all that apply.)**
   1. Apply lubricating lotion
   2. Administer prescribed antihistamine
   3. Use tepid water for bathing
   4. Vigorously massage affected areas
   5. Administer prescribed antibiotics

   NCLEX Client Need: Physiological Integrity: Reduction of Risk Potential

3. **Nursing students are required to have certain immunizations. Vaccination for which of the following is required because health care providers are often in contact with body fluids?**
   1. Hepatitis A
   2. Hepatitis B
   3. Hepatitis C
   4. Hepatitis D

   NCLEX Client Need: Physiological Integrity: Reduction of Risk Potential

4. **A patient with cirrhosis has esophageal varices and hemorrhoids. The nurse understands that varices and hemorrhoids are caused by:**
   1. Blood vessels weakened by malnutrition.
   2. Inability to conjugate and excrete bilirubin.
   3. Elevated pressure in GI blood vessels.
   4. Fluid retention associated with excess aldosterone.

   NCLEX Client Need: Physiological Integrity: Physiological Adaptation

5. **SLO/Objective:** Explain the pathology, signs and symptoms, diagnosis, complications, and medical treatment of selected disorders of the pancreas.

   NGN Item Type: Enhanced Hot Spot

   Cognitive Skill: Recognize Cues
   A 52-year-old female patient comes to the clinic for follow-up 1 month after liver transplantation. The nurse's focused assessment data are as follows:
   - Oral temperature 100.4°F
   - Heart rate 92 beats per minute
   - Respiratory rate 16 breaths per minute
   - Blood pressure 128/70 mm Hg
   - Skin warm and dry
   - Reports having heartburn; treated with Tums

   Which one of the assessment findings would concern the nurse *most*?

   NCLEX Client Need: Physiological Integrity: Reduction of Risk Potential

6. **Which of the following structures comprise the common bile duct? (Select all that apply.)**
   1. Duodenum
   2. Cystic duct
   3. Hepatic bile ducts
   4. Main pancreatic duct
   5. Ductus arteriosis

   NCLEX Client Need: Physiological Integrity: Physiological Adaptation

7. **A patient returns from surgery for an incisional cholecystectomy with a T-tube. The nurse understands that the purpose of the T-tube is to:**
   1. Maintain bile flow in the common bile duct.
   2. Relieve pressure on the liver.
   3. Divert intestinal contents from the surgical site.
   4. Prevent bile leakage into the abdomen.

   NCLEX Client Need: Physiological Integrity: Reduction of Risk Potential

8. **The endocrine functions of the pancreas include which of the following? (Select all that apply.)**
   1. Storage and secretion of insulin in response to high blood glucose levels
   2. Conversion of excess blood glucose to glycogen for storage
   3. Breakdown of excessive fats and carbohydrates in the intestine
   4. Production and secretion of digestive enzymes into the duodenum through a duct
   5. Manufacture and storage of bile

   NCLEX Client Need: Physiological Integrity: Physiological Adaptation

9. A 60-year-old male patient with chronic pancreatitis is taking pancreatic enzyme tablets. To assess the effectiveness of the tablets, the nurse would teach the patient to:

1. Monitor daily weights.
2. Examine the stools for steatorrhea.
3. Record intake and output.
4. Report increasing pain.

NCLEX Client Need: Physiological Integrity: Physiological Adaptation

10. The nurse is teaching a health promotion class. The participants should be told that they can reduce the risk of pancreatic cancer by:

1. Smoking cessation.
2. Increased dietary protein.
3. Regular exercise.
4. Stress reduction activities.

NCLEX Client Need: Physiological Integrity: Reduction of Risk Potential

41 Urologic System Introduction

http://evolve.elsevier.com/Linton/medsurg

Objectives

1. List the data to be collected when assessing a patient who has a urologic disorder.
2. Describe the diagnostic tests and procedures for patients with urologic disorders.
3. Explain the nursing responsibilities for patients who are having tests and procedures to diagnose urologic disorders.
4. Describe the nursing responsibilities for common therapeutic measures used to treat urologic disorders.

Key Terms

anuria (ă-NŪ-rē-ă)
cystectomy (sĭs-TĔK-tō-mē)
dysuria (dĭs-Ū-rē-ă)
hematuria (hĕm-ă-TŪ-rē-ă)
lithotripsy (LĬTH-ō-trĭp-sē)
nephrotoxic (nĕf-rō-TŎK-sĭk)
nocturia (nŏk-TŪ-rē-ă)
oliguria (ŏlĭ-GŪ-rē-ă)
osmolality
polyuria (pŏl-ē-Ū-rē-ă)
stress incontinence
urge incontinence

The urinary tract has a vital role in maintaining homeostasis and removing metabolic wastes. Because body systems are interdependent, disease processes in other body systems may have a direct and harmful effect on the urinary system. Similarly, urinary system diseases may affect the respiratory and circulatory systems significantly. Serious alterations in urinary function eventually affect all other systems. A person can live with one functioning kidney, but the body cannot live if both kidneys are lost.

ANATOMY OF THE URINARY SYSTEM

The normal urinary system consists of two kidneys, two ureters, the bladder, and the urethra (Fig. 41.1).

KIDNEYS AND URETERS

The kidneys are bean-shaped organs located just under and below the 12th rib near the waist of the body trunk called the *flank* (Fig. 41.2). They each are surrounded by fibrous capsules and layers of fat. They are tightly wedged between the peritoneum, a membrane that separates them from the digestive system, and a layer of muscle in the back. Slightly displaced by the liver, the right kidney is situated slightly lower than the left.

The hilum, or entry, to the kidney is located on the concave surface of the kidney near the spine (Fig. 41.3). The right and left renal arteries branch off from the abdominal artery and enter the kidneys at the hilum. The entire blood supply circulates through the kidneys every 4 to 5 minutes. Each renal vein returns filtered blood directly to the inferior vena cava. The kidney is divided into an outer layer called the *cortex* and an inner layer called the *medulla*. The cortex receives a large blood supply and is very sensitive to changes in blood pressure (BP) and blood volume. The medulla is organized into pyramid-shaped structures that concentrate and collect urine and drain it into the calyces, which drain urine into the renal pelvis. The renal pelvis is at the center of the kidney and forms the funnel-shaped proximal end of the ureter. The ureter carries urine from the renal pelvis to the bladder.

The nephron is the functional unit of the kidney. Each kidney has 1 to 1.25 million nephrons. The nephron is a vascular tubular system consisting of a glomerulus, a Bowman capsule, and a tubule. The glomerulus is a mass of blood vessels tucked into the cuplike Bowman capsule. Each tubular system consists of a proximal tubule, the loop of Henle, a distal tubule, and collecting tubules (Fig. 41.4). The nephron is located mostly in the cortex of the kidney, with the loop of Henle dipping into the medulla. A single collecting duct is formed by several tubules and travels through the medulla to the calyces.

BLADDER AND URETHRA

The bladder, made of smooth muscle that stretches to store urine, rests on the floor of the pelvic cavity behind the peritoneum. It is located in front of the rectum in men and in front of the vagina and uterus in women. The upper portion of the bladder is called the *apex* and the base, or *fundus*, is close to the pelvic floor. The bladder neck, containing the internal sphincter, is the most inferior portion. The trigone is a triangular-shaped area on the posterior wall, as seen in Fig. 41.5. The trigone muscles help to close the junction of the ureters and the bladder during urination, preventing backflow of urine into the ureters.

The urethra is a muscular tube lined with mucous membranes that carries urine from the bladder out of the body. The urethra functions as a sphincter, meaning that it contracts to hold urine in the bladder and relaxes to allow urine to flow from the bladder. Approximately 3 cm of the proximal male urethra is encircled by the prostate gland. The urethra is about 18 to 20 cm long in men and 3 to 4 cm long in women. The short length and proximity of the urethra to the female anus are two reasons that women experience an increased incidence of urinary infections.

PHYSIOLOGY OF THE URINARY SYSTEM

The functions of the urinary system are regulatory, excretory, and hormonal. Regulatory functions are performed by the formation of urine and the secretion of renin, which affects BP. Regulatory processes maintain fluid balance, keep electrolytes within normal range, and maintain acid-base balance. The excretory function of the kidney is the elimination of urine. The hormonal function is to stimulate red blood cell (RBC) production.

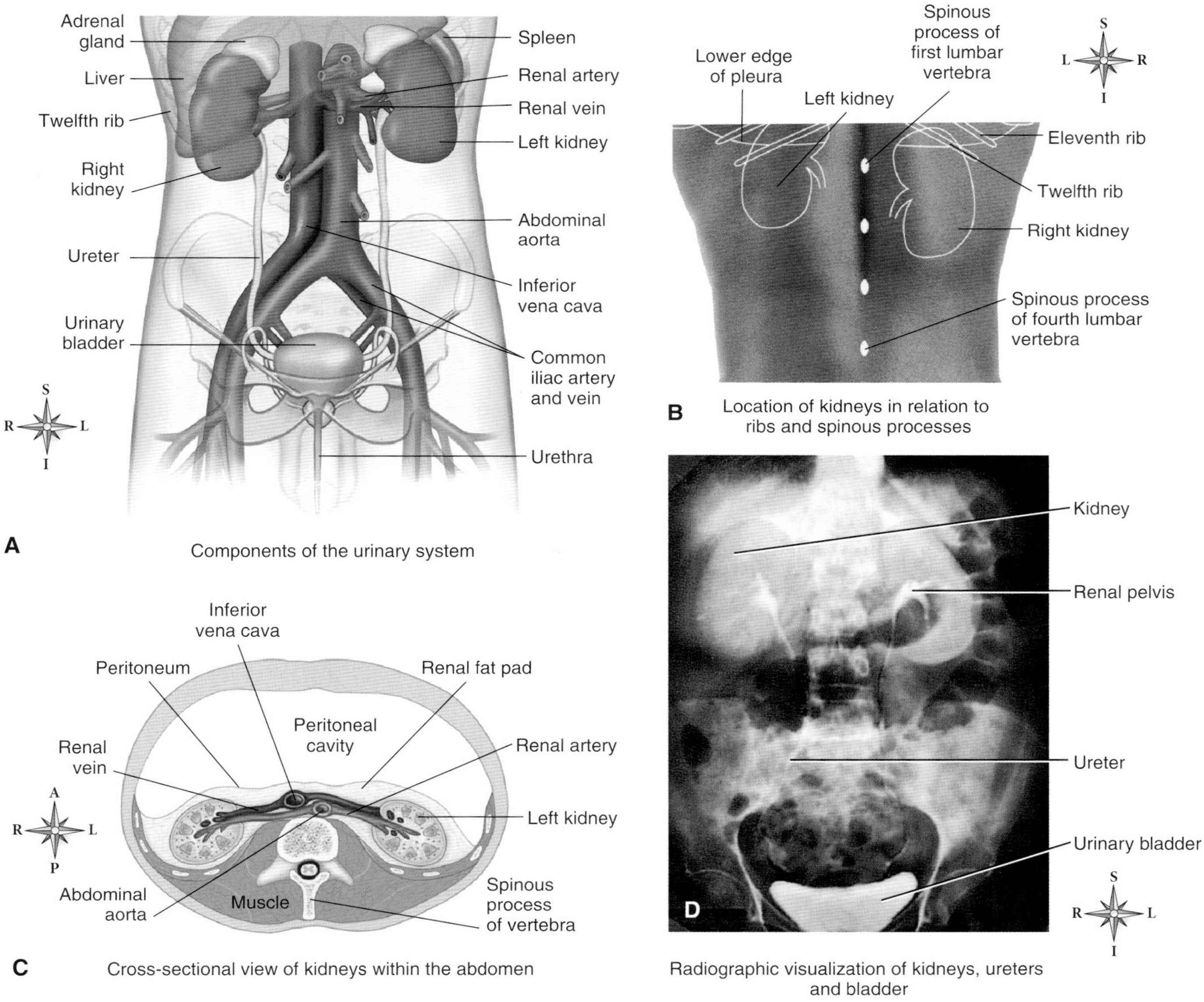

Fig. 41.1 The kidneys and related structures. (A) Components of the urinary system. (B) Location of kidneys in relation to ribs and spinous processes. (C) Cross-sectional view of kidneys within the abdomen. (D) Radiographic visualization of kidneys, ureters and bladder. (From Patton KT, Thibodeau GA: *Human body in health & disease*, ed 7, St. Louis, 2018, Elsevier.)

REGULATION AND EXCRETION

Urine Production

Three processes occur in urine production: (1) glomerular filtration, (2) tubular reabsorption, and (3) tubular secretion.

Glomerular filtration. Glomerular filtration is an ultrafiltration process in the glomerular capsule. Fluids, electrolytes, and other substances are filtered out of the blood as it passes through the glomerulus. Plasma proteins are too large to pass through the glomerulus and therefore remain in the blood. The ultrafiltration process requires adequate blood volume and BP. The product of glomerular filtration is called the *glomerular filtrate*. It contains water, electrolytes (i.e., sodium, potassium, calcium, magnesium, chloride, bicarbonate, phosphate, other anions), glucose, urea, creatinine, uric acid, and amino acids. Glomerular filtrate and blood plasma are essentially the same, except that the filtrate does not have proteins. Most of the filtrate is returned to the blood from the tubules by reabsorption.

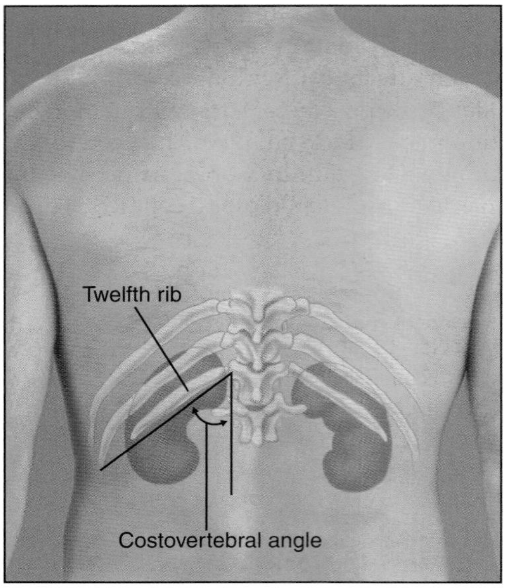

Fig. 41.2 The kidneys are located just under and below the 12th rib. The costovertebral angle is illustrated here. (From Monahan FD, Drake DT, Neighbors M, editors: *Medical-surgical nursing: foundations for clinical practice*, ed 2, Philadelphia, 1998, Saunders.)

Tubular reabsorption. Water, some electrolytes, and nonelectrolytes are reabsorbed from the tubules of the kidney into the blood as needed to maintain normal fluid balance. Reabsorption occurs through diffusion, active transport, and osmosis. Some nonelectrolytes (i.e., urea, creatinine, uric acid) are not readily reabsorbed and are excreted in the urine. The reabsorption of water reflects the ability of the kidney to concentrate or dilute urine as necessary. The amount of water reabsorbed is influenced by antidiuretic hormone (ADH) and aldosterone. ADH, stored in the posterior pituitary, affects the amount of water reabsorbed in the distal tubules and the collecting ducts. If blood volume decreases or blood osmolality (concentration) increases, ADH is secreted from the posterior pituitary. The distal tubules and collecting ducts of the kidney become more permeable to water so that reabsorption into the circulating blood increases and urine becomes more concentrated.

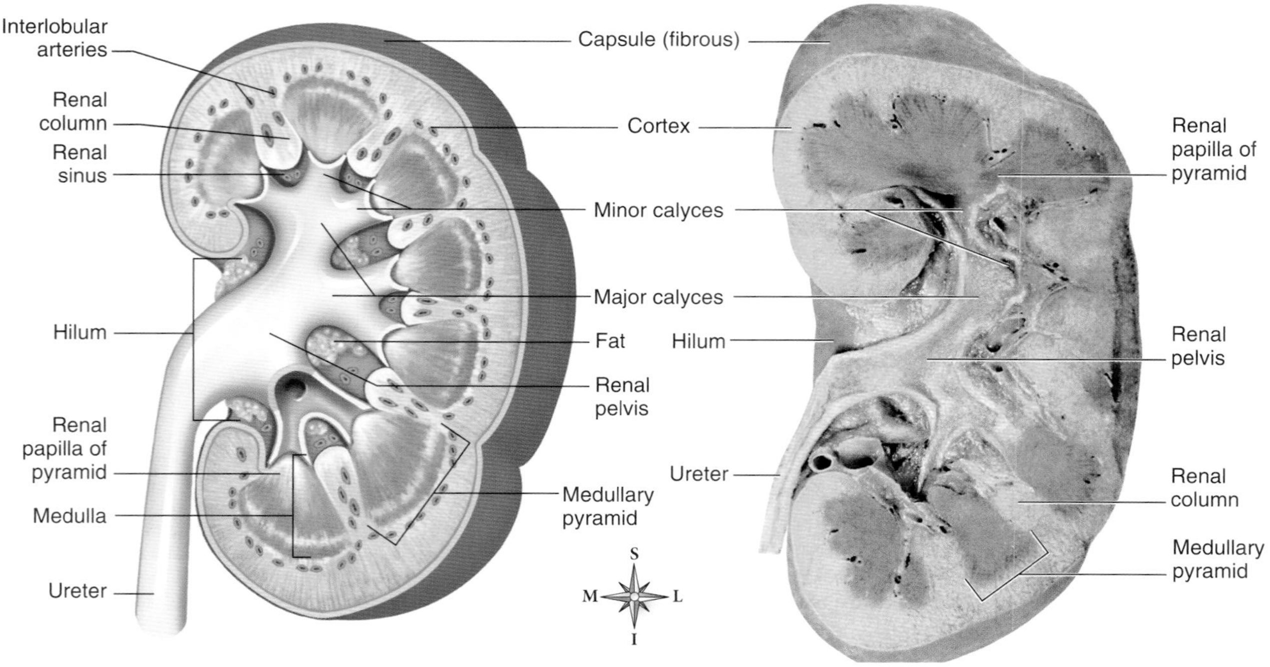

Fig. 41.3 View of interior kidney structures. (From Patton KT, Thibodeau GA: *Human body in health & disease*, ed 7, St. Louis, 2018, Elsevier.)

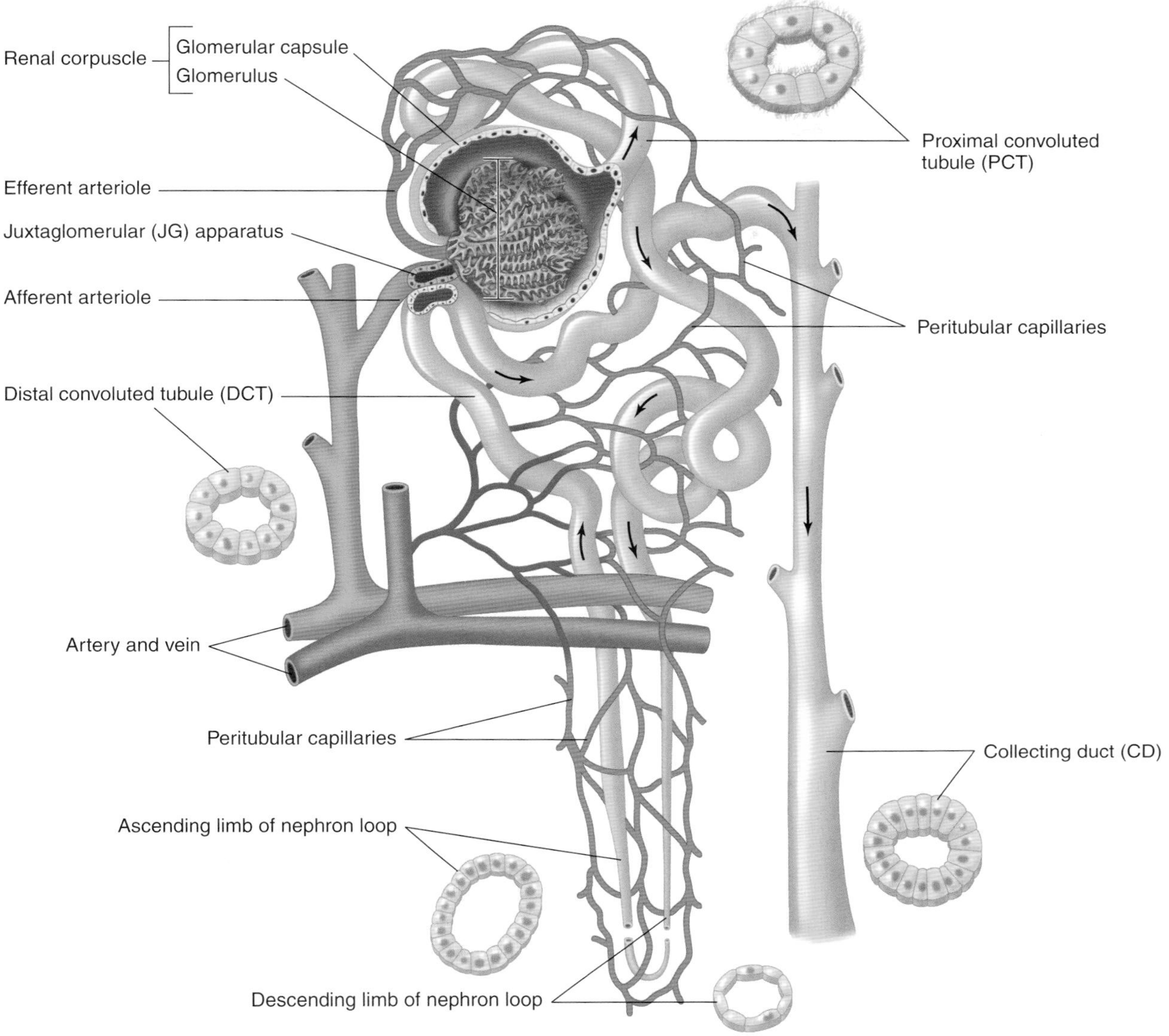

Fig. 41.4 Details of a nephron. (From Patton KT, Thibodeau GA: *Human body in health & disease*, ed 7, St. Louis, 2018, Elsevier.)

Tubular secretion. Potassium and hydrogen ions are secreted into the tubules from the blood. This secretion process regulates serum potassium levels and is the basis for the kidney's acid-base regulating mechanism. The normal pH of urine is 4.6 to 8.0, with an average of 6.0 (Pagana et al., 2017).

The kidneys and lungs work together to maintain the acid-base balance of the body. The lungs excrete carbon dioxide (CO_2), a volatile acid, and the kidneys excrete fixed acids produced by normal metabolism. Base levels are maintained by renal conservation of bicarbonate, excretion of sodium for hydrogen, and excretion of ammonia.

The end product of glomerular filtration, tubular reabsorption, and tubular excretion is urine. Urine is composed mostly of water, sodium, potassium, chloride, urea, creatinine, and uric acid. The body normally excretes 1 to 2 L of urine each day (~30 mL/h minimum), which is approximately 1% of the blood filtered by the glomeruli in the same period of time. Glucose and proteins are substances present in blood but not normally present in the urine. Normally, glucose is completely reabsorbed in the tubules. The presence of proteins in urine indicates glomerular damage. Urine is delivered to the renal pelvis, where it flows into the ureter. The production of urine is illustrated in Fig. 41.6.

Urine Elimination

Peristaltic waves move urine from the kidney through the ureter to the bladder. The presence of 250 to 300 mL of urine in the bladder causes the urge to urinate although the bladder can distend to hold several times that amount. Urination is a complex process that is under a variety of neural controls and is voluntary for the toilet-trained person with intact motor and sensory nerve pathways. Urination generally occurs 5 to 6 times a day and may occur once at night. The amount

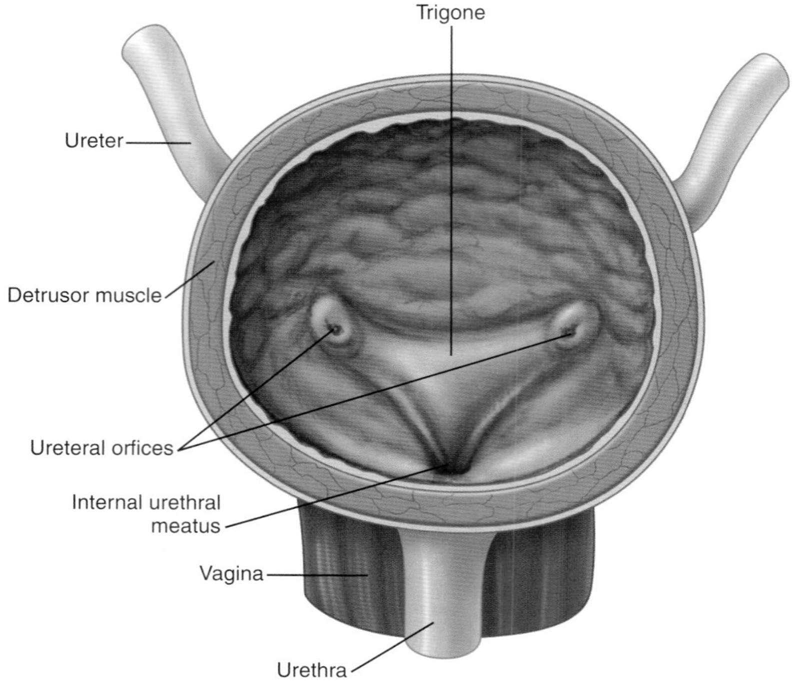

Fig. 41.5 The urinary bladder cut to reveal the interior. (From Walters MD, Barber MD: *Hysterectomy for benign disease*, Philadelphia, 2010, Saunders.)

of urine produced is affected by fluid intake, temperature, diaphoresis, vomiting, diarrhea, and medications such as diuretics as well as some medical conditions.

A series of events allow the release of urine from the bladder. The pelvic floor muscles and the urethral sphincter relax. The trigonal muscles contract, closing the ureters to prevent backflow of urine into the ureters. The bladder muscle (detrusor) contracts and urine is forced through the urethra (see Fig. 41.6). After the bladder empties, the bladder muscle relaxes, the bladder neck closes, the trigonal muscles relax, and the perineal muscles resume resting tone. Voiding is primarily a reflex act. Voluntary control of voiding is exhibited in the initiation, restraint, and interruption of urine flow.

Regulation of Serum Calcium and Phosphate

Parathyroid hormone (PTH) is a hormone secreted by the parathyroid glands to maintain serum calcium levels. When serum calcium is low, PTH is secreted and acts on the tubules to promote reabsorption of calcium ions. At the same time, tubular reabsorption of phosphate is decreased. This mechanism helps to maintain normal serum calcium and phosphate levels.

Regulation of Blood Pressure

BP is regulated through fluid volume maintenance and release of the hormone renin from the kidneys. One way to raise or lower BP is to change blood volume. This can be done by retaining additional fluid or by eliminating excess fluid. For example, suppose that a patient has had severe vomiting and diarrhea resulting in dehydration and low BP. Hypertonic plasma caused by dehydration stimulates the release of ADH from the posterior pituitary. ADH causes reabsorption of water from the renal tubules, decreasing urine volume. The retained fluid expands blood volume, with a subsequent rise in BP.

A second mechanism by which the kidneys affect BP is the secretion of renin. Renin is released in response to inadequate renal blood flow or low arterial pressure. Renin acts on angiotensinogen, a hormone produced by the liver, and converts it to angiotensin I. A lung enzyme converts angiotensin I to angiotensin II. Angiotensin II is a powerful peripheral vasoconstrictor. In addition, angiotensin II triggers the release of aldosterone from the adrenal cortex. Aldosterone stimulates tubular reabsorption of sodium and water and plasma volume is expanded.

With severely decreased cardiac output, as seen in hemorrhage and shock, the renal arteries constrict to prevent fluid loss and to shunt blood to more vital organs (i.e., heart, lungs, brain). This vasoconstriction limits renal blood flow. If blood flow is not restored, renal tissue death may occur.

HORMONAL STIMULATION OF RED BLOOD CELL PRODUCTION

Erythropoietin is secreted in the kidneys and stimulates the bone marrow to produce RBCs. This process is triggered by decreased oxygen (O_2) in renal blood. Patients in renal failure have a deficiency of erythropoietin, which causes them to become anemic.

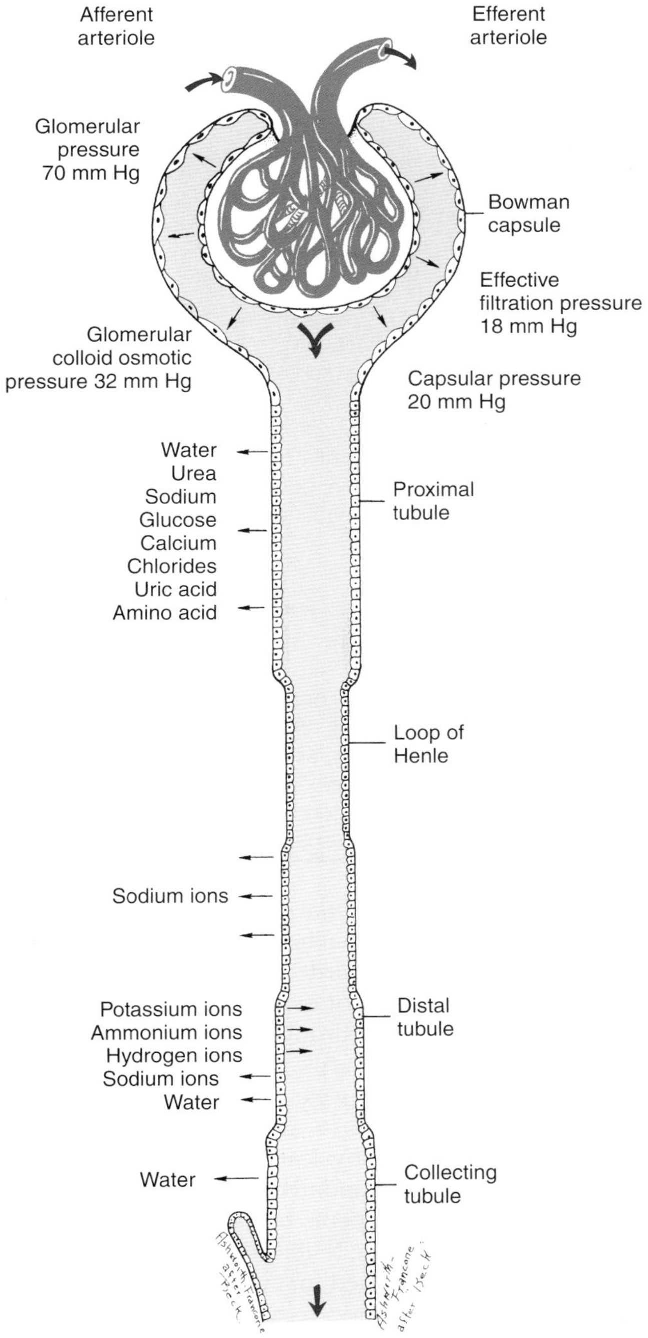

Fig. 41.6 Urine production. (From Jacob WW, Francone CA: *Elements of anatomy and physiology*, ed 2, Philadelphia, 1989, Saunders.)

AGE-RELATED CHANGES IN THE URINARY SYSTEM

As people age, significant changes occur in the urinary system. Fortunately, the kidneys have enough reserve that normal function is usually maintained. However, when older people are stressed, the kidneys do not adapt as well as they do in younger people. Changes include the following:

- Decline in renal blood flow and glomerular filtration
- Decreased ability to concentrate and dilute urine as needed
- Slowed clearing of wastes
- Higher threshold for glucose to appear in the urine when hyperglycemic
- **Nocturia** (common)
- Increased risk of infection resulting from incomplete bladder emptying

Incontinence is not a normal consequence of age, but it is common. Female urinary incontinence is often caused by relaxed pelvic muscles related to childbirth trauma and lack of estrogen after menopause. For detailed information on incontinence, see Chapter 14. In men, urethral obstruction is more often a problem. It is often caused by the enlarged prostate closing in on the urethra. Prostate enlargement is discussed in Chapter 54.

NURSING ASSESSMENT OF THE URINARY SYSTEM

Elimination is a very personal activity, and some people are not accustomed to discussing it with others. Therefore, assessment of urinary function and problems may be embarrassing for the patient. Privacy and a calm, nonjudgmental attitude can help to put the patient at ease.

HEALTH HISTORY

Reason for Seeking Care

Patients with urinary problems often report changes in urine quality or quantity, pain, or changes in urination.

Present Health

Ask about the patient's usual pattern of urination. Important data include frequency, volume, and urine appearance. The patient may have difficulty estimating the amount of urine voided but can usually recognize an increase or decrease from their baseline. If intake and output records are available, note the recent pattern. Document urine volume as ***polyuria*** (a large urine output), ***oliguria*** (a low output), or ***anuria*** (the absence of output). Record urine characteristics including color, clarity (clear or cloudy), presence of particles, odor, and ***hematuria*** (the presence of blood in the urine).

Pain may or may not occur, but it is more common with acute conditions. Painful urination is called ***dysuria***. Ask the patient to describe the presence and characteristics of the pain: intensity, location, distribution, onset, duration, frequency, relationship to urination, precipitating factors, and measures that provide relief. Urologic conditions may also cause pain in the flank, abdomen, pelvic area, and genitalia. The pain may be so severe that it causes nausea and vomiting.

Document problems the patient has had with initiating or controlling urination, and the circumstances under which these problems occur. For example, involuntary loss of urine with laughing or sneezing is typical of ***stress incontinence***. ***Urge incontinence*** is the inability to hold urine when feeling the need to void.

Past Health History

After the present illness has been fully described, the patient's past medical history should be explored. Significant findings include a history of streptococcal infections, recurrent urinary tract infections (UTIs), renal calculi ("stones"), diabetes mellitus, gout, and/or hypercalcemia. Ask if the patient has had urologic surgery, catheterization, examination (e.g., cystoscopy, radiography), or trauma, and if the patient uses any type of urinary diversion or collection device. Document recent and current medications, including prescription and over-the-counter (OTC) drugs, vitamin and herbal remedies, because some of these are ***nephrotoxic*** (harmful to the kidneys). Document exposure to toxic chemicals in the home or the workplace.

Family History

Important family medical history data include congenital problems such as polycystic kidneys or urinary tract malformations, diabetes mellitus, and hypertension.

Review of Systems

Assess all body systems to detect other problems that may be related to the urinary tract complaints. Ask if the patient has had changes in skin color, respiratory symptoms, edema, fatigue, nausea, vomiting, chills, and fever.

Functional Assessment

The functional assessment includes information about habits and practices that might affect or contribute to urinary tract disorders. Inquire how the chief concern has affected the patient's daily life. Ask about daily fluid consumption, because urine production varies with fluid intake. Determine the patient's usual exercise pattern because excessive exercise or prolonged immobility affects the urinary system.

Pharmacology Capsule

Nephrotoxic drugs are harmful to the kidneys.

PHYSICAL EXAMINATION

The physical examination begins with inspection of the skin for color (i.e., ashen, yellow) and the presence of crystals on the skin (i.e., uremic frost). Evaluate tissue turgor to detect signs of dehydration or edema. Examine the area around the eyes for periorbital edema, which may suggest fluid retention. Inspect the mouth and mucous membranes for moisture and odor. Patients in renal failure may have an odor of urine on their breath.

Observe respiratory rate, pattern, and effort. Respirations may be rapid with metabolic acidosis, infection, and fluid overload. Kussmaul respirations, seen with metabolic acidosis, are rapid and deep. Dyspnea may be evident with fluid overload. Auscultate the lungs for abnormal sounds that may indicate fluid overload. Heart rhythm irregularities may be noted with potassium imbalances.

Inspect the abdomen for scars and contours and palpate for tenderness and bladder distention. Auscultate the kidney area over the costovertebral angle (see Fig. 41.2) to detect renal bruits (swishing sounds caused by turbulent blood flow). Renal bruits indicate renal artery stenosis (narrowing). Then percuss the abdomen. A dull sound may be heard over a full bladder. Pain may be elicited over one or both kidneys.

Observe for edema throughout the examination. With renal failure, edema is generalized rather than dependent. The skin may be dry, flushed, and shiny over the edematous area.

The last part of the physical examination is inspection of the genitalia. Standard precautions should be observed. Examine the penis for lesions, scars, or discharge. If there are penile lesions or urethral discharge, smears should be obtained for culture. The health care provider may also perform rectal and pelvic examinations, especially if symptoms suggest problems of the reproductive system. The pelvic examination may reveal gynecologic rather than urologic problems. The male rectal examination helps to detect prostate enlargement, which often creates problems with voiding. Nursing assessment of urologic function is outlined in Box 41.1. The licensed vocational nurse/licensed practical nurse (LVN/LPN) assists with positioning and draping the patient and sending specimens for study.

Box 41.1 Assessment of the Patient With a Urologic Disorder

HEALTH HISTORY

Present Illness

Changes in urine quality or quantity, voiding pattern, pain

Past Health History

Streptococcal infections, urinary tract infections (UTIs) or calculi, gout, hypercalcemia, urologic surgery or instrumentation, urinary diversion, recent and current medications

FAMILY HISTORY

Urinary disorders, diabetes mellitus, hypertension

Review of Systems

Fatigue, pruritus, dyspnea; urine quantity: polyuria, oliguria, anuria; urine quality: color, odor, components; frequency of voiding; pain: onset, intensity, frequency, location, duration, precipitating and relieving factors

Functional Assessment

Fluid intake, diet, activity

PHYSICAL EXAMINATION

Vital signs

Height and weight

General appearance: Level of consciousness, orientation

Skin: Color, moisture, turgor, crystals

Respirations: Rate, pattern, effort, breath sounds

Circulation: Dysrhythmias, blood pressure (BP) alterations

Abdomen: Scars, contour, tenderness, bruits

Genitalia: Lesions, scars, discharge

DIAGNOSTIC TESTS AND PROCEDURES

Diagnostic tests and procedures for urinary disorders are described here. Related nursing care is presented in Table 41.1.

Table 41.1 Diagnostic Tests and Procedures: Urinary Disorders

TEST AND PURPOSE	PATIENT PREPARATION	POSTPROCEDURE CARE
Laboratory Studies		
General considerations: Check agency manual for specific instructions. Determine if patient needs to be fasting before sample is obtained. Explain which sample (e.g., blood, urine) is needed and why. For blood studies, apply a small dressing to venipuncture site. Apply pressure if oozing persists or if the patient's blood does not clot normally. For urine samples, provide instructions or assist the patient in sample collection. Urine specimens should be sent to the laboratory promptly; refrigerate in a specimen-only refrigerator if a delay occurs.		
Urine culture and sensitivity: Culture identifies microorganisms in urine. Sensitivity determines which antibiotic will be effective. Normal: No growth occurs; results are obtained in 24–36 hours.	Collect a specimen of the first voided urine of the day. Teach midstream, clean-catch technique: cleanse the penis or vulva thoroughly, void a small amount, stop the urine stream, and then void into a sterile container. Collect the specimen before starting antibiotic therapy. If catheterization is necessary, collect the specimen after discarding a small amount of urine.	Unless the specimen container has a preservative, cap the specimen and refrigerate it or send promptly to the laboratory.
Blood urea nitrogen (BUN): Measures amount of urea nitrogen in the blood. Normal: 10 to 20 mg/dL (Pagana et al., 2017). Increases with renal failure, gastrointestinal (GI) bleeding, shock, dehydration, and when taking certain drugs. Decreases with liver failure, overhydration (fluid overload or SIADH), malnutrition or malabsorption, nephrotic syndrome (Pagana et al., 2017).	No special preparation is required.	No special care needed. See general considerations.
Urine creatinine clearance: Measures glomerular filtration rate. Decreases with renal disease. Normal value: 107 to 139 mL/min (male) or 87 to 107 mL/min (female) (Pagana et al., 2017).	Provide a specimen container. Document the first void and save all urine for the next 12 or 24 hours as ordered. Keep the specimen refrigerated. If the patient has a Foley catheter, place the drainage bag in a basin of ice and empty it into a refrigerated container hourly.	No special care needed. See general considerations.
Serum creatinine: Measures the kidneys' ability to excrete waste based on the amount of creatinine in the blood. Normal values: 0.6 to 1.2 mg/dL (male) or 0.5 to 1.1 mg/dL (female) (Pagana et al., 2017). Increased with impaired renal function, urinary obstruction, and muscle disease. Decreased with debilitation, muscular dystrophy, myasthenia gravis.	Usually no preparation is needed.	No special care needed. See general considerations.
Serum electrolytes: Detects alterations reflecting the inability of kidneys to retain or excrete electrolytes. Sodium and potassium are elevated and calcium is decreased in renal failure. Normal values: See Chapter 6.	No special preparation is required.	Check laboratory reports and notify the health care provider of abnormalities. Electrolyte imbalances can be life threatening. See Chapter 6 for details on specific electrolytes.

Continued

Table 41.1 Diagnostic Tests and Procedures Urinary Disorders—cont'd

TEST AND PURPOSE	PATIENT PREPARATION	POSTPROCEDURE CARE
Ultrasound		
Abdominal and renal ultrasound: Uses sound waves to detect cysts, tumors, urinary calculi, and urinary tract malformations or obstructions. Can be used to guide needle insertion for closed biopsy. For the transabdominal route, gel is applied to the skin and an instrument is moved over the lubricated skin surface. Images are recorded for study. To study the rectum or prostate, the instrument is inserted into the rectum.	Patient may be asked to drink a specified amount of water (typically 3 to 4 8-oz glasses of water within 2 hours of the procedure) so that the bladder will be full during ultrasound. The procedure takes about 15 minutes and is painless except for discomfort of full bladder. An enema is usually given if the transrectal route is to be used.	Wash gel off the skin if the transabdominal route is used.
Radiographic Studies		
General interventions: Explain the test to the patient. Radiation exposure is generally contraindicated during pregnancy. Patients should be asked about allergies, especially any previous reactions to contrast dye. Special premedication may be ordered for those patients reporting an allergy to iodine, or an alternative contrast medium may be used. Itching, hives, wheezing, and respiratory distress are symptoms of an allergic reaction. Allergic reactions are treated by discontinuing the administration of the contrast, giving antihistamines, and administering cardiopulmonary resuscitation (CPR) if necessary. The patient can expect a flushed, warm feeling; a salty taste in the mouth; and possible nausea when the contrast medium is injected.		
KUB provides a radiographic view of the kidneys, ureters, and bladder.	No special preparation is required. Schedule this test before studies that use contrast media.	No special care is required.
Intravenous pyelogram (IVP): Uses radiographs and a fluoroscope to outline the kidneys. Uses contrast medium to show urine flow and obstructions. Detects urinary abnormalities, calculi, ureters, and bladder. Laxatives can cause gas that obscures the visualization of stones.	Tell the patient that "dye" (the contrast medium) will be injected and radiographs taken to study the urinary tract. Give laxatives and enemas as ordered before the test. The patient should be placed on nothing-by-mouth (NPO) status 8 to 10 hours before the test.	Encourage fluids to flush contrast medium from the body after the procedure. Monitor for signs of iodine allergy: urticaria, rash, nausea, and swollen parotid glands. Check the injection site for inflammation.
Arteriogram: Used to examine blood vessels of kidney, and to differentiate cysts and tumors. Contrast medium is injected into a catheter (usually placed in the groin) and radiographs are taken as the dye circulates through the kidneys.	NPO for 8 to 12 hours and laxatives and enemas are given. Follow the health care provider's order for medications to be taken or avoided before procedure. Anticoagulant drugs are likely to be withheld before the test to reduce the risk of bleeding. Signed informed consent is required. Have the patient void before sedation.	Monitor the patient for signs of bleeding: tachycardia, dyspnea, restlessness, and abdominal or flank pain. Check the injection site for bleeding. A pressure dressing should be in place. Monitor respiratory status if the patient is sedated. Electrocardiogram (ECG) monitoring may be ordered. Monitor pulse, color, warmth and sensation of the extremity in which the catheter was inserted. Maintain bed rest as ordered. Encourage fluids to eliminate the dye. Measure intake and output.
Computed tomography (CT): Creates cross-sectional images of the kidneys and other organs to reveal abnormalities.	Inform the radiologist if the patient is allergic to contrast media, iodine, or shellfish. Inform the patient that the procedure is painless and noninvasive. NPO status may be ordered. Explain that the patient will lie still on a stretcher while a donut-shaped machine moves around them. Contrast dye is sometimes injected intravenously, which can cause a feeling of warmth, a salty taste, and nausea. Sedation can be ordered if the patient has difficulty lying still.	No special care is usually needed. Inform the health care provider of any signs of allergic response to the contrast dye. Give antihistamines as ordered for allergy.

Table 41.1 Diagnostic Tests and Procedures Urinary Disorders—cont'd

TEST AND PURPOSE	PATIENT PREPARATION	POSTPROCEDURE CARE
Magnetic resonance imaging (MRI): This painless, noninvasive procedure creates soft-tissue images using magnets and radio waves. A contrast medium may be injected intravenously.	Tell the patient that they must lie still for 30 minutes or more. Thumping sounds are heard as the machine operates. Earplugs or headphones may be provided. Some equipment has videos that the patient can view to reduce anxiety. Ask whether the patient is claustrophobic. Give sedation as ordered for agitated or anxious patients. An open MRI machine can be used for claustrophobic patients. Remove any metallic objects such as jewelry. Inquire whether the patient has any implanted devices such as cardiac pacemaker or intracranial aneurysm clips and notify the radiologist. This procedure is contraindicated with some implants. Metal may not be a problem with some newer equipment.	No special postprocedure care is required. Safety precautions should be taken if the patient is sedated.
Renal scan: Uses radioisotopes and radiographs to study renal blood flow. Detects infarctions, trauma, atherosclerosis, transplant rejection, and some renal diseases.	Explain that an isotope will be injected and radiographs taken. This procedure takes about 1 hour. The radiation dose is small and quickly eliminated.	No special care is required unless the patient is incontinent. If so, wear gloves to handle urine; change linens and discard per agency protocol. Continent patients can use a toilet. Pregnant caregivers should avoid these patients for 24 hours.
Invasive Procedures		
Renal biopsy: Excision of a small amount of kidney tissue is done for examination. This may be obtained through an incision (open biopsy) or with a special needle (closed biopsy).	The health care provider explains the procedure selected. For closed biopsy, the patient is positioned prone with a rolled blanket under the abdomen for approximately 45 minutes. Ensure that reports of clotting studies (i.e., prothrombin time [PT], partial thromboplastin time [PTT], platelets) are in the chart. Report elevated blood pressure (BP), which increases the risk of bleeding. Patient should be NPO for 6 hours or as ordered. Signed informed consent is required.	Check the pressure dressing for bleeding. Monitor vital signs for hemorrhage: tachycardia, restlessness, and flank pain radiating to abdomen. Position the patient supine with a blanket roll or sandbag under the flank area. Patient should be on bed rest for 24 hours. Advise the patient to do no heavy lifting, exercise, or sports for 1 to 2 weeks. Hemoglobin (Hgb) and hematocrit (Hct) are checked at 6 and 24 hours after the biopsy.
Cystoscopy: Uses lighted cystoscope inserted through the urethra to visualize urethra, bladder, and ureteral openings. Allows diagnosis of problems, removal of bladder calculi, biopsy, and some treatments. Local or general anesthesia may be used. Dye may be injected into the kidneys through ureters (retrograde pyelography).	Signed informed consent is required. Inform that procedure is done in the operating room or special room under sterile conditions. For local anesthesia, liquids may be allowed; patient should be NPO before general anesthesia. Give laxatives or enemas as ordered. Give medications as ordered to reduce anxiety and bladder spasms. Antibiotics may be ordered 2 to 3 days before procedure and continued several days afterward.	Safety precautions should be used because orthostatic hypotension is common. Monitor intake and output, vital signs, and urine color; urine may initially be pink tinged to wine colored but should lighten to its usual color in 24 to 48 hours. Report severe pain to the health care provider. Advise that: (1) analgesics or antispasmodics may be prescribed for pain, (2) sitz baths help to relieve pain and urinary frequency, (3) patient should drink 2 to 3 L of fluids daily unless contraindicated, and (4) urine will be pink tinged for 1 to 2 days.

Continued

Table 41.1 Diagnostic Tests and Procedures Urinary Disorders—cont'd

TEST AND PURPOSE	PATIENT PREPARATION	POSTPROCEDURE CARE
Urodynamic Studies		
Cystogram and cystourethrogram: Uses dye injected into the bladder through a catheter followed by radiographs to outline the bladder and demonstrate reflux of urine from bladder to ureters.	For a voiding cystourethrogram, the bladder and urethra are radiographed during urination. Rate of urine flow is measured. Inform that a catheter will be inserted and dye instilled into the bladder.	Monitor urine output and vital signs. Encourage increased fluids unless contraindicated. Observe for allergic reaction to dye. Assess for urinary retention.
Cystometrogram: Evaluates bladder tone.	Inform that fluid will be instilled into the bladder through a urethral catheter. When the patient feels the urge to void, the catheter will be removed. After the patient voids, residual urine is measured. Drugs may be given to test bladder response.	Encourage increased fluids unless contraindicated. Monitor intake and output. Administer drugs as ordered for bladder spasms.

KUB, Kidneys, ureters and bladder; *SIADH*, syndrome of inappropriate antidiuretic hormone.

URINE TESTS

Urinalysis

A urine specimen is examined for color, pH, specific gravity, glucose, protein, blood, ketones, and bilirubin. Normal urine is straw colored and slightly acidic. Microscopic examination is used to assess for cells, casts, bacteria, and crystals. Chemical examination to assess electrolytes and ***osmolality*** (concentration) of the urine determines the ability of the kidneys to excrete or conserve electrolytes and water. By comparing the osmolality of urine with serum osmolality, it is possible to know if the kidneys are functioning appropriately. If serum osmolality is elevated, the kidneys should reabsorb or conserve water to dilute the serum and excrete more concentrated urine (i.e., urine with high osmolality). If serum osmolality is low (urine is dilute), the kidneys should reduce reabsorption of water to increase serum concentration and produce more dilute urine (i.e., urine with low osmolality). Specific gravity is a measure of osmolality. Data reported from a routine urinalysis are summarized in Table 41.2.

Urine Culture and Sensitivity

Normal urine is sterile. A urine culture permits identification of microorganisms present in the urine. Sensitivity testing determines which antibiotics will be most effective against the specific organisms. The specimen can be obtained by the patient, if able, or the nurse. If an antibiotic is ordered, collect the urine specimen before starting the antibiotic drug. Instructions are given in Table 41.1.

Creatinine Clearance

Creatinine clearance, the rate at which the kidney removes creatinine from the blood, is the best test of overall kidney function. It serves as an estimate of glomerular filtration rate. This test requires collection of all urine for 12 or 24 hours, as ordered. Normal levels vary for men and women. Because values depend on muscle mass, they are usually lower in women. Urine and serum creatinine levels are compared to determine kidney function. If serum creatinine rises and urine creatinine falls, anticipate decreased kidney function and glomerular filtration rate.

BLOOD TESTS

Blood Urea Nitrogen

The blood urea nitrogen (BUN) test is a general indicator of the kidneys' ability to excrete urea, an end product of protein metabolism. In addition to renal failure, factors that increase BUN are nephrotoxic drugs, a high-protein diet (especially with renal disease), gastrointestinal (GI) bleeding, dehydration, myocardial infarction, shock, burns, and sepsis (Pagana et al., 2017).

Serum Creatinine

Creatinine is a waste product of skeletal muscle breakdown. The level of creatinine in the blood is an indication of the kidneys' ability to excrete wastes. Serum creatinine is elevated primarily in renal disorders and is a better measurement of kidney function than BUN. Unlike BUN, creatinine is not influenced by diet, hydration, nutritional status, or liver function. With normally functioning kidneys, the serum creatinine level is very low and the urine level is high. The normal ratio of BUN to creatinine is 6 to 25, with 15.5 being considered optimal (Pagana et al., 2017).

Serum Electrolytes

Serum electrolytes must be monitored in the renal patient because imbalances can have very serious consequences. In renal failure, sodium and potassium levels are elevated and calcium levels are decreased.

Table 41.2 Urinalysis Data

COMPONENTS	NORMAL VALUES	IMPLICATIONS OF ABNORMAL VALUES
Color	Amber yellow	Dilute, colorless: overhydration, diabetes insipidus, diabetes mellitus, chronic renal failure Concentrated dark amber: dehydration, some medications or foods Bright red: Bleeding from lower urinary tract Dark red: Bleeding from kidney Green urine: *Pseudomonas* bacteria
Appearance	Clear	Cloudy, hazy: may indicate bacteria, RBCs, pus (may also be from certain foods)
pH	4.6 to 8.0	<4.0: acidosis, starvation, diarrhea >7.0: alkalosis, bacteriuria, UTI
Specific gravity	1.005 to 1.030	<1.003: diabetes insipidus, overhydration, renal disease, severe hypokalemia >1.030: dehydration, diabetes mellitus
Protein	0 to 8 mg/dL 50–80 mg/24 h at rest <250 mg/24 h exercise	Persistent proteinuria: renal disease, preeclampsia in pregnant women; complications of diabetes mellitus
Glucose	Negative	Positive: diabetes mellitus, stroke, Cushing syndrome, anesthesia, severe stress
Ketones	Negative	Positive: diabetes mellitus, starvation, excessive protein ingestion, alcoholism, isopropanol ingestion
Bilirubin	Negative	Positive: liver disease (jaundice)
Microscopic Examination		
RBCs	≤2	>4.0 (hematuria): kidney trauma, renal disease, anticoagulants
WBCs	0 to 4	>5.0: UTI, strenuous exercise
WBC Casts	Negative	Positive: fever, renal disease, heart failure
Crystals	Negative	Positive: renal stone formation
Bacteria	Negative	Positive: UTI

RBCs, Red blood cells; *UTI*, urinary tract infection; *WBCs*, white blood cells.

RADIOGRAPHIC TESTS AND PROCEDURES

Kidneys, Ureters, and Bladder

A KUB (for kidneys, ureters, and bladder) is a radiograph that provides a general outline of the kidneys, revealing their approximate size and contour. Tumors, malformations, and calculi may be found with this type of radiograph. This procedure requires no special preparation or aftercare. It is not done on pregnant patients and it should be done before any other studies that require contrast media.

Intravenous Pyelogram/Urogram

An intravenous pyelogram (IVP) is a diagnostic procedure in which a radiographic contrast medium ("dye") is injected intravenously. Radiographs of the KUB are taken at 5- to 15-minute intervals. As the contrast is concentrated by the kidneys and excreted through the ureters into the bladder, kidney function and structures, ureter size and patency, bladder size and shape, and presence of calculi (stones) or other obstructions can be assessed. The procedure is contraindicated in older adult patients with known renal insufficiency and in patients with diabetes mellitus or multiple myeloma. Use of the IVP is declining in favor of safer imaging procedures.

Renal Arteriogram

A renal arteriogram permits study of the renal blood vessels. It is used to diagnose renal artery stenosis, aneurysms, vascular tumors, renal cysts, and renal infarctions. A catheter is inserted through the femoral artery and threaded into the aorta. A contrast medium is injected into each renal artery and radiographs are taken as the contrast passes through the kidneys.

Cystogram

Contrast media can be instilled in the bladder using a catheter or a cystoscope. Films are then taken to visualize the bladder. This procedure is useful in detecting reflux of urine from the bladder into the ureters.

Renal Scan

A renal scan indicates the size, shape, and location of the kidneys; detects renal infarction, atherosclerosis, trauma, or rejection of a transplant; and identifies primary renal disease. An intravenous radioisotope is injected, and radiographs are taken to demonstrate blood flow to each kidney. The test is not done on pregnant women but can be used for patients who are allergic to contrast that contains iodine.

Computed Tomography and Magnetic Resonance Imaging

A computed tomography (CT) scan is useful in detecting kidney size, tumors, abscesses, obstruction, and adrenal masses and tumors. Contrast media may be used to clarify details; assess the patient for iodine sensitivity. Magnetic resonance imaging (MRI) may also be used to visualize the kidneys.

ULTRASOUND

Ultrasonography (ultrasound) uses high-frequency sound waves to create images of the bladder. It is used to detect urinary tract malformations and obstructions, tumors, renal calculi, perineal fluid accumulation, and cysts. Ultrasound may also be used to guide a needle inserted to aspirate specimens from cysts or tumors. The bladder should be full for visualization of abdominal organs and tissues. The procedure may be done through the abdominal wall (transabdominal), the rectum (transrectal), the urethra (transurethral), or the vagina (transvaginal). Preparation and patient instructions are specific for each approach.

INVASIVE PROCEDURES

Renal Biopsy

A renal biopsy is performed to obtain a specimen of renal tissue for direct microscopic examination. It is usually done to evaluate conditions leading to renal failure. The procedure may be done through open or closed methods. The open method is a surgical procedure in which an incision is made in the flank and a specimen of kidney tissue is removed. The closed procedure involves insertion of a needle under fluoroscopy or ultrasonography to aspirate the tissue specimen. For the closed procedure, the patient must be able to lie in the prone position with a blanket roll under the lower abdomen for up to 45 minutes. Patients with breathing problems may not be able to tolerate this position or alter their breathing patterns as needed during the procedure.

The most serious complication of a renal biopsy is hemorrhage. If bleeding is suspected, the patient is given intravenous fluids to restore fluid volume. Persistent bleeding may require surgery.

Cystoscopy

Cystoscopy is the direct visualization of the interior of the urethra, bladder, and ureteral orifices. The procedure may be done in the health care provider's office for diagnostic reasons or in an outpatient facility for diagnostic or treatment purposes under local or general anesthesia. As a diagnostic procedure, the cystoscopy allows the health care provider to observe lesions, locate sources of bleeding, and take biopsy samples. Treatments that can be performed with this procedure include cauterization of lesions; removal of calculi, tumors, or foreign materials; implantation of radium seeds; insertion of ureteral catheters; and control of bleeding. A lighted tube called a *cystoscope* is inserted through the urethra into the bladder under sterile conditions. Retrograde pyelography, which involves injecting contrast into the ureters, can also be done during cystoscopy.

Back pain, bladder spasms, urinary frequency, and burning on urination are common after cystoscopy. Mild analgesics may bring relief. Belladonna and opium suppositories may be ordered to reduce bladder spasms. Bladder perforation is rare but should be suspected if the patient has severe abdominal pain.

URODYNAMIC STUDIES

Urodynamic studies are performed to determine the physiology of urination. The studies assess innervation of the bladder, incontinence, and other variations in urinary patterns. Urodynamic studies measure the rate and volume of urine flow during voiding. The rate of flow is decreased with obstruction or decreased innervation.

Cystogram and Voiding Cystourethrogram

The cystogram involves placing a catheter into the bladder and filling the bladder with contrast material, followed by radiographs. This outlines the contour of the bladder and shows reflux or backflow of urine from the bladder into the ureters. Cystograms are useful in diagnosing neurogenic bladders, fistulas, tumors, and ruptured bladders.

A voiding cystourethrogram gives the health care provider additional information on urethral disorders during voiding. The bladder is filled with contrast and radiographs are taken during and after urination. This procedure may be embarrassing for the patient. Provide support, explain the need for the test, and provide privacy during the procedure.

Cystometrogram

The cystometrogram is used to evaluate bladder tone in the patient with incontinence or with a neurogenic bladder. A catheter is inserted in the bladder and fluid is instilled until the patient reports the urge to void. When the patient feels urgency, the catheter is removed, the patient voids, and residual urine is measured. Drugs may be given to see if they effectively enhance or relax bladder tone in the individual patient.

COMMON THERAPEUTIC MEASURES

CATHETERIZATION

Catheterization is the introduction of a catheter through the urethra into the bladder for draining urine. Urethral catheters are inserted when patients are unable to void as a result of the effects of anesthesia, paralysis, trauma, unconsciousness, certain surgical procedures, and other factors that inhibit voiding. The major concern with catheterization is the potential for introduction of bacteria in the normally sterile bladder. Catheterization is the primary cause of health care–associated infections (HAIs). It is essential that strict aseptic techniques be followed when catheterization is necessary.

Urinary catheters are available in a variety of sizes for adults. The most commonly used sizes for adult urethral catheterization range from the small 12 French (Fr) to the larger 18 Fr. Catheters may be of a retaining or nonretaining design. A retaining catheter is one that has a device, such as an inflatable balloon, that anchors the catheter in the bladder. Examples of retaining catheters are the coudé, Foley, Malecot, and Pezzer. Nurses are most familiar with Foley catheters that have either double or triple lumina. Malecot and Pezzer catheters are used most often as suprapubic catheters. Robinson and whistle-tip catheters are nonretaining or straight catheters.

To determine whether a patient is emptying their bladder, the amount of urine remaining in the bladder after voiding (residual urine) must be measured. A bladder scanner can be used to measure postvoid residual (PVR). This procedure may be diagnostic and may also be used as part of a bladder training program for patients who have lost control over bladder function. Residual volume should be measured immediately after voiding. Occasionally, patients are catheterized to measure residual urine. Less than 50 mL of residual urine is considered normal.

The reader should refer to a fundamentals nursing textbook for detailed information on the insertion and care of urethral catheters. Key points to remember when catheterization is necessary are the following:

1. Catheterize only after other noninvasive measures have failed or when absolutely necessary for diagnostic purposes. If possible, have the patient shower or bathe before catheterization.
2. Wash hands thoroughly, and use sterile technique and equipment to insert the catheter.
3. With an indwelling catheter:
   a. Secure the tubing to the female patient's inner thigh or the male patient's upper thigh or lower abdomen.
   b. Handle the catheter gently to avoid trauma to the urethra.
   c. Keep the urine collection bag below the level of the patient's bladder and the tubing in a circular fashion on the bed.
   d. Keep the drainage system closed as much as possible.
   e. Empty the bag before it is full. A full bag inhibits urine drainage, which could cause bladder spasms.
   f. Provide perineal care twice daily. (Note: antibiotic ointments are not recommended.)
   g. Use Standard Precautions before and after handling the catheter.

URETERAL CATHETER

A ureteral catheter is threaded through a ureter into the renal pelvis. It can be inserted through the bladder during cystoscopy or through an abdominal incision. A ureteral catheter permits urine to flow through the swollen ureter after traumatic surgery. The catheter is connected to a drainage system and output is measured every 1 to 2 hours. Record output from this catheter separately from other urine output. Make certain that the catheter is not kinked or clamped because pressure would build up in the kidney, causing tissue damage. The capacity of the renal pelvis is only 3 to 5 mL. If irrigation is ordered, slowly instill no more than 5 mL (or less, as ordered) of lukewarm, sterile normal saline. Use strict aseptic technique for the irrigation. Unless both ureters are completely obstructed, urine continues to drain into the bladder. Remember to document urine from each source on the output record.

The patient with a ureterostomy tube is usually kept on bed rest unless a double-J catheter is used. The double-J catheter has one coiled end in the renal pelvis and the other coiled end in the bladder.

NEPHROSTOMY TUBE

When a ureter is completely obstructed, the health care provider may insert a nephrostomy tube through a flank incision directly into the kidney pelvis. The tube is connected to a drainage system and assessed frequently. Ensure that the tube is not kinked or clamped at any time, because drainage must be continuous. Some urine usually leaks around the tube and flows through the flank incision. Perform sterile dressing changes and skin care as needed. Irrigation with a small amount of sterile normal saline, using strict aseptic technique, may be ordered. Because of the small capacity of the renal pelvis, no more than 5 mL of irrigating fluid is used.

URINARY STENT

A stent is a hollow tube that is placed in a structure to give it support and allow fluid to flow through. A urinary stent may be placed in the ureter to maintain alignment or to provide a route for urine drainage. The health care provider inserts the stent; it may be completely internal, or it may extend through the urethra or skin. Several types of stents are available.

UROLOGIC SURGERY

Urologic surgery may be done on any part of the urinary tract. Nephrectomy is removal of the kidney because of cancer, massive trauma or bleeding, severe chronic failure with infection, or polycystic kidney disease, or for donation. Many types of surgery are used to remove calculi, depending on their location. A surgical opening may be made in the renal tissue, renal pelvis, ureter, or bladder. ***Lithotripsy*** is a noninvasive procedure used to break up calculi, but patient care is similar to that of the surgical patient. Bladder surgery may be necessitated by bleeding, functional problems, or cancer. Removal of the bladder is a ***cystectomy***; an incision in the bladder is a *cystotomy*. Some surgical procedures can be done through a cystoscope, so no external incision exists. Surgical procedures that reroute the flow of urine are called *urinary diversions*. A cystostomy is the formation of an opening or stoma on the abdomen for catheterization or to enable the collection of urine in an external reservoir. Prostate surgery is discussed in Chapter 54.

Preoperative Care

Preparation for urologic surgery includes a complete diagnostic workup to rule out other medical problems. Fluid status is evaluated and any imbalances are corrected. Usual preoperative care measures are taken as described in Chapter 17. Bowel cleansing may be ordered before some procedures. If the patient will have a stoma for urine drainage, an enterostomal therapist is usually consulted to identify the optimal stoma site as well as for patient counseling and teaching.

Postoperative Care

After surgery, particular attention is given to urine output, respirations, and bowel function. Output is closely monitored, with drainage from various tubes recorded separately. Urine output of less than 30 mL per hour should be reported to the health care provider. Flank or abdominal incisions cause pain on deep breathing. Adequate pain management and support of the patient for coughing and deep breathing decrease the risk of atelectasis and pneumonia. Auscultate lungs frequently to assess breath sounds. Urologic surgery often involves manipulation of the bowel, which can lead to paralytic ileus, so food and fluids are usually withheld until bowel sounds are present.

DRUG THERAPY

A number of drugs are available to treat urinary tract disorders. Major classifications of commonly used drugs are diuretics, antihypertensives, phosphate binders, hormones, vitamin and mineral supplements, and immunosuppressants. These classifications, specific drugs, their actions and adverse effects, and nursing interventions are summarized in Table 41.3. Immunosuppressant drugs are addressed separately in Table 41.4. In addition, see the Complementary and Alternative Therapies box.

Complementary and Alternative Therapies

Herbal remedies, like medications, can be harmful to the kidney. For example, aloe can cause nephritis and ephedra (*má huáng*) can cause kidney stones. Teach patients to always disclose complementary and alternative remedies used in their medication histories.

Table 41.3 Medications for Urinary Disorders

General Considerations

- Drugs are selected carefully for patients with urologic disorders because many drugs are nephrotoxic.
- Drug dosages may need to be reduced if renal function is impaired and the drug is excreted in the urine.

DRUG	USE AND ACTION	SIDE EFFECTS	NURSING INTERVENTIONS
Diuretics and Antihypertensive Agents			
Diuretics: general information. Specific classes follow	Cause kidneys to excrete water and sodium and lower blood pressure (BP)	Dehydration, electrolyte imbalances	Monitor the patient's intake and output, BP, and weight. Administer the drug in the morning to minimize nocturia. Assess for electrolyte imbalances. Monitor serum potassium level. Potassium supplements may be ordered except with potassium-sparing drugs.
Osmotic diuretic: mannitol (Osmitrol)	Increases osmolarity of glomerular filtrate which inhibits the reabsorption of water and increases urine output	Edema, dehydration, electrolyte imbalances	Monitor for circulatory overload (increased BP, bounding pulse) and extravasation during infusion. Administer only freshly prepared solutions.

Table 41.3 Medications for Urinary Disorders—cont'd

DRUG	USE AND ACTION	SIDE EFFECTS	NURSING INTERVENTIONS
Thiazide diuretics: hydrochlorothiazide (Microzide) methyclothiazide (Enduron) chlorothiazide (Diuril) Thiazide-type diuretics: metolazone (Zaroxolyn)	Increase renal excretion of sodium, chloride, potassium, and water	Hypokalemia, hypercalcemia, hypotension, hyponatremia	Monitor patients with diabetes for hyperglycemia. Monitor patients taking digoxin for low potassium levels. Encourage potassium-rich foods.
Loop diuretics: furosemide (Lasix)	Blocks reabsorption of sodium and chloride in the loop of Henle, which prevents reabsorption of water and increases urine output	Orthostatic hypotension, hypokalemia, hyponatremia, hearing loss	Monitor patients with diabetes for hyperglycemia. Encourage potassium-rich foods. Teach patients how to prevent orthostatic hypotension by changing position slowly and avoiding prolonged standing.
Potassium-sparing diuretics: spironolactone (Aldactone), triamterene (Dyrenium), amiloride (Midamor)	Promotes retention of potassium and excretion of sodium	Hyperkalemia, drowsiness, gynecomastia in men on long-term therapy, menstrual irregularities, impotence	Institute and maintain safety measures. Assess for hyperkalemia (nausea, diarrhea, muscle weakness, electrocardiogram [ECG] changes). Use with caution with angiotensin-converting enzyme inhibitors (ACEIs), angiotensin receptor blockers, and direct renin inhibitors.
Antihypertensive agents: general information. See specific classes subsequently	Lower BP	Orthostatic hypotension. Reflex tachycardia and fluid retention with some types. Rebound hypertension if stopped suddenly	Monitor BP. Do not discontinue the drug suddenly. For orthostatic hypotension, teach patients to change position slowly and avoid prolonged standing.
Centrally acting $alpha_2$ agonists: methyldopa, clonidine (Catapres)	Reduce sympathetic stimulation	Drowsiness, hemolytic anemia, liver damage	Institute and maintain safety measures. May cause sedation; administer at bedtime. Can cause dry mouth. Advise the patient to discontinue the drug only under medical direction.
$Alpha_1$ adrenergic antagonists: prazosin doxazosin (Cardura) terazosin	Increase kidney perfusion; block sympathetic stimulation of blood vessels, permitting vasodilation	Orthostatic hypotension (especially with initial dose)	Give the first dose or increased dose at bedtime. Teach the patient how to prevent orthostatic hypertension.
Beta-adrenergic blockers/ antagonists: propranolol (Inderal), metoprolol (Lopressor et al.)	Inhibit the renin-angiotensin-aldosterone system	Bronchoconstriction, bradycardia, hypoglycemia, heart failure. Masks symptoms of low blood glucose.	Monitor respirations in patients with asthma and chronic obstructive pulmonary disease. Assess for edema. Monitor glucose levels.
Direct-acting vasodilators: hydralazine	Relaxation of blood vessels lowers peripheral resistance	Tachycardia, palpitations, headache, lupus-like syndrome	Report lupus-like symptoms: fever, sore throat, skin rash.

Continued

Table 41.3 Medications for Urinary Disorders—cont'd

DRUG	USE AND ACTION	SIDE EFFECTS	NURSING INTERVENTIONS
Vitamin and Mineral Supplements			
ferrous sulfate	Treats iron deficiency anemia	Constipation or diarrhea, dark stools	Administer on an empty stomach with water. Can give the liquid with water or fruit juice to disguise taste.
folic acid, calcium gluconate	Supplements dietary intake. Treats hypocalcemia	Although few adverse effects are produced by these supplements, occasional side effects include hypercalcemia and constipation	Monitor for occasional hypersensitivity. Monitor blood studies. Administer in divided doses with or after meals. Do not give with other drugs.
Hormone			
Erythropoietic growth factors: erythropoietin	Improve red blood cell (RBC) formation. Reverse anemia. Require adequate serum iron and ferritin to be effective	Headache, tachycardia, hypertension, dyspnea, diarrhea, hyperkalemia, nausea, vomiting, clotted vascular assess, seizures	Monitor BP. Contraindicated in uncontrolled hypertension. Dosage is adjusted to maintain hemoglobin between 10 and 11 g/dL.
Antibiotics			
Sulfonamides: trimethoprim/sulfamethoxazole (Bactrim, Septra)	Used to treat acute or chronic UTIs, otitis media, bronchitis, pneumocystis pneumonia, and to prevent pneumocystis pneumonia in patients with AIDS	Hypersensitivity (Stevens-Johnson syndrome: severe skin lesions; can be fatal), blood dyscrasias (hemolytic anemia), renal damage related to crystalluria, hyperkalemia, birth defects. Enhances warfarin, phenytoin, and glipizide	Teach to report any skin rash (which may be an allergic response). Encourage good hydration—at least 1500 mL daily to prevent kidney damage. Monitor serum potassium. Avoid sunlight or wear sunscreen when outdoors.
Beta Lactams Penicillin: ampicillin/sulbactam Cephalosporins: ceftriaxone, ceftazidime	Effective against most gram-positive and some gram-negative pathogens	Anaphylaxis, gastrointestinal (GI) distress, rash, blood dyscrasias	Monitor for allergic reaction: rash, itching, wheezing. Report any evidence of an allergic reaction to the health care provider immediately.
Fluoroquinolones: ciprofloxacin norfloxacin levofloxacin	Broad-spectrum antibiotics that are effective against many gram-positive and gram-negative pathogens	Drowsiness, headache, agitation, seizures, cardiac dysrhythmias, hepatotoxicity, pseudomembranous colitis. Anaphylaxis, severe skin reactions, crystalluria	Notify the health care provider immediately of possible allergic reaction: rash, pruritus, urticaria, wheezing. Monitor liver function tests. Advise to drink 1500 to 2000 mL of fluid each day to prevent crystal formation. Do not give the drug within 2 hours of antacids, iron, or zinc. Check for many other drug-drug interactions. Implement and maintain safety measures because of possible drowsiness.
Bacterial MurA Inhibitor: fosfomycin (Monurol)	Single dose therapy for uncomplicated UTI in women	Diarrhea, headache, sore throat, back pain, vaginitis, nausea	Single dose regimen: 3-g water-soluble sachet.

Table 41.3 Medications for Urinary Disorders—cont'd

DRUG	USE AND ACTION	SIDE EFFECTS	NURSING INTERVENTIONS
Urinary Antiseptics			
methenamine	An antibacterial agent that is effective in chronic lower UTIs	Nausea, vomiting, diarrhea	Give with meals to reduce GI effects. Encourage adequate fluids. Discourage large intake of milk products. Do not use in combination with sulfonamides.
nitrofurantoin (Furadantin, Macrodantin)	Treat acute and chronic UTIs. Often used for lower UTIs in women	Dyspnea, cough. Nausea and vomiting. Numbness and tingling of legs. Hematologic reactions. Headache, vertigo, drowsiness.	Administer with food or milk to reduce gastric distress.
Urinary Antispasmodic Agents			
oxybutynin (Ditropan et al): oral, topical, and transdermal forms.	Inhibits neurogenic bladder, overactive bladder	Anxiety, seizures, palpitations, blurred vision, dry mouth, nausea, vomiting, diarrhea or constipation, urinary retention, fever, anaphylaxis	Monitor voiding pattern. Avoid hazardous activities. Report chest pain, palpitations, dyspnea. Instruct patient in use of topical and transdermal drugs.
Urinary Analgesic			
phenazopyridine (Pyridium)	Relieves symptoms of urinary tract infection. Does NOT treat the infection	Nausea, vomiting, headache, dizziness, stomach cramps. May cause bluish skin appearance. Most serious: acute renal failure, hemolytic anemia.	Manufacturer advises to limit drug use to 2 days. Tell patient to notify health care provider of rapid weight gain, decreased (or no) urine output.

AIDS, Acquired immunodeficiency syndrome; *UTI*, urinary tract infection.

Table 41.4 Immunosuppressant Drugs

General Considerations

- Patients on immunosuppressant drugs have reduced resistance to infection, so they must be monitored for even subtle signs of infection.
- Protect patients from infections.
- Teach patients the importance of taking drugs as prescribed and keeping follow-up appointments.
- Immunosuppressants increase the risk of malignancies.

DRUG	USE AND ACTION	SIDE EFFECTS	NURSING INTERVENTIONS
Corticosteroids			
prednisone, methylprednisolone (Medrol), methylprednisolone sodium succinate (Solu-Medrol)	Antiinflammatory agents that prevent movement of leukocytes into transplanted tissue	Retention of water and sodium; loss of potassium, elevated blood glucose, hypertension, GI bleeding, mood swings, psychosis, infections, and impaired healing	Monitor intake and output. Assess for fluid and electrolyte imbalances: edema, increased BP, cardiac dysrhythmias, muscle weakness, confusion. Antacids are often ordered to protect the stomach.
Cytotoxic Agents			
cyclophosphamide	Alkylating neoplastic agent	Diarrhea, bone marrow suppression, vomiting, sepsis, sterility, hemorrhagic cystitis	Ensure negative pregnancy test before starting therapy. Assess patient for thrombocytopenia (i.e., bruising, bleeding) and leukopenia (i.e., frequent infections).

Continued

Table 41.4 Drugs for Suppressing Immunity—cont'd

DRUG	USE AND ACTION	SIDE EFFECTS	NURSING INTERVENTIONS
Monoclonal and Polyclonal Antibodies			
muromonab-CD3, basiliximab (Simulect), daclizumab antithymocyte globulin (Thymoglobulin), antilymphocyte globulin	Reacts with T-cell antigens and destroys them. Used to prevent or reverse acute rejection in renal transplant recipients	Numerous side effects including fever, chills, headache, tremor, dyspnea, flushing, anaphylaxis, nausea, vomiting, diarrhea, chest pain. Potentially fatal anaphylaxis. Bleeding risk with Thymoglobulin. See pharmacology reference for more complete information	Monitor closely for anaphylaxis, especially with the first dose. Monitor for fluid overload. Check infusion site. Change site if evidence of extravasation exists. With Thymoglobulin, assess for bleeding: gums, stools, urine. Caution to avoid injury.
T-Cell Suppressors			
cyclosporine (Sandimmune and Neoral are *not* interchangeable!), tacrolimus (Prograf)	Interferes with T-lymphocyte activity. Enhances transplant survival with less risk of infection	Nephrotoxicity (elevated serum creatinine), fluid retention, hypertension, hyperkalemia, hirsutism, venous thrombosis, gingival hyperplasia, tremors, infections, anemia, leukopenia, thrombocytopenia, anaphylaxis with intravenous administration, hepatotoxicity	Monitor serum creatinine and electrolytes. Check for edema. Monitor BP. Have epinephrine available during intravenous administration. Monitor liver function studies. Mix the oral form with food or chocolate to disguise unpleasant oiliness.
azathioprine (Imuran), mycophenolate (CellCept)	Inhibits B and T lymphocytes	Teratogenic. Neutropenia, thrombocytopenia, diarrhea, sepsis	Assess CBC results, bleeding. Ensure pregnancy is ruled out before starting therapy.

BP, Blood pressure; *CBC*, complete blood count; *GI*, gastrointestinal.

Get Ready for the NCLEX® Examination!

Key Points

- The urinary system eliminates metabolic wastes in urine; stimulates RBC production; and maintains fluid, electrolyte, and acid-base balance.
- Age-related changes in the urinary system include reduced ability to concentrate or dilute urine, nocturia, and decreased bladder capacity.
- To diagnose urologic disorders, the physician may order urine tests, blood tests, imaging procedures, endoscopic examinations, and/or urodynamic studies.
- It is essential that strict aseptic techniques be followed when catheterization is necessary, because this procedure is the primary cause of health care–associated infections (HAIs).
- Residual volume refers to the amount of urine remaining in the bladder after voiding. The volume may be assessed with a Doppler ultrasound or by catheterization. Less than 50 mL of residual urine is considered normal.
- When a patient has a ureteral catheter or a nephrostomy tube, make certain it is draining freely to prevent urine from backing up and damaging the kidney.
- The capacity of the renal pelvis is only 3 to 5 mL. If irrigation of a ureteral catheter or nephrostomy is ordered, slowly instill no more than 5 mL (or less, as ordered) of lukewarm, sterile normal saline.
- Nephrectomy is removal of the kidney for donation or because of cancer, massive trauma or bleeding, severe chronic failure with infection, or polycystic kidney disease.
- Lithotripsy is a noninvasive procedure used to break up renal calculi.
- Surgical procedures that reroute the flow of urine are called *urinary diversions*.
- After urologic surgery, particular attention is given to urine output, respirations, and bowel function.
- Drug classifications used to treat urinary tract disorders include diuretics, antihypertensives, phosphate binders, hormones, antibiotics, urinary antiseptics and analgesics, vitamin and mineral supplements, and immunosuppressants.

Additional Learning Resources

SG Go to your Study Guide for additional learning activities to help you master this chapter content.

Go to your Evolve website (http://evolve.elsevier.com/Linton/medsurg) for the following learning resources and much more:

- Fluid & Electrolyte Tutorial
- Review Questions for the NCLEX® Examination

Clinical Judgment and Next-Generation NCLEX® Examination-Style Questions

1. **An 86-year-old woman was seen by her primary care provider four times last year for kidney infections. Which age-related factors does the nurse identify that may contribute to these frequent infections? (Select all that apply.)**
   1. Incomplete bladder emptying
   2. Decreased renal blood flow
   3. Decreased creatinine clearance
   4. Reflux of urine into the ureters
   5. Decreased bladder capacity

   NCLEX Client Need: Physiological Integrity: Physiological Adaptation

2. **A client reports a painful, burning sensation during urination. Which term should the nurse use to document this symptom?**
   1. Polyuria
   2. Anuria
   3. Hematuria
   4. Dysuria

   NCLEX Client Need: Physiological Integrity: Physiological Adaptation

3. **The first time that a client voids after cystoscopy, the nurse observes pink-tinged urine. What is the appropriate nursing response?**
   1. Promptly notify the health care provider
   2. Restrict fluids
   3. Document normal findings
   4. Contact the Rapid Response Team

   NCLEX Client Need: Physiological Integrity: Reduction of Risk Potential

4. **SLO/Objective: Explain the nursing responsibilities for patients who are having tests and procedures to diagnose urologic disorders.**

   NGN Item Type: Enhanced Hot Spot

   Cognitive Skill: Recognize Cues

   A 50-year-old male patient who has been having urinary symptoms comes into the clinic for an outpatient cystoscopy that will be done under intravenous sedation. On arrival, he is alert and oriented. His admission vital signs are as follows: BP 130/84 mm Hg, Pulse 78 beats per minute, Repirations 16 breaths per minute, Temperature 98º F. He reports no pain but states he is "a little nervous" about the procedure. After the cystoscopy, he is received in a recovery area. The following data are collected in the postprocedure assessment:
   - Very drowsy but responds appropriately
   - Pain in penis and lower abdomen at 6 on a 10 point scale
   - BP 120/74 mm Hg
   - Pulse 102 beats per minute
   - Respirations 20 breaths per minute
   - Temperature 97°F
   - Voided 150 mL bright red urine with blood clots
   - Bowel sounds present in all four quadrants

   Highlight or place a check mark next to the assessment finding(s) that require follow-up by the nurse.

   NCLEX Client Need: Physiological Integirty: Reduction of Risk Potential

5. **Which of these patients is at greatest risk for developing a health care–associated infection?**
   1. A 70-year-old woman having a cystoscopy
   2. A 25-year-old man receiving intravenous antibiotics
   3. A 90-year-old man who requires catheterization for urinary retention
   4. A 50-year-old woman being treated with lithotripsy for kidney stones

   NCLEX Client Need: Physiological Integrity: Reduction of Risk Potential

6. **Which interventions are appropriate when a patient is taking a sulfonamide for a UTI? (Select all that apply.)**
   1. Monitor bowel movements.
   2. Advise patient to avoid exposure to sunlight.
   3. Encourage at least 1.5 quarts (1500 mL) of fluids daily.
   4. Tell patient that urine will be orange.
   5. Inspect the skin for lesions.

   NCLEX Client Need: Physiological Integrity: Pharmacological Therapies

7. **An order is written to irrigate a ureteral catheter. The nurse knows that the maximum amount of irrigating fluid is:**
   1. 5 mL.
   2. 10 mL.
   3. 15 mL.
   4. 30 mL.

   NCLEX Client Need: Physiological Integrity: Reduction of Risk Potential

42 Urologic Disorders

http://evolve.elsevier.com/Linton/medsurg

Objectives

1. Explain the pathophysiology, signs and symptoms, complications, and treatment of disorders of the kidneys, ureters, bladder, and urethra.
2. Contribute to the development of the nursing plan of care for patients with urologic disorders.

Key Terms

calculus (pl. calculi) (KĂL-kŭ-lŭs, KĂL-kŭ-lī)
dialysis
hemodialysis
lithotomy (lĭ-THŎT-ō-mē)
osteitis fibrosa
uremic frost
urolithiasis

In health, the kidneys do a remarkable job of regulating fluid and electrolyte and acid-base balance, removing metabolic waste products, controlling red blood cell (RBC) production, and maintaining normal blood pressure (BP). Therefore, urologic disorders deserve prompt attention to prevent serious complications and disruptions in homeostasis. This chapter addresses the major pathologic processes that can affect the urologic system including infection, lithiasis (stones), structural abnormalities, and renal failure.

URINARY TRACT INFLAMMATION AND INFECTIONS

Urinary tract infections (UTIs) are common, especially among women. They can involve any part of the urinary tract (upper or lower) and can be acquired through the blood or lymph or may enter through the urethra. UTIs are the most common health care–associated infections (HAIs). Most UTIs are bacterial, but they can be caused by viruses, yeasts, and fungi. It is important to treat UTIs to prevent renal scarring that can lead to failure. Risk factors for UTI are listed in Box 42.1.

URETHRITIS

Urethritis is inflammation of the urethra. Inflammation may be caused by microorganisms, trauma, or hypersensitivity to chemicals in products such as vaginal deodorants, spermicidal jellies, or bubble bath detergents. The most frequently identified causative microorganisms are *Escherichia coli*, *Chlamydia*, *Trichomonas*, *Neisseria gonorrhoeae*, and herpes simplex virus type 2.

Clinical Manifestations

Signs and symptoms of urethritis include dysuria, frequency, urgency, and bladder spasms. A urethral discharge may be noted.

Medical Diagnosis

Urethritis is diagnosed based on patient signs and symptoms, urinalysis, and urethral smear. Cystitis (bladder inflammation) may be present at the same time.

Medical Treatment

Antimicrobials are used to treat the condition when it is caused by microorganisms. If the patient is sexually active, the patient and the sexual partner may be treated with antimicrobials to prevent reinfection.

NURSING CARE OF THE PATIENT WITH URETHRITIS

Focused Assessment

Assessment of the patient with a urologic disorder is outlined in Chapter 41, Box 41.1. Important aspects of assessment for the patient with urethritis include comfort, possible causative factors, and understanding of treatment and prevention.

Patient Problems, Goals, and Outcome Criteria: Urethritis

Patient Problems	Goals and Outcome Criteria
Acute pain related to tissue inflammation	Pain relief: patient states pain is relieved, reports pain is decreased from prior assessment
Ineffective self-care management related to lack of knowledge of cause, treatment, and prevention of urethritis	Patient manages treatment plan effectively: patient accurately describes treatment and preventive measures, has no recurrence of urethritis

Box 42.1 Risk Factors for Urinary Tract Infections

- Use of indwelling or intermittent catheters
- Urinary or kidney stones
- Compromised immunity
- Female anatomy
- Vaginal infections
- Use of bubble baths and vaginal deodorant sprays
- Dehydration
- Use of tight-fitting, synthetic undergarments
- Infrequent voiding
- Pregnancy
- Menopause

Interventions

Sitz baths are soothing and may reduce the pain of urethritis. Instruct female patients to wipe from front to back after toileting, and to void before and after sexual intercourse as a means of preventing urethritis. Discourage bubble baths and vaginal deodorant sprays. Instruct uncircumcised male patients to clean the penis under the foreskin regularly. Advise patients to void after swimming.

CYSTITIS

Cystitis is inflammation of the urinary bladder. The most common cause is bacterial contamination. Other risk factors for cystitis include prolonged immobility, renal calculi, urinary diversion, indwelling catheters, radiation therapy, and treatment with some types of chemotherapy. Women are more susceptible than men because the female urethra is shorter and closer to the vagina and rectum. The longer urethra and antibacterial substances in prostatic fluid are thought to decrease the incidence of UTIs in men. Cystitis in the absence of other pathology of the urinary tract is said to be *uncomplicated* or *acute simple* cystitis. Recurring UTIs are more likely to be associated with urinary tract pathology.

Clinical Manifestations

Symptoms of cystitis include urgency, frequency, dysuria, hematuria, nocturia, bladder spasms, incontinence, and low-grade fever. Urine may be dark, tea-colored, or cloudy. Fever, fatigue, and pelvic or abdominal discomfort may indicate that the infection extends beyond the bladder. Bladder spasms may be experienced as pain behind the symphysis pubis. Spasms may occur during or after urination. Some patients have bacteria in the urine but no symptoms at all, a situation that does not always warrant the use of antibiotics.

Medical Diagnosis

The health care provider may diagnose cystitis based on the symptoms alone. A urine specimen may be obtained for urinalysis, culture, and sensitivity. The presence of bacteria does not mean that the patient has an infection unless the patient also has white blood cells (WBCs) in the urine. The presence of WBCs reflects bacterial tissue invasion—an indicator of infection. Other diagnostic procedures may be indicated to rule out pathology that might be responsible for the infection.

Medical Treatment

Cystitis is treated with antibiotics that concentrate in the urine. The health care provider may order an antibiotic while awaiting the results of the culture and sensitivity. The order is changed if the results show that another antibiotic would be more effective. For uncomplicated cystitis, treatment may be given in a single dose or in a 1- to 3-day or 1- to 5-day regimen. Patients with recurrent cystitis may be placed on continuous prophylactic antibiotics. A mild analgesic such as acetaminophen is useful for relieving discomfort. Phenazopyridine (Pyridium) may be ordered to decrease discomfort and bladder spasms, however, it can have serious side effects, so the use is limited to 2 days. Oxybutynin chloride (Ditropan) may also be ordered to decrease bladder spasms.

NURSING CARE OF THE PATIENT WITH CYSTITIS

Focused Assessment

General assessment of the patient with a urinary tract disorder is outlined in Chapter 41, Box 41.1. The nursing assessment of the patient with cystitis focuses on patient symptoms, possible causative factors, and understanding of treatment and prevention.

Patient Problems, Goals, and Outcome Criteria: Cystitis

Patient Problems	Goals and Outcome Criteria
Acute pain related to tissue inflammation	Pain relief: patient states pain is relieved, reports pain is decreased from prior assessment
Ineffective self-care management of condition related to lack of knowledge of cause, treatment, and prevention of cystitis	Patient effectively manages treatment plan: patient accurately describes treatment and preventive measures, has no recurrence of cystitis

Put On Your Thinking Cap!

Using the recommended fluid intake for a person with cystitis, calculate how much fluid you would need to take in 24 hours based on your body weight.

Interventions

Cystitis is usually treated on an outpatient basis. Advise the patient to take analgesics as ordered for pain. Warm sitz baths are also comforting. Patient teaching should emphasize the need for high fluid intake, instructions about prescribed drugs, and measures to avoid future infections (see the Patient Teaching box). The patient needs to consume at least 30 mL/kg of fluid per day and void frequently. Fluids should be consumed during the day and at night so that the urinary tract is continually flushed. Instruct the patient to complete the entire course of prescribed antibiotics. Also advise the patient taking phenazopyridine, a drug that relieves burning on urination, that the drug causes an orange-red urine color that may stain skin and clothing.

Patient Teaching

Cystitis

To reduce the risk of future infections, teach patients to:

- Wear cotton undergarments because they keep the perineum drier than synthetic materials. Moisture encourages bacterial growth.
- Avoid tight-fitting clothing in the perineal area.
- Take showers instead of tub baths.
- Avoid coffee, tea, carbonated beverages with caffeine, and apple, grapefruit, orange, and tomato juices because these irritate the bladder.
- Maintain a high fluid intake and empty the bladder often.
- Drink cranberry juice, as this is sometimes recommended to make the urine more acidic and discourage bacterial growth. Although research has not agreed on the value of this juice and the amount needed to be effective, it is a safe, simple measure to try.
- Wipe from front to back after bowel movements or voiding (for females).
- Drink a glass of water after swimming and before and after intercourse to "flush" the urethra.
- Keep appointments for follow-up urinalyses to ensure that the infection has been eliminated.

Pharmacology Capsule

Instruct patients to complete the entire course of antimicrobial therapy to ensure that the infection is eradicated.

INTERSTITIAL CYSTITIS/BLADDER PAIN SYNDROME

Pathophysiology and Diagnosis

Interstitial cystitis is an inflammatory disease of the bladder that is usually chronic. The cause of the disease, which usually affects females, is unknown. The patient typically reports moderate to severe bladder and pelvic pain, as well as urinary frequency and urgency. Chronic inflammation can cause the bladder to become scarred and stiff, which reduces its capacity. Ulcers may form in the bladder lining, and bleeding may occur. The condition is diagnosed by cystoscopy. Other diagnostic measures may be performed to rule out other pathologic conditions such as cancer.

Medical Treatment

Treatment is directed toward symptom management and attempts to treat possible causes. Among the drugs that sometimes are helpful are tricyclic antidepressants, antispasmodics, antihistamines if the patient has allergies, bladder anesthetics, calcium-channel blockers, urine alkalinizers, and nonsteroidal antiinflammatory drugs (NSAIDs). A drug that brings symptomatic relief is pentosan polysulfate (Elmiron). Other treatments include stretching the bladder under anesthesia; instillation of various medications, including dimethyl sulfoxide, into the bladder; and electrostimulation. Some sources advise dietary and activity changes and heat application. Cystectomy (surgical removal of the bladder) is an extreme measure that is necessary in some cases (see the Complementary and Alternative Therapies box).

◆ NURSING CARE OF THE PATIENT WITH INTERSTITIAL CYSTITIS

Interstitial cystitis is usually treated in the community setting, so you are more likely to encounter patients in clinic or home settings than in hospitals. It is important to show acceptance of the patient and demonstrate empathy for the disruption of life caused by this disease. It is a physiologic illness, not a psychologic one. Your primary role is teaching and support. The Interstitial Cystitis Association (www.ichelp.com) is a source of general information, as well as dietary advice to avoid bladder irritation (see the Patient Teaching box).

Patient Teaching

Interstitial Cystitis

- Avoid foods that cause symptoms (e.g., acidic foods, coffee, tea, citrus products, hot peppers, alcohol, artificial sweeteners, and carbonated drinks).
  The Interstitial Cystitis Association provides excellent dietary guidance online at http://ichelp.org/living-with-ic/interstitial-cystitis-and-diet/
- Wear clothing that fits loosely around the waist and lower abdomen.
- A local support group may be available for education and encouragement.
- Consult with your urologist before taking any medications along with those you take for your IC.

Complementary and Alternative Therapies

Biofeedback may help some patients to deal with the symptoms of interstitial cystitis.

PYELONEPHRITIS

Pyelonephritis is inflammation of the renal pelvis. It may affect one or both kidneys. Acute pyelonephritis is most often caused by an ascending bacterial infection, but it may be bloodborne. Chronic pyelonephritis may be persistent or recurrent and result in damage to the renal parenchyma (functional tissue). It most often is the result of reflux of urine from inadequate closure of the ureterovesical junction during voiding. Progressive scarring results in atrophy of the affected kidneys and development of hypertension and renal ischemia.

Chronic pyelonephritis, usually caused by long-standing UTIs with relapses and reinfections, may lead to chronic renal failure. If the patient progresses to renal atrophy and end-stage renal disease (ESRD), **dialysis** or transplantation is the only means of keeping the patient alive. Several types of dialysis procedures exist; all are used to remove wastes or toxins and to restore fluid and electrolyte balance. Detailed information about dialysis is presented later in this chapter.

Clinical Manifestations

Signs and symptoms of acute pyelonephritis include high fever, chills, nausea, vomiting, and dysuria. Severe pain or a constant dull ache occurs in the flank area. The patient with chronic pyelonephritis often reports bladder irritation, chronic fatigue, and a slight aching over one or both kidneys.

Medical Treatment

The goal of treatment for pyelonephritis is to prevent further damage. Mild to moderate symptoms can usually be managed on an outpatient basis. Severe symptoms are commonly treated in the hospital. Antibiotics, urinary tract antiseptics, analgesics, and antispasmodics may be ordered. Long-term antibiotic therapy may be prescribed for patients who have repeated acute infections or chronic infection. Specific antibiotics are selected based on the severity of the infection and individual patient factors. Additional medications may be needed to treat hypertension. Adults are advised to drink at least eight 8-oz glasses of fluids daily. Intravenous fluids may be ordered if the patient has nausea and vomiting. Dietary salt and protein restriction may be imposed on the patient with chronic disease. If an obstruction or congenital anomaly is present, it should be treated. Urine samples must be obtained for follow-up cultures to determine whether the infection has been resolved.

NURSING CARE OF THE PATIENT WITH PYELONEPHRITIS

Focused Assessment

General assessment of the patient with a urinary tract disorder is outlined in Chapter 41, Box 41.1. When caring for the patient with pyelonephritis, record the presence of signs and symptoms, history of previous urinary tract disorders, predisposing factors, and the effects of the infection on activities of daily living (ADLs).

Patient Problems, Goals, and Outcome Criteria: Pyelonephritis

Patient Problems	Goals and Outcome Criteria
Acute pain related to inflammation	Pain relief: patient states pain relieved, reports pain is decreased from prior assessment
Decreased activity tolerance related to fatigue	Improved activity tolerance: completes activities of daily living (ADL) without reporting excessive fatigue
Fluid volume deficit related to vomiting, anorexia	Adequate hydration: fluid intake and output equal, pulse and blood pressure (BP) consistent with patient's baseline values
Inadequate nutrition related to anorexia, nausea, vomiting	Adequate nutrition: stable body weight
Ineffective self-care management related to lack of knowledge of treatment and future prevention of pyelonephritis	Effectively manages treatment plan: accurately describes prescribed treatment and preventive measures, has no recurrence of infection

Interventions

Acute pain. Administer analgesics, usually NSAIDs or antipyretics, as ordered for pain. Antibiotics do not provide direct pain relief but eventually help by eliminating the cause of the inflammation.

Reduced activity tolerance. The pain and systemic symptoms of infection can contribute to fatigue and activity intolerance. Assist with ADLs and schedule activities to allow for periods of uninterrupted rest. If the patient is being treated at home, advise family members of the patient's need for additional rest, and to limit responsibilities until recovered.

Fluid volume deficit and inadequate nutrition. Adequate food and fluids are very important for the patient with pyelonephritis. If nausea and vomiting occur, inform the health care provider and administer antiemetics as ordered. Record food and fluid intake and fluid output. If the patient is unable to take in the recommended 2 to 3 L of fluid daily, intravenous fluids may be ordered. Monitor fluid intake to avoid circulatory overload. In the older patient, a sudden increase in fluid volume may result in heart failure (HF). Possible signs of HF include bounding pulse, rising BP, dyspnea, and edema.

Ineffective self-care management. If the infection is not adequately treated, the condition may progress to sepsis and death. The hospitalized patient will usually be given antibiotics intravenously. Administer drugs on time, and monitor patients for adverse effects. Upon discharge, the patient is usually changed to oral antibiotics. Emphasize the importance of completing the full course of therapy to prevent recurrence.

When the patient will be taking medications at home, review the drugs and stress the importance of taking them as prescribed. Explain the importance of follow-up evaluation to assess effects of treatment and the need to report suspected recurrence to the health care provider immediately (see the Patient Teaching box).

Patient Teaching

Pyelonephritis

- Take your medications exactly as prescribed. Report side effects (for specific drugs) to your health care provider. Be sure to complete the course of therapy.
- Limit physical activity and exercise as advised by your health care provider.
- Even after this infection has been treated, drink at least eight 8-oz glasses of fluids each day to dilute urine and to reduce the risk of recurrence.
- If advised, follow dietary protein and sodium restrictions.

HEREDITARY RENAL DISEASE

POLYCYSTIC KIDNEY DISEASE

Polycystic kidney disease is a hereditary disorder. It is characterized by grapelike cysts in place of normal kidney tissue (Fig. 42.1). The cysts enlarge, compress functional renal tissue, and eventually result in renal failure. They may also create pressure on nearby organs. As the kidneys lose the ability to concentrate urine, hypertension, and HF develop. Often, cystic lesions are found on other organs. Chronic infection contributes to progressive loss of function.

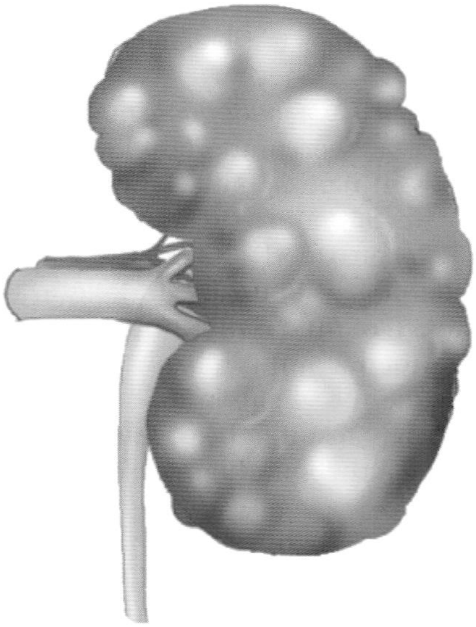

Fig. 42.1 Polycystic kidney. (From Hagen-Ansert SL: *Textbook of diagnostic sonography*, ed 8, St. Louis, 2018, Elsevier.)

Signs and Symptoms

This slowly progressive disorder begins with various types of pain, sometimes described as dull, aching abdominal, lower back, or flank pain; or it starts with colicky pain that begins abruptly.

Medical Treatment

Supportive treatment is recommended to preserve kidney function, treat UTI, and control hypertension. Infections should be treated promptly with appropriate antibiotics. The preferred antihypertensive agent is an ACE inhibitor or an angiotensin receptor blocker. Dietary sodium may be restricted to 2 g or less per day, and fluid may be limited to 3 L/day. Genetic counseling is advised for these patients because each of their children has a 50% chance of inheriting the condition.

◆ NURSING CARE OF THE PATIENT WITH POLYCYSTIC KIDNEY DISEASE

See the sections on nursing care of patients with ESRD and those having renal surgery, dialysis, and transplantation in this chapter.

IMMUNOLOGIC RENAL DISEASE

ACUTE GLOMERULONEPHRITIS

Pathophysiology

Glomerulonephritis is an immunologic disease characterized by inflammation of the capillary loops in the glomeruli. Several immunologic mechanisms can cause acute glomerulonephritis. The patient may develop antibodies against antigens in the glomeruli. A common type of glomerulonephritis follows an infection of the respiratory tract caused by group A–negative hemolytic streptococcus. An antigen-antibody reaction results in inflammation of the glomeruli and scar tissue forms. Glomerular permeability increases, allowing proteins to leak into the urine. The glomerular filtration rate decreases, and nitrogenous wastes accumulate in the blood. Blood urea nitrogen (BUN) and serum creatinine levels rise. Acute glomerulonephritis usually resolves completely, yet some patients develop chronic glomerulonephritis or progress to irreversible renal failure. Rapidly progressing glomerulonephritis (RPGN) is one type that quickly results in end-stage renal failure.

Clinical Manifestations

Urine becomes tea-colored as output decreases. Peripheral and periorbital (around the eye) edema is evident. As glomerular filtration decreases, mild to severe hypertension occurs and hypervolemia (increased blood volume) results.

Medical Diagnosis

Diagnosis is based on patient assessment and laboratory tests. A urinalysis is done to detect proteinuria and

RBC casts. Blood studies measure BUN, creatinine, and albumin. Streptococcal antibody tests indicate whether the patient has had a streptococcal infection. Findings in blood and urine studies tend to vary from one patient to another. Renal ultrasound, renal biopsy, or both may also be ordered.

Medical Treatment

Acute glomerulonephritis is treated with a diuretic such as furosemide, which helps eliminate excess fluid and lower blood pressure. Antibiotics are indicated if evidence of current streptococcal infection exists. In the acute phase, bed rest may be ordered to prevent or treat HF and severe hypertension from fluid overload. Activity restriction is usually continued as long as urine tests show blood or protein or if BP is elevated. Fluids, sodium, potassium, and protein may be restricted until sufficient recovery of kidney function occurs. When fluid overload has been corrected, moderate activity is permitted, but the patient still needs sufficient rest to allow the kidneys to heal.

Because some patients with acute glomerulonephritis develop renal insufficiency, follow-up is essential. If renal failure develops, dialysis is necessary. Patients who progress to chronic glomerulonephritis acquire ESRD in 1 to 30 years. (See the section entitled "Chronic Kidney Disease.")

NURSING CARE OF THE PATIENT WITH ACUTE GLOMERULONEPHRITIS

Focused Assessment

Assessment of patients with urinary tract disorders is outlined in Chapter 41, Box 41.1. For the patient with acute glomerulonephritis, it is especially important to note signs and symptoms, recent infections (especially sore throat or skin lesions), and changes in urine characteristics.

During the physical examination, inspect the area around the eyes, the extremities, and the abdomen for fluid accumulation. Assess tissue turgor. Evaluate respiratory and cardiac function for evidence of excess fluid volume: dyspnea, tachycardia, hypertension. Accurate intake and output records and daily weights help to assess the kidneys' ability to excrete excess fluid.

Patient Problems, Goals, and Outcome Criteria: Acute Glomerulonephritis

Patient Problems	Goals and Outcome Criteria
Fluid volume excess related to renal dysfunction	Restoration of normal fluid balance: balanced fluid intake and output, vital signs consistent with patient's baseline, absence of edema
Decreased activity tolerance related to retention of chemical wastes, fatigue, prescribed bed rest	Improved activity tolerance: patient reports less fatigue with physical activity
Ineffective self-care management related to prescribed bed rest, lack of knowledge of treatment measures of care	Patient adheres to plan of care: self-care is accomplished within activity restrictions, patient adheres to plan
Anxiety related to possibility of chronic illness	Reduced anxiety: patient states anxiety is lessened, appears calm

Interventions

Fluid volume excess. Administer diuretics as ordered. Maintain accurate records of fluid intake and output. Instruct patients and family members about the importance of carefully keeping track of intake and output. If fluids are restricted, explain the need for the restriction, and help the patient to plan the timing and amounts of allowed fluids. Fluid restriction can be very distressing. It helps to present fluids in small containers rather than serving an ounce or two in a large glass. If the patient has edema, special skin care is needed. Handle the patient gently because taut, swollen tissue is damaged easily and heals slowly.

Reduced activity tolerance. Activity intolerance may occur because of infection, accumulated toxins, or anemia. During the acute illness, discourage activity to allow the kidneys to heal. Explain the importance of rest for recovery. Schedule activities to allow for periods of uninterrupted rest. The patient on bed rest is at risk for complications of immobility: skin breakdown, pneumonia, muscle weakness, joint stiffness, constipation, and thrombus formation. Have the patient change positions, cough and deep breathe, and gently exercise joints periodically, at a minimum of every 2 hours. Nursing measures to prevent the complications of immobility are discussed in Chapter 12.

Ineffective self-care management. The patient needs to understand that rest, dietary restrictions, and medications promote recovery. Provide assistance with ADLs. Emphasize the need for follow-up care. When the patient is discharged, reinforce the importance of reporting signs of recurrence, such as changes in urine characteristics or edema. Instruct the patient to increase activities gradually as the edema and fatigue resolve.

Anxiety. The patient with acute glomerulonephritis may be very concerned about the possibility of developing a chronic, life-threatening condition. Give the patient an opportunity to ask questions and share concerns. Helpful interventions may include empathetic listening, providing factual information, and appropriately referring to other professionals.

URINARY TRACT OBSTRUCTIONS

RENAL CALCULI

Urolithiasis is the formation of **calculi** (stones) in the urinary tract and are often called *"kidney stones."* The prevalence of urolithiasis in the United States has been rising. In their lifetime, 19% of men and 9% of women are predicted to have stone formation (National Kidney Foundation, 2016). Kidney stones have a high incidence of recurrence (see the Cultural Considerations box).

Cultural Considerations

What Does Culture Have to Do With Urinary Calculi?

Urinary calculi are most common among non-Hispanic White peoples, followed by Hispanic White peoples. They are least common among Black and Asian peoples (Curhan, 2020).

Pathophysiology

Most calculi are precipitations of calcium salts (calcium oxalate or calcium phosphate), uric acid, magnesium ammonium phosphate (struvite), or cystine. All of these substances are normally found in the urine. Factors that foster the development of calculi include:

- Concentrated urine
- Excessive intake of vitamin D, animal protein, oxalates, sodium, sucrose, vitamin C, calcium-based antacids
- Low dietary calcium intake
- Familial history
- Hyperparathyroidism, gout, diabetes, obesity, gastric bypass procedure, inflammatory bowel disease, renal tubular acidosis
- Immobility, urinary stasis
- Sedentary lifestyle
- Altered urine pH
- Lack of kidney substance that inhibits calculi formation

Evidence indicates that low calcium intake is associated with calculi formation. Urine is normally acidic, with a pH ranging from 4.6 to 8.0 (Pagana et al., 2017). Some substances tend to precipitate in acid urine, causing calculus formation; others precipitate in alkaline urine. UTIs, particularly those caused by *Proteus*, *Klebsiella*, and *Pseudomonas*, are associated with calculi because these organisms cause the urine to become alkaline. The kidneys excrete substances that are believed to inhibit calculi formation, so a decrease in these substances may contribute to calculus formation.

Most calculi originate in the kidney (nephrolithiasis) and travel through the ureters to the bladder (urolithiasis).

Clinical Manifestations

The patient's reason for seeking care is usually pain. The location and characteristics of the pain may provide clues to the site of the calculus. Dull flank pain suggests a calculus in the renal pelvis or stretching of the renal capsule from urine retention (hydronephrosis). If a calculus lodges in a ureter, the patient usually has excruciating pain in the abdomen that radiates to the groin or the perineum. The ureter goes into spasm (colic) in an attempt to move the calculus along and relieve the obstruction. Nausea, vomiting, and hematuria may accompany the pain. The patient may also show signs and symptoms of UTI.

Medical Diagnosis

A computed tomography (CT) scan without contrast is the usual imaging procedure when stones are suspected. Other diagnostic tools are KUB (kidneys, ureters, bladder) radiography, kidney and bladder ultrasound, and abdominopelvic radiography. A routine urinalysis and culture and sensitivity are usually ordered as well. If a calculus can be obtained, its composition can be determined by laboratory analysis. Therefore, the patient is asked to strain all urine and save any stones or fragments that pass. Knowing the stone composition guides treatment and other measures to reduce the risk of recurrence. Additional diagnostic procedures may be done to rule out other causes of pain such as acute cholecystitis, pyelonephritis, musculoskeletal pain, duodenal ulcer, and abdominal aortic aneurysm.

Medical Treatment

Treatment is based on the type, location, and size of the stone. Often, small calculi pass spontaneously. Ambulation may facilitate the passage of some calculi. Most patients can be treated at home, although hospitalization may be needed if the patient cannot tolerate oral intake or has uncontrollable pain or fever. Parenteral NSAIDs such as ketorolac and antispasmodics are ordered to relieve the intense, colicky pain. Opioid analgesics may be needed in some cases. Medical expulsive therapy (MET) is the use of drugs that promote passage of kidney stones. The alpha adrenergic blocker tamsulosin is the preferred drug for MET. Intravenous fluids are commonly given to dilute the urine and reduce the risk of additional stone formation. Antibiotics are ordered if infection is present or if internal manipulation of the calculus is necessary. If the calculus does not pass, several procedures may be used to destroy or remove it. Options include shock wave lithotripsy (SWL), ureteroscopic lithotripsy, laparoscopic stone removal, and percutaneous nephrolithotomy.

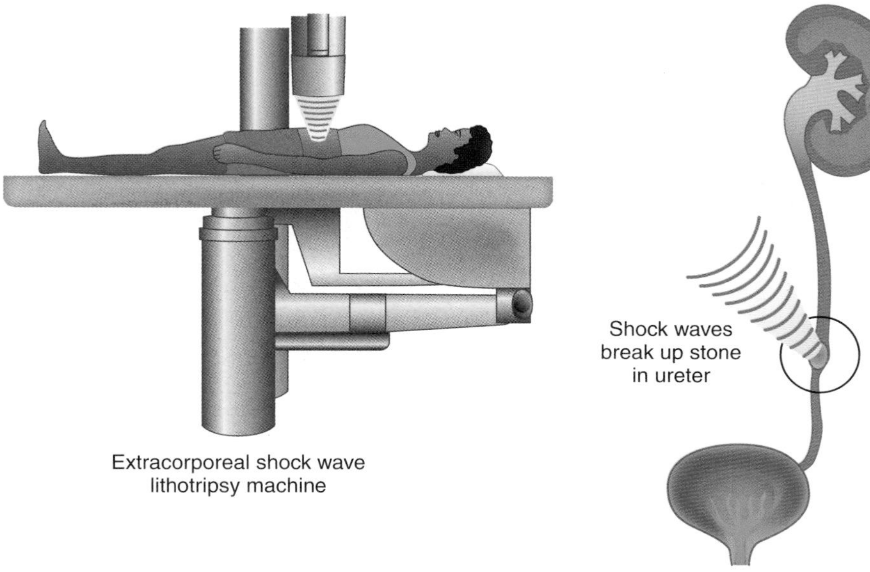

Fig. 42.2 Extracorporeal shock wave lithotripsy. (From Monahan FD, Drake DT, Neighbors M, editors; *Medical-surgical nursing: foundations for clinical practice*, ed 2, Philadelphia, 1998, Saunders.)

Lithotripsy. Lithotripsy (shattering of the calculus) may be accomplished by extracorporeal shock wave lithotripsy (ESWL), which uses sound, laser, or dry shock wave energy (electrohydraulic, electromagnetic, piezoelectric) to shatter the stones. ESWL uses a lithotripter to deliver a series of shock waves to disintegrate calculi. Guided by an ultrasound probe, the energy is directed to the stone through a water-filled cushion. Depending on the type of energy used, conscious sedation, preoperative sedation, or analgesics may be given because the series of 1000 to 1500 shocks is painful (Fig. 42.2). The shocks are coordinated with the patient's cardiac cycle. The pulverized calculus is excreted in the urine over 1 to 4 weeks. After lithotripsy, the urine is often a bright-red color at first, gradually turning to a dark-red or smoky shade. A stent may be placed in the ureter before treatment to facilitate passage of the stone fragments. The stent is usually removed in several weeks. Possible complications of lithotripsy include injury to the kidney and adjacent organs, hypertension, and diabetes mellitus. Patients taking anticoagulants may hemorrhage. Most patients are able to resume normal activities on the day after the procedure. Antibiotics may be given for up to 2 weeks to prevent UTI.

Endourologic procedures. Stones in the bladder can often be crushed and removed using cystoscopic techniques. A ureteroscope and other accompanying instruments can be passed through the bladder to reach stones located in the renal pelvis and ureters. In lasertripsy, the calculus is visualized and destroyed with a laser. Like ESWL, fragments are usually passed in the urine. General anesthesia is used, but premedication is commonly omitted because radiographs must be obtained immediately before the procedure. When stones are large or cannot be broken with lithotripsy, a percutaneous nephrolithotomy may be done. The surgeon creates a tunnel directly through the flank into the kidney, and then uses ultrasound or electrohydrolysis to break the stone into pieces. Some pieces are removed through the tunnel with a nephroscope. A nephrostomy tube is placed and left for 1 to 2 weeks to promote healing. The urine will be blood tinged for several days. Encourage oral fluid intake and record intake and output, including urine passed through the tube.

Surgical procedures. If calculi are not passed spontaneously or crushed with a lithotriptor, surgery may be necessary. The incision of an organ or a duct to remove a calculus is a **lithotomy**. A nephrolithotomy is the surgical procedure used if the calculus is in the kidney. The removal of a calculus from the renal pelvis is a *pyelolithotomy*. A ureterolithotomy is removal of a calculus from a ureter (Fig. 42.3).

Prevention

Prevention of recurrence of renal calculi is an important goal. Long-term management of these patients includes a high fluid intake to keep urine dilute, dietary restrictions for specific elements depending on the type of stones (e.g., animal protein, purines), regular exercise, and occasionally medications to alter the urine pH. An appropriate fluid intake is judged by a urine output of at least 2 L a day. Fluid intake may need to be increased during hot weather because of fluid loss through perspiration. Drugs that may be used include thiazide diuretics for elevated urine calcium and allopurinol for elevated urine uric acid. For individuals with oxalate stones, potassium citrate and magnesium supplement may be ordered. Medications are less effective than dietary management.

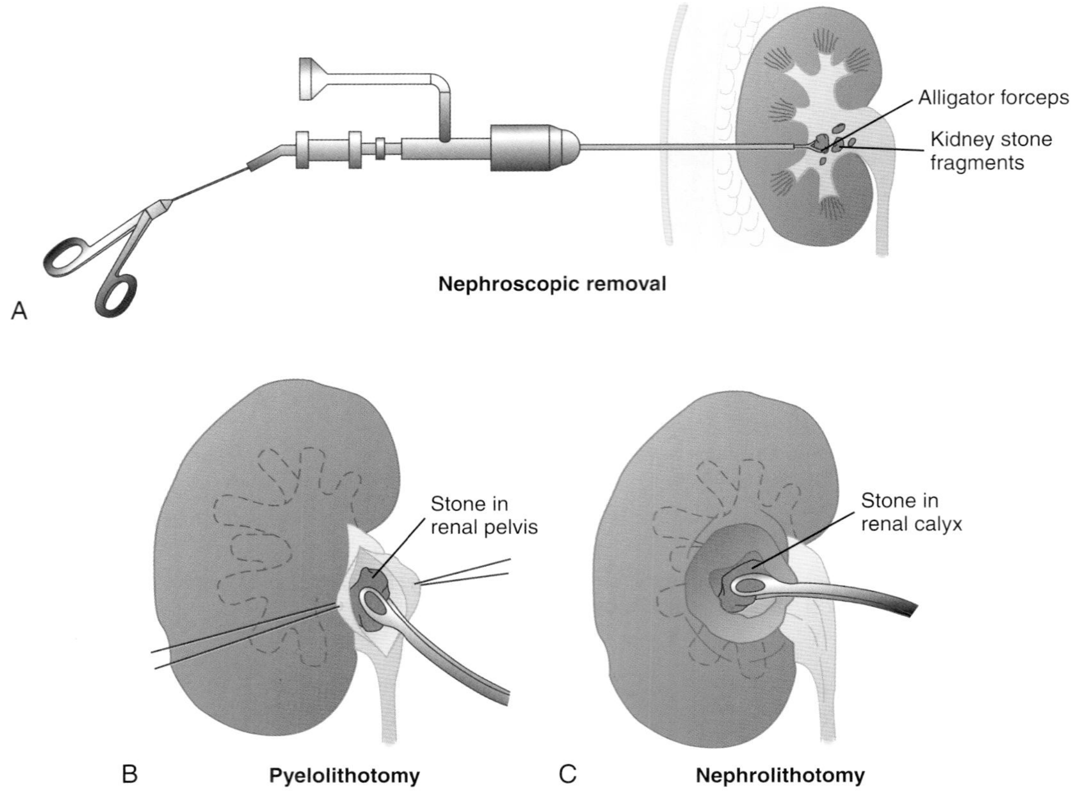

Fig. 42.3 Surgical procedures for renal calculi. (A) Nephroscopy. (B) Pyelolithotomy. (C) Nephrolithotomy. (From Black JM, Hawks JH: *Medical-surgical nursing: clinical management for positive outcomes*, ed 8, St. Louis, 2009, Saunders.)

NURSING CARE OF THE PATIENT WITH RENAL CALCULI

Focused Assessment

Assessment of the patient with a urinary tract disorder is summarized in Chapter 41, Box 41.1 (see also Nursing Care Plan: Patient With Renal Calculi). When the patient has known or suspected urinary calculi, assess for personal or family history of calculi. Describe the patient's usual fluid intake and diet, including use of vitamin, mineral, and/or herbal supplements. Assess the duration, location, severity, type, and modifying factors that exacerbate or relieve pain. Record changes in urine amount or characteristics. Assess temperature to detect fever. The health care provider will palpate and percuss the flanks and abdomen, noting the presence of pain, tenderness, or a distended bladder.

Patient Problems, Goals, and Outcome Criteria: Renal Calculi

Patient Problems	Goals and Outcome Criteria
Acute pain related to obstruction, trauma, and renal colic	Pain relief: patient states pain has been alleviated or relieved, reports pain is decreased from prior assessment
Reduced urinary output related to obstruction	Unobstructed urine elimination: urine output equal to fluid intake

Patient Problems, Goals, and Outcome Criteria: Renal Calculi—cont'd

Patient Problems	Goals and Outcome Criteria
Potential for fluid and electrolyte imbalance related to anorexia, nausea, and vomiting	Normal fluid balance: fluid intake and output approximately equal, pulse and blood pressure (BP) consistent with patient baseline
Ineffective self-care management related to lack of knowledge of prevention and treatment of calculi	Patient accurately describes prevention and treatment, adheres to preventive measures, has no recurrences
If surgery is performed, additional patient problems and goals may include the following.	
Potential for infection related to invasive procedures	Absence of infection: normal body temperature and white blood cell (WBC) count, clear urine
Decreased cardiac output related to blood loss	Adequate cardiac output: pulse and BP consistent with patient baseline
Potential for inadequate ventilation related to splinting of painful incision	Adequate ventilation: clear breath sounds throughout lung fields, respiratory and depth consistent with patient baseline; O_2 saturation of 95% or higher

Nursing Care Plan Patient With Renal Calculi

FOCUSED ASSESSMENT

Health History

A 40-year-old woman was admitted with excruciating flank and abdominal pain, nausea, and vomiting. Past medical history included hypertension, for which she takes amlodipine 5 mg once daily, and high cholesterol, which is managed with lovastatin, 20 mg at bedtime. She has no other medical history other than frequent urinary tract infections (UTIs) when she was very young. Her most recent UTI was at 34 years of age when she was pregnant. She has been a frequent drinker of diet soda since 18 years of age. Radiologic studies showed a calculus lodged in the right ureter. Extracorporeal shock wave lithotripsy (ESWL) was done to shatter the calculus. Because of her vomiting and need for IV fluids, she was admitted to the hospital. The patient has returned to her hospital room and now reports right lower abdominal pain at a level of "5" on a 1–10 pain scale.

Physical Examination

Vital signs: blood pressure 126/66 mm Hg, pulse 90 beats per minute, respiration 180 breaths per minute, oral temperature 100°F (37.8°C). Ht. 5′6″, Wt. 200 lb. She is oriented to time, place, person, and situation but is drowsy. Her abdomen is soft; no bladder distention is noted. She has just voided 350 mL of pink-tinged urine, and reports soreness in her right lower abdomen at a level of "5" on a 1–10 pain scale, intravenous fluids are infusing at 125 mL/h.

Patient Problems	Goals and Outcome Criteria	Interventions
Acute pain related to ESWL.	Patient will report pain decrease to a level of "3" or below on a 1–10 pain scale.	Assess pain characteristics. Administer analgesics and antispasmodics as ordered. Assist with ambulation when fully alert to promote passage of calculus fragments. Position changes, back rubs, relaxation, and imagery may be used to relieve pain. Document effects of pain relief interventions.
Potential for urinary obstruction related to trauma and obstruction by stone fragments.	Patient's urine output will be approximately equal to fluid intake (e.g., 1 L input approximately equal to 1 L output).	Measure all fluid intake and output. Report low output to health care provider. Strain all urine to collect calculi fragments. Send fragments to laboratory for analysis. Maintain intravenous fluids as ordered.
Potential for fluid and electrolyte imbalances nausea and vomiting.	Patient will be adequately hydrated as evidenced by moist mucous membranes, urine with normal urine specific gravity value, and vital signs consistent within what is expected for the average healthy 40-year-old female.	Administer intravenous fluids as ordered. Assess for deficient fluid volume: hypotension, tachycardia, sticky mucous membranes, and concentrated urine. Encourage oral fluids when permitted. Administer antiemetics as ordered for nausea and vomiting.
Potential for decreased cardiac output related to dehydration, possible blood loss caused by ESWL trauma.	Patient's cardiac output will remain normal, as evidenced by vital signs consistent within what is expected for the average healthy 40-year-old female and by absence of tachycardia, hypotension, or restlessness.	Assess the abdomen and groin area for bruising; some is expected; document increased redness and bruising. Note color of urine, which is normally red initially after ESWL, and report increased viscosity of urine associated with bleeding. Monitor vital signs to detect signs of decreasing cardiac output: tachycardia, restlessness, and hypotension.
Inability to manage self-care after lithotripsy related to lack of knowledge of prevention and treatment of calculi, self-care after lithotripsy.	Patient will manage self-care, as evidenced by correct description of self-care after lithotripsy and measures to prevent recurrence of calculi.	Tell the patient that the fragments of the stones are usually passed in the urine over a period of several weeks and may cause some pain. Administer antibiotics as ordered and emphasize the importance of treating any new urinary tract infections to reduce the risk of calculi formation. Advise the patient to consume enough fluid daily to produce at least 2 L of output unless the health care provider prescribes less. Fluids should be consumed around the clock to prevent concentration during the night. If any dietary restrictions are imposed, request a dietary consultation to explain them to the patient.

CRITICAL THINKING QUESTIONS

1. Why would the patient continue to have pain after the stones have been shattered with lithotripsy?
2. When might 3 to 4 L/day of fluid intake be contraindicated?

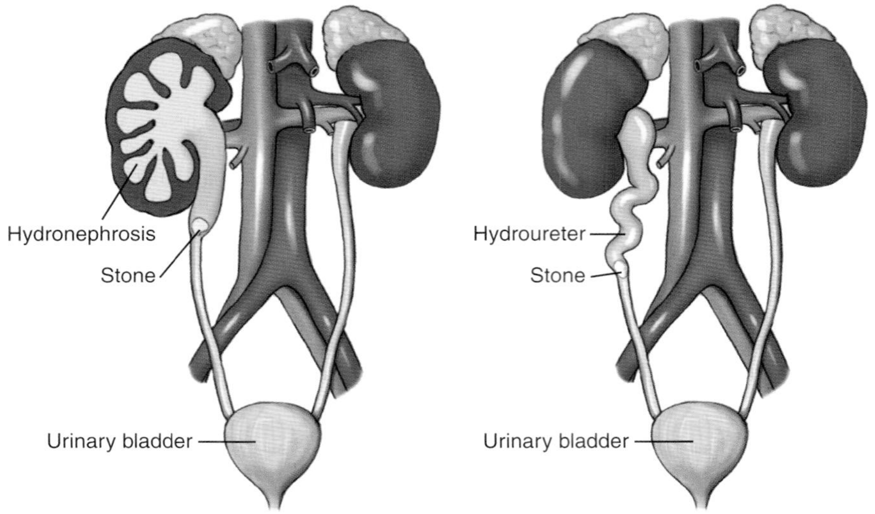

Fig. 42.4 Hydronephrosis caused by obstruction of the upper portion of the ureter. Hydroureter caused by obstruction of the lower portion of the ureter. (From Leonard PC: *Building a medical vocabulary with Spanish translations*, ed 10, St. Louis, 2018, Elsevier.)

Interventions

Acute pain. Because calculi in the urinary tract can cause excruciating pain (renal colic), pain relief is a priority. Initially intravenous NSAIDs are commonly ordered. If pain is not relieved, intravenous opioid analgesics may be ordered. Antispasmodics are usually ordered to reduce the smooth muscle spasms in the ureters. If pain is intermittent, the patient may be permitted to ambulate when comfortable because this may help the calculus to move through the urinary tract. Safety precautions are needed if opioids have been given. Pain may resolve suddenly if the calculus moves into the bladder or is passed through the urethra.

Reduced urinary elimination. Depending on its size and location, a calculus may obstruct urine flow. If urine backs up into the kidney, hydronephrosis—distention of the kidney with urine—may develop. This condition can cause permanent damage (Fig. 42.4). Maintain accurate records of fluid intake and output and report low output to the health care provider. In addition, all urine is strained and examined for calculi. If any calculi are recovered, send them to the laboratory for analysis.

Potential for electrolyte imbalance. Renal colic is often accompanied by nausea and sometimes vomiting. Give antiemetics promptly as ordered. The health care provider may order intravenous fluids to maintain dilute urine and to flush the urinary tract. A fluid intake to maintain an output of 2 L/day is recommended. Large volumes of fluids must be given carefully to the older patient, in whom fluid volume excess can develop easily. Monitor for signs of circulatory overload, such as tachycardia, bounding pulse, dyspnea, edema, and hypertension. Although dilute urine decreases the risk of stone recurrence (Prezioso et al., 2015), increased fluids do not necessarily facilitate the passage of existing stones.

Ineffective self-care management. When the patient is discharged, reinforce the need to continue to consume adequate amounts of fluid daily. The fluid needs to be consumed over the 24-hour period so that urine does not become concentrated at night. Advise the patient to drink two glasses of water before bed and another two glasses when awakening at night to void. This pattern should be followed for life to reduce the risk of calculus formation in the future. If the health care provider has prescribed a special diet or dietary restriction, provide instructions or have the dietitian do so. Dietary guidelines vary with the type of stone (e.g., calcium, uric acid).

Postoperative Care

Procedures to remove kidney stones may be minimally invasive or require an open incision that will affect specific nursing interventions. Before surgery, explain the expected procedure to the patient and answer questions. Goals of postoperative care are maintenance of urine drainage, prevention of UTI, and prevention of pulmonary and circulatory complications.

Potential for infection. To maintain alignment and urine flow, the patient may have drains, catheters, a ureteral stent, or a combination of these. Each tube is connected to its own closed drainage system. Position tubes for free flow of urine at all times. Keep accurate accounts of drainage from each tube. If the patient has a flank incision, frequently check the area around the dressing for drainage because urine tends to leak from the incision. A large amount of serosanguinous drainage is normal immediately after surgery. In approximately

2 days, the drainage changes to serous. Frequent dressing changes using sterile technique may be required. In some cases, an ostomy appliance is used to collect drainage and to permit accurate measurement of the drainage.

Some patients have nephrostomy tubes placed directly in the kidney. The tube is placed for drainage or for instillation of irrigating fluid. It also diverts urine flow from the ureter until adequate healing has occurred. If irrigations are ordered, use strict aseptic technique and not more than 5 mL of warm, sterile normal saline at a time.

Decreased cardiac output. The patient is at risk for the same postoperative complications as any surgical patient. Monitor for signs of excessive bleeding, infection, or pulmonary complications. To detect bleeding, inspect the dressing and drainage hourly for the first 24 hours. Immediately report bright red blood, excessive serosanguinous drainage, increasing pulse, restlessness, or decreasing BP to the health care provider. Indications of infection, such as odor, cloudy drainage, or temperature above 100°F should also be reported. Measures to reduce the risk of infection include maintaining a closed drainage system, changing wet dressings promptly, and using strict aseptic technique when handling tubes or dressings.

Potential for inadequate ventilation. Monitor the patient's pulmonary status carefully. A flank incision can make taking a deep breath very painful. Assist the patient to turn, cough, and deep breathe at least every 2 hours. An incentive spirometer helps to determine how much the patient is able to inflate the lungs. When the patient coughs, the incision needs to be splinted with pillows. For the first postoperative days, administer analgesics before turning, coughing, and deep breathing to make the patient as comfortable as possible before performing these activities. Adequate fluid intake thins respiratory secretions and makes them easier to expectorate. Early and frequent ambulation promotes improved respiratory function. All of these efforts help to prevent atelectasis and pneumonia.

UROLOGIC TRAUMA

The kidneys sustain 50% of all urologic injuries. Trauma may be penetrating or blunt. Penetrating injuries most often result from knives or guns. Blunt trauma occurs when a force is applied to the abdominal wall and the energy is diffused into the abdominal cavity. Examples of blunt-force trauma include motor vehicle accidents, contact sports injuries, falls, and intentional injuries. Blunt injuries to the kidneys can produce lacerations or contusions. The ureters are rarely injured with blunt trauma; they are disrupted most often by penetration and require surgical anastomosis. The bladder may rupture from blunt trauma if full, but it is rarely harmed when empty. The urethra is most apt to be injured in men because of its unprotected anatomic location.

When blunt trauma is suspected, the patient is observed for bruising on the abdomen or in the flank area. Assess for signs of shock (tachycardia, restlessness, hypotension, pallor), pain, and a palpable abdominal or flank mass. Bruising over the flank and lower back that occurs with retroperitoneal bleeding is called *Grey Turner sign*. Immediately report these findings to the registered nurse or health care provider.

The health care provider may order a kidney, ureter, and bladder (KUB) urography, CT scan, or ultrasound to determine the extent of injury. Diagnostic peritoneal lavage may be performed to determine whether there is bleeding in the peritoneal cavity. Surgery is required to determine the cause of bleeding if the peritoneal lavage is positive.

The most common indication of urologic trauma is hematuria. Depending on the extent of injuries, it may not be possible for the patient to void. Before catheterizing a patient with suspected trauma, carefully inspect the urethral meatus. If there is blood in or around the meatus, a urologist should perform the catheterization or insert a suprapubic catheter.

If the injury is not severe, if there is little bleeding, and if there are no signs of shock, continue to monitor the patient closely. More severe injuries may require surgery to repair damage. Postsurgical care of these patients is similar to the care of the patient with a nephrectomy, urinary calculi, or cystectomy.

CANCERS OF THE URINARY SYSTEM

Care of the patient with cancer is discussed in Chapter 7. This section focuses on the specific needs of the patient with cancer of the urinary tract.

RENAL CANCER

Malignancies of the kidney are expected to account for approximately 73,750 new cases of cancer in the United States in 2021 (National Cancer Institute, 2021). The incidence is higher in Black Americans and Native American/Alaska Natives than in other ethnicities (National Cancer Institute, 2017c). Risk factors include smoking, obesity, hypertension, family history of renal cancer, long-term misuse of acetaminophen or aspirin, and environmental exposures (asbestos, cadmium, gasoline).

A renal tumor may reach considerable size before it is detected. Renal malignancies metastasize to the liver, lungs, long bones, and the other kidney. Direct extension of the tumor may be found in the ureter. Early symptoms are anemia, weakness, and weight loss. Painless, gross hematuria is the classic sign, usually in the advanced stage of the disease, as is a dull ache in the flank.

Medical Diagnosis

The health care provider may be able to palpate a mass in the flank area. CT scan is the primary diagnostic tool for renal cell cancer. Other diagnostic tests and procedures to study the mass may include ultrasonography and magnetic resonance imaging (MRI), results of which can provide additional information that helps in making treatment decisions. Care of the patient undergoing these procedures is detailed in Chapter 41, Table 41.1.

Medical Treatment

Removal of a kidney, the treatment of choice for renal cancer, is called a *nephrectomy*. Radical nephrectomy involves removal of the kidney and its adjacent tissue, adrenal gland, renal artery and vein, and local lymph glands. Before nephrectomy, the renal artery may be occluded to reduce the blood supply to the tumor. Partial nephrectomy may be an option when the tumor is small. Laparoscopic complete or partial nephrectomy has largely replaced open surgical approaches. Although renal tumors are not generally responsive to radiation or chemotherapy, immunotherapy, antiangiogenetic therapy, or thermal ablation may be used for the patient with metastatic disease.

◆ NURSING CARE OF THE PATIENT WITH RENAL CANCER

Focused Assessment

Nursing assessment of the patient with a urologic disorder is outlined in Chapter 41, Box 41.1. Inquire about weakness, fatigue, and any changes observed in the urine. Explore the patient's emotional status, usual coping strategies, and support systems.

Preoperative care. General preoperative nursing care is discussed in detail in Chapter 17. Before renal surgery, the patient's primary problems are inadequate coping related to potentially fatal disease and lack of knowledge of tests, procedures, and effects of renal surgery. The goals of nursing care are effective patient use of coping mechanisms and understanding of what is being done and what to expect.

Thorough explanations of diagnostic tests and preoperative teaching provide important information. Assure the patient that one functioning kidney can sustain adequate kidney function. Tests are done to confirm that the unaffected kidney functions adequately before a nephrectomy. Serum and urine laboratory tests are ordered to serve as baseline data for postoperative comparison. Older patients are more likely to have renal insufficiency, and they eventually may need renal dialysis after nephrectomy. The teaching plan includes what to expect in the postoperative period and how to turn, cough, and deep breathe. Other preoperative care is the same as that for any other major surgery.

Postoperative care. Common aspects of postoperative care are discussed in Chapter 17. After nephrectomy, monitor vital signs to detect fluid volume alterations related to blood loss or fluid retention. Record intake and output as another measure of fluid balance and renal function. Routinely check drains and tubes to ensure proper function. Monitor dressings for drainage. Inspect the wound for intactness and signs of infection (excessive redness or swelling, purulent drainage). Determine and address the patient's comfort level. Auscultate breath sounds and bowel sounds. Anticipate emotional distress, and encourage the patient to express thoughts and feelings about having cancer.

Patient Problems, Goals, and Outcome Criteria: Renal Cancer, Postoperative

Patient Problems	Goals and Outcome Criteria
Acute pain related to incisional tissue trauma	Pain relief: patient states pain is lessened or relieved, reports pain is decreased from prior assessment
Potential for fluid volume deficit related to dehydration, blood loss	Normal hydration and blood volume: pulse and blood pressure (BP) consistent with patient baseline, elastic skin turgor
Inadequate ventilation related to proximity of incision to diaphragm	Adequate ventilation: clear breath sounds throughout lung fields
Potential for injury related to decreased peristalsis caused by bowel manipulation during surgery	Absence of abdominal distention: active bowel sounds, abdomen soft
Potential for infection related to break in skin	Absence of infection: normal body temperature and white blood cell (WBC) count
Inadequate coping related to diagnosis of cancer	Effective coping: patient practices strategies that reduce anxiety but do not interfere with therapeutic plan
Inability to manage self-care related to lack of knowledge of postoperative limitations related to lack of information	Patient understands postoperative restrictions and accurately describes and adheres to activity limitations

Interventions

Acute pain. Obtain a complete description of the patient's pain. Incisional pain is intense at first and requires prompt administration of prescribed analgesics. Because of the patient's position during surgery, there may be muscle aches in the opposite side and flank area. Medication can be supplemented with position changes and back rubs. Other comfort measures are described in Chapter 8.

Potential for fluid volume deficit. Intravenous fluids are given initially. The health care provider normally orders approximately 3 L of fluid daily. Maintain accurate intake and output records. At first, urine may be measured every 1 to 2 hours. Notify the health care provider if less than 30 mL is produced in an hour. Daily weights are a preferable measure of fluid balance than intake and output. BUN, serum creatinine, serum electrolytes, and urine specific gravity are assessed and compared with preoperative values.

Monitor the nephrectomy patient for bleeding. Frequently check the dressing drainage. Be careful to check *under* the patient because blood flows to the most dependent area. Sometimes the dressing is dry and intact, but the patient may be lying in a pool of blood.

Inadequate ventilation. The location of the flank incision causes pain with expansion of the thorax. Patients tend to protect the area by not breathing deeply. This may lead to pneumonia and atelectasis. It is especially important to have the patient turn, cough, and deep breathe every 1 to 2 hours. You can help by supporting the incision during respiratory exercises. Supervise use of an incentive spirometer to encourage deeper inspiration. As soon as ambulation is permitted, assist the patient out of bed. Be careful not to place tension on tubes and drains. Gradually increase the time and distance walked.

Potential for injury. Anesthesia and manipulation of abdominal organs cause temporary cessation of peristalsis in the intestines. Until peristalsis returns, the patient is not permitted to take anything by mouth. If peristalsis does not return within 3 to 4 days, the patient is said to have *paralytic ileus*. Because paralytic ileus is common after nephrectomy, a nasogastric tube may be inserted and attached to suction during surgery. Suction keeps the stomach empty, reducing the risk of nausea and abdominal distention. The return of peristalsis is detected by active bowel sounds and the passage of flatus (gas). Auscultate the abdomen for bowel sounds and observe for abdominal distention. Ambulation promotes the return of peristalsis.

Potential for infection. During dressing changes, use strict aseptic technique. Montgomery straps may decrease irritation from the adhesive tape if frequent dressing changes are required.

Inadequate coping. The patient facing cancer may fear the possibility of death, mourn the loss of an organ, and/or dread additional cancer therapy. You can help by encouraging the patient to talk and voice concerns, listening empathetically, providing requested information, and referring the patient to expert counselors. Explore usual coping strategies and sources of support. Chapter 7 provides additional details on nursing care of the patient with cancer.

Inability to manage self-care. Before discharge, teach the patient not to lift or participate in strenuous activities for 8 weeks. Contact sports are prohibited for life because trauma to the remaining kidney could eliminate all kidney function.

BLADDER CANCER

Cancer of the bladder is the most common malignancy of the urinary tract, with more than 83,000 new cases predicted in the United States in 2021 (American Cancer Society). Over the years, chemical agents have been suspected as carcinogens (see the Cultural Considerations box). The tars found in smoking tobacco, aniline dyes found in industrial compounds, and tryptophan all have been implicated in the development of bladder cancer.

> **Cultural Considerations**
>
> **What Does Culture Have to Do With Bladder Cancer?**
>
> Risk factors for bladder cancer include cigarette smoking and exposure to chemicals used in the rubber and cable industries. Historically, men have been more likely than women to smoke and to work in industry, which may explain why this cancer is 3 times as common among men as among women (National Cancer Institute, 2017a).

Clinical Manifestations

The most common sign of bladder cancer is painless, intermittent hematuria. Other signs and symptoms include bladder irritability; infection with dysuria, frequency, and urgency; and decreased stream of urine.

Medical Diagnosis

When the patient's signs and symptoms suggest bladder cancer, the health care provider may order a urinalysis with urine cytology and cystoscopy. Cystoscopy is done to visualize the bladder and permit biopsy of any observable lesions. Depending on the initial findings, additional studies may be done, including CT, MRI, intravenous pyelogram (IVP), CT-urogram, chest radiograph, and radionuclide bone scan. Details of these tests and procedures and nursing implications are provided in Chapter 41, Table 41.1.

Medical Treatment

Surgery is the treatment of choice for bladder malignancies. The type of surgery depends on whether the cancer is superficial, invasive, or metastatic. Superficial cancers involve only the bladder mucosa or submucosa, or sometimes both. Superficial lesions with low recurrence rates may be treated with cystoscopic resection and fulguration or with laser photocoagulation. Cystoscopic resection is the removal of tissue through a cystoscope with a special cutting instrument. Fulguration is the use of electric current to burn and destroy tissue. Laser photocoagulation is the use of an intense beam of light (argon laser) to destroy tissue.

Two other surgical procedures for bladder cancer include segmental bladder resection and radical cystectomy with pelvic lymphadenectomy (excision of lymph nodes). A segmental bladder resection is done for a single, primary tumor too large to remove by cystoscopic resection. It involves removal of the tumor and adjacent bladder muscle, a procedure that decreases the size of the bladder. A radical cystectomy is removal of the entire bladder and adjacent structures with diversion of the ureters. In men, the prostate is removed. In women, the urethra, uterus, fallopian tubes, ovaries, and anterior vaginal wall are removed. This procedure is reserved for malignancies that are untreatable with less conservative measures. Because this is a very extensive surgery, an optimal state of health before surgery is desirable. In addition to surgery, treatment may include chemotherapy, radiation, immunotherapy, or targeted therapy depending on the extent of the malignancy. Sometimes chemotherapeutic drugs or immune-stimulating agents are instilled directly into the bladder. This procedure is called *intravesical therapy*. A drug such as bacillus Calmette-Guérin (BCG) is administered into the bladder through a urinary catheter. The patient's position is changed at 15-minute intervals to ensure that the drugs reach the site of the lesion. After about 2 hours, the drugs are drained from the bladder. Treatment may be repeated weekly for 6 to 12 weeks, followed by a program of maintenance therapy.

Urinary diversion. When the bladder and urethra must be removed completely, urine must be allowed to drain through another route, called *urinary diversion*. Several types of urinary diversions exist with the most common being the ileal and sigmoid (colon) conduit, orthoptic neobladder, and the cutaneous ureterostomy. Ureterosigmoidoscopy is used less now because it has been associated with deterioration of renal function, metabolic disturbances, and secondary cancer of the sigmoid colon. The neobladder is a reservoir that is attached to the urethra so that the patient voids through the urethra. These diversions are illustrated in Fig. 42.5 and Chapter 18, Fig. 18.7 and discussed in detail in Chapter 18.

To form an ileal conduit, a portion of the ileum is resected from the small bowel. The ureters are implanted in the ileum, one end of the ileum is closed, and the open end is implanted on the abdominal surface as a stoma. Urine is excreted through the ileal conduit rather than the urethra. A urinary drainage pouch is attached to the skin to collect the urine. A sigmoid conduit is formed by the same procedure, except that a section of sigmoid colon instead of ileum is used. A continent reservoir is an internal pouch created from a segment of bowel. Urine collects in the pouch and is drained with a catheter at intervals. A ureterostomy brings the ureter to the abdominal surface, where urine is eliminated through a stoma. A nephrostomy is the placement of a tube in the kidney so that urine may drain through the tube into an external collection device. Detailed information about urinary diversion is presented in Chapter 18.

◆ NURSING CARE OF THE PATIENT WITH BLADDER CANCER

Focused Assessment

Assessment of the patient with possible or confirmed bladder cancer includes a complete description of urinary signs and symptoms. Fatigue and weight loss are significant and should be noted. The health history may reveal use of tobacco or exposure to carcinogenic chemicals. Explore the patient's emotional state, coping strategies, and sources of support.

Preoperative care. In addition to the common nursing care described in Chapter 17, important preoperative patient problems for the patient facing segmental resection for cancer may be fear related to life-threatening diagnosis and inadequate coping related to anticipated lifestyle change. The goals of nursing care are reduced fear and effective coping strategies. To accomplish these goals, explore the patient's feelings and provide information and encouragement. The thought of having cancer is frightening, and nurses must educate the public about multiple treatments available. Assess coping strategies and provide resources as needed. The patient needs support to accept the diagnosis and follow through with the treatment.

Unless a neobladder is constructed, the patient having radical cystectomy faces a more difficult adjustment—that of permanent urinary diversion. The patient needs to be prepared psychologically, as well as physically, to cope with a change in body image. The enterostomal therapist is a valuable resource to both you and the patient in preparing for this surgery. The therapist selects the stoma site with the patient. The patient may be advised to wear a water-filled pouch for several days before surgery to help ensure proper stoma placement (see the Patient Teaching box). If the patient would like to talk to someone who has had a cystectomy, this often can be arranged through a local ostomy club or chapter of the American Cancer Society.

Patient Teaching

Urinary Diversion

- Proper stoma care reduces the risk of complications.
- Notify your health care provider for signs of infection: fever; increasing redness, swelling, and tenderness of incisions.
- Restrict activity as prescribed by your health care provider to avoid strain on the surgical site.
- If you have a ureterosigmoidostomy, you will need a colonoscopy at regular intervals to assess for a malignancy.
- Resources include the enterostomal therapist, the American Cancer Society, and the United Ostomy Association (email: info@uoaa.org; telephone: 1-800-826-0826).

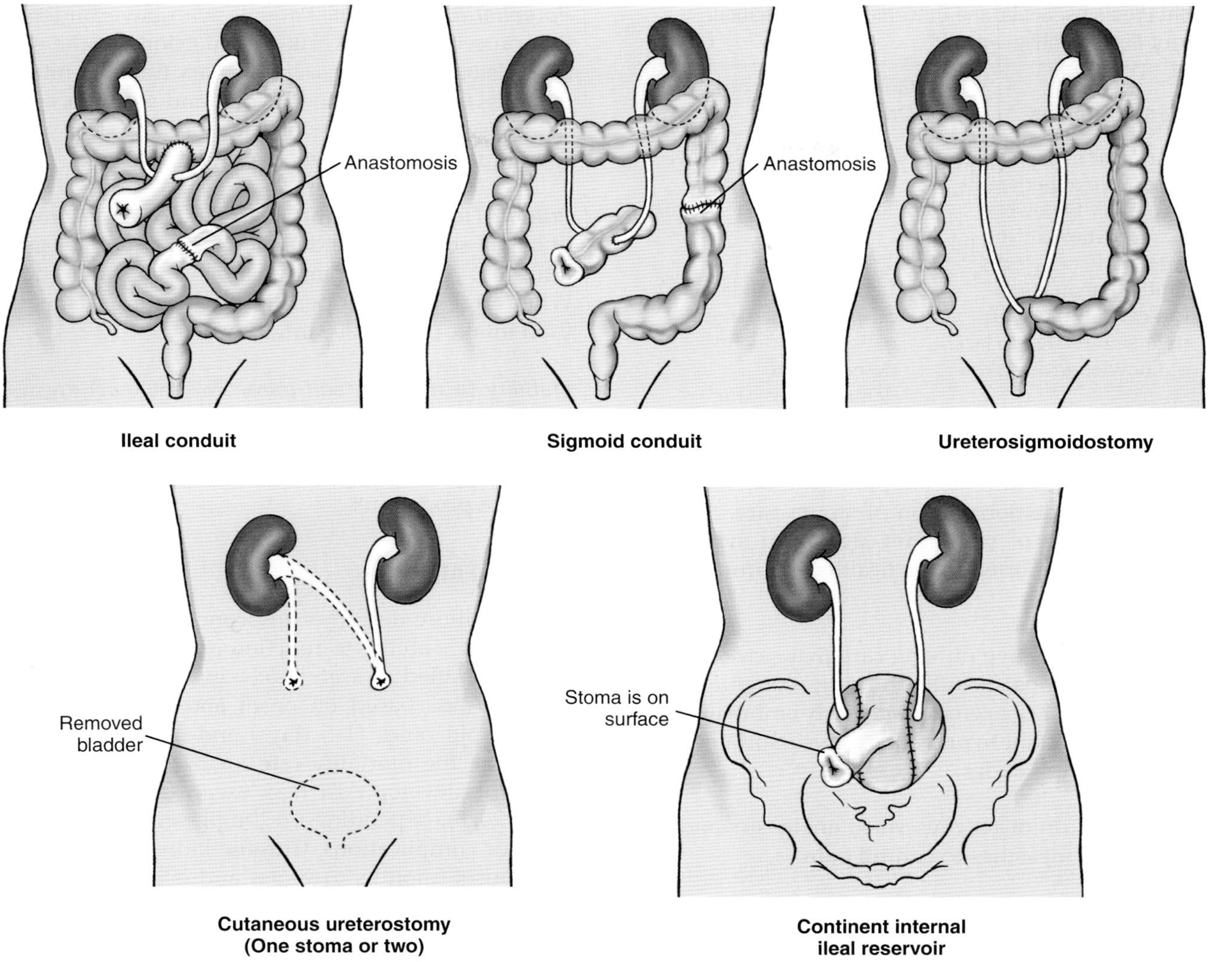

Fig. 42.5 Types of urinary diversion procedures. (From Monahan FD, Drake DT, Neighbors M, editors: *Medical-surgical nursing: foundations for clinical practice*, ed 2, Philadelphia, 1998, Saunders.)

Preoperative care for an ileal or sigmoid conduit includes thorough preparation of the intestinal tract. Bowel preparation requires several days. The patient begins with a low-residue diet, and then a clear-fluid diet. Oral neomycin, an antibiotic that is not absorbed from the intestinal tract, is ordered to reduce bacteria in the bowel. Enemas are also ordered before surgery.

The patient who has received effective preoperative nursing interventions demonstrates reduced fear and effective coping strategies.

Postoperative care. Postoperative assessment includes vital signs, intake and output, patency of tubes, bowel sounds, comfort, and appearance of the drainage, stoma, and wound.

Additional patient problems such as altered body image and lack of knowledge of stoma care are appropriate if the patient has ostomy surgery.

Patient Problems, Goals, and Outcome Criteria: Bladder Surgery, Postoperative

Patient Problems	Goals and Outcome Criteria
Acute pain related to tissue trauma	Pain relief: patient states pain is relieved, reports pain is decreased from prior assessment
Altered urinary elimination related to urinary diversion	Unobstructed urine drainage: urine clear, flows freely, output equal to fluid intake
Disrupted skin integrity related to surgical incision	Well-healed incision: wound margins intact, decreasing redness and swelling
Potential for infection related to tissue trauma	Absence of infection: normal body temperature and white blood cell (WBC) count

Continued

Patient Problems, Goals, and Outcome Criteria: Bladder Surgery, Postoperative—cont'd

Patient Problems	Goals and Outcome Criteria
Potential for injury related to absence of peristalsis secondary to bowel manipulation during surgery	Normal peristalsis: active bowel sounds, soft abdomen
Inability to manage self-care with urinary diversion related to lack of knowledge and skill	Patient understands self-care after discharge: patient accurately describes and demonstrates care

For the patient with urinary diversion, the outcomes of nursing care are adaptation to altered body image, patient demonstration of stoma care, and patient knowledge of significant signs and symptoms that should be reported to the health care provider.

Interventions

Routine postoperative nursing care that serves to prevent complications includes turning, coughing, and deep breathing. Leg exercises and early ambulation are especially important to prevent edema associated with excision of lymph nodes.

Acute pain. Administer prescribed analgesics and use other comfort measures to control pain.

Altered urinary elimination. Inspect urethral and suprapubic catheters and provide wound care as detailed in Chapter 17. Urine should be free of sediment, blood, or casts. Once the catheters are removed, encourage frequent voiding in the patient who has had a segmental resection. Bladder capacity will increase up to 250 to 300 mL over several months.

If a patient has had a radical cystectomy with urinary diversion, inspect the stoma for inflammation and irritation. Details of stoma care are provided in Chapter 18. The patient with a neobladder will have a catheter and a suprapubic drain. Irrigations are ordered to remove mucus. The catheter is left in place for several weeks. Once the catheter is removed, the patient is taught to empty the bladder by relaxing the external sphincter and straining to increase abdominal pressure. The patient is also taught self-catheterization in case the bladder cannot be emptied by voiding.

Disrupted skin integrity. Monitor the surgical incision to ensure that it is healing without increasing redness, swelling, or purulent drainage. Provide wound care as ordered or per agency protocol. Sites of urine drains and the stoma must also receive care to prevent skin irritation and breakdown.

Potential for infection. Patients who have undergone this procedure are at risk for infections in the surgical incisions, drain sites, and urinary tract. Monitor the patient's vital signs, blood work, and wounds, continually assessing for signs of infection. Use strict aseptic technique when providing wound care.

Potential for injury. Withhold oral fluids as ordered until bowel sounds provide evidence that peristalsis has returned. Administer intravenous fluids as ordered. When oral intake is permitted, encourage adequate fluid intake (2500–3000 mL/day).

Inability to manage self-care. Patient teaching must begin in the early postoperative period because the patient needs to learn self-care before discharge. Allow time for the patient or a caregiver to practice self-care procedures.

KIDNEY FAILURE

Kidney failure describes any condition that decreases the kidney's ability to function normally. Kidney failure is classified as *acute kidney injury* (AKI) or *chronic kidney disease* based on onset and reversibility. AKI has a rapid onset (1–7 days) and may be reversible. However, the mortality rate for patients in intensive care who develop AKI may exceed 60% (Lianglos & Jaber, 2020), depending on the presence of other diseases or complications. Chronic kidney disease has a slow onset (months to years) and is characterized by progressive, irreversible damage.

ACUTE KIDNEY INJURY

Causes

Causes of AKI can be prerenal, intrarenal, or postrenal. Prerenal failure results from decreased blood flow to the glomeruli. A systolic BP of 70 mm Hg or greater is necessary to sustain glomerular filtration. If the systolic pressure drops to less than 70 mm Hg and is not corrected, renal failure may develop.

Intrarenal failure may be caused by nephrotoxic drugs, kidney infections, occlusion of intrarenal arteries, hypertension, diabetes mellitus, or direct trauma to the kidney. Antibiotics (particularly the "mycins"), heavy metals (lead and mercury), cleaning compounds, pesticides, and poisonous mushrooms may be toxic to the kidneys. Pyelonephritis, glomerulonephritis, renal tuberculosis, and polycystic kidney disease are examples of kidney conditions that may lead to kidney failure. The arteries in the renal parenchyma may become narrowed as a result of atherosclerosis, hypertension, nephrosclerosis, or blood components (sickled red cells, hemoglobin [Hgb], or myoglobin). Trauma from motor vehicle accidents, contact sports injuries, and other direct blows may also be intrarenal causes of failure.

Postrenal causes of AKI are obstructions beyond the kidneys causing urine to back up into the renal pelvis, resulting in *hydronephrosis*. Ureteral calculi, benign prostatic hypertrophy, prostate cancer, and trauma are the most common causes.

Patients at risk for AKI include those having major surgery, experiencing major trauma, or receiving large doses of nephrotoxic drugs. These patients should have their BP and fluid balance assessed frequently. Older adults are at risk for AKI because they are less able to adapt to alterations in fluid balance or cardiac output. Renal function should always be assessed with any acute condition in the older patient. Early detection and treatment may significantly decrease the risk of death from AKI.

Pharmacology Capsule

Nonsteroidal antiinflammatory drugs and nephrotoxic antibiotics can lead to acute kidney injury (AKI).

Stages of Acute Kidney Injury

The four phases of AKI are (1) onset, (2) oliguric (anuric), (3) diuretic (increased production of urine), and (4) recovery.

Onset phase. The onset phase is short, with a duration between hours to days. It is characterized by increasing BUN and serum creatinine with normal to decreased urine output. The primary treatment goal during this stage is reversal of failing renal function to prevent further damage.

Oliguric (anuric) phase. During the oliguric (anuric) phase, the urine output decreases to 400 mL/day or less. The serum values for BUN, creatinine, potassium, and phosphorus increase. Serum calcium and bicarbonate decrease. The oliguric phase follows the initial stage and continues between 8 and 14 days. Urine specific gravity becomes fixed at 1.010 (normal range: 1.003–1.030), indicating the inability of the tubules to concentrate urine. The patient becomes hypervolemic, meaning that the blood volume is greater than normal. Urine osmolality decreases and serum osmolality increases as waste products are retained.

Diuretic phase. The diuretic phase begins when the cause of AKI is corrected. Urine output exceeds 400 mL/day and may rise above 4 L/day. Despite the production of large quantities of urine, few waste products are excreted and wastes accumulate in the blood. Toward the end of the diuretic stage, the kidneys begin to excrete BUN, creatinine, potassium, and phosphorus and retain calcium and bicarbonate. This is an indication of return of kidney function. It is important to monitor for electrolyte depletion during this phase.

Recovery phase. As renal tissue recovers, serum electrolytes, BUN, and creatinine return to normal, and the glomerular filtration rate returns to 70% to 80% of normal. This recovery stage lasts several months to a year. If complete recovery does not occur, renal insufficiency or chronic renal failure may develop. Renal insufficiency is indicated by loss of approximately 80% of function. It is possible to lead a relatively normal life with renal insufficiency unless other illnesses place an additional burden on kidney function.

Medical Treatment

The primary goal of treatment for AKI is to prevent further damage. Supportive measures, including fluid and dietary restriction, restoration of electrolyte balance, and possible dialysis, are implemented to control symptoms and to prevent complications. Nephrotoxic drugs and drugs that reduce renal blood flow must be avoided. Additional treatment depends on the cause of the failure. For prerenal AKI, BP and blood volume must be restored. Treatment of intrinsic AKI is based on efforts to stimulate urine production with intravenous fluids and with dopamine, furosemide, or both. Postrenal AKI is treated by removal of the cause (typically an obstruction).

Drug therapy. Oliguria is treated with diuretics, most often a loop diuretic such as furosemide (Lasix). Hyperkalemia, which typically accompanies oliguria, is treated aggressively because it can be life threatening. Among the drugs given intravenously to lower serum potassium are glucose and insulin, and calcium gluconate. Sodium polystyrene sulfonate (Kayexalate), given orally or rectally, also lowers serum potassium.

Pharmacology Capsule

Oliguria may be treated with diuretics such as furosemide.

Diet. Dietary modifications for AKI are individualized based on consideration of serum electrolytes and urea. Sodium, potassium, and phosphorus may be restricted. Adequate carbohydrates and fats are provided to prevent the breakdown of fat and protein. Essential amino acid supplements may be ordered. If the patient's nutritional needs are not being met by oral intake, enteral nutritional support is instituted. If the gastrointestinal (GI) tract is not functioning, total parenteral nutrition (TPN) is necessary.

Fluids. Daily fluid calculations will be made by the health care provider based on clinical presentation. Close monitoring is important for any patient receiving fluid replacement to be sure that the patient does not experience volume overload, and that fluid administration sufficiently covers fluid losses.

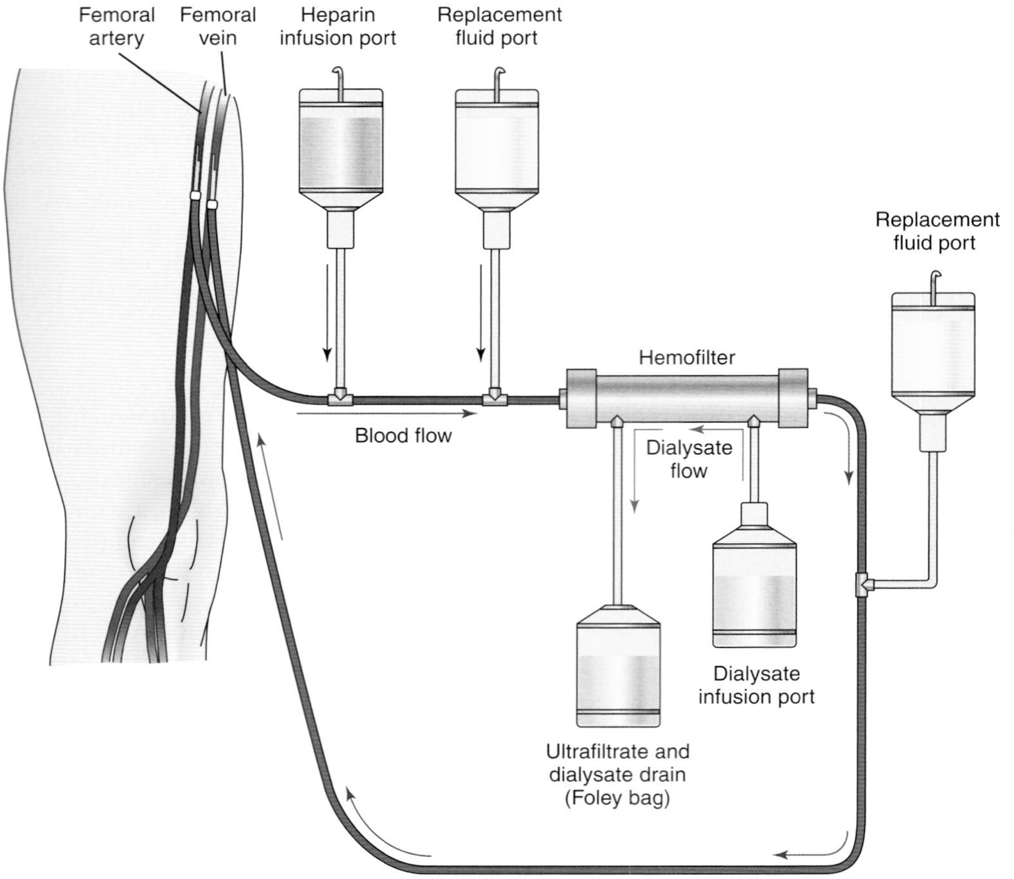

Fig. 42.6 Continuous renal replacement therapy. (From Lewis SM, Heitkemper MM, Dirksen SR: *Medical-surgical nursing: assessment and management of clinical problems*, ed 5, St. Louis, 2000, Mosby.)

Hemodialysis and peritoneal dialysis. **Hemodialysis** may be required if other conservative measures fail to treat hyperkalemia, severe metabolic acidosis, pulmonary edema, and rising BUN. A temporary cannula can be placed in the jugular, femoral, or subclavian vein. Disadvantages of a femoral cannula include that the patient must be immobile between dialysis treatments, and the risk for infection increases. However, if the cannula is removed and replaced repeatedly, a risk of hematoma formation exists. A subclavian cannula can be left in place between treatments but can cause thrombosis, stenosis, pneumothorax, hemothorax, and brachial nerve damage. Per agency policy, only trained dialysis staff should draw blood or administer medications through the temporary cannula. Peritoneal dialysis is also an option, especially for the patient with HF. The section entitled "Chronic Kidney Disease" describes these procedures in more detail.

Continuous renal replacement therapy. Continuous renal replacement therapy (CRRT) offers additional options for treating the patient with AKI. A cannula placed in an artery and a vein (arteriovenous therapy) or two veins (venovenous therapy) is connected to tubing that contains a blood filter and a collection device. The patient's blood flows through the tubing, and excess fluids, electrolytes, and wastes are filtered into the collection device. The blood is then returned to the patient. This procedure does not require dialysate, has little effect on cardiovascular stability, and is continuous. It can be used alone or with hemodialysis (Fig. 42.6).

◆ NURSING CARE OF THE PATIENT WITH ACUTE KIDNEY INJURY

Focused Assessment

Complete assessment of the patient with a urinary disorder is summarized in Chapter 41, Box 41.1. For the patient with AKI, monitoring fluid status is critical. Precise intake and output records must be recorded. Daily weights are an effective means of assessing changes in fluid status (500 mL of fluid weighs approximately 1 lb). Daily weights must be done at the same time each day, using the same scale, and with the patient wearing the same amount of clothing. Because hypervolemia (fluid volume excess) is a major problem during the oliguric phase, assess for signs and symptoms of impending HF: hypertension, bounding pulse, edema, cough, dysrhythmias.

Electrolyte imbalances can include alterations in serum potassium, sodium, calcium, phosphate, and magnesium. Signs and symptoms of each of these imbalances are discussed in Chapter 6. General assessment of electrolyte balance includes cardiac rate and rhythm, neuromuscular status, edema, and mental status. The acutely ill patient must also be monitored for signs and symptoms related to immobility (i.e., pressure injuries, impaired circulation, constipation, atelectasis).

Also determine the patient's understanding of the condition and its treatment. Identify fears, anxiety, coping strategies, and sources of support.

Patient Problems, Goals, and Outcome Criteria: Acute Kidney Injury

Patient Problems	Goals and Outcome Criteria
Fluid volume excess related to impaired kidney function (oliguric stage)	Normal fluid and electrolyte balance: normal tissue turgor, absence of dyspnea, normal serum electrolyte values
Decreased cardiac output and fluid volume deficit related to high-output renal failure (diuretic stage)	Normal cardiac output: pulse and blood pressure (BP) consistent with patient baseline
Anxiety related to life-threatening illness	Decreased anxiety: patient states anxiety is reduced, reports anxiety is lessening
Potential for complications of immobility related to therapeutic restrictions on activity	Absence of complications associated with immobility: intact skin, regular bowel movements without difficulty, breath sounds clear to auscultation
Inability to manage self-care with acute kidney injury related to lack of knowledge of condition and treatment	Patient understands condition, treatment, and self-care: patient accurately describes and participates in self-care as allowed

Interventions

Fluid volume excess. Continually assess and document fluid status. In the oliguric phase, fluid is likely to be restricted. Explain and reinforce fluid restrictions. Measures to help the patient cope with fluid limitations include considering patient preferences in fluid selection and carefully planning fluid intake throughout waking hours. Remember to plan for fluids needed to take medications. When only a few ounces of fluids are allowed at a time, a small juice cup should be used rather than a large glass that is only one-quarter full. This creates an illusion of volume that may make the patient feel less deprived. To obtain patient cooperation, it is essential for the patient and family to understand the importance of adhering to the fluid restriction.

Give diuretics as ordered and monitor the patient for adverse effects. A fluid challenge of normal saline may be rapidly infused while diuretics are given to promote improved renal perfusion.

Decreased cardiac output and fluid volume deficit. During the diuretic phase, patients produce large volumes of dilute urine. Deficient fluid volume becomes a possibility. The heart rate must increase to make up for the diminished blood volume. Because eventually the heart may fail, it is important to monitor for cardiac dysrhythmias, changes in BP, and shortness of breath. Give oral and intravenous fluids as ordered with careful monitoring of output at the same time.

Anxiety. Anxiety is understandable when a vital organ fails. The patient may fear death or chronic illness, with the potential for financial ruin, loss of vitality, and dependence on medical care. Provide honest responses to questions about renal failure and its treatment. Refer specific questions about the patient's prognosis to the health care provider.

The patient with AKI may experience a complete recovery. This may take up to 1 year. Unfortunately, some patients do not recover and progress to chronic kidney disease. These patients need special support to help them learn to accept and deal with this major health deviation.

Potential for complications of immobility. The patient with AKI is very ill and may be immobilized. Prevent complications of immobility by providing skin care, turning, coughing, deep breathing, leg exercises, and measures to promote bowel elimination. Care of the immobilized patient is described in Chapter 12.

Inability to manage self-care. When the patient is acutely ill, provide basic information about the disease, diagnostic tests and procedures, and treatments. Explain the reasons for interventions, such as fluid restrictions, turning, deep breathing, and leg exercises. As the patient improves, patient teaching should include management of fluids, diet, drug therapy, activity, and signs and symptoms that should be reported to the health care provider (i.e., dyspnea, edema, fever).

CHRONIC KIDNEY DISEASE

Chronic kidney disease is characterized by progressive destruction of the nephrons of both kidneys that results in elevated urine albumin and decreased GFR for 3 or more months. The severity is described in stages, with the final stage (stage 5) being ESRD. The healthy kidneys comprise far more nephrons than needed. Therefore a person can lose about 80% of the nephrons before kidney function becomes impaired. Creatinine clearance is an important measure of renal function. When it falls below 15 mL/min, dialysis or transplantation becomes necessary.

Chronic kidney disease is characterized by azotemia (i.e., increased nitrogenous waste products in the blood). *Uremia* is the term used for the symptoms that develop when the condition advances to the point of ESRD, when the kidneys are unable to maintain fluid and electrolyte or acid-base balance. Uremic symptoms may include nausea, vomiting, anorexia, peripheral neuropathy, and central nervous system abnormalities. All of the causes of AKI listed earlier may lead to chronic kidney disease. In addition, chronic renal infections may predispose the patient to progressive renal failure. However, the most common causes are hypertension, diabetes mellitus, and atherosclerosis.

Clinical Manifestations

Azotemia. The first function lost in chronic kidney disease is the ability to concentrate urine. This results in an increase of waste products in the blood, despite producing large amounts of dilute urine. As the disease progresses, urine output typically declines until very little to no urine is produced.

BUN is an approximate estimate of the glomerular filtration rate (GFR). It is affected by protein breakdown. Normal BUN ranges from 10 to 20 mg/dL, although it may be a bit higher in older adult patients (Pagana et al., 2017). When BUN reaches or exceeds 70 mg/dL, dialysis is needed to reduce it.

Serum creatinine is a waste product of skeletal muscle breakdown. It is a more reliable measure of kidney function than BUN. It is not affected by diet, hydration, hepatic function, or metabolism. Normal serum creatinine is 0.5 to 1.1 mg/dL in female patients, and 0.6 to 1.2 mg/dL in male patients (Pagana et al., 2017). A serum creatinine level that is twice the normal level reflects a 50% loss of function. When the value reaches or exceeds 10 times normal, 90% of function has been lost. The kidneys are able to adapt to a loss of up to 80% of function. The kidneys increase in size to maintain function.

Creatinine clearance (a urine test) is the best indicator of renal function. This requires collection of all urine in a 12- or 24-hour period. Normal creatinine clearance is 107 to 139 mL/min in males, and 87 to 107 mL/min in females (Pagana et al., 2017).

Insulin resistance. In renal failure, cells become resistant to the action of insulin. As a result, blood insulin and glucose levels rise. Hyperinsulinemia (high blood insulin) stimulates the liver to produce triglycerides. Patients with chronic kidney disease have high serum levels of very-low-density lipoproteins (VLDLs). Elevated lipids in the blood contribute to atherosclerosis.

Electrolyte and Acid-Base Imbalances

Hyperkalemia. The primary means of potassium excretion is through the kidneys. As kidney function fails, potassium is retained, which results in hyperkalemia, the most life-threatening effect of renal failure. The normal range for serum potassium is 3.5 to 5.0 mEq/L (Pagana et al., 2017). Elevated serum potassium interferes with normal cardiac function, causing cardiac dysrhythmias. Dysrhythmias are potentially fatal. The patient becomes apathetic and confused and may have nausea, abdominal cramps, muscle weakness, and numbness of the extremities. Serum potassium greater than 6 mg/dL requires cardiac monitoring. If the serum potassium is not reduced, bradycardia (pulse ≤50 beats per minute) or asystole (no heartbeat) may develop.

Hyperkalemia is treated with intravenous glucose and insulin or intravenous 10% calcium gluconate. These drugs drive potassium back into the cells, reducing the serum potassium level. They are used as temporary emergency measures. Kayexalate, given orally or rectally, causes potassium to be drawn into the bowel and eliminated in the feces. The method used most often to reduce elevated serum potassium is dialysis.

Hypocalcemia. Diseased kidney tissue lacks the enzyme that activates vitamin D. Without active vitamin D, calcium absorption from the bowel decreases. The body tries to compensate by shifting calcium from the bones to the blood. Serum phosphate binds with calcium, further depleting calcium levels. The normal total serum calcium level is 9 to 10.5 mg/dL, and the normal ionized calcium is 4.5 to 5.6 mEq/L (Pagana et al., 2017). Abnormally low serum calcium is called *hypocalcemia*. Patients with hypocalcemia experience tingling sensations, muscle twitches, irritability, and tetany. Tetany is sustained, painful muscle contraction. Hypocalcemia is treated with calcium supplements, active vitamin D, and phosphate binders. Phosphate binders include calcium carbonate, calcium acetate, or sevelamer (Renagel). Side effects of phosphate binders include hypophosphatemia and constipation. Antacids with aluminum or magnesium, such as milk of magnesia, magnesium carbonate, magnesium oxide, and magnesium trisilicate, should be avoided.

Metabolic acidosis. Failure of the renal tubules to excrete acid ions and acid waste products causes the body's acid level to rise. Decreased bicarbonate reabsorption renders the body unable to neutralize the excess acid. Excess acid leads to metabolic acidosis. The lungs attempt to compensate by eliminating more carbon dioxide (CO_2) through hyperventilation. Symptoms associated with metabolic acidosis include headache, lethargy, and delirium.

Fluid balance. Most patients with chronic kidney disease retain sodium and water, causing hypernatremia and hypervolemia. Elevated BP and edema are signs of hypervolemia. HF may develop in the hypervolemic patient because the patient's heart cannot handle the high fluid volume. Prevention and treatment of hypervolemia include fluid restriction, diuretics, and dialysis if necessary. Some patients lose excess sodium and water in the urine and become hyponatremic and hypovolemic.

Hematologic System

Anemia. Kidneys of patients with chronic kidney disease produce less erythropoietin, a hormone necessary for RBC production. Even the RBCs that are produced have a shorter life span than usual because of the toxic environment in which they live. Therefore, patients with chronic kidney disease have anemia. Iron supplements and folic acid may be ordered. Transfusions may be required if the hematocrit (Hct) drops below 20%. Normal Hct values are 37% to 47% for women and 42% to 52% for men (Pagana et al., 2017). A genetically engineered erythropoietin (epoetin alfa) can be administered intravenously after hemodialysis or subcutaneously for patients on peritoneal dialysis. This product improves RBC formation and has reversed anemia and the need for transfusions in some patients with chronic kidney disease.

Infection. Because the inflammatory response diminishes with chronic kidney disease, fewer WBCs gather at the site of an infection or injury. The general immune response is suppressed, and antibody production declines. Therefore, the patient has a reduced ability to resist infections.

Cardiovascular system. The cardiovascular system is affected by hypervolemia, hyperkalemia, and hypocalcemia. Hypervolemia increases the workload of the heart, possibly leading to HF. Symptoms of HF include moist breath sounds, bounding pulse, dependent edema, and dyspnea. Dysrhythmias may be caused by hyperkalemia or hypocalcemia.

Neurologic system. Neurologic effects of chronic kidney disease are mental status changes (i.e., lethargy, irritability, confusion) and peripheral neuropathy. Peripheral neuropathy may be evident initially as a restless feeling and later as foot drop, loss of feeling in the legs, or paralysis of the legs. Some health care providers may consider the development of peripheral neuropathy as a sign to begin dialysis.

Disequilibrium syndrome may occur with hemodialysis. The rapid removal of urea from the blood leaves an increased concentration of solutes in the brain and the cerebrospinal fluid (CSF). The solutes increase the osmotic pressure, which draws fluid from the bloodstream into the CSF and brain tissue. Confusion, lethargy, headache, nausea, and vomiting may progress to coma or seizures if not treated. Disequilibrium is corrected with the administration of hypertonic glucose.

Integumentary system. The integumentary system is also affected by the accumulation of waste products. Calcium phosphate crystals and urea accumulate in the skin, causing itching. Dryness results from decreased oil gland production and decreased perspiration. Skin may appear to be yellow or pale grey as a result of anemia and from unexcreted bilirubin and uremic pigments. Hair and nails become dry and brittle. **Uremic frost** is the term used when whitish crystals composed of urea and other salts precipitate on the skin and around the mouth. It is a very late sign in chronic kidney disease.

Gastrointestinal system. Ammonia is a breakdown product of urea. When ammonia accumulates in the GI tract, it causes irritation, nausea, vomiting, a metallic taste in the mouth, and bleeding. Antacids administered every 2 hours help to relieve the irritation. A diet high in carbohydrates and low in protein is prescribed to reduce the accumulation of urea. Other common GI disturbances with chronic kidney disease include stomatitis (i.e., inflammation of the mouth), anorexia, nausea, vomiting, constipation, and diarrhea.

Musculoskeletal system. Renal osteodystrophy, the skeletal changes characteristic of chronic kidney disease, includes: (1) metastatic calcification, (2) bone demineralization, and (3) osteitis fibrosa. Metastatic calcification is deposition of calcium phosphate complexes in blood vessels and in joints, lungs, muscles, and eyes. Deposits in blood vessels can impair blood flow so severely that fingers and toes may become gangrenous. Bone demineralization is directly related to hypocalcemia. Low serum calcium triggers increased production of parathyroid hormone by the parathyroid glands. Parathyroid hormone mobilizes calcium from the bone and shifts it into the blood. Over time, loss of bone mass can be significant. When calcium is lost from bones, it is replaced with fibrous tissue, a condition known as **osteitis fibrosa**.

Reproductive system. Chronic kidney disease affects the male and female reproductive systems. The production of sex hormones declines and libido is diminished. Ovulation and menstruation usually cease in women. Men may have low sperm counts and erectile dysfunction. The general effects of a chronic illness may also affect sexual desire and function.

Endocrine function. Patients with chronic kidney disease usually appear hypothyroid. Hyperparathyroidism occurs in response to the chronically low serum calcium and high serum phosphates. Patients with diabetes require less exogenous insulin because the enzyme that normally breaks down insulin (renal insulinase) is reduced. Oral hypoglycemics also place the patient at risk for hypoglycemia because the drugs are normally excreted by the kidneys.

Emotional and psychologic effects. Emotional and psychologic effects of chronic kidney disease include emotional lability, depression, anxiety, and slowed intellectual functioning.

Medical Treatment

Treatment of chronic kidney disease promotes elimination of wastes, maintenance of fluid balance, and

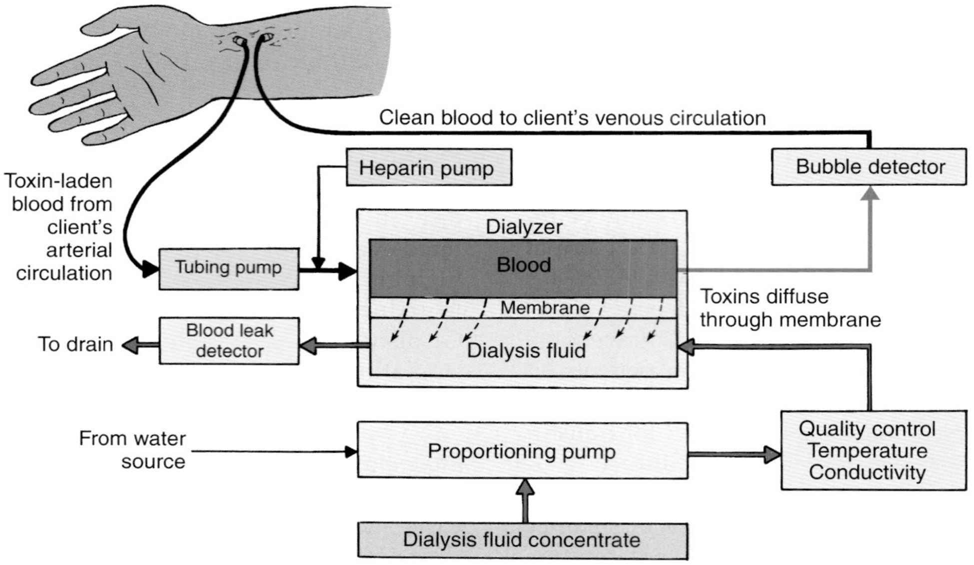

Fig. 42.7 Schematic diagram of hemodialysis. As the patient's blood passes through the dialyzer, toxins diffuse into the dialysis fluid. (From Black JM, Hawks JH: *Medical-surgical nursing: clinical management for positive outcomes*, ed 8, St. Louis, 2009, Saunders.)

management of the systemic effects of the disease. Conservative treatment of the systemic effects of chronic kidney disease includes:

- Intravenous glucose and insulin, calcium salt (e.g., carbonate; oral or rectal sodium polystyrene sulfonate to treat hyperkalemia
- Statins in the early stages of renal failure to decrease the risk of cardiovascular complications
- Calcium, active vitamin D, and phosphate binders to treat hypocalcemia
- Fluid and sodium restriction to treat hypervolemia
- Diuretics, angiotensin-converting enzyme (ACE) inhibitors, angiotensin-receptor blockers (ARBs), and calcium channel blockers to treat hypertension
- Water-soluble vitamins to replace those lost in dialysis
- Iron supplements, folic acid, and synthetic erythropoietin to treat anemia
- Hypertonic glucose to treat disequilibrium syndrome
- Diet tailored to chronic kidney disease stage and type of dialysis treatment

Kidney replacement therapy. When kidney failure can no longer be managed conservatively, dialysis is required to sustain life. Dialysis is the passage of molecules through a semipermeable membrane into a special solution called *dialysate solution*. Dialysis operates like the kidney. Small molecules such as urea, creatinine, and electrolytes pass out of the blood, across a membrane, and into a solution.

The goals of dialysis include:

- Remove the end products of protein metabolism from the blood
- Maintain safe concentrations of serum electrolytes
- Correct acidosis and replenish the body's bicarbonate buffer system
- Remove excess fluid from the blood

Dialysis enables many patients to maintain or regain self-esteem and to feel productive. Others may feel depressed because of the frequency with which dialysis takes place. Two primary means of dialysis are (1) hemodialysis and (2) peritoneal dialysis.

Hemodialysis. Hemodialysis is a process by which blood is removed from the body and circulated through an "artificial kidney" for removal of excess fluid, electrolytes, and wastes. The dialyzed blood is then returned to the patient (Fig. 42.7). Hemodialysis requires vascular access (i.e., access to the patient's bloodstream). This may be accomplished by catheter, cannula, graft, or fistula. Subclavian or femoral catheters can be used for temporary access for dialysis during AKI while a graft or fistula matures (dilates and toughens), or for patients on peritoneal dialysis who need immediate access for hemodialysis.

Internal connections between veins and arteries do not require dressings. An internal connection between the patient's artery and vein is called a *fistula*. A fistula requires approximately 6 to 8 weeks to mature and may be used for 3 to 5 years. Connections may also be made using bovine or synthetic grafts that require 2 to 4 weeks to heal before use and last for 7 to 9 years. Grafts have an increased rate of thrombosis and infection compared with fistulas.

An arteriovenous shunt or cannula is an external connection between an artery and a vein (Fig. 42.8). By connecting the external ends of the synthetic tubing

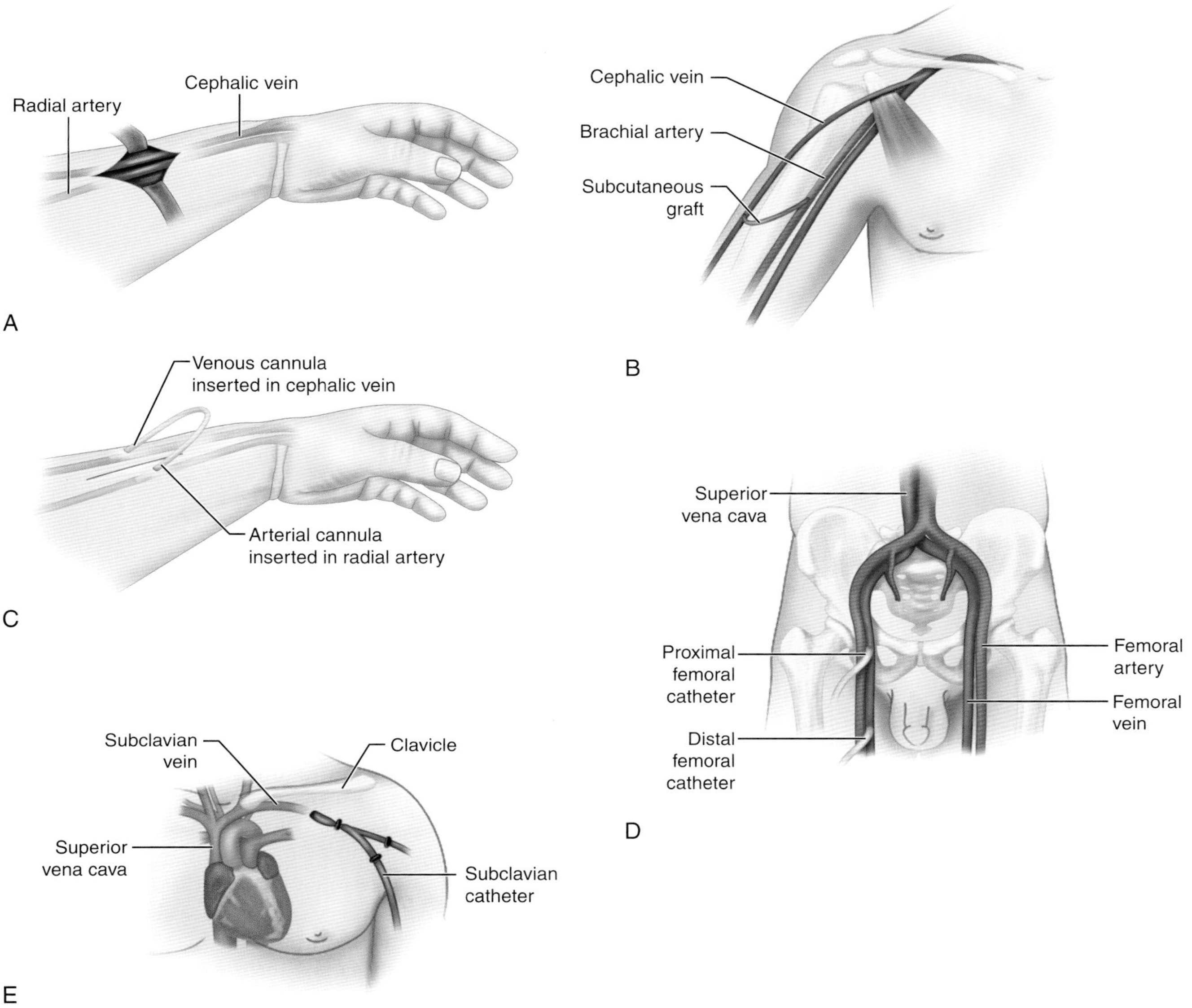

Fig. 42.8 Frequently used means for gaining vascular access for hemodialysis include arteriovenous fistula (A), arteriovenous graft (B), external arteriovenous shunt (C), femoral vein catheterization (D), and subclavian vein catheterization (E). (A) and (B) are options for long-term vascular access for hemodialysis. (C), (D), and (E) are used for short-term access for intermittent hemodialysis or for continuous renal replacement therapy in acute care. (From Ignatavicius DD, Workman ML, Rebar CR, Heimgartner NM: *Medical-surgical nursing: concepts for interprofessional collaborative care*, ed 10, St. Louis, 2021, Elsevier.)

for dialysis, venipuncture is not necessary. However, because the cannula is external, danger of hemorrhage, risk of skin breakdown, restriction of activities, and risk of site infection exist. The arteriovenous shunt is very rarely used because of the potential complications.

All vascular access sites must be assessed for patency. Check pulses below the shunt to ensure that circulation is adequate. Steal syndrome occurs when too much arterial blood is diverted from the extremity by the access device. Palpate the venous side of the shunt for a thrill or rippling sensation caused by movement of blood through a changed pathway. A bruit or swoosh may be heard through a stethoscope with each heartbeat. Absence of these signs may indicate occlusion of the vessel, making it unsuitable for hemodialysis.

Once vascular access is established, the patient may be hemodialyzed. Blood flows from the artery through the vascular access device, circulates through the dialyzer, and returns through the venous line. Heparin is used as an anticoagulant to prevent blood from clotting. Hemodialysis requires specially trained personnel and specialized equipment. Although dialysis for chronic kidney disease is usually performed in a dialysis center, home dialysis is available. The hemodialysis process takes approximately 4 hours and is usually done 3 times weekly.

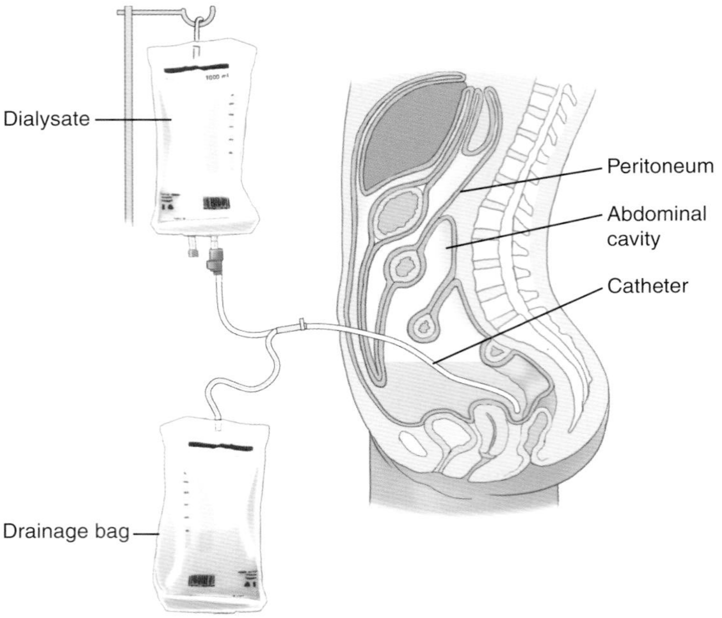

Fig. 42.9 Peritoneal dialysis. (From Shiland BJ: *Medical terminology & anatomy for coding*, ed 3, St. Louis, 2018, Elsevier.)

Advantages of hemodialysis include its usefulness in emergencies and the rapid removal of wastes, electrolytes, and fluid. Disadvantages include the need for vascular access, the use of an anticoagulant, and the potential for hemorrhage, anemia, rapid fluid and electrolyte shifts (dialysis disequilibrium syndrome), muscle cramps, nausea and vomiting, and air emboli.

Complications of hemodialysis include atherosclerotic cardiovascular disease, anemia, gastric ulcers, disturbed calcium metabolism, and hepatitis. The leading causes of death for patients being treated with hemodialysis are related to cardiovascular disease, infection, and dialysis withdrawal (Mailloux & Heinrich, 2017). The care of patients during hemodialysis is beyond the scope of this text. Nurses who work in this field require specialized training.

Peritoneal dialysis. Peritoneal dialysis uses the patient's own peritoneum as a semipermeable dialyzing membrane. A catheter is inserted through the abdominal wall and anchored with cuffs. Dialysis fluid is instilled into the peritoneal cavity through the catheter; waste products are drawn into the fluid, which is then drained from the peritoneal cavity (Fig. 42.9).

Peritoneal dialysis may be done temporarily or on a permanent basis. For temporary use, a catheter is inserted in the peritoneal cavity through the abdominal wall. For long-term use, a catheter is implanted in the peritoneal cavity. Over time, a fibrous tissue barrier forms at the insertion site and provides some protection against infection. After the catheter insertion site is healed, patients can shower and care for the site as directed by the health care provider.

Advantages of peritoneal dialysis over hemodialysis include less anemia, reduced cost of equipment, fewer dietary and fluid restrictions, independence, and closer resemblance to normal kidney function. It can also be initiated in almost any hospital. Disadvantages include the risk of peritonitis (the major complication) and catheter site infection, hyperglycemia, elevated serum lipids, and body image disturbance. In addition, peritoneal dialysis cannot be used for patients with recent abdominal surgery, extensive abdominal trauma, or open abdominal wounds.

Peritoneal dialysis has three phases: (1) inflow, (2) dwell, and (3) drain. The three phases comprise one exchange. During inflow, fluid (commonly 2 L) is allowed to drain into the peritoneal cavity through an established catheter over about 10 minutes. During the dwell time, fluid remains in the cavity for a specified period of time while ultrafiltration, osmosis, and diffusion occur. The fluid bearing wastes and excess water is then drained from the cavity over 20 to 30 minutes.

Continuous ambulatory peritoneal dialysis (CAPD) allows the patient freedom from a machine and the independence to perform dialysis alone. The exchange process is usually repeated 4 times each day by outpatients. It may be done more often in patients who are acutely ill and hospitalized. Strict aseptic technique must be used with the initiation of the process and with each exchange. The patient or a reliable caregiver must be taught the process by someone who understands it well.

Continuous cycling peritoneal dialysis uses a device called a *cycler* to perform the automated peritoneal dialysis (APD) during the night. This allows the patient freedom during the day. It also reduces the risk of infection because the system is interrupted less often. Several variations of this procedure exist that may be done from 5 to 7 times a week and may or may not leave the fluid in the abdomen during the waking hours.

Peritonitis (i.e., infection of the peritoneum) is the most serious complication of peritoneal dialysis. Infections may also develop at the catheter exit site and tunnel where the catheter is placed under the skin. Cloudiness and particles in the fluid in the outflow container are evidence of infection. Redness, swelling, and purulent drainage are signs of infection at the exit site. Immediately report any signs of infection to the health care provider. Peritonitis is usually treated with antibiotics administered through the peritoneal catheter. Other complications include bleeding, abdominal pain, hernias, low back pain, respiratory distress, and decreased serum albumin. Encapsulating sclerosing peritonitis is a condition in which a thick membrane develops around the bowel. The thickened membrane can obstruct the intestines and interfere with ultrafiltration.

NURSING CARE OF THE PATIENT WITH CHRONIC KIDNEY DISEASE

Focused Assessment

General assessment of the patient with a urologic disorder is outlined in Chapter 41, Box 41.1. For the patient with chronic kidney disease, frequent monitoring for changes in status is especially important. Fluid balance is evaluated closely. During hospitalization, strict intake and output records must be kept. Be alert for signs and symptoms of excess fluid volume that can lead to cardiac failure, such as increasing edema, dyspnea, tachycardia, bounding pulse, and rising BP.

Serum electrolytes are measured frequently, but you must still be alert for signs and symptoms of electrolyte imbalances such as hyperkalemia and hypocalcemia, and metabolic acidosis. Hyponatremia and hypovolemia are less common. Assessment of fluid and electrolyte imbalances includes monitoring pulse and respirations, BP, mental status, and neuromuscular activity.

Data related to nutrition includes appetite, usual daily intake, weight gain or loss pattern, and prescribed diet. Determine how well the patient understands and follows the prescribed diet (see the Nutrition Considerations box).

Carefully observe mental and emotional status. Increasing confusion or loss of consciousness can be caused by accumulated toxins or electrolyte imbalances. Emotional responses to a diagnosis of chronic kidney disease vary. Determine the patient's perceptions of the situation and identify usual coping strategies. Anxiety, fear, disturbed body image, depression, and lowered self-esteem are common.

The long-term effects of chronic kidney disease and its treatment put the patient at risk for many complications. Monitor bowel elimination for constipation or diarrhea. Monitor for signs and symptoms of local or systemic infections (redness, swelling, foul drainage, fever, increased WBC count). Inspect the skin for bruising, bleeding, or trauma. Evaluate sensation in the extremities. Ask if sexual dysfunction has been a problem, and obtain a description of the problem.

Explore patient understanding about chronic kidney disease, its treatment, and self-care measures. Document the patient's ability to perform ADL.

Specific patient problems and goals vary based on the individual patient data. Many diagnoses and interventions discussed in the section entitled "Acute Kidney Injury" also apply to the patient with chronic kidney disease. The emphasis in this section is on the common problems experienced by the patient with chronic renal failure.

Patient Problems, Goals, and Outcome Criteria: Chronic Kidney Disease

Patient Problems	Goals and Outcome Criteria
Fluid volume excess related to fluid retention because of kidney dysfunction	Reduced fluid volume and absence of symptoms of heart failure: normal tissue turgor, blood pressure (BP) at patient baseline, no dyspnea
Inadequate nutrition related to anorexia, nausea, vomiting, stomatitis, dietary restrictions	Adequate nutrition: consumption of prescribed diet, serum albumin and total protein within acceptable limits
Potential for acute confusion related to effects of uremia on the nervous system	Normal cognitive function: alert and oriented
Inadequate coping related to multiple life changes	Effective coping: patient uses healthy coping strategies that decrease anxiety without compromising care
Low self-esteem related to change in appearance, loss of kidney function, venous access devices, inability to fulfill usual roles and responsibilities	Improved self-esteem: positive statements of confidence
Potential for infection related to impaired immune response, malnutrition, break in skin integrity	Absence of infection: normal body temperature and white blood cell (WBC) count
Potential for injury related to coagulation disorder, impaired wound healing, bone demineralization, peripheral neuropathy	Absence of injury: no bruises, bleeding, fractures

Continued

Patient Problems, Goals, and Outcome Criteria: Chronic Kidney Disease—cont'd

Patient Problems	Goals and Outcome Criteria
Constipation related to inactivity, drug side effects, fluid restriction, electrolyte imbalances	Normal bowel elimination: regular formed stools passed without straining
Diarrhea related to electrolyte imbalances, drug side effects	Normal bowel elimination: formed stools
Impaired sexual function related to fatigue, drug side effects, hormone deficiencies, altered self-image	Satisfactory sexual function: patient states intimate relationship is satisfactory
Inability to manage self-care related to lack of knowledge, confusion, anemia, fatigue	Accomplishment of self-care: patient performs activities of daily living (ADL) within limitations imposed by renal failure and treatments

Interventions

Fluid volume excess. As renal failure progresses, the patient's ability to excrete excess fluids continually declines. In the early stages, diuretics may be used to treat fluid retention, but they are not used once dialysis is begun. Fluid intake may be restricted. If intravenous fluids are ordered, closely monitor the rate of infusion. Antihypertensive drugs may be needed to control BP, and digoxin may be given to support cardiac function. Dosage adjustments are often needed because kidney failure affects the ability to excrete these drugs. Administer medications, monitor for side effects, and teach the patient how to take them after discharge and what adverse effects to report.

Patients with fluid volume excess require comfort and safety measures. Edematous legs are injured easily and heal slowly. Protect them from pressure or trauma. If cardiac failure and dyspnea develop, position the patient with the head elevated to ease breathing. Cerebral edema causes confusion and decreasing consciousness. Implement safety measures to protect the confused or semiconscious patient from injury.

Pharmacology Capsule

Because most drugs are excreted in the urine, people with impaired renal function are at risk for drug toxicity.

Inadequate nutrition. Maintaining adequate nutrition can be a challenge for the patient with chronic kidney disease. Anorexia, nausea, vomiting, and stomatitis interfere with food intake. Restrictions in sodium, potassium, protein, and sometimes fat can make the diet less appealing. Measures to encourage food intake include frequent mouth care and small feedings. Explain the importance of good nutrition to the patient and family. The person who prepares the patient's food at home should be included in dietary instructions. Vitamin supplements are routinely ordered because of dietary restrictions. Monitor weight to evaluate both fluid and nutritional status. Teach the patient and the caregivers about medications and status monitors. The dietitian can help the patient learn to cope with the diet.

Nutrition Considerations

1. Renal failure results in an inability of the kidneys to excrete wastes and maintain fluid and electrolyte balance.
2. The nutritional goal is to modify the diet so that the work of the kidneys is reduced.
3. Fluid intake may be restricted to 1000 to 1500 mL/day for patients with renal disease.
4. Sodium and potassium intakes are restricted (including medications) to maintain electrolyte balance in patients who require dialysis.
5. Protein is restricted in patients with renal disease; any protein ingested should be high in essential amino acids. Examples of these proteins include eggs, meat, poultry, fish, and milk products.
6. People with renal calculi should increase fluid intake to maintain at least 2 L of urine output daily and should avoid foods that lead to the formation of calculi.
7. Remember that people with low serum calcium are at increased risk for formation of calculi.

Potential for acute confusion. Renal failure affects the central nervous system (CNS) and the peripheral nervous systems. Cerebral edema and elevated metabolic wastes in the blood can cause confusion, slowed thought processes, lethargy, and loss of consciousness. Protect confused patients and orient them to person, place, and time. Present information simply and repeat as needed. Avoid sensory overload by reducing environmental stimuli and demands on the patient. For safety reasons, assign the patient to a room close to the nurses' station. Put the bed in the low position, and keep the call bell within reach.

The effects of renal disease on the peripheral nerves can lead to loss of sensation in the extremities (peripheral neuropathy). These patients are at risk for injury. Inspect the affected areas daily for any signs of injury. Pressure, ill-fitting shoes, or external heat or cold can cause serious injury before the patient is aware of it. Teach the patient about peripheral neuropathy and how to prevent injuries.

Ineffective coping. Patients with chronic kidney disease often experience anxiety and fear. They face life-threatening illness, endure invasive treatments and procedures, and undergo radical changes in lifestyle. Explore the patient's coping strategies and identify factors that interfere with adjustment to renal disease. It helps for the patient to have a regular primary nurse so that a therapeutic relationship can develop. You can help by talking to patients and having them focus on the sources of their distress. It is important to be accepting of the patient's thoughts and feelings. Do not give false reassurance or tell patients not to worry. Explain routines and procedures and provide practical teaching on the management of everyday problems. Many patients benefit from talking to a mental health professional or attending support groups for people with similar problems. While encouraging patients to adjust to treatment, respect their rights to be informed and to refuse treatment if they so choose.

People on dialysis typically go through stages of adjustment. When dialysis is first started, they usually feel much better. They may feel encouraged and view dialysis positively. This might be described as a "honeymoon period." At this stage, the patient is most receptive to teaching. Use this opportunity to educate the patient.

After several months of treatment, patients may tire of the routine. Depression and disappointment are common. Some cope by denying the need for treatment. They may omit medications or fail to keep appointments for follow-up. Be accepting of the patient but not the behavior at this stage. Confront the patient when ineffective coping behaviors are identified.

Eventually, most patients accept the need for ongoing treatment. They may try to resume their former levels of activity. Use this opportunity to guide the patient in realistic goal setting.

Low self-esteem. The patient's self-esteem may suffer because of changes in body image and role performance. Encourage patients to talk about the changes they are experiencing and what those changes mean to them. Therapeutic communication and touch convey acceptance to patients. Help the patient with grooming to enhance appearance if they desire.

Encourage patients to examine their daily routines and look for ways to conserve time and energy. Sources of help and support need to be identified (see the Complementary and Alternative Therapies box). Family functions may have to be redistributed. It is important for the patient to continue to have roles in the family and to be seen as a contributing family member.

Complementary and Alternative Therapies

Patients with irreversible chronic diseases are vulnerable to claims of miracle cures. Caution patients to discuss alternative therapies with the health care provider to prevent potentially harmful outcomes.

Potential for infection. Patients with chronic kidney disease must avoid exposure to others with infections. Be sure that they know how to take their own temperatures. Instruct them to report fever or other signs of infection to the health care provider. Practice good hand washing and aseptic technique for invasive procedures.

Potential for injury. The patient is susceptible to injury because of impaired coagulation and wound healing, bone demineralization, and peripheral neuropathy. Calcium, vitamin D, and phosphate binders are ordered to reduce loss of calcium from the bones. Encourage ambulation, which helps to strengthen bones. Assess and protect body parts that lack sensation. Provide an environment with adequate support equipment and remove obstacles that might cause bruises or falls.

Constipation. Constipation is a common problem with chronic kidney disease because of inactivity, fluid restriction, electrolyte imbalances, and drug side effects. Encourage activity within the patient's tolerance level. Stool softeners are often ordered to prevent constipation.

Diarrhea. Diarrhea may be caused by drugs or anxiety. Measure liquid stools and record this as fluid output. Give antidiarrheals as ordered. Provide perianal care after each stool.

Impaired sexual function. Sexual dysfunction is attributed to physical and emotional causes. Remind patients that it is acceptable to express concerns related to intimacy. Explain how kidney disease affects sexual function and explore what this means to the patient. Alternative means of sexual expression may enable the patient to continue to feel loved and to maintain intimacy. Referral to a counselor who specializes in treatment of sexual dysfunction may be appreciated.

Inability to manage self-care. Patients with chronic kidney disease spend more time at home than they do in the hospital. Nurses need to prepare them for self-care.

RENAL TRANSPLANTATION

KIDNEY DONATION

In 2020, 22,817 kidney transplants were done in the United States (United Network for Organ Sharing [UNOS], 2021). A healthy kidney may be obtained from a live donor (usually a relative) or from a cadaver. The tissues of the donor and the recipient must match or the recipient will reject the new kidney. Matching is based on ABO blood groups and human leukocyte antigens. Crossmatching between the blood of the prospective donor and recipient reveals any cytotoxic preformed antibodies that would certainly result in organ rejection. A national network maintains lists of people awaiting donor kidneys. When a cadaver kidney is available, the network tries to locate the best match for the kidney to improve the chances of success.

Kidney donors must be at least 18 years of age, be in good physical and mental health, be free of systemic disease (such as hypertension, diabetes, cancer, and other organ-specific diseases) or infection (such as hepatitis and human immunodeficiency [HIV]), have no history of renal disease, and have normal renal function (United Network for Organ Sharing, 2017).

Cadavers must meet the same criteria as living donors. Many people carry signed donor cards indicating their willingness to have organs used for transplantation in the event of brain death. If brain death does occur, written permission is still sought from the family of the potential donor before organs are removed. The vital organs of the person who experienced brain death must be kept functioning until the kidney is removed.

PREOPERATIVE NURSING CARE OF THE RENAL TRANSPLANT RECIPIENT

Preoperative care of the renal transplant recipient is similar to that of any other patient facing major surgery (see Chapter 17). The patient must be prepared mentally and physically for the procedure. The unique aspect of this situation is that the patient awaits an organ from another human being. If a relative is the donor, the surgery can be planned and both people prepared emotionally. Counseling is advised for both the donor and the recipient. The patient may be ambivalent about receiving a relative's organ. The gift of a kidney can restore health, but the recipient may feel guilty about asking a loved one to endure surgery and to give up an organ. The donor faces the stress of surgery and a future with only one kidney. The donor also has to accept that the kidney could be rejected. Both recipient and donor face the threat of surgical complications.

If awaiting a cadaver kidney, the patient must face the idea that someone must die for a kidney to become available. These potential recipients are on call and must be ready to report to the hospital at any time.

Preoperatively, the recipient and the live donor have complete diagnostic workups to rule out other medical problems and to evaluate the function of the urinary tract. Normal function of both donor's kidneys must be affirmed. The recipient is given medications to bring BP within normal limits. Immunosuppressant drugs are started to control the body's response to foreign tissue (i.e., the donated kidney; see Chapter 41, Table 41.4). The recipient may also be given a transfusion of the donor's blood, a measure that has been found to reduce rejection. If the recipient has severe hypertension or a UTI, bilateral nephrectomies may be done before transplantation. The patient is dialyzed shortly before transplantation.

Focused Assessment

In the preoperative period, a complete assessment is done as outlined in Chapter 17. Before renal transplantation, explore the patient's understanding of the surgery. Document baseline vital signs. Identify any specific fears or questions that need to be addressed.

Patient Problems, Goals, and Outcome Criteria: Renal Transplantation, Preoperative

Patient Problems	Goals and Outcome Criteria
Fear related to perceived threat of death	Reduced fear: patient states fear is lessened
Inability to manage self-care related to lack of knowledge of preoperative and postoperative care	Patient understands preoperative and postoperative care: patient verbalizes accurate information, cooperates in care

Interventions

Preoperative teaching begins when the patient is identified as a candidate for transplantation. To achieve these goals, acknowledge and encourage the patient to discuss concerns. Accept fear as understandable and natural. Provide factual information to help the patient to cope by reducing fear of the unknown. Involve the patient in planning and self-care. When patients are active participants in their care, they feel less helpless and less anxious. Reinforce information that has been taught when the actual surgery is imminent.

SURGICAL PROCEDURE

The donor kidney is removed from the live donor in an operating room and taken to an adjacent room where the recipient has been prepared to receive it. A cadaver kidney is removed under sterile conditions and transported to the hospital where the recipient is waiting. The donor kidney is placed in the recipient's abdomen and anastomosed (attached) to the bladder via the ureter and also to the blood vessels (Fig. 42.10).

Complications

Complications after renal transplantation include acute tubular necrosis (ATN), rejection, renal artery stenosis, hematomas, abscesses, and leakage of ureteral or vascular anastomoses. When the time between organ harvest and implantation is delayed, a risk of ATN exists. With ATN, urine output may decline and metabolic wastes may not be eliminated. This condition requires dialysis until renal function improves. Rejection of the new organ by the recipient is a major problem with most tissue transplants. Rejection is characterized by fever, elevated BP, and pain over the location of the new kidney. Three types of rejection can occur: (1) hyperacute, (2) acute, and (3) chronic. Hyperacute rejection occurs within 48 hours after transplantation. It is not reversible, and the kidney must be removed. Acute rejection develops between 1 week and 2 years after transplantation and is treated with increased immunosuppressant drugs. Chronic rejection develops and

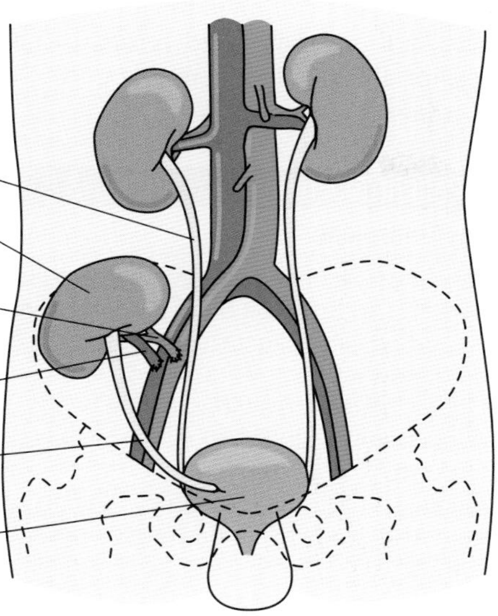

Fig. 42.10 Placement of a transplanted kidney. (From Monahan F, Sands J, Neighbors M, et al.: *Phipps' medical-surgical nursing: health and illness perspectives*, ed 8, St. Louis, 2007, Mosby.)

progresses slowly. Chronic rejection eventually mimics chronic kidney disease and dialysis may become necessary.

Immunosuppressant drugs, begun before surgery, are continued in the postoperative period to reduce the risk of rejection. These drugs include (1) T-cell suppressors: cyclosporine, tacrolimus, or sirolimus; (2) cytotoxic drugs: cyclophosphamide; and (3) corticosteroids. Antibodies are drugs that are used primarily for short periods to prevent or reverse acute rejection. Those used for transplant patients include polyclonal antibodies (antithymocyte globulin, antilymphocyte globulin) and monoclonal antibodies (muromonab-CD3, daclizumab). Examples of immunosuppressant agents, their actions and adverse effects, and nursing interventions are provided in Chapter 41, Table 41.4. They are called *immunosuppressants* because they inhibit the body's immune response to foreign tissue. This action is intended to prevent the donor kidney from being destroyed by the recipient's defenses. The action of immunosuppressants also reduces the body's response to pathogens, so patients who take these drugs are at increased risk for infection.

POSTOPERATIVE NURSING CARE OF THE RENAL TRANSPLANT RECIPIENT

Focused Assessment

General postoperative care is described in Chapter 17. This section emphasizes care that is unique to the renal transplant recipient. For the renal transplant recipient, it is especially important to monitor and accurately document fluid intake, urine output, weight changes, and vital signs. Patients are usually in a critical care unit for at least the first 24 hours because circulatory status requires constant monitoring, including central venous pressure readings.

Patient Problems, Goals, and Outcome Criteria: Renal Transplantation, Postoperative

Patient Problems	Goals and Outcome Criteria
Decreased urinary elimination related to rejection of transplanted kidney, renal failure	Adequate urine elimination: fluid intake and output equal
Fluid volume deficit related to diuresis, blood loss	Normal fluid volume: pulse and blood pressure (BP) consistent with patient baseline
Potential for infection related to suppression of immune response	Absence of infection: normal body temperature and white blood cell (WBC) count
Inability to manage self-care following transplantation related to lack of information	Effective management of self-care: patient accurately describes and carries out plan of care
Anxiety related to possibility of organ rejection	Reduced anxiety: patient states anxiety is lessened

Interventions

Immediately after surgery, the transplant patient is taken to a special care unit for close monitoring for circulatory and respiratory complications. Assist the patient with turning, coughing, deep breathing, and leg exercises. Institute pain control measures.

Decreased urinary elimination. The patient has an indwelling catheter for 3 to 5 days to permit constant observation of urine output. Urine is pink to bloody initially, and then gradually clears. Maintain catheter patency at all times. The health care provider may give orders to gently irrigate the catheter if obstruction by blood clots is suspected. Closely monitor the patient for signs that the transplanted organ is functioning: increasing urine output, normal BP, decreasing BUN and serum creatinine, stable weight. Commonly, the patient begins to diurese (i.e., eliminate excess fluid) as soon as blood flow to the donor kidney is established. The output may be as high as 1 L/h until BUN and serum creatinine return to normal.

If the patient is oliguric, a fluid challenge and diuretics are prescribed. In addition to the possibilities of renal failure and rejection, be alert for signs and symptoms of cardiac failure related to excess fluid volume (i.e., dyspnea, edema, bounding pulse, cardiac dysrhythmias).

Put On Your Thinking Cap!

What are some measures that you can take to maintain catheter patency in the posttransplant patient?

Fluid volume deficit. Massive postoperative diuresis causes fluid volume deficit in some patients. With excessive fluid loss, the patient is at risk for electrolyte imbalances and decreased cardiac output. A thready pulse, low BP, and poor tissue turgor suggest dehydration. Serum electrolyte studies are ordered to identify specific imbalances. Intravenous fluid orders must be carefully individualized.

Potential for infection. Because the immunosuppressant drugs that protect the new kidney also inhibit the body's ability to resist pathogens, monitor the transplant recipient carefully for signs and symptoms of infection (i.e., fever, elevated WBC count, cough, purulent wound drainage). Signs and symptoms may be very subtle despite development of a major infection. Maintain good hand washing and aseptic technique when working with the patient. Separate the patient from others who have infections. Teach the patient and family members the importance of protecting the patient from exposure to infections. Give prophylactic antibiotics as prescribed. Clarify and reinforce these restrictions on diet, fluids, and activity. It is critical that the patient knows the signs and symptoms of infection, rejection, and renal failure.

Inability to perform self-care and manage condition. Ideally, patient teaching begins before the transplant so that it can be reinforced after the procedure (see the Patient Teaching box).

Anxiety. Anxiety may lessen as renal function improves, but the patient always lives with the possibility of rejection. It is helpful for the patient to talk about feelings and explore ways to deal with them. Some patients find comfort in a support group of people who have had similar experiences, or in spiritual resources. Others may need referral to a mental health professional to help them cope constructively with their stress.

Patient Teaching

Kidney Transplant

- Take medication exactly as prescribed to control rejection and prevent other complications.
- Report adverse effects (specific to drugs) to the health care provider.
- Follow the diet prescribed by the health care provider.
- Avoid people with infections because resistance is lowered.
- Increase activity as ordered by the health care provider.
- Immediately notify the health care provider of signs and symptoms of infection (i.e., fever, cough, increasing wound drainage) and rejection (i.e., fever, pain in kidney area).

KIDNEY DONOR

Physical care of the donor is similar to that described earlier for nephrectomy, which may be conventional or laparoscopic. Pain is considerably worse with the conventional approach, so provide thorough pain control measures. With the conventional approach, the donor will be hospitalized 4 to 7 days and return to work in 6 to 8 weeks. With the laparoscopic approach, the donor is hospitalized 2 to 4 days and can return to work in 4 to 6 weeks.

Emotionally, the donor usually feels very good about the experience because of the value of the kidney to the recipient. If the kidney fails, however, the donor may be very disappointed. Be sensitive to the emotional needs of the donor.

Get Ready for the NCLEX® Examination!

Key Points

- Untreated or repeated UTIs can result in renal scarring and lead to renal failure.
- Inflammatory conditions of the urinary tract include cystitis (bladder inflammation), urethritis (urethral inflammation), glomerulonephritis (glomerular inflammation), and pyelonephritis (inflammation of the renal pelvis).
- Risk factors for UTI include female gender, prolonged immobility, dehydration, infrequent voiding, tight fitting synthetic undergarments, bubble baths and vaginal deodorants, renal calculi, urinary diversion, and indwelling urinary catheters.
- UTIs are treated with antibiotics, urinary tract antiseptics, analgesics, and antispasmodic agents.
- Acute glomerulonephritis commonly follows a streptococcal infection and results in an immune response that scars the glomeruli.
- Patients with renal disorders are at risk for fluid volume excess, hypertension, and heart failure.
- Management of renal disorders requires attention to pain management, fluid balance, activity intolerance, and patient education.
- Urinary obstructions anywhere in the urinary tract can lead to hydronephrosis and kidney damage.
- Urinary calculi (stones) form in the urinary tract and may move through the tract with the flow of urine.
- Although most calculi pass spontaneously, some require surgical removal or disintegration by lithotripsy.
- Nursing care of the patient with renal calculi focuses on acute pain, reduced urinary elimination, potential for electrolyte imbalance, and inability to manage self-care.
- Complications of urinary tract surgery include urinary tract and wound infection, atelectasis, paralytic ileus, and hemorrhage.

- Renal tumors are often large before they are detected because early symptoms are subtle.
- Cystectomy (bladder removal) requires urine to be diverted to an alternate drainage or collection system. Types of urinary diversion used include ileal and sigmoid conduits, ureterostomy, and nephrostomy.
- A neobladder is created from a segment of bowel and connected to the urethra for normal voiding.
- Nursing care after bladder surgery focuses on pain management, unobstructed urine flow, skin integrity, bowel function, and self-care.
- Renal failure can result from hypotension, toxins, infections, impaired blood flow, trauma, and obstructions.
- The four stages of AKI are (1) onset, (2) oliguria, (3) diuresis, and (4) recovery.
- Management of AKI emphasizes fluid and dietary restrictions, restoration of fluid balance, waste elimination, and maintenance of cardiac output.
- When 90% to 95% of kidney function is lost, the patient is considered to have chronic kidney disease.
- Effects of chronic kidney disease include excess fluid volume, hyperkalemia, hypocalcemia, hyperuricemia, and anemia.
- Dialysis uses a semipermeable membrane to draw excess water, electrolytes, and wastes into a special solution called *dialysate.*
- Renal transplantation is the only alternative to dialysis for the patient with ESRD.
- Signs and symptoms of rejection of a transplanted kidney are fever, increased BP, and pain over the location of the new kidney.

Additional Learning Resources

SG Go to your Study Guide for additional learning activities to help you master this chapter content.

Go to your Evolve website (http://evolve.elsevier.com/Linton/medsurg) for the following learning resources and much more:
- Fluid & Electrolyte Tutorial
- Review Questions for the NCLEX® Examination

Clinical Judgment and Next-Generation NCLEX® Examination-Style Questions

1. **Ms. P, 85 years of age, is hospitalized with pyelonephritis. She is receiving intravenous fluids because she is unable to take adequate fluids orally. About an hour after the intravenous fluids are initiated, she complains of feeling short of breath. Her pulse is 90 beats per minute and bounding. What action should the nurse take?**
   1. Elevate the foot of the bed
   2. Discontinue the intravenous fluids
   3. Assure Ms. P that this is normal with pyelonephritis
   4. Notify the registered nurse that Ms. P. may have fluid overload

   NCLEX Client Need: Physiological Integrity: Reduction of Risk Potential

2. **Ms. P, 25 years of age, has been recently diagnosed with polycystic kidney disease. She reports that her mother died of kidney disease, but she does not know much about it. What information should be included in the teaching plan?**
   1. Polycystic kidney disease occurs randomly, so it is probably unrelated to her mother's kidney failure
   2. Prompt treatment of UTIs helps to prevent progressive kidney damage
   3. Repeated childhood urinary infections cause polycystic kidney disease
   4. Polycystic kidney disease is an autoimmune condition in which the body's immune system damages the kidneys

   NCLEX Client Need: Health Promotion and Maintenance

3. **Which of the following contribute to the development of renal calculi? (Select all that apply.)**
   1. Sedentary lifestyle
   2. High calcium intake
   3. Inadequate fluid intake
   4. Family history of calculi
   5. Excessive vitamin D supplements

   NCLEX Client Need: Physiological Integrity: Physiological Adaptation

4. **Mr. C has been admitted through the emergency department with a diagnosis of renal calculi. While awaiting several diagnostic tests, Mr. C. cries out and asks for "something for pain." Which nursing action is most appropriate?**
   1. Encourage fluid intake to promote passage of calculi
   2. Coach him to remain calm and breathe deeply
   3. Administer opioid analgesics as ordered
   4. Assist him to ambulate in the room

   NCLEX Client Need: Physiological Integrity: Pharmacological Therapies

5. **When a ureter is obstructed by a renal calculus, which complication may occur?**
   1. Extracellular fluid excess
   2. Hydronephrosis
   3. ESRD
   4. Nephrotoxicity

   NCLEX Client Need: Physiological Integrity: Physiological Adaptation

6. **Following a nephrectomy, which of the following patient needs takes priority?**
   1. Breathing exercises
   2. Fluid intake
   3. Relief of anxiety
   4. Prevention of thrombi

   NCLEX Client Need: Physiological Integrity: Reduction of Risk Potential

7. **The nurse is preparing to teach a group of women about reducing the risk of cystitis. Which teaching will the nurse include? (Select all that apply.)**
   1. Avoid caffeine
   2. Take tub baths instead of showers
   3. Drink a glass of water before and after intercourse
   4. Cleanse the perineum from front to back after elimination
   5. Wear synthetic undergarments that serve as a barrier to moisture

   NCLEX Client Need: Health Promotion and Maintenance

8. **Glomerulonephritis is caused by which of the following?**
   1. Bacteria
   2. Viruses
   3. Urinary obstruction
   4. Immunologic processes

   NCLEX Client Need: Physiological Integrity: Physiological Adaptation

9. **The maximum amount of fluid that can be used to irrigate a nephrostomy tube is ___________ mL.**

   NCLEX Client Need: Physiological Integrity: Reduction of Risk Potential

10. **After a nephrectomy, the nurse assesses that a patient has eliminated 25 mL in the past hour. Which nursing action is appropriate?**
    1. Have the patient change positions
    2. Give the patient an 8-oz glass of water every 2 hours
    3. Increase the flow rate of the patient's intravenous fluids.
    4. Notify the health care provider that the patient's urine output is too low

11. **SLO/Objective: Contribute to the development of the nursing plan of care for patients with urologic disorders.**

    NGN Item Type: Cloze

    Cognitive Skill: Prioritize Hypotheses

    The nurse is caring for a 45-year-old man who had a left nephrectomy 24 hours ago. The assessment data at this time include:
    - Alert and oriented
    - Pain in left flank rated 3 on a 10-point scale
    - Temperature 101°F
    - Heart rate 92 beats per minute
    - Respirations 24 breaths per minute
    - Breath sounds diminished in left lung
    - Oxygen saturation 90% on room air
    - Surgical dressing dry
    - 24 hour fluid intake 2300 mL
    - 24 hour urine output 2100 mL
    - Bowel sounds present all four quadrants

    Choose the *most likely* options for the information missing from the statements below by selecting from the list of options provided.

    The nurse recognizes that elevated _________, increased _________ and _________, and decreased _________ and ___________ may be signs of complications. Failure to recognize and treat this health problem can most likely lead to _________ and ___________.

OPTIONS
Pain level = 3 on 10-point scale
Temperature
Heart rate
Respiratory rate
Oxygen saturation
Urine output
Breath sounds
Acute renal injury
Atelectasis
Chronic renal disease
Pneumonia
Heart failure

    NCLEX Client Need: Physiological Integrity: Reduction of Risk Potential

12. **A patient with chronic kidney disease becomes confused and reports nausea, abdominal cramps, and lack of sensation in the legs. Upon assessment, the heart rate is found to be irregular. Which condition does the nurse suspect?**
    1. Increased BUN
    2. Hyperkalemia
    3. Metabolic acidosis
    4. Hypocalcemia

    NCLEX Client Need: Physiological Integrity: Physiological Adaptation

Musculoskeletal System Introduction

43

http://evolve.elsevier.com/Linton/medsurg

Objectives

1. Describe the structure and function of the musculoskeletal system.
2. Identify the data to be collected to assist with a comprehensive nursing assessment of a patient with a musculoskeletal condition.
3. Describe the nurse's responsibilities for diagnostic tests and procedures used for assessing patient with musculoskeletal conditions.
4. Discuss the drugs used to treat conditions associated with the musculoskeletal system.

Key Terms

goniometer (gō-nē-ŎM-ĕ-tĕr)
intraarticular (ĭn-tră-ăr-TĬK-ū-lăr)
crepitus (KRĔP-ĭ-tŭs)

More than 50 million people in the United States report having been diagnosed with a condition that affects the bones, joints, and muscles, including fractures, amputations, osteoarthritis, rheumatoid arthritis (RA), gout, lupus, and fibromyalgia. These conditions may cause pain, depression, immobility, decreased ability to carry out activities of daily living, and social isolation.

ANATOMY AND PHYSIOLOGY OF THE MUSCULOSKELETAL SYSTEM

The musculoskeletal system is made up of voluntary (skeletal) muscle and connective tissues that bind structures together and provide a framework for the body as a whole. The components of the musculoskeletal system store fat, transport substances, provide protection, and play a role in repair of damaged tissue. The types of muscle and connective tissue are loose (areolar, adipose, reticular), dense (tendons, fascia, dermis, gastrointestinal [GI] tract submucosa, fibrous joint capsules), elastic (aortic walls, vocal cords, parts of trachea and bronchi, some ligaments), hematopoietic (blood), and strong supportive (cartilage, bone, ligaments).

BONE

Bone is the hard tissue that makes up most of the skeletal system. The functions of the bones are support, protection, movement, storage of calcium and other ions, and manufacture of blood cells.

CARTILAGE

Cartilage is a specialized fibrous connective tissue. It provides firm but flexible support for the embryonic skeleton and part of the adult skeleton. Cartilage differs from bone in that its matrix has the consistency of a firm plastic or gristle-like gel. Cartilage cells are called *chondrocytes* and are located in tiny spaces that are distributed throughout the matrix.

LIGAMENTS

Ligaments are strong and flexible fibrous bands of connective tissue that link bones and cartilage and support muscles. Yellow ligaments and white ligaments have distinctively different functions. Yellow ligaments, located in the vertebral column, are elastic and allow for stretching. White ligaments connect articulating joints, such as the knee, provide stability, and do not stretch.

TENDONS

Tendons are composed of very strong and dense fibrous connective tissue. They are in the shape of heavy cords and anchor muscles firmly to bones. One of the most prominent tendons is the Achilles tendon, which can be felt at the back of the ankle just above the heel.

JOINT STRUCTURE AND FUNCTION

A joint is the site at which two or more bones of the body are joined. Joints permit motion and flexibility of the rigid skeleton. The only bone in the human body that does not articulate with at least one other bone is the hyoid bone, to which the tongue is attached.

Classified on the basis of the extent of movement, joints include synarthroses (fixed joints), amphiarthroses (slightly movable joints), and diarthroses (freely movable joints). Synarthroses, such as those in the skull, allow no movement at all. An example of an

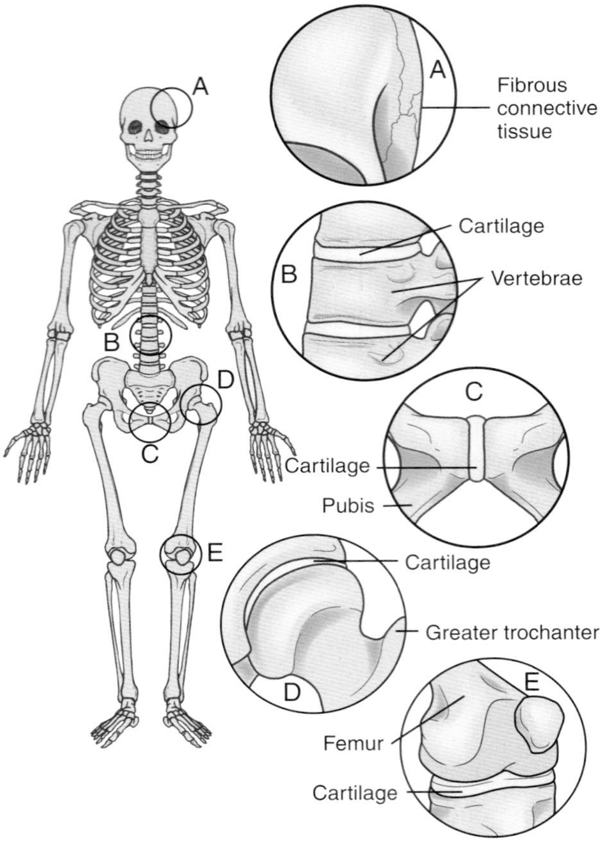

Fig. 43.1 Classification of joints. (A to C) Synarthrotic (immovable) and amphiarthrotic (slightly movable) joints. (D and E) Diarthrodial (freely movable) joints. (From Lewis et al.: *Medical-surgical nursing*, ed 10, St. Louis, 2017, Elsevier.)

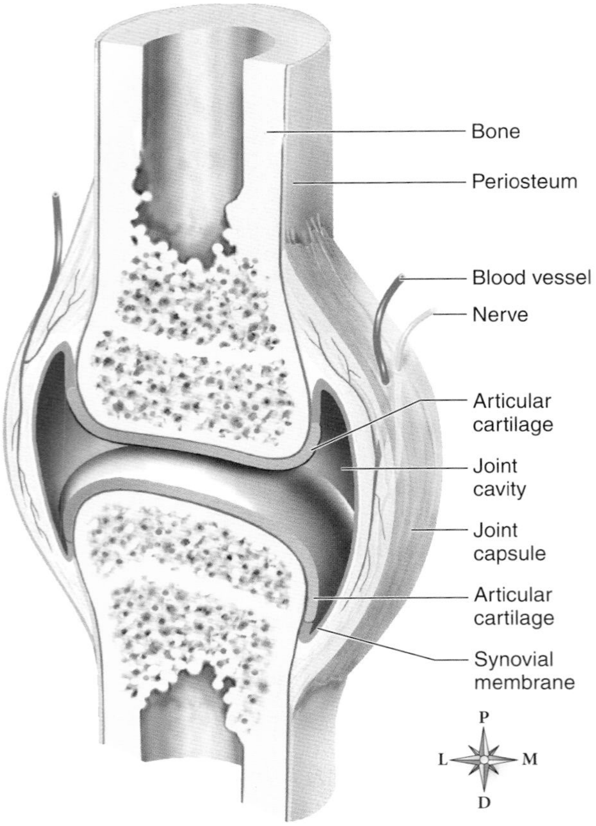

Fig. 43.2 Structure of diarthrodial (synovial) joint. (From Patton KT, Thibodeau GA: *The human body in health & disease*, ed 7, St. Louis, 2018, Elsevier.)

amphiarthrosis is the juncture of the ulna and radius in the forearm. Diarthroses, also called *synovial joints*, found in the elbows, shoulders, fingers, hips, and knees, allow considerable movement. They are encased in a fibrous capsule made of strong cartilage and lined with a synovial membrane (Fig. 43.1).

The synovial membrane is smooth, thus permitting structures to move without friction. A smooth layer of cartilage also covers the ends of the bones, where it serves as a kind of shock absorber. Synovial fluid fills and lubricates the space in the middle of the joint. Bursae are sacs of synovial fluid found in joints that also promote smooth articulation of joint structures. The bursae permit tendons to slide easily with movement of the bones (Fig. 43.2).

SKELETAL MUSCLE

The primary function of skeletal (voluntary, striated) muscle tissue is to contract and cause movement. Muscles work to keep joints stable by preventing excess movement of the bones and joints, maintaining skeletal stability, and preventing skeletal structural damage or deformation. Skeletal muscles also protect internal organs (particularly abdominal and pelvic organs) by acting as an external barrier or shield to external trauma and by supporting the weight of the organs.

Skeletal muscles are located throughout the body for voluntary control of functions such as swallowing, urination, and defecation. The only way to functionally contract a skeletal muscle is through signaling from the nervous system. In skeletal muscles that work with tendons to pull on bones, the muscle collagen intertwines with the collagen of a tendon. At the other end of the tendon, it fuses with the periosteum coating the bone.

Skeletal muscles contractions are called either *isometric* or *isotonic*. Isometric contractions increase tension within a muscle but do not produce movement; isotonic contractions produce movement. Immobility reduces muscle contractions and can produce muscle atrophy (decrease in size), whereas exercise and activity increase muscle contractions to produce muscle hypertrophy (increase in size).

A layer of fascia called the *epimysium* covers skeletal muscles. Individual muscle cells are bundled together by collagen to form a *fascicle*. Because muscle cells are elongated and cylindrical, each muscle cell is called a *muscle fiber*. The fiber bundles are covered by *perimysium* and an inner layer of connective tissue called the *endomysium*. Almost the entire cross-section of the muscle fiber is taken up by hundreds of long, cylindrical strands of contractile proteins called *myofibrils*. Each myofibril is divided into segments called *sarcomeres* (Fig. 43.3).

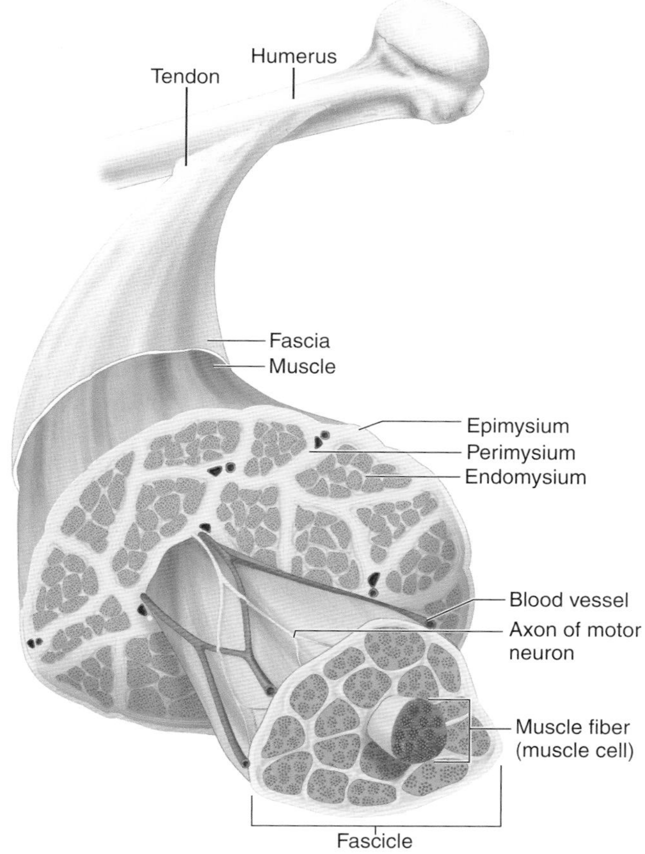

Fig. 43.3 Structure of a muscle. (From Patton KT, Thibodeau GA, Douglas M. *Essentials of anatomy and physiology*, St. Louis, 2012, Mosby.)

AGE-RELATED CHANGES IN THE MUSCULOSKELETAL SYSTEM

Age-related changes in the musculoskeletal system can cause pain, limited mobility, and impaired function, contributing significantly to a loss of independence. Box 43.1 provides a list of changes with aging.

NURSING ASSESSMENT OF THE MUSCULOSKELETAL SYSTEM

The licensed vocational/practical nurse (LVN/LPN) collects data to assist the registered nurse (RN) with a comprehensive assessment related to a musculoskeletal disorder.

HEALTH HISTORY

Reason for Seeking Care

Determine why the patient is seeking health care. Possible reasons related to musculoskeletal disorders are aches, pain, joint swelling or stiffness, generalized weakness, a change in appearance that is significant to the patient, and a change in ability to carry out activities of daily living (ADLs).

Box 43.1 Age-Related Changes in the Musculoskeletal System

- Loss of bone mass and density
- Decrease in bone strength
- Loss of elasticity and water in joint cartilage, resulting in softening, fraying, and ulceration
- Loss of cartilage in joints resulting in osteophytes (bony spurs) and friction during joint movement
- Decline in muscle mass, especially in the extremities

Present Health

Ask about the patient's general health status to determine the patient's perception of well-being. Specifically, ask whether the patient has had fatigue, malaise, anorexia, weight loss, pain, stiffness, edema, dysphagia, or dyspnea. Be aware that many cultures react differently to pain and disability; some may be stoic, whereas others are very expressive.

Past Health History

The nursing assessment requires a detailed health history because many of the signs and symptoms of musculoskeletal disorders are insidious. In addition, patients with chronic conditions may come to accept their symptoms as a way of life and fail to report them to the nurse. Thus it may be helpful to have a family member present to assist the patient as historian. The family member may provide a clearer picture of how the changes in health have evolved.

Inquire about past medical and surgical conditions. Ask whether a history of tuberculosis, poliomyelitis, diabetes mellitus, gout, arthritis, rickets, infection of bones or joints, autoimmune diseases, and neuromuscular disabilities exists. Also determine whether the patient has ever had phlebitis, varicosities, thromboses, emboli, or stasis ulcers in either the affected or the unaffected extremities. Record the dates of immunizations for polio and tetanus because postpolio syndrome and tetanus are characterized by musculoskeletal symptoms. Note preexisting cardiovascular problems because hypertension, coronary artery disease (CAD), congestive heart failure (CHF), and cardiac defects can greatly affect the patient's ability to tolerate surgery and recover successfully.

A review of the patient's psychosocial background may offer insight into how the patient can tolerate treatments and procedures. Knowledge of how the patient copes with stress may help in planning care to reduce anxiety and fear. The patient about to undergo an amputation may have a number of fears and concerns about the surgical procedure, the loss of a body part, the potential loss of independence, and pain and disfigurement. Open discussion of these concerns may help to alleviate those fears.

Accidents and injuries. Accidents and injuries, even in the distant past, may be significant because they could be related to the patient's current problem. For example, low back pain in the present may be the result of an injury sustained several years ago. Inquire about participation in sports and the type of work the patient has done. Many types of sports injuries result in osteoarthritis in later life.

Current and past medications. Record the patient's use of prescription and over-the-counter (OTC) drugs. Self-medication is common with musculoskeletal pain, and patients may fail to report it unless specifically asked. Inquire about the use of alternative therapies, including herbal supplements and home remedies. Many herbal supplements interact with traditional medications and have significant side effects. It is important to list all medications prescribed previously and describe their effectiveness. Note any problems associated with current medications and whether the patient thinks that these medications are effective. Some drugs, including corticosteroids and antiseizure drugs, can contribute to bone loss. Record any allergies.

Family History

Record a family history of conditions that may be causes of amputation, including diabetes, hypertension, and vascular diseases. Determine whether the patient or any relative has had osteoporosis, osteoarthritis, rheumatoid arthritis, gout, or scoliosis, because these conditions appear to have some genetic basis. In addition, note any history of other autoimmune diseases, such as thyroid disorders.

Functional Assessment

Data collected for the functional assessment include usual diet and fluid intake, intake of salt and alcohol, and use of tobacco. Describe exercise, rest, and sleep habits, as well as the effects of the current symptoms on the patient's usual activities. Identify the patient's occupation and responsibilities to determine how the disorder will affect that aspect of their life.

The following questions may be used to determine the patient's functional status and the significance of any changes to the patient.

- How does this problem affect the way you live?
- Have you had to change your everyday activities?
- How do you feel about any changes that you have had to make?
- What have you found helpful in adapting to these changes?
- How do you carry out the treatment program prescribed by your physician?
- Has your treatment plan been effective for you?
- What type of support systems do you have at home?

PHYSICAL EXAMINATION

A total physical examination should be done, with special attention to the neurologic, cardiovascular, and integumentary systems. Measure height and weight and vital signs to uncover factors that may affect circulation, including obesity and hypertension. Be aware that many patients with arthritis have limited physical abilities to stand, step up, or get onto an examination table. A chair scale is very useful for these patients. Compare findings with the patient's norms, if available.

Throughout the examination, evaluate neurovascular status. Record the patient's skin color, texture, temperature, and turgor. The overall color, condition, and temperature of the skin are good indicators of blood supply to the extremities. Cool or cold, clammy, mottled skin that is pale or cyanotic may indicate a poor blood supply. Palpating both legs simultaneously can help to detect circulatory differences between the two legs. In addition, there may be open areas on the skin. Describe any skin lesions and drainage from them. Wounds to the extremities are common when blood supply is inadequate.

Palpate the peripheral pulses for presence, quality, and symmetry. If pulses are not palpable, a Doppler ultrasound device can be used. Determine capillary refill by applying pressure to the nail bed of a finger or toe until it blanches (i.e., turns white). When the pressure is released, the nail bed normally regains its normal pink color within 3 seconds. In extremities with a diminished supply of blood, capillary refill may take 5 seconds or longer. Check sensation by asking the patient to identify touch on the extremities. Experienced examiners may evaluate the patient's ability to sense sharp, dull, warm, and cold stimuli.

Inspect the skin for color, rashes, lesions, scars, or any signs of injuries. Inspect joints for swelling and deformity, and check for warmth and tenderness. Assess joint pain and range of motion by asking the patient to move each extremity through the normal range of motion. Take care not to extend joints beyond their range or point of comfort. Inflamed joints are extremely sensitive to movement and pressure. During the movement, watch for signs of pain and listen for the crackling sound called ***crepitus***. The health care provider may make a more precise measurement of joint motion using an instrument called a ***goniometer***, which measures the range of movement of the joints. Measurement of limb length and muscle strength may also be done.

Collect data about the patient's mental and emotional status and general cognitive abilities to determine the patient's understanding of the condition.

Nursing assessment of the patient with a musculoskeletal disorder is outlined in Box 43.2.

Box 43.2 Focused Assessment of the Patient With a Musculoskeletal Disorder

HEALTH HISTORY

Reason for Seeking Care

Problem related to specific musculoskeletal disorder

Present Health

Changes in movement, activities of daily living (ADLs); areas of pain, swelling, or tenderness; fatigue; past or recent injuries because of accidents or falls, use of assistive devices

PAST HEALTH HISTORY

Previous illnesses, operations, hospitalizations, trauma, hypertension, coronary artery disease (CAD), congestive heart failure (CHF), cardiac murmurs or defects, phlebitis, varicosities, thromboses, emboli, stasis ulcers, diabetes mellitus, tuberculosis, poliomyelitis, gout, arthritis, rickets, neuromuscular disabilities

Past Health History

Diabetes mellitus, hypertension, vascular diseases, rheumatoid arthritis (RA), degenerative arthritis (need for joint replacement surgery), gout, scoliosis, other autoimmune disorders

FUNCTIONAL ASSESSMENT

Usual diet and fluid intake; intake of salt and alcohol; use of tobacco; exercise, rest, and sleep habits; occupation, roles, and responsibilities; ability to carry out ADLs

PHYSICAL EXAMINATION

Height and weight
Vital signs
Posture, balance, gait
Skin: Color, texture, temperature, turgor, capillary refill, bruising, swelling, lesions, nodules, ulcers (location, size, color, drainage), scars
Peripheral pulses: Presence, quality, symmetry
Pain: Nature, location, severity, precipitating factors, alleviating factors
Sensation: Loss or change, abnormal perception of heat and cold
Joints: Warmth, redness, swelling, tenderness, nodules, range of motion, crepitus, function of hands
Upper extremities: Symmetry, swelling, tenderness, pain, range of motion, posture
Lower extremities: Movement of hips, knees, and ankles; pain; skin condition
Mental status: Level of consciousness, emotional state, ability to follow directions
Emotional status: Coping strategies, fears and concerns

DIAGNOSTIC TESTS AND PROCEDURES

Procedures used to diagnose musculoskeletal disorders are primarily laboratory studies of blood and urine and radiologic imaging studies of the bones and joints. Routine blood studies include a complete blood count (CBC), the erythrocyte sedimentation rate (ESR), and C-reactive protein (CRP) determination. These studies help to determine whether a connective tissue disorder is inflammatory or noninflammatory. Other blood studies are the Venereal Disease Research Laboratory (VDRL), rheumatoid factor (RF), creatinine, and antinuclear antibody (ANA) tests. Urine may be tested for creatinine and uric acid levels. Fluids aspirated from joints may be studied to detect uric acid crystals or white blood cells (WBCs). Most laboratory tests are not diagnostic for a single condition because many factors can cause an increase in inflammation. The health care provider may rely on multiple diagnostic procedures along with the health history and physical examination to reach a diagnosis.

Radiologic imaging studies include radiography, ultrasonography, arthrography, nuclear scintigraphy, magnetic resonance imaging (MRI), discography, tomography, and computed tomography (CT). Other useful measures are biopsy and arthroscopy.

VASCULAR STUDIES

Vascular studies may be done for a patient with compromised circulation, such as in trauma or vascular disease. Angiography is a procedure that involves the injection of a radiopaque dye into blood vessels, which are then viewed radiographically to determine their patency.

PULSE VOLUME RECORDING

Pulse volume recording uses a noninvasive device that gives general information about the volume of blood flow to an extremity. Another name for this procedure is *plethysmography.*

THERMOGRAPHY

Thermography involves the use of a device that detects and records heat in various parts of the body. Hot or cold spots are revealed, indicating the amount of blood flow to that part of the body. Cool areas generally indicate less blood flow than warm areas.

DOPPLER ULTRASOUND

Doppler ultrasound uses sound waves to determine the presence of pulses in the extremities. This technology is much more sensitive than using the fingertips to try to palpate a pulse. The adequacy of circulation can also be assessed with transcutaneous tissue oxygen (O_2) measurement.

BIOPSY

In patients with tumors, a biopsy may be done to determine the nature of the tumor. A biopsy involves removing a small portion of tissue, which is then examined for malignancy.

Table 43.1 summarizes commonly used diagnostic studies and related nursing care. Agency procedure manuals provide more specific information on preparation and postprocedure care.

Table 43.1 Diagnostic Tests and Procedures for Musculoskeletal Disorders

General Interventions: Check your agency procedure manual for diagnostic tests and procedures. Always tell the patient what to expect when tests are ordered. Explain if nothing-by-mouth (NPO) status is necessary. Document the care provided and relevant assessment data. If venipuncture is done, apply a dressing and check for the site oozing. Apply pressure and elevate the arm if patient's blood clotting is impaired.

TEST AND PURPOSE	PATIENT PREPARATION	POSTPROCEDURE NURSING CARE
Blood Studies		
Antinuclear Antibodies (ANAs) Positive in SLE, RA, SSc, Raynaud phenomenon, Sjögren syndrome, and necrotizing arteritis.	Fast 8 hours before test.	See General Interventions.
C-Reactive Protein (CRP) Detects active inflammation as in RA and disseminated lupus erythematosus.	Restrict food and fluids for 4 hours.	See General Interventions.
Creatinine Assesses renal function. Increased with SLE, SSc, and polyarteritis.	Fasting is not required.	See General Interventions.
Erythrocyte Sedimentation Rate (ESR) Determines the presence of inflammation. Increased with RA and rheumatic fever; decreased with osteoarthritis.	Fasting is not required.	See General Interventions.
Red Blood Cell (RBC) Count Detects and differentiates blood dyscrasias. Decreased in RA and SLE.	Fasting is not required.	See General Interventions.
Rheumatoid Factor (RF) Detects antibodies in patients with RA.	Fasting is not required.	See General Interventions.
Venereal Disease Research Laboratory (VDRL) Test Measures antibodies to syphilis. Sometimes decreased in SLE.	Fasting is not required.	See General Interventions.
White Blood Cell (WBC) Count Increased in infection, tissue necrosis, and inflammation; may decrease in SLE.	Fasting is not required.	See General Interventions.
Urine Studies		
24-Hour Urine for Creatinine Measures renal function and status of muscle diseases.	Instruct the patient to collect a 24-hour urine specimen. Discard the first morning specimen. Save the rest of urine voided over a 24-hour period in a clean, refrigerated 3-L container with or without preservative. Include urine voided at end of 24-hour period. Fasting not required.	See General Interventions.
Urinary Uric Acid (24-Hour Collection) Measures uric acid metabolism; increased in gout, liver disease, chronic myelogenous leukemia, and fever.	Requires 24-hour urine specimen (as described earlier). Fasting not required.	See General Interventions.

Table 43.1 Diagnostic Tests and Procedures for Musculoskeletal Disorders—cont'd

TEST AND PURPOSE	PATIENT PREPARATION	POSTPROCEDURE NURSING CARE
Radiologic Studies		
Arthrography Uses contrast medium to show soft-tissue joint structures.	[a]Dye precautions. Tell the patient that needle insertion may cause discomfort and swelling that lasts several days.	[a]Dye precautions. Assess and document discomfort and swelling. Instruct the patient to avoid strenuous activity for 12 to 24 hours after test. Joint may be wrapped.
Computed Tomography (CT) Detects tumors and some spinal fractures.	Tell the patient that the procedure may be lengthy (up to 30 minutes per body part). Patient lies on a stretcher while a machine scans the area being studied.	See General Interventions.
Discography Visualizes the vertebral disk after contrast medium is injected into the disk.	Same as for arthrography.	Same as for arthrography.
Magnetic Resonance Imaging (MRI) Visualizes soft tissue. May detect avascular necrosis, disk disease, tumors, osteomyelitis, and torn ligaments.	Tell the patient that the procedure is painless; must lie still for 30 minutes or more. Some equipment includes videos that the patient can view to reduce anxiety. Ask whether the patient is claustrophobic. Give sedation if ordered for agitated or anxious patients. Remove any metallic objects such as jewelry. Inquire whether the patient has any implanted devices such as cardiac pacemaker or intracranial aneurysm clips, and notify the radiologist. Procedure is contraindicated with some implants. Metal may not be a problem with some newer equipment.	See General Interventions. Take safety precautions if the patient is sedated.
Nuclear Scintigraphy (Bone Scan) Detects bone malignancies, osteoporosis, osteomyelitis, and some fractures.	Contraindicated during pregnancy. Tell the patient that a small amount of radioactive material will be injected intravenously; then a scanner will move slowly back and forth over the body as the patient lies on a stretcher. May take 1 hour. Procedure is painless except for venipuncture. Radioactive isotopes are not harmful except to fetus. Empty bladder immediately before procedure for comfort and to prevent blocked view of pelvis.	See General Interventions. No special precautions are required for handling urine or stool.
Radiography Shows density, texture, and alignments of bones; reveals soft tissue involvement.	Tell the patient to expect to lie on a radiograph table or to stand next to a special device while films are taken. Remove any radiopaque objects (e.g., jewelry) that can interfere with results. Advise radiology of the patient's physical limitations related to moving, turning, and climbing.	See General Interventions.

Continued

Table 43.1 Diagnostic Tests and Procedures for Musculoskeletal Disorders—cont'd

TEST AND PURPOSE	PATIENT PREPARATION	POSTPROCEDURE NURSING CARE
Tomography		
Provides details of structures otherwise hidden by bone.	Requires lying in a cylindrical scanner; assess for claustrophobia and inform the radiologist.	See General Interventions.
Ultrasonography		
Reveals masses or fluid in soft tissue.	No preparation is required.	See General Interventions.
Special Tests		
Arthroscopy		
A surgical procedure to visualize a joint cavity and structure and to obtain fluid, tissue, or both for study.	Inform the patient that the procedure is performed in an operating room under local or general anesthesia.	The patient will have a sterile dressing applied to the wound, which will also be wrapped with a compression dressing. Report any drainage of blood or fluid to the physician. Instruct the patient to limit activity for a few days.
Joint Aspiration		
Examination of fluid taken from a joint to diagnose inflammation.	Procedure is usually done at bedside or in examination room. Tell the patient that a local anesthetic is used to minimize discomfort.	Apply pressure dressing to the joint. Instruct the patient to rest the joint for 8 to 24 hours. Record on patient's chart, and report to the physician or nurse supervisor any leakage of blood or fluid. Apply a pressure dressing to the affected area, and keep it immobilized for 12 to 24 hours.
Bone Densitometry (DXA and DPA)		
Determines bone mineral content and density to detect osteoporosis. Screening procedures may scan the finger, heel, or radius. If abnormal, the more conclusive scan of the pelvis and hips is advised.	No special advance preparation is required. Patient will need to remove any metallic objects (e.g., zippers, belts) in the area being examined. Explain that the patient will be positioned on an imaging table and an instrument will pass over the pelvic and hip region. A computer will record density measurements. Radiation exposure is minimal. The procedure is painless.	See General Interventions.
Muscle Biopsy		
A sample of muscle tissue is taken to detect inflammatory reaction, as in polymyositis or myopathic disease.	May be performed under local or general anesthesia.	Apply a pressure dressing to the affected area, and keep it immobilized for 12 to 24 hours.
Skin Biopsy		
Studies excised skin to confirm inflammatory connective tissue diseases such as SLE and SSc.	Tell the patient a local anesthetic will be injected; slight discomfort may be felt when the skin sample is obtained.	Keep the biopsy site clean and dry with a small adhesive bandage until a scab develops. Patients who are taking aspirin or NSAIDs are at risk for bleeding, bruising, or both at the biopsy site.

[a]**General Interventions**

When contrast dye used: *Before procedure*—assess patient allergy to dye, iodine, or shellfish. If patient reports allergy, notify radiology. Tell patient that injection of contrast dye can create a feeling of warmth, a salty taste, and nausea. *After procedure*—inform the physician of any signs of allergic response to the contrast dye. Administer antihistamines as ordered for allergy.

DPA, Dual-photon absorptiometry; *DXA*, dual-energy x-ray absorptiometry; *NSAIDs*, nonsteroidal antiinflammatory drugs; *RA*, rheumatoid arthritis; *SLE*, systemic lupus erythematosus; *SSc*, systemic sclerosis.

Note: See agency laboratory manual for specific preparation and norms. Results vary with different types of tests and may be reported in different units of measurement.

COMMON THERAPEUTIC MEASURES

Management of the patient with a musculoskeletal condition requires the services of a multidisciplinary team that includes the patient, nurse, physician, social worker, nutritionist, physical therapist, and occupational therapist. The goals of therapy are to reduce inflammation and pain, promote functional abilities, and foster adaptation to the condition or disability. Therapeutic measures may include physical and occupational therapy, modification of ADLs, patient education and support, nutritional counseling, drug therapy, psychologic and emotional support, and surgical intervention. Although none of these measures is curative, they can greatly enhance the patient's function and quality of life. Various sources suggest that dietary modifications for inflammatory conditions may be helpful; research is ongoing to determine valid recommendations. Some patients report that specific foods increase or decrease their symptoms.

PHYSICAL AND OCCUPATIONAL THERAPY

Physical therapy uses exercise and positioning to help preserve functional capability and minimize disability. For many patients, braces and splints help support inflamed joints, protect the patient from further injury, and relieve discomfort. Occupational therapy assists the patient in making adaptations in work and personal life that allow maximal possible function.

EDUCATION AND SUPPORT

Education is focused on the treatment plan and the patient's understanding of how to comply with it. Team members must be sensitive to the inconvenience and discomfort that a condition causes and should provide psychological support to identify coping mechanisms. Patients and their families need information about community support groups that can offer encouragement, information, and resources. Many research studies have demonstrated a connection between a patient's positive attitude and a successful outcome of a chronic condition.

DRUG THERAPY

Drug therapy for musculoskeletal disorders has traditionally included nonsteroidal antiinflammatory drugs (NSAIDs) and glucocorticoids to reduce inflammation and pain. When glucocorticoids are indicated, occasional local injections or short-term systemic therapy is preferred over long-term therapy. For many patients already on NSAIDs, acetaminophen is often prescribed as a safe analgesic. Other less safe drugs are gold salts, azathioprine, penicillamine, and cyclosporine.

Three categories of drugs are used in the treatment of arthritis: (1) NSAIDs, (2) glucocorticoids, and (3) disease-modifying antirheumatic drugs (DMARDs). NSAIDs are the safest type of these; they relieve pain and reduce inflammation but do not prevent joint damage or slow the progress of the disease. First-generation NSAIDs include salicylates (e.g., aspirin) and nonsalicylates such as ibuprofen. The only available second-generation NSAID, also called a *selective cyclooxygenase (COX)-2 inhibitor*, is celecoxib (Celebrex). Major side effects of celecoxib include GI bleeding/perforation and increased risk of thromboembolism, myocardial infarction, and stroke.

Glucocorticoids relieve symptoms, reduce inflammation, and may slow disease progression. Oral glucocorticoids such as prednisone are used for generalized symptoms, whereas ***intraarticular*** injections may be used when only one or two joints are affected. Long-term glucocorticoid therapy is discouraged because of adverse effects.

DMARDs reduce joint destruction and slow disease progression. They are classified as *nonbiologic DMARDs* or *biologic DMARDS*. DMARDs may be prescribed with a COX-2 inhibitor to obtain rapid symptom relief as well as joint preservation. The first choice among the DMARDs is usually the nonbiologic methotrexate. Other choices are leflunomide, hydroxychloroquine, cyclosporine, and sulfasalazine. Although all can have serious side effects, they generally are the safest of the DMARDs. The biologic DMARDs (biologic response modifiers, or BRMs) are immunosuppressive drugs that are usually given in combination with methotrexate. Biologic DMARDs work by interfering with some aspect of the inflammatory process. Examples of these drugs are etanercept (Enbrel), infliximab (Remicade), adalimumab (Humira), rituximab (Rituxan), and abatacept (Orencia). The nonbiologic agents are far less expensive than the biologic agents. Additional drugs will be noted with the conditions for which they are used. The DMARDs can generally have very serious adverse effects. Drugs that suppress the immune response put the patient at risk for overwhelming infection, so patients must be monitored for even mild symptoms. Patients should have immunizations updated before beginning therapy and should not receive immunizations while taking these drugs. Many of these drugs can be harmful to a developing embryo, so pregnancy should be avoided during and for a specified time after therapy (Table 43.2).

SURGICAL TREATMENT

Surgical interventions may be indicated for musculoskeletal disorders, such as degenerative joint disease and arthritis, fractures, and amputations. Specific interventions are discussed with the particular conditions in Chapters 44 to 46.

Table 43.2 Drugs Used to Treat Musculoskeletal Disorders

DRUG	USE AND ACTION	SIDE EFFECTS	NURSING INTERVENTIONS
First-Generation Nonsteroidal Antiinflammatory Drugs (NSAIDs)			
aspirin diclofenac sodium (Voltaren) ibuprofen (Motrin, Rufen) indomethacin (Indocin) naproxen (Naprosyn) nabumetone (Relafen)	Analgesic Antipyretic Antiinflammatory (inhibits prostaglandin synthesis) Decreases pain and deformity Inhibits platelet aggregation (clumping)	Gastrointestinal (GI) upset, GI bleeding because of anticoagulation (may be silent in older adults). Increased blood pressure (BP) because of fluid retention. Ototoxicity. Some may cause drowsiness.	Instruct patient to take with food or to take enteric-coated aspirin and report ringing in ears (tinnitus), abdominal pain, dark stools. Assess for bruising and bleeding. Caution patient not to take aspirin and NSAIDs concurrently and not to drive if drowsy.
Second-Generation NSAIDs: Selective Cyclooxygenase (COX)-2 Inhibitor			
celecoxib (Celebrex)	Analgesic Antipyretic Antiinflammatory (inhibits prostaglandin synthesis)	GI bleeding (less risk than first-generation NSAIDs), fatigue, dependent edema, nausea, increased BP because of fluid retention. Dizziness. FDA is studying for possible increased risk of MI, CVA, and death.	Administer with food or full glass of water. Remain in upright position 15 to 30 minutes after taking. Safety precautions if dizzy. Do not confuse with Celexa (antidepressant) or Cerebyx (injectable fosphenytoin to treat seizures). Do not use with aspirin, alcohol, or acetaminophen concurrently.
Glucocorticoids			
hydrocortisone (Cortef, Hydrocortone) hydrocortisone sodium succinate (Solu-Cortef, cortisol) cortisone acetate (Cortone) prednisone (Deltasone) prednisolone (Delta-Cortef)	Suppress normal immune response and inflammation Used in inflammatory and allergic conditions	Muscular weakness, nausea, anorexia, hypotension; sodium retention, hypokalemia; insomnia; nervousness; euphoria; rise in serum glucose. Osteoporosis. Increased susceptibility to infections.	Highest dose usually given in early morning; lowest dose given later in day to mimic normal secretion in body. Stress to patient need to adhere to prescribed schedule. Remember that glucocorticoids mask signs of infection. Observe for any unusual drainage, odors, and elevated temperatures. Must be tapered off rather than stopped abruptly.
Disease-Modifying Antirheumatic Drugs (DMARDs)			
Nonbiologic (First Choice) DMARDs			
methotrexate (Folex)	Treats rheumatoid (RA) and psoriatic arthritis. Mild immunosuppressant	Anorexia, nausea, vomiting, diarrhea. Toxic effects on oral tissues, liver, lungs, bone marrow, skin, and kidneys. Hemorrhage; hair loss.	Monitor periodic blood and urine studies to detect abnormalities of toxicity. Encourage fluid intake. Tell patient to avoid trauma because of risk of bleeding; to avoid people with infections; and to report bruising, bleeding, or signs of infection promptly.
hydroxychloroquine sulfate (Plaquenil)	Basis of antirheumatic effects unknown; may suppress antigens that trigger hypersensitivity reactions	Headache, nausea, vomiting, anorexia. Ocular toxicity. With prolonged therapy: bone marrow suppression, psychosis. Instruct patient to see an eye doctor while taking this drug.	Ask about known allergy to drug. Tell patient to report visual or hearing disturbances promptly. Monitor complete blood cell count (CBC) and liver function studies.

Table 43.2 Drugs Used to Treat Musculoskeletal Disorders—cont'd

DRUG	USE AND ACTION	SIDE EFFECTS	NURSING INTERVENTIONS
sulfasalazine (Azulfidine)	Antimicrobial, antiinflammatory Used to treat RA	Anorexia, nausea, vomiting, headache, oligospermia. Toxic effects on bone marrow, liver, kidneys. Rarely: anaphylaxis.	Monitor liver and kidney function. Ensure urine output of at least 1500 mL/day. Assess for bruising, jaundice, fever, sore throat. Tell patient to avoid direct sunlight.
leflunomide (Arava)	Treats active RA, retards structural damage Slows disease progression	Diarrhea, liver toxicity, hair loss. Teratogenic.	Monitor liver studies. Tell patient to report severe diarrhea. Known to cause fetal harm; women of childbearing age should avoid conception. Avoid alcohol consumption while on medication.
cyclosporine (Neoral)	Treats RA and psoriasis Also used to prevent rejection of transplanted organs Works by suppressing immune response	Tremors, oral candida, gum hyperplasia, hirsutism, infection, renal failure, electrolyte imbalances.	Monitor renal and liver function studies. Carefully follow directions for preparation of oral dose. Do not give with grapefruit juice. IV drug must be administered via glass container only. Advise patient to report any signs of infection, even if minor. Avoid pregnancy during and 12 weeks after therapy.
Biologic DMARDs (BRMs)			
etanercept (Enbrel)	Used to treat severe RA in adults who do not respond to other DMARDs Binds tumor necrosis factor (TNF), which is involved in immunity and inflammation	Injection site reaction, abdominal pain, heartburn, headache, dizziness, upper respiratory infections, cough.	Reconstitute supplied diluent, add to powder, swirl to mix (do not shake), and administer immediately. Use only clear, colorless solution. Do not mix with other drugs. Administer SC in upper arm, abdomen, or thigh. Rotate sites. Check injection site for redness, itching. Caution in people with recurring infections or people at risk for infections.
infliximab (Remicade)	A monoclonal antibody that neutralizes activity of TNF, which decreases inflammation Used to treat RA, Crohn disease	Anaphylaxis, anemia, tachycardia, GI distress, skin rash, headache, dizziness, depression, upper respiratory infections, muscle aches, painful urination, chest pain, hypotension, hypertension.	Given IV every 1 to 2 months in combination with methotrexate. 2-hour infusion. Reconstitute and use immediately. Monitor for signs of infection, especially upper respiratory tract infections. Cannot be infused in IV line with other agents.

Continued

Table 43.2 Drugs Used to Treat Musculoskeletal Disorders—cont'd

DRUG	USE AND ACTION	SIDE EFFECTS	NURSING INTERVENTIONS
adalimumab (Humira)	A monoclonal antibody that inhibits structural damage by blocking the action of TNF Used to treat rheumatoid and psoriatic arthritis	Injection site reaction (swelling and pain at injection site may last 4–5 days), flu-like symptoms, infection, headache, sinusitis, abdominal pain, nausea.	Stop treatment and notify physician if any signs of infection occur. For SC injection, do not mix with other drugs, do not use filter. DO protect from light. Rotate injection sites between abdomen, upper arms, and thighs; inject at 45-degree angle. Caution patient not to take immunizations while on Humira therapy.
anakinra (Kineret)	Decreases cartilage damage and bone loss by blocking action of interleukin-1 Used to treat severe RA	Injection site reaction (swelling and pain for 4–5 days), flu-like symptoms, infection, headache, sinusitis, abdominal pain, nausea, worsening of RA symptoms.	For SC injection, do not mix with other drugs, do not use filter. DO protect from light. Rotate injection sites between abdomen, upper arms, and thighs. Do not use if cloudy or discolored. No concurrent immunizations.
abatacept (Orencia)	Inhibits activation of T lymphocytes, which are necessary for inflammatory process in RA	Headache, dizziness, cough, back pain, nausea, hypertension. Serious infections.	Monitor for hypersensitivity (rare): dyspnea, hypotension. IV and SC routes. Prefilled syringes should be refrigerated. SC injection in anterior thigh, outer upper arm, or abdomen.
Antigout Medications			
allopurinol (Zyloprim) febuxostat (Uloric)	Inhibits synthesis of uric acid	Drowsiness. Toxicity: maculopapular rash, fever, chills, joint pain. Rarely: bone marrow depression, nausea, diarrhea.	Tell patient to drink 8 to 10 glasses of fluid daily to maintain output of at least 2000 mL/day. Assess urine for abnormal characteristics. Safety precautions if drowsy. Tell patient it takes several weeks for full effects. Assess and record response.
probenecid (Benemid)	Increases urinary excretion of uric acid	Headache, urinary frequency, GI distress. Rarely: anaphylaxis. Toxicity: maculopapular rash, fever, joint pain, leukopenia, GI distress. Urinary calculi (stones).	Assess allergies. Do not give with penicillin. Use caution with renal impairment. Encourage fluid intake to maintain output of at least 2000 mL/day. Tell patient it takes several weeks for full therapeutic effect.

Table 43.2 **Drugs Used to Treat Musculoskeletal Disorders—cont'd**

DRUG	USE AND ACTION	SIDE EFFECTS	NURSING INTERVENTIONS
Uricolytic			
pegloticase (Krystexxa)	Breaks uric acid down to readily excreted end product	Gout flare during initial treatment. Anaphylaxis. Infusion reaction: urticaria, dyspnea, pruritis, chest discomfort.	Administer only in a setting equipped to handle emergencies. Premedicate with an antihistamine and glucocorticoid to prevent anaphylaxis. If mild or moderate infusion reaction occurs, slow rate of infusion. If severe reaction, stop infusion.
Bone Resorption Inhibitors			
ibandronate sodium (Boniva)	Used to prevent and treat osteoporosis in postmenopausal women	Abdominal pain, hypertension, dyspepsia, arthralgia, nausea, diarrhea.	Main advantage is monthly dosing. Instruct patient to take on empty stomach upon arising. Do not eat or drink anything and remain upright for at least 60 minutes after each dose. Does not replace the need for adequate calcium and vitamin D intake. Contraindicated with uncorrected hypocalcemia.
alendronate sodium (Fosamax)	Increases bone mineral density by impairing bone resorption	Abdominal pain, muscle pain, diarrhea, constipation, severe GI disturbances with overdose, hypocalcemia.	Take with 6 to 8 oz water upon arising, nothing else by mouth for 30 minutes. Patient should not lie down for 30 minutes after taking.
calcitonin (Miacalcin)	Impairs bone resorption	With injections: hypotension, flushing, nausea, vomiting, sweating. With oral form: constipation, edema.	Monitor for hypercalcemia (dry mouth, constipation, headache, depression, weakness). Take tablets with full glass of water ½ to 1 hour after meals. Not to be taken with other oral medications, alcohol, or foods with fiber. Patient must avoid excess tobacco use and caffeine.
raloxifene (Evista)	Prevents bone loss and lowers cholesterol without stimulating endometrium Used to prevent osteoporosis in postmenopausal women	Frequent side effects: infection, flu syndrome, nausea, hot flashes, weight gain, joint pain, sinusitis, thrombosis.	Seek medical care for chest pain, dyspnea, changes in vision. Should not be taken during pregnancy, before menopause, or during periods of immobility.

BRM, Biologic response modifier; *CVA*, cerebrovascular accident; *FDA*, U.S. Food and Drug Administration; *IV*, intravenous; *MI*, myocardial infarction; *SC*, subcutaneous.

Get Ready for the NCLEX® Examination!

Key Points

- Major connective tissues are bone, blood, cartilage, ligaments, skin, and tendons.
- Age-related changes in connective tissue can have a significant effect on function and quality of life.
- Three categories of drugs are used in the treatment of arthritis: (1) NSAIDs, (2) glucocorticoids, and (3) DMARDs.
- Management of the patient with a musculoskeletal condition requires the services of a multidisciplinary team that includes the patient, nurse, physician, social worker, nutritionist, physical therapist, and occupational therapist.

Additional Learning Resources

SG Go to your Study Guide for additional learning activities to help you master this chapter content.

Go to your Evolve website (http://evolve.elsevier.com/Linton/medsurg) for the following learning resources and much more:
- Fluid & Electrolyte Tutorial
- Review Questions for the NCLEX® Examination

Clinical Judgment and Next-Generation NCLEX® Examination-Style Questions

1. **The joints between the bones of the skull are classified as which type of joint?**

   ____

   NCLEX Client Need: Physiological Integrity

2. **Age-related changes in connective tissue include which of the following? (Select all that apply.)**
   1. Hardening of bone tissue
   2. Decreased water content
   3. Loss of cartilage elasticity
   4. Development of bone spurs
   5. Loss of bone mass and density

   NCLEX Client Need: Physiological Integrity

3. **Take Action Using Matrix Test Item**

   A 63-year-old woman was seen at her health care provider's office because of pain in her left knee that was causing difficulty in getting up out of a chair, walking, and doing housework. A radiograph revealed that she had reduced amounts of cartilage that caused irritation and inflammation. The health care provider administered a glucocorticoid steroid injection into the joint to help relieve the pain and increase mobility.

   Use an X for the health teaching below that is *Indicated* (appropriate or necessary), *Contraindicated* (could be harmful), or *Nonessential* (makes no difference or not necessary) before the patient's discharge at this time.

HEALTH TEACHING	INDICATED	CONTRAINDICATED	NONESSENTIAL
"Take your antiinflammatory medications as prescribed"			
"Do deep knee bends to strengthen muscles and ligaments"			
"Try to rest. Don't overexert yourself"			
"Drink at least 8 glasses of water per day"			
"Maintain a positive attitude"			
"Adding carbohydrates to your diet will give you added energy"			
"Be aware of stressors in your life; here are a couple of relaxation techniques that you can use"			

Connective Tissue Disorders

44

http://evolve.elsevier.com/Linton/medsurg

Objectives

1. Describe the characteristics and prevalence of connective tissue diseases.
2. Describe the pathophysiology and treatment of osteoarthritis (degenerative joint disease), rheumatoid arthritis, osteoporosis, gout, progressive systemic sclerosis, polymyositis, bursitis, carpal tunnel syndrome, ankylosing spondylitis, polymyalgia rheumatica, Reiter syndrome, Behçet syndrome, and Sjögren syndrome.
3. Assist in developing a nursing care plan for a patient whose life has been affected by a connective tissue disease.

Key Terms

ankylosis (ăng-kĭ-LŌ-sĭs)
arthroplasty (ĂR-thrō-plăs-tē)
hyperuricemia (hī-pĕr-ŭr-ĭ-SĒ-mē-ă)
intraarticular (ĭn-tră-ăr-TĬK-ū-lăr)
rheumatoid nodule (ROO-mă-toyd NŎD-ūl)
tophi (TŌ-fī)
vasculitis (văs-kū-LĪ-tĭs)

According to the Centers for Disease Control and Prevention (CDC, 2020) data, an estimated 22.7% (54.4 million) adults aged 18 and older in the United States have been diagnosed with arthritis. There is a significantly higher prevalence in women (23.5%) than in men (18.1%), and the prevalence increases with age. Often called *rheumatoid disorders,* these conditions are chronic and are characterized by alternating exacerbations and remissions, with progressive deterioration. Many have no known cause or cure. Rheumatoid disorders challenge the body and spirit of a person. They dramatically alter the patient's lifestyle, self-image, employability, and hope for the future. A number of the conditions discussed in this chapter are classified as *autoimmune disorders.* They are included here because their primary effects are on connective tissue. For a thorough explanation of autoimmunity, see Chapter 5.

OSTEOARTHRITIS

Osteoarthritis (OA) is the most common type of arthritis affecting about 32.5 million Americans (CDC, 2020). Sometimes called *degenerative joint disease* or *"wear and tear" arthritis,* OA most frequently occurs in the hands, hips, knees, and spine. The cartilage and bones within a joint begin to break down, causing pain, stiffness, and swelling. These changes usually develop slowly and get worse over time. Risk factors for OA include:

- Joint injury or overuse, such as knee bending and repetitive stress on a joint
- Increased age
- Gender: women are more likely to develop OA than men, especially after age 50
- Obesity: extra weight puts more stress on weight-bearing joints, especially hips and knees; obesity may have metabolic effects that increase risk
- Genetics: family history of OA increases likelihood of occurrence; people with hand OA more likely to develop knee OA
- Race: some Asian populations have lower risk for OA

The most common source of major disability is osteoarthritis of the knee.

Osteoarthritis may be classified as *primary* or *secondary,* depending on the cause. In primary osteoarthritis, an unknown factor triggers the release of chemicals that break down joint cartilage. Osteoarthritis that occurs with aging is generally considered to be primary and may have a genetic basis (see the Cultural Considerations box). Secondary osteoarthritis may be associated with trauma, infection, congenital deformities, corticosteroid therapy, and a variety of other conditions including diabetes mellitus.

Cultural Considerations

What Does Culture Have to Do With Osteoarthritis?

The sites affected most often by osteoarthritis vary with ethnic background. For example, osteoarthritis of the hips is more common among people who live in Japan and Saudi Arabia than among Caucasians living in the United States.

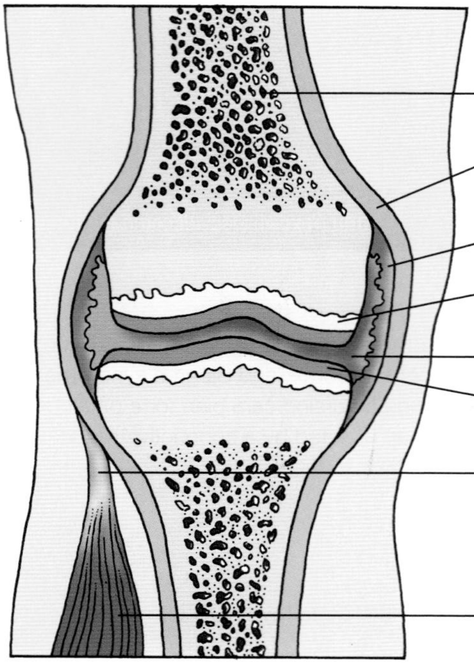

Fig. 44.1 The structure of a diarthrodial joint. Synovium lines the joint capsule but does not extend into the articular cartilage. (From Ignatavicius DD, Workman ML: *Medical-surgical nursing: patient-centered collaborative care*, ed 8, St. Louis, 2016, Saunders.)

PATHOPHYSIOLOGY

Osteoarthritis is characterized by the degeneration of articular cartilage with hypertrophy of the underlying and adjacent bone. Normally, the articular cartilage provides a smooth surface for one bone to glide over another (Fig. 44.1). The cartilage transfers the weight of one bone to another so that the bones do not shatter. Deterioration of the articular cartilage means that the shock-absorbing protection is gradually lost. New bone growth is stimulated by exposed bone surfaces, causing bone spurs to develop. Although osteoarthritis generally is classified as a *noninflammatory condition*, tissue breakdown can cause inflammation of the joint in advanced conditions.

CLINICAL MANIFESTATIONS

Joint pain is the primary symptom of OA and is what usually brings the patient to the health care provider. The pain commonly is associated with activity and relieved by rest. However, in advanced disease, the pain may occur at rest and can interfere with sleep. A fall in barometric pressure in the atmosphere before the onset of severe weather also may precipitate pain. Along with pain in the affected joint, the patient with osteoarthritis may complain of stiffness, limitation of movement, mild tenderness, swelling, and deformity or enlargement of the joint (Fig. 44.2).

Unlike joint pain, joint stiffness occurs after periods of rest, especially in the morning, and is relieved by activity within about 30 minutes. OA usually is asymmetrical, that is, occurring on one side of the body. For

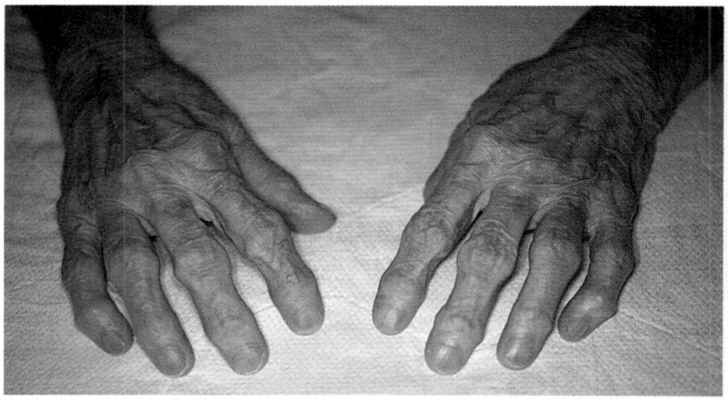

Fig. 44.2 Osteoarthritis (degenerative joint disease): Heberden nodes at the distal interphalangeal joints and Bouchard nodes at the proximal interphalangeal joints. (From Swartz M: *Textbook of physical diagnosis: history and examination*, ed 6, Philadelphia, 2009, Saunders.)

example, a patient may experience OA in the left knee and the right hip, or in the third finger of the right hand and the second finger in the left. Sometimes the symptoms subside for long periods of time, and then return. The disease may affect a single joint or only a few joints.

MEDICAL DIAGNOSIS

The diagnosis of osteoarthritis is based on the health history and radiographic studies. In the early stages of the disease, the patient may have no symptoms, even though radiographs reveal classic joint changes. From radiographic evidence, 68% of women older than 65 years of age have osteoarthritis. The incidence is slightly lower for men of the same age. The extent of the disease process is not necessarily related to the severity of symptoms.

Because plain radiographs do not always reveal cartilage abnormalities, arthroscopy, magnetic resonance imaging (MRI), scintigraphy, and ultrasonography may be used. Synovial fluid may be aspirated to assess the presence of leukocytes. With OA, there should be a normal erythrocyte sedimentation rate (ESR), negative rheumatoid factor (RF) assay, and synovial fluid with few or no leukocytes. However, it is not unusual for a healthy older person to have a slightly elevated ESR and low titers of RF and antinuclear antibody (ANA).

MEDICAL TREATMENT

No known cure exists for osteoarthritis, but much can be done to make the patient more comfortable. The goals of patient therapy are to reduce the pain to a manageable level, maintain as much mobility as possible, and minimize disability.

Medical treatment includes physical measures, education, drug therapy, and surgery. For some patients, diet and counseling are indicated. Referral to a pain specialist may be indicated if conservative measures are not effective. The course of the treatment is dictated by the individual patient's condition and response.

Physical Measures

A physical therapy program uses measures to improve range of motion and to maintain muscle mass and strength. Maintaining muscle mass reduces the load on joint cartilage. Most patients, especially those with mild osteoarthritis, benefit from such a program. Isometric exercises are recommended over isotonic exercises because isotonic movements place increased strain on the joints. Exercise should be followed by periods of rest during the day. When the hips or knees are affected, some activity restriction may be advised. Wearing cushioned shoes and using a cane to walk reduces the stress on the affected joints.

Cold compresses and moist heat applications can be used to help relieve pain, depending on patient preferences. Heat also prepares the muscles and joints for exercise. Transcutaneous electrical nerve stimulation (TENS) devices often are effective for treating back pain.

Drug Therapy

Although drug therapy is not curative, the pain of osteoarthritis frequently can be controlled with nonopioid analgesics such as acetaminophen or nonsteroidal antiinflammatory drugs (NSAIDs). NSAIDs may decrease pain and improve mobility in patients with osteoarthritis, but their side effects are more dangerous than those of acetaminophen. People who should be cautioned about taking NSAIDs are those over age 65 years; have asthma; have had an allergic reaction to NSAIDs in the past; have hypertension; have had stomach ulcers; or have any cardiac, renal, liver, circulatory or bowel problems. Possible side effects of NSAIDs are indigestion, stomach ulcers, headaches, drowsiness, dizziness, and allergic reactions. NSAIDs are especially effective when the patient shows signs of inflammation, such as warmth, swelling of joints, and erythema (redness). Similar to NSAIDs, indomethacin (Indocin) is effective in reducing inflammation but may cause serious adverse effects.

Salicylates are relatively inexpensive, but a risk of toxicity exists. The symptoms of salicylate intoxication in older adults may be atypical. Instead of the common gastrointestinal (GI) complaints or ototoxicity, the older person may exhibit confusion, slurring of speech, agitation, or seizures.

Complementary and Alternative Therapies

Glucosamine and chondroitin supplements are popular with the public; however, studies of their effectiveness in treating osteoarthritis have had inconsistent results. Turmeric (curcumin) may help to alleviate pain or discomfort. Topical treatments include capsaicin, Voltaren (diclofenac sodium), and Arnica gel or cream.

Pharmacology Capsule

First-generation nonsteroidal antiinflammatory drugs (NSAIDs) can cause significant gastrointestinal (GI) ulcers and bleeding.

Pharmacology Capsule

Salicylate toxicity may be manifested by tinnitus or, in older adults, by confusion, agitation, slurred speech, or seizures.

Injections. When oral medications do not relieve knee pain, but a patient is not ready to have surgery, **intraarticular** injections can be beneficial.

Hyaluronic acid supplements. Hyaluronic acid is injected into knee joints to supplement naturally occurring hyaluronic acid that may break down. In healthy joints, hyaluronic acid acts as a shock absorber and lubricant, allowing joints to move smoothly over each other. Injecting it into a joint may lessen pain and inflammation. The injections are given weekly for 3 or 5 weeks, depending on the product (examples are Synvisc and Hyalgan). A small amount of joint fluid is removed first to make room for the hyaluronic acid.

Corticosteroid injections. Corticosteroids are injected directly into the knee joint for quick relief of pain and inflammation. Their benefits may last anywhere from a few days to more than six months. With repeated injections, the corticoid steroids may contribute to cartilage breakdown, so that they may be limited to 3 to 4 times a year.

Arthrocentesis. Also called joint fluid aspiration, arthrocentesis is removal of fluid from the joint space of the knee. Removing the excess fluid can ease pain and swelling.

◆ NURSING CARE OF THE PATIENT WITH OSTEOARTHRITIS

ASSESSMENT

General nursing assessment of the patient with a connective tissue disorder is summarized in Chapter 43, Box 43.2. When a patient has osteoarthritis, ask about joint pain or tenderness and examine the joints for crepitus, enlargement, deformity, and decreased range of motion. It is helpful to compare affected and unaffected joints to detect abnormalities. Gently support joints during the examination to minimize the patient's discomfort. Observe the patient's movements and gait, noting abnormalities, and record the location and severity of any problems. Determine how the disease affects the patient's mobility and ability to perform activities of daily living (ADLs) (Box 44.1).

Patient Problems, Goals, and Outcome Criteria: Osteoarthritis

Patient Problems	Goals and Outcome Criteria
Chronic pain with motion related to loss of smooth joint surfaces	Pain relief: patient states pain is reduced or relieved, as noted on a 1 to 10 pain scale; relaxed manner
Decreased mobility related to pain, limited range of motion	Improved functional mobility: patient accomplishes activities of daily living (ADLs) with minimal discomfort

Continued

Patient Problems, Goals, and Outcome Criteria: Osteoarthritis—cont'd

Patient Problems	Goals and Outcome Criteria
Inadequate coping related to pain, discomfort, disability	Adequate coping: patient states is able to make adaptations to cope with condition, makes positive comments about ability to manage
Lack of knowledge related to lack of understanding of osteoarthritis management and self-care	Patient manages disease appropriately: patient demonstrates self-care measures and describes prescribed regimen

Box 44.1 Nursing Assessment for Osteoarthritis

SUBJECTIVE
- Pain (severity, occurrence)
- Stiffness
- Rest and activity
- Sleep disturbance
- Stress and coping
- Knowledge of condition

OBJECTIVE
- Joint crepitus, enlargement, deformity
- Range of motion
- Comparison of affected and unaffected joints
- Movements and gait
- Mobility
- Joint swelling and warmth
- Ability to perform activities of daily living

Interventions

Chronic pain. With good pain management, a patient can be more active and have a better quality of life. Administer analgesic and antiinflammatory drugs as prescribed, or instruct the patient in self-medication. In addition, instruct the patient in heat or cold treatments as ordered, and monitor and record the effects of interventions designed to relieve pain. It is important to inform the physician if pain relief measures are ineffective. Measures that protect the joint, discussed in the next section ("Decreased Physical Mobility"), also help to reduce chronic pain. Although it is not unusual for hospitalized patients to have osteoarthritis, most patients manage their own symptoms at home (see the Cultural Considerations box). Thus everyday management depends on good patient teaching.

Cultural Considerations

What Does Culture Have to Do With Chronic Illness?

How people react to chronic illness, disability, and dependence is related to their cultural values and beliefs. Consider an older Japanese American patient who values family interdependence over independence, a Mexican American patient who accepts illness as God's will, or a person of German heritage who faces pain stoically. Each of these may handle osteoarthritis differently. Nurses must consider these factors when planning patient care.

Decreased mobility. Decreased physical mobility can significantly interfere with the patient's ability to carry out usual activities in the home or work setting. Modification of daily activities and joint protection measures can help to maintain function. Recommend a regular program of exercise to maintain muscle mass. Aerobic, muscle-strengthening, and water-based exercises are appropriate. The patient who is overweight can benefit from weight loss to reduce stress on joints. Emphasize the importance of balancing rest and activity to avoid becoming overly tired. The household may need to be reorganized to reduce demands on the patient. Everyday tasks such as dressing and bathing may be affected by the disorder. If the patient's hands are affected, suggest clothing with Velcro closures rather than buttons, pants with an elastic waist, and slip-on shoes. Bathroom grab bars, a shower seat, and a raised toilet seat may promote independence and safety for the patient with poor hip mobility.

Inadequate coping. Give the patient an opportunity to discuss concerns about osteoarthritis and its effects on lifestyle. Help the patient to prioritize activities and plan how to continue those activities that are most valued. Practical suggestions for managing the condition help the patient to feel a sense of control and confidence in their ability to live with the condition.

Lack of knowledge. Determine what the patient already knows about osteoarthritis and correct any misconceptions. Design and implement an individualized teaching plan (see the Patient Teaching box).

Patient Teaching

Osteoarthritis

To reduce joint strain and pain, tell the patient the following:
- Maintain proper posture and body alignment.
- Attain and maintain a healthy body weight.
- Identify activities that take a long time to do or for which you need assistance.
- Plan activities when help is available or when time is not a major concern and take periodic rest breaks.
- Wear splints or support devices that rest or relieve painful, unstable joints.
- Push or slide heavy objects rather than pull them.
- Wear shoes with low heels and shock-absorbent soles to help decrease stress on the knee joints.
- Avoid stairs whenever possible.
- Sit rather than stand.
- Use high stools when sitting at a counter.
- Use higher chairs rather than low sofas.
- When rising from a chair, inch to the edge of the seat, and then use the armrests to push up from the seat.
- Use large-diameter pencils and pens, and use eating utensils with large, round handles.

SELF-MEDICATION
- Analgesics are usually more effective if taken routinely as prescribed rather than only when you have pain.
- Identify the side effects of your medications, and notify your physician if they occur (provide specific list).
- Resource: Arthritis Foundation (www.arthritis.org; telephone: 1-800-283-7800).

Surgical management. Surgical management usually is reserved for persons with persistent pain and disability despite conservative treatment. Arthroscopic surgery that removes loose bodies and repairs defects may be useful for patients with osteoarthritis of the knee, shoulder, ankle, and spine. The surgical treatment of choice for osteoarthritis of the hip or knee is total joint replacement (**arthroplasty**). The primary indication for total joint replacement is intractable pain that disrupts sleep and daily activities. Total hip or knee arthroplasty usually relieves pain and restores function to the joint (Fig. 44.3). Some experts recommend delaying joint replacement until 60 years of age because of the risk of prosthesis failure during the expected lifetime. Others believe that most modern prostheses are durable enough to be implanted in younger persons. Prosthesis failure is most often characterized by loosening of the joint implant. A recent development is minimally invasive joint replacement surgery. This type of procedure requires a much smaller incision than the traditional approach. Some minimally invasive joint replacement procedures are done in outpatient surgical settings.

TOTAL JOINT REPLACEMENT

Although joints that can be replaced include the elbow, shoulder, phalangeal finger joints, hip, knee, and ankle, knee and hip arthroplasty are the most common.

TOTAL KNEE ARTHROPLASTY

Total knee arthroplasty (TKA), also known as total knee replacement, is one of the most common joint replacement procedures. The surgery can result in significant pain relief, as well as improved function and quality of life. Over 95% of TKAs in the United States are performed for osteoarthritis.

The surgical procedure is done with general anesthesia or neuraxial anesthesia (i.e., spinal, epidural, or combined spinal epidural). The prosthesis is composed of metal and polyethylene, and consists of three components: femoral, tibial, and patellar. Cement is used to fix the prosthesis to the bone. During the surgery, a large tourniquet is used to control bleeding and to provide a drier area for cement fixation at the surgical site. The risks postoperatively for tourniquet use are venous thrombosis, increased pain, and reduced early range of motion with a potential delay in early rehabilitation. The site of the tourniquet placement on the thigh above the surgical site may appear massively bruised with blue/black coloration. Postoperative management focuses on pain management, prevention of venous thromboembolism (VTE), and appropriate physical therapy to achieve the best possible knee motion and return to full function as safely as possible.

Patients usually are mobilized the day of surgery, and with the aid of a physical therapist, can walk with assistive devices the day after surgery. Hospitalization can vary from 0 to 5 days, depending on the patient and the surgeon. Recently, TKA is being performed on an outpatient basis for selected low-risk patients, who are then discharged directly to their home. A well-structured rehabilitation program with range of motion exercises, gait training, quadriceps strengthening, and training in activities of daily living is required for a successful outcome following a TKA. Clinical improvement generally occurs between 6 and 12 weeks postoperatively; a full recovery occurs between 1 and 2 years postoperatively.

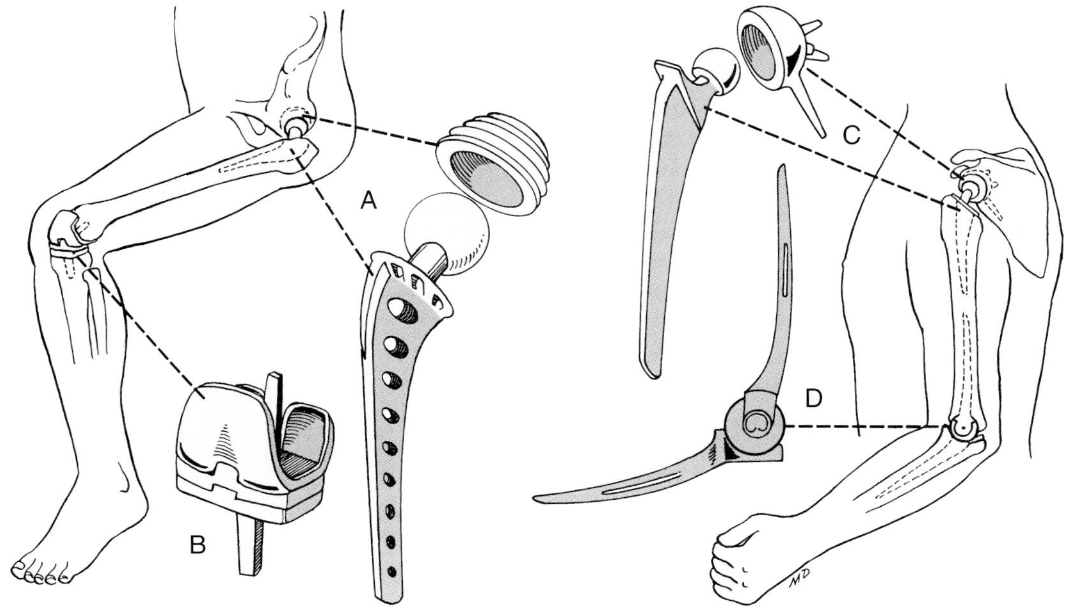

Fig. 44.3 Total joint replacements. (A) Hip. (B) Knee. (C) Shoulder. (D) Elbow. (From Black JM, Matassarin-Jacobs E: *Luckmann and Sorenson's medical-surgical nursing: a psychophysiologic approach*, ed 4, Philadelphia, 1993, Saunders.)

TOTAL HIP ARTHROPLASTY

Total hip arthroplasty (THA), also known as total hip replacement, is one of the most successful orthopedic procedures performed today. Over 370,000 THAs are performed in the United States each year. THA is an elective surgery that can relieve pain, restore function, and improve quality of life.

All patients undergoing THA usually receive prophylactic antibiotics and thromboprophylaxis to prevent infection and thrombi. Surgery is performed with general, regional, or neuraxial anesthesia (i.e., spinal, epidural, or combined spinal epidural). The hip arthroplasties consist of femoral and acetabular components, and a bearing surface, that are made up of metal and metal and polyethylene. Cement may or may not be used for fixation of the prosthesis. Substantial blood loss is estimated at approximately 1000 mL during hip replacement surgery, so tranexamic acid, an antifibrinolytic agent may be given intravenously at the start of the surgery and/or postoperatively. Postoperative management is focused on pain management and prevention of venous thromboembolism. The hospital length of stay is typically 1 to 3 days postoperatively; however, the surgery is increasingly performed in an outpatient setting. Rehabilitation generally is started immediately to promote mobilization, recovery of function, and prevention of deep vein thrombosis (DVT). Exercises to restore normal hip motion and strength and a gradual return to normal activities are initiated in the hospital and continued upon discharge. Improvement and minimal pain take place about 3 months postoperatively; further improvement can occur up to a year after surgery.

◆ NURSING CARE AFTER TOTAL JOINT REPLACEMENT

Preoperative care prepares the patient for the surgical procedure and the postoperative period. Nurses and physical therapists may instruct the patient in postoperative exercises. It is helpful to advise the patient and family of postoperative limitations and encourage planning to adapt the home and work environment as needed.

General nursing care of the surgical patient is discussed in Chapter 17. This section describes the postoperative nursing care needs of the patient who has had a joint replacement. Surgical orders or protocols are usually very specific for each type of joint surgery and may vary somewhat among surgeons. Common postoperative measures for specific procedures are presented in Box 44.2.

FOCUSED ASSESSMENT

Routine postoperative care includes monitoring vital signs, level of consciousness, intake and output, respiratory and neurovascular status, urinary function, bowel elimination, wound condition, comfort, and preventing complications of immobility. After total joint replacement, it is especially important to monitor circulation and sensation in the affected extremity and to determine the need for assistance with ADLs.

Box 44.2 Guidelines for Nursing Care After Replacement of Specific Joints

HIP REPLACEMENT

1. Do not flex hip more than 90 degrees.
2. Avoid flexion, adduction, and internal rotation.
3. Place a large pillow between the patient's legs when turning the patient, when the patient is supine, and when the patient is lying on unaffected side.
4. Advise the patient not to cross the legs or feet and not to put on their own shoes, socks, or stockings for 6 weeks to 2 months, as directed by the surgeon.
5. Apply leg abductor splints as ordered.
6. Do not turn onto the operative side unless specifically ordered to do so by the surgeon.
7. Have the patient sit in a chair that has arms to facilitate rising without extreme hip flexion.
8. Arrange for a raised toilet seat to allow toileting without extreme hip flexion.
9. Permit weight bearing as ordered, depending on type of prosthesis used and whether cement was used.
10. Encourage the patient to exercise the unaffected extremities to maintain strength.

KNEE REPLACEMENT

1. Encourage quadriceps-setting exercises and straight leg lifts beginning on postoperative day 2 to 5, as ordered.
2. Monitor weight bearing with walker or crutches as ordered.

FINGER JOINT REPLACEMENT

1. Instruct the patient to elevate the affected hand.
2. Assess sensation and warmth in the affected fingers.
3. Instruct the patient to use splints during sleep as ordered.
4. Reinforce exercises taught by the physical therapist—must be continued for 10 to 12 weeks.
5. Advise the patient not to lift heavy objects with the affected hand.

Patient Problems, Goals, and Outcome Criteria: Total Joint Replacement, Postoperative

Patient Problems	Goals and Outcome Criteria
Acute pain related to tissue trauma	Pain relief: patient states pain is reduced and less than 4 on a 1 to 10 pain scale; relaxed expression
Potential for injury related to improper alignment, dislocated prosthesis, weakness	Prevent injury: patient maintains proper alignment of operative joint
Decreased mobility related to immobilization, pain, weakness	Maintain mobility without complications of immobility: patient is increasingly mobile without excess fatigue or injury, absence of pressure injuries

Patient Problems, Goals, and Outcome Criteria: Total Joint Replacement, Postoperative—cont'd

Patient Problems	Goals and Outcome Criteria
Inadequate peripheral circulation related to peripheral trauma, hemorrhage, thrombi, compression of blood vessels	Normal circulation to affected extremity: symmetric color and warmth of extremities, palpable pulse in affected limb
Potential for infection related to invasive procedure, prosthesis placement	Absence of infection: normal body temperature, decreasing wound redness, normal white blood cell (WBC) count
Anxiety related to outcome of procedure	Reduced anxiety: patient states anxiety is reduced, calm manner
Ineffective self-care management related to postoperative care needs	Patient manages postoperative self-care: patient describes and demonstrates self-care

Interventions

Acute pain. To assist with assessment of the patient's pain, ask about pain location, nature, and severity. Surgical pain is expected, but the patient with osteoarthritis may also have pain in other joints. If the patient has patient-controlled analgesia, reinforce instructions for its use. Administer analgesics as ordered, and document their effects. Reposition the patient as permitted by physician's orders. Use massage, relaxation techniques, imagery, or other strategies to help the patient deal with pain. Notify the surgeon of any sudden, severe pain in the surgical area, which may signal prosthesis dislocation. Uncontrolled pain may make the patient reluctant to participate in rehabilitation measures. Administer analgesics 30 minutes to 1 hour before painful exercises to improve patient participation.

Potential for injury. Prosthetic joints can become dislocated if they are not maintained in proper alignment. For example, after hip replacement, the affected leg must be kept in a position of abduction to prevent dislocation. Instruct patients not to cross the legs or flex the hip more than 90 degrees. Splints or traction may be used if ordered to maintain the desired position. Progressive exercises are usually prescribed and may be done by the physical therapist. As the patient's activity is increased, teach and reinforce precautions. Instruct the patient to recognize signs and symptoms of dislocation, including an audible pop, pain in the affected joint, loss of function, and shortening or deformity of the extremity.

Decreased mobility. The degree of mobility depends on which joints are affected, as well as on the patient's general physical state. In general, early mobility is encouraged. When mobility is severely decreased, the patient is at risk for pulmonary and circulatory complications, urine retention, constipation, and skin breakdown. In addition, unused muscles weaken, and unused joints stiffen. Reposition the patient as allowed, carefully inspecting pressure areas for redness caused by circulatory impairment. In addition, coach and support the patient during coughing and deep-breathing exercises and use of the incentive spirometer. Auscultate for breath sounds to detect atelectasis or retained secretions and inspect and palpate the abdomen for bladder or bowel distention. Administer intravenous fluids as ordered until the patient takes adequate oral fluids. Give stool softeners and laxatives as ordered.

The patient may have self-care deficits related to mobility impairments or restrictions. It is vital to identify activities the patient cannot do alone and to provide appropriate assistance. As the patient progresses, encourage increasing independence. Rehabilitation requires patient participation in the prescribed exercise program. The patient may need reassurance that the joint can and should be exercised. Patients are discharged as soon as 1 day after joint replacement surgery. Individuals who may have difficulty at home may go to a rehabilitation facility initially.

Inadequate peripheral circulation. DVT is the most serious postoperative complication of hip and knee replacement surgery. Signs and symptoms of DVT include tenderness, swelling, redness, warmth, and firm, palpable blood vessels called *cords*. Monitor body areas distal to the operative joint for circulatory adequacy by collecting data about skin temperature, color, and peripheral pulses. To reduce the risk of DVT in the legs, antiembolic stockings or pneumatic compression devices may be ordered in addition to anticoagulant drugs. Check splints, dressings, and stockings to ensure that they are not restricting circulation. Do not place pillows or pads under the legs. Determine the specific exercises that may be done, based on the health care provider's orders and protocols. For example, after hip replacement, the patient should flex and extend the toes, feet, and ankles hourly to promote venous return. Coach the patient in prescribed exercises.

The patient is at risk for hemorrhage after joint replacement. Check the dressings and wound drainage for increasing bleeding. In addition, monitor vital signs for tachycardia and hypotension, and observe for restlessness and anxiety. Inspect and measure wound drainage in suction devices at least every 8 hours. A risk of fat embolus exists, which can produce signs of local or cerebral blood vessel occlusion (i.e., petechial [pinpoint] hemorrhage of the upper chest and conjunctiva, fat globules in the urine, headache, irritability, confusion, loss of consciousness).

Pressure caused by edema or constrictive dressings can cause nerve damage, which may be manifested by anesthesia (lack of sensation) or paresthesia (abnormal sensation). Thus monitor sensation distal to the joint and report symptoms of impairment to the surgeon.

In addition, check dressings, stockings, and splints to ensure that they are not too tight.

Supervise ambulation until the patient is steady and clearly understands their limitations. Keep the environment free of clutter to prevent falls.

Potential for infection. Monitor the patient's temperature for elevation that may indicate infection. Check the surgical wound for redness, swelling, warmth, and foul-smelling drainage. Use strict sterile technique when handling the wound, drains, or dressings, and keep wound dressings clean and dry. Administer antimicrobials as ordered, and instruct the patient in hand washing and wound care.

Anxiety. Total joint replacement is usually done after conservative treatments have failed to maintain joint mobility. The patient is typically hopeful but anxious about the outcome of the surgery. Tell the patient what to expect, explain procedures and equipment, and offer to answer questions. Responding promptly to the patient's needs and checking on them frequently is reassuring.

Inadequate self-care. From admission through discharge, teach the patient about self-care, wound care, and signs of possible infection (see the Patient Teaching box). Ensure understanding by having patients repeat important information in their own words. Before teaching, assess for pain, fatigue, or communication barriers. Recognizing cultural differences in lifestyle, diet, and care issues is important. Assist patients in planning for care at home, and involve family members in teaching sessions.

Patient Teaching

Total Joint Replacement

Specifics of the teaching plan depend on which joint was replaced, but all patients need to know the following:

- Activities that are permitted
- Activities that are contraindicated
- Directions for drug therapy
- Wound care
- Signs and symptoms to be reported to the health care provider
- When to return for follow-up care
- Sources of assistance such as home health care

INTERVERTEBRAL OSTEOARTHRITIS

Osteoarthritis may cause changes in the structure of the spinal vertebrae and discs, particularly at L5–S1 and C3–C7. Arthritic changes include spinal stenosis (narrowing of the spinal canal), bone spurs, calcification of spinal ligaments, and disc degeneration. A degenerated disc can lead to a herniation (herniated or slipped disc), in which a spinal disc bulges outward between the vertebrae. These changes can narrow the space around the spinal canal and nerve roots, producing compression and inflammation. The inflammation precipitates pain, weakness, and numbness. The pain in the lumbar region starts in the lower back and radiates to the buttocks and legs. In the cervical region, the pain radiates to the arms and hands.

Medical diagnosis is achieved by means of history and physical exam, radiography, CT scan, MRI, discography, myelogram or electromyogram (EMG) (see Chapter 43, Table 43.1). Medical treatment is similar to other joint problems associated with osteoarthritis, including mild analgesics such as NSAIDs for pain and stiffness; antidepressants, particularly duloxetine (Cymbalta) for pain and sleep problems; and the antiseizure medication, gabapentin (Neurontin) for possible improvement in walking and to relieve leg symptoms (see Chapter 43, Table 43.2). Also recommended are weight reduction, rest periods, local heat and cold application, and exercise and activity. Biofeedback, acupuncture, and yoga are complementary therapies that may help to relieve pain. Epidural corticosteroid injections provide some pain relief as well.

Surgery is performed if the medical interventions fail to provide adequate pain relief and mobility. Minimally invasive spinal surgery (MISS) has become the surgical treatment of choice for qualified patients in recent years. MISS is used for conditions such as herniated disc, spinal stenosis, spinal deformities (scoliosis), spinal instability, spondylolysis in the lower vertebrae, fractured vertebrae, excision of spinal tumor, and spinal infection. With open surgery, a long vertical incision is made, and the muscles and soft tissue around the spine are moved away with possible tissue excision. During MISS, a smaller incision is made, after which a tubular retractor (a stiff, tube-shaped tool) is inserted that creates a tunnel to the problem area of the spine. Muscle and soft tissue around the area are gently pushed aside, then small tools are put through the tunnel to work on the spine. This procedure is called microdiscectomy tubular retraction (MITR). A discectomy to remove a damaged or herniated disc as well as scraping or removing burn spurs can be performed. MISS and MITR frequently are executed in an outpatient setting, although some patients may be hospitalized for 1 or 2 days.

Patients may go home about 2 hours postoperatively. They should eat a well-balanced diet and drink plenty of fluids. A back brace may be worn when the patient is out of bed. Some health care providers may encourage the use of Plasma Flow calf sleeves for the first 2 to 3 days postoperatively to prevent deep vein thromboses. This is accomplished by pumps that deliver a set amount of air to the leg cuffs that compress the calves to aid blood flow. The sleeves also may be worn on airplane or long road trips to prevent thrombi. All heavy activity should be avoided, with no bending, lifting, or twisting (easily remembered with the acronym BLT). Patients are encouraged to take short walks, gradually building up time and distance. Driving is off-limits until the health care provider gives approval.

Pain management is important because healing is faster when pain is kept under control. Pain may be dull, stabbing, cramping, throbbing, constant, or intermittent. The health care provider may prescribe a strong pain medication such as morphine, but NSAIDs or acetaminophen may be sufficient. Other pain management measures include application of heat or cold compresses to the surgical site, relaxation techniques, aromatherapy, and pillows for added support.

RHEUMATOID ARTHRITIS

Rheumatoid arthritis (RA) is a chronic, progressive inflammatory disease. Although it is a systemic disorder, the most notable effect of RA is on diarthroses (synovial joints). The disease may occur at any time but has a peak onset in people 30 to 60 years of age and is more common in women than in men. It affects over 1.3 million Americans and as much as 1% of the worldwide population. The course of the disease is variable, ranging from minimal symptoms to severe debilitation.

PATHOPHYSIOLOGY

No single cause of RA is known, but it is considered an autoimmune disorder. Among the proposed triggers for RA are antigens in the patient's system, viruses or bacteria, genetic predisposition, environmental factors, and hormonal factors. Smoking appears to be a factor contributing to RA for people with a certain antigen. Research to determine the exact cause continues, but many recent discoveries have improved the lives of RA patients.

Onset of the disease symptoms is characterized by synovitis (inflammation of the synovial tissues, which hold the lubricating fluid of the joints). In RA, the synovium becomes thickened and fluid accumulates in the joint space. Vascular granulation tissue, called *pannus*, forms in the joint capsule and breaks down cartilage and bone. Fibrous tissue invades the pannus, converting it first to rigid scar tissue, and finally to bony tissue. These changes result in **ankylosis** (loss of joint mobility) (Fig. 44.4). Other than joint effects,

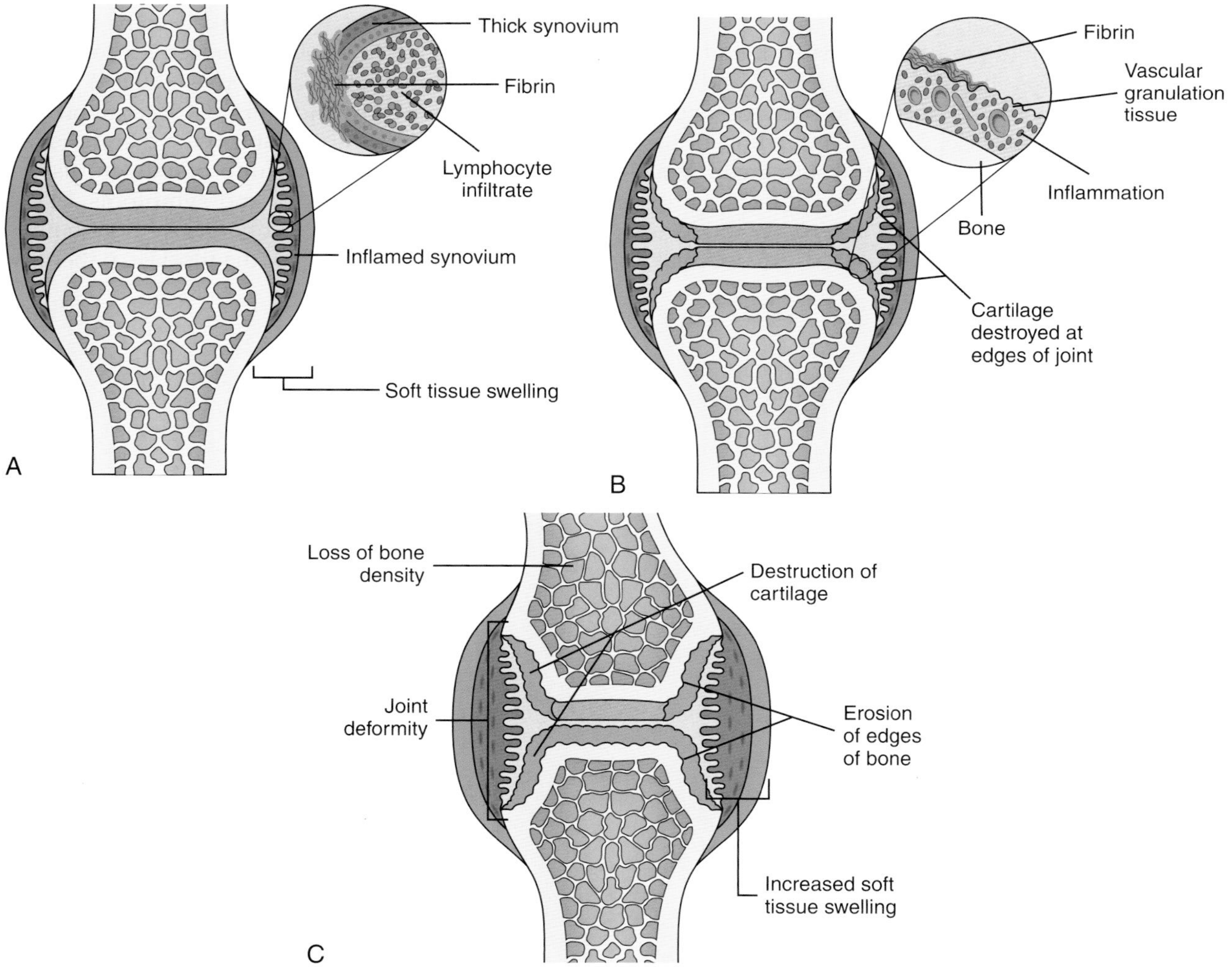

Fig. 44.4 Phases in the progression of rheumatoid arthritis. (A) Early phase: leukocytes increase in inflamed synovium. (B) Pannus grows over the cartilage; bone edges erode; destruction of articular tissue. (C) Destruction of bone. (From Stevens A, Lowe J: *Pathology: illustrated review in color*, ed 2, London, 2000, Mosby.)

RA can be manifested in rheumatoid nodules, diminished lacrimal and salivary secretions, inflammation of the eye, enlargement of the spleen and lymph nodes, pulmonary disease, and blood dyscrasias. **Rheumatoid nodules** are firm, nontender masses that develop on the fingers, elbows, base of the spine, back of the head, sclera, and lungs.

CLINICAL MANIFESTATIONS

The most common symptom of RA is pain in the affected joints that is aggravated by movement. Morning stiffness lasting more than 1 hour is almost always a feature of RA, unlike the stiffness of osteoarthritis, which is relieved within minutes. Other symptoms include weakness, easy fatigability, anorexia, weight loss, muscle aches and tenderness, and warmth and swelling of the affected joints. Joint changes are usually symmetric, meaning that the same joints in both extremities are affected simultaneously. The distal interphalangeal and metacarpophalangeal joints are affected most often. The wrist, elbow, knee, and ankle are other possible areas affected. Rheumatoid nodules, which are subcutaneous nodules over bony prominences, also may be present (Fig. 44.5).

RA can affect any organ of the body. If blood vessels are affected, they become inflamed, a condition called **vasculitis**. The blood supply to body organs is impaired, with possible ischemia or infarction of affected organs. Ischemic lesions of the skin are brownish spots most often seen around the nail beds. Large lesions that tend to ulcerate may appear on the legs. Secondary effects on bone can cause osteoporosis, making the bones susceptible to fractures. The disease may produce inflammatory changes in the tissues of the heart, lungs, kidneys, and eyes. Pleural effusions and pulmonary fibrosis can lead to respiratory impairment or pulmonary hypertension and eventual heart failure.

Some patients with RA develop clusters of symptoms, including Sjögren syndrome, Felty syndrome, or Caplan syndrome. Sjögren syndrome is characterized by dryness of the mouth, eyes, and vagina. Felty syndrome, characterized by liver and spleen enlargement and neutropenia, is less common. Caplan syndrome, marked by rheumatoid nodules in the lungs, occurs most often in coal miners and asbestos workers.

MEDICAL DIAGNOSIS

The diagnosis of RA is based on the health history and physical examination, laboratory findings, and changes detected on radiographic and other imaging studies. No single test diagnoses RA, but groups of tests and radiographic findings help to confirm the disorder. See Chapter 43, Table 43.1 for common studies for connective tissue disorders.

Laboratory studies that are likely to be ordered include rheumatoid factor, ESR, C-reactive protein (CRP), anticitrullinated protein antibodies (ACPA), and anticyclic citrullinated peptide (anti-CCP) antibodies. The presence of RF does not establish the diagnosis of RA; however, its presence may support a diagnosis in persons who have other signs and symptoms. The CRP level, ESR, and anti-CCP antibodies, although not specific, also help to support the diagnosis in patients with

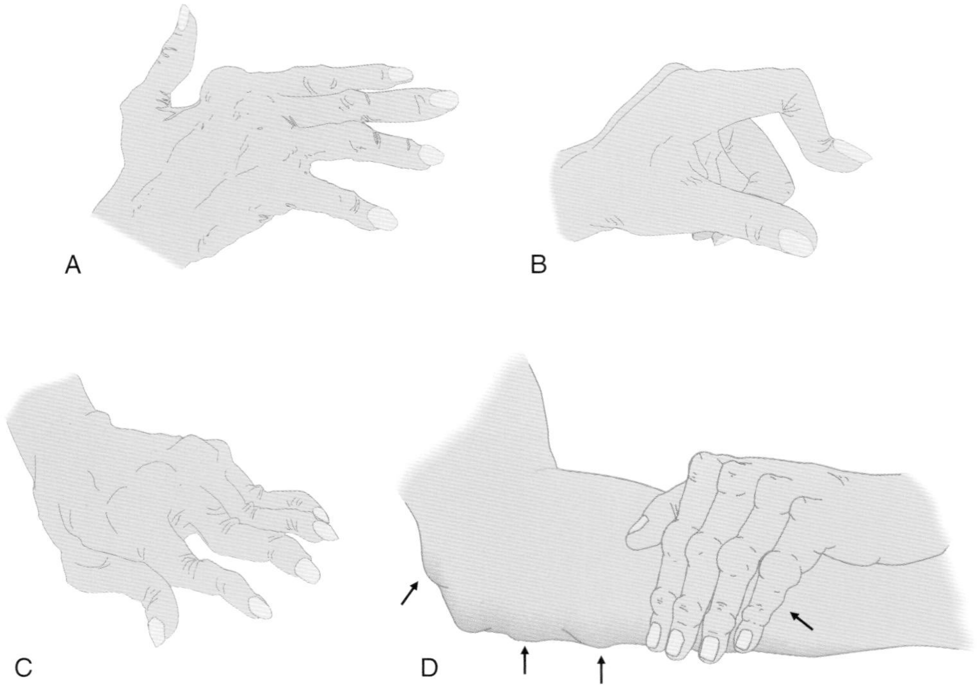

Fig. 44.5 Four types of hand deformity characteristics of patients with rheumatoid arthritis. (A) Ulnar drift. (B) Boutonnière deformity. (C) Swan-neck deformity. (D) Rheumatoid nodules. (From Black JM, Hawks JH: *Medical-surgical nursing: clinical management for positive outcomes*, ed 8, St. Louis, 2009, Saunders.)

other suggestive symptoms. Synovial fluid is analyzed for viscosity, WBCs, and glucose and is subjected to a mucin clot test.

The primary purpose of radiographs is to detect changes brought about by RA and to determine the potential usefulness of disease-modifying drugs or surgery. MRI, bone scans, and dual-energy x-ray absorptiometry (DXA) scans provide more detailed information that may be used to monitor disease progression and response to treatment.

MEDICAL TREATMENT

The treatment of RA involves combined efforts of medicine, nursing, physical therapy, occupational therapy, and social services. Treatment options include rest, drug therapy, physical and occupational therapy, and surgery. The focus of medical treatment is the "treat to target principle" to determine whether a specific goal for a positive outcome has been achieved. The primary target in RA is remission. Measures such as the Clinical Disease Activity Index (CDAI) are used to determine whether or not the goal has been achieved.

Drug therapy is aimed at controlling the local inflammatory process and providing symptomatic relief. Five types of medication are used to treat RA: (1) NSAIDs, (2) steroids (corticosteroids), (3) methotrexate and other traditional *disease-modifying antirheumatic drugs* (DMARDs), (4) biologic response modifiers that are a subset of DMARDs, and (5) Janus Kinase (JAK) inhibitors. Aggressive therapies are used to relieve inflammation within a 3-month period and to prevent deformities. Combinations of NSAIDs, glucocorticoids, and DMARDs are prescribed to meet the individual patient's therapeutic goal. Leflunomide (Arava) is a DMARD that can reportedly slow the progression of the disease. Etanercept (Enbrel) and infliximab (Remicade) have shown great success in rheumatoid patients, with some patients having a remission of the disease. Joint injections of corticosteroids can also be given 2 or 3 times a year and may provide significant symptomatic relief. A nonbiologic DMARD such as methotrexate sodium (Folex) often is very effective in the symptomatic treatment of RA. Systemic glucocorticoids are used to control inflammation initially; then they are gradually reduced to the lowest effective dose as the DMARDs take effect. Maximal effects of DMARDs may require 2 to 6 months of therapy. Patients on glucocorticoid therapy should receive bisphosphonates to prevent osteoporosis associated with glucocorticoid therapy. The newest medications are JAK inhibitors, or "Jakinibs," that act on the immune system to stop the inflammatory process. Tofacitinib (Xeljanz) is the only JAK inhibitor approved by the United States (U.S.) Food and Drug Administration (FDA) at this time (see Chapter 43, Table 43.2).

In addition to drug therapy, supportive treatments may be used—including rest, joint splints to reduce motion that aggravates the inflammation, orthotic devices to support deformed joints, and assistance in modifying ADLs. Afternoon rest periods may reduce the fatigue often felt late in the day. Temporary immobilization may be prescribed during acute episodes. However, long-term immobilization contributes to decreased joint flexibility. Types of exercise that may benefit the patient with RA include walking, cycling, aerobics, yoga, and aquatics. A physical therapist can recommend the exact exercise program for each patient. Some resources recommend heat treatments before exercise. Because vitamin D is thought to play a role in reducing inflammation, some health care providers may recommend supplements.

Surgical management of RA is reserved for those patients with severe pain and deformities. Among the options are arthroplasty (total joint replacement), synovectomy (removal of synovial tissue around the joint), tenosynovectomy (surgical excision of the tendon sheath, a layer of membrane surrounding the tendon, to reduce joint inflammation and pain), and arthrodesis (joint fusion). The most successful procedures are those performed on the knees and hips.

◆ NURSING CARE OF THE PATIENT WITH RHEUMATOID ARTHRITIS

FOCUSED ASSESSMENT

General assessment of the patient with a connective tissue disorder is summarized in Chapter 43, Box 43.1. When a patient has RA, collect data related to pain, joint swelling, tenderness, joint deformities and limitation of movement, fatigue, and decreased ability to perform ADLs (e.g., dressing, grooming, eating and toileting).

Patient Problems, Goals, and Outcome Criteria: Rheumatoid Arthritis

Patient Problems	Goals and Outcome Criteria
Chronic pain related to swelling and tenderness	Reduced pain: patient reports decreased pain, relaxed manner
Decreased mobility related to fatigue	Improved mobility: performance of small tasks without needing a rest period
Inadequate coping related to frustration, embarrassment, inability to do activities independently	Effective coping: patient identifies ways to deal with physical changes
Decreased socialization related to physical impairment and poor body image	Increased social activity: patient resumes at least one social activity that had been abandoned, has realistic view of physical abilities

Continued

Patient Problems, Goals, and Outcome Criteria: Rheumatoid Arthritis—cont'd

Patient Problems	Goals and Outcome Criteria
Inability to manage self-care related to lack of knowledge of rheumatoid arthritis (RA), its treatment, and self-care	Patient effectively manages self-care and treatment regimen: patient describes and demonstrates correct self-care and treatment regimen

Pharmacology Capsule

Aspirin and nonsteroidal antiinflammatory drugs (NSAIDs) prolong bleeding time; therefore, patients must be monitored for bruising and bleeding.

Interventions

Chronic pain. Chronic pain imposes a terrible burden on the patient. Administer prescribed drugs and teach outpatients about their drug therapy. Teach the patient other measures to control pain, including application of heat or cold and administration of medications as ordered. A warm shower on arising may relieve morning pain and stiffness (see the Complementary and Alternative Therapies box). Maintaining a program of exercise and rest can also help to manage joint pain and relieve stress. Care of the patient with pain is discussed in Chapter 8.

Complementary and Alternative Therapies

Nonpharmacologic approaches to pain management include application of heat or cold, balanced exercise and rest, relaxation exercises, meditation, imagery, Tai chi, yoga, acupuncture, massage, and mindfulness. Participation in support groups can increase knowledge of RA, increase confidence in managing it, and increase quality of life. Diet has been found to slow RA progression and decrease damage to joints. Foods with antioxidants and antiinflammatory properties (raw or lightly cooked vegetables; spices, including turmeric and ginger; fruit; and yogurt) are recommended, and processed foods, sugar, and animal products should be avoided. Supplements such as probiotics, fish oil, evening primrose, and thunder god vine have been helpful for some patients. Topical agents such as creams, gels and lotions containing menthol, benzocaine and procaine hydrochloride, as well as lemongrass essential oil may provide relief. Topical ointments that come in spray form or patches, including products that contain capsaicin, salicylates, camphor, or menthol are standard for treating RA.

Decreased mobility. With the patient, develop a plan of activities around periods of rest and activity. Provide assistance with changing positions, getting in and out of bed, toileting, bathing, and dressing as needed. Patients who are severely disabled may need help with all ADLs. Physical and occupational therapy may be ordered. Encourage the patient to follow the prescribed therapy program.

Inadequate coping. A trusting, collaborative relationship is a prerequisite to providing therapeutic care. Spend time with the patient exploring concerns, answering questions, teaching skills, and planning care. It is vital to emphasize the patient's strengths and explore previously used coping skills. Some patients respond to their physical and functional losses with demanding behavior that others see as manipulative. Patients from some cultures may deal with the pain and disability differently; some are more stoic and reserved, while others are demanding or helpless (see the Cultural Considerations box). Caregivers must recognize this as an attempt by the patient to maintain some control in their life. An important part of coping is learning to maintain maximal possible independence despite the crippling effects of RA. Adaptations in the home and workplace and the use of appropriate assistive devices can promote independence and an improved sense of well-being. Provide information about community resources, such as the local chapter of the Arthritis Foundation. If indicated, consult with a health care provider about a referral to a home care agency to help the patient learn to manage better at home.

Cultural Considerations

What Does Culture Have to Do With Pain?

The way in which people deal with pain may be culturally based. For example, many people of German, Japanese, and Irish heritage try to be stoic and are reluctant to express pain, whereas many people from Italy and the Dominican Republic are more likely to express pain openly. Nurses should not make assumptions about a patient's pain based only on their behavior.

Because a chronic illness affects the family as well as the patient, support family members, by offering information, encouragement, problem solving, and resources. Recognize that the family structure differs from one culture to another; the patient's role in the family plays an important part in how they view the effects of the disease.

Decreased socialization. Physical deformities that alter appearance and impair function evoke a great sense of loss in the patient with RA. The resulting depression, irritability, and feelings of helplessness can have a devastating effect on the patient's interpersonal relationships. In addition, patients who take corticosteroids often have mood swings, which make their behavior unpredictable. These emotional changes may result in discouraging staff and family visits, which increase the patient's isolation. Visit the patient often so that they do not feel isolated and lonely. Explain the patient's irritability and mood swings to family and friends. In addition, emphasize the importance of their continued support to the patient, and encourage the patient to identify appropriate social activities in which they can remain involved.

Inability to manage self-care. The teaching plan should include information about the disease process, drug therapy, and the need for balanced rest and activity (see the Patient Teaching box).

Patient Teaching

Rheumatoid Arthritis

- Take your medications exactly as prescribed and notify your physician of any adverse effects (provide drug names, dosage, schedule, side and adverse effects).
- Keep follow-up appointments; the effects of many drugs need to be monitored with periodic blood studies.
- Balance activity and rest.
- Avoid prolonged bed rest, which can lead to further loss of function.
- Use assistive devices as needed to maintain safe mobility.
- Support your joints in functional positions to reduce the risk of contractures.
- Do as much as you can for yourself but do not hesitate to ask for help with difficult tasks.
- Avoid heavy lifting that may cause strain on your joints.

Put on Your Thinking Cap!

A 30-year-old mother of a 6-month-old infant and a 5-year-old child has just been diagnosed with rheumatoid arthritis (RA). She is married and works full time as a teacher. Identify ways in which she can modify strain on her joints in both the home setting and the work setting.

GOUT

Gout is an inflammatory arthritis characterized by sudden, severe attacks of pain, redness, and tenderness in joints, especially the joint at the base of the big toe. Gout is more prevalent among men than women, with a peak onset in men between the age of 30 and 45 years. Women are more likely to be affected after menopause. Gout is particularly common among people older than 65 years regardless of gender, and it affects nearly 4% of adults in the United States. Risk factors for developing gout include obesity, hypertension, chronic kidney disease, overeating or prolonged fasting, consuming excessive amounts of alcohol (particularly beer, whiskey, gin, vodka, or rum) on a regular basis, consuming large amounts of meat or seafood, consuming beverages containing high amounts of fructose corn syrup (such as soda), and taking medications that affect blood levels of urate (especially diuretics). In people already diagnosed with gout (*established gout*), an increased risk of repeated flares can be caused by injury or recent surgery, fasting, consuming excessive amounts of alcohol, overeating, taking medications that induce sudden changes in blood urate levels, and dehydration.

PATHOPHYSIOLOGY

Gout is characterized by **hyperuricemia** (i.e., excess uric acid in the blood) that occurs because of excessive production or decreased excretion of uric acid by the kidneys. The result is an accumulation of urate crystals in and around the joints. When crystals are deposited, painful inflammation known as *gouty arthritis* results. Infection may develop if the skin breaks open. Kidney stones develop in about 20% of patients with gout.

CLINICAL MANIFESTATIONS

Three phases of gout exist: (1) *gout flare*, (2) *intercritical gout*, and (3) tophaceous gout.

- Phase 1: Gout flare. Characterized by severe, crushing pain usually affecting a single joint, most often the big toe or knee. People with osteoarthritis in their fingers may experience their first flares in their fingers rather than their toe or knee. The symptoms usually disappear within a few days and joint function is completely restored until the next attack. With more frequent episodes, flares may be more severe and prolonged with less time between episodes.
- Phase 2: Intercritical gout. Occurs between periods of gout flares. The second flare may occur within 2 years, and the frequency increases thereafter. With untreated gout, the time between gout flares may shorten and flares become increasingly severe and prolonged involving multiple joints.
- Phase 3: Tophaceous gout. Caused by **tophi** that develop after repeated gout flares or persistent hyperuricemia in advanced gout. Tophi are deposits of sodium urate crystals in joints, bursae, bones, cartilage, or under the skin that are visible as small white nodules. (Fig. 44.6). They may cause erosion of the bone and eventually joint damage or deformity, which may contribute to restricted movement and disability.

MEDICAL DIAGNOSIS

Gout is diagnosed through history and physical examination, as well as a joint fluid test that reveals urate crystals in synovial fluid. Blood tests measure the levels of uric acid and creatinine, although the results may be misleading and do not always indicate the presence of gout. A musculoskeletal ultrasound can detect urate crystals in a joint or tophus. Joint x-rays may rule out other causes of joint inflammation. The criteria for suspected gout are:

- Rapidly developing pain and inflammation, especially in the big toe
- Complete resolution of symptoms between flares
- High levels of urate in the blood

MEDICAL TREATMENT

The goal of treatment for a gout flare is prompt and safe termination of pain, inflammation, and disability. Although symptoms usually resolve within a few days

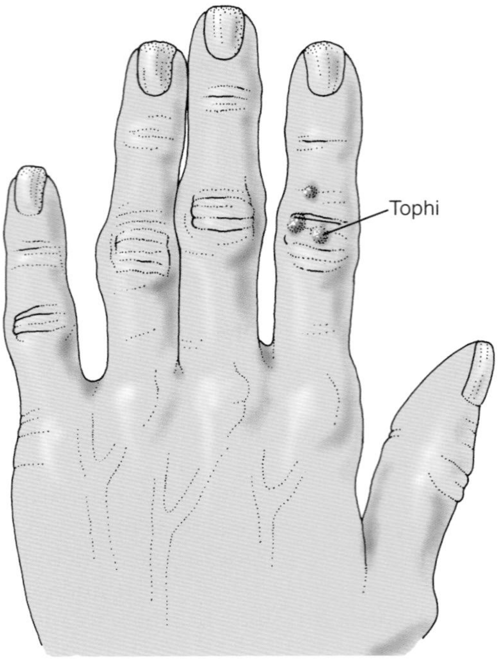

Fig. 44.6 Typical appearance of tophi, which may occur in chronic gout on an index finger. (From Ignatavicius DD, Workman ML, Mishler MA: *Medical-surgical nursing across the health care continuum*, ed 3, Philadelphia, 1999, Saunders.)

without treatment, with early administration of anti-inflammatory drugs, symptoms improve more quickly and completely. The primary drugs used to treat attacks of acute gouty arthritis are NSAIDs, corticosteroids, and oral colchicine. Potent oral NSAIDs, such as naproxen or indomethacin are recommended for a gout flare, and they are best given within 48 hours of the onset of symptoms. Patients taking NSAIDs may be given a proton-pump inhibitor to prevent gastric ulcers and bleeding. When a single joint is affected, prednisone may be injected into the joint. This is particularly useful for patients who are unable to take oral medications. Oral glucocorticoids (prednisone or prednisolone) may be prescribed if injections into the joint or NSAIDs are contraindicated. Colchicine is an option instead of glucocorticoids and NSAIDs and is most effective when given within 24 hours of onset of a gout flare. Colchicine in low doses is the drug of choice for preventive treatment of gout flares. Some sources recommend indomethacin and NSAIDs instead of colchicine in older adults.

To manage chronic tophaceous gout and prevent future attacks, three types of drugs are available. Uricostatic agents, which include allopurinol and febuxostat, prevent urate formation. Probenecid is a uricosuric agent, meaning that it increases the renal excretion of uric acid. Pegloticase is a uricolytic agent; that is, it breaks down uric acid to a soluble product for elimination (see Chapter 43, Table 43.2).

Patients who are on antigout medications do not have to severely restrict their diets. They are advised to avoid foods high in purines (liver, kidney, sweetbreads, etc.) and to limit animal proteins, alcohol, and fructose. Fructose is commonly used as a sweetener in prepared foods and drinks. If the patient is obese, weight loss is recommended.

Pharmacology Capsule

Patients taking antigout drugs need to maintain urine output of at least 2000 mL/day to reduce the risk of urinary calculi formation.

◆ NURSING CARE OF THE PATIENT WITH GOUT

FOCUSED ASSESSMENT

Complete assessment of the patient with a connective tissue disorder is summarized in Chapter 43, Box 43.2. When the patient has gout, collect data specifically about pain; joint swelling; tophi; uric acid stones; fever; and a history of trauma, injury, or surgery.

Patient Problems, Goals, and Outcome Criteria: Gout

Patient Problems	Goals and Outcome Criteria
Acute pain related to joint inflammation	Pain relief: patient states there is pain reduction as measured on a 1 to 10 pain scale, pain relief, or both; appears relaxed
Decreased mobility related to painful joint movement	Improved mobility: patient gradually resumes activities without unbearable pain
Fluid volume imbalance related to urate kidney stones	Normal urine output without symptoms of urinary obstruction: fluid intake and output equal, no flank or abdominal pain, no hematuria
Inability to manage treatment regimen related to lack of knowledge of gout, its treatment, and self-care measures	Patient effectively manages condition; correctly describes and follows plan of care

Interventions

Acute pain. Nursing care to decrease discomfort includes elevating the affected extremity, administering prescribed medications, encouraging rest, and avoiding pressure on the area. Because even bed sheets may cause pain, a bed cradle should be used. Hot or cold packs may be ordered. Splints or bandages may be used to immobilize the affected joint. When a patient is taking colchicine, always check laboratory results for abnormalities in blood cell counts. Fatal blood dyscrasias have occurred in patients taking this drug.

Decreased mobility. Bedrest usually is recommended during gout flares. Provide assistance with ADLs as needed. When ambulation is permitted, advise the patient to protect affected joints from trauma by wearing supportive, firm shoes and by keeping walking pathways clearly lighted and free of obstacles that might cause falls.

Fluid volume imbalance. When the serum uric acid level is elevated, the excess acid is excreted in the urine, where it may form uric acid stones. Urinary stones can obstruct urine flow from the kidney, causing renal damage. To prevent this complication, advise the patient to drink 8 to 16 8-oz cups of fluid daily unless contraindicated. Drugs may be prescribed to make the urine alkaline, because uric acid stones precipitate in acid urine. During hospitalization, intravenous fluids may be given. Monitor intake and urine output, and promptly report signs and symptoms of urinary stones (i.e., pain in the flank, lower abdomen, or genitals; fever; hematuria; decreased urine output) to a health care provider.

Inability to manage treatment regimen. Instruct the patient in measures to prevent or decrease future attacks (see the Patient Teaching box).

Patient Teaching

Gout

Consult a dietitian to help the patient plan a well-balanced diet and give the patient information about foods high in purines (Box 44.3). Maintain a fluid intake of 8 to 16 8-oz glasses daily to reduce the risk of uric acid stone formation in the urinary tract.

- Take your drugs as prescribed (provide specific dosage, schedule, list of side effects).
- To prevent severe attacks, report early joint or urinary symptoms to the physician. Severe attacks may be averted if treatment is begun soon after symptoms develop.
- If you are overweight, weight loss may help by reducing stress on joints.

Put On Your Thinking Cap!

Explain how increased fluid intake will help to prevent kidney stones in the patient with gout.

OSTEOPOROSIS

PATHOPHYSIOLOGY

Bone is constantly being formed and absorbed. Until adolescence, bone formation exceeds bone absorption so that bones grow and strengthen. The processes remain equal through a person's 20s, but beginning around 30 years of age, bone absorption surpasses bone formation. Loss of trabecular bone, the innermost

Box 44.3 Purine Content of Selected Foods

HIGH PURINE CONTENT

Avoid these foods during both acute and remission stages of gout:

Anchovies	Bouillon	Brains	Broth
Consommé	Goose	Gravy	Heart
Herring	Kidney	Mackerel	Meat extracts
Mincemeat	Mussels	Partridge	Roe
Sardines	Scallops	Sweetbreads	Yeast (baker's and brewer's as supplement)

MODERATE PURINE CONTENT

One serving (2–3 oz) meat, fish, or poultry or one serving (1/2 cup) of vegetable from these groups is allowed daily (depending on condition) during remissions:

- Fish, poultry, meat, shellfish
- Asparagus, dried beans, lentils, mushrooms, dried peas, spinach

(Modified from Mahan LK, Escott-Stump S, Raymond JL. *Krause's food and the nutrition care process*, 13th ed. St. Louis, Elsevier-Saunders, 2012.)

layer, occurs first. The loss of cortical bone, the hard outer shell, begins later in life. The loss of cortical bone begins earlier and progresses faster in women than in men. The net result is loss of bone mass, which leaves the patient susceptible to fractures. The most common sites of fractures caused by osteoporosis are the wrist, vertebrae, and hip, followed by the pelvis and the humerus. Most cases of osteoporosis are related to aging and estrogen deprivation without other apparent causes. Other cases of osteoporosis are secondary to a wide range of disorders and other variables.

RISK FACTORS

At greatest risk are older women who have small frames, who are White or of northern European heritage, and who have fair skin and blond or red hair (see the Cultural Considerations box). Other risk factors are estrogen deficiency; physical inactivity; low body weight; inadequate calcium, protein, or vitamin D intake; long-term therapy with corticosteroids or heparin; and excessive use of cigarettes, caffeine, and alcohol. A number of disorders, such as Cushing disease, hyperparathyroidism, hypogonadism, cirrhosis, leukemia, and diabetes mellitus, are also associated with osteoporosis.

Cultural Considerations

What Does Culture Have to Do With Osteoporosis?

Small, fair-skinned women of northern European descent are at greatest risk for osteoporosis. These women should be targeted early for bone-building dietary and exercise programs.

CLINICAL MANIFESTATIONS

Signs and symptoms of osteoporosis may include back pain, fractures, loss of height because of vertebral compression, and kyphosis. Bone deterioration in the jaw can cause dentures to fit poorly. Collapsed vertebrae can cause chronic pain and decline in function. Often the patient has no symptoms of osteoporosis until a fracture occurs.

MEDICAL DIAGNOSIS

A variety of noninvasive tools can be used to assess bone mineral density. The most accurate and precise diagnostic study is the dual energy x-ray absorptiometry (DEXA) of the spine, hip, radius, finger, or total body. Radiographs show bone fractures but do not reveal decreased bone density until loss of 30% to 50% of the bone mass occurs. Blood studies are usually normal with primary osteoporosis, but a battery of tests may be ordered to rule out possible secondary causes of osteoporosis. Several markers of bone turnover have been identified in the blood and urine, but these are not routinely assessed.

MEDICAL TREATMENT

The incidence and severity of osteoporosis may be reduced by identifying high-risk people and taking steps to promote healthy bone development. Preventive measures include calcium and vitamin D supplementation, physical activity, smoking cessation, limited alcohol intake, and, in some cases, estrogen replacement. Regular exercise promotes bone formation and improves strength, balance, and reaction time, thereby reducing the risk of falls and fractures. Aerobic exercise at least three times a week is encouraged.

Medical treatment is aimed at preventing fractures and stimulating bone formation. Some types of osteoporosis drugs slow bone breakdown; others spur new bone growth. Drugs that may be used to prevent or treat osteoporosis include:

- Bisphosphonates, such as Fosamax, Boniva, Actonel, and Reclast
- Calcitonin, sold as Fortical and Miacalcin
- Hormone therapy or estrogen
- SERMs (selective estrogen receptor modulators), such as Evista (raloxifene)
- Parathyroid hormone Forteo (teriparatide), Tymlos (abaloparatide), and Evenity (romosozumab)
- Prolia, a biologic drug

Prolia, the newest osteoporosis drug, targets a chemical in the immune system. It may cause low blood calcium levels and could increase the risk of infection.

Calcium supplementation and estrogen replacement for postmenopausal women is generally thought to slow bone loss. The recommended elemental calcium intake is 1000 mg per day for premenopausal women and for postmenopausal women who are on estrogen replacement therapy. Postmenopausal women who are not on estrogen replacement therapy need 1200 to 1500 mg/day of calcium. The only contraindications to supplementary calcium are hypercalcemia, hypophosphatemia, or a history of kidney stones. Vitamin D supplements are also advised. Estrogen replacement in women is controversial, but if it is not contraindicated, it may have beneficial effects on the bones for up to 15 years after the onset of menopause. The patient should discuss the issue with their health care provider. A physical therapist may be consulted to develop an appropriate exercise program for the patient. Although osteoporosis is more common in women, it affects men as well. Treatment options might include androgen replacement, hydrochlorothiazide, and alendronate (see Chapter 43, Table 43.2).

Patients who have spinal fractures caused by osteoporosis may be considered for vertebroplasty, an outpatient procedure in which bone cement is injected into a cracked or broken vertebra. After the cement hardens, it stabilizes the fractures and supports the spine. This procedure can relieve pain, increase mobility, and reduce the use of pain medication in patients with a compression fracture who have severe, disabling pain. Kyphoplasty is a similar procedure in which special balloons are inserted into the vertebra to create spaces that are filled with cement. This procedure helps to correct spinal deformity and restore lost height.

◆ NURSING CARE OF THE PATIENT WITH OSTEOPOROSIS

FOCUSED ASSESSMENT

Nursing assessment of the patient with a connective tissue disorder is summarized in Chapter 43, Box 43.2. When a patient has osteoporosis, collect data specifically about the patient's diet, calcium intake, and exercise pattern. Note whether a female patient is menopausal or has had an oophorectomy (i.e., surgical removal of the ovaries) and is taking estrogen replacement therapy. Measure the patient's height, and compare it with previous measurements. Describe the patient's posture, clearly noting the presence and degree of deformity. Finally, assist the patient with changes in position during the examination for safety and comfort.

Patient Problems, Goals, and Outcome Criteria: Osteoporosis

Patient Problems	Goals and Outcome Criteria
Potential for injury related to loss of bone strength	Maintain safety: performance of daily activities without falls or other injuries
Acute pain related to fractures, pressure on nerves because of vertebral compression	Pain relief: patient states pain is relieved, relaxed manner
Inability to manage treatment regimen related to lack of knowledge of measures to promote bone formation and prevent bone loss	Effective patient management of condition: patient describes and demonstrates activities to improve bone mass

Interventions

Potential for injury. Determine the patient's ability to carry out ADLs, and provide assistance if necessary. Tell ambulatory patients to wear good supportive shoes, and provide canes or walkers to improve balance if needed. Keep the environment free of hazards that might cause the patient to fall. Place personal articles within reach. In the home setting, look for possible hazards, and take steps to provide a safer environment. Evaluate the patient's gross visual acuity. To maneuver safely, the patient must be able to see. If indicated, recommend an eye examination.

Acute pain. Obtain a complete description of the patient's pain. Administer analgesics as ordered, but consider nonpharmacologic interventions as well (see Chapter 8). Some patients, especially those with vertebral compression, may have chronic pain that is difficult to manage. A referral to a clinic that specializes in pain management may be suggested. Document the effects of pain management strategies.

Inability to manage treatment program. Patient teaching is key to helping the patient learn to manage osteoporosis (see the Patient Teaching box).

Patient Teaching

Osteoporosis

- Women need 1000 mg of calcium daily before menopause and while on hormone replacements.
- Women need 1200 mg of calcium daily after 50 years of age.
- Men require 1000 mg every day up to 71 years of age, when the amount should be increased to 1200 mg per day.
- Approximately 300 mg of calcium are found in each of the following: 1 cup of milk, 1 cup of yogurt, 1 oz of Swiss cheese.
- Nonfat and skim milk have as much calcium as whole milk.
- Increase your fluid intake if you are taking calcium supplements unless advised not to do so by your health care provider.
- You need at least 600 IU of vitamin D every day up to 71 years of age, when your physician may advise an increase.
- Taking excessive amounts of calcium and/or vitamin D can cause kidney stones.
- Limit your intake of alcohol and caffeine.
- If Fosamax is prescribed, take it in the morning with a full glass of water on an empty stomach; sit or stand for 30 minutes after taking it.
- Regular weight-bearing exercise helps to maintain bone strength.
- Avoid activities that might lead to falls and fractures.

Put On Your Thinking Cap!

List two ways in which a premenopausal woman can obtain her recommended daily calcium intake without supplements.

SYSTEMIC SCLEROSIS (SCLERODERMA)

Systemic sclerosis (SSc) or scleroderma is a chronic autoimmune disease of unknown origin that takes its name from the characteristic hardening of the skin. When systemic sclerosis is confined to the skin and/or muscles, it is usually relatively mild and is called localized SSc. In addition to the skin, SSc can affect the GI tract, lungs, heart, kidneys, muscles, joints, and blood vessels. The course of the disease varies among individuals, depending on the severity of involvement of the internal organs. The onset of disease is usually between 30 and 50 years of age, with more women than men affected. Death may occur because of infection or cardiac or renal failure. An estimated 300,000 individuals in the United States have SSc.

Two types of SSc exist: (1) diffuse sclerosis and (2) limited sclerosis, also called CREST syndrome. Diffuse sclerosis is characterized by thickening of the skin and systemic effects, specifically, hardening of internal organs. CREST syndrome consists of five features: (1) calcinosis (calcium deposits in the tissues), (2) Raynaud phenomenon (vascular spasms), (3) esophageal dysfunction, (4) sclerodactyly (scleroderma of the digits), and (5) telangiectasis (dilated superficial blood vessels).

PATHOPHYSIOLOGY

Systemic sclerosis is thought to be the result of environmental factors and genetic susceptibility. Environmental factors that may serve as triggers include infectious agents and occupational, dietary, medical, and lifestyle exposures. The manifestations of the disease follow a chain of events from inflammation to degeneration of tissues that results in decreased elasticity, stenosis, and occlusion of vessels.

CLINICAL MANIFESTATIONS

The signs and symptoms of SSc reflect problems of the blood vessels, skin, joints, and internal organs. Common manifestations are Raynaud phenomenon; symmetric, painless swelling or thickening of the skin; taut and shiny skin; morning stiffness; frequent reflux of gastric acid; difficulty swallowing; weight loss; dyspnea; pericarditis; and renal insufficiency. Raynaud phenomenon is manifested by episodes of vasoconstriction in the extremities, especially in response to cold exposure. Affected areas appear pale, then cyanotic, and finally red as blood flow returns.

MEDICAL DIAGNOSIS

Findings in the health history and physical examination may lead the health care provider to suspect SSc. However, it is difficult to differentiate from other autoimmune conditions at the earliest stage. A positive ANA serum assay result supports the diagnosis.

MEDICAL TREATMENT

Even though no cure exists for SSc, treatment with immunosuppressive (e.g., cyclophosphamide, methotrexate) and antifibrotic drugs (e.g., D-penicillamine) may help. Low-dose, short-term corticosteroid therapy alleviates joint pain and stiffness, but glucocorticoids are discouraged because they present a risk for renal complications. Various drugs are used to treat the symptoms of SSc, although results have been variable. The management of Raynaud phenomenon is aimed at eliminating anything that causes vasospasm: smoking, cold environmental temperature, and vasoconstricting drugs. Angiotensin II receptor blockers such as losartan often are effective. A variety of other vasodilators may be used if losartan is not sufficient. Angiotensin-converting enzyme (ACE) inhibitors are used to control hypertensive crisis and to avert sclerodermal renal crisis (see Chapter 43, Table 43.2).

Additional aims of treatment are management of symptoms and prevention of complications. Treatment includes physical therapy to maintain joint mobility and preserve muscle strength. Esophageal reflux may be treated with proton-pump inhibitors to decrease the acidity of gastric secretions, periodic dilation of the esophagus, and other measures, such as small, frequent feedings and elevation of the head of the bed.

◆ NURSING CARE OF THE PATIENT WITH PROGRESSIVE SYSTEMIC SCLEROSIS

FOCUSED ASSESSMENT

General assessment of the patient with a connective tissue disorder is summarized in Chapter 43, Box 43.2. When a patient has SSc, the health history should document pain and stiffness in the fingers and intolerance for cold. Record signs and symptoms suggestive of cardiovascular, respiratory, renal, and GI problems.

During the physical examination, inspect for skin rash, loss of wrinkles on the face, limitations of joint range of motion, muscle weakness, and dry mucous membranes. Carefully examine the hands for contractures of the fingers and for color changes or lesions on the fingertips. Palpate the fingers to determine warmth.

Patient Problems, Goals, and Outcome Criteria: Systemic Sclerosis

The patient problems and goals for patients with systemic sclerosis (SSc) are similar to those of patients with other connective tissue diseases. The following are the major diagnoses.

Patient Problems	Goals and Outcome Criteria
Disrupted skin tissue integrity related to thickening	Optimal tissue integrity: warm, intact skin with normal color and texture
Impaired performance of activities of daily living (ADLs) (bathing, feeding, toileting) related to pain, contractures of fingers, discomfort	Independent self-management: patient performs ADLs without excessive discomfort
Chronic pain related to swelling and stiffness, vasospasm	Pain relief: patient states pain is relieved, relaxed manner
Decreased socialization related to poor self-concept, changes in physical appearance	Decreased social isolation: patient maintains or increases social interactions
Inadequate nutrition related to esophageal dysfunction	Adequate nutrition: stable body weight, maintains weight within standards recommended for height
Potential for fluid and electrolyte imbalance related to diminished renal blood flow	Maintain adequate fluid and electrolyte balance: blood pressure (BP) consistent with patient norms, urine intake and output equal
Inability to manage treatment regimen related to lack of knowledge of SSc, medical management, and self-care	Effective management of condition: patient correctly describes and follows plan of care

Interventions

Disrupted tissue integrity. Keep the patient's skin clean and dry. Encourage the patient to wear protective clothing as needed to maintain warmth and reduce skin discomfort. Cool baths with mild soaps followed by emollient skin lotions may be soothing. Meticulous mouth care is warranted to prevent oral lesions. Administer antifibrotic and vasodilating drugs if ordered, and advise the patient to avoid practices that trigger vasospasm, such as exposure to cold and smoking.

Impaired ability to carry out activities of daily living (bathing, feeding, toileting). Encourage the patient to participate in self-care as much as possible. Monitor the patient's tolerance for activity and provide assistance as needed. Schedule rest periods after activities to prevent overtiring. Encourage the hospitalized patient to maintain independence in activities within their abilities.

Chronic pain. The patient with SSc usually has chronic joint pain and episodes of severe pain in the hands and feet associated with Raynaud phenomenon. Measures to treat joint pain are like those described for rheumatoid arthritis. During acute episodes of Raynaud phenomenon, the patient may be unable to tolerate anything touching the affected skin. A bed cradle can be used to keep the linens off the body. Adjust the room temperature to prevent chilling, which could provoke vasospasm, and ensure that the patient is aware that smoking and severe stress can also trigger vasospasm.

Decreased socialization. Swelling of the hands and facial changes can create a birdlike appearance that may cause the patient to withdraw from social interactions (Fig. 44.7). Explore the patient's concerns about the altered appearance, and help the patient to anticipate how to deal with various social situations. Demonstrate acceptance of the patient by expressing concern and using touch.

Inadequate nutrition. If the patient has esophageal involvement, suggest smaller, more frequent meals, which may be better tolerated. A relaxing environment before and after meals is helpful. Spicy foods, alcohol, and caffeine are discouraged because they stimulate gastric secretions. Because esophageal reflux is common, a proton-pump inhibitor may be ordered to reduce the risk of esophagitis and ulceration. After meals, the head of the bed should remain elevated for 1 to 2 hours to discourage reflux. Monitor and assess the adequacy of nutritional intake.

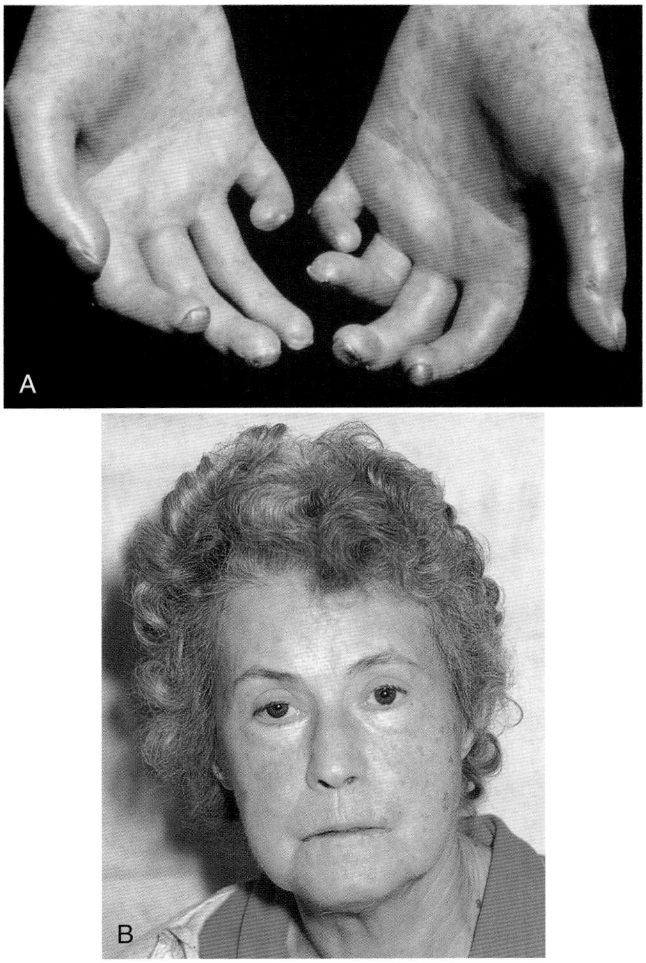

Fig. 44.7 Late-stage skin changes seen in patients with progressive systemic sclerosis. (A) Edema of the hands and fingers. (B) Typical facial appearance. (A, From Ignatavicius DD, Workman ML, Mishler MA: *Medical-surgical nursing across the health care continuum*, ed 3, Philadelphia, 1999, Saunders. B, From Swartz M: *Textbook of physical diagnosis: history and examination*, ed 6, Philadelphia, 2009, Saunders.)

Potential for fluid and electrolyte imbalance. Scleroderma renal crisis is a life-threatening complication of SSc, resulting in constricted blood vessels gradually reducing blood flow to the kidneys. Increased renin secretion triggers vasoconstriction in a cycle that can result in malignant hypertension. This is a medical emergency that requires hospitalization and treatment with ACE inhibitors. Teach patients to monitor their blood pressure (BP) and to seek medical care if there is a sudden increase in BP.

Inability to manage treatment regimen. As with other chronic illnesses, the patient must learn to implement the medical plan and manage the signs and symptoms of the condition. Patient teaching with SSc includes the nature of the disease, measures to prevent episodes of Raynaud phenomenon, measures to maintain good nutrition and prevent esophageal reflux, signs and symptoms that should be reported to the physician, and self-medication. (Key points are listed in the Patient Teaching box.)

Patient Teaching

Systemic Sclerosis

- To prevent vasospasm, keep your hands warm and reduce stress and exhaustion.
- Take drugs as prescribed and report adverse effects to your physician (provide specific information about drug names, dosage, schedule, and adverse effects).
- Esophageal reflux can be managed with drug therapy; relaxing meals; avoiding spicy foods, caffeine, and alcohol; and maintaining an upright position for 1 to 2 hours after eating.

Nutrition Considerations

Connective Tissue Disorders

1. A daily intake of 1000 to 1200 mg/day of calcium and 600 IU/day of vitamin D is important for the prevention of osteoporosis.
2. Eight ounces of milk (whole, low fat, or skim) provides 300 mg of calcium.
3. A well-balanced diet, including foods high in vitamin E and zinc, is recommended for persons with rheumatoid arthritis (RA).
4. A weight loss program for persons with arthritis reduces stress on weight-bearing joints.
5. Patients with gout are advised to limit intake of animal foods, alcohol, and fructose.
6. The patient with esophageal involvement of systemic sclerosis (SSc) needs small, frequent meals and limited spicy foods, alcohol, and caffeine.

OTHER CONNECTIVE TISSUE DISORDERS

Other connective tissue disorders are bursitis, carpal tunnel syndrome, ankylosing spondylitis, polymyalgia rheumatica, Reiter syndrome, Behçet syndrome, Sjögren syndrome, and periarteritis nodosa as described in Table 44.1. Systemic lupus erythematosus (SLE) is an important autoimmune disorder that is discussed in Chapter 32. The term *mixed* (or *overlapping*) *connective tissue disease* may be used when patients have features of multiple rheumatic diseases. These patients typically progress to develop SLE, SSc, or polymyositis.

Table 44.1 Other Connective Tissue Disorders

DISORDER	PATHOPHYSIOLOGY	MANAGEMENT
Bursitis	Description: Acute or chronic inflammation of the bursae caused by trauma, strain, or infection. Calcification of bursae may occur. Cause: Usually excessive use of joint. Signs and symptoms: Pain and limited movement in affected joints. Shoulder and hip most often affected.	NSAIDs, rest, and splinting; cold compresses for the first 24 hours and heat thereafter; lidocaine injections for temporary pain relief. Once pain resolves, progressive range of motion, such as "walking" the fingers of the affected arm up the wall, is helpful.
Carpal tunnel syndrome	Description: Common condition in which the median nerve in the wrist becomes compressed, causing pain and numbness. Cause: Caused by pressure on median nerve as it passes through structures of the wrist. People who do repetitive wrist movements such as typing are at risk. Signs and symptoms: Pain and numbness in palmar side of fingers, weakness of thumb.	Splinting to prevent flexion and hyperextension, glucocorticoid injections, and surgical release of transverse carpal ligament. Postoperatively, assess color and temperature of hand. Notify surgeon of pallor, cyanosis, or numbness.
Ankylosing spondylitis	Description: Chronic inflammatory disease that affects vertebral column, causing spinal deformities. Cause: Unknown but appears to be linked to human leukocyte antigen (HLA)-B27 antigen. Signs and symptoms: First symptom usually dull, aching pain in buttocks. In addition, low-back morning stiffness of several hours' duration that improves with activity; fatigue. Complications: Spinal fractures, iritis (inflammation of the iris of the eye), arthritis.	NSAIDs, DMARDs, monoclonal antibodies. Physical therapy.
Polymyalgia rheumatica and giant cell arteritis (GCA)	Description: Rheumatic disease. Cause: Unknown but likely has hereditary link. Signs and symptoms: Aching and morning stiffness in neck, shoulders and hips, proximal extremities, and torso. Symptoms resolve in 1 to 2 hours and return after a period of inactivity. Fatigue, weight loss, low-grade fever, anemia. Risk of vision loss with GCA.	Corticosteroids.
Reactive arthritis (Reiter syndrome)	Description: Connective tissue disease. Cause: Often follows infection of GI or GU tract (esp. *Chlamydia trachomatis*); incidence increased in people with certain familial tendencies. Signs and symptoms: Triad of arthritis, urethritis, conjunctivitis. Fever, malaise, fatigue, anorexia, weight loss, conjunctivitis, heel pain, skin lesions.	Antibiotic, NSAIDs, and physical therapy.
Behçet syndrome	Description, signs, and symptoms: Chronic systemic autoimmune syndrome. Classic signs: oral and genital ulcers, eye inflammation. Other: large joint arthritis, GI lesions. Cause: Not considered hereditary, but there seems to be a familial link.	Treatment varies based on specific manifestations. May include colchicine, thalidomide, anticoagulants, glucocorticoids, cyclosporine, tumor necrosis factor inhibitors (e.g., infliximab), chlorambucil, azathioprine, methotrexate, and retinal proteins.
Sjögren syndrome	Description: Inflammatory disease that obstructs secretory ducts in the eyes, mouth, and vagina. Cause: Autoimmune disorder; often seen with rheumatoid arthritis (RA), polymyositis, scleroderma, or systemic lupus erythematosus (SLE). Classic signs and symptoms: Dry eyes, mouth, and vagina. Can affect joints, lung, liver, nervous system, blood, and kidney.	Artificial tears and lubricant ointments; artificial saliva, pilocarpine hydrochloride to stimulate salivary flow, and dental care; vaginal lubricants, perineal hygiene; and glucocorticoids. Other agents based on additional manifestations.

Table 44.1 Other Connective Tissue Disorders—cont'd

DISORDER	PATHOPHYSIOLOGY	MANAGEMENT
Polyarteritis nodosa	Description: A form of systemic necrotizing vasculitis. Inflammation of small- and medium-sized arteries; can result in thrombosis, infarction, and hemorrhage. Affects mainly skin, peripheral nerves, GI tract, and kidneys. May be associated with hepatitis B. Signs and symptoms: Onset insidious. Fever, weight loss, skin lesions, hypertension, joint swelling, malaise, abdominal pain, change in urinary pattern, anemia, ischemia of fingers, pleuritis. Symptoms of renal, GI, and cardiac involvement.	Glucocorticoids, methotrexate, cyclophosphamide, antihypertensive agents, lamivudine or entecavir, and diuretics. Other drugs are prescribed for specific manifestations of the disorder.
Dermatomyositis and Polymyositis *Polymyositis* is applied to the condition when no skin involvement exists, and the term *dermatomyositis* is used when a characteristic skin rash occurs.	Description: Relatively rare acute or chronic inflammatory diseases that affect primarily the skeletal muscle. Infiltration of inflammatory cells, causing destruction of muscle fibers and inflammation of tissues surrounding blood vessels Cause: Unknown, but frequently seen in patients with scleroderma, RA, vasculitis, systemic lupus erythematosus, or Sjögren syndrome. Sometimes associated with malignancy. Signs and symptoms: Muscle weakness, reflected in inability to do normal activities like climbing stairs, raising the arms over the head, and turning over in bed; Raynaud phenomenon; joint pain and inflammation. With dermatomyositis, periorbital edema (i.e., swelling around the eyes). Slow or abrupt onset may occur.	High-dose glucocorticoids such as prednisone and chemotherapeutic drugs such as methotrexate. Balance rest and exercise to prevent contractures, which is difficult to achieve because range-of-motion exercises may aggravate the condition. Polymyositis is seen in conjunction with other connective tissue diseases, see earlier sections of the chapter for applicable nursing interventions.

DMARDs, Disease-modifying antirheumatic drugs; *GI*, gastrointestinal; *GU*, genitourinary; *NSAIDs*, nonsteroidal antiinflammatory drugs.

Nursing Care Plan: Patient With a Total Hip Replacement

FOCUSED ASSESSMENT

Health History

A 74-year-old homemaker has had osteoarthritis for 10 years, with progressive loss of function in both hips. She had a left total hip replacement (arthroplasty) 2 days ago. Her medical history reveals no other major health problems except poor vision. She lives with her daughter and helps with household chores, which gives her some satisfaction. Postoperatively, she is alert and participates in her exercises. She was assisted out of bed this morning. She was somewhat weak but was able to walk a short distance.

Physical Examination

Vital signs: blood pressure 148/66 mm Hg, pulse 82 beats per minute, respiration 16 breaths per minute, temperature 98°F (36.7°C) measured orally. Height 5′9″, weight 162 lb. Patient is positioned on her right side with an abductor cushion in place. Breath sounds are clear on auscultation. Abdomen is soft and bowel sounds are present. No bladder distention or redness exists over bony prominences on back and left side. Warmth, color, and peripheral pulses are symmetrical in both legs. She has good sensation in affected leg. The dressing on the surgical incision is dry and intact.

Patient Problems	Goals and Outcome Criteria	Interventions
Inadequate peripheral circulation related to deep vein thrombosis (DVT), decreased mobility, and surgical trauma.	The patient will have adequate circulation in the affected extremity, as evidenced by warmth, normal color, and palpable pulses.	Assess neurologic and circulatory status. Check vital signs at least every 4 hours (q4h). Report and record any abnormalities. Observe for excess swelling or bleeding at operative site. Assist with exercises as prescribed by physical or occupational therapist. Record and report any change in condition of skin at operative site and pressure areas.
Potential for injury related to unsteady gait.	The patient will experience no falls during hospitalization.	Assist patient in and out of bed. Place call bell within easy reach. Check frequently for patient's need to toilet and need for change of position. Provide assistive devices as ordered.

Continued

Nursing Care Plan — Patient With a Total Hip Replacement—cont'd

Patient Problems	Goals and Outcome Criteria	Interventions
Potential for injury related to subluxation (dislocation) of joint prosthesis because of improper position, movement, or activity.	The patient will maintain proper body alignment and hip positioning and will not exhibit signs of prosthesis dislocation: sudden, severe pain; abnormal position.	Instruct patient to keep legs slightly abducted. May place pillows between legs to achieve abduction while supine and during turning. Turn only to unaffected side. Tell patient not to cross legs or put on own shoes, socks, or stockings for 2 months. Assess for pain and loss of function. Make home health referral if needed to facilitate transition to home setting.
Potential for infection related to break in skin integrity from surgical hip replacement procedure.	The patient will be free of infection during hospitalization, as evidenced by orientation to person, place, and time; normal body temperature, intact wound with decreasing redness, minimal edema, and no purulent drainage.	Encourage fluids and activity when appropriate. Observe for change in mental status or confusion, which may be first signs of infection in older adults. Keep in mind that previous administration of prednisone may mask symptoms of infection. Turn at least every 2 hours (q2h) from back to unaffected side only. Use aseptic technique for wound care. Offer fluids at least q2h.

CRITICAL THINKING QUESTIONS

1. Describe at least two behaviors that could reflect a change in this patient's mental status.
2. What data would suggest the need for a home health referral?

Get Ready for the NCLEX® Examination!

Key Points

- Osteoarthritis is characterized by degeneration of articular cartilage, hypertrophy of underlying and adjacent bone, and inflammation of surrounding synovium that leads to pain with joint movement.
- Osteoarthritis may be treated with drug therapy, education, physical therapy, modification of daily activities, and surgery.
- Nursing care of the patient with osteoarthritis focuses on pain, immobility, inadequate coping, and inability to perform self-care.
- Total joint replacement can be done on the elbow, shoulder, phalangeal finger joints, hip, knee, and ankle.
- Nursing care after total joint replacement addresses pain, potential injury, immobility, inadequate peripheral circulation, potential for infection, anxiety, and inadequate knowledge of postoperative self-care.
- RA, a chronic, progressive inflammatory disease that leads to deformity and loss of joint mobility, is treated with drug therapy, supportive treatments, and modification of ADLs.
- Gout, a systemic disease characterized by the deposition of urate crystals in the joints and other body tissues, usually responds to drug therapy that lowers the serum uric acid level.
- Systemic sclerosis (SSc), commonly called *scleroderma*, is characterized by thickening of the skin and may affect the blood vessels, GI tract, lungs, heart, and kidneys.
- Nursing care for the patient with SSc addresses loss of protective barrier; impaired ability to carry out activities of daily living (bathing, feeding, toileting); pain; decreased socialization; inadequate nutrition; inability to manage treatment program; and potential for injury.
- Less common connective tissue disorders are polymyositis, ankylosing spondylitis, polymyalgia rheumatica, Reiter syndrome, Behçet syndrome, Sjögren syndrome, and periarteritis nodosa.
- Most connective tissue disorders are chronic and, although they are not specifically curable, can be improved with symptomatic treatment.

Additional Learning Resources

SG Go to your Study Guide for additional learning activities to help you master this chapter content.

Go to your Evolve website (http://evolve.elsevier.com/Linton/medsurg) for the following learning resources and much more:

- Fluid & Electrolyte Tutorial
- Review Questions for the NCLEX® Examination

Clinical Judgment and Next-Generation NCLEX® Examination-Style Questions

1. **A patient who has gout calls the clinic to report having flank pain and blood in her urine. Which of the following actions should you take?**
   1. Report signs and symptoms of urinary stones to the physician immediately
   2. Tell her that these symptoms are normal with gout and that they will improve soon
   3. Make an appointment for her to see the physician within 1 week
   4. Document her complaints in her record and ask her to call the next day if symptoms continue

   NCLEX Client Need: Health Promotion and Maintenance

2. **One week after total hip replacement surgery, a patient complains of sudden severe pain in the affected hip and inability to bear weight on that leg. Which of the following should be suspected?**
   1. Wound dehiscence
   2. Prosthesis rejection

3. A new hip fracture
4. Prosthesis dislocation

NCLEX Client Need: Physiological Integrity: Reduction of Risk Potential

3. **The licensed vocational nurse/licensed practical nurse (LVN/LPN) is assisting in developing a care plan for a patient with RA. Which patient problems are likely to be appropriate? (Select all that apply.)**

1. Impaired mobility related to fatigue
2. Social isolation related to physical impairment and poor body image
3. Ineffective perfusion related to vasoconstriction
4. Pain related to joint inflammation and swelling
5. Risk for injury related to loss of bone strength

NCLEX Client Need: Physiological Integrity: Reduction of Risk Potential

4. **A women's club has asked the nurse to explain how osteoporosis can be prevented. The nurse should inform the club members that recommended daily calcium intake for women 50 years of age and older is:**

1. 200 mg
2. 500 mg
3. 1000 mg
4. 1200 mg

NCLEX Client Need: Physiological Integrity: Physiological Adaptation

5. **When probenecid (Benemid) is prescribed for a patient with gout, patient teaching should include which of the following points? (Select all that apply.)**

1. Avoid people who have infections because your immune system is depressed
2. Drink enough fluid each day to maintain urine output of at least 2 L
3. It takes several weeks for this medication to be fully effective
4. Go to an emergency room if your BP suddenly increases
5. Remain in an upright position for at least 30 minutes after taking this medication

NCLEX Client Need: Health Promotion and Maintenance

6. **Which statement should be included in the teaching plan for a patient with systemic sclerosis?**

1. Keep the temperature in your home below 70°F
2. Remain upright for 1 to 2 hours after meals
3. This is an acute condition that will improve over time
4. Systemic sclerosis affects only the skin

NCLEX Client Need: Physiological Integrity: Pharmacological Therapies

7. **A patient being admitted for surgery reports that she has Sjögren syndrome. The nurse should anticipate a need for:**

1. Dim lighting in her room
2. Oral moisturizer
3. Assistance with meals
4. Hand splints

NCLEX Client Need: Physiological Integrity: Physiological Adaptation

8. **Take Action Using Matrix Test Item**

A 58-year-old woman had an appointment with her primary care provider for ongoing treatment of rheumatoid arthritis. She has been receiving a combination of NSAIDs, corticosteroids, and DMARDS (methotrexate) to control inflammation and provide symptomatic relief.

Use an X for the health teaching below that is *Indicated* (appropriate or necessary), *Contraindicated* (could be harmful), or *Nonessential* (makes no difference or not necessary) during the patient's appointment.

HEALTH TEACHING	INDICATED	CONTRAINDICATED	NONESSENTIAL
"Take a warm shower in the morning to relieve stiffness and pain"			
"Alternate rest and activity to for comfort and mobility"			
"You may have to wear splints indefinitely to immobilize your joints"			
"Drink at least 8 glasses of water per day"			
"Aerobic exercises may increase mobilization of joints"			
"Adding carbohydrates to your diet will give you added energy"			
"Be aware of stressors in your life; here are a couple of relaxation techniques that you can use"			

45 Fractures

http://evolve.elsevier.com/Linton/medsurg

Objectives

1. Identify the types of fractures.
2. Describe the five stages of the healing process.
3. Discuss the clinical manifestations of the major complications of fractures.
4. Compare the types of medical treatment for fractures, particularly reduction and fixation.
5. Describe common therapeutic measures for fractures, including casts, traction, crutches, walkers, and canes.
6. Discuss the nursing care of a patient with a fracture.
7. Describe specific types of fractures, including hip fractures, Colles fractures, and pelvic fractures.

Key Terms

bone remodeling
closed reduction or manipulation
comminuted fracture (KŎM-ĭ-nūt-ĕd)
compartment syndrome
complete fracture
delayed union
fat embolism (ĔM-bō-lĭzm)
fixation (fĭx-SĀ-shŭn)
fracture
greenstick fracture
incomplete fracture
malunion (măl-ŪN-yŏn)
nonunion (nŏn-ŪN-yŭn)
open or compound fracture
open reduction
reduction
stress fracture

A **fracture** is defined as a break or disruption in the continuity of a bone. When a fracture occurs, surrounding soft tissue is also injured. The severity of soft tissue injury depends on the location and severity of the break.

All fractures are either complete or incomplete. A **complete fracture** is one in which the break extends across the entire bone, dividing it into two separate pieces. An **incomplete fracture** is one in which the bone breaks only partway across, leaving some portion of the bone intact. The term **greenstick fracture** has been used to describe the incomplete fractures most commonly seen in children. In this case, the bone is splintered on one side but only bent on the other.

CLASSIFICATION OF FRACTURES

Fractures may be classified as *open* or *closed*, depending on the type and extent of soft tissue damage. A closed or simple fracture is one in which the broken bone does not break through the skin (Fig. 45.1). In an **open or compound fracture**, the fragments of the broken bone break through the skin. Open fractures have three grades of severity:

- Grade I: least severe injury, with minimal skin damage
- Grade II: moderately severe injury, with skin and muscle contusions (bruises)
- Grade III: most severe injury (wound larger than 6 to 8 cm), with skin, muscle, blood vessel, and nerve damage.

Fractures may also be classified as *stress* or *pathologic fractures*, depending on their cause. A **stress fracture** is caused by either repeated or prolonged stress. Stress fractures are often related to sports such as track or basketball. A pathologic fracture occurs because of a pathologic condition in the bone such as a tumor or disease process that causes a spontaneous break. Fig. 45.2 illustrates common types of fractures.

CAUSE AND RISK FACTORS

Fractures are caused most commonly by trauma to the bone, especially from automobile accidents and falls. Bone disease such as bone cancer can also lead to a fracture. Hip fractures in older adults are usually associated with falls. Risk factors for hip fractures include osteoporosis, advanced age, Caucasian race, and female gender (see the Cultural Considerations box).

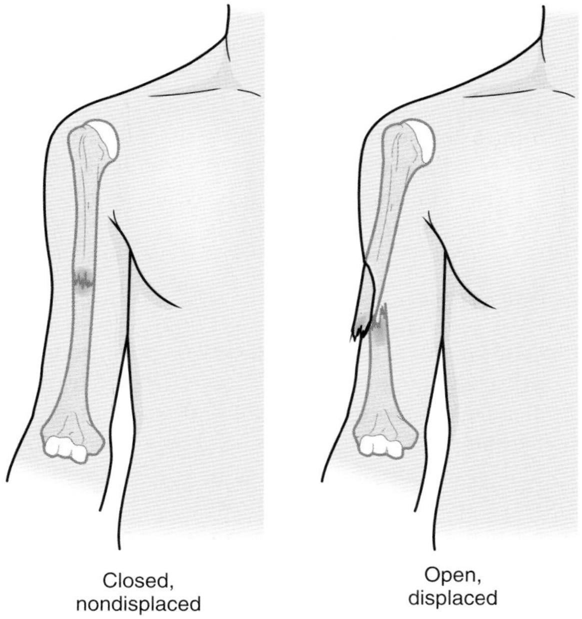

Fig. 45.1 Common classification of fractures. (From Ignatavicius DD, Workman ML, Rebar CR, Heimgartner NM: *Medical-surgical nursing: concepts for interprofessional collaborative care*, St. Louis, 2021, Elsevier.)

Cultural Considerations

What Does Culture Have to Do With Fractures?

Older White women have a high incidence of osteoporosis and therefore are at increased risk for fractures. To reduce the risk, preventive measures should be taken throughout life. Osteoporosis is easier to prevent than to treat.

In adults, the bones most commonly fractured are the ribs. Fractures of the femur are most common in young and middle-aged adults, whereas hip, wrist, and vertebral fractures are most common in older adults. In 2010 hip fractures accounted for more than 258,000 hospital admissions among persons 65 years of age and older.

FRACTURE HEALING

A bone begins to heal as soon as an injury occurs. New bone tissue is formed to repair the fracture, resulting in a sturdy union between the broken ends of the bone. Healing occurs in the following five stages:

- Stage 1: Hematoma formation. Immediately after a fracture, bleeding and edema occur. In 48 to 72

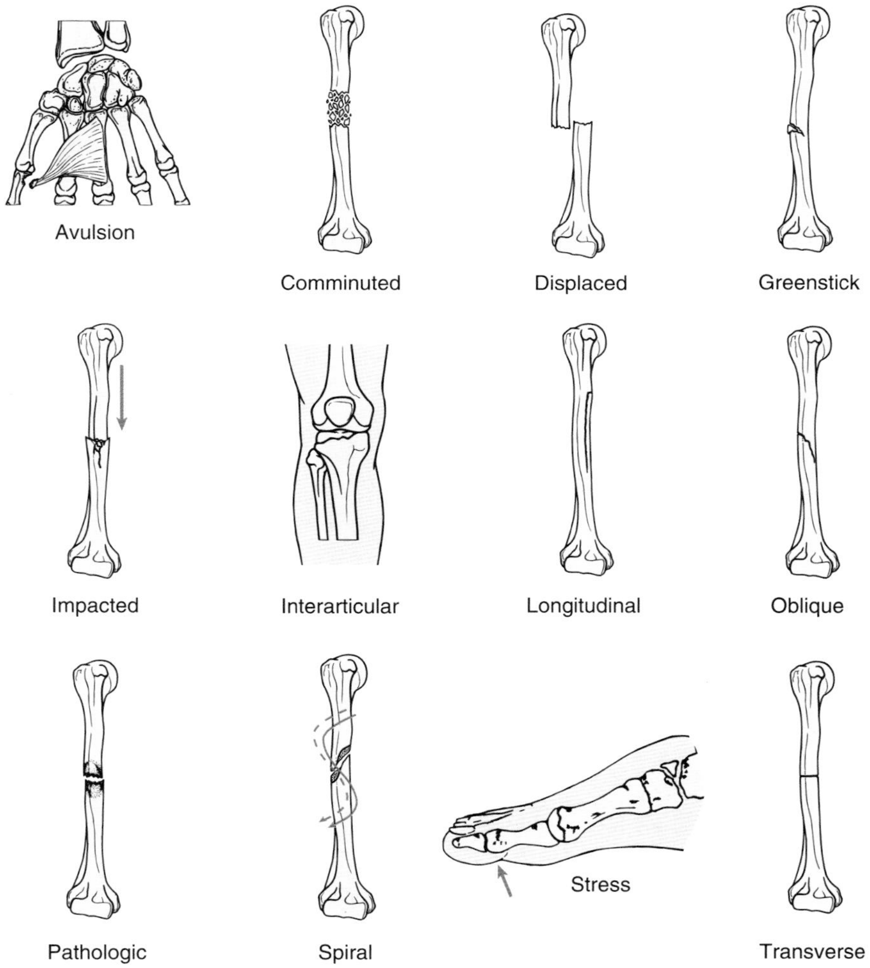

Fig. 45.2 Common types of fractures. (From Lewis SM, Heitkemper MM, Dirksen SR, et al.: *Medical-surgical nursing: assessment and management of clinical problems*, ed 7, St. Louis, 2007, Mosby.)

hours, a clot or hematoma forms between the two broken ends of the bone.

- Stage 2: Fibrocartilage formation. The hematoma that surrounds the fracture does not resorb as does a hematoma in other parts of the body. Instead, other tissue cells enter the clot and granulation tissue forms, replacing the clot. The granulation tissue then forms a collar around each end of the broken bone, gradually becoming firm and forming a bridge between the two ends.
- Stage 3: Callus formation. Within 1 to 4 weeks after injury, the granulation tissue changes into a callus formation. Callus is made up of cartilage, osteoblasts (i.e., bone cells that form new bone), calcium, and phosphorus. The callus is larger than the diameter of the bone and serves as a temporary splint.
- Stage 4: Ossification. Within 3 weeks to 6 months after the break, a permanent bone callus, known as *woven bone*, forms. It is during this stage that the ends of the broken bone begin to knit.
- Stage 5: Consolidation and remodeling. Consolidation occurs when the distance between bone fragments decreases and eventually closes. During **bone remodeling**, the immature bone cells are gradually replaced by mature bone cells. The excess bone is naturally chiseled away by stress to the affected part from motion, exercise, and weight bearing. The bone then takes on its original shape and size (Fig. 45.3).

Healing is affected by many factors, including the location and severity of the fracture, the type of bone, other bone pathology, blood supply to the area, infection, and the adequacy of immobilization. Other factors that affect healing include age, endocrine disorders, and some drugs. The healing time for fractures increases with age, and it may take 6 times longer for the same type of fracture to heal in an older adult as in an infant. In the absence of bone disease, the majority of older adults eventually heal as well as younger adults. However, many older adults, especially women, have a loss of bone mass.

COMPLICATIONS

Complications of a fracture can delay or impede healing and may even be life threatening. Short-term complications include infection, fat embolism, deep vein thrombosis (DVT), compartment syndrome, and shock. Long-term complications include joint stiffness and contractures, malunion, nonunion, delayed union, posttraumatic arthritis, avascular necrosis, and complex regional pain syndrome.

INFECTION

Infection of the bone, called *osteomyelitis*, can result from contamination of the open wound associated with a fracture, from contamination of the indwelling hardware used to repair the broken bone, or through the blood from a distant infection. When an infection is inadvertently introduced by surgery or other treatment, it is known as an *iatrogenic* or *health care–associated infection*. Any infection can interfere with normal healing. Osteomyelitis occurs most commonly after an open fracture and surgical repair and may become chronic. In deep, grossly contaminated wounds, gas gangrene may develop.

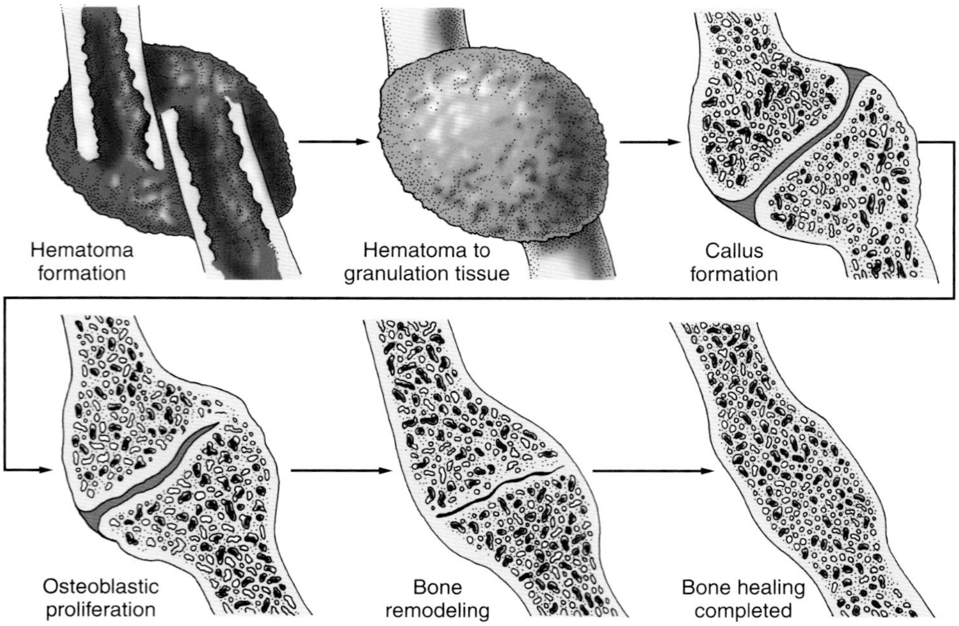

Fig. 45.3 Stages of fracture healing. (From Ignatavicius DD, Workman ML: *Medical-surgical nursing: patient-centered collaborative care*, ed 8, St. Louis, 2016, Saunders.)

Signs and symptoms of bone infection are local pain, redness, purulent wound drainage, chills, and fever. With gas gangrene, a foul-smelling watery drainage is seen, with significant redness and swelling of affected tissue. A diagnosis is based on clinical findings supported by culture of drainage or material obtained by needle aspiration. Imaging procedures—computed tomography (CT), magnetic resonance imaging (MRI), positron emission tomography (PET) scan—may be helpful. Radiographic changes typically are not seen until 10 to 14 days after the onset of infection.

Osteomyelitis requires aggressive antibiotic therapy. Intravenous antibiotics may be given for 4 to 8 weeks, followed by an additional 4 to 8 weeks of oral drug therapy. Chronic infection may require continuous, long-term antimicrobials. Wound care may include irrigation, treatment with antibiotic beads, and surgical removal of dead bone tissue, hardware, or both.

FAT EMBOLISM

Fat embolism is a condition in which fat globules are released from the marrow of the broken bone into the bloodstream. Once the fat droplets enter the circulation, they migrate to the lungs. Because they are too large to pass through the pulmonary circulation, they lodge in the capillaries and obstruct blood flow. The fat particles break down into fatty acids, which inflame the pulmonary blood vessels, leading to pulmonary edema.

Fat embolism syndrome is associated most commonly with fractures of the long bones, multiple fractures, and severe trauma. It occurs 24 to 72 hours after injury, most often in young men 20 to 40 years of age and in older adults 70 to 80 years of age. An older patient with a hip fracture is at highest risk. The most important preventive action is careful immobilization of fractures.

Respiratory distress is the first sign of a fat embolism, followed by tachycardia, tachypnea, fever, confusion, and decreased level of consciousness. Another characteristic feature is petechiae, a measles-like rash over the neck, upper arms, chest, or abdomen. Treatment of fat embolism consists of bed rest, gentle handling, oxygen (O_2), and ventilatory support. Other specific interventions will be needed if the patient develops hypovolemic shock, acidosis, and/or pulmonary edema. Although controversial, corticosteroids are sometimes used. The prognosis is generally good; however, the condition can be fatal.

DEEP VEIN THROMBOSIS

Venous stasis, vessel damage, and altered clotting mechanisms contribute to the formation of blood clots (thrombi), most commonly in the deep veins of the legs. This complication is increased with immobility often associated with a fracture. Like fat particles, thrombi can break off and travel to the lungs, causing a pulmonary embolism. The prevention and treatment of DVT and pulmonary embolism are discussed in Chapters 27 and 35.

COMPARTMENT SYNDROME

Compartment syndrome is a serious complication that results from internal or external pressure on the affected area. Compartments are located in the muscles of the extremities. They are enclosed spaces made up of muscle, bone, nerves, and blood vessels wrapped by a fibrous membrane, or fascia. External pressure caused by a cast or tight dressing can decrease blood flow to the area. Internal pressure can be caused by edema or bleeding into a compartment. Fluid trapped in the compartment puts pressure on the tissues, nerves, and blood vessels, decreasing blood flow and resulting in pain and tissue damage.

Although compartment syndrome is relatively rare, it is a serious condition and can create an emergency situation. Within 4 to 6 hours after the onset of compartment syndrome, irreversible muscle and nerve damage can occur. Paresis (i.e., partial paralysis) can result if the condition is not treated within 24 hours. In 24 to 48 hours, the limb can become useless.

A primary symptom of compartment syndrome is pain, especially with touch or movement that cannot be relieved with opioid analgesia. Other signs and symptoms are edema, pallor, weak or unequal pulses, cyanosis, tingling, numbness, and paresthesia.

The goal of treatment is to relieve pressure. When internal pressure exists, a surgical fasciotomy, which entails making linear incisions in the fascia, may be done to relieve pressure on the nerves and blood vessels. For external pressure, the cast or dressings are removed and replaced.

SHOCK

After a fracture, there is a risk of excessive blood loss. Tissue trauma may rupture local blood vessels and vascular internal organs may be punctured, with resultant internal bleeding. Loss of blood leads to shock, which is evidenced by tachycardia, anxiety, pallor, and cool, clammy skin. Careful immobilization of fractures reduces the risk of hemorrhage. If severe external bleeding is evident, external pressure should be applied and medical assistance summoned immediately. Management of hypovolemic shock is discussed in Chapter 9.

Put On Your Thinking Cap!

A 16-year-old male patient was admitted after a motorcycle accident. He had a compound fracture of the femur with severe soft tissue injury. After surgery, he has an external fixation device on the affected leg. A Jackson-Pratt drain is in place. Daily wound care is ordered. List all potential sources of bone infection.

JOINT STIFFNESS AND CONTRACTURES

Joint fractures or dislocations may be followed by stiffness or contractures, especially in older persons, because of immobility often associated with a fracture. Prevention requires appropriate positioning and progressive exercise programs as prescribed. Treatment may include the use of splints, traction, casts, surgical manipulation, and aggressive physiotherapy.

MALUNION, NONUNION, AND DELAYED UNION

Malunion takes place when expected healing time is appropriate, but unsatisfactory alignment of bone results in external deformity and dysfunction. **Nonunion** occurs when a fracture never heals. Failure of a fracture to heal in the expected time is called **delayed union**. With delayed union, the bone usually heals eventually—it may just be slower. These complications can be caused by inadequate immobilization or excess movement, poor alignment of the bone fragments, infection, or poor nutrition.

When nonunion of a fracture exists, a variety of methods may be used to stimulate fracture healing. The implantation of bone grafts is an *osteogenic method*. Osteoconductive methods use synthetic materials to provide a matrix for bone growth. The use of substances such as platelet-derived growth factor is called *osteoinduction*. In addition, devices that deliver electric stimulation or pulsed electromagnetic fields may be used to stimulate bone growth. The stimulation may be internal or external and is done up to 10 hours a day for 3 to 6 months. Although the procedure is time consuming, it can prevent further surgery and bone grafts. Hyperbaric O_2 therapy has been used, but its value in treatment of nonunion has not been confirmed.

POSTTRAUMATIC ARTHRITIS

Weight-bearing joints are most vulnerable to posttraumatic arthritis. Excessive stress and strain on the joint or fracture must be avoided to reduce the risk of this complication. Posttraumatic arthritis can be a result of nonunion of a fracture.

AVASCULAR NECROSIS

A fracture or bone infection can interfere with the blood supply to the bone. Once bone cells are deprived of O_2 and nutrients, they die and their cell walls collapse. This condition is called *avascular necrosis*. Signs and symptoms include increasing pain, instability, and decreased function in the affected area. Treatment measures include relief of weight bearing and removal of part of the bone to decrease pressure. If conservative measures fail, a variety of surgical procedures may be recommended. Sometimes amputation is necessary.

COMPLEX REGIONAL PAIN SYNDROME

Complex regional pain syndrome (CRPS) type 1 is usually precipitated by a fracture or other trauma. It is characterized by severe pain at the injury site despite no detectable nerve damage, edema, muscle spasm, stiffness, vasospasms, increased sweating, atrophy, contractures, and loss of bone mass. Symptoms persist longer than expected with the type of injury suffered. The condition is treated with nerve blocks; physical therapy; transcutaneous electrical nerve stimulation (TENS); and drugs, including analgesics, antiseizure drugs, antidepressants, and alpha-1 adrenergic agonists. Various nonopioid infusions such as lidocaine and ketamine have been used with some success. The effects and treatment of CRPS type 2, also called *causalgia*, are similar but nerve damage can be detected.

CLINICAL MANIFESTATIONS

The signs and symptoms of a fracture depend on the type and location of the break. Some fractures have so few clinical manifestations that they can be detected only with a radiograph. The most common signs and symptoms are swelling, bruising, pain, tenderness, loss of normal function, abnormal position, and decreased mobility. Box 45.1 lists various signs and symptoms of fractures and their causes.

DIAGNOSTIC TESTS AND PROCEDURES

A thorough history and physical are important when fracture is suspected because they may provide valuable information, such as mechanism of injury, and often help to direct treatment. The most common diagnostic tests used to confirm the presence of a fracture are radiologic studies. Standard radiographs are used first to reveal bone disruption, deformity, or malignancy. CT may be used to detect fractures of complex structures, such as the hip and pelvis, or compression fractures of the spine. MRI aids in the assessment of soft tissue damage. A bone scan may be useful for detecting small bone fractures or fractures caused by stress or disease. Diagnostic tests for fractures are described in Chapter 43, Table 43.1.

MEDICAL TREATMENT

The goals of medical treatment for a fracture are to realign the bone fragments, establish a sturdy union between the broken ends of the bone, and restore function. The most common therapeutic techniques to accomplish these goals are closed or open reduction and internal or external fixation.

REDUCTION

Reduction is the process of bringing the ends of the broken bone into proper alignment. **Closed reduction or manipulation** is the nonsurgical realignment of the bones that returns them to their previous anatomic position. No surgical incision is made; however,

Box 45.1 Signs and Symptoms of Fractures and Their Causes

PAIN
Immediate, severe pain is felt at the time of injury. After injury, pain may result from muscle spasm, overriding of the fractured ends of the bone, or damage to adjacent structures.

DEFORMITY
Strong muscle pull may cause bone fragments to override; therefore alignment and contour changes occur, such as (1) angulation, rotation, and limb shortening; (2) bone depression; or (3) altered curves in the injured site, especially when compared with the opposite site. Swelling (edema) may appear rapidly from localization of serous fluid at the fracture site and extravasation of blood into adjacent tissues. Bruising (ecchymosis) may result from subcutaneous bleeding. Muscle spasms—involuntary muscle contractions near the fracture—may occur.

TENDERNESS
Tenderness over the fracture site is caused by underlying injuries.

IMPAIRED SENSATION (NUMBNESS)
Sensation may be impaired as a result of nerve damage or nerve entrapment from edema, bleeding, or bony fragments.

LOSS OF NORMAL FUNCTION
Normal function may be lost because of instability of the fractured bone, pain, or muscle spasm.

PARALYSIS
Paralysis may be caused by nerve damage.

ABNORMAL MOBILITY
Movement of a part that is normally immobile is caused by instability when the long bones are fractured.

CREPITUS
Crepitus results from broken bone ends rubbing together. Grating sensations or sounds are felt or heard if the injured part is moved.

HYPOVOLEMIC SHOCK
Hypovolemic shock may result from blood loss or other injuries.

Modified from Black JM, Hawks JH, Keene AM: *Medical-surgical nursing: clinical management for positive outcomes*, ed 6, Philadelphia, 2001, Saunders.

general or local anesthesia is given. Closed reduction may be done by using traction, manual pressure, or a combination of these (Fig. 45.4). After reduction of a fracture, a radiograph is taken, and the injured part is immobilized.

Open reduction is a surgical procedure in which an incision is made at the fracture site. It is usually done for open (i.e., compound) or **comminuted fractures** (i.e., bone is broken or crushed into small pieces) to clean the area of fragments and debris.

Effective pain management of a fracture is essential for patient mobilization and healing. Once the fracture is aligned, immobilization is necessary for healing to occur. Immobilization of the bones is important because it prevents movement and increases union. It can be accomplished in many ways such as fixation, casts, splints, and traction.

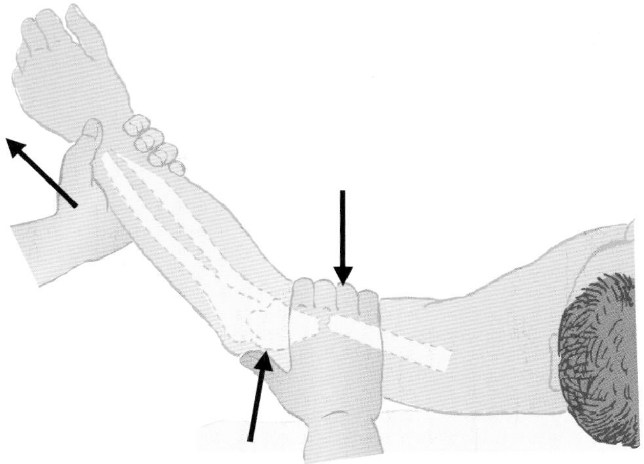

Fig. 45.4 Closed (manipulative) reduction to realign a fracture of the arm. (From Black JM, Hawks JH: *Medical-surgical nursing: clinical management for positive outcomes*, ed 8, St. Louis, 2009, Saunders.)

FIXATION

Fixation is an attempt to attach the fragments of the broken bone together when reduction alone is not feasible because of the type and extent of the break. Internal fixation is done during the open reduction surgical procedure. Internal fixation includes the use of rods, pins, nails, screws, or metal plates to align bone fragments and keep them in place for healing (Fig. 45.5). Fig. 45.5C illustrates an open reduction and internal fixation of a fractured femur in which a nail is used to maintain alignment. Internal fixation promotes early mobilization and is often preferred for older adults who have brittle bones that may not heal properly or who may suffer the consequences of immobility.

External fixation is similar to internal fixation, but the pins are inserted directly into the bone, above and below the fracture. The pins are then attached to an external frame and adjusted to align the bone (Fig. 45.6). When extensive soft tissue damage or infection occurs, external fixation allows easier access to the site and facilitates wound care. In addition, the device allows for early ambulation and mobility while relieving pain. Pin track infection occurs in approximately 10% of patients with external fixation. Pin care is extremely important to prevent the migration of organisms along the pin from the skin to the bone. Patients should be taught to do their own pin care and to recognize signs of infection.

COMMON THERAPEUTIC MEASURES

CASTS, SPLINTS, AND IMMOBILIZERS

Casts, splints, and other immobilizers are used to secure the position of the body parts being treated as

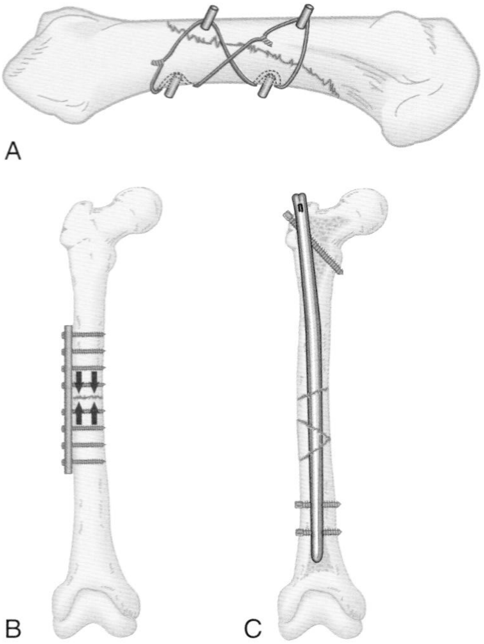

Fig. 45.5 Examples of different types of internal fixation devices. (A) Tension band wiring technique using Kirschner wires for fracture of a phalanx. (B) Compression plate applied to the lateral aspect of the femur. (C) Intramedullary nail fixed to both proximal and distal fragments of the femur. (From Black JM, Hawks JH: *Medical-surgical nursing: clinical management for positive outcomes*, ed 8, St. Louis, 2009, Saunders.)

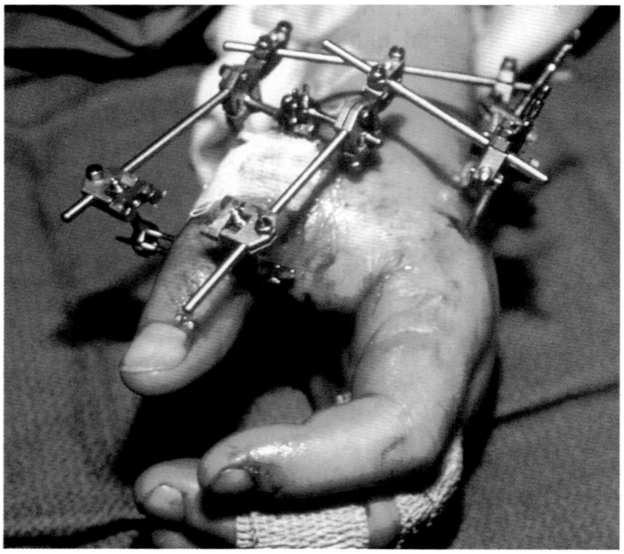

Fig. 45.6 External fixators. Mini Hoffman system in place on hand. (Image reprinted with permission from Stryker Corporation. Copyright © 2018 Stryker Corporation. All rights reserved.)

well as to reduce pain. They hold the bone in alignment while allowing enough movement of other parts of the body to carry out activities of daily living (ADLs).

Fiberglass, a waterproof synthetic casting material, is most frequently used for fracture immobilization. After the cast is applied, drying time is 10 to 15 minutes, and the cast can withstand weight bearing 30 minutes after application (Fig. 45.7).

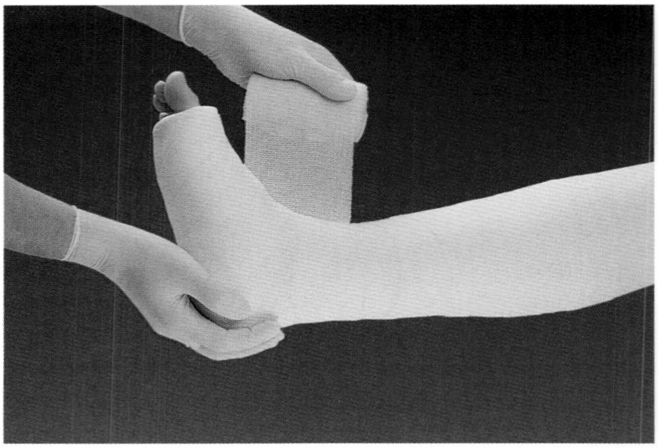

Fig. 45.7 Application of a fiberglass synthetic cast. (From Perry AG, Potter PA, Elkin MK: *Nursing interventions & clinical skills*, ed 5, St. Louis, 2012, Mosby, in Ignatavicius DD, Workman ML, Rebar CR, Heimgartner NM. *Medical-surgical nursing: concepts for interprofessional collaborative care*, St. Louis, 2021, Elsevier.)

Plaster, the least expensive type of cast traditionally employed in the past, is used less frequently today. After a well-fitting stockinette has been applied, the gauze is immersed in water and wrapped around the affected part. The stockinette must not be too tight because it may impair circulation. A stockinette that is too loose can wrinkle and result in pressure sores. The number of layers of wrapped gauze and the technique of application determine the strength of the cast.

Initially the wet cast is hot, and the heat may cause edema of the underlying tissues from the increased circulation. The cast quickly becomes damp and cool. It dries after about 24 to 72 hours, depending on the size and location. When the cast is dry and strong, it can withstand weight bearing and other stresses. The underlying stockinette covers the edges of the cast to prevent scratching and irritation from the rough plaster. Short pieces of tape are sometimes placed over the edges of the casts to prevent skin irritation by rough edges and to protect the cast from moisture and soiling. This is referred to as *petaling*.

Sometimes the cast is split down the front to allow the casting material and padding to spread. This is referred to as a *univalved cast*. A bivalved cast is cut down both sides so that the front portion can be removed while the back portion maintains immobilization. When an opening is cut into the cast to allow inspection of the body area or to relieve pressure, it is said to be a *windowed cast*. It is important to save the cut-out "window" because it may be reinserted later.

The four main groups of casts are (1) upper extremity, (2) lower extremity, (3) cast brace, and (4) body or spica cast. Various types of casts and their uses are illustrated in Table 45.1. Cast care may vary according to the type of material used (see the Patient Teaching box).

Table 45.1 Cast Types and Common Uses

TYPE	ILLUSTRATION	FEATURES
Short arm cast	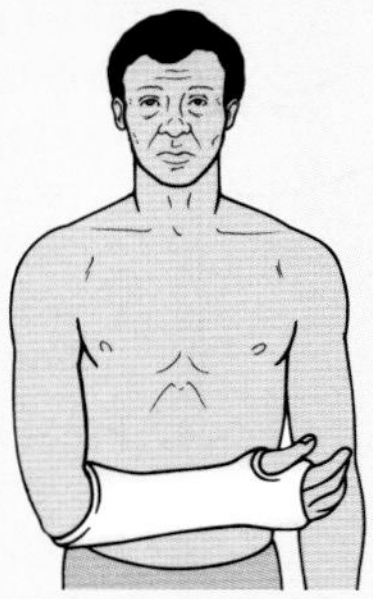 Short arm cast	Fracture of hand or wrist Postoperative immobilization after open reduction and internal fixation. Can be weighted to create traction Keep arm elevated above the heart when lying in bed to prevent swelling
Long arm cast	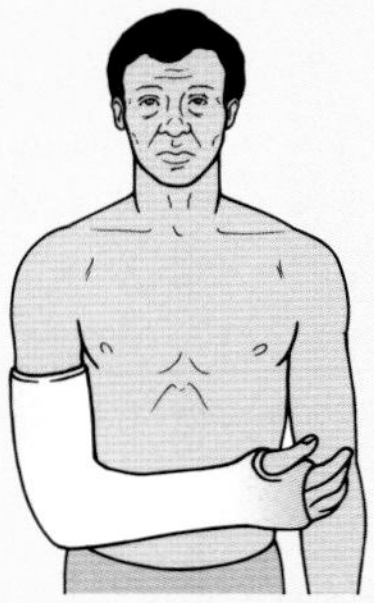 Long arm cast	Fracture of forearm, elbow, or humerus Postoperative immobilization after open reduction and internal fixation Can be weighted to create traction Arm supported by sling when up and out of bed
Body jacket cast	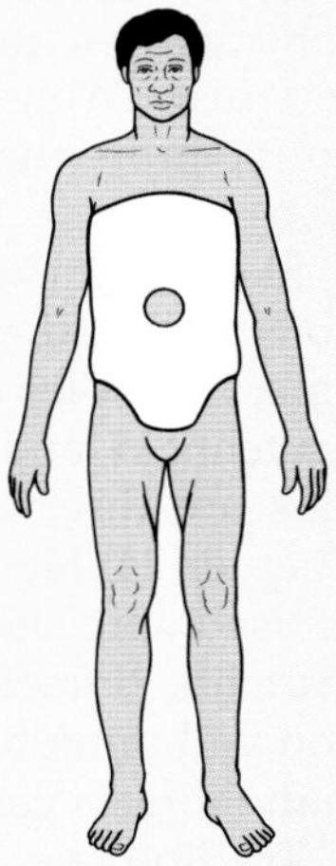 Body jacket cast	Stable spine injuries of the thoracic or lumbar spine Severely limits mobility that may cause pressure injuries, respiratory problems, constipation, joint contractures
Bilateral long leg hip spica cast	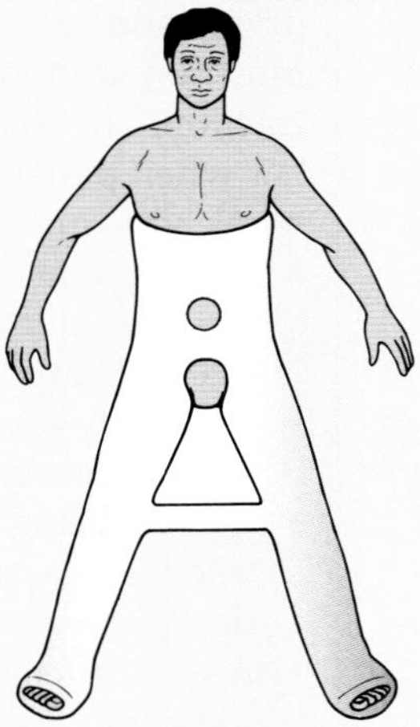 Double hip spica	Fractures of femur, acetabulum, or pelvis Postoperative immobilization after open reduction and internal fixation Limited mobility; turning requires several people Nausea and abdominal distention can result from *cast syndrome* (compression of a portion of the duodenum between the superior mesenteric artery and aorta and vertebral column)

Continued

Table 45.1 Cast Types and Common Uses—cont'd

TYPE	ILLUSTRATION	FEATURES
Long leg cast	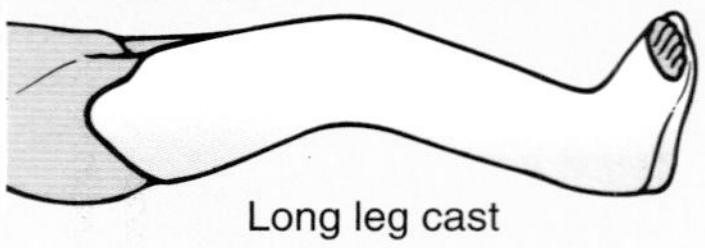	Fracture of distal femur, knee, or lower leg Soft tissue injury to knee or knee dislocation Postoperative immobilization after open reduction and internal fixation Allows mobility with crutches Elevate affected extremity on several pillows first few days to prevent swelling
Short leg cast	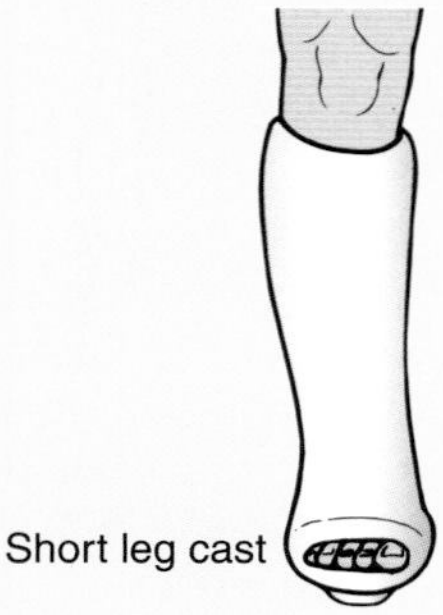	Fracture of foot, ankle, or distal tibia or fibula Severe sprain or strain Postoperative immobilization after open reduction and internal fixation Correction of deformity, such as talipes equinovarus Allows mobility with crutches Elevate affected extremity on several pillows first few days to prevent swelling

Illustrations from Lewis SM, Dirksen SR, Heitkemper MM, et al.: *Medical-surgical nursing: assessment and management of clinical problems*, ed 9, St. Louis, 2015, Mosby.

Patient Teaching

Cast Care

- Keep plaster casts dry; follow the physician's instructions regarding wetting fiberglass casts.
- Do not remove any padding.
- Do not insert any foreign object inside the cast.
- Do not bear weight on a new plaster cast for 48 hours (with fiberglass, may be less than 1 hour).
- Do not cover a plaster cast with plastic for prolonged periods.
- Report the following to a health care provider: swelling, discoloration of toes or fingers, pain during motion, and burning or tingling under the cast.

The cast is removed only on the health care provider's orders. A special device called a *cast cutter* is used to cut the cast. Blunt scissors are then used to cut the padding. Tell the patient that the cutter blade is noisy but will not cut the skin. When the cast is removed, the skin under the cast will be tender and dry and may have crusts of dry skin. Gently wash the area and explain that the skin will regain its normal appearance after a few days. Muscle atrophy may be apparent. Assure the patient that muscle mass will be restored with use of the limb.

TRACTION

Traction exerts a pulling force on a fractured extremity to provide alignment of the broken bone fragments. It is also used to prevent or correct deformity, decrease muscle spasm, promote rest, and maintain the position of the diseased or injured part.

Traction may be applied directly to the skin (i.e., skin traction) or attached directly to a bone by means of a metal pin or wire (i.e., skeletal traction). Examples of skin traction, such as Buck traction, are shown in Fig. 45.8. It is used for hip and knee contractures, muscle spasms, and alignment of hip fractures. Weight used during skin traction should not be more than 5 to 10 lb. to prevent injury to the skin.

Skeletal traction provides a strong, steady, continuous pull and can be used for prolonged periods of time. Examples of skeletal traction are Gardner-Wells, Crutchfield, and Vinke tongs and a halo vest, in which pins are inserted into the skull on either side (see Chapter 24, Figs. 24.6 and 24.7). Heavier weights can be used with skeletal traction, usually from 15 to 30 lb. Crutchfield traction and a halo vest are used for reduction and immobilization of fractures of the cervical or high thoracic vertebrae.

Traction may cause complications such as impaired circulation, inadequate fracture alignment, skin breakdown, and soft tissue injury. As noted earlier, pin track infection and osteomyelitis can occur with skeletal traction. The following are important points to remember when patients are in traction:

- Weights must always hang freely.
- Ensure that the amount of weight used is correct as ordered, clamps are tight, and ropes move freely over pulleys.
- Maintain good body alignment so that the line of pull is correct.
- Use padding to prevent trauma to the skin where traction is applied. Report skin breakdown or irritation to the physician.
- Assess affected extremities for temperature, pain, sensation, motion, capillary refill time, and pulses.
- With skeletal traction, assess pin sites for redness, drainage, or odor, which may indicate infection.

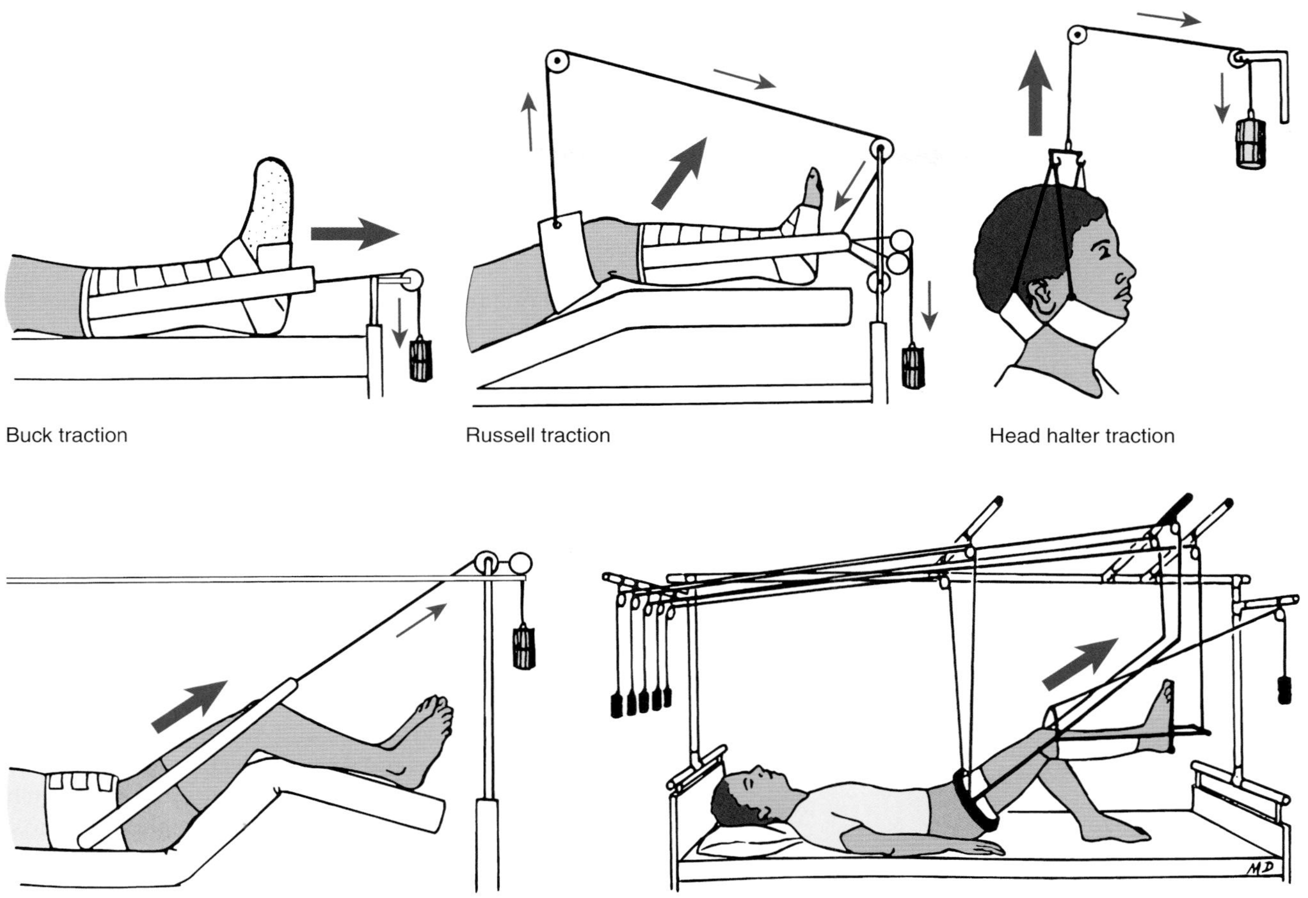

Fig. 45.8 Examples of skin traction. (Redrawn from Polaski AK, Tatro SE: *Luckmann's core principles and practice of medical-surgical nursing*, Philadelphia, 1996, Saunders.)

ELECTRICAL STIMULATION AND PULSED ELECTROMAGNETIC FIELDS

Electrical stimulation may be used to promote bone healing by promoting bone growth. An electrical current is delivered through a surgically implanted device, a device applied to the skin, or a device that uses pins inserted through the skin. Electrical bone stimulators are successful in approximately 80% of cases, with an average healing time of 16 weeks. Pulsed electromagnetic fields (PEMFs) are noninvasive devices that include a control box and a pad that induces electrical changes around and within the cell. In theory, the electrical changes activate and regenerate cells, which promotes healing and reduces pain.

ASSISTIVE DEVICES

CRUTCHES

Crutches increase mobility and assist with ambulation after a fracture of the lower extremity. Success in crutch walking depends on many factors, including the patient's motivation, age, interests and activities, and ability to adjust to the crutches. Crutch use requires good upper body strength, so it may not be appropriate for older or frail patients.

In most cases, a physical therapist measures the patient for proper fit and instructs the patient in crutch-walking techniques. The nurse reinforces the instructions and evaluates whether the crutches are being used properly. A properly fitted crutch should reach to about two finger widths below the axilla to avoid pressure on the axilla and nerves when walking (Fig. 45.9). Axillary pressure could result in temporary or permanent numbness in the hands. When walking, the patient's weight should rest on the handgrips. The handgrips are adjusted so that the elbow is slightly flexed, enough so that the elbow may be fully extended when taking a step. The total crutch length should equal the distance from the armpit to about 6 inches in front of a shoe.

The "Tripod Position"

The tripod position is the position in which the patient stands and begins to walk. To get into the tripod position, place the crutch tips about 4 to 6 inches to the side and in front of each foot. Stand on the "good" foot (the one that is weight bearing) (Fig. 45.10).

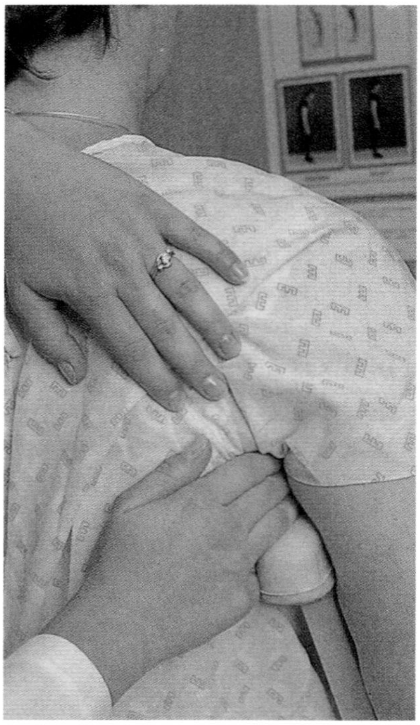

Fig. 45.9 The distance between the crutch pad and the patient's axilla should be 3 to 4 fingerbreadths. (From Potter PA, Perry AG, editors: *Fundamentals of nursing*, ed 7, St. Louis, 2009, Mosby.)

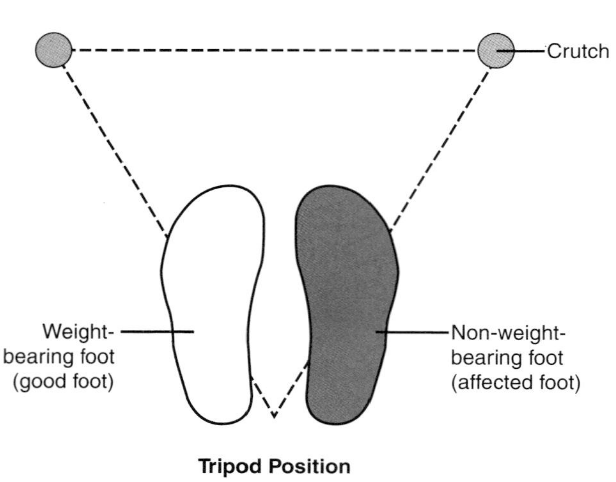

Fig. 45.10 The tripod position. (From the American College of Foot and Ankle Surgeons [ACFAS], All Rights Reserved © 2017.)

Gait Patterns

Several types of gait patterns are used with crutches. The type of gait used depends on the severity of the patient's disability and the patient's physical condition, trunk strength, upper and lower extremity strength, and balance. All of the gaits begin with the tripod position.

The five types of gait patterns used with crutches are as follows:

1. Two-point gait: The crutch on one side and the opposite foot are advanced at the same time. This gait is used with partial weight-bearing limitations and with bilateral lower extremity prostheses.
2. Three-point gait: Both crutches and the foot of the affected extremity are advanced together, followed by the foot of the unaffected extremity. This gait requires strength and balance. It is used for partial weight bearing or no weight bearing on the affected leg.
3. Four-point gait: The right crutch is advanced, then the left foot, then the left crutch, and then the right foot. This gait is used if weight bearing is allowed and one foot can be placed in front of the other.
4. Swing-to gait: Both crutches are advanced together and then both legs are lifted and placed down again on a spot behind the crutches. The feet and crutches form a tripod.
5. Swing-through gait: Both crutches are advanced together and then both legs are lifted through and beyond the crutches and placed down again at a point in front of the crutches. This gait is used when adequate muscle power and balance in the arms and legs exist.

To get into and out of a chair safely, make sure the chair is stable and will not roll or slide. It must have arms and back support. The patient walks up to a chair, turns using the crutches, and backs up until the unaffected leg touches the seat of the chair. One hand then grips both crutches by the handgrips and the crutches are placed to the unaffected side. The patient bends at the waist, places the hand on the affected side on the seat, moves the affected leg forward, and lowers onto the seat slowly (Fig. 45.11). To get up from a sitting position, the patient pushes off against the chair with the hand of the affected side and pushes down with the other hand, which is holding both crutches by the handgrips.

Going up and down stairs on crutches is challenging. For stair climbing, the unaffected leg goes up the step first while the crutches support the body. The full body weight is transferred to the unaffected leg, followed by movement of the crutches and the affected leg to the step. To descend stairs, the affected leg and the crutches move down one step first and then the unaffected leg follows. So, when climbing stairs, the good leg goes first and when descending stairs, the bad leg goes first. ("The good leads up and bad leads down.")

The safest way to go up and down stairs is without crutches in a sitting position. To go up the stairs, the patient sits on a low step and places the crutches as far up the stairs as possible, gradually moving them to the top. While sitting, the arms are placed behind on the stair above. The arms and weight-bearing foot are then used to lift the patient up one step. The process is repeated one step at a time. To go down the stairs, the patient is seated on the top step. The crutches are moved downstairs by continually sliding them to the lowest possible point on the stairway. While sitting, both arms are placed behind the patient. The arms and weight-bearing foot/leg are used to lift the patient down one step at a time.

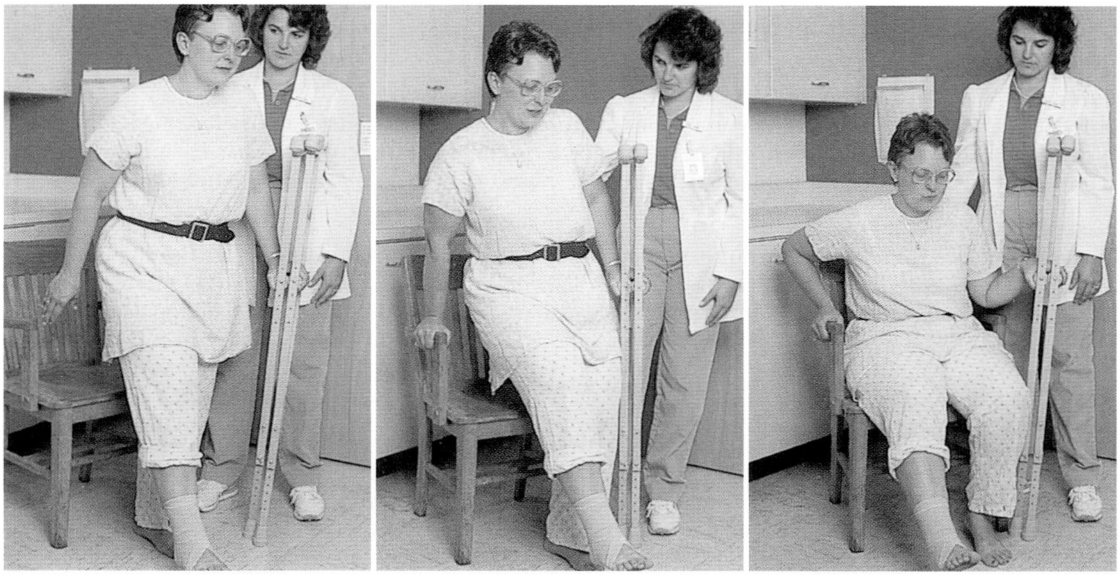

Fig. 45.11 Standing to sitting with crutches. (From Potter PA, Perry AG, editors: *Fundamentals of nursing*, ed 7, St. Louis, 2009, Mosby.)

Patient Teaching

Follow These Rules for Safety and Comfort

- Don't look down. Look straight ahead as you normally do when you walk.
- Don't use crutches if you feel dizzy or drowsy.
- Don't walk on slippery surfaces. Avoid snowy, icy, or rainy conditions.
- Don't put any weight on the affected foot if your doctor has so advised.
- Do make sure your crutches have rubber tips.
- Do wear well-fitting, low-heel shoes (or shoe).
- Do position the crutch hand grips correctly (see "Sizing Your Crutches")
- Do keep the crutch pads 1½ to 2 inches below your armpits.
- Do call your foot and ankle surgeon if you have any questions or difficulties.

WALKERS

A walker is used for support and balance. A modified swing-to gait is used with a walker so that the walker is pushed or lifted forward and then the legs are brought up to it. Rather than lifting both legs forward together, as with crutch walking, one foot is brought forward at a time.

CANES

Canes are used to provide minimal support and balance and to relieve pressure on weight-bearing joints. The cane is placed on the unaffected side with the top of the cane even with the patient's greater trochanter. The elbow should be flexed to approximately 30 degrees. A two-point or four-point gait is used with a cane. The cane should be held close to the body on the unaffected side and advanced along with the affected leg. When walking, it is better to lift the cane rather than slide it along to prevent catching the cane tip and tripping or falling.

NURSING CARE OF THE PATIENT WITH A FRACTURE

Once the initial emergency treatment and medical management of a patient with a fracture have been provided, nursing care becomes very important. The focus of nursing care is on preventing complications and restoring the patient to independent function. (See Nursing Care Plan: Patient With a Fracture. For a discussion of emergency care, see Chapter 63.)

FOCUSED ASSESSMENT

Health History

Even after the initial medical care has been given and the fracture has been set, it is helpful to gather information on the cause, type, and extent of the injury. This information is important because the nurse may observe for complications or other injuries that may have been overlooked during the emergency situation. Ask the patient, family members, or witnesses about the events leading up to the accident and exactly what happened during it. In addition, describe symptoms associated with the injury, including the type and extent of pain, the presence of numbness or tingling or both, the loss of motion and sensation, and the complaint of muscle spasms.

Document the number and types of prescription and over the counter (OTC) medications taken by the patient to determine whether they played any role in the development of the fracture or will affect recovery and rehabilitation. It is also helpful to find out about other medical problems that may either have been related to the cause of the fracture, such as a pathologic

Nursing Care Plan — Patient With a Fracture

FOCUSED ASSESSMENT

Health History

Mrs. Jacobson, 80 years of age, was admitted for a Colles fracture in the left wrist 2 days ago. Before the injury, she lived alone and cared for herself. She was active, alert, and independent. Since the fracture repair, she has complained of pain over the area of the break but has had no signs of infection. Her physician is ready to discharge her home.

Physical Examination

Vital signs: blood pressure 165/95 mm Hg, pulse 98 beats per minute with slight irregularity, respiration 20 breaths per minute, temperature 97.4°F (36.3°C) measured orally. Height 5′3″, weight 132 lb. Alert and oriented to time, place, and person. Needs assistance with activities of daily living (ADLs), particularly bathing, dressing, and toileting. Cast on left arm from above her elbow to her fingers.

Patient Problems	Goals and Outcome Criteria	Interventions
Acute pain related to bone fracture, edema, soft tissue damage, muscle spasm	The patient's pain will be relieved, as evidenced by absence of verbal complaints, anxiety, and moaning or wincing; patient confirms pain relief.	Provide adequate pain relief using medications and other comfort measures such as positioning and massage.
Inadequate peripheral circulation related to decreased blood flow caused by injury	The patient will have adequate tissue perfusion, as evidenced by normal skin color in areas distal to the fracture, adequate capillary refill, and adequate sensation.	Relieve edema by elevating the affected limb above the level of the patient's heart while she is lying in bed and applying cold for brief periods of time; encourage patient to wiggle fingers to increase circulation to the area.
Decreased mobility related to pain and treatment modalities for fracture	The patient will maintain as much mobility as possible, as evidenced by independence in ADLs and absence of secondary complications.	Encourage regular movement, including passive or active range-of-motion exercises. Reinforce activity and exercise program for the patient. Seek referral to home health for assistance at home.
Potential for disrupted skin tissue integrity related to cast	The patient will maintain skin integrity, as evidenced by intact skin.	Inspect the skin around cast edges for pressure or irritation. Monitor circulation and sensation in the fingers.
Inability to manage treatment regimen related to lack of experience with immobilization devices (e.g., casts)	The patient will demonstrate knowledge of the immobilization device and will describe its proper care and complications that could arise.	Teach the patient interventions that promote bone and tissue healing; teach the patient to recognize signs and symptoms of complications that should be reported to the physician. Instruct the patient in cast care.
Inability to perform ADLs independently (bathing, feeding, dressing, toileting) related to immobilization of wrist	The patient performs ADLs independently or with assistance.	Assess the patient's ability to do ADLs and to perform tasks such as cooking and grocery shopping. Determine whether she has anyone to assist her if needed. If not, request a home health or social work evaluation so that home care or assistance can be provided.

CRITICAL THINKING QUESTIONS

1. What activities can the patient perform that will promote bone and tissue healing?
2. What signs and symptoms require physician intervention?

fracture, or may affect healing. Determine the patient's occupation and usual roles and responsibilities and discuss with the patient and family the effects of the injury on usual activities.

Physical Examination

Because fractures usually involve some type of accidental injury, be alert for signs of serious complications, such as head, thoracic, or abdominal injuries. In addition, examine the patient for associated tissue trauma, such as bleeding, bruising, and lacerations.

When inspecting the suspected fracture area, observe for deviations in bone alignment. The limb may appear to be deformed. The length of the extremity may change, usually becoming shorter. Inspect the skin over the fracture for lacerations, bruising, or swelling.

Compare the affected extremity with the unaffected extremity. Do neurovascular checks (i.e., pulse, skin color, capillary refill time, sensation) in the areas distal to the wound to compare circulation and sensation. Assess pulse rate and volume as well as capillary refill time in the nails distal to the injury. Observe capillary refill time by applying pressure to the nail and checking the time required for color to return to the area. Skin color is a good indication of circulation to the extremity, and pallor indicates poor circulation. Determine sensation by pinprick, especially in the web space between the first and the second toes or between the thumb and the forefinger.

Patient Problems, Goals, and Outcome Criteria: Fracture

Patient Problems	Goals and Outcome Criteria
Acute pain related to bone fracture, edema, soft tissue damage, or muscle spasm	Pain relief: relaxed manner, patient statement of pain relief
Inadequate peripheral circulation related to tissue trauma or pressure caused by edema, bone fragments, hemorrhage, or therapeutic devices	Adequate circulation: affected tissue warm, normal pulses, normal skin color, minimal edema
Potential for infection related to break in skin, bone trauma, soft tissue damage	Absence of infection: normal body temperature and white blood cell (WBC) count, clear wound drainage, decreasing edema and redness
Decreased mobility related to pain and immobilization	Improved mobility: patient performs daily activities as permitted while protecting fracture
Potential for disrupted skin tissue integrity related to injury, immobility, and immobilizing devices	Intact or healing skin: absence of open wounds, redness, or pallor because of pressure; skin warm
Potential for activity intolerance related to prolonged immobilization	Improved activity tolerance: performance of daily activities without fatigue

Additional patient problems may include inadequate nutrition related to additional metabolic needs of healing bone and soft tissues (see the Nutrition Considerations box); constipation related to prolonged immobility and pain medication; inadequate self-care related to pain and immobility; inadequate coping related to prolonged immobility, hospitalization, or altered lifestyle; sleep disturbance related to pain or immobility; and decreased diversional activity related to immobility.

Nutrition Considerations

1. Calcium in the diet and calcium supplements are recommended to help prevent fractures because of osteoporosis in older age.
2. Prolonged immobilization, which is often required after multiple fractures, contributes to the loss of calcium and protein.
3. Essential nutritional elements for optimal bone healing are protein, calcium, and vitamins D, B, and C.
4. Supplemental feedings that are high in calories, protein, and calcium, such as milkshakes, may be served between meals to promote healing.
5. During periods of immobilization, a daily fluid intake of 2000 to 3000 mL is recommended (unless contraindicated) to promote bowel and bladder function.
6. Advise the patient in a hip spica that overeating may cause abdominal pressure and cramping.

Interventions

Acute pain. Fractures are painful. The degree of pain experienced depends on the extent and type of injury and the pain tolerance of the patient. The primary method of pain relief is immobilization of the affected part. Elevating the affected area will help to manage edema. Analgesic medications and muscle relaxants, as well as cold therapy, can be helpful. Other methods of pain relief include repositioning, massage, and diversion. General pain management is discussed in more detail in Chapter 8.

Inadequate peripheral circulation. Factors that cause ineffective peripheral tissue perfusion are soft tissue injury resulting from trauma, fracture fragments, hemorrhage, edema, compartment syndrome, and positioning. The treatment of the fracture can also interfere with peripheral circulation, including moving or splinting the fracture, manipulation during reduction, and application of a cast, a splint, traction, or a brace.

Frequent neurovascular checks determine whether circulation is adequate and detect signs of pressure on nerves. For patients at risk for circulatory impairment, elevate the affected part above the level of the heart, apply cold packs as ordered to minimize edema, and encourage finger and toe movement. Evidence of impaired circulation includes abnormal coolness or warmth, weak or absent pulses, pale or bluish skin color, and sluggish capillary refill. Pressure on a nerve can cause pain, tingling, numbness, or motor impairments. Immediately report signs of impaired circulation to the physician. If a cast is too tight, it may need to be cut or replaced.

Potential for infection. Disruption of skin integrity may occur with a fracture, and when there is open reduction with external fixation, the potential for infection always exists. Infection can delay healing and rehabilitation. Bone infections are especially difficult to treat. Use strict aseptic technique for dressing changes, wound irrigations, and care of pins and drains. Observe wounds and pin sites for signs of infection, such as drainage, redness, swelling, and warmth, and monitor the patient's temperature for fever. If an infection develops, use standard infection control precautions and administer antibiotics as prescribed. The management of infection is discussed in more detail in Chapter 5.

Decreased mobility. Interventions for immobility are aimed at promoting independence and preventing related complications. Patients may experience anxiety and powerlessness when their activity is restricted because of the enforced immobilization related to traction, casts, or other equipment. In addition, they may experience secondary complications of immobility such as DVT, pulmonary embolism, contractures or muscular atrophy, skin breakdown, and gastrointestinal (GI) problems, especially constipation. Older individuals are particularly vulnerable to the effects of immobility. Adequate hydration and nutrition are important.

Encourage all patients with fractures to engage in regular movement of some kind. Passive or active range-of-motion exercises are helpful for both bedridden and ambulatory patients. Support the joints above and below the injury in functional positions. Periodic elevation of the affected limb promotes venous return and reduces edema. Gait training with crutches, walkers, and canes promotes mobility and independence. A physical therapist usually works out an activity and exercise program for patients recovering from fractures, and the role of the nurse is to reinforce and encourage patients to carry out the program. More discussion of immobility appears in Chapter 12.

If patients are unable to care for themselves independently at home, assistance from formal agencies such as home health services or social services may be needed. Areas to be assessed for home care needs include ability to carry out ADLs, mobility, mental status, and skilled nursing needs. If you think home care will be needed, consult the case manager or social worker about the appropriate referral.

Potential for disrupted skin tissue integrity. Disrupted skin integrity can be a result of the injury itself or the treatment of the injury. A compound fracture causes a break in the skin, and soft tissue injury occurs with almost every kind of fracture. Treatment measures such as immobilization or devices such as casts or traction may cause pressure on areas of the skin and result in pressure sores. In addition, the improper use of equipment can cause pressure on certain areas of the skin. Individuals who are at highest risk for skin breakdown are older adults, people with preexisting conditions such as diabetes mellitus, and people whose general condition was poor before the injury.

To prevent skin breakdown, patients should begin moving around as soon as possible after the fracture has been treated. Proper positioning and frequent turning are essential for the prevention of skin *breakdown*. Guidelines for proper positioning are listed in Table 45.2. Good nutrition and fluid intake help to maintain healthy tissues.

Put On Your Thinking Cap!

Assume that you are going home with a walker. Assess the barriers in your home and modifications that would be needed for you to get around safely in it.

Potential for activity intolerance. With prolonged immobility, people become weaker and their ability to participate in activities diminishes. Encourage patients to keep their strength up by carrying out range-of-motion exercises, resistance exercises of the unaffected extremities, and, when possible, ambulation. Participation in ADLs and recreational activities is also helpful. Rest periods between activities help to preserve strength.

Teaching should take place in the hospital immediately after the fracture is treated to prepare for the patient's discharge home. Assess the patient and family members for their readiness and ability to learn. Patient teaching after fractures should include the types of medical and nursing interventions that will be carried out to promote bone and tissue healing, signs

Table 45.2 Tips on Positioning

FRACTURE	POSITIONING
Cervical	Before treatment: with patient supine, immobilize neck with sandbags or Philadelphia collar If patient must be turned, be sure head and neck alignment is maintained
Thoracic spine	Position of comfort
Lumbar spine	Avoid high sitting positions, logroll
Pelvis	Stable fracture or after fixation: turn to side opposite fracture Unstable: do not turn
Hip	Before surgical treatment: turn toward fracture (avoid dislocation or further displacement of fragments) with pillows between legs Postoperatively: turn away from fracture until comfortable enough to turn on operative side, with pillows between legs Arthroplasty: maintain abduction at all times with abduction pillow or regular pillows between legs
Shoulder/humerus	Elevate head of bed to comfort Turn to side opposite fracture
Forearm/foreleg	Elevate distal portion of extremity higher than heart

From Maher AB, Salmond SW, Pellino TA: *Orthopedic nursing*, Philadelphia, 1994, Saunders.

and symptoms of complications that should be reported to a physician, how to use equipment and assistive devices, and techniques for managing ADLs.

Pharmacology Capsule

Patients who administer their own pain medications are more in control and better able to manage their pain successfully.

MANAGEMENT OF SPECIFIC FRACTURES

HIP FRACTURE

By 90 years of age, 17% of men and more than 30% of women have sustained a hip fracture. Most hip fractures are in the femoral neck and intertrochanteric regions (Fig. 45.12). The most common direct cause is a fall on a hard surface; however, it is thought that many fractures in older individuals result from decreased bone mass or brittle bones associated with osteoporosis (see the Health Promotion box). Among older adults, 3% to 5% of all falls result in fractures. Signs and symptoms of a hip fracture are a recent fall, severe pain and tenderness in the region of the fracture site, evidence of soft tissue trauma, the affected leg shorter than the unaffected leg, and the hip on the affected side is rotated externally.

Health Promotion

Once Is Enough: Preventing Future Fractures in Patients With Osteoporosis

Osteoporosis is a public health threat that affects 9% of Americans 50 years of age and older. The disease makes bones more prone to fractures, especially of the hip, spine, and wrist. One in two women and one in four men will have an osteoporosis-related fracture in their lifetime. Women near or past menopause who have sustained a fracture in the past are twice as likely to experience another fracture. However, unfortunately only 5% of patients with osteoporotic fractures are referred for an osteoporosis evaluation and medical treatment.

Ensure that your patients receive the necessary referrals for bone mineral density testing and other appropriate evaluations. Patients may be reluctant to exercise for fear of breaking another bone. Explain that engaging in weight-bearing exercises and resistance exercises preserves bone density and prevents falls by enhancing balance, flexibility, and strength. As appropriate, you can recommend the following activities to your patients:

- Walking
- Strength training
- Dancing
- Tai Chi
- Stair climbing
- Hiking
- Bicycling
- Swimming
- Gardening

Modified from National Institute of Arthritis and Musculoskeletal and Skin Diseases: *Once is enough: a guide to preventing future fractures*, July 2014 (website): www.niams.nih.gov/bone/hi/prevent_fracture.htm.

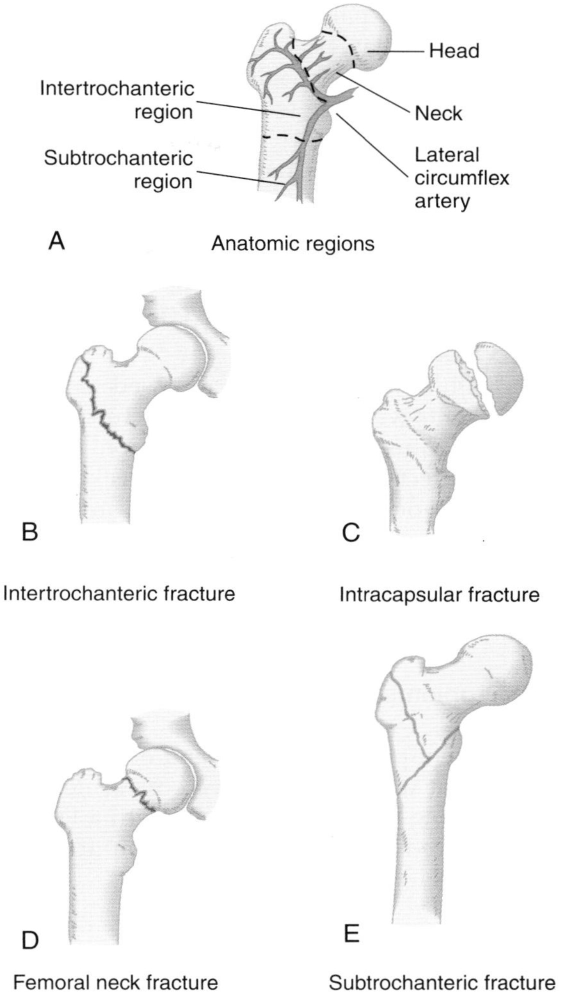

Fig. 45.12 Femoral fractures. (A) Anatomic regions of the proximal end of femur. (B) Intertrochanteric fracture. (C) Intracapsular fracture. (D) Femoral neck fracture. (E) Subtrochanteric fracture. (From Black JM, Hawks JH: *Medical-surgical nursing: clinical management for positive outcomes*, ed 8, St. Louis, 2009, Saunders.)

Medical Diagnosis

Hip fracture should be suspected any time an older adult falls on a hard surface. The first health care provider on the scene should assess for external rotation (turning outward) of the hip, muscle spasm, shortening of the affected extremity, and severe pain and tenderness at the affected site. The diagnosis of hip fracture is confirmed by radiography. Other studies, such as a complete blood count (CBC), a urinalysis, and electrocardiography, may be done in preparation for surgery.

Medical Treatment

Traction and surgical repair (internal fixation, femoral head replacement, or total hip replacement) are the standard treatments for hip fracture. For older patients, surgical repair of the fracture is often the treatment of choice because it allows them to move around sooner and results in fewer complications related to immobility. Traction may require 12 to 16 weeks of immobilization for healing.

Postoperatively, patients may begin physical therapy as early as 1 day after surgery, depending on the type of repair. They may begin by sitting in a chair and then progress to walking with a walker. After internal fixation, weight bearing on the affected side is limited initially and then gradually increased as tolerated. After total hip replacement, weight bearing can begin almost immediately.

❖ POSTOPERATIVE NURSING CARE OF THE PATIENT WITH A HIP FRACTURE

Focused Assessment

Patients with a hip fracture are assessed in the same way as patients with other types of fractures. Monitor for pain, impaired peripheral circulation on the affected side, effects of immobility, skin breakdown, and ability to carry out ADLs. Older patients are especially prone to developing delirium after a broken hip, particularly from the use of anesthesia during surgery; note mental status and problem behaviors related to confusion.

Patient Problems, Goals, and Outcome Criteria: Hip Fracture

General patient problems, goals, and outcome criteria for the patient with a fracture were presented earlier under "Nursing Care of the Patient With a Fracture." The special needs of the patient with a hip fracture are discussed here.

Interventions

Nursing interventions are geared toward relieving pain, promoting mobility and independence, and preventing complications. Older patients have special nursing care needs because they are vulnerable to complications of immobility and confusion. Pain management is of utmost importance. Confused patients may not be able to tell you the extent or degree of their pain and, many times, they may be undermedicated. Problem behaviors such as agitation, trying to climb out of bed, pulling out intravenous tubes or other tubes, and alterations in sleep patterns may be related to pain. Use comfort measures such as repositioning, body massage, and diversional activities to enhance the effect of medications.

Proper body alignment is extremely important in preventing injury to the fracture area after it has been treated. Turn patients from side to side as ordered. After total hip replacement, the affected hip must not be adducted and must not be flexed more than 90 degrees because excessive flexion or adduction can dislocate the prosthesis. Instruct these patients to use elevated toilet seats, sit in supportive chairs with straight backs and seats, and avoid crossing their legs even at the feet. Care of the patient who has undergone joint replacement surgery is detailed in Chapter 44, and fall prevention is discussed in Chapter 11.

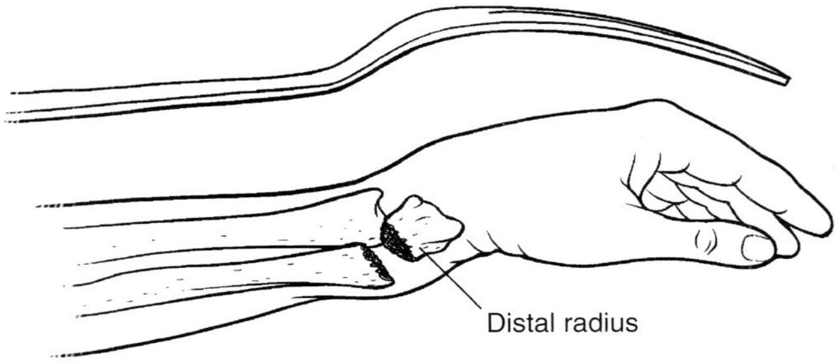

Fig. 45.13 Appearance of dinner fork displacement of distal radius in a Colles fracture. (From Freer L, Constance BB, Auerbach PS: *Field guide to wilderness medicine*, ed 5, St. Louis, 2019, Elsevier.)

COLLES FRACTURE

Fractures of the wrist, or distal radius, are the most common in the upper extremities, accounting for about one-sixth of all fractures treated in emergency departments in the United States. People with the highest occurrence of wrist fractures are youth involved in sports who sustain a high-energy fall, and elders with osteoporosis who sustain a low-energy fall.

A Colles fracture, often called a "dinner fork" fracture, occurs when there is a break and displacement of the distal radius bone in which the wrist has the appearance of a dinner fork (Fig. 45.13). These fractures frequently occur in older women when an outstretched hand is used to break a fall. The major signs and symptoms are pain, especially when flexing the wrist, tenderness, bruising and swelling, as well as the dinner fork deformity in the area of the injury. The most common complication is impaired circulation in the area resulting from edema.

Medical Diagnosis

The diagnosis is confirmed by the characteristic bone deformity of the wrist and by radiography.

Medical Treatment

Colles fractures are managed by closed reduction or manipulation of the bone and immobilization in either a splint or a cast. The elbow is immobilized as well, to prevent misalignment.

❖ NURSING CARE OF THE PATIENT WITH A COLLES FRACTURE

Focused Assessment

Assess patients for pain and swelling following medical treatment of the fracture.

Patient Problems, Goals, and Outcome Criteria: Colles Fracture

General patient problems, goals, and outcome criteria for the patient with a fracture were presented earlier under "Nursing Care of the Patient With a Fracture." The special needs of the patient with a Colles fracture are discussed here.

Interventions

Interventions are aimed at relieving pain and preventing or reducing edema. The extremity should be supported and protected and can be elevated on a pillow during the first few days. Encourage patients to move their fingers and thumb to promote circulation and reduce swelling, and to move their shoulders to prevent stiffness and contracture. In addition, teach proper cast care.

PELVIC FRACTURE

Although pelvic fractures account for a small percentage of total fractures (3%), they are the second leading cause of death from trauma, after head injury. Motor vehicle accidents are the most common cause of pelvic fractures in young adults, and falls are the main cause in older adults. The extent of the injury can range from minimal to life threatening. Internal trauma, such as laceration of the colon, hemorrhage, or rupture of the urethra or bladder, often accompanies a pelvic fracture. The patient may have local swelling, tenderness, bruising, and deformity. Pelvic fractures typically heal within 6 to 8 weeks.

Medical Diagnosis

As with other fractures, the diagnosis and severity of the injury are confirmed by radiography.

Medical Treatment

Medical treatment depends on the severity of the fracture. A less severe nondisplaced fracture is usually treated with bed rest on a firm mattress or bed board for a few days to 6 weeks. A more severe fracture may require one or more of the following: a pelvic sling, skeletal traction, a double hip spica cast, or external fixation.

❖ NURSING CARE OF THE PATIENT WITH A PELVIC FRACTURE

Focused Assessment

Observe for signs of bleeding, swelling, infection, thromboembolism, and pain. Because of the high risk of internal trauma, closely monitor the patient so that specific injuries can be treated immediately. Check for the presence of blood in the urine and stool and assess the abdomen for any signs of rigidity or swelling. Assess urine output because the absence of urine may indicate a perforated bladder.

Patient Problems, Goals, and Outcome Criteria: Pelvic Fracture

General patient problems, goals, and outcome criteria for the patient with a fracture were presented earlier under "Nursing Care of the Patient With a Fracture." The special needs of the patient with a pelvic fracture are discussed here.

Interventions

Interventions are designed to alleviate pain, promote mobility, and prevent complications. When handling patients, take extreme care to prevent displacement of fracture fragments. Move the patient gently and turn only as ordered by the physician. Have the patient pull up on the trapeze so that back care can be given. Encourage ambulation as soon as ordered to prevent the serious consequences of immobility.

Get Ready for the NCLEX® Examination!

Key Points

- A fracture is a break or disruption in the continuity of a bone, usually causing injury to surrounding soft tissue.
- Open or compound fractures have three grades of severity, ranging from least severe injury with minimal skin damage to most severe injury with skin, muscle, blood vessel, and nerve damage.
- Fractures of the femur are most common in young and middle-aged adults, and fractures of the hip, wrist, and vertebrae are most common in older adults.
- Fractures are usually caused by trauma to the bone, especially as a result of falls and automobile accidents.
- Risk factors for hip fractures include osteoporosis, advanced age, Caucasian race, use of psychotropic drugs, and female gender.
- The most common signs and symptoms of a fracture are swelling, bruising, pain, tenderness, loss of normal function, and abnormal mobility.
- Bone healing occurs in five stages: (1) hematoma formation, (2) fibrocartilage formation, (3) callus formation, (4) ossification, and (5) consolidation and remodeling.
- Healing time for fractures increases with age; it may take 6 times as long for the same type of fracture to heal in an older person as it does in an infant.
- Complications of a fracture include infection, fat embolism, DVT and pulmonary embolism, joint stiffness and contractures, posttraumatic arthritis, compartment syndrome, malunion, nonunion, delayed union, avascular necrosis, and complex regional pain syndrome.
- The goals of medical treatment for a fracture are to realign the bone fragments, establish a sturdy union between the broken ends of the bone, and restore function.
- The most common therapeutic techniques used to treat a fracture are closed and open reduction and internal and external fixation.
- Casts are used for external fixation of extensive fractures and fractures of the extremities.
- Traction provides alignment of the broken bone fragments, prevents or corrects deformity, decreases muscle spasm, promotes rest and exercise, and maintains the position of a diseased or injured part.
- Crutches increase mobility and assist with ambulation after a fracture of the lower extremity.

- A walker is used for support and balance, usually by older patients.
- Canes provide minimal support and balance and relieve pressure on weight-bearing joints.
- Common patient problems for the patient with a fracture include pain, inadequate peripheral circulation, potential for infection, immobility, potential skin breakdown, and potential activity intolerance.

Additional Learning Resources

SG Go to your Study Guide for additional learning activities to help you master this chapter content.

Go to your Evolve website (http://evolve.elsevier.com/Linton/medsurg) for the following learning resources and much more:

- Fluid & Electrolyte Tutorial
- Review Questions for the NCLEX® Examination

Clinical Judgment and Next-Generation NCLEX® Examination-Style Questions

1. **A patient is brought to the emergency department with an injury to his arm that was incurred in a fall. A bone end protrudes from his forearm. The surrounding skin is bruised and swollen. Exposed muscle tissue is also swollen. The patient has normal sensation in his fingers. His injury is best described as which of the following?**
   1. Closed complete fracture
   2. Grade III incomplete open fracture
   3. Grade I complete closed fracture
   4. Grade II complete open fracture

   NCLEX Client Need: Physiological Integrity: Physiological Adaptation

2. **The ends of a broken bone begin to knit during which stage of healing?**

   NCLEX Client Need: Physiological Integrity: Physiological Adaptation

3. **A patient with a femoral fracture suddenly complains that he cannot catch his breath. His pulse is 106 beats per minute and respiration is 30 breaths per minute. You notice a measles-like rash on his neck and chest. You should suspect which of the following?**
   1. Shock
   2. Fat embolism
   3. Avascular necrosis
   4. Compartment syndrome

   NCLEX Client Need: Physiological Integrity: Physiological Adaptation

4. **A patient's femoral fracture is not healing as rapidly as hoped. Methods that might be used to stimulate bone growth and healing include: (Select all that apply.)**
   1. Traction
   2. Pulsated electromagnetic fields
   3. Bone grafts
   4. Fixation
   5. Electrical stimulation

   NCLEX Client Need: Physiological Integrity: Physiological Adaptation

5. **A patient is being discharged with a plaster of Paris cast on her arm. Patient teaching should include which of the following? (Select all that apply.)**
   1. Notify the physician if your fingers become discolored.
   2. Do not insert any objects under the cast.
   3. After the cast dries, you can take a shower without damaging it.
   4. Loss of sensation is normal; it will return when the cast is removed.
   5. The cast dries completely within 8 hours.

   NCLEX Client Need: Physiological Integrity: Reduction of Risk Potential

6. **A patient with a foot injury is leaving the clinic with crutches. The nurse knows that the crutches are properly fitted when:**
   1. The patient says that they are comfortable
   2. The elbows are bent at 45-degree angles
   3. The crutch is 75% of the patient's height
   4. The crutch pad is about two finger widths below the axilla

   NCLEX Client Need: Physiological Integrity: Reduction of Risk Potential

7. **Which of the following is the main advantage of surgery over traction for older patients with hip fractures?**
   1. Traction is more expensive because a longer hospitalization is required.
   2. Surgery allows earlier mobilization, which results in fewer complications.
   3. After a few days, surgical treatment is generally less painful than traction.
   4. Bones of older people heal better with surgery than with traction.

   NCLEX Client Need: Physiological Integrity: Reduction of Risk Potential

8. **Which of the following is the most common cause of Colles fracture?**
   1. Using an outstretched hand to break a fall
   2. Jumping from a high place onto a hard surface
   3. Landing in a sitting position after falling
   4. Falling with the leg in a position of outward rotation

   NCLEX Client Need: Physiological Integrity: Physiological Adaptation

9. **Mr. J. was recently discharged to home health care after treatment for a pelvic fracture. The nurse is encouraging a diet to promote healing of the fracture, which should include: (Select all that apply.)**
   1. Reduced fat and calories to prevent weight gain
   2. High-calorie meal supplements
   3. Increased protein and calcium to build new bone
   4. Supplementary doses of vitamins B, C, and D
   5. Decreased fluid intake to prevent bladder distention

   NCLEX Client Need: Physiological Integrity: Basic Care and Comfort

10. **A patient comes to the clinic after a fall at home. When he moved his injured arm, a grating sound was heard. How should the nurse document this sound?** ________________________

    NCLEX Client Need: Physiological Integrity: Physiological Adaptation

11. **SLO/Objective: Prioritize nursing care for patients with a hip fracture.**

    NGN Item Type: Extended Multiple Response

    Cognitive Skill: Prioritize Hypotheses

    A 75-year-old woman has been hospitalized after sustaining a right hip fracture. She has a history of osteoporosis, hypertension, poor balance, and mild memory loss. She is receiving metoprolol and hydrochlorothiazide to treat hypertension and alendronate sodium (Flomax) for osteoporosis. She is one day postop for a total hip replacement.

    When planning care for this patient, for which *priority* potential complications would the nurse monitor. (Select all that apply.)

    - Delirium
    - Urinary incontinence
    - Orthostatic hypotension
    - Head injury
    - Pneumonia
    - Impaired right sided peripheral circulation
    - Disrupted skin integrity

46 Amputations

http://evolve.elsevier.com/Linton/medsurg

Objectives

1. Identify the clinical indications for amputations.
2. Describe the various types of amputations.
3. Discuss the medical and surgical management of the patient undergoing amputation.
4. Identify appropriate nursing interventions during the preoperative and postoperative phases of care.
5. Assist in developing a nursing care plan for the amputation patient.

Key Terms

amputation
amputee
closed amputation
congenital amputation
gangrene
guillotine amputation
open amputation
phantom limb
replantation
residual limb
staged amputation
stump

Derived from the Latin word-meaning "cutting around," the term **amputation** refers to the removal of body limbs or parts of limbs. Amputations have been performed since the beginning of humankind, according to findings by archeologists. Ancient amputations, originally performed to remove gangrenous or damaged limbs, were also performed for ritual sacrifice, punishment, exorcism of evil spirits, and, in some cases, beautification.

In the past two decades, many advances have been made in surgical amputation and replantation (i.e., limb reattachment) techniques, prosthetic devices (i.e., artificial limbs), and rehabilitation programs. Advances have allowed many **amputees** (i.e., people with amputations) to remain active and productive despite their disabilities. In the United States, the vast majority of amputees have had lower extremity amputations.

Amputation can occur through a joint or through a bone itself. *Disarticulation* is the term used for an amputation through the joint. The amputation is identified by means of its location to the nearest joint. For example, removal of the lower leg at the middle of the shin or calf is called a *below-knee* amputation. Some of the most common sites of amputation are shown in Fig. 46.1.

INDICATIONS AND INCIDENCE

Four categories of conditions or situations that are primary reasons for amputations are: (1) trauma, (2) disease, (3) tumors, and (4) congenital defects.

TRAUMA

In some serious accidents, a traumatic amputation may occur in which part or all of a limb may be detached. In other situations, the limb may be damaged so severely that it must be removed surgically. Common types of accidents and injuries leading to amputation include those involving motorcycles and automobiles, farm machinery, firearms and explosives, electrical equipment, power tools, and frostbite. Trauma tends to be the most common reason for upper extremity amputations.

DISEASE

Vascular diseases account for the majority of the estimated 185,000 lower extremity amputations performed in the United States each year. In these cases, blood supply to the tissues is inadequate and the tissues become deprived of oxygen and other important nutrients. Without these nutrients, necrosis or death of the tissue occurs, resulting in gangrene. **Gangrene** is the death of tissue caused by inadequate circulation followed by infection. Some examples of diseases leading to impaired circulation are peripheral vascular disease, diabetes mellitus, and arteriosclerosis. Circulation problems are more common in the lower extremities among older adults. Chronic osteomyelitis, an infection of the bone, bone marrow, or surrounding soft tissue, also can lead to amputation. Sometimes when disease leads to severe necrosis, autoamputation can occur; the limb, most often a toe, self-amputates itself without surgery.

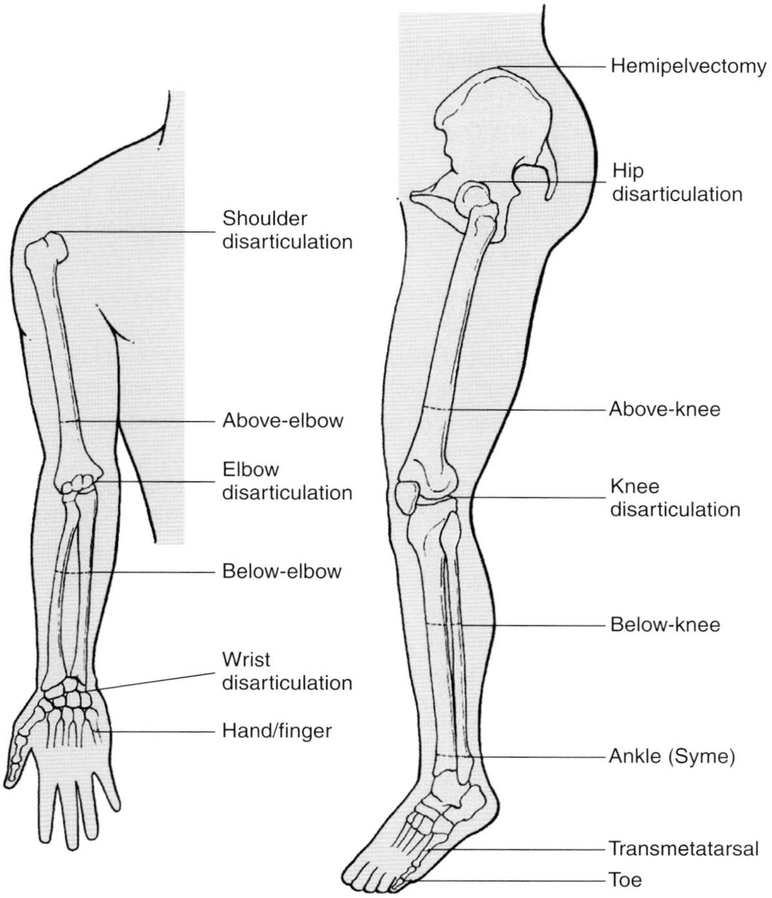

Fig. 46.1 Common sites of amputation in the upper and lower extremities. (From Monahan FD, Drake DT, Neighbors M, editors: *Medical-surgical nursing: foundations for clinical practice*, ed 2, Philadelphia, 1998, Saunders.)

TUMORS

Amputations may be performed for bone tumors that are very large and invasive. Treatment may require amputation and disarticulation of an entire limb. Although primary bone tumors can occur at any age, they are seen most frequently in adolescents, with approximately one-third of all cases occurring at 11 to 20 years of age.

CONGENITAL DEFECTS

In some situations, a limb or part of a limb may be absent or deformed at birth, sometimes called **congenital amputations**. They result from factors that affect the developing fetus in such a way that the infant is born with a missing, deficient, or abnormal limb. Sometimes surgery is performed to convert a deformed limb into a more functional one that can be fitted with a prosthetic device.

DIAGNOSTIC TESTS AND PROCEDURES

The types of diagnostic studies done for a patient requiring amputation depend on the underlying disease or injury. For example, in a patient with vascular disease, tests to assess circulation are indicated. An elevated white blood cell (WBC) count is consistent with infection. Chapter 43, Table 43.1 lists examples of diagnostic findings associated with some of the contributing factors in amputations.

MEDICAL TREATMENT

The medical care of the patient undergoing amputation must include the appropriate treatment and control of any underlying diseases or injuries. For example, diet, medication, and exercise are used to help patients with diabetes and poor peripheral circulation to attain good control of their diabetes. Patients with peripheral vascular disease are encouraged to stop smoking because nicotine causes vasoconstriction. The patient who has experienced trauma may have to be stabilized with measures that will maintain their heart rate and blood pressure within a normal range.

SURGICAL TREATMENT

Amputation is recommended only when other options are not possible or have failed. To avoid amputation, the health care provider may perform angioplasty or surgical bypass of obstructed vessels.

Table 46.1 Complications of Amputation

COMPLICATION	DESCRIPTION AND CONTRIBUTING FACTORS
Hematoma and hemorrhage	Bleeding into tissue in and around residual limb because of inadequate hemostasis
Necrosis	Tissue destruction and death because of ongoing disease; requires surgical debridement or revision, or both
Wound dehiscence	Opening of suture line because of early removal of sutures or trauma; requires reclosure
Gangrene	Death of tissue associated with inadequate blood supply and bacterial destruction of tissue; requires reamputation
Edema	Swelling and discomfort in residual limb because of dependent position or incorrect wrapping; requires elevation and rewrapping
Contracture	Flexion of joints with loss of range of motion because of prolonged elevation or immobilization of extremities; may be prevented by frequent position changes and range-of-motion exercises
Pain	Extreme, sharp pain at incision site because of scar formation on nerve fibers (neuroma); may require surgical treatment
Infection	Redness, warmth, swelling, and exudate formation at residual limb site because of invasion of tissues by pathogens; may require antibiotics and surgical drainage
Phantom limb sensation	Patient experiences sensations (tingling, numbness, itching, warmth/cold) as if the limb were still present; caused by stimulation along a nerve pathway in which sensory endings were in the amputated part
Phantom limb pain	Patient experiences pain as if the limb were still present; more common when patient had pain in limb before amputation; pain may be enhanced by anxiety and depression; usually diminishes over time but may become chronic

Surgical amputation is performed at the lowest level of the limb to preserve healthy tissue and favor wound healing. The surgeon chooses one of two basic types of surgical procedures, depending on the condition of the extremity and the reason for the surgery: (1) closed amputations and (2) open amputations.

CLOSED AMPUTATIONS

Closed amputations are performed on lower extremity amputations to create a weight-bearing residual limb or stump. A long skin flap with soft tissue and muscle is positioned over the severed end of the bone and sutured in place. The sutures are positioned so that they do not bear the full weight of the patient. This technique has many variations.

OPEN AMPUTATIONS

In **open amputations**, the severed bone or joint is left uncovered by a skin flap. This type of amputation is required when an actual or potential infection exists, as may occur with gangrene or trauma. The wound is left open for 5 to 10 days, sometimes longer, and is closed surgically when infection no longer poses a problem. Another term for this procedure is a **staged amputation** or **guillotine amputation**.

COMPLICATIONS

Complications associated with amputations include hemorrhage and hematoma, necrosis, wound dehiscence, gangrene, edema, contracture, pain, infection, phantom limb sensation, and phantom limb pain. Factors contributing to each of these complications are listed in Table 46.1.

PROSTHESES

Prostheses are artificial substitutes for missing body parts. A prosthetist creates the prosthesis, fits the patient, and instructs the patient in its use. In some situations, the prosthesis may be placed while the patient is still in the operating room. In other cases, particularly with lower extremity amputations, older or debilitated patients, and infection, fitting of the prosthesis is delayed until the remaining part of the limb heals. Provided that no problems occur, a patient can usually bear full weight on a permanent prosthesis approximately 3 months after amputation (Fig. 46.2). Advances in prosthesis design and surgical muscle reinnervation are producing significant improvements in function.

❖ NURSING CARE OF THE PATIENT HAVING AMPUTATION SURGERY

Routine preoperative and postoperative care are detailed in Chapter 17. This section focuses on the specific needs of the patient having an amputation (see also Nursing Care Plan: Patient With an Upper Extremity Amputation).

PREOPERATIVE CARE

Before having a lower limb amputation, patients should be encouraged to carry out upper extremity muscle strengthening exercises to promote arm strength for crutch walking and gait training. For example, push up exercises can be carried out in a bed or wheelchair. When appropriate, teach the patient about the anticipated type of prosthesis that will be used and when it

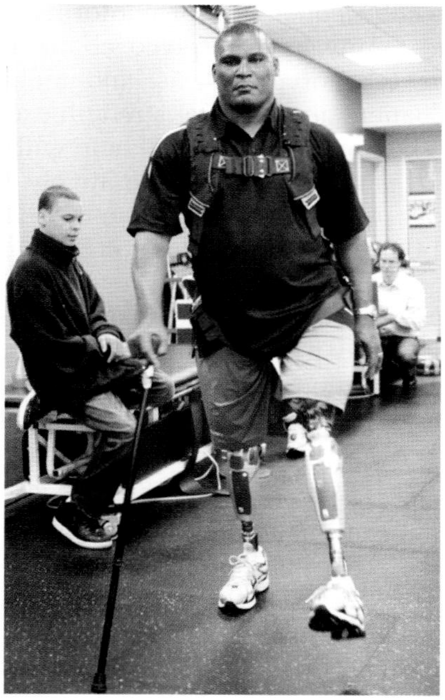

Fig. 46.2 Lower extremity prostheses. (From Harding MM, Kwong J, Roberts D, Hagler D, Reinisch C: *Lewis's medical-surgical nursing: assessment and management of clinical problems*, ed 11, St. Louis, 2020, Elsevier.)

would be applied. Teach patients that the amputated limb may feel as though it is still present after surgery, called *phantom limb sensation.* In addition, the psychological and social implications of an amputation present opportunities for the nurse to support the patient who may experience anxiety or anticipatory grief.

POSTOPERATIVE CARE

The postoperative phase begins immediately after the surgical amputation and includes both immediate care and long-term rehabilitation. Priorities for the postoperative patient are (1) pain relief, (2) restored function, and (3) avoidance of complications.

Monitor vital signs frequently in the first 48 hours postoperatively to detect early signs of complications. Inspect the dressing frequently for any bleeding. Some nurses try to monitor the amount of oozing by marking the stained area on the dressing with a pen, although this is a very rough assessment of bleeding. Sometimes the dressing is dry, but blood is draining around the dressing and under the patient. If a drain receptacle is present, note the color and amount of the drainage. The drainage should gradually decrease in amount and lighten in color. Monitor the patient's temperature for elevations that may indicate infection. Also note any foul odor from the dressing. After the dressing is removed, inspect the **residual limb (stump)** for edema. Document the patient's pain, including type, location, severity, and response to treatment. Other aspects of postoperative assessment are detailed in Chapter 17.

Focused Assessment

Patient Problems, Goals, and Outcome Criteria: Amputation

Patient Problems	Goals and Outcome Criteria
Anxiety related to anticipated change in body image and in function	Decreased anxiety: relaxed manner, patient statement that anxiety is reduced
Anticipatory grief related to expected loss of body part and function	Progress toward grief resolution: expresses feelings about impending losses, demonstrates healthy coping strategies
Lack of knowledge related to self-care of the residual limb, phantom limb sensation, and prosthetic use	Knowledge of self-care of amputated limb: verbalizes self-care of residual limb; describes phantom limb sensation; discusses prosthetic use
Patient Problems: Postoperative	Goals and Outcome Criteria
Inadequate circulation related to blood loss	Normal circulation: pulse and blood pressure (BP) consistent with patient norms, skin warm and dry
Acute pain related to surgical wound	Pain relief: relaxed manner, patient statement that pain is relieved; less than 4 on a 1–10 pain scale
Potential for infection related to surgical disruption of skin integrity	Absence of infection: normal body temperature, decreasing redness and edema of wound margins, drainage that decreases in volume and becomes clear
Disrupted skin tissue integrity related to incision	Healed wound: incision margins intact without drainage, excessive swelling, or warmth
Potential disrupted skin tissue integrity related to advanced age and decreased mobility	Absence of new skin lesions: skin intact, no redness because of pressure
Inadequate knowledge regarding phantom limb sensations or phantom limb pain related to lack of information	Demonstrates knowledge of phantom limb sensation/pain: acknowledges that phantom limb sensation/pain is normal after amputation, states that pain or other sensation is reduced
Potential for injury related to loss of a limb or part of a limb, weakness, debilitation	Absence of injury: no falls or evidence of injury because of weakness or problems with balance
Decreased mobility related to loss of a limb or part of a limb	Restored mobility: patient performs activities of daily living (ADLs), gradually returns to preoperative level of functioning

Continued

Patient Problems, Goals, and Outcome Criteria: Amputation—cont'd

Patient Problems	Goals and Outcome Criteria
Activity intolerance related to weakness	Improved ability to tolerate activity: patient carries out daily activities without excessive fatigue, gradual increase in activity level
Ineffective self-care management related to loss of limb	Resumed self-care: patient performs self-care within limits imposed by limb loss, learns new ways to care for self
Anxiety or stress related to perceived threat of disability, possibility of death	Decreased anxiety, stress, or both: calm manner; patient statement of lessened anxiety, stress, or both
Inadequate coping related to difficulty accepting loss of limb	Effective coping with loss: patient talks about loss, participates in rehabilitation efforts and self-care
Grief related to loss of limb and altered sense of self	Resolution of grief: accepts new functional abilities and self-image with a more positive outlook
Altered body image related to loss of a body part or residual limb	Positive body image: patient accepts limb loss, demonstrates proper care, makes positive remarks about self and abilities

Interventions

Anxiety. Emotional support is important throughout all phases of care of the patient with an amputation. The patient needs time to prepare psychologically and emotionally for the surgery. Encourage the patient to express thoughts and concerns about the impending amputation. Accept the patient's responses. Allow the patient to express anger or to cry without being judged or given false reassurances. Tell the patient about physical and occupational therapy programs designed to restore maximal independent function.

Anticipatory grief. Recognize that the loss of a limb or part of a limb as well as the loss of functional abilities is stressful. Patients commonly experience anticipatory grief and mourn the impending loss. The patient may be concerned about altered physical appearance as well as loss of function. Explore the patient's expectations and fears about these changes. Gently encourage the patient to focus on what they will be able to do despite physical limitations. Allowing patients to grieve is an important part of their recovery and rehabilitation. Nursing care of the grieving patient is discussed in Chapter 19.

Inadequate knowledge. Reinforce information that the patient and family have received about the level of amputation, type of prosthesis, and mobility training. Teach patient about upper strength exercises (i.e., pushups in bed or chair) that will help with the use of crutches and gait training postoperatively. Inform the patient about *phantom limb sensation,* in which the amputated limb feels as though it is still there.

Inadequate circulation. Hemorrhage is the greatest danger in the early postoperative period. It may be detected by observations of excessive bleeding or changes in vital signs and behavior. Restlessness and increasing pulse and respiratory rates may be early signs of hemorrhage. Hypotension and cyanosis are late signs. If an immediate prosthesis had been applied while in surgery, the dressing may be difficult to observe, so monitoring vital signs is even more critical.

A portable wound suction system, such as a Jackson-Pratt drain, may be placed to collect drainage. Inspect the dressing and the bed linens under the patient. Bright red bleeding, either from the drains or from the dressing itself, is not normal. Apply a pressure dressing over the existing dressing, elevate the residual limb, and notify the surgeon immediately. A large BP cuff may be placed at the bedside for emergency use as a tourniquet.

Put On Your Thinking Cap!

Sometimes an immediate postoperative prosthesis is applied to the residual limb while the patient is in surgery. The surgical site is heavily covered and makes it difficult to assess the condition of the wound, so you must rely on other assessment data. What data would cause you to suspect excessive blood loss in that situation?

Acute pain. Postoperatively, the patient has incisional pain that is treated with prescribed pain medications, usually opioid analgesics. After giving analgesics, document the effects and notify the physician if pain is not relieved. For a thorough discussion of pain management, see Chapter 8.

Potential for infection. Use aseptic technique when handling the residual limb, the dressing, and the drains to help reduce the risk of infection. Monitor for signs and symptoms of infection. The incision should be dry, intact, and only slightly red. Suspect infection if a foul or unpleasant odor comes from the dressing, if the patient has a sudden temperature elevation, or if the residual limb is red, excessively warm, or edematous. Laboratory results may also detect an elevated WBC count. Treatment for infection may include antibiotics and incision and drainage of the infected residual limb. In severe cases, the infection may cause further tissue damage and require reamputation at a higher level. Thus it is very important to take measures to prevent infection and to act promptly if there is evidence of infection.

Disrupted Skin Tissue Integrity/Potential for Disrupted Skin Tissue Integrity

The care of the residual limb depends on the overall condition of the patient and the type of prosthesis. If the amputation is closed, some type of compression dressing with elastic bandages is used, as well as a cast in some cases. The residual limb is bandaged to promote healing and to shrink and shape the residual limb to a tapered, round, smooth end that will fit the prosthesis. Wrap the bandage smoothly with even, moderate tension to all parts of the residual limb. Rewrap the residual limb as needed to maintain pressure. It is very important to avoid a tourniquet-like effect caused by pulling the bandage too tightly or unevenly. Fig. 46.3 illustrates the correct bandaging of a residual limb. Commercial "shrinker socks" are available that maintain compression; however, they are expensive, and it is difficult to find the right size and length for many patients.

Inspect the residual limb frequently for irritation and edema. Edema in the residual limb is most common during the first 24 hours postoperatively. To minimize this, a heavy cast or pressure dressing is applied in the operating room. Elevate the affected lower extremities by raising the foot of the bed. Pillows can be placed under a below-knee amputation, although the use of pillows is discouraged with lower extremity amputations because it can cause contractures of the hip. For the same reason, position the patient in a low Fowler rather than a high Fowler position. After the fifth to seventh postoperative day, the residual limb can be massaged to promote circulation. If permitted, a patient with a lower extremity amputation should lie prone for 30 minutes 3 or 4 times a day.

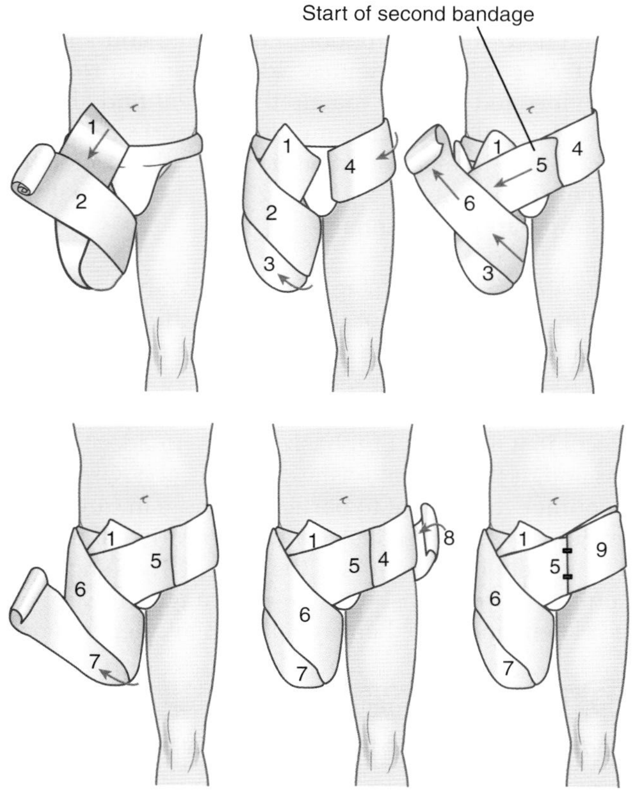

Fig. 46.3 Bandaging for the above-the-knee amputation residual limb. Figure-8 style covers progressive areas of the residual limb; 2 elastic wraps used. (From Harding MM, Kwong J, Roberts D, Hagler D, Reinisch C: *Lewis's medical-surgical nursing: assessment and management of clinical problems*, ed 11, St. Louis, 2020, Elsevier.)

Inadequate knowledge. Pain or a phantom limb sensation is common. It is often described as a burning, stinging, or crushing pain. It tends to lessen with activity, weight bearing, and exercise. If the patient reports such pain, notify the surgeon. Reassure the patient that this is common after amputation and that various treatments are available. Treatment for this type of pain may include diversional activities, whirlpool, massage, injection of the residual limb with an anesthetic, or transcutaneous electrical nerve stimulation (TENS). A properly fitting dressing helps some patients. Drugs that are sometimes helpful include beta-blockers, anticonvulsants, neuroleptics, benzodiazepines, and antidepressants (see the Complementary and Alternative Therapies box).

Complementary and Alternative Therapies

Many complementary therapies may be used with analgesics to control pain. Examples are imagery, relaxation, meditation, and acupuncture.

Put On Your Thinking Cap!

The home health nurse is visiting an older woman who had a lower leg amputation 1 month ago. The wound appears to be well healed, but the woman complains of pain that is sometimes severe in the amputated limb. She asks if she is going crazy. What would you tell her?

Potential for injury. The patient must learn to function without the amputated limb (see the Patient Teaching box). They must also learn to compensate for the lost extremity in unexpected ways, such as maintaining balance in sitting and standing positions. After lower extremity amputation, safe mobility is a priority. Reinforce the proper use of assistive devices (e.g., crutches, walkers) as taught by the physical therapist. Also encourage and assist the patient to do exercises to strengthen remaining limbs. Keep the environment free of clutter to prevent tripping. Patients with upper limb amputations must learn adaptations to perform activities of daily living (ADL). Everyday activities such as cooking may result in injury. The occupational therapist helps the patient learn to perform these tasks safely. Rehabilitation centers typically have demonstration homelike settings that allow patients to practice meal preparation and other daily activities. Occupational therapy services also extend to the home, where the therapist helps the patient and family to plan for any needed environmental alterations.

Patient Teaching

Amputation

- A rehabilitation team, including a prosthetist (if applicable), physical therapist, and occupational therapist, will work with you to help you regain the best function possible.
- If a prosthetic device is appropriate for you, the prosthetist will fit the device and teach you about it.
- Many modern prostheses are nearly lifelike in appearance and function.
- **Phantom limb** sensations are sensations perceived in the limb that has been removed; they are commonly experienced by amputees and may disappear spontaneously or continue for years.
- Medications and other treatments can be used to treat phantom pain.
- With lower extremity amputation, upper body training is important to strengthen your arms.
- If you will be using crutches, we will teach you crutch walking and you will need to practice.
- We can arrange for a person who has recovered after an amputation like yours to visit, if you would like that.

Decreased mobility. The physical therapist usually initiates an exercise program. An important goal is the prevention of contractures. These are most common in the knee, hip, and elbow. The patient with a lower extremity amputation may be instructed to lie prone (if tolerable), with the head turned away from the affected side for 30 minutes three or four times a day. Traction, trochanter rolls, and a firm mattress may keep the body in alignment while the patient is in bed. An overbed trapeze may be ordered to facilitate moving back and forth between the bed and the chair. Avoid prolonged flexion of the hip (as when propped on a pillow). Prolonged sitting can lead to hip and knee contractures. Active and passive range-of-motion exercises also are an important part of maintaining mobility and preventing debilitation. Explain the value of exercises to the patient to encourage cooperation and participation.

The patient may have either an immediate or a delayed prosthetic fitting. An immediate fitting allows the patient to become accustomed to weight bearing, ambulation, and balance shortly after surgery. A delayed fitting is usually performed in above-knee amputations, bilateral extremity amputations, or cases of infection in which an open amputation has been performed. The appropriate time frame for fitting a prosthetic device in these situations depends on the healing of the residual limb and the overall condition of the patient. When the residual limb has healed well, the patient is fitted for the prosthesis. A suitable choice for prosthesis is based on the site of the amputation and the age, intelligence, health, motivation, occupation, and financial status of the patient.

Activity intolerance. Surgery and bed rest may adversely affect the patient's tolerance for any type of sustained activity. It is extremely important to plan care to avoid too much patient exertion. Encouraging the patient to resume the preoperative level of activity too soon can impair physical and psychological healing. A typical activity order is for the patient to be assisted out of bed 2 or 3 times on the first postoperative day for 1 hour at a time. Over the next few days, the patient with a lower extremity amputation is usually encouraged to remain out of bed for longer periods and to begin to practice ambulation gradually. This may initially involve only a few steps, but these will gradually be increased over time. The patient's level of activity and the rate at which they regain endurance depend on many individual factors.

Inability to manage self-care. During the immediate postoperative period, assist the patient in performing ADLs as needed. Gradually guide the patient to adapt to the lost limb and encourage more independence. Patients feel less helpless when they regain the ability to provide self-care.

Anxiety or stress and inadequate coping. Provide opportunities for patients to talk about their concerns. Explore how the patient's usual coping strategies can be used in this situation. Encourage and support effective coping strategies. Identify inappropriate behaviors and attempt to help the patient find alternatives. Referral to a local amputee support group may be helpful. As mentioned earlier, it is normal for the patient to experience a grieving process, especially if the amputation is traumatic.

Altered body image. The patient may have difficulty looking at and caring for the affected extremity (see the Cultural Considerations box). It takes time for the patient to incorporate the change into their body image. Encourage the patient to talk about the change and the effects it will have. Emphasize ways to adapt to the loss and, if the patient wishes, to conceal it. Gradually encourage the patient to participate more in care of the residual limb. Patient instruction for residual limb care is extremely important (see the Patient Teaching box). Family and friends should be encouraged to support the patient and help them avoid excessive dependence.

Cultural Considerations

What Does Culture Have to Do With Amputations?

Values related to body appearance, function, and independence are culturally influenced and will affect the way in which individuals react to amputation. In addition, religious beliefs may dictate the disposal of amputated body parts by burial or cremation. For example, Orthodox Jews require that such body parts be made available for burial.

Patient Teaching

Care of Residual Limbs and Prostheses

RESIDUAL LIMBS

- Wash the residual limb with soap and water every night. Rinse and dry the skin thoroughly.
- Using a mirror to assist, inspect the *entire* residual limb, especially the incision, daily for irritation, redness, and edema.
- Expose the residual limb to air when possible.
- Residual limb socks should be hand washed, rinsed well, and dried flat. A clean sock should be used every day. Having several socks will allow time for the socks to dry between washings.
- Mended socks should not be worn because a seam is irritating and creates pressure.
- Shoes with uneven heels will change the weight distribution of the residual limb and lead to irritation and possible skin breakdown.
- Lotions, ointments, or powders should not be used unless prescribed by the physician.
- If redness or irritation develops on the residual limb, discontinue use of the prosthesis until you have the area checked.

PROSTHETIC DEVICES

- Keep the prosthetic socket (the opening in which the residual limb is seated) clean.
- The residual limb may shrink in size for up to 2 years after surgery. Annual visits to the prosthetist are recommended for necessary adjustments (these visits are more frequent for children, as their residual limb grows in size with them).
- Wipe the inside of the prosthesis socket daily with a damp, soapy cloth, then remove the soap with a clean, damp cloth. Dry thoroughly.
- Consult a prosthetist if any problems occur with the prosthesis. Do not attempt to make adjustments yourself.

OLDER ADULT WITH AN AMPUTATION

The older adult with an amputation may have some additional needs that should be considered when planning and providing care. For example, when constructing a teaching plan for the older adult, keep in mind that the healthy older person is completely capable of learning but often requires smaller units of information, more repetition, and more time. Skip unnecessary details and make sure that patients with glasses or hearing aids have them in place during the teaching process.

It is also important to clearly explain phantom sensations to older adults. Some may not wish to report phantom sensations or phantom pain for fear of seeming foolish. Reminding the older patient that phantom sensations are not uncommon or bizarre can reduce the fear or anxiety that these sensations can cause.

Many older adults have one or more chronic health problems. This factor should be considered in the selection of a prosthetic device. For example, a patient with diabetes is prone to circulation problems and poor wound healing and may need a prosthetic device with extra padding or support. Poor vision and decreased sensation may keep the older person from recognizing complications.

Because many older adults have decreased appetites, their nutritional status may be poor. Emphasizing high-calorie and high-protein intake is essential to promote healing and to maintain or build strength (see the Nutrition Considerations box).

Nutrition Considerations

1. A nutritional assessment should be made preoperatively for patients undergoing surgical amputation, especially for older, immobilized, or chronic alcoholic patients.
2. Patients undergoing surgical amputation should be well hydrated; intravenous fluids may be given if oral fluids are not tolerated.
3. Surgical amputation is accompanied by a stress response, resulting in an increased need for calories and protein for healing.
4. Dietary supplements may be needed for patients whose intake of regular foods is inadequate for healing.
5. Patients are encouraged to become mobile as soon as possible after an amputation to prevent loss of calcium and protein.
6. Dietary choices high in protein, zinc, and vitamin C promote wound healing.

Because many older individuals have had to deal with other losses in their lives, such as the loss of loved ones, the loss of independence, and the loss of income associated with retirement, it is important to provide psychologic support after the additional loss associated with an amputation. In addition, elders may lack confidence that they can adapt and gain strength.

Empathy, patience, and respect toward older patients should be maintained.

If the patient is unable to participate fully in their care, instruct family members along with the older patient. Home health nursing services may be arranged to facilitate adaptation in the home setting and to monitor for complications. Building strength and activity tolerance is vital to walking with lower extremity prostheses. Some frail older adults may need to use a wheelchair rather than a prosthetic device.

REPLANTATION

In some amputation injuries, a type of surgical technique called **replantation** may be performed. This involves the use of a microscope and highly specialized instruments to reanastomose (reconnect) blood vessels and nerve fibers in a severed limb. The limb is then sutured into its correct anatomic position. Advances in microsurgical techniques and preservation of severed limbs have made this technique increasingly successful. Attachment of donor limbs (transplantation) is gaining acceptance and achieving success as more effective drugs are being developed to control rejection. However, lifelong immunosuppression creates new risks and challenges.

INDICATIONS

The surgeon considers a number of factors before performing replantation surgery—for example, the type of injury and location and the extent of limb ischemia. Replantation surgery is most likely to be performed for amputations through the hand or wrist. Amputated thumbs are reattached whenever possible because of the thumb's importance in total hand function. In a severely injured hand in which two or more fingers are detached, an attempt is made by the surgeon to restore as many fingers as possible. In general, the greater the muscle mass injury, the less likely that replantation will be successful or even possible.

EMERGENCY CARE

Proper handling of amputated parts is extremely important for successful replantation. Current preservation techniques include wrapping the amputated parts in a clean cloth saturated with normal saline or lactated Ringer solution. These parts are then placed in a sealed plastic bag that is placed in ice water. Direct contact between the amputated part and the ice can lead to further tissue damage and cell death. Partially amputated parts should remain attached to the patient and should also be kept cool if possible. Extra care should be taken to avoid detaching any parts, because even small connections increase the chances for successful repair.

The patient may require treatment for shock because of blood loss. This may include intravenous fluids and blood products. Applying a clean, dry dressing, which can be reinforced as needed, may minimize blood loss. Tourniquets should not be used unless absolutely necessary because they can cause ischemia of the residual limb.

SURGICAL CARE

Preoperative and postoperative care is discussed in detail in Chapter 17. This section emphasizes the special needs of the replantation patient.

PREOPERATIVE CARE

General preoperative care of the replantation patient includes careful assessment of circulatory status, close monitoring of vital signs, and inspection of the residual limb (or dressing) for bleeding. Ask about pain at the site of the injury and at other locations. Measure and record fluid intake and output. Note the patient's emotional status and assess understanding of the preoperative activities and postoperative routines. Identify sources of support.

POSTOPERATIVE CARE

Postoperative assessment includes monitoring vital signs, intake and output, and level of consciousness. An essential aspect of care after replantation is hourly neurovascular assessment of the replanted limb. A Doppler device or pulse oximeter may be used to evaluate circulation. When the patient arrives on the nursing unit, immediately assess and document circulatory status to establish a baseline for comparison. Note and record the limb's color, capillary refill, turgor, temperature, and sensation. Signs of arterial occlusion are pale or blue color, slow capillary refill, shriveled appearance, and coolness. Signs of venous congestion are cyanosis, rapid capillary refill, edema, and warmth. Assess the limb for edema because massive edema often accompanies replantation.

FOCUSED ASSESSMENT

Patient Problems, Goals, and Outcome Criteria: Replantation

Patient Problems	Goals and Outcome Criteria
PREOPERATIVE	
Inadequate circulation related to decreased blood volume	Normal circulation: pulse and blood pressure (BP) within patient norms, skin warm and dry
Stress related to severe injury or possible failure of replantation	Reduced stress: calm manner, patient statement of less stress
Anxiety related to lack of knowledge of surgical routines	Decreased anxiety: relaxed manner, patient statement of reduced anxiety
Acute pain related to injury to affected limb	Decreased pain: patient statement of less pain, relaxed manner, pulse and BP within patient norms
POSTOPERATIVE	
Inadequate peripheral circulation related to trauma, edema, compensatory vasoconstriction	Adequate circulation to replanted limb: warmth, normal skin color, arterial pulses
Acute pain related to postoperative tissue trauma	Pain relief: relaxed expression, statement of less pain; pain rated less than 4 on a 1 to 10 pain scale
Altered body image related to disfigurement, loss of function	Improved body image: patient touches and looks at affected part, makes positive statements about self

INTERVENTIONS

Preoperative

Administer intravenous fluids and blood as ordered. If the dressing becomes saturated with blood, reinforce the dressing. Report continued or excessive bleeding to the health care provider. Even though preparations for replantation are hurried, be sensitive to the patient's fear and anxiety. Accept the patient's feelings. Provide brief, simple explanations. Administer analgesics as ordered for pain.

Postoperative

Measures to promote circulation to the replanted limb include elevation of the limb and microvascular precautions. Elevation of the limb promotes venous and lymphatic drainage. Take care not to elevate the limb above the level of the heart because this may impair arterial flow. Several soft pillows or a stockinette connected to an intravenous pole may help to achieve this. Microvascular precautions include avoiding any substances or conditions that contribute to blood vessel spasm or constriction. Encourage the patient to abstain from nicotine- and caffeine-containing products for 7 to 10 days postoperatively. In addition, maintain room temperature at 80°F to prevent compensatory vasoconstriction of the peripheral tissues in response to cold. Loosen tight or restrictive gowns or pajamas. Explain the importance of these measures to the patient and family (see the Patient Teaching box).

Patient Teaching

Postoperative Replantation

- Avoid nicotine and caffeine for 7 to 10 days or as directed by the surgeon.
- Avoid tight clothing that might impair circulation to the replanted limb or digit.
- Keep the limb positioned as instructed.
- A rehabilitation team will teach you proper care to promote improved function.
- Inform your health care provider of changes in the color or warmth of the replanted limb or digit immediately.

Administer intravenous low-molecular-weight dextran (Dextran 40), aspirin, or heparin as ordered to reduce the risk of thrombosis. Monitor for adverse effects. Inadequate arterial blood flow to the replanted limb is a medical emergency. If evidence of inadequate arterial circulation exists (i.e., no pulse, pallor or cyanosis, cool skin), immediately notify the health care provider and prepare the patient for a return to the operating suite. In some facilities, venous congestion is treated with leeches (hirudotherapy). Leeches are attached to a selected area of the replanted limb. The saliva of the leeches contains an anticoagulant, a local vasodilator, and a local anesthetic. The leech extracts excess blood, reducing venous congestion.

Provide the patient with an opportunity to discuss thoughts and feelings about the replantation, disfigurement, and loss of function. It may take time before the patient is able to look at and touch the replanted limb. Support and demonstrate acceptance of the patient. Your comfort with handling the limb can help the patient to feel accepted. The rehabilitation team works with the patient to restore maximum possible function.

If the replantation is not successful, the limb is surgically removed. This represents a significant loss to the patient. Recognize this loss and support the patient.

Other essential aspects of care include routine postoperative measures such as frequent position changes, pulmonary hygiene, and pain management.

Put On Your Thinking Cap!

What could you do or say to support the patient whose replanted limb must be amputated?

Nursing Care Plan — Patient With an Upper Extremity Amputation

FOCUSED ASSESSMENT

Health History

A 32-year-old man sustained an injury in an industrial accident that required amputation of his right forearm just below the elbow. The patient's right hand was his dominant hand. He has had no other serious physical injuries or illnesses. He is a machinist who is a senior employee in his department. He is married and is the father of three children. His wife is a homemaker who has never worked outside the home.

Physical Examination

Vital signs: blood pressure 126/68 mm Hg, pulse 80 beats per minute, respiration 16 breaths per minute, temperature 98.2°F (36.8°C) measured orally. Alert. A bulky dressing is in place on the residual limb of the right arm; dressing is dry and intact. A Jackson-Pratt drain is in place and the receptacle contains approximately 30 mL of sanguineous fluid. Intravenous fluids are infusing into the left arm. Up in chair for breakfast. Using left arm for self-feeding. Expresses intent to remain independent.

Patient Problems	Goals and Outcome Criteria	Interventions
Inadequate circulation related to blood loss	The patient's blood volume will remain normal, as evidenced by stable vital signs, urine output equal to fluid intake, and absence of restlessness or frank bleeding.	Reinforce dressing, apply pressure, and elevate residual limb if bleeding is apparent. Monitor for signs of hypovolemia: tachycardia, restlessness, and decreased urine output. Check brachial pulse on the affected arm if dressing allows.

Continued

Nursing Care Plan — Patient With an Upper Extremity Amputation—cont'd

Patient Problems	Goals and Outcome Criteria	Interventions
Acute pain related to surgical incision, trauma, edema	The patient will state that pain is relieved and will appear more relaxed.	Have the patient describe pain nature, location, and severity. Administer analgesics as ordered. Provide comfort measures such as back rub, distraction, and imagery. Inform the surgeon if pain is not relieved.
Potential for infection related to surgical wound, traumatic injury	The patient will remain free of infection, as evidenced by normal body temperature and absence of foul drainage, excessive redness, warmth, or edema.	Monitor temperature for elevation. Assess the dressing for foul drainage. When the dressing is removed, inspect the residual limb for excessive redness, warmth, or edema. Use Standard precautions when handling the dressing and residual limb. Teach the patient good hygiene to decrease the risk of infection. Administer antimicrobials as ordered.
Disrupted skin tissue integrity related to incision	The patient's residual limb will heal completely.	Keep the residual limb dressing smooth and snug to mold the residual limb for future prosthesis use. Use caution not to impair blood flow. Check the residual limb for irritation or signs of pressure. Maintain elevation as ordered to minimize edema and pressure on the suture line. Apply cold to the residual limb dressing as ordered. After the first week, massage the residual limb as ordered to promote circulation.
Inadequate knowledge regarding phantom limb sensation or phantom limb pain related to lack of information	The patient will report phantom limb sensations or pain if they occur.	Tell the patient that these sensations sometimes follow amputation. Notify the surgeon. Medicate as ordered. Advise the patient that several therapies are available for the treatment of this problem.
Potential for injury related to loss of part of limb, weakness	The patient will identify activities requiring adaptation and will avoid dangerous activities.	Help the patient to identify usual activities that cannot be done safely without the dominant hand or that require modification. Discuss strategies to adapt activities or to learn to use the left hand. Consult a rehabilitation specialist for adaptation in work setting.
Inability to manage self-care related to need for assistance from caregivers	The patient will accomplish self-care with minimal assistance from others.	Assist the patient with self-care but encourage increasing effort on his part. Praise efforts. Organize the environment to facilitate self-care (e.g., place bedside objects on the patient's left). Teach the patient to care for the residual limb and any prosthesis. 1. Wash residual limb with soap and water daily, rinse, and dry. 2. Inspect residual limb daily for irritation, redness, and edema. 3. Keep prosthetic socket and residual limb sock clean and dry. 4. Do not apply lotions, powders, or creams except as prescribed by the physician. 5. If residual limb is red or irritated, temporarily remove the prosthesis; see physician. 6. Prosthesis will require periodic adjustments.
Anxiety related to perceived threat of disability	The patient will verbalize concerns about injury.	Explore the patient's fears and anxiety. Encourage the patient to talk about the loss. Express concern but not pity. Request the services of a mental health or spiritual counselor if the patient desires. Include family in care and explore their needs as well.
Inadequate coping related to overwhelming injury	The patient will demonstrate realistic goal setting and express intent to participate in rehabilitation program.	Explain the importance of proper residual limb care in preparing for rehabilitation. Consult a social worker to assist the patient in obtaining rehabilitation services.
Altered body image related to loss of body part	The patient will express feelings about loss of the hand and will consider strategies to improve function and appearance.	Gradually encourage the patient to take more responsibility for care of the residual limb. Counsel family members to demonstrate acceptance of the injury and not to promote excessive dependence. Facilitate a meeting with prosthetist to discuss cosmetic and functional options.

CRITICAL THINKING QUESTIONS

1. What data should you collect to assess the patient's pain?
2. What sensations might this patient feel after the amputation?
3. List three activities that are likely to require modification after loss of the dominant hand.
4. How would you help this patient to explore his fears and anxieties?

Get Ready for the NCLEX® Examination!

Key Points

- Amputation is the surgical removal of body limbs or parts of limbs.
- Conditions or situations that can lead to an amputation include trauma, disease, tumors, and congenital problems.
- Medical management of patients who have amputations involves the appropriate treatment and control of underlying diseases such as diabetes mellitus and peripheral vascular disease.
- Complications of amputation include hemorrhage, hematoma, necrosis, wound dehiscence, gangrene, edema, contracture, pain, and infection.
- Preoperatively, the patient needs to prepare physically and psychologically for an impending amputation.
- Postoperative nursing care focuses on inadequate circulation, pain, potential for infection, loss of protective barrier (skin), potential for loss of protective barrier (skin), knowledge deficit, potential for injury, impaired mobility, inability to tolerate activity, desire for self-care, anxiety or stress, inadequate coping, and altered self-concept.
- Replantation of severed limbs is sometimes possible.
- Focus care on preserving the severed part and managing the patient's blood loss before replantation.
- Priorities after replantation include assessing for and managing inadequate tissue perfusion, pain, and altered body image.
- Immediately notify the surgeon and prepare the patient for a return to the operating suite if evidence exists of inadequate arterial circulation in a replanted limb.

Additional Learning Resources

SG Go to your Study Guide for additional learning activities to help you master this chapter content.

Go to your Evolve website (http://evolve.elsevier.com/Linton/medsurg) for the following learning resources and much more:
- Fluid & Electrolyte Tutorial
- Review Questions for the NCLEX® Examination

Clinical Judgment and Next-Generation NCLEX® Examination-Style Questions

1. **Which of the following is the most common cause of lower extremity amputation?**
   1. Trauma
   2. Vascular disease
   3. Tumors
   4. Congenital defects

   NCLEX Client Need: Physiological Integrity: Physiological Adaptation

2. **The nurse is teaching a patient who had a finger replanted. The teaching plan should explain that smoking is contraindicated after replantation because nicotine causes ________________.**

   NCLEX Client Need: Physiological Integrity: Reduction of Risk Potential

3. **In which of the following situations would an *open* amputation be most likely?**
   1. A teenager with bone cancer
   2. A diabetic patient with poor arterial blood flow
   3. A child with a congenital deformity
   4. An accident victim with a crushing injury

   NCLEX Client Need: Physiological Integrity: Reduction of Risk Potential

4. **A patient complains that her amputated foot itches and feels hot. The nurse should recognize that this represents which of the following?**
   1. Poor psychologic adjustment
   2. Phantom limb sensation
   3. Early symptoms of infection
   4. Denial of the amputation

   NCLEX Client Need: Physiological Integrity: Physiological Adaptation

5. **In the early postoperative period, what is the greatest danger to the patient who has had an amputation?**
   1. Pneumonia
   2. Pain
   3. Hemorrhage
   4. Anxiety

   NCLEX Client Need: Physiological Integrity: Physiological Adaptation

6. **A patient who had a below-knee amputation this morning has a cast on the residual limb. The nurse knows that the purpose of the cast in this case is to:**
   1. Reduce pain.
   2. Shape the residual limb.
   3. Prevent wound contamination.
   4. Prevent stimulation of nerve endings.

   NCLEX Client Need: Physiological Integrity: Reduction of Risk Potential

7. **When caring for a patient who has had an above-knee amputation, the nurse implements measures to prevent contractures in the residual limb. These measures should include: (Select all that apply.)**
   1. Keep the patient up in a chair as much as possible.
   2. Guide the patient through active range-of-motion exercises.
   3. Have the patient lie supine for 30 minutes 3 or 4 times a day.
   4. Prop the residual limb on a pillow when the patient is supine.
   5. Encourage the patient to sleep on the side of the amputation.

   NCLEX Client Need: Physiological Integrity: Reduction of Risk Potential

8. **Patient teaching related to care of a residual limb and prosthesis should include which of the following statements? (Select all that apply.)**
   1. Wear a clean residual limb sock every day.
   2. Wash, rinse, and dry the prosthetic socket every day.
   3. Apply lotion to the residual limb only if ordered to do so.
   4. Redness and irritation of the residual limb are normal.
   5. Wash the residual limb with soap and water daily.

   NCLEX Client Need: Physiological Integrity: Reduction of Risk Potential

9. **While on a camping trip, a camper accidentally cut off a finger while chopping wood. A nurse provided first aid and summoned emergency medical care. Meanwhile, how should the amputated finger be handled for possible replantation?**
   1. Cover the finger with ice
   2. Wrap the finger in a clean, dry cloth
   3. Wash the part carefully, dry it, and wrap it in plastic
   4. Seal the part in a plastic bag and put it in ice water

   NCLEX Client Need: Physiological Integrity: Reduction of Risk Potential

10. **When you examine a patient's replanted hand, it is slightly bluish, swollen, and warm. These findings indicate which of the following?**
    1. Arterial occlusion
    2. Rejection of the replanted hand
    3. Venous congestion
    4. That the replantation was successful

    NCLEX Client Need: Physiological Integrity: Physiological Adaptation

11. **SLO/Objective:** Determine appropriate nursing actions for clients experiencing postoperative complications.

    NGN Item Type: Extended Drag and Drop

    Cognitive Skill: Take Action

    A 45-year-old man with a history of diabetes mellitus is one-day postoperative for a below knee amputation after his left leg was severely damaged in an automobile accident. He has not yet been fitted with a prosthesis, and his residual limb is wrapped in a figure-8 bandage.

    Indicate which nursing action listed in the far left column is appropriate for the potential postoperative complication. Note that not all nursing actions will be used.

NURSING ACTION	POTENTIAL POSTOPERATIVE COMPLICATION	APPROPRIATE NURSING ACTION FOR POSTOPERATIVE COMPLICATION
Administer opioids as prescribed	Hemorrhage	
Encourage patient to discuss feelings about loss of limb	Edema	
Help patient to get out of bed 2–3 times a day	Contracture	
Observe for restlessness, cyanosis, increased pulse and respiratory rate	Acute Pain	
Note an increase in temperature or redness, soreness, or edema in residual limb	Infection	
Wrap elastic smoothly with even, moderate tension	Phantom limb sensation	
Place in prone position three times a day, if possible		
Massage residual limb; provide diversional activities		/

Endocrine System Introduction

47

http://evolve.elsevier.com/Linton/medsurg

Objectives

1. Identify data to be collected for the nursing assessment of the patient with an endocrine disorder.
2. Describe the tests and procedures used to diagnose disorders of the endocrine system, and related nursing care.
3. Identify the classes of drugs used to treat endocrine disorders including actions, uses, and side effects.
4. Describe the nursing responsibilities when administering endocrine drugs.

Key Terms

adrenaline (ă-DRĔN-ă-lĭn)
androgens (ĂN-drō-jĕnz)
catecholamines (kăt-ĕ-KŌL-ă-mēnz)
Chvostek sign (KVŎS-tĕk)
endocrine glands (ĔN-dŏ-krĭn)
estrogens (ĔS-trō-jĕnz)
exophthalmos (ĕk-sŏf-THĂL-mŏs)
glucocorticoid (gloo-kō-KŎR-tĭ-koyd)
mineralocorticoids (mĭn-ĕr-ăl-ō-KŎR-tĭ-koyd)
Trousseau sign (troo-SŌZ)

The endocrine system is a complex communication network composed of glands and glandular tissue that make, store, and secrete chemical messengers called *hormones*. It affects virtually every cell in the human body. Hormones are delivered to tissues by the bloodstream to target organs and body. The **endocrine glands** are depicted in Fig. 47.1.

Another class of glands includes the exocrine glands. The exocrine glands pass secretions through ducts or tubes that empty outside the body or into the lumen or opening of other organs. Examples of this type of gland are sweat glands and the portion of the pancreas that secretes digestive enzymes.

HORMONE FUNCTIONS AND REGULATION

The term *hormone* was coined in 1905. It is derived from the Greek word meaning "I arouse to activity." This definition is appropriate because hormones are normally released in response to the body's needs. Hormones are responsible for important functions related to reproduction, fluid and electrolyte balance, host defenses, responses to stress and injury, energy metabolism, and growth and development. The overall mission of the endocrine system is to maintain homeostasis. Homeostasis is the maintenance of physiologic stability despite the constant changes that occur in the environment. A hormone is a substance composed of amines, peptides, or steroids. These substances bind to receptors located inside the cell nucleus or on the cell membranes of target organs or tissues. Receptors are specific for certain kinds of hormones. Once the hormones bind with their receptors, they exert their effects on the organ or tissue.

Regulation of endocrine activity is controlled by mechanisms, called *feedback mechanisms*, that either stimulate or inhibit hormone synthesis and secretion. Feedback mechanisms are triggered by blood levels of specific substances. These substances may be hormones or other chemical compounds regulated by hormones. Feedback may be either positive or negative (Fig. 47.2).

In negative feedback, high levels of a substance inhibit hormone synthesis and secretion whereas low levels stimulate hormone synthesis and secretion. A simple example of this is the household thermostat. As the environmental temperature rises, the production of heat is decreased or stopped; however, as the temperature drops, heat production increases. In positive feedback, high levels of a substance stimulate hormone synthesis and secretion whereas low levels inhibit additional hormone synthesis and secretion.

Hormones have specific rates and rhythms of secretion. Three basic secretion patterns are (1) circadian or diurnal pattern, (2) pulsatile and cyclic patterns, and (3) patterns that depend on levels of circulating substances (e.g., calcium, sodium, potassium, or the hormones themselves).

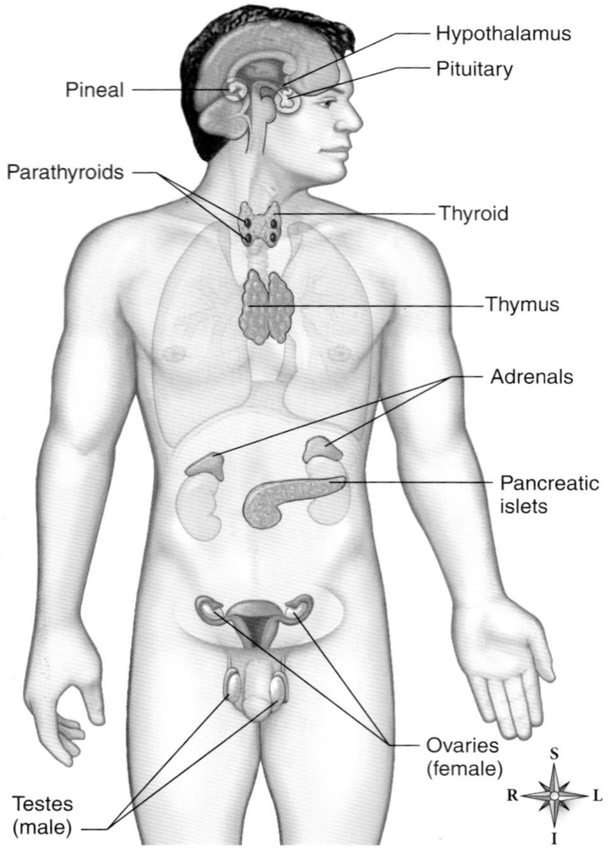

Fig. 47.1 The endocrine system. The organs of the endocrine system include the pituitary gland, thyroid gland, parathyroid glands, adrenal glands, pancreas, testes (in the man), and ovaries (in the woman). (From Patton KT, Thibodeau GA: *The human body in health & disease*, ed 7, St. Louis, 2018, Elsevier.)

ANATOMY AND PHYSIOLOGY OF THE ENDOCRINE SYSTEM

PITUITARY GLAND

The pituitary gland, also called the *hypophysis*, is a structure that weighs approximately 0.6 g and is located in the sella turcica, a small indentation in the sphenoid bone at the base of the brain. It is connected to the hypothalamus by the infundibular (hypophyseal) stalk. The pituitary gland is small and oval and has a diameter of approximately 1 cm. It consists of two parts, or lobes. The larger of the two lobes, which accounts for 70% to 80% of the gland's weight, is the anterior lobe. The anterior lobe is also called the *adenohypophysis*. The hormones of the anterior pituitary and their actions are as follows:

1. Growth hormone (GH), or somatotropic hormone: stimulates the growth and development of bones, muscles, and organs. GH stimulates the release of insulin-like growth factor 1 (IGF-1) by the liver and other tissues. IGF-1 promotes tissue growth.
2. Adrenocorticotropic hormone (ACTH): controls the growth, development, and function of the cortex of the adrenal glands; controls release of glucocorticoids and adrenal androgens; is necessary for secretion of aldosterone but does not control rate of aldosterone secretion.
3. Thyroid-stimulating hormone (TSH), or thyrotropic hormone: controls the secretory activities of the thyroid gland.
4. Follicle-stimulating hormone (FSH): stimulates the development of the eggs in the ovaries and estrogen production in the woman; stimulates sperm production in the man.
5. Luteinizing hormone (LH): controls progesterone production and ovulation or egg release in the woman; controls testicular growth and testosterone production in the man.
6. Prolactin, or lactogenic hormone: stimulates breast milk production in the woman.
7. Melanocyte-stimulating hormone (MSH): promotes pigmentation.

The smaller lobe of the pituitary is known as the *posterior pituitary* because it is located behind the anterior lobe in the sella turcica. It is sometimes referred to as the *neurohypophysis*. The hormones secreted by the posterior pituitary and their actions are as follows:

1. Antidiuretic hormone (ADH), or arginine vasopressin: causes the reabsorption of water from the renal tubules of the kidney. By doing so, water excretion from the body in the form of urine is decreased.
2. Oxytocin: causes contractions of the uterus in labor and the release of breast milk.

ADRENAL GLANDS

The adrenal glands are a pair of small, highly vascularized, triangular-shaped organs. They are located in the retroperitoneal cavity on the superior poles of each kidney, lateral to the lower thoracic and upper lumbar vertebrae. Each gland weighs approximately 4 g and measures 3.3 cm in length. The adrenal gland itself is composed of two parts: (1) an outer portion called the *cortex* and (2) an inner portion called the *medulla*. The cortex and medulla have very different, independent functions.

Adrenal Medulla

The medulla constitutes 20% of the adrenal gland and contains sympathetic ganglia (i.e., groups of nerve cell bodies) with secretory cells. Stimulation of the sympathetic nervous system causes the medulla to secrete two types of **catecholamines**: (1) norepinephrine (i.e., noradrenaline) and (2) epinephrine (i.e., **adrenaline**). Both of these substances act as neurotransmitters. They are released into the circulation and transported to target organs or tissues, where they exert their effects by binding to adrenergic receptors. Catecholamine effects vary depending on the specific receptor in the cell membrane of the target organ. Multiple adrenergic receptors exist, including $alpha_1$, $alpha_2$, $beta_1$, and $beta_2$ receptors. Norepinephrine binds to $alpha_1$, $alpha_2$, and $beta_1$ adrenergic receptors

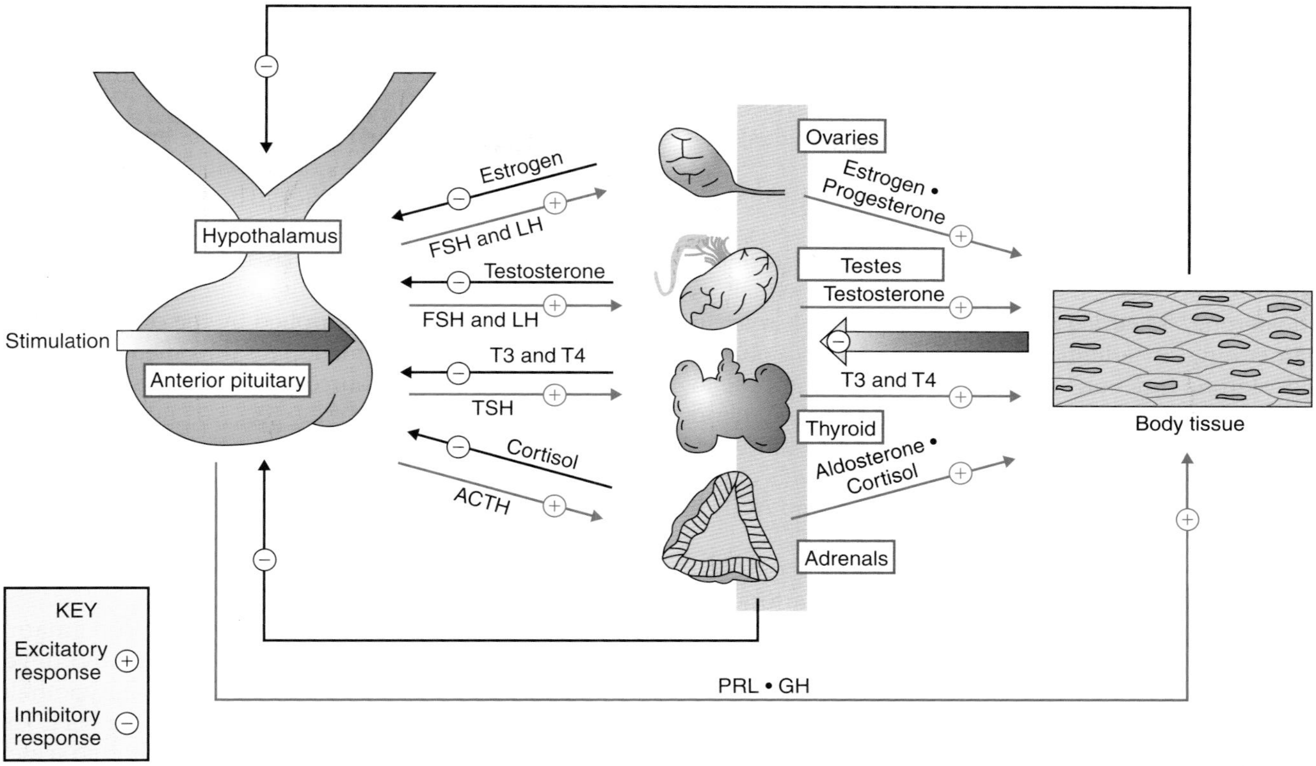

Fig. 47.2 The feedback system of the hypothalamus, pituitary, and target glands. *ACTH*, Adrenocorticotropic hormone; *FSH*, follicle-stimulating hormone; *GH*, growth hormone; *LH*, luteinizing hormone; *PRL*, prolactin; *T3*, triiodothyronine; *T4*, thyroxine, *TSH*, thyroid-stimulating hormone. (From Ignatavicius DD, Workman ML, Mishler MA: *Medical-surgical nursing across the health care continuum*, ed 3, Philadelphia, 1999, Saunders.)

Table 47.1 Receptors and Effects of Adrenal Medullary Hormones on Selected Locations

RECEPTOR SUBTYPE	LOCATION	RESPONSE TO RECEPTOR ACTIVATION
$alpha_1$	1. Arterioles: skin, viscera, mucous membranes 2. Veins 3. Eye 4. Male sex organs 5. Prostate 6. Bladder	1. Constriction 2. Constriction 3. Contraction of radial muscle in iris = mydriasis 4. Ejaculation 5. Contraction 6. Contraction of trigone and sphincter
$alpha_2$	Presynaptic nerve terminals	Inhibits neurotransmitter release
$beta_1$	1. Heart 2. Kidney	1. Inotropism: increased heart rate, force of contraction, increased AV conduction rate 2. Release of renin
$beta_2$	1. Arterioles: heart, lung, skeletal muscle 2. Bronchi 3. Uterus 4. Liver 5. Skeletal muscle	1. Dilation 2. Dilation 3. Relaxation 4. Glycogenolysis[a] 5. Enhanced glycogenolysis[a]

[a]Breaks down glycogen into glucose.
Modified from Table 13.3, p. 114, Burchum JR, Rosenthal LD. *Lehne's pharmacology for nursing* care, 10th ed. St. Louis, MO, Elsevier, 2019.

whereas epinephrine affects $alpha_1$, $alpha_2$, $beta_1$, and $beta_2$-adrenergic receptors. Table 47.1 lists the specific effects of these catecholamines and the types of receptors with which they bind. The major function of these substances is adaptation to stress, as characterized by the "fight-or-flight response," and maintenance of homeostasis.

Adrenal Cortex

The adrenal cortex, which comprises 80% of the adrenal gland, is the outer portion of the gland. This is the portion that is considered to be a part of the endocrine system. The cortex is essential for maintenance of many life-sustaining physiologic activities. The cells of the cortex are organized into three distinct layers or zones. Proceeding from the outermost to innermost layers, they are (1) the zona glomerulosa, (2) the zona fasciculata, and (3) the zona reticularis. The hormones synthesized and secreted by the cortex are known as *steroids* and consist of mineralocorticoids, glucocorticoids, and androgens or estrogens.

Function of the Adrenal Glands

Mineralocorticoids. The zona glomerulosa produces mineralocorticoids, the most abundant of which is aldosterone. **Mineralocorticoids** play a key role in maintaining an adequate extracellular fluid volume. Aldosterone functions at the renal collecting tubule to promote the reabsorption of sodium and the excretion of potassium by the kidney. The secretion of aldosterone is regulated by several factors: serum levels of potassium, the renin-angiotensin mechanism, and ACTH.

Renin, angiotensin, and aldosterone. Renin is produced by the juxtaglomerular cells of renal afferent arterioles. Its release is stimulated by a decrease in extracellular fluid volume. Any factor that can cause this decrease (blood or fluid loss, sodium depletion, or changes in body position or posture) can stimulate renin release. Renin acts on plasma proteins to release angiotensin I, which is catalyzed in the lung to angiotensin II. Angiotensin II stimulates the secretion of aldosterone, which results in sodium and water retention. Retention of sodium and water preserves or increases extracellular fluid volume and subsequently increases blood pressure (BP). This compensatory mechanism plays a very important role in maintaining intravascular volume in shock states.

Glucocorticoids. The **glucocorticoids** are produced by the zona reticularis and zona fasciculata. The most abundant and potent of the glucocorticoids is cortisol. Approximately 92% of circulating cortisol is bound to a plasma protein. Free cortisol (8%) binds with receptors in the cytoplasm and nuclei of target cells. Cortisol has a permissive effect on other physiologic processes, meaning that the glucocorticoid must be present for other processes, such as catecholamine activity and excitability of the myocardium, to occur. Glucocorticoid functions include control of carbohydrate, lipid, and fat metabolism; regulation of antiinflammatory and immune responses; and control of emotional states by the following:

- Increasing hepatic gluconeogenesis and inhibiting peripheral glucose use to maintain glucose levels
- Increasing lipolysis and release of glycerol and free fatty acids
- Increasing protein catabolism
- Degrading collagen and connective tissue
- Increasing polymorphonuclear leukocytes released from bone marrow
- Decreasing capillary permeability, movement of white blood cells (WBCs) into the injured tissue, and phagocytosis
- Stabilizing lysosomal membranes
- Suppressing lymphocyte reproduction
- Maintaining behavioral and cognitive functions

Sex hormones. Adrenal **androgens** are another class of steroids produced in the zona fasciculata and zona reticularis of the adrenal cortex. Their primary function is masculinization in men. Other sex hormones include **estrogen** and progesterone. In men, these substances contribute little to reproductive maturation. In women, however, estrogens are supplied by the ovaries and the adrenal glands. In postmenopausal women, the adrenal cortex is the primary source of endogenous estrogen.

THYROID GLAND

The thyroid gland is located in the lower portion of the anterior neck. It consists of two lobes, one on each side of the trachea. The lobes are connected in front of the trachea by a narrow bridge of tissue called the *isthmus* (Fig. 47.3).

The thyroid gland plays a major role in regulating the body's rate of metabolism and growth and development. When the metabolic rate falls, the hypothalamus stimulates the pituitary gland to secrete TSH. This hormone in turn stimulates the thyroid gland to secrete hormones that affect the production and use of energy.

The hormones produced by the thyroid gland are thyroid hormone, triiodothyronine, and calcitonin. Each of these is known by several names. Thyroid hormone is also called *thyroxine, tetraiodothyronine,* or T_4. Triiodothyronine is referred to as T_3. Both T_4 and T_3 increase the body's metabolic rate. Calcitonin, or thyrocalcitonin, plays a role

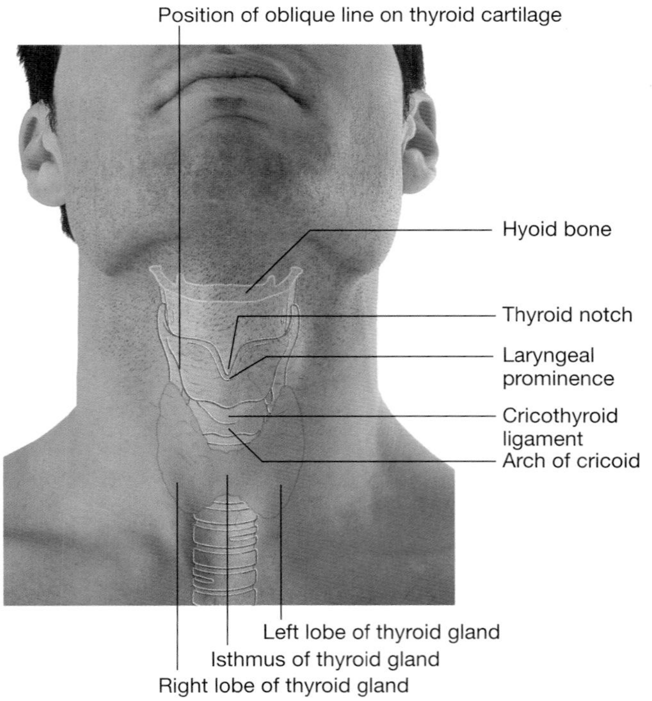

Fig. 47.3 The thyroid gland. (From Drake RL, Vogl AW, Mitchell AWM: *Gray's anatomy for students*, ed 3, Philadelphia, 2015, Churchill Livingstone.)

in regulating the serum calcium level. It is secreted when serum calcium levels are high, limiting the shift of calcium from the bones into the blood.

PARATHYROID GLANDS

The parathyroid glands are small glands usually located on the back of the thyroid gland (see Fig. 47.1). Occasionally some glands are found in the mediastinum as well. Most people have four parathyroids, but some people have more. Although they are typically embedded in the thyroid, the parathyroids function independently. They secrete only one hormone, but it is a vital one, *parathormone* (PTH). Parathormone plays a critical role in regulating the serum calcium level.

Calcium is an essential component of strong bones and plays a vital role in the functions of nerve and muscle cells. When the serum calcium level falls, PTH is secreted. PTH increases the absorption of calcium from the intestines, transfers calcium from the bones to the blood, and signals the kidneys to conserve calcium. In general, calcium retention by the kidney is balanced by phosphate loss.

PANCREAS

Introductory information about the exocrine functions of the pancreas is found in Chapter 37. Pancreatitis and pancreatic cancer are addressed in Chapter 40. Diabetes mellitus and hypoglycemia are discussed in Chapter 50.

AGE-RELATED CHANGES IN THE ENDOCRINE SYSTEM

In healthy older adults, endocrine function usually remains adequate. However, small changes may be important when homeostasis is altered by illness. Changes include the following:

- Diminished response to ADH so the older person is less able to compensate for inadequate fluid intake or excessive fluid loss and is at risk for dehydration.
- Decline in GH and IGF-1, resulting in reduced protein synthesis, decreased lean body and bone mass, and reduced immune function.
- Decline in cortisol secretion; usually balanced by decreased cortisol metabolism.
- Decline in secretion of aldosterone and plasma renin activity, which decreases the efficiency of sodium conservation and adaptation to position changes.
- Although not normal, hypothyroidism is more common, especially among women.

NURSING ASSESSMENT OF THE PATIENT WITH AN ENDOCRINE DISORDER

The nursing assessment of the patient with an endocrine disorder is outlined in Box 47.1. The licensed vocational nurse/licensed practical nurse (LVN/LPN) assists with the collection of relevant data.

Box 47.1 Nursing Assessment of the Patient With an Endocrine Disorder

HEALTH HISTORY

Reason for Seeking Care

Fatigue, headache, weight changes.

Present Health/History of Present Illness

Changes in energy level, weight, height, appearance, skin color, sleep pattern, sexual function, and urinary function. Also gastrointestinal (GI) disturbances, vision disturbances, mental/emotional changes, and musculoskeletal symptoms (weakness, twitching, bone pain).

Past Health History

Diabetes mellitus, brain tumor, head trauma, central nervous system (CNS) infection, vascular disorders, renal calculi ("stones"), chronic renal failure, tuberculosis, hypothyroidism. Diseases of the pancreas, liver, or bone. Intracranial surgery or radiation to the head, neck, or abdomen. All recent or current medications including calcium and vitamin D supplements.

Family History

Diabetes mellitus, thyroid disease, other endocrine disorders, cancer.

Review of Systems

General health state: fatigue, headache, weakness, restlessness, changes in appearance, personality changes. Changes in skin color, texture, and moisture; pruritus; sensory changes, that is, blurred vision and diplopia; changes in the breasts, genitalia, body hair distribution. Increased appetite, thirst, and urine volume. Chest pain, orthostatic hypotension, constipation, polyuria, sexual dysfunction, joint pain, abnormal sensations, muscle cramps, edema, seizures, intolerance of heat or cold. Change in stool color.

Functional Assessment

Sleep disturbances. Usual diet; changes in appetite. Fat intolerance. Alcohol intake. Effects of symptoms on self-concept and usual activities.

PHYSICAL EXAMINATION

Height and weight

General Survey: mental alertness, orientation

Vital Signs: blood pressure sitting and standing

Skin: bronzed or smoky pigmentation, bruising, petechiae, vitiligo, pallor. Texture and turgor.

Head and neck: facial expression, thickened lips, broad nose, prominent forehead and jaw, excess facial hair on females. Visual acuity; exophthalmos. Neck enlargement. Color and moisture of oral cavity. Chvostek sign.

Thorax: fat pads under the clavicles, "buffalo hump," male breast enlargement, darkening of areola

Abdomen: striae, discoloration, distention, guarding, obesity.

Extremities: muscle wasting, edema; joint range of motion, limitations, crepitus; reflexes, muscle strength, hand tremor. Trousseau sign.

External genitalia: atrophy, hair loss, appropriateness for age.

HEALTH HISTORY

Reason for Seeking Care

Because hormones affect all body tissues, patients with endocrine disorders often report vague symptoms such as fatigue, headache, or weight changes.

Present Health/History of Present Illness

An exploration of the patient's concerns may reveal more specific data such as changes in energy level, weight, height, appearance, skin color, sleep pattern, sexual function, and urinary function. Gastrointestinal (GI) disturbances, problems with vision, mental/emotional changes, and musculoskeletal symptoms (weakness, twitching, bone pain) may be noted.

Past Health History

A history of diabetes mellitus, brain tumors, head trauma, central nervous system (CNS) infection, vascular disorders, renal calculi ("stones"), chronic renal failure, tuberculosis, and hypothyroidism, as well as disease of the pancreas, liver, or bone, should be documented. Note if the patient has had intracranial surgery or radiation to the head, neck, or abdomen. List all recent or current medications including calcium and vitamin D supplements.

Family History

Note a family history of endocrine disorders.

Review of Systems

Ask about the patient's general health state and note fatigue, headache, weakness, restlessness, or personality changes. Inquire about changes in skin color, texture, and moisture as well as changes in appearance. Note reports of significant sensory changes such as blurred vision and diplopia (i.e., double vision). Increases in appetite, thirst, and urine volume are especially important as they suggest possible diabetes mellitus. For both men and women, ask about changes in the breasts, genitalia, and body hair distribution. Also inquire whether the patient has experienced chest pain, dizziness with position changes, constipation, polyuria, sexual dysfunction, joint pain, abnormal sensations, muscle cramps, edema, seizures, and intolerance of heat or cold.

Functional Assessment

In the functional assessment, determine whether the patient has had sleep disturbances or changes in appetite. Obtain a description of usual diet and note the effects of symptoms on the person's self-concept and usual activities.

PHYSICAL EXAMINATION

Measure the patient's height, weight, and vital signs. Take the BP when the patient is reclining and after the patient has moved to an upright position to detect a significant decrease. Note patient responses and ability to follow instructions. Inspect the skin for a bronzed or smoky pigmentation (especially in surgical scars, the skin over the knuckles, skinfolds, and the areola), bruising, petechiae, vitiligo (i.e., loss of pigmentation), and pallor. Palpate the skin texture and turgor.

Note the facial expression and characteristics as well as the mental alertness. Inspect the head and face for thickened lips, broad nose, and prominent forehead and jaw. Test visual acuity. Inspect the face of the female patient for excess facial hair. Examine the eyes for **exophthalmos** (bulging). Inspect the neck for enlargement typical of goiter. Nurses with advanced physical examination skills may palpate the neck for thyroid enlargement or nodules. Examine the oral mucous membranes for color changes and moisture.

Inspect the anterior thorax for fat pads under the clavicles and the posterior thorax for the "buffalo hump." Note obesity of the trunk. Examine the breasts for enlargement in men and for striae ("stretch marks") and darkening of the areola in both men and women. Inspect the abdomen for striae and the extremities for muscle wasting and edema. Perform joint range of motion, noting any limitations or crepitus. Test reflexes for slowness of response and evaluate muscle strength. Observe the hands for tremor. Simple tests are used to elicit Chvostek sign and Trousseau sign, which are both indicative of hypocalcemia. **Chvostek sign** is a spasm of the facial muscle when the face is tapped over the facial nerve. **Trousseau sign** is a carpopedal spasm that occurs when a BP cuff is inflated above the patient's systolic BP and left in place for 2 to 3 minutes (Fig. 47.4). During examination of the external genitalia, assess for atrophy, hair loss, and appropriateness for age.

DIAGNOSTIC TESTS AND PROCEDURES

RADIOGRAPHIC STUDIES

Conventional radiographs, computed tomography (CT) scans, and magnetic resonance imaging (MRI) may be used to detect structural abnormalities (e.g., nodules, tumors, enlargement, atrophy) of the pituitary, adrenals, thyroid, parathyroid glands, and the pancreas. Angiography, in which a radiopaque dye is injected into the arteries, may reveal the presence of vascular anomalies associated with pituitary or adrenal disorders. Ultrasound is useful in assessing adrenal, thyroid, and parathyroid conditions.

For a thyroid scan, the patient ingests radioactive iodine (RAI); then a specialized instrument is used to scan the area of the thyroid gland. It creates an image of the gland based on the distribution of the iodine. The image aids in diagnosing cancer because the patterns of iodine concentration in normal and malignant tissue are different. The scan may be repeated at specific intervals. The low dose of radiation used for diagnostic purposes poses no danger to the patient or others. However, pregnancy is a contraindication because of possible harm to the fetus.

LABORATORY STUDIES

Because hormones are circulating in very small quantities, tests to identify normal levels must be sensitive and precise. The radioimmunoassay and the enzyme-linked immunosorbent assay (ELISA) are tests that measure levels of hormones in the blood.

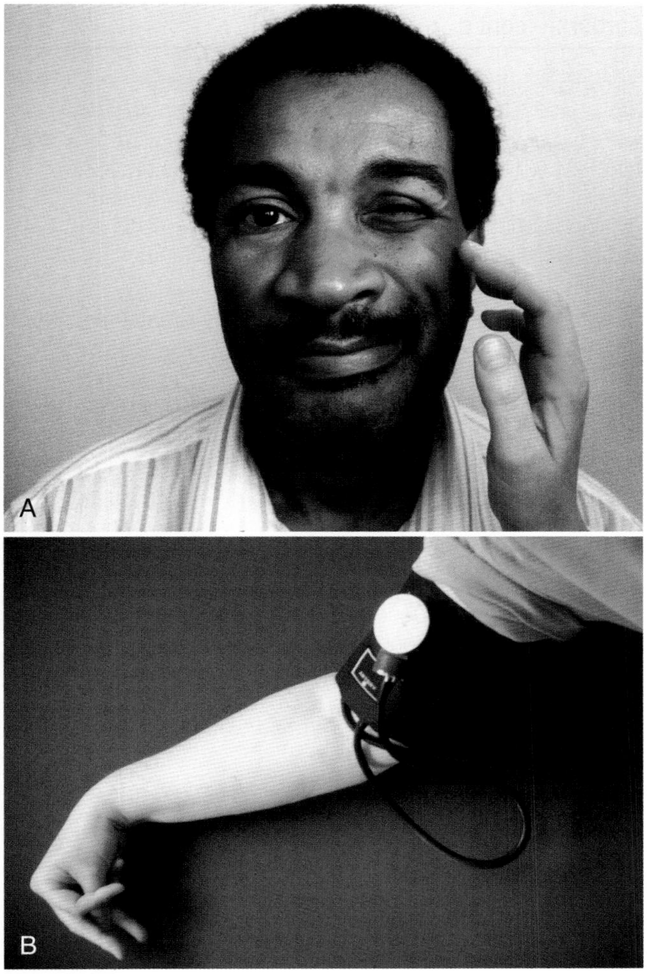

Fig. 47.4 Signs of hypocalcemia. (A) Chvostek sign (facial twitch). (B) Trousseau sign (carpopedal spasm). (From Ignatavicius DD, Workman ML. *Medical-surgical nursing: patient-centered collaborative care*, 8th ed. St. Louis, Elsevier, 2016.)

Hormone reserve activity can also be measured using a number of "suppression" or "stimulation" tests. In these tests, hormone levels are measured after administration of an agent that stimulates or suppresses hormonal function. Stimulation will cause a healthy endocrine gland to increase hormone production. Suppression will cause a healthy endocrine gland to decrease hormone production. The response helps the physician to determine whether the target gland (e.g., thyroid, adrenal, gonads) or the hypothalamic-pituitary regulatory mechanism is responsible for abnormal hormone levels.

A GH suppression test may be done by measuring blood glucose levels before and after a dose of a glucose solution. The glucose will suppress GH levels through a negative-feedback process. In normal patients, GH levels fall to less than 5 mg/mL. However, in patients with hyperpituitarism, large decreases in GH occur. This constitutes a positive result. Other studies measure serum levels of GH, IGF-1, and gonadotropins (FSH, LH). A 6-hour water deprivation test is done to determine the cause of diabetes insipidus (DI). ADH is administered and urine and blood samples are taken at intervals.

The most useful tests of thyroid function are measurements of serum TSH and free T4. The thyroid-releasing hormone (TRH) stimulation test measures the blood level of TSH after administration of TRH. This test shows whether thyroid hormone abnormalities are caused by a disorder of the thyroid gland itself or by altered production of stimulating hormones by the hypothalamus or the pituitary. Additional blood tests may help to determine the type of dysfunction.

The thyroid gland uses iodine to manufacture hormones. Therefore RAI isotopes (iodine-131 [^{131}I], iodine-123 [^{123}I], and technetium-99m [99mTc]) are useful for diagnostic purposes because they concentrate in the thyroid. The amount of iodine taken up by the thyroid is measured to assess the activity level of the gland. This test is called an *RAI uptake test.*

Additional information about diagnostic tests and procedures for endocrine disorders and related nursing care is presented in Table 47.2.

DRUG THERAPY

In general, endocrine drugs are given to replace or supplement deficient hormones, to stimulate or suppress hormone secretion, or to manage symptoms of endocrine disorders. Table 47.3 lists types of endocrine drugs with uses, actions, side effects, and nursing interventions. Additional specific drugs including insulin are discussed with the conditions for which they are prescribed in the remaining chapters of this unit.

Table 47.2 Diagnostic Tests and Procedures for Endocrine Disorders

General interventions for radiologic studies with contrast dye. *Before procedure:* Ask about patient allergy to dye, iodine, or shellfish. If patient reports allergy, notify radiology. Tell patient that injection of contrast dye can create a feeling of warmth, a salty taste, and nausea. *After procedure:* Inform the physician of any signs of allergic response to the contrast dye. Administer antihistamine as ordered for allergy.
General interventions for laboratory studies: Check agency procedure manual for diagnostic tests and procedures. Always tell the patient what to expect when tests are ordered. Explain if nothing by mouth (NPO) status is necessary. Document the care provided and relevant assessment data. If venipuncture is done, apply a dressing and check the site for oozing. Apply pressure and elevate arm if patient's blood clotting is impaired.

Continued

Table 47.2 Diagnostic Tests and Procedures for Endocrine Disorders—cont'd

TEST AND PURPOSE	PATIENT PREPARATION	POSTPROCEDURE CARE
Pituitary Studies		
Radiologic Studies		
Cerebral CT scan: Uses radiographs to create images of internal structures; detects tumors, edema, and structural abnormalities.	Dye precautions. Tell the patient they will lie still on a stretcher while a circular scanner moves around the head. Clicking sounds are heard but no sensations are felt. Remove jewelry and hairpins.	Dye precautions. If contrast medium is used, assess for side effects: nausea, vomiting, headache, and delayed allergic reaction.
MRI scan with gadolinium infusion: Gadolinium is a contrast medium used with MRI to enhance brain imaging. No radiation exposure.	Dye precautions. Nonfasting. Tell the patient an intravenous (IV) injection may be given. All metal, including medication patches with metallic backing, must be removed. Encourage the patient to void in advance to avoid discomfort of a full bladder. During the scan, the patient must remain still. A loud thumping noise will be heard during the procedure.	Dye precautions. General interventions.
Blood Studies		
Growth hormone stimulation: Arginine is infused followed by insulin. Both stimulate growth hormone (GH) secretion. Low serum GH level in response indicates GH deficiency.	NPO per laboratory manual except for water. Tell patient an IV line will be used to give medications and withdraw blood samples. Blood glucose will be monitored.	General interventions. Send blood specimen to the laboratory immediately after collection.
Somatomedin C (IGF-1): IGF-1 provides more accurate measure of mean serum GH concentration than random blood sample.	NPO overnight before blood drawn.	General interventions.
Gonadotropins: Follicle stimulating hormone (FSH) and luteinizing hormone (LH). Helps determine whether gonadal insufficiency is caused by gonads or pituitary insufficiency.	No fasting required. General interventions for blood tests. For urine tests, instruct patient in collection of 24-hour specimen. Refrigerate container. If home urine tests are done, a kit with instructions is provided.	General interventions.
Water deprivation test: Differentiates types of polyuria by assessing urine and serum osmolality according to specific guidelines while fasting.	NPO period depends on patient's 24-hour urine volume. Tell patient that hourly weights and urine samples will be taken over several hours, as well as some blood samples.	Provide fluids for rehydration. Monitor vital signs reclining and sitting to detect orthostatic hypotension.
Adrenal Studies		
Radiologic Studies		
See General Interventions for Radiologic Studies (previously)		
CT scan: Preferred abdominal scan to detect adrenal tumors and metastases. Oral or IV contrast medium may be used.	Dye precautions. Tell patient they will need to lie still during scan.	Dye precautions.
MRI: Useful in imaging the adrenal glands	Dye precautions. Nonfasting. Tell the patient an intravenous (IV) injection may be given. All metal, including medication patches with metallic backing, must be removed. Encourage the patient to void in advance to avoid discomfort of a full bladder. During the scan, the patient must remain still. A loud thumping noise will be heard during the procedure.	

Table 47.2 Diagnostic Tests and Procedures for Endocrine Disorders—cont'd

TEST AND PURPOSE	PATIENT PREPARATION	POSTPROCEDURE CARE
Blood Studies		
Cortisol: Used to evaluate adrenal function for hypersecretion or hyposecretion of cortisol.	Tell patient blood samples will be taken around 8 AM and 4 PM. Notify the health care provider if the patient is stressed emotionally or acutely ill.	General interventions.
Aldosterone: Used to diagnose hyperaldosteronism and determine whether primary or secondary.	Tell the patient they will need to remain upright for 2 hours before blood is drawn. Determine whether any drugs need to be withheld (e.g., propranolol) and for what period of time.	General interventions.
Adrenocorticotropic hormone (ACTH): When cortisol is overproduced or underproduced, this test reveals whether the basic pathology is in the pituitary or adrenal glands.	NPO overnight. Notify health care provider if patient is stressed (stress can affect results). Determine whether patient is on any drugs that need to be withheld.	After blood is drawn, place the tube in ice water and send it to the laboratory immediately.
ACTH stimulation with cosyntropin (rapid test): For adrenal insufficiency, determines whether the basic pathology is in the pituitary or the adrenal glands.	NPO overnight. Tell patient a blood sample will be drawn, then an IV drug will be injected and additional blood sample drawn 30 and 60 minutes later.	General interventions.
Dexamethasone ACTH suppression (rapid test): Used to diagnose adrenal hyperfunction, and its cause.	Tell patient dexamethasone will be given with milk or an antacid at 11 PM, then NPO overnight. At 8 AM, a blood sample will be drawn. If cortisol not suppressed, test may be repeated with higher dose. Determine whether any drugs should be withheld.	General interventions.
ACTH stimulation with metanephrine: Used to differentiate adrenal tumors from ACTH overproduction.	Caffeine, alcohol, and some drugs may need to be withheld. Tell patient metyrapone will be given at 11 PM and a blood sample drawn the next morning. Contraindicated with adrenal insufficiency; could cause adrenal crisis.	Monitor for signs of Addisonian crisis: deficient fluid volume, hyperkalemia.
Petrosal sinus sampling: Used to determine whether increased ACTH is caused by a pituitary or other site tumor.	After a fast of 4 or more hours, an injection of corticotropin-releasing hormone (CRH) is given. Blood samples are drawn from petrosal sinuses (veins that drain the pituitary and from a more distant site).	Tell patient an IV will be started. Blood samples will be drawn at intervals before and after CRH is given IV. Patient may have facial flushing and metallic taste when drug administered.
Pheochromocytoma suppression testing: Assesses adrenal response to clonidine; no response is diagnostic for pheochromocytoma.	The patient needs to recline and relax for 30 minutes. A baseline blood sample is drawn, PO clonidine given, and another blood sample obtained 3 hours later. Monitor for hypotension throughout test period.	Monitor vital signs for at least 1 hour after last blood sample drawn.
Urine Studies		
17-ketosteroids: Used to evaluate adrenal cortex function.	Instruct patient in 24-hour urine collection. Patient should drink fluids during the collection. Withhold all drugs per health care provider orders, usually several days.	Note start and stop times on collection container. Specimen should be kept refrigerated or on ice and sent to the laboratory as soon as completed.
Cortisol (free): Used to assess adrenal gland function.	Same as 17-ketosteroids (earlier).	Same as 17-ketosteroids (earlier).

Continued

Table 47.2 Diagnostic Tests and Procedures for Endocrine Disorders—cont'd

TEST AND PURPOSE	PATIENT PREPARATION	POSTPROCEDURE CARE
Thyroid Studies		
Radiologic Studies and Ultrasonography		
Radioactive iodine (RAI) uptake test: After RAI is given orally, the amount of iodine-131 (^{131}I) taken up by thyroid is measured with a special instrument. High uptake is seen with hyperthyroidism and low uptake is seen with hypothyroidism.	Tell the patient that the procedure is painless. Ask about pregnancy, in which case radiation is contraindicated. Advise the patient that the radiation dose is small and will not harm others.	For 24 hours after the test, the patient should practice thorough handwashing with soap and water after voiding. If a caregiver discards the patient's urine, gloves should be worn; the used gloves should be washed, removed, and the caregiver's bare hands washed. Pregnant women should avoid patient contact for 24 hours.
Thyroid scan: ^{131}I, iodine-123 (^{123}I), or technetium-99m (99mTc) is given orally and a scanner is used to detect the pattern of uptake by the thyroid gland. This test can differentiate benign and malignant nodules as well as other abnormalities.	Tell the patient an isotope will be given and scans performed afterwards. The waiting period varies with the type of isotope used. For the scan, the patient must lie still on their back for 20 minutes. For 1 week before the test, the patient should not consume iodine. Iodine is in radiographic dyes, some oral contraceptives, weight control drugs, multivitamins, all thyroid drugs, and some food (especially seafood).	Postprocedure care is the same as for the RAI uptake test.
Thyroid ultrasonography: Provides high-quality images of the thyroid and any nodules.	Advise the patient that the procedure is painless and noninvasive. An instrument is moved over the neck area and uses sound waves to create an image of the gland.	General interventions.
Blood Studies		
Serum T3 (triiodothyronine) and serum T4 (thyroxine): Measurements of free and total T4 detect abnormal levels of thyroid hormones. Elevated T3 indicates possible Graves disease, toxic adenoma, and toxic nodular goiter. Elevated T4 indicates hyperthyroidism or excessive thyroid hormone replacement. T3 and T4 decrease with hypothyroidism.	General interventions. No fasting required. Some medications may be withheld before blood is drawn.	General interventions.
Serum thyroid-stimulating hormone (TSH): Increases with hypothyroidism and decreases with hyperthyroidism.	General interventions.	General interventions.
Thyroid-releasing hormone (TRH) stimulation test: Assesses the response of the pituitary to TRH and differentiates the types of hypothyroidism. TSH normally increases after TRH is given intravenously.	Tell the patient that a drug will be given intravenously; then several blood samples will be drawn.	General interventions.
Antithyroglobulin antibody: Aids in diagnosis of autoimmune thyroid disease.	Nonfasting. Blood sample drawn.	General interventions.
Biopsy		
Fine-needle aspiration biopsy: Material from thyroid nodules can be aspirated using a needle and guided by ultrasonography.	Give the patient the same instructions as for thyroid ultrasonography. Tell the patient that the physician will use a small needle to remove a tissue sample.	Assess the patient for any signs of bleeding: swelling in the area of the biopsy site, bleeding from the puncture site, increasing pulse.

Table 47.2 Diagnostic Tests and Procedures for Endocrine Disorders—cont'd

TEST AND PURPOSE	PATIENT PREPARATION	POSTPROCEDURE CARE
Parathyroid Studies		
Scan		
Parathyroid scan (STDP method): Uses radioactive isotopes and scanning to locate glands, obtain images, and reveal abnormally active areas.	Dye precautions. Tell patient an isotope will be injected and scans done 15 minutes and 3 hours later. Some drugs may need to be restricted before test. Assure patient that the dose of radiation is very small. Usually not done during pregnancy unless benefits perceived to outweigh risks.	Dye precautions. No radiation precautions needed.
Blood Studies		
Parathyroid hormone (PTH) and serum calcium (total[a]): Done together to detect bone and parathyroid disorders.	NPO overnight. Tell patient a blood sample will be drawn at 8 AM. Specimen must be kept cold and transported on dry ice. Note time of blood draw on laboratory slip.	General interventions.
Calcium (ionized): Measures only ionized (free) serum calcium.	General interventions. Nonfasting.	General interventions.
Phosphate: Used in diagnosis of parathyroid and calcium abnormalities.	General interventions. Nonfasting.	General interventions.
Pancreatic Studies		
Blood Studies		
Fasting blood glucose: Most often used to screen for diabetes and guide insulin dosing in people with diabetes. Personal glucometers and glucose sensors are discussed in Chapter 50.	NPO 8 to 12 hours (except water).	General interventions.
Oral glucose tolerance test (OGTT): Data contributes to diagnosis of diabetes mellitus. Blood and urine specimens are taken to measure glucose levels before and after consuming a glucose solution.	12-hour fast. Provide written instructions about pretest dietary requirements. Record patient weight. Transient dizziness, sweating, and weakness may occur. If persistent, check blood glucose.	General interventions.
Glycosylated hemoglobin (A1C): Provides a long-term index of the patient's average blood glucose level.	Nonfasting. General interventions. Tell the patient that the result indicates how well diabetes is being controlled. Target level is <7%.	General interventions.
Urine Studies		
Glucose: Screening test for diabetes mellitus.	Nonfasting. Use fresh double-voided specimen.	General interventions.
Ketones: Part of routine urinalysis; presence of ketones reflects massive breakdown of fatty acids, usually caused by poorly controlled diabetes with hyperglycemia.	Instruct patient in collection of urine specimen in a urine container. Take to laboratory immediately or refrigerate.	No special care required. Recognize critical values: Adult male: <50 and >450 mg/dL Adult female: <40 and >450 mg/dL
Radiologic Studies		
CT scan: Preferred tool to identify pancreatic cysts or tumors.	Dye precautions if IV or PO contrast used. Check renal function tests before contrast. Tell the patient they will lie still on a stretcher while a circular scanner moves around the head. Clicking sounds are heard but no sensations are felt.	Dye precautions if used.

[a]Total includes ionized and protein bound Ca^{2+}.

Ca^{2+}, Calcium; *CT*, computed tomography; *MRI*, magnetic resonance imaging; *PO*, orally; *STPD*, single tracer double phase.

Modified from Kelly KA: Assessment of endocrine system. In: Lewis SL, Bucher L, Heitkemper MM, Harding MM, Kwong J, Roberts D, editors: *Medical-surgical nursing: assessment and management of clinical problems*, St. Louis, Elsevier, 2017; Pagana, KD, Pagana TJ: *Mosby's manual of diagnostic and laboratory tests*, ed 5, St. Louis, 2014, Elsevier

Table 47.3 Drug Therapy for Endocrine Disorders

DRUG	USE AND ACTION	SIDE EFFECTS	NURSING INTERVENTIONS
Drugs for Adrenal and Pituitary Conditions			
ADH Hormone Preparations			
	All promote conservation of water.	All can cause water intoxication, inadequate tissue perfusion because of vasoconstriction.	Monitor for early signs and symptoms of water intoxication: drowsiness, listlessness, headache. Patient should reduce fluid intake first few days of treatment.
Desmopressin (DDAVP, Stimate, et al.) nasal spray, parenteral, oral preparations	Treats DI, hemophilia (increases production of clotting factor VIII), nocturnal diuresis, headache.	Rhinorrhea, nasal irritation, and congestion. Rarely: dyspnea, hypertension, coronary vasoconstriction.	Teach patient use of intranasal inhaler: hold bottle upright, place nozzle in nostril, spray prescribed number of times, do not inhale. Explain how to monitor intake and output. With DI, stress need for lifelong therapy. Monitor BP, pulse.
Pituitary Hormone Suppressants (Somatostatin Analogs)			
Octreotide acetate (Sandostatin), lanreotide (Somatuline Depot)	Suppresses secretion of growth hormone. Used to treat acromegaly.	Nausea, vomiting, diarrhea, headache, flushing, edema, dizziness, altered blood glucose, drowsiness, orthostatic hypotension, visual disturbances, cholelithiasis.	Monitor weight, BP, pulse, respirations, urine output. Assess for edema. Refrigerate ampules. Discard if discolored or contains visible particles. Teach patient to give self-injections; advise to take exactly as prescribed and never take double doses. Assess for changes in blood glucose. Caution about drowsiness and dizziness. Very expensive.
Dopamine agonist: cabergoline (Dostinex)	Prevents/inhibits secretion of prolactin. May lower GH secretion in some patients with acromegaly.	Nausea, constipation, abdominal pain, headache, dizziness, asthenia, fatigue, drowsiness.	Contraindicated with uncontrolled hypertension.
GH receptor antagonist: pegvisomant (Somavert)	Used to treat acromegaly. Prevents GH from exerting effects on body tissues.	Infection, pain, injection site reaction, chest pain, back pain, flu syndrome, abnormal liver function tests, diarrhea, dizziness, edema, sinusitis.	Contraindicated with latex allergy because vial stopper contains latex. Teach patient or family member to prepare and give SC injections. Do not shake vial when reconstituting drug. Solution should be clear. Discard leftover reconstituted drug.
Vasopressin receptor antagonists: tolvaptan (Samsca), conivaptan (Vaprisol)	Used to treat hyponatremia in patients with normal blood volume. May be used for SIADH.	Atrial fibrillation, nausea, vomiting, dry mouth, constipation, hematuria, anemia, dehydration, electrolyte imbalances (low sodium, potassium, magnesium). Pain and redness at injection site.	Fluid status must be monitored closely. Avoid pregnancy and breastfeeding. Report neurologic changes: confusion, headache, insomnia.
Adrenal Hormones: Glucocorticoids			
Dexamethasone (e.g., Decadron) prednisolone (Econopred))	All stimulate formation of glucose, promote storage of glucose as glycogen, affect fluid and electrolytes, increase hemoglobin, suppress inflammation. Used to treat adrenal insufficiency. Some also have mineralocorticoid effects.	All: hypokalemia, hypocalcemia, nausea and vomiting, edema, hypertension, increased risk of infection, hyperglycemia, muscle wasting, osteoporosis, ulcer development, acne, pathologic fractures. May cause death if suddenly discontinued.	Monitor weight, intake and output, BP, blood glucose. Assess for edema. Protect from sources of infection. Report signs of infection even if subtle. Assess for hypocalcemia: muscle weakness and twitching. Assess for hypokalemia: muscle weakness and tingling, cardiac dysrhythmias, irritability. Protect from falls and possible fractures. Give oral drugs with food or milk. Many patients with adrenal insufficiency manage with only glucocorticoids.

Table 47.3 Drug Therapy for Endocrine Disorders—cont'd

DRUG	USE AND ACTION	SIDE EFFECTS	NURSING INTERVENTIONS
Adrenal Hormones: Mineralocorticoids			
Fludrocortisone (Florinef, Florinef Acetate)	Stimulates reabsorption of sodium and excretion of potassium and hydrogen ions in renal tubules. Used to treat adrenal insufficiency.	Hypokalemia, nausea and vomiting, edema, hypertension, muscle weakness, dizziness, tendon contractures, CHF.	Monitor weight, intake and output, BP, heart rate and rhythm, serum electrolytes. Assess for hypokalemia-prescribed sodium intake. Do not discontinue suddenly. Tell patient to carry drug identification card.
Adrenocortical Cytotoxic Agent			
Mitotane (Lysodren)	Suppresses adrenocortical function.	Nausea and vomiting, diarrhea, lethargy, dizziness, hypouricemia, hearing and vision disturbances, BP changes, dyspnea.	Monitor BP. Report infections or trauma so drug can be discontinued temporarily. Tell patient not to have immunizations without physician approval and to avoid contact with people who have recently had polio or DPT vaccine. Increase fluid intake and monitor uric acid.
Antifungal Agent			
Ketoconazole (Nizoral)	Fungistatic. Suppresses adrenocortical function.	Nausea and vomiting, pruritus, diarrhea or constipation, GI bleeding, lethargy, headache, dizziness, adrenocortical insufficiency. Occasionally: thrombocytopenia, hemolytic anemia, hepatotoxicity.	Monitor stools. Administer antipruritics or apply topical agents as ordered. Safety measures if dizzy or drowsy. Monitor liver function tests and assess for pale stools, dark urine, fatigue, and anorexia. Avoid alcohol.
Drugs for Thyroid Conditions			
Thyroid Hormone Replacement Drug			
Levothyroxine (Synthroid) **Note:** Generic products may not all be truly equivalent. Patients are usually maintained on the same brand-name product to avoid fluctuations in blood levels.	Treat hypothyroidism and thyroiditis (increases the metabolic rate).	Overdose: irritability, insomnia, nervousness, tachycardia, diarrhea, and weight loss may occur.	Older patients are more susceptible to toxicity. Low doses are given initially and gradually increased. Lifelong therapy usually required. Monitor the pulse and BP of older patients. Withhold drug and notify the physician if the older patient's pulse >100 bpm or if chest pain occurs.Thyroid preparations affect metabolism of many other drugs.
Antithyroid Drugs: Thionamides			
Methimazole (Tapazole), propylthiouracil (PTU)	Treat hyperthyroidism by interfering with the synthesis of thyroid hormones.	Agranulocytosis, rash, thrombocytopenia, skin discoloration, fever, headache, drowsiness, diarrhea, nausea, and vomiting.	Contraindicated during pregnancy. Monitor for bleeding, liver toxicity (jaundice, abdominal pain), agranulocytosis (fever, sore throat, malaise), and hypothyroidism (weight gain, fatigue). Tell the patient to report any of these signs and symptoms to the health care provider. Safety precautions if drowsy. Stress importance of follow-up.
Iodides			
Saturated solution of potassium iodide (SSKI)	Reduces size and vascularity of the thyroid gland in hyperthyroidism. May be used before thyroidectomy.	Excess iodine: fever, rash, oral lesions, metallic taste, diarrhea, parotitis, hypothyroidism.	Dilute liquids in water, fruit juice, or milk. Give SSKI after meals. Have the patient use a straw to reduce the unpleasant taste and prevent tooth-staining Monitor for symptoms of excess iodine.

Continued

Table 47.3 Drug Therapy for Endocrine Disorders—cont'd

DRUG	USE AND ACTION	SIDE EFFECTS	NURSING INTERVENTIONS
Radioactive iodine (RAI): iodine-131 (^{131}I)	Used in thyroid scans (concentrates in thyroid tissue). A higher therapeutic dose destroys thyroid tissue in hyperthyroidism and thyroid malignancies.	1. Diagnostic dose: no side effects. Therapeutic dose: nausea, vomiting.	Diagnostic dose usually requires no radiation precautions except precautions with urine for 24 hours after the test (see Table 47.2). Therapeutic dose requires isolation measures. Monitor the patient for signs of hypothyroidism (e.g., fatigue, weight gain).
Drugs for Parathyroid Conditions			
Drugs for Hypoparathyroidism			
Vitamin D (e.g., calcitriol)	Treatment of hypoparathyroidism, osteomalacia; prevention of vitamin D deficiency.	Early toxicity: weakness, fatigue, GI disturbances, anorexia, and constipation. Severe hypercalcemia: polyuria, nocturia, proteinuria, seizures, confusion, ataxia, cardiac dysrhythmias	Caution patients not to exceed recommended dose and to have regular serum calcium tests.
Calcium salts: acetate, carbonate, citrate, glubionate, gluconate, lactate; tricalcium phosphate. **NOTE:** Percentage of calcium in different preparations varies.	Treatment of hypoparathyroidism, along with vitamin D	High doses can cause hypercalcemia (previous symptoms)	Caution patients to have periodic serum calcium measurements and not to exceed recommended dosage. Stay on one type to maintain even blood level.
Calcitriol vitamin D_3 (Rocaltrol)	Increases calcium absorption in intestines. Treats hypocalcemia in chronic renal disease and other conditions.	Dysrhythmias, anaphylaxis, drowsiness, myalgia, headache, edema, nausea, vomiting, constipation	Do NOT confuse with calcitonin! Monitor for hypercalcemia. Teach dietary restrrictions if ordered. Some electrolytes may be restricted.
Drug for Hyperparathyroidism			
Calcium receptor agonist: cinacalcet (Sensipar)	Lowers parathyroid hormone level in hyperparathyroidism; lowers serum calcium.	Dizziness, seizures, dysrhythmias, hypotension, hypocalcemia, myalgia	Monitor for hypocalcemia: tetany, tingling, cramping, seizures. Report immediately. Take with food or after eating, not with other meds. Do not break or chew.
Parathyroid agent: calcitonin (Calcimar, Miacalcin)	Treats hypercalcemia by decreasing bone resorption. Opposes parathyroid hormone. Inceases bone mass in osteoporosis.	Nasal spray: headache, eye pain. IM/SUBCUT: myalgia, nocturia, dyspnea, flushing, bronchospasm, nausea, vomiting, diarrhea.	Rotate injection sites. Teach self- medication if appropriate. Apply nasal spray at room temperature to alternating nostrils.
Drugs For Diabetes Mellitus (DM)			
Oral Hypoglycemic Agents			
Sulfonylureas (second generation): glipizide (Glucotrol), glyburide (Diabeta), glimepiride (Amaryl)	Stimulates pancreatic secretion of insulin	Hypoglycemia, weight gain, sulfa allergy, hepatotoxicity, blood dyscrasias, photosensitivity, serious hypersensitivity	Inform patient to take in the morning. Do not take with alcohol. Do not discontinue abruptly. Use sunscreen when outdoors.
Biguanides: metformin (Glucophage, Fortamet, Riomet)	Inhibits hepatic glucose production; increases insulin sensitivity. Often initial therapy for type 2 DM	Common: nausea, diarrhea, decreased appetite. Life-threatening lactic acidosis (rare).; hypoglycemia when used with sulfonylurea or meglitinide	Monitor for lactic acidosis; provide list of symptoms to patient: hyperventilation, fatigue, chills, myalgia, somnolence, et al Teach patient symptoms of hypoglycemia

Table 47.3 Drug Therapy for Endocrine Disorders—cont'd

DRUG	USE AND ACTION	SIDE EFFECTS	NURSING INTERVENTIONS
Meglitinides: repaglinide (Prandin), nateglinide (Starlix)	Stimulates pancreatic secretion of insulin	Hypoglycemia, weight gain	Teach patient signs of hypoglycemia. Have glucagon emergency kit. Do not stop abruptly.
Thiazolidinediones: pioglitazone (Actos); rosiglitazone (Avandia)	Increases insulin sensitivity in the tissues	Hypoglycemia when used with sulfonylurea or meglitinide, weight gain, decreased effectiveness of oral contraceptives, possible liver dysfunction; risk of heart failure and death in geriatric patients	Advise patient to report signs of hepatic dysfunction, Nausea, vomiting, abdominal pain, fatigue, anorexia, dark urine, jaundice. Report signs of heart failure: weight gain, edema. Dyspnea.
Alpha-glucosidase inhibitors: acarbose (Precose), miglitol (Glyset)	Delays absorption of carbohydrates in the intestine	GI side effects May cause hypoglycemia if taken with insulin or sulfonylureas: weakness, hunger, tremors, sweating, tachycardia	Teach patient symptoms of hypoglycemia if applicable. Take glucose to treat hypoglycemia.
Dipeptidyl peptidase-4 (DPP-4) Inhibitors (Glyptins)			
DPP-4 inhibitors: sitagliptin (Januvia), saxagliptin (Onglyza), alogliptin (Nesina), linagliptin (Trajenta)	Increases insulin production and decreases hepatic glucose production	Occasional stomach upset and diarrhea, headache, peripheral edema, hypoglycemia Can cause pancreatitis, acute renal failure, anaphylaxis	Teach recognition and management of hypoglycemia. Report skin reactions, severe abdominal pain.
Sodium glucose co-transporter-2 (SGLT-2) inhibitor:			
SGLT-2 Inhibitors: canagliflozin (Invokana), dapagliflozin (Farxiga), empagliflozin (Jardiance)	Inhibition of SGLT2 reduces renal resorption of glucose resulting in increased urinary glucose excretion	Hypotension, hyperkalemia, renal impairment, increased incidence of vulvovaginal candidiasis, increased risk of diabetic ketoacidosis	Teach patient how to monitor blood pressure, teach recognition of signs/symptoms of hyperkale mia (nausea, fatigue, muscle weakness, irregular heartbeat, or tingling sensations). Advise patient to stay properly hydrated.
Insulin			
Various preparations are presented in Table 50.1.	Used to treat DM. Decreases blood glucose by transporting glucose into cells and converting glucose to glycogen. Also see Box 50.1.	Hypoglycemia, blurred vision, dry mouth, flushing, rash, urticaria, lipodystrophy, lipohypertrophy, peripheral edema	Confirm correct insulin preparation and dosage. Monitor for signs of hypoglycemia: sweating, weakness, confusion, tachycardia, tremors. See Patient Teaching in Chapter 50.
Non-Insulin Injectable Drugs for Diabetes Mellitus			
Amylin Mimetic			
pramlintide (Symlin)	Treats types 1 and 2 DM. May decrease amount of insulin needed before meals. Decreases glucose production by liver and increases uptake of glucose by muscle. Slows movement of food through digestive tract, which slows rate of glucose absorption.	Increases risk of GI side effects (decreased appetite, nausea, diarrhea, flatulence, cramps, abdominal distention, borborygmus) and hypoglycemia (but only in the presence of excessive insulin). Lactic acidosis (rarely).	Injected at mealtimes at same time as insulin but the two cannot be mixed in the same syringe. Caution patient about increased risk of hypoglycemia.

Continued

Table 47.3 Drug Therapy for Endocrine Disorders—cont'd

DRUG	USE AND ACTION	SIDE EFFECTS	NURSING INTERVENTIONS
Incretin Mimetics			
Glucagon-like peptide-1 receptor agonists (GLP-1 agonists): Dulaglutide (Trulicity), Exenatide (Bydrueon), Liraglutide (Victoza), Lixisenatide (Lyxumia), albiglutide (Tanzeum)	Treats type 2 DM Increases insulin secretion but does not replace the need for insulin in patients who require it. Slows gastric emptying, stimulates glucose-dependent release of insulin, inhibits the postprandial rise in blood glucose, and suppresses appetite.	Initially: nausea, vomiting, and diarrhea. Increases the risk for pancreatitis, pancreatic cancer, and renal failure. Hypoglycemia when given with sulfonylureas. GI side effects: weight loss (common), diarrhea, nausea, vomiting. Dizziness, headache, edema. Thyroid cancer. Renal damage. Small risk of liver damage.	Teach patient to use prefilled syringe. Monitor liver function. Discontinue if anaphylaxis, angioedema, or severe abdominal pain occurs (possible pancreatitis). Drug is expensive without insurance. Given by injection once daily. Easy dosing: doses are not based on glucose levels, meal intake, or activity. Tell patient to report severe abdominal pain

ADH, Antidiuretic hormone; *BP*, blood pressure; *bpm*, beats per minute; *CAD*, coronary artery disease; *CHO*, carbohydrates; *DI*, diabetes insipidus; *DM*, diabetes mellitus; *DPT*, diphtheria, pertussis, tetanus; *GH*, growth hormone; *GI*, gastrointestinal; *IM*, intramuscular; *MI*, myocardial infarction; *SC*, subcutaneous; *SIADH*, syndrome of inappropriate antidiuretic hormone, *SGTL*, sodium glucose cotransporter.
Data from American Diabetes Association. Pharmacologic approaches to glycemic treatment, *Diabetes Care,* 2017;40 (Suppl 1):S68–S70. Burchum JR, Rosenthal JR. *Lehne's pharmacology for nursing care*, 9th ed. St. Louis: Elsevier; 2016. Skidmore-Roth L: *2017 Nursing drug reference*, 30th ed. St. Louis: Elsevier; 2017.

Get Ready for the NCLEX® Examination!

Key Points

- The endocrine system is composed of glands and glandular tissue that make, store, and secrete hormones; it affects virtually every cell in the human body.
- The exocrine glands such as sweat glands pass secretions through ducts or tubes that empty outside the body or into the lumen or opening of other organs.
- The overall mission of the endocrine system is to maintain homeostasis despite the constant changes that occur in the environment.
- Feedback mechanisms control the production and secretion of hormones.
- In negative feedback, high levels of a substance inhibit hormone synthesis and secretion whereas low levels stimulate hormone synthesis and secretion.
- In positive feedback, high levels of a substance stimulate hormone synthesis and secretion whereas low levels inhibit additional hormone synthesis and secretion.
- The anterior pituitary gland secretes GH, ACTH, TSH, FSH, LH, prolactin, and MSH.
- The posterior pituitary secretes ADH and oxytocin.
- Stimulation of the sympathetic nervous system causes the adrenal medulla to secrete two types of catecholamines: (1) norepinephrine and (2) epinephrine.
- Aldosterone is the primary mineralocorticoids that plays a key role in maintaining an adequate extracellular fluid volume.
- Renin, angiotensin, and aldosterone are vital to restoring and maintaining intravascular fluid volume.
- Glucocorticoids control carbohydrate, lipid, and fat metabolism; regulate antiinflammatory and immune responses; and control emotional states.
- The thyroid gland plays a major role in regulating the body's rate of metabolism and growth and development.
- Parathormone, which is secreted by the parathyroid glands, plays a critical role in regulating the serum calcium level.
- With aging, endocrine function is generally adequate to meet physiologic needs.
- The nursing assessment of the patient with an endocrine disorder is very comprehensive because of the many systemic effects of endocrine disease.
- Conventional radiographs, CT scans, MRI, angiography, and ultrasound may be used to detect structural abnormalities of the endocrine glands.
- In addition to the radioimmunoassay and ELISA tests that measure levels of hormones in the blood, tests that stimulate or suppress hormone secretion may be used to assess gland function.
- In general, endocrine drugs are given to replace or supplement deficient hormones, to stimulate or suppress hormone secretion, or to manage symptoms of endocrine disorders.

Additional Learning Resources

SG Go to your Study Guide for additional learning activities to help you master this chapter content.

Go to your Evolve website (http://evolve.elsevier.com/Linton/medsurg) for the following learning resources and much more:
- Fluid & Electrolyte Tutorial
- Review Questions for the NCLEX® Examination

Clinical Judgment and Next-Generation NCLEX® Examination-Style Questions

1. **Which of the following is the overall mission of the endocrine system?**
   a. To maintain electrolyte balance
   b. To control metabolic rate
   c. To maintain homeostasis
   d. To resist infection

   NCLEX Client Need: Physiological Integrity: Physiological Adaptation

2. **Hormones secreted by the anterior pituitary include which of the following? (Select all that apply.)**
   1. ADH
   2. ACTH
   3. GH
   4. LH
   5. TSH

   NCLEX Client Need: Physiological Integrity: Physiological Adaptation

3. **Older adults have a reduced renal response to ADH. What is the significance of this age-related change?**
   1. Increased risk for dehydration
   2. Decreased resistance to infection
   3. Inappropriate breast milk production
   4. Elevated blood glucose level

   NCLEX Client Need: Physiological Integrity: Physiological Adaptation

4. **Which of the following hormones is involved in the process of reproduction? (Select all that apply.)**
   1. ADH
   2. FSH
   3. LH
   4. GH
   5. MSH

   NCLEX Client Need: Physiological Integrity: Physiological Adaptation

5. **The major function of catecholamines is:**
   1. Conservation of body water.
   2. Adaptation to stress.
   3. Reduction of blood pressure.
   4. Prevent physiologic exhaustion.

   NCLEX Client Need: Physiological Integrity: Physiological Adaptation

6. **How do the neurotransmitters epinephrine and norepinephrine exert effects on body tissues?** ______________________________
   ____

7. **SLO/Objective: Identify the classes of drugs used to treat endocrine disorders including actions, uses, and side effects.**

   NGN Item Type: Cloze

   Cognitive Skill: Prioritize Hypotheses

   A 65-year-old woman patient has been on oral corticosteroids to treat an autoimmune disorder for several years. She is seen in the clinic because she "is not feeling well." The nurse's assessment includes:

   - Temperature 100.4°F
   - Heart rate 82 beats per minute regular
   - Respirations 18 breaths per minute
   - Blood pressure 162/86 mm Hg
   - Weight 175 lb
   - Height 5′3″
   - Round face
   - Multiple bruises on forearms
   - Enlarged knuckles of fingers of both hands
   - 2+ edema in both ankles

   Choose the *most likely* options for the information missing from the statements below by selecting from the list of options provided.

   The data requiring the *most immediate* follow-up by the nurse is elevated __________. Failure to investigate this finding could lead to severe_______. The patient's edema and elevated ______ are *most likely* related to ___________.

OPTIONS
Temperature
Blood pressure
Heart failure
Fluid retention
Infection
Joint enlargement
Fragile skin

   NCLEX Client Need: Physiological Integrity: Physiological Adaptation

9. **Which of the following are physiologic effects of glucocorticoid drugs? (Select all that apply.)**
   1. Increased formation of glucose
   2. Suppression of inflammation
   3. Storage of glucose as glycogen
   4. Increase in serum potassium
   5. Increased risk for infection

   NCLEX Client Need: Physiological Integrity: Pharmacological Therapies

10. **Which isotope is used for diagnosis and treatment of thyroid disorders because it concentrates in the thyroid gland?**

    NCLEX Client Need: Reduction of Risk Potential

11. **A 90-year-old patient with hypothyroidism has been on levothyroxine for 6 months. Which patient data may indicate excessive hormone replacement and should be reported promptly to the primary care provider?**
    1. Respiratory rate of 14 breaths per minute
    2. Complaints of excessive sleepiness
    3. Apical heart rate of 110 beats per minute
    4. Weight gain of 5 pounds in last 6 months

    NCLEX Client Need: Physiological Integrity: Pharmacological Therapies

12. **The primary function of thyroid hormones is to regulate** ____________.

    NCLEX Client Need: Physiological Integrity: Physiological Adaptation

48 Pituitary and Adrenal Disorders

http://evolve.elsevier.com/Linton/medsurg

Objectives

1. Describe the pathophysiology and medical treatment of adrenocortical insufficiency, excess adrenocortical hormones, hyperpituitarism, hypopituitarism, diabetes insipidus, and pituitary tumors.
2. Assist in developing nursing care plans for patients with selected disorders of the adrenal and pituitary glands.

Key Terms

acromegaly
Addison disease
Cushing disease
Cushing syndrome
diabetes insipidus
estrogen
gigantism
hypophysectomy
syndrome of inappropriate antidiuretic hormone

Because the endocrine system affects virtually every cell in the human body, it is vital that normal function be maintained. However, dysfunction may occur, most often in the form of excess or deficient hormone production. This chapter covers a variety of disorders that can affect the pituitary and adrenal glands.

DISORDERS OF THE PITUITARY GLAND

Dysfunction of the pituitary gland can result from a problem in the gland itself or from a problem in the hypothalamus. The hypothalamus is an organ in the brain that secretes factors that can directly inhibit or stimulate the pituitary (see Chapter 47, Fig. 47.2). Pituitary disease is usually manifested by excess or deficient production and secretion of a specific hormone. These hormone imbalances lead to disorders that can be manifested in a variety of ways, including changes in physical appearance, emotional state, mental status, metabolism, and homeostatic mechanisms essential for survival. The pituitary disorders discussed in this chapter are hyperpituitarism, hypopituitarism, diabetes insipidus (DI), and syndrome of inappropriate antidiuretic hormone (SIADH).

HYPERPITUITARISM

Cause

Hyperpituitarism is a pathologic state caused by excess production of one or more of the anterior pituitary hormones. Growth hormone (GH), prolactin, follicle-stimulating hormone (FSH), luteinizing hormone (LH), and adrenocorticotrophic hormone (ACTH) are the hormones most often produced in excess. GH is responsible for the growth and development of the body's muscles, bones, and other tissue. Overproduction of GH can lead to gigantism or acromegaly. Overproduction of prolactin causes hyperprolactinemia.

The most common factor in hyperpituitarism is the presence of a pituitary adenoma. An adenoma is a benign tumor composed of epithelial tissue. It may vary in size and invasiveness. Those that are larger than 10 mm are called *macroadenomas*; those that are smaller than 10 mm are called *microadenomas*. Adenomas tend to occur most commonly in young women in their teens through early 30s. Pituitary adenomas that secrete hormones may cause amenorrhea, galactorrhea (i.e., abnormal milk secretion), hyperthyroidism, and Cushing syndrome, in addition to gigantism or acromegaly.

GH, in addition to regulating tissue growth, mobilizes stored fat for energy. As a result of lipolysis of body adipose, excess levels of GH elevate free fatty acids in the bloodstream. This can stimulate the development of atherosclerosis, which causes coronary artery disease (CAD) and cerebrovascular disease over time. Excess GH also antagonizes insulin and interferes with its effects, leading to hyperglycemia and possibly diabetes mellitus (DM).

Prolactinemia. Excess prolactin can cause prolactinemia, characterized by abnormal lactation (galactorrhea), amenorrhea, decreased vaginal lubrication, impotence and decreased libido in men, depression, anxiety, and visual loss.

Gigantism. **Gigantism** is a rare condition that occurs in early childhood or puberty, while the long bones of the body are still growing. The long bones consist of epiphyses, which are the end portions of the bone, and a diaphysis, which is the middle or shaft of the bone. Toward the end of puberty or in early adulthood, the line between these structures seals or closes, preventing further growth. Before the epiphyseal plates on the ends of these bones close, the diaphysis or long shaft of the bone may continue to grow to great lengths when stimulated by excess GH. The growth in these bones is usually proportional and may cause affected people to reach heights of up to 8 feet or more and weights of more than 300 lb. A rapid gain in weight typically occurs shortly before the abnormal growth begins. Mild to moderate obesity is common. These people tend to have multiple health problems and often die in early adulthood.

Acromegaly. **Acromegaly**, although also rare, is more common than gigantism. Most patients with acromegaly are found to have pituitary adenomas that secrete excess GH. Symptoms usually appear in the fourth or fifth decade of life and affect men and women equally. In these people, excess GH production occurs after epiphyseal closure. The closed epiphyses prevent longitudinal growth of the bones; instead, bones increase in thickness and width. Acromegaly also affects the cardiovascular, digestive, nervous, and genitourinary systems.

Clinical Manifestations

Visual deficits and headaches are common in hyperpituitarism and may be the first symptoms of a problem. Visual problems are most often a result of pressure on optic nerves where they are joined near the pituitary gland. Physical features of the disease include enlargement of the hands, feet, and paranasal and frontal sinuses and deformities of the spine and mandible. In addition, soft tissues may become enlarged, especially the tongue, skin, liver, and spleen. This may in turn lead to speech impediments, coarse or distorted facial features, abdominal distention, and sleep apnea. People with acromegaly may also report excessive perspiration (diaphoresis), oily skin, peripheral neuropathies, degeneration of the joints, and proximal muscle weakness. The effects of excess GH impede the activity of insulin, causing patients to have symptoms of DM.

In addition to the features described, patients with gigantism and acromegaly initially have increased strength, progressing rapidly to complaints of weakness and fatigue. The skilled examiner may also detect organomegaly (i.e., enlargement of internal organs), hypertension, dysphagia, and a deep voice because of hypertrophy of the larynx. Those patients who also have elevated levels of prolactin may have galactorrhea (in women) or hypogonadism (in men). Fig. 48.1 provides a dramatic illustration of the progression of acromegaly.

Medical Diagnosis

The diagnosis of hyperpituitarism is based on a number of data sources, including physical assessment, radiographic and other imaging studies, and laboratory findings.

Radiographic and imaging studies. Radiographic films of the skull may show a large sella turcica and increased bone density. Enhanced computed tomography (CT) scans using a water-soluble dye or magnetic resonance imaging (MRI) scans with gadolinium infusion may be performed to locate and evaluate potential intracellular or extracellular lesions or tumor formation. Angiography may also be of use to rule out any vascular abnormalities such as aneurysms or arteriovenous malformations.

Laboratory studies. As mentioned earlier, in hyperpituitarism usually only one pituitary hormone such as GH or prolactin is produced in excess. Pathologic conditions producing elevated levels of LH or FSH are extremely rare. In patients with possible hyperpituitarism, levels of anterior pituitary hormones are measured. Elevation of any hormone level requires further evaluation and follow-up. It is normal for LH and FSH to be slightly elevated in postmenopausal women. Excess GH stimulates the liver to secrete insulin growth factor (IGF-1). Therefore, an elevated level of insulin growth factor-1 (IGF-1) in the presence of clinical manifestations strongly suggests acromegaly. The GH suppression test may help to support a diagnosis of acromegaly. The patient is given intravenous glucose and blood samples are drawn to measure GH. Although the GH concentration normally falls in response to glucose, it is unchanged in the patient with acromegaly.

Medical Treatment

Hyperpituitarism that is manifested as acromegaly or gigantism causes skeletal changes and disfigurement that cannot be reversed with treatment. However, soft tissue hypertrophy can improve with treatment. Treatment options to prevent further changes include surgery, radiation, and drug therapy.

Surgical management. For patients diagnosed with pituitary tumors, the surgical removal of the adenoma or of the pituitary itself **(hypophysectomy)** is the treatment of choice. A transsphenoidal approach is the most commonly used surgical method. A transsphenoidal hypophysectomy is a microsurgical procedure performed under general anesthesia with the patient in the semi-Fowler position. An incision is made at the inner aspect of the upper lip through the maxillary bone, and the sella turcica is entered through the sphenoid

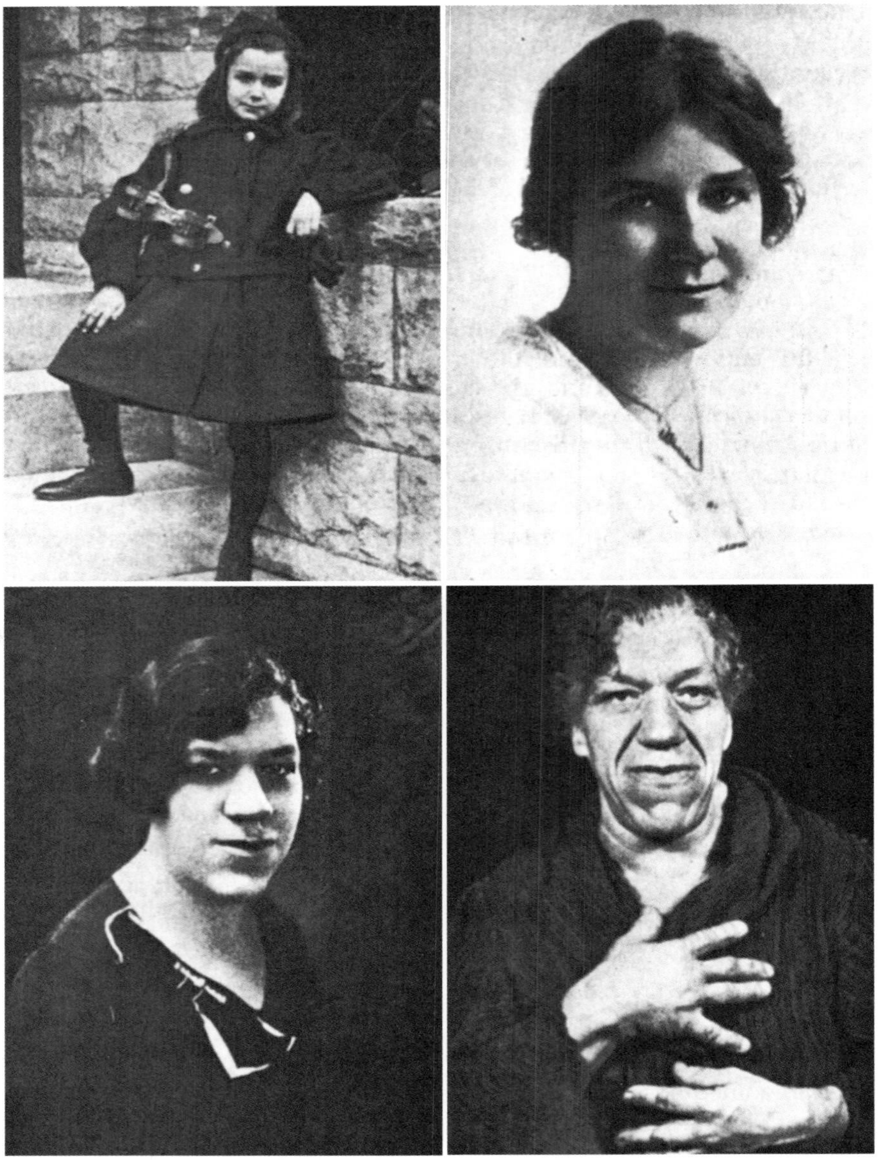

Fig. 48.1 The progression of acromegaly. A series of photographs of the same person over the course of her lifetime depict the physical changes that occurred. The woman was affected after reaching maturity. (From Mendeloff A, Smith DE: Acromegaly, diabetes, hypermetabolism, proteinuria and heart failure, *Am J Med.* 1956; 20:133.)

sinus (Fig. 48.2). A newer procedure is performed endoscopically through the nasal cavity. After the gland or a portion of it is removed, a small piece of adipose tissue is harvested from the abdomen and is used to pack the dura mater (one of the meningeal layers) to prevent leakage of cerebrospinal fluid (CSF). An absorbent gauze or similar dressing is used to pack the nasal passages and an external nasal dressing is applied to keep the packing in place. If the entire pituitary is removed, the patient will require lifelong replacement of glucocorticoids, thyroid hormone, and sex hormones.

Radiation. Radiation therapy is sometimes used to treat tumors that produce excess GH, but the overall response is slow and numerous complications, such as hypopituitarism, optic nerve damage, cognitive dysfunction, and visual defects, can occur. It may be used in combination with surgery or drug therapy. Gamma Knife radiosurgery (stereotactic radiosurgery), which uses radiation delivered to the site from multiple angles, is the most common method used to treat acromegaly. Patients usually require hormone replacement after radiosurgery.

Drug therapy. Several types of drugs are effective in the treatment of acromegaly. These include somatostatin analogs, dopamine agonists, and GH receptor antagonists. Octreotide (Sandostatin, Sandostatin Depot), a somatostatin analog, is the most commonly prescribed drug for patients with acromegaly. Sandostatin, a short-acting preparation, is given every 8 hours by subcutaneous injection. Sandostatin Depot is long acting and

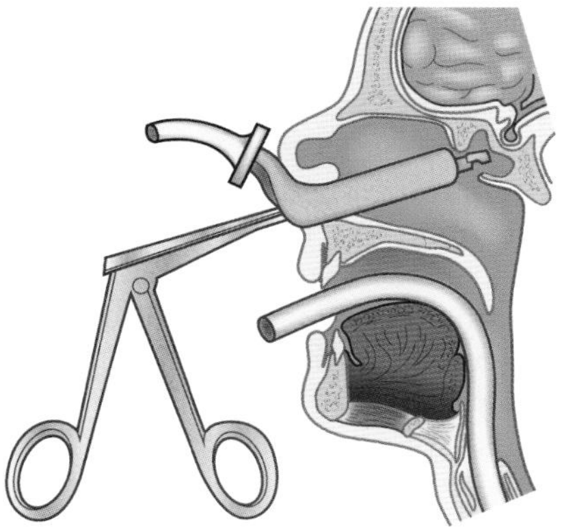

Fig. 48.2 The transsphenoidal surgical approach to the pituitary gland. (From Lewis SL, Bucher L, Heitkemper MM, Harding MM, editors: *Medical-surgical nursing: assessment and management of clinical problems*, ed 10, St. Louis, 2017, Elsevier.)

is given by intramuscular (IM) injection every 4 weeks. Common side effects of octreotide acetate are headache, changes in cardiac conduction, nausea, vomiting, diarrhea, abdominal pain, gallstones, reduction in insulin release, hyper or hypoglycemia, and transient pain at the injection site. Because this drug also suppresses insulin secretion, the patient's blood glucose must be monitored. Blood pressure (BP) and weight are monitored to detect fluid retention. Dopamine receptor agonists such as cabergoline (Dostinex) suppress the secretion of GH. Pegvisomant (Somavert) is a GH receptor antagonist. It is most often used after radiotherapy and pituitary surgery. Bromocriptine (Parlodel) was once the primary drug, but it has been largely replaced by the newer options that have fewer side effects. Some of the most common side effects of bromocriptine are headache, dizziness, drowsiness, confusion, nausea, vomiting, dry mouth, and urticaria.

Chapter 47, Table 47.2 provides additional information about drugs used to treat hyperpituitarism.

Pharmacology Capsule

Drugs used to treat gigantism and acromegaly decrease hormone secretion and may improve soft tissue changes, but do not reverse the existing skeletal effects of the condition.

NURSING CARE OF THE PATIENT WITH HYPERPITUITARISM

Education and emotional support are vital components in the nursing care of the patient with hyperpituitarism. Patients with hyperpituitarism need to know that many body changes, such as visual disturbances and visceral enlargement, are not reversible. Surgical treatment is aimed primarily at preventing further symptoms and complications.

Focused Assessment

Assessment of the patient with an endocrine disorder is summarized in Chapter 47, Box 47.1. When a patient has gigantism or acromegaly, areas that merit special attention are energy level, height and weight, vital signs, contours of the face and skull, visual acuity, speech, voice quality, and abdominal distention. If surgical intervention is planned, determine what the patient knows and expects.

Patient Problems, Goals, and Outcome Criteria: Hyperpituitarism

Patient Problems	Goals and Outcome Criteria
Altered body image related to changes in physical appearance	Adjustment to physical changes: patient verbalizes feelings about body and indicates acceptance of changes
Reduced activity tolerance related to fatigue	Improved activity tolerance: accomplishment of daily activities without excessive tiring
Pain related to musculoskeletal overgrowth, headache	Pain relief: patient verbalizes relief of pain, appears relaxed
Ineffective management self-care related to lack of knowledge of condition, treatment, and expected outcomes	Patient manages own treatment with realistic expectations: patient correctly describes self-medication, therapeutic effects, and drug adverse effects

Interventions

Altered body image. Demonstrate acceptance of the patient and provide opportunities for the patient to share feelings and concerns. Encourage the patient to pay attention to grooming. If they have difficulty adjusting, a referral to a support group or mental health professional may be appropriate.

Reduced activity tolerance. Because the patient with acromegaly tires quickly, help the patient to develop a daily schedule that permits achievement of necessary activities balanced with rest requirements.

Pain. Monitor and document pain. Teach relaxation techniques as discussed in Chapter 8 (see the Complementary and Alternative Therapies box). Administer prescribed analgesics and evaluate effects.

Put On Your Thinking Cap!

Explain why some people with excess growth hormone (GH) develop gigantism and other people with excess GH develop acromegaly.

Ineffective management self-care. Advise patients on drug therapy to take medications exactly as prescribed and not to take double doses if a dose is missed. Assess the patient's ability to self-medicate. Other nursing implications are noted in Chapter 47, Table 47.2.

◆ POSTOPERATIVE NURSING CARE OF THE PATIENT WITH HYPERPITUITARISM

If the patient has surgery (in this case, hypophysectomy), general preoperative and postoperative care is provided, as described in Chapter 17. This section describes specific nursing care of the patient having pituitary surgery. The patient may be admitted to a critical care unit for the first 24 hours after surgery because of the risk for a number of complications.

Focused Assessment

Although the registered nurse (RN) is responsible for the complete assessment, the licensed vocational nurse/licensed practical nurse (LVN/LPN) collects data that are essential to caring for the patient during the postoperative period. Neurologic status and vision must be monitored closely, with particular attention to level of consciousness, pupil size and equality, and vital signs. Changes in data that may indicate edema caused by the manipulation of tissues or intracranial bleeding are decreasing alertness, slow pupil response to light, and decreased or asymmetric muscle strength. Prompt recognition and reporting of these changes may enable the health care provider to intervene and avert serious complications including loss of vision.

Strict documentation of intake and output and measurement of specific gravity are important because these patients are at risk for DI or possibly SIADH. These disorders are discussed in detail in sections "Diabetes Insipidus" and "Syndrome of Inappropriate Antidiuretic Hormone." Urine output in excess of 200 mL/h for more than 3 consecutive hours or a urine specific gravity less than 1.005 are consistent with DI. These data must be reported immediately so measures can be taken to prevent serious fluid and electrolyte imbalances (i.e., fluid volume deficit, hypernatremia). SIADH may develop around the fourth postoperative day. It results in fluid retention and hyponatremia.

Inspection of the nasal dressing for drainage is important because CSF leaks may sometimes occur. Document clear, colorless drainage and notify the surgeon. To confirm whether the drainage is CSF, a specimen of the drainage should be sent to the laboratory for glucose testing. A high level of glucose supports the diagnosis of a CSF leak. A bedside test using a testing strip is no longer recommended. CSF leaks often resolve within 72 hours with rest and head elevation; however, severe, persistent headaches may be treated with a spinal tap to reduce CSF pressure. A return to surgery is rarely indicated.

Monitoring the patient for signs and symptoms of infection is also an important aspect of nursing care. An elevated white blood cell (WBC) count, sudden rise in temperature, headache, or nuchal rigidity may be indications of meningitis (i.e., inflammation of the meninges, the protective layer of membranes that cover the brain and spinal cord). When meningeal inflammation is present, the patient experiences severe head or neck pain when touching the chin to the chest.

The patient who has had Gamma Knife radiosurgery (stereotactic radiosurgery) will return from the procedure with a stereotactic frame in place. Because the frame is secured to the skull with pins, pin care is needed. If the patient has a history of seizures, they are at increased risk for seizures for at least 24 hours. In an emergency, the frame may have to be removed quickly by trained personnel. The nursing unit should have a protocol for this procedure.

Patient Problems, Goals, and Outcome Criteria: Hypophysectomy, Postoperative

Patient Problems	Goals and Outcome Criteria
Anxiety related to lack of knowledge of surgical postoperative care and routines	Reduced anxiety: patient calm, states they feel less anxious
Visual disturbance related to intracranial tissue trauma and swelling	Absence of visual disturbances: patient reports no change in vision
Pain related to tissue trauma	Pain relief: patient statement of pain relief, relaxed manner
Disrupted oral tissue integrity related to surgical incision	Healed surgical incision: incision closed, minimal swelling and redness
Potential for injury related to disruption of packing	Absence of cerebrospinal fluid (CSF) drainage: no clear nasal drainage
Fluid volume excess or fluid volume deficit related to abnormal antidiuretic hormone (ADH) production	Normal fluid balance: fluid intake and output approximately equal, normal tissue turgor
Potential for infection related to impaired tissue integrity, pins for stereotactic frame	Absence of infection: normal white blood cell (WBC) count; no neck stiffness, fever, or headache; pin insertion sites clean without drainage or excessive redness or swelling

Interventions

Anxiety. Orient the patient to the environment and explain all procedures. Give drugs as ordered to replace pituitary hormones. When the patient is well enough, provide information about drug therapy and self-medication. The patient who has a total hypophysectomy requires hormone replacements for the rest of their life. Replacement therapy typically includes antidiuretic hormone (ADH), cortisol, and thyroid hormone (see section "Disorders of the Adrenal Glands" for a more detailed discussion of glucocorticoids).

Visual disturbance. Be aware of existing visual disturbances and collect data to identify new disturbances that might indicate increased intracranial pressure or pressure on the optic nerve. Treatment does not usually correct existing disturbances but can prevent further harm.

Pain and disrupted oral tissue integrity. The immediate postoperative period is uncomfortable, especially when nasal packing is present, and the patient is forced to breathe through the mouth. Administer analgesics as ordered, and follow up to see if the medication was effective. The presence of a "mustache" dressing may also make the patient feel uncomfortable. Frequent mouth care with moistening of the lips increases comfort. If a gingival incision was done, tooth brushing is not permitted until the incision heals. With Gamma Knife radiosurgery, the pin insertion sites may cause discomfort.

Potential for injury. To prevent dislodgment of the fat pad or adipose graft at the surgical site, instruct the patient to avoid any activities that can cause a Valsalva maneuver. Coughing, straining, vomiting, or sneezing can create enough intracranial pressure to disrupt the surgical site and cause CSF leakage or even bleeding. Stool softeners and laxatives may be ordered to prevent straining. Instead of coughing, incentive spirometry and deep-breathing exercises help to maintain pulmonary function without increasing intrathoracic and intracranial pressure. Advise the patient to avoid lifting heavy objects and bending from the waist. Instruct patients to avoid these activities at home as the physician directs (usually for 2 to 3 months after surgery) (see the Patient Teaching box).

Patient Teaching

Hypophysectomy, Postoperative

- If the anterior pituitary is removed, you will need hormone replacements for the rest of your life.
- For 3 months (or as advised by your physician), avoid any activities that cause straining, heavy lifting, and bending from the waist.
- It is important to prevent constipation because straining increases intracranial pressure.
- Numbness of the incision area and decreased sense of smell are temporary.
- Follow-up care is essential to monitor for any signs of tumor recurrence.

Fluid volume excess or fluid volume deficit. Provide intravenous fluids as ordered and monitor pulse, BP, and intake and output. Monitor for transient DI (i.e., large volume of dilute urine). Notify the physician of excessive fluid retention or diuresis. Changes in vital signs, mental status, and neuromuscular status suggest fluid and electrolyte imbalances.

Potential for infection. Administer antibiotics as ordered. Monitor body temperature. Be especially alert for stiffness of the neck and headache because these are symptoms of meningitis (infection of the membranes covering the brain and spinal cord). The patient with a stereotactic frame will require pin care. If the patient will be discharged with the frame in place, teach a family member how to perform pin care.

HYPOPITUITARISM

Cause and Pathophysiology

Hypopituitarism is characterized by a deficiency of one or more pituitary hormones, most often GH and gonadotropins. When inadequate secretion of GH occurs during preadolescence, short stature may result. The causes of this condition may be hereditary or may be related to damage to the anterior portion of the pituitary gland. The anterior pituitary may be damaged by necrosis after hemorrhage, trauma, infection, radiation, or autoimmune disorders. Inadequate secretion of GH or an inability of the target organs to respond to GH is usually considered to be the major cause. In rare instances, hypothalamic dysfunction can lead to short stature as well. It is important to note that although an actual or relative deficiency of GH may exist, other anterior pituitary hormones may also be deficient.

Complementary and Alternative Therapies

Imagery, relaxation exercises, and massage can all be used with analgesics to manage pain.

If growth has been completed and some pathologic process impairs the function of the pituitary, a syndrome known as *panhypopituitarism* can occur. In this situation, all hormones of the anterior pituitary are usually affected. A number of causes exist for panhypopituitarism, which include :

1. Sheehan syndrome: shock and hypotension during the postpartum period leading to infarction of the pituitary gland
2. Tumors of the pituitary gland itself or cranial tumors that impinge on the pituitary
3. Chronic recurrent infections
4. Total or subtotal destruction or removal of the pituitary as a result of trauma, surgery, or radiation therapy
5. Suppression of pituitary tropic hormones by excess target gland hormones (e.g., as seen in patients on prolonged corticosteroid therapy)

Clinical Manifestations

The manifestations of hypopituitarism depend on the stage of life when the deficiency occurs and which hormones are deficient. If GH is deficient early in life, the person is remarkably short in stature, but with proportional physical characteristics.

When a state of panhypopituitarism exists, the patient has muscle and organ wasting and disruptions of digestion and metabolism. Decreased muscle and organ size is attributed to decreased GH. An absence of ACTH affects the person's ability to cope effectively with stress (see section "Adrenal Hypofunction"). This, in turn, affects the person's ability to metabolize glucose, and hypoglycemia may result. Because thyroid-stimulating hormone (TSH) is depleted, the thyroid is not stimulated to produce thyroid hormone. A lack of thyroid hormone produces a state referred to as *hypothyroidism.* In hypothyroidism, insufficient thyroid hormone is available for normal metabolism and thermogenesis, or heat production. Consequently, people who are hypothyroid may be unable to maintain a normal basal metabolic rate (BMR) or body temperature.

If a lack of melanocyte-stimulating hormone (MSH) exists, decreased pigmentation of the skin occurs. This results in extreme pallor. Finally, with the absence of gonadotropins, gonads may become atrophied. In both men and women, loss of libido, decreased body hair, and sexual dysfunction may occur; in women, amenorrhea (i.e., absence of menstruation) may be seen.

General signs and symptoms may include fatigue, weakness, malaise, cold intolerance, and lethargy. Again, the type and degree of symptoms vary greatly depending on the specific hormones affected. If the pituitary dysfunction is caused by a tumor, the patient may have headaches, vision disturbances, seizures, and loss of the sense of smell.

Medical Diagnosis

A diagnosis of panhypopituitarism is based on the health history, physical examination, and diagnostic tests. Diagnostic tests and procedures may include MRI and CT scans to detect pituitary or cranial tumors. Cerebral angiography may be ordered to detect malformed blood vessels. Serum levels of pituitary hormones may be measured as well.

Medical and Surgical Treatment

Deficient hormones are replaced as needed, depending on the specific deficiencies of the patient. Deficiency of thyroid-stimulating hormone necessitates thyroid replacement with levothyroxine (Synthroid), usually for the rest of the person's life. Gonadotropin deficiency requires lifelong therapy. To produce or maintain libido, secondary sexual characteristics, and well-being, men should also receive testosterone and women should receive **estradiol** and a progestin. In patients for whom childbearing is desirable, FSH and LH are administered to both men and women. However, gonadotropin replacement is contraindicated in some conditions, including breast cancer in women and prostate cancer in men. GH replacement is necessary for growth in children. In most instances, GH is administered until the epiphyses (endplates) of the long bones close or the person no longer responds to the drug. Replacement of GH in adults with a GH deficiency produces improved energy, increased lean body mass, and a general feeling of well-being. Negative effects include increased fasting blood glucose. The use of human GH produced by bacteria through recombinant deoxyribonucleic acid (rDNA) technology such as somatropin (Humatrope and others) is considerably safer than products used previously. The annual cost of therapy with GH is very expensive. ACTH deficiency is managed with hydrocortisone on a schedule that mimics the natural pattern of secretion. If a tumor is causing hypopituitarism, surgery or radiation is the treatment of choice (see "Surgical Management" in the Hyperpituitarism section). Chapter 47, Table 47.2 provides additional information about drug therapy for hypopituitarism.

◆ NURSING CARE OF THE PATIENT WITH HYPOPITUITARISM

Focused Assessment

The general assessment of the patient with an endocrine disorder is summarized in Chapter 47, Box 47.1. When collecting data for assessment of the patient with hypopituitarism, be especially aware of mental acuity, emotional stability, and affect. Document the patient's general sense of well-being, energy level, and appetite. In reviewing the systems, ask the patient about changes in skin texture, body temperature, hair, and libido. Determine the patient's usual activities and whether there has been any difficulty carrying out those activities.

In the physical examination, measure height and weight and compare with previous measurements. Inspect the hair for distribution, texture, and thickness. Inspect and palpate the skin and nails for color, texture, and moisture. Document the development of secondary sex characteristics, including axillary and pubic hair, genital maturity, breast development, and onset of menarche.

Patient Problems, Goals, and Outcome Criteria: Hypopituitarism

Patient Problems	Goals and Outcome Criteria
Altered body image related to lack (or loss) of secondary sex characteristics	Improved body image: patient makes positive statements about self and takes measures to improve appearance
Sexual dysfunction related to hormone deficiency	Enhanced sexual development and function: secondary sex characteristics and satisfying sexual function
Inadequate nutrition or excessive calorie intake related to hormone imbalance	Adequate nutrition: normal body weight for height

Continued

Patient Problems, Goals, and Outcome Criteria: Hypopituitarism—cont'd

Patient Problems	Goals and Outcome Criteria
Fluid volume deficit related to hormone deficiency, impaired homeostasis	Normal fluid balance: normal tissue turgor, pulse, and blood pressure (BP)
Ineffective management self-care related to lack of understanding of condition, treatment, and self-care	Patient follows prescribed treatment regimen: correctly demonstrates self-care, diminishing signs and symptoms of hormone deficiency

Interventions

Patient education is the most important aspect of nursing care because disturbances in body image, sexual function, nutritional status, and fluid balance all can be improved if the patient understands and follows the prescribed therapy. Meanwhile, acknowledge the patient's feelings and encourage expression of concerns (see the Patient Teaching box). Referral to a mental health counselor is appropriate if the patient has difficulty dealing with the effects of the disease. Good teaching is essential for patients and families to understand hypopituitarism and to participate in the treatment plan.

Patient Teaching

Hypopituitarism

- It will be necessary for you to take medications for the rest of your life to replace the pituitary hormones.
- You must become familiar with the signs and symptoms of inadequate or excessive hormone replacement (provide written descriptions) and appropriate actions.
- You must have periodic follow-up care.
- Wear a medical alert bracelet or necklace so that your condition can be recognized quickly in an emergency.
- Carry a card that lists prescribed drugs and dosages and your physician's name and phone number.

POSTERIOR PITUITARY DISORDERS

Disorders of the posterior pituitary or neurohypophysis are characterized by deficient or excess ADH production. Another name for ADH is *vasopressin.* ADH helps to maintain fluid balance by promoting reabsorption of water in the renal tubules when body water is decreased or very concentrated. The amount of ADH secreted is reflected in the amount of water retained by the kidneys. Increased ADH release causes increased water retention. This results in increased intravascular volume and decreased urine output.

Two disorders are associated with dysfunction of the neurohypophysis: (1) DI and (2) SIADH. DI is the more common of the two disorders.

DIABETES INSIPIDUS

Cause

Diabetes insipidus is characterized by excessive output of dilute urine. It can be caused by a number of factors. Thus DI is classified as nephrogenic, neurogenic (central or hypothalamic), or dipsogenic DI (primary polydipsia). Nephrogenic DI is an inherited defect in which the renal tubules of the kidney do not respond to ADH, resulting in inadequate water reabsorption by the kidneys. In this case, ADH is produced in sufficient amounts, but the kidneys do not respond to it appropriately. Some cases are caused by drugs such as lithium carbonate (Eskalith-CR) or demeclocycline (Declomycin), which affect the kidney by inhibiting its response to ADH. In neurogenic DI, a defect in either the production or the secretion of ADH exists. Neurogenic DI can result from hypothalamic tumors, head trauma, infection, surgical procedures (hypophysectomy), or metastatic tumors originating in the lung or breast. It can also be triggered by a cerebrovascular accident (CVA), aneurysm, or intracranial hemorrhage. Dipsogenic DI is a disorder of thirst stimulation. When the patient ingests water, serum osmolality decreases, which causes reduced vasopressin secretion. Other factors that may be associated with dipsogenic DI are habitual excessive water intake and psychiatric conditions. The severity of symptoms in dipsogenic DI varies.

Pathophysiology

ADH deficiency or an inability of the kidneys to respond to ADH results in the excretion of large volumes of very dilute urine, a symptom referred to as *polyuria.* The distal tubules and collecting ducts do not reabsorb sufficient water. Massive diuresis occurs, resulting in increased plasma osmolarity, which stimulates the osmoreceptors. The osmoreceptors, in turn, relay information to the cerebral cortex, causing the person to feel thirsty. Increased thirst serves as a compensatory mechanism, in that it causes the person to increase water ingestion. Unfortunately, this compensatory mechanism cannot keep up with the demand for water, and diuresis continues. Massive dehydration ensues, which leads to decreased intravascular volume, hypotension, and circulatory collapse. This is accompanied by neurologic changes such as a decreased level of consciousness and severe electrolyte imbalances. Electrolyte imbalances contribute to circulatory collapse by causing dysrhythmias and impaired contractility of the heart. If left untreated, severe cases of DI can lead to cardiac arrest and death.

When DI follows intracranial surgery, a typical pattern occurs. The initial acute phase is marked by the sudden onset of polyuria. In the next phase, urine volume returns to normal. Then the third phase, which occurs 10 to 14 days postoperatively, results in permanent DI. When DI is associated with head trauma, it is more likely to resolve with treatment.

Clinical Manifestations

Common signs and symptoms of DI are massive diuresis, dehydration, and thirst. Dehydration is characterized by hypotension, tachycardia, dizziness, decreased skin turgor, weakness, and possible fainting episodes. Additional findings include malaise, lethargy, and irritability. An irregular heartbeat may be detected.

Medical Diagnosis

The diagnosis of DI is made primarily on the basis of the health history, physical examination, and laboratory findings. A history of any known cause, such as surgery, infection, injury, or medication ingestion, should be noted.

The loss of free water is apparent in laboratory studies of blood and urine. An initial diagnosis of DI is made based on a 24-hour urine output greater than 4 L, without food or fluid restrictions. Patients with DI can excrete up to 30 L/day, depending on the severity of the ADH deficiency or relative deficiency. Because the urine is very dilute, the specific gravity is also extremely low and the osmolarity of the urine is decreased. For the water deprivation test, water is withheld for 8 to 16 hours, during which time, BP, weight, and urine osmolality are measured each hour. The test is stopped when the osmolalities stabilize, the patient loses 5% of their body weight, or the patient develops orthostatic hypotension. A dose of ADH is then given, and the urine osmolality is measured 1 hour later. If the patient has neurogenic DI, the urine osmolality should increase (i.e., the urine is more concentrated).

Medical Treatment

Management of DI is geared to controlling the signs and symptoms of the disease and possibly reversing the cause of the syndrome. Intravenous fluid volume replacement and vasopressors are often required to maintain adequate BP. Treatment also includes a variety of pharmacologic therapies. A list of these agents can be found in Chapter 47, Table 47.2. Most of these agents act by augmenting existing ADH or replacing it. The most common hormone replacement drug for neurogenic DI is desmopressin acetate (DDAVP), which can be given orally, intravenously, or by nasal inhalation. Short-term therapy is usually managed with subcutaneous injections of aqueous vasopressin. This is usually indicated in situations in which the cause of DI is reversible, such as infection- or medication-related DI. Patients on long-term therapy are placed on nasal spray (lypressin), which may be required for life. This long-term therapy may be necessary after hypophysectomy or other surgical procedures. Patients with primary polyuria related to a psychiatric condition may require ADH supplementation while psychotherapy is used to treat the underlying disorder.

The administration of ADH does not help with nephrogenic DI because the kidneys do not respond to the hormone. Sodium intake may be restricted and thiazide diuretics prescribed for nephrogenic DI. This depletes sodium and decreases the glomerular filtration rate, which increases the reabsorption of water in the proximal tubules.

Pharmacology Capsule

Adverse effects of vasopressin administered as a nasal spray are mucous membrane ulcers, chest tightness, and upper respiratory infections.

◆ NURSING CARE OF THE PATIENT WITH DIABETES INSIPIDUS

Focused Assessment

A complete history of the patient's symptoms, medical history, and drug history should be obtained by the RN. The LVN/LPN can assist by monitoring for thirst, change in urine appearance or volume, dizziness, weakness, fainting, and palpitations. The physical examination focuses on the symptoms of DI. Monitor hydration, including skin turgor, moisture of mucous membranes, pulse rate and quality, BP, and mental status. Maintain records of intake and output, daily weights, and urine specific gravities.

Patient Problems, Goals, and Outcome Criteria: Diabetes Insipidus

Patient Problems	Goals and Outcome Criteria
Anxiety related to physical symptoms and diagnosis	Decreased anxiety: patient states anxiety is reduced, appears calm
Altered body image related to altered function	Adaptation to physical changes: patient adjusts routines to minimize symptoms
Fluid volume deficit related to excessive urine output	Normal fluid balance: fluid intake approximately equal to fluid output
Decreased activity tolerance related to fatigue and weakness	Improved activity tolerance: patient performs activities of daily living (ADLs) without tiring
Inability to manage self-care related to lack of understanding of symptom management and treatment of diabetes insipidus (DI)	Effective self-care: patient describes and demonstrates self-care and self-medication

Interventions

The patient with a pituitary disorder may be experiencing mild to moderate symptoms or may be critically ill. Specific nursing care depends largely on the type of DI, the severity of the symptoms, and the needs identified in the nursing assessment.

Anxiety and altered body image. The patient who is able must be allowed adequate time to express feelings and discuss the disorder. Changes in body function can be very disturbing. Assure the patient that some changes can be controlled with proper treatment. Be alert to the patient's emotional status and provide support and make referrals as necessary.

Fluid volume deficit. Carefully measure intake and output. When the urine output is excessive, as in DI, the physician may order measurement of output at 15- to 30-minute intervals. Because adequate hydration is essential, administer intravenous fluid replacements as ordered. Encourage oral intake, with the prescribed amount based on the volume of urinary output. In addition, weigh the patient at least once daily to identify significant weight loss secondary to water loss.

In situations in which the patient is experiencing excessive fluid loss, administer exogenous ADH as ordered (see Chapter 47, Table 47.2). Be familiar with routes of administration, side effects, and contraindications associated with the use of these agents. Be aware that reversal of the fluid volume deficit with ADH can result in water intoxication. Continued monitoring of urine output and osmolality is essential.

Reduced activity tolerance. Extreme fatigue or muscle weakness can interfere with the patient's ability to participate in activities of daily living (ADLs), such as hygiene and grooming. Frequently observe the functional ability of these patients, and address the amount of assistance required in the patient's care plan.

Inability to manage self-care. Patients who require long-term treatment of DI must learn to manage their symptoms and medications. If the patient has difficulty doing this, a family member or friend may be included in the teaching sessions. Some patients are taught to adjust dosages based on urine output, specific gravity (using a hydrometer), and thirst. If the patient's self-care abilities are in doubt, initiate a referral to a home nursing service (see the Patient Teaching box).

Patient Teaching

Irreversible Diabetes Insipidus

- Continue your prescribed drug therapy and notify your physician of any side or adverse effects (provide written details).
- Notify your physician if you have increased urine output, thirst, weight loss, and general feelings of malaise or weakness. You may need additional treatment.
- Prolonged use of nasal sprays can cause ulceration of mucous membranes, chest tightness, upper respiratory infections, and respiratory problems.
- Keep office or clinic appointments to identify any changes in pituitary function.
- Schedule activities and regular rest periods to avoid excessive fatigue.
- Wear a medical alert bracelet.
- Drowsiness, listlessness, and headache are signs of water intoxication, which may result from vasopressin therapy.

SYNDROME OF INAPPROPRIATE ANTIDIURETIC HORMONE

Cause

Syndrome of inappropriate antidiuretic hormone (SIADH) is characterized by a water imbalance related to an increase in ADH synthesis, ADH secretion, or both. Factors that may cause or contribute to the development of SIADH include brain trauma, surgery, tumors, and infection; some drugs, including vasopressin, general anesthetics, oral hypoglycemics, and tricyclic antidepressants; some pulmonary diseases; hypothyroidism; lupus erythematosus; and some types of cancer, including small cell lung cancer, duodenal cancer, and pancreatic cancer.

Pathophysiology

When ADH is elevated despite normal or low serum osmolality, the kidneys retain excessive water. Plasma volume expands, causing the BP to rise. Body sodium is diluted (hyponatremia), and water intoxication develops. Several types of SIADH exist, with various patterns of abnormal ADH secretion.

Clinical Manifestations

The main symptoms of SIADH initially reflect the effects of dilutional hyponatremia and water retention: weakness, muscle cramps or twitching, anorexia, nausea, diarrhea, irritability, headache, and weight gain without edema. When the central nervous system (CNS) is affected by water intoxication, the level of consciousness deteriorates. The patient may have seizures, lapse into a coma, or experience respiratory arrest.

Medical Diagnosis

The diagnosis of SIADH is confirmed by laboratory tests of serum and urine electrolytes and osmolality. Simultaneous measurements of urine and serum osmolality are especially useful. When measured simultaneously, urine osmolality much higher than that of the serum is consistent with SIADH. In this case, the serum is very dilute, and the urine is very concentrated. Major characteristics include hyponatremia, hypochloremia, hypouricemia, reduced blood urea nitrogen (BUN) and creatinine clearance, increased urine sodium, and fluid volume excess without edema. Urine osmolality may be high, considering the level of serum osmolality, or it may be extremely dilute. Radiographic studies of the brain and lungs may also be done to detect causative factors.

Medical Treatment

Treatment is intended to correct the cause, if possible, to promote elimination of excess water, and to normalize serum sodium. Acutely ill patients (i.e., those with neurologic symptoms and serum sodium of 120 mEq/L) are treated with intravenous hypertonic saline given either in bolus doses or by continuous infusion. The specific fluid orders depend on the duration and severity of the condition. Serum sodium is monitored hourly. Once neurologic symptoms resolve, principles of chronic therapy are instituted. Patients with chronic SIADH are treated on an inpatient basis if the serum sodium is less than 120 mEq/L. Fluids may be restricted to 800 to 1000 mL/day with a high intake of dietary sodium. For severe hyponatremia, normal saline may be administered with loop diuretics. A diuretic can be used only if the serum sodium is at least 125 mEq/L because the diuretic will cause further loss of sodium. Patients on diuretic therapy may require sodium and potassium supplements. Patients who cannot adhere to fluid restriction with high sodium intake may be given a vasopressor receptor antagonist, such as conivaptan or tolvaptan, which block the effects of ADH in the renal collecting ducts, thereby increasing water excretion. Adverse effects of these drugs can cause complications (see Chapter 47, Table 47.2).

◆ NURSING CARE OF THE PATIENT WITH SYNDROME OF INAPPROPRIATE ANTIDIURETIC HORMONE

Focused Assessment

The health history records the presence of anorexia, nausea, vomiting, diarrhea, headache, irritability, and muscle cramps and weakness. Document a history of head trauma, cancer, pulmonary disease, nervous system disorders, hypothyroidism, or lupus erythematosus. Note any prescription drugs the patient is taking. Measure the patient's vital signs, weight, intake and output, and urine specific gravity. Palpate the skin for moisture. Test muscle strength by having the patient grip your hands and push and pull against resistance. Document seizures and muscle weakness, twitching, or cramps. Describe mental status (level of consciousness, orientation) at least every 4 hours in the alert, oriented patient and hourly if there is evidence of impairment. Monitor serum sodium tests and notify the health care provider of results.

Patient Problems, Goals, and Outcome Criteria: Syndrome of Inappropriate Antidiuretic Hormone

Patient Problems	Goals and Outcome Criteria
Potential for injury related to confusion, seizures associated with hyponatremia, fluid retention, cerebral edema	Absence of injury: no seizures or associated trauma
Fluid volume excess related to excess antidiuretic hormone (ADH) secretion	Normal fluid balance: normal tissue turgor, fluid intake and output approximately equal
Inability to manage self-care related to lack of understanding of management of chronic syndrome of inappropriate antidiuretic hormone (SIADH)	Patient effectively manages prescribed therapy: takes drugs correctly, monitors for and reports adverse effects

Interventions

Potential for injury. If the patient becomes confused, take measures to ensure safety, including putting the bed in a low position and checking on the patient frequently. Intravenous saline solutions must be infused very slowly using an infusion pump. Rapid infusion could cause hypernatremia. In general, the head of the bed should be elevated no more than 10 degrees. This position improves the return of blood to the heart and reduces the release of ADH. However, in the presence of cerebral edema, position the patient with the head elevated 30 to 45 degrees or as specified by the health care provider. Institute seizure precautions per agency policy.

Fluid volume excess. Advise the physician of declining neurologic status. Enforce fluid restrictions, which may be as little as 500 mL/24 h. Explain the restriction to the patient and family. Remove the large water pitcher. Space fluids over waking hours to reduce thirst and feelings of deprivation. Serve oral fluids in small containers to create the illusion of volume. Encourage frequent mouth care. Patients with chronic SIADH who are managed at home can weigh daily to assess for changes in fluid status. They should report a weight gain in excess of 2 lb/day.

Inability to manage self-care. Although SIADH is usually temporary, it may not resolve during hospitalization, and the patient may need to learn how to manage the condition at home. Provide verbal and written information about prescribed drugs, dosages, and adverse effects. Be sure the patient has a scale at home to monitor weight (see the Patient Teaching box).

Patient Teaching

Syndrome of Inappropriate Antidiuretic Hormone

- Weigh daily and notify the physician if you gain 2 lb or more in 1 day.
- In addition to weight gain, signs and symptoms of excessive water retention (water intoxication) are drowsiness, listlessness, and headache.
- Do not take any nonprescription drugs without consulting your physician or pharmacist.
- See your physician on a regular basis.
- If taking demeclocycline or lithium carbonate, report adverse effects to your physician (provide specifics).
- Maintain a daily fluid intake of 800 to 1000 mL/day or as advised by your physician.
- Ice chips and sugarless chewing gums may help you to manage thirst.

DISORDERS OF THE ADRENAL GLANDS

ADRENAL HYPOFUNCTION (ADDISON DISEASE)

Pathophysiology

Adrenal insufficiency may be classified as either *primary* or *secondary*. Primary adrenal insufficiency, which is also called **Addison disease**, is frequently the result of a destructive disease process affecting the adrenal glands that causes deficiencies of cortisol and aldosterone. The most common cause of Addison disease is an autoimmune disease in which adrenal tissue is destroyed by antibodies formed by the patient's own immune system. Other causes of Addison disease include adrenalectomy; infections such as tuberculosis and HIV, and fungal infections (i.e., histoplasmosis, coccidioidomycosis); hemorrhage related to anticoagulant therapy; physical trauma, sepsis, or severe stress; and metastatic cancer.

Pharmacology Capsule

Adrenal insufficiency can be caused by drugs that inhibit synthesis of cortisol, increase metabolism of cortisol, or decrease ACTH production.

Secondary adrenal insufficiency is a result of dysfunction of the hypothalamus or pituitary (decreased corticotropin, ACTH), which leads to decreased androgen and cortisol production. Unlike primary adrenal insufficiency, in which all steroids are affected, aldosterone may or may not be affected. Causes of secondary adrenal insufficiency include pituitary tumors; postpartum necrosis of the pituitary (Sheehan syndrome); hypophysectomy; radiation therapy; pituitary or intracranial lesions; or high-dose, long-term glucocorticoid treatment, which suppresses the adrenal glands' intrinsic activity. Some sources categorize adrenal insufficiency because of hypothalamic dysfunction resulting in inadequate corticotropin secretion as *tertiary* adrenal insufficiency.

Clinical Manifestations

Insufficiency of adrenocortical steroids causes defects associated with the loss of mineralocorticoids and glucocorticoids. The signs and symptoms vary greatly depending on the rate and extent of loss of adrenal function. Impaired secretion of cortisol results in decreased gluconeogenesis and decreased liver and muscle glycogen. This, in turn, decreases supplies of available glucose, causing hypoglycemia. In addition, the glomerular filtration rate of the kidneys and gastric acid production by the parietal cells of the stomach both slow significantly. The cumulative effects of these processes cause decreased urea nitrogen excretion, irritability, anorexia, weight loss, nausea, vomiting, and diarrhea.

Decreased levels of aldosterone alter the clearance of potassium, water, and sodium by the kidney. Potassium excretion is decreased, and hyperkalemia may occur. Because hyperkalemia promotes hydrogen ion retention, metabolic acidosis can also occur. Hypovolemia and hyponatremia may result from accelerated sodium and water excretion.

Other manifestations of adrenal insufficiency are progressive weakness, lethargy, unexplained abdominal pain, and malaise. Skin hyperpigmentation, particularly in sun-exposed areas, pressure points, joints, and creases of the body, is another possible sign. It is most likely the result of increased secretion of a beta-lipoprotein or an MSH, which is released by a part of the pituitary. This is a direct result of hypercortisolism and a lack of negative feedback. Hyperpigmentation, orthostatic hypotension, and salt craving are more common with primary rather than secondary adrenal insufficiency.

If adrenal androgen levels are lowered, a decrease or loss of body, axillary, and pubic hair may occur. In prepubescent people, facial, pubic, and axillary hair may fail to grow entirely. The severity of these symptoms is linked to the degree of hormone deficiency. This lack of secondary sex characteristics tends to be seen in primary adrenal insufficiency rather than in secondary adrenal insufficiency.

Symptoms of chronic insufficiency are generally less dramatic and life threatening than symptoms presented during acute adrenal crisis, which is discussed later.

Put On Your Thinking Cap!

Explain how a pituitary disorder could cause adrenal insufficiency.

ACUTE ADRENAL CRISIS (ADDISONIAN CRISIS)

Patients with either primary or secondary adrenal insufficiency are at risk for episodes of acute adrenal crisis, also called *addisonian crisis*, which is a life-threatening emergency. This usually results from a sudden marked decrease in available adrenal hormones. Precipitating factors are adrenal surgery, pituitary destruction, abrupt withdrawal of steroid therapy (often a result of a patient unwittingly stopping medications), and stress. Any factor that causes stress in the person can initiate a crisis. Examples of stressors include infection, illness, trauma, and emotional or psychiatric disturbances.

Manifestations of an addisonian crisis include more severe symptoms of mineralocorticoid and glucocorticoid deficiency: hypotension, tachycardia, dehydration, confusion, hyponatremia, hyperkalemia, hypercalcemia, and hypoglycemia. If left untreated, fluid and electrolyte imbalances can lead to circulatory collapse, cardiac dysrhythmias, cardiac arrest, coma, and death. The management of an addisonian crisis is outlined in Table 48.1.

Pharmacology Capsule

When steroid therapy is discontinued, the drug is tapered gradually. An abrupt decline in adrenal hormones could precipitate acute adrenal crisis.

Medical Diagnosis

Laboratory studies. Addison disease is diagnosed on the basis of clinical manifestations and a variety of laboratory studies beginning with measures of 8 AM serum cortisol and plasma ACTH, and the ACTH stimulation test. Measurement of plasma ACTH concentration before treatment helps to define the basis of the patient's symptoms. If the plasma ACTH level is low, the pituitary is not producing adequate ACTH. An increased

Table 48.1 Emergency Medical Care for Acute Adrenal Crisis

INTERVENTION	RATIONALE
1. Blood sample collected to determine plasma cortisol level	To establish a baseline and obtain data to guide treatment
2. Intravenous (IV) infusion of normal saline with 5% dextrose	To provide access for administration of fluids and drugs
3. Initial dose of hydrocortisone (Solu-Cortef) IV push, followed by infusion of saline and dextrose over 8 hours	To provide a loading dose and maintenance infusion
4. Additional doses of hydrocortisone per infusion at rate of 100 mg every 8 hours	To ensure continuous source of glucocorticoids

plasma ACTH level suggests that the adrenal glands are unable to respond to stimulation to produce corticoids. An ACTH stimulation test is necessary for a definitive diagnosis of adrenal insufficiency. One common technique used in this test is the administration of a dose of synthetic ACTH (cosyntropin), which is given intramuscularly or intravenously. Plasma cortisol levels are measured at onset of administration and at 30 and 60 minutes after administration. In primary adrenal insufficiency, the cortisol response is absent or markedly decreased despite a high ACTH level. In secondary insufficiency, a less dramatic decrease in serum cortisol occurs; however, the ACTH level is low. An eosinophil count may be performed during ACTH stimulation. The eosinophil count drops significantly after ACTH administration in normal people. Patients with Addison disease show little or no change in the number of circulating eosinophils. If a glucose fasting test is performed, the serum glucose does not rise as high as it would in normal people and returns to a fasting level more rapidly.

In addition, 24-hour urine tests may be performed. This type of testing reflects cortisol secretion over a 24-hour period and is the most accurate measurement of cortisol secretion, which varies with the diurnal rhythm. Based on results of these tests, a corticotropin stimulation test may be indicated to determine whether the basic problem lies in the adrenals, the pituitary, or the hypothalamus. Various other laboratory tests may be done including fasting glucose, electrolytes, BUN, and urinary 17-hydroxycorticosteroids. Common findings with adrenal insufficiency may include low fasting glucose, hyponatremia, hyperkalemia, increased BUN, and low or borderline androgen metabolites.

Nursing responsibilities for these tests are provided in Table 47.1.

Electrocardiogram. Alterations in electrolyte levels often are reflected as deviations in the normal electrocardiogram (ECG). For example, hyperkalemia results in peaked T waves, a widened QRS complex, and an increased PR interval.

Radiographic studies. Skull films, an arteriogram, CT scan, and MRI may be performed to rule out causative factors in secondary adrenal insufficiency. They may reveal intracranial lesions that impinge on the pituitary, aneurysms, or other defects. Abdominal imaging may detect atrophy of the adrenal glands and identify a possible cause of primary insufficiency.

Medical Treatment

The mainstay of treatment of patients with Addison disease is replacement therapy with glucocorticoids and mineralocorticoids. Hydrocortisone is commonly used because it contains both. If glucocorticoids, such as cortisone are given, they may be given in a single morning dose or divided into doses with two-thirds of a daily dose taken in the morning and one-third taken in the evening. The divided dosage schedule is based on human hormonal variations. Glucocorticoids normally peak in the early morning and are at their lowest level in the afternoon. A mineralocorticoid (fludrocortisone), if needed, is typically given each morning or every other morning. See Table 47.2 for details. Secondary adrenal insufficiency is treated with glucocorticoids, but mineralocorticoids are usually unnecessary. If the patient has an acute illness, additional glucocorticoids are needed to prevent a life-threatening condition (i.e., addisonian crisis). Addisonian crisis is treated with intravenous fluids, hydrocortisone, electrolytes, and dextrose to restore normal BP.

Patients with Addison disease are not at great risk for harmful side effects of corticosteroids because the goal is only to restore the blood level to normal.

Pharmacology Capsule

Addison disease is treated with glucocorticoids given in a single morning dose or in divided doses to mimic the body's normal hormonal cycles.

◆ NURSING CARE OF THE PATIENT WITH ADDISON DISEASE

Focused Assessment

Assessment of the patient with an endocrine disorder is summarized in Chapter 47, Box 47.1 (see also Nursing Care Plan: Patient With Addison Disease). Details of the health history that are especially relevant to Addison disease are weight loss, salt craving, nausea and vomiting, abdominal cramping and diarrhea, muscle weakness and aches, poor stress response, decreased libido, and amenorrhea. The patient may be irritable or confused. The physical examination may reveal pale skin with bronzed areas, emaciation, sparse body hair, poor skin turgor, hypotension, and muscle wasting. The patient with an acute episode of Addison disease requires ongoing monitoring of fluid and electrolyte levels and measurement of daily weights.

Nursing Care Plan Patient With Addison Disease

FOCUSED ASSESSMENT

Health History

A 52-year-old White man is admitted with recently diagnosed primary Addison disease. He considers himself healthy but has had some joint pain in his knees. He had an appendectomy 20 years ago. The patient complains of weight loss, anorexia, weakness, and darkening of the skin on his face and arms. His usual weight is 170 lb. He has had bouts of nausea, vomiting, and diarrhea accompanied by vague abdominal pain. The patient is a salesman and reports that his symptoms are making it difficult for him to keep up with his work. He is embarrassed about the change in his skin color.

Physical Examination Vital signs: blood pressure 110/80 mm Hg (sitting) and 88/42 mm Hg (standing), pulse 102 beats per minute with slight irregularity, respiration 20 breaths per minute, temperature 98°F (36.7°C) measured orally. Height 5′8″, weight 155 lb. The patient is oriented but somewhat lethargic. The skin on his face and arms and his abdominal scar are darkly pigmented. His body hair is sparse. The patient's oral mucous membranes are slightly dry.

Patient Problems	Goals and Outcome Criteria	Interventions
Inadequate peripheral circulation related to electrolyte imbalance, fluid volume deficit, and cardiac dysrhythmias	The patient will have improved peripheral circulation, as evidenced by warm, dry skin, strong peripheral pulses, and fluid output equal to fluid intake.	Monitor for signs and symptoms of inadequate tissue circulation: confusion, disorientation, tachycardia, hypotension, apical-radial pulse deficit, fluid output exceeding intake. Administer intravenous fluids (normal saline, plasma expanders) and vasopressors, as ordered. Monitor for hyperkalemia: weakness, paresthesia, dizziness. Report evidence of inadequate tissue perfusion or hyperkalemia to the physician.
Potential for injury related to acute adrenal insufficiency, impaired stress response, postural hypotension	The patient will remain free of injury because of hypotension, shock, or falls.	Monitor for orthostatic hypotension. If the patient has dizziness with position changes, instruct him to exercise his legs before rising, to rise slowly, and to call for help when getting out of bed. Administer fluids and hormones as ordered.
Inadequate nutrition related to impaired metabolism, inability to ingest sufficient nutrients, and lack of interest in eating	The patient will be adequately nourished, as evidenced by weight within 5 lb of baseline.	Weigh daily to monitor fluid balance and nutritional status. Request dietary consult for patient education so that his food preferences can be respected. Provide a high-protein, low-carbohydrate diet as ordered. Tell the patient that salt may be used freely. Provide a pleasant atmosphere for meals. Report signs of hypoglycemia: headache, trembling, tachycardia, sweating.
Fatigue related to fluid, electrolyte, and glucose imbalances	The patient will report improved stamina.	Explain medically prescribed activity limitations. Plan care to allow for periods of rest. Discuss energy conservation after discharge.
Altered body image related to changes in appearance and function	The patient will adapt to altered physical appearance and function, as evidenced by efforts to improve appearance and positive comments about self.	Explore how the patient feels about skin changes. Discuss strategies to deal with changes: long sleeves, avoidance of excess sunlight. Inform him that the skin pigmentation will improve with medical therapy. Advise the patient to arrange work with rest periods. Encourage attention to grooming. Compliment his efforts.
Inability to manage self-care related to lack of understanding of long-term glucocorticoid therapy	The patient will manage self-care and prescribed treatment; correctly explain the disease, its treatment, and medication therapy; state intent to adhere to prescribed regimen.	Implement a teaching plan for Addison disease to include the following: • Wear a medical alert tag and carry an emergency kit with dexamethasone. • Take glucocorticoids as directed, either a single morning dose or in divided doses in the morning and afternoon with food. • Increase medication dosage as ordered when under stress. • Notify the physician or go to the emergency room if unable to take oral medications for more than 24 hours. • Remember that lifelong therapy and monitoring are needed. Report signs and symptoms of inadequate and excessive hormone replacement.

CRITICAL THINKING QUESTIONS

1. Name three strategies for energy conservation.
2. How might you encourage the patient to share his feelings about the skin changes?

Patient Problems, Goals, and Outcome Criteria: Addison Disease

Patient Problems	Goals and Outcome Criteria
Inadequate peripheral circulation related to electrolyte imbalance, hypovolemia, cardiac dysrhythmias	Improved tissue perfusion: warm, dry skin with strong peripheral pulses
Potential for injury related to acute adrenal insufficiency, orthostatic hypotension, impaired physiologic response to stress	Decreased risk for injury: blood pressure (BP) within patient norms, absence of faintness with position changes
Inadequate nutrition related to impaired metabolism, inability to ingest sufficient nutrients, lack of interest in eating	Adequate nutrition: weight within 5 lb of patient's baseline
Fatigue related to fluid, electrolyte, and glucose imbalances	Improved stamina: patient states fatigue is lessened, performs activities of daily living (ADLs) without tiring
Altered body image related to changes in appearance and function	Adaptation to physical changes: patient makes efforts to improve appearance, makes positive comments about self
Inability to manage self-care related to lack of knowledge about long-term glucocorticoid and mineralocorticoid replacement	Patient manages self-care and prescribed treatment: patient explains disease process and treatment with stated intent to adhere to prescribed regimen

Interventions

Inadequate peripheral circulation. Monitor for signs and symptoms of inadequate tissue perfusion: confusion, disorientation, tachycardia, apical-radial pulse deficit, general weakness and malaise, and hypotension (including orthostatic changes). Administer prescribed intravenous normal saline, plasma expanders, and vasopressors to maintain blood pressure. The patient whose fluid output is greater than intake is at risk for hypovolemia. Because the patient is at risk for hyperkalemia, monitor serum electrolytes and assess for weakness, paresthesia, dizziness, and ECG changes. Promptly report these signs and symptoms of hyperkalemia to the physician (see the Patient Teaching box).

Patient Teaching

Addison Disease

- Wear a medical alert tag and carry an emergency kit with dexamethasone.
- Take glucocorticoids exactly as ordered: timing is vital to restore normal blood levels around the clock.
- Increase your medication dosage as ordered when under stress.
- Notify the physician or go to the emergency department if you are unable to take oral medications for more than 24 hours.
- Remember that lifelong therapy and monitoring are needed.
- Report signs and symptoms of inadequate and excessive hormone replacement.

Potential for injury. Be alert for orthostatic hypotension and other signs of hypovolemia. Instruct the patient who has dizziness with position changes to call for help when getting out of bed and to rise slowly to prevent falls. Exercising the legs before standing promotes venous return and may minimize the drop in BP.

Sudden profound weakness with orthostatic hypotension is characteristic of acute addisonian crisis and leads to shock and death if not corrected. Administer fluid replacement and hormones as ordered to treat addisonian crisis.

Inadequate nutrition. Daily weights provide important data to assess fluid balance. Weight changes also provide information about the adequacy of the patient's diet (see the Nutrition Considerations box). If nutrition is a problem, consult the dietitian. Salt is not restricted because patients with Addison disease tend to lose sodium. People who live in hot climates may actually need to increase their salt intake to make up for losses through perspiration. Respect the patient's food preferences as much as possible. The mealtime atmosphere should be conducive to eating.

Hypoglycemia may develop as a result of decreased cortisol secretion. Encourage frequent rest periods to avoid depletion of glycogen stores. Meals should be taken regularly, and between-meal snacks may be needed to maintain blood glucose. Monitor for (and teach the patient) symptoms of hypoglycemia: headache, tachycardia, trembling, and sweating. Keep appointments for periodic laboratory studies needed to monitor your condition.

Fatigue. Explain any prescribed activity limitations to the patient. Encourage the patient to plan specific rest periods to conserve energy. He may need assistance with ADLs at times. If the patient is on bed rest, intervene to prevent complications of immobility as described in Chapter 12.

Altered body image. Explore the patient's reaction to the physical changes experienced. Discuss strategies to cope with changes. When the patient's condition has stabilized, encourage attention to grooming and compliment the patient's efforts. Inform him that the skin changes will diminish with medical therapy.

Inability to manage self-care. Care of the patient with a chronic disease requires in-depth education and information about stress management. It is critical for the patient to understand Addison disease and to know how to recognize the effects of the disease, as well as those of overmedication. The patient must learn to make adjustments in replacement hormones depending on various stressors. To confirm understanding, encourage the patient to teach-back. Provide written material to supplement the teaching sessions.

ADRENAL HYPERSECRETION (CUSHING SYNDROME)

Cause

Hypersecretion of the adrenal cortex may result in the production of excess amounts of corticosteroids, particularly glucocorticoid. The condition that results from excessive cortisol is called **Cushing syndrome**. The overproduction of adrenocortical hormones may result from endogenous (internal) as well as exogenous (external) causes.

Endogenous causes include corticotropin-secreting pituitary tumors, a cortisol-secreting adrenal tumor, and excess secretion of corticotropin by a carcinoma of the lung or other tissues. The incidence of Cushing syndrome caused by disease is infrequent, affecting women 8 times more often than men. Approximately 25% of cases of Cushing syndrome are caused by adrenal tumors.

The most common and single exogenous cause of Cushing syndrome is prolonged administration of high doses of corticosteroids.

Excessive production of ACTH because of a pituitary tumor is called **Cushing disease**.

Pathophysiology

Clinical manifestations of Cushing syndrome affect most body systems and are related to excess levels of circulating corticosteroids. In some instances, signs and symptoms of mineralocorticoid and androgen excess may appear; however, signs and symptoms of glucocorticoid excess usually predominate.

Hyperadrenalism produces marked changes in the personal appearance of the affected person, including obesity, facial redness, hirsutism (i.e., excess hair), menstrual disorders, hypertension of varying degrees, and muscle wasting of the extremities (Fig. 48.3). Additional findings include delayed wound healing, insomnia, irrational behavior, and mood disturbances, such as irritability and anxiety. The following are hallmark findings that lead to a diagnosis of Cushing syndrome:

- Truncal obesity (excess adipose in body trunk)
- Protein wasting (slender extremities and very thin and friable skin)

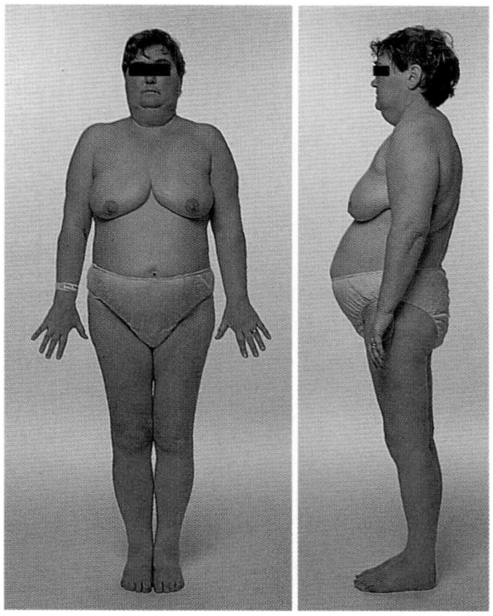

Fig. 48.3 Clinical manifestations in a patient with Cushing syndrome. (From Forbes CH, Jackson WF: *Color atlas and text of clinical medicine*, ed 3, St. Louis, 2003, Elsevier Science Limited/Mosby.)

- Facial fullness, often called a *moon face*
- Purple striae on the abdomen, breasts, buttocks, or thighs
- Osteoporosis (a significant finding in premenopausal women)
- Hypokalemia of uncertain cause

Medical Diagnosis

In addition to physical signs and symptoms, some laboratory, radiographic, and imaging results may be useful in determining a diagnosis.

Laboratory studies. When Cushing syndrome is suspected, initial testing may include a 24-hour urine collection for free cortisol, an overnight dexamethasone suppression test, and/or a late night salivary cortisol level. Based on results of these tests, a corticotropin stimulation test may be ordered to determine whether the problem is originating in the adrenals, the pituitary, or the hypothalamus.

Abnormal laboratory findings include polycythemia, hypokalemia, hypernatremia, hyperglycemia, leukocytosis, glycosuria, hypocalcemia, and elevated plasma cortisol. ACTH may be high or low, depending on whether the basic problem lies in the adrenals or in the pituitary.

Radiographic studies. If a tumor is suspected as a causative factor in Cushing syndrome, a pituitary MRI may be done to confirm and localize the site of the tumor. Radiographic films may also reveal osteoporosis of the spinal column, especially in women.

Medical Treatment

Depending on the specific patient and the cause of the disease, various therapies may be used. These include drug therapy, radiation, and surgery. If Cushing syndrome is caused by administration of synthetic glucocorticoids, the physician may gradually withdraw them. Most patients affected with hyperadrenalism because of a single benign adrenal tumor undergo surgical intervention. Bilateral benign tumors are more often treated with an aldosterone antagonist agent (i.e., a drug that reduces aldosterone secretion or blocks its effects). An example of an aldosterone antagonist is the potassium-sparing diuretic spironolactone (Aldactone). Patients with metastatic adrenal cancer are usually treated with surgery and chemotherapy. However, a cure for metastatic adrenal cancer is yet to be found. When Cushing syndrome is caused by a pituitary tumor, removal of part of the pituitary or radiation may reduce ACTH secretion without disturbing other pituitary functions. If this fails, the remaining pituitary tissue may be removed.

Drug therapy. When surgery is contraindicated, certain agents that interfere with ACTH production or adrenal hormone synthesis may be administered. One example is mitotane (Lysodren), a cytotoxic substance that is used as a palliative treatment for inoperable adrenal tumors. Agents that interfere with cortisol production include ketoconazole (Nizoral) and metyrapone (Metopirone). Metyrapone is also used in combination with mitotane for enhanced effects. A risk of acute adrenal crisis occurs when patients are on drugs that suppress adrenal function. In addition, the drugs must be promptly discontinued if trauma or shock occurs because the patient's ability to adapt is diminished. Table 47.2 provides additional information.

Pharmacology Capsule

Drugs that suppress adrenal function can lead to acute adrenal crisis and must be promptly discontinued if shock or trauma occurs.

Radiation. In cases in which a pituitary adenoma causes excessive secretion of ACTH, the adenoma may be treated with radiation therapy. Radiation can be administered either externally or internally. Internal radiation involves the transsphenoidal implantation of a radioactive material that remains in place for a specified period of time. Radiation therapy is not always effective, requires a long period of treatment, and can destroy healthy tissue. If radiation therapy is being used to treat a patient with a pituitary adenoma, you must be alert for any significant changes in the patient's neurologic status, such as a complaint of headache or a change in mental status or pupillary responses. In addition, the patient may experience side effects associated with radiation therapy. These include alopecia (i.e., hair loss) and dry, red, or irritated skin. The patient must be educated about these drug effects.

Surgical management. The surgical treatment of hyperadrenalism depends on the specific cause of the disorder. For example, if adrenal hypersecretion is caused by a pituitary adenoma that is producing ACTH, a transsphenoidal hypophysectomy is performed (see "Surgical Management" in the Hyperpituitarism section). If adrenal adenoma or carcinoma is the cause of the adrenal hypersecretion, an adrenalectomy (i.e., removal of the adrenal gland) is performed. If only one gland is removed, the procedure is referred to as a *unilateral adrenalectomy*; the removal of both glands is called a *bilateral adrenalectomy*. An adrenalectomy may be performed in situations in which drug and radiation therapies are unsuccessful. Patients who are undergoing a unilateral adrenalectomy can expect to require replacement therapy for up to 2 years after surgery. A bilateral adrenalectomy necessitates lifelong replacement of both glucocorticoids and mineralocorticoids. Depending on the tumor size, a laparoscopic procedure may be an option. Surgery and chemotherapy are indicated for metastatic adrenal cancer. These treatments may induce remission but are not curative.

◆ NURSING CARE OF THE PATIENT WITH CUSHING SYNDROME

Focused Assessment

Initial assessment of the patient with Cushing syndrome includes a detailed history and physical examination done by the RN. The LVN/LPN may collect specific information about the onset of symptoms, prior treatments, drug allergies, and current medications (see the Complementary and Alternative Therapies box). The complete nursing assessment of the patient with an endocrine disorder is summarized in Chapter 47, Box 47.1.

Complementary and Alternative Therapies

Patients with Cushing syndrome should be cautioned that long-term use of some herbs, including celery, juniper, licorice, and parsley, can cause hypokalemia.

Patient Problems, Goals, and Outcome Criteria: Cushing Syndrome

Patient Problems	Goals and Outcome Criteria
Potential for infection related to high serum cortisol levels	Absence of infection: normal body temperature and white blood cell (WBC) count
Anxiety related to depression, mood swings, anxiety, irrational behavior	Decreased anxiety: stable mood, calm demeanor
Potential for disrupted skin tissue integrity related to changes in skin and connective tissue and edema	Absence of injury to skin: skin intact with minimal or no bruising

Patient Problems, Goals, and Outcome Criteria: Cushing Syndrome—cont'd

Patient Problems	Goals and Outcome Criteria
Potential for injury (fracture) related to osteoporosis	Absence of fractures: no skeletal trauma or fractures
Altered body image related to changes in physical appearance and function	Adaptation to altered body image: patient attends to appearance, grooming; makes positive comments about self
Inability to manage self-care related to lack of understanding of disease, drug therapy, diet, and self-care	Patient follows prescribed treatment: verbalizes and demonstrates self-care, condition stabilizes

Interventions

Potential for infection. Exposure to people with infections should be avoided because of the patient's decreased resistance to infection. Minor symptoms, such as a low-grade fever (≥99.5°F), sore throat, or aches, can indicate the onset of a potentially serious infection. Any symptoms indicative of a cold or other problem should be brought to the attention of the physician.

Anxiety. Personality changes often accompany adrenal disorders. When they do occur, discuss them with the patient and the family. Understanding that mood swings are a part of this disorder may help the patient and family to cope more effectively. If the emotional changes, particularly depression, become severe, carefully monitor the patient. A psychiatric referral may be necessary.

Potential for disrupted skin integrity. The skin of the patient with Cushing syndrome is extremely fragile. Inspect the skin daily to detect early signs of pressure or injuries. Assist the patient with limited mobility to change positions at least every 2 hours. Keep bed linens clean and dry. Advise the patient to wear shoes when out of bed to reduce the risk of foot injuries. During transfers and position changes, be careful to prevent trauma to the skin.

Potential for injury. Because fractures occur very easily, protect the patient with Cushing syndrome from falls or trauma. Keep the bed in low position and the call bell within reach. If the patient is very weak or confused, raise the side rails. Instruct the patient to call for assistance when getting in and out of bed.

Altered body image. Bruises, abnormal fat distribution, and hirsutism may embarrass the patient. Provide an opportunity for the patient to share thoughts and concerns about these changes. If they are distressing, suggest clothing to conceal them. Encourage and assist patients to be well groomed. Women may choose to shave or to use depilatories to remove unwanted hair. Reassure the patient that physical changes usually improve gradually after medical or surgical treatment.

Inability to manage self-care. To manage Cushing syndrome, the patient must understand the condition, complications, treatment, and self-care. Provide written information to supplement verbal teaching about drugs, including drug names and dosages, schedules, and adverse effects. A referral may be made to the dietitian for nutritional counseling. The diet is typically low in calories with sufficient protein and calcium. (For key teaching points, see the Patient Teaching box.)

Patient Teaching

Cushing Syndrome

- Avoid people with infections because you have increased risk of infections; report any temperature elevation to your physician.
- Mood swings and changes in appearance are usually corrected with treatment.
- Avoid activities that could result in trauma because you have increased risk of bleeding and fractures.
- It is critical that you continue drug therapy under medical supervision.

NURSING CARE OF THE ADRENALECTOMY PATIENT

General nursing care of the surgical patient is discussed in Chapter 17. This section addresses the specific needs of the adrenalectomy patient.

PREOPERATIVE NURSING CARE

Preoperative care of the patient undergoing an adrenalectomy involves monitoring for and correcting any existing electrolyte imbalances. Strict hand washing and observance of aseptic technique are key in the prevention of infections in these susceptible patients. Preoperative education involves a discussion of glucocorticoid replacement therapy, including dosage, side effects, and complications.

POSTOPERATIVE NURSING CARE

After adrenalectomy, the patient is sent to a critical care unit for at least 1 to 2 days for close observation and assessment. During this period, monitor vital signs for signs and symptoms of impending shock, which may be evident as hypotension, a weak or thready pulse, decreased urinary output, and changes in level of consciousness. Pulse and BP may be unstable for 24 to 48 hours after surgery and vasopressors may be needed to maintain BP in the immediate postoperative period.

A patient problem specific to the adrenalectomy patient is potential for injury related to addisonian crisis as a result of the sudden decrease in adrenal hormone secretion. Assess for signs and symptoms of acute adrenal insufficiency: vomiting, weakness, hypotension, joint pain, pruritus, and emotional disturbances. Closely monitor fluid and electrolyte balance. Intravenous fluids may be prescribed to restore or maintain balance. High doses of cortisol are given intravenously during and for several days after surgery to enable the patient to deal with the physical stress of surgery. The dosages are adjusted on the basis of the BP, blood glucose, serum electrolytes, and serum cortisol levels. Later, glucocorticoids are administered orally.

Because the patient's resistance to infection is lowered, be especially careful to protect the patient by using strict aseptic technique for wound care and invasive procedures. Signs of infection may be very subtle.

Assess comfort at frequent intervals, and treat pain with opioid analgesics. Document the effects of treatment. To minimize the risk of pulmonary complications, such as stasis of secretions and pneumonia, instruct the patient to turn, cough, deep breathe, or use an incentive spirometer.

Nutrition Considerations

1. Early symptoms of Addison disease may include anorexia, nausea, vomiting, diarrhea, and weight loss, resulting in impaired nutrition.
2. Patients with Addison disease are advised not to restrict salt intake.
3. Patients with Cushing syndrome may experience sodium and water retention.
4. Diet therapy for Cushing syndrome may include decreased caloric and sodium intake and increased potassium intake.
5. Reducing sodium intake can decrease edema and related weight gain with Cushing syndrome.
6. Patients with diabetes insipidus (DI) usually experience excessive thirst or urination, so they must drink liquids almost continuously to avoid dehydration and hypovolemic shock.

PHEOCHROMOCYTOMA

A pheochromocytoma is a tumor, usually benign, of the adrenal medulla that causes secretion of excessive catecholamines (i.e., epinephrine, norepinephrine). Patients with a pheochromocytoma exhibit episodes of severe hypertension, hypermetabolism, and hyperglycemia. The classic clinical findings are hypertension with a diastolic pressure of 115 mm Hg or higher; severe, pounding headache; and diaphoresis (profuse sweating). Other signs and symptoms include flank pain, elevated heart rate, palpitations, anxiety (often resembling a panic attack), pallor, dilated pupils, orthostatic hypotension, and blurred vision. Episodes may be triggered by emotional distress, exercise, manipulation of the tumor, postural changes, and major trauma, including surgery.

The condition usually is treated by surgical removal of the tumor. Before surgery, the surgeon attempts to stabilize the patient's fluid status and to normalize vital signs first with alpha adrenergic antagonists, and then with beta adrenergic antagonists to block the effects of catecholamines. An example of an alpha adrenergic antagonist is phenoxybenzamine; propranolol and metoprolol are examples of beta adrenergic antagonists. The nurse monitors cardiovascular status and prepares the patient for surgery as detailed in Chapter 17.

Postoperative nursing care is generally the same as that described for the patient having an adrenalectomy. However, special postoperative problems in the patient with pheochromocytoma include a greater risk for fluctuations in blood pressure and hypoglycemia. These problems require close monitoring and treatment.

Get Ready for the NCLEX® Examination!

Key Points

- Hyperpituitarism, caused by excess anterior pituitary hormones, leads to gigantism or acromegaly depending on the age of onset.
- Hyperpituitarism is treated with drugs or surgery to remove the tumor or the entire pituitary (hypophysectomy).
- Treatment of hyperpituitarism can prevent further changes and complications. Soft tissue hypertrophy may be reduced, but existing skeletal changes are not reversible.
- Inadequate GH in children results in short stature.
- Panhypopituitarism is a deficiency of all anterior pituitary hormones and is treated with replacement hormones.
- DI, caused by a deficit in ADH, results in massive diuresis and is treated with vasopressin.
- SIADH, caused by excess ADH, results in fluid retention and is treated with a vasopressor receptor antagonist, such as conivaptan or tolvaptan and diuretics.
- Primary adrenal insufficiency (Addison disease) causes hypoglycemia, hyperkalemia, hyponatremia, and hypovolemia and requires lifelong replacement of glucocorticoids and mineralocorticoids.
- Acute adrenal crisis is a life-threatening emergency caused by a sudden marked decrease in adrenal hormones that can lead to circulatory collapse and death.
- Cushing syndrome results from hypersecretion of cortisol, a glucocorticoid, or from prolonged administration of corticosteroids.
- Cushing syndrome is characterized by polycythemia, hypokalemia, hyperglycemia, leukocytosis, and glycosuria.
- Cushing syndrome is treated with drug therapy, radiation, and hypophysectomy or adrenalectomy.
- Nursing care for the patient with Cushing syndrome is concerned with potential for infection, anxiety, potential for

disrupted skin tissue integrity, potential for injury, altered body image, and Inability to manage self-care.
- All chronic pituitary and adrenal conditions require patient teaching to enable the patient to manage the condition by taking medications properly and recognizing the need for medical intervention.
- A pheochromocytoma is an adrenal tumor that increases secretion of catecholamines, causing hypertension, hypermetabolism, and hyperglycemia.

Additional Learning Resources

SG Go to your Study Guide for additional learning activities to help you master this chapter content.

Go to your Evolve website (http://evolve.elsevier.com/Linton/medsurg) for the following learning resources and much more:
- Fluid & Electrolyte Tutorial
- Review Questions for the NCLEX® Examination

Clinical Judgment and Next-Generation NCLEX® Examination-Style Questions

1. **A patient who has recently started treatment for acromegaly says, "I will be so glad to look like myself again!" Which of the following is the most appropriate response?**
   1. "I know you are looking forward to that."
   2. "The process of reversing the effects of acromegaly is very slow."
   3. "Treatment will keep your symptoms from getting worse but will not reverse all of them."
   4. "These drugs can slow down the progression of acromegaly, but you will have additional bone enlargement."

   NCLEX Client Need: Physiological Integrity: Physiological Adaptation

2. **After surgery to remove a pituitary adenoma, a patient complains of neck stiffness. Which of the following actions would the nurse take?**
   1. Give a gentle neck massage
   2. Administer a prescribed analgesic
   3. Lower the head of the bed
   4. Look for other signs of infection

   NCLEX Client Need: Physiological Integrity: Reduction of Risk Potential

3. **Which of the following is the main symptom of SIADH?**
   1. Increased blood glucose
   2. Water retention
   3. Generalized edema
   4. Hypotension

   NCLEX Client Need: Physiological Integrity: Physiological Adaptation

4. **To regulate drug dosages for the patient with DI, which of the following records must be maintained?**
   1. Daily diet
   2. Sodium intake
   3. Urine specific gravity
   4. BP and pulse

   NCLEX Client Need: Physiological Integrity: Reduction of Risk Potential

5. **Fluid and electrolyte imbalances associated with Addison disease include which of the following? (Select all that apply.)**
   1. Hyperkalemia
   2. Hyponatremia
   3. Hypervolemia
   4. Metabolic alkalosis
   5. Hypercalcemia

   NCLEX Client Need: Physiological Integrity: Physiological Adaptation

6. **SLO/Objective: Assist in developing nursing care plans for patients with adrenal disorders.**

   NGN Item Type: Enhanced Hot Spot

   Cognitive Skill: Recognize Cues

   A patient is brought to the emergency department by a coworker who said the patient was not "making sense." A medical alert bracelet states that he takes drugs for Addison disease. The nurse's assessment data include:
   - Temperature 98°F
   - BP 88/40 mm Hg
   - Heart rate 108 beats per minute, thready, irregular
   - Respirations 20 breaths per minute
   - Lethargic and confused
   - Mucus membranes dry
   - Dark pigmentation of arms and face

   Highlight or place a check mark next to the assessment findings that require follow up by the nurse.

7. **SLO/Objective: Assist in developing nursing care plans for patients with adrenal disorders.**

   NGN Item Type: Enhanced Hot Spot

   Cognitive Skill: Recognize Cues

   The patient in question 6 is confused. The nurse would recognize the signs and symptoms of which of the following?
   1. Acute adrenal crisis.
   2. Cushing syndrome
   3. Diabetic ketoacidosis
   4. Cushing disease

   NCLEX Client Need: Physiological Integrity: Physiological Adaptation

8. **Nursing care of the patient with Cushing syndrome should include which of the following? (Select all that apply.)**
   1. Apply moisturizers to dark, toughened areas of skin
   2. Protect the patient from visitors and other patients with infections
   3. Tell the patient that mood swings and irritability will lessen with treatment
   4. Encourage the patient to use salt liberally to offset excessive loss in the urine

   NCLEX Client Need: Physiological Integrity: Physiological Adaptation and Reduction of Risk Potential

49 Thyroid and Parathyroid Disorders

http://evolve.elsevier.com/Linton/medsurg

Objectives

1. Describe the pathophysiology, signs and symptoms, complications, and treatment of hyperthyroidism, hypothyroidism, thyroid cancer, hyperparathyroidism, and hypoparathyroidism.
2. Assist in the development of nursing care plans for patients with disorders of the thyroid or parathyroid glands.

Key Terms

goitrogen (GOI-trō-jĕn)
laryngospasm (lă-RĬNG-gō-spăzm)
myxedema (mĭk-sĕ-DĒ-mă)
nodule (NŎD-ūl)
parotiditis (pă-rŏt-ĭ-DĪ-tĭs)
tetany (TĔT-ă-nē)
thyroiditis (thī-roid-Ī-tĭs)
thyrotoxicosis (thī-rō-tŏk-sĭ-KŌ-sĭs)

THYROID DISORDERS

❖ NURSING ASSESSMENT OF THE PATIENT WITH A THYROID DISORDER

Thyroid disorders may escape detection until they are rather severe because the symptoms are often vague. Periodic assessment of the patient with a thyroid disorder is necessary for the health care provider to evaluate the response to treatment and make adjustments if needed. Data collected by the registered nurse (RN) and the licensed vocational nurse/licensed practical nurse (LVN/LPN) contribute to this assessment and evaluation. The complete assessment of the patient with an endocrine disorder is presented in Chapter 47 and summarized in Box 47.1.

HEALTH HISTORY

When collecting data from the patient with a thyroid disorder, the focused assessment should include any changes in energy level, sleep patterns, personality, mental function, emotional state, or weight. Fatigue may be found with both hypothyroidism and hyperthyroidism. Because thyroid hormones affect the metabolic rate, patients may have unexplained weight changes. Hormone deficiency lowers the metabolic rate, so patients may gain weight. At the other extreme, hormone excess increases the metabolic rate, often causing weight loss.

In the review of systems, pay particular attention to changes in menstrual cycles, sexual function, hydration (i.e., thirst, changes in urine output, tissue turgor, moisture of mucous membranes), bowel elimination pattern, and tolerance of heat and cold.

PHYSICAL EXAMINATION

Measure the patient's vital signs and height and weight. Note the facial expression and characteristics as well as the mental alertness. Vital signs are important because they reflect the metabolic rate. Thyroid disorders may cause increased or decreased heart rate, respirations, blood pressure (BP), and temperature as well as irregular heart rhythms. Inspect and palpate the skin for moisture, temperature, and texture. In the head and neck examination, note the hair texture. Examine the eyes for exophthalmos (bulging). Inspect the neck for enlargement typical of goiter. Observe the hands for tremor. Nurses with advanced physical examination skills may palpate the neck for thyroid enlargement or nodules.

DIAGNOSTIC TESTS AND PROCEDURES

Diagnostic studies of the thyroid gland include laboratory blood tests and studies using radioactive iodine (RAI). Chapter 47, Table 47.1 summarizes the use of each test and identifies nursing implications.

The most useful tests of thyroid function are measurements of serum thyroid-stimulating hormone (TSH), serum triiodothyronine (T_3), and thyroxine (T_4). The thyroid-releasing hormone (TRH) stimulation test measures the blood level of TSH after administration of TRH. This test shows whether thyroid hormone abnormalities are caused by a disorder of the thyroid gland itself or by altered production of stimulating hormones by the hypothalamus or the pituitary. Additional blood tests may help to determine the type of dysfunction.

The thyroid gland uses iodine to manufacture hormones. Therefore radioisotopes (iodine-123 [^{123}I, and technetium-99m [^{99m}Tc]) are useful for diagnostic purposes because they concentrate in the thyroid. The amount of iodine taken up by the thyroid is measured to assess the activity level of the gland. This test is called a *RAI uptake test.*

For a thyroid scan, the patient ingests the radioisotope, then a specialized instrument is used to scan the area of the thyroid gland. It creates an image of the gland based on the distribution of the iodine. The image aids in diagnosing cancer because the patterns of iodine concentration in normal and malignant tissue are different. The scan may be repeated at specific intervals. The low dose of radiation used for diagnostic purposes poses no danger to the patient or others. However, pregnancy is a contraindication because of possible harm to the fetus.

Thyroid ultrasonography yields very clear images of the thyroid gland and any nodules present. This technology can be used to guide a needle for aspiration of samples from the nodules. For evaluation of metastatic disease or to image the portion of the thyroid concealed by the sternum, a PET scan or computed tomography (CT) is used.

Put On Your Thinking Cap!

A patient's blood studies show a high level of TSH and a low level of T_4. Explain what this finding means.

DISORDERS OF THE THYROID GLAND

HYPERTHYROIDISM

Hyperthyroidism, or **thyrotoxicosis**, is characterized by abnormally increased synthesis and secretion of thyroid hormones. The most common types of hyperthyroidism are Graves disease and multinodular goiter.

Graves disease is thought to be an autoimmune disorder triggered by genetic and/or environmental factors. Antibodies activate TSH receptors, which in turn stimulate thyroid enlargement and hormone secretion. Graves disease develops most often in women. Whether treated or not, the condition tends to have periods of remission and exacerbation. Some patients with Graves disease eventually develop hypothyroidism.

Multinodular goiter occurs most often in women in their sixth and seventh decades. It is most likely to develop in people who have had goiter for a number of years. Hyperthyroidism in this case is caused by thyroid **nodules** that secrete excess thyroid hormone without TSH stimulation. There may be multiple hyperfunctioning small nodules or a single nodule (toxic adenoma). The nodules can be benign or malignant. Symptoms of hyperthyroidism are usually less severe with multinodular goiter than with Graves disease.

Because all types of hyperthyroidism have many common features and because Graves disease is the most common form, it will be used as the example of hyperthyroidism.

Clinical Manifestations

Many of the signs and symptoms of hyperthyroidism are caused by an increased metabolic rate and can range from mild to severe. Weight loss and nervousness may be the only symptoms in patients with a mild form of the disease. In more severe cases, the patient's history may reveal restlessness, irritable behavior, sleep disturbances, emotional lability, personality changes, hair loss, and fatigue. Weight loss, even when the patient is eating well, is common. Some patients overcompensate for the increased metabolism, overeat, and gain weight. Many patients report poor tolerance of heat and excessive perspiration. Changes in menstrual and bowel patterns may occur. Examination findings may include warm, moist, velvety skin; fine tremors of the hands; swelling of the neck; and exophthalmos (protruding eyeballs). Exophthalmos (also called *ophthalmopathy*) is a classic sign of Graves disease. It is caused by fat accumulation, edema, and inflammation of the orbital contents. Tearing, light sensitivity, decreased visual acuity, and swelling around the orbit of the eye occur as well (Fig. 49.1). If severe, it may cause corneal ulcerations and visual disturbances because of pressure on the optic nerve.

Excess thyroid hormones stimulate the heart, causing tachycardia, increased systolic BP, and sometimes atrial fibrillation. The heart rate may be as rapid as 160 beats per minute. Even during sleep, the pulse may remain above 80 beats per minute.

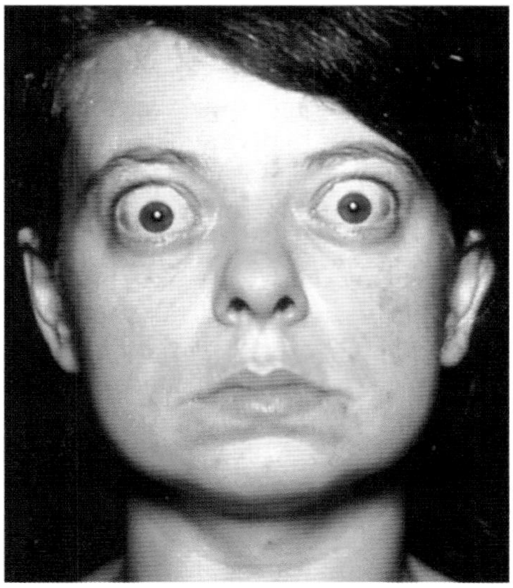

Fig. 49.1 This patient has exophthalmos, bulging eyes, associated with Graves disease. (From Ignatavicius DD, Workman ML: *Medical-surgical nursing: patient-centered collaborative care*, ed 8, St. Louis, 2016, Saunders.)

Some patients with Graves disease develop dermopathy, also called pretibial myxedema. Dermopathy is manifested as itching and thickening on the anterior aspect of the shins. Occlusive wraps with topical glucocorticoids may limit the progression of dermopathy, but there is no definitive cure.

Complications

Severe thyrotoxicosis, referred to as *thyrotoxic storm* or *thyroid crisis*, is a medical emergency requiring intensive monitoring and treatment. Excessive stimulation caused by elevated thyroid hormone levels can produce dangerous tachycardia and hyperthermia. It may be triggered by a variety of factors including trauma, surgery, and infection. A risk of heart failure exists. The patient is restless and agitated and may lapse into a coma. Fortunately, modern treatment of hyperthyroidism makes this complication rare.

Medical Diagnosis

Laboratory findings consistent with Graves disease are decreased TSH and elevated serum T_4. TSH can be so low that it cannot be detected in the blood. Measurement of thyroid-stimulating antibodies and results of an radioisotope uptake test are useful in specifically diagnosing Graves disease.

Medical Treatment

Three methods are used to treat hyperthyroidism: (1) drug therapy, (2) radiation therapy, and (3) surgery. In addition, beta-adrenergic blockers such as propranolol (Inderal) may be given to relieve some of the cardiovascular symptoms associated with hyperthyroidism. In addition, patients in crisis may require intravenous fluids and glucocorticoids.

Drug therapy. Hyperthyroidism may be treated initially with antithyroid drugs (i.e., drugs that block the synthesis, release, or activity of thyroid hormones) and beta-adrenergic blockers. Thionamides and iodides are antithyroid drugs. Although these drugs can be used for long-term treatment of hyperthyroidism, they are more often used temporarily to lower the level of hormones in the blood before surgery or radiation therapy. This process reduces the risk of bleeding and lowers the danger of releasing large amounts of thyroid hormones into the bloodstream during surgery. When a patient is on drugs that interfere with T_4 secretion, monitor for symptoms of hypothyroidism (e.g., cold intolerance, edema, weight gain). Beta blockers help to control palpitations, tremor, and anxiety caused by excessive sympathetic stimulation.

Pharmacology Capsule

Patients on antithyroid drugs must be monitored for hypothyroidism.

Thionamides. Methimazole (Tapazole) and propylthiouracil (PTU) are thionamides currently in use. It can take up to 8 weeks before the effects of thionamides are noticeable. The drugs may be given for months or years. The goal is to induce a remission that will allow the drugs to be discontinued. Thyroid function tests must be done regularly to prevent hypothyroidism.

Rare but serious adverse effects of thionamides are liver failure, and agranulocytosis. Agranulocytosis is a condition in which the production of neutrophils is suppressed. Without adequate neutrophils, the patient is unable to resist infection. Any signs of infection, such as sore throat or fever, should be reported to the physician immediately. Signs of liver inflammation include abdominal pain and jaundice. The risk of liver of damage is greater with PTU than with methimazole.

Iodides. Iodides are useful because iodine inhibits the synthesis of thyroid hormones. They are used most often after a course of PTU to suppress hormone secretion before thyroidectomy. The iodides may also be used to treat thyrotoxicosis. Saturated solution of potassium iodide (SSKI) can be given to people who have been exposed to radiation to prevent damage to the thyroid gland.

The iodides most often used to treat hyperthyroidism are Lugol solution (5% iodine and 10% SSKI) and SSKI. Iodides may bring some relief within 24 hours, but it takes several weeks for maximum effect. The effect does not last as long as that of thionamides; therefore iodides are not generally used as the sole treatment for hyperthyroidism.

Iodine solutions can cause discoloration of the teeth and gastric upset. These effects are minimized if the iodine solution is diluted with milk, fruit juice, or some other beverage and sipped through a straw. Signs of iodine toxicity include swelling and irritation of the mucous membranes and increased salivation.

Pharmacology Capsule

Iodine solutions can stain the teeth! They should be mixed with a beverage and sipped through a straw.

Radioactive iodine (radioiodine). Radioactive iodine (sodium iodide 131/^{131}I) can be used alone or with antithyroid drugs to treat hyperthyroidism. It quickly accumulates in the thyroid gland, where it destroys thyroid tissue. However, the resulting decrease in thyroid hormone production is not evident for several months. Meanwhile, beta-adrenergic blockers can be given to control cardiac symptoms.

The radiation dose used to treat hyperthyroidism does not pose a threat to others. However, it should not be used during pregnancy or lactation because it affects the thyroid gland of the fetus/infant. Side effects of the treatment are minimal. Inflammation of the thyroid gland **(thyroiditis)** and the parotid glands **(parotiditis)** may occur. Parotiditis causes the mouth to be dry and irritated. Hypothyroidism may develop years after treatment. Drugs used to treat thyroid disorders are summarized in Chapter 47, Table 47.2.

Surgical treatment. Graves disease is often treated by removing most of the thyroid gland. This procedure is called a *subtotal thyroidectomy.* The procedure may be done endoscopically or through a larger incision across the top of the clavicles. As mentioned earlier, patients are commonly given antithyroid drug therapy for several weeks before surgery. Before these drugs were commonly used, patients often had dramatic postoperative responses because of the escape of thyroid hormones into the bloodstream during surgery. This severe episode of hyperthyroidism, called *thyroid storm* or *thyroid crisis,* is a medical emergency because it is potentially fatal.

NURSING CARE OF THE NONSURGICAL PATIENT WITH HYPERTHYROIDISM

Most patients with hyperthyroidism are treated as outpatients. Therefore the nurse in the community or long-term care setting may need to help the patient learn to adapt until treatment brings relief.

Focused Assessment

Complete assessment of the patient with an endocrine disorder is summarized in Chapter 47, Box 47.1. Data collected by the LVN/LPN help to provide a detailed picture of the patient's status. For the patient with hyperthyroidism, significant data would include activity tolerance, heat tolerance, bowel elimination pattern, appetite, weight changes, and food intake. Also consider the patient's mental-emotional state, adaptation to the condition, and understanding of the treatment. Measure vital signs and height and weight. Document skin texture and edema. Note bulging of the eyes.

Patient Problems, Goals, and Outcome Criteria: Hyperthyroidism

Patient Problems	Goals and Outcome Criteria
Decreased cardiac output related to cardiac dysrhythmias or heart failure caused by excessive thyroid hormone stimulation	Normal cardiac output: pulse and blood pressure (BP) within patient norms, no edema or dyspnea (signs and symptoms of heart failure)
Sleep disturbance related to metabolic disturbance	Improved sleep: absence of insomnia, patient describes feeling rested on awakening
Heat intolerance related to increased metabolic energy production, hyperthermia	Improved heat tolerance: patient statement of comfort in relation to environmental temperature, no excess perspiration
Inadequate nutrition related to increased metabolic requirements	Adequate nutrition: stable body weight if no significant recent loss, weight gain if underweight

Patient Problems, Goals, and Outcome Criteria: Hyperthyroidism—cont'd

Patient Problems	Goals and Outcome Criteria
Potential for injury related to exophthalmos	Decreased risk of eye injury: lids cover eyeball, eyeball is moist, no pain associated with corneal injury
Discomfort related to ophthalmopathy	Improved comfort: patient reports less eye pain, photosensitivity
Diarrhea related to excessive thyroid hormone stimulation	Normal bowel elimination: formed stools at regular intervals

Put On Your Thinking Cap!

Explain why people with hyperthyroidism do not tolerate heat well.

Interventions

When a person is treated as an outpatient, teaching should focus on self-care. In the unlikely event that a patient is hospitalized for hyperthyroidism, the nurse provides more direct care.

Decreased cardiac output. Monitor the patient's pulse and blood pressure for elevations. Beta-adrenergic blockers should be taken as ordered to counteract the stimulant effects of the elevated thyroid hormones. Signs of heart failure include tachycardia, tachypnea, dyspnea, confusion, and edema. Older adults require especially careful monitoring because they are more susceptible to cardiovascular stress with thyroid disease. Immediately report any signs of heart failure to the health care provider. Medical treatment of heart failure usually includes oxygen, intravenous fluids, sedatives, and cardiac drugs.

Sleep disturbance. Despite fatigue and weakness, the hyperthyroid patient often feels restless and has trouble sleeping. Encourage the patient to arrange the day to allow periods of rest. Caffeine should be avoided because of its stimulating effects. Encourage bedtime rituals, which may be helpful in preparing for sleep. For the hospitalized patient, provide a restful environment and a soothing back rub to promote relaxation. Give sedatives as ordered to promote sleep.

In addition to physical rest, patients need emotional rest. The patient and the family may be able to cope better if they understand the reason for the patient's irritability and nervousness. Patients need to recognize stressful situations and avoid them.

Heat intolerance. Hyperthyroid patients usually have some heat intolerance because of their high metabolic rate. They tend to feel too warm even when others are comfortable. Only light clothing may be needed. Adjust the environmental temperature as much as possible for comfort. A private room allows the patient more freedom to select the room temperature. If the patient perspires heavily, frequent bathing and clothing changes help to promote comfort.

Inadequate nutrition. Despite a normal dietary intake, the patient may not be meeting the increased caloric needs (see the Nutrition Considerations box). Weigh daily to monitor nutritional adequacy. A diet high in calories, vitamins, and minerals is recommended. Depending on the severity of the condition, the patient may need additional full meals or between-meal snacks. Some patients require as many as 4000 to 5000 calories daily to maintain body weight. The physician may order supplementary vitamins. Additional fluids are recommended to replace fluids lost through increased insensible loss (i.e., fluid lost through the skin and the lungs).

Nutrition Considerations

1. Hypothyroid and hyperthyroid patients may require adjustments in calorie intake that are appropriate to metabolic needs.
2. Lack of iodine is associated with the development of a goiter (enlargement of the thyroid gland) in adults and cretinism in infants.
3. Iodized salt is the best way to obtain an adequate amount of iodine in the diet.
4. Another important source of iodine is saltwater seafood.
5. Parathyroid hormone (PTH), secreted by the parathyroid gland, and thyrocalcitonin, secreted by the thyroid gland, maintain serum calcium levels.

Potential for injury. Exophthalmos is a condition in which deposits of fat and fluid behind the eyeballs make them bulge outward (see Fig. 49.1). Both eyes are usually affected. If the condition is severe, the eyelids do not cover the eyeballs. The eyeballs are not kept moist and are susceptible to injury. It may be necessary to tape the lids shut. Lubricated eye pads or artificial tears may be used. Raising the head of the bed at night and limiting salt intake may be helpful.

The patient with exophthalmos has a startled appearance. This may make the person self-conscious and embarrassed. Dark glasses help to conceal the eyes. For these patients, altered body image is an important additional patient problem. Reassure the patient that the condition usually improves after treatment of hyperthyroidism.

Discomfort. In addition to exophthalmos, the hyperthyroid patient has a variety of eye symptoms that may include double vision, periorbital edema, tearing, photosensitivity, and a feeling of "sand" in the eyes. It helps to elevate the head of the bed, reduce bright lighting, and advise use of tinted glasses. Methylcellulose eye drops and diuretics may be ordered to decrease inflammation and swelling. Severe inflammation is treated with a 2- to 4-week course of prednisone. After acute inflammation subsides, surgical procedures on the eyeball muscles and the eyelids may be needed to eliminate double vision and to restore coverage of the eye.

Diarrhea. If the patient has diarrhea, electrolyte imbalances and skin irritation may result. Give antidiarrheal medications as ordered and monitor the effect. Thorough perianal cleansing after each stool reduces the risk of skin breakdown.

Patient Teaching

Hyperthyroidism

- This is a chronic condition that requires long-term care.
- You must take your medications exactly as prescribed.
- Notify your physician of excessive fatigue and depression, which may indicate hypothyroidism caused by your antithyroid drug.

◆ NURSING CARE OF THE PATIENT HAVING A THYROIDECTOMY

General care of the surgical patient is discussed in Chapter 17. This section covers the special needs of the patient having a thyroidectomy.

Focused Assessment

Preoperative care. The preparation of the patient undergoing thyroid surgery is essentially the same as for any major surgery. Ask what the patient knows about surgery and what to expect before and after the procedure. Patient problems may include those listed earlier for hyperthyroidism, but the condition is usually brought under control before surgery is scheduled. In addition, identify and address learning needs (see the Patient Teaching box). Teaching is the primary preoperative nursing intervention. The goals of preoperative teaching are patient understanding of the usual preoperative and postoperative procedures and decreased anxiety. Tell the patient to expect a dressing on the front of the neck. The size of the incision will depend on the surgical approach used. Demonstrate how to avoid straining the neck incision by supporting the head when rising. To evaluate the effectiveness of preoperative teaching, ask the patient to repeat the information presented. Ask patients to return demonstrations of activities such as deep breathing and supporting the head during position changes.

Postoperative care. The patient usually recovers quickly from a thyroidectomy and may be discharged in 1 or 2 days. Rare but serious complications are airway obstruction, recurrent laryngeal nerve damage, hemorrhage, and tetany (a sign of hypocalcemia associated with damage to the parathyroids). One other complication, thyroid storm, is usually prevented by preoperative treatment with antithyroid drugs.

If part of the thyroid gland is left (i.e., subtotal thyroidectomy), it should eventually regenerate and produce adequate hormones. The patient may be somewhat hypothyroid at first, but replacement therapy is not recommended. Giving thyroid hormone would interfere with the regeneration of thyroid tissue.

Immediately after thyroidectomy, it is especially important to monitor and document respiratory status, level of consciousness, wound drainage or bleeding, voice quality, comfort, and neuromuscular irritability (muscle twitching, spasms).

Patient Problems, Goals, and Outcome Criteria: Thyroidectomy

Patient Problems	Goals and Outcome Criteria
Potential for airway obstruction related to laryngeal nerve damage, laryngeal spasm, or pressure on trachea	Effective airway clearance: normal breath sounds, respiratory rate of 12 to 20 breaths per minute, no dyspnea
Decreased cardiac output related to blood loss, heart failure (HF) secondary to thyroid crisis	Normal cardiac output: pulse and blood pressure (BP) within normal limits, no edema
Altered body image related to surgical scar	Adaptation to change in appearance: looks at scar, verbalizes acceptance of scar
Acute pain related to tissue trauma	Pain relief: patient statement of less or no pain, relaxed manner
Potential for infection related to impaired skin integrity	Absence of infection: wound margins intact, minimal redness, no purulent drainage, normal body temperature

Interventions

Potential for airway obstruction. Turning and deep breathing are recommended to prevent respiratory complications, as with any other surgical patient. However, the surgeon may not want the patient to cough because of possible stress on the suture line.

It is especially important to monitor and document the rate and ease of respirations after thyroidectomy. Respiratory distress can result from compression of the trachea or from a spasm of the larynx because of nerve damage or hypocalcemia. Before the patient returns from surgery, suction equipment, a laryngoscope, an endotracheal tube, oxygen (O_2), and an emergency tracheostomy tray must be available. Your agency may require the tracheostomy tray at the bedside. Elevate the head of the bed to decrease edema. Use pillows to prop and support the head to avoid stress on the suture line.

Because of the location of the thyroidectomy incision, edema or bleeding can cause pressure on the trachea. Signs and symptoms of poor oxygenation because of airway obstruction or blood loss include restlessness, increasing pulse and respiratory rates, and dyspnea. Without prompt intervention, the patient with airway obstruction could die.

The laryngeal nerve innervates the vocal cords. If it is damaged during surgery, vocal cord paralysis can occur. Paralysis of both cords may cause spasms (**laryngospasm**) that close the airway. An emergency tracheostomy is needed to restore the airway. Signs of laryngeal nerve damage are hoarseness and inability to speak. This is more severe than the usual hoarseness most people have after general anesthesia. Ask the patient to respond verbally to simple questions to determine voice quality.

Before the function of the parathyroid glands was understood, patients having a thyroidectomy often experienced unexplained muscle contractions and respiratory difficulty that sometimes led to death. Eventually, it was determined that the symptoms were caused by hypocalcemia because of a deficiency of parathyroid hormone (PTH). Surgeons are now careful to locate and spare the small parathyroid glands. Occasionally, however, the parathyroid glands are injured or accidentally removed during thyroidectomy.

Without PTH, the serum calcium level falls, thus causing **tetany**. Muscle contractions begin as twitches around the mouth and eyes. The face, fingers, and toes begin to tingle. The patient may have painful "cramps," including the classic signs depicted in Fig. 49.2. The most serious effect of hypocalcemia is spasm of the larynx. As the larynx closes, the patient has difficulty breathing and can suffocate. Cardiac dysrhythmias and seizures can also occur.

Tetany is treated with calcium salts given intravenously or orally. The condition usually improves as the injured parathyroid glands recover. Rarely is hypoparathyroidism permanent. If it is, lifetime treatment is required, as described later in the section on "Hypoparathyroidism."

Decreased cardiac output. Frequently inspect the dressing to detect bleeding and take the vital signs. Because the dressing is on the front of the neck, blood might flow under the dressing to the back of the neck. Therefore be sure to check behind the patient's neck and upper back to detect this.

Complementary and Alternative Therapies

Position changes and back rubs enhance the effects of prescribed analgesics.

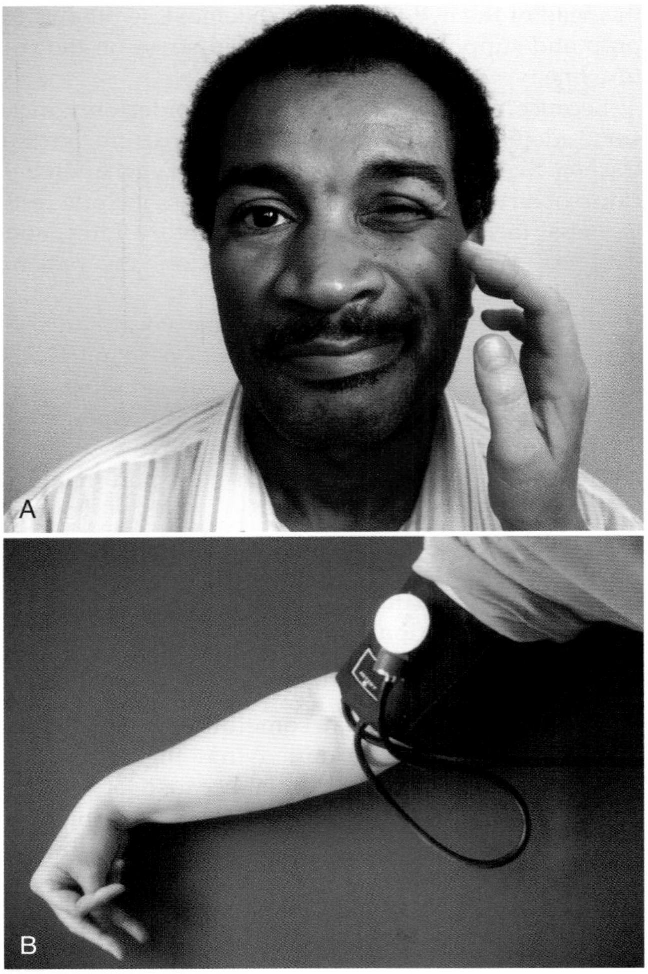

Fig. 49.2 Signs of hypocalcemia. (A) Chvostek sign (facial twitch). (B) Trousseau sign (carpopedal spasm). (From Ignatavicius DD, Workman ML: *Medical-surgical nursing: patient-centered collaborative care*, ed 8, St. Louis, 2016, Saunders.)

Thyroid storm can develop when large amounts of thyroid hormone enter the bloodstream during surgery or when patients with severe hyperthyroidism develop a severe illness or infection. This postoperative complication is rare because surgery is typically delayed until serum hormone levels are reduced. However, a brief description follows. Approximately 12 hours after surgery, the patient in thyroid crisis shows signs of severe hyperthyroidism (e.g., tachycardia, cardiac dysrhythmias, vomiting, fever, confusion).

If not treated promptly, the patient will die as a result of heart failure (HF). Early detection of thyroid crisis requires careful monitoring of vital signs during the first postoperative day. Treatment of thyroid crisis consists of antithyroid drugs, intravenous sodium iodide, corticosteroids, beta-adrenergic blockers, antipyretics, intravenous fluids, O_2, and a hypothermia (cooling) blanket or other measures to reduce body temperature.

Altered body image. The patient may be worried about the appearance of the surgical scar. Thyroidectomy incisions follow the natural contours of the neck. Once the scar fades, it usually is not noticeable. Meanwhile, it is easy to conceal the fresh scar with clothing. If an endoscopic procedure is used, the incisions will be very small.

Acute pain. Frequently inquire about the postoperative patient's comfort level. Promptly administer prescribed analgesics and evaluate and document effects. Chapter 8 discusses pain management in detail.

Potential for infection. Whenever the skin is broken, the potential for infection exists. Practice good hand washing and use aseptic technique when handling dressings. Tell the patient to avoid touching the fresh incision and to report any signs and symptoms of infection (i.e., fever, increasing wound redness and swelling, foul drainage). Inform the patient about wound care after discharge. Protect the incision from strain and possible dehiscence by supporting the neck when rising and reclining (see the Patient Teaching box).

Patient Teaching

Thyroidectomy

- If all of your thyroid gland was removed, you will need lifelong replacement of thyroid hormones.
- If only part of your thyroid gland was removed, you may feel tired for a while; however, this should improve as the remaining gland increases hormone production.
- Thyroidectomy scars usually heal so that they are eventually barely noticeable; they are easily concealed with clothing.
- Take your drugs exactly as prescribed.
- Nervousness and palpitations may be adverse effects of thyroid replacement drugs (hyperthyroidism); notify the physician if they occur.

HYPOTHYROIDISM

Hypothyroidism is the result of inadequate secretion of thyroid hormones. It is seen in infants, children, and adults. If not treated early, hypothyroidism during infancy causes congenital iodine deficiency syndrome characterized by permanent retardation of physical and mental development (see the Cultural Considerations box). The effects in adults can be quite serious but usually are reversible with treatment. The term *myxedema* is sometimes used for hypothyroidism. **Myxedema** actually refers to edema that develops in the hands, face, feet, and area around the eyes with severe, long-term hypothyroidism (Fig. 49.3). Not all hypothyroid patients have myxedema.

Cultural Considerations

What Does Culture Have to Do With Cretinism?

Neonatal hypothyroidism, which causes cretinism if not corrected early, is much more common among European heritage than among those of African heritage.

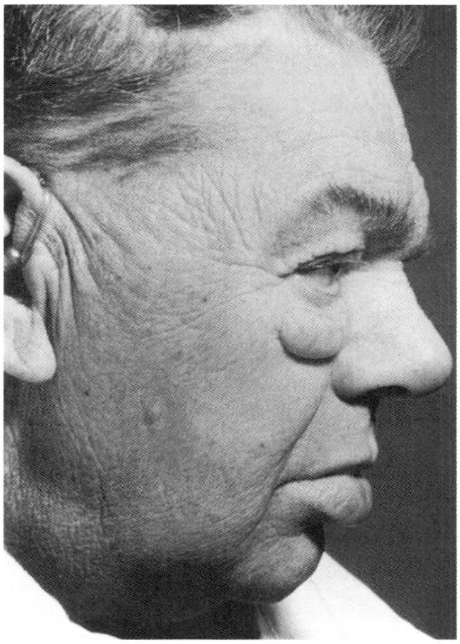

Fig. 49.3 Typical appearance of the patient with myxedema. (From Jacob WW, Francone CA: *Elements of anatomy and physiology*, ed 2, Philadelphia, 1989, Saunders.)

Cause and Risk Factors

Hypothyroidism has many causes, including atrophy of the thyroid gland after years of Graves disease or thyroiditis, treatment for hyperthyroidism, dietary iodine deficiency, high intake of goitrogens, and defects in thyroid hormone synthesis. These are examples of primary hypothyroidism. They account for 90% to 95% of all cases of hypothyroidism. Some foods and drugs act as **goitrogens**, meaning that they suppress thyroid hormone production. Examples of foods that are goitrogens if taken in large quantities are soybeans, turnips, and rutabagas. Goitrogenic drugs that are often used to treat hyperthyroidism are methimazole, propylthiouracil, and iodine (see the Cultural Considerations box).

> **Cultural Considerations**
>
> **What Does Culture Have to Do With Hypothyroidism?**
>
> The incidence of hypothyroidism is 10 to 20 times higher in iodine-deficient parts of the world (e.g., Democratic Republic of Congo, Nepal) than in the United States.

Hypothyroidism caused by a deficiency of the pituitary hormone TSH is called *secondary hypothyroidism.* Deficiency of TSH lowers the secretion of thyroid hormones even though the thyroid gland itself remains normal. When the hypothalamic hormone thyrotropin-releasing hormone is deficient, the patient is said to have tertiary hypothyroidism. Of course, patients who have had their entire thyroid or pituitary gland surgically removed will also be hypothyroid. Hypothyroidism can also result from tissue resistance to thyroid hormone (i.e., the hormone is present, but the body cells are unable to use it normally).

Clinical Manifestations

The signs and symptoms of hypothyroidism in general are the opposite of those of hyperthyroidism (Table 49.1). The onset is usually gradual. The metabolic rate slows, often causing weight gain even with decreased food intake. Hypothyroid patients commonly report lethargy, forgetfulness, and irritability. They may experience frequent headaches, constipation, menstrual disorders, numbness and tingling in the arms and legs, and intolerance to cold. The pulse tends to be slow and dyspnea may be present.

Examination may reveal swelling of the lips and eyelids; dry, thick skin; bruising; thin, coarse hair; and hoarseness. Generalized nonpitting edema and facial edema may be present. The patient may seem slow, depressed, or apathetic. Pallor may be present, associated with anemia. Signs and symptoms may be more subtle in the older patient or may be masked by signs and symptoms of other acute or chronic disorders. Therefore thyroid function in older adults should be assessed as part of routine checkups.

Medical Diagnosis

Hypothyroidism is diagnosed based on the laboratory determination of free T_4 and TSH. A TRH stimulation test may also be ordered. Free T_4 is low with hypothyroidism, except when the problem is tissue resistance to the hormone. TSH level enables the physician to determine whether the basic problem is primary, secondary, or tertiary hypothyroidism.

Complications

Severe, untreated hypothyroidism can progress to myxedema coma. Infection, trauma, excessive chilling, and some drugs (opioids, sedatives, and tranquilizers) may precipitate myxedema coma in a hypothyroid patient. The main signs of this life-threatening condition are hypothermia, hypotension, and hypoventilation.

Medical Treatment

Hypothyroidism is treated with hormone replacement therapy, most commonly levothyroxine (Synthroid). Patients should be monitored periodically to evaluate the response to therapy. A patient with heart disease may have difficulty adapting to a sudden increase in metabolic rate. For that reason, replacement therapy for older patients or those with heart disease is usually started with a very low dose and gradually increased. If these patients have any chest pain once therapy is started, the health care provider should be notified immediately so that steps can be taken to prevent cardiac complications. Because of variations between brands, patients should consistently take the same brand. If a brand change is required, the serum TSH should be checked in 6 weeks and dosage adjusted as needed.

> **Pharmacology Capsule**
>
> Opioids, sedatives, and tranquilizers can precipitate potentially fatal myxedema coma in a severely hypothyroid person.

Table 49.1 Comparison of Signs and Symptoms of Hypothyroidism and Hyperthyroidism

SYSTEM	HYPOTHYROIDISM	HYPERTHYROIDISM
Integumentary	Coarse, dry skin and hair; thick nails	Smooth, moist skin; silky hair; diaphoresis
Musculoskeletal	Muscle aches and pains, weakness, slow movements	Weakness
Cardiovascular	Bradycardia, dysrhythmias, hypotension, anemia, capillary fragility	Tachycardia, dysrhythmias, palpitations, systolic hypertension, angina
Respiratory	Hypoventilation, dyspnea	Increased respiratory rate, dyspnea
Gastrointestinal (GI)	Anorexia, nausea and vomiting, constipation, weight gain	Increased appetite, increased bowel sounds, diarrhea, weight loss
Neurologic	Apathy, lethargy, slowed mental function, depression, slow speech, paresthesias, decreased tendon reflexes	Nervousness and irritability, insomnia, personality change, agitation, inability to concentrate, fine tremor of fingers and tongue, hyperreflexia
Reproductive	Women: amenorrhea or prolonged menses, infertility, decreased libido Men: decreased libido, erectile dysfunction	Women: menstrual irregularities, decreased libido Men: decreased libido, erectile dysfunction, gynecomastia
Other	Cold intolerance, decreased body temperature, facial puffiness or coarseness, thick tongue, nonpitting edema of hands and feet, sensitivity to central nervous system (CNS) depressants	Increased body temperature, exophthalmos, goiter, sensitivity to CNS stimulants

◆ NURSING CARE OF THE PATIENT WITH HYPOTHYROIDISM

Hypothyroidism usually does not require hospitalization, but it may be detected when patients are hospitalized for other reasons. Because the onset of symptoms is often subtle, the nurse in the community or long-term care setting must be alert for signs and symptoms of hypothyroidism (see Nursing Care Plan: Patient With Hypothyroidism).

Focused Assessment

General assessment of the patient with an endocrine disorder is summarized in Chapter 47, Box 47.1. Relevant data for thyroid patients include measurement of vital

Nursing Care Plan Patient With Hypothyroidism

FOCUSED ASSESSMENT

Health History

A 53-year-old woman comes to the physician's office complaining of fatigue and irritability. Her symptoms have gradually worsened and are now interfering with her work as an executive assistant. She reports that her health has generally been good, with only one hospitalization for an appendectomy 7 years ago. The review of systems reveals frequent headaches, anorexia, constipation, menstrual irregularity, numbness and tingling in the legs, and intolerance to cold. She has noticed a 10-lb weight gain over the past 6 months without a change in diet or exercise.

Physical Examination

Vital signs: blood pressure 90/60 mm Hg, pulse 56 beats per minute, respiration 18 breaths per minute, temperature 97°F (36.1°C) measured orally. Height 5′5″, weight 155 lb. Patient's record indicates that her previous blood pressure was 128/76 mm Hg and previous pulse was 74 beats per minute. She is oriented but lethargic. Her hair is coarse, and her skin is dry.

Patient Problems	Goals and Outcome Criteria	Interventions
Decreased activity tolerance related to decreased metabolic energy production	The patient will report less fatigue with activities of daily living (ADL).	Advise the patient to schedule additional rest periods until the condition improves. Assure her that these symptoms are temporary.
Inadequate nutrition related to intake greater than metabolic needs	The patient's weight will stabilize within 2 lb of her usual 145 lb.	Weigh the patient during each office visit. Encourage a balanced diet. Tell her that her weight should normalize when the condition is corrected.
Cold intolerance related to slow metabolic rate	The patient will report adequate warmth and increased tolerance of cool temperatures.	In inpatient settings, adjust the room temperature for comfort. In the clinic, provide adequate covering during physical examination. For home care, inform the patient of the cold intolerance.

Nursing Care Plan Patient With Hypothyroidism—cont'd

Patient Problems	Goals and Outcome Criteria	Interventions
Constipation related to decreased peristalsis	The patient will have regular bowel movements passed without straining.	Encourage increased fluid intake and a high-fiber diet with fresh fruits and raw vegetables. Instruct the patient in taking stool softeners if advised by physician. Encourage a gradual increase in physical activity as tolerance improves.
Potential for disrupted skin integrity related to dryness	The patient's skin will remain intact and usual moisture will be restored.	Advise the patient to decrease bathing frequency and to use moisturizing creams or lotions. Advise her to avoid scratching.
Decreased cardiac output related to cardiovascular changes secondary to hypothyroidism	The patient's cardiac output will improve, as evidenced by improved stamina, regular pulse between 60 and 100 beats per minute, blood pressure (BP) consistent with patient norms, and no dyspnea.	Monitor the patient for tachycardia, hypertension, and dysrhythmias after hormone replacement therapy is begun. Tell her to notify the physician if she has palpitations.
Inability to manage condition related to lack of knowledge of mental and emotional effects of hypothyroidism	Improved self-care: The patient acknowledges that her mental and emotional symptoms will improve with treatment; patient will identify strategies to reduce workplace demands.	Explain that mental slowness is related to hypothyroidism and that it will improve with treatment. Do not overload the patient with information. Teach only the critical information initially and supplement it with written information. Ask her how her work expectations could be adjusted temporarily to accommodate her symptoms.
Fatigue related to slow metabolism	Less fatigue: The patient's ADLs will be accomplished with only normal fatigue.	Ask the patient to consider her daily activities and set priorities. Encourage rest periods. Delay difficult or strenuous tasks until her condition improves.

CRITICAL THINKING QUESTIONS

1. What is the most critical information you should teach the patient about hypothyroidism?
2. How can you help the patient to set priorities and determine daily activities?

signs, height, and weight. In addition, ask about activity and temperature tolerance, voice quality, bowel elimination pattern, and changes in weight and dietary intake. Inspect and palpate the skin for turgor, texture, and moisture. Note level of consciousness and emotional state. Ask if the patient has noticed a change in mental alertness. Also explore the patient's understanding of hypothyroidism and its treatment.

Patient Problems, Goals, and Outcome Criteria: Hypothyroidism

Patient Problems	Goals and Outcome Criteria
Reduced activity tolerance related to decreased metabolic energy production	Improved activity tolerance: patient report of less fatigue with daily activities
Weight gain related to decreased metabolism	Appropriate calorie intake: stable body weight or gradual return to weight before thyroid disorder
Cold intolerance related to slow metabolism	Improved cold tolerance: warm hands and feet, no complaints of coldness
Constipation related to decreased peristalsis	Normal bowel function: regular stools without difficulty
Potential for disrupted skin integrity related to dryness and edema	Decreased risk of skin breakdown: skin moist, intact

Patient Problems, Goals, and Outcome Criteria: Hypothyroidism—cont'd

Patient Problems	Goals and Outcome Criteria
Decreased cardiac output related to cardiovascular changes secondary to hypothyroidism	Normal cardiac output: improved stamina, pulse and blood pressure (BP) within normal limits; no dyspnea, edema, or dysrhythmias
Altered body image related to altered physical appearance, disturbed thought processes, lack of energy	Improved body image: patient makes positive statements about appearance, tends to personal appearance
Fatigue related to slow metabolism	Less fatigue: patient gradually resumes responsibility for personal care, completes care with less fatigue
Inability to manage condition related to lack of knowledge of effects of hypothyroidism treatment and self-care	Improved self-care: patient describes therapy, self-care, and intent to comply with instructions; patient understands that changes in mental and emotional status are symptoms of their condition and that they will improve with treatment

Interventions

Decreased activity intolerance. The hypothyroid patient lacks energy and tires easily. Arrange the schedule to allow for rest periods. Sedatives and barbiturates should be avoided because they may cause excessive sedation. If they are given, lower dosages are recommended. Monitor and document the patient's respirations and level of consciousness. Families and employers need to understand the patient's fatigue and make adjustments until the patient recovers. Improvement is gradual but is usually evident after 2 to 3 weeks.

Weight gain. Despite having a poor appetite, the patient may have gained weight. Weekly weights are helpful in evaluating the effects of hormone replacement therapy. Calorie reduction may be prescribed for the patient who is overweight. Encourage a balanced diet.

Cold intolerance. Cold intolerance is a very uncomfortable effect of hypothyroidism. Provide extra clothing and blankets as needed. Maintain the room temperature at a level comfortable to the patient. This is easier to manage if the patient has a private room. Once thyroid replacement is initiated, cold intolerance gradually improves.

Constipation. Constipation is a common problem. Until the hypothyroidism is corrected, take measures to promote normal elimination. Adequate fluids, dietary fiber, and physical activity all help to reduce constipation. Bulk laxatives or stool softeners may be indicated if other measures do not solve the problem. Remember that adequate fluids are essential to prevent bowel obstruction with bulk laxatives. Older patients should increase activity levels gradually to avoid excessive stress on the heart.

Potential for disrupted skin tissue. Dry skin, which is common with hypothyroidism, is prone to breakdown. Liberally apply lotions and creams to help maintain moisture and control itching. Reduce the frequency of bathing to prevent additional drying of the skin.

Decreased cardiac output. Atherosclerosis and heart disease develop in patients whose hypothyroidism is uncorrected for a long time. Monitor these patients for any signs and symptoms of HF, such as dyspnea and increasing edema. After hormone replacement therapy is begun, some risk of excessive cardiac stimulation exists. Tell the patient that any chest pain should be reported promptly. Monitor the pulse to detect potentially serious changes in rhythm or rate. Remember that the older adult's circulatory system adapts more slowly to increased thyroid hormone.

Pharmacology Capsule

Any older adult who is taking more than 0.15 mg of L-thyroxine daily is at risk for hyperthyroidism.

Confusion. Mental dullness and depression can significantly affect the patient's life. Explain that these symptoms are related to hypothyroidism and that correction of hypothyroidism usually results in marked improvement. (An exception is the person who has congenital iodine deficiency syndrome caused by untreated hypothyroidism during fetal development or early infancy. The mental retardation of cretinism is not reversible.) Until mental function improves, be careful not to demand too much of the patient. Break teaching into small units and reinforce at intervals.

Altered body image. The puffy, apathetic look and weight gain associated with hypothyroidism can be very distressing to the patient. Be accepting of the patient's concerns but encourage good grooming and attention to appearance. Tell the patient that treatment will gradually eliminate these changes.

Fatigue. Encourage the patient to examine daily activities to make a schedule that conserves energy. Assure them that fatigue gradually lessens with treatment. Educate the family about the patient's need for extra rest and relief from some responsibilities at this time.

Inability to manage self-care. The hypothyroid patient can expect to need lifelong hormone replacement therapy. Explain this to the patient and stress the need for periodic medical evaluation. Describe the name, dosage, and adverse effects of the prescribed drug therapy. Teach the patient the symptoms of hyperthyroidism that might occur with excessive hormone replacement (tachycardia, weight loss, nervousness). Document patient teaching.

Put On Your Thinking Cap!

A patient who was recently diagnosed with hypothyroidism complains that she has no appetite but has gained 20 lb over the past few months. How would you explain this to her?

GOITER

Goiter is the term used to describe enlargement of the thyroid gland. Enlargement may be diffuse (distributed throughout the gland) or nodular (clustered in nodes that secrete excess thyroid hormone). Patients with goiters may have normal, decreased, or increased thyroid hormone production. The management of goiter depends upon the cause.

Thyroid enlargement with normal thyroid hormone production (Fig. 49.4) may be caused by iodine deficiency and long-term exposure to goitrogens. The gland may enlarge to compensate for hypothyroidism. Sometimes the enlarged gland produces excess hormones, making the patient hyperthyroid.

The type of treatment depends on the degree of enlargement and level of thyroid hormone production. If enlargement is mild and hormones are normal, no intervention is required. Some patients need hormone replacement therapy. Surgery is indicated if pressure is

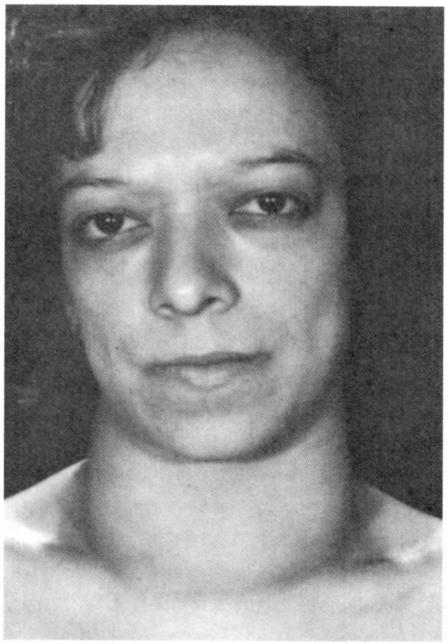

Fig. 49.4 Goiter. (From Wilson J, Foster D: *Williams textbook of endocrinology*, ed 7, Philadelphia, 1985, Saunders.)

noted on the trachea or esophagus or if the condition is disfiguring.

Nodules

Multinodular goiter is discussed earlier with "Hyperthyroidism." As noted, nodules can be benign or malignant. To help determine whether cancer is present, the physician may order a scan that uses radioisotopes. Nodular goiters are usually removed surgically. In benign conditions, only the nodule may be removed.

THYROID CANCER

Thyroid cancer is not common. It is fatal in less than 1% of all cases. In the early stages, the only sign may be a nodule that can be felt on the thyroid gland. Later, if the cancer spreads, enlarged lymph nodes are felt in the neck. The patient may not show dramatic changes in thyroid hormone levels. Total thyroidectomy is the usual treatment. Nursing care of the thyroidectomy patient is covered in the section on "Hyperthyroidism." If the malignancy has spread beyond the thyroid gland, more radical surgery may be indicated.

Surgery may be followed with radioactive iodine treatment to destroy any remaining tissue that might harbor malignant cells. This is the same type of iodine used in diagnostic studies, but a larger dose is used. The patient needs to be isolated and on radiation precautions. Body fluids must be handled according to radiation precaution guidelines because they are contaminated. The care of the patient receiving internal radiation therapy is discussed in Chapter 7.

The patient is likely to be alarmed at the diagnosis of cancer. They may find some comfort in knowing that the 5-year survival rate for thyroid cancer is among the highest of all types of cancer. Long-term care after thyroid cancer includes management of hypothyroidism and monitoring for recurrence. Scans using radioactive iodine are sometimes ordered at intervals to detect the presence of any remaining cancerous tissue. Periodic TSH and thyroglobulin tests may be ordered. Thyroglobulin rises if thyroid cancer recurs. Thyroid replacement therapy is based on the TSH level.

PARATHYROID DISORDERS

NURSING ASSESSMENT OF PARATHYROID FUNCTION

HEALTH HISTORY

Although the RN is responsible for the complete assessment, the LVN/LPN may assist with data collection. Relevant data from the health history include changes in mental and emotional status, such as memory problems, irritability, or personality changes. Ask about a history of musculoskeletal problems, including weakness, skeletal pain, backache, and muscle twitching or spasms. Note if the patient has experienced urinary frequency, polyuria, urinary calculi (stones), or constipation. Document a past medical history of head or neck radiation, renal calculi, or chronic renal failure. List medications, including calcium and vitamin D supplements.

PHYSICAL EXAMINATION

Important data in the physical examination include heart rate and rhythm, BP, respiratory effort, muscle strength, muscle twitching, and hair and skin texture. Chvostek sign and Trousseau sign may be elicited to detect hypocalcemia as depicted in Fig. 49.2.

Nursing assessment of the patient with an endocrine disorder is outlined in Chapter 47, Box 47.1. Data specific to parathyroid disorders is described above.

DIAGNOSTIC TESTS AND PROCEDURES

The diagnosis of parathyroid disorders is based on blood and urine studies and skeletal radiographs. Blood tests include measurements of calcium, phosphate, creatinine, uric acid, magnesium, alkaline phosphatase, and PTH. The presence of parathyroid antibodies may also be identified through blood studies. A 24-hour urine specimen may be collected to determine how much calcium is being excreted in the urine.

If excessive calcium has been drawn from bones, demineralization will be apparent on radiographs. Bone cysts and tumors may be found. A dental examination may be done to detect changes in the teeth consistent with parathyroid dysfunction. An electrocardiogram (ECG) may also be ordered because calcium imbalances can cause alterations in the electrical activity in the heart.

DISORDERS OF THE PARATHYROID GLANDS

HYPERPARATHYROIDISM

The secretion of excess PTH is called *hyperparathyroidism*. It is caused most often by a tumor called an *adenoma*. The tumors can be benign or malignant. Other factors that may stimulate excess PTH secretion are vitamin D deficiencies, malabsorption, chronic renal failure, exposure to neck radiation in childhood, and elevated serum phosphate. People who receive a kidney transplant after having been on dialysis for a long time may also have hyperparathyroidism.

The most notable effect of hyperparathyroidism is elevation of serum calcium (i.e., hypercalcemia). High levels of PTH cause calcium to shift from the bones into the bloodstream. Excess PTH also promotes retention of calcium and loss of phosphate by the kidneys. If hyperparathyroidism is untreated, severe demineralization of bone tissue occurs. Bones can become brittle, resulting in serious fractures. The high level of calcium in the urine can lead to the formation of urinary calculi. Obstruction of the urinary tubules by calculi can quickly cause severe kidney damage. The effects of hyperparathyroidism on the heart can cause dysrhythmias and hypertension.

Clinical Manifestations

Because hyperparathyroidism usually develops gradually, symptoms are vague at first. The patient may report weakness, lethargy, depression, anorexia, and constipation. Other findings might include mental and personality changes, cardiac dysrhythmias, weight loss, and urinary calculi. Additional signs and symptoms of hyperparathyroidism are outlined in Table 49.2.

Medical Diagnosis

The diagnosis of hyperparathyroidism is based primarily on blood and urine studies. Typical findings include elevated serum calcium and decreased serum phosphate, elevated PTH, and elevated 24-hour urine calcium. Skeletal radiographs and bone density studies reveal bone demineralization if the condition is severe. Sometimes the condition is not recognized until the patient has a spontaneous fracture. Other diagnostic procedures that may be used include renal CT and ultrasound, MRI, fine-needle aspiration, and selective arteriography.

Medical Treatment

Surgical intervention. If a tumor is causing hyperparathyroidism, it is usually removed surgically. In some cases, more than one gland is removed. The surgeon attempts to leave some parathyroid tissue to prevent hypoparathyroidism. It is often possible for the procedure to be done with an endoscope. However, parathyroidectomy can be a complicated procedure because some parathyroid glands may be located in the mediastinum. Sometimes a remnant of the patient's normal parathyroid tissue is transplanted to a muscle in the forearm or the neck where it will continue to secrete PTH. This procedure may be indicated when a patient with end-stage kidney disease requires parathyroidectomy to control calcium and PTH metabolism.

Drug therapy. If the condition is mild or the patient is not a good candidate for surgery, medical treatment is aimed at lowering the serum calcium level. The patient is instructed to maintain a high fluid intake to dilute the urine. Calcium intake may be restricted. Sodium and phosphorus replacements may be ordered. When it is necessary to lower the calcium level quickly, an infusion of normal saline is often prescribed. Several drugs can be used to treat hypercalcemia. Calcitonin (Calcimar), bisphosphonates (zoledronate), and estrogen inhibit the release of calcium from bones. Cinacalcet (Sensipar) suppresses PTH secretion. Oral phosphates inhibit the absorption of calcium from the digestive tract. Furosemide (Lasix) may be given to promote the excretion of calcium in the urine. If hypercalcemia is caused by vitamin D intoxication, glucocorticoids are highly effective. Drugs used to treat parathyroid disorders are described in Chapter 47, Table 47.2.

Table 49.2 Comparison of Signs and Symptoms of Hypoparathyroidism and Hyperparathyroidism

SYSTEM	HYPOPARATHYROIDISM	HYPERPARATHYROIDISM
Musculoskeletal	Fatigue, weakness, cramps, twitching	Poor muscle tone, weakness, bone pain, demineralization, fractures
Urinary	Frequency	Polyuria, renal calculi
Cardiovascular	Decreased cardiac output, dysrhythmias	Hypertension, dysrhythmias
Neurologic	Hyperactive reflexes, memory impairment, depression, anxiety, irritability, personality changes, confusion, numbness and tingling of hands and feet and around mouth, muscle spasms	Depressed reflexes, decreased mental function, depression, mood swings, confusion, coma, poor coordination
Gastrointestinal (GI)	Abdominal cramps	Anorexia, nausea and vomiting, constipation
Integumentary	Brittle nails, dry skin	Moist skin
Temperature tolerance	Cold intolerance	Heat intolerance

Pharmacology Capsule

Furosemide (Lasix) is a diuretic that promotes the excretion of calcium in the urine.

NURSING CARE OF THE PATIENT WITH HYPERPARATHYROIDISM

Focused Assessment

The complete assessment of the patient with an endocrine disorder is summarized in Chapter 47, Box 47.1. When caring for the patient with hyperparathyroidism, the focused assessment requires you to monitor vital signs, urine output, weight, muscle strength, neuromuscular irritability, bowel elimination, and digestive disturbances.

Patient Problems, Goals, and Outcome Criteria: Hyperparathyroidism

Patient Problems	Goals and Outcome Criteria
Decreased activity tolerance related to weakness and fatigue	Improved activity tolerance: patient reports performing daily activities with less fatigue
Potential for injury related to weakness and decreased bone mass	Reduced risk for injury: improved muscle strength, no falls
Potential for urinary obstruction related to urinary calculi	Normal urinary output: urine output equal to fluid intake
Constipation related to altered intestinal motility	Normal bowel elimination: regular stools without straining
Inability to manage self-care related to lack of knowledge of hypercalcemia and its treatment	Improved knowledge of effects of hypercalcemia: patient understands that irritability and depression are symptoms that will improve with treatment.
Inadequate nutrition related to nausea and vomiting	Adequate nutrition: stable body weight, no nausea or vomiting

Interventions

Decreased activity tolerance and potential for injury. Determine the patient's ability to perform self-care safely and provide help as needed. Move and handle the patient gently. Evaluate the environment for any safety hazards and take corrective measures. Plan care to allow for periods of rest. If the patient is being treated at home, stress the need to plan for rest periods. Assure the patient that weakness and fatigue are caused by the parathyroid disorder and will improve as the condition is corrected.

Potential for urinary obstruction. Maintain accurate intake and output records because hypercalcemia can cause urinary calculi and serious kidney damage. Decreasing urine output; sharp pain in the flank (kidney area), lower abdomen, or genitalia; and hematuria are consistent with urinary calculi and should be reported to the physician. A high fluid intake, sometimes as much as 4000 mL/day, may be ordered. Closely monitor urine output and vital signs when large volumes of fluid are administered. Older adults and people with heart disease are at risk for excess fluid volume and HF. Patients with cardiac or renal disease may be unable to tolerate this much fluid. Urine may be strained and examined for crystals or calculi. A low-calcium diet and urine acidifiers may be ordered to decrease the risk of calculi formation.

Constipation. Chart bowel movements, including frequency and characteristics of stools. Constipation can often be managed with adequate fluids and fiber in the diet. If these measures are not effective, the physician may order bulk laxatives or stool softeners. It is especially important to monitor bowel elimination in the older patient. Illness, inactivity, and multiple medications combine to increase their risk of constipation and even fecal impaction.

Inability to manage self-care. Recognize that irritability, personality changes, and depression are common with hyperparathyroidism. Patients and their families appreciate knowing that these symptoms are caused by an elevated blood calcium level and that they will improve with treatment (see the Patient Teaching box).

Inadequate nutrition. Take measures to control nausea and vomiting if present. Monitor weight to detect inadequate nutrition if the patient's intake is poor. Small feedings may be better tolerated. Provide a pleasant mealtime environment.

Patient Teaching

Hyperparathyroidism

- Take drugs exactly as ordered and report adverse effects to the physician.
- Eat a balanced diet with moderate calcium and high fluid intake. Notify the physician of bloody urine or pain in the kidney area or groin.
- Increase fluid intake to the amount recommended by the physician.

Postoperative Care

After parathyroidectomy, the patient requires the same care as any surgical patient, as detailed in Chapter 17. Two potential complications specific to parathyroidectomy are (1) airway obstruction and (2) hypocalcemia. When the patient has a neck incision, accumulated fluid and blood in the surgical site can compress the trachea and cause airway obstruction. Monitor and document the respiratory rate and effort and the pulse rate. Increasing pulse and respiratory rates, especially accompanied by restlessness, suggest inadequate oxygenation. The surgeon should be notified of any indications of respiratory distress. Keep an emergency tracheostomy tray on hand in the event of acute airway obstruction.

A second possible cause of airway obstruction is related to severe hypocalcemia. Be alert for tetany, a symptom of hypocalcemia, caused by the postoperative decrease in PTH. A tingling sensation around the mouth and in the fingers is an early symptom of tetany. It may progress to severe muscle spasms or cramps and even to laryngospasm. To prevent this from happening, calcium and other electrolytes are monitored closely in the postoperative period. Promptly inform the RN or physician of signs of tetany or abnormal electrolyte values. Tetany is treated with oral or intravenous calcium supplements. Treatment of hypocalcemia is discussed in detail in the subsequent "Hypoparathyroidism" section.

Sometimes the procedure can be performed in an outpatient setting using endoscopy. The incisions created by an endoscopic surgical procedure are small. After the procedure, inspect the dressing and the back of the patient's neck for bleeding. Elevate the patient's head to help reduce swelling. When a classic approach is used, the incision may be on the front of the neck, the upper chest, or both and usually is covered with a bulky pressure dressing. As with the thyroidectomy patient, this patient's suture line should be protected from stress. Show the patient how to support the head when changing positions.

HYPOPARATHYROIDISM

Hypoparathyroidism is a deficiency of PTH. It is an uncommon condition, usually caused by unintentional removal of or damage to parathyroid glands during surgery. Primary hypoparathyroidism can be caused by an autoimmune process and by several conditions, including Wilson disease (copper overload). Inadequate secretion of PTH leads to hypocalcemia. Severe hypocalcemia can progress to convulsions and respiratory obstruction because of spasms of the larynx. Laryngospasm can be fatal.

Clinical Manifestations

The possibility of parathyroid dysfunction requires close monitoring after thyroid surgery. Trauma or accidental removal of one or more parathyroid glands may lead to symptoms of hypoparathyroidism, as discussed in the section titled "Nursing Care of the Patient Having a Thyroidectomy."

Signs and symptoms of hypocalcemia are painful muscle cramps, fatigue and weakness, tingling and twitching of the face and hands, mental and emotional changes, dry skin, and urinary frequency. With severe hypocalcemia, the patient may have difficulty breathing, convulsions, and cardiac dysrhythmias.

Medical Diagnosis

The diagnosis of hypoparathyroidism is based on patient signs and symptoms and blood studies. Typical findings include low serum calcium, elevated serum phosphate, low urine calcium, and sometimes low serum magnesium. Two classic signs of hypocalcemia that support a diagnosis of hypoparathyroidism are Chvostek sign and Trousseau sign (see Fig. 49.2).

Medical Treatment

Mild hypocalcemia may be treated with oral calcium salts. Severe hypocalcemia is treated with intravenous calcium salts. Acute hypoparathyroidism is sometimes treated with parenteral PTH, which is not practical for chronic management. Other electrolyte imbalances must be treated as well.

On a long-term basis, the patient with chronic hypoparathyroidism is treated with oral calcium salts and a form of vitamin D, most often calcitriol. Chronic hypoparathyroidism that is normally well controlled may be affected when the patient is under severe stress or is very ill. If the patient is unable to take oral calcium, hypocalcemia can develop quickly. Temporary intravenous calcium may be needed.

Pharmacology Capsule

Lifelong calcium supplementation is required to treat chronic hypoparathyroidism.

◆ NURSING CARE OF THE PATIENT WITH HYPOPARATHYROIDISM

Focused Assessment

Assessment of the patient with an endocrine disorder is summarized in Chapter 47, Box 47.1. When the patient has hypoparathyroidism, be especially alert for signs and symptoms of neuromuscular irritability: paresthesia (numbness) of fingers, toes, area around mouth; tetany, muscle cramps, carpopedal spasm; positive Chvostek and Trousseau signs; seizures; laryngospasm; and bronchospasm.

Patient Problems, Goals, and Outcome Criteria: Hypoparathyroidism

Patient Problems	Goals and Outcome Criteria
Potential for injury related to hypocalcemia	Decreased risk for injury: serum calcium level within normal limits; no muscle spasms, convulsions, or respiratory distress; negative Chvostek and Trousseau signs
Decreased cardiac output related to dysrhythmias and heart failure (HF) secondary to hypocalcemia	Normal cardiac output: normal pulse rate and rhythm, normal blood pressure (BP), no dyspnea or edema

Interventions

Administer drugs as ordered for hypoparathyroidism and hypocalcemia. When administering calcium salts intravenously, monitor the infusion site carefully because the leakage of calcium salts into body tissues causes inflammation. The infusion site should be changed if extravasation occurs. Frequently assess the patient for signs and symptoms of calcium imbalances. Hypocalcemia may appear as a result of inadequate calcium supplementation. Hypercalcemia can result from excessive calcium intake.

If there has been any recent seizure activity or if the patient shows severe neuromuscular irritability, follow seizure precautions. Any signs of respiratory distress may suggest laryngospasm and should be documented and reported to the surgeon immediately. Monitor the pulse and BP to detect dysrhythmias and HF. Report cardiac irregularities, edema, and dyspnea to the physician.

Teach patients with chronic hypoparathyroidism the signs and symptoms of calcium imbalances and provide instructions for self-medication. Advise them to carry medical identification cards to alert health care providers to the disorder in the event of an emergency.

Get Ready for the NCLEX® Examination!

Key Points

- Hyperthyroidism is the abnormally increased production of thyroid hormones that may be treated with antithyroid drugs, surgery, or radiation therapy.
- Nursing care of the patient with hyperthyroidism may address sleep disturbance, heat intolerance, inadequate nutrition, decreased cardiac output, potential for injury, and diarrhea.
- Nursing care after thyroidectomy is concerned with potential for airway obstruction, decreased cardiac output, altered body image, pain, and potential for infection.
- Hypothyroidism is inadequate secretion of thyroid hormones that is treated with hormone replacement therapy.
- Nursing care of the patient with hypothyroidism addresses decreased activity tolerance, inadequate nutrition, cold intolerance, constipation, potential for disrupted tissue integrity, decreased cardiac output, altered body image, and inability to manage self-care.
- Goiter is enlargement of the thyroid gland that may be associated with hypothyroidism or hyperthyroidism.
- Hyperparathyroidism raises the serum calcium level and may cause bone demineralization and obstruction of kidney tubules.
- Nursing care of the patient with hyperparathyroidism focuses on decreased activity tolerance, potential for injury, potential for urinary obstruction, constipation, lack of knowledge, and inadequate nutrition.
- Hypoparathyroidism, a deficiency of PTH that sometimes follows thyroidectomy, causes the serum calcium level to fall, producing neuromuscular irritability that can progress to seizures, cardiac dysrhythmias, and laryngospasm.
- Patient problems for the patient with hypoparathyroidism are potential for injury and decreased cardiac output.

Additional Learning Resources

SG Go to your Study Guide for additional learning activities to help you master this chapter content.

Go to your Evolve website (http://evolve.elsevier.com/Linton/medsurg) for the following learning resources and much more:

- Fluid & Electrolyte Tutorial
- Review Questions for the NCLEX® Examination

Clinical Judgment and Next-Generation NCLEX® Examination-Style Questions

1. Which of the following statements made by a patient who is being treated for hypothyroidism indicates the need for additional teaching? (Select all that apply.)

1. I need to take my levothyroxine only when I feel unusually tired.
2. Shortness of breath is a sign of too much levothyroxine.
3. Levothyroxine can cause me to have a rapid heart rate.
4. I will only need levothyroxine until my thyroid gland returns to normal.
5. I should take my levothyroxine about the same time each day.

NCLEX Client Need: Physiological Integrity: Pharmacological Therapies.

2. You are notified that a patient with severe hypothyroidism is being admitted to your nursing unit. Which of the following action(s) is/are appropriate?

1. Obtain an emergency tracheostomy tray
2. Close the blinds to dim the light in the room
3. Have extra blankets put in the room
4. Pad the side rails on the bed
5. Set the room temperature to 68°F

NCLEX Client Need: Physiological Integrity: Basic Care and Comfort

3. Which of the following findings are most likely in a patient with severe hyperthyroidism? (Select all that apply.)

1. Respiratory rate of 12 breaths per minute
2. Heart rate of 120 beats per minute
3. Fine tremors of the hands
4. BP of 160/90 mm Hg
5. Oral temperature of 96°F

NCLEX Client Need: Physiological Integrity: Physiological Adaptation

4. **You observe that a hyperthyroid patient has prominent, bulging eyeballs. What term is used to describe this condition? ________________________**

   NCLEX Client Need: Physiological Integrity: Physiological Adaptation

5. **A course of treatment with methimazole is prescribed for a patient who is scheduled for a thyroidectomy. The patient asks why she has to take this medication. Which of the following is the best response?**
   1. "Methimazole will help you to eliminate excess thyroid hormone."
   2. "It reduces your thyroid activity, which makes surgery safer for you."
   3. "Methimazole will provide replacement thyroid hormones after your thyroid gland is removed."
   4. "This drug will cause your thyroid gland to shrink, which will reduce pressure on your airway."

   NCLEX Client Need: Physiological Integrity: Pharmacological Therapies

6. **SLO/Objective: Assist in the development of nursing care plans for patients with disorders of the thyroid gland.**

   NGN Item Type: Enhanced Hot Spot

   Cognitive Skill: Recognize Cues

   A 33-year-old woman comes into the postoperative care unit following a thyroidectomy for treatment of thyroid cancer. The nurse documents these findings one hour later:
   - Heart rate 90 beats per minute and regular
   - Respiration rate 28 breaths per minute
   - BP 136/86 mm Hg
   - Dressing dry and intact
   - Oxygen saturation 92%
   - Drowsy but responsive
   - Reports feeling pressure on neck

   Highlight or place a check mark next to the assessment findings that require follow up by the nurse.

   NCLEX Client Need: Physiological Integrity: Reduction of Risk Potential

7. **Which of the following is the purpose of measuring serum thyroglobulin in a patient who has had thyroid cancer?**
   1. To determine adequacy of thyroid hormone replacement
   2. To detect any recurrence of the thyroid cancer
   3. To see whether all radioisotopes have been eliminated
   4. To determine whether parathyroid function is normal

   NCLEX Client Need: Physiological Integrity: Reduction of Risk Potential

8. **A patient who is hypoparathyroid after thyroidectomy asks what the parathyroids do and why she needs calcium. Which of the following statements by the nurse accurately describe the relationship between PTH and serum calcium? (Select all that apply.)**
   1. The secretion of PTH increases when serum calcium is low.
   2. Increased secretion of PTH causes the kidneys to retain calcium.
   3. Chronically decreased PTH can lead to bone demineralization.
   4. Decreased serum PTH causes calcium to shift from the bones to the blood.
   5. PTH regulates the level of calcium in the blood.

   NCLEX Client Need: Physiological Integrity: Physiological Adaptation

9. **A patient had a parathyroid adenoma removed 3 days ago. She is now complaining of muscle cramps in her hands and feet. Which of the following should you suspect?**
   1. Poor circulation
   2. Thyroid storm
   3. Hypocalcemia
   4. Metabolic acidosis

   NCLEX Client Need: Physiological Integrity: Physiological Adaptation

10. **Nursing implications for administering iodide solutions to a patient include which of the following?**
    1. Dilute in milk or juice and provide a straw
    2. Take the patient's pulse and BP before each dose
    3. Tell the patient to report any changes in hearing acuity
    4. Carefully maintain accurate intake and output records

    NCLEX Client Need: Physiological Integrity: Pharmacological Therapies

Diabetes and Hypoglycemia

50

http://evolve.elsevier.com/Linton/medsurg

Objectives

1. Explain the pathophysiology, clinical manifestations, complications, diagnostic tests, and treatment of diabetes mellitus and hypoglycemia.
2. Explain the difference between type 1 and type 2 diabetes mellitus.
3. Describe the role of insulin in the body.
4. Differentiate between acute hypoglycemia and diabetic ketoacidosis.
5. Describe the treatment of a patient experiencing acute hypoglycemia or diabetic ketoacidosis.
6. Identify nursing interventions for a patient diagnosed with diabetes mellitus or hypoglycemia.
7. Assist in developing a nursing care plan for patients with diabetes mellitus, hypoglycemia, or ketoacidosis.

Key Terms

endogenous (ĕn-DŎJ-ĕn-ŭs)
exogenous (ĕks-ŎJ-ĕn-ŭs)
glycosuria (glī-kō-SŪ-rē-ă)
hyperglycemia (hī-pĕr-glī-SĒ-mē-ă)
hypoglycemia (hī-pō-glī-SĒ-mē-ă)
ketoacidosis (kē-tō-ă-sĭ-DŌ-sĭs)
ketone bodies (KĒ-tōn)
lipoatrophy (lĭp-ō-ĂT-rō-fē)
lipohypertrophy (lĭp-ō-hī-PĔR-trō-fē)
macrovascular (MĂK-rō-văs-cū-lăr)
microvascular (MĪK- rō-văs-cū-lăr)
nephropathy (nĕ-FRŎP-ă-thē)
neuropathy (nū-RŎP-ĕ-thē)
polydipsia (pŏl-ē-DĬP-sē-ă)
polyphagia (pŏl-ē-FĂ-jē-ă)
polyuria (pŏl-ē-Ū-rē-ă)
retinopathy (rĕt-ĭ-NŎP-ă-thē)

DIABETES MELLITUS

Symptoms of diabetes mellitus (DM) have been reported in the literature throughout history, but the cause was not identified until the early 20th century. In an experiment, the pancreata of several sheep were removed, resulting in the development of diabetes. Through this experiment, insulin and the role it plays in the body was discovered. The search then began for a way to provide insulin to people whose bodies did not produce enough. Before insulin became available for commercial use in 1921, people with diabetes were placed on high-protein diets until they went into acidosis and died, usually a short time after the onset of the disease. The 2020 National Diabetes Statistics report from the Centers of Disease Control and Prevention (CDC) estimates that 43.2 million people in the United States have DM, which is 10.5% of the total population. This estimate includes 7.3 million people with undiagnosed diabetes. It is estimated that an additional 88 million have prediabetes (34.5% of the adult population in the United States). Diabetes remains a major health problem and the seventh leading cause of death by disease. People with diabetes are at increased risk for heart disease, renal disease, blindness, amputation, and complications during pregnancy. Fortunately, with early diagnosis and better management, it is possible to reduce the risk of serious complications.

PATHOPHYSIOLOGY

DM is a chronic disorder characterized by impaired metabolism and by vascular and neurologic complications. A key feature of diabetes is elevated blood glucose, called **hyperglycemia**. The blood glucose level is normally regulated by insulin, a hormone produced by the beta cells in the islets of Langerhans located in the pancreas. In healthy individuals, small amounts of insulin are secreted continuously (basal secretion) into the bloodstream. The ingestion of carbohydrates triggers the secretion of a larger volume of insulin (bolus secretion). Insulin that is produced in one's own body is called **endogenous**, meaning that it is produced internally. Insulin that is obtained from other sources and administered to a person is called **exogenous**, meaning that it comes from an external source.

DM is classified as *type 1* or *type 2*. Both types have a genetic component, but many people with diabetes have no genetic predisposition.

Type 1 DM, characterized by the absence of endogenous insulin, was previously called *juvenile-onset diabetes* because it occurs most commonly in juveniles and young adults. However, it can also occur in middle-aged and older adults. There is a debate on whether this is because of a progression of autoimmune disease, and the term latent autoimmune diabetes in adults (LADA) may be used instead of type 1 diabetes. Regardless, type 1 diabetes is an autoimmune process, possibly triggered by a viral infection that causes destruction of the beta cells, the development of insulin antibodies, and the production of islet cell antibodies (ICAs). People with type 1 diabetes require exogenous insulin for the rest of their lives.

Type 2 DM, previously referred to as *noninsulin-dependent diabetes mellitus (NIDDM),* is characterized by inadequate endogenous insulin and the body's inability to use insulin properly. Initially, blood glucose rises but beta cells do not respond with adequate insulin, resulting in chronically elevated blood glucose. The continuous high glucose level in the blood desensitizes the beta cells so that they become progressively less responsive to the elevated glucose. A second problem is that specific insulin receptor sites become insensitive to insulin (i.e., "insulin resistance"). So, despite the presence of some insulin, glucose is unable to enter the cells where it is needed for normal function. Although type 2 DM is more common among adults, it is increasingly found in children as well. One inherited form is maturity-onset diabetes of the young (MODY) or monogenic diabetes, which causes type 2 DM among all age groups in affected families.

Type 2 DM may be controlled by diet and exercise alone or may require oral hypoglycemic agents or exogenous insulin. Some patients are treated with insulin initially to normalize blood glucose and then are treated with diet, exercise, and perhaps oral agents.

Gestational diabetes mellitus (GDM) is diagnosed when a woman is found to have glucose intolerance for the first time during pregnancy. After delivery, the condition resolves. (See a maternity nursing text for information on the management of GDM.)

Role of Insulin

Insulin is considered a critical hormone for glucose metabolism. However, insulin is also needed for the synthesis of fatty acids and proteins (Box 50.1).

Glucose. Insulin stimulates the active transport of glucose into the cells. When insulin is absent, glucose cannot enter most cells, so it remains in the bloodstream. The blood then becomes thick with glucose, which increases the osmolality of the blood. Increased osmolality stimulates the thirst center, causing the patient to experience **polydipsia** (i.e., excessive thirst) and take in additional fluid. The increased fluid does not pass into body tissues, however, because the high serum osmolality retains the fluid in the bloodstream. As the blood passes through the kidneys, some excess glucose is eliminated. The osmotic force created by the glucose draws extra fluid and electrolytes with it, causing abnormally increased urine volume (**polyuria**).

Box 50.1 Insulin: Actions and Effects of Deficiency

INSULIN

- Increases the transport of glucose into the resting muscle cell
- Regulates the rate at which carbohydrates are used
- Promotes the conversion of glucose to glycogen
- Inhibits the conversion of glycogen to glucose
- Promotes fatty acid synthesis
- Spares fat
- Inhibits the breakdown of adipose tissue
- Inhibits the conversion of fats to glucose
- Stimulates protein synthesis in the tissues
- Inhibits the conversion of protein into glucose

LACK OF INSULIN

- Stimulates the conversion of glycogen to glucose
- Permits fat stores to break down
- Increases triglyceride storage in the liver
- Halts the storage of proteins
- Causes protein to be dumped into the bloodstream

Because most cells are not able to use glucose without insulin, stored fat is broken down to provide fuel for heat and energy. Tissue breakdown and loss of lean body mass send hunger signals to the hypothalamus. The patient experiences excessive hunger (**polyphagia**). The patient may take in more food, but unfortunately the cells of the body cannot use the extra glucose without insulin. Weight loss often occurs despite increased appetite and food ingestion.

Insulin is needed to transport glucose into resting muscle cells. During heavy exercise, however, muscle fibers are highly permeable to glucose even in the absence of insulin. Therefore exercise must be considered in the regulation of serum glucose levels. Other tissues that can use glucose without insulin are the brain, nerves, heart, and lens of the eye.

Insulin regulates the rate of glucose metabolism. The more insulin released, the faster carbohydrates are metabolized. In a healthy person, when blood glucose falls, insulin production is inhibited and stored glycogen is converted to glucose by a process called *glycogenolysis.* When blood glucose rises, insulin production is stimulated and the glycogenolysis is inhibited. This process usually maintains the blood glucose within a normal range. However, when insulin secretion is inadequate, glycogenolysis continues to elevate the blood glucose in an attempt to nourish glucose-starved tissues, but the cells cannot use the glucose.

Fatty acids. Insulin promotes fatty acid synthesis and the conversion of fatty acids into fat, which is stored as adipose tissue. Insulin spares fat by inhibiting the breakdown of adipose tissue and the mobilization of fat. It also inhibits the conversion of fats to fatty acids and glycerol.

Without adequate insulin, fat stores break down and increased triglycerides are stored in the liver. Increased fatty acids in the liver can triple the production of lipoproteins, which promotes the development of atherosclerosis. This helps to explain why people with DM have a high incidence of cardiovascular disease.

Protein. Insulin enhances protein synthesis in tissues and inhibits the conversion of protein into glucose. Amino acids are allowed into cells, which enhances the rate of protein formation while preventing the degradation of proteins. Without adequate insulin, the storage of proteins halts and large amounts of amino acids are dumped into the bloodstream. High levels of plasma amino acids place people with diabetes at risk for development of gout. Changes in protein metabolism lead to extreme weakness and poor organ functioning.

CAUSE OF DIABETES MELLITUS

Type 1 DM has been attributed to genetic, immunologic, and environmental (i.e., viruses, toxins) factors. The tendency toward type 1 DM is found in families with a genetic predisposition. Evidence of a strong genetic component in type 2 DM is seen as well.

It is possible that an autoimmune disorder triggers the sudden onset of diabetes. Our bodies are guarded by an elaborate and extensive immune system. When foreign antigens enter the body, several mechanisms are activated to prevent the antigen from harming tissues. Sometimes the protective mechanisms react to a person's normal tissue forming antibodies (in this case, autoantibodies) that attack and destroy the target tissue. Autoantibodies are present in most individuals that develop type 1 DM.

CLINICAL MANIFESTATIONS

Type 1 Diabetes

Type 1 diabetes is characterized by a rapid onset with "the 3 Ps": polyuria, polyphagia, and polydipsia. The mechanisms that cause these classic symptoms were described under "Pathophysiology." Weakness and fatigue are common.

Type 2 Diabetes

Whereas the onset of type 1 DM is rather dramatic, the symptoms of type 2 DM may be somewhat vague. Often patients report that they have blurred vision, fatigue, recurrent yeast infections, and slow wound healing. The "3 Ps" are less common than with type 1 DM.

RISK FACTORS

Risk factors for type 1 DM, other than genetic ones, are not known. According to the National Institute of Diabetes and Digestive and Kidney Disease (NIDDK), which is part of the National Institutes of Health (NIH), risk factors for type 2 DM include the following:

- Obesity
- Sedentary lifestyle
- Family history of diabetes
- Age 45 years and older
- History of GDM
- History of delivering infants weighing more than 9 lb
- Ethnicity derived from Alaskan Native, Native American, Asian American, Hispanic/Latino, African descent, Native Hawaiian or Pacific Islander (see the Cultural Considerations box)
- Polycystic ovary syndrome
- Cardiovascular disease and hypertension
- Presence of acanthosis nigricans (a deeply pigmented skin thickening, commonly in the neck, axilla, and groin) or other conditions associated with insulin resistance

Cultural Considerations

What Does Culture Have to Do With Diabetes?

The risk of diabetes mellitus (DM) is the highest among Native Americans and Alaskan Natives, followed closely by Hispanic and non-hispanic Black Americans. Effective measures to decrease this risk must be sensitive to cultural practices and values.

Pharmacology Capsule

Pharmacologic use of glucocorticoids can elevate the blood glucose level. Although unlikely to cause DM in people with normal pancreatic function, glucocorticoid therapy may unmask latent diabetes. It also complicates management of known DM.

Metabolic Syndrome

Metabolic syndrome is the term used to describe a syndrome that is thought by many to be a precursor to diabetes. This syndrome is also referred to as *syndrome X*, *insulin resistance syndrome*, and *cardiovascular dysmetabolic syndrome*. Patients with metabolic syndrome typically have:

- impaired glucose tolerance (IGT)
- high serum insulin
- hypertension
- elevated triglycerides
- low high-density lipoprotein (HDL) cholesterol
- altered size and density of low-density lipoprotein (LDL) cholesterol.

It is believed that metabolic syndrome represents a chronic low-grade inflammatory process affecting endothelial tissue (the lining of the heart, blood and lymph vessels). The long-term effects include atherosclerosis, ischemic heart disease, left ventricular hypertrophy, and sometimes type 2 DM. Research is now focused on early detection of this syndrome and interventions that might slow or arrest the progress.

COMPLICATIONS

Long-Term Complications

The duration of diabetes and poor control of blood glucose are the best predictors of the severity of complications. These complications affect almost every organ of the body. They may be classified as microvascular, macrovascular, or *neuropathic.*

Microvascular complications. **Microvascular** complications result from changes in small blood vessels that are unique to diabetes and occur in both type 1 and type 2 diabetes. The basement membrane of capillaries thickens, which impairs the exchange of nutrients, gases, and wastes. Tissues that are most vulnerable to microvascular complications are the eyes (**retinopathy**) and the kidneys (**nephropathy**). Changes in the capillaries appear to be related to persistent hyperglycemia and are aggravated by hypertension and smoking. Neuropathy is sometimes classified with microvascular complications; it is discussed later.

Retinopathy. Among people between 25 to 74 years of age, DM is the leading cause of new-onset blindness. People with diabetes are at increased risk for retinopathy, cataracts, and glaucoma. *Diabetic retinopathy* is a term used to describe pathologic changes in the retina that are associated with DM. Two types of diabetic retinopathy have been identified: (1) nonproliferative and (2) proliferative. Both types may be present at the same time. Manifestations of nonproliferative disease include small hemorrhages and aneurysms in the retina, hard lipid and protein exudates that leak from the blood vessels, infarcted nerve fibers (described as "*cotton wool spots*"), and changes in retinal veins. Proliferative disease is characterized by the growth of abnormal capillaries on the retina and the optic disc. These fragile vessels can penetrate the vitreous humor and rupture. When hemorrhaging into the vitreous occurs, it becomes cloudy and vision is lost. The blood is eventually reabsorbed but scars may remain, which places traction on the retina and may result in retinal detachment.

Macular edema occurs with both types of diabetic retinopathy. The macula is the center of vision and edema causes loss of central vision. To illustrate the effect, imagine this page with only the outer margins clearly visible. The center would be clouded.

Signs and symptoms that suggest impending eye problems are the presence of spots ("floaters") in the field of vision, seeing "cobwebs," or sudden visual changes. Often no warning signs of retinal changes exist. Therefore patients with diabetes should have an eye examination at least once a year so that early changes in the eye can be detected and measures taken to try to prevent further deterioration and possible blindness. One strategy that may reduce the risk of injury to the eye is control of hypertension. Early laser treatment of macular edema can halt the progression of retinopathy and may even improve vision.

Nephropathy. Diabetes is the most common cause of end-stage renal disease (ESRD) in the United States. It is estimated that almost 36% of individuals diagnosed with DM also have chronic kidney disease. Black Americans, Native Americans, and Hispanic Americans have a 4 to 6 times greater risk for developing ESRD (see the Cultural Considerations box). Factors that contribute to the development of nephropathy (i.e., kidney damage) include poor control of blood glucose, hypertension, long-standing diabetes, and genetic susceptibility. High concentrations of **glycosuria** (i.e., glucose in the urine), along with hypertension, gradually destroy the capillaries that supply the renal glomeruli. Increased permeability of the glomeruli permits serum proteins to be lost in the urine. No symptoms are seen in the early stages, but rising microalbuminuria (i.e., small amounts of albumin in the urine) signals the onset of kidney damage. When the level of protein in the urine exceeds 300 mg per day of albumin or 500 mg per day of total protein, the condition will likely progress to ESRD. Signs and symptoms of kidney failure include persistent proteinuria, elevated blood pressure (BP) and serum creatinine, hematuria, and oliguria or anuria. Diagnosis is based on laboratory values (see Chapters 41 and 42).

Cultural Considerations

What Does Culture Have to Do With Nephropathy?

Genetic factors increase the risk for nephropathy among Black Americans, Native Americans, Hispanics, and Asian Americans.

Measures to reduce the risk of damage to the kidneys include good glycemic control, control of hypertension, use of angiotensin-converting enzyme (ACE) inhibitors or angiotensin receptor blockers (ARBs), maintaining good hydration, and avoiding nephrotoxic chemicals, including drugs. Modest protein restriction may be recommended. Screening for microalbuminuria can detect early renal changes that may be reversible. Early detection and treatment may slow the development and progression of ESRD.

Macrovascular complications. Atherosclerotic plaque development occurs earlier and is more severe and more extensive in people with diabetes than in other people. Atherosclerosis affects the peripheral, carotid, cerebral, and coronary blood vessels. The accelerated atherosclerotic changes associated with diabetes are called **macrovascular** *complications*.

Chronic hyperglycemia as a result of poor blood glucose control may play an important role in the premature development of atherosclerosis in patients with diabetes. However, evidence indicates that the elevated insulin levels occurring with insulin resistance also play a role in the development of atherosclerosis. This is especially apparent in White middle-aged men. Hyperinsulinemia damages the endothelium of blood vessels, permitting lipids to be easily deposited on the cell walls of the blood vessels. Other risk factors for macrovascular complications are central obesity, hyperlipidemia, hypertension, genetics, sedentary lifestyle, and smoking.

Macrovascular changes are associated with coronary heart disease (CHD); cerebrovascular accidents (CVAs), or stroke; and peripheral vascular disease (PVD). The risk for heart disease, stroke, and PVD is 2 to 4 times higher for individuals with diabetes. Because of these risks, aspirin therapy may be considered for individuals with diabetes. Signs and symptoms of PVD may include diminished pedal pulses and claudication (i.e., pain in the calf, back, or buttocks while walking). When arteries in the lower extremities can no longer deliver oxygen (O_2) and nutrients to peripheral tissues, gangrene may develop, necessitating amputation of affected parts of extremities.

Treatment for macrovascular disease is directed toward weight loss and exercise. Patients who smoke are strongly encouraged to quit because of vasoconstriction caused by nicotine. With weight loss, insulin uptake improves and circulating insulin levels decrease. As a result of aerobic exercise, insulin receptor sites become more sensitive and serum insulin levels decrease. Exercise, in conjunction with weight loss, reduces the amount of exogenous insulin needed. Because it is thought that exogenous insulin may create immune complexes that damage arterial walls, reduced exogenous insulin needs may reduce the risk for macrovascular disease in DM.

For additional information about CHD, CVA, and PVD, see Chapters 23, 34, and 35.

Neuropathic complications. Pathologic changes in nerve tissue, called **neuropathy**, are related to poor glucose control, ischemic lesions of nerves, and chemical changes in peripheral nerve cells. Almost 30% of individuals with diabetes over 40 years of age have impaired sensation in at least one area of the foot. It is estimated that 50% of individuals with diabetes have some form of neuropathy. Neuropathy can be classified as *mononeuropathy*, *polyneuropathy*, or *autonomic neuropathy*.

Mononeuropathy. Mononeuropathy affects a single nerve or group of nerves. It results from inadequate blood supply and is experienced as sharp, stabbing pain. Pain and atrophy occur in muscles enervated by the affected nerve. Sometimes the pain is relieved by walking.

Polyneuropathy. Polyneuropathy involves sensory and autonomic nerves. Sensory polyneuropathy commonly affects both legs symmetrically. Symptoms range from tingling, numbness, and burning sensations to complete loss of sensation. Pain is often worse during the night. Sometimes polyneuropathy resolves spontaneously. All patients with DM should have a comprehensive foot examination annually, including testing for loss of protective sensation.

Autonomic neuropathy. Autonomic neuropathy affects the sympathetic and parasympathetic nervous systems. It can affect the pupillary response and functions of the cardiovascular, gastrointestinal (GI), and genitourinary systems. Cardiovascular involvement may be manifested as postural hypotension, resting tachycardia, exercise intolerance, and failure of the heart rate to increase with vigorous exercise. Common GI symptoms include constipation or, less commonly, diarrhea as well as anorexia, nausea, vomiting, gastric reflux, and bloating after meals. The stomach may dilate and lose muscle tone so that gastric emptying is delayed, a condition called *gastroparesis*.

The patient may have urinary problems such as an atonic bladder, in which the bladder capacity increases and eventually causes retention with overflow. Sexual problems in men such as erectile dysfunction and retrograde ejaculation are common. Women may have painful intercourse.

Diabetic amyotrophy (i.e., loss of muscle mass) causes pain in the muscles of the pelvic girdle and thighs. This pain may be so severe that it interferes with activity and sleep. The muscles look wasted, and fasciculation (i.e., involuntary twitching of muscle fibers) may be visible under the skin. These contractions do not produce movement.

Hypoglycemic unawareness. Normally, patients recognize signs and symptoms of **hypoglycemia** (i.e., abnormally low level of glucose in the blood) so that they can take corrective action. With hypoglycemic unawareness, the usual symptoms of tachycardia, palpitations, tremor, sweating, and nervousness may be absent. Without this "early warning system," the patient suddenly may have changes in mental status as the first sign of hypoglycemia. This phenomenon may be related to autonomic neuropathy.

Foot complications of diabetes. People with diabetes may have foot problems associated with neuropathy, inadequate blood supply, or a combination of both. When neurologic function is impaired but blood flow is adequate, the foot is warm and pink with good pulses but lacks normal sensation. The patient may have a foot injury but fail to recognize it in the absence of pain.

If the blood supply is impaired but neurologic function is adequate, the foot is cold but sensation is normal. When the foot is raised, it turns pale. When the foot is lowered, it becomes red. Pulses are weak or absent.

Neuropathic ulcers can result from injury to the foot caused by the following:

- Mechanical irritation, such as that caused from rough shoe linings or amateur attempts at shaving calluses or cutting toenails
- Thermal injury, such as burns caused from heat exposure such as heating pads and sitting too close to a fire or radiator
- Chemical irritation caused by substances such as salicylic acid, found in many corn plasters

Patients who cannot see or feel their feet may fail to notice injuries or dangerous situations (see the Patient

Teaching box). A neglected callus may become inflamed, allowing blood and fluid to accumulate beneath the lesion, which can create a site for infection. Poor perfusion caused by PVD can make these injuries worse. An abscess may form that ruptures to create an ulcer. Treatment is difficult and not always effective, so the best treatment is prevention. Some 60% of nontraumatic limb amputations are caused by complications of DM.

Patient Teaching

"Dos and Don'ts" Regarding Foot Care

DO

- Control your blood sugar, blood pressure, and cholesterol.
- Be physically active.
- Check your feet every day.
- Wash your feet every day.
- Test the water before putting your feet in to make sure the water is not too hot.
- Wear shoes at all times.
- Wear shoes that fit well.
- Trim your toenails across and file the edges with an emery board.
- Buy shoes at the end of the day when your feet are at their largest.
- See your physician regularly and ask them to examine your feet at each visit.

DON'T

- Smoke.
- Walk barefoot, even in the house.
- Soak your feet in hot water.
- Remove corns or calluses yourself. See a podiatrist for their removal.
- Wear shoes without socks.

For more details, see *Diabetes and Your Feet* from Centers for Disease Control and Prevention: https://www.cdc.gov/features/diabetesfoothealth/index.html.

Prevention of long-term complications. The landmark Diabetes Control and Complications Trial (DCCT) found that intensive treatment of type 1 DM delayed the onset or slowed the progress of diabetic retinopathy, nephropathy, and neuropathy. Treatment that maintained tight control of blood glucose levels used multiple daily insulin injections or programmable external insulin pumps. The United Kingdom Prospective Diabetes Study (UKPDS) demonstrated similar benefits of tight control with type 2 DM. Tight control means that the blood glucose is maintained in the normal range with carefully balanced drugs, diet, and exercise.

Despite the benefits of tight control, it does increase the risk for hypoglycemia, especially if the patient is also taking beta-blockers. Target glucose levels may need to be adjusted if frequent hypoglycemia occurs, which underlines the need for individualized treatment goals for each patient with diabetes. Other major studies have shown that intensive glucose control may increase cardiovascular complications. These studies highlight the need to individualize target glucose levels for patients with a long duration of diabetes, recurrent hypoglycemia, severe cardiovascular disease, and advanced age.

Box 50.2 Recommendations for Glycemic, Blood Pressure, and Lipid Control for Adults With Diabetes

Glycosylated hemoglobin ($HgbA_{1c}$)	<7% (more stringent goals may be appropriate for selected individuals)
Preprandial capillary plasma glucose	80–130 mg/dL
Peak postprandial capillary plasma glucose	<180 mg/dL
Blood pressure (BP)	<130/80 mm Hg for those with DM, HTN and increased CVD risk, <140/90 mm Hg for those with DM, HTN and low CVD risk
Total cholesterol	<200 mg/dL
Low-density lipoprotein (LDL) cholesterol	<100 mg/dL
High-density lipoprotein (HDL) cholesterol	>50 mg/dL
Triglycerides	<150 mg/dL

Note: More stringent lipid control is advised for individuals with multiple risk factors for cardiovascular disease.
Data from American Diabetes Association: Standards of medical care in diabetes, *Diabetes Care* 44 (suppl 1):S73–S87, 2021.

The American Diabetes Association acknowledges that other factors increase the risk for developing complications. Box 50.2 lists recommendations to reduce the risks of complications. In addition, individuals with diabetes should be given information regarding smoking cessation. Use of aspirin and ACE inhibitors is recommended for those with increased cardiovascular and renal risk factors.

Acute Emergency Complications

Acute hypoglycemia. Patients being treated with insulin or other hypoglycemics are at risk for acute hypoglycemia. Events that may trigger this dangerous drop in blood glucose include taking too much insulin, not eating enough food, not eating at the right time, and an inconsistent pattern of exercise. Other variables that lower blood glucose are gastroparesis, renal insufficiency, and certain drugs, including aspirin and beta-adrenergic blockers (see the Complementary and Alternative Therapies box). A glucose level less than 70 mg/dL is considered hypoglycemia and a level between 50 and 70 mg/dL is considered moderate hypoglycemia. However, some people with hypoglycemia unawareness have been known to have serum glucose levels below 50 mg/dL without signs and symptoms.

Complementary and Alternative Therapies

Among the many herbal supplements that may lower blood glucose are dandelion, onion, garlic, and ginseng. Patients should consult with their physician if they consider using these products.

The signs and symptoms of hypoglycemia are classified as *adrenergic* and *neuroglucopenic.* Adrenergic symptoms appear first and reflect the response of the nervous system to inadequate glucose for cell function. These symptoms are shakiness, nervousness, irritability, tachycardia, anxiety, lightheadedness, hunger, tingling or numbness of the lips or tongue, and diaphoresis. Beta-adrenergic blockers may mask the adrenergic symptoms of hypoglycemia, delaying the diagnosis and treatment of hypoglycemia.

If treatment is delayed, a second set of symptoms may appear. These symptoms are called *neuroglucopenia* or *neuroglycopenia* because they are caused by a shortage of glucose to the brain. If the glucose level has fallen rapidly, however, these symptoms may be the first signs of hypoglycemia. They include drowsiness, irritability, impaired judgment, blurred vision, slurred speech, headaches, and mood swings progressing to disorientation, seizures, and unconsciousness. Even more severe hypoglycemia progresses to loss of consciousness, convulsions, coma, and death. It is important to remember that individuals who are experiencing severe hypoglycemia may not be able to recognize and treat the hypoglycemia without assistance.

Treatment. To treat hypoglycemia, follow the 15/15 rule. Give the conscious patient 15 g of quick-acting carbohydrate, wait 15 minutes, and retest the blood glucose. Examples of 15 g carbohydrate:

- 4 oz of undiluted orange or apple juice or soft drink (not sugar-free)
- 8 oz of skim milk
- 1 tablespoon of sugar, honey, or syrup
- 4 to 5 Life Savers or other hard candies
- 3 to 4 glucose tablets or 15 g of glucose gel

Repeat every 15 to 30 minutes until the blood glucose is above 80 mg/dL for adults and above 80 to 100 mg/dL for older adults and children. Once the blood glucose level returns to normal, a meal or snack should be consumed to prevent recurrence of hypoglycemia.

Individuals who are taking insulin should always have injectable glucagon on hand. If the patient is unable to swallow, an intramuscular or subcutaneous injection of 1 mg of glucagon or an intravenous dose of 50 mL of 50% dextrose should be given as ordered or per protocol. On regaining consciousness, the patient should be given an additional treatment of some form of glucose. If it will be 1 hour or more until the next meal, give the patient some form of complex carbohydrate and protein, such as a slice of cheese or meat with crackers.

Diabetic ketoacidosis. Diabetic **ketoacidosis** (DKA) is a life-threatening emergency caused by insulin deficiency in addition to elevated glucagon, catecholamines, cortisol, and growth hormone (GH). This results in disorders in the metabolism of carbohydrates, fats, and proteins. The sequence of events is as follows:

1. Tissues cannot use glucose without insulin, resulting in an increase in serum glucose levels.
2. Excess glucose entering the renal tubules increases osmotic pressure. This results in the reabsorption of water, increasing urine output (i.e., osmotic diuresis). As glucose is eliminated in the kidneys, so are large amounts of water and electrolytes.
3. The patient voids large amounts of dilute urine (i.e., polyuria).
4. To make matters worse, the sympathetic nervous system responds to the cellular need for fuel by converting glycogen to glucose and manufacturing additional glucose.
5. As glycogen stores are depleted, the body begins to burn fat and protein for energy.
6. The breakdown of fat and protein for energy produces acidic substances called **ketone bodies**. As the ketones accumulate, the pH of the blood decreases and results in severe acidosis, which can be fatal.
7. Protein metabolism results in the loss of lean muscle mass and a negative nitrogen balance (the amount of nitrogen being excreted is greater than the amount of nitrogen ingested).

Early signs and symptoms of DKA are anorexia, headache, and fatigue. As the condition progresses, the classic symptoms of polydipsia, polyuria, and polyphagia develop. If untreated, the patient becomes dehydrated, weak, and lethargic with abdominal pain, nausea, vomiting, fruity breath (because of ketone production), increased respiratory rate, tachycardia, blurred vision, and hypothermia. Late signs are air hunger (seen as Kussmaul respirations: rapid and deep), coma, and shock. Death can result if prompt medical care is not instituted.

The patient with ketoacidosis has hyperglycemia (≥300 mg/dL), ketonuria, and acidosis, with a pH of less than 7.3 or a bicarbonate level of less than 15 mEq/L.

The mortality rate is 2% to 5% for DKA, and DKA accounts for half of all deaths in diabetes patients younger than 24 years of age. It is most likely to occur when diabetes is undiagnosed; when the patient does not take enough insulin; when the patient with uncontrolled type 1 DM exercises too vigorously; or when the patient experiences stress linked to illness, infection, surgery, or emotions. Some drugs such as corticosteroids, sympathomimetics, and thiazide diuretics can also raise serum glucose. In about one-quarter of patients with DKA, no cause is identified. Early identification of DKA and prompt treatment are aimed at correction of the three main problems: (1) dehydration, (2) electrolyte imbalance, and (3) acidosis.

Dehydration. The patient with ketoacidosis may have lost a large volume of fluid as the result of vomiting, polyuria, and hyperventilation. Volume deficits may be estimated at 100 mL/kg of body weight. In addition to the risk of shock because of depleted blood volume, the patient is at risk for development of blood clots.

The first need is to replace the fluid, which will aid the kidneys in eliminating excess glucose. The physician usually orders 1000 mL of normal saline to run over the first hour, followed by an additional 2000 to 8000 mL of intravenous fluids for the next 24 hours. If the patient has hypertension or hypernatremia or is at risk for heart failure (HF), 0.45% saline solution may be ordered instead of normal saline. In addition, the rate and total amount of fluid may be decreased in older patients who may not tolerate rapid changes in fluid volume.

Electrolyte imbalance. The electrolyte of primary concern in ketoacidosis is potassium. Potassium shifts out of the cells, causing transient (temporary) hyperkalemia. The hyperkalemia associated with hyperglycemia should be treated with fluid replacement and insulin administration. Medications (e.g., cation-exchange resins) should not be used to lower potassium levels. As the patient is rehydrated and normal urine output is reestablished, potassium is lost in the urine. Also, insulin replacement enhances the movement of potassium from the extracellular compartment back into the cells. During this time, the patient is at risk for developing severe hypokalemia that can cause life-threatening cardiac dysrhythmias.

Replacement of potassium is initiated only after adequate urine output is established. During potassium replacement, you must monitor the patient closely. Large doses of potassium may be required even though the serum potassium level is normal at the onset of treatment, because the plasma level will drop during treatment. Because potassium is irritating to the veins and a potassium drip must be carefully regulated, it is better to run the intravenous fluid containing potassium by the piggyback method at a prescribed rate, which is slower than the hydration rate. Remember that potassium must always be diluted before intravenous administration.

Sodium deficiency is generally corrected by infusion of normal saline. Phosphate, magnesium, and calcium levels should also be monitored. Once therapy begins, phosphate and magnesium may fall and calcium can rise to dangerous levels.

Pharmacology Capsule

When a patient is given insulin to treat diabetic ketoacidosis (DKA), monitor for hypokalemia because insulin causes potassium to move from the extracellular fluid into the cells.

Acidosis. Ketoacidosis is a problem primarily with type 1 DM. It occurs when ketone bodies accumulate as the result of the breakdown of fats for energy associated with inadequate insulin. In addition, ketoacidosis can occur in individuals with type 2 DM when severe hyperglycemia is associated with another acute condition, such as sepsis or a myocardial infarction.

Ketoacidosis is treated with the slow intravenous infusion of insulin. When the serum glucose level reaches 250 to 300 mg/dL, dextrose solution is added. The intravenous insulin is given continuously or as a bolus until subcutaneous insulin can be given or else the patient may become ketoacidotic again. The serum glucose level returns to normal several hours before the serum bicarbonate level. As long as the serum glucose level is normal but the serum bicarbonate level remains abnormal, the insulin drip must be maintained and glucose level corrected. More glucose is added to the intravenous fluid to cover the insulin. Normal levels of glucose do not mean that the acidosis has been corrected. The insulin drip must be maintained until the serum bicarbonate is 15 to 18 mEq/L. When the patient is able to eat and all laboratory values are normal, subcutaneous insulin can be given and the insulin drip discontinued.

Pharmacology Capsule

For continuous intravenous infusion, insulin is usually diluted in a 100-mL bag of solution. Because insulin binds with plastic, flush plastic tubing with the intravenous solution before adding insulin to the solution.

Hyperosmolar hyperglycemic nonketotic syndrome. Hyperosmolar hyperglycemic nonketotic syndrome (HHNS) is a condition in which a patient goes into a coma from extremely high glucose levels (≥600 mg/dL) but no evidence exists of elevated ketones. With HHNS, the patient's pancreas produces just enough insulin to prevent the breakdown of fatty acids and the formation of ketones but not enough insulin to prevent hyperglycemia. Mortality rates for HHNS are as high as 15%.

The basic defect is the lack of effective insulin or the inability to use available insulin. The patient's persistent hyperglycemia causes osmotic diuresis, resulting in the loss of fluid and electrolytes. To maintain osmotic equilibrium, fluid shifts from the intracellular fluid space to the extracellular space. Dehydration and hypernatremia develop. Dehydration and neurologic changes may be more pronounced with HHNS than with DKA. Patients with HHNS do not experience GI symptoms, nor do they experience Kussmaul respirations because they lack significant lactic acid levels. These patients often tolerate polyuria and polydipsia for weeks before seeking treatment. For some patients, HHNS is the first sign of diabetes. Others have been previously diagnosed with borderline diabetes.

HHNS may be caused by the same factors that trigger ketoacidosis. It can also be brought about by total parenteral nutrition (TPN) or dialysis. In both of these procedures, intravenous solutions that contain large amounts of glucose are administered to the patient.

Because the digestive system is bypassed, no stimulus triggers the pancreas to release insulin. Treatment of HHNS is similar to the treatment of DKA, except for the fact that no ketoacidosis is associated with HHNS. Older patients should be monitored carefully for signs of fluid overload during the rehydration phase of treatment.

MEDICAL DIAGNOSIS

The diagnosis of DM is based on serum glucose levels. Normal fasting serum glucose levels are between 70 and 100 mg/dL. The most recent official criteria for a diagnosis of DM were published in 2017 by the Expert Committee on the Diagnosis and Classification of Diabetes Mellitus. A patient who meets one or more of the following criteria on two separate occasions is considered to have DM:

1. Fasting serum glucose level 126 mg/dL or more (after at least an 8-hour fast)
2. A_{1c} 6.5% or more. The test should be performed in a laboratory using a method that is certified by the National Glycohemoglobin Standardization Program (NGSB) and standardized to the DCCT assay.
3. Symptoms of diabetes (polyuria, polydipsia, polyphagia, unexplained weight loss) plus random glucose level 200 mg/dL or more. (A random reading is based on a blood sample drawn any time of day without regard to mealtimes.)
4. Two-hour postprandial glucose level 200 mg/dL or more during an oral glucose tolerance test (OGTT) under specific guidelines. (The test must use a glucose load of 75 g of anhydrous glucose dissolved in water.)

Prediabetes

Individuals with impaired fasting glucose (IFG), impaired glucose tolerance (IGT), or both are referred to as having *prediabetes.* IFG and IGT are risk factors for developing diabetes and cardiovascular disease. The individuals should receive education on weight reduction and increasing physical activity. Diagnostic criteria for prediabetes include:

- IFG: fasting plasma glucose level from 100 to 125 mg/dL
- IGT: 2-hour plasma glucose between 140 and 199 mg/dL during OGTT
- A_{1c}: 5.7% to 6.4%

Testing for diabetes or prediabetes should begin at at 45 years of age and sooner for those with risk factors such as obesity, high risk ethnicity, first degree relative with diabetes, history of CVD or HTN, and for women with polycystic ovary syndrome.

MEDICAL TREATMENT

The goals of managing diabetes are to normalize the blood glucose, serum lipids, and body weight while meeting energy needs and achieving healthy body weight.

Nutritional Management

Medical nutrition therapy (MNT) is an important part of diabetes management and should be included in diabetes self-management education (see the Nutrition Considerations box). Because of the complexity of nutritional management, a registered dietitian should be part of the diabetes management team and the individual with diabetes should be included in decision making. According to the ADA 2021 Standards of Medical Care in Diabetes, the goals of MNT are the following:

1. Support and promote healthy eating patterns including nutrient-dense foods in appropriate portions to:
   - Achieve and maintain body weight goals
   - Attain individualized glycemic, blood pressure, and lipid goals
   - Delay or prevent the complications of diabetes.
2. Address individual nutritional needs while considering lifestyle, personal and cultural preferences, and the willingness to change.
3. Maintain the pleasure of eating by limiting food choices only when indicated by scientific evidence.
4. Provide practical tools for developing healthy eating habits rather than focusing on individual macro/micronutrients or foods.
5. Provide self-management training for safe exercise, including prevention and treatment of hypoglycemia and management during acute illness.

Nutrition Considerations

1. Diet is an essential component in the management of type 1 and type 2 diabetes mellitus (DM).
2. The goal of the diabetic diet is to maintain plasma glucose as near to the normal physiologic range as possible.
3. A person who requires insulin to control DM should coordinate insulin administration with mealtime patterns.
4. Distribute food intake throughout the day to avoid large concentrations of calories, carbohydrates, and sugar.
5. Diet plans are individualized based on glucose and lipid levels, weight management goals, medical history, lifestyle, physical activity, and readiness to change.
6. When hypoglycemia is attributed to an overproduction of insulin in response to carbohydrate ingestion, a low-carbohydrate, high-protein diet with smaller meals may control the condition.

To maintain weight, a caloric intake of 28 calories/kg of body weight is required. To reduce weight, the caloric intake is calculated based on 15 to 20 calories/kg body weight. To arrive at a person's weight in kilograms, divide the weight in pounds by 2.2. For example, if a woman weighs 110 lb, her weight in kilograms is 50 kg. To maintain her weight, she needs to consume 1540 calories daily. Diets that advocate extreme reductions in carbohydrates (<130 g/day) are not recommended for individuals with diabetes.

Several nutrition planning approaches are in use. Carbohydrate counting is particularly useful for people who use intensive insulin therapy or pumps. In addition to basal insulin requirements, bolus insulin doses are based on the total grams of carbohydrate ingested because carbohydrates have a greater effect on blood glucose levels than fat or protein. An emphasis is placed on maintaining a consistent carbohydrate intake each day but also allowing for insulin adjustments when carbohydrate intake is increased or decreased. Successful carbohydrate counting depends on understanding what foods are considered carbohydrates, how much of the food is considered a serving, reading labels, and knowing how much insulin is required for each serving of carbohydrate. Usually, 15 grams of total carbohydrate is considered a serving. Carbohydrates include starchy vegetables, fruits, bread, cereal, pasta, milk and milk products, and sweets. The amount of rapid-acting insulin required for each carbohydrate serving varies according to an individualized insulin-to-carbohydrate ratio (ICR) that is determined by a physician or diabetes educator. For example, if the ICR is 1 unit of rapid-acting insulin per carbohydrate serving, a carbohydrate intake of 45 grams would require a 3-unit bolus of rapid-acting insulin. The complexities of carbohydrate counting require motivation of the person using the system and thorough self-management education by a registered dietitian and/or a certified diabetes educator.

For most patients, a more simplified meal plan with the emphasis on a well-balanced diet within the prescribed distribution of proteins, fats, and carbohydrates is useful. The American Diabetes Association supports use of the Create Your Plate method. The American Dietetic Association advocates using the MyPlate food guide. For further explanation of these methods, see the Health Promotion box.

Patient teaching should include sample menus that include as many favorite foods as possible. People with diabetes require considerable education and support to learn to manage the dietary guidelines (see the Complementary and Alternative Therapies box). It is vital to consider their personal and ethnic choices. Most nursing care situations do not lend themselves to the in-depth teaching, planning, and reinforcement needed. Outpatient education and visits with a

Health Promotion

Recommended Calorie Distribution for Patients Who Take Insulin

The American Diabetes Association recommends that the daily calorie intake be distributed as a mix of carbohydrates, protein, and fat adjusted to meet the metabolic goals of the individual. Saturated fat (animal fats, egg yolks, coconut oil, palm kernel oil, palm oil, and hydrogenated vegetable oils) intake should be less than 7% of the total calories. Reduction of trans fat is recommended to lower low-density lipoprotein (LDL) cholesterol and increase high-density lipoprotein (HDL) cholesterol.

High-protein diets are not recommended for weight loss because of the increased risk for kidney damage. Increased protein intake may increase the glomerular filtration rate (GFR). Sustained increases in the GFR cause renal and retinal vasodilation, leading to renal damage and retinopathy. Protein choices should come from lower fat sources, such as nonfat dairy products, legumes, skinless poultry, fish, and lean meats.

Carbohydrates should come from whole-grain breads, cereals, pasta, beans, brown rice, fruits, and vegetables. Learning to read food labels is essential because carbohydrate sources vary in calorie and fat content. Key strategies for glycemic control include carbohydrate counting, exchanges, and estimation. High-calorie food with low nutritional value should be limited. Foods containing sugar should be substituted for other carbohydrates (e.g., potatoes). Short-term (up to 1 year) use of low-carbohydrate or low-fat diets may be helpful for weight loss but potential health risks should be considered. Lipid levels and renal functions should be monitored, and patients should be advised on the increased risk for hypoglycemia. Sodium intake may be restricted for individuals with hypertension or renal insufficiency.

The addition of water-soluble fibers in the daily diet may lower total cholesterol and LDL levels. In addition, the lower fat intake improves lipid levels which improves insulin sensitivity in skeletal muscle. Foods containing soluble fibers include oatmeal, rice, dried beans, oat bran, lentils, squash, whole wheat breads, and some fruits. Fiber intake should come from soluble and insoluble sources. When fiber is added to the diet, it should be done gradually. A sudden addition of large amounts of fiber to the diet may reduce the amount of glucose available for the exogenous insulin or hypoglycemic agent taken by the patient and may result in hypoglycemic episodes. Foods with a lower glycemic index that are rich in fiber, vitamins, and other nutrients are encouraged.

Limiting saturated fat to less than 7% of the total intake and minimizing *trans* fats are essential for controlling lipid levels. Elevated serum cholesterol and triglyceride levels are often associated with type 2 DM, increasing the risk of cardiovascular disease. Cholesterol should not exceed 200 mg/day. Research in the past several years has indicated that replacing some of the allotted fat calories with calories from carbohydrates and fiber has a positive effect on the lipid profile.

A simplified method of meal planning for people with diabetes has been designed by the American Diabetes Association. The Create Your Plate plan focuses on reducing starchy foods and meat and increasing intake of nonstarchy vegetables. The plate is divided in half and then one half is divided again into two sections. The largest section is filled with nonstarchy vegetables. One of the smaller sections is for starchy foods and the other smaller section is for protein. This plan is finished off with a serving of milk and a piece of fruit. The American Dietetic Association advocates a similar approach called MyPlate. The plate is divided into four sections, each of which represents a different food (protein, whole grains, fruits, and vegetables), with the addition of a serving of milk.

certified diabetes educator (CDE) can help to meet this need.

Complementary and Alternative Therapies

Caution patients who take herbal supplements for diabetes that the supplements should not be used to replace conventional therapy. Ensure that the physician is aware of supplements being used.

Exercise

Exercise is a very effective treatment adjunct for people with diabetes. It aids weight loss in obese patients, improves cardiovascular conditioning, improves insulin sensitivity, and promotes a sense of well-being. Exercising muscle uses glucose at 20 times the rate of a muscle at rest and does not require insulin. Much of the morbidity and mortality in patients with type 2 DM occurs because of the atherosclerosis that accompanies long-term uncontrolled diabetes, which places the patient at risk for CVA (stroke) and cardiovascular disease. Exercise is known to improve LDL cholesterol, serum glucose, BP, some blood coagulation parameters, and triglycerides. People with diabetes are advised to exercise at least 150 minutes each week (see the Patient Teaching box). However, exercise must be accompanied by appropriate nutrition to have long-term beneficial results.

Patient Teaching

Exercise and Diabetes

- Have a complete medical examination before initiating a new exercise program.
- Because circulating insulin may be inadequate to ensure glucose uptake, avoid exercise when your serum glucose is elevated and ketosis is present.
- Exercise with caution if your serum glucose is greater than 300 mg/dL and no ketosis is present.
- Wear comfortable athletic shoes that provide good support.
- Before every exercise session, warm up with 5 to 10 minutes of slow, continuous aerobic exercise and stretching.
- Discuss with your physician whether to alter food or insulin intake before exercise. A general recommendation is to exercise shortly after eating or to have a small snack before exercising if your serum glucose is less than 100 mg/dL.
- Avoid exercise during the peak action of insulin and oral hypoglycemics when hypoglycemia is more likely to occur.
- Carbohydrate snacking may be necessary with prolonged or intense exercise.
- If you take insulin, inject it in the abdomen rather than in an extremity before a workout because the drug is absorbed much more quickly from the abdomen.
- Some people experience hypoglycemia several hours after exercise; have food available for these situations.

The metabolic adjustments that maintain glucose levels during exercise are regulated largely by hormones. A decrease in plasma insulin levels and the presence of glucagon is necessary for the liver to produce glucose during physical activity. Increased plasma glucagon and catecholamines are required for hepatic glucose release during prolonged exercise. Exercise affects individuals with type 1 DM differently from those with type 2 DM who do not require insulin. Hyperglycemia may occur with exercise in the patient with type 1 DM when insulin levels are inadequate. An excessive release of glucagon, catecholamines, cortisol, and growth hormone along with mobilization of free fatty acids result in ketone production, which can lead to the development of DKA. In patients with type 2 DM, exercise makes insulin receptor sites more sensitive to insulin and lowers plasma glucose levels, which can result in hypoglycemia.

Because of this, it is important for individuals with diabetes to monitor blood glucose levels before and after exercise. Individuals taking insulin may also need to monitor blood glucose levels during prolonged exercise. Exercising during peak activity of injected insulin increases the risk of hypoglycemia. Additional carbohydrate intake may be needed during prolonged exercise and any time glucose levels are less than 100 mg/dL. Physical activity should be avoided if the fasting glucose levels are more than 250 mg/dL and ketones are present. Caution should be used if glucose levels are more than 300 mg/dL in the absence of ketones.

An appropriate combination of aerobic and anaerobic exercises should be determined. Aerobic exercise produces the most therapeutic effect. The patient should exercise for 30 to 60 minutes 3 to 4 times a week. Warm-up exercises such as stretching and walking are recommended before exercise, followed by cool-down exercises afterward. The best aerobic exercises are walking, swimming, bicycle riding, and jogging. Anaerobic exercises such as weight lifting, yoga, and sit-ups build muscle mass. Very strenuous exercises can raise BP, which is undesirable with retinopathy and nephropathy. Eventually, the patient with type 2 disease who adheres to a sound nutritional plan and exercise regimen may be able to decrease the amount of exogenous insulin or oral hypoglycemics needed (see the Health Promotion box).

Insulin Therapy

All patients with type 1 DM need insulin injections and some patients with type 2 DM may eventually need insulin. Insulin is classified by onset and duration of action.

The insulin currently in use is identical to endogenous insulin, which eliminates some of the problems with earlier insulin that was obtained from animal sources. Insulin can be classified as *rapid acting*, *short acting*, *intermediate acting*, and *long acting*. Rapid-acting insulins include insulin lispro (Humalog, Admelog), insulin aspart (NovoLog, Fiasp), insulin glulisine (Apidra), and inhaled regular insulin (Afrezza). Regular insulin (Humulin R, Novolin R) is classified as

Health Promotion

Physical Activity for People With Prediabetes and Diabetes

Research has shown that physical activity has the following benefits for patients with diabetes—and for the rest of us:

- Lowers blood glucose and blood pressure (BP)
- Lowers low-density lipoprotein (LDL) cholesterol and raises high-density lipoprotein (HDL) cholesterol
- Improves the body's ability to use insulin
- Lowers the risk of heart disease and stroke
- Strengthens bones
- Keeps joints flexible
- Lowers the risk of falling
- Aids in weight loss
- Reduces body fat
- Increases energy level and reduces stress

Physical activity also plays an important part in preventing type 2 DM. A major government study, the Diabetes Prevention Program, showed that a healthy diet and a moderate exercise program resulting in a 5% to 7% weight loss can delay and perhaps prevent the onset of type 2 diabetes.

For those who already have diabetes, physical activity offers all of the benefits listed previously. However, because some exercises may worsen diabetic complications, care should be taken in starting and maintaining an exercise program. For example, activities that increase the ocular blood pressure (BP), such as lifting heavy weights, can worsen any existing ophthalmologic complications.

To avoid blisters that go unnoticed, leading to a serious infection, patients who walk or engage in other aerobic activities should wear cotton socks and shoes that are designed for the activity. After exercise, the feet should be checked for cuts, sores, bumps, or redness. Patients with numbness in their feet might try swimming instead of walking for aerobic exercise.

Because exercise can cause hypoglycemia, the following precautions are recommended.

BEFORE EXERCISE

- Patients should be careful about exercising after skipping a recent meal.
- Patients who take insulin should ask their health care team whether they should change their dosage before engaging in physical activity.

DURING EXERCISE

- Patients should wear a medical identification bracelet or other form of identification.
- Patients with type 2 DM should always carry food or glucose tablets so that they are prepared to treat hypoglycemia.
- If patients exercise for more than 1 hour, blood glucose should be checked at regular intervals.

AFTER EXERCISE

- Patients should check to see how exercise affected their blood glucose level.

Modified from American Diabetes Association, *Diabetes Care.* 44(1): 17–19, 2021.

short-acting insulin. Intermediate-acting insulins are NPH (Humulin N, Novolin N). Long-acting insulins are insulin glargine (Lantus, Basaglar, Toujeo), insulin detemir (Levemir), and insulin degludec (Tresiba). All rapid-acting and short-acting insulins are clear. Intermediate-acting and long-acting insulins have traditionally been cloudy but Lantus and Levemir are clear. Insulin vial labels should be read carefully to prevent errors. Onset, peak, and duration for various insulin preparations are compared in Table 50.1. The effect of insulin on blood glucose levels is shown in Fig. 50.1.

Route. Insulin cannot be given orally because it is rendered useless in the GI tract. All insulins can be given subcutaneously. Historically, only Regular insulin was given intravenously; however, intravenous administration of rapid-acting insulin has become a common practice. A form of inhaled insulin was approved by the U.S. Food and Drug Administration (FDA) in 2015.

Concentrations. Insulins are available in varying concentrations. U-100 insulin has a concentration of 100 U/mL and U-500 has 500 U/mL. U-100 is most commonly used. U-500 insulin is used only in emergencies and for patients who are extremely insulin resistant.

Premixed insulin products. Premixed insulins that contain two types of insulins are available. Four mixtures are commonly used: (1) 70% NPH and 30% Regular insulin (Humulin 70/30, Novolin 70/30), (2) 50% lispro protamine and 50% insulin lispro (Humalog Mix 50/50), (3) 75% lispro protamine and 25% lispro (Humalog Mix 75/25), and (4) 70% aspart protamine and 30% aspart (NovoLog Mix 70/30). Premixed solutions are easier to prepare, and they decrease the risk of errors associated with drawing up two types of insulin in the same syringe. The downside to use of premixed insulin is that you cannot adjust each type of insulin individually to fine-tune glucose control.

Dosing schedules. The pancreas secretes minute amounts of insulin continuously except after the ingestion of a meal, when it secretes a bolus of insulin into the system. Exogenous insulin is administered to mimic the action of a normal pancreas. Therefore the person with diabetes requires a bolus of rapid-acting or short-acting insulin before meals to prevent too rapid a rise in glucose. A long-acting or intermediate-acting insulin may be prescribed as well to keep glucose levels even at other times.

Pharmacology Capsule

Insulin lispro, insulin aspart, and insulin glulisine act rapidly. Regular insulin is short acting, NPH is intermediate acting, and insulin glargine, insulin detemir, and insulin degludec are long acting. Be sure to administer the correct type!

Conventional therapy. Conventional therapy uses one of several dosage schedules and typically uses a

Table 50.1 Drug Therapy: Insulin Preparations: Time Course of Action

INSULIN TYPE	APPEARANCE	ONSET	PEAK	DURATION
Rapid-Acting Insulin				
Insulin lispro (Humalog, Admelog) Insulin aspart (NovoLog, Fiasp) Insulin glulisine (Apidra)	Clear	10 to 30 minutes	120 minutes	3 to 5 hours
Inhaled Regular insulin (Afrezza)		15 to 30 minutes	60 minutes	2 to 3 hours
Short-Acting Insulin				
Regular insulin (Humulin R, Novolin R)	Clear	30 minutes to 1 hour	2 to 3 hours	5 to 8 hours
Intermediate-Acting (NPH) Insulin				
Humulin N Novolin N	Cloudy	2 to 4 hours	4 to 12 hours	12 to 16 hours
Long-Acting Insulin				
Insulin glargine (Lantus, Basaglar) Insulin detemir (Levemir)	Clear	1 hour	Minimal	Up to 24 hours
Ultra-Long Acting				
Insulin degludec (Tresiba) Insulin glargine (Toujeo) (u 300)	Clear Clear	1 hour 6 hours	Minimal Minimal	At least 42 hours 36 hours

Modified from US Pharmacist.com and the *American Diabetes Association Standards of Care* 44 (suppl 1); S111–S124, 2021.

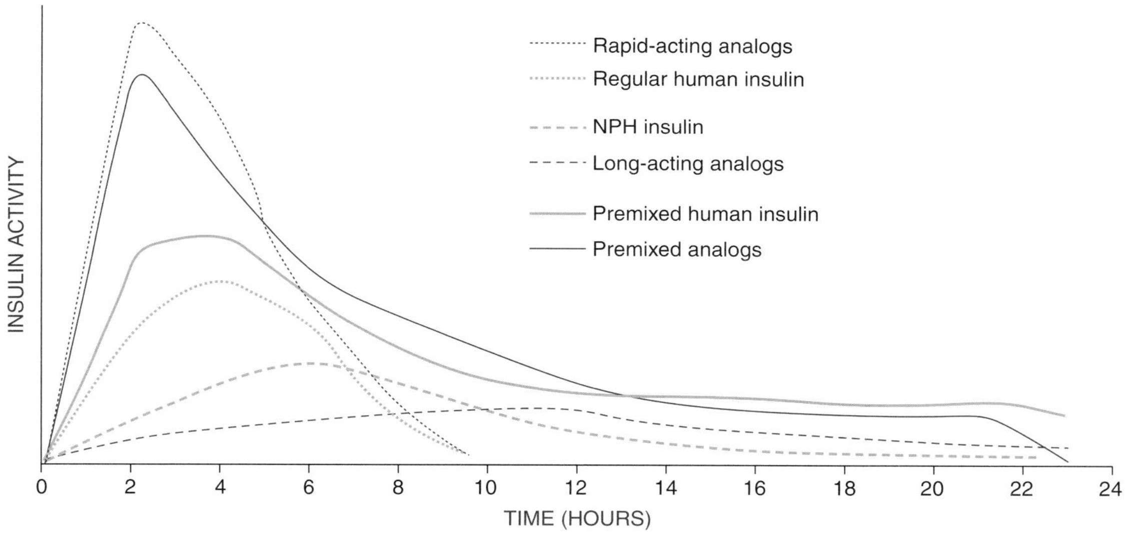

Adapted from product label information approved by the Food and Drug Administration.

Fig. 50.1 Effect of insulin on blood glucose levels. (From Agency for Healthcare Research and Quality. Clinician's guide: premixed insulin analogues, a comparison with other treatments for type 2 diabetes. 08(09)-EHC017-3, 2009. Used with permission.)

combination of a rapid-acting and an intermediate-acting or long-acting insulin. One example is the one-fifth rule that some physicians use for prescribing insulin. In the morning, the patient takes two-fifths of the day's supply in an intermediate-acting insulin such as NPH. In addition, the patient takes one-fifth of the daily requirement of insulin as Regular insulin. The latter dose covers breakfast glucose. Because the NPH peaks at lunchtime, the patient does not need Regular insulin for this meal. At suppertime, the patient takes one-fifth of the daily insulin requirement in the form of an intermediate-acting insulin and one-fifth as rapid-acting insulin to cover supper carbohydrates. For example, a patient who is prescribed 50 units of insulin a day might take it as follows:

- AM: 20 units of NPH insulin
- AM: 10 units of Regular insulin
- PM: 10 units of NPH insulin
- PM: 10 units of Regular insulin

Patients on conventional therapy should monitor their blood glucose before meals at least two times each day. A major problem with conventional therapy is nocturnal hypoglycemia: blood glucose falls between 3 AM and 4 AM. Because of this, intermediate-acting and long-acting insulin may be administered at bedtime.

Basal-bolus insulin therapy. Research supports the use of basal-bolus insulin therapy (also called *intensive insulin therapy*) for improved glycemic control. This regimen requires the use of:

- Basal insulin (long-acting insulin) to counteract hepatic glucose production. Dosing is based on weight and estimated insulin sensitivity. Basal insulin is usually given once daily, most often at bedtime.
- Rapid-acting insulin before each meal to blunt postprandial glucose spikes. Dosing is based on weight, insulin sensitivity, and carbohydrate intake. The bolus dose can also be adjusted to treat premeal hyperglycemia.

An example of basal-bolus insulin therapy would be the following:

- Premeal: Rapid-acting insulin, usually started at 0.05 U/kg/meal (2–10 units per meal) plus correctional insulin for hyperglycemia.
- Bedtime: Long-acting insulin, usually started at 0.2 to 0.3 U/kg/day (20–50 units/day) in a single dose at bedtime. Sometimes this basal insulin is divided into two injections.

Home blood glucose monitoring is essential with this regimen. The intensified program permits more flexibility in meal composition and timing. Basal-bolus insulin therapy does increase the risk for hypoglycemia, which underlines the importance of consistent blood glucose monitoring. It is important to note that studies like the RABBIT 2 Trial (Umpierrez, 2011) show that basal-bolus insulin therapy provides better glycemic control in hospitalized patients undergoing surgery when compared with standard sliding scale or PRN insulin. The positive results of this study have led many practitioners to advocate the use of basal-bolus insulin therapy in the outpatient setting.

Continuous subcutaneous insulin infusion. The last dosing schedule uses continuous subcutaneous insulin infusion. The patient has an indwelling subcutaneous catheter connected to an external portable infusion pump. The pump delivers rapid-acting or regular insulin continuously at basal rates set by the user. Before meals, the patient activates the pump to provide the appropriate amount of insulin bolus for the meal to be consumed. Patients who use pumps must also do self-monitoring of blood glucose (SMBG). Newer versions of insulin pumps allow for multiple settings for basal insulin dosages as well as transmission of blood glucose levels to the insulin pump for more precise insulin dosing. Some insulin pump users can also perform continuous glucose monitoring (CGM) with a separate sensing device that automatically transmits glucose levels to the insulin pump for immediate adjustments in insulin dosages.

Pharmacology Capsule

Remember "clear to cloudy!" When mixing short-acting (clear) and longer-acting NPH (cloudy) insulins, draw the short-acting insulin into the syringe first to avoid contaminating the short-acting insulin with NPH insulin. Only NPH insulin should be mixed with short-acting insulins (Regular, lispro, aspart and glulisine). Note: Insulin glargine (Lantus) and insulin detemir (Levemir) cannot be mixed with other insulin types!

Insulin injection. The suggested sites for subcutaneous insulin injections are illustrated in Fig. 50.2. Site rotation helps to prevent **lipohypertrophy** (i.e., swelling or lumps) or **lipoatrophy** (i.e., hollowing or pitting of the subcutaneous tissue). Because lipohypertrophy interferes with the absorption of insulin, affected areas should be avoided as injection sites.

The absorption rate of insulin varies with different body sites. The rate of absorption from the abdomen is approximately 50% faster than from the thighs. For this reason, the American Diabetes Association recommends rotating sites within one anatomic area rather than moving among all areas. Heat and massage increase the absorption rate, as does exercise. As mentioned earlier, if insulin is injected into the thigh before exercise, such as jogging, the absorption rate is greatly increased.

Insulin pump. An external insulin pump looks much like a pager. It consists of a battery-driven syringe with a long piece of tubing (usually made of Teflon) that is attached to a small needle. The needle is inserted subcutaneously in an appropriate part of the anatomy (Fig. 50.3). The syringe usually contains a 2- to 3-day supply of insulin. The pump is programmed to deliver a steady trickle of insulin throughout the day and can provide a bolus of insulin at mealtimes. In this manner, the unit mimics the pancreas. The patient calculates the bolus based on self-monitored blood glucose levels. Every 2 to 3 days, the syringe, needle, and tubing are replaced.

One advantage of the external insulin pump is that patients do not have to use intermediate-acting or long-acting insulin, with their uncertain fluctuations in glucose. Other advantages are that it gives the patient more flexibility regarding mealtimes, travel, and exercise. Potential problems with the pump are occlusion of the tubing or the needle and infection at the site of needle insertion. To use the pump, the patient must undergo intensive education and be willing to self-monitor blood glucose levels several times a day if the pump does not monitor blood glucose levels. Some medical insurance companies do not cover the cost of the pump or pump therapy, which makes the cost prohibitive to many. Efforts to develop an "artificial pancreas" are underway. The device would be implanted under the skin and would dispense insulin in response to changing blood glucose levels.

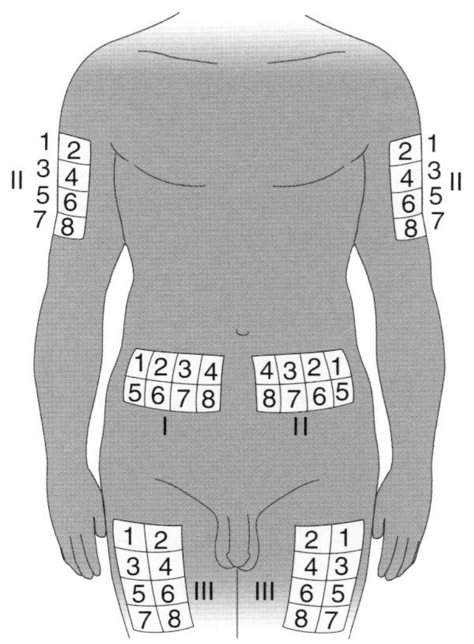

Fig. 50.2 Insulin injection sites. (From Shiland BJ: *Mastering healthcare terminology*, ed 5, St. Louis, 2016, Mosby.)

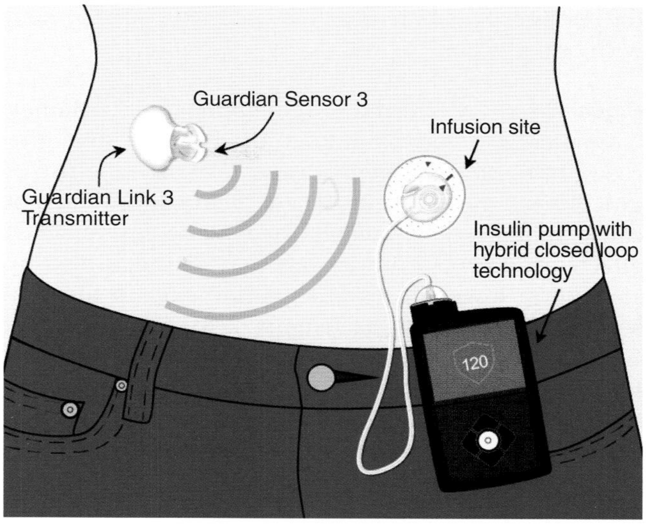

Fig. 50.3 The MiniMed 670G is a Hybrid Closed Loop system that monitors the patient's glucose and adjusts the amount of insulin delivered to the patient every five minutes. (From Medtronic, Inc., Northridge, CA.)

Other less commonly used devices for insulin administration are the jet injector, pen injector, and implanted insulin pump. The jet injector delivers insulin through the skin without a needle. The injection does sting and may bruise thin and older people. The high cost of the jet injector is a deterrent to its use. The pen injector looks like a fountain pen and holds preloaded cartridges with the prescribed insulin dose. These prefilled insulin pens are very convenient and easy to use because the insulin dose is dialed in. The insulin pens are easy to transport and work well for individuals who are on the go.

Other Non-Insulin Antidiabetic/Antihyperglycemic Drugs

If patients with type 2 DM are unable to control their blood glucose with a nutrition program and exercise, the physician may prescribe one or more oral hypoglycemics. If the serum glucose level stays elevated, insulin may be prescribed temporarily until the blood glucose levels decrease below 200 mg/dL. Oral hypoglycemics include sulfonylureas, alpha-glucosidase inhibitors, biguanides, thiazolidinediones, meglitinides and D-phenylalanines, dipeptidyl peptidase-4 (DPP-4) inhibitors, and sodium glucose cotransporter-2 inhibitors.

Sulfonylureas. Sulfonylureas lower blood sugar by stimulating the pancreas to secrete more insulin and increasing the sensitivity of insulin receptors. First- and second-generation sulfonylureas are equally effective in controlling serum glucose but have some important differences, as shown in Chapter 47, Table 47.2. Because of the long duration of action, first-generation sulfonylureas are not often used now.

A significant adverse effect of the sulfonylureas is the risk of hypoglycemia. First-generation sulfonylureas also have the potential for interactions with many other drugs, which is problematic in the patient who is taking multiple medications. First-generation drugs are not recommended in patients with liver or renal disease. Because the sulfonylureas are chemically similar to sulfonamide antibacterials, patients who are allergic to one may also be allergic to the other. Be sure to assess for allergy to sulfonamides before a patient starts taking a sulfonylurea.

The second- and third-generation drugs are more potent (so require lower dosage), pose less risk of hypoglycemia, have fewer other side effects, and have fewer drug interactions. Many older people have diminished renal and liver function, which affects metabolism and elimination of drugs and increases the risk of hypoglycemia. When a sulfonylurea is ordered for the older patient, it is usually glipizide (Glucotrol), which must be taken on an empty stomach; glyburide (DiaBeta, Micronase); glimepiride (Amaryl), or Gliclazide (Diamicron). Drugs with long durations of action are more likely to accumulate and cause toxic effects in older patients.

Alpha-glucosidase inhibitors. Examples of alpha-glucosidase inhibitors are acarbose (Precose) and miglitol (Glyset). These drugs delay digestion of complex carbohydrates into glucose and other simple sugars. Sometimes they are given in combination with insulin or a sulfonylurea. Side effects include abdominal cramping and distention, flatulence, and diarrhea. Alpha-glucosidase inhibitors are contraindicated with inflammatory bowel disease (IBD) or other intestinal diseases. Acarbose and miglitol do not cause hypoglycemia when used alone. However, if the patient becomes hypoglycemic because of another hypoglycemic agent taken in combination with the alpha-glucosidase inhibitor, oral sucrose will not effectively raise the blood sugar because of the decreased absorption of the sucrose. The patient will instead require treatment with oral glucose.

Biguanides. Metformin (Glucophage, Fortamet, Glumetza, Riomet) is a biguanide that decreases glucose production by the liver and increases the use of glucose by muscle cells. These medications do not cause hypoglycemia when used alone. Adverse GI effects are fairly common but may be decreased by starting at lower doses and working up to the prescribed dose. Dosing is usually 2 to 3 times a day. Glucophage XR is an extended-release form of metformin that is taken only once a day. A rare but potentially fatal adverse effect is lactic acidosis, which usually occurs in the presence of impaired renal function. Biguanides should not be used in the very old or when severe kidney, cardiovascular, or respiratory conditions are present. This medication should also be held after procedures or tests that require the use of intravenous dye.

Thiazolidinediones. Thiazolidinediones include rosiglitazone maleate (Avandia) and pioglitazone HCl (Actos). Classified as *insulin-sensitizing agents*, they increase the uptake of glucose by skeletal muscle and fat tissue. These drugs do not cause hypoglycemia when used alone but may when used with a sulfonylurea. Because the first drug in this class (Rezulin) was found to have serious adverse effects on the liver, liver function must be monitored when this class of drugs is used. To date, Avandia and Actos appear to pose a low risk of liver damage. Side effects include weight gain, edema, and mild transient anemia. Patients should be aware that these drugs decrease the effectiveness of oral contraceptives. They are contraindicated with class III or IV HF and during pregnancy.

Meglitinides and D-phenylalanines. Repaglinide (Prandin) is a meglitinide and nateglinide (Starlix) is a D-phenylalanine. Because of the similarity of these two types of drugs, called *mealtime insulin secretagogues*, they will be discussed together. Meglitinides and D-phenylalanine stimulate the release of insulin from the pancreas. Taken before each meal, they prevent postprandial blood glucose elevations and prolonged hypoglycemia. Patients should omit the medications if they skip a meal. Hypoglycemia may occur with strenuous exercise or alcohol consumption. Weight gain is a side effect. They are used cautiously with moderate to severe liver failure.

Dipeptidyl peptidase-4 inhibitors. Dipeptidyl peptidase-4 (DPP-4) inhibitors stimulate pancreatic release of insulin and inhibit hepatic glucose production. They include sitagliptin (Januvia), saxagliptin (Onglyza), alogliptin (Nesina), and linagliptin (Tradjenta). These medications can be taken alone or with other oral diabetes medications. Neither should be taken with insulin. Side effects include stomach upset, diarrhea, and headache. Possible adverse reactions are elevated liver enzymes and inflamed pancreas. Dose adjustments of DPP-4 inhibitors are necessary for individuals with moderate to severe renal disease.

Sodium glucose cotransporter-2 inhibitors. Canagliflozin (Invokana) was the first in a new class of glucose-lowering drugs, an oral inhibitor of sodium glucose cotransporter-2 (SGLT2). This class now includes dapagliflozin (Farxiga), empagliflozin (Jardiance), and ertugliflozin (Steglatro). Inhibition of SGLT2 reduces the resorption of glucose in the kidney, resulting in increased urinary glucose excretion, lowering of plasma glucose levels, and weight loss. Side effects include hypotension, hyperkalemia, yeast infections, urinary tract infections, and decreased urination. These side effects and the link to increased risk for cardiovascular events and strokes may limit the use of this medication.

Combination medications. With increasing use of combination therapy, patients must take more medication doses—a factor that often reduces compliance. A number of combination drugs have been released that help to simplify dosing schedules. These medications are listed in Table 50.2. The actions and side and adverse effects are the same as for each individual drug. In 2005 two new injectable medications to treat diabetes were approved by the FDA. The first was pramlintide (Symlin), which suppresses postprandial glucagon secretion, slows gastric emptying, and suppresses appetite. Pramlintide, used to treat type 1 and type 2 diabetes (requiring insulin), increases the risk for hypoglycemia and GI side effects. It is administered by injection before each meal and cannot be mixed with insulin. The second was exenatide (Byetta, Bydureon), classified as an *incretin mimetic* or glucagon-like peptide -1 (GLP-1) receptor agonist that is used only with type 2 diabetes. GLP-1 receptor agonists now include liraglutide (Victoza), albiglutide (Tanzeum), dulaglutide (Trulicity), lixisenatide (Adlyxin), and semaglutide (Ozempic, Rybelsus). They lower blood glucose levels by increasing insulin secretion, suppressing postprandial glucagon secretion, slowing gastric emptying, and suppressing appetite. GLP-1 receptor agonists work only in the presence of elevated glucose levels, so no increased risk for hypoglycemia exists unless the patient is also on sulfonylureas or insulin. Most individuals on GLP-1 receptor agonists experience a decreased appetite and weight loss, as well as nausea and vomiting when initiating new therapy. These medications have somewhat complex dosing schedules and require injections before each meal. They are also expensive and not covered by many insurance companies. Additional details about these injectable medications are included in Chapter 47, Table 47.2.

Approximately 30% to 40% of patients with type 2 diabetes fail to respond to oral agents. Another 10%

Table 50.2 Combination Oral Diabetes Drugs

TRADE NAME	COMPONENT DRUGS
Actoplus Met	pioglitazone and metformin
Avandamet	rosiglitazone and metformin
Avandaryl	rosiglitazone and glimepiride
Duetact	pioglitazone and glimepiride
Glucovance	glyburide and metformin
Invokamet	canagliflozin and metformin
Janumet	sitagliptin and metformin
Jentadueto	linagliptin and metformin
Kazano	aloplitpin and metformin
Kombiglyze	saxagliptin and metformin
Metaglip	glipizide and metformin
Oseni	alogliptin and pioglitazone
PrandiMet	metformin and repaglinide
Segluromet	ertugliflozin and metformin
Steglujan	ertugliflozin and sitagliptin
Xigduo	dapagliflozin and metformin

cease to respond after a period of successful treatment. To maintain optimal glucose control, it is beneficial for these patients to use insulin. Some of them may have to take one dose of insulin, often at night, and then are able to control serum glucose for the rest of the day with oral drugs. A variety of combination regimens (using oral agents and insulin) are being studied.

Self-Monitoring of Blood Glucose

People with diabetes need to monitor their blood glucose levels so that they can regulate their diet, exercise, and medication regimens to maintain normal blood glucose levels and lead lifestyles that are as normal as possible. SMBG is seen as the greatest breakthrough in managing diabetes since the advent of insulin. It reduces the complications of long-term diabetes by helping the patient to normalize blood glucose levels. The frequency of blood glucose monitoring depends on individualized treatment plans and patient goals. More frequent monitoring (3–6 times a day) is required for patients on insulin or using insulin pumps. Monitoring of postprandial glucose levels may also be appropriate when postmeal glucose targets are not being met.

The use of portable electronic glucose meters has largely replaced other methods of self-monitoring. The patient puts a drop of blood on a special reagent strip and inserts the strip in the meter. In less than 1 minute, the glucose level appears on a monitor. Some meters give plasma glucose values, whereas others give whole blood readings. Factors that may affect the use of these meters include cost, comfort with technology, fine-motor coordination, intellectual ability, and willingness to use the meter. SMBG is a useful tool in managing diabetes during pregnancy when glucose levels may change frequently. It is also a must in managing unstable diabetes and for patients who are prone to sudden hypoglycemic episodes or ketoacidosis or who have abnormal renal glucose thresholds.

Advances in technology allow for continuous glucose monitoring (CGM), which measures the interstitial glucose levels. The popularity of CGM has increased because of the convenience, ease of use, and the ability to sync readings with smart phones and smart watches. Testing sensors are inserted into the abdomen almost painlessly and can be worn for 10 to 14 days. Continuous readings are available every 5 minutes. This allows users to view real-time effects of food and exercise on blood glucose levels. Some devices allow for parameter alarms to be set, warning the user of high or low blood glucose readings. Most devices allow the user to easily individualize glucose target parameters and quickly monitor their "time in range." Periodic finger sticks are still required for calibration to validate CGM results and as a backup if the CGM fails.

Ketone testing is also recommended when symptoms of illness, such as nausea, vomiting, or abdominal pain, are present. Ketones are produced when the body breaks down fat for energy instead of using carbohydrates. Presence of ketones, along with hyperglycemia and illness, may indicate the development of DKA. Ketones can be detected in the blood before ketones spill over into the urine, so blood testing is preferred. Some more advanced home glucose monitors can also measure ketones. Otherwise, urine ketone testing is recommended.

Goals for glycemic control should be clearly set with consideration to age and comorbidities (i.e., medical conditions in addition to DM). For nonpregnant adults, preprandial plasma glucose levels should be between 80 and 130 mg/dL. Peak postprandial plasma glucose levels should be less than 180 mg/dL. Results falling outside of these recommended parameters warrant alterations in the diabetes regimen. It is important to note that glycemic control during hospitalization must be adjusted. Insulin therapy should be initiated for persistent glucose levels greater than 180 mg/dL, with a goal of maintaining glucose levels between 140 and 180 mg/dL. More stringent glucose control during acute illness increases the risk for hypoglycemic episodes.

Glycosylated Glucose Levels

Determination of glycosylated hemoglobin ($HgbA_{1c}$) or fructosamine levels every 2 to 3 months is an essential check of glycemic control. The $HgbA_{1c}$ reflects glucose levels over the past few months, whereas the fructosamine levels reflect those over several weeks. When the glucose level is elevated, a certain percentage of the glucose molecules bind to the hemoglobin on the red blood cell (RBC). The glucose stays on the cell for the life of the cell, which is approximately 3 months. By measuring $HgbA_{1c}$ or fructosamine levels, the physician is able to determine how well the blood glucose has been regulated in the recent past. It also allows patients who monitor their own blood glucose levels to evaluate their methods of control. For example, an HgbA1c result of 6.0% reflects a 3-month average blood glucose level of 126 mg/dL, whereas a result of 9.0% reflects a 3-month average blood glucose of 212 mg/dL. The American Diabetes Association recommends an $HgbA_{1c}$ level less than 7% as a treatment goal—or as close to normal as possible without risking hypoglycemia. Less stringent control is advocated for those with episodes of severe hypoglycemia, those who are very young or very old, and those with increased comorbidities. The American Diabetes Association offers a $HgbA_{1c}$ converter on the ADA website: https://www.diabetes.org/diabetes/a1c-test-meaning/a1c-and-eag

Complications of Therapy

Hypoglycemia. A common complication of diabetes management is hypoglycemia. Hypoglycemia can be the result of excessive insulin or oral hypoglycemic agents, inadequate food intake, delayed or missed meals, and inconsistent or excessive exercise. Treatment of hypoglycemia is discussed in the section titled "Acute Emergency Complications," but the main thing for the nurse to remember is that the patient needs some form of glucose immediately.

Somogyi phenomenon. Too much insulin can actually cause hyperglycemia. The Somogyi phenomenon is characterized by rebound hyperglycemia that occurs in response to hypoglycemia. The phenomenon begins with an episode of hypoglycemia, often during the night. Hypoglycemia triggers the body's stress response to restore homeostasis. Epinephrine is secreted, which stimulates the liver to convert stored glycogen to glucose, thereby raising the blood glucose level to the point of hyperglycemia.

The Somogyi phenomenon should be suspected when a patient reports awakening with a headache and complains of restless sleep, nightmares, enuresis (involuntary voiding during sleep), and nausea and vomiting. The blood glucose records reflect fluctuation between hypoglycemia and hyperglycemia. The patient may have tried without success to correct the hyperglycemia by increasing the insulin.

To confirm suspected Somogyi phenomenon, the patient's blood glucose needs to be measured between 2 AM and 4 AM and again at 7 AM. The 2 AM and 4 AM levels below 60 mg/dL and a 7 AM level above 180 mg/dL support the diagnosis of Somogyi phenomenon. This vicious cycle can be broken by gradually decreasing the evening dose of exogenous insulin by 2 or 3 units every 3 or 4 days until the rebound hyperglycemia is brought under control. A bedtime snack may also be helpful.

Dawn phenomenon. Some people with diabetes who are insulin dependent experience an increase in fasting blood glucose levels between 5 AM and 9 AM that is not related to a period of hypoglycemia. The most likely cause is the release of GH and cortisol, which increase blood glucose during early-morning rapid eye movement sleep. The blood glucose level is typically normal at 3 AM but elevated at 6 AM or 7 AM. The condition may be treated with a bedtime snack and delay of the evening intermediate-acting insulin until 10 PM.

❖ NURSING CARE OF THE PATIENT WITH DIABETES MELLITUS

FOCUSED ASSESSMENT

When a person with diabetes seeks medical care in an emergency situation, a complete assessment must be delayed until the patient is stable. The licensed vocational nurse/licensed practical nurse collects data that assist in the management of this situation. If the patient is in ketoacidosis, the assessment is likely to show ketonuria, Kussmaul respirations, orthostatic hypotension, hypertension (at times), nausea, vomiting, and lethargy or change in level of consciousness. In the hypoglycemic patient, expect to find tachycardia, anxiety, trembling, and decreasing level of consciousness. Be alert for indications of HHNS (decreased level of consciousness, polyuria, and polydipsia in the absence of ketosis).

In each of these situations, attempt to determine the following:

- Type of diabetes
- Hypoglycemics: name, dosage, when last dose was taken
- Food and fluid intake for the past 3 days
- Relevant laboratory values: blood glucose, blood pH, bicarbonate levels, electrolytes, and serum and urine osmolality

Once the patient is stabilized, a complete health history and physical examination should be done by the registered nurse.

Health History

The data collection focuses on the signs and symptoms of chronic hyperglycemia and possible complications. Physical and psychosocial factors that may have an effect on the patient's capacity to learn and perform self-care activities should be documented.

Reason for seeking care. Ask the patient to describe the signs and symptoms that prompted them to seek medical care. The patient might report unexplained weight loss, dryness of skin, vaginal itching, or sores that are slow in healing. Polyphagia, polydipsia, and polyuria, known as the *three Ps*, are classic signs of DM.

Present health/history of present illness. If the patient is known to have DM, note the type and duration. Document the name and dosage of prescribed medications and when they were last taken. If the patient monitors blood glucose, record the type of equipment used, the testing schedule, and recent test results.

Past health history. The history should note diagnoses of circulatory, cardiac, or renal problems. Previous hospitalizations and surgeries are noted. If the patient is a woman, record an obstetric history, including number of pregnancies (if any), outcomes of all pregnancies, and birth weights of full-term infants. For patients who had GDM, ask whether insulin was required or if diet and exercise maintained adequate control. Other important data to collect are immunization records and allergies.

Family history. A family history of diabetes, heart disease, stroke, hypertension, and hyperlipidemia is significant when a person has or is suspected of having DM.

Review of systems. The review of symptoms begins with a description of the patient's general health. Note changes in skin moisture or turgor. To detect possible changes in the eyes associated with diabetes, inquire whether the patient has had floaters (i.e., dark spots that cross the field of vision), diplopia (i.e., double vision), or blurred vision or has seen white halos around objects. Document significant abdominal symptoms including diarrhea, abdominal bloating, and gas. Problems passing or holding urine should be noted. If the patient has had any pain in the legs, note when the pain occurs. Describe any numbness, tingling, or burning sensations in the extremities. Last, the patient should be asked if they have experienced changes in mental alertness or seizures.

Functional assessment. The functional assessment explores factors that can affect the patient's ability to perform self-care, including literacy, financial resources such as health insurance, and family support. Ask the patient to describe the usual pattern of activity and rest. A typical 24-hour dietary history is useful in evaluating how well the patient understands and adheres to the prescribed diet. Explore the effect of diabetes on the patient's life, including self-concept, social relationships, and employment.

Physical Examination

In the general survey, note the patient's level of consciousness, posture and gait, and apparent well-being. Record vital signs, including BP, height, and weight. Throughout the examination, note the skin color, warmth, turgor, and lesions.

The trained examiner inspects the eyegrounds for evidence of diabetic retinopathy or cataracts. The vision assessment is important because visual defects may affect the patient's ability to read vital medication instructions or labels. Gross visual acuity may be assessed by having the patient read available print. A Snellen test and other more sophisticated measures may also be used to evaluate the function of the eyes. During the examination of the head and neck, the examiner should be alert for a sweet, fruity odor to the patient's breath that is common with ketoacidosis.

The feet receive special attention. Document blisters, lesions, pallor, discoloration, deformities, and edema. Document the condition of the nails, particularly thickened or ingrown nails. Palpating both ankles and feet simultaneously for warmth and pedal pulses helps to identify poor circulation in either or both extremities. Evaluate strength in the legs by having the patient sit and try to raise and lower each foot while applying pressure to it. Assess range of motion in the ankles and feet.

Testing gait, balance, and motor coordination provides data about neurologic integrity. This is important because patients who have problems walking or feeding themselves have problems manipulating syringes and glucose monitors. In addition, test the lower extremities for the ability to perceive hot, cold, sharp, and dull sensations as well as painful stimuli.

Assessment of the patient with DM is outlined in Box 50.3.

The following diagnoses are not an exhaustive list because many other patient problems may be made if a patient has complications associated with DM. The nursing care plan must be individualized based on the assessment. Management of emergencies is discussed in the section titled "Acute Emergency Complications."

Patient Problems, Goals, and Outcome Criteria: Diabetes

Patient Problems	Goals and Outcome Criteria
Ineffective self-care management related to lack of knowledge of diabetes, dietary management of glucose, faulty metabolism, nausea and vomiting, imbalance between food intake and activity expenditure	Effective management of diabetes: patient correctly describes self-care measures, maintains blood glucose within limits of 70 and 130 mg/dL, achieves optimal weight
Altered family dynamics related to financial, personal, family pattern disruption associated with diabetes management	Patient and family adapt to changes required to manage diabetes using prescribed treatment regimen: patient and family verbalize understanding of and intent to adhere to treatment regimen, patient uses resources needed for diabetes mellitus (DM) management

Continued

Patient Problems, Goals, and Outcome Criteria: Diabetes—cont'd

Patient Problems	Goals and Outcome Criteria
Potential for fluid volume deficit related to hyperglycemia, alterations in urine output	Normal extracellular fluid volume: patient correctly describes fluid needs, recognizes the significance of polyuria and oliguria; pulse and blood pressure (BP) remain within patient norms
Potential for injury related to adverse effects of drugs, diminished alertness, increased susceptibility to infection	Decreased potential for injury: blood glucose 70 to 130 mg/dL and absence of signs of infection (normal body temperature and white blood cell [WBC] count)
Decreased activity tolerance related to impaired tissue perfusion, decreased mobility	Stable or improved activity tolerance: patient performs daily activities without excess fatigue
Chronic pain related to neuropathy	Pain relief or reduction: patient states pain is relieved or reduced, appears relaxed
Disrupted skin tissue integrity related to neurologic and circulatory changes	Absence of injury associated with sensory loss: skin intact, no redness or blisters
Potential for acute confusion related to abnormal blood glucose, metabolic imbalances	Normal thought processes: patient is alert and oriented to person, place, and time
Inadequate coping related to diagnosis, dietary restrictions, disturbed body image, sexual dysfunction, anxiety, fear	Adequate coping: patient verbalizes feelings about diabetes and expresses willingness to follow plan of care and to use resources as needed

INTERVENTIONS

Immediate nursing care of the patient with DM is geared toward urgent needs and complications. After urgent needs are met, nursing care focuses on teaching the patient to manage diabetes (see Nursing Care Plan 50.1 and Nursing Care Plan 50.2).

Ineffective Self-Care Management

Patient education requires that the patient understand the physiology of glucose metabolism and the signs and symptoms of hypoglycemia, DKA, and HHNS. Teach the patient how and when to monitor blood glucose and urine ketone levels, how to interpret the results, and the appropriate actions to take based on the results. If the patient is using a glucose meter, explain and demonstrate calibration and operation of the device, collection of blood samples, and disposal of lancets.

The teaching plan also prepares the patient for self-medication as prescribed. Explain drug names, dosages, actions, and adverse effects. If insulin is prescribed, demonstrate proper techniques for drawing up and injecting insulin and explain site rotation. Explain how adjustments in insulin or diet and exercise are used to maintain blood glucose levels between 70 and 130 mg/dL before meals and less than 180 mg/dL after meals. Not only provide verbal instruction but also allow the patient to handle equipment and demonstrate skills multiple times. If the patient cannot correctly draw up insulin, a caregiver can prepare the syringes in advance. If the insulin is refrigerated in prefilled syringes, it is stable for 1 week. The syringes should be stored in a vertical or tilted position (needle up) to

Box 50.3 Assessment of the Patient With Diabetes Mellitus

HEALTH HISTORY

Reason for Seeking Care/Present Health

Polydipsia, polyuria, polyphagia, unexplained weight loss, dry skin, vaginal itching, delayed healing, blood glucose, urine ketones

Past Health History

Established diagnosis of diabetes mellitus (DM): type, onset; cardiovascular or renal disorders; previous hospitalizations; obstetric history: number of pregnancies, outcomes, birth weights, gestational diabetes mellitus (GDM); immunizations; allergies; and current medications: drug names, dosages, schedules, time last dose of each drug taken

Family History

Diabetes, heart disease, stroke

Review of Systems

Changes in skin moisture or turgor; changes in vision; diarrhea, abdominal bloating, gas; urine retention or incontinence; pain, tingling, or numbness in extremities; changes in mental status; seizures

Functional Assessment

Literacy, financial resources, usual activity and rest pattern, diet, personal effect of diabetes on life; self-monitoring of blood glucose (SMBG): type of equipment used, testing schedule, recent test results

Physical Examination

General Survey: Level of consciousness, posture and gait, well-being

Vital Signs: Tachycardia, hypertension, hypotension, Kussmaul respirations

Height and Weight: Current and usual

Skin: Color, warmth, turgor, lesions

Eyes: Changes in eyegrounds, acuity

Mouth: Sweet, fruity breath odor

Lower Extremities: Blisters, lesions, color, edema, pulses, deformities, strength, range of motion

Neurologic: Gait and balance; motor coordination; perception of temperature, touch, and pain

Nursing Care Plan 50.1 Patient With Type 1 Diabetes Mellitus

FOCUSED ASSESSMENT

Health History

A 17-year-old woman who has recently been diagnosed with type 1 diabetes mellitus (DM) is hospitalized to begin her insulin therapy and stabilize her blood glucose. She sought medical attention because of persistent thirst and increased urination. She has no other health problems but has had frequent upper respiratory infections the past few years. The review of systems reveals periodic blurred vision, itching, increased appetite, weight loss of 7 lb in 3 months, and fatigue.

Physical Examination

Vital signs: blood pressure 92/58 mm Hg, pulse 88 beats per minute, respiration 14 breaths per minute, temperature 98.4°F (36.9°C) measured orally. Height 5′2″, weight 107 lb. Physical findings are all within normal limits (WNL).

Patient Problems	Goals and Outcome Criteria	Interventions
Ineffective management of diabetes related to lack of knowledge of diabetes and its treatment	The patient will correctly describe type 1 diabetes mellitus (DM) and its treatment. The patient will demonstrate self-medication, meal planning, and understanding of management of exercise and drug effects.	Explain the physiology of glucose metabolism, signs and symptoms of ketoacidosis, and hypoglycemia. Teach the patient to perform self-monitoring of blood glucose (SMBG), urine ketone testing, and how to interpret results. Explain the insulin types, their actions, and their administration. Have the patient practice insulin injection. Explain the relationship between diet, exercise, insulin, and blood glucose. Obtain a dietary consult regarding diet. Monitor food intake and replace food not eaten with a substitute identified by the dietitian.
Altered family dynamics related to financial, personal, or family pattern disruption	The patient and family will express making alterations in lifestyle to adhere to prescribed regimen of care.	Request patient and family education by certified diabetes educator (CDE), if available. If not, present information in a positive manner and in small units. Identify barriers to self-management. Determine resources and sources of support. Have the patient repeat aspects of care and consequences of nonadherence to the program. Acknowledge the difficulty of making major changes in eating and activity patterns and in administering self-injections. Identify community resources such as the local chapter of the American Diabetes Association. Teach the patient and family members to recognize and respond to hypoglycemia and ketoacidosis.
Potential for fluid volume deficit related to altered urine output	The patient will maintain normal blood volume, as evidenced by normal tissue turgor, pulse, and blood pressure (BP).	Stress the importance of drinking at least eight glasses of water daily. Point out that excessive urine output may indicate hyperglycemia. Assess hydration, including tissue turgor, mucous membrane moisture, and vital signs.
Potential for injury related to adverse effects of drugs, increased susceptibility to infection	The patient's blood glucose will remain within goal range established by the physician. The patient will state measures to reduce risk of infection and will identify symptoms that should be reported to the physician.	Teach the patient to recognize the signs and symptoms of hypoglycemia: shakiness, nervousness, irritability, tachycardia, anxiety, lightheadedness, hunger, tingling or numbness of lips and tongue. Instruct the patient to take concentrated sugar if hypoglycemia occurs, followed by a complex carbohydrate (e.g., milk, bread) to prevent rebound hypoglycemia. The patient should contact the physician if ill and unable to take food or fluids. Caution the patient that impaired sensation could develop in the extremities and that healing of injuries may be impaired. Encourage the patient to avoid trauma and to inspect the feet daily to detect any injuries.
Decreased activity tolerance related to metabolic imbalance	The patient will perform usual activities of daily living (ADL) and carry out planned exercise program without excess fatigue.	An exercise regimen is built into the plan of care. Exercise must be done as part of a regular routine. Tell the patient to avoid injecting insulin into a body area that will be affected by exercise soon after the injection. Patient should not exercise during peak insulin activity and should eat a snack before or during exercise if the blood glucose is <100 mg/dL to avoid hypoglycemia.
Visual disturbance related to abnormal serum glucose	The patient will report correction of blurred vision.	Advise the patient that blurred vision may be caused by hyperglycemia. Encourage an annual ophthalmologic examination to detect vision changes or problems.
Potential for acute confusion related to abnormal serum glucose	The patient will continue to be alert and fully oriented.	Monitor the patient's mental status. Recognize confusion as a sign of abnormal serum glucose. Tell the patient and family that mental changes are best treated with carbohydrates. If the patient does not improve, the blood glucose should be measured and medical attention must be sought.

Continued

Nursing Care Plan 50.1 Patient With Type 1 Diabetes Mellitus—cont'd

Patient Problems	Goals and Outcome Criteria	Interventions
Inadequate coping related to diagnosis, dietary restrictions, disturbed body image, anxiety, and fear	The patient will identify concerns about living with DM and plan strategies for dealing with it.	Encourage the patient to express feelings about DM and to ask questions. Assure her that most regular activities can be resumed. Identify the patient's strengths and resources. Explore her knowledge about DM and any misconceptions. Tell her that pregnancy must be carefully monitored but is a future option. Offer support groups if available.

CRITICAL THINKING QUESTIONS

1. How are type 1 and type 2 DM alike and how are they different?
2. Diagram the mechanisms by which the body tries to adapt to (1) high blood glucose and (2) low blood glucose.
3. Describe the signs and symptoms of ketoacidosis and hypoglycemia.

Nursing Care Plan 50.2 Patient With Type 2 Diabetes Mellitus

FOCUSED ASSESSMENT

Health History

An 80-year-old Latina was seen in her physician's office and diagnosed with type 2 diabetes mellitus (DM). A referral has been made to a home health agency. The assessment was done in the patient's home. She lives three blocks from a grocery store, which also has a pharmacy. Her physician prescribed glyburide (Micronase), 2.5 mg daily before breakfast. The patient sought medical treatment for fatigue, weight loss (10 lb in 2 months), and symptoms of a urinary tract infection (UTI). She has a history of hypertension, which is treated with verapamil, and venous insufficiency. When asked, she states that she has had some problems with her vision and vaginal pruritus. She reports that her appetite is very good, so she could not understand why she was losing weight. Her usual diet is primarily Mexican-American food, but she reports trying not to eat "too much fat." She expresses concern that a diabetic diet will be too expensive because she has only Social Security income. She says that her father died of a heart attack at 57 years of age; her mother died at 73 years of age from kidney failure. One of her brothers has DM, one is deceased from heart disease, and a third is alive and well at 70 years of age. The patient says her symptoms have interfered with performance of usual daily activities and that she is getting up frequently during the night to void, which has affected the quality of her rest. She is a widow who lives alone. She has four adult children, but only one lives in the same city and visits her on weekends.

Physical Examination

Vital signs: blood pressure 160/95 mm Hg, pulse 86 beats per minute, respiration 16 breaths per minute, temperature 97°F (36.1°C) measured orally. Height 5′2″, weight 150 lb. Patient is alert and oriented. Her skin is dry and tissue turgor is poor. She has kyphosis and walks slowly. Heart and breath sounds are normal; 2+ edema in both legs. Popliteal pulses are weak; pedal pulses are not palpable. Skin is dark around the ankles. Feet are cool. Capillary return in toenails is 4 seconds. Toenails are unevenly cut. A reddened area is seen on one heel, but the patient says it is not painful.

Patient Problems	Goals and Outcome Criteria	Interventions
Ineffective self-care management related to lack of knowledge of dietary management of diabetes mellitus (DM), drug therapy, and self-monitoring	The patient will demonstrate the ability to adhere to the prescribed diet and drug therapy and to monitor blood glucose.	Assess the patient's understanding of her condition and treatment and explore her attitude toward managing type 2 DM. Assess gross visual acuity and assist her to get an eye examination and corrective lenses as needed. Contact local Lions Club if she cannot afford prescribed lenses. Design a teaching plan to explain key aspects of care. Emphasize skills needed immediately: how to take medications, what foods to avoid, and how to recognize and treat hypoglycemia. If home blood glucose monitoring is prescribed, practice the process with her and evaluate her ability to perform the test and interpret the results. Develop a plan with her to cover additional topics. Discuss home health referral with physician.
Altered family dynamics related to financial limitations and difficulties with transportation for food, drugs, and medical care	The patient will manage her prescribed diet and drug therapy with support from family.	Assess any barriers the patient and family perceive to managing her prescribed diet and drug therapy. If financial problems exist, consult a social worker or determine what assistance is available. If transportation and shopping are difficult, explore how the daughter who lives locally can help or provide information about public transportation available for older adults and the disabled. Provide dietary information that incorporates Mexican-American dishes. Discuss the advantages of using senior nutrition programs or Meals on Wheels to provide some meals and ease the burden of food preparation. Monitor weight and blood glucose to assess effects of treatment.

Nursing Care Plan 50.2 Patient With Type 2 Diabetes Mellitus—cont'd

Patient Problems	Goals and Outcome Criteria	Interventions
Potential for injury related to adverse effects of drugs, circulatory impairment, decreased sensation, and increased susceptibility to infection	The patient will take measures to reduce the risk of injury associated with hypoglycemia, inadequate circulation, and diminished sensation; the patient will remain free of fever.	Explain the importance of eating properly while on oral medications that lower the blood glucose. Describe the related signs and symptoms and advise the patient to consume a glucose source such as sweetened orange juice to reverse hypoglycemia. Stress the importance of contacting the physician if ill and unable to take oral food and fluids. Explain how DM affects the blood vessels and nerves, making the extremities especially vulnerable to injury. Emphasize the importance of protecting the feet from injury by wearing properly fitting shoes and keeping the nails trimmed correctly. She should be told to avoid heating pads and to test bath water with a bath thermometer. Advise her to have foot care done by a physician or other specialist (see the Patient Teaching box earlier in this chapter).
Decreased activity tolerance related to fatigue, venous insufficiency, and circulatory impairment	The patient will resume her previous level of activity without excessive fatigue.	Assess the patient's energy level. Explore her usual day and discuss ways to conserve energy.
Inadequate coping related to diagnosis of serious chronic illness that requires alterations in daily life	The patient will demonstrate effective coping with management of diabetes.	Encourage the patient to share her thoughts and feelings about having diabetes and her ability to deal with it. Assure her that many older people learn to manage quite well and that resources are available to help her. Communicate with her frequently until her confidence increases. Let her know how she can reach ready sources of information.

CRITICAL THINKING QUESTIONS

1. What effect does nutrition have with regard to blood glucose?
2. What barriers might the patient perceive to managing diet and drug therapy?

reduce clogging of the needle. Before administering, tell the patient to pull back the plunger slightly and gently rock the syringe to remix the solution. Follow manufacturer guidelines for storage of prefilled insulin pens.

Advise the patient to consult the physician or pharmacist before taking new medications, because many medications interact with drugs given for diabetes.

Consult the dietitian regarding diet and reinforce nutritional information. During hospitalization, record food intake. Details of medical and dietary management are presented in the section titled "Medical Treatment."

Ideally, you should present small units of content in each teaching session. Unfortunately, there may be time to provide the patient only with "survival skills" during a brief or busy hospitalization. Therefore verbal instructions should be accompanied by other sources of information, such as written materials, compact discs (CDs), or digital video discs (DVDs), as well as by information about local resources such as the hospital's CDE and the local chapter of the American Diabetes Association. Office nurses, community health nurses, and home health nurses also often participate in teaching the patient with diabetes.

Instruct the patient on the importance of having yearly eye examinations. The patient should inform the ophthalmologist of the diagnosis of diabetes. If the patient has impaired vision, audiotapes, CDs, special reading materials, and special devices for preparing and administering insulin and for testing blood glucose may be needed.

If the patient has a hearing problem, give directions while facing the patient at eye level and speak clearly. Ask the patient to repeat or demonstrate instructions to make sure that they were heard correctly. Supplement verbal information and demonstrations with written material.

Pharmacology Capsule

Many drugs can affect blood glucose. For example, beta-adrenergic blockers lower the blood glucose and hydrochlorothiazides raise it.

Altered Family Dynamics

When a patient has had diabetes education but does not follow the prescribed plan, explore possible barriers to carrying out the plan. Some patients may think that the program is too hard to follow and not even try. Others may think that complications are inevitable and that treatment will not really make a difference. Other reasons for noncompliance can include lack of financial resources (for medications, testing supplies, and nutrient rich foods), food insecurity, homelessness, limited access to care, health literacy, and language barriers. Nursing interventions depend on the barriers identified. They are designed to provide practical help, support, and encouragement.

Teach family members how to support and help the family member with diabetes. Treat the family as integral members of the health care team. It is especially important in the nutrition teaching to include the person who does the shopping and cooking. A referral to social services is necessary if the patient cannot afford syringes and insulin. A referral to a diabetes educator, home health nurse, or community health nurse for follow-up teaching and monitoring is also recommended.

Potential for Fluid Volume Deficit

Teach the patient the relationship between blood glucose and urine output. Explain that abnormally increased output may signal hyperglycemia and may eventually lead to dehydration and DKA or HHNS.

Potential for Injury

Advise the patient to keep immunizations current because of increased susceptibility to infection and impaired healing. Teach patients to see a physician promptly if they have signs and symptoms of infection such as fever, cough, painful urination, or lesions with purulent drainage.

On sick days, insulin or oral agents should be taken as usual and blood glucose checked every 2 to 4 hours. If the blood glucose exceeds 250 mg/dL, the blood or urine should be tested for ketones. Glucose levels greater than 300 mg/dL and the presence of ketones in the blood or urine should be reported to the physician. Patients with type 1 DM may need additional insulin. To prevent dehydration and ketoacidosis, the patient should eat 10 to 15 g of carbohydrates every 1 to 2 hours and drink small amounts of fluid every 15 to 30 minutes: 4 oz of orange or apple juice, non-diet soda, or Jell-O provides approximately 15 g of carbohydrates. If nausea and vomiting occur, suggest soft foods or liquids instead of solid foods. Tell the patient to report nausea, vomiting, and diarrhea to the physician at once, because severe fluid loss may occur. The patient who is unable to retain oral fluids may require hospitalization to restore fluid and electrolyte balance.

Decreased Activity Tolerance

An exercise regimen can be designed with the hospital rehabilitation department. "All things in moderation" is the best rule of thumb. Lack of exercise or too vigorous activity just before bedtime may contribute to sleeplessness. Details about the effects of exercise on blood glucose and activity recommendations are discussed in the section titled "Exercise."

Chronic Pain

Leg pain as the result of long-term complications may require analgesics. Document pain, administer medications as ordered, and evaluate the effects of interventions. If the patient is taking analgesics at home, explain how the medication is to be taken and any significant side effects such as drowsiness.

Potential for Disrupted Skin Tissue Integrity

Alterations in tactile sensations may result in burns or frostbite. The patient and the family need to be aware of the danger of impaired sensation. Instruct the patient to avoid injury from heat or cold when outdoors in extreme weather. Caution the patient about the possibility of burns when using heating pads or electric blankets, working around a hot stove, or sitting next to a hot radiator. When taking a bath, measure the temperature of the bath water with a bath thermometer. The temperature should not exceed 43° C (109.4° F). Tissue may be burned before the patient is aware of the excessive heat.

The patient or someone else should examine the patient's feet daily for signs of trauma. A physician should see injuries or blisters promptly. Foot care for the diabetic is summarized in the Patient Teaching box.

Potential for Acute Confusion

Acute confusion may be caused by hypoglycemia, ketoacidosis, or HHNS. Without treatment, the hypoglycemic patient may be irritable at first, then confused, irrational, lethargic, and eventually comatose. In ketoacidosis, the patient becomes drowsy and the level of consciousness decreases and may progress to coma. HHNS is also characterized by altered levels of consciousness, progressing from confusion to coma. Emergency and medical treatments are covered in the section titled "Acute Emergency Complications."

When the patient is confused or disoriented, first initiate actions to determine the cause and seek appropriate medical care. Meanwhile, have someone remain with the patient to ensure safety until the condition improves. Because of the risk of disturbed thought processes, people with diabetes should wear a medical alert tag. The tag identifies the patient as having diabetes so that medical attention will be sought.

Inadequate Coping

Patients may be anxious about the immediate and long-term effects of diabetes and how it will affect their lives. They may be overwhelmed by what they need to learn for self-care. They also may be fearful about lifestyle changes, self-medication, glucose testing, adverse drug effects, and possible complications. Encourage patients to express these concerns so that they can be addressed. Talking with other people who are coping successfully with diabetes can have positive effects.

Encourage patients to express their feelings regarding diabetes and to ask for help or advice when needed. Make every effort to encourage them to resume normal activities and to continue their usual social activities. Help patients to identify their strengths and weaknesses and explore coping strategies for managing areas of concern.

One source of stress to some patients is altered sexual function. Listen to the patient's concerns and encourage consultation with the physician on the matter. Altered sexual function may be the result of diabetes, but other causes are possible. Some diagnostic procedures may be done to assess erectile dysfunction. For irreversible erectile dysfunction, the physician can offer the male patient several options (see Chapter 54). Research is ongoing into treatments for female dysfunction. You can explore with the patient the importance of sexual intercourse and their willingness to consider alternative means of sexual expression. Patients and their partners may wish to seek counseling from therapists with expertise in sexual dysfunction.

Patient Teaching

Diabetes Mellitus

- Learn the names of your prescribed drugs, dosages, schedule, and (if on insulin) technique for injections.
- Take some form of carbohydrate if you have symptoms of hypoglycemia: nervousness, palpitations, hunger.
- Monitoring your blood glucose helps you to see how well your diabetes is being controlled.
- We will teach you how to check your blood glucose, how to interpret the findings, and what actions, if any, to take.
- Nutrition is an important part of managing your diabetes. The dietitian will discuss dietary guidelines with you.
- Regular exercise helps to control your blood glucose and improves circulation.
- Because your feet are susceptible to injury and may not heal well, wear properly fitting shoes, inspect your feet daily, and immediately seek medical care for wounds, blisters, and calluses.
- When you are sick, monitor your blood glucose and ketones; continue your insulin (if taking), take in carbohydrates that provide 10 to 15 g of carbohydrates every 1 to 2 hours, and take small amounts of fluids every 15 to 30 minutes.
- Although no cure for diabetes exists at this time, you can reduce your risk of complications with good management.

HYPOGLYCEMIA UNRELATED TO DIABETES

The management of hypoglycemia in the patient with diabetes is addressed earlier under "Acute Emergency Complications." This section addresses hypoglycemia resulting from causes other than the pharmacologic treatment for diabetes.

PATHOPHYSIOLOGY

Hypoglycemia is defined as a syndrome that develops when the blood glucose level falls to less than 70 mg/dL. Hypoglycemia may result from abnormalities in insulin levels, available glucagon, and the secretion of catecholamines, GH, and cortisol. Symptoms can occur at different blood levels according to individual tolerances and how rapidly the level falls. The causes of hypoglycemia may be divided into three categories: (1) exogenous, (2) endogenous, and (3) functional. Summaries of each of these three categories are presented in Table 50.3.

Exogenous hypoglycemia results from outside factors acting on the body to produce a low blood glucose. These include insulin, oral hypoglycemic agents, alcohol, or exercise.

Endogenous hypoglycemia occurs when internal factors cause an excessive secretion of insulin or an increase in glucose metabolism. These conditions may be related to tumors or genetics.

Functional hypoglycemia may result from a variety of causes, including gastric surgery, fasting, or malnutrition. Alimentary hypoglycemia occurs in a patient who has undergone gastric surgery. The gastric contents empty rapidly, resulting in increased glucose absorption. In response to the increased glucose, excessive insulin production occurs, causing the hypoglycemia. In impaired glucose tolerance (IGT) hypoglycemia, an excessive response of insulin to glucose occurs. Spontaneous reactive hypoglycemia has received much publicity by the lay and medical communities alike. Symptoms occur as a result of an extreme insulin response to ingestion of foods containing carbohydrates. Low blood glucose levels need to be verified for the diagnosis to be accepted.

CLINICAL MANIFESTATIONS

Signs and symptoms of hypoglycemia vary according to how quickly the blood glucose levels are falling. When the levels fall rapidly, epinephrine, cortisol, glucagon, and GH are secreted by the body to increase glucose levels. Adrenergic symptoms that result from these physiologic responses include weakness, hunger, diaphoresis, tremors, anxiety, irritability, headache, pallor, and tachycardia. If the blood glucose level falls over several hours, symptoms are attributed to lack of essential glucose to brain tissue. These symptoms include confusion, weakness, dizziness, blurred or double vision, seizure, and, in severe cases, coma.

MEDICAL DIAGNOSIS

The diagnosis of hypoglycemia not associated with diabetes can be based on fasting blood glucose, OGTT, intravenous glucose tolerance test, and 72-hour inpatient fasting. The diagnosis should be based on three criteria known as *Whipple's triad:* (1) the presence of symptoms, (2) documentation of low blood glucose when symptoms occur, and (3) improvement of these symptoms when blood glucose rises. These criteria must occur in the absence of sulfonylurea treatment or abnormal plasma insulin and C peptide (which indicates levels of endogenous insulin being produced).

MEDICAL TREATMENT

Treatment of hypoglycemia depends on the cause of the problem and the patient's condition. In an unconscious patient who has diabetes, hypoglycemia

Table 50.3 Exogenous, Endogenous, and Functional Causes of Hypoglycemia in Adults

CAUSES	PREDISPOSING FACTORS	OCCURRENCE
Exogenous Causes		
Insulin	Intentional or accidental overdose; may be combined with inadequate food intake, usually increased exercise, decrease in insulin requirement, or potentiating medications	Most frequent cause of hypoglycemia
Oral hypoglycemic agents	Intentional or accidental overdose; may be combined with inadequate food intake, increased exercise, or potentiating medications	Frequent cause of hypoglycemia with sulfonylureas and meglitinides
Alcohol	Particularly likely in chronically malnourished or acutely food-deprived people	Occurs within 6 to 36 hours of ingesting moderate to large amounts of alcohol
Exercise	Increased duration and intensity of exercise increases glucose uptake and normally decreases insulin secretion	Occurs with both insulin sulfonylurea administration and intense exercise but may be unpredictable in onset
Endogenous Causes		
Organic hypoglycemia	Insulinoma (a tumor of the beta cells of the pancreatic islets of Langerhans)	Uncommon neoplasm of beta cells of the islets of Langerhans
Extrapancreatic neoplasms	May be mesenchymal tumors, hepatomas, adrenocortical carcinomas, gastrointestinal (GI) tumors, lymphomas, or leukemias	Rare; most common in adults 40 to 70 years of age
Functional Causes		
Alimentary hypoglycemia	Rapid dumping of carbohydrates into upper small intestine	Post gastrectomy
Drug-related (ethanol, haloperidol, pentamidine, salicylates) reactive hypoglycemia	Syndrome with symptoms such as diaphoresis, tachycardia, tremulousness, headache, fatigue, drowsiness, and irritability	Rarely diagnosed throughout the world; widely diagnosed in the United States, prompting American Diabetes Association and Endocrine Society to issue statement that entity is probably over diagnosed
Drinking alcohol on empty stomach	Impaired hepatic glycogen stores	More common with drinks containing saccharin (e.g., beer, gin and tonic, rum and cola, whiskey and ginger ale)
Rapid discontinuation of total parenteral alimentation	Endocrine deficiency states (cortisol, growth hormone [GH], glucagon, epinephrine)	Easily prevented
Glucocorticoid deficiency	Critical illness (cardiac, hepatic, and renal disease)	A danger for any person with adrenal insufficiency
Severe liver deficiency	Insufficient glucose output by liver	Fasting hypoglycemia
Lack of body stores for protein, fat, and carbohydrates	Profound malnutrition	Common; also found with relative frequency in kwashiorkor
Prolonged muscular exercise	Metabolism of energy-producing substances	Occurs if exercise is too prolonged or severe or if nutritional intake and carbohydrate stores are insufficient

Data from Desimone ME, Weinstock RS: Non-diabetic hypoglycemia. In DeGroot, LS, Chrousos, G, Dungan, K, et al.: *Endotext*. South Dartmouth, MA, 2017.

should be suspected until it is ruled out as a cause of the patient's symptoms. Fifty milliliters of 50% glucose solution should be administered intravenously immediately. The patient with a milder form of hypoglycemia is treated following the 15/15 rule as described earlier

Prevention of hypoglycemia by proper food intake is an important treatment component. The diet is directed by the underlying cause. If the cause is related to an overproduction of insulin after carbohydrate ingestion, a low-carbohydrate, high-protein diet is commonly ordered. The health care provider or nutritionist will recommend the appropriate daily calorie intake and distribution among the food groups. General guidelines are listed in the Patient Teaching box.

Patient Teaching Box

Dietary Guidelines for Hypoglycemia Unrelated to Diabetes

- Restrict carbohydrates to no more than 100 g/day
- Avoid simple sugars; eat complex carbohydrates instead
- A high-protein diet is recommended
- Include fats to obtain remaining calories in the diet
- Smaller, more frequent meals may be better tolerated.
- Avoid alcohol

NURSING CARE OF THE PATIENT WITH HYPOGLYCEMIA

FOCUSED ASSESSMENT

Health History

Reason for seeking care. Begin by asking why the patient has sought medical care.

Present health/history of present illness. The present health history is especially important in the diagnosis of hypoglycemia. Describe the present illness, which may include the following symptoms: shakiness, nervousness, irritability, tachycardia, anxiety, lightheadedness, hunger, tingling or numbness of the lips or tongue, nightmares, and crying out during sleep. Note when the episodes occur in relation to meals and particular food intake.

Past health history. The past medical history documents diabetes, previous gastric surgery, abdominal cancer, or adrenal insufficiency. Record medications, paying particular attention to any drugs that lower blood glucose. Note the drug names, prescribed dose, and the time that the last dose was taken. The functional assessment elicits information about current diet, exercise, alcohol intake, and the effects of symptoms on daily activities.

Physical Examination

Important aspects of the physical examination include general behavior, appearance, pulse, and BP.

Patient Problems, Goals, and Outcome Criteria: Hypoglycemia Unrelated to Diabetes

Patient Problems	Goals and Outcome Criteria
Inability to manage condition related to lack of knowledge of hypoglycemia prevention and treatment	Patient is prepared to manage hypoglycemic episodes appropriately: patient accurately describes and demonstrates self-care measures
Potential for injury related to episodes of dizziness and weakness	Decreased potential for injury: no falls or injuries as a result of hypoglycemic episodes
Inadequate coping related to perceived effects of illness on lifestyle	Patient adapts to changes required to manage hypoglycemia: patient describes and practices measures to manage hypoglycemia, integrates dietary guidelines into usual eating habits

INTERVENTIONS

Inability to Manage Condition

Patient education is a priority after a confirmed diagnosis to prevent future occurrences. Teach patients to recognize the signs and symptoms and to treat them promptly. Advise the patient of factors that may trigger hypoglycemic episodes, such as foods, medications, alcohol, fasting, and exercise. Basic concepts of the diet described earlier need to be stressed and reinforced. A referral for a consultation with a registered dietitian may be helpful for the patient. Because hypoglycemia is commonly treated in an out-patient setting, nurses in those settings need to reinforce patient teaching and encourage self-management.

Potential for Injury

The hypoglycemic patient is at risk for injury as a result of weakness and dizziness. In the health care setting, monitor for signs and symptoms of hypoglycemia. Monitor serum glucose levels. Administer carbohydrates as prescribed by the physician. Until the episode passes, the patient should lie down and should not get up unassisted.

Inadequate Coping

Emotional support for the patient with hypoglycemia is necessary during diagnosis and treatment. Prepare the patient for diagnostic tests and tell the patient what to expect. Once the diagnosis is made, explore the patient's feelings and concerns. Support the patient in learning to incorporate the management of hypoglycemia into their lifestyle. Guide the patient to anticipate problem situations and possible solutions.

Get Ready for the NCLEX® Examination!

Key Points

- DM is a condition characterized by impaired metabolism related to tissue resistance to insulin or insulin deficiency.
- DM is managed with diet, exercise, and insulin or oral hypoglycemic agents (or with both).
- The major complications of DM are ketoacidosis, hyperosmolar nonketotic coma, vascular changes, and neuropathy.
- Ketoacidosis causes dehydration, electrolyte imbalance, and metabolic acidosis and is treated with fluid and electrolyte replacement and insulin.
- Hyperosmolar nonketotic coma is loss of consciousness caused by extremely high serum glucose without ketoacidosis.
- The major complications of insulin therapy are hypoglycemia, insulin shock, and hyperglycemia (Somogyi effect).
- Nursing care of the patient with DM focuses on ineffective management self-care, inadequate family coping, fluid volume deficit, potential for injury, decreased activity tolerance, chronic pain, disrupted skin tissue integrity, acute confusion, and inadequate coping.
- Hypoglycemia (low serum glucose) in the absence of DM can be caused by pancreatic tumors, adrenal insufficiency, liver disease, and pituitary disorders, but sometimes no specific cause is identified.
- Nursing care of the nondiabetic patient who has hypoglycemia focuses on inability to manage self-care, potential for injury, and ineffective coping.

Additional Learning Resources

SG Go to your Study Guide for additional learning activities to help you master this chapter content.

Go to your Evolve website (http://evolve.elsevier.com/Linton/medsurg) for the following learning resources and much more:
- Fluid & Electrolyte Tutorial
- Review Questions for the NCLEX® Examination

Clinical Judgment and Next-Generation NCLEX® Examination-Style Questions

1. **Functions of insulin include which of the following? (Select all that apply.)**
   1. Serves as an energy source
   2. Helps to transport glucose into cells
   3. Metabolizes glucose for energy
   4. Synthesizes fatty acids and proteins
   5. Stimulates excretion of excess glucose

   NCLEX Client Need: Health Promotion and Maintenance

2. **Of the following ethnic groups, which has the highest incidence of DM?**
   1. Hispanic/Latino
   2. Native American
   3. European

   d. Asian

   NCLEX Client Need: Physiological Integrity: Reduction of Risk Potential

3. **Macrovascular complications of diabetes include which conditions? (Select all that apply.)**
   1. Retinopathy
   2. ESRD (end-stage renal disease)
   3. Stroke
   4. Heart failure
   5. Peripheral vascular disease

   NCLEX Client Need: Physiological Integrity: Reduction of Risk Potential

4. **You are collecting data from a patient who has had type 2 DM for 10 years. He complains of dizziness when rising to a standing position and increasing fatigue with his usual exercise program. His vital signs are normal except for a heart rate of 108 beats per minute. You should report these data to the registered nurse (RN) because these findings are consistent with which of the following?**
   1. CHD
   2. Inadequate control of blood glucose
   3. Autonomic neuropathy
   4. Hyperglycemic episodes

   NCLEX Client Need: Physiological Integrity: Reduction of Risk Potential

5. **A patient who has just been diagnosed with diabetes and started on oral medications says, "I feel strange and my mouth feels numb. Something is wrong!" You note that his hands are trembling and that he is perspiring. What is your best response?**
   1. "These are common symptoms of diabetes. They will go away soon."
   2. "Let's check your blood sugar. It is probably low."
   3. "Your physician will probably need to increase your medication dose."
   4. "This is very unusual. I will call your physician."

   NCLEX Client Need: Physiological Integrity: Pharmacological Therapies

6. **A patient recently diagnosed with DM asks why he should limit his protein intake. The nurse's response should be based on which of the following?**
   1. Metabolism of excess protein causes ketoacidosis.
   2. Protein needs are decreased because excess glucose meets metabolic needs.
   3. High protein intake interferes with absorption of other nutrients.
   4. High protein intake indirectly contributes to the development of nephropathy.

   NCLEX Client Need: Physiological Integrity: Reduction of Risk Potential

7. **SLO/Objective:** Explain the pathophysiology, signs and symptoms, complications, diagnostic tests, and treatment of diabetes mellitus and hypoglycemia.

   NGN Item Type: Cloze

   Cognitive Skill: Prioritize Hypotheses

   A patient with type 1 diabetes is being seen by the home health nurse. He is disabled because of poor vision and peripheral vascular disease. He is 68 years old, lives alone, and takes NPH and Regular insulin. His daughter lives nearby and brings his lunch and dinner daily. The nurse's assessment data are:

- BP: 96/54 mm Hg
- Heart rate: 88 beats per minute, weak, regular
- Respirations: 18 breaths per minute
- Blood glucose: 160 mg/dL
- 5 lb weight loss in past 2 weeks
- Good appetite
- Reports urinary frequency and urgency
- Feels lightheaded when rising from reclining position

Choose the *most likely* options for the information missing from the statements below by selecting from the list of options provided.

The nurse would suspect that the lightheadedness, urinary symptoms, and weight loss are related to __________. The nurse would also recognize that a low ________, increased __________, and ______blood glucose may indicate complications of diabetes. Failure to address these findings could lead to _________.

OPTIONS
High
Low
Blood pressure
Heart rate
Respiratory rate
Blood glucose
Weight loss
Dehydration
Renal failure
Hypoglycemia
Ketoacidosis

NCLEX Client Need: Physiological Integrity: Physiological Adaptation

8. **A patient with type 2 diabetes is taking Precose, an alpha-glucosidase inhibitor. The nurse knows this drug does not cause hypoglycemia unless:**
   1. A dose is omitted
   2. The patient does not eat after taking the drug
   3. Precose is taken along with a sulfonylurea
   4. The patient engages in strenuous physical activity

   NCLEX Client Need: Physiological Integrity: Pharmacological Therapies

9. **Which of the following comprises the classic signs and symptoms of DM? (Select all that apply.)**
   1. Polydipsia
   2. Polyhidrosis
   3. Polyphagia
   4. Polyuria
   5. Polycythemia

   NCLEX Client Need: Physiological Integrity: Physiological Adaptation

10. **A patient who was newly diagnosed with diabetes says, "Everyone I know with diabetes has had one or both legs amputated." What is the most appropriate reply?**
    1. "Try not to think about that."
    2. "Most people with diabetes eventually have to have amputations."
    3. "The ones who had amputations did not follow their physician's orders."
    4. "You can do many things to reduce your risk of future amputations."

    NCLEX Client Need: Physiological Integrity: Reduction of Risk Potential

51 Female Reproductive System Introduction

http://evolve.elsevier.com/Linton/medsurg

Objectives

1. List data to be collected related to the assessment of the female reproductive system.
2. Describe the nursing interventions for women who are undergoing diagnostic tests and procedures for reproductive system disorders.
3. Identify the classes of drugs used for female reproductive disorders, and related nursing care.
4. Identify the nursing interventions associated with douche, cauterization, heat therapy, and topical medications used to treat disorders of the female reproductive system.

Key Terms

dysplasia (dĭs-PLĀ-sē-ă)
hysterectomy (hĭs-tĕr-ĔK-tō-mē)
menarche (mĕ-NĂR-kē)
menopause (MĔN-ō-păwz)

The female reproductive system includes external and internal genitalia and the breasts. The term *vulva* refers to the external genitalia, which comprise the mons pubis, labia majora, labia minora, clitoris, and clitoris (Fig. 51.1). In addition, included in the vulva are mucus-secreting glands. Bartholin glands are located on both sides of the posterior edge of the vaginal opening, and Skene glands are located just inside the urethral opening. The perineum is the area between the posterior junction of the labia minora and the anus. The internal genitalia include two ovaries, two fallopian tubes, the uterus, and the vagina (Fig. 51.2).

ANATOMY AND PHYSIOLOGY OF THE FEMALE REPRODUCTIVE SYSTEM

EXTERNAL GENITALIA

The mons pubis is a pad of fatty tissue that covers and protects the symphysis pubis. The labia majora are extensions of the fatty tissue that cover and protect inner vulvar structures. The labia majora extend from the mons pubis to the perineum. The inner folds of the labia majora are smooth and moist.

The labia minora are thin folds of smooth skin that form a hood, called the *prepuce*, over the clitoris. The clitoris is a small structure that corresponds to the male penis. Like the penis, the clitoris is composed of erectile tissue with sensory nerve endings that are responsive to psychologic and physical stimuli. The labia minora are richly endowed with sebaceous glands, nerves, and blood vessels that also respond to psychologic and physical stimulation. The labia minora may be entirely covered by the labia majora or may be visible between the outer labia.

The urethral (urinary) meatus is below the clitoris. The openings of Skene glands are located on both sides of the urinary meatus. The vaginal opening, the introitus, is partially or entirely covered by a thin fold of tissue called the *hymen.* The hymen may be intact, distended, or ruptured. The size of the introitus varies from very small to large and gaping.

INTERNAL GENITALIA

The vagina is a canal that extends from the vulva to the uterus. This structure has the ability to expand and lengthen to accept an erect penis and to provide an exit for a term fetus. The mucous membranes of the vaginal walls secrete lubricating fluid that cleanses the vagina and interacts with bacteria to maintain an acid pH.

The uterus is a firm, muscular organ that is pear shaped and hollow. Its lower segment is called the *cervix.* The end of the cervix extends into the upper aspect of the vagina. The os is the opening of the cervix into the vagina. The inner lining of the uterus is called the *endometrium.* The upper segment of the uterine body, or corpus, is called the *fundus.*

The two fallopian tubes are thin, hollow, cilia-lined, tubular structures that extend from the uterine fundus. The fallopian tubes have funnel-shaped ends that partially surround the ovaries, and that receive the ovum from the ovary. The fallopian tubes serve as passages for ova from the ovaries and for sperm that travel through the vagina and into the tubes. Fertilization, the union of sperm and ovum, takes place in the fallopian tubes.

The two ovaries are almond-shaped structures located on each side of the uterus. They correspond to the male testes. Ovarian functions include maturation and

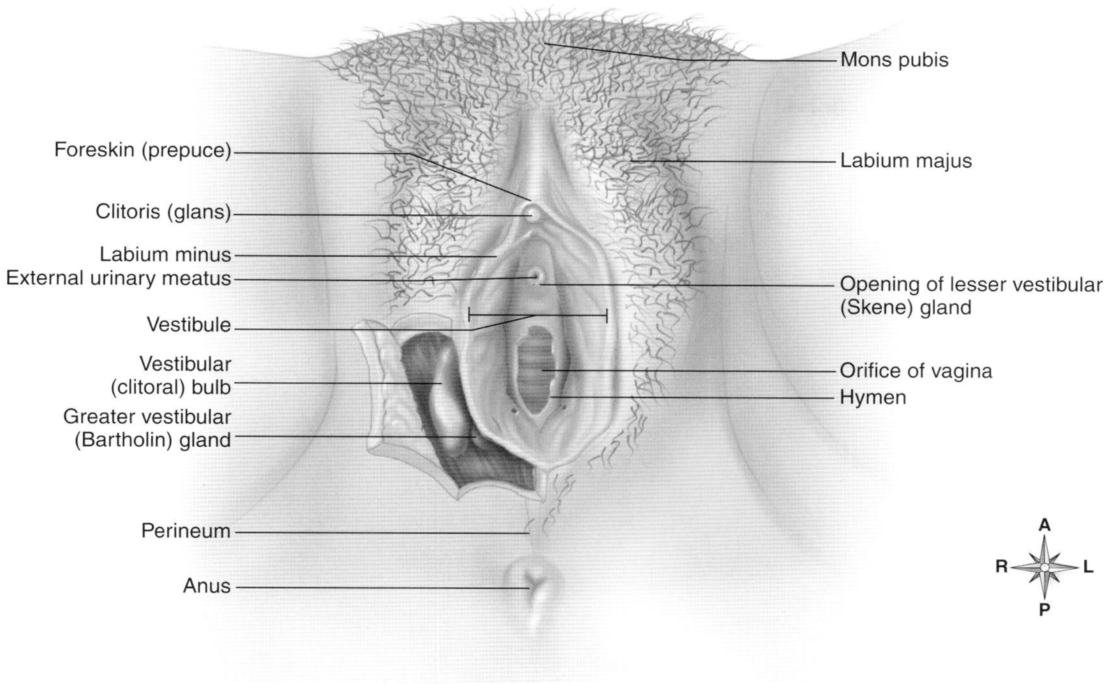

Fig. 51.1 External female genitalia. (From Patton KT, Thibodeau GA: *Human body in health & disease*, ed 7, St. Louis, 2018, Elsevier.)

release of ova (ovulation) and secretion of hormones—estrogens, progesterone, androgens, and relaxin.

It is important to note that the pathway through the female reproductive tract, intended to serve as a route for reproduction, also provides a route for infectious organisms to access the pelvic cavity and its organs.

BREASTS

Although the breasts are not directly involved in the reproductive process, they are addressed as accessories to reproduction because of their function: to nourish the infant after birth. Breast structure is illustrated in Fig. 51.3. The inner structure is composed of glandular and ductal tissue, fibrous tissue, and fat. (The fat is responsible for most of the variation in breast size and shape.) The breast is divided into several lobes, each divided into lobules. Lobules contain many hollow, grape-shaped alveoli that produce milk when stimulated by the pituitary hormone *prolactin.* Ducts carry milk from the lobules, through the lobes, to the opening in the nipple.

The nipple with its surrounding areola is a pigmented structure located at the midline of each breast. Breast milk passes through the openings of the lactiferous ducts. Small, round sebaceous glands called *Montgomery tubercles* are visible under the skin of the areolae. These glands produce a lubricating secretion that protects nipple tissue. Except during normal lactation, no discharge from the nipple should occur.

MENSTRUAL CYCLE

The menstrual cycle, or female reproductive cycle, consists of the ovarian cycle and the uterine cycle. It results from a complex interaction of the hypothalamus, anterior pituitary, and ovary (Fig. 51.4). The interaction causes the ovary to release a mature ovum (i.e., ovulation) and prepares the uterine lining to receive and nourish the ovum if it is fertilized. If the ovum is not fertilized, the menstrual cycle begins with the onset of menstruation. Menstruation is the passage through the vagina of a mixture of blood, other fluids, and tissue formed in the lining of the uterus to receive the fertilized ovum.

The length of the menstrual cycle averages 28 to 30 days, but the range may be 21 to 40 days and may be affected by various factors such as stress, physical activity, and illness. Regardless of the length of the cycle, the progression is the same:

1. Menstruation (day 1 through days 4 to 7) occurs
2. Maturation of an ovarian follicle occurs, with subsequent rupture and release of an ovum in response to follicle-stimulating hormone (FSH) and luteinizing hormone (LH) from the anterior pituitary (days 1 to 14 in a 28-day cycle)
3. Estrogen production (days 6 to 14) by the maturing follicle occurs; progesterone production (days 15 to 26) by the corpus luteum that is formed from the ruptured follicle occurs
4. Preparation of the uterine lining for implantation of the fertilized ovum occurs, stimulated by estrogen and progesterone from the follicle and corpus luteum (days 6 to 26)

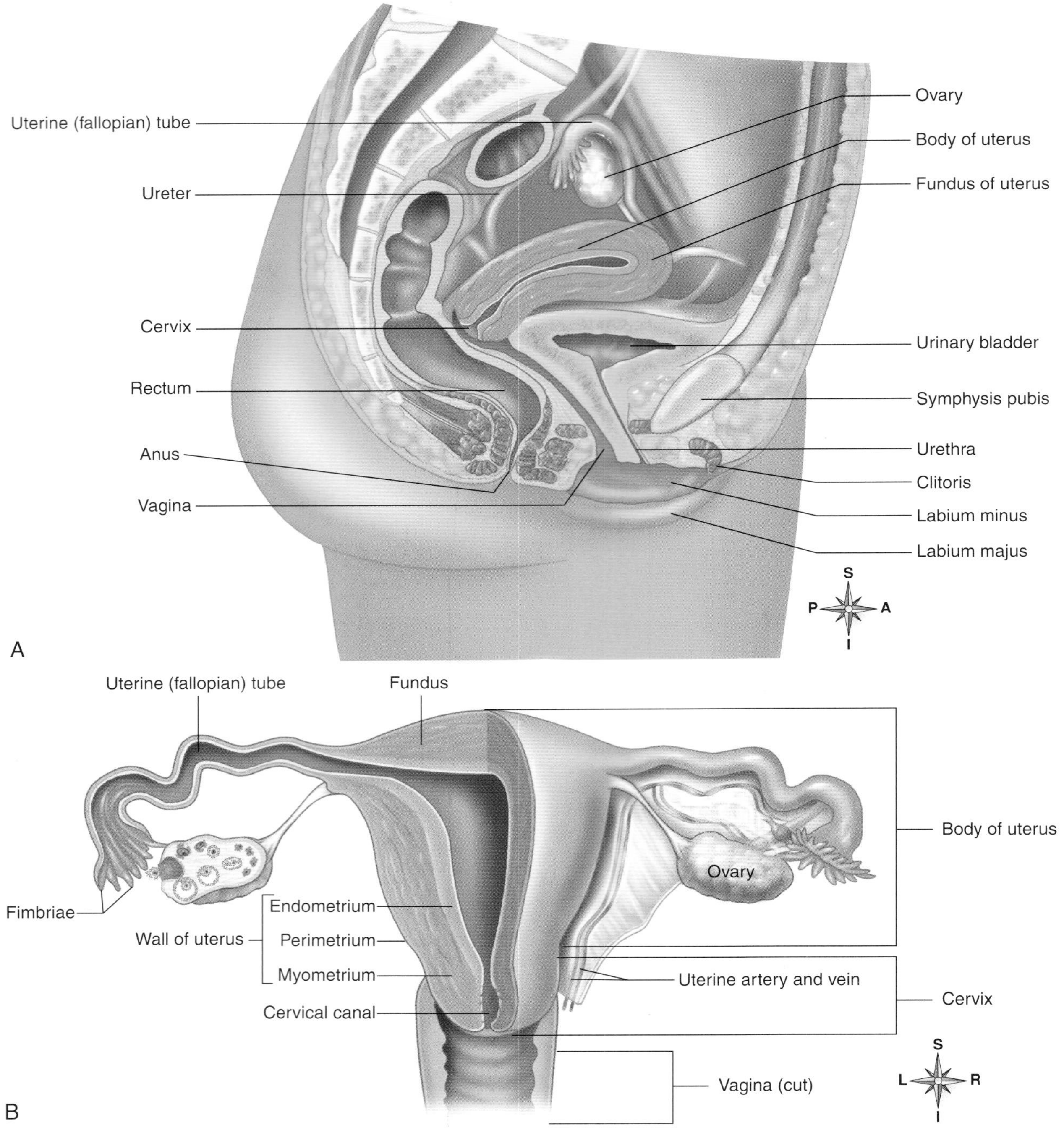

Fig. 51.2 Internal female genitalia. (A) Cross-sectional view of female reproductive organs. (B) Detailed uterine structure. (From Patton KT, Thibodeau GA: *Human body in health & disease*, ed 7, St. Louis, 2018, Elsevier.)

5. The fertilized ovum implants in the uterine lining and secretes human chorionic gonadotropin (HCG), which maintains the corpus luteum and estrogen and progesterone levels; menstruation does not occur (day 14)
   Or
   The unfertilized ovum does not implant. Absence of HCG causes the corpus luteum to degenerate, which, in turn, causes a drop in estrogen and progesterone levels and necrosis of the uterine lining (days 27 to 28). The necrotic lining is shed as menstrual flow and begins another cycle at day 1.

NURSING ASSESSMENT OF THE FEMALE REPRODUCTIVE SYSTEM

HEALTH HISTORY

Reason for Seeking Care

The licensed vocational nurse/licensed practical nurse (LVN/LPN) collects data that contribute to the professional nurse's complete assessment. The complete assessment is described here even though the LVN/LPN would not be responsible for all of it.

The basic assessment begins with the patient's reason for seeking medical care. "What is the reason for your visit?" is an opening question that allows the patient to describe in her own terms the reason for the visit and to include related information that may guide subsequent questions.

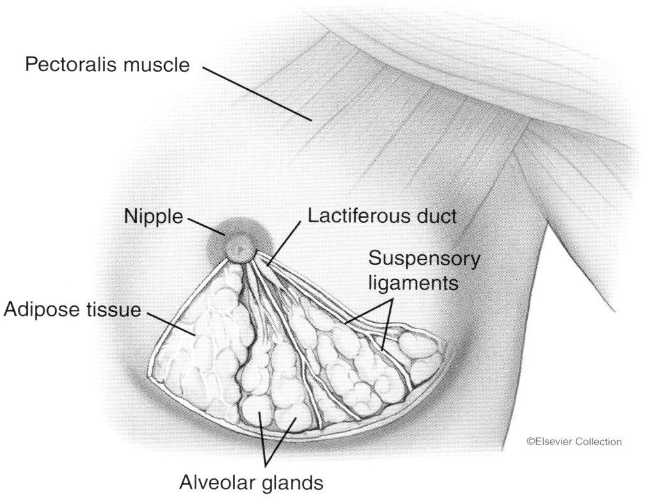

Fig. 51.3 Structure of the mature female breast. (Copyright © Elsevier Collection.)

Present Health/History of Present Illness

If the reason for the visit is an existing problem, include related signs and symptoms and their onset, frequency, and effect on normal functioning.

Past Health History

Menstrual history. Record the age at which menstruation began (**menarche**), the date of the onset of the last menstrual period, the usual number of days between the onset of one period and the onset of the next, the total amount of menstrual flow, the usual number of days of menstrual flow per period, and the use of tampons.

"Many women experience problems with their periods. What problems have you noticed?" is a questioning technique that implies acceptance of a wide variety of problems and invites the patient to provide additional relevant information. Problems commonly reported include spotting or frank bleeding between periods, abdominal pain at the time of ovulation, abdominal cramping or pain before or during periods (or both), and premenstrual mood changes.

For women who have stopped menstruating owing to **menopause** (cessation of menses), important data include the age at which menstruation ceased and related

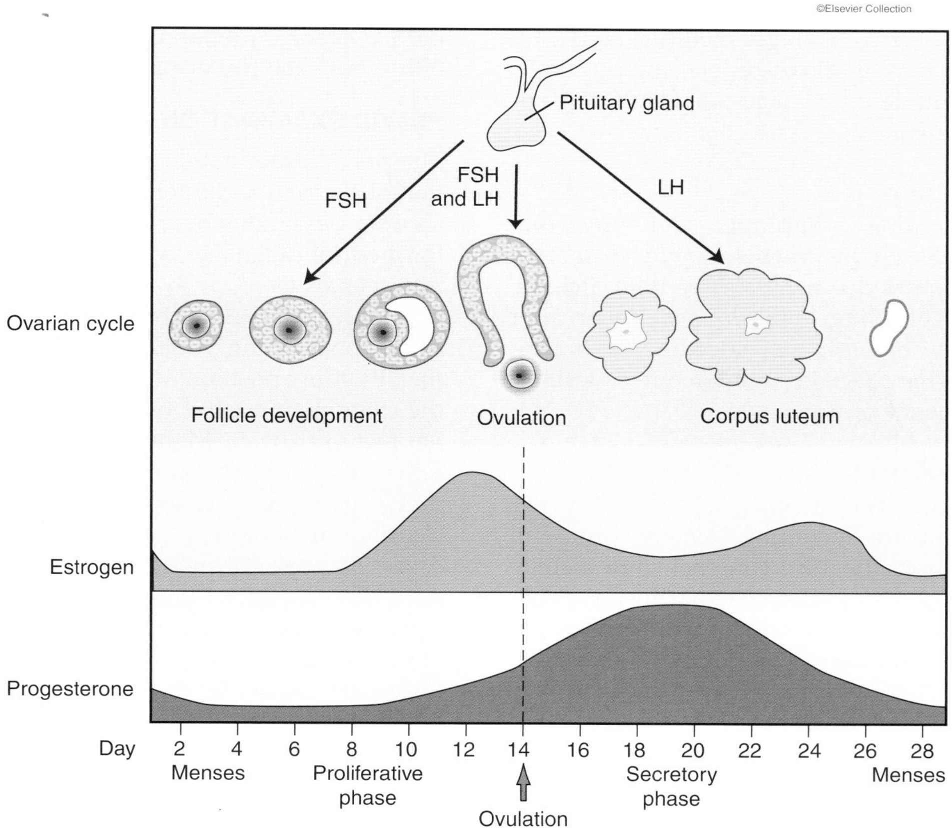

Fig. 51.4 Female hormonal cycle. *FSH*, Follicle-stimulating hormone; *LH*, luteinizing hormone. (Copyright © Elsevier Collection.)

details, such as whether menopause occurred naturally or resulted from surgery, chemotherapy, or radiation therapy. Include information about menopausal symptoms and prescribed or over-the-counter (OTC) medications taken to relieve menopausal symptoms.

Obstetric-gynecologic history. "Have you ever been pregnant?" is an appropriate opening question for the obstetric history. If the response indicates that the woman has been pregnant, inquire about the number of term and preterm births, number of living children, number of abortions (spontaneous or induced), and number of multiple pregnancies (e.g., twins, triplets). Note blood type and Rhesus (Rh) factor, as well as any history of rubella or rubella immunization. Terms related to obstetric history are *gravidity* and *parity.* Gravidity refers to the total number of pregnancies. Parity refers to the number of pregnancies reaching 20 weeks of gestation, which is considered the "age of viability." Parity may be recorded according to a number of different codes that use one- to five-digit numbers. Each institution provides direction on how parity is to be coded for obstetric histories.

The gynecologic history addresses such problems as infections and sexually transmitted infections (STIs), cysts and tumors, structural and functional abnormalities, birth control, infertility, sexual trauma and rape, and stress incontinence.

Family History

Record a family history of diabetes mellitus (DM), cancer, heart disease, psychiatric disorders, complications of pregnancy, multiple pregnancies, genetic disorders, or congenital anomalies.

Review of Symptoms

Information regarding symptoms and any prescribed or self-selected treatments should be recorded. Commonly reported symptoms are pain, itching, burning, vaginal bleeding between periods or after menopause, heavy or prolonged bleeding with periods, vaginal discharge, painful intercourse, lesions, and urinary frequency or urgency.

Functional Assessment

The functional assessment includes a diet history; use of dietary supplements including calcium, iron, and botanical medications; health maintenance to include immunizations; exercise pattern; sexual history; substance use; disabilities; occupational exposure to potential teratogens; and effects of symptoms on usual activities.

PHYSICAL EXAMINATION

In the general survey, important data include the patient's appearance, facial expression, and any obvious signs of distress. Measure vital signs, including height, weight, and blood pressure (BP). Note skin color, texture, and moisture. Examine the breasts for dimpling and abnormal skin texture. With the patient leaning forward, observe for asymmetry in the breasts. Ask the patient about changes from usual contours. Palpate all breast tissue for thickening or lumps (see the section titled "Breast Self-Examination").

Inspect the abdomen for distention and palpate for tenderness. Inspect the legs for swelling and palpate for tenderness. The pelvic examination may be done by the physician or a nurse with advanced training. Therefore, it is discussed in detail with other diagnostic tests and procedures. Basically, the examiner assesses the external genitalia for lesions, lumps, swelling, and discharge. The vagina and uterine cervix are inspected for lesions, growths, discharge, and redness. The vagina, abdomen, and rectum are palpated for abnormalities. Assessment of the female reproductive system is summarized in Box 51.1.

DIAGNOSTIC TESTS AND PROCEDURES

The physician or nurse practitioner performs most diagnostic tests and procedures. The responsibilities of the nurse usually focus on patient instruction regarding the procedure, preparation of the patient, support of the patient throughout the tests and procedures, and assistance to the physician or nurse practitioner. Regardless of the test or procedure to be performed, provide anticipatory guidance by telling the patient what to expect. Check the institution's procedure manual for specific preparations and assistants' responsibilities for each test or procedure.

PELVIC EXAMINATION

The pelvic examination allows inspection and palpation of external and internal reproductive structures to identify deviations from normal, provide information for medical diagnoses, and collect specimens for laboratory analysis.

Slightly elevate the head of the examination table before positioning your patient. The patient assumes the lithotomy position, with her buttocks at the edge of the examination table, her hips and knees flexed, and her feet in stirrups. Many women report that the position is unpleasant because of the sense of vulnerability they experience. To decrease this effect, delay positioning until just before the examination begins, carefully drape to preserve modesty, and provide verbal and nonverbal support. Remember to take care in positioning older patients who have osteoarthritis or have had prior hip surgery to avoid excessive hip rotation and knee movement. To decrease physical discomfort associated with use of the stirrups, cover them with thick footlets or encourage the patient to continue to wear her socks or shoes.

The pelvic examination is divided into three parts: (1) visual inspection and palpation of the external genitalia, (2) visual inspection of the vagina and uterine

Box 51.1 Assessment of the Female Reproductive System

HEALTH HISTORY
Present Health/History of Present Illness
Reason for visit, related signs and symptoms, onset and frequency of symptoms, effects on normal functioning

PAST HEALTH HISTORY
Menstrual History
Age at menarche, date of onset of last menstrual period, duration of menstrual period, amount of menstrual flow, use of tampons, pain, bleeding between periods, premenstrual mood changes; for menopausal women: age at which menopause occurred, whether menopause was natural or surgical, related symptoms, medications taken to relieve symptoms
Obstetric and Gynecologic History
Number of pregnancies, number of term and preterm births, number of living children, number of abortions (spontaneous and induced), number of multiple pregnancies, past problems with reproductive organs, fertility, stress incontinence, sexual trauma and rape, history of rubella or rubella immunization, frequency of breast self-examination (BSE), contraception use
Family History
Diabetes, cancer, complications of pregnancy, heart disease, psychiatric disorders, genetic disorders, multiple pregnancies, congenital anomalies
Review of Systems
Pain, itching, burning, vaginal bleeding between periods or after menopause, heavy or prolonged bleeding with periods, vaginal discharge, urinary frequency or urgency
Functional Assessment
Diet; use of dietary supplements including calcium, iron, and botanical medications; health maintenance to include immunizations; exercise pattern; sexual history; substance use; disabilities; occupational exposure to potential teratogens
Physical Examination
General Survey: Appearance, facial expression, obvious distress

VITAL SIGNS
Height and Weight
Skin: Texture, moisture, color
Breasts: Dimpling, texture changes in skin, asymmetry when leaning forward, changes from usual contours, changes in texture, vascular pattern changes, lumps, nipple discharge
Extremities: Temperature, rashes, swelling, tenderness
Abdomen: Contour, distention, vascular pattern changes, tenderness
Pelvic Examination
External Genitalia: Appearance, lesions, lumps, swelling, discharge
Vagina and Uterine Cervix: Appearance, lesions, growths, discharge, redness
Rectal Examination: Appearance, lesions, growths

cervix after introduction of a plastic or metal speculum (Fig. 51.5), and (3) bimanual palpation of the vagina and abdomen. The latter procedure may be performed with two fingers of one gloved hand in the vagina or with one finger in the vagina and one finger in the rectum (Fig. 51.6) and the other hand on the abdomen to allow compression of internal structures between the two hands. The final step is a rectal examination with a gloved finger.

The examiner can do much to decrease the patient's anxiety if this is her first pelvic examination by explaining each step in advance using models or showing equipment before the examination. Discomfort varies among women. Some women report no discomfort other than feelings of pressure; other women report pain. One common discomfort is related to a cold speculum. This can be prevented by warming the speculum in water or by wrapping the packaged speculum in the folds of a heating pad. Supportive measures include talking to the patient and directing breathing and relaxation techniques to relieve pain and tension. After the pelvic examination, assist the patient to sit up and to get off the table. Provide tissues to wipe the perianal area and, if possible, an adhesive panty liner to absorb lubricant as it is expelled from the vagina.

STAINS AND CULTURES

Collection of specimens for laboratory analysis is one of the purposes of the pelvic examination (see Fig. 51.5D). Institutional policy specifies the necessary equipment and the care of slides for each specimen.

Specimens are routinely collected for a Papanicolaou (Pap) test for detection of cervical cancer and other abnormal cervical cells (**dysplasia**). Additional specimens may be collected for the identification of possible infections, such as herpes, *Chlamydia*, and gonorrhea. The examiner may swab vaginal and cervical fluid to identify bacterial-, fungal-, or trichomonal-related infections, as well as to assess pH.

ENDOMETRIAL AND CERVICAL BIOPSIES

Endometrial biopsies are generally performed for four reasons: (1) to assess the endometrium for readiness to accept and nourish a fertilized ovum, (2) to indirectly assess corpus luteum function in cases of possible infertility, (3) to diagnose irregular uterine bleeding patterns, and (4) to diagnosis uterine cancer. The nurse's responsibilities are similar to those for a pelvic examination and collection of specimens for stains and cultures. The physician or nurse practitioner dilates the cervix and scrapes tissue specimens from the endometrium. The procedure may cause cramping so severe that an anesthetic is necessary.

Cervical biopsies are used to remove suspicious tissue and rule out cervical cancer. Two types of biopsy exist: (1) multiple punch and (2) cone. Multiple punch biopsies are done in a physician's office or an outpatient clinic. Because several specimens are obtained by punching out small samples of cervical tissue, the process is usually painful. The nurse's responsibilities are similar to those for endometrial biopsies. You can

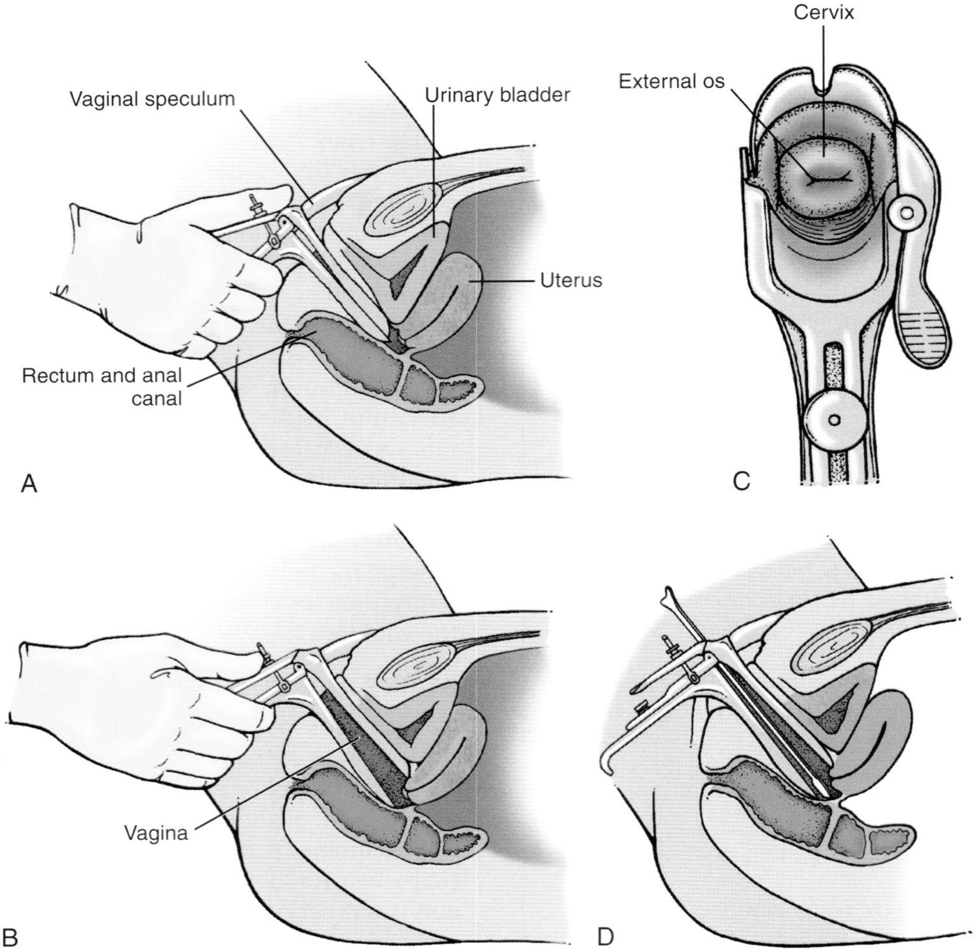

Fig. 51.5 Internal examination of the cervix. (A) Insertion of the speculum. (B) Open speculum within the vagina. (C) Examiner's view of the cervix through an open speculum. (D) An instrument called an *Ayre spatula* is inserted through the speculum to obtain a cervical specimen for a Papanicolaou (Pap) test. (From Monahan FD, Drake DT, Neighbors M, editors: *Medical-surgical nursing: foundations for clinical practice*, ed 2, Philadelphia, 1998, Saunders.)

support the patient by coaching her to use breathing and relaxation techniques to minimize discomfort.

The cone biopsy is invasive surgery and requires admission to an outpatient surgery facility or a hospital. Under general anesthesia, a large amount of cervical tissue is removed. Although the cone biopsy is rarely used to diagnose cancer, its advantage lies in its potential to diagnose and remove cancerous tissue.

COLPOSCOPY

An instrument called a *colposcope* is used to inspect the cervix under magnification and to identify abnormal and potentially cancerous tissue. Colposcopy is commonly done before cervical biopsies. Patient preparation and nursing care are similar to those for a pelvic examination.

CULDOSCOPY

A culdoscopy is an invasive surgical procedure usually performed with light sedation and local anesthetic on an outpatient basis. When performed by a skillful physician, culdoscopy is the simplest way to directly visualize the female pelvic cavity. With the patient in the knee-chest or lithotomy position, the culdoscope is inserted through a small incision in the posterior vagina. The culdoscope permits examination of the patient's uterus, ovaries, and fallopian tubes. It is performed to obtain tissue specimens and to identify ectopic pregnancy, pelvic masses, and causes of infertility or pain.

The nurse's responsibilities are similar to those for other outpatient procedures, with details specified by institutional policies. Scrupulous asepsis must be maintained. Many women consider the knee-chest position physically uncomfortable, embarrassing, and humiliating. Assure the patient that she will be draped throughout the procedure and be conscientious about following through with that assurance. When the procedure is completed, help the patient to get out of the knee-chest position without exposure. Advise her that she may experience shoulder pain caused by air entering the pelvic cavity during the procedure. In addition, reassure her that the incision will close and heal without sutures, but that nothing should be inserted in

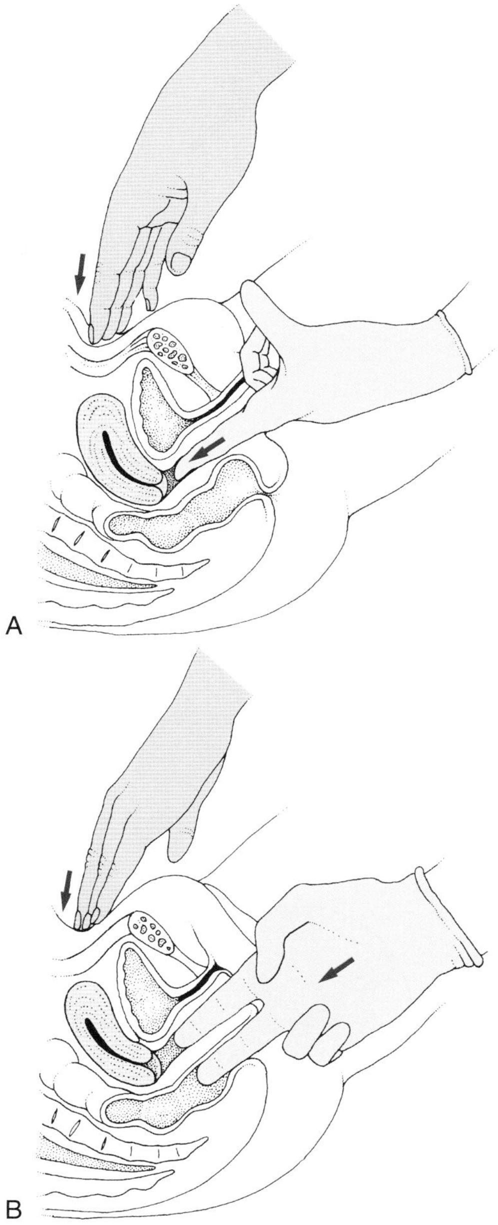

Fig. 51.6 Bimanual palpation. (A) Bimanual pelvic examination. (B) Bimanual rectovaginal examination. (From Ignatavicius DD, Workman ML, Mishler M: *Medical-surgical nursing: a nursing process approach*, ed 2, Philadelphia, 1995, Saunders.)

the vagina (e.g., no vaginal intercourse, douching, or tampons) for the period of time the physician specifies.

LAPAROSCOPY

Laparoscopy (Fig. 51.7) is a surgical procedure that may be performed under local anesthesia on an outpatient basis or under general anesthesia in an outpatient surgical facility or hospital. The physician uses an instrument called a *laparoscope* to visualize abdominal organs and perform minor surgery, such as a tubal ligation. The laparoscope is inserted through a small abdominal incision. Instruments may be inserted through the laparoscope itself or through a small second incision. Before the laparoscope is inserted, a small quantity of gas is injected into the abdomen to create a pocket in which to insert the laparoscope and to allow a clear view of the organs. This gas eventually is absorbed, but in the immediate postoperative period, it tends to cause shoulder pain, pain below the rib cage, or both. Inform and reassure the patient that the discomfort is expected and is temporary.

DILATION AND CURETTAGE

Dilation and curettage (D&C) is used for diagnostic and treatment purposes. The D&C is used to diagnose uterine cancer and causes of abnormal uterine bleeding. It may also be used to treat some causes of bleeding.

D&C is performed in two steps. The first is dilation of the cervix by insertion of a series of progressively larger rods. The second step is endometrial curettage, or scraping of the entire uterine lining. The scraped tissue sample is removed by vacuum aspiration (suction). Tissue samples are prepared for laboratory analysis according to institutional procedures.

Most D&Cs can be performed under local anesthesia in the physician's office or outpatient clinic. Patient preparation and positioning are similar to those used for the pelvic examination. As for all procedures, institutional policy directs the nurse's role and responsibilities.

MAMMOGRAPHY

Mammography is a radiologic test used to detect breast cysts or tumors, especially those not palpated on physical examination. The test used most often in the United States is full field digital mammography. The newest innovation is the digital breast tomosynthesis (DST) three-dimensional (3D) mammography. The 3D test may be more sensitive in young women and women with very dense breast tissue; however, it has a slightly higher rate of false-positive results. The American Cancer Society (ACS) recommends that mammograms be obtained in women at average risk for breast cancer at the age of 40 to 44 years, with subsequent testing done annually thereafter until 55 years of age, at which time, the woman may be transitioned to biennial screening or continued annually for as long as she is otherwise in good health (ACS, 2021). Women in their 40s should consult with their health care provider to see if they would benefit from screening. The ACS website (cancer.org) should be accessed to confirm the society's latest recommendations. Mammography takes only a few minutes and is performed by a trained technician. For the procedure, each breast is compressed in a mammography machine and two views are taken of each breast, one from above and one from the side. The images are usually available immediately, allowing a radiologist to view them before the patient leaves the setting. Most mammograms are obtained in

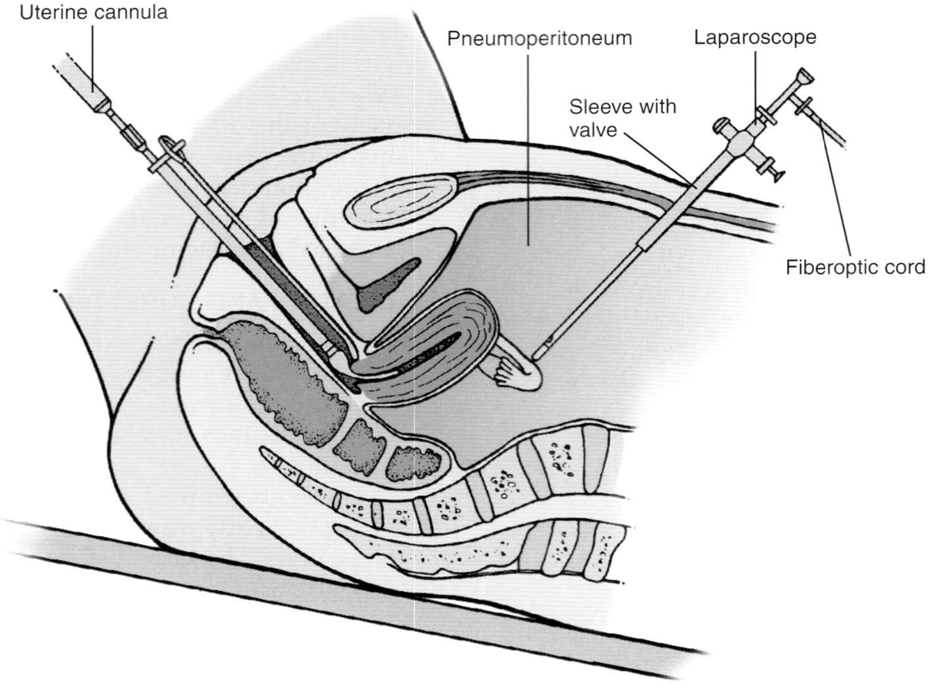

Fig. 51.7 Laparoscopy. (From Monahan FD, Drake DT, Neighbors M, editors: *Medical-surgical nursing: foundations for clinical practice*, ed 2, Philadelphia, 1998, Saunders.)

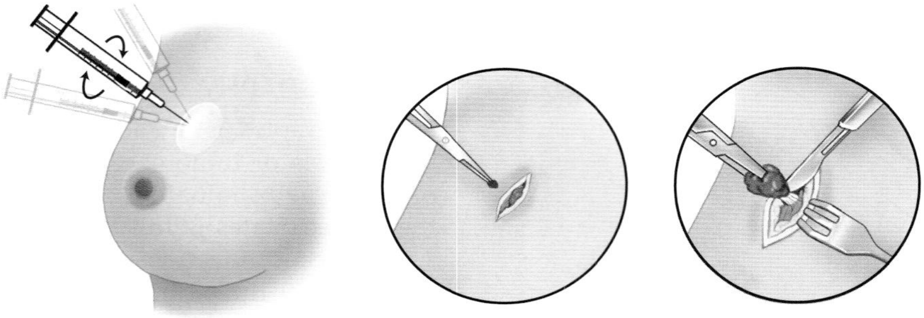

Fig. 51.8 Breast biopsy techniques. (From Leonard PC: *Building a medical vocabulary with Spanish translations*, ed 10, St. Louis, 2018, Elsevier.)

settings that do not routinely employ nurses. However, you need to be familiar with the process so that you can prepare the patient.

Put On Your Thinking Cap!

A 53-year-old woman who has never had a mammogram states that her friends have told her it is very painful. What approaches might you use in encouraging her to have a mammogram?

BREAST SELF-EXAMINATION

In the past, women were encouraged to examine their breasts monthly to detect changes that might include malignant growths. However, newer guidelines do not endorse this procedure as a means of finding breast lumps. Instead, periodic mammograms are recommended. This is based on findings that only 10% of malignant lesions are detected by palpation.

BREAST BIOPSY

When breast changes are discovered, a breast biopsy may be done to determine the reason for the change. A biopsy is the definitive test for diagnosing breast cancer.

The physician decides which diagnostic procedures are appropriate. Breast biopsies for palpable small lumps can be performed under local anesthesia on an outpatient basis (Fig. 51.8). A needle may be used to aspirate fluid from cysts. Solid masses require a surgical approach to obtain a specimen of the questionable tissue or to remove the mass. Biopsies of large masses are generally performed under general anesthesia in a hospital setting. All removed tissue and aspirated fluid are sent to the laboratory for analysis. Decisions for further treatment are based on biopsy reports.

The patient admitted to the health care setting for a breast biopsy needs a great deal of supportive care. She needs an opportunity to talk about her fears and a thorough explanation of what she can expect during the preoperative, operative, and postoperative periods.

Information about diagnostic tests and procedures is summarized in Table 51.1.

COMMON THERAPEUTIC MEASURES

DOUCHING

Douching is a procedure in which the vagina is flooded with fluid containing various cleansing or perfumed agents. Douching is not recommended for regular hygiene because it washes away some of the elements that maintain the normal acidic pH. The acidic environment helps the vagina to maintain its self-cleansing properties and fight off pathogenic organisms.

Douching is potentially dangerous because it may force tissue and microorganisms up into the uterus. In addition, cleansing and perfumed agents may cause allergic or irritant reactions. Contrary to common belief, douching is not an effective contraceptive practice.

The physician or nurse practitioner may order douching to wash the vagina with a bactericidal solution in preparation for surgery, radiation therapy, or other treatment. If ordered, prepare the douche solution using exact measures of the prescribed ingredients; administer the douche according to your institutional procedure.

Because it is also the nurse's responsibility to teach the patient about appropriate vaginal hygiene, you can teach while the douche is administered (see the Patient Teaching box).

Table 51.1 Diagnostic Tests and Procedures: Female Reproductive System

TEST AND PURPOSE	PATIENT PREPARATION	POSTPROCEDURE NURSING CARE
Pelvic examination includes assessment of external genitalia, vagina, uterine cervix, abdomen, and rectum: to identify abnormalities and to collect fluid or tissue specimens.	Explain the examination; then assist the patient into the lithotomy position immediately before the examination. Drape for privacy. Warm the vaginal speculum. Encourage relaxation.	Assist the patient to assume a sitting position and to get down from the examining table. Offer tissues to wipe the perineal area and a panty liner to absorb lubricant as it drains.
Papanicolaou (Pap) test: to detect abnormalities of cervical cells, including cervical cancer. Cultures: to detect pathogens that cause herpes, *Chlamydia*, gonorrhea, etc. Wet prep/potassium hydroxide (KOH): to detect organisms that cause vaginitis and cervicitis. Human papilloma virus (HPV) DNA Testing: may be combined with conventional Pap testing to screen for high-risk HPV types.	Obtain appropriate equipment for specimen collection and preparation. Position and drape the patient.	Same as for pelvic examination. Proper handling of specimens is essential for accurate studies. Prepare specimens, label, and send to the laboratory. Properly dispose of used supplies.
Endometrial biopsy: to study fertility or to detect cancer. Cervical biopsy: to detect cancer.	Endometrial and cervical biopsies: assist the patient into the lithotomy position; drape for privacy. Procedure is painful; encourage breathing and relaxation exercises.	Same as for pelvic examination.
Breast biopsy (or fluid aspiration): to diagnose breast cancer. (Done under local or general anesthesia.)	Recognize patient anxiety about outcome and possible implications. Explain procedure.	Check incision for bleeding. Safety precautions if sedated. Provide opportunity to express fears.
Mammography: to diagnose breast cysts or tumors.	Explain that each breast is compressed and images taken. Mildly uncomfortable, but brief, pressure. Do not use underarm deodorants before procedure.	No special care needed. Patient usually asked to wait until images are viewed by radiologist. Repeat testing may be requested.
Colposcopy: a colposcope is used to inspect the cervix under magnification to identify abnormal tissue. Usually done before cervical biopsy.	Same as for pelvic examination.	Same as for pelvic examination.

DNA, Deoxyribonucleic acid.

CAUTERIZATION

Cauterization is a method of deliberate tissue destruction by means of heat, electricity, or chemicals. The physician or nurse practitioner may cauterize small growths or polyps during the pelvic examination.

APPLICATION OF HEAT

Heat is used as treatment for many reproductive system conditions and disorders. Dry and moist heat are used to relieve pain, promote healing by increasing blood flow and tissue metabolism, and stimulate rupture of abscesses. Because potential damage is associated with excessively high temperature and with conditions such as impaired circulation, edema, and bleeding disorders, any form of heat must be used judiciously.

Patient Teaching

Genital Hygiene

- Wash the external genitalia with plain soap and water at least once a day.
- Keep the genital area clean and dry.
- Wear cotton panties.
- Do not douche unless ordered to do so by the physician or nurse practitioner.

Dry heat in the form of a hot water bottle, a disposable chemical pack, an electric heating pad, or an aquathermia pad (K-pad) may be applied to the breasts or abdomen to relieve pain and to enhance circulation. The commonly recommended temperature range for most of these devices is 40°C to 56°C (104°F to 133°F). Institutional policy and physician's orders dictate the exact temperature and the duration of application time. Although the exact procedure for each method varies among institutions, key points when applying dry heat are as follows:

1. A physician's order is required.
2. Protect the skin by using a barrier between the heating device and the skin.
3. Monitor the patient's response.
4. Maintain the dry heat source temperature in the appropriate range.

Moist heat in the form of hot compresses and sitz baths is used for the same general purposes as dry heat. Hot compresses are particularly useful for applying heat to small areas, such as the vulva or perineum. Depending on the purpose of treatment, the acceptable temperature range for hot compresses is 40.5°C to 46.0°C (105°F to 115°F).

Sitz baths provide heat to the perianal area to relieve pain, cleanse the area, promote healing or drainage, or stimulate urination. The patient sits in warm water that may be in a special tub or in a disposable plastic device that fits on the rim of a regular toilet bowl. A continuous flow of fresh, temperature-controlled warm water is provided by the plumbing apparatus of the sitz bathtub or by a suspended plastic water bag with tubing extended to the disposable device. Water temperature is maintained within 38°C to 46°C (100°F to 115°F); the treatment is used for a maximum of 25 minutes; and the patient is monitored closely for signs of faintness, shock, or severe pain. Because dilation of large pelvic blood vessels by heat may cause hypotension, the patient should not be left alone. Disposable devices are usually taken home by the patient, so it is your responsibility to give detailed instructions on their use.

DRUG THERAPY

Among the many drugs used to treat conditions of the female reproductive system are ovarian hormones (estrogens and progestins), selective estrogen receptor modulators (SERMs), androgens, gonadotropin-releasing hormone (GnRH) agonists, contraceptives, and ovulatory stimulant and fertility drugs.

The use of hormones (estrogen and progestin) to treat menopausal symptoms has had an interesting history. Like any drug therapy, estrogen poses benefits and risks depending on the individual patient profile. For years, hormones were readily prescribed for most postmenopausal women. Then, concerns about adverse effects caused hormone prescription to be drastically curtailed. Currently, only three indications (Lehne, 2019) for hormone therapy are generally supported:

- Treatment of moderate to severe vasomotor symptoms associated with menopause
- Treatment of moderate to severe symptoms of vulvar and vaginal atrophy associated with menopause
- Prevention of postmenopausal osteoporosis

Treatment of the vasomotor, vulvar, and vaginal symptoms is usually limited to 3 to 4 years, which minimizes risk factors. Therapy to prevent osteoporosis needs to be continued long-term and therefore carries more risk. For that reason, health care providers are encouraged to consider nonestrogen treatments such as raloxifene (Evista).

When estrogen is used, it is used alone for women who have had a **hysterectomy** (i.e., surgical removal of the uterus). A combination of estrogen and progestin is used if the woman still has her uterus, because it was found that estrogen alone ("unopposed") increased the risk of uterine cancer. Many authorities agree that decisions about hormone replacement therapy must be based on assessment of individual risk profiles. In general, short-term use of low-dose hormone therapy to manage menopausal symptoms (e.g., moderate to severe hot flashes and vaginal atrophy) is still considered appropriate. The transdermal route is thought to pose less risk for DVT and stroke than oral estrogen.

Medications for application to the vulva or vagina are in the forms of tablets, creams, and suppositories. Because mucous membranes are delicate and highly vascular, a risk of injury exists, and there is a chance of excessive drug effects associated with high drug absorption. The application hand should be gloved for protection of the patient and nurse. Whether inserted with a finger or an applicator, tablets and suppositories are positioned with a down-and-backward motion into the vagina of the supine woman. Cream is administered through an applicator packaged with the cream. Direct the patient to remain supine for at least 15 minutes after application of either medium to allow the medication to disperse throughout the vagina and be absorbed. The medication will dribble out over time, so advise the patient to use a sanitary pad to protect underclothing from staining. Drugs commonly used to treat disorders of the female reproductive system are listed in Table 51.2.

Table 51.2 Drug Therapy: Drugs Used to Treat Disorders of the Female Reproductive System

DRUG	USE AND ACTION	SIDE EFFECTS	NURSING INTERVENTIONS
Ovarian Hormones			
Conjugated estrogens: estradiol (Estrace, Depogen, Dioval, Estinyl, Premarin, Cenestin). Intravaginal tablets: (Vagifem) Transdermal estradiol patch (Minivelle, Climera, et al) Estradol gel (Eiviget, et al) Estradiol spray (Evamist) Estradiol vaginal ring (Estring, Femring).	Replacement of natural hormones after menopause, palliative treatment of advanced breast cancer, treatment of osteoporosis caused by estrogen deficiency. Stimulates endometrial growth and thickening. Enhances bone formation. Depresses beta-lipoprotein and cholesterol plasma levels. Estradiol patch applied to trunk of body; replaced as ordered.	Breast tenderness, breakthrough bleeding, vaginal candidiasis, headache, dizziness, depression, elevated blood pressure (BP), thromboembolism, stroke, myocardial infarction (MI), nausea, skin hyperpigmentation, and decreased glucose tolerance. Increased risk of endometrial cancer, especially in postmenopausal women who take estrogens continuously for ≥ 1 year.	Advise patients to report signs and symptoms of the following: 1. Thromboembolism: calf pain or swelling, chest pain, numbness, visual disturbances. 2. Cardiovascular problems: weight gain, edema. 3. Liver disorders: abdominal pain, jaundice. 4. Breast lumps. 5. Vaginal bleeding. Discourage smoking, which increases risk of adverse effects. Take with evening meal to reduce nausea. Review directions for use of specific drug preparation
Estradiol transdermal spray (Evamist)	Applied between elbow and wrist to provide estradiol.	Hormonal effects may occur in children or pets who are exposed to Evamist.	Prime the applicator before the first use only. Apply to clean, dry, and unbroken skin of the forearm. Let the spray dry for at least 2 minutes before dressing and 30 minutes before washing the area. Provider prescribes number of sprays per day.
Oral progestins: medroxyprogesterone acetate (Provera), norethindrone (Micronor), norethindrone acetate (Aygestin), micronized progesterone (Prometrium)	Promote secretory function in endometrium. Influence uterine contractile activity. Uses: treat uterine bleeding, some types of amenorrhea, and premenstrual syndrome (PMS). Palliative treatment of endometriosis and some cancers. Used with estrogens as oral contraceptives.	Breakthrough bleeding, amenorrhea, breast tenderness, edema, pruritus, increased BP, thromboembolism, depression, photosensitivity.	Monitor weight and BP. Assess for pruritus. Tell patient to report signs of circulatory impairment: swelling, numbness, pain in calf or thigh. Advise patient to avoid excessive sun exposure. Assess mental state. Contraindicated with history of thromboembolism, undiagnosed vaginal bleeding, liver dysfunction, cerebral hemorrhage.

Continued

Table 51.2 Drug Therapy: Drugs Used to Treat Disorders of the Female Reproductive System—cont'd

DRUG	USE AND ACTION	SIDE EFFECTS	NURSING INTERVENTIONS
Parenteral progestin contraceptives: medroxyprogesterone acetate (Depo-Provera) IM and SubQ preparations	Depo-Provera protects against pregnancy for ≥3 months.	Irregular bleeding, breast tenderness, skin rash, weight gain or loss, depression, acne, altered sex drive, bone density loss.	Encourage calcium intake. Monitor for depression and other side effects. To rule out pregnancy, the first dose should be given during the first 5 days of the normal menstrual period, in the first 5 days postpartum if not breastfeeding, or at 6 weeks postpartum if breastfeeding.
Parenteral progestin: hydroxyprogesterone caproate (IM) (Makena)	Used to prevent preterm birth in selected women who have a history of preterm birth.	Injection site reactions, nausea, diarrhea, fluid retention, depression, glucose intolerance.	Inject over at least 1 minute. Monitor blood glucose in women with diabetes. Assess emotional state.
Intravaginal progestin: progesterone (Crinone)	Contraception. Treatment of abnormal uterine bleeding, amenorrhea.	Thromboembolism, stroke, MI, cholestatic jaundice, spontaneous abortion, anaphylaxis.	Intravaginal instructions: use applicator to apply cream or tablet high in vagina.
Transdermal estrogen/progestin combination: norethindrone with estradiol (CombiPatch)	Menopausal hormone therapy.	Skin irritation at patch site. Abdominal pain, nausea and vomiting, bloating, breast tenderness, headache, back pain, weight changes.	Transdermal instructions: apply to clean, dry skin (not on breast or waistline), press for 10 seconds. Replace once or twice weekly as ordered or if patch falls off. Rotate sites.
Selective Estrogen Receptor Modulators (SERMs)			
tamoxifen (Nolvadex) toremifene (Fareston) raloxifene (Evista)	Stimulate estrogen receptors in some tissues, and block them in other tissues. Intended to provide benefits of estrogen with fewer risks. Tamoxifen and toremifene used to treat breast cancer. Raloxifene is the only approved SERM to prevent osteoporosis.	Hot flashes, fluid retention, vaginal discharge, nausea, vomiting, blurred vision, bone pain, menstrual irregularities, confusion. Increases risks of endometrial cancer, stroke, thromboembolism. Teratogenic.	Do not double up if a dose is missed. Tell patient to report severe bone pain to physician so analgesics can be prescribed. Pain is evidence of drug effectiveness; resolves over time. Also report weight gain, edema, or dyspnea. Patient should use nonhormonal barrier method of contraception during and for 1 month after therapy.
Androgens			
danazol (Danocrine)	Inhibits production of pituitary gonadotropins. Used to treat endometriosis and fibrocystic breast disease. Causes atrophy of uterine tissue and endometrial implants.	Acne, oily skin and hair, hirsutism, edema, weight gain, nervousness, deepening of the voice, decreased breast size, muscle cramps, sleep disorders, hot flashes, vaginal dryness.	Monitor weight and BP. Assess for signs of liver dysfunction: jaundice, abdominal pain, light-colored stools. Explain side effects to patient. Contraindications: undiagnosed vaginal bleeding; severe cardiovascular, renal, or hepatic disorders.

Table 51.2 Drug Therapy: Drugs Used to Treat Disorders of the Female Reproductive System—cont'd

DRUG	USE AND ACTION	SIDE EFFECTS	NURSING INTERVENTIONS
Gonadotropin-Releasing Hormone (GnRH) Agonists			
leuprolide acetate (Lupron) goserelin acetate (Zoladex) nafarelin acetate (Synarel)	Initially increases, then decreases, testosterone levels. Used to treat endometriosis (see Chapter 52) and advanced prostate cancer (see Chapter 54).	Hot flashes, decreased libido, dizziness, headache, nausea, constipation or diarrhea.	Lupron should be discarded if discolored or if precipitate forms. Use only diluent provided to reconstitute. Administer immediately after reconstituting. Zoladex is gradually dispersed from an implant placed under the skin. Synarel is inhaled nasally. Tell patient to expect hot flashes that usually decrease with time. Pregnancy should be ruled out before giving any of these drugs because they may cause abortion.
Oral Contraceptives			
Estrogen-progestin combinations (Ortho-Novum, Norinyl, Loestrin, Ovral) Progestin only (Micronor) Estrogen only (diethylstilbestrol)	Suppress ovulation to prevent pregnancy, alter the endometrium and cervical mucus.	Nausea, vomiting, headache, edema, weight gain, breast tenderness. Increased risk of thromboembolism (especially among smokers). Severe nausea and vomiting.	Reinforce instructions for self-medication. Monitor weight. Tell patient to report signs of circulatory impairment: swelling, pain, numbness in an extremity. Contraindicated during pregnancy and in patient with history of thromboembolism, MI. Patient should follow manufacturer's instructions if a dose is missed.
Vaginal Contraceptive			
Etonogestrel/ethinyl estradiol (NuvaRing) vaginal contraceptive device		Vaginal ulceration or irritation may occur with NuvaRing.	Should not use with a diaphragm. Expulsion of the ring is possible.
Subdermal Contraceptive			
Etonogestrel (Nexplanon) subdermal contraceptive	A rod containing a synthetic progesterone is implanted in the upper arm. The drug is slowly dispensed over 3 years. The rod is then removed.	Irregular vaginal bleeding.	Implanted contraceptive may be less effective in overweight women. Rod needs to be removed if thromboembolic event or jaundice occurs and after 3 years of use.
Intrauterine Contraceptive Device			
Intrauterine copper contraceptive device (IUD) (Paragard)	Hormone-free IUD used for contraception. Effective for emergency contraception if inserted within 5 days of unprotected sex.	Insertion may be uncomfortable or painful. Menstrual flow may be lighter or heavier. Although pregnancy is highly unlikely, it may occur, and result in tubal pregnancy or loss of the embryo. Rarely: attaches to or perforates uterine wall.	IUDs are indicated for women in a mutually monogamous/stable relationship. Replaced every 10 years but can be removed at any time if desired. Each month, patient should check for the thread that remains outside the uterus to be sure the device is in place.

Continued

Table 51.2 **Drug Therapy: Drugs Used to Treat Disorders of the Female Reproductive System—cont'd**

DRUG	USE AND ACTION	SIDE EFFECTS	NURSING INTERVENTIONS
Levonorgestrel Intrauterine Contraceptive Devices			
Kyleena, Liletta, Mirena, Skyla	Used for contraception. Mirena also used for menorrhagia.	Risk of PID, especially with STIs. Can cause cramping and altered menstrual patterns. Rarely, perforation of uterine wall can occur.	Must be replaced every 3 to 5 years but can be removed at any time if desired. Presence of threads in the vagina should be checked monthly to confirm placement.
Ovulatory Stimulant and Fertility Drugs			
Clomiphene citrate (Clomid)	All stimulate or mimic actions of natural pituitary gonadotropins. All can result in multiple births.	Hot flashes, breast tenderness, nausea, vomiting, visual disturbances, headache, depression, fatigue, reversible hair loss, weight gain, dizziness, ovarian enlargement.	Contraindicated with liver dysfunction, pregnancy, abnormal bleeding. Safety precautions if patient is dizzy or has visual disturbances. Stop drug and contact physician if visual disturbances occur. Tell patient to report vaginal bleeding or weight gain, signifying ovarian hyperstimulation, in which case, monitor fluid status, weight, and possible signs of internal bleeding. Tell patient to avoid sexual intercourse with ovarian enlargement because of possible rupture.
Menotropins (Repronex, Menopur)	Promotes follicular maturation and ovulation. After follicle matures, hCG is given to promote ovulation.	Ovarian hyperstimulation with sudden enlargement of ovaries. If severe, ascites, pleural effusion, and pain require hospitalization. Pain and irritation at injection site. Rarely, flu-like symptoms: nausea, vomiting, fever.	Reconstitute per directions and administer immediately. Patient should know that menotropin therapy often results in multiple births.
Urofollitropin (Metrodin)	Stimulates ovarian follicular growth. Used to treat selected patients who have not responded to clomiphene citrate.	Same as with menotropins.	
Emergency Contraceptive Drugs			
Levonorgestrel emergency contraception (Plan B) vaginal contraceptives	Plan B used as emergency postcoital contraceptive ("morning-after pill"); taken within 72 hours after unprotected intercourse to prevent implantation of fertilized ovum.	Heavier menstrual bleeding, nausea, abdominal pain, headache, dizziness, vomiting.	
Selective progesterone receptor modular emergency contraception: ulipristal acetate (ella)	ella is used within 120 hours (5 days) after unprotected intercourse. Prevents ovulation.	Headache, nausea, dysmenorrhea, abdominal pain.	

hCG, Human chorionic gonadotropin; *PID*, pelvic inflammatory disease; *STI*, sexually transmitted disease.
NOTE: Research evidence has revealed increased risks of coronary heart disease and invasive breast cancer when combination estrogen and progestin therapy is used in women with an intact uterus.

SURGICAL PROCEDURES

Many disorders of the female reproductive system are treated surgically. Specific examples are given in Chapter 52. Abdominal procedures may be performed through an abdominal incision, vaginally, or endoscopically. The surgeon selects the specific approach according to the diagnosis and the patient's condition. Nursing care varies with each approach. An abdominal approach results in an external excision that requires assessment and care. You must also assess vaginal discharge in these patients because the vagina provides an exit route for blood and other fluids. Vaginal procedures leave no visible incisions, so the patient must be assessed for excessive bleeding through the vagina or for indications of infection such as purulent or foul-smelling vaginal discharge. Laparoscopic procedures require care similar to that for abdominal incisions, but the incisions are much smaller. Again, the patient may have vaginal discharge that should be assessed after laparoscopic pelvic procedures.

Get Ready for the NCLEX® Examination!

Key Points

- The female reproductive system includes the external and internal genitalia and the breasts.
- The female reproductive tract can provide a route for infectious organisms to access the pelvic cavity and its organs.
- Common therapeutic measures for the female reproductive system include douche, cauterization, heat application, topical medications, and surgical procedures.
- The length of the menstrual cycle averages 28 to 30 days; it may be affected by various factors, such as stress, physical activity, and illness.
- Menarche is the age at which menstruation began.
- Common problems related to the menstrual cycle include spotting or frank bleeding between periods, abdominal pain with ovulation, abdominal cramping or pain before or during periods (or both), and premenstrual mood changes.
- Gravidity refers to the total number of pregnancies.
- Parity refers to the number of pregnancies reaching 20 weeks of gestation, which is considered the "age of viability."
- Actions to decrease discomfort during the pelvic examination include delaying positioning until just before the examination begins, carefully draping to preserve modesty, warming the speculum, and providing verbal and nonverbal support.
- The Pap test is done to detect cervical cancer and other abnormal cervical cells (dysplasia).
- Culdoscopy is an invasive surgical procedure performed to obtain tissue specimens and to identify ectopic pregnancy, pelvic masses, and causes of infertility or pain.
- During a laparoscopy, gas that is injected into the abdomen may cause temporary postprocedure pain in the shoulder and/or below the rib cage.
- Mammography is the only screening tool for breast cancer that is recommended by the American Cancer Society.
- Although it may be used for some therapeutic purposes, douching is not recommended for regular hygiene because it washes away some of the elements that maintain the normal acidic pH of the vagina.
- Drugs used to treat conditions of the female reproductive system include ovarian hormones (estrogens and progestins), SERMs, androgens, GnRH agonists, contraceptives, and ovulatory stimulant and fertility drugs.
- Short-term use of low-dose hormone therapy to manage menopausal symptoms is still considered appropriate.
- According to Lehne (2019), the only indication for long-term hormone replacement therapy is for the prevention of postmenopausal osteoporosis.
- Effective alternatives to hormone therapy to prevent postmenopausal osteoporosis include raloxifene, bisphosphonates, calcitonin, and teriparatide.

Additional Learning Resources

SG Go to your Study Guide for additional learning activities to help you master this chapter content.

Go to your Evolve website (http://evolve.elsevier.com/Linton/medsurg) for the following learning resources and much more:

- Fluid & Electrolyte Tutorial
- Review Questions for the NCLEX® Examination

Clinical Judgment and Next-Generation NCLEX® Examination-Style Questions

1. **Fertilization occurs in which site?**
   1. Uterus
   2. Ovary
   3. Fallopian tube
   4. Vagina

   NCLEX Client Need: Health Promotion and Maintenance

2. **Which question collects data about the patient's menarche?**
   1. "At what age did you begin menstruating?"
   2. "Would you describe your menstrual flow as light or heavy?"
   3. "What was your age when you first experienced hot flashes?"
   4. "Do you usually have any changes in mood before your menstrual period?"

   NCLEX Client Need: Health Promotion and Maintenance

3. **Which of the following statements are appropriate to prepare a patient for culdoscopy? (Select all that apply.)**
   1. "You will need to be in a knee-chest or lithotomy position."
   2. "You will have no restrictions after the procedure."
   3. "You will need to return in 1 week to have your sutures removed."
   4. "You may have shoulder pain caused by air entering the pelvic cavity."
   5. "You will be given general anesthesia for this procedure."

   NCLEX Client Need: Reduction of Risk Potential

4. **You are teaching a class on early detection of breast cancer to women of various ages. Which of the following information should be included? (Select all that apply.)**
    1. "Only women with a family history of breast cancer need periodic screening."
    2. "Periodic mammograms are the best tests to detect breast cancer early."
    3. "Women who examine their breasts regularly do not need other screening tests."
    4. "Mammograms are needed only after menopause"
    5. "Breast examinations by the health care provider detect most malignant lumps."

    NCLEX Client Need: Physiological Integrity: Reduction of Risk Potential

5. **SLO/Objective:** List data to be collected related to the assessment of the female reproductive system.

    NGN Item Type: Enhanced Hot Spot

    Cognitive Skill: Recognize Cues

    A young woman has come to the physician's office with gynecologic symptoms. The health history elicits these data:
    - First menstrual period at age 12 years
    - Abdominal cramps before and during menstrual period
    - Irritable around time of menstrual period
    - Douches after period to cleanse vagina
    - Sexually active since age 17 years
    - Takes oral contraceptives
    - Painful intercourse last 2 weeks
    - Burning on urination

    Highlight or place a check mark next to the assessment findings that require follow up by the nurse.

    NCLEX Client Need: Health Promotion and Maintenance

6. **A patient is scheduled for a Pap test as part of her annual checkup. The nurse can explain that this test is used to detect abnormalities in which tissue?**
    1. Breast
    2. Cervix
    3. Lymph nodes
    4. Ovaries

    NCLEX Client Need: Physiological Integrity: Reduction of Risk Potential

7. **When assisting with a pelvic examination, the role of the LVN/LPN includes which of the following? (Select all that apply.)**
    1. Assist the patient onto the examination table
    2. Warm the speculum before use
    3. Encourage breathing and relaxation
    4. Collect vaginal specimens
    5. Assist the patient to get off the examination table

    NCLEX Client Need: Physiological Integrity: Reduction of Risk Potential

8. **The term *gravidity* refers to a patient's total number of:**
    1. Living children
    2. Pregnancies
    3. Live deliveries
    4. Pregnancies reaching 20 weeks of gestation

    NCLEX Client Need: Health Maintenance and Promotion

9. **Plan B and ella are examples of which class of drugs?**
    1. Emergency contraceptives
    2. Hormone replacement drugs
    3. Ovulatory stimulants
    4. Selective estrogen receptor modulators

    NCLEX Client Need: Physiological Integrity: Pharmacological Therapies

10. **A 40-year-old patient asked when she should begin having regular mammograms. What should she be told?**
    1. She should have a mammogram every 2 years between 40 and 60 years of age.
    2. Routine mammograms are no longer recommended for women with no family history of breast cancer.
    3. She should consult with her primary care provider about the appropriate schedule for mammograms.
    4. Ideally, she should have had a baseline screening before 40 years of age.

    NCLEX Client Need: Physiological Integrity: Reduction of Risk Potential

Female Reproductive Disorders

52

http://evolve.elsevier.com/Linton/medsurg

Objectives

1. Explain the pathophysiology, clinical manifestations, complications, diagnostic procedures, and medical or surgical treatment for selected disorders of the female reproductive system.
2. Assist in developing a nursing care plan for patients with common disorders of the female reproductive system.
3. Describe the nursing interventions for the patient who is having symptoms related to menopause.

Key Terms

cystocele (SĬS-tō-sēl)
dysmenorrhea (dĭs-mĕn-ō-RĒ-ă)
dyspareunia (dĭs-pă-ROO-nē-ă)
dysplasia (dĭs-PLĀ-sē-ă)
endometriosis (ĕn-dō-mē-trē-Ō-sĭs)
hysterectomy (hĭs-tĕr-ĔK-tō-mē)
mastitis (măs-TĪ-tĭs)
menorrhagia (mĕn-ō-RĀ-jă)
metrorrhagia (mĕ-trō-RĀ-jă)
rectocele (RĔK-tō-sēl)
retroversion (RĔT-rō-vĕr-zhŭn)
salpingo-oophorectomy (săl-pĭng-gō-ō-ŎF-ō-RĔK-tō-mē)
vaginitis (vă-jĭ-NĪ-tĭs)

UTERINE BLEEDING DISORDERS

PATHOPHYSIOLOGY

Normal menstrual patterns vary widely in length of cycles (21–40 days), duration of menstruation (2–8 days), and amount of blood lost (40–100 mL). Bleeding patterns that are irregular in the spacing and amount are common in the first 2 years after the onset of menarche and in the 5-year period before menopause. Deviations from the normal cycles are viewed as uterine bleeding disorders. Two of the most common abnormal bleeding patterns, **metrorrhagia** (i.e., bleeding or spotting between menstrual periods) and **menorrhagia** (i.e., menstrual periods characterized by profuse or prolonged bleeding), are addressed in Table 52.1. Amenorrhea is the absence of menses.

CAUSES AND RISK FACTORS

Metrorrhagia and menorrhagia are symptoms of underlying factors rather than being specific definable conditions in themselves. Underlying causes for each vary widely. Common causes include hormonal dysfunction, benign and malignant tumors, coagulation disorders, systemic diseases, use of some contraceptives, endometrial hyperplasia, and inflammatory processes. The amount of blood loss varies with the type of disorder. Causes of amenorrhea include pregnancy; excessive weight gain or loss, physical activity, or stress; pituitary, hypothalamic, thyroid, or adrenal disorders; ovarian failure; and uterine abnormalities.

MEDICAL DIAGNOSIS AND TREATMENT

The diagnosis of uterine bleeding is based on the health history and physical examination as well as on the results of various diagnostic tests and procedures. Ultrasonography, dilatation and curettage, and biopsy, as well as laboratory analyses of blood components, hormone levels, and tissue specimens or stains, provide diagnostic information. Because anemia may result from excessive bleeding, hemoglobin (Hgb) and hematocrit (Hct) levels are usually measured as well. Endometrial ablation is another common procedure often completed as outpatient surgery to treat perimenopausal and postmenopausal menorrhagia. The treatment of amenorrhea depends on the cause and whether the patient desires pregnancy. Pharmacologic treatment can include oral contraceptives or progestins in either oral or intrauterine devices. Surgery is also used if abnormal uterine structures need to be removed.

◆ NURSING CARE OF THE PATIENT WITH UTERINE BLEEDING

Focused Assessment

Complete assessment of the female patient with a disorder affecting the reproductive system is summarized in Chapter 51, Box 51.1. When a patient has metrorrhagia or menorrhagia, the menstrual history is especially important.

Table 52.1 Uterine Bleeding Disorders

CAUSE	SIGNS AND SYMPTOMS	MEDICAL TREATMENT
Metrorrhagia		
Ovulation	Spotting with regularity 14 days before menses	None—this is regarded as a normal deviation.
Intrauterine contraceptive device	Intermittent spotting between menses	None if bleeding is not severe and if other causes are ruled out. Monitor serum hemoglobin; iron supplements if hemoglobin low. Intrauterine device removed if bleeding is severe.
Oral contraceptive use	Irregular spotting early or late in menstrual cycle	Patient is directed to take pill at same time each day. Oral contraceptive changed to adjust estrogen or progestin component.
Trauma; introduction of foreign objects	Sudden onset of frank bleeding or spotting	Foreign object is removed. Tissue damage is repaired.
Vaginitis, cervicitis	Spotting combined with vaginal discharge characteristic of infectious organism	Treatment based on cause determined by vaginal examination and laboratory tests.
Ectopic or molar pregnancy	Spotting or frank bleeding in addition to symptoms specific to molar pregnancy, ectopic pregnancy	Ultrasonography and laboratory tests (serum human chorionic gonadotropins level) done. Products of conception removed surgically. Methotrexate may be used to stop cell growth in an ectopic pregnancy.
Reproductive tract pathology: Endocervical polyps Cervical eversion Cervical dysplasia Endometriosis Salpingitis Ovarian cyst Benign neoplasm Malignant neoplasm	Spotting or frank bleeding in addition to other symptoms characteristic of specific pathology	Diagnostic procedures and treatment specific to identified pathologic condition: hormone therapy, antimicrobial or other drug therapy, surgery.
Menorrhagia		
Intrauterine contraceptive device	For all: By definition, profuse or prolonged bleeding during menstruation in addition to other symptoms characteristic of specific cause	Removal and/or replacement of intrauterine device. Alternative contraceptive methods considered. PGSIs may reduce menstrual blood loss. Treatment for remaining causes is specific for each cause.
Hormonal disturbances		Hormone therapy or other drug therapy initiated based on assessment of hormone status.
Endometrial hyperplasia		Endometrial hyperplasia may be diagnosed and treated by dilation and curettage. For women past childbearing age, hysterectomy may be performed.
Benign neoplasm		Benign tumors may be left alone and monitored.
Malignant neoplasm		Malignant tumors require a combination of surgical and medical interventions.
Inflammatory process		Specific cause is treated.
Systemic diseases		Specific cause is treated.

PGSI, Prostaglandin synthesis inhibitor.

Patient Problems, Goals, and Outcome Criteria: Metrorrhagia or Menorrhagia

Patient Problems	Goals and Outcome Criteria
Inability to manage self-care related to lack of knowledge about condition and treatment	Patient understands condition and treatment: patient accurately describes condition and treatment
Anxiety related to unknown cause of menorrhagia or metrorrhagia	Reduced anxiety: patient states that they feel less anxious, calm manner

Interventions

Inability to manage self-care. When the course of treatment has been selected, it may be your responsibility to

Table 52.2 Vaginitis: Infectious Causes

CAUSE	SIGNS AND SYMPTOMS	TREATMENT
Fungus: *Candida albicans*	Itching, redness, painful urination, painful intercourse. If discharge present, usually white, thick, clumpy.	Oral: fluconazole. Intravaginal: clotrimazole, miconazole, nystatin, terconazole, tioconazole, butoconazole
Protozoa: *Trichomonas vaginalis*	May be asymptomatic. When symptoms present in females: purulent malodorous discharge, dysuria. In males: clear or mucopurulent urethral discharge.	Metronidazole single dose or 7-day course
Bacterial overgrowth: Bacterial vaginosis	Mostly asymptomatic; may have thin, off-white discharge with unpleasant odor.	If symptomatic: metronidazole or clindamycin, tinidazole. Oral or vaginal preparations available.

teach the patient her role in the treatment process and ensure that she is able to follow through appropriately.

Anxiety. You can be a source of emotional support for the patient, who is often fearful or anxious about the unidentified cause of abnormal bleeding. The underlying causes of abnormal uterine bleeding may be relatively simple and easily treatable or complex and life threatening. Therefore, you must be prepared to help patients cope with all eventualities. Supportive measures such as encouraging the patient to express their feelings, use of touch, and listening convey concern to the patient. In general, it is your responsibility to provide information regarding procedures to be done. Give explanations in terms the patient can understand.

INFECTIONS AND INFLAMMATION

Most infections covered in this chapter are often transmitted through unprotected sexual activity (oral, genital, and rectal). In addition, the causative organisms are often those associated with sexually transmitted infections (STIs), which are discussed in Chapter 55. However, this chapter focuses primarily on the effects of the microorganisms on the female reproductive tract and subsequent medical and nursing interventions rather than on the specific disease processes.

Infections of the female reproductive tract affect patients physiologically and psychologically. The physiologic effects range from short-term reversible changes to long-term changes that result in infertility. The potential psychologic effects are numerous. Changes in relationships, feelings of distrust toward sexual partners, shame, embarrassment, and diminished self-esteem are but a few. When interacting with patients who have reproductive tract infections or their effects (e.g., infertility), you must be sensitive, tactful, and absolutely nonjudgmental.

VAGINITIS

Pathophysiology

Vaginitis is characterized by a local inflammatory response to infectious agents, chemical irritants, or age-related factors.

Infectious Vaginitis

Anything that alters the normal ecosystem of the vagina may invite infection. This includes diabetes mellitus, broad-spectrum antibiotics, altered level of estrogen, vaginal hygiene products, sexual activity, and some contraceptives. The most common vaginal infections are *Candidal* vulvovaginitis, *Trichomonis vaginalis*, and bacterial vaginosis. Information about these infections is summarized in Table 52.2.

A second cause of vaginitis is exposure to chemical irritants, douches, perfumed soaps, scented toilet tissue and perineal pads, feminine hygiene sprays, laundry detergent residues, and spermicides are a few examples of common irritants.

Estrogen deficiency associated with the aging process frequently results in nonpathogenic vaginitis because of a combination of tissue atrophy and a decrease in the acid vaginal secretions that normally maintain healthy mucous membranes.

Clinical Manifestations

Many vaginal infections are asymptomatic. However, common signs and symptoms include local swelling, redness, itching, and distinctive discharge

Complications

Ascending infection (an infection that moves through the vagina to internal structures) is a potential complication of vaginitis. Infection confined to the lower reproductive tract seldom poses a threat to life or fertility.

Medical Diagnosis

The diagnosis is based on the patient's symptoms and on inspection of the vulva and vagina. Discharge specimens may be collected to aid in identification of specific microbes if microbial infection is suspected.

Medical Treatment

Treatment specific to the causative agent may include topical/intravaginal antifungal creams, oral antiprotozoals or antibiotics, vaginal suppositories to reestablish normal vaginal flora, topical or systemic estrogen replacement therapy (ERT), improved diabetes control, and avoidance of offending chemical agents. Symptoms are managed with frequent cleansing with neutral agents; wearing cotton panties, cotton-crotched pantyhose, and nonconstricting clothing; and heat in the form of sitz baths and perineal irrigations. Advise the patient not to scratch the itching tissues, which can cause further mechanical trauma and infection. During the course of treatment, the patient should avoid sexual intercourse or use of condoms. The patient's sexual partner or partners may be treated for some infections to avoid reinfection. See Table 52.2.

◆ NURSING CARE OF THE PATIENT WITH VAGINITIS

Vaginitis is usually diagnosed and treated on an outpatient basis. Because patients usually manage their own treatment, you may be responsible for ensuring that the patient understands all self-care instructions and reinforcing the health care provider's other instructions. General nursing care of patients with reproductive tract infections is addressed in Table 52.3.

BARTHOLIN GLAND ABSCESS

Pathophysiology

Bartholin glands are mucus-secreting structures located on either side of the vaginal opening. Because of their location, these glands are vulnerable to a wide variety of infectious microorganisms. If the resultant edema and pus occlude the duct of the affected gland, an abscess forms.

Cause and Risk Factors

Although various microorganisms can be transmitted from the anus, vulva, or vagina to the Bartholin gland duct, *E. coli* is the most common cause of infection. The organisms are often introduced through improper perineal hygiene (i.e., wiping from the anus toward the vagina).

Clinical Manifestations

Perineal pain is the symptom that most commonly motivates the woman to seek medical assistance. Additional signs and symptoms include fever, labial edema, chills, malaise, and purulent discharge.

Complications

Without proper treatment, bartholinitis may progress from a local infection to a systemic infection.

Medical Diagnosis

Visual inspection reveals a swollen, often reddened mass on the affected side of the vaginal introitus. Gentle palpation causes pain, tenderness, or both. If drainage is seen, a specimen may be obtained for culture and sensitivity testing. Because causative microorganisms may include those responsible for transmission of STIs, the patient is usually screened for these diseases (see Chapter 55).

Table 52.3 Care of Patients With Reproductive Tract Infections

PATIENT PROBLEM	NURSING INTERVENTIONS
Denial, embarrassment related to questions about infection	Convey acceptance. Tactfully elicit information about hygiene and sexual practices: • All products applied on or near the vulva or in the vagina, such as feminine hygiene products and "love potions" (i.e., flavored or scented lubricants, massage oils) • Anal contact with penis, fingers, or other objects before contact with vulva or vagina • Number of sexual partners; accessibility to partners if their treatment is indicated
Inability to manage self-care related to lack of knowledge regarding condition and treatment	Explanation of teaching about use of creams, jellies, and suppositories: • Purpose • Position for application or insertion • Application or insertion method • Position after insertion • Care of equipment (i.e., applicator) • Use of tampon or perineal pad to hold medication in place Instructions about perineal hygiene: • Frequent washing with neutral soap • Thorough rinsing • No douching unless specifically ordered • No commercial perineal deodorants • Frequent change of underpants (preferably cotton) • Sitz baths to relieve pain, itching • Wiping perineal-anal area from front to back; one stroke per tissue • Complete full course of prescribed drug therapy

Medical Treatment

Conservative treatment consists of oral analgesics and moist heat in the form of frequent sitz baths or hot wet packs. The moist heat relieves pain and facilitates spontaneous rupture and drainage of the abscess. The health care provider may do a surgical incision and drainage of the abscess. More aggressive treatment with broad-spectrum antibiotics is indicated if symptoms of systemic infection are present. Surgical excision of the gland is reserved for situations that do not respond to conservative treatment.

◆ NURSING CARE OF THE PATIENT WITH BARTHOLIN ABSCESS

Basic nursing interventions are outlined in Table 52.3. Provide the appropriate instruction to help the patient comply with the prescribed treatment. Tactful instruction in basic perineal hygiene principles is in order if the evidence indicates that inappropriate or inadequate practices are being followed. Basic practices include soap-and-water cleansing at least once daily and wiping the perineal area with a clean tissue from front to back after urination or defecation.

CERVICITIS

Pathophysiology

Cervicitis is inflammation of the cervix. It may be acute or chronic.

Cause and Risk Factors

Cervicitis is caused by pathogenic organisms and mechanical or chemical trauma. The most common infectious agents are *Chlamydia trachomatis* and *Neisseria gonorrhoeae*. Mechanical trauma may be caused by scraping of cells for diagnostic tests, cryosurgery, childbirth, and the use of tampons or condoms. Chemical irritants might be medications or spermicides. Decreased estrogen levels after menopause may also contribute to cervicitis.

Clinical Manifestations

Cervicitis is usually asymptomatic, although it may cause pain. Vaginal discharge, bleeding, or dysuria may be reported. Unsuspected cervicitis may be detected on a routine pelvic examination or on routine Papanicolaou (Pap) tests. When viewed via a speculum, the cervix appears swollen and reddened; gentle touch may precipitate bleeding. Mucopurulent discharge and vesicular or ulcerated lesions are most often associated with STIs.

Complications

Cervicitis itself is a relatively benign condition. However, if the causative agent is an infection, the infection may ascend through the reproductive tract and cause pelvic inflammatory disease (PID). Certain microorganisms that cause cervicitis also alter the vaginal pH and exert a spermicidal effect that can result in infertility.

Medical Diagnosis and Treatment

Cervicitis may be diagnosed on the basis of the history, pelvic examination, and culture of discharge, if present. Treatment depends on the cause. Infections are treated with systemic or topical antimicrobials. Cervicitis related to menopause is treated with topical or oral estrogen. Additional treatment options exist for specific patient situations.

> **Pharmacology Capsule**
>
> Instruct patients to complete the full course of antimicrobial therapy to treat infections.

NURSING CARE OF THE PATIENT WITH CERVICITIS

Cervicitis is usually diagnosed and treated in outpatient settings. In most cases, the health care provider or the patient administers treatment. Nursing care is limited to assisting with assessment procedures, patient support, and teaching the patient to carry out the prescribed treatment and posttreatment procedures.

MASTITIS

Pathophysiology

Mastitis is an infection-induced inflammation of breast tissue most commonly occurring in the lactating woman. Mastitis is associated with a combination of ineffective breastfeeding techniques that result in poor drainage of mammary ducts and alveoli, lowered resistance to infection because of stress and fatigue, and exposure of breast tissue to infection-causing organisms.

Cause and Risk Factors

S. aureus is the microorganism most commonly associated with mastitis; however, *Escherichia coli* and streptococci may also be the agents of infection. The nipple serves as the portal of entry for the organism. Cracked nipples are especially susceptible. A common mechanism of organism transmission is touching the nipples with unclean hands.

Clinical Manifestations

Mastitis is usually confined to one breast and may be asymptomatic except for breast tenderness and low-grade (and often unsuspected) fever. The infection therefore may be undetected if frequent breastfeeding empties breast ducts and alveoli and if the woman's natural immune response prevents spread of the infection. In symptomatic mastitis, the causative organism invades the breast connective tissue or the lobes and ducts and stimulates an inflammatory response that results in localized pain, fever, tachycardia, general malaise, and headache. The affected breast tissue feels hard and warm on palpation; the skin over the infected area is reddened.

Complications

Untreated symptomatic mastitis may result in abscess formation as the sepsis becomes localized. Enlargement of axillary lymph nodes may also result.

Medical Diagnosis and Treatment

The diagnosis is based on presenting symptoms. Symptomatic mastitis is unmistakable. If a purulent discharge from the nipple is noted, a specimen can be collected for culture and sensitivity testing. However, treatment is initiated based on the symptoms alone and consists primarily of immediate and aggressive antibiotic therapy.

Symptoms are managed by complete emptying of the breast, cold compresses, rest, and NSAIDs for pain. The question of whether to empty the breast by breastfeeding or by artificial pumping is controversial. Many broad-spectrum antibiotics are tolerated well by the mother and the infant. This is significant because antibiotics taken by the mother will be present in her breast milk.

If an abscess forms, surgical incision and drainage of the abscess may be necessary and a longer period of antibiotic therapy will be required.

◆ NURSING CARE OF THE PATIENT WITH MASTITIS

The most effective nursing intervention is teaching patients how to prevent mastitis (see the Patient Teaching box).

Focused Assessment

Explore the breastfeeding woman's knowledge of measures to prevent mastitis. Take the patient's temperature. Palpate the breasts for pain, tenderness, warmth, and hardness and inspect for purulent discharge from the nipple.

Patient Problems, Goals, and Outcome Criteria: Mastitis

Patient Problems	Goals and Outcome Criteria
Potential for injury related to possible abscess formation	Recovery without complications: absence of fever, pain, redness, and purulent drainage
Inability to manage self-care related to lack of knowledge of mastitis prevention and treatment	Patient understands how to treat mastitis and prevent recurrence: patient accurately describes and demonstrates self-care measures

Interventions

Potential for injury. If mastitis or breast abscess occurs, reinforce the prescribed treatment. If heat treatments or drug therapy are prescribed, ensure that the patient understands the instructions.

Inability to manage self-care. The points commonly addressed in breastfeeding education are those that also prevent the infectious process from occurring.

Patient Teaching

Mastitis

- Be sure to complete your course of antibiotics as prescribed.
- Report continued or additional symptoms.
- Pain can usually be managed with analgesics as prescribed.
- Allow for extra rest periods.
- To prevent recurrence during breastfeeding, do the following:
  - Breast-feed frequently and completely empty the breasts.
  - Wash hands thoroughly before handling breasts.
- To avoid cracked nipples, do the following:
  - Make certain that the infant's lips and gums are around the areola and not on the nipple itself.
  - Break suction before removing the nipple from the infant's mouth.
  - Cleanse with plain water to prevent chemical trauma from soap, alcohol, and other drying agents.
  - Leave milk on nipples and expose them to the air or a heat lamp after breastfeeding.
- Wear a supportive but nonconstrictive bra.
- Get adequate rest, nutrition, and fluids.
- Promptly report early symptoms of breast infection to a health care provider.

PELVIC INFLAMMATORY DISEASE

PATHOPHYSIOLOGY

Pelvic inflammatory disease (PID) is an infectious process that may affect any or all structures in the pelvic portion of the reproductive tract and peritoneal cavity. It is called an *ascending infection* because causative organisms migrate upward from the vulva or vagina.

PID is a major female reproductive health problem and a major cause of infertility in the United States. The infectious process results in scarring and adhesions in the fallopian tubes that can cause total or partial obstruction. Total obstruction results in infertility. Partial obstruction often results in ectopic pregnancy, in which the fertilized ovum implants in a site other than the uterus, usually in the fallopian tube or pelvic cavity. Unfortunately, the incidence of PID is particularly high in adolescent girls.

CAUSE AND RISK FACTORS

The majority of PID cases are caused by sexually transmitted organisms. *N. gonorrhoeae, C. trachomatis,* and *M. genitalium* are recognized as the organisms most associated with PID, although multiple pathogens may be present. *Chlamydia* infection is thought to be the most commonly occurring STI and the one most often responsible for PID. As such, it is often implicated in infection of the fallopian tubes (salpingitis) and is considered the primary cause of ectopic pregnancy and infertility associated with tubal obstruction.

Not all PID is associated with STI organisms. Sources of non–STI-associated PID include contaminated hands or instruments during gynecologic surgery, childbirth, abortion, and pelvic examinations. IUDs and other intravaginal devices have been implicated as well. Women with compromised resistance to infection and women who are poorly nourished are particularly prone to developing non–STI-associated PID.

The risk of PID increases as the number of sexual partners increases. This factor is most applicable to PID caused by organisms implicated in STIs.

Vaginal douching is also considered to be a possible risk factor for PID. It is thought that the force of the fluid used in douching may propel microorganisms from the vagina through the cervical os (opening) and into the uterus, fallopian tubes, and pelvic cavity.

CLINICAL MANIFESTATIONS

PID may be a silent infection with no symptoms. As a result, it may remain untreated while causing damage to pelvic structures. Symptomatic PID may appear with either the gradual onset of dull, steady, low abdominal pain or the sudden onset of severe abdominal pain, chills, and fever. Other symptoms may include dysuria, irregular bleeding, a foul-smelling vaginal discharge that may cause inflammation and skin breakdown of the vulva, and **dyspareunia** (pain during sexual intercourse).

Symptomatic PID is much more likely to be diagnosed and treated than asymptomatic PID. In many instances, evidence of PID is first discovered during surgery for ectopic pregnancy, blocked fallopian tubes, ovarian abscess, or other pelvic disorders.

COMPLICATIONS

The risk of complications of PID increases with each repeated infection. Common effects of PID include ectopic pregnancy, infertility, and chronic abdominal discomfort. Without prompt diagnosis and aggressive treatment, infection of the entire peritoneal cavity (i.e., peritonitis) and systemic septic shock are also potential complications.

MEDICAL DIAGNOSIS

The diagnosis is based on the presenting symptoms (if any) and the pelvic examination. The definitive diagnosis is based on culture of the causative organism or organisms. Sonography, laparoscopy, and culdocentesis are additional diagnostic procedures that may be used.

MEDICAL TREATMENT

PID can usually be treated at home. However, very acute symptoms and severe pain may require inpatient care. Treatment includes rest; application of heat via warm compresses, a heating pad, or sitz baths; and a regimen of analgesics and broad-spectrum antibiotics. Depending on the severity and extent of the infection, oral or parenteral antibiotics (or both) are prescribed. Directly observed therapy is generally recommended because some patients do not take prescribed drugs as ordered. The patient should avoid sexual intercourse for at least 3 weeks. If the causative organism is thought to have been transmitted sexually, the patient's sexual partner or partners should be treated to avoid repeated infection. Expedited partner therapy in which the patient is provided with a prescription or additional drugs for their partner has been found to be more effective than referring partners for treatment. Follow-up is recommended to ensure successful treatment.

NURSING CARE OF THE PATIENT WITH PELVIC INFLAMMATORY DISEASE

Focused Assessment

Nursing assessment of the woman with a disorder of the reproductive system is summarized in Chapter 51, Box 51.1. Preparation of the patient for physical examination includes anticipatory guidance, positioning and draping, and emotional support. You need to simultaneously assist the examiner and provide support for the patient. Precautions to avoid reproductive tract infections and transmission of infection are summarized in the Patient Teaching boxes.

Patient Problems, Goals, and Outcome Criteria: Pelvic Inflammatory Disease

Patient Problems	Goals and Outcome Criteria
Pain related to inflammation	Pain relief: patient states that pain is relieved
Disrupted skin integrity related to infectious drainage	Restored skin integrity: intact skin without excessive redness or edema
Inability to manage self-care related to lack of knowledge of treatment and prevention of reinfection	Patient understands and carries out treatment and preventive measures: patient verbalizes instructions and states intent to follow prescribed measures

Patient Teaching

Precautions to Avoid Reproductive Tract Infection

- Maintain optimum general health: adequate nutrition and sleep, good stress management.
- Cleanse the perianal area daily with neutral soap followed by thorough rinsing; apply no other products unless ordered to do so by your health care provider.
- Wipe the perianal area with one front-to-back swipe per tissue.
- Avoid sharing of any equipment (including washcloths) used for perineal or vaginal hygiene.
- Change perineal pads or tampons frequently during menses even when flow is slight. Increase soap-and-water cleansing to at least twice per day.
- Inspect the genitalia of your partner before intercourse or other contact with the perianal area. Avoid contact if any lesions or discharge is noted. The same precautions should be followed for any part of the partner's anatomy (e.g., mouth, hands, fingers) that will contact the perianal area during a sexual encounter.
- Wash the penis, hands, or other objects that contact the anus with soap and water before contact with the vulva or vagina.
- Use condoms with spermicidal cream or jelly for penis-vulva-vaginal contact when a monogamous relationship is not well established.
- Avoid intercourse during treatment for a reproductive tract infection. Use a condom if intercourse cannot be avoided.

Interventions

Care of the patient with PID includes rest with limited activity, application of heat as ordered, administration of prescribed antibiotics, patient education, and recognizing and reporting signs and symptoms of the side effects of antibiotics.

Pain.. Prescribed analgesics are administered for pain control. Additional pain relief measures are discussed in Chapter 8. Monitor and record the efficacy of analgesics.

Disrupted skin integrity. If perineal pads are needed for collection of vaginal discharge, change them frequently. Note the character, amount, color, and odor of vaginal discharge. Frequent perineal cleansing is done with mild soap and water, followed by rinsing and patting dry. Inspect the vulva for signs of inflammation or excoriation and monitor and record the temperature.

Patient Teaching

Prevention of Pelvic Inflammatory Disease

When teaching prevention of pelvic inflammatory disease (PID) to the sexually active woman with multiple partners or with a single partner with an unknown sexual history, include the following:

- During sexual intercourse, always use protective mechanical or chemical barriers such as a condom, diaphragm, vaginal sponge, and spermicidal vaginal jelly or cream.
- Recognize the signs and symptoms of common sexually transmitted infections (STIs).
- Seek prompt medical diagnosis and treatment of STIs or other possible reproductive tract infections.
- Have a routine yearly pelvic examination by a physician or nurse practitioner, with testing done to detect *Neisseria gonorrhoeae*, *Chlamydia trachomatis*, and other organisms.
- Routinely inspect the sexual partners' genitalia for signs of infection before each contact for sexual intercourse.

Inability to manage self-care. Nurses play a significant role in the primary prevention of PID and in fostering early diagnosis and treatment of reproductive tract infections so that they do not result in PID. Primary prevention includes measures to reduce risk factors. All women should practice good reproductive tract hygiene habits. The patient with PID needs to understand the importance of taking antibiotics as prescribed. Failure to complete the course of therapy encourages the development of resistant strains of bacteria. Other teaching points include the need to abstain from intercourse for the prescribed period and the need for the sexual partner to be treated if advised.

FIBROCYSTIC BREAST CHANGES

PATHOPHYSIOLOGY

Fibrocystic breast changes represent an exaggerated response to hormonal influences. Excess fibrous tissue develops accompanied by overgrowth of the lining of the mammary ducts, proliferation of mammary ducts, and the formation of cysts. Fibrocystic nodules do not "become cancerous," but their presence may make it more difficult to detect malignant tumors by palpation.

CAUSE AND RISK FACTORS

Fibrocystic changes are more common among women who have never given birth, have had a spontaneous abortion, and had an early menarche and late menopause. The risk is also greater for women who have premenstrual abnormalities and do not use oral contraceptives.

CLINICAL MANIFESTATIONS

This painful condition usually affects both breasts. Smooth round lumps that are freely movable may be felt. Sometimes milky yellow or green discharge from the nipple is seen. Symptoms are commonly most apparent during the premenstrual phase of the menstrual cycle and typically improve after the menstrual period.

MEDICAL DIAGNOSIS AND TREATMENT

Diagnosis is based on the physical examination and health history. A mammogram or ultrasound can help to distinguish lumps as fibrocystic changes rather than cancer. If indicated, fluid for study may be aspirated from a mass or the mass may be surgically removed for examination. Women with fibrocystic changes should have regular mammograms as recommended by their health care providers.

No specific cure exists for fibrocystic changes. Danazol reduces symptoms by decreasing estrogen production. However, it is no longer recommended by the FDA because of the side effects (i.e., acne, edema, excess hair growth).

Complementary and Alternative Therapies

Although research evidence is lacking, some women with fibrocystic changes seem to find these strategies helpful: vitamin E supplements, diuretics, a low-salt diet, wearing a good support bra, stress reduction, and restriction of coffee and chocolate.

◆ NURSING CARE OF THE PATIENT WITH FIBROCYSTIC CHANGES

Fibrocystic breast changes are treated on an outpatient basis. Therefore, the primary role of the nurse is to instruct the patient in self-examination and to encourage scheduled mammograms.

BENIGN GROWTHS

ENDOMETRIOSIS

Pathophysiology

The cause of endometriosis is uncertain. It may involve retrograde menstruation, metaplasia, or altered

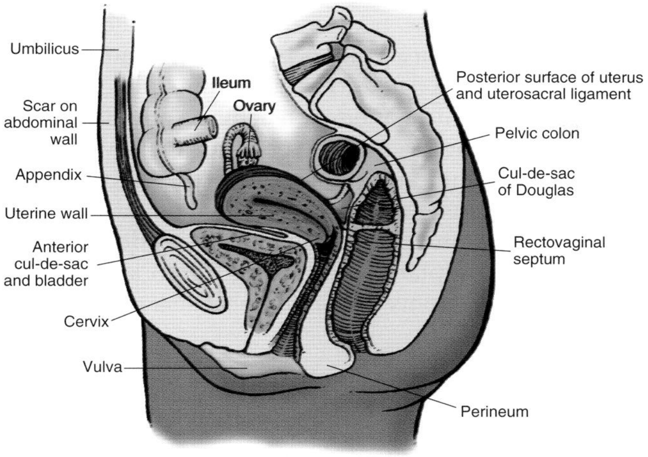

Fig. 52.1 Common sites of endometriosis. (From Monahan FD, Drake DT, Neighbors M, editors: *Medical-surgical nursing: foundations for clinical practice*, ed 2, Philadelphia, 1998, Saunders.)

function of immune-related cells (or a combination of these conditions). The most popular theory (the Sampson theory) suggests that retrograde menstruation seeds the peritoneal cavity with endometrial cells. Endometrial tissue that lines the uterus responds to hormonal influences during the menstrual cycle. During menstruation, small amounts of menstrual fluid are thought to be ejected through the fallopian tubes into the pelvic cavity rather than through the cervical os into the vagina. In some women, the endometrial cells deposited in the pelvic cavity implant on structures within the cavity; once there, they continue to respond to menstrual cycle hormonal stimulation. The result is the periodically painful and potentially destructive condition called **endometriosis**. In women with endometriosis, the ectopic (out of place) endometrial tissue behaves in the pelvic cavity as it does in the uterus: it proliferates and then bleeds if fertilization of the ovum does not occur. As a result, more and more endometrial cells attach to pelvic structures and may form cell clusters called *implants*. When in the ovaries, the implants are sometimes referred to as *chocolate cysts* because of their color and cystic quality. The implants are thought to migrate to other areas of the body, possibly transported by blood or lymph. Bleeding by endometrial tissue causes local inflammation and pain wherever the site of implantation may be located. The number of implants gradually increases, creating multiple sites of inflammation and pain. In response to the inflammation, fibrous tissue that results in scarring and adhesions forms (Fig. 52.1).

Cause and Risk Factors

Although it is known that almost all women experience retrograde menstruation to some degree, it is not known why some women develop endometriosis and others do not. Several theories have been explored; one is that endometriosis may be linked to a defect in the immune system of its sufferers. The disease is believed to occur in 10% of all women of reproductive age. The incidence and severity are greatest in women with relatives who have endometriosis.

Clinical Manifestations

As noted previously, the major symptom is pain, although some women are asymptomatic. Because the uterine endometrial tissue is bleeding simultaneously, pain appears as **dysmenorrhea** and may extend to a feeling of general pelvic heaviness. Additional symptoms can include pain with defecation, dyspareunia, and abnormal bleeding. Emotional symptoms, including anger and depression, are also common. Infertility may be a sign of endometriosis when adhesions affect uterine position or fallopian tube patency, movement, or both.

Complications

The most common complication of endometriosis is constriction of pelvic structures by endometriosis-related adhesions. Constriction of the bowel, ureters, or both may cause partial or complete obstruction within the affected structure, creating a medical emergency.

Medical Diagnosis

Visualization and excision of endometrial implants via laparoscopy provide specimens for laboratory analysis and are the primary diagnostic procedures for endometriosis. Ultrasonography may be used as a preliminary diagnostic tool to determine the presence of pelvic masses.

Medical Treatment

The treatment of endometriosis varies with the severity of the condition. For mild to moderate pain, nonsteroidal antiinflammatory drugs (NSAIDs) are used. Oral contraceptives may be prescribed on a long-term basis to inhibit endometrial proliferation, thereby relieving symptoms. If this approach is not effective, the health care provider may prescribe gonadotropin-releasing hormone (GnRH) agonists, a synthetic androgenic steroid, or an aromatase inhibitor. See Table 51.2 for details.

Pharmacology Capsule

Androgens have masculinizing effects on women. The effects usually resolve when the drugs are discontinued.

Pharmacology Capsule

Oral contraceptives are contraindicated in a woman with a history of cardiovascular disease, cerebrovascular disease, or thrombophlebitis.

Surgical management is commonly used and includes laparoscopy for diagnosis and removal of endometrial implants via resection, electrocauterization, or laser vaporization. Because it is difficult to visualize and remove all implants and because the underlying cause continues to exist, such surgery does not constitute a permanent cure and may need to be repeated at intervals. When fertility is no longer desired or complications develop, total abdominal **hysterectomy** with bilateral **salpingo-oophorectomy** (i.e., excision of the uterus, fallopian tubes, and ovaries) may be performed. Removal of the ovaries prevents the production of estrogen that would stimulate endometrial tissue. However, ERT is not an option to relieve menopausal effects for these women as long as endometrial implants remain, because the implants continue to respond to the estrogen and symptoms return.

◆ NURSING CARE OF THE PATIENT WITH ENDOMETRIOSIS

Endometriosis is usually treated on an outpatient basis, so nursing care is limited unless the patient is admitted for surgery. Perhaps the most significant nursing interventions are validating that the pain is real and providing information about pain relief measures (see Chapter 8). The office or clinic nurse may be involved in patient teaching. Specific patient teaching depends on the treatment method selected and includes anticipatory guidance and treatment-specific instructions. Because periodic bleeding of all endometrial sites may cause anemia, teaching should include symptoms of anemia and the need for dietary or supplemental vitamin and mineral therapy. Preoperative and postoperative nursing care of the patient who has had a hysterectomy for endometriosis is addressed in the nursing care plan (see Nursing Care Plan: Patient Having Hysterectomy for Endometriosis).

CYSTS

A cyst is a closed, saclike structure that is lined with epithelium and contains fluid, semisolid, or solid material. Cysts are classified as *neoplasms* and may be benign or malignant; the majority are benign. The most common ovarian and breast cysts are covered individually in Table 52.4.

For women with ovarian or breast cysts, nursing intervention focuses on teaching. Instruct the patient to keep a diary of symptoms, detailing when they occur and any factors that may be associated with the symptoms. Teaching is specific to the prescribed therapy.

Nursing Care Plan: Patient Having Hysterectomy for Endometriosis

FOCUSED ASSESSMENT

Past Health History

A 42-year-old married woman has been pregnant three times and has three living children. She was diagnosed with endometriosis ten years ago that was initially treated with oral contraceptives. When the symptoms returned, she was treated with Lupron which controlled her symptoms. However, she found the side effects to be intolerable and stopped taking it. She has since tried to manage her pain with NSAIDs, which have become increasingly ineffective. Her menstrual periods have been regular, with onset every 30 days and lasting for 6 days. She describes her menstrual flow as heavy with severe pain that begins several days before her menstrual period and lasts for the duration of the period. The pain is centered in the lower abdomen, the outer quadrants of her left side, and her lower back. She relates the left side pain to constipation that occurs around the time of her menstrual period. On a scale of 1 to 10, she rates her pain as ranging from 5 to a peak of 8. Diagnostic studies reveal endometrial implants scattered throughout her abdomen with several compressing the descending colon. She reports that her health has been very good except for the endometriosis symptoms.

She has been admitted for a total abdominal hysterectomy with bilateral salpingo-oophorectomy and excision of obstructive implants. This will be her first experience with surgery.

Physical Examination

Vital signs: blood pressure 126/74 mm Hg, pulse 72 beats per minute, respiration 18 breaths per minute, temperature 97.8°F (36.6°C) measured orally. Height 5′3″, weight 166 lb. Lungs clear on auscultation. Skin color medium tan; nail beds pink with rapid capillary refill.

Laboratory

Urinalysis, complete blood count (CBC): All reports indicate no deviation from normal ranges except for hemoglobin (Hgb) concentration 10.4 g/dL (normal: 11–16 g/dL) and hematocrit (Hct) 30% (normal: 31%–44%). She has been typed and cross-matched for 2 U of whole blood "on hold" for surgery.

Patient Problems	Goals and Outcome Criteria	Interventions
PREOPERATIVE PATIENT PROBLEMS		
Anxiety about outcomes of surgical experience	Reduced anxiety: patient states she is less anxious	1. Encourage her to verbalize sources of anxiety and to identify usual effective coping strategies. 2. Respect her concerns with empathy 3. Answer her questions or refer them to surgeon as appropriate.

Nursing Care Plan **Patient Having Hysterectomy for Endometriosis—cont'd**

Patient Problems	Goals and Outcome Criteria	Interventions
Potential for low self-esteem related to perceived potential loss of reproductive capacity and femininity, possible negative effect on sexual relationship	Stable or improved self-esteem: patient verbalizes understanding of expected changes in anatomy and physiology and of ability to resume a satisfying sexual relationship with her husband after recovery from surgery.	Explain the following: 1. The only expected noticeable effects of loss of the uterus and ovaries will be cessation of menstrual periods and ability to become pregnant, in addition to cessation of symptoms for which she is seeking surgery. 2. She may experience vaginal numbness for a short period of time. 3. Many women experience improved libido and sexual satisfaction after hysterectomy; sexual spontaneity may increase with the lack of need for contraception. 4. Although penile or vaginal intercourse should not be resumed until at least 6 weeks after surgery, oral sex and masturbation to orgasm are safe. 5. Positions for sexual intercourse should avoid pressure on the abdominal incision for as long as incisional tenderness persists. 6. Orgasmic contractions of the uterus will no longer be present; this change of uterine sensation is noted by some but not most women. 7. Removal of ovaries results in loss of hormones. Whether hormone replacement therapy is an option depends on presence of implants. Discuss plans with health care provider.
POSTOPERATIVE PATIENT PROBLEMS		
Acute pain related to surgical tissue trauma	Patient's pain will be reduced: patient rates pain level at 4 or less	Assess pain location, character, and severity. Provide comfort measures: reposition, give back rub, encourage breathing exercises. Administer analgesics as ordered. Document response. See Chapter 8 for additional pain management interventions.
Inadequate peripheral circulation related to anemia, surgical trauma, effects of anesthesia, thrombus formation	The patient will have adequate oxygenation of tissues, as evidenced by a pulse rate of 66 to 80 beats per minute, respiratory rate of 12 to 20 breaths per minute, stable skin color, and alert mental status; no pain or tenderness in calves.	Monitor pulse, respirations, blood pressure, and oxygen saturation, Auscultate lung sounds. Assist patient to turn, deep breathe, cough on schedule; assist with incentive spirometer if ordered. Monitor skin color, temperature, and capillary refill, including lower extremities. Instruct and assist with foot and leg exercises; encourage and assist with ambulation when allowed. Assess ability to answer questions appropriately. If elastic hose are ordered, ensure they are applied and removed according to schedule when patient is in bed and at all times when out of bed; instruct patient in self-application. If intermittent pneumatic compression is used, be certain they are applied correctly. Monitor laboratory reports.
Potential for fluid volume deficit related to postoperative bleeding	The patient will maintain adequate fluid volume, balanced fluid intake and output, moist mucous membranes, stable pulse and blood pressure	Check abdominal dressing and perineal pad at least every hour for the first 12 hours; report any drainage observed on dressing, excessive vaginal bleeding. Should saturate less than one perineal pad per hour. Compare fluid intake (intravenous, oral) with urinary output (indwelling catheter collection bag or voided); report discrepancies. Monitor intravenous infusion; carry out related responsibilities according to institutional policy. Encourage fluid intake when allowed. Check mucous membranes for moisture; offer frequent mouthwashes during nothing-by-mouth status. Monitor pulse and blood pressure; compare with baseline levels; report deviations from acceptable ranges.

Continued

Nursing Care Plan **Patient Having Hysterectomy for Endometriosis—cont'd**

Patient Problems	Goals and Outcome Criteria	Interventions
Urinary retention related to surgical manipulation, local tissue edema, temporary sensory or motor impairment	The patient will empty bladder at regular intervals without catheterization.	Assist patient to bathroom or commode; use bedpan only if absolutely necessary. Assist patient to assume comfortable position. Provide privacy but remain within calling distance. If patient is unable to void without assistance, use assistive measures: run water in sink or shower; pour warm water over perineum. Teach or assist patient to perform perineal hygiene at least every 8 hours: wash vulva with warm, soapy water; rinse with warm water from irrigating apparatus; rinse perineum after every voiding. Measure and record urine output; note color, clarity, and odor of urine. Palpate for bladder fullness above symphysis pubis to assess for urinary retention. If patient is unable to void or is retaining urine, allow her to rest for 30 minutes and repeat attempt for spontaneous voiding. Follow order for intermittent catheterization or repeat insertion of indwelling catheter if patient is unable to void a sufficient quantity. Continue to monitor and to assist with voiding until patient consistently empties her bladder without assistance.
Constipation related to weakening of abdominal musculature, abdominal pain, decreased physical activity, dietary changes, drug side effects	The patient will have bowel movement on or before the fourth day after surgery.	Auscultate abdomen for bowel sounds, palpate for distention. Insert rectal tube as ordered, if appropriate. When oral intake is allowed, administer antiflatulent if ordered; teach patient self-administration if allowed. Encourage early and frequent ambulation. Encourage oral intake of fluids, especially of fruit juices. Assess for nausea and vomiting; administer antiemetic if nausea and vomiting are present. Follow protocol for diet; encourage selection of high-fiber foods when patient is allowed options. Administer stool softener or laxative if ordered. Assist patient to splint abdomen while attempting to pass feces. Report inability to have a bowel movement within the allotted time period.

CRITICAL THINKING QUESTIONS

1. Explain the potential complications that may occur after an abdominal hysterectomy and how they are prevented and detected.
2. Outline your strategy for helping a patient who is distressed about the loss of reproductive capacity.

FIBROID TUMORS (MYOMAS, LEIOMYOMAS)

Cultural Considerations

What Does Culture Have to Do With Uterine Fibroid Tumors?

The incidence of fibroid tumors is increased among Black American women. These women should be advised to report menstrual irregularities and pain so that the condition can be diagnosed early and treatment can be initiated.

Pathophysiology

Uterine fibroid tumors are benign and common. It is predicted that at least 20% to 30% of all women will develop fibroid tumors during their reproductive periods. Fibroid tumors grow slowly during the reproductive years but tend to atrophy after the onset of menopause.

Cause and Risk Factors

Although the exact cause is unknown, it is widely thought that fibroid tumors form and grow in response to stimulation by estrogen, primarily estradiol. Human growth hormone and human placental lactogen may also promote the tumors' development and growth.

Clinical Manifestations

Fibroid tumors may be asymptomatic, but the most common symptoms are menstrual irregularities: menorrhagia and dysmenorrhea. Discomfort from pressure on pelvic structures and dyspareunia may be associated with a large tumor. For some women, the initial hint that something is wrong is the gradual enlargement of the lower abdomen, which may be mistaken for pregnancy.

Complications

A very large fibroid tumor may compress the urethra, obstructing urine flow and causing secondary hydronephrosis. More common complications include infertility, crowding and malpositioning of the fetus during pregnancy, and degenerative changes related to interruption of blood supply.

Medical Diagnosis

On pelvic examination, the uterus is found to be enlarged and distorted. Ultrasound, a pregnancy test,

Table 52.4 Common Ovarian and Breast Cysts

TYPE OF CYST	PATHOPHYSIOLOGY	SIGNS AND SYMPTOMS	DIAGNOSIS AND MANAGEMENT
Follicular ovarian cyst	Forms when a dominant follicle fails to rupture and release its ovum and thus continues to grow. Occasionally formed in response to ovarian hyperstimulation by fertility drugs. May rupture and bleed into the pelvic cavity, causing sudden, severe abdominal pain.	Usually asymptomatic unless very large; then pelvic heaviness or congestion and an aching feeling are noted.	Usually detected during a pelvic examination. Most disappear in 2 to 3 months without treatment. If cyst remains after 6 to 10 weeks, may be drained or removed laparoscopically
Corpus luteum ovarian cyst	Forms after ovulation; characterized by excessive bleeding into the luteal cavity and by increased progesterone secretion. Use of fertility drugs is associated with ovarian hyperstimulation and formation of multiple cysts. Associated with more complications than follicular cysts. May rupture and hemorrhage into the pelvic cavity, causing a degree of pain related to the amount of bleeding.	Initial symptom is delayed onset of the menstrual period, followed by irregularities in menstrual amount and duration of flow. Patient may have dull, aching pelvic pain or cramping.	Is palpable as a small, tender mass on the affected ovary. If severe abdominal pain exists, ectopic pregnancy should be ruled out as a cause. May be visualized via laparoscopic or culdoscopic examination. Usually no treatment indicated. Normally disappears spontaneously.
Dermoid ovarian cyst	Composed of tissue from the three embryonic germ cell layers. May contain remnants of fat, hair, teeth, cartilage, and nerve tissue. Usually arises from the ovary on a pedicle (stalk). A small number (3%–5%) of dermoid cysts become malignant.	Asymptomatic when small. Pelvic aching or heaviness when large . Moderate to severe pain if pedicle becomes twisted.	Palpated as a dense, firm mass during pelvic examination. With a long pedicle, the mass may be found some distance from the ovary to which it is attached. A pregnancy test is needed to rule out ectopic pregnancy. If radiographs show teeth in the mass, the diagnosis of dermoid cyst is confirmed. Any dermoid cyst should be removed surgically because of the potential for malignancy.
Breast cyst	Most commonly identified cause is ovarian estrogen secretion. Additional contributing factors may be stress and caffeine. Is an exaggerated response to hormonal influence. May enlarge during the premenstrual period and shrink from the onset of menstruation until the next ovulation. Commonly called *fibrocystic disease.* Controversial: Some fibrocystic subtypes are considered precancerous.	Most are round, freely movable, benign cysts. May be soft or firm, depending on the contents. Small cysts are numerous; breasts have lumpy "cottage cheese" consistency. Varying degrees of pain are noted between ovulation and menstruation.	Methods of preliminary diagnosis include palpation, mammography, and ultrasonography (useful for initial study). Contents of fluid-filled cysts may be aspirated for laboratory study or observed over time. Accurate diagnosis of a solid cyst requires surgical biopsy. Treatment includes oral analgesics and heat application. Dietary measures include caffeine restriction, decreased salt intake, and supplementary vitamins and fatty acids. Most aggressive surgical treatment is mastectomy, which occasionally is an option selected by women who undergo repeated surgical biopsies. Hormone therapy: 1. Danazol (Danocrine): Decreases secretion of estrogen. Dosage is generally low enough to avoid serious side effects. 2. Low-dose estrogen with progesterone or progestins.

Pap stain analysis, and complete blood count (CBC) should be done to rule out other conditions.

Medical Treatment

Many women need no treatment and their tumors atrophy after menopause. Treatment options include various surgical procedures and drug therapies based on fibroid type, symptom severity, and whether a patient desires future pregnancy. Treatment options include

- Myomectomy to remove the tumor alone, usually by laser surgery.
- Endoscopic excision of small tumors
- Cryosurgical destruction of small tumors
- Uterine artery embolization to block blood flow to the tumor resulting in tissue destruction
- Hysterectomy for tumors that are very large or associated with complications when conservation measures have failed

Commonly used drugs include:

- Combined estrogen-progestin contraceptive (oral tablet, transdermal patch, vaginal ring)
- Leuprolide (Lupron), a GnRH agonist, may be ordered to shrink large tumors before surgery. However, concerns exist that this drug causes bone demineralization.

◆ NURSING CARE OF THE PATIENT WITH FIBROID TUMORS

Assist the physician or nurse practitioner with diagnostic procedures and provide support to the patient. Patients tend to equate the word *tumor* with malignancy. Therefore you may need to reinforce that the fibroid tumor is benign. Patients with fibroid tumors who have heavy bleeding should avoid NSAIDs and other drugs that enhance bleeding.

PELVIC ORGAN PROLAPSE ANTERIOR AND POSTERIOR VAGINAL

Wall Prolapse Pathophysiology

Pelvic organ prolapses are vaginal disorders caused by weakness of supportive structures between the vagina and bladder (cystocele) or the vagina and rectum (rectocele). They typically occur together. Bulging of the bladder and rectum through the vaginal wall is visible and palpable on vaginal examination. An enterocele is the herniation of intestines through the vaginal wall. Although small cystoceles and rectoceles may cause no problems, larger herniations may cause problems with emptying of bladder and bowel. Stress incontinence, incomplete bladder emptying, difficulty with expulsion of fecal matter collected in the area of herniation, and incontinence of gas or liquid feces are problems typically reported.

Cause and Risk Factors

During pregnancy and childbirth, the muscles that support the pelvic floor may be weakened. Repeat pregnancies result in further weakening that may eventually allow the bladder and the bowel to press through the vaginal wall. Other contributing factors are advancing age and obesity.

Clinical Manifestations

Symptoms other than the already described common bladder and bowel problems include dyspareunia, lower back and pelvic discomfort, and recurrent bladder infections.

Medical Diagnosis and Treatment

The diagnosis is made on the basis of inspection and palpation. Small cystoceles and rectoceles may be treated with pelvic floor (Kegel) exercises, which improve muscle tone. (See Chapter 14 for Kegel exercises.) ERT or hormone therapy (HT) may be prescribed to improve tone and vascularity of supportive tissues. A pessary may be helpful with cystocele. A pessary is a device that is inserted into the vagina to provide support.

Surgical intervention via anterior colporrhaphy and posterior colporrhaphy (A&P) repair to tighten the vaginal wall is an option for larger or symptomatic cystoceles and rectoceles. An anterior colporrhaphy tightens the anterior vaginal wall and is used to treat a cystocele. Posterior colporrhaphy tightens the posterior vaginal wall and is used to treat a rectocele. A risk of vaginal stenosis exists, which results in painful intercourse after posterior repair. These procedures are usually not done during the childbearing years because vaginal delivery would disrupt the repair.

It is interesting to note that nurse researchers who use noninvasive methods based on pelvic floor exercises report long-term success rates comparable to those found with colporrhaphy.

◆ NURSING CARE OF THE PATIENT WITH PELVIC ORGAN PROLAPSE

Focused Assessment

Assessment of the female patient with a disorder of the reproductive system is outlined in Chapter 51, Box 51.1. When a patient has a pelvic organ prolapse, also record problems related to urinary and bowel function. If surgery is planned, assess the patient's understanding of the procedure, the preoperative and postoperative care, and the patient's concerns.

Patient Problems, Goals, and Outcome Criteria: Pelvic Organ Prolapse (Cystocele and Rectocele)

Patient Problems	Goals and Outcome Criteria
Urinary incontinence related to pelvic muscle weakness	Control of urine elimination: patient reports improved bladder control
Constipation related to collection of feces in herniated bowel	Normal bowel elimination: regular bowel movements without straining

Patient Problems, Goals, and Outcome Criteria: Pelvic Organ Prolapse (Cystocele and Rectocele)—cont'd

Patient Problems	Goals and Outcome Criteria
Altered sexual function related to painful intercourse	Satisfying sexual practices without pain: patient's statement of lack of pain during intercourse
Potential for infection related to incomplete bladder emptying	Absence of urinary tract infections (UTIs): normal body temperature, no pain on urination
After surgical intervention, additional patient problems and goals are the following.	
Pain related to Acute pain tissue trauma	Reduced pain: patient states pain is relieved, relaxed manner
Potential for injury related to infection and stress on surgical incisions	Wound healing without disruption or infection: intact surgical incisions without increasing redness or purulent drainage
Inability to manage self-care related to lack of knowledge of postoperative recovery needs	Patient understands surgical routines and self-care: patient accurately describes postoperative self-care

Interventions

Nursing interventions vary depending on the medical treatment.

Urinary incontinence. For conservative treatment, you can teach Kegel exercises (see Chapter 14). The exercise is viewed as a preventive measure that can be adopted in early adulthood to maintain optimum pelvic floor muscle support throughout life.

Constipation. For the patient who reports problems with expelling feces, teaching includes directions to maintain soft stool consistency and regular bowel elimination. Dietary support focuses on frequent ingestion of fluids and a wide variety of high-fiber foods such as fruits, vegetables, and grains. Regular use of bulk stool softeners may be necessary.

Altered sexual function. For the patient who is treated with colporrhaphy, preoperative nursing care includes anticipatory guidance regarding the impending surgery and postsurgical period and carrying out the physician's orders. The patient may fear painful intercourse postoperatively or may be concerned about the effects of surgery on sexual function. Explain that intercourse should be delayed for a prescribed period of time for healing to occur. No permanent impairment of sexual function is expected.

Potential for infection. Depending on the specific surgical procedure, preoperative orders may include a vaginal douching with an antibacterial solution, a cleansing enema, and hair removal according to agency procedure. Postsurgical nursing care is directed at preventing infection and protecting the suture line. Perineal care is provided at regular intervals. In addition to incisional infections, the patient is at risk for urinary tract infections (UTIs). An indwelling urethral or suprapubic catheter is commonly left in place for several days to keep the bladder empty and thus prevent strain on sutures and to let local edema subside. Instruct the patient to report urinary frequency, burning, or foul odor, which suggests infection of the urinary tract.

Acute pain. Postoperative perineal care includes cleansing of the perineum at regular intervals, initial application of cold to reduce pain and swelling, and subsequent application of heat via sitz baths and heat lamps. Because postoperative pain may be severe, administer analgesics as ordered. Assess the effects of comfort measures and inform the physician if pain is not relieved.

Potential for injury. A low-residue diet reduces fecal bulk, and stool softeners are recommended to prevent straining during defecation after surgery. Encourage adequate fluids and ambulation.

Inability to manage self-care. Discharge teaching focuses on the patient's responsibility for continued self-care as the physician orders. Reinforce instructions regarding diet, medications, activity restrictions, and avoidance of sexual intercourse for the time the physician specifies. Reassure the patient that loss of vaginal sensation is expected and will resolve after a few months. To minimize vaginal stenosis after posterior repair, the surgeon may instruct the patient to use dilators and vaginal lubricants and to resume intercourse 6 weeks after surgery.

UTERINE PROLAPSE

Uterine prolapse is a condition in which the uterus descends into the vagina from its usual position in the pelvis (Fig. 52.2). Descent is rated as *first degree* if the cervix is above the vaginal introitus, *second degree* if the cervix protrudes from the introitus, and *third degree* if the vagina is inverted and the cervix and the body of the uterus protrude from the introitus. If the vagina inverts, it carries with it the adjacent bladder and rectum. Although uterine prolapse can occur in women who have never been pregnant, it is most common in postmenopausal women who have had multiple pregnancies.

Cause and Risk Factors

The structures that support the uterus in its anatomic position may be congenitally weak or may become stretched during pregnancy or injured

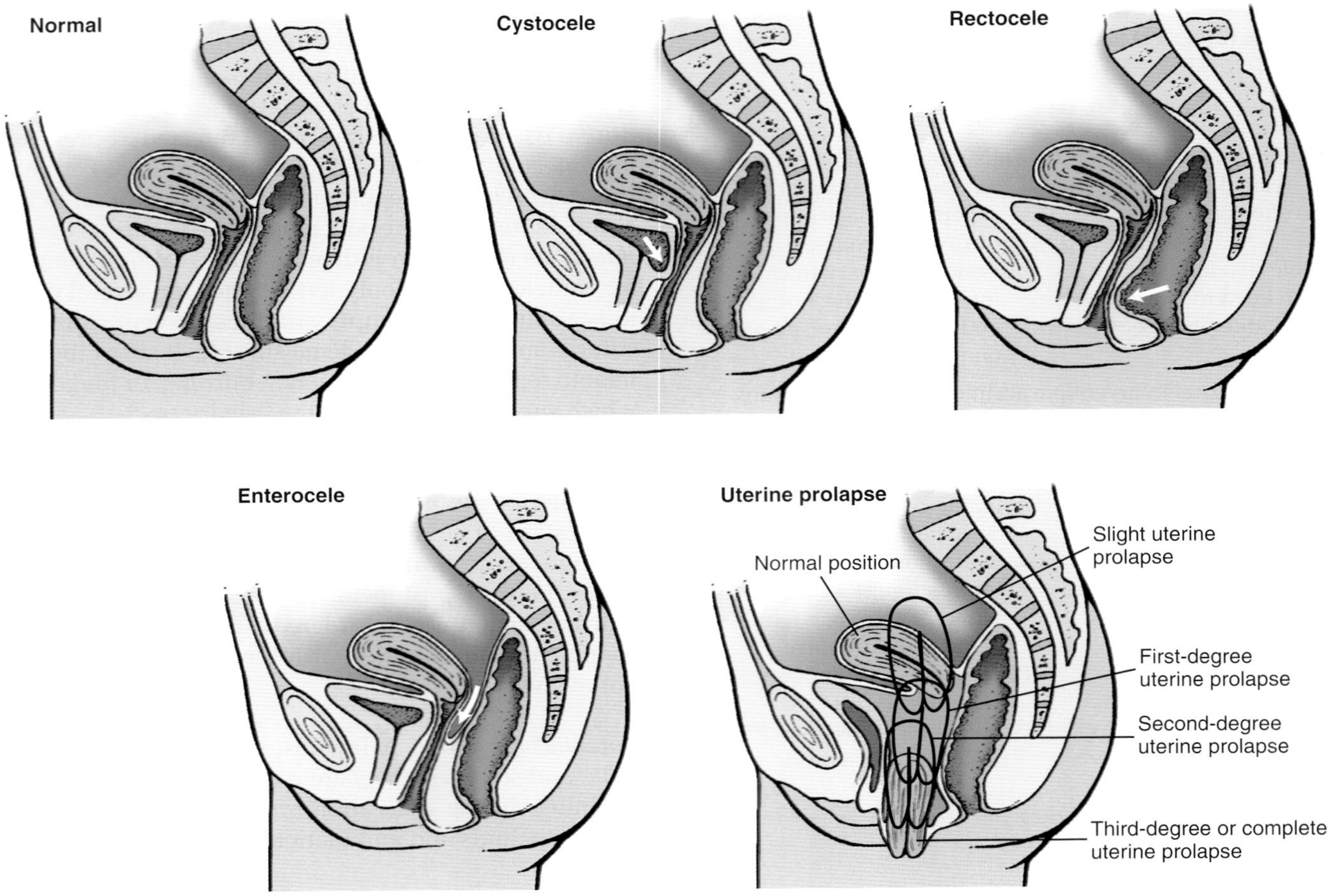

Fig. 52.2 Types of genital prolapse. (From Monahan FD, Drake DT, Neighbors M, editors: *Medical-surgical nursing: foundations for clinical practice*, ed 2, Philadelphia, 1998, Saunders.)

during childbirth. Pelvic trauma, connective tissue diseases, and medical conditions that increase abdominal pressure (e.g., obesity) are also risk factors. As a woman ages, supportive structures and uterine walls tend to relax, resulting in some degree of uterine prolapse.

Clinical Manifestations

Dyspareunia, backache, and a feeling of pelvic heaviness and pressure are commonly reported symptoms. Cystocele and rectocele usually accompany uterine prolapse.

Complications

In second-degree and third-degree prolapse, the protruding uterine portion is subject to trauma and may become eroded and necrotic.

Medical Diagnosis

Second-degree and third-degree prolapse are readily detected by visual inspection. First-degree prolapse is diagnosed through pelvic examination, although early first-degree prolapse may escape detection because the uterine descent is not evident when the patient is supine.

Medical Treatment

Vaginal hysterectomy with anterior and posterior colporrhaphy is the most common surgical treatment for uterine prolapse. For the woman who desires to preserve childbearing capability, it is possible to shorten the supportive ligaments surgically and return the uterus to the correct anatomic position.

For women who are poor surgical risks or who refuse surgical treatment, pessaries may be used. Pessaries are instruments that are inserted into the vagina to apply pressure on the vaginal wall, thereby supporting the uterus in the pelvis. Several types of pessaries exist, including ring ("donut") pessary and lever pessary. After placement of a pessary, advise the patient to return within 24 hours for the physician to assess placement, effectiveness, and problems related to pressure on surrounding structures. Pessaries must be removed, cleaned, and replaced periodically. If they are not maintained or are fitted improperly, they may act as irritants and cause tissue erosion, malignant tissue changes, or both. Be sure to document that the patient has a pessary so that it will not be forgotten and neglected. Topical estrogen creams or vaginal tablets may improve the tone of the muscles in the pelvic floor.

NURSING CARE OF THE PATIENT WITH UTERINE PROLAPSE

Focused Assessment

Nursing assessment of the female patient with a disorder of the reproductive system is outlined in Chapter 51, Box 51.1. When the patient has uterine prolapse, record related symptoms. If the prolapsed uterus is visible, note any signs of trauma or tissue breakdown.

Patient Problems, Goals, and Outcome Criteria: Second- or Third-Degree Uterine Prolapse

Patient Problems	Goals and Outcome Criteria
Altered body image related to interference of uterine prolapse with daily activities	Improved body image: positive patient remarks about self and ability to manage uterine prolapse
Altered sexual function related to abnormal uterine position	Satisfying sexual function: patient states sexual activity is satisfying and without pain
Potential for injury related to trauma of the exposed uterus	Absence of uterine trauma: no breaks in tissue integrity of uterus
Inability to manage self-care related to lack of knowledge	Patient understands and practices self-care: patient accurately describes self-care, keeps follow-up appointments

Interventions

You can serve as a source of emotional support and information for the patient. Nursing care depends on the treatment selected. Proper use of a pessary can reduce the risk of uterine trauma. When a pessary is the treatment of choice, explain the importance of frequent examinations by a physician or nurse practitioner, the need to report pessary-related discomfort to the health care provider, and the need for pessary care. Although some primary health care providers prefer to remove, clean, and replace pessaries, capable patients can be taught to do this themselves.

Put On Your Thinking Cap!

A newly hired nurse in a long-term care facility is surprised to learn that some patients have pessaries. The nurse says, "Nobody uses those things any more!" How would you explain the use of pessaries in this population?

ANTEFLEXION, ANTEVERSION, RETROFLEXION, AND RETROVERSION

The position of the uterus relative to the vagina has common variations. Positions of the uterus are stable throughout a woman's lifetime unless trauma or disease conditions arise. Displacements are classified as *anteflexion*, *anteversion*, *retroflexion*, or *retroversion*. The uterus is commonly positioned at a 45-degree angle anterior to the vagina, with the cervix pointed downward toward the posterior vaginal wall (Fig. 52.3). With anteversion, the entire uterus tilts forward at a sharper angle to the vagina. With anteflexion, the uterus bends forward as if folding on itself. **Retroversion** is a backward tilt of the uterus. With retroflexion, the body of the uterus bends backward on itself. Displacement from the woman's normal uterine position may be related to a number of other factors (Fig. 52.4). The uterus may become fixed and immobile if trapped by disease or scar tissue.

Cause and Risk Factors

Weakening and stretching of the ligaments and weakened pelvic floor musculature related to childbearing are the most common causes of uterine displacement. Other causes include surgical trauma, pelvic tumors, PID, and endometriosis.

Clinical Manifestations

Most uterine displacement is asymptomatic, although dyspareunia and low back pain may occur with retroversion.

Complications

Difficulty with conception has been associated with uterine displacement, particularly with retroversion. However, most complications are now thought to be associated with an underlying pathology (e.g., endometriosis, PID) rather than with displacement itself.

Medical Diagnosis and Treatment

The pelvic examination reveals uterine displacement. Treatment is seldom used, although some women find relief from backache by assuming a knee-chest position. Kegel exercises may be used to strengthen the pelvic floor muscular support system. For patients who are not candidates for surgery, a pessary may be used (see the section titled "Uterine Prolapse").

NURSING CARE OF THE PATIENT WITH ANTEFLEXION, ANTEVERSION, RETROFLEXION, AND RETROVERSION

The nurse's role is usually limited to history taking and providing information. If a pessary is inserted, provide instructions similar to those described in the section titled "Uterine Prolapse."

VAGINAL FISTULAS

Vaginal fistulas are abnormal passageways between the vagina and other pelvic organs. A fistula between the vagina and the urinary bladder is called a *vesicovaginal fistula;* a urethrovaginal fistula is located between the urethra and the vagina. Both of these fistulas permit urine to flow into the vagina. A rectovaginal fistula is located between the vagina and the rectum and

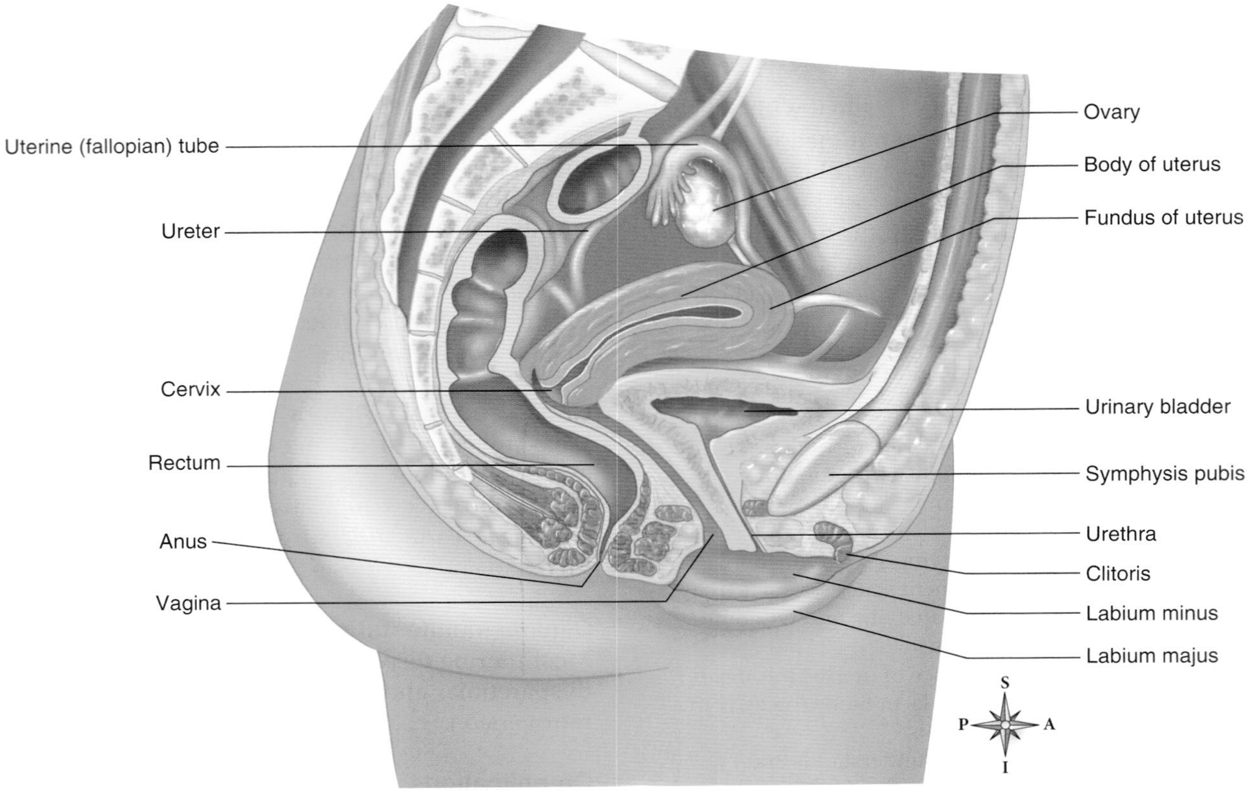

Fig. 52.3 Normal position of the uterus. (From Patton KT, Thibodeau GA: *The human body in health & disease*, ed 7, St. Louis, 2018, Elsevier.)

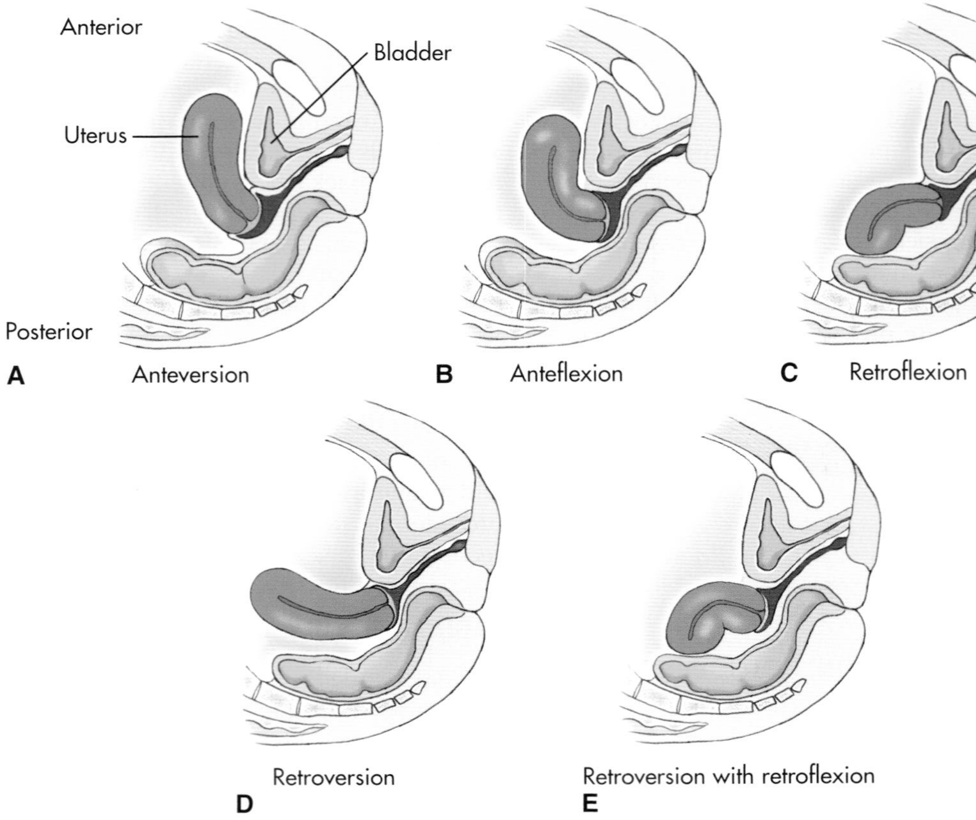

Fig. 52.4 Types of uterine displacement. (From Hagen-Ansert SL: *Textbook of diagnostic sonography*, ed 8, St. Louis, 2018, Elsevier.)

permits flatus and feces to pass into the vagina. Urine or fecal matter in the vagina can lead to severe vaginal and vulvar irritation and infection. Vaginal fistulas can often be diagnosed on the basis of the health history and physical examination findings. Dye may be injected into the vagina and radiographs may be made to locate the fistula.

Surgical correction is often needed, although some small fistulas close spontaneously. Preoperatively, instruct the patient in perineal hygiene and measures to control odor. Encourage fluid intake to reduce the risk of infection. The physician may prescribe sitz baths and deodorizing douches. Remember that excessive pressure during douching may force fluid through the fistula. Perineal pads are needed but must be changed frequently, and perineal care should be done every 4 hours.

After repair of a urinary fistula, the patient will have a urinary catheter that must be kept patent. Encourage fluids to promote urine output and to maintain catheter patency. After repair of a rectovaginal fistula, a liquid, low-residue diet is ordered initially to delay the need for a bowel movement so that the surgical site can heal. After several days, stool softeners and laxatives may be ordered to promote bowel elimination. Enemas are contraindicated because they may disrupt the sutured area. Unfortunately, surgical correction is not always successful.

CANCER

A diagnosis of cancer of the female reproductive system can have profound psychologic effect. For example, cancer implies threats to personal survival, sexual relationships, family integrity, and a woman's concept of herself as a woman. You can play a potentially significant role in helping the patient to cope with decision making, treatment methods and their effects, the inevitable grieving process, and the reactions of family members and friends.

BREAST CANCER

Breast cancer is the most prevalent form of cancer in American women; the current prediction is that 1 in every 8 or 9 women will develop breast cancer at some point in their life. It is the second leading cause of cancer deaths in women. Men can have breast cancer also, although it accounts for only 0.22% of all cancer deaths among men. It once was thought that survival rates were poorer for men, but that is not true.

For early detection of breast cancer, the American Cancer Society (ACS) recommends periodic mammography beginning between ages 40 and 45 for women of average risk and at age 30 for women at high risk. In addition, women at high risk should have an annual breast MRI. High risk is determined by a formula that uses personal health history, family history, and genetic testing results. Breast self-exams (BSE) and clinical breast exams are not a substitute for regular mammograms. Although it is estimated that 80% of breast lumps prove to be benign, those that are malignant must be identified and treated aggressively to prevent invasion of surrounding tissue, metastasis to distant structures, and death.

The three major types of breast cancer, according to the type of cells undergoing malignant changes, are (1) ductal, (2) lobular, and (3) nipple. Malignant growths are usually singular and affecting only one breast. Although they can be found in any part of the breast, nearly one-half of all malignant breast tumors are located in the upper outer quadrant and nearly one-fourth are located in the nipple-areolar complex. Most are painless and are palpated as firm, irregularly shaped, and fixed to underlying structures or skin. However, they sometimes resemble benign lumps: soft or semifirm, symmetric in shape with discrete borders, and freely movable. Therefore no lump should be ignored because it "feels" benign. Prompt evaluation is vital and may include tissue examination of cells obtained by needle aspiration or surgical biopsy.

Box 52.1 Established Risk Factors for Breast Cancer

- Sex: female
- Family history: mother, sister, or daughter diagnosed with breast cancer
- Age: 50 years or older
- Age at menarche: 11 years or younger
- Age at first childbirth: 30 years or older (or nulliparous)
- Personal medical history: atypical hyperplasia in the breast, breast cancer
- *BRCA1* or *BRCA2* gene mutation

Cause and Risk Factors

White, non-Latina women have the highest incidence of breast cancer. Black American women are most likely to die from it (see the Cultural Considerations box). Women who drink alcohol, are overweight after menopause, or have not had their first child before age 30 years may be at higher risk for breast cancer as well.

Cultural Considerations

What Does Culture Have to Do With Breast Cancer?

Some genetic factors increase the risk of breast cancer. Other potential risk factors, including high-fat diet, obesity, and sedentary lifestyle, may be culturally based. No race or culture is free of breast cancer.

Although no cause has been identified for breast cancer, the American Cancer Society (2021) indicates the existence of a number of risk factors (Box 52.1). Women who have a mutation of the breast cancer (*BRCA*) genes have a 50% to 85% lifetime risk of developing breast cancer. However, these women account for only 5% to 10% of all breast cancers.

Family history is important. The risk rises if one or more first-degree family members (mother, sister, daughter) have had breast cancer and if that cancer was premenopausal and bilateral. Additional risk factors reported in some studies are radiation of the chest between ages 10 and 30 years, menopause onset after age 50 years, obesity, alcohol intake, hormone therapy, sedentary lifestyle, being childless or having first child after age 30 years and oral contraceptives. The risk of developing breast cancer rises as the number of factors rise. However, it is important to remember that most women who are diagnosed with breast cancer have none of these known risk factors (see the Nutrition Considerations box).

Nutrition Considerations

1. Long-term dieting is associated with amenorrhea and reduced fertility.
2. Factors that may interfere with optimal nutrition for women of childbearing age include lack of resources, lack of nutrition knowledge, self-imposed dietary restrictions, and genetic idiosyncrasies.
3. High dietary fat intake (especially animal fat) has been associated with higher risk for developing breast cancer.

Prognosis

When cancer is confined to the breast, the 5-year relative survival rate is 99%. When cancer has spread to surrounding tissue, the 5-year survival rate is 86%; when the disease has metastasized, the 5-year survival rate is 28%. See the Cultural Considerations box.

Cultural Considerations

What Does Culture Have to Do With Breast Cancer Survival?

Low-income Black American women more often have advanced disease when diagnosed and are more likely than White women to die from breast cancer. This population should be targeted for education and screening and screening. Resources for evaluation and treatment that are available to these women must be identified.

Clinical Manifestations

Painless breast tissue thickening or lump is the initial sign best visualized on a mammogram. Most late symptoms—dimpling of the skin, nipple discharge, nipple or skin retraction, edema, dilated blood vessels, ulceration, and hemorrhage—are associated with the tumor's invasion of surrounding tissues. Dry, patchy nipple skin is suggestive of Paget disease, an uncommon cancer of the nipple and areola. Chest pain may be associated with metastasis to the lung.

Complications

Infiltration of adjacent breast and axillary tissue and metastasis to distant sites are the major complications of advanced breast cancer.

Medical Diagnosis

Tools employed to diagnose breast cancer include ultrasound, (three-dimensional [3D]) mammography, and magnetic resonance imaging (MRI) for questionable mammogram readings. Procedures to biopsy suspicious tissue include fine-needle aspiration, core-needle aspiration, incisional biopsy, and excisional biopsy. If malignancy is confirmed, additional studies will be done to determine whether the tumor is confined to the local area or has spread.

Medical Treatment

If tissue examination confirms the malignancy, the patient and physician consider surgical options based on the type, size, and extent of the cancerous growth. Women are playing increasingly active roles in the decision-making process and may "shop" for surgeons with whom they can agree on the selected surgical method. An oncologist may serve as a consultant in the decision-making process. Surgical options include lumpectomy, simple mastectomy, and modified radical mastectomy. Lumpectomy is removal of the tumor with a margin of surrounding healthy tissue but with preservation of most of the breast. A simple mastectomy is removal of the entire breast which is rarely done now. A modified radical mastectomy removes breast tissue and lymph nodes. leaving the pectoral muscles intact. Three commonly used options are depicted in Fig. 52.5. Lymphatic mapping and sentinel node biopsy uses dye or radioactive material to locate the lymph node that drains first from the site of the tumor. Study of this node enables the surgeon to determine whether and how far the cancer has spread. This procedure may avoid more extensive and unnecessary node dissection. For treatment of early-stage cancer, evidence indicates that lumpectomy plus radiotherapy offers the same long-term survival rate as more extensive surgery with radiotherapy. Additional treatment options depend on staging. Breast cancer is staged according to the American Joint Committee on Cancer (AJCC) tumor-node-metastasis (TNM) classification explained in Chapter 7. The stages are summarized in Fig. 52.6.

Hormone receptor assays are important tests that reveal whether a tumor needs estrogen or progesterone for growth. A tumor that needs estrogen is described as estrogen receptor positive (ER+); if it does not need estrogen, it is estrogen receptor negative (ER–). Likewise, a tumor that needs progesterone is progesterone receptor positive (PR+) and a tumor that does not need progesterone is progesterone receptor negative (PR–). These findings have implications for the best therapy. If cells are ER+, indicating that the tumor needs estrogen for growth, the drug *tamoxifen citrate* may be prescribed. Tamoxifen is a selective estrogen receptor modulator (SERM). SERMs block circulating estrogen from reaching the receptor cells.

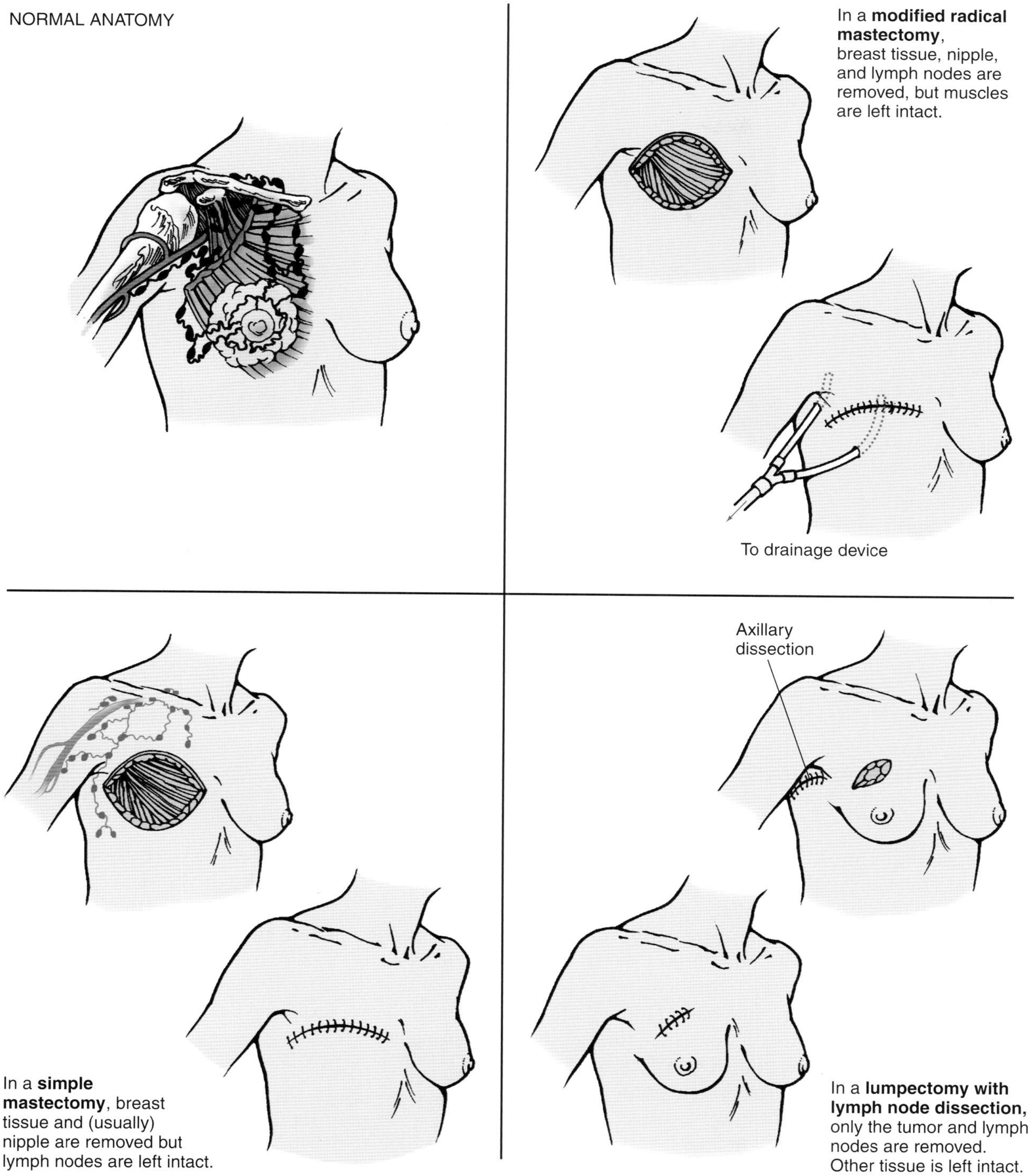

Fig. 52.5 Options in the surgical management of breast cancer. (From Ignatavicius DD, Workman ML: *Medical-surgical nursing: patient-centered collaborative care*, ed 6, St. Louis, 2010, Saunders.)

The oncologist plays a critical role in continued management of care. Chemotherapy, hormone therapy, radiation therapy, biologic therapy, or a combination of these may be used before, during, or after surgery. Most physicians routinely follow lumpectomy with radiation therapy, even when evidence indicates that all malignant cells were removed. Radiation therapy is used because small metastases may exist without nodal involvement. See Chapter 7 for a discussion of treatment modalities.

Many women elect to have breast reconstruction after mastectomy. Reconstruction is performed by a plastic surgeon and may be initiated immediately after the mastectomy and before closure of the wound or may be delayed. Implant reconstruction usually begins with placement of of a tissue expander placed

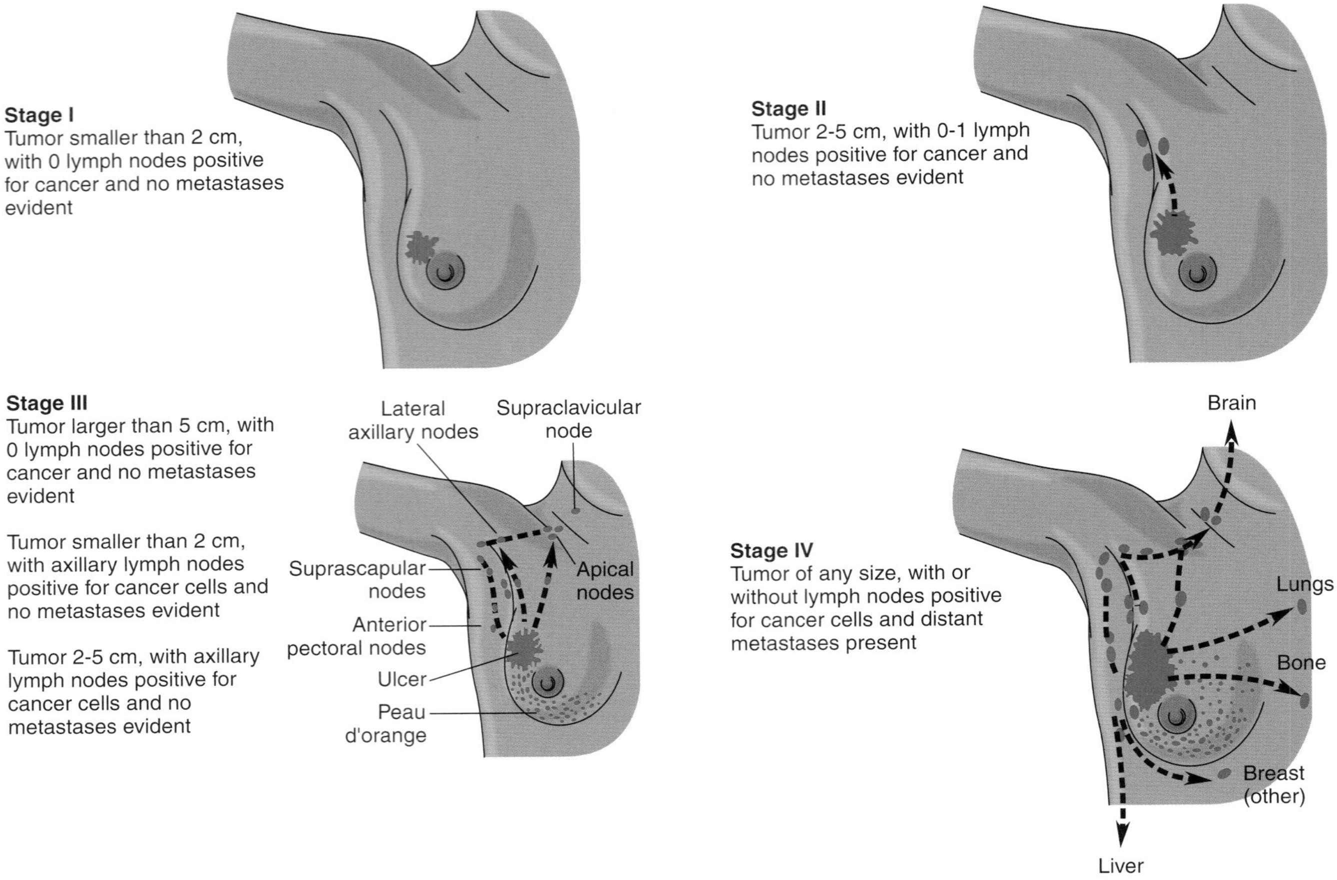

Fig. 52.6 Stages of breast cancer. (From Ignatavicius DD, Workman ML, Mishler MA: *Medical-surgical nursing across the health care continuum*, ed 3, Philadelphia, 1999, Saunders.)

under the pectoralis muscle. Small amounts of normal saline are injected periodically into the expander until it creates a space the size of the prosthesis that will replace the expander in a future surgical procedure. Other reconstruction methods use transfer of tissue from other areas of the patient's own body, including the abdomen and back (Table 52.5). The last stage of breast reconstruction is creation of a natural-appearing nipple. The new nipple is constructed from tissue taken from the other breast or the upper, inner thigh. Permanent pigment may be used to create the appearance of the nipple and areola.

◆ NURSING CARE OF THE PATIENT WITH BREAST CANCER

Focused Assessment

Nursing assessments are focused on physical manifestations of disease, physical and psychologic responses to treatments, review of all body systems, presence of pain, psychosocial factors, and level of knowledge. In the immediate postoperative period, the licensed vocational nurse/licensed practical nurse (LVN/LPN) may monitor the patient's vital signs, the wound dressings and drainage, and the arm on the affected side for edema.

Care of the surgical patient is discussed in Chapter 17 and care of the patient who has cancer is discussed in Chapter 7. Additional specific patient problems and goals for the mastectomy patient are listed in the following box.

Patient Problems, Goals, and Outcome Criteria: Mastectomy, Postoperative

Patient Problems	Goals and Outcome Criteria
Altered body image related to change in appearance, loss of breast, perceived loss of attractiveness	Improved body image: patient demonstrates comfort with the new body image
Potential for injury related to lymphedema secondary to excision of lymph nodes	Decreased risk for injury: absent or minimal lymphedema, arm circumference unchanged
Potential limited range of motion of affected arm related to axillary lymph node dissection	Normal mobility of affected arm: patient has full range of motion in affected arm within 6 weeks

Patient Problems, Goals, and Outcome Criteria: Mastectomy, Postoperative—cont'd

Patient Problems	Goals and Outcome Criteria
change to Inability to manage condition related to lack of knowledge of self-care and resources	Patient understands self-care: patient demonstrates self-care and identifies resources

Interventions

Altered body image. The breasts are an important part of a woman's self-image. To many women, loss of a breast represents loss of femininity. Even with immediate reconstruction, the breasts do not look completely normal. The patient may see herself as sexually unattractive and fear rejection by her sexual partner. These feelings are superimposed on the fear created by a diagnosis of cancer.

Be accepting of the patient, whose feelings may surface in a variety of ways, including anger, denial, and depression. From the early postoperative period, encourage the patient to attend to her appearance. Provide information about breast prostheses and clothing designed for women who have had mastectomies. If the patient has had chemotherapy, hair loss may also contribute to her body image disturbance. Strategies and resources for the cancer patient with a body image disturbance are discussed in Chapter 7 (see the Cultural Considerations box).

Cultural Considerations

What Does Culture Have to Do With Body Image After Mastectomy?

The importance of reproductive capacity as a measure of a woman's value depends on cultural values. In cultures that associate the breasts with sexuality, the loss of a breast can cause a woman to feel undesirable.

Potential for injury. A radical mastectomy includes the removal of lymph nodes in the axilla on the affected side. Because lymph nodes normally help to return tissue fluid to the bloodstream, their removal can result in lymphedema (i.e., the accumulation of fluid in the affected area). Fibroadipose tissue accumulates along with protein rich lymph fluid causing the limb to swell and resulting in discomfort and limited range of motion. An important aspect of postoperative care after mastectomy is directed toward preventing and minimizing lymphedema in the arm on the affected side. Interventions to manage lymphedema include the following:

- Elevate the arm to a height above the level of the heart.
- Measure blood pressure (BP) on the arm on the unaffected side, never on the affected side.
- Do not use the affected arm for venipuncture, injections, or parenteral fluid administration.

Table 52.5 Examples of Breast Reconstruction Procedures

PROCEDURE	DESCRIPTION
Implantation	An implant matching the size of the other breast is placed under the muscle of the operative side to create a breast mound.
Tissue expansion	A tissue expander is placed under the muscle and gradually expanded with saline to stretch the overlying skin and create a pocket. After several weeks, the tissue expander is exchanged for an implant.
Myocutaneous flaps	A flap of skin, fat, and muscle is transferred from the donor site to the operative area. The flap contains an appropriate amount of fat to match the other breast and is similar in appearance to breast tissue. A blood supply is established by reanastomosis of vessels from the operative area to those with the flap when possible. A new nipple may be created with tissue from the other nipple, labia, or thigh. Nipples can also be created by tattooing.

- Do not apply deodorant to or shave the axilla on the affected side.
- Frequently measure the circumference of the affected arm; immediately report an increase.
- Encourage frequent and progressive exercise of the arm on the affected side.
- Encourage the patient to use the arm for as many activities of daily living (ADLs) as possible.

Position the patient alternately on her unaffected side and her back, observing regular postoperative care as described in Chapter 17. If lymphedema develops, it may be managed with a compression garment, self-massage, manual lymphatic drainage by a certified therapist, and/or intermittent pneumatic compression. Some patients are candidates for surgical procedures to improve lymphatic drainage. Fortunately, the incidence of lymphedema has been reduced by surgical procedures that dissect fewer lymph nodes (i.e., sentinel node biopsy).

Potential for limited range of motion. If lymph nodes in the axilla are dissected, the patient is at risk for contractures unless proper positioning is maintained, and exercises are begun as soon as the surgeon permits. Postoperatively, place the patient in semi-Fowler position with the affected arm elevated on a pillow. Encourage her to flex and extend her fingers. Offer analgesics 30 minutes ahead of time so that the exercises can be done more comfortably. The exercises should be done 3 to 5 times each day until full arm and shoulder range of motion is restored (Fig. 52.7).

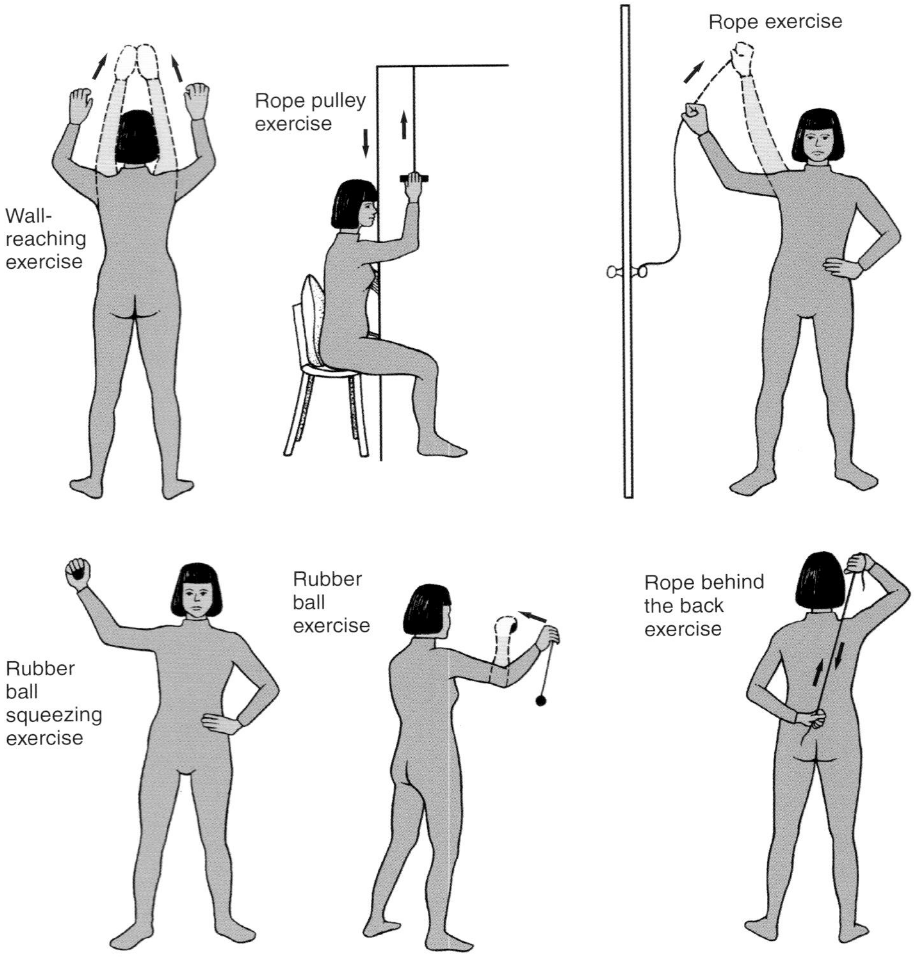

Fig. 52.7 Arm exercises for mastectomy patients. (From Monahan FD, Drake DT, Neighbors M, editors: *Medical-surgical nursing: foundations for clinical practice*, ed 2, Philadelphia, 1998, Saunders.)

Inability to manage self-care.. With the patient's permission, arrangements can be made for visits from a representative of the ACS's Reach for Recovery program. The representatives are volunteers who have experienced breast cancer themselves and learned to cope successfully with the diagnosis, treatment, and related stressors. They assist patients by providing information, anticipatory guidance, and emotional support.

Patient teaching should have begun preoperatively but must be reinforced postoperatively. Content to cover includes signs and symptoms of infection, wound care, arm exercises, prevention of lymphedema, resources, and (if appropriate) management of the effects of chemotherapy or radiotherapy. With the patient's permission, include their significant other in the teaching process. This provides an opportunity for the partner to understand the patient's experience, demonstrate support, and participate in their recovery. With simple mastectomies, patients are sometimes discharged in less than 24 hours. This makes patient teaching especially challenging. Be sure to provide written information and resources along with verbal instructions.

CERVICAL CANCER

Cervical cancer generally grows slowly. For patients who have regular pelvic examinations and Pap tests, cervical cancer is usually diagnosed and treated in its early stage. Advanced cervical cancer may invade such surrounding structures as pelvic walls, bowel, and bladder.

Cause and Risk Factors

Research indicates that the risk for cervical cancer is increased in women who have been infected with certain human papillomavirus (HPV) subtypes or who have a compromised immune response, as in HIV. Additional factors associated with cervical cancer are cigarette smoking, initial sexual intercourse in early adolescence, and multiple sexual partners. Two vaccines, Gardasil and Gardasil 9 are available to protect against HPV infection and therefore dramatically reduce cervical cancer. These vaccines are now available for both young men and young women. It is hoped that by vaccinating all teens before they are sexually active, the rates of cervical cancer will be reduced dramatically.

Clinical Manifestations

Early cervical cancer is asymptomatic. Advanced cancer may also be asymptomatic or may be associated with blood-tinged or frank bloody vaginal discharge, menstrual irregularities, or bleeding after intercourse.

Complications

Invasion of cervical cancer into adjacent structures causes site-related symptoms such as pain, backache, and bleeding. Anemia may develop because of chronic bleeding.

Medical Diagnosis

Cervical cancer is often first suspected when a positive Pap test result reveals atypical cells. Tissue specimens are studied for microscopic evidence of malignancy. Cervical cancer is preceded by changes in cells called **dysplasia**.

Cervical cancer is staged according to the extent of invasion, with stage IA1 signifying limitation to the cervical epithelium and stage IVB indicating metastasis to distant organs.

Medical Treatment

Treatment depends on the stage of the tumor and on various general health factors. Sometimes monitoring without immediate intervention is appropriate. Mild dysplasia may be treated with conization which is excision of the affected tissue or ablation. Ablative techniques destroy abnormal tissue using a CO_2 laser, cryotherapy, or diathermy. Localized carcinoma (in situ) may be treated with laser destruction, cryosurgery, or conization alone; total hysterectomy may be performed if childbearing is not desired.

Invasive cancer is treated with radiation, surgery, or chemotherapy (or a combination of treatments). Radiotherapy may be external or internal. Internal therapy (brachytherapy) can be delivered with several options including the placement of a sealed radiation source in the vagina for a specified period of time and the insertion of needles into the affected area. Because effective treatment requires proper placement, the patient who had a sealed source is immobilized as much as possible for the duration of the treatment. Radiotherapy and related nursing care are discussed in detail in Chapter 7.

If surgery is elected, the extent of the surgery depends on the extent of invasion. It ranges from radical hysterectomy (removal of the uterus, fallopian tubes, upper third of the vagina, and usually the ovaries) to total pelvic exenteration (removal of the uterus, ovaries, fallopian tubes, vagina, bladder, urethra, descending colon, rectum, anal canal, and pelvic lymph nodes). Nursing care of the patient with cervical cancer is discussed in the section titled "Nursing Care of the Patient With Cancer of the Cervix, Ovaries, Vulva, or Vagina."

OVARIAN CANCER

Ovarian cancer occurs most often in women between 55 and 65 years of age. Although the incidence is relatively low compared with that of other cancers, the mortality rate from ovarian cancer is the highest of all female reproductive system cancers. The high mortality is because ovarian cancer is asymptomatic until it is advanced, so it usually grows for an extended period of time before it is diagnosed. In most cases, abnormal cell growth occurs in both ovaries.

Cause and Risk Factors

No specific causes have been found for ovarian cancer. However, risk factors include a family or personal history of ovarian cancer; a personal history of ovarian dysfunction or of breast, endometrial, or colorectal cancer; obesity; nulliparity (i.e., has not produced a viable offspring); and early menarche and late menopause. Ovarian cancer is rarely found in women who have had children or who have used hormonal contraceptives. Prophylactic bilateral oophorectomy (i.e., surgical removal of the ovaries) may be suggested for women at high risk for ovarian cancer.

Signs and Symptoms

Ovarian cancer is asymptomatic in its early stage. Symptoms of even advanced ovarian cancer tend to be vague and nonspecific, usually attributed to various other conditions before ovarian cancer is considered. Abdominal pain and bloating, heavy feeling in the pelvis, unexplained and worsening back pain, gastrointestinal (GI) tract symptoms such as flatulence, and urinary tract complaints may be reported. Abnormal uterine bleeding is not common. In extremely advanced cancer, ascites may be noted.

Complications

Ovarian cancer can spread to the peritoneum, omentum, and bowel surface via direct invasion, peritoneal fluid, and the lymphatic and venous systems.

Medical Diagnosis

Palpable tumors may be discovered on pelvic and rectal examinations. Abdominal and transvaginal ultrasound with color Doppler imaging may be used as diagnostic tools. Blood may be drawn for a cancer antigen 125 (CA-125) serum marker test which may be elevated in the presence of ovarian epithelial cancer. If evidence supports a diagnosis of ovarian cancer, an exploratory laparotomy or laparoscopy is done to visualize the tumor or tumors directly and to obtain tissue for definitive diagnosis and for staging and grading of the malignancy.

Some practitioners advocate routine screening of blood serum for CA-125 for early detection of ovarian cancer. However, elevated CA-125 levels can be caused by other factors in addition to ovarian cancer. Also, some patients with ovarian cancer have normal

CA-125 levels. The test may be most useful in assessing tumor progression or regression during treatment.

Medical Treatment

Treatment depends on the staging of the tumor or tumors. Options include surgery (usually total abdominal hysterectomy and bilateral salpingo-oophorectomy), systemic or intraperitoneal chemotherapy, intraperitoneal radioisotope instillation, and external radiation therapy. Even with advanced disease, treatment can improve comfort. Nursing care of the patient with ovarian cancer is discussed in the section titled "Nursing Care of the Patient With Cancer of the Cervix, Ovaries, Vulva, or Vagina."

VULVAR CANCER

Cancer of the vulva is relatively rare but also one of the most visible of the cancers of the female reproductive system. It may appear as a visible and palpable lump on the vulva or as a deviation from the normally pink, moist mucosa. The lesion may be scaly; red, white, or irregularly pigmented; and edematous. Drainage from the lesion may be pink (serosanguinous) or bloody. The most common site is the labia majora. Although it is rare, malignant melanoma may occur in the vulva. Its incidence is highest in postmenopausal women. The symptoms are similar to those of the more common vulvar cancers.

Cause and Risk Factors

More than half of these cancers are linked to having had an infection with a high-risk type of HPV. Other risk factors are smoking, having vulvar neoplasia (abnormal cells that are not cancerous), or having had other genital cancers such as cervical cancer.

Clinical Manifestations

The most commonly reported symptom is pruritus (itching). Pain and bleeding are additional symptoms.

Complications

Although cancer of the vulva generally remains localized, it may become invasive if not discovered and treated. It can invade adjacent structures or metastasize via the lymphatic system.

Medical Diagnosis

A preliminary diagnosis is made through palpation of a mass or by visualization of tissue that appears suspicious. Biopsy is necessary for definitive diagnosis.

Medical Treatment

Treatment depends on the extent to which the malignant cells have spread. For localized lesions, conservative removal by laser surgery or topical chemotherapy may be used. For wider, deeper, or invasive lesions, radical procedures may be indicated. Surgical procedures include hemivulvectomy or vulvectomy with bilateral dissection of groin lymph nodes and pelvic exenteration. Radical hemivulvectomy is generally preferred because radical vulvectomy results in greater scarring and loss of function and is more prone to wound breakdown. Pelvic exenteration is the removal of all pelvic organs, including the bladder; the descending colon and anal canal may or may not be removed. Chemotherapy, radiation therapy, or both may follow surgery. Nursing care of the patient with vulvar cancer is discussed in the section titled "Nursing Care of the Patient With Cancer of the Cervix, Ovaries, Vulva, or Vagina."

VAGINAL CANCER

The vagina is an extremely rare primary site for reproductive tract cancer; rather, it is the site for the extension of cancer that originates in the vulva, cervix, or endometrium. Vaginal cancer is found most commonly in postmenopausal women.

Cause and Risk Factors

Although, no definite cause has been identified for vaginal cancer, the following risk factors have been identified: STIs, vaginal neoplasia (noncancerous lesions), younger age at initial sexual intercourse, greater number of lifetime sexual partners, smoking, HPV infection, a previous diagnosis of cervical or vulvar cancer, and previous radiation therapy

Clinical Manifestations

In its early and most easily treated form, vaginal cancer is usually asymptomatic. Later symptoms include a burning sensation, vaginal discharge that may have a foul odor, dyspareunia, spotting after intercourse, and vaginal bleeding. Pelvic pain, if present, is usually associated with invasion of adjacent structures.

Complications

Invasion of adjacent structures and metastasis are the most common complications of epithelial vaginal cancer. The prognosis is poor for vaginal malignant melanoma, with an extremely low 5-year survival rate.

Medical Diagnosis and Treatment

Most cases are detected during inspection of the vagina and from routine Pap tests. A definitive diagnosis is made via colposcopy and biopsy of suspicious areas followed by tissue studies. Treatment of vaginal cancer depends on the extent of invasion. In situ (localized) cancer may be treated relatively simply with local laser surgery or cryosurgery. More radical treatment is indicated if the cancer is more invasive. Possible treatments used either alone or in combination include topical chemotherapy, internal or external radiotherapy, partial or total vaginectomy, and pelvic exenteration.

◆ NURSING CARE OF THE PATIENT WITH CANCER OF THE CERVIX, OVARIES, VULVA, OR VAGINA

The patient with cancer of the cervix, ovaries, vulva, or vagina presents many challenges. They have a life-threatening condition whose treatment very often threatens not only the patient's self-concept but also their sexual function. Treatments beyond local excision of affected tissue may result in disfigurement or in anatomic changes that hinder penile-vaginal intercourse, or both. The patient's psychosocial needs are as critical as their physical needs.

Focused Assessment

Complete assessment of the patient with a disorder of the female reproductive system is summarized in Chapter 51, Box 51.1. When the patient has or may have cancer, the health history documents signs and symptoms and possible risk factors. When reviewing the systems, describe changes or problems that may be related such as fatigue, pain, infection, and bowel or bladder dysfunction. Explore the effects of the symptoms on normal functioning. The patient may react to the diagnosis with anxiety, fear, depression, anger, or withdrawal. A complete physical examination should be done. The physician or nurse practitioner performs a pelvic examination that may reveal lesions, masses, and lymph node enlargement.

Patient Problems, Goals, and Outcome Criteria: Cancer of the Cervix, Ovaries, Vulva, or Vagina

Patient Problems	Goals and Outcome Criteria
Anxiety and fear related to threat to health and lack of knowledge about the cancer and prescribed treatment	Reduced anxiety and fear: patient's statement of reduced anxiety and fear, calm manner
Altered body image related to change in body appearance or function	Positive body image: patient makes positive statements about self, makes efforts to maintain or improve appearance
Potential for impaired sexual function related to physical and emotional effects of cancer of the reproductive system	Satisfactory sexual activity: patient's discussion of effects of disease or treatment on sexuality and coping strategies
Inadequate family coping related to lack of knowledge, situational crisis, role changes, or patient preoccupation with self	Appropriate family and patient interactions: family demonstration of support and positive coping
Potential for injury (to patient and others) related to effects of radiotherapy, chemotherapy	Decreased risk of injury from treatment: maintenance of applicator position and adherence of patient and others to radiation precautions

Interventions

Anxiety and fear. The patient needs to be able to express their feelings about their diagnosis and prescribed treatment without being judged. Listen carefully to determine any knowledge deficits or misconceptions. Provide information or sources of information as appropriate. Many patients of all ages are computer literate and therefore have access to endless sources. However, patients should be cautioned that not all information on the internet is accurate or appropriate for their situations. National organizations such as the ACS have excellent patient education materials. Community agencies may have a lending library of books and videotapes. Support groups are often helpful because patients learn from others who have had similar experiences. Many patients appreciate follow-up phone calls or the ability to call a resource person when needed.

Altered body image. The patient may be distressed if appearance or function is altered by the cancer or the treatment. Loss of reproductive capacity can be especially painful for those who still wish to bear children. You can listen kindly when the patient wishes to express their thoughts. Patients who are severely distressed should be offered the benefit of a mental health professional or spiritual counselor. Encourage measures to improve the appearance and praise the patient's positive efforts. Management of alopecia (i.e., hair loss) associated with cancer therapy is discussed in Chapter 7.

Potential for impaired sexual function. The health care provider should present realistic expectations for future sexual functioning. The patient may be advised to abstain from sexual intercourse during the treatment and healing. Permanent effects of the disease and treatment may require alternative sexual practices. The patient may wish to discuss this topic with you. It is critical that you show an accepting attitude toward sexuality in general and toward any specific sexual practices acceptable to the patient and their partner. A psychiatric nurse practitioner or counselor may be consulted to help the patient adapt.

Inadequate family coping. Include the family or identified support system in the patient's care. The family needs to understand the effects of the cancer and the treatments. They also need to understand the patient's need for support and for assistance during therapy and recovery. Encourage members of the household to consider ways to reduce demands on the patient. In addition, be sensitive to the needs of family members who may fear losing a loved one. Inclusion of the patient's sexual partner is particularly critical if altered sexual expression is expected after treatment.

Potential for injury. Physical care of the patient varies with the prescribed treatment and is based on the physician's orders, institutional policies and procedures, and patient problems. Care of the patient who is having internal or external radiotherapy is detailed in Chapter 7.

Put On Your Thinking Cap!

A patient with pelvic cancer has had a surgical procedure that includes removal of the vagina. She tearfully says, "I will never be able to make love to my husband again." What are some things you could say or do to show acceptance of her feelings at this time?

Care of the patient admitted for a pelvic exenteration is exceptionally complex and beyond the scope of this text. Expert nursing staff are essential to provide the emotional support and physical care demanded for this patient.

INFERTILITY

Infertility is generally defined as the inability to conceive within 1 year of regular unprotected sexual intercourse. Infertility is categorized as *primary infertility* if the woman has never conceived or if the man has never impregnated a woman. *Secondary infertility* refers to the woman who has conceived at least one time but is not able to conceive again. An estimated 10% of American females from 15 to 44 years of age (or 15% of couples) are infertile. Treatment enables approximately 60% of those couples to conceive and carry pregnancies to term.

CAUSE AND RISK FACTORS

Causes of infertility may be related to the woman, the man, or both. Sometimes the cause cannot be determined. Conception depends on a number of factors, broadly categorized as follows:

1. Timing and techniques used for sexual intercourse:
   - Impregnation of ovum by the sperm must occur within 24 hours after ovulation. Intercourse should be scheduled for every other day around ovulation time to optimize the potential for fertilization of the ovum.
   - Semen should be deposited deeply in the vagina, in proximity to the cervical os.
2. Production and release of a healthy ovum by the woman and of numerous (~20–150 million per ejaculate) healthy sperm by the man.
3. Anatomically and physiologically correct female and male reproductive systems:
   - The woman should have patent fallopian tubes with active fimbriated ends and uterine endometrium prepared for reception and implantation of a fertilized ovum.
   - The man should have an epididymis temperature that maintains sperm viability during storage, patent seminiferous tubules, and a vas deferens with enervated musculature.
4. Biochemical compatibility between female vaginal-cervical-fallopian environment and male ejaculate.

Box 52.2 Causes of Infertility

FEMALE
- Developmental: uterine abnormalities
- Endocrine: pituitary, thyroid, and adrenal dysfunctions; ovarian dysfunctions (inhibit maturation and release of ova)
- Diseases: pelvic inflammatory disease (PID), especially from gonococcus; fallopian tube obstructions; diseases of cervix and uterus that inhibit passage of active sperm
- Other: malnutrition, severe anemia, anxiety

MALE
- Developmental: undescended testes, other congenital anomalies (inhibit development of sperm)
- Endocrine: hormonal deficiencies (pituitary, thyroid, adrenal) (inhibit development of sperm)
- Diseases: testicular destruction from disease, orchitis from mumps, prostatitis
- Other: excessive smoking, fatigue, alcohol, excessive heat (hot baths), marijuana use

BOTH MALE AND FEMALE
- Diseases: sexually transmitted infections (STIs), cancer with obstructions (inhibit transport of ovum or sperm)
- Other: immunologic incompatibility (inhibit sperm penetration of ovum), marital problems
- Diethylstilbestrol exposure in utero (suggested but not proved as a cause of male infertility)

From Phipps WJ, Monahan FD, Sands JK, et al.: *Medical-surgical nursing: health and illness perspectives*, ed 7, St. Louis, 2003, Mosby

Faulty timing or technique for sexual intercourse is easily corrected through patient education. Many other causes for infertility exist. Untreated STIs can impair fertility by altering anatomy, physiology, and patency of the reproductive tracts of either or both partners. Additional causes include hypothalamic-pituitary-endocrine system dysfunction, malnutrition or obesity, smoking, drug and alcohol use, exposure to toxic chemicals or radiation, nervous system disorders that affect reproductive structures that transfer ova and sperm, and male practices that maintain above-normal epididymal temperature (i.e., wearing tight underwear and pants, frequent and prolonged immersion in hot water or sauna). Causes of infertility are summarized in Box 52.2.

MEDICAL DIAGNOSIS

The diagnosis of infertility is based on extensive psychosocial and physical health and sexual health histories of both partners. If the histories provide clues that may explain possible detriments to fertility, such as poor timing or techniques of sexual intercourse or habitual epididymal exposure to high temperatures, then further diagnostic attempts may be delayed until the couple has had time to remediate the potential problem or problems. If such simple factors are not identified, systematic, comprehensive physical examinations and laboratory tests are conducted.

The male partner is usually the initial focus of diagnostic procedures because tests for diagnosis of male-associated infertility problems are generally easier, less invasive, less expensive, and (unlike a complete female fertility workup) not cycle dependent. A semen specimen for analysis is collected by masturbation after a period of sexual abstinence (usually 2–3 days) that approximates the man's average frequency interval for intercourse. The specimen is then assessed for volume and for sperm count, morphology (shape), duration of viability, motility, and liquefaction. A second specimen is examined if variations from normal are found. He may be referred to a urologist or endocrinologist for further diagnosis and possible treatment.

Evaluation of the female partner includes a battery of tests. The woman may be instructed to maintain a record of her basal body temperature each morning on awakening and to monitor for daily symptoms. The basal body temperature rises when ovulation occurs, which suggests the timing of intercourse. She may also assess for cervical mucus changes that occur in response to ovulation. The woman will note the change from cervical mucus that is thick (pre- and postovulatory) to a slippery, stretchy, and thin quality that peaks during ovulation. She also may sense a cramping sensation in the lower abdomen as the ovum ruptures, referred to as *mittelschmerz*.

Another tool is the ovulation prediction kit that measures luteinizing hormone (LH) in the urine. Daily measurements detect a rise in LH, which is usually followed by ovulation in 28 to 36 hours. Other diagnostic data are obtained using a variety of tools and tests including cervical and vaginal stains, endometrial biopsy, and measurement of plasma progesterone. The assessment of ovarian reserve, which determines the quality and quantity of oocytes and reproductive potential, is expected to be a valuable component of infertility assessment. However, no ideal test exists at this time.

Pharmacology Capsule

Ovulatory stimulants can cause ovarian hyperstimulation with possible rupture of the enlarged ovary.

If the diagnostic tests indicate normal hormonal functions, a postcoital test may be done. The couple has intercourse around the expected time of ovulation and 2 to 12 hours before the scheduled test. The physician or nurse practitioner aspirates a specimen of cervical and vaginal secretions from the cervix. The specimen is examined for mucus characteristics and for sperm number and motility. If a previous test of the male's semen indicated normal motility and viability of sperm but the postcoital test indicates nonviable sperm, this suggests that the cervical mucus is not conducive to sperm survival, perhaps because of an antigen-antibody response to the semen.

Table 52.6 Common Causes of Female Infertility and Related Medical Treatment

CAUSE	MEDICAL TREATMENT
Failure to ovulate, associated with the following: Delayed follicular maturation Hypogonadotropin secretion Hypothalamic-pituitary dysfunction Elevated prolactin level Hypothyroidism Ovarian tumors	Clomid (clomiphene citrate) Letrozole (aromatase inhibitor) Pergonal (menotropins) Gonadotropin-releasing hormone (GnRH) Parlodel (bromocriptine mesylate) Thyroid-stimulating hormone (TSH) Surgical excision
Inadequate endometrial development	Progesterone therapy
Endometriosis	Lupron therapy; surgery Gamete intrafallopian transfer
Reproductive tract infections	Antimicrobial therapy
Tubal obstruction	Hysterosalpingogram
Sperm-inhospitable cervical mucus	Therapeutic intrauterine insemination In vitro fertilization
Immunologic reaction to sperm	Use of condoms to reduce antibody titer, followed by unprotected intercourse at time of ovulation only In vitro fertilization

Determination of fallopian tube patency is usually accomplished with hysterosalpingography. A radiopaque dye is injected through the cervix. Radiographs are then taken to visualize the uterus and tubes. Physical assessment of the peritoneal cavity, if required, uses laparoscopy or culdoscopy. Ultrasonography may be used for additional assessment.

Women are considered to be sterile and thus are not candidates for infertility diagnosis and treatment if they have congenital reproductive tract anomalies that cannot be corrected by surgery. Absence of one or more reproductive tract structures is also untreatable.

MEDICAL TREATMENT

Treatment for infertility depends on specific diagnostic findings. A brief overview of specific problems and related treatments is presented in Table 52.6 .

◆ NURSING CARE OF THE PATIENT WITH AN INFERTILITY DISORDER

Focused Assessment

Assessment of the female reproductive system is summarized in Chapter 51, Box 51.1. The LVN/LPN assists with data collection for the assessment.

Patient Problems, Goals, and Outcome Criteria: Infertility

Patient Problems	Goals and Outcome Criteria
Low self-esteem related to inability to conceive or feeling of failure	Improved self-esteem: positive expressions about self
Altered sexual function related to structured efforts to conceive or loss of spontaneity	Acknowledgment of the effects of the situation on one's sexual relationship: patient identifies ways to maintain a satisfying sexual relationship
Inadequate coping related to unmet expectations or feelings of loss	Effective coping: patient uses healthy coping strategies
Lack of knowledge of diagnostic and treatment procedures	Patient understands diagnostic and treatment procedures: patient verbalizes diagnostic and treatment procedures

Interventions

Fertility tests and treatments are generally done on an outpatient basis. The woman who undergoes the process usually has a prolonged relationship and frequent contacts with the nurse in the outpatient setting.

Low self-esteem. Invasion of personal privacy is necessarily greater in fertility diagnosis and treatment than in any other condition. Gently explore the feelings of the patient and partner about their difficulty conceiving. An open, empathetic attitude is vital if the patient is to be open. Support groups or professional counselors may help the couple to maintain self-esteem.

Altered sexual function. The most intimate details of the patient's sexual relationship with their partner are elicited, and diagnostic and treatment procedures repeatedly violate the desire for modesty. Intercourse becomes scheduled rather than spontaneous.

Inadequate coping. You may be the only person with whom the woman shares her psychologic reactions to the diagnosis of infertility and her subsequent emotional highs and lows throughout diagnosis and treatment. You therefore play a critical role in assisting the patient to cope with infertility. Give the patient the opportunity to discuss her thoughts and feelings about infertility and to explore coping strategies.

Inability to manage self-care. The needs of the patient's sexual partner must be considered as well and they should be included in patient teaching. Patient teaching includes information about diagnostic procedures, treatments, causes of infertility, and resources.

MENOPAUSE

Menopause is the cessation of menstruation that marks the end of a woman's reproductive capacity. Natural menopause is part of normal aging, but surgical menopause results from removal of the ovaries. Natural menopause occurs gradually and may permit better adaptation than surgical menopause, which suddenly eliminates the source of natural estrogen. Diminished ovarian function associated with aging causes ovulation to cease and estrogen production to decline. The onset of menopause may begin as early as 35 years of age but more commonly occurs between 45 and 55 years of age, with the average age of menopause being 51 years of age. With natural menopause, the woman's first sign may be menstrual irregularity. Menstrual periods tend to be spaced farther apart and the amount of bleeding gradually diminishes. The entire process from earliest signs to complete cessation of menstruation usually is 2 years or less. A woman is said to be *menopausal* when she has not had a menstrual period for 1 year. Some women experience a surgical menopause brought on by the surgical removal of the ovaries. Unless estrogen replacement is begun promptly, the patient develops the signs and symptoms of menopause rapidly.

CLINICAL MANIFESTATIONS

The signs and symptoms of menopause may include hot flashes, a warm feeling caused by vasodilation that affects the face, neck, and upper body. Hot flashes are typically accompanied by perspiration and sometimes by a feeling of faintness. Other common symptoms are vaginal dryness, insomnia, joint pain, headache, and nausea. Without estrogen, the uterus becomes smaller, the vagina shortens, and vaginal tissues become drier. Breast tissue may lose its firmness and pubic and axillary hair become sparse. Supporting pelvic structures relax, causing some women to have stress incontinence. Significant loss of bone mass may occur, leading to fragile bones, a condition called *osteoporosis.* Some women report emotional instability, irritability, and depression, but the effect of menopause on a woman is very individualized. Some grieve for the loss of reproductive capacity and some feel a loss of femininity and sexual attractiveness. Others welcome the end of menstrual periods and no longer having to worry about the risk of pregnancy.

Complementary and Alternative Therapies

Black cohosh is sometimes used to treat menstrual cramps and as an alternative to estrogen for treatment of menopausal symptoms. In general, research has not found it to be more effective in reducing hot flashes than placebo. The two most common side effects are headache and gastrointestinal (GI) upset. It should not be used by people with liver disease or during pregnancy.

MEDICAL TREATMENT

Estrogen therapy decreases the risk of osteoporosis but, if taken for more than 5 years, may increase the risk of breast cancer. Therefore each woman's health history must be considered so that she and her physician can decide whether menopausal HT (MHT) will be used. Estrogens are contraindicated with estrogen-dependent cancer, undiagnosed abnormal vaginal bleeding, and current or past thromboembolic disorders.

Many drug regimens exist. The patient who still has her uterus and ovaries has typically been treated with estrogens and progestins (compounds that have actions like progesterone). Because progestin decreases the risk of endometrial cancer related to estrogen therapy, it is not needed in women who no longer have a uterus. Findings from the Women's Health Initiative indicate that combination therapy in women with an intact uterus increases the risk of invasive breast cancer and coronary heart disease.

Oral drug therapy is most commonly used, but transdermal forms of estrogen are also available. The transdermal drug is delivered by an adhesive bandage-like patch or spray. Estrogen creams, vaginal tablets, and suppositories may be used to relieve vaginal dryness. Drugs used to control "hot flashes" include clonidine patches, gabapentin, Bellergal-S, and several antidepressants such as venlafaxine and paroxetine (see the Complementary and Alternative Therapies box).

Complementary and Alternative Therapies

Over-the-counter (OTC) options to sustain the patient's well-being in menopause include natural vitamin E with mixed tocopherols (400–800 IU PO [by mouth] daily), vitamin B complex (200 mg PO daily), and calcium (1500 mg with vitamin D per manufacturer's instructions).

◆ NURSING CARE OF THE MENOPAUSAL PATIENT

Focused Assessment

Assessment of the woman with a disorder of the reproductive system is summarized in Chapter 51, Box 51.1. When a woman has menopausal symptoms, record them and explore how the patient is coping with this significant life change.

Patient Problems, Goals, and Outcome Criteria: Menopause

The primary patient problem for the menopausal patient is usually ineffective management of symptoms related to lack of understanding of the effects and treatment of menopause. The goals of nursing care are effective management of prescribed therapy and decreased signs and symptoms of menopause. The outcome criterion is the patient's report of reduced symptoms.

Interventions

Assess the patient's understanding of menopause and how she feels about it. The patient may need reassurance that her symptoms and responses are normal and common. If drug therapy is used, instruct the patient regarding self-medication. Caution patients on estrogen to report any signs of circulatory disorders (i.e., numbness, pain in calf, shortness of breath) to the physician immediately. Additional information about drug therapy is summarized in Chapter 51, Table 51.2. The patient who cannot (or chooses not to) take hormone therapy needs additional assistance to cope with the symptoms of menopause. Women who wish to prevent "menopausal" pregnancy should use a reliable form of contraception for at least 1 year after cessation of menses.

Get Ready for the NCLEX® Examination!

Key Points

- Two common uterine bleeding disorders are metrorrhagia (bleeding or spotting between menstrual periods) and menorrhagia (menstrual periods characterized by profuse bleeding).
- The primary patient problems for the patient with a uterine bleeding disorder are inability to manage self-care and anxiety related to unknown cause of bleeding.
- The effects of reproductive tract infections may include infertility, changes in relationships, feelings of distrust toward sexual partners, shame, embarrassment, and diminished self-esteem.
- Because most infections are treated on an outpatient basis, the nurse's primary role is to educate the patient in preventing and treating infections.
- Benign growths of the female reproductive system include cysts of the breasts and ovaries and endometriosis.
- The two primary patient problems for the patient with endometriosis, a disorder marked by the growth of endometrial tissue outside the uterus, are pain and inability to manage self-care.
- Cysts are saclike structures that contain fluid, semisolid, or solid material and are usually benign.
- Fibroid tumors are benign but may have to be removed because they can compress abdominal structures and lead to infertility, crowding, and malpositioning of the fetus during pregnancy, as well as to degenerative changes related to interruption of blood supply.
- Pelvic organ prolapse (i.e., herniation of the bladder or of the rectum into the vagina) can disrupt urinary and bowel function and is often corrected surgically.
- Patient problems after surgery for correction of a cystocele or rectocele may include urinary obstruction, potential for injury, and pain.

- Uterine prolapse, the descent of the uterus into the vagina, may be treated with corrective surgery or vaginal hysterectomy.
- Breast cancer is the most common form of cancer in American women. It has a 5-year survival rate of 99% when detected while still localized.
- After mastectomy, patient problems may include potential for injury, potential for limited range of motion, potential for infection, altered body image, and altered sexual function.
- Cervical cancer can be detected early by regular pelvic examinations and Pap tests. Prompt treatment is usually curative.
- Ovarian cancer has the highest mortality rate of all female reproductive system cancers because it is asymptomatic in the early stages.
- Patient problems for the patient with cancer of the reproductive system may include anxiety, fear, altered body image, altered sexual function, inadequate family coping, and (if treated with radiotherapy) potential for injury.
- Infertility, the inability to produce viable offspring, can sometimes be treated medically or surgically.

Additional Learning Resources

SG Go to your Study Guide for additional learning activities to help you master this chapter content.

Go to your Evolve website (http://evolve.elsevier.com/Linton/medsurg) for the following learning resources and much more:
- Fluid & Electrolyte Tutorial
- Review Questions for the NCLEX® Examination

Clinical Judgment and Next-Generation NCLEX® Examination-Style Questions

1. **Widespread immunization against the HPV is anticipated to greatly reduce the occurrence of which of the following?**
   1. Breast cancer
   2. Endometriosis
   3. Cervical cancer
   4. Infertility

   NCLEX Client Need: Health Maintenance and Promotion

2. **Which measures are appropriate to manage lymphedema after mastectomy? (Select all that apply.)**
   1. Immobilize the affected arm as much as possible.
   2. Avoid venipunctures on the affected arm.
   3. Elevate the affected arm above the level of the heart.
   4. Do not shave the axilla of the affected arm.
   5. Take blood pressures on the unaffected arm.

   NCLEX Client Need: Physiological Integrity: Reduction of Risk Potential

3. **What is the most prevalent type of cancer in American women?**
   1. Uterine
   2. Ovarian
   3. Vulvar
   4. Breast

   NCLEX Client Need: Physiological Integrity: Physiological Adaptation

4. **Which of the following statements made by a patient with endometriosis indicates that she correctly understands her condition?**
   1. HPV increases the risk of endometriosis.
   2. Endometriosis is a type of uterine cancer.
   3. Endometriosis may contribute to infertility.
   4. Estrogen therapy effectively destroys endometrial implants.

   NCLEX Client Need: Physiological Integrity: Physiological Adaptation

5. **A patient comes to the clinic with complaints of a "yeast" infection. Which information from the health history is especially relevant to this diagnosis?**
   1. Recently started taking an oral contraceptive drug.
   2. Takes daily antibiotics for acne.
   3. Prefers hot tub baths over showers.
   4. Uses feminine hygiene sprays.

   NCLEX Client Need: Physiological Integrity: Physiological Adaptation

6. **Which organism is *not* commonly associated with PID?**
   1. *Neisseria gonorrhoeae*
   2. *Chlamydia trachomatis*
   3. *Mycoplasma genitalium*
   4. *Escherichia coli*

   NCLEX Client Need: Physiological Integrity: Physiological Adaptation

7. **A patient completed a 6-month course of danazol (Danocrine) for treatment of endometriosis. She would like to become pregnant. Which of the following is it important for her to understand?**
   1. She will begin menstrual bleeding within 1 week after stopping the danazol.
   2. Her best chances of pregnancy are in the first month after completing danazol therapy.
   3. She should not become pregnant for 1 month because danazol can cause birth defects.
   4. She is unlikely to become pregnant for at least 1 year after taking danazol.

   NCLEX Client Need: Physiological Integrity: Pharmacological Therapies

8. **An older woman with uterine prolapse is being fitted with a pessary. What information should be included in the teaching plan?**
   1. The pessary permanently corrects the uterine prolapse.
   2. Once the pessary is in place, no further care is needed.
   3. No complications are associated with pessaries.
   4. The position of the pessary must be checked in 24 hours.

   NCLEX Client Need: Physiological Integrity: Reduction of Risk Potential

9. **A 30-year-old woman who reports menarche at 12 years of age, first sexual intercourse at 14 years of age, and a history of treatment for HPV infection at 15 years of age is at increased risk for which of the following?**

   1. Breast cancer
   2. Uterine prolapse
   3. Cervical cancer
   4. Fibroid tumors

   NCLEX Client Need: Physiological Integrity: Reduction of Risk Potential

10. **SLO/Objective: Assist in developing a care plan for patients with common disorders of the female reproductive system.**

    NGN item Type: Enhanced Hot Spot

    Cognitive Skill: Recognize Cues

    A 30-year-old woman is being treated for PID. She comes into the community clinic for a follow-up visit. The assessment data on this visit are:

    - Stopped antibiotics after four days because she felt better
    - Abdominal pain has decreased from 6 to 0 on pain scale
    - Resumed sexual intercourse after stopping antibiotics
    - Perineum washed after sexual intercourse
    - Condom used for penile/vaginal contact
    - Has burning on urination
    - douched after intercourse to prevent pregnancy

    Highlight or place a check mark next to the assessment findings that require follow up by the nurse.

53 Male Reproductive System Introduction

http://evolve.elsevier.com/Linton/medsurg

Objectives

1. Describe the major structures and functions of the normal male reproductive system.
2. Identify data to be collected when assessing a male patient with a reproductive system disorder.
3. Explain commonly performed diagnostic tests and procedures for male reproductive disorders and the nursing implications of each.
4. Identify common classes of drugs used to treat disorders of the male reproductive system and the nursing implications of each.

Key Terms

cryptorchidism (krip-TAWR-ki-diz-uhm)
ejaculation
emission
hematocele (HĔM-ăh-tō-sēl)
hydrocele (HĪ-drō-sēl)

ANATOMY OF THE MALE REPRODUCTIVE SYSTEM

The male reproductive system consists of the scrotum, testes, epididymis, vas deferens, seminal vesicles, prostate gland, ejaculatory duct, internal urethra, and penis (Fig. 53.1).

SCROTUM

The scrotum is a thin, pendulous sac on the outside of the body that encloses each of the two testicles (testes) in separate compartments. Sperm production and survival require a temperature 3°C lower than the core body temperature. Therefore, the scrotum helps to regulate testicular temperature. The scrotum contracts into thick folds (i.e., rugae) during fear, anger, arousal, or cold, drawing the testes close to the body for protection and insulation. On warm days, the scrotal muscles relax and allow the scrotum to hang free of the body. Sweat glands may be activated to cool the testes and maintain a testicular temperature that is below body temperature.

TESTES

The two testes are the male reproductive organs. They lie within the scrotum, suspended from the spermatic cord (Fig. 53.2). They are composed of numerous highly coiled seminiferous tubules that produce spermatozoa and the male hormone testosterone. The testicles develop in the embryo at about the seventh week of gestation and begin producing small amounts of testosterone. Secretion of this male hormone results in the development of other male reproductive organs and causes the testes to descend into the scrotum during the last 2 months of gestation. At around 10 to 13 years of age, during puberty, the increased production of testosterone results in the production of sperm and the development of body hair, muscle mass, and other secondary sex characteristics.

EPIDIDYMIS

Newly developed sperm move from each testicle through the epididymis, a coiled tubule almost 20 feet long that rests along the top and side of the testes. This passage may take several days and allows the sperm to mature and develop the capability for motility (movement) and fertilization (see Fig. 53.2).

VAS DEFERENS

As mature sperm leave the epididymis, they enter the vasa deferentia (*sing.*, vas deferens), which are tubes of secretory ducts that serve as the primary storage sites for sperm, contribute to the fluid content of semen, and contract to help propel the mature sperm into the urethra during ejaculation. The vas deferens is bundled together with the spermatic artery and veins, lymphatic vessels, and nerves by the spermatic cord; the bundle exits the scrotum and enters the pelvic cavity via the inguinal canal (see Figs. 53.1 and 53.2).

SEMINAL VESICLES

The seminal vesicles are hollow, twisted, tubular secretory glands located on the posterior surface of the bladder. They produce a mucoid fluid that constitutes about 60% of the volume of the semen and provides

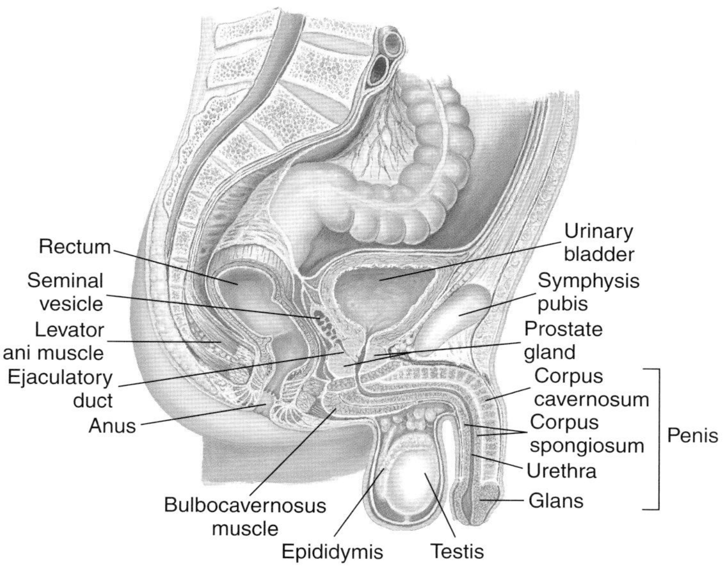

Fig. 53.1 Male reproductive system. (From Seidel HM, Ball JW, Dains JE, et al.: *Mosby's guide to physical examination*, ed 7, St. Louis, 2010, Mosby.)

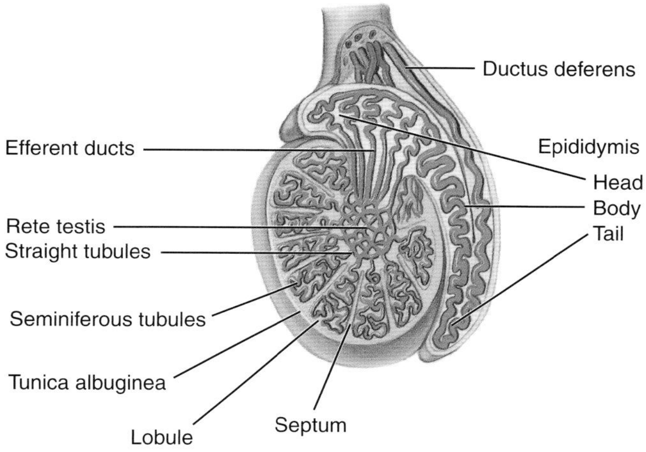

Fig. 53.2 Basic structures of a testis. (From Applegate EJ: *The anatomy and physiology learning system*, ed 4, St. Louis, 2011, Saunders.)

nutrients and hormones important for motility and successful fertilization (Fig. 53.3 and see Fig. 53.1).

PROSTATE GLAND

The prostate is a walnut-sized fibromuscular gland that surrounds the neck of the urinary bladder and the first inch of the internal urethra. The prostate produces a thin, milky, alkaline liquid that enhances the motility and fertility of the sperm and contracts to propel semen into the urethra during ejaculation (see Fig. 53.3).

COWPER GLANDS

Cowper glands (bulbourethral glands) are pea-sized structures, located just below the prostate, that secrete a clear mucus into the urethra. The secretion contributes little to semen volume but provides lubrication during sexual arousal.

URETHRA

The urethra extends from the bladder to the urinary meatus at the end of the penis. The vas deferens and the seminal vesicles come together to form the ejaculatory duct, which passes through the prostate and empties into the internal urethra. The sperm and fluids from the vasa deferentia, seminal vesicles, and prostate are propelled through the ejaculatory duct into the penile urethra during ejaculation. The urethra serves to empty urine from the bladder and provide outflow for semen during ejaculation. However, urine and semen are never in the urethra at the same time because the sphincter flap between the bladder and urethra closes during ejaculation.

PENIS

The external penis in its flaccid state is a soft, round cylinder of spongy tissue ending in an acorn-shaped tip known as the *glans*. The glans has a sensitive ridge at its base called the *corona* that gives rise to a hood or foreskin. In uncircumcised men, the foreskin can be rolled back to expose the glans. About one-half of the penis extends within the body toward the anus and attaches to the pelvis. Two corpora cavernosa lie on the upper side of the penis. These erectile chambers provide a huge surface area for the inflow of blood and blood storage, which results in expansion of the penis during sexual arousal, called an *erection*. The corpus spongiosum on the underside of the penis surrounds the urethra and supplies blood to the glans (Fig. 53.4).

PHYSIOLOGY OF THE MALE REPRODUCTIVE SYSTEM

SPERMATOGENESIS

Sperm are produced in the seminiferous tubules of the testes from about age 13 years throughout the

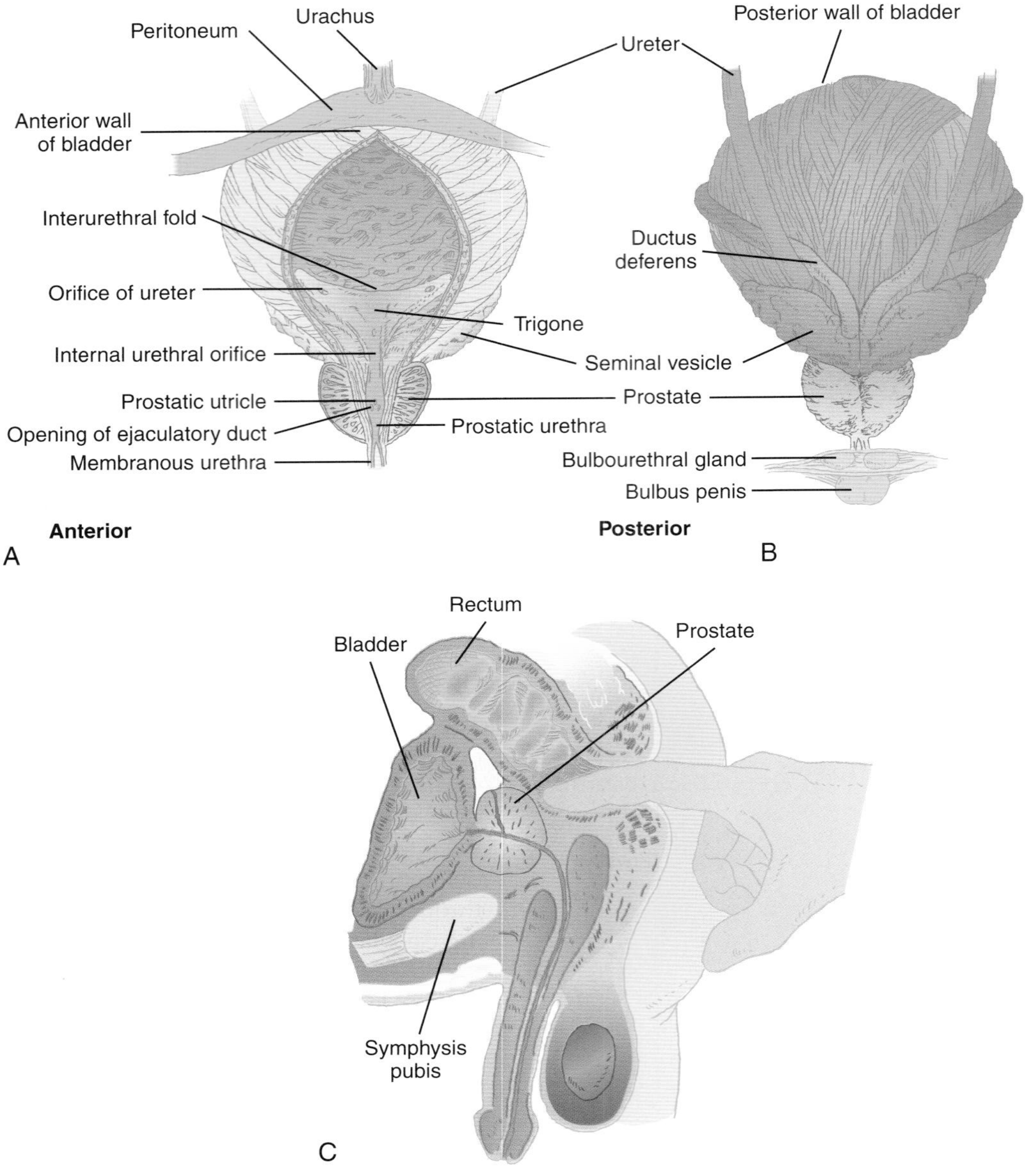

Fig. 53.3 (A and B) Anterior and posterior views of the prostate gland. (C) Diagrammatic representation of the anatomic position of the prostate gland. It surrounds the urethra at the base of the bladder. (From Black JM, Hawks JH, Keene AM: *Medical-surgical nursing: clinical management for continuity of care*, ed 6, Philadelphia, 2011, Saunders.)

remainder of life. Testosterone is believed to set in motion the division of germinal cells into spermatocytes, which subsequently develop into sperm. The process may take 75 days.

The cooling function of the scrotum is essential for spermatogenesis. An increase in testicular temperature may cause degeneration of some of the cells of the seminiferous tubules and may contribute to sterility.

Cryptorchidism, or failure of the testicles to descend from the abdomen into the cooler scrotum, may result in sterility. Incomplete or partial descent of the testicles may be resolved by surgical assistance before maturity but if fetal testes are abnormally formed and do not secrete enough testosterone to cause the testicles to descend into the scrotum, surgical intervention is unlikely to be successful. The tubular epithelium of testes that remains in the warm abdomen degenerates completely and is incapable of producing sperm.

ERECTION

For the penis to become erect, it must have a high-pressure supply of arterial blood, a means of relaxing the smooth muscle tissue of the cavernosal arterioles, and a functioning blood storage mechanism to keep the blood in the penis long enough for sexual function. The blood pressure (BP) in the flaccid corpus cavernosa is about 6 to 8 mm Hg—very low when compared with the 120/90 mm Hg BP in the arm or cavernosal artery.

During sexual arousal, parasympathetic nerves release neurotransmitters that cause the cavernosal arteriole walls to relax. This allows the relatively high-pressure arterial blood to flood the sinuses of the

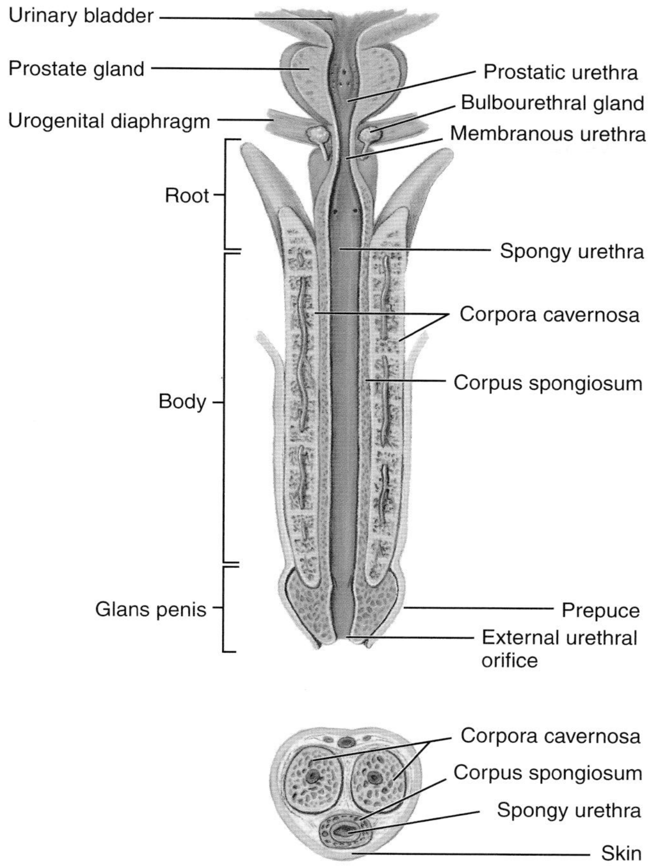

Fig. 53.4 Cross-section of the penis. (From Applegate EJ: *The anatomy and physiology learning system*, ed 2, Philadelphia, 2000, Saunders.)

erectile chambers, increasing the blood volume of the penis to 8 to 10 times the flaccid volume and raising the cavernosal BP to approximately the same as arterial BP.

The blood storage mechanism for the penis is unique. The cavernosal artery is buried deep in the erectile chambers, causing them to fill from the inside. The venules that drain blood from the erectile chambers are near the surface and are compressed against the outer coat of the chambers during engorgement. The elastic limitations of this covering severely decrease the drainage of blood from the chamber sinuses and maintain the erection. After stimulation ceases or ejaculation occurs, sympathetic nerves release constricting neurotransmitters that narrow the arteriole walls and decrease the inflow of blood. As the cavernosal pressure decreases, drainage increases and the penis returns to a flaccid state.

EMISSION AND EJACULATION

The male sex act culminates in emission and ejaculation. **Emission** is the result of sympathetic stimulation leaving the spinal cord at L1 and L2. The pudendal nerve communicates with the spinal cord at S2 and S3 and affects motor responses for ejaculation. Physical stimulation of internal and external sex organs initiates

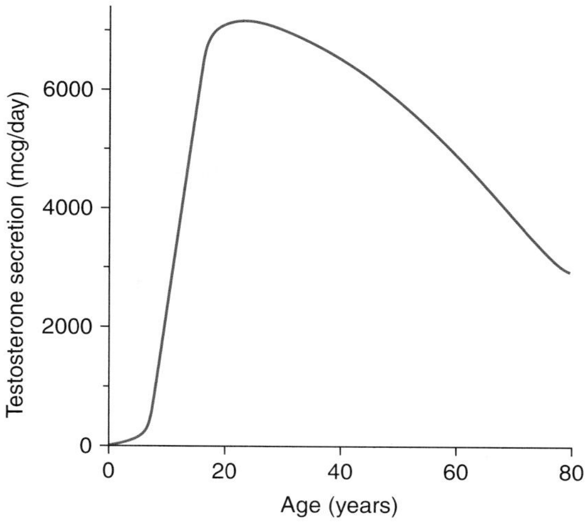

Fig. 53.5 Testosterone secretion by age. (From Guyton AC, Hall JE: *Textbook of medical physiology*, ed 9, Philadelphia, 1996, Saunders.)

contractions of the vasa deferentia and prostatic capsule. The contractions move sperm to the ejaculatory ducts and expel them into the internal urethra. There they mix with prostatic and seminal fluids and are propelled forward through the penile urethra. The filling of the urethra excites nerves in the sacral region of the spinal cord to initiate rhythmic muscular contractions of the internal genital organs, pelvis, and body trunk and results in **ejaculation** (expulsion) of semen.

Although psychic stimulation is not essential to the male sex act, it is an enhancing factor and should be considered in the physiology. Experience, culture, and self-development influence the effect of visual, fantasy, and dream stimulation on sexual sensation and nocturnal erections and emissions.

AGE-RELATED CHANGES IN THE MALE REPRODUCTIVE SYSTEM

As described in Chapter 10, normal aging produces several changes in the male reproductive system. These include:

- Rapid decrease in testosterone production after 50 years of age (Fig. 53.5).
- Male climacteric may be associated with hot flashes, feelings of suffocation, and psychic disorders similar to those of menopause.
- Changes in sexual response occur: slower arousal and longer can refractory period between erections.

In a healthy man, spermatogenesis and the ability to have erections last a lifetime.

◆ NURSING ASSESSMENT OF THE MALE REPRODUCTIVE SYSTEM

Assessment of the male reproductive system should include information on changes in the patient's health status, sexual function, and sexual relationships as well as the patient's knowledge level and ability for self-care. The extent of the nursing assessment of the male reproductive system depends on the nurse's education, experience, and role in the setting. This section describes a complete nursing assessment, although some aspects may be performed only by an examiner with advanced training. The licensed vocational nurse/licensed practical nurse (LVN/LPN) contributes data for the overall assessment.

The interview and physical assessment may be particularly difficult for some male patients because of health beliefs, the need for privacy, or defensiveness about behaviors. It is important to allow the patient to tell his own story and maintain as much control over the environment and experience as possible. Establishing a comfortable relationship with the patient is most successful if open-ended questions are used. The examiner should avoid questions beginning with "why?" and leave sensitive questions until later in the interview. Although it is helpful to empathize with the patient and gently press for important details, comments on how he should feel or behave are inappropriate. The assessor should not jump to conclusions too early or bias the patient's story by expressing a personal opinion.

Health History

Reason for seeking care and present health. The health history begins with a detailed description of the current problem. Complaints may include pain, weight loss, infertility, erectile dysfunction (impotence), alteration in self-image, scrotal masses, penile discharge, or skin lesions. If the symptoms are acute, include detailed information about the onset and development of the problem and about activities related to the symptoms. If the patient has pain, tools such as pain scales provide objective data.

Past health history. The medical history helps to link the current problem with previous symptoms, injuries, diseases, operations, or allergies and the treatments or medications prescribed for them. Question the patient about his management of chronic health problems such as diabetes, thyroid or pituitary dysfunction, cardiovascular disease, neurologic injury or disease, and addictive behavior. Because disorders of the urethra or penile circulation (or both) may be related to trauma to the groin or perineum, document childhood injuries or accidents. Spinal cord injuries are significant because the level of the injury is associated with specific types of sexual dysfunctions.

Patients who are reluctant to discuss what many consider to be the most private part of their lives may also be unwilling to do regular self-examinations or follow recommended self-care regimens. Thoughtfully planned questioning provides clues about knowledge deficits and patient participation in health management. This information is important in developing plans for care that include the patient and his significant other and require their cooperation.

Family history. In the family history, note the age and health or age at death of parents, grandparents, and siblings. In addition, record any family history of cancer, diabetes, hypertension, stroke, and blood disorders such as sickle cell anemia and hemophilia.

Review of systems. Review of all systems with a focus on male reproductive system disorders begins with an assessment of the patient's general health. Questions focus on changes in appetite, weight, exercise or activity level, and the management of daily self-care. These data may reveal general changes in health status that may affect the reproductive system.

Describe changes in the skin, including lesions, drainage, bleeding, itching, or pain. If the patient has itching or pain, note whether it is intermittent or continuous and whether it has any relationship to specific activities or time. Encourage the patient to use descriptive terms, such as *stinging* or *aching*. When assessing pain, having the patient describe the intensity on a scale from 1 to 10 is helpful.

A review of the circulatory and pulmonary systems provides data about hypertension, cardiac or pulmonary disease, and exercise tolerance.

Symptoms of possible endocrine dysfunction are important because undiagnosed or poorly managed endocrine disorders may have a direct and devastating effect on sexual function, sterility, and self-image for the male patient. Questions about fatigue, nervousness, heat or cold intolerance, polyphagia, polydipsia, polyuria, and medications taken for pituitary or thyroid conditions may yield important clues.

Review of the musculoskeletal and nervous systems should include questions about weakness, paralysis, coordination problems, joint pain or stiffness, mood changes, and depression.

The health history should note medications the patient is taking because many drugs, including a number of antihypertensive agents, can impair sexual function.

Functional assessment. The functional assessment elicits information about diet, usual activities, sleep and rest, medications, and the use of tobacco, alcohol, and illicit drugs. Record sources of stress and coping strategies. Once a therapeutic relationship is established, the patient's interest level and satisfaction of sexual relationships can be assessed. Questions may include the frequency of intercourse, the ability to have and maintain an erection, the desire and ability to have children, and the relationship of sexual function to self-image.

Physical Examination

The physical examination of the male reproductive system is usually done by the physician or nurse practitioner. Gloves are always worn to examine the genitals. The LVN/LPN may prepare the patient for the examination, collect some data, and see that specimens are processed properly. Instruct the patient to empty

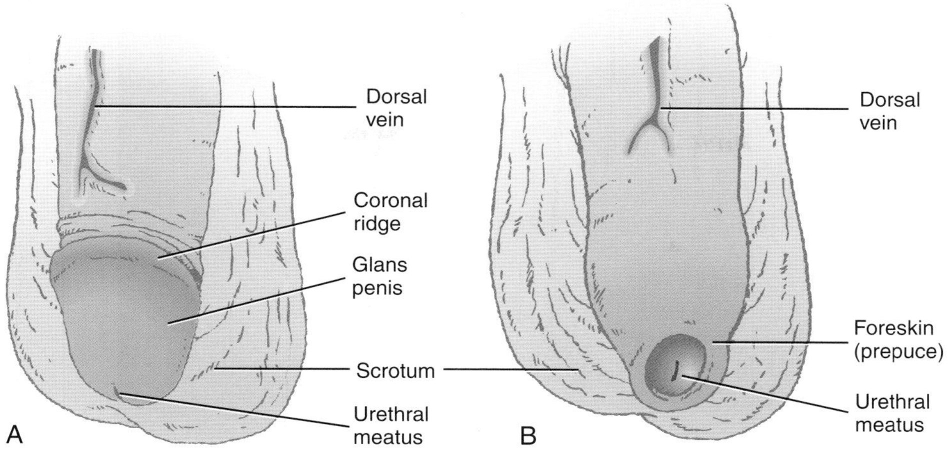

Fig. 53.6 Appearance of the penis. (A) Circumcised. (B) Uncircumcised. (From Black JM, Hawks JH, Keene AM: *Medical-surgical nursing: clinical management for continuity of care*, ed 6, Philadelphia, 2001, Saunders.)

the bladder before the examination and to collect a urine specimen if needed. The patient should be properly draped for privacy.

Record the patient's height, weight, and vital signs and note his general appearance. Inspect the skin for lesions or discolorations and the breasts for gynecomastia (enlargement). For the examination of the genitals, the patient may be standing or supine with the legs slightly spread. The skin of the external organs and perineum should be warm, dry, and free of lesions, edema, and odor. The pubic hair is normally distributed in a diamond-shaped area across the symphysis pubis, covering the base of the penis and spreading along the inner thighs. The lower abdomen and groin are palpated for masses.

Penis. The normal flaccid penis is semisoft and straight. The size, shape, and appearance are noted. The examiner palpates for nodules, swelling, and lesions. If the patient is uncircumcised, the foreskin is retracted to inspect the glans (Fig. 53.6). A small amount of white, thick, odoriferous smegma (sebaceous secretion) may be seen between the glans and the foreskin. The urethral meatus should be at the tip of the penis. If any discharge from lesions or the urethra is seen, a specimen may be collected for culture.

Scrotum. The skin of the scrotum should be slightly darker in color, wrinkled, and loose. Because the scrotum is close to the body and may not be well ventilated, it is susceptible to irritation from heat and moisture, fungal infections, abscesses, and parasites.

Each side of the scrotum should be palpated for the right and left testes, epididymis, and vasa deferentia. It is normal for the testes to retract temporarily when the scrotum is touched or cooled; they will reappear with relaxation or rewarming. The left testicle hangs lower than the right. Both should be oval in shape, smooth, firm, and without masses or tenderness. Older patients may have smaller, softer testes. It is important, especially in the young patient, to note that two testes exist.

The examiner proceeds to palpate the epididymis and the vas deferens. If scrotal thickening, nodules, masses, or asymmetric conditions are discovered, they can be further investigated by shining a light through the scrotum in a darkened room, a technique called *transillumination* (Fig. 53.7). **Hydrocele**, a mass filled with serous fluid, glows red in the light. If the mass is solid (e.g., a **hematocele** or tumor), no light passes through it, making it appear as a dark shadow.

The examiner inspects for hernias, which are protruding segments of the bowel through the abdominal wall. The most common sites for hernia are the lower abdomen, groin, and upper scrotal area. The examination is done first with the patient standing quietly and again when straining as if to have a bowel movement. The practitioner with advanced training is able to palpate inguinal hernias by reaching up through the scrotum into the inguinal canal. Abnormal findings should be noted and referred to a physician.

The advanced practitioner or physician also examines the prostate gland by inserting the examining finger through the anus toward the anterior wall of the rectum. Variations in the firmness and size of the prostate may be associated with benign hyperplasia, chronic prostatitis, or malignancy.

The skin of the perineum is darker than the skin on the buttocks and should be intact. The anal area has more coarse skin and is moist and without hair. Inspect the area for lesions, irritation, inflammation, fissures, abscesses, and dilated veins (hemorrhoids). With the patient bearing down, the examiner again inspects the anus for rectal prolapse or internal hemorrhoids. The advanced practitioner or physician examines the anal canal with an index finger to assess for resistance, bleeding, sphincter tone, nodules, or polyps. A stool specimen may be tested for occult blood when appropriate.

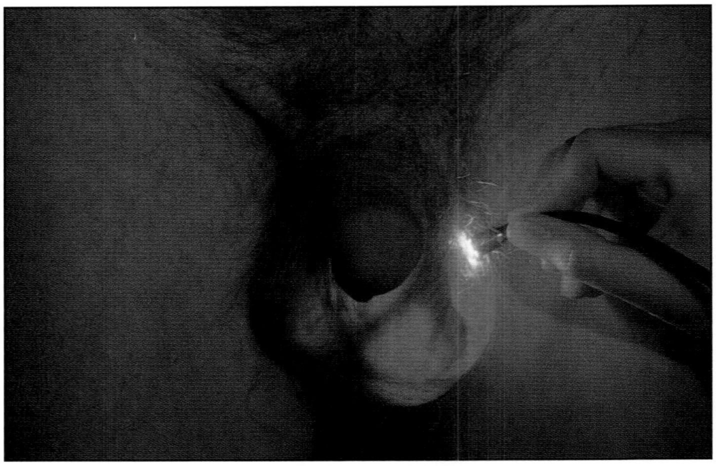

Fig. 53.7 Transillumination of the scrotum. (From Swartz MH: *Textbook of physical diagnosis*, ed 7, Philadelphia, 2014, Saunders.)

The assessment of the male reproductive system is summarized in Box 53.1.

DIAGNOSTIC TESTS AND PROCEDURES

Diagnostic tests and procedures for disorders of the male reproductive system include laboratory studies and radiologic imaging procedures.

Laboratory Studies

Semen analysis. Analysis of the semen may be done to assess male fertility or to document sterilization after a vasectomy. The analysis may include gross evaluation of semen for volume, thickness, color, and pH and microscopic evaluation of the sperm for count, motility, shape, and ability to penetrate cervical mucus. The patient is instructed to abstain from sexual activity for 2 to 3 days and then collect a semen specimen in a clean container. Discourage patients from prolonged abstinence because it may result in diminished quality and motility of the sperm. If the patient is unable to collect the specimen in the physician's office or laboratory by masturbating, it may be collected at home by using a plastic condom or coitus interruptus. Rubber condoms should not be used because the powders and lubricants used in their manufacture may be spermicidal. The specimen should be kept at room temperature, protected from heat or cold, and brought to the laboratory within 1 hour after collection.

Endocrinologic studies. The endocrine system secretes hormones that regulate metabolism, growth, stress response, and reproduction (gonadotropins) directly into the blood. The serum levels of these hormones can be determined from blood drawn from the patient without special preparation.

Testosterone is secreted by Leydig cells in the interstitium of the testes. Below-normal levels of testosterone may be the result of hypothalamic or pituitary dysfunction or seminiferous tubule destruction. Among the causes of increased levels of testosterone in the adult male are testicular tumor, adrenal tumor, adrenal dysfunction, and some drugs (anticonvulsants and barbiturates). Lower serum levels of testosterone may be related to gonad hypofunction, orchidectomy, hepatic cirrhosis, and some drugs (androgens, alcohol, phenothiazines, spironolactone, and corticosteroids). Testosterone levels fall with age, beginning around 30 years of age.

Follicle-stimulating hormone (FSH) is secreted by the anterior pituitary gland and causes stimulation of Sertoli cells in the testes to complete the formation and maturation of sperm. The negative-feedback system prevents oversecretion of FSH and maintains a constant level of sperm production. Below-normal levels of sperm result in increased secretion of FSH from the pituitary gland and high serum levels of FSH. Spermatogenesis results in decreased excretion of FSH and normal serum levels.

Luteinizing hormone (LH) is secreted by the anterior pituitary gland and causes stimulation of special cells (i.e., Leydig cells) in the testes to produce testosterone. As testosterone is produced, a negative-feedback system reduces the amount of LH secreted by the pituitary. Low levels of testosterone result in high levels of serum LH. This indicates an effort by the pituitary to stimulate Leydig cell function and return testosterone levels to normal.

Prolactin, another hormone secreted by the anterior pituitary gland, is closely related to LH. It has a potentiating effect on testosterone production. In some patients, when endocrine function is in question, serum prolactin levels may be tested. Secretion of prolactin is controlled by a negative-feedback system. Above-normal levels of prolactin may be caused by a benign pituitary tumor and may result in gynecomastia in the male patient.

Tumor markers. Tumor markers are substances found in the serum of cancer patients. When used in conjunction with other diagnostic tools, they can be helpful in diagnosing cancer, estimating the degree of cancer development, predicting the effect of

Box 53.1 Assessment of the Male Reproductive System

HEALTH HISTORY

Reason for Seeking Care and Present Health
Pain, weight loss, infertility, erectile dysfunction (ED), scrotal mass, penile discharge, lesions

Past Health History
Previous injuries, diseases, or surgeries
Chronic Illnesses: Diabetes mellitus (DM), cardiovascular disease, addictive behavior
Allergies
Current medications

FAMILY HISTORY
Diabetes, hypertension, stroke, blood disorders, cancer

Review of Systems
General Health State: Changes in appetite, weight, activity, self-care
Skin: Lesions, drainage, bleeding, itching, pain
Cardiovascular System: Edema
Respiratory System: Cough, dyspnea
Endocrine System: Fatigue, heat or cold intolerance, nervousness
Nervous System: Paralysis
Genitourinary System: Changes in urination or urine characteristics
Sexual Function: Interest in sexual relationship, frequency of intercourse, ED, desire to have children, effect of sexual function on self-image

Functional Assessment
Usual Day: Occupation, home roles and responsibilities, diet, rest
Use of tobacco and alcohol
Stressors and coping strategies
Sexual relationships

Physical Examination
Vital signs
General Appearance of Genitalia: Skin lesions or discoloration, hair distribution
Penis: Size, shape, skin lesions, discharge, position of urinary meatus, nodules, swelling
Scrotum: Color, edema, irritation, presence of testicles, testicular tenderness or masses
Inguinal hernia
Prostate: Size, texture, masses
Perineum: Color, lesions
Anus: Lesions, irritation, inflammation, fissures, abscesses, hemorrhoids, rectal prolapse

treatment, and monitoring the effect of treatment on the cancer or the return of cancer after treatment. The use of prostate-specific antigen (PSA) testing as a screening tool to detect prostate cancer is controversial. PSA may be elevated by many factors other than cancer. Also, some prostate cancers grow so slowly that they are unlikely to cause problems during the patient's lifetime. The treatment of prostate cancer can have serious side effects (e.g., urinary incontinence, sexual dysfunction) that affect quality of life. Therefore, the health care provider and the patient should explore the risks and benefits of testing to determine whether testing will be done. When screening results are elevated, experts recommend that two PSA confirmatory results should be done before any action is taken. A referral to a urologist is advised. Current American Cancer Society recommendations for PSA screening are listed in Box 53.2. No special preparation is needed for these tests. Scientists have developed a number of modified PSA tests and combination tests in hopes of finding one that is more specific to prostate cancer.

Box 53.2 American Cancer Society Recommendations for Early Detection of Prostate Cancer

- Men should be informed about the uncertainties, risks, and potential benefits of prostate cancer screening **before** deciding whether to be screened or not. The discussion about screening should take place:
  - At age 50 for men at average risk with a life expectance of at least 10 years
  - At age 45 for men at high risk: Black Americans, men with a first degree relative (brother or father) who was diagnosed with prostate cancer before age 65
  - At age 40 for men at even higher risk: those with more than one first-degree relative diagnosed with prostate cancer before age 65.

If screening results are normal, future screenings may be recommended based on the prostate-specific antigen (PSA) levels.

General laboratory studies. Urinalysis provides information about genitourinary tract infections as well as measures of kidney function. Clean-catch samples can usually be used unless the patient is unable to collect the urine without contamination. If appropriate instruction is given for collection, no other patient preparation is needed. If the patient is unable to clean himself properly, cannot see well enough, or is not able to understand the instructions, it may be necessary to obtain a specimen by catheterization.

Blood studies may include a complete blood count (CBC) to establish baseline data and provide information in forming a diagnosis when anemia or bone metastases are suspected. Alkaline phosphatase and serum calcium levels may also be measured because they increase with metastasis to bone (Table 53.1). Thyroid function studies and tests for diabetes mellitus (DM) may be done in patients with erectile dysfunction. No special preparation for these tests is usually necessary.

Radiologic Imaging Studies

Computed tomography (CT) may be used in assessing metastatic testicular and prostatic tumors. Ultrasound may be used to examine scrotal masses or define prostatic lesions. Examination of the prostate is done via the rectum. Magnetic resonance imaging (MRI) is used to stage prostate cancer.

Radionuclide imaging may be done to assess testicular abnormalities such as torsion, tumors, abscesses, epididymitis, or hydroceles. Radioactive substances are injected intravenously or given orally. After a waiting period to allow for distribution of the substance throughout the body, scans are done to locate organs and tissues that have increased concentrations of the isotopes because of abnormal tissue metabolism. Diagnostic tests and procedures and related nursing care are summarized in Table 53.2.

Ultrasound. Transrectal ultrasound is the most accurate method for obtaining anatomic details of the prostate. A biopsy specimen may be obtained, guided by the transrectal ultrasound image.

COMMON THERAPEUTIC MEASURES

Drug Therapy

Classes of drugs used to treat disorders of the male reproductive system include androgens, drugs used to treat benign prostatic hypertrophy (5-alpha reductase inhibitors, alpha-1 adrenergic antagonists), testosterone inhibitors, gonadotropin-releasing hormone agonists, agents used to treat erectile dysfunction, and miscellaneous others for various purposes. These drugs are included in Table 53.3 and discussed in Chapter 54 with conditions for which they are used.

Table 53.1 Laboratory Tests for Male Reproductive Disorders

TEST	REFERENCE VALUES	CONDITION IN WHICH LEVELS ARE ALTERED
Hematologic Tests (CBC)		
Hemoglobin (Hgb)	14–18 g/dL	↓ In anemia; nonspecific; may indicate malignancy
Hematocrit (Hct)	40%–50%	↓ In anemia; nonspecific; may indicate malignancy
Leukocytes (WBCs)	4800–11,000/mm^3	↓ In metastatic bone disease
Neutrophils	54%–62%	↓ In bone marrow depression
Lymphocytes	25%–30%	↓ In bone marrow depression
Eosinophils	1%–3%	↓ In bone marrow depression
Platelets	150,000–300,000/mm^3	↓ In bone marrow depression
Blood/Serum Tests		
Acid phosphatase	0.11–0.60 mU/mL	↑ In metastatic prostate cancer
Alkaline phosphatase	20–90 mU/mL	↑ In cancer of bone or bone metastases, liver cancer
Calcium	9.0–11.0 mg/dL	↑ In bone metastasis
Tests for Tumor Markers		
AFP	<10 ng/mL	↑ In nonseminomatous testicular cancer
CEA	0–2.5 ng/mL nonsmokers	↑ In prostate cancer
HCG	0.5 IU/L	↑ In germ cell testicular cancer
Prostatic acid phosphatase	0.26–0.83 U/L	↑ In metastatic prostate cancer
PSA	0–4 ng/mL	↑ In prostate cancer

AFP, Alpha-fetoprotein; *CBC*, complete blood count; *CEA*, carcinoembryonic antigen; *HCG*, human chorionic gonadotropin; *PSA*, prostate-specific antigen; *WBC*, white blood cell.

Table 53.2 Diagnostic Tests and Procedures: Male Reproductive System

TEST AND PURPOSE	PATIENT PREPARATION	POSTPROCEDURE NURSING CARE
General Nursing Actions: Confirm orders and check agency protocol. Tell patient any required preparation (i.e., fasting), what to expect before, during, and after procedure. When venipuncture is required, apply pressure and Band-Aid to site. If contrast media will be used, report iodine allergy to radiologist.		
Urethral Smears and Stains		
A small specimen is obtained for microscopic study to identify pathogens, including STIs.	The specimen should be obtained before voiding. Tell the patient a sterile swab will be inserted into the urethra to obtain a specimen. Have the patient lie down because the instrument may trigger a hypotensive episode with fainting. Specimens may also be obtained from the anal canal and pharynx. Collect the specimen for culture before beginning prescribed antimicrobials.	Assess for hypotension, bradycardia, and pallor before assisting the patient to rise. Use Standard Precautions to handle body fluids and contaminated instruments. Prepare specimens and send them to the laboratory.

Table 53.2 Diagnostic Tests and Procedures: Male Reproductive System—cont'd

TEST AND PURPOSE	PATIENT PREPARATION	POSTPROCEDURE NURSING CARE
Cultures of Organisms		
Permit identification of pathogens and susceptibility to various antimicrobials.	Explain the specimen collection process.	Prepare specimens according to laboratory protocol. Send them to the laboratory.
Semen Analysis		
Examines a semen specimen to assess male fertility or to document sterilization after vasectomy. In a fertility workup, repeated testing is advised because sperm count varies from day to day.	Instruct the patient to abstain from sexual activity and alcoholic beverages for 2–3 days; then collect the specimen in a clean container. Rubber condoms should not be used. The best specimen is obtained in the office or laboratory by masturbation. If the specimen is collected at home, it should be kept at room temperature and brought to the laboratory within 1 h. When the specimen will be used to evaluate the effects of vasectomy, the patient should ejaculate several times before the day on which the specimen is collected to clear the distal portion of the vas deferens.	No special care is needed.
Endocrinologic Studies		
Studies include measurement of LH, prolactin, FSH, and testosterone. Assess level of hormones needed for sexual development and function.	Tell the patient that a venous blood sample will be drawn.	Assess the venipuncture site for bleeding. Apply a small dressing.
Tumor Markers for Prostate Cancer		
Studies measure markers that change with prostate cancer. Elevated serum PSA may rise with prostate cancer, but also with prostatic hyperplasia, cirrhosis, osteoporosis and a number of other conditions. Modifications of the test (Percent free PSA, percent [-2] proPSA, et al.) are intended to be more specific to prostatic cancer.	Tell the patient a venous blood sample will be drawn. Fasting is not necessary.	Assess the venipuncture site for oozing or hematoma. Apply a small dressing. For some modified tests, the sample must be handled per specific laboratory guidelines.
Cystoscopy		
Uses a lighted instrument inserted through the urethra to visualize the urethra, bladder, and prostatic urethra. May detect prostatic hyperplasia and bladder tumors.	Routine preoperative measures are indicated (i.e., signed consent form, skin scrub, food restriction). Antibiotics may be prescribed. Inform the patient the procedure is done in a special room under sterile conditions. Local anesthetic is instilled in the urethra and a sedative is given intravenously.	Measure the patient's urine output for 24 h. Urine will be pink tinged. Report excessive bleeding or inability to void promptly. Encourage fluid intake when the patient is voiding well. Burning and hesitancy are common for several days. Give antibiotics as ordered.
Computed Tomography		
Creates images of internal structures to locate or assess testicular and prostatic tumors.	Assess allergy to iodine or previous contrast reactions if contrast dye will be injected. Report allergy to the radiologist. Tell the patient he will lie on a movable table while a machine moves around him. No sensations occur unless dye is injected. Some patients react to dye with nausea, vomiting, flushing, itching, or a bitter taste. Claustrophobic patients may need mild sedation.	No special postprocedure care is required. If dye is injected, the patient is encouraged to drink fluids to flush the dye from the body.

Continued

Table 53.2 Diagnostic Tests and Procedures: Male Reproductive System—cont'd

TEST AND PURPOSE	PATIENT PREPARATION	POSTPROCEDURE NURSING CARE
Ultrasonography		
Uses sound waves to create images of internal structures; used to study the prostate for enlargement or lesions.	Tell the patient an instrument will be inserted in the rectum to study the prostate. A full bladder is no longer required. Tell the patient the procedure is uncomfortable.	No special care is needed.
Radionuclide Imaging		
Uses radioactive substances injected intravenously or given orally followed by imaging to assess testicular abnormalities (i.e., torsion, tumors, abscesses, epididymitis, hydrocele).	Assess allergies to radioactive substance and inform the radiologist if allergic. Reassure the patient that the radiation dose is low and does not cause cell destruction.	Fluid intake is encouraged to promote elimination of the isotope.

FSH, Follicle-stimulating hormone; *LH*, luteinizing hormone; *PSA*, prostate-specific antigen; *STI*, sexually transmitted infection.
From Pagana KD, Pagana TJ: *Mosby's manual of diagnostic and laboratory tests*, ed 5, St. Louis, 2014, Mosby.)

Table 53.3 Drug Therapy: Disorders of the Male Reproductive System

DRUG	USE AND ACTION	SIDE EFFECTS	NURSING INTERVENTION
Androgens: Testosterone			
Testosterone is a schedule III controlled substance **Oral preparations:** methyltestosterone (Methitest, Testred), fluoxymesterone (Androxy) **Intramuscular preparations:** testosterone cypionate (Depo-Testosterone), testosterone enanthate (Delatestryl) **Transdermal patch:** Androderm **Transdermal gel:** AndroGel, Testim, Fortesta **Transdermal topical (underarm) solution:** Axiron **Implantable pellets:** Testopel **Buccal system:** Striant **Nasal gel:** Natesto	Treats hormone deficiency caused by developmental disorders, testicular diseases, or removal of testicles. Increases testosterone level. Treats symptoms of menopause in females. Treats anemias and catabolic states in males and females. The use of androgens to enhance athletic performance is *contraindicated!*	Risk of thrombosis resulting in stroke, myocardial infarction, and death. Retention of water, sodium, potassium, and chloride. Jaundice, GI distress. Virilization in females. Increased effects of anticoagulants and oral hypoglycemics. Androderm patches may irritate skin. Buccal tablets may irritate the mouth and gums. Gels and underarm solution can be transferred to others via intimate contact. Females and children should not have contact with these.	Assess for hypertension and edema. IM injections should be given deeply in the gluteus muscle using the Z-track technique. Androderm patches are applied to the arm, back, abdomen, or thigh; not to the scrotum. AndroGel and Testim can be applied to the upper arm and shoulder. AndroGel can also be applied to the abdomen; none should be applied to the scrotum. Axiron is applied to one or both armpits at same time each morning. Pellets are implanted subcutaneously. Follow directions on nasal gel applicator.
Drugs Used to Treat Benign Prostatic Hypertrophy/Hyperplasia (BPH)			
5-Alpha reductase inhibitors: finasteride (Proscar), dutasteride (Avodart)	Reduce prostate size, which decreases urethral obstruction. Effects not evident for several months.	Decreased ejaculate volume and libido. Decreases PSA, which must be considered in interpreting PSA screening results. Teratogenic for male fetus.	Females who are or might become pregnant should not handle medication with bare hands or be exposed to patient's semen. Tell patient that effects are not immediate.

Table 53.3 Drug Therapy: Disorders of the Male Reproductive System—cont'd

DRUG	USE AND ACTION	SIDE EFFECTS	NURSING INTERVENTION
Alpha-1 adrenergic antagonists (blockers): tamsulosin (Flomax), doxazosin (Cardura), terazosin (Hytrin), silodosin (Rapaflo), alfuzosin (Uroxatral), tadalafil (Cialis) Tamsulosin/dutasteride (Jalyn) is a combination of an alpha-1 antagonist and an alpha-reductase inhibitor.	Relaxes smooth muscle in bladder neck, prostate capsule, and prostatic urethra, which reduces urethral obstruction.	Doxazosin, terazosin, alfuzosin: lower BP, dizziness, sleepiness, rhinitis. Silodosin and tamsulosin: abnormal ejaculation. All: risk of complications of cataract surgery; possible floppy iris syndrome.	Therapy must be continued lifelong to maintain benefit. Best taken at bedtime. Monitor BP. Caution with other drugs that lower BP. Tell patient if changes in ejaculation may occur.
Testosterone Inhibitors (Androgen Receptor Blockers)			
flutamide (Eulexin) bicalutamide (Casodex) nilutamide (Nilandron)	Decreases testosterone level. Used with LHRH (later) to treat advanced prostate cancer.	Nausea, constipation, pain, weakness, hepatotoxicity, gynecomastia, ED, hot flashes, edema, hypertension, anxiety, confusion, mental depression. Nilutamide may cause interstitial pneumonitis.	Liver function must be monitored. Do not double up if a dose is missed. Be sure patient understands that drug must be taken with LHRH. Advise of effects on sexual function. Tell patient to report dyspnea, GI distress, pain in right side, dark urine, yellowish color of skin or sclera which may indicate liver toxicity.
abarelix (Plenaxis)	Suppresses testosterone production. Used for palliative therapy for advanced prostate cancer.	Risk of severe immediate allergic reactions with hypotension and fainting, hot flashes, sleep disturbances, gynecomastia, breast pain/nipple tenderness, pain, constipation, peripheral edema.	IM injection. Monitor BP for 30 min after injection.
Gonadotropin-Releasing Hormone Agonists (LHRH Analogs)/LHRHs			
leuprolide (Eligard, Lupron, Viadur) triptorelin (Trelstar Depot, Trelstar LA) goserelin (Zoladex), histrelin (Vantas)	Leuprolide desensitizes pituitary receptors for GnRH; testosterone release rises at first, then declines. Used for advanced prostate cancer. May be given with an androgen receptor blocker to reduce adverse effects.	Hot flashes, impotence, loss of libido, reduced muscle mass, increased adipose mass. May cause increased pain initially; usually resolves over time.	Leuprolide can be given daily (subcutaneously), monthly or quarterly (IM), or yearly (implant). Triptorelin given IM monthly or quarterly. Goserelin comes as a pellet that is injected into the upper abdominal wall with a 16-gauge needle; a local anesthetic may be given first.
CYP17 Inhibitor			
abiraterone	Inhibits androgen production to treat metastatic prostate cancer in selected patients.	Hepatotoxicity, hypokalemia, edema, joint pain, muscle discomfort, hot flashes, diarrhea, urinary tract infection, cough, hypertension; decreased libido, muscle mass, and bone mass.	Liver function should be monitored. Prednisone may reduce some adverse effects. Tell patient to take with water 1 h before or 2 h after meals. Presence of food greatly increases absorption.

Continued

Table 53.3 Drug Therapy: Disorders of the Male Reproductive System—cont'd

DRUG	USE AND ACTION	SIDE EFFECTS	NURSING INTERVENTION
Immunotherapy			
sipuleucel-T (Provenge)	Stimulates immune response against prostate cancer cells. Made from patient's immune cells. Improves survival in select patients with prostate cancer.	Chills, fatigue, fever, back pain, nausea, joint pain, headache, constipation, acute infusion reactions are common: fever, chills, nausea, vomiting, hypertension, tachycardia, respiratory distress.	Before each dose, macrophages must be collected from venous blood. Premedication with acetaminophen and an antihistamine may reduce infusion reaction.
Gonadotropin-Releasing Hormone Antagonist			
degarelix (Firmagon)	Palliative therapy for advanced prostate cancer. Suppresses testosterone production by the testes. Given subcutaneously; long half-life.	Pain at injection site, weight gain, hot flashes, reduced libido, erectile dysfunction, decreased bone and muscle mass, gynecomastia.	Inform patient of usual side/adverse effects. Monthly maintenance injections are required.
Agents Used to Treat Erectile Dysfunction			
PDE5 Inhibitors: (all oral) sildenafil (Viagra) vardenafil (Levitra) tadalafil (Cialis) avanafil (Stendra)	Relaxes smooth muscle in corpus cavernosum, which increases blood flow with subsequent erection. Tadalafil, which persists longer than the other preparations, is available for PRN or daily use.	Headache, dizziness, abnormal vision, diarrhea, dyspepsia, priapism, UTI, flushing, rash. Sudden death, cardiovascular collapse if taken with organic nitrate therapy. Numerous other contraindications including MAO inhibitors, severe hepatic or renal impairment, pregnancy or lactation (not recommended for women), history of coronary artery disease, CHF, dysrhythmias, or stroke. *Many interactions*; refer to a drug handbook when administering.	Do not take if taking organic nitrates (e.g., nitroglycerin) combination can be fatal. Drug is only effective with sexual stimulation. Patients over 65 years of age may be started on the lowest dose and increased if necessary. If on PRN tadalafil, instruct patient to take 1 h before sexual activity and not to take more than once daily.
Vasodilator + alpha-adrenergic antagonist (intracavernosal injection): papaverine plus phentolamine	Increases arterial blood flow to penis and decreases venous outflow. Produces erection within 10 min that lasts 2–4 h. Sometimes given in combination with alprostadil.	Priapism (erection lasting more than 6 h), painless fibrotic nodules at injection sites, orthostatic hypotension, transient numbness, bruising at injection site.	Injected directly into the corpus cavernosum. Advise patient to seek medical attention for priapism.
Prostaglandin E_1 alprostadil intracavernosal injection (Caverject) and intraurethral suppositories (MUSE)	Increases blood flow to penis.	Injection: priapism, fibrotic nodules. Suppository: urethral pain, inflammation.	Teach patient self-administration. Advise to seek treatment for persistent erection.
Other Drugs for Disorders of the Male Reproductive System			
estramustine (Emcyt) (a hybrid of estrogen and an alkylating agent)	Palliative therapy for advanced prostate cancer.	Gynecomastia, heart failure, thrombosis causing stroke or MI, fluid retention, nausea, vomiting, diarrhea, hypercalcemia.	Monitor for heart failure: dyspnea, edema, fatigue. Inform patient not to take with milk or other high-calcium food.

BP, Blood pressure; *CHF*, congestive heart failure; *ED*, erectile dysfunction; *GI*, gastrointestinal; *GnRH*, gonadotropin-releasing hormone; *IM*, intramuscular; *LHRH*, luteinizing hormone–releasing hormone; *MAO*, monoamine oxidase; *MI*, myocardial infarction; *PRN*, as needed; *PSA*, prostate-specific antigen; *UTI*, urinary tract infection.

Get Ready for the NCLEX® Examination!

Key Points

- The male reproductive system consists of the scrotum, testes, epididymis, vasa deferentia, seminal vesicles, prostate gland, ejaculatory duct, Cowper glands, internal urethra, and penis.
- Despite normal age-related changes in the reproductive systems, in a healthy male spermatogenesis and the ability to have erections may last a lifetime.
- Laboratory tests and imaging procedures are the primary diagnostic tools to evaluate the male reproductive system.
- Analysis of the semen may be done to assess male fertility or to document sterilization after a vasectomy.
- For semen analysis, the patient is instructed to abstain from sexual activity for 2 to 3 days and then collect a semen specimen in a clean container.
- PSA is used as a screening tool to detect prostate cancer; however, its use is controversial.
- PSA can be elevated by many factors other than cancer. Modified PSA tests are being designed that are more specific to prostate cancer.
- CT, MRI, ultrasound, and radionuclide imaging may be used to diagnose disorders of the male reproductive system.
- Classes of drugs used to treat disorders of the male reproductive system include androgens, drugs to treat benign prostatic hypertrophy (5-alpha reductase inhibitors, alpha-1 adrenergic antagonists), testosterone inhibitors, gonadotropin-releasing hormone agonists, agents used to treat erectile dysfunction, and miscellaneous others.

Additional Learning Resources

SG Go to your Study Guide for additional learning activities to help you master this chapter content.

Go to your Evolve website (http://evolve.elsevier.com/Linton/medsurg) for the following learning resources and much more:

- Fluid & Electrolyte Tutorial
- Review Questions for the NCLEX® Examination

Clinical Judgment and Next-Generation NCLEX® Examination-Style Questions

1. **The school nurse is teaching students about normal growth and development. The nurse should inform the students that the hormone responsible for male sexual development is:**
   1. LH
   2. Testosterone
   3. Gonadotropin
   4. Progesterone

   NCLEX Client Need: Health Promotion and Maintenance

2. **A health class for older adults should include which of the normal age-related changes in the reproductive system of a healthy man? (Select all that apply.)**
   1. Decreasing production of testosterone beginning at 50 years of age
   2. Longer refractory period between erections
   3. Loss of ability to maintain an erection by 70 years of age
   4. Increased time needed for sexual arousal
   5. Lack of interest in sexual activity

   NCLEX Client Need: Health Promotion and Maintenance

3. **The nurse is teaching a class on normal fetal development to pregnant women. Which statement is accurate regarding the expected descent of testes into the scrotum in males?**
   1. The testes should descend by puberty.
   2. The testes normally descend shortly after birth.
   3. The testes should descend by the third month of gestation.
   4. The testes usually descend within the last 2 months of gestation.

   NCLEX Client Need: Health Promotion and Maintenance

4. **A patient's health history includes the fact that he had cryptorchidism. The nurse understands that this refers to:**
   1. Erectile dysfunction
   2. Undescended testes
   3. A scrotal cyst
   4. Obstruction of the vas deferens

   NCLEX Client Need: Physiologic Integrity: Physiologic Adaptation

5. **Patients taking androgen receptor antagonists (blockers) such as bicalutamide (Casodex) should know that they may experience which drug effects?**
   1. Hot flashes
   2. Hypotension
   3. Agitation
   4. Headache

   NCLEX Client Need: Physiological Integrity: Pharmacological Therapies

6. **Students in the health class ask if there is a "male menopause"? What is the most appropriate response by the school nurse?**
   1. There is no physiologic basis for a "male menopause."
   2. Only men who have had a prostatectomy have symptoms of hormone deficiency.
   3. Testosterone production normally continues at the same level throughout life.
   4. The symptoms of the male "menopause," or climacteric, are similar to those of the female menopause.

   NCLEX Client Need: Health Promotion and Maintenance

7. **The clinic nurse is teaching a class on healthy aging. One of the participants asks if it is true that BP medications cause erectile dysfunction. What is the best response by the nurse?**
   1. Many BP medications can interfere with sexual function.
   2. Erectile dysfunction is an expected aging change, not a drug effect.
   3. It is dangerous for men with high BP to engage in sexual activity.
   4. BP medications have no effect on sexual function.

   NCLEX Client Need: Physiological Integrity: Pharmacological Therapies

8. **The nurse in the fertility clinic is instructing a patient in the collection of a semen specimen. The patient should be told:**
   1. Use a rubber condom to collect the specimen.
   2. Abstain from sexual activity for 2 to 3 days before collecting a specimen.
   3. Refrigerate the specimen until it can be delivered to the laboratory.
   4. Deliver the specimen to the laboratory within 24 hours of collection.

   NCLEX Client Need: Physiological Integrity: Reduction of Risk Potential

9. **A young man who is training for an athletic event asks if he could get testosterone to enhance his performance. What is the nurse's best response?**
   1. Supplementary hormones have no effect on physical abilities.
   2. Testosterone can be purchased in stores that sell fitness products.
   3. If taken under supervision, testosterone can be safe and effective.
   4. The use of male hormones to enhance athletic performance is NOT recommended.

   NCLEX Client Need: Physiological Integrity: Pharmacological Therapies

10. **Patients who take testosterone should know that the most serious adverse effect is:**
    1. Electrolyte imbalance
    2. Possible liver damage
    3. Gastrointestinal distress
    4. Thrombosis

    NCLEX Client Need: Physiological Integrity: Pharmacological Therapies

11. **SLO/Objective:** **Identify common classes of drugs used to treat disorders of the male reproductive system and the nursing implications of each.**

    NGN Item Type: Enhanced Hot Spot

    Cognitive Skill: Recognize Cues

    The nurse in a clinic for men with erectile dysfunction is doing an initial assessment of a 72-year-old patient. The patient requests a prescription for sildenafil (Viagra). The history data include:

- Prostate cancer treated with radiation 1 year ago
- Sexually active until prostate cancer treatment
- Difficulty achieving erection adequate for penetration
- sildenafil (Viagra) obtained from a friend was effective
- Hypertension managed with a calcium channel blocker
- Diagnosed with type 2 diabetes mellitus 3 years ago
- Takes nitroglycerin sublingual tablets occasionally for angina pectoris.

Highlight or place a check mark next to the assessment findings that require follow up by the nurse.

NCLEX Client Need: Physiological Integrity: Pharmacological Therapies

Male Reproductive Disorders

54

http://evolve.elsevier.com/Linton/medsurg

Objectives

1. For selected disorders of the male reproductive system, explain the pathophysiology, signs and symptoms, complications, medical diagnosis, and medical treatment.
2. Identify common therapeutic measures used to treat disorders of the male reproductive system and the nursing implications of each.
3. Assist in developing a nursing care plan for a male patient with a reproductive system disorder.

Key Terms

epididymitis (ĕp-ĭ-dĭd-ĕ-MĪ-tĭs)
erectile dysfunction (ĕ-RĔK-tīl dĭs-FŬNK-shŭn)
infertility
paraphimosis (păr-ă-phī-MŌ-sĭs)
phimosis (fī-MŌ-sĭs)
prostatectomy (prŏs-tă-TĔK-tō-mē)
prostatitis (prŏs-tă-TĪ-tĭs)
sterile

INFECTIONS AND INFLAMMATORY CONDITIONS

Infections of the male reproductive system may be caused by bacteria, viruses, protozoa, fungi, and ectoparasites that can be acquired through sexual contact. The most common inflammatory conditions are prostatitis and epididymitis. Orchitis is rare but important because it can cause sterility. Sexually transmitted infections (STIs) are discussed in Chapter 55.

PROSTATITIS

Prostatitis is inflammation of the prostate gland. The types of prostatitis are acute bacterial prostatitis (type I), chronic bacterial prostatitis (type II), chronic prostatitis/chronic pelvic pain syndrome (type III), and asymptomatic inflammatory prostatitis (type IV). Clinical manifestations may include pelvic, perineal, penile, or ejaculatory pain; voiding problems; and sexual dysfunction. With severe infections, fever and chills may be present. Diagnosis is based on the patient's reported symptoms, confirmed by laboratory studies including analysis of cultures from prostatic secretions and urine obtained before and after prostatic massage. Imaging studies using computed tomography (CT) or transrectal ultrasound may be done as well.

When inflammation is caused by bacterial infection, oral or intravenous antibiotics are required.

Prostatitis without infection is treated with adrenergic antagonists/alpha blockers, and antiinflammatory drugs. Alpha adrenergic antagonists improve voiding by relaxing the bladder neck and prostate. Symptoms may be managed with analgesics, muscle relaxants, and sitz baths. The patient is advised to rest, increase fluid intake, and avoid spicy foods, caffeine, and alcohol. For patients with voiding problems, stress reduction, relaxation, and pelvic floor muscle exercises may be helpful.

Stool softeners may be prescribed to prevent constipation, which is especially painful with prostatitis. Urethral catheterization is contraindicated with urethral inflammation, but suprapubic catheterization may be necessary if the patient has difficulty voiding. Prostate massage and ejaculation may be helpful with some types of prostatitis because they drain excess prostatic secretions.

Most patients with prostatitis are treated as outpatients, but hospital admission may be indicated if a high fever is present, the patient has urinary retention, or intravenous antibiotic therapy is needed. Ask the hospitalized patient about pain and administer analgesics and other treatments as ordered. If the patient is discharged with medications, provide instructions and information about the drugs. Features of each type of prostatitis are described in Table 54.1.

EPIDIDYMITIS

Epididymitis, inflammation of the epididymis, may be caused by infections, trauma, or the reflux of urine from the urethra through the vas deferens. Signs and symptoms are painful scrotal edema, nausea, vomiting, chills, and fever. Epididymitis is treated with bed rest, ice packs, sitz baths, analgesics, antibiotics,

Table 54.1 Prostatitis: Types, Manifestations, Treatments

TYPE AND CAUSE	MANIFESTATIONS	TREATMENTS
I. Acute prostatitis	Pelvic, penile, perineal, or ejaculatory pain. Fever and chills with severe infection	Oral or intravenous (IV) antibiotics
II. Chronic bacterial prostatitis	Some patients have no symptoms. Others have recurrent symptoms of urinary tract infection	Antibiotics: fluoroquinolones or trimethoprim-sulfamethoxazole. Usually 4–6 weeks of therapy
IIIA. Chronic prostatitis/pelvic pain syndrome, inflammatory	Chronic or recurrent urogenital symptoms *with* inflammation, but no bacterial infection	Adrenergic antagonists, alpha blockers, NSAIDs
IIIB. Chronic prostatitis/pelvic pain syndrome, noninflammatory	Chronic or recurrent urogenital symptoms *without* inflammation or bacterial infection	
IV. Asymptomatic inflammatory prostatitis	No symptoms. Inflammatory cells in prostate tissue or secretions	Alpha-adrenergic blocker

antiinflammatory drugs, and scrotal support. A bridge made of tape and gauze or a rolled towel can be placed across the patient's thighs while in bed to elevate the scrotum and reduce pain. If the condition is associated with an STI, the patient's sexual partner is treated with antibiotic therapy as well. Nursing care involves monitoring temperature, edema, and comfort. Carry out prescribed treatments and record their effects.

ORCHITIS

Orchitis is inflammation of one or both testes. It may be related to trauma or to infections such as mumps, pneumonia, or tuberculosis. Signs and symptoms of orchitis include fever, tenderness and swelling of the affected testicle, and scrotal redness. The inflammation can lead to reduced fertility, although sterility is uncommon. Orchitis is treated with analgesics, antipyretics, bed rest, scrotal support, and local heat to the scrotum. Nursing care includes pain management, assistance with activities of daily living (ADLs), patient teaching, and anxiety reduction.

BENIGN PROSTATIC HYPERPLASIA

Benign prostatic hyperplasia (BPH) is enlargement of the prostate gland. It is a common age-related change.

CLINICAL MANIFESTATIONS

Signs and symptoms of benign prostatic hyperplasia can be classified as *voiding*, *storage*, or *postmicturition*. Voiding symptoms include hesitancy, weak urinary stream, straining, and prolonged voiding. Frequency, urgency, nocturia, urge incontinence, and voiding small volumes are storage symptoms. Postmicturition symptoms are postvoid dribbling and incomplete emptying of the bladder. Patients typically have a combination of these symptoms. Symptoms may be triggered by bladder irritants as well as some drugs. Bladder irritants include alcohol, caffeine, and artificial sweeteners. Drugs that may aggravate the condition are diuretics, decongestants, and antihistamines.

MEDICAL DIAGNOSIS

A diagnosis of benign prostatic hyperplasia is based on reported symptoms and findings from a digital rectal examination, and a urinalysis. The patient may be asked to keep a voiding diary that documents fluid intake, voiding frequency, symptoms, and urine volumes. Additional studies that may be done to rule out other conditions that could cause the symptoms include cystoscopy, transrectal ultrasound, measurement of residual urine volume by ultrasound, and sometimes urodynamic testing and serum prostate specific antigen (PSA) (see Chapter 53).

MEDICAL TREATMENT

Conservative measures can decrease urinary symptoms. These include maintaining fluid intake of 1500 to 2000 mL/day, fluid restriction for 2 hours before bedtime, avoidance of caffeine and alcohol, and some bladder training exercises (see Chapter 14). Drugs that may be prescribed to treat benign prostatic hyperplasia and related symptoms include 5-alpha-reductase inhibitors, alpha$_1$-adrenergic receptor antagonists (alpha$_1$ blockers), and anticholinergics. 5-Alpha-reductase inhibitors suppress prostatic tissue growth by decreasing testosterone levels. Examples are finasteride (Proscar) and dutasteride (Duagen). Alpha$_1$ blockers such as tamsulosin (Flomax), doxazosin (Cardura), terazosin (Hytrin), silodosin (Rapaflo), and extended-release alfuzosin (Uroxatral) are used to relax smooth muscle in the bladder neck and prostate, thereby reducing obstruction to urinary flow. Anticholinergics include tolterodine (Detrol), solifenacin (VESIcare), and fesoterodine (Toviaz). Combinations of drugs are proving more effective than either type of drug alone (see the Complementary and Alternative Therapies box).

Complementary and Alternative Therapies

Saw palmetto is claimed to relieve urinary symptoms associated with benign prostatic hyperplasia. However, it is not recommended because well designed research has not found it to be effective.

Table 54.2 Treatment for Benign Prostatic Hyperplasia

DESCRIPTION	ADVANTAGES	DISADVANTAGES
Minimally Invasive		
Transurethral microwave thermotherapy (TUMT): use of microwave radiating heat to produce coagulative necrosis of the prostate	Outpatient procedure Erectile dysfunction, urinary incontinence, and retrograde ejaculation are rare	Potential for damage to surrounding tissue Urinary catheter needed after procedure
Transurethral needle ablation (TUNA): low-wave radiofrequency used to heat the prostate, causing necrosis	Outpatient procedure Erectile dysfunction, urinary incontinence, and retrograde ejaculation are rare Precise delivery of heat to desired area Very little pain experienced	Urinary retention common Irritative voiding symptoms Hematuria
Laser prostatectomy: procedure uses a laser beam to cut or destroy part of the prostate. Different techniques are available: Visual laser ablation of prostate (VLAP) Contact laser Photovaporization of prostate (PVP) Interstitial laser coagulation (ILC)	Short procedure Comparable results with TURP Minimal bleeding Fast recovery time Rapid symptom improvement Very effective	Catheter (up to 7 days) needed after procedure because of edema and urinary retention Delayed sloughing of tissue Take several weeks to reach optimal effect Retrograde ejaculation
Transurethral electrovaporization of prostate (TUVP): electrosurgical vaporization and desiccation are used together to destroy prostatic tissue	Minimal risks Minimal bleeding and sloughing	Retrograde ejaculation
Invasive (Surgery)		
Transurethral resection of prostate (TURP): use of excision and cauterization to remove prostate tissue via cystoscope. Remains the standard for treatment of benign prostatic hyperplasia (BPH)	Erectile dysfunction unlikely	Bleeding Retrograde ejaculation
Transurethral incision of the prostate (TUIP): involves transurethral incisions into prostatic tissue to relieve obstruction. Effective for men with small to moderate prostates	Outpatient procedure Minimal complications Low occurrence of erectile dysfunction or retrograde ejaculation	Urinary catheter needed after procedure
Open prostatectomy: surgery of choice for men with large prostates, bladder damage, or other complicating factors. Involves external incision with two possible approaches	Complete visualization of prostate and surrounding tissue	Erectile dysfunction Bleeding Postoperative pain Risk of infection

From Quallich SA. Male reproductive and genital problems. In: Lewis SL, Bucher L, Heitkemper MM, Harding MM, editors: *Medical-surgical nursing*, ed 10, St. Louis, MO; 2017, Elsevier, p. 1272.

SURGICAL AND INVASIVE TREATMENTS

Surgical or other invasive intervention is usually advised if complete urinary obstruction develops, if evidence of existing or impending renal damage exists, if the patient has repeated urinary tract infections (UTIs), or if significant bleeding occurs. In general, invasive procedures involve surgical removal of all or part of the prostate (**prostatectomy**) or ablation (destruction) of prostate tissue.

Types of Prostatectomy

A number of procedures to remove prostate tissue and relieve urethral obstruction are available. These are summarized in Table 54.2. Minimally invasive procedures are performed through the urethra and use various techniques to destroy prostate tissue. Some of the options are transurethral microwave thermotherapy (TUMT), transurethral needle ablation (TUNA), transurethral laser enucleation (HoLEP and ThuLEP), and photoselective vaporization of prostate tissue (PVP).

Although the trend is toward minimally invasive approaches, surgical intervention may be needed when the prostate is very large or complications such as bladder damage exist. The standard surgical procedure is the transurethral resection of the prostate (TURP). During a TURP, an instrument is inserted into the urethra and various techniques are used to destroy or remove portions of the enlarged prostate. No external incision is made. A standard or triple-lumen urinary catheter is commonly used to maintain continuous irrigation and bladder drainage. Continuous irrigation is intended to clear the bladder of blood and debris. If the catheter output is less than the irrigating fluid delivered, the catheter may be obstructed. Manual irrigation may be needed as ordered to clear the clots and restore drainage. If drainage cannot be restored, the physician should be notified immediately. Pressure in the bladder is one cause of painful bladder spasms. When only part of the gland is removed, the remaining tissue can continue to grow and obstruction may recur.

A simple prostatectomy is the removal of the prostate by way of an open incision, laparoscopic procedure, or robotic approach. It may be selected when the prostate is very large or when bladder abnormalities also exist that require surgical correction. Simple prostatectomy requires hospitalization and convalescence is longer than with a transurethral prostatectomy.

Complications

Depending on the type of prostatectomy, the patient is at risk for urinary infection and incontinence, hemorrhage, urinary leakage, inflammation of the pubic bone, and erectile dysfunction (ED). Retrograde ejaculation may occur, meaning that semen enters the bladder instead of being ejected through the urethra. The semen is then voided later with urine. This is not harmful to the patient but does render him **sterile** (infertile).

NURSING CARE OF THE PATIENT WITH BENIGN PROSTATIC HYPERPLASIA

Focused Assessment

The complete assessment of the male reproductive system is summarized in Chapter 53, Box 53.1. Data needed for assessment of the patient with benign prostatic hyperplasia include a complete description of urinary symptoms: frequency, urgency, hesitancy, a change in stream size or force, and nocturia. Record the presence of pain or hematuria and palpate the lower abdomen or use a Doppler to detect bladder distention. If ordered, residual urine volume is measured, preferably with ultrasound rather than catheterization.

Patient Problems, Goals, and Outcome Criteria: Benign Prostatic Hyperplasia

Patient Problems	Goals and Outcome Criteria
Urinary obstruction related to enlarged prostate	Normal bladder emptying: no distention on palpation, urine output approximately equal to fluid intake
Fear related to invasive diagnostic and therapeutic procedures	Reduced fear: patient states fear is reduced, appears calm
Ineffective self-care management related to lack of knowledge of BPH and treatment, limited resources	Patient understands condition and treatment and follows prescribed plan of care: patient correctly describes condition and treatment, demonstrates self-care

Interventions

Urinary obstruction. Instruct the patient to void promptly when the urge is felt and to space fluid intake throughout the day rather than consuming large amounts of liquids at one time. A daily total fluid intake of 1500 to 2000 mL is recommended. Fluid restriction is not recommended because it increases the risk of UTI. However, avoiding fluids for 2 hours before bedtime may reduce nighttime voiding. Scheduled voiding in which the patient voids every 90 to 120 minutes while awake may avoid urge incontinence. Another strategy is double voiding in which the person voids, waits several minutes, and voids again to empty the bladder.

The patient should notify the physician if unable to void and the bladder becomes distended. The patient may have to come into the clinic or emergency department for catheterization. It may be difficult to pass the catheter because of the enlarged prostate. If the catheter does not pass easily, it should not be forced. Forcing the catheter could damage the urethra. The physician should be notified. A urologist using special instruments may have to insert the catheter.

Pharmacology Capsule

Common nonprescription drugs, including many cold remedies, may cause urinary retention in the patient with prostatic hyperplasia.

Put On Your Thinking Cap!

Draw an illustration that you could use to teach a patient the effects of prostate enlargement.

Fear. Explore the patient's fears and provide information about anticipated procedures and effects.

Ineffective management self-care. Because this condition requires long-term management, the patient or a caregiver must understand how to manage the condition. Advise the patient that over-the-counter (OTC) drugs containing antihistamines or pseudoephedrine, which are commonly found in cold remedies, can aggravate urinary symptoms (see the Patient Teaching box). The patient should avoid caffeine and alcohol, which have a diuretic effect.

Patient Teaching

Prostatic Hyperplasia

- An enlarged prostate compresses the urethra, which interferes with passage of urine.
- To prevent urinary retention, drink fluids throughout the day.
- Avoid caffeine and alcohol.
- Consult your physician or pharmacist about nonprescription drugs. Common drugs such as antihistamines (e.g., cold remedies) can cause urinary retention.
- Report signs and symptoms of infection (i.e., burning on urination, foul urine odor, cloudy urine) and obstruction (i.e., feeling of bladder fullness, inability to empty bladder, lower abdominal pain).
- Take your medications as prescribed and notify your physician of any adverse effects. (Provide the patient with information about specific drugs.)
- Try scheduled voiding or double voiding to improve bladder emptying.

NURSING CARE OF THE PATIENT WITH A PROSTATECTOMY

Detailed care of the surgical patient is presented in Chapter 17. This section addresses the specific needs of the postoperative prostatectomy patient (see Nursing Care Plan: Patient With a Prostatectomy).

Focused Assessment

When the patient returns to the nursing unit, measure his vital signs and compare them with preoperative measurements. Inspect urine, dressings, and wound drainage for excess bleeding. Maintain accurate records of fluid intake and output to avoid overdistention

Nursing Care Plan Patient With a Prostatectomy

FOCUSED ASSESSMENT

Health History

The patient is a 77-year-old retired radio announcer who underwent a transurethral prostatectomy this morning. He returned to the nursing unit 3 hours ago. He complains of genital pain and states that he feels like he needs to empty his bladder. He appears tense and is clenching the side rails.

Physical Examination

Vital signs: blood pressure 132/70 mm Hg, pulse 84 beats per minute, respirations 18 breaths per minute, temperature 98°F (36.7°C) measured orally. Height 5′11″, weight 165 lb. Alert and oriented. Breath sounds clear on auscultation. Intravenous fluids infusing at 100 mL per hour. Three-way Foley catheter in place, taped to inner thigh and draining freely into collection bag. Irrigation fluid set at the prescribed flow rate. Urine pink, not viscous. Several clots observed in bag.

Patient Problems	Goals and Outcome Criteria	Interventions
Potential for fluid volume deficit related to blood loss	The patient will have balanced fluid intake and output without signs of hypovolemia (i.e., tachycardia, decreased urine output, hypotension, restlessness).	Monitor the patient's urine for excessive bleeding: thick, bright blood with clots. Assess for signs of hypovolemia. Ensure that traction is maintained on catheter by keeping tape in place until surgeon removes it. Maintain flow of irrigating fluid as ordered. If urine flow decreases or bladder distention is detected, irrigate the catheter manually as ordered. Turn off the irrigating fluid and inform the surgeon if unable to irrigate or urine output remains low.
Pain related to tissue trauma and bladder spasms	The patient will verbalize relief from pain and will appear more relaxed.	Check tubing to ensure that urine is draining freely. If not, reposition the tubing and irrigate it as ordered or per agency policy. Notify the surgeon immediately if unable to clear tubing. Administer analgesics and antispasmodics as ordered. Reposition the patient. Give back rubs. Use distraction. Assess the effects of pain-relief interventions.
Potential for infection related to invasive procedures of the urinary tract or catheterization	The patient will remain free of infection, as evidenced by normal body temperature, normal white blood cell (WBC) count, and absence of confusion or cloudy, foul urine.	Use strict aseptic techniques when handling the urinary drainage system. Keep closed system intact. Monitor temperature and urine characteristics. Report fever (>101°F), confusion, and cloudy or foul urine.
Potential for injury related to obstructed urine flow or trauma to urinary sphincter	The patient will have no injuries, as evidenced by continuous urine flow	Maintain flow of isotonic irrigating fluid as ordered. Monitor output and assess bladder for distention. Monitor vital signs. Administer stool softeners as ordered to prevent constipation. Encourage oral fluid intake when permitted.
Potential for altered sexual function (retrograde ejaculation) related to removal of prostate	The patient will correctly describe the physiologic effects of prostatectomy and potential for altered sexual function.	Be open to the patient's questions about the effects of surgery on sexual function. Reinforce preoperative teaching that erectile dysfunction is not common after transurethral prostate resection. Retrograde ejaculation may occur but is not harmful. Offer to include the sex partner in teaching. Be sensitive to possible feelings about loss of masculinity. The patient may demonstrate some anger or sadness related to a sense of loss.
Inability to manage self-care related to lack of knowledge of postoperative routines and self-care	The patient will demonstrate understanding of postoperative exercises and procedures. The patient will state changes that should be reported to the surgeon.	Support and encourage the patient to turn and deep breathe at least every 2 hours (q2h). Explain the catheter and the irrigation system. Tell him that some blood is normal the first few days after surgery. Encourage early ambulation as soon as permitted and explain the benefits of activity to recovery. Before discharge, advise the patient to restrict strenuous activity and heavy lifting (no more than 10–20 lb as specified by the physician) for 4–6 weeks. If he will go home with a catheter, discuss catheter care.

CRITICAL THINKING QUESTIONS

1. Describe the application of strict aseptic technique in the care of this patient.
2. Why might this surgery affect sexual function?

of the bladder; input and output should be balanced. Record the color of the urine and any clots present. Check intravenous fluids and regulate the rate of flow. Monitor the patient's level of comfort for incisional pain and bladder spasms.

Patient Problems, Goals, and Outcome Criteria: Prostatectomy

Patient Problems	Goals and Outcome Criteria
Potential fluid volume deficit related to blood loss	Normal fluid balance: balanced fluid intake and output, stable vital signs consistent with patient norms
Acute pain related to tissue trauma and bladder spasms	Pain relief: patient states pain is relieved, relaxed expression
Potential for infection related to invasive procedures of the urinary tract and surgical incision	Reduced risk of infection: freely flowing, clear urine
Potential for injury related to obstructed urine flow, excessive absorption of irrigating fluids, trauma to the urinary sphincter	Absence of complications because of obstruction, water intoxication, or sphincter injury
Urge incontinence related to poor urinary sphincter control, bladder contractions	Improved control of urine elimination: patient controls urine passage; has decreasing incidents of incontinence
Altered sexual function related to removal of prostate, retrograde ejaculation, possible neurologic injury	Management of sexual dysfunction: patient states he understands sexual dysfunction and identifies appropriate adaptations and resources
Low self-esteem related to anticipated alteration in sexual function	Improved self-esteem: patient makes positive statements about self
Inability to manage self-care related to lack of knowledge of postoperative needs	Patient understands routines and self-care: patient correctly describes limitations and demonstrates self-care activities

Interventions

Potential for fluid volume deficit. Restlessness and an increasing heart rate are early signs of fluid volume deficit. Blood in the urine is expected for several days after a prostatectomy; however, the drainage should be light pink within 24 hours. Bleeding with clots can signal hemorrhage and must be reported to the surgeon immediately. Bright-red blood may indicate arterial bleeding that requires surgical intervention. Dark blood may require pressure on the surgical area at the neck of the bladder. To apply pressure, the surgeon may inject additional fluid into the balloon that anchors the indwelling catheter. The catheter is then pulled so that the balloon fits tightly against the neck of the bladder and various forms of traction are used, including taping the catheter to the thigh. This traction may be maintained for several hours or more and then released by the surgeon.

Continuous bladder irrigation helps to prevent clot formation and subsequent obstruction that can cause bladder spasms and infection. Hang irrigating fluids (usually normal saline) and regulate flow at the prescribed rate.

Acute pain. Pain after prostatectomy may be associated with urinary obstruction, bladder spasms, and surgical trauma. If urine is not draining freely, reposition the tubing and irrigate according to agency policy or surgeon's orders. Antispasmodic agents such as oxybutynin chloride (Ditropan), belladonna and opium suppositories, or propantheline bromide (Pro-Banthine) are usually effective in relieving bladder spasms. Administer analgesics as ordered and assess effectiveness (see the Complementary and Alternative Therapies box).

Complementary and Alternative Therapies

In addition to analgesics, try nonpharmacologic interventions for postoperative pain such as repositioning, back rubs, and relaxation exercises.

Potential for infection. To reduce the risk of infection, use strict aseptic technique when handling urinary drainage, wound drains, and dressings. Keep closed urinary drainage systems intact to prevent the introduction of pathogens. Following an open prostatectomy, provide wound care in accordance with the physician's orders or the agency's policy. Monitor for signs of infection, including temperature above 101°F (38.3°C), purulent wound drainage, and confusion in older patients.

Potential for injury. Urinary obstruction and bladder distention can lead to renal complications (i.e., hydronephrosis), infection, and increased bleeding. Therefore it is critical to maintain urine flow. If urine flow ceases, assess the bladder for distention. If the bladder is distended, temporarily turn off the irrigating fluid and manually irrigate the bladder as ordered. If you cannot clear the tubing, notify the surgeon immediately. After the catheters are removed, you must continue to monitor output because edema or scarring may occur and obstruct the urethra.

Urge incontinence. Urinary incontinence or dribbling is common immediately after the catheter is removed. In most cases, control can be improved with perineal exercises. Instruct patients to contract and relax the perineal muscles 10 to 20 times each hour. If control does not improve, the surgeon may recommend biofeedback, a penile clamp, a condom catheter, or incontinence briefs. In severe cases, an artificial sphincter may be surgically implanted. Some patients never regain full control of urination. For additional information, see Chapter 14.

Altered sexual function and low self-esteem. Alterations in sexual function that may distress the patient include sterility, retrograde ejaculation, and ED. The patient should be encouraged to discuss these concerns with the surgeon before surgery. Potential complications of a planned procedure should be included in the Informed Consent document signed by the patient. ED is not common after surgical treatment of benign prostatic hyperplasia but if it does occur, the patient may need counseling, as described in **Erectile Dysfunction** section. No treatment for retrograde ejaculation exists but you can reassure the patient that it is not harmful. All of these alterations, along with urinary control problems, can threaten the patient's self-image and self-esteem. Be sensitive to the patient's feelings of loss and need to assert a masculine image. The patient may wish to include his sex partner in teaching and counseling sessions.

Inability to manage self-care. Teaching for postoperative care must begin in the preoperative period because patient hospitalizations are usually short, and the patient may be discharged with a catheter. Verbal instructions should be accompanied by written material (see the Patient Teaching box).

Patient Teaching

Postprostatectomy

- After a prostatectomy, semen may be ejaculated into the bladder (retrograde ejaculation). This is not harmful.
- Signs and symptoms of complications that should be reported include inability to pass urine, bladder distention, renewed bleeding, fever, and cloudy or foul-smelling urine.
- Practice perineal exercises as instructed to reduce the risk of incontinence.
- Walking is encouraged but avoid strenuous activity or heavy lifting until approved by the physician.
- Drink one and one half to two quarts of fluids each day.
- To prevent constipation and straining, which could cause bleeding, take stool softeners as prescribed and consume a high-fiber diet.
- Keep your urinary drainage system closed except when emptying it. Wash your hands before and after handling the system.
- Do not resume driving or sexual intercourse until directed by the surgeon (usually about 6 weeks).

PROSTATIC CANCER

Cancer of the prostate is found on postmortem examination in 30% of men over 50 years of age and the incidence increases steadily with each decade to 100% of men in the 10th decade. More than 248,000 new cases were expected to be diagnosed in the United States in 2021 and more than 34,000 deaths from prostate cancer were predicted in that year. Although the cause is unknown, the risk factors include age over 50 years, of African origin, family history of prostate cancer, and ingestion of a high-fat diet (see the Cultural Considerations box).

Cultural Considerations

What Does Culture Have to Do With Prostate Cancer?

The incidence of prostate cancer among Black American men is nearly twice that among White Americans. High-risk groups should be targeted for education about the importance of early evaluation of urinary symptoms.

EARLY DETECTION

Serum PSA increases with prostate cancer but also with a variety of other conditions. Whether PSA should be used as a screening tool is controversial. In 2018 the US Preventive Services Task Force (USPSTF) recommended that the decision to be screened for prostate cancer should be an individual one for men aged 55 to 69 years. This decision should be based on consultation with the health care provider and identification of the benefits and risks associated with screening. The USPSTF recommended that men aged 70 years and over not be screened. The Task Force indicated that elevated PSA often led to cancer treatment with serious complications for many men whose cancer never would have become life threatening. On the other hand, the American Cancer Society (ACS) recommends that by 50 years of age, all men discuss with their physician the pros and cons of periodic screening (PSA with or without rectal examination) so that they can make a decision that is right for them. The ACS recommends that Black American men and other men with increased risk for prostate cancer initiate this discussion by 40 to 45 years of age. Men at high risk are those with first-degree relatives (father, brother, son) who have had prostate cancer before the age of 65 years.

MEDICAL DIAGNOSIS

Prostatic lesions are typically slow growing and confined to the prostatic capsule. However, younger men tend to have very aggressive tumors. Prostatic tumors may go undetected until the disease is advanced and has metastasized to bone or liver. Large tumors may cause bladder outlet obstruction, rectal pressure, stool changes, painful defecation, or painful ejaculation. Because early diagnosis may improve treatment results, methods to permit early detection may be advised.

The diagnosis may be based on rectal examination, transrectal ultrasound, PSA level, and needle aspiration and biopsy. If a diagnosis of prostate cancer is made, additional procedures may be done to identify the stage of the disease. These may include radiographs, radionuclide imaging, bone scans, excretory urography, transurethral ultrasound, CT, and MRI.

MEDICAL TREATMENT

The treatment of prostate cancer is controversial because of the difficulty in staging tumors and the unpredictable biologic behavior of the disease. Treatment options include "watchful waiting," radiotherapy, brachytherapy, cryosurgery, and radical surgery. Chemotherapy is useful in limited cases. Often, combinations of treatments are used. Sometimes "watchful waiting" is recommended for patients with a life expectancy of less than 10 years who have small cancers or who are not good surgical risks. The patient is monitored frequently and treatment is initiated if the tumor begins to enlarge.

Radical prostatectomy includes removal of the prostate gland, the outer capsule, the seminal vesicles, sections of the vas deferens, and sometimes a portion of the bladder neck. Most operations include removal of the pelvic lymph nodes to check for metastasis. The surgical approach is usually perineal or retropubic. The latter approach permits an autonomic nerve-sparing technique, which may preserve erectile function. The urinary incontinence that occurs in 10% to 15% of men who undergo radical prostatectomy subsides within 6 months in 85% to 90% of those affected. Minimally invasive radical prostatectomy using a laparoscope and robot-assisted technology is available in some settings. It is believed that less invasive techniques will result in less blood loss and less postoperative pain.

Radiation alone is often effective when the cancer is confined to the prostate. Radiation can be delivered by external beam or by implanting seeds (brachytherapy) of radioactive gold, iodine, or iridium in the prostate through hollow needles inserted under anesthesia. External beam radiation requires only a few minutes, 5 days a week for 6 to 8 weeks. Side effects include skin dryness and irritation; diarrhea, cramping, and gastrointestinal (GI) bleeding; sexual dysfunction; fatigue; bone marrow suppression; and various urinary symptoms such as dysuria, frequency, hesitancy, urgency, and nocturia. The radioactive seeds affect surrounding tissues less than external beam radiation. Patients often have some urinary symptoms of irritation or obstruction after the seeds are implanted. Newer radiation options include three-dimensional conformal radiation therapy or intensity-modulated radiation therapy. The new procedures deliver higher doses to the target tissue with less toxicity.

Prostate cancer growth is influenced by hormones. Therefore androgen deprivation therapy (ADT) is used to eliminate the effects of androgens by interfering with androgen production or blocking receptors for the androgens. Testosterone reduction can also be achieved by removing the testicles. Many men elect drug therapy over the surgical option. Types of drugs used in ADT include luteinizing hormone–releasing hormone (LHRH) agonists and androgen receptor blockers. LHRH analogs include leuprolide (Lupron), goserelin acetate (Zoladex), histrelin (Vantas), and triptorelin (Trelstar). These agents inhibit the release of pituitary hormones necessary for testosterone production. They are given intramuscularly or subcutaneously. One form is available in pellets that are implanted subcutaneously and deliver medication for 1 year. With initial therapy, patients may experience bone pain, which resolves over time. Drugs that inhibit the action of testosterone include flutamide (Eulexin), bicalutamide (Casodex), and nilutamide (Nilandron). They may be used in combination with LHRH agonists (see Chapter 53, Table 53.3).

The adverse effects of all of these agents can include hot flashes and ED. When these agents are no longer effective, other drugs may be used that reduce testosterone production in the adrenals. Examples are spironolactone (Aldactone), aminoglutethimide (Cytadren), and glucocorticoids. Hormonal therapy is usually effective for a limited period of time, generally 1 to 3 years. Bone pain and fractures are complications of prostate cancer. Bisphosphonates such as alendronate (Fosamax) may be ordered to help relieve bone symptoms. PSA is a useful tool for the follow-up of patients who have undergone treatment. Persistent or rising PSA levels indicate advancing or recurrent tumor growth.

NURSING CARE OF THE PATIENT WITH PROSTATIC CANCER

Details of the assessment of the male reproductive system are summarized in Chapter 53, Box 53.1. Nursing care of male patients should include encouragement to discuss whether to have periodic screenings for prostate cancer with the health care provider. If the patient has undergone surgery, nursing care is similar to that described in the section titled "Nursing Care of the Patient With Benign Prostatic Hyperplasia." Nursing care of the patient with cancer is discussed in Chapter 7, and the care of patients having urologic surgery is discussed in Chapters 41 and 42. Specific problems that may require special interventions after prostate surgery are bladder spasms, ED, urinary incontinence, and body image disturbances associated with changes in the reproductive system. Newer techniques have reduced the risk of urinary incontinence and ED.

ERECTILE DYSFUNCTION

Erectile dysfunction (ED), which is the inability to produce and maintain an erection for sexual intercourse,

Table 54.3 Factors Related to Erectile Dysfunction

FACTOR	DESCRIPTION	TREATMENTS
Psychologic factors	Depression, fear, grief, anxiety, interpersonal problems with partner	Psychotherapy, marital therapy, group therapy, sex therapy.
Medical conditions	Cardiovascular disease, diabetes mellitus (DM), stroke, osteoarthritis, Parkinson disease, back pain, chronic obstructive pulmonary disease (COPD)	Management of underlying condition. Erectile dysfunction (ED) drug therapy, vacuum therapy, penile implant. Adaptation of sexual practices to accommodate disabilities.
Medical and surgical interventions	Medication side effects Pelvic radiation Perineal surgery, ostomy, mastectomy	Alternative drug therapy. Counseling. ED drug therapy, vacuum therapy, penile implant. Adaptation of sexual practices to accommodate disabilities.
Lifestyle	Tobacco use Excessive alcohol intake Lack of physical conditioning Obesity	Minimize or cease use of tobacco and alcohol. Regular exercise. Weight control.

can be devastating for a man and his partner. An adequate erection requires intact neurologic function, sufficient inflow of blood to fill the corpus cavernosa, and a leak-proof storage mechanism for maintaining the erection. Factors that contribute to ED and related treatments are summarized in Table 54.3.

CONTRIBUTING FACTORS

A number of vascular, endocrine, neurologic, and psychologic factors may cause or contribute to ED.

Vascular Disorders

Systemic or local changes in blood flow can impair the ability to achieve an erection. Generalized atherosclerosis may be a factor in inadequate filling of the corpus cavernosa. Many modifiable factors contribute to the development of atherosclerosis. These include high cholesterol levels, smoking, excessive alcohol consumption, illicit drug use, and inadequate exercise. The cavernosal artery in the perineum between the scrotum and the anus may be damaged by physical injury to the pelvis, falls on the crossbar of a bicycle, horseback riding, or other blows. Significant damage to the artery limits the inflow of blood to the corpus cavernosa.

Endocrine Disorders

Endocrine disorders that affect sexual function include diabetes mellitus (DM) and low testosterone. Patients with DM are at risk for ED because of atherosclerosis and autonomic neuropathy. Autonomic neuropathy is the dysfunction of some aspect of the autonomic nervous system, which is essential to normal sexual response.

Men who have diabetes, regardless of type of treatment, are at very high risk of developing ED, making diabetes the most common cause of ED. Diabetes is believed to interfere with blood supply to the penis when arterial walls lose flexibility, or distensibility, as a result of hardening of the arteries (atherosclerosis). Atherosclerosis may be accelerated by diabetes.

Autonomic neuropathy in patients with diabetes affects the ability of nerves to relax the smooth muscle surrounding the tiny sinuses (lacunar spaces) of the erectile chambers. Without relaxed muscle tone and expansion of the sinuses, adequate filling with blood for an erection may not be possible.

Factors that are associated with increased risk of ED in men with DM include neuropathy, retinopathy, long duration of DM, and poor glycemic control. Although the primary cause of ED related to DM is physiologic, the psychologic reaction to the problem is an important factor. Cognitive behavioral therapy may be used to teach the patient to manage negative thinking.

Vascular surgery to clear blocked arteries is not usually recommended for people with diabetes because they often have complicating problems with nerves, cells, erectile tissue, and blood vessels throughout the penis.

A penile implant (Fig. 54.1) may be recommended for a patient with failure to initiate (nerve damage) or failure to fill (artery damage), which are related to diabetes. As many as one-third of penile implant patients have diabetes.

Phosphodiesterase type 5 (PDE5) inhibitors such as sildenafil (Viagra), tadalafil (Cialis), vardenafil (Levitra), and avanafil (Stendra) are oral drugs that may be effective. They all may be taken 20 to 60 minutes before intercourse; tadalafil may also be taken on a daily basis rather than "on demand." Papaverine plus phentolamine self-injection is indicated as a second-line treatment for failure to initiate or fill. Alprostadil (prostaglandin E_1) is available in an injectable form and as a pellet that is inserted into the urethra. Patients need training in self-injection and must have hand dexterity and adequate vision.

Neurologic Disorders

Spinal cord injuries and other neurologic disorders may cause ED. If communication between the spinal

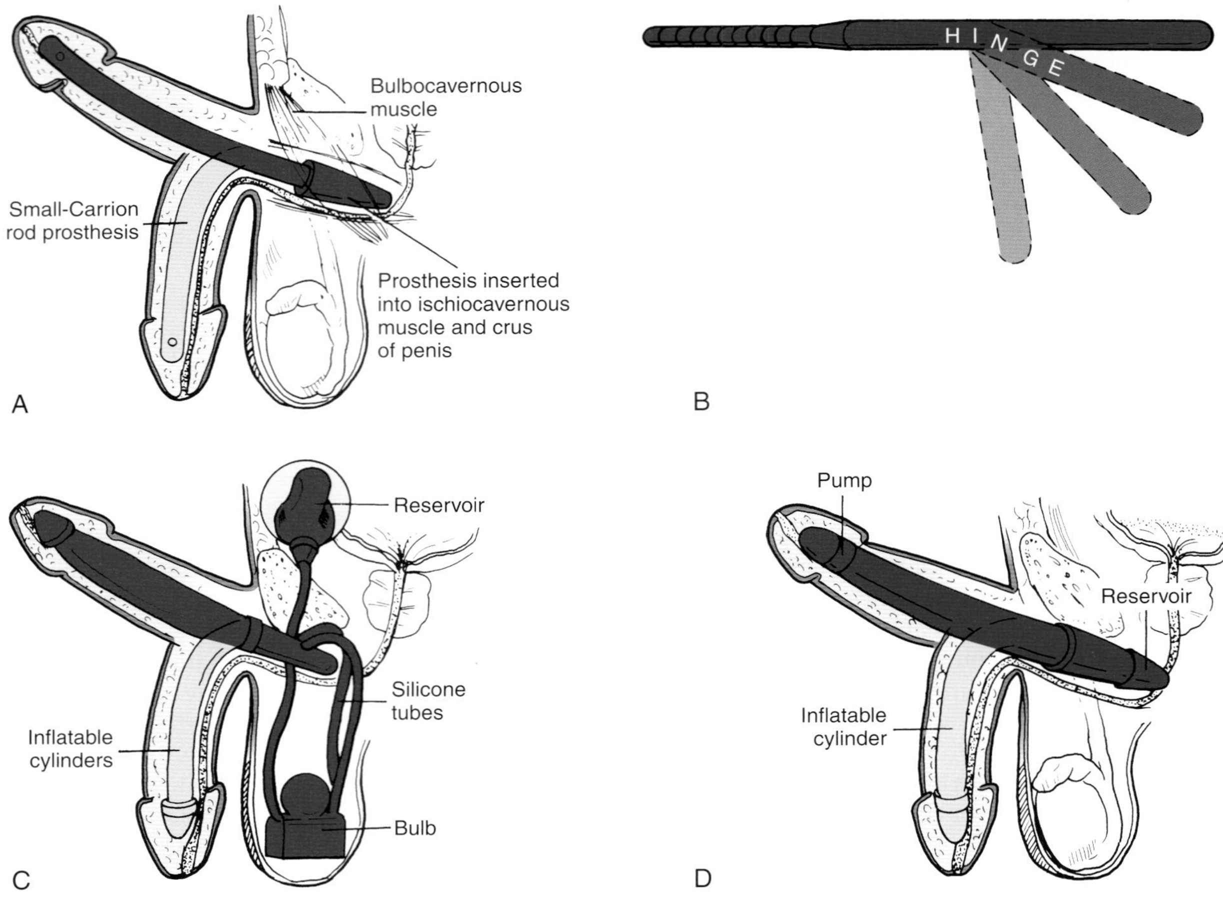

Fig. 54.1 Penile prostheses. (A) Small-Carrion prosthesis. (B) Flexi-rod semirigid implant. (C) Inflatable prosthesis. (D) Self-contained prosthesis. (From Black JM, Matassarin-Jacobs E: Luckmann and Sorenson's medical-surgical nursing: clinical management for continuity of care, ed 5, Philadelphia, 1997, Saunders.)

cord and the penis remains intact, the penis becomes erect with direct stimulation. For the penis to remain erect, smooth muscle relaxation is necessary and, in some way, relies on communication between the brain and the spinal cord. The more complete the injury and the lower the injury, the more likely it is that erection will be affected, even though higher injuries tend to cause more paralysis and loss of sensation. In addition to spinal cord injuries, perineal and rectal surgery can damage nerves involved in erectile function.

Treatment of ED related to spinal cord injuries or neurologic disorders such as multiple sclerosis (MS) may include phosphodiesterase type 5 inhibitors, papaverine, or alprostadil; vacuum constriction devices; or penile implants.

Medication Side Effects

Medications used to treat a variety of conditions may cause or contribute to ED. Drugs used to reduce high blood pressure (BP) (antihypertensive agents) are the most likely to interfere with erection. If systemic hypertension is accompanied by blockages and stiffening in the arterial walls of the penis, antihypertensives that lower the BP in all arteries of the body may reduce the BP in penile arteries to the extent that failure to fill occurs. Digoxin, which is used to treat heart conditions, may increase levels of estrogen and decrease levels of testosterone; medications for stomach ulcers, such as cimetidine; and anticancer drugs may decrease libido; and anticholinergics and antihistamines may block neurotransmitters that cause relaxation of smooth muscle (see the Complementary and Alternative Therapies box).

Complementary and Alternative Therapies

National Center for Complementary and Integrative Health (last updated April 2019). Erectile Dysfunction/Sexual Enhancement. Retrieved May 29, 2021 from: ncchi.nih.gov/health/erectile-dysfunctionsexual-enhancement

Treatment for ED related to these drugs' side effects may include changes in drugs or dosage, but such changes can be made only on a physician's order (see the Complementary and Alternative Therapies box). Counseling or sex therapy, vacuum constriction devices, drug therapy, or penile implants may be appropriate for these patients.

Complementary and Alternative Therapies

Nonprescription products marketed to enhance sexual performance have been found to be tainted with drug ingredients or related substances, sometimes with excessive high doses or combinations of multiple ingredients.

Pharmacology Capsule

Antihypertensive drugs are among those most likely to interfere with erection.

Psychologic Factors

The psychologic aspects of ED are extremely important and should be included in the medical history. Psychogenic ED is often the result of anxiety about performance. Problems may arise with aging, sexual beliefs, or behavior; communication patterns or relationships with sex partners; changes in lifestyle; changes in medications; or chronic or poorly managed disease processes. Anxiety may cause constriction of smooth muscle tissue in the penis and its arteries, reducing inflow and increasing outflow of blood from the penis, leaving it flaccid. Sex therapy that includes behavior modification techniques may be able to restore potency.

MEDICAL TREATMENT

Drug Therapy

Phosphodiesterase type 5 inhibitors. Examples are sildenafil (Viagra), tadalafil (Cialis), vardenafil (Levitra), and avanafil (Stendra). These oral vasodilators may be prescribed for failure to fill or store. They must be prescribed with care in patients with cardiovascular disease because of the risk of myocardial infarction and sudden death. Research has suggested that cardiac events are not caused by PDE5 inhibitors, but by the underlying cardiovascular pathology. They are contraindicated for patients taking nitrate vasodilators or alpha-adrenergic antagonists because of the risk of hypotension and cardiovascular collapse.

Alprostadil. Alprostadil can be used for intracavernosal injection (Caverject) or urethral suppositories (MUSE). It has been successful for some men. It is a vasodilator but produces a more localized effect on arteriole filling and improved storage. Urethral pain and urethritis are possible complications.

Papaverine. Self-injection of intracavernosal papaverine may be recommended for failure to initiate, fill, or store or for psychogenic causes. Papaverine is injected with a small needle into the erectile chambers, with relatively little pain. Erection is achieved within 10 to 15 minutes and lasts 30 to 60 minutes. Papaverine acts on smooth muscles to relax arterial walls and erectile tissue, increasing blood flow into the penis. Papaverine is often mixed with phentolamine, which blocks the constriction of erectile tissue, making it possible to sustain the erection.

Testosterone. Testosterone replacement for men with low hormone levels may improve libido but is unlikely to improve ED (see Chapter 53, Table 53.3).

Pharmacology Capsule

PDE5 inhibitors are absolutely contraindicated in men taking any nitrates such as nitroglycerin for angina pectoris. The combination can cause life-threatening hypotension.

Psychotherapy

When psychological factors cause or contribute to ED, the condition is described as psychogenic. ED is often associated with depression which may respond well to treatment for depression. The patient should be referred to a certified sex therapist. Psychotherapy may reveal other issues that need to be addressed.

Vacuum Constriction Devices

Vacuum constriction devices may be prescribed for failure to initiate, fill, or store or for psychogenic causes. The flaccid penis is slipped into a cylinder and then the patient squeezes a pump that removes all of the air from the space in the cylinder around the penis, creating a vacuum that draws blood into the penis. When the erection has been achieved, a rubber ring is slipped off the bottom of the cylinder onto the penis near the base, trapping the blood safely for up to about 30 minutes. When air is again allowed into the cylinder, the cylinder can be removed.

Revascularization

Revascularization is a surgical procedure that bypasses blocked arteries, removes or ties off incompetent veins, and tightens the surrounding tissue. This procedure is not commonly done. Few men qualify for it, and the long-term success rate is 50% to 65%. Factors associated with failure of penile revascularization include smoking, diabetes mellitus, hypertension, hyperlipidemia, history of radiation therapy, coronary artery disease, alcohol abuse, obesity, cavernosal fibrosis, and distal arterial disease.

Penile Implants

Penile implants (see Fig. 54.1) may be prescribed for patients with failure to initiate or failure to fill or store and for some patients with psychogenic problems that are not appropriate for or responsive to counseling or sex therapy. Semirigid implants are silicon cylinders placed in the erection chambers that keep the penis firm at all times but without increasing circumference. Rigid models can be bent downward but still may not be easily concealed under clothing. Hydraulic implants have cylinders that can be inflated by squeezing a pump in the scrotum or at the end of the penis behind the glans. The pumping action causes the cylinders to fill with fluid from a reservoir in the abdomen or the scrotum. These implants more closely replicate the natural states of flaccidity and erection.

NURSING CARE OF THE PATIENT WITH ERECTILE DYSFUNCTION

Focused Assessment

The nursing assessment of a man with ED includes a health history that elicits information about the frequency of intercourse and satisfaction with sexual relations (see the Cultural Considerations box). The licensed vocational nurse/licensed practical nurse (LVN/LPN) may collect data that contribute to the complete assessment. The interviewer should not assume that sexual activity is no longer important to older adults. ED may be the first sign of DM, so a complete exploration of the patient's general health and family history to look for diabetes is important. Surgical procedures, injuries, illness, cancer, and medications used regularly should be recorded. The patient's habits and lifestyle, including daily activities, diet, use of alcohol and illicit drugs, exercise habits, lifestyle, health care beliefs, interpersonal relationships, capability for self-care, age, physical condition, and educational needs, should be explored.

Cultural Considerations

What Does Culture Have to Do With Erectile Dysfunction?

Beliefs and values related to sexual function, as well as acceptable forms of sexual expression, are largely learned in one's culture. If a cultural belief is that older adults lose interest in sex as their abilities decline, older adults may try to act accordingly. That is, they may accept erectile dysfunction as "normal" and not seek treatment.

Patient Problems, Goals, and Outcome Criteria: Erectile Dysfunction

Patient Problems	Goals and Outcome Criteria
Impaired sexual function related to erectile dysfunction	Improved sexual function or satisfying alternatives to sexual intercourse: patient states function has improved or he is satisfied with alternatives
Low self-esteem related to impaired sexual function	Improved self-esteem: patient makes more positive comments about self
Ineffective management self-care related to lack of knowledge of factors contributing to erectile dysfunction and measures to improve sexual function or related to reluctance to seek help	Patient understands factors contributing to erectile dysfunction and uses measures to improve sexual function: patient states management is satisfactory

Interventions

The management of ED requires sensitivity and knowledge. When a therapeutic relationship has been established with the patient, he may choose to share his concerns with you. Listen and be careful not to dismiss the issue as unimportant. Provide factual information and resources. If you are not well informed about ED, you should refer patients to the physician, advanced practice nurse, or a counselor with training in this area.

PEYRONIE DISEASE

Peyronie disease is the development of a hard, nonelastic, fibrous tissue (plaque) just under the skin on the dorsal surface of the penis. The plaque develops spontaneously or as a result of an injury. It interferes with the ability to fill during an erection. The plaque is usually located on the dorsal midline surface of the penis and results in an upward bending of the penis during erection that may be painful and interfere with successful vaginal penetration (Fig. 54.2). In a small percentage of patients, the condition resolves spontaneously. More likely, it will remain stable or progress. The choice of treatment for Peyronie disease depends on the size of the plaque and the curvature and resultant degree of dysfunction. A variety of drugs (e.g., collagenase *Clostridium histolytica*) have been used with varying degrees of success. Radiation therapy may reduce pain and penile curvature; however, it may also compromise erectile function, especially in the aging male. Surgical correction involves excision of the plaque with procedures that address the individual's pathology.

PRIAPISM

Priapism is a prolonged penile erection unrelated to sexual stimulation or desire. It is classified as ischemic or nonischemic. Nonischemic priapism is usually related to trauma and resolves spontaneously. Ischemic

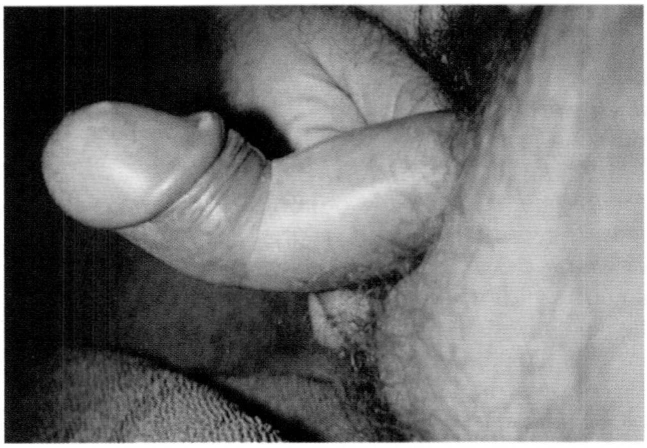

Fig. 54.2 Peyronie disease. (Courtesy Dr. Hans Stricker, Department of Urology, Henry Ford Hospital, Detroit, MI.)

priapism is very painful. It is a medical emergency because it may lead to ischemia of the penis, gangrene, fibrosis, and ED if not treated promptly. Urine flow may be obstructed, causing hydronephrosis. Priapism is associated with many factors, including sickle cell crisis, injury to the penis, leukemia, and malignant tumors. Drugs that may be responsible include cocaine, phosphodiesterase type 5 inhibitors (sildenafil, vardenafil, tadalafil, avanafil), and papaverine plus phentolamine intracavernosal injections.

Immediate removal of blood may be accomplished by aspirating blood from the erectile chambers or by injecting drugs that cause contraction of smooth muscle (e.g., phenylephrine), inhibiting inflow of blood and allowing outflow. If these efforts fail, emergency surgery may be needed.

Nursing care must be particularly sensitive to the embarrassment the patient may experience. Understanding the condition and alleviating pain are important.

PHIMOSIS AND PARAPHIMOSIS

Normally the penile foreskin in the uncircumcised male can be retracted, exposing the glans. Uncircumcised men need to retract the foreskin for cleaning as part of daily hygiene. As a result of poor hygiene, the foreskin may become inflamed and swollen, preventing retraction of the foreskin. This condition, called **phimosis**, is treated with proper cleansing using saline baths twice a day. Drug therapy may include antimicrobial agents, antifungal agents, and/or topical steroids. Circumcision is sometimes recommended to prevent recurrences. **Paraphimosis** is just the opposite in that the foreskin is retracted and cannot be moved over the glans. Constriction of the penis causes the glans to swell. If the foreskin cannot be reduced to cover the glans, prompt surgical intervention is necessary.

INFERTILITY

Infertile is a term used to describe couples who have had unprotected intercourse over a 12-month period and have been unable to become pregnant. **Infertility** may be caused by a reproductive problem in the man, the woman, or both.

CAUSE AND RISK FACTORS

Male infertility may be related to endocrine disorders, testicular problems, or abnormalities of the ejaculatory system. Correction of endocrine disorders may restore fertility. Infections can affect testicular and ejaculatory function. Structural factors that can affect testicular function are cryptorchidism, testicular torsion, and varicocele (dilation of the veins that drain the testes). Drug therapy, radiation, substance abuse, and environmental hazards can also affect the testes. In addition to infection, the ejaculatory mechanism can be disrupted by obstruction and some surgical procedures.

Infections

Destruction of the seminiferous tubular epithelium results in failure or reduced ability to produce sperm. Mumps may result in acute orchitis and epididymitis, accompanied by fever and debilitating pain, bilateral swelling, and redness of the testicles. If damage to seminiferous epithelium occurs, the size of the testes will be reduced. Other infections such as tuberculosis, pneumonia, and syphilis may affect the testes but less dramatically than mumps.

Genitourinary tract infections can cause infertility in men. *Chlamydia trachomatis* is sexually transmitted and is most prevalent in young adults with multiple sex partners. The infection is most commonly limited to the urethra and causes varying degrees of painful urination and discharge. Progressive infection may include the epididymis and prostate gland. *Neisseria gonorrhoeae* is a common urethral infection in the United States. It is sexually transmitted and may cause extremely painful urination and a purulent discharge. Infections that ascend to the epididymis may result in decreased fertility.

Cryptorchidism

Cryptorchidism is defined as any testis located in other than a dependent scrotal position. It is a common congenital condition, being found in approximately 30% of preterm male infants and in 1.0% to 3.4% of full-term male infants (Fig. 54.3). Although genetic disorders can cause cryptorchidism, the cause is usually

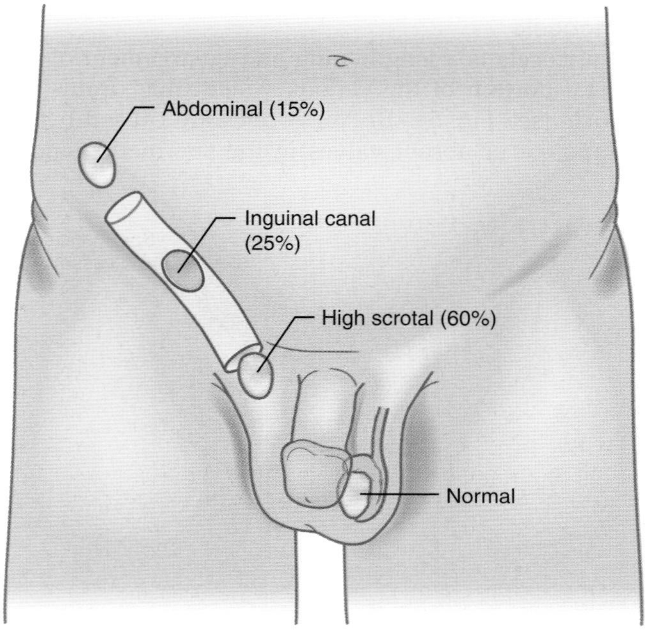

Fig. 54.3 Common sites of undescended or mispositioned testicles. (From Proctor D, Niedzwiecki B, Pepper J, et al: *Kinn's the medical assistant: an applied learning approach*, ed 13, St Louis, 2017, Elsevier.)

unknown. Because the abdominal cavity is warmer than the scrotum, excessive warmth can damage the seminiferous epithelium of undescended testes and result in decreased spermatogenesis.

Medical treatment. Cryptorchidism must be corrected within the first 18 months of life to give the best chance for fertility. Men with undescended testes have a 10 to 30 times higher incidence of testicular cancer than men whose testes descended normally. The risk remains higher even if the condition is subsequently corrected. If the testes are within the normal path but do not descend or cannot be pulled into the scrotum, they usually do not respond to hormonal therapy, and surgery is needed. Whether medical or surgical therapy is indicated, it is performed after the first birthday and before the second birthday. Untreated bilateral cryptorchidism results in sterility. Unilateral cryptorchidism may result in a low sperm count but spermatogenesis continues and pregnancies are sometimes initiated without difficulty.

Testicular Torsion

Testicular torsion occurs when the spermatic cord twists, cutting off the blood supply to a testicle (Fig. 54.4A). It most commonly occurs in adolescents. Symptoms are intense pain, often accompanied by nausea and vomiting. If it does not resolve spontaneously, emergency surgery is required to untwist the cord and restore blood flow. If the testicle is deprived of blood for more than 4 hours, it may become necrotic and require removal. After testicular torsion is corrected, lowered sperm counts and infertility may follow.

Varicocele

A varicocele is a lengthening and enlargement of the scrotal portion of the venous system that drains the testicle (see Fig. 54.4B). Varicoceles are caused by incompetent or absent valves in the spermatic venous system, which allows pooled blood and the resulting increased pressure to dilate the veins. Most often, only the left testicle is affected. Affected testicles may be smaller and may have reduced spermatogenesis. Varicoceles are a factor in about half of male infertility cases. Treatment includes surgical ligation or injection of a sclerosing agent into the dilated vein. Varicoceles may reappear after surgery and fertility may or may not improve.

Put On Your Thinking Cap!

A couple visits the clinic seeking help for infertility. During the initial interview, one of them says, "My brother and his wife couldn't get pregnant either. Then he switched from briefs to boxer shorts. Within a few months, his wife was pregnant! Do you think his underwear could have had anything to do with that?" How would you reply appropriately and accurately?

Vasectomy

Vasectomy is the surgical removal or tying of a portion of the vasa deferentia for sterilization purposes (Fig. 54.5). Erection, ejaculation, and intercourse are unaffected. Vasectomy is usually performed as an outpatient procedure in a physician's office or outpatient clinic. Postoperative pain or swelling can be managed with application of an ice bag, mild analgesics, and scrotal support. The patient can resume intercourse as soon as he feels comfortable, but it is important that he uses other methods of birth control until analysis of the semen determines that a complete absence of sperm exists. The patient can expect the analysis to be done after about 15 ejaculations postvasectomy.

The physician should explain the procedure, but the nurse can tell the patient what to expect and reinforce postoperative self-care. Although a vasectomy can sometimes be successfully reversed, it should be considered permanent. The reversal procedure

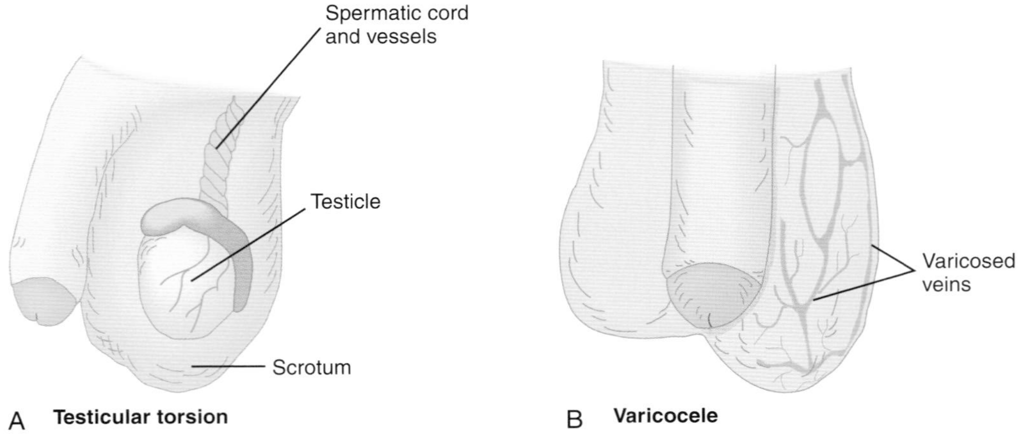

Fig. 54.4 Disorders of the testes. (A) Torsion of the testis. (B) Varicocele. (From Black JM, Hawks JH: *Medical-surgical nursing: clinical management for positive outcomes*, ed 8, St. Louis, 2009, Saunders.)

in which the severed ends of the vas deferens are anastomosed (surgically joined) is called a *vasovasectomy.* The nurse should be sensitive to the readiness of the male patient to undergo this procedure. Fears related to postoperative loss of sexual function may cause anxiety in some men, even though they desire the procedure. Acceptance and reassurance are important.

PENILE CANCER

Cancer is a frightening diagnosis for any patient. Cancer of the male reproductive system may arouse the worst fears about sexual dysfunction, disfigurement, and diminished self-esteem. Penile cancer is relatively rare in the United States. Risk factors include not being circumcised in early life (especially if phimosis is present), infection with some types of human papillomavirus (HPV) or human immunodeficiency virus (HIV), and smoking. Cancer may appear as a shallow ulcer or dry, painless growth on the penis that is easily confused with a wart. It can be removed surgically if treated in early stages. Growths in advanced stages may ulcerate and involve the foreskin and penile shaft. Extensive resection or amputation as well as resection of nearby lymph nodes may be necessary. Radiotherapy or chemotherapy may be used for advanced cases.

TESTICULAR CANCER

Testicular germ cell carcinoma occurs most often in young men between the ages of 15 and 35 years. Among the risk factors for this type of cancer are cryptorchidism, a genetic abnormality, HIV infection, and acquired immunodeficiency syndrome (AIDS) (see the Cultural Considerations box). A painless palpable mass or enlargement of one testis is the most common symptom of testicular cancer. A feeling of heaviness and pain in the testicle occurs as the tumor grows (Fig. 54.6). The diagnosis is often delayed because patients do not seek medical help.

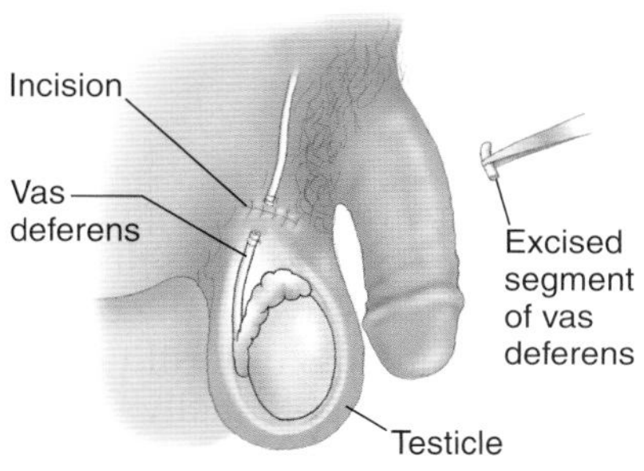

Fig. 54.5 Vasectomy. The vas deferens is located and exposed. Then a small segment of vas deferens is removed and severed ends are tied. Finally, the scrotal wound is closed. (From Leonard PC: *Building a medical vocabulary with Spanish translations*, ed 10, St. Louis, 2018, Elsevier.)

Cultural Considerations

What Does Culture Have to Do With Testicular Cancer?

Young White males are at highest risk for testicular cancer. Therefore education in testicular self-examination should target these individuals.

EARLY DETECTION

Self-examination and early diagnosis offer the highest chance of finding early-stage disease and subsequent cure. Therefore men need to be educated about the need for self-examination. Self-examination includes monthly examination of the penis, scrotum, and perineal area. The individual should use a mirror to visualize areas that he cannot see and look for any changes from normal such as swelling, lumps, tenderness, lesions, asymmetry, discoloration, or discharge. The examination is best done after a warm bath or shower, when he is warm and the scrotum is relaxed. The scrotum is held in the palm of his hands with the index and middle fingers on the underside of the testicle and the thumb on top (Fig. 54.7). Each testicle is palpated between the thumbs and forefingers of both hands, with the testicle rolled gently between the fingers. The left testicle is usually lower than the right. The testicles are egg shaped and should feel firm but not hard and smooth without lumps. The epididymis, located on the top and posterior side of each testicle, feels soft and spongy. The spermatic cords are smooth, firm, tubular structures that run upward from the testicles on the back side.

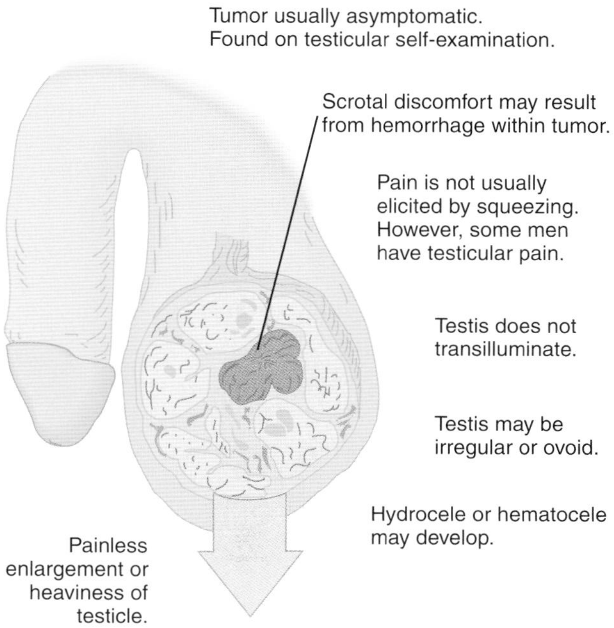

Fig. 54.6 Characteristics of testicular tumors. (From Black JM, Hawks JH, Keene AM: *Medical-surgical nursing: clinical management for continuity of care*, ed 6, Philadelphia, 2001, Saunders.)

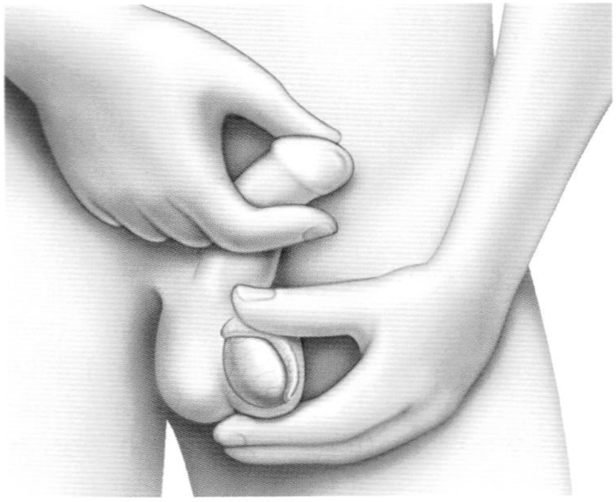

Fig. 54.7 Testicular self-examination. (From Harkreader H, Hogan, MA, Thobaben M: *Fundamentals of nursing: caring and clinical judgment*, ed 3, St. Louis, 2007, Saunders.)

MEDICAL DIAGNOSIS

Diagnostic procedures include ultrasound and blood studies to measure tumor markers: alpha-fetoprotein and human chorionic gonadotropin. If the diagnosis is in doubt, surgical exploration is done. Radiographs, CT scans, and bone scans may be done to assess for metastasis.

MEDICAL AND SURGICAL TREATMENT

Treatment for testicular cancer is designed according to the type of cancer and the stage. Treatment options are active surveillance, orchiectomy (i.e., surgical excision of the testis), retroperitoneal lymph node dissection, radical orchiectomy, radiation, and chemotherapy. If treated in stage 1, orchiectomy alone is curative for most patients. If desired, a testicular prosthesis may be placed at the time of orchiectomy or later. Follow-up includes monitoring tumor marker levels and abdominal and chest scans for a period of 5 years from diagnosis. Treatment of testicular cancer may affect fertility and erections. The physician will inform the patient of the option of banking sperm before treatment begins.

❖ NURSING CARE OF THE PATIENT WITH TESTICULAR CANCER

Nursing care of the surgical patient is discussed in Chapter 17 and care of the patient who has cancer is discussed in Chapter 7. Therefore this discussion is limited to nursing care specific to the patient with testicular cancer.

Focused Assessment

The nursing assessment of the male reproductive system is outlined in Chapter 53, Box 53.1. When a patient has testicular cancer, fears or concerns related to the effects of surgery and other treatment must be assessed.

Patient Problems, Goals, and Outcome Criteria: Testicular Cancer, Postoperative

Patient Problems	Goals and Outcome Criteria
Anxiety related to the diagnosis of cancer and the anticipation of side effects of treatments	Reduced anxiety: patient states anxiety is reduced, calm manner
Acute pain related to surgical incision	Pain relief: patient states pain is relieved, relaxed manner
Impaired urinary elimination related to the effects of anesthesia and abdominal or pelvic surgery	Normal urine elimination: no bladder distention
Potential for injury (shock, infection, fluid and electrolyte imbalances) related to surgery	Absence of excess bleeding or infection and normal fluid balance: vital signs consistent with patient norms, oral temperature less than 101°F (38.3°C), electrolytes within normal ranges and fluid output approximately equal to fluid intake
Constipation related to diminished or absent peristalsis caused by bowel manipulation during surgery (with abdominal procedure)	Normal bowel elimination: no abdominal distention, bowel sounds present, bowel movements resume
Low self-esteem and body image disturbance related to potential loss of reproductive capacity and loss of one or both testes	Improved self-esteem: patient makes positive remarks about self
Inability to manage self-care related to lack of knowledge of disease and treatment	Patient understands disease, treatment, and self-care: patient accurately describes condition, treatment, side effects, and management of side effects; patient demonstrates self-care

Interventions

Anxiety. From the time cancer is suspected, the patient faces anxiety-producing threats to self-image and self-esteem. You must be sensitive to the patient's fears of altered sexual function, loss of fertility, stressful treatments, and the threat of a potentially fatal disease. You can help the patient through listening actively, providing information, and referring him for counseling if needed. The patient may wish to have a significant other included in interactions with you and other health professionals.

Acute pain. The amount of postoperative pain will vary with the type of procedure done. Assess pain with each vital sign check and take steps to treat it promptly. In addition to analgesics, you can use other pain control techniques such as mental imagery and relaxation exercises (see Chapter 8).

Impaired urinary elimination. Radical orchiectomy usually requires a short hospitalization and has few complications. Nevertheless, monitor the patient's urinary status to confirm normal function before discharge. If the patient has a radical retroperitoneal lymph node dissection, he probably will have a catheter immediately after surgery.

Potential for injury. Some patients with testicular cancer undergo radical retroperitoneal lymph node dissection. These patients have extensive surgical incisions and usually need intensive nursing care initially. As with any major abdominal surgery, the patient is at risk for shock, infection, bowel and bladder dysfunction, and fluid and electrolyte imbalances. Shock can result from fluid loss and the effects of anesthesia during the lengthy surgery. Measure and evaluate vital signs and fluid intake and output. Monitor the patient's electrolyte levels and administer intravenous fluids as ordered to maintain fluid and electrolyte balance. The patient is likely to have a urinary catheter in place and a nasogastric tube attached to suction.

Constipation. Palpate the abdomen for bowel or bladder distention and auscultate for bowel sounds. When permitted, encourage ambulation, increased fluid intake unless contraindicated, and a diet with adequate fiber to promote bowel elimination. Administer stool softeners as ordered.

Low self-esteem and body image disturbance. The patient may or may not be rendered sterile as a result of the treatment used. Radical orchiectomy results in sterility but does not impair erection and orgasm. If radiotherapy is used, the patient's sperm count typically declines at first but usually returns to normal by 2 to 3 years after treatment is completed. The effects of chemotherapy on fertility vary with the drug used. Retroperitoneal lymph node dissection often causes ED and problems with ejaculation. Help the patient to formulate questions for the physician about the effects of specific treatments on sexual function and fertility. If sterility is anticipated, the patient should be counseled preoperatively about the possibility of banking sperm for future use. Because this type of cancer commonly affects young men, the potential to father a child at a later date may be very important to them.

Inability to manage self-care. Teaching is essential to prepare the patient for treatment and to provide the tools needed for him to cope with the diagnosis. The patient teaching plan will vary greatly with the extent of the cancer and the type of treatment given. Include the type of therapy prescribed, the side effects, the management of side effects, and available resources.

Get Ready for the NCLEX® Examination!

Key Points

- Prostatitis is an inflammation of the prostate gland that is treated with antimicrobials, analgesics, and sitz baths.
- Epididymitis is an inflammation of the epididymis that is treated with bed rest, cold packs, sitz baths, analgesics, antibiotics, and scrotal support.
- Benign prostatic hyperplasia—enlargement of the prostate gland that may lead to obstruction of the urethra—may be treated with drugs or surgical intervention.
- Nursing care after prostatectomy addresses potential for fluid volume deficit, acute pain, potential for infection, potential for injury, urge urinary incontinence, impaired sexual function, low self-esteem, and lack.
- ED, the inability to achieve or maintain an erection adequate for sexual intercourse, may be treated with psychologic intervention, oral drug therapy, vacuum constriction devices, self-injection therapy, intraurethral pellets, or penile implants.
- Nursing care of the patient with ED may focus on impaired sexual function, low self-esteem, and ineffective management of condition.
- Peyronie disease is the formation of fibrous tissue in the penis that causes it to bend upward during erection, causing pain and interfering with vaginal penetration.
- Priapism is prolonged penile erection not related to sexual desire that requires emergency treatment to prevent ischemia, gangrene, fibrosis, and future ED.
- Infertility is the inability to impregnate despite unprotected intercourse over a 12-month period.
- Causes of infertility include endocrine or testicular dysfunction and disorders of the ejaculatory system.
- Cancer of the male reproductive system may affect the penis, testicles, or prostate gland.
- Nursing care of the patient with testicular cancer focuses on anxiety, acute pain, potential for injury, impaired urine elimination, constipation, low self-esteem, and lack of knowledge.
- Other disorders affecting the male reproductive system are hydrocele, phimosis, and paraphimosis.

Additional Learning Resources

SG Go to your Study Guide for additional learning activities to help you master this chapter content.

Go to your Evolve website (http://evolve.elsevier.com/Linton/medsurg) for the following learning resources and much more:

- Fluid & Electrolyte Tutorial
- Review Questions for the NCLEX® Examination

Clinical Judgment and Next-Generation NCLEX® Examination-Style Questions

1. **A resident of a retirement center had a hypotensive episode. Once his BP stabilized, he informed the nurse that he had "borrowed" a sildenafil (Viagra) tablet provided by a friend shortly before he became dizzy. What data would be most significant for the nurse to collect?**
   1. When the patient last engaged in sexual activity
   2. The name of the person who provided the sildenafil to the patient
   3. Documentation of the effects of the sildenafil
   4. A list of all the patient's usual medications

   NCLEX Client Need: Physiologic Adaptation: Pharmacological Therapies

2. **The nurse is teaching a class on ED to a group of retirement center residents. The nurse should include which of the following measures that may help to treat ED? (Select all that apply.)**
   1. Ask your health care provider if any of your drugs cause ED.
   2. Engage in physical activity to improve conditioning.
   3. Use alcohol to relax before sexual activity.
   4. Seek counseling to address stress and anxiety.
   5. Attain or maintain ideal weight.

   NCLEX Client Need: Health Promotion and Maintenance

3. **Which of the following should be included when teaching a patient about benign prostatic hyperplasia? (Select all that apply.)**
   1. Moderate use of alcohol will promote emptying of the bladder.
   2. Void promptly when you feel the urge to empty your bladder.
   3. Limit your daily fluid intake to six glasses of water.
   4. Medications that contain antihistamines may cause you to retain urine.
   5. Prolonged exposure to warm temperatures promotes bladder spasms.

   NCLEX Client Need: Physiological Integrity: Reduction of Risk Potential

4. **Bleeding after a transurethral prostatectomy is *most likely* to be detected by inspection of which of the following?**
   1. Abdominal dressing
   2. Perineal drainage
   3. Urine characteristics
   4. Suprapubic drain

   NCLEX Client Need: Physiological Integrity: Reduction of Risk Potential

5. **When preparing to irrigate a urinary catheter for a patient who had a prostatectomy this morning, the nurse checks to be certain that normal saline solution is available. Why is normal saline preferable for urinary catheter irrigation?**
   1. It is isotonic and will not cause water intoxication.
   2. It is less expensive than sterile water for irrigation.
   3. It is absorbed into the bloodstream to maintain blood volume.
   4. Sterile water stings when it comes in contact with the surgical sites.

   NCLEX Client Need: Physiological Integrity: Reduction of Risk Potential

6. **A couple has come to the fertility clinic for evaluation. During the health history, the husband reports having had all of the childhood diseases listed subsequently. Which may be significant in relation to infertility in men?**
   1. Measles
   2. Chickenpox
   3. Mumps
   4. Diphtheria

   NCLEX Client Need: Physiological Integrity: Physiological Adaptation

7. **A nurse in the newborn nursery assesses a newborn male for the presence of the testes in the scrotum. The nurse knows that failure of the testes to descend into the scrotum (cryptorchidism) must be treated early in life to prevent:**
   1. Testicular torsion
   2. Varicocele
   3. Chronic infection
   4. Sterility

   NCLEX Client Need: Health Promotion and Maintenance

8. **Patient teaching related to vasectomy should include which of the following?**
   1. You will be sterile immediately after the procedure.
   2. Vasectomy is easily reversible if you wish to father a child later.
   3. Postoperative problems with erection and ejaculation are common.
   4. You will need to have a semen analysis to determine if sperm are present.

   NCLEX Client Need: Physiological Integrity: Reduction of Risk Potential

9. **A patient is undergoing treatment for prostate cancer. The clinic nurse reminds him that he will need to come in periodically for which of the following to determine the effectiveness of his treatment?**
   1. Measurement of the PSA level
   2. Periodic biopsies of perineal tissue
   3. Studies of urine flow rates
   4. Radiographs of the abdomen

   NCLEX Client Need: Physiological Integrity: Reduction of Risk Potential

10. **A 75-year-old patient is brought to the emergency department after a fainting episode. Admission data include:**
    - BP 90/60
    - Heart rate 96 beats per minute
    - Respirations 18 breaths per minute
    - Height 5′10″
    - Weight 190 lb
    - Past medical history: MI 5 years ago, hypothyroidism, hypertension, erectile dysfunction last year
    - EKG normal sinus rhythm
    - Active lifestyle
    - Felt faint during sexual intercourse
    - Medications include
        - doxazosin (an $alpha_1$ blocker) for hypertension
        - levothyroxine for hypothyroidism
        - tadalafil for erectile dysfunction
        - paroxetine for depression

    Choose the most likely options for the information missing from the statements below by selecting from the list of options provided.

    The nurse recognizes that a low ____________ may be related to the interaction of ________ and ___________.

    The patient needs to be referred to the health care provider for an evaluation of current medications. Failure to do so could result in ____________.

OPTIONS
heart rate
blood pressure
respiratory rate
levothyroxine
tadalafil
doxazosin
thyroid crisis
renal failure
hypotensive shock

NCLEX Client Need: Physiological Integrity: Pharmacological Therapies, Reduction of Risk Potential

55 Sexually Transmitted Infections

http://evolve.elsevier.com/Linton/medsurg

Objectives

1. Describe tests used to diagnose sexually transmitted infections and the nursing considerations associated with each.
2. Explain why specific sexually transmitted infections must be reported to the health department.
3. List infectious diseases classified as *sexually transmitted infections.*
4. Describe the pathophysiology, signs and symptoms, complications, and medical treatment for selected sexually transmitted infections.
5. Explain the importance of the nurse's approach when dealing with patients who have sexually transmitted infections.
6. List nursing considerations when a patient is on drug therapy for a sexually transmitted infection.
7. Identify data to be collected when assessing a patient with a sexually transmitted infection.
8. Assist in developing a nursing care plan for a patient with a sexually transmitted infection.
9. Design a teaching plan on the prevention of sexually transmitted infections.

Key Terms

chancre (SHĂNG-kĕr)
latent (LĀ-tĕnt)
opportunistic infections
pelvic inflammatory disease (PID)
sexually transmitted infections (STIs)

Sexually transmitted infections (STIs) include several conditions that can be transmitted from one person to another during intimate contact. The term *sexually transmitted disease (STD)* is commonly used to describe these same conditions as well. The difference in the two terms is that a disease, by definition, has recognizable signs and symptoms, whereas infections may or may not manifest specific signs and symptoms.

Despite medical advances, STIs continue to be a serious public health problem in the United States. Worldwide the incidence of STIs increases every year. More than 1 million STIs are acquired every day worldwide. Each year, there are an estimated 357 million new infections with 1 of 4 STIs: chlamydia, gonorrhea, syphilis, and trichomonas. In the United States, an estimated 26 million new infections occur each year. Almost half of these are in persons between 15 and 24 years of age. Although STIs are more common in people of lower socioeconomic status and in those with less education and limited access to health care, all segments of the population are represented. Drug abuse and having multiple sexual partners are also risk factors. In the United States, STI rates are highest among Black Americans, followed by Latino Americans and then by non-Latino White Americans (see the Cultural Considerations box).

Cultural Considerations

What Does Culture Have to Do With Sexually Transmitted Infections?

The incidence of sexually transmitted infections (STIs) varies among races, but poverty, lack of education, and limited access to health care probably play a larger role than race and ethnicity. In addition, cultural beliefs about sexual practices, use of condoms, and educating children about STI prevention may all affect the incidence of STIs in any given population.

Despite public education efforts, some people resist taking preventive measures. Infected people do not always inform their sexual partners, so the disease continues to be passed on to others. In addition, symptoms are sometimes absent or subtle; thus STIs that go undetected can spread and invade other parts of the body. These infections may have serious and permanent consequences.

Nurses must be aware of their feelings about working with people who have STIs. A stigma is associated with these infections, and we must ensure the same quality of care to patients with an STI that we give to patients with any other diagnoses. Judgmental behavior on the part of health care providers discourages people from seeking appropriate medical care. In this chapter, specific diseases are explained, followed by a general discussion of nursing care appropriate for all patients with STIs.

DIAGNOSTIC TESTS AND PROCEDURES

Individuals who engage in high-risk sexual behaviors are at increased risk for each of the STIs. Therefore patients diagnosed with one STI should be evaluated for others as well. Infections with some STIs appear to increase the risk of human immunodeficiency virus (HIV) infection. The primary measures used to diagnose STIs are serologic tests and studies of smears and cultures. Some over-the-counter (OTC) or mail service tests can be purchased for home use. Concerns with this type of testing include possible false-negative or false-positive results, uncertainty about the reliability of a specific product or laboratory, and possible delayed treatment of serious infections.

SEROLOGIC TESTS

Serologic tests may be ordered to detect infections with hepatitis A, B, C, D, and E; syphilis; HIV; herpes simplex; and cytomegalovirus. These tests are designed to detect infections by measuring antigens or antibodies in the blood. Many factors can cause inaccurate results, especially with older tests. Agency laboratory procedures specify the patient preparation for specific tests.

SMEARS, SWABS, AND CULTURES

Patients with gonococcal, chlamydial, herpes simplex, *Trichomonas*, or yeast infections often have discharge from the vagina or penis. In addition to this discharge, exudate from lesions can be collected and studied to determine the exact infecting organism. For women, the sample may be collected from the vagina or cervix. The procedure varies with the type of organism suspected. To collect a sample from a male patient, a swab or special loop may be used. The person who collects the sample wears gloves and treats the sample as a potential source of infection. The sample may be submitted for microscopic examination or for culture and sensitivity tests.

Pharmacology Capsule

When you have an order to obtain a specimen for culture and another order to administer antiinfective agents, collect the specimen before giving the first dose of the antiinfective.

PATHOPHYSIOLOGY

Although more than 30 different bacteria, viruses, and parasites are known to be transmitted through sexual contact, the World Health Organization identifies eight that account for the greatest number of infections. These are syphilis, gonorrhea, chlamydia, trichomonas, hepatitis B, herpes simplex virus (HSV) or herpes, HIV, and human papillomavirus (HPV). The first four listed are curable with treatment, whereas the latter four are not curable at this time.

DRUG THERAPY

The drugs recommended by the Centers for Disease Control and Prevention (CDC) are noted with the discussion of each specific infection. The CDC also recommends alternative drugs for people who are allergic to the primary drugs, pregnant women, infants and children, and people who are being treated for multiple infections. Details are available at the CDC website: https://www.cdc.gov/std/treatment-guidelines/default.htm. Examples of drugs commonly used to treat STIs are presented in Table 55.1.

REPORTING SEXUALLY TRANSMITTED INFECTIONS

Confirmed cases of HIV, acquired immunodeficiency syndrome (AIDS), gonorrhea, syphilis, chlamydia, chancroid, and viral hepatitis are among the infections that must be reported to the local health department. A current list is posted yearly at https://wwwn.cdc.gov/nndss/conditions/notifiable/2021/. An investigator asks the patient to name their contacts. Those individuals are contacted and advised that they have been exposed to the disease and are encouraged to seek medical evaluation. The purpose of this process is to identify and treat infected individuals so that transmission of the infection can be slowed. Another approach is to provide the patient with a prescription or additional drugs for their sexual partner without examination of the partner. This approach, which is legal in some but not all states, is called *expedited partner therapy (EPT)*.

SPECIFIC SEXUALLY TRANSMITTED INFECTIONS

CHLAMYDIAL INFECTION

Chlamydial infection is thought to be the most common bacterial STI in the United States. In 2019, over two million new cases were reported to the CDC. Chlamydia is an intracellular bacterium that comprises multiple genera and species. The specific species that causes the infection classified with STIs is *Chlamydia trachomatis*. This infection is transmitted by contact with the mucous membranes in the mouth, eyes, urethra, vagina, or rectum. Newborns of infected women may have eye infections (conjunctivitis) or pneumonia. Therefore erythromycin ophthalmic ointment may be ordered for the newborn because it is effective against chlamydial infection as well as gonorrhea.

Table 55.1 Drug Therapy: Drugs Used to Treat Sexually Transmitted Infections

General Considerations

- Always assess for history of allergies before giving any antimicrobial.
- If the patient reports being allergic to the prescribed drug, withhold it and notify the physician.
- Observe all patients for possible allergic responses: rash, difficulty breathing, hypotension.
- Obtain specimens for culture before administering the first dose of the antimicrobial.
- When giving intravenous antimicrobials through a secondary line, check compatibility with primary fluid.
- Tell the patient it is important to complete the full course of treatment to prevent organisms from becoming resistant and to prevent relapse because all organisms had not been killed.
- Tell the patient that the sexual partner or partners should be treated at the same time to prevent infection.
- Assess for drug interactions.

DRUG	USE AND ACTION	SIDE EFFECTS	NURSING INTERVENTIONS
Antibacterial Agents			
Beta-Lactams			
penicillin G (Bicillin, Pfizerpen, benzathine)	First choice for treatment of syphilis. Primary Secondary Tertiary	Ulcer or chancre at infection site. Nausea, vomiting, diarrhea, pain at injection site. Skin rash, mucocutaneous lesions, and lymphadenopathy. Cardiac, gummatous lesions, tabes dorsalis, and general paresis anaphylaxis. Jarisch-Herxheimer reaction: headache, fever, chills, diaphoresis, tachycardia, muscle and joint pain. If allergic to cephalosporins, may also be allergic to penicillins.	Scratch test may be ordered to assess allergy. Alternative drugs are available if allergic. Check drug insert for preparation of injection. (Given by deep injection in large muscle. Do not pause during injection; needle may clog. Massage site.) Have patient wait 30 minutes after injection in case there is allergic reaction. Tell patient Jarisch-Herxheimer reaction may occur; resolves within 24 hours.
ceftriaxone sodium (Rocephin)	Effective against organism that causes gonorrhea.	Nausea, vomiting, headache, dizziness, and (rarely) bleeding. Allergic reactions, including anaphylaxis. Patients allergic to penicillin may have cross-sensitivity to cephalosporins. Nephrotoxicity with high doses or renal disease. Superinfections: diarrhea, candidiasis. Intravenous (IV) route: pain, thrombophlebitis. Intramuscular (IM) route: pain, induration at injection site.	Notify physician of profuse, watery diarrhea. Report vaginal or anal itching. Assess for bruising, bleeding. An injection given intramuscularly (IM) is painful.
Tetracyclines			
doxycycline (Vibramycin)	Effective against organisms that cause gonorrhea (in combination with ceftriaxone), chlamydia, granuloma inguinale, syphilis, and lymphogranuloma venereum.	Anorexia, nausea, vomiting, diarrhea, dysphagia, fungal infections, anaphylaxis, increased intracranial pressure, photosensitivity. Rarely: rash, urticaria, hemolytic anemia.	Assess allergies to tetracycline and to sulfites. Monitor food intake and stools. Assess blood pressure and level of consciousness. Report genital or anal itching. Give with full glass of water, not dairy products.
Macrolides			
erythromycin (E-Mycin, Ilosone, Erythrocin Stearate)	Effective against organisms that cause chlamydial infection, syphilis, and gonorrhea. Ophthalmic ointment used in newborn to prevent eye infection.	Nausea, vomiting, diarrhea, phlebitis at infusion site, allergic reactions, hepatitis, ototoxicity.	Report tinnitus or jaundice. Give oral drug on empty stomach with full glass of water—no fruit juice.

Table 55.1 Drug Therapy: Drugs Used to Treat Sexually Transmitted Infections—cont'd

DRUG	USE AND ACTION	SIDE EFFECTS	NURSING INTERVENTIONS
azithromycin (Zithromax)	Effective against *Chlamydia* (which causes urethritis and cervicitis). Used in combination with ceftriaxone for gonorrhea.	Diarrhea, nausea, vomiting, abdominal pain, vaginitis.	Caution if patient has liver impairment. Do not give with antacids. Give 1 hour before meals or 2 hours after meals.
Miscellaneous Antiinfective			
tinidazole (Tindamax) metronidazole (Flagyl)	Tinidazole is first choice for *Trichomonas.* Metronidazole is used to treat bacterial vaginosis and is second choice for treating *Trichomonas.*	Headache, dizziness, nausea, vomiting, abdominal pain, anorexia, diarrhea, skin irritation, peripheral neuropathy, leukopenia.	Give with food or milk. Instruct patient not to take a double dose if a dose is missed. Tell patient to avoid alcohol. Advise patient to follow safety precautions if dizziness occurs. Monitor fluid status because drug contains sodium. Urine may be dark. Monitor blood cell counts. Severe reaction with alcohol.
clindamycin vaginal cream	Used to treat bacterial vaginosis.	Headache, dizziness, abdominal pain, nausea, vomiting.	Advise patient that cream weakens latex condoms and diaphragms, which may interfere with their effectiveness. Instruct in use of applicator. Should be used at bedtime. Wash hands after use. Avoid sexual intercourse during treatment. Advise sanitary napkin to prevent stains on clothing.
Antivirals			
acyclovir (Zovirax) valacyclovir (Valtrex) famciclovir (Famvir)	Decreases frequency and severity of genital herpes infections. Is not curative.	Dizziness, headache, diarrhea, nausea, vomiting, renal failure, seizures.	Apply ointment with gloved finger. Do not double up if an oral dose is missed. Tell patient drug is not curative. Condoms should be used during sexual contact and sexual contact should be avoided when lesions are present.
Dermatologic Agents			
podophyllin (Podocon-25)	Topical agent used to remove genital warts.	Highly caustic; can be applied directly on warts. Excessive application can cause kidney damage, neuropathy, blood dyscrasias. Teratogenic; contraindicated during pregnancy.	Should be applied only by physician. Treated area must be washed with alcohol or soap and water within 1–4 hours.
imiquimod (Aldara)	Used to treat genital warts and actinic keratoses.	Erythema, erosion, flaking. Local itching, burning, pain. No systemic effects.	Instruct patient to apply at bedtime and wash off in morning. Usual application is 3 times/week for 16 weeks or until warts are gone.

Continued

Table 55.1 Drug Therapy: Drugs Used to Treat Sexually Transmitted Infections—cont'd

DRUG	USE AND ACTION	SIDE EFFECTS	NURSING INTERVENTIONS
podofilox (Condylox)	Used to treat genital warts.	Local inflammation, erosion, pain, itching, bleeding. Causes more discomfort than imiquimod but costs less and treatment is shorter.	Instruct patient to apply twice daily for 3 consecutive days, then take 4 days off. The cycle can be repeated if needed for a maximum of 4 cycles until the warts are gone. Does not have to be washed off. Advise patient not to use more than 0.5 mg/d and apply only to warts, not to normal skin.
kunecatechins (sinecatechins)	Used to treat genital warts.	Erythema, pruritus, burning, pain, ulceration, edema, rash.	Must be applied 3 times a day or for 16 weeks until warts clear. Advise patient to avoid sexual contact when gel is applied. Do not apply to vagina, rectum, or open wounds.
Antiretroviral Therapy (ART)			
ART uses various combinations of nonnucleoside reverse transcriptase inhibitors, nucleoside reverse transcriptase inhibitors, and protease inhibitors to treat HIV. See details in Chapter 32.			

Lymphogranuloma venereum (LGV) is a more invasive systemic infection caused by the LGV strain of *C. trachomatis*. Lesions may affect the inguinal lymph nodes and the rectal mucosa.

Clinical Manifestations

One reason chlamydial infection is so common is that most people have no symptoms. Symptoms, if any, are generally noted 1 to 3 weeks after being infected. Symptoms are more noticeable in men and include penile discharge, which is initially thin and becomes creamy later. Another common complaint among men is painful or frequent urination. Epididymitis is manifested by testicular pain, swelling, and tenderness. Women may experience vaginal discharge, painful urination, nausea, fever, painful intercourse, bleeding between menstrual periods, and lower abdominal pain. Rectal infection is characterized by pain, discharge, bleeding, or a combination of these problems. Unlike other forms of chlamydial infection, LGV patients have fever, muscle aches, swollen inguinal lymph nodes, and elevated white blood cell (WBC) count.

Complications

If left untreated, chlamydial infection can result in sterility in men and women. The sperm ducts can become inflamed and blocked. In women, **pelvic inflammatory disease (PID)**, which involves the ovaries, fallopian tubes, and pelvic area, can block the fallopian tubes and damage the uterus. The risk of ectopic pregnancy (i.e., the fertilized ovum develops outside the uterus) is increased in the presence of chlamydial infection. In addition, chlamydial infection may increase one's risk of becoming infected with HIV if exposed to it.

Medical Diagnosis and Treatment

The diagnosis is based on the individual's sexual history and the results of laboratory studies. The nucleic acid amplification test (NAAT) is the most effective diagnostic tool; it has largely replaced the cell tissue culture.

The infection is usually treated with a 7-day course of doxycycline (Vibramycin). Other antimicrobials may also be administered because patients with chlamydial infection may have gonorrhea as well. The test should be repeated 3 to 4 months after treatment to confirm successful results of treatment. The patient is advised to avoid all sexual contact (genital, oral, anal) until a cure has been achieved. When sexual activity is resumed, condom use is recommended to prevent reinfection.

Nursing care of the patient with chlamydial infection and other STIs is discussed in the section titled "Nursing Care of the Patient With a Sexually Transmitted Infection." Information about chlamydial infection is summarized in Table 55.2.

GONORRHEA

Gonorrhea is one of the most commonly reported STIs in the United States. The CDC (last reviewed 2021) estimated that 1.6 million new cases of gonorrhea were reported in 2018. Gonorrhea is transmitted most often through direct sexual contact. Cases have been reported of transmission to newborn infants by infected mothers and to medical personnel with skin lacerations who have come in contact with infected fluids. The infection is not picked up from toilet seats, doorknobs, or towels. Neonates may acquire a gonococcal infection during delivery from an infected mother.

Table 55.2 Chlamydial Infection

SIGNS AND SYMPTOMS	POSSIBLE COMPLICATIONS	MEDICAL TREATMENT	NURSING CONSIDERATIONS
Sometimes no signs or symptoms. *Males:* penile discharge (thin at first, then creamy); painful, frequent urination. *Females:* vaginal discharge, lower abdominal pain.	Sterility in both sexes. Transmission to newborn infants, causing eye infections or pneumonia.	azithromycin (Zithromax) or doxycycline (Vibramycin).	Counsel about importance of treatment to prevent complications. Advise of need for follow-up to ensure that infection has been treated successfully. Tell patient to avoid sexual contact until cured.

The bacterium that causes this disease is *Neisseria gonorrhoeae*. This organism lives in warm, moist areas of the body such as the cervix and the urethra. Areas affected by local gonorrhea infections may include the pharynx, rectum, urethra, prostate, epididymis, uterus, and fallopian tubes. A high incidence of rectal gonorrhea exists among men who have sex with men. The presence of bacteria in the throat is common among individuals who perform oral sex (fellatio) on an infected partner. With systemic (disseminated) infection, the heart, joints, skin, and meninges may become involved. Drug resistance, especially for gonorrhea, is a major threat to efforts to reduce the impact of STIs worldwide.

Clinical Manifestations

Many people with gonorrhea have no symptoms. When present, symptoms typically occur 2 to 10 days after exposure and are generally more apparent in men than in women. Men who do have symptoms often have whitish or greenish discharge from the penis and often complain of a burning sensation during urination. Testicular pain and swelling may be present. Women may experience vaginal discharge, bleeding during sexual intercourse, redness and swelling of the external genitalia, a burning sensation during urination, abdominal pain, or abnormal menstruation. A rectal infection may cause discharge, anal itching, soreness, bleeding, or painful bowel movements. Symptoms of rectal infection usually occur 2 to 5 days after infection but may be as long as 30 days later. Throat infections usually have no symptoms, but a sore throat may be present. Symptoms generally disappear after a few weeks, but if the infection is untreated, the bacteria remain in the body and the person remains highly infectious.

Complications

If untreated, gonorrhea can cause sterility in both sexes and infections that may lead to damage to heart tissue and joints. Men may develop epididymitis and prostatitis. Women may develop PID and ectopic pregnancy. People with gonorrhea are at increased risk for HIV; people with HIV and gonorrhea are more likely to transmit HIV to another person.

Medical Diagnosis

The diagnosis is based on the individual's health history and physical examination findings as well as on laboratory studies. Although smears and cultures of exudate from infected body parts or urinalysis are still used in some settings, NAAT is now the preferred diagnostic tool.

Medical Treatment

Treatment is usually initiated based on the physical examination without waiting for laboratory results. This is because many patients will not return for follow-up and immediate treatment has been highly effective. Treatment usually consists of a single dose of intramuscular ceftriaxone sodium (Rocephin). One treatment cures most cases of gonorrhea quickly and safely. Erythromycin ophthalmic ointment may be ordered for the newborn to prevent eye infection caused by exposure to gonococci during delivery.

Follow-up examination is essential after antimicrobial therapy for gonorrhea to ensure that the infection has been eradicated. Additional information about drug therapy for gonorrhea is provided in Table 55.1.

Nursing care of the patient with gonorrhea and other STIs is discussed in the section titled "Nursing Care of the Patient With a Sexually Transmitted Infection." Table 55.3 summarizes information related to the signs and symptoms of gonorrhea, the possible complications, the medical treatment, and the nursing considerations.

SYPHILIS

Syphilis is caused by a spirochete (coiled bacterium) called *Treponema pallidum*. The organism is generally transmitted by sexual contact but can also be spread through breaks in the skin. It can also be passed through the placenta, thus causing an infant to be born with the disease (i.e., congenital syphilis). In the United States in 2019; 129,813 new cases of primary and secondary syphilis and 1870 new cases of congenital syphilis were reported (CDC, last reviewed Apr 13, 2021).

Clinical Manifestations

Signs and symptoms change throughout the course of the disease. If untreated, syphilis progresses through four stages: (1) primary, (2) secondary, (3) latent, and (4) late (tertiary).

Table 55.3 Gonorrhea

SIGNS AND SYMPTOMS	POSSIBLE COMPLICATIONS	MEDICAL TREATMENT	NURSING CONSIDERATIONS
Men: Thick urethral discharge (purulent green or yellow), swelling and redness of the meatus, urinary urgency and dribbling.	Epididymitis, urethritis, infections of Cowper and Tyson glands.	Treated with ceftriaxone (Rocephin).	Send specimen to laboratory for culture. Instruct the patient that all sexual partners should also be treated. Instruct the patient to take complete prescription of the drug (if receiving ciprofloxacin [Cipro] or tetracycline for self-medication), even if symptoms have disappeared. Stress abstinence or condom use.
Women: Increased, foul-smelling vaginal discharge; dysuria (difficulty urinating); fever; abnormal or painful menstruation; vulval soreness; peritonitis; backache; lower back pain (usually involving only one side).	Infertility, urethral and labial infection, risk of tubal pregnancy, pelvic inflammatory disease (PID), septicemia.	Same as for male patients.	Counsel the patient about potential complications.

Primary stage. A typical lesion, called a **chancre**, is the first sign of syphilis. The chancre is generally first noticed 1 to 12 weeks after contact. During the primary stage, a reddish papule appears where the organism entered the body, usually on the genitals, anus, or mouth. Within 1 week, the papule becomes a painless red ulcer. Lymph nodes in the area of the chancre may be enlarged but are not tender. The chancre may last from 1 to 5 weeks. When it disappears, patients may assume that they are cured when in fact the infecting organism has moved into the blood (Fig. 55.1).

Secondary stage. The secondary stage occurs 1 to 6 months after contact. Symptoms may include a rash on the extremities, chest or back, palms of the hands, and soles of the feet. Pustules that contain highly contagious material often develop. Fever, sore throat, and generalized aching are also seen in this stage. The patient is contagious during the first and second stages.

Latent stage. The **latent** stage, in which no symptoms exist, follows the secondary stage. Although no symptoms are present, the organisms are invading the major organs. The infection is not spread by sexual contact during the latent stage but may be transmitted by blood exposure.

Late ("tertiary") stage. It is generally 3 years after contact before late syphilis develops, although it may be decades. Even without treatment, most patients never advance to this stage. Signs and symptoms of late syphilis include arthritis, numbness of the extremities, lesions of the skin and internal organs (called *gummas*), and pain because of damage to the heart, blood vessels (especially the aorta), or central nervous system.

Complications

The patient with untreated syphilis may develop severe, potentially fatal complications, including neurosyphilis (meningitis, blindness, paralysis) and cardiovascular disease. An infected woman who becomes pregnant has a greatly increased risk of fetal infection, deformities, or death. The lesions also make it easier for a person to transmit and contract HIV infection.

Medical Diagnosis

The diagnosis is based on physical examination findings and a blood test to detect the presence of antibodies. Tests for syphilis include screening (nontreponemal) and confirmation (treponemal) tests. Two screening tests are (1) the Venereal Disease Research Laboratory (VDRL) test and (2) the rapid plasma reagin (RPR) test. Both detect a protein that appears in the blood when a person has syphilis. Screening tests can be inaccurate because other factors can cause false-positive reactions. In addition, the tests are not effective until antibodies for *T. pallidum* are present in the blood. This may not occur until 3 to 4 weeks after exposure.

Confirmation tests, those that specifically detect *T. pallidum*, are needed to confirm the disease. A number of confirmation tests exist including the fluorescent treponemal antibody absorption (FTA-ABS) test, chemiluminescence, and immunoassays. Because patients with syphilis often have multiple infections, HIV testing is often recommended as well.

Pharmacology Capsule

Patients who do not complete the prescribed course of anti-infective therapy may not be cured of the infection.

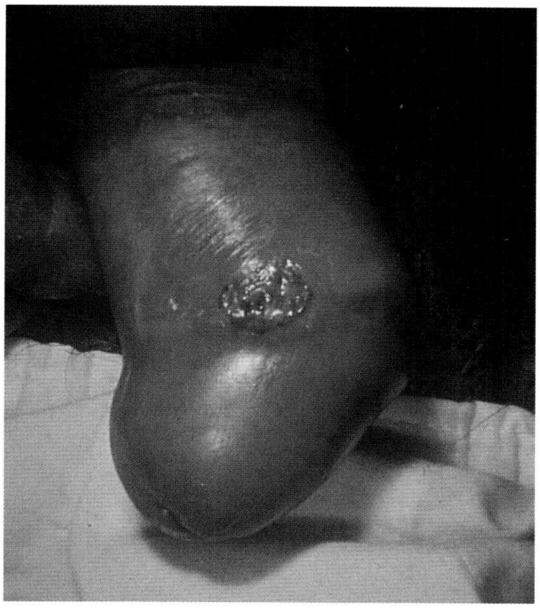

Fig. 55.1 Chancre typical of primary syphilis. (Courtesy New York City Health Department.)

Medical Treatment

Treatment of syphilis (drug, dosage, length of treatment) varies with the stage and clinical manifestations of the infection. The treatment of choice for syphilis is parenteral benzathine penicillin G unless contraindicated. For a primary, secondary, or early latent infection, a single dose is usually sufficient. For more advanced infections, a longer course of therapy is indicated. Neurosyphilis and ocular syphilis require aqueous crystalline penicillin G. Information about drug therapy for syphilis is presented in Table 55.1. Advise the patient to make a follow-up appointment with a health care provider to determine whether the treatment was effective. In addition, advise the patient not to engage in sexual activity until 1 month after completing treatment for primary or secondary syphilis.

Nursing care of the patient with syphilis and other STIs is discussed in the section titled "Nursing Care of the Patient With a Sexually Transmitted Infection." Table 55.4 summarizes the signs and symptoms of syphilis, possible complications, medical treatment, and nursing considerations.

GENITAL HERPES

The herpes virus has plagued humans for many centuries. Several different types of the virus are passed easily from person to person. The virus that causes cold sores (*herpes febrilis* or herpes simplex virus-1 [HSV-1]) was first described in AD 100 and is transmitted through contact with open lesions, usually on the lips or inside the mouth. Prevention strategies generally focus on avoiding direct contact (kissing). Nurses should use good hand washing technique when caring for infected persons.

The incidence of genital herpes (caused by herpes simplex virus-2 [HSV-2]) has been on the rise since the 1960s. HSV-2 is generally transmitted by sexual contact. Vaginal or anal intercourse and oral-genital contact are the primary transmission modes, but HSV-2 can be transferred by hand contact as well.

Although HSV-1 and HSV-2 are similar, type 1 is usually nongenital, with lesions typically above the waist. Type 2 is considered an STI because it is most often below the waist and is transmitted by genital contact. However, type 1 is being found in increasing numbers of genital infections, presumably transmitted by oral-genital contact. A characteristic of herpes viruses is the ability to become latent. The virus can remain in the tissues in an inactive state for long periods of time and then be reactivated.

Clinical Manifestations

Most patients with genital herpes have no symptoms. When symptoms are present, they typically begin with a rash, followed by small blisters that eventually ulcerate creating painful, itching sores on or around the genitals. The symptoms appear 2 to 20 days after infection, and last about 2 to 3 weeks. People often complain of flu-like symptoms and a burning sensation during urination. Episodes of active symptoms may recur, especially with type 2 infections, and are frequently precipitated by anxiety (Fig. 55.2). Recurrent episodes, or "outbreaks," are commonly preceded by prodromal symptoms such as genital pain, and tingling or shooting pains in the legs, hips, and buttocks. These episodes tend to be less severe than the initial infection.

Complications

An increased risk of cervical cancer exists in women who have genital herpes. An infected woman should be taught to have a Papanicolaou (Pap) test done annually to detect cervical cancer early. If she is pregnant, a physician should supervise her closely. Various guidelines are used to determine whether the patient should have a vaginal delivery or a cesarean section. The goal is to decrease the risk of transmission to the baby. New diagnostic procedures allow the physician to detect active disease more accurately than in the past. Herpes simplex encephalitis is a dangerous complication, usually caused by HSV-1. It has a mortality rate of 20% to 30% and a significant proportion of survivors have moderate to severe neurologic impairment. Other neurological complications such as Bell palsy may occur as well.

Medical Diagnosis and Treatment

A diagnosis of HSV-2 may be suspected based on the appearance of genital lesions. Laboratory tests are used to confirm the diagnosis. These include antigen detection tests and NAAT using tissue or fluid specimens. Exudate from lesions can be examined under a microscope and cultured to reveal the virus.

Table 55.4 Syphilis

SIGNS AND SYMPTOMS	POSSIBLE COMPLICATIONS	MEDICAL TREATMENT	NURSING CONSIDERATIONS
Primary Syphilis			
Chancre (round ulcer with well-defined margin): lesion thickened, rubbery, and painless. (If untreated, the lesion persists only for 3–6 weeks and heals.) Regional lymphadenopathy: enlarged lymph nodes only in the area of the chancre.	Prompt, effective treatment can result in complete recovery without complications. Otherwise, the infection progresses to the secondary stage.	Parenteral benzathine penicillin G is given IM in a single dose. If the patient is unable to take penicillin, PO tetracycline or doxycycline is used.	Ensure that ordered blood studies are done: VDRL, RPR, FTA-ABS. Assess for transient fever, flulike symptoms, and malaise. Provide rest periods. Wear gloves to assess the skin and mucous membranes. Inspect for skin changes and lesions. Provide medications. After administration of parenteral antibiotics, observe the patient for 30 minutes for allergic reactions such as rash, fever, or chills. Have emergency drugs on hand in the event of anaphylaxis.
Secondary Syphilis			
Sore throat, malaise, rash, fever, weight loss, headaches, musculoskeletal pain.	May become latent without further problems or may progress to tertiary stage.	Parenteral benzathine penicillin.	
Tertiary Syphilis			
Pain, areas that lack sensation, loss of position sense, abnormal gait, foot deformity and ulcerations.	Irreversible complications: arthritis, bursitis, osteitis, liver enlargement, heart disease, meningitis, CNS disorders.	Benzathine penicillin doses at 1-week intervals.	

CNS, Central nervous system; *FTA-ABS*, fluorescent treponemal antibody absorption; *IM*, intramuscularly; *IV*, intravenously; *PO*, by mouth; *RPR*, rapid plasmin reagin; *VDRL*, Venereal Disease Research Laboratory.

No cure for HSV infection exists but the oral antiviral drugs acyclovir (Zovirax), valacyclovir (Valtrex), and famciclovir (Famvir) help by partially controlling the signs and symptoms during initial and recurrent episodes. Patients should know to start the drug when preliminary (prodromal) symptoms of recurrence are experienced or within 1 day of the outbreak of lesions. This treatment routine is called episodic therapy. Some patients with especially disabling recurrences take one of these drugs continuously to reduce the frequency of outbreaks, an approach called chronic suppressive therapy. Choice of the specific therapy depends on the frequency of recurrences and the patient's desire to prevent transmission to a partner. Patients with severe clinical complications are treated with intravenous antiviral drugs.

Nursing care of the patient with HSV and other STIs is discussed in the section titled "Nursing Care of the Patient With a Sexually Transmitted Infection." Table 55.5 summarizes the signs and symptoms of HSV infections, possible complications, medical treatment, and nursing considerations.

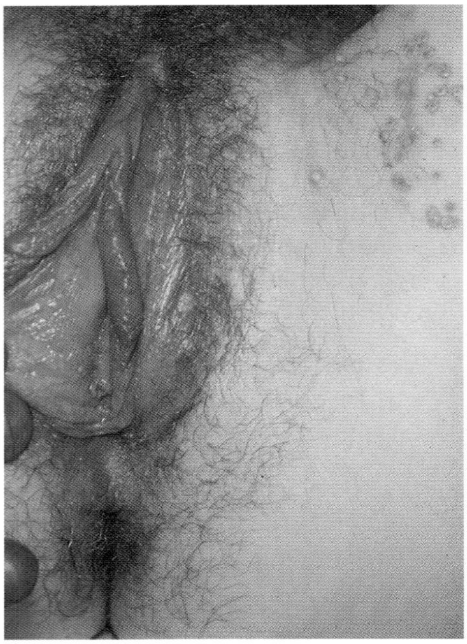

Fig. 55.2 Genital herpes lesions on the vulva and inner thigh. (Courtesy Leonard Wolf, MD, New York, NY.)

TRICHOMONIASIS

Trichomoniasis is caused by the protozoan parasite *Trichomonas vaginalis* and is virtually always sexually transmitted. Although the parasite can survive for hours on damp cloths and clothing, there is no proof of transmission because of this type of contact. The CDC estimates that more than 7 million new cases occur each year. This infection usually affects the vagina in women and the urethra in men. Trichomoniasis is associated with an increased risk of HIV transmission. During pregnancy, it may cause premature birth or low birth weight.

Clinical Manifestations

Women typically complain of a frothy, yellowish vaginal discharge that has a foul odor; however, some women have no symptoms. Vaginal irritation and itching may also be present. Urinary frequency and burning suggest that the infection has invaded the urethra (Fig. 55.3). If the infection becomes chronic, bladder and anal involvement are possible. Although the incidence of trichomoniasis is less common in men, it can certainly occur. Men usually have no symptoms, although some have a mild discharge or slight burning after urination or ejaculation.

Medical Diagnosis and Treatment

The organism may be detected by microscopic study of vaginal discharge or urine (in men). The discharge can also be cultured to reveal the organism.

Metronidazole (Flagyl) is the drug of choice. for treating trichomoniasis with tinidazole (Tindamax) is an alternative. A single dose is usually effective. It is important that the patient and any sexual partners be treated at the same time to avoid reinfection.

Nursing care of the patient with trichomoniasis and other STIs is discussed in the section titled "Nursing Care of the Patient With a Sexually Transmitted Infection."

HUMAN PAPILLOMAVIRUS

Infection with human papillomavirus (HPV) is the most common STI in the United States, with more than 14 million new cases reported every year. More than 200 types of HPV exist, some classified as *low-risk* types and others as *high-risk* types. High-risk types have been associated with cervical, vulvar, vaginal, anal, penile, oral, and oropharyngeal cancer, whereas low-risk types of HPV are associated with condylomata acuminata, or genital warts. Although not always seen, the presence of genital warts is the most easily recognized sign of HPV infection. They generally affect the genital and anal regions of both men and women. Transmission of the virus is by vaginal, anal, or genital contact with an infected person. Incidents of transmission have been reported from persons who had no visible signs of infection. The incubation period usually ranges from 3 weeks to 8 months.

Fortunately, three vaccines are available. Gardasil protects against four types of HPV, including types 6 and 11 that cause 90% of all genital warts and types 16 and 18 that cause 70% of cervical cancers. Gardasil 9, which is used in the U.S., protects against types 6, 11, 16, 18, 31, 33, 45, 52, and 58. Cervarix protects against types 16 and 18 only but is believed to confer protection for a longer period of time. The CDC (2021) recommends that girls and boys who begin the vaccination series between ages 9 and 14 years receive two doses. Those who initiate the series between ages 15 and 26 years and individuals who are immunocompromised should have the three-dose series.

Clinical Manifestations

Condylomata warts are generally pink or red and soft, with a cauliflower-like appearance. These lesions may

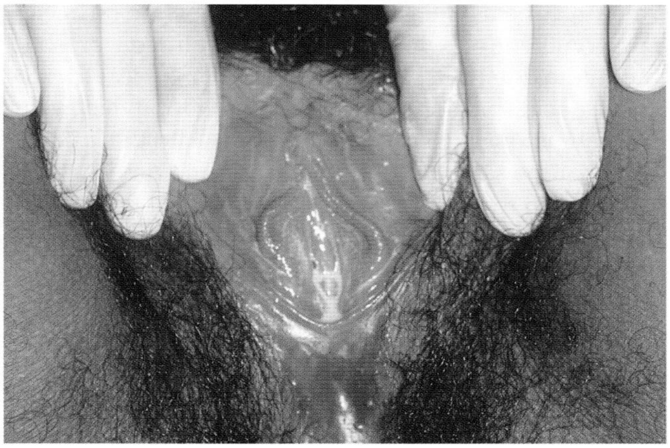

Fig. 55.3 Trichomonas vaginal discharge is profuse and watery and appears purulent. (Courtesy Leonard Wolf, MD, New York, NY.)

Table 55.5 Herpes Simplex Infections

SIGNS AND SYMPTOMS	POSSIBLE COMPLICATIONS	MEDICAL TREATMENT	NURSING CONSIDERATIONS
Painful genital lesions, burning during urination.	Localized infections; risk of infecting baby on delivery.	Treatment is basically symptomatic and includes sitz baths. Acyclovir may minimize symptoms; however, no cure for herpes exists. Recurrences may be treated with acyclovir, valacyclovir, or famciclovir.	Ensure that the patient notifies sexual contacts. Inform the patient that the virus can survive on objects such as towels. Assist in decreasing the patient's anxiety by allowing them to verbalize feelings. Instruct the patient to avoid sexual contact when lesions are present and to use condoms at other times.

be single or multiple. Men generally have warts on the glans, foreskin, urethral opening, penile shaft, or scrotum. These lesions may be single or multiple. In women, warts generally appear in or around the vulva, vagina, cervix, perineum, anal canal, and urethra.

Less often, the lesions are seen on the labia and deep within the vaginal canal and endocervix. In men who have sex with men and women who engage in anal intercourse, warts are common in the anal area. Oral, pharyngeal, and laryngeal lesions occur as well. Multiple warts can become so large that they obstruct the vaginal opening or rectal canal. Genital warts tend to grow large if they are in an area that is kept moist by vaginal or urethral discharge. For unknown reasons, pregnancy can stimulate genital warts to grow very large (Fig. 55.4).

Medical Diagnosis

The diagnosis is usually made based on a simple observation of the warts. A biopsy of the lesions is necessary to make a definitive diagnosis. When genital warts are present, the physician will usually screen for cervical cancer as well as for HPV.

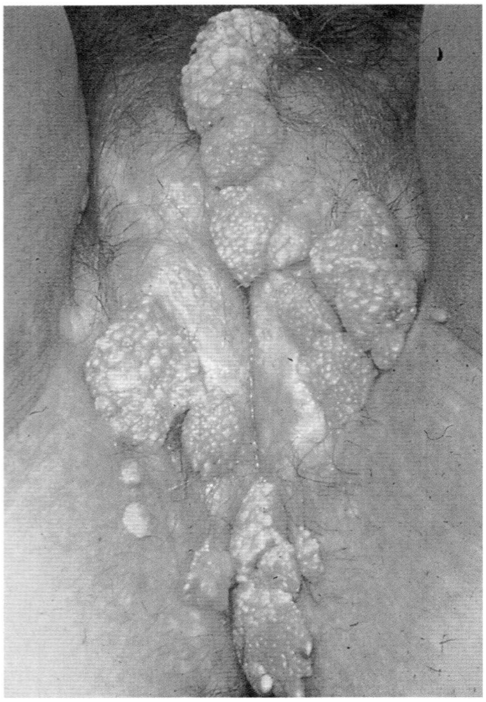

Fig. 55.4 Condylomata acuminata in a female patient. (Courtesy New York City Health Department.)

Medical Treatment

Genital warts may or may not disappear spontaneously. Although no cure for condylomata acuminata exists, removal of visible warts provides symptomatic relief. Some treatments, such as the application of podofilox, imiquimod, or kunecatechins, can be managed by the patient. Other treatments must be administered by the physician (i.e., cryotherapy, which uses liquid nitrogen or solid carbon dioxide [CO_2] to freeze the warts; topical trichloroacetic acid, bichloroacetic acid, or podophyllin resin; surgical removal; injection of interferon into the lesions). Note that the safety of podofilox and imiquimod and of podophyllin resin during pregnancy has not been established. None of these methods has proven totally effective in all cases. The recurrence rate is very high.

Nursing care of the patient with condylomata warts and other STIs is discussed in the section titled "Nursing Care of the Patient With a Sexually Transmitted Infection."

BACTERIAL VAGINOSIS

Bacterial vaginosis (BV) is caused by *Gardnerella vaginalis* and other anaerobic bacteria. The infectious bacteria tend to emerge when the normal bacteria in the vagina are suppressed. Risk factors include having a new sex partner or multiple sex partners, douching, and cigarette smoking. BV can be transmitted by sex toys, oral-genital contact, and fingers. Recurrences are fairly common and may be related to incomplete initial treatment. The usual signs and symptoms are genital irritation and itching, painful urination, a thin gray discharge, and a fishy odor; however, some women report no symptoms. The infection is diagnosed by microscopic examination of the discharge fluid and by culture. Some commercially available card tests are also available. The condition is treated with a course of metronidazole (Flagyl) administered orally or vaginally; or clindamycin vaginal cream. The patient is advised not to consume alcohol while taking metronidazole. The combination of alcohol and metronidazole may trigger a disulfiram-like reaction, with vomiting, tachycardia, and hypotension. When using clindamycin cream, the patient should know that the cream can weaken latex condoms and diaphragms. Treatment of sex partners has not been found to affect relapse or recurrence. (For a discussion of the potential complications of bacterial vaginosis, see the Health Promotion box.)

Pharmacology Capsule

If alcohol is consumed when taking metronidazole (Flagyl), the patient may experience vomiting, tachycardia, and hypotension as a result of an alcohol-drug interaction.

Health Promotion

Preventing Complications of Bacterial Vaginosis

In most cases, bacterial vaginosis causes no complications. However, an association has been documented between bacterial vaginosis and conditions such as pelvic inflammatory disease (PID), gonorrhea, and human immunodeficiency virus (HIV) infection. Bacterial vaginosis can also cause premature birth and low-birth-weight infants. Therefore some health experts recommend that all pregnant women be assessed for bacterial vaginosis if they have previously delivered a premature baby. A pregnant woman who has not delivered a premature baby should be treated if she has symptoms and laboratory evidence of bacterial vaginosis.

No longer considered merely a harmless annoyance, this condition is the object of serious study as research nurses and other scientists try to clarify its role in such conditions as PID and pregnancy-related complications.

HUMAN IMMUNODEFICIENCY VIRUS INFECTION

Many diseases that cause illness or death have plagued Americans, but it is likely that none of these has had the profound medical, social, economic, and psychologic effects as has the HIV infection known as *AIDS.* This syndrome is a disorder of the immune system caused by HIV. HIV gradually destroys T4 lymphocytes, which are essential for resisting pathogens. As the number of T4 lymphocytes declines, the patient becomes increasingly susceptible to opportunistic infections. An opportunistic infection is one that thrives when the immune system is impaired. HIV is transmitted through exposure to body fluids. No cure for the infection exists, although combination drug therapy can delay progress of the disease. Chapter 32 provides a thorough discussion of HIV infection and drugs used to treat it.

Put On Your Thinking Cap!

Consider this situation: A 30-year-old minister's wife is admitted after being injured in an automobile accident. While hospitalized, she is diagnosed with gonorrhea. You recognize that staff members are treating her differently since the gonorrhea was diagnosed. What behaviors would indicate lack of acceptance of the patient?

Do you think you would feel differently about this patient? What could you do to demonstrate acceptance and caring?

NURSING CARE OF THE PATIENT WITH A SEXUALLY TRANSMITTED INFECTION

FOCUSED ASSESSMENT

Assessment of the female and male reproductive systems is discussed in Chapters 51 and 53 and outlined in Boxes 51.1 and 53.1. When a patient has an STI, certain aspects of that assessment are especially important (see Nursing Care Plan: Patient With Gonorrhea). The licensed vocational nurse/licensed practical nurse (LVN/LPN) may be responsible for collecting important data to contribute to the assessment.

Health History

A thorough history is necessary to identify high-risk behaviors. A discussion of sexual behavior can be awkward for the nurse and the patient. Before nurses can deal with patients' sexuality, they must be aware of their own feelings and values. Privacy is essential for the patient interview. Questions about sexuality should be addressed in a straightforward manner. The interviewer should keep in mind that many patients lack scientific knowledge about the reproductive system and sexual activity. The patient may use some words that are considered crude by professionals, but the nurse must be careful not to embarrass or shame the patient. Many outpatient settings use computer programs to allow patients to respond to checklists and to describe their concerns either online or with a handheld device. Some patients may find this more comfortable than discussing their sexual history verbally. The health care provider can then scan the document to identify data that require exploration.

Present health/history of present illness. The history begins with an exploration of the patient's reason for seeking medical care. With an STD, common reasons include pain, fever, lesions, or genital discharge. Obtain a thorough description of the signs and symptoms, including onset, duration, and severity.

Past health history. In the discussion of past health, document serious conditions or chronic illnesses. The obstetric history may be significant as well. If the patient is of childbearing age, record the date of the last menstrual period. Record recent and current medications and note drug allergies.

Review of systems. The review of systems elicits potentially significant signs and symptoms, including weight change; fever; weakness; fatigue; skin rashes or lesions; oral lesions; dysuria; whether the patient is sexually active; pain, lesions, or lumps in the genitals; vaginal or penile discharge; and altered sexual functioning. It is important to document a history of blood transfusions.

Functional assessment. Relevant aspects of the functional assessment include frequency and variety of sexual behaviors, intravenous drug use, past infections with STIs, and sexual contact with a person known to have an STI. In addition, determine whether the patient may be classified as an *at-risk patient* because age (e.g., an adolescent experimenting with sexuality), sexual preference (men who have sex with men), or habits (drug use) place them at a higher risk for acquiring an STI. Victims of sexual abuse (of all ages) may have been exposed to STIs. Occupation may also be significant if the patient comes into contact with potentially infected body fluids. Health care providers at risk for exposure include nursing personnel, physicians, emergency medical technicians, operating room technicians, housekeepers in health care facilities, and medical laboratory technicians.

Physical Examination

The physical examination begins with inspection of the patient's skin for rashes and lesions. During the head and neck examination, the mouth is inspected for lesions. Palpate the neck for enlarged lymph nodes. Inspect the abdomen for distention and palpate for

Nursing Care Plan Patient With Gonorrhea

FOCUSED ASSESSMENT

Health History

A 23-year-old woman comes to the physician's office because of painful urination, abdominal pain, and vaginal discharge of 3 days' duration. She has had no serious illnesses or injuries. She has had two sexual partners in the past 6 months, with her most recent contact 2 weeks ago, when a condom was not used. The patient expresses concern about sexually transmitted infections (STIs) and human immunodeficiency virus (HIV). She states that she cannot believe she was "so stupid" and is very embarrassed about these symptoms.

Physical Examination

Vital signs: blood pressure 130/82 mm Hg, pulse 84 beats per minute and regular, respiration 14 breaths per minute. Temperature 98°F orally. Height 5′3″, weight 110 lb. The physical examination findings are all normal except for the genital and pelvic examination. The vaginal tissues are red and edematous, with a whitish discharge. A smear is taken for examination. The nurse practitioner makes a preliminary diagnosis of gonorrhea. A single dose of intramuscular ceftriaxone sodium (Rocephin) is ordered. The patient is also given a prescription for 7 days of oral doxycycline calcium (Vibramycin) because chlamydia often accompanies gonorrhea.

Patient Problems	Goals and Outcome Criteria	Interventions
Disrupted tissue integrity and acute pain related to infection and inflammation	The patient will report decreased pain and redness, and discharge will diminish.	Tell the patient that the symptoms should improve with treatment. Mild analgesics may be needed as ordered. Sitz baths may be soothing.
Potential for injury related to disease process	The patient will report for follow-up examination and remain free of signs and symptoms of complications.	Explain that persistent infection can lead to sterility and affect the heart and joints. Emphasize the importance of completing medications and returning for an examination to ensure successful treatment.
Anxiety related to possible complications of gonorrhea or stigma of sexually transmitted infection (STI)	The patient will express reduced anxiety and will be calm.	Provide opportunity to talk. Help the patient focus on the source of anxiety. For example, if she does not know what to expect, information is needed. If she is trying to decide how to discuss the condition with her sexual partners, help her solve the problem. Assure her that proper treatment is usually effective and prevents complications.
Low self-esteem related to diagnosis	The patient's self-image will improve, as evidenced by positive comments about self.	Be accepting and nonjudgmental. Assure the patient that she has done the right thing by seeking medical attention.
Inability to manage self-care related to lack of knowledge of disease process, treatment, or prevention of future infections	The patient will verbalize the importance of treatment, complications of untreated infection, and measures to prevent future infections.	Explore her understanding of gonorrhea. Provide information as needed. Emphasize use of condoms in sexual contacts to reduce risk of future infections with gonorrhea or other STIs. Ask about drug allergies before giving antimicrobials. Explain self-medication dosage, side effects, and adverse effects.

CRITICAL THINKING QUESTIONS

1. How can you help this patient to decide how to discuss this condition with her sexual partner?
2. Describe the best approach in addressing the patient's embarrassment about her condition. How might you put her at ease?

tenderness. Depending on the setting and your specialized education, you may examine the genitals or assist the physician or nurse practitioner in the examination. The examiner wears gloves to examine the genitals. A good light source is essential for thorough inspection. In the male patient, the examiner notes the general appearance of the penis, scrotum, and anal area. Any skin breaks, rashes, or redness is noted.

The LVN/LPN may prepare the female patient for a pelvic examination. While the patient is on the examination table and properly draped, the genitalia and the perianal area are inspected. The labia are separated and inspected for skin breaks, redness, or rashes. If a vaginal examination is to be done, ensure that the speculum and other supplies are ready. The speculum is warmed and lubricated before insertion in the vagina. Tissue and fluid specimens may be taken, including tissue scrapings for a Pap test. You may be responsible for preparing the specimen and sending it to the laboratory.

In cases of sexual assault, it is especially important that the examiner be specially trained to deal with such situations. Not only does the patient need a great deal of support, but the examination may produce evidence that must be preserved for legal purposes.

If a discharge is present, its color, amount, and consistency are recorded. Specimens may be collected for laboratory study. The specimen is handled as infective material, prepared according to agency procedures, labeled, and sent to the laboratory.

Assessment of the patient with an STI is outlined in Box 55.1. Most patients with STDs are treated as outpatients, and able to carry out their own treatments.

Patient Problems, Goals, and Outcome Criteria: Sexually Transmitted Infection

Patient Problems	Goals and Outcome Criteria
Disrupted tissue integrity related to lesions, rash	Restored tissue integrity: healed, intact skin and mucous membranes
Acute pain related to lesions, inflammation	Pain relief: patient reports pain is relieved, relaxed manner
Potential for injury related to disease process, complications, potential adverse effects of drugs	Freedom from additional injury: absence of signs and symptoms of complications
Anxiety related to possible effects of sexually transmitted infection (STI), reaction of partner	Reduced anxiety: patient reports anxiety is reduced, calm manner
Low self-esteem related to diagnosis of STI	Improved self-esteem: increased positive comments about self, confident manner
Altered social relationships related to presence of communicable disease, social stigma	Resumption of satisfying social interactions: patient states is satisfied with socialization
Impaired sexual function related to fear of transmission, impaired tissue integrity	Practices safe sexual behaviors: patient accurately describes safe behaviors, indicates will not engage in unsafe behavior
Inadequate coping related to stigma associated with STI, shame, anger	Effective coping: patient states is better able to deal with stress of condition
Ineffective management self-care related to denial, embarrassment, lack of understanding of disease process, mode of transmission, treatment, and prevention	Effective management of therapeutic plan: patient seeks medical care and follow-up, accurately describes self-care measures, expresses intent to follow plan of care and preventive measures

Box 55.1 Assessment of the Patient With a Sexually Transmitted Infection

HEALTH HISTORY

Reason for Seeking Care/Present Health

Pain, fever, lesions, genital discharge

Past Health History

Serious conditions, chronic conditions, hemophilia, obstetric history, date of last menstrual period, recent and current medications

Review of Systems

Weight change, fever, weakness, fatigue, skin rashes or lesions, oral lesions, dysuria, whether sexually active, sexual contact with a person known to have a sexually transmitted infection (STI), sexual dysfunction, history of blood transfusions

Functional Assessment

Frequency and variety of sexual behaviors, intravenous drug use, past STIs, sexual preference, occupational exposure to infective material

Physical Examination

General Survey: Distress, lethargy

Skin: Rashes, lesions

Mouth: Lesions

Abdomen: Distention, tenderness

Genitals: General appearance; lesions; rashes; redness; color, amount, odor, and consistency of discharge

Interventions

Disrupted tissue integrity. Ensure that patients who will treat themselves at home understand the prescribed therapy and how to protect others from infection.

If the patient has visible lesions, advise them to monitor the condition and contact the health care provider if there is no improvement with treatment. Signs of systemic infection including fever, chills, and flu-like symptoms also should be reported. Explain prescribed treatments such as oral and topical medications, and sitz baths.

If you have daily contact with the patient, assess the skin on a daily basis. Record changes in lesions. Carry out orders for treatments or instruct the patient, including topical medications and sitz baths for patients in health care settings. Monitor the patient's temperature at regular intervals to detect fever that may accompany acute infection. Handle soiled clothing and bed linens in accordance with agency policy.

Acute pain. Some STIs are painless, but patients may have pain associated with pelvic infection, oral lesions, or rectal lesions. The lesions of HSV are especially painful. Instruct the patient in use of analgesics, topical medications, ice packs, or warm compresses as ordered.

Potential for injury. Untreated STIs can lead to serious complications such as PID and sterility. The patient with AIDS is at high risk for secondary infections (called *opportunistic infections*) because of impaired immune function. Infected patients also pose a threat to their sexual partners. An STI may be passed to the fetus in utero or transmitted during delivery. Therefore it is important for the patient to receive the entire course of prescribed therapy. In addition, stress the importance of notifying sexual contacts so that they can be tested and treated as well, if necessary.

Drug therapy has the potential for injury. Before administering medications, assess the patient's allergies. When injections are given to an outpatient, ask the patient to remain for 30 minutes afterward in case an allergic reaction occurs. Emergency drugs, including epinephrine, corticosteroids, and diphenhydramine hydrochloride (Benadryl), must be readily available. Information about drugs commonly used to treat STIs is presented in Table 55.1.

Anxiety. The patient may be anxious about the outcome of treatment and the potential complications of the disease. Anxiety may be heightened by the stigma associated with having contracted an STI and the patient may feel ashamed. Encourage the patient to verbalize fears and frustrations. Provide accurate information and teach the patient how to avoid reinfection and infecting others. Patients with HIV infections also must deal with a potentially life-threatening illness.

Low self-esteem. The patient's self-esteem may suffer because of a diagnosed STI. Provide an opportunity for the patient to talk about the effects of the disease on self-concept. Try to guide the patient to focus on their positive attributes. If the patient's self-esteem remains low despite nursing intervention, a referral to a mental health counselor may be suggested.

Altered social relationships. A diagnosis of STI can be very distressing to the patient, who may fear rejection by others. The patient may be angry at the person who transmitted the infection and may be concerned about infecting others. Because STIs must be reported to public health authorities who attempt to trace all sexual contacts, the patient may also fear reprisals. One way you can help is by demonstrating acceptance of the patient through kindness and touch.

Impaired sexual function. Patients with STIs may experience sexual dysfunction related to fear of transmission, the presence of lesions, or anxiety. In addition, precautions that should be taken to prevent transmission of the disease may require changes in sexual practices. In general, sexual activity should be avoided until the infection is cured. Chronic infections such as HSV and HIV require permanent alterations in sexual activity. Explore the importance of sexual activity to the patient. Accept the patient's feelings in a nonjudgmental way. Explain that emotions and sexual function are closely related and that dysfunction may be overcome by dealing with the emotional reactions to the disease. For persistent dysfunction, advise the patient to discuss the problem with the health care provider who may make a referral to a therapist who specializes in sexual dysfunction. Encourage the patient to communicate openly with the sexual partner about the difficulties experienced. Alternative means of sexual expression (other than intercourse) may be suggested. Box 55.2 compares the relative safety of various sexual practices.

Box 55.2 Sex Practices to Reduce the Risk of Disease Transmission

SAFER SEX PRACTICES: Reduce the risk of mucous membranes or broken skin being exposed to the infected body fluids:

- Use latex or polyurethane condom for genital and anal intercourse
- Use a condom or latex barrier over the genitals or anus during oral-genital or oral-anal sexual contack
- Wear gloves for finger or hand contact with the vagina or rectum
- Practice abstinence
- Practice mutual monogamy
- Decrease the number of sexual partners

Modified from Rebar, CR: Concepts of care for patients with sexually transmitted infections. In Ignatavicius DD, Workman ML, Rebar CR., & Heimgartner N M, editors: *Medical-Surgical Nursing,* (10th ed.). St. Louis, 2021, Elsevier

Inadequate coping. Ineffective coping may be related to guilt, shame, anger, actual or anticipated rejection, or a combination of these reactions. Behaviors associated with ineffective coping include failure to adhere to the prescribed treatment, failure to exercise precautions to prevent spread of the disease or reinfection, chronic anxiety or depression, and inability to cope. The patient with an HIV infection must also deal with the potential for developing AIDS, sometimes with inadequate personal support. Show support for the patient by being sensitive, courteous, and nonjudgmental. Point out dangerous behaviors. Encourage the patient to evaluate their lifestyle and to identify modifications that could reduce future risks (see the Nutrition Considerations box). You may refer patients who have HSV and HIV infections to support groups. A spiritual counselor may also be suggested if the patient desires.

Nutrition Considerations

1. Persons with oral lesions may require modified diets.
2. Patients who are taking antibiotics are generally advised to drink at least 2000 mL of fluids each day to prevent harm to the kidneys.

Ineffective management self-care. Patient teaching is essential for effective treatment and prevention of future infections. Explain to the patient what causes the infection, how it is transmitted, how it can be prevented (including "safer sex" practices), and why treatment and follow-up care are important. (See the Patient Teaching box.) The term *safer sex* is considered more accurate than *safe sex* because no sex with a partner can be guaranteed to be safe. However, there are precautions people can take to reduce the risk of disease transmission.

Patient Teaching

Sexually Transmitted Infections

- Be sure to complete the prescribed course of antibiotics and return so that the physician can determine whether the treatment has been effective.
- Sexually transmitted infections (STIs) are transmitted by sexual contact. Avoid sexual contact with high-risk individuals: people who have had multiple sex partners, prostitutes, and those with known human immunodeficiency virus (HIV) or hepatitis B virus (HBV).
- Avoid sexual activity until your infection is cured.
- If you engage in sexual activity that involves any genital contact, use condoms.
- If you have sexual contact with high-risk individuals, people you do not know well, or persons who do not use condoms, you should have periodic medical examinations.
- Use condoms if you have condylomata (genital warts).
- If you have herpes simplex virus (HSV) infection, you should abstain from sexual activity when lesions are present. Use condoms always. It is important to realize that although periods of remission are seen, the condition is chronic and transmissible.
- Women with HPV, HSV, or condylomata are advised to have annual Papanicolaou tests because they are at increased risk of cervical cancer.
- If you have HIV infection, medical treatment may prevent or delay the development of acquired immunodeficiency syndrome (AIDS). Precautions must be taken to prevent infecting sexual partners even though you may not have signs and symptoms of disease.
- Because HIV is transmitted through body fluids, you cannot donate blood if you are HIV positive.
- Drugs that help to prevent HIV (PrEP) must be taken regularly.
- Postexposure HIV prophylaxis (PEP) must be taken within 72 hours of exposure.

Knowledge does not guarantee compliance, but patients cannot comply unless they understand what they need to do to care for themselves. Determine what the patient knows about the infection. Provide information about the disease and its treatment in terms the patient can understand. If the patient can read, include supplementary written material. Stress the importance of completing the course of therapy and returning for follow-up to reduce the risk of complications associated with untreated disease. Evaluate the patient's understanding of the material covered and explore any barriers that might prevent the patient from following the instructions.

CONDOM USE

Many people do not know how to use condoms correctly. At this time, only male condoms are in common use, although female condoms are available. Dental dams are used for oral sex.

Illustrated instructions of the use of male and female condoms and dental dams can be seen at:

- https://www.cdc.gov/condomeffectiveness/dental-dam-use.html
- https://www.cdc.gov/condomeffectiveness/male-condom-use.html
- https://www.cdc.gov/condomeffectiveness/female-condom-use.html

See the Patient Teaching boxes.)

Patient Teaching

Use of a Male Condom

- Condoms do not provide 100% protection against disease transmission.
- Latex condoms are preferred because some pathogens can pass through natural membrane condoms.
- Protect condoms from heat and sunlight to keep them from deteriorating.
- Do not use condoms that are brittle, discolored, or in damaged packages.
- Use only water-based lubricants because other lubricants can cause the condom to break. Spermicides may be used.

Place the condom on the head of the erect, hard penis. If uncircumcised, pull back the foreskin first.

- Hold the condom by the tip and unroll it onto the penis.
- Leave a space of about 1 inch at the tip for semen. Pinch the air out of the tip
- Withdraw the penis carefully after ejaculation to prevent the condom from slipping off and spilling the contents and to avoid unprotected contact.
- Always discard used condoms for sanitary disposal.

DENTAL DAM USE

Dental dams are latex or polyurethane sheets used to prevent contact between the mouth and vagina or anus during oral sex.

Patient Teaching

Use of a Dental Dam

- Use a new latex or polyurethane dental dam with every oral sex encounter.
- Read the package and check for expiration date.
- Use only water-based or silicone-based lubricant to prevent breakage.
- Make sure there are no tears or defects.
- Put the dental dam on before starting oral sex and keep it on until finished.
- Carefully open the dental dam from the package.
- Place the dental dam flat to cover the vaginal opening or anus.
- When finished, throw away used dental dam in trash.

Patient Teaching

Use of a Female Condom

- The female condom has a thick inner ring that is placed in the vagina and holds the condom in place.
- The thin outer ring remains outside the body and covers the vaginal opening.
- Hold the outside of the condom at the closed end. Squeeze the sides of the inner ring together with the thumb and forefinger and insert into the vagina.
- Use a finger to push the inner ring up as far as it will go until it rests against the cervix.
- Be sure the condom is not twisted.
- Insert the partner's penis into the opening of the condom.
- Stop intercourse if the penis slips outside the condom or the outer ring is pushed into the vagina.
- When finished, twist the outer ring and pull the condom out of the vagina. Discard.

Get Ready for the NCLEX® Examination!

Key Points

- One factor contributing to increased rates of STIs in women is reinfection from an untreated sexual partner.
- EPT (expedited partner therapy) is an approach to treating partners of persons with STIs. The infected patient is provided with a prescription or extra medications to give to the partner.
- EPT is being used by many clinicians in the United States for gonorrhea and chlamydial infection.
- Gonorrhea is one of the most commonly reported STIs in the United States, but it often has no symptoms.
- Gonorrhea can lead to damage to the heart and joints as well as to PID.
- Chlamydial infection is diagnosed in more than 1 million people in the United States each year; it can result in sterility in both sexes.
- Syphilis, if untreated, progresses through four stages, with eventual damage to the cardiovascular and nervous systems, the skin, and the joints.
- Newborns of women with gonorrhea or chlamydial infection may acquire eye infections during birth.
- HSV can be transmitted by sexual contact; however, it can also be transmitted by hand contact.
- Because HSV increases the risk of cervical cancer in infected women, they are advised to have annual Pap tests.
- Condylomata acuminata (genital warts) is caused by HPV and has a high rate of recurrence despite drug therapy, cryotherapy, cautery, and surgical or laser excision.
- Infection with HIV leaves the patient unable to resist opportunistic infections.
- HIV is transmitted through exposure to body fluids and no cure exists for the infection, although combination drug therapy can delay progress of the disease.
- Most STIs, except HSV infection and HIV infection, can be cured by antimicrobials.
- HSV infection is minimized but not cured by acyclovir sodium (Zovirax).
- Abstinence from sexual contact is the best way to prevent transmission of STIs but use of condoms during sexual contact also reduces the risk.
- Standard Precautions prescribe specific protective measures for health care providers to take when working with people who have infections that can be transmitted through body fluids.
- The nursing care of patients with STIs may address disrupted tissue integrity, pain, potential for injury, anxiety, low self-esteem, altered social relationships, impaired sexual function, inadequate coping, and ineffective management self-care.
- Patient teaching is essential for patients with STIs and should include information about drug therapy and other treatment options, disease transmission, abstinence during treatment, and preventive measures.

Additional Learning Resources

SG Go to your Study Guide for additional learning activities to help you master this chapter content.

Go to your Evolve website (http://evolve.elsevier.com/Linton/medsurg) for the following learning resources and much more:

- Fluid & Electrolyte Tutorial
- Review Questions for the NCLEX® Examination

Clinical Judgment and Next-Generation NCLEX® Examination-Style Questions

1. Which of the following is the purpose of reporting STIs?

1. To prosecute the individuals who are transmitting the disease to others
2. To emphasize to infected persons the importance of practicing safe sex

3. To reduce transmission of the infection by treating all infected persons
4. To teach the public about measures to prevent STIs

NCLEX Client Need: Safe and Effective Care Environment: Safety and Infection Control

2. **Nurses in the newborn nursery anticipate that erythromycin ophthalmic ointment will be ordered for the newborn of a mother who has: (Select all that apply.)**
    1. Genital warts
    2. Chlamydia
    3. Gonorrhea
    4. Hepatitis B
    5. Syphilis

    NCLEX Client Need: Physiological Integrity: Pharmacological Therapies

3. **A patient who was diagnosed with gonorrhea did not return for treatment. When contacted, she reported that her symptoms had gone away, so she thought she had recovered from the infection. The most appropriate response by the nurse would be which of the following?**
    1. "Without treatment, the bacteria remain in your body and you remain highly infectious."
    2. "If your symptoms have cleared up, no reason exists to treat you now."
    3. "If you have symptoms in the future, come to the clinic immediately."
    4. "Fortunately, gonorrhea has no serious complications, but I must advise you to seek treatment anyway."

    NCLEX Client Need: Health Promotion and Maintenance

4. **A patient who was admitted to the hospital after an injury is diagnosed with syphilis in the primary stage. During the nursing assessment, the nurse is likely to find:**
    1. A rash on the extremities, chest or back, palms of the hands, and soles of the feet
    2. A reddish papule or painless red ulcer on the genitals, anus, or mouth
    3. Tender lymph nodes in the area of the skin lesion
    4. Fever, sore throat, and generalized aching

    NCLEX Client Need: Physiological Integrity: Physiological Adaptation

5. **The patient with untreated syphilis may develop which of the following? (Select all that apply.)**
    1. Blindness
    2. Mental illness
    3. Paralysis
    4. Heart disease
    5. Osteoporosis

    NCLEX Client Need: Physiological Integrity: Reduction of Risk Potential

6. **In a health education class, the nurse is teaching the students about HSV infection. Which statements are true regarding the HSV-1 and HSV-2? (Select all that apply.)**
    1. "Type 2 is most often transmitted by genital contact."
    2. "The modes of transmission of both types 1 and 2 are the same."
    3. "Both types 1 and 2 can be treated with antiviral drugs."
    4. "Type 1 only affects the genitals and type 2 only affects the mouth."
    5. "Vaccines are available to prevent HSV-1 but not HSV-2."

    NCLEX Client Need: Physiological Integrity: Physiological Adaptation

7. **A young woman is being treated at the university clinic for a genital HSV-2 infection. The teaching plan for her should include which of the following statements? (Select all that apply.)**
    1. "You should have yearly Pap tests because you are at increased risk for cervical cancer."
    2. "You should not become pregnant because the herpes infection causes fetal deformities."
    3. "Once you have finished taking your medicine, you will be cured of the herpes infection."
    4. "Your partner must use a condom for intercourse even when lesions are not present."
    5. "Medications may reduce the frequency and severity of your symptoms."

    NCLEX Client Need: Physiological Integrity: Physiological Adaptation

8. **The teaching plan for a patient with genital warts should include which of the following statements?**
    1. "This condition cannot be transmitted to a sexual partner."
    2. "Genital warts are caused by poor personal hygiene."
    3. "A topical medication can remove the warts but is not curative."
    4. "Once the warts are removed, they are unlikely to come back."

    NCLEX Client Need: Physiological Integrity: Physiological Adaptation

9. **Information for effective use of condoms should include which of the following statements? (Select all that apply.)**
    1. "Condoms provide 100% protection against disease transmission."
    2. "Latex condoms are preferred over natural membrane condoms."
    3. "Use only oil-based lubricants to prevent breakage of the condom."
    4. "Leave a space of about 1 inch at the tip for semen."
    5. "Remove the used condom carefully to prevent spillage of contents."

    NCLEX Client Need: Health Promotion and Maintenance

10. **Which of the following STIs can usually be cured with antimicrobials? (Select all that apply.)**
    1. Gonorrhea
    2. Herpes simplex
    3. Syphilis
    4. Trichomonas
    5. Chlamydia

    NCLEX Client Need: Physiological Integrity: Pharmacological Therapies

11. **SLO Objective:** List nursing considerations when a patient is on drug therapy for a sexually transmitted infection.

NGN Item Type: Cloze

Cognitive Skill: Prioritize Hypotheses

A 25-year-old female graduate student is seen in the Student Health Clinic for an ulcer on her labia minora that appeared about a week ago. The lesion is red, but painless. The patient reports that she had a sexual encounter with an old boyfriend about one month ago. She has had no other sexual activity in the past 6 months. The health care provider suspects syphilis and draws a blood sample for testing. The patient has no chronic health problems and no history of surgery. She smokes one pack of cigarettes per day, and drinks alcohol occasionally. Vital signs: BP 126/72, Heart rate 74 beats per minute, Respirations 14 breaths per minute, Temperature 97.8°F.

Her tests confirm syphilis, and she returns to the center where she is given an IM injection of benzathine penicillin G. She is asked to remain in the waiting room for 30 minutes. Ten minutes later, the patient asks to speak to the nurse. The nurse collects the following data:

- BP 90/50
- Heart rate 104 beats per minute, regular
- Respirations 24 breaths per minute
- Temperature 98°F
- Pounding headache
- Sweating
- Feeling short of breath

Choose the *most likely* options for the information missing from the statements below by selecting from the list of options provided.

The nurse recognizes that a/an _______ blood pressure, __________ respiratory rate, and __________ are consistent with a/an __________. Failure to treat this health problem can *most likely* lead to __________.

OPTIONS
low
high
rapid
slow
allergic reaction
Jarisch-Herxheimer reaction
disulfiram reaction
dehydration
anaphylaxis
heart failure
dyspnea

Integumentary System Introduction

56

http://evolve.elsevier.com/Linton/medsurg

Objectives

1. Describe the structure and functions of the skin.
2. Define terms used to describe the skin and skin lesions.
3. List the components of the nursing assessment of the skin.
4. Explain the tests and procedures used to diagnose skin disorders.
5. Clarify the nurse's responsibilities regarding the tests and procedures for diagnosing skin disorders.
6. Explain the therapeutic benefits and nursing considerations for patients who receive dressings, soaks and wet wraps, phototherapy, and drug therapy for skin problems.

Key Terms

acrochordons
angiomas (ăn-jē-Ō-mă)
debridement (dă-BRĒD-mĕnt)
dermatitis (dĕr-mă-TĪ-tĭs)
keratolytics (kĕr-ă-tō-LĬT-ĭks)
lentigines
nevi (*sing.* nevus) (NĒ-vŭs, NĒ-vī)

ANATOMY AND PHYSIOLOGY OF THE SKIN

ANATOMY OF THE SKIN

The skin is an organ that covers the body surface. The anatomy of the skin is illustrated in Fig. 56.1. It is composed of two distinct layers: (1) the epidermis and (2) the dermis. The epidermis is the outermost layer that covers the dermis. The base of the epidermis continually produces new cells to replace those at the surface. Epidermal cells produce melanin, a dark pigment that helps to determine the color of the skin. Strong ultraviolet light, such as in sunlight, stimulates the production of melanin.

The dermis is strong connective tissue that contains nerve endings, sweat glands, and hair roots. The dermis is well supplied with blood vessels, causing the skin to redden when surface vessels are dilated. Subcutaneous tissue lies beneath the dermis.

The hair, nails, and sebaceous glands are appendages (or derivatives) of the skin. The hair root is located in a tube in the dermis called a *hair follicle.* The arrector muscles of the hair (i.e., arrectores pilorum), located around the hair follicles, can contract, causing the hairs to stand erect and the skin to take on a gooseflesh appearance. Also around the hair follicles are sebaceous glands that secrete an oily substance called *sebum.* Sweat glands, found in most parts of the skin, secrete water through the skin surface that contains salts, ammonia, amino acids, lactic acid, ascorbic acid, uric acid, and urea.

FUNCTIONS OF THE SKIN

The functions of the skin are protection, body temperature regulation, secretion, sensation, and synthesis of vitamin D. In addition, the blood vessels of the skin can serve as a blood reservoir.

Protection

The skin performs its protective function by shielding underlying tissues from trauma and pathogens, and by preventing excess loss of fluids from those tissues. A second type of protective function is fulfilled by Langerhans cells, which initiate an immune response when foreign substances invade the epidermis.

Temperature Regulation

The skin participates in temperature regulation by altering the diameter of surface blood vessels and through sweating. To dissipate heat, the blood vessels dilate. As the blood flows close to the body surface, heat is lost through the surface. To retain heat, blood vessels constrict, and heat loss is minimized. Sweating helps to cool the body because heat is lost as sweat evaporates from the skin.

Secretion

Sweat is one skin secretion; sebum is another. Sebum coats the skin, creating an oily barrier that holds in water. Sweat promotes loss of body heat through evaporation, as noted previously, and plays a role in excretion of wastes.

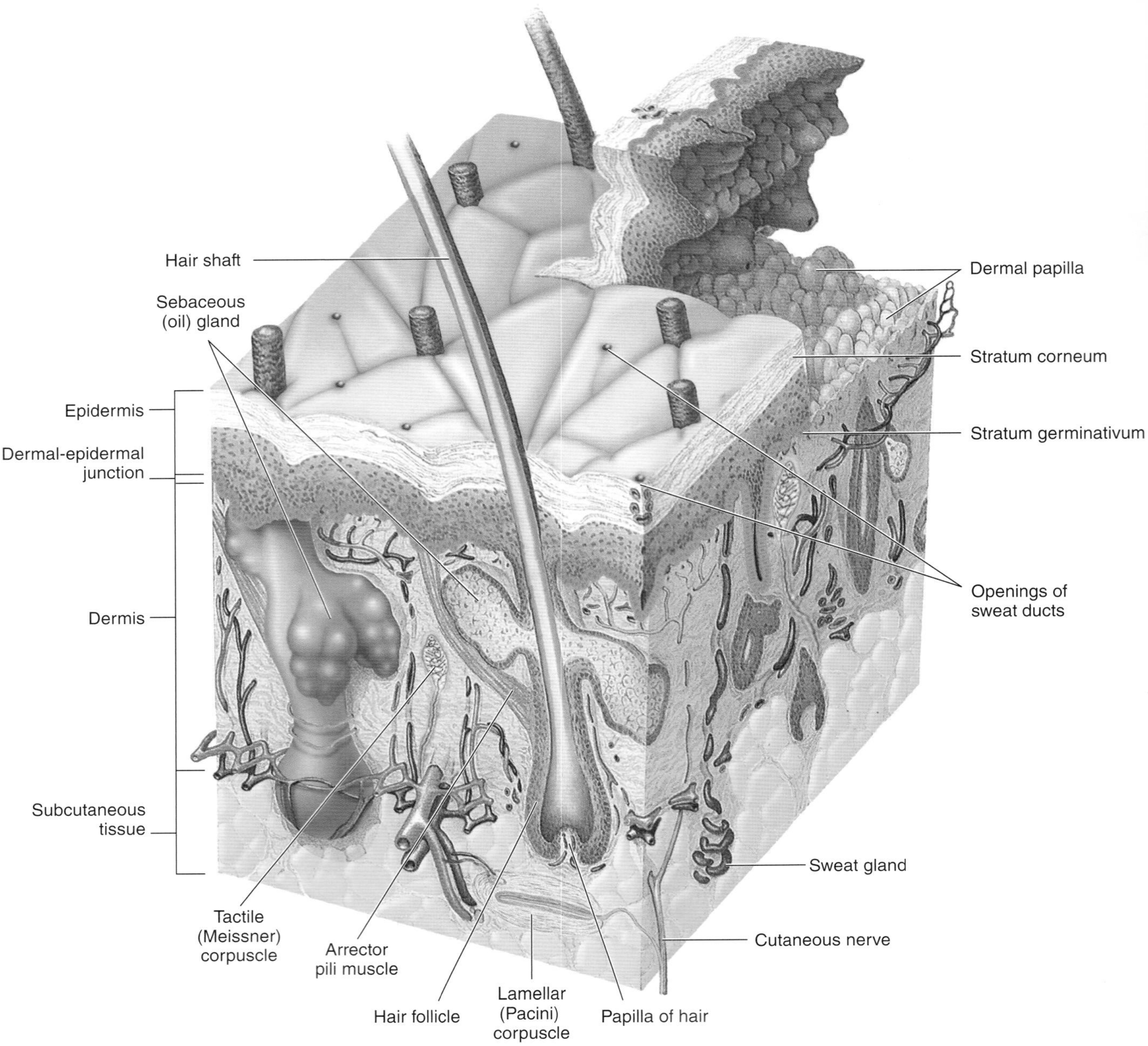

Fig. 56.1 Anatomy of the skin. (From Patton KT, Thibodeau GA: *Human body in health & disease*, ed 6, St. Louis, 2018, Elsevier.)

Sensation

The skin is heavily endowed with sensory receptors for touch, pressure, pain, and temperature. When these sensory receptors are stimulated, nerves convey messages to the brain for interpretation.

Synthesis of Vitamin D

Ultraviolet rays in sunlight activate a substance in the skin called *7-dehydrocholesterol* that undergoes a series of changes that eventually convert it into vitamin D.

Blood Reservoir

The skin contains an extensive blood vessel network that can store as much as 10% of the body's total blood volume. Constriction of these superficial blood vessels shunts blood to vital organs when needed.

NURSING ASSESSMENT OF THE SKIN

HEALTH HISTORY

Reason for Seeking Care and Present Health

When a patient has a skin disorder, the reason for seeking care may be discomfort, pruritus, color changes, lesions, hair loss, or abnormal hair growth. The onset of the condition and any precipitating and alleviating factors should be determined. Precipitating factors include any new medications, soaps, laundry detergent, or perfumes that may have been added within the last

Box 56.1 Assessment of the Patient With a Skin Disorder

HEALTH HISTORY

Reason for Seeking Care and Present Health

Pruritus, skin color changes, lesions, hair loss, abnormal hair growth

Past Health

Skin diseases or problems; drug therapy; allergies; chronic illnesses: diabetes mellitus (DM), cancer, kidney failure, thyroid disease, liver disease, anemia

Family History

Family history of asthma, hay fever, eczema, food allergies, or skin cancer

Functional Assessment

Occupation, exposure to chemicals or other irritants, skin care habits, extent of sun exposure, dietary habits

Physical Examination

Skin: Color, pigmentation, dilated blood vessels, angiomas, nevi, lesions, rash, drainage, temperature, texture, moisture, thickness, edema, mobility, turgor, scars. Change in skin color or pigmentation, change in a mole, sores that heal slowly, itching, dryness or scaliness, excessive bruising, changes in nails

Hair: Color, distribution, oiliness, texture, nits

Scalp: Scaliness, lesions

Nails: Shape, contour, color of nail bed, blanching with pressure, capillary refill, angle of nail base

week. The progression of symptoms and changes in the distribution or appearance of lesions may be helpful in the diagnostic process.

Past Health

Document previously diagnosed skin diseases or problems, current and recent medications (including nonprescription drugs), and allergies.

Family History

Determine whether there is a family history of asthma, hay fever, eczema, food allergies, or skin cancer.

Functional Assessment

Because the functional assessment can provide important clues to skin problems, record the patient's past and present occupations, exposure to chemicals or other irritants, skin care habits, and extent of sun exposure. Note recent changes in the work or living environment. Also inquire about current stressors and sources of anxiety.

The nursing assessment of the patient with a skin disorder is outlined in Box 56.1.

The link between nutrition and skin health is discussed in the Nutrition Considerations box.

Nutrition Considerations

1. Vitamin A is essential for healthy skin.
2. Food sources of vitamin A are liver, avocado, pumpkin, sweet potatoes, carrots, spinach, broccoli, cantaloupe, and apricots.
3. Food allergies can cause atopic dermatitis.
4. Skin changes associated with malnutrition include cracked skin, dermatitis, xerosis (i.e., dry skin), purpura, and petechiae (i.e., purple or red spots).

REVIEW OF SYSTEMS

Inspect the skin with attention to the color and variations in pigmentation. Sun-exposed areas are typically darker than protected areas. Document dilated blood vessels and **angiomas** (i.e., benign tumors composed of blood vessels). Table 56.1 describes variations in skin color and the significance of each.

Cultural Considerations

It may be more difficult to assess some skin characteristics in dark-skinned people. To inspect for cyanosis, jaundice, and pallor, check the oral mucous membranes, the conjunctivae, the palms of the hands, nailbeds, and the soles of the feet. Look for differences in color between the area affected and the surrounding skin. Check skin temperature and assess for pain or itching.

Note changes in a mole, sores that have been slow to heal, itching, dryness or scaliness, excessive bruising, rashes, lesions, hair loss, unusual hair growth, and changes in nails.

The physical examination also may reveal other disorders that cause changes in the skin. Specific signs and symptoms may be associated with circulatory, respiratory, renal, hepatic, gastrointestinal (GI), and endocrine conditions. For example, skin manifestations may occur with diabetes mellitus (DM), cancer, kidney failure, thyroid disease, liver disease, and anemia.

Carefully inspect **nevi** (i.e., moles) for irregularities in shape, pigmentation, and ulcerations or changes in surrounding skin. **Nevi** are also palpated for tenderness and measured in centimeters. If a rash is present, describe the location, distribution, and characteristics. If any drainage exists, note the color, amount, and odor. Terms used to describe skin lesions are defined in Table 56.2.

Inspect the hair for color, distribution, and oiliness and palpate to determine the texture. Inspect the scalp for scaliness, infestations, and lesions. The term *lesion* is a general term that applies to wounds, sores, ulcers, tumors, and any other tissue damage. Examples of various skin lesions are pictured in Fig. 56.2.

Note the shape and contour of the fingernails and toenails and the color of the nail bed. Check capillary refill by applying pressure to the nail, enough to cause blanching, and then releasing the pressure. The color should return to normal within 3 to 5 seconds.

Palpating the skin is a way to collect data about the temperature, moisture, texture, thickness, edema, mobility, and turgor. Assessment of mobility and turgor is illustrated in Fig. 56.3.

Table 56.1 Variations in Skin Color

COLOR CHANGE	DESCRIPTION	CAUSES
Pallor	White or pale in light-skinned people, yellowish-brown in brown-skinned people, ashen in black-skinned people; may be evident in mucous membranes, lips, and nail beds as well as skin	Vasoconstriction because of acute anxiety or fear, cold, some drugs, cigarette smoking; edema
Erythema	Bright red	Increased local blood flow because of inflammation, fever, or emotions such as embarrassment or anger
Cyanosis	Bluish	Excess deoxygenated blood in the tissue because of anemia, respiratory disorders, or cardiovascular disorders
Jaundice	Golden or greenish yellow	Reflects increased bilirubin in the blood because of liver disease or destruction of red blood cells (RBCs)

Table 56.2 Common Skin Lesions

LESION	CHARACTERISTICS	EXAMPLES
Macule	Distinct flat area with color different from surrounding tissue	Freckle, petechiae, hypopigmentation
Papule	Any raised, solid lesion with clearly defined margins; <1 cm in diameter	Mole, wart
Vesicle	Raised, fluid-filled cavity; <1 cm in diameter	Herpes simplex, herpes zoster
Pustule	Raised, well-defined cavity that contains pus	Acne, impetigo
Patch	Macule >1 cm	Vitiligo
Plaque	Combined papules that form a raised area >1 cm in diameter	Psoriasis
Nodule	Raised, solid lesion >1 cm in diameter; may be hard or soft and may extend deeper into dermis than papule	Fibroma, xanthoma
Wheal	Superficial, irregular swelling caused by fluid accumulation	Allergic response, insect bite
Tumor	Firm or soft lesion that extends deep into dermis	Lipoma, hemangioma
Bulla	Thin-walled, fluid-filled chamber >1 cm in diameter	Blister
Crust	Thick, dried exudate remaining after vesicles rupture	Impetigo, weeping eczematous dermatitis
Scale	Dry or greasy skin flakes	Psoriasis, seborrheic dermatitis, eczema
Fissure	Distinct linear crack extending into dermis	Cheilosis, tinea pedis
Erosion	Shallow, superficial depression	Impetigo, herpes zoster, or herpes simplex lesions after vesicles rupture
Ulcer	Depression deeper than erosion; may bleed	Pressure injury, chancre
Excoriation	Abrasion caused by scratching	Scratching with insect bites, scabies, dermatitis
Nevus (mole)	Flat or raised; color darker than surrounding skin	
Cyst	Fluid-filled cavity in dermis or subcutaneous tissue	Sebaceous cyst

AGE-RELATED CHANGES IN THE SKIN

Changes in the skin are probably the most readily recognized of all signs of physical aging. Specific changes are listed in Box 56.2.

Fig. 56.4 illustrates some age-related changes in the skin.

The risk of premalignant and malignant skin lesions also increases with age. These are discussed along with other pathologic conditions in Chapter 57 under the section titled "Cancer."

By 50 years of age, approximately half of all people have some gray hair. Men commonly begin to lose some hair from the scalp in their fourth decade, and by 80 years of age many men are almost bald. Scalp hair thins in women as well, but usually this is less obvious. Many older women and men have an increase in facial hair and a decrease in body hair, especially the legs and underarms. Men may also have increased hair in the nares, eyebrows, or helix of the ear. In addition to aging changes in the skin and hair, the nails flatten and become dry, brittle, and discolored.

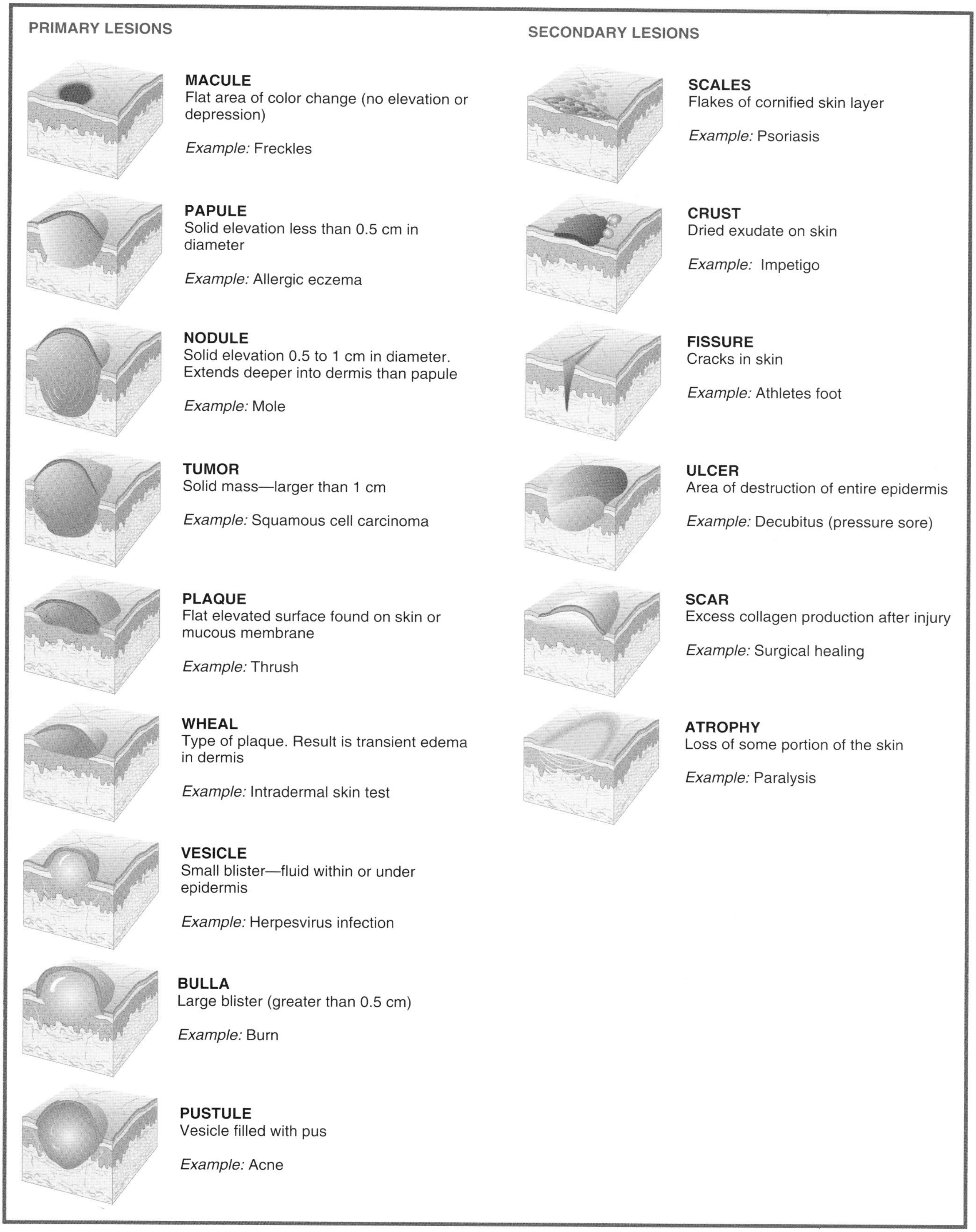

Fig. 56.2 Skin lesions. (From Proctor D, Niedzwiecki B, Pepper J, et al: *Kinn's the medical assistant: an applied learning approach*, ed 13, St. Louis, 2017, Elsevier.)

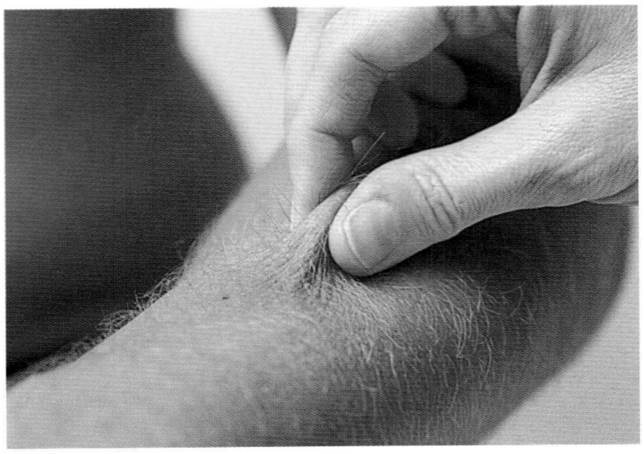

Fig. 56.3 Skin mobility is determined by assessing how easily a large fold of skin is pinched up. Skin turgor is evaluated by observing how quickly the fold returns to the previous position. (From Ball JW, Dains JE, Flynn JA, et al: *Seidel's guide to physical examination: an interprofessional approach*, ed 9, St. Louis, 2019, Elsevier.)

Box 56.2 Aging Changes in the Skin

- Thinning of skin layers and degeneration of elastin fibers resulting in wrinkling
- Decrease in size and number of sweat glands
- Decrease in production of sebum by sebaceous glands
- Dryness and pruritus (i.e., itching) increase
- Decrease in production of melanin resulting in increased paleness
- Development of skin lesions including:
  1. Lentigines: pigmented spots (liver spots) on sun-exposed areas (*sing.* lentigo).
  2. Senile purpura: large, purplish bruises resulting from minor trauma that resolve very slowly.
  3. Senile angiomas: bright-red papules.
  4. Seborrheic keratoses: waxy, raised lesions that are flesh colored to dark brown or black and variously sized from small and nearly flat to large and prominent.
  5. **Acrochordons** (skin tags): small, soft, raised lesions that are flesh colored or pigmented.

DIAGNOSTIC TESTS AND PROCEDURES

CULTURE AND MICROSCOPIC EXAMINATION OF SKIN SPECIMENS

Studies of skin specimens that are used to diagnose skin conditions include the following:

- Potassium hydroxide (KOH) examination is done to diagnose fungal infections of the skin, hair, or nails by studying a skin specimen. For a culture, a skin scraping or a nail clipping is implanted in medium.
- Tzanck test is used to diagnose viral skin infections.
- Scabies scraping is used to detect scabies (mites), eggs, or feces excreted by mites.
- Skin specimens may be cultured to identify fungal, bacterial, and viral infections.

WOOD'S LIGHT EXAMINATION

In a Wood's light examination, a black light is used to assess for pigmentation changes and superficial skin infections. It may also be used to examine the vulva after a sexual assault because it may reveal traces of saliva or semen.

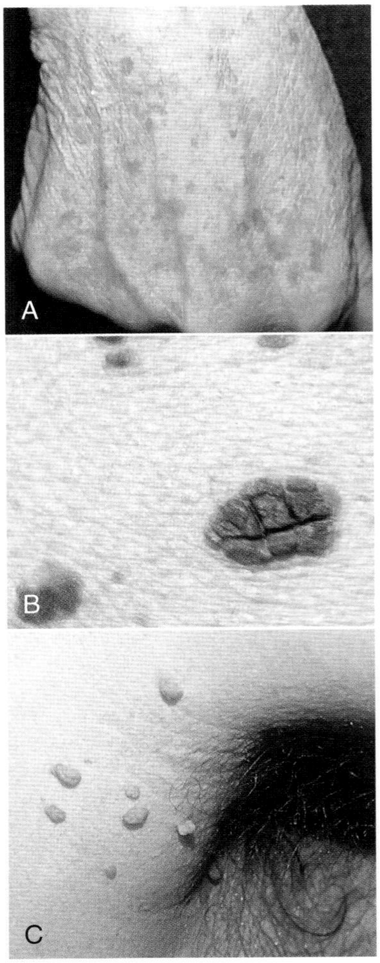

Fig. 56.4 Common skin changes in the older adult. (A) Lentigines. (B) Seborrheic keratoses. (C) Skin tags. (From Lookingbill DP, Marks JG: *Principles of dermatology*, ed 2, Philadelphia, 1993, Saunders.)

PATCH TESTING FOR ALLERGY

To identify allergens, very small amounts of common irritants are applied to the skin, covered, and later examined for allergic reactions. Assessment and treatment of allergies are discussed in detail in Chapter 5.

BIOPSY

A biopsy is the removal of tissue for microscopic examination. The types of skin biopsies (Fig. 56.5) are as follows:

- Shave biopsy: A specimen no deeper than the dermis is obtained with a scalpel or other specialized instrument. Bleeding usually is minimal and controlled with pressure, cautery, or chemicals.
- Punch biopsy: A circular tool cuts around the lesion, which is then lifted up and severed. Pressure or chemicals usually control bleeding, but suturing

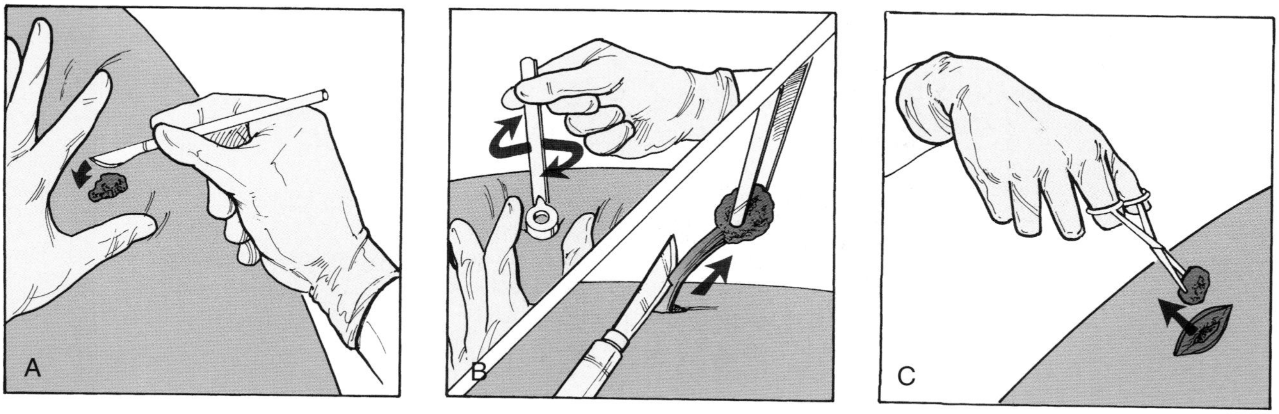

Fig. 56.5 Types of biopsy procedures. (A) Shave. (B) Punch. (C) Surgical excision. (From Black JM, Matassarin-Jacobs E: *Luckmann and Sorenson's medical-surgical nursing: clinical management for continuity of care*, ed 5, Philadelphia, 1997, Saunders.)

may be needed to close the site. The excision is relatively shallow.

- Incisional biopsy: A wedge of tissue is removed from the lesion.
- Excisional biopsy: For deep specimens, surgical excision biopsy is indicated. The entire lesion is removed. Sutures are required to close the defect left by the procedure.

Table 56.3 presents additional details and nursing interventions for patients undergoing diagnostic procedures.

COMMON THERAPEUTIC MEASURES

DRESSINGS

Dressings are used to protect healing wounds and to retain surface moisture to promote healing. Types of dressings include wet, dry, absorptive, and occlusive dressings. Dry dressings protect wounds and absorb drainage. Wet dressings are used to decrease inflammation, soften crusts, and promote tissue granulation. Absorptive dressings are used to promote removal of excess exudate and are especially useful in wounds with necrotic tissue. Occlusive dressings protect wounds and maintain moisture to promote healing.

NEGATIVE PRESSURE WOUND THERAPY

Negative pressure wound therapy, such as the V.A.C. systems, appears to reduce the time required for healing of traumatic wounds, dehisced surgical wounds, skin grafts, pressure injuries, and chronic ulcers. The wound is first cleansed with normal saline. Then a skin preparation product is applied around the wound to receive the adhesive dressing. The wound is then filled with one of two types of sponges, depending on the wound characteristics. A tube in the sponges is used to exert negative pressure. A transparent adhesive dressing is applied over the sponges and around the tubing so that the wound closure is airtight. The tubing is connected to suction that is set at a prescribed negative pressure. Suction may be applied intermittently or continuously as ordered. Continuous suction is less painful than intermittent suction. A small suction canister attached to the machine collects drainage from the wound. The suction canister needs to be checked periodically, as once the container is full, the suction will not function. Notify the enterostomal therapist, wound care specialist, or health care provider if the pain is distressing. The pressure may have to be reduced or converted from intermittent to continuous suction. Because dressing changes are painful, give the patient an analgesic about 1 hour before the procedure. When the suction is discontinued, the sponges are moistened with normal saline before removal to prevent the sponge from adhering to the wound.

SOAKS AND WET WRAPS

Soaks and wet wraps are used to soothe, soften, and remove crusts, debris, and necrotic tissue. Warm water is used, and various agents may be added for specific skin conditions. After a soak, gently dry the treated area. A wet wrap may be applied to a single affected area or to the entire body. It is usually covered by a dry dressing and left in place for 15 to 20 minutes. Moisten the wet dressing again before removal. Otherwise, healthy tissue may adhere to the dry material and be traumatized. If **debridement** is intended, the gauze is not moistened before removal because the purpose of a wet-to-dry dressing is to remove debris and drainage. Once a wound is clean, wet-to-dry dressing is no longer appropriate. After various soaks and dressings, topical medications are applied if ordered.

PHOTOTHERAPY

Phototherapy is the use of light in combination with photosensitive drugs to promote shedding of the epidermis. Types of ultraviolet light are ultraviolet A (UVA), ultraviolet B (UVB), and ultraviolet C (UVC). Phototherapy may be used in the treatment of

Table 56.3 Diagnostic Tests and Procedures for Skin Disorders

TEST AND PURPOSE	PATIENT PREPARATION	POSTPROCEDURE CARE
Potassium hydroxide (KOH) examination is used along with a culture to diagnose fungal infections of the skin and nails.	Inform the patient that a small scraping of skin will be taken from the affected area for microscopic examination. The skin scrapings and a nail clipping are used for cultures to determine the exact cause of the lesion. The procedure is painless.	Inform the patient when results will be available.
Tzanck test is used to diagnose viral infections.	Tell the patient the lesion will be washed and opened to obtain a fluid sample, which will be examined microscopically. The procedure may cause mild discomfort. The results may be available immediately.	No special care is required.
Scabies scraping is used to assess skin lesions for the presence of scabies (i.e., mites), eggs, or feces excreted by the mites.	Inform the patient that the top of a lesion will be taken off for microscopic examination. The procedure is briefly uncomfortable but requires no anesthesia.	No special care is required.
Wood's light examination uses black light to reveal superficial skin infections and changes in pigmentation.	Tell the patient the procedure is done in a dark room. The skin will be inspected carefully under black light. The procedure is noninvasive and painless.	No special care is required.
Patch testing is used to identify substances to which patients are allergic.	Inform the patient that various common irritants are applied to the skin and covered with special patches or tape. The patches must be left in place and examined ("read") after 48, 72, and 96 hours and sometimes after 1 week. Skin reactions that indicate allergy include redness, swelling, and blisters. Patch testing is painless.	No special care is required.
Biopsy is the removal of tissue for microscopic examination.	Tell the patient the physician will remove some tissue for diagnostic evaluation. Small, shallow biopsies usually require only a dressing. Deeper biopsies require sutures. Patients are usually advised to avoid aspirin or other nonsteroidal antiinflammatory drugs (NSAIDs) for 48 hours before the biopsy to prevent excessive bleeding.	Inspect the site for bleeding. Apply direct pressure if necessary to control bleeding. If sutures are used, instruct the patient to return on a specified date for suture removal. Tell the patient how to care for the biopsy site (protocols vary) and when results are expected.

psoriasis, vitiligo, and chronic eczema. It is contraindicated in patients with a history of herpes simplex infection, skin cancer, cataracts, and lupus erythematosus because it aggravates these conditions. After phototherapy, the patient may have pruritus and dry skin. Assess for signs and symptoms of phototoxicity (redness, vesicles, pain).

Phototherapy with a psoralen and UVA (PUVA) is a treatment that uses a combination of oral or topical 8-methoxypsoralen and UVA (long-wave ultraviolet light). It is used to treat vitiligo, psoriasis, and cutaneous T-cell lymphoma. For 8 hours before and after the treatment, the patient is instructed to wear sunscreen, protective clothing, and dark glasses to decrease exposure to other sources of ultraviolet light. The Goeckerman regimen is a type of phototherapy specifically used to treat psoriasis and atopic **dermatitis**. The patient first bathes in a tar emulsion bath. Then a topical tar product is applied, and the patient is exposed to ultraviolet light.

DRUG THERAPY

A number of topical and oral drugs are used to treat skin disorders and skin manifestations of other conditions. Topical drugs include **keratolytics** (capable of dissolving keratin), antipruritic agents, emollients, lubricants, sunscreens, tars, antiinfectives, glucocorticoids, antimetabolite agents, antihistamines, antiseborrheic agents, and vitamin A derivatives. Examples of selected drug classifications and their actions, side effects, and nursing interventions are presented in Table 56.4.

For topical application, drugs are combined with various substances in forms called *vehicles*. Topical medication vehicles include powders, lotions, aerosols, gels, creams, and ointments (see the Complementary and Alternative Therapies box).

Complementary and Alternative Therapies

Topical herbal preparations that are used as emollients include balm of Gilead, coltsfoot, and comfrey.

Table 56.4 Drug Therapy: Skin Disorders

DRUG	USE AND ACTION	SIDE EFFECTS	NURSING INTERVENTIONS
Keratolytics			
benzoyl peroxide (also an antimicrobial) salicylic acid sulfur coal tar	Dissolve keratin and slow bacterial growth. Used to treat dandruff, acne, and psoriasis.	Excessive dryness, irritation, scaling, edema, photosensitivity.	Advise patient to avoid excessive sun exposure. Assess effects.
Oral Antibiotics			
doxycycline minocycline tetracycline erythromycin	Acne	Sensitivity to UV light.	Ask about allergies. Wear protective clothing or use sunscreen. Report allergic reactions to antibiotics.
Topical Antibacterials			
bacitracin Polysporin (bacitracin and polymyxin B)	Destroy microorganisms. Used to treat skin infections. Also used on partial-thickness (first-degree) burns.	Contact dermatitis. Allergy (rare): itching, burning, anaphylaxis.	Ask about allergies before applying. Apply as prescribed after allergy ruled out. Report itching, burning, rash, redness.
silver sulfadiazine (Silvadene)	Bactericidal. Used to prevent and treat wound infection with serious burns.	Rash, pruritus, burning, pain. Rare: nephritis, anorexia. Can cause blood dyscrasias, hepatitis, nephrosis, hypoglycemia.	Apply to clean burn surface with gloved hands. Use a 4 × 4 or a tongue blade to remove the cream from the jar. Do not reinsert 4 × 4 in the jar. Cover burn completely and continuously. Monitor renal and GI distress, headache, joint pain, hepatic function. Monitor vital signs, CBC, serum glucose.
Antivirals			
acyclovir (Zovirax) famciclovir valacyclovir foscarnet	Interfere with viral replication. Used to treat infections caused by herpes simplex virus types 1 and 2 and herpes zoster. Not curative but may reduce severity and duration of symptoms.	Topical form: burning, stinging, pruritus. Oral form: nausea and vomiting. IV form: phlebitis, rash, urticaria, hypotension, hematuria, diaphoresis. Rare: confusion, agitation, seizures. Nephrotoxicity with high IV doses.	Ask about allergies. Monitor closely if patient has renal impairment. Measure I&O. Monitor infusion site for redness. Monitor neurologic status. Use gloved finger to apply ointment. Encourage adequate fluid intake.
Topical Antifungals			
nystatin clotrimazole (Mycostatin, Mycelex) oxiconazole (Oxistat) naftifine (Naftin) terbinafine (Lamisil)	Effective against fungi. Used to treat fungal infections.	Irritation, erythema, burning, rash. Abdominal cramps and cystitis with vaginal preparations.	Apply as directed. Do not apply occlusive dressings without order.
Oral Antifungals			
terbinafine (Lamisil) griseofulvin (Fulvicin P/G) ketoconazole (Nizoral)	Used to treat fungal infections that do not respond to topicals. Common use: nail infections.	Terbinafine: hepatotoxicity, headache, diarrhea, GI distress. Griseofulvin: headache, rash, insomnia, GI distress. Ketoconazole: hepatotoxicity.	Give ketoconazole with food or milk to minimize GI effects and 2 hours apart from any drugs that reduce gastric acidity. Monitor liver function with ketoconazole and terbinafine. Griseofulvin decreases effects of warfarin.

Continued

Table 56.4 Drug Therapy: Skin Disorders—cont'd

DRUG	USE AND ACTION	SIDE EFFECTS	NURSING INTERVENTIONS
Topical Antiinflammatory Agents			
hydrocortisone (e.g., Cortizone) triamcinolone (e.g., Aristocort) fluocinolone (e.g., Bio-Syn)	Reduce inflammation in various skin disorders.	Itching, erythema, irritation. Severe allergic reactions rare. Systemic absorption varies with specific drug preparation and size of area treated.	Do not apply occlusive dressing without order. Apply sparingly and rub in thoroughly.
Topical Antimicrobials			
azelaic acid (Azelex) clindamycin (e.g., Cleocin) erythromycin (e.g., Eryderm) benzoyl peroxide	Antimicrobial against *Propionibacterium acnes* and *Staphylococcus epidermidis.*	Pruritus, burning, stinging, tingling. Allergy: mild to moderate inflammatory acne vulgaris.	Avoid occlusive dressings. Keep away from mouth, eyes. Temporary skin irritation common. Two antiinfectives needed to prevent *P. acnes* resistance.
Vitamin A Derivative			
Topical: tretinoin (Retin-A) Oral: isotretinoin (Accutane)	Reduces formation of comedones. Increases mitosis of epithelial cells. Used to treat acne. Decreases size of sebaceous glands. Decreases sebum production. Used to treat severe acne. May decrease risk of skin cancer and PUVA.	Stinging, erythema, scaling expected. Allergy rare. Occasionally severe erythema, blistering. Excessive dryness of skin, nose, mouth. Conjunctivitis, vomiting, elevated serum triglycerides, bone or joint pain, muscle aches. Rare: hepatitis, IBD, depression. Cases of suicide have been reported in people on isotretinoin. Risk for major fetal deformities with isotretinoin. See www.ipledgeprogram.com for details of a program intended to ensure that pregnant women never take isotretinoin.	Tell patient not to use with keratolytics or other topical antiacne drugs. Do not apply tretinoin to eyes, mouth, angles of nose. Patient should avoid sun exposure, use sunscreen. If dryness is excessive, decrease frequency of use. Tell patient to expect symptoms to worsen at first, then improve. Report severe GI symptoms. Avoid sun exposure because of photosensitivity. With isotretinoin: Promptly notify prescriber if symptoms of depression occur. Because the drug is teratogenic, two negative serum pregnancy tests must be obtained before starting therapy. Explain importance of testing for pregnancy every month when taking therapy. Two reliable forms of contraception must be used simultaneously beginning 1 month before starting therapy and continuing for 1 month after therapy is completed.
tazarotene (Tazorac) adapalene (Differin)	Tazarotene and adapalene both are topical agents used to treat acne. Tazarotene is also used to treat psoriasis.	Both can cause itching, burning, and stinging. More serious skin reactions sometimes occur.	Advise patients to avoid direct sunlight and use sunscreens because of photosensitivity. Acne may worsen before beneficial results occur. Instruct patient on correct application (see instructions for each drug).
Pediculicides and Scabicides			
crotamiton (Eurax) permethrin (Nix)	Kill parasites and their eggs. Used to treat pediculosis (lice) and scabies (mite) infestations.	Skin and eye irritation. Systemic effects with excessive use.	Follow directions specifically. Avoid contact with eyes. Most products are effective with one application but a repeat treatment may be recommended. Clothing and bed linens must be treated to prevent reinfestation.

Table 56.4 Drug Therapy: Skin Disorders—cont'd

DRUG	USE AND ACTION	SIDE EFFECTS	NURSING INTERVENTIONS
Antipsoriatics			
anthralin and tar (Estar gel)	Used to treat psoriasis.	Anthralin: erythema, inflamed eyes, staining. Tar: skin irritation, photosensitivity, staining.	Protect skin and clothing from preparations that stain. Most have unpleasant odor.
Retinoid Antipsoriatic			
acitretin (Soriatane)	Decreases proliferation of epidermal cells; antiinflammatory, immunomodulatory. For severe psoriasis only.	Hair loss, skin peeling, dry mouth, rhinitis, gingivitis, elevated liver enzymes and triglycerides. Many other side and adverse effects.	*Contraindicated during pregnancy!* Ensure that patient understands risk to fetus and uses contraception if sexually active for at least 3 years after therapy is completed. Should be taken with meals. Monitor for all side effects.
Photosensitivity Drug			
methoxsalen (Oxsoralen)	Decreases proliferation of epidermal cells in psoriasis.	Nausea, headache, vertigo, rash, pruritus, burning and peeling of skin. Can cause anemia, leukopenia, thrombocytopenia, ulcerative stomatitis, bleeding, alopecia, cystitis.	Encourage patient to return for periodic blood tests as ordered and to report easy bruising or excessive bleeding.
Biologic Agents			
etanercept (Enbrel)	Used in the treatment of rheumatoid arthritis, psoriasis arthritis, plaque psoriasis. Neutralizes tumor necrosis factor.	Infection, Stevens-Johnson syndrome, heart failure, cancer, neutropenia, tuberculosis, thrombocytopenia, liver failure	

CBC, Complete blood count; *GI*, gastrointestinal; *I&O*, intake and output; *IBD*, inflammatory bowel disease; *IV*, intravenous; *PUVA*, psoralen and ultraviolet A; *UV*, ultraviolet.

Get Ready for the NCLEX® Examination!

Key Points

- The functions of the skin are protection, body temperature regulation, secretion, sensation, synthesis of vitamin D, and blood storage.
- A skin assessment may detect skin disorders and systemic disorders that affect the skin.

Additional Learning Resources

SG Go to your Study Guide for additional learning activities to help you master this chapter content.

Go to your Evolve website (http://evolve.elsevier.com/Linton/medsurg) for the following learning resources and much more:
- Fluid & Electrolyte Tutorial
- Review Questions for the NCLEX® Examination

Clinical Judgment and Next-Generation NCLEX® Examination-Style Questions

1. **You are caring for several clients with skin disorders. You understand that the skin regulates body temperature by which of the following?**
   1. Reacting to foreign substances that invade the epidermis
   2. Dilating and constricting surface blood vessels
   3. Secreting sebum to insulate the outer layers of skin
   4. Reacting to sunlight by producing vitamin C

   NCLEX Client Need: Physiological Integrity: Reduction of Risk Potential

2. **When inspecting the skin of an older adult, you observe flat, pigmented spots on the backs of both hands. You should recognize these as ______________________.**

   NCLEX Client Need: Physiological Integrity: Physiological Adaptation

3. SLO/Objective: Apply knowledge of anatomy and physiology and pathophysiology to determine which assessment data require follow-up from the nurse.

NGN Item Type: Enhanced Hot Spot

Cognitive Skill: Recognize Cues

A 75-year-old man is hospitalized for evaluation and treatment of atrial fibrillation. He has a history of hypertension and peripheral vascular disease. The patient states that he has minimal feeling in his lower legs and feet. He is constantly scratching his calves and ankles.

- Blood pressure 156/90 mm Hg
- Pulse 92 beats per minute, irregular
- Respirations 18 breaths per minute
- Temperature 99.6°F
- Dry mouth
- Fatigue and weakness
- Weak peripheral pulses
- Pruritus in lower legs
- Reddened areas in lower legs
- Nailbeds in feet unreactive to pressure
- Lack of hair on lower legs
- Skin on lower legs and feet is dry and flaky

Highlight or place a check mark next to the assessment findings that require follow up by the nurse.

Skin Disorders

57

http://evolve.elsevier.com/Linton/medsurg

Objectives

1. Identify and describe common skin disorders.
2. Describe the medical interventions and nursing considerations for patients with skin disorders.
3. Assist in developing a nursing care plan for the patient with a skin disorder.

Key Terms

acne (ĂK-nē)
debridement (dă-BRĒD-mĕnt)
dermatitis (dĕr-mă-TĪ-tĭs)
intertrigo (ĭn-tĕr-TRĪ-gō)
keratolytics (kĕr-ă-tō-LĬT-ĭks)
pemphigus (PĔM-fĭ-gŭs)
pruritus (proo-RĪ-tŭs)
psoriasis (sō-RĪ-ă-sĭs)

The skin or *integument* is an organ that covers the outer surface of the body. The functions of the skin are protection, body temperature regulation, secretion, sensation, and synthesis of vitamin D. In addition, the blood vessels of the skin can serve as a blood reservoir. Skin disorders, although not always life threatening, can be a great source of discomfort, have an impact on body image, and produce psychologic consequences.

PRURITUS

Pruritus or itching, is a symptom rather than a disease and is very common with many skin and systemic disorders. Therefore, an overview of pruritus is presented here.

CAUSE AND RISK FACTORS

The sensation of itching is not completely understood, but it may be triggered by touch, temperature changes, emotional stress, and chemical, mechanical, and electrical stimuli. The severity of the response to stimulation is enhanced by emotional stress, anxiety, and fear.

Pruritus is a prominent symptom with dermatitis, eczema, psoriasis, and insect bites. It also may be seen with the following systemic conditions: urticaria, some cancers, renal failure, diabetes mellitus (DM), thyroid disorders, liver disease, and anemia. Among the drugs that can cause pruritus are opiates and phenothiazines.

MEDICAL TREATMENT

To help soothe itchy skin, health care providers recommend the following:

- Apply a cold, wet cloth, or ice pack to itchy skin for about five to 10 minutes or until the itch subsides.
- Take an oatmeal bath.
- Use a moisturizer free of additives, fragrances and perfumes
- Apply topical anesthetics that contain pramoxine (bacitracin, neomycin, polymyxin, Neosporin, cortisone)
- Apply cooling agents such as menthol or calamine

To help prevent itching, health care providers recommend the following:

- Bathe with lukewarm water (not hot) and limit bath or shower to 10 minutes.
- Use fragrance-free lotions, soaps, and detergents.
- Wear loose-fitting cotton clothes rather than wool or rough feeling fabrics.
- Avoid extreme temperature changes; maintain a relatively cool, neutral humidity environment.
- Reduce stress, which can make itching worse.

(From American Academy of Dermatology Association, 2021. Retrieved from aad.org.)

Medications frequently ordered for pruritus include corticosteroids, antihistamines, and local anesthetics. In some situations, antidepressant and antiserotonin drugs may be prescribed.

Complementary and Alternative Therapies

When a patient has an allergic skin reaction, be sure to assess for topical use of herbal products. For example, aloe can cause allergic dermatitis in susceptible persons and angelica can cause a skin rash if a patient is exposed to sunlight.

INFLAMMATORY CONDITIONS AND INFECTIONS

ATOPIC DERMATITIS (ECZEMA)

Pathophysiology

Atopic **dermatitis** is one of several disorders referred to as *eczema*. Eczema has three stages. The *acute stage* is characterized by a red, oozing, crusty rash and intense pruritus.

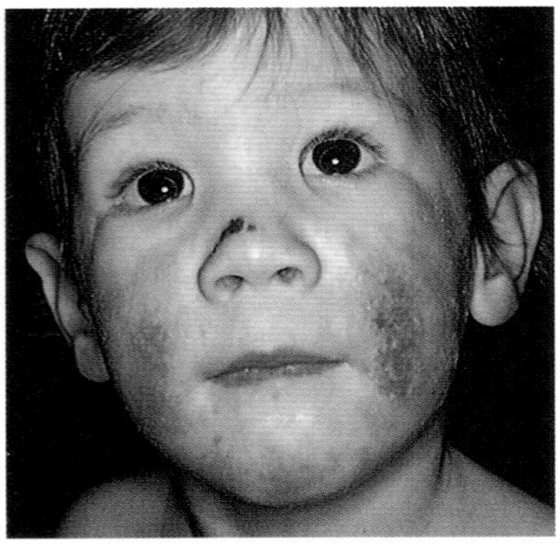

Fig. 57.1 Atopic dermatitis. (From Hurwitz S: *Clinical pediatric dermatology: a textbook of skin disorders of childhood and adolescence*, ed 2, Philadelphia, 1999, Saunders.)

The *subacute stage* is identified by redness, excoriations, and scaling plaques or pustules (Fig. 57.1). Fine scales may give the patient's skin a silvery appearance. In the *chronic stage*, the skin becomes dry, thickened, scaly, and brownish gray in color. Open lesions invite infection and scarring may occur. Multiple stages may be present at the same time. The areas most affected by eczema are the back of the neck, the elbow creases, and the backs of the knees. Other areas may include the face, trunk, wrists and forearms.

Cause and Risk Factors

Genetics plays a strong role in the development of atopic dermatitis, and most patients have a personal or family history of eczema and allergic conditions. There appears to be a genetic abnormality in the epidermis, so that the skin is less strong and more permeable. Therefore, the skin is less able to prevent environmental irritants, allergens and microbes from entering the body; in addition, the compromised skin is unable to prevent water from exiting the body. People with atopic dermatitis have an immune dysfunction, but it is not known whether that dysfunction is a cause or an effect of the disorder.

Medical Diagnosis

A medical diagnosis of atopic dermatitis is based primarily on the health history and physical examination. Determining factors include long-term and recurrent itching, symptoms that began at a young age, and symptoms that get worse after exposure to certain triggers such as cold or dry environments, sweating, emotional stress or anxiety, rapid temperature changes, and exposure to particular chemical agents or cleaning solutions. Procedures that might be done to confirm the diagnosis are skin biopsy, serum immunoglobulin E levels, and cultures to diagnose secondary infections. If allergy is suspected as a cause of dermatitis, the health care provider may perform allergy tests to identify allergens.

Medical Treatment

Emollients moisturize the skin and prevent it from drying out. Thick creams such as Eucerin, Cetaphil and Nutraderm, and ointments such petroleum jelly and Vaseline, can be used several times a day if needed and are most effective when applied after bathing. Lotions are less effective for moisturizing the skin than creams and ointments because they contain more water. Wet dressings can soothe and hydrate the skin, reduce itching and redness, loosen crusted areas, and prevent skin damage caused by scratching. Dressings should be changed every 8 hours. Lukewarm soaks, baths, or showers may hydrate and cool the skin and temporarily relieve the itching. Some health care providers recommend dilute bleach baths to help decrease the number of bacteria on the skin and to prevent worsening symptoms or infections. The bleach bath is prepared using ¼ to ½ cup of bleach in a full tub of lukewarm water (~40 gallons). The bath usually is taken for 5 to 10 minutes twice a week, followed by the application of an emollient.

Topical corticosteroids and moisturizers provide the best control of inflammation. However, steroids can cause skin atrophy, loss of pigmentation, permanent red lesions, and, with high doses, adrenal suppression. In severe cases that do not respond to topical agents, a short course of systemic corticosteroids may be ordered.

Oral antihistamines, such as over-the-counter diphenhydramine (Benadryl) or prescription antihistamines, such as hydroxyzine (Vistaril, Atarax), may be ordered to relieve itching. Because they cause drowsiness, they may be especially helpful when itching interferes with sleep. Nondrowsy over-the-counter antihistamines such as cetirizine (Zyrtec) or loratadine (Alavert, Claratin) can relieve itching during the day. Patients who do not respond to safer therapies may be treated with the immunosuppressants tacrolimus ointment (Protopic) or pimecrolimus cream (Elidel). These drugs may increase the risk of skin cancer and lymphoma, as well as an increased risk for infection. Treatment of allergic disorders is discussed in Chapter 5.

◆ NURSING CARE OF THE PATIENT WITH ATOPIC DERMATITIS

Focused Assessment

When the patient has atopic dermatitis, specifically inquire about known allergies, bathing practices (i.e., frequency, water temperature, use of soaps), and current medications to identify possible contributing factors. The physical examination includes inspection and palpation of the skin for lesions, moisture, and abrasions.

Patient Problems, Goals, and Outcome Criteria: Atopic Dermatitis

Patient Problems	Goals and Outcome Criteria
Disrupted skin tissue integrity related to plaques, open lesions, and pustules	Improved skin integrity: intact, moist skin
Potential for infection related to break in skin, decreased resistance to infection	Absence of infection: no fever, decreased redness and drainage

Patient Problems, Goals, and Outcome Criteria: Atopic Dermatitis—cont'd

Patient Problems	Goals and Outcome Criteria
Altered self-concept related to lesions	Improved self-concept: positive statements about self

Interventions

Disrupted skin tissue integrity. Use measures that decrease itching and moisturize the skin to maintain tissue integrity. Encourage the patient to keep the room temperature at 68°F to 75°F with 45% to 55% humidity. Advise the patient to avoid possible irritants. New clothing should be washed with mild detergent before it is worn, and clothes should be rinsed twice. Recommend open-weave fabrics and loose clothing. Advise the use of moisturizers and sunscreens. If drugs are ordered for pruritus, administer them as directed or instruct the patient in self-medication. Evaluate skin integrity and hydration on an ongoing basis

Potential for infection. Any break in the skin presents an entry for pathogens. Inspect the skin and report new lesions to the health care provider. Monitor the patient's temperature for elevation that may indicate a systemic infection. Teach the importance of protecting the skin from trauma. If scratching is a problem, the fingernails need to be cut short and kept smooth (see the Patient Teaching box). Gloves or mittens may help to prevent traumatic scratching during sleep or in the confused person. Administer antibiotics as ordered.

Patient Teaching

Atopic Dermatitis

- Avoid known irritants and constrictive clothing.
- Use moisturizers and sunscreens.
- Take drugs as prescribed: name, dosage or application instructions, adverse effects.
- After swimming in chlorinated water, shampoo and bathe or shower using a mild soap. Then apply a moisturizer.

Altered self-concept. Demonstrate acceptance of the patient's appearance through attentive care and touch. Teach the patient and family that atopic dermatitis is not contagious and is not caused by poor hygiene. Explore the patient's concerns about the skin disorder. If the patient is very stressed, the nurse can discuss coping strategies or request a referral for professional counseling.

CONTACT DERMATITIS

Contact dermatitis is an inflammatory condition caused by contact with a substance that triggers an allergic response. Allergic and immune disorders are discussed in Chapter 5.

SEBORRHEIC DERMATITIS

Pathophysiology

Seborrheic dermatitis is a chronic, relapsing inflammatory condition that may last for decades. It usually affects areas that are rich in sebaceous glands, including the scalp (most common form known as *dandruff*), forehead below the hairline, eyebrows, eyelids, external ears, sternal area, axillae, umbilicus, groin, gluteal crease, and area under the breasts. The mustache and beard areas in men also may be affected. Seborrheic dermatitis is characterized by fine, powdery scales; thick crusts; or oily patches. Scales may be white, yellowish, or reddish. Pruritus is common.

Cause and Risk Factors

The cause of seborrheic dermatitis is unknown; however, the condition may be an inflammatory reaction to the fungus *Malassezia* that grows easily in the *sebaceous* glands. People with HIV infection are more susceptible to seborrheic dermatitis, and there is an increased prevalence among people with Parkinson disease. The condition is aggravated during the cold, dry winter months and by emotional stress.

Medical Diagnosis

Diagnosis of seborrheic dermatitis is based on the health history and physical examination.

Medical Treatment

The goal of treatment is to clear the visible signs of the condition and to reduce symptoms such as erythema and pruritis. Seborrheic dermatitis is a chronic condition that may require long time maintenance treatment. Topical antifungal agents and antiinflammatory agents usually are prescribed. Antifungal agents such as ketoconazole (Nizoral) and ciclopirox are effective for the treatment of the scalp and face. Topical corticosteroids (e.g., hydrocortisone) reduce inflammation, erythema, and pruritis. Dandruff is treated with medicated shampoos used 2 or 3 times a week. Appropriate shampoos are those that contain selenium sulfide (Selsun), ketoconazole, tar, zinc pyrithione, salicylic acid, or resorcin. Some corticosteroid solutions also may be prescribed.

◆ NURSING CARE OF THE PATIENT WITH SEBORRHEIC DERMATITIS

Although seborrheic dermatitis does not require inpatient treatment, it is a common condition encountered among patients in the community and long-term care settings and among those hospitalized for other reasons.

Focused Assessment

Relevant data include symptoms and identification of treatments being used. Inspect and describe the affected areas.

Patient Problems, Goals, and Outcome Criteria: Seborrheic Dermatitis

Patient Problems	Goals and Outcome Criteria
Inability to manage treatment program related to lack of knowledge about disease process	Implements the prescribed treatment plan: correctly describes plan and self-care treatment
Altered self-concept related to altered appearance (lesions)	Improved self-concept: decreasing signs of the condition, patient's statements reflect a positive view of self

Interventions

Explain the condition and reinforce the health care provider's instructions for treatment. Suggest measures to relieve pruritus, as described earlier. Discuss the patient's concerns about the condition and emphasize that seborrheic dermatitis can be controlled with treatment. Demonstrate acceptance of the patient through genuine interest and use of touch.

ACNE

Pathophysiology

Acne is a skin condition that affects the hair follicles and sebaceous glands. The chief characteristics are comedones (whiteheads and blackheads), pustules, and cysts. The lesions develop most often on the face, neck, and upper trunk. Acne commonly begins in adolescence and may last throughout a lifetime. Most cases are mild, but serious cases with extensive inflammation can cause permanent scarring.

Cause and Risk Factors

Acne lesions develop when androgenic hormones cause increased sebum production and a proliferation of bacteria *(Propionibacterium acnes)*, resulting in blocked and inflamed sebaceous follicles. Despite popular opinion, acne is not caused by fatty foods, chocolate, or poor hygiene. In addition to androgenic hormones, exacerbations of acne can be triggered by high levels of progestin in birth control pills, oil-based cosmetics, high doses of systemic corticosteroids, hormonal changes associated with the menstrual period, and some endocrine disorders.

Pharmacology Capsule

Accutane can cause mental depression, possibly leading to suicidal ideation. Should depression develop, contact the health care provider immediately to have the drug discontinued. Depression should resolve once the drug is stopped. Should depression continue, the patient should be referred for additional counseling.

Medical Diagnosis

Acne is diagnosed on the basis of the health history and physical examination findings.

Medical Treatment

Treatment varies with the severity of the condition. Mild cases may respond very well to topical antimicrobials or retinoids (vitamin A preparations). Topical antimicrobials include azelaic acid (Azelex) and benzoyl peroxide; topical retinoids include tretinoin (Retin-A) or tazarotene (Tazorac). If these agents do not adequately control acne, oral antibiotics (i.e., tetracycline, doxycycline, azithromycin, erythromycin) may be given over a period of several months. Estrogen may be prescribed to counteract the effects of androgenic hormones, as well as spironolactone for its antiandrogenic effects. If acne is severe and unresponsive to all of these treatments, isotretinoin (Accutane), a derivative of vitamin A, may be prescribed.

Nonpharmacologic treatment may include comedone extraction or cryotherapy. Dermabrasion may be used to reduce scarring.

Pharmacology Capsule

Isotretinoin (Accutane) can cause severe fetal deformities. Thus, women who take the drug must prevent pregnancy until at least 1 month after therapy has been completed.

◆ NURSING CARE OF THE PATIENT WITH ACNE

Assessment

Explore the patient's concerns and knowledge about acne. Document any treatments being used. Note all medical conditions and medications because some contribute to or aggravate acne. Inspect the skin to determine the extent and severity of the condition.

Patient Problems, Goals, and Outcome Criteria: Acne

Patient Problems	Goals and Outcome Criteria
Altered self-concept related to acne lesions	Improved self-concept: fewer lesions and patient's expression of improved body image
Inability to manage treatment program related to lack of understanding of causes and treatment of acne	Effective treatment management: patient correctly describes and demonstrates prescribed skin care and self-medication

Interventions

Altered self-concept. Because acne almost always affects the face, most patients with moderate or severe acne suffer changes in self-concept. Be sensitive to this concern and encourage the patient to see a dermatologist for treatment. This condition can be harmful to the patient's self-esteem and should not be dismissed as a minor problem.

Inability to manage treatment program. Explain the causes of acne as well as the many myths about the disease. Assure the patient that acne does not reflect poor hygiene, but that cleanliness does reduce the risk of infections. Dietary interventions are no longer thought to be useful. Discourage picking or squeezing lesions because it may force infected material deeper into the follicle. Advise the patient that harsh cleansers and vigorous scrubbing have no therapeutic value.

Explain prescribed drugs and discuss any adverse effects. Patient teaching is especially important if isotretinoin is used. Isotretinoin is an oral medication that has a drying effect on the skin. Tell the patient to expect the condition to worsen initially and then begin to improve. Advise the patient that the drug is teratogenic, meaning that it is harmful to a developing fetus. Thus, two forms of effective contraception must be used if the patient is sexually active while taking the drug. When isotretinoin is prescribed for females, the patient must have two negative pregnancy tests within 2 weeks of starting therapy and one negative test before each monthly refill. The drug should be started on the third or fourth day of the next normal menstrual period. Because of the very high risk of fetal deformity, patients must agree to the terms of the iPLEDGE program to receive the drug. See www.ipledgeprogram.com for detailed information about this program.

FUNGAL INFECTIONS

Pathophysiology

Superficial infections of the skin and mucous membranes caused by fungi include tinea pedis (athlete's foot), tinea manus (hand), tinea cruris (groin), tinea capitis (scalp), tinea corporis (body), tinea barbae (beard), and candidiasis, which can affect the skin, mouth, vagina, gastrointestinal (GI) tract, and lungs.

Cause and Risk Factors

The organisms that cause tinea infections take advantage of trauma in moist, warm tissue. Some organisms can be spread through direct contact or by inanimate objects. Lesions vary but may be scaly patches with raised borders. The lay term *ringworm* is sometimes used to describe circular lesions. Pruritus is a common symptom of tinea. Scratching that breaks the skin may lead to a secondary bacterial infection. Tinea capitis, tinea corporis, and tinea pedis are easily spread by sharing contaminated objects.

Candidiasis, commonly called a *yeast infection*, is caused by *C. albicans.* Patients at risk for candidiasis include those with diabetes mellitus, who are pregnant, malnourished, immunosuppressed, and taking antibiotics or oral contraceptives. Common sites affected are the mouth, vagina, and skin. The skin around an ostomy site also is susceptible to candidiasis because of the constant moisture in the area. Infections of the mucous membranes are manifested as red lesions with white plaques. Skin infections with *C. albicans* are seen as moist, red lesions (Fig. 57.2). The lesions often are found in folds of body tissue (see section titled "Intertrigo").

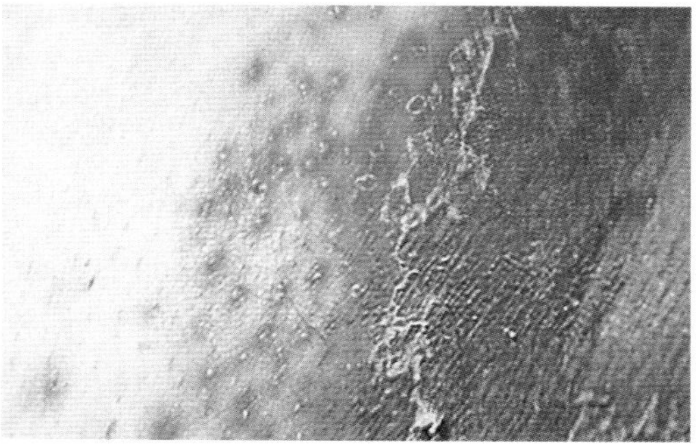

Fig. 57.2 Candidiasis. (From Lookingbill DP, Marks JG: *Principles of dermatology*, ed 2, Philadelphia, 1993, Saunders.)

> **Pharmacology Capsule**
>
> Antibiotic therapy eliminates the microorganisms that normally control fungal growth, making the patient susceptible to fungal infections.

Medical Diagnosis

Fungal infections are diagnosed on the basis of the history and physical examination but may be confirmed by microscopic examination of scrapings from a lesion using a KOH wet mount preparation.

Medical Treatment

Fungal infections of the skin and mucous membranes are treated with antifungal powders and creams. Wet compresses and **keratolytics** may be ordered to soften scales with some tinea infections. Butenafine (Lotrimin) is used for tinea pedis, tinea corporis, tinea cruris, and tinea versicolor. Oral candidiasis is treated with clotrimazole troches, oral amphotericin B, or nystatin mouthwash or lozenges. For acquired immunodeficiency syndrome (AIDS) patients, clotrimazole is superior to nystatin. Candidiasis of the vulva and vagina may be treated with topical azoles (e.g., clotrimazole, miconazole, tioconazole) or oral fluconazole (Diflucan). Systemic fungal infections require intravenous amphotericin B, an effective but very toxic drug. Patients receiving amphotericin B are pretreated with an antihistamine and a nonopioid analgesic to reduce the risk of chills, fever, and headache. Patients with severe adverse effects may be given a glucocorticoid and either meperidine or dantrolene for rigors (i.e., shaking chills).

> **Pharmacology Capsule**
>
> Systemic amphotericin B is highly toxic to the kidneys. An infusion of 1 L of saline on the day of treatment helps to reduce renal damage.

◆ NURSING CARE OF THE PATIENT WITH A FUNGAL INFECTION

Focused Assessment

Identify conditions that might make a person susceptible to fungal infections, including diabetes mellitus, malnutrition, and immunosuppression. Note antibiotic therapy, another risk factor. During the physical examination, inspect the skin and mucous membranes for lesions. Creamy white lesions that can be scraped off easily are characteristic of oral candidiasis.

Patient Problems, Goals, and Outcome Criteria: Fungal Infection

Patient Problems	Goals and Outcome Criteria
Disrupted oral tissue integrity related to oral candidiasis	Healthy oral mucous membranes: absence of oral lesions, infection
Disrupted skin tissue integrity related to skin lesions	Improved skin tissue integrity: absence of skin lesions
Altered self-concept related to skin lesions	Improved self-concept: absence of skin lesions, patient's positive statements about appearance

Interventions

Disrupted oral tissue integrity. Teach the patient with oral candidiasis the proper use of prescribed medications. Mouthwashes may be swished to coat all oral surfaces before swallowing. Lozenges should be dissolved in the mouth. If the patient wears dentures, they should be soaked in an antifungal solution.

Disrupted skin tissue integrity. Teach the patient the proper use of prescribed medications. Instruct the patient to keep the affected areas of the skin as clean and dry as possible. A cool environment helps by reducing perspiration. Advise patients with tinea infections to avoid sharing personal items such as hairbrushes and clothing. They should also dry thoroughly after bathing and wear absorbent underwear and socks. Eradication of candidiasis infections in bedridden patients can be especially challenging. Frequently reposition the patient to permit evaporation of moisture. The thighs can be separated by using a pillow between the knees and a folded cloth may be placed beneath pendulous breasts.

Altered self-concept. Be sensitive to the patient's reaction to a skin infection; visible lesions may be especially embarrassing. If the genitalia are affected, the patient may think that the symptoms are caused by a sexually transmitted infection (STI). Explain the cause of the infection, how it is treated, whether it is contagious, and how transmission and reinfection can be avoided.

DISORDERS OF THE NAILS

The two major conditions affecting the nails are (1) infections (fungal or bacterial) and (2) inflammation caused by ingrown nails. Infections are characterized by redness, swelling, and pain around the margin of the nail. They are treated with warm soaks and topical or systemic antiinfective agents. Fungal infections of the nail, called *onychomycosis*, are treated with a 3- to 6-month course of oral terbinafine (Lamisil) and itraconazole (Sporanox). Incision and drainage may be necessary.

Complementary and Alternative Therapies

A Listerine foot soak can be used at home to treat athlete's foot and onychomycosis (toenail fungus). Soak feet in one part Listerine and two parts of water or white vinegar for 45 to 60 minutes once a day. Listerine also may be applied with a cotton ball twice a day.

An ingrown toenail causes painful inflammation at the distal corner of the nail. The usual cause is trimming the nail too short at the corners or wearing shoes that are too tight on the toes. The ingrown nail should be protected from pressure as it grows out. Warm soaks may be soothing. Sometimes surgical excision of the ingrown portion of the nail is needed.

◆ NURSING CARE OF THE PATIENT WITH A NAIL DISORDER

Nail disorders rarely require inpatient care unless complications exist. However, nurses may be the first to detect nail problems and are in a position to teach patients how to prevent or treat them.

Focused Assessment

In the health history, document the diagnoses of diabetes mellitus (DM) or peripheral vascular disease (PVD). In the physical examination, inspect around the nails for redness, swelling, or pain. Inquire about the use of artificial nails and professional manicures and pedicures. Artificial nails carry a high incidence of fungal infections, and some nail salons do not follow aseptic practices. Inspect the extremities for lesions and abnormal color; palpate for warmth and peripheral pulses. Teach the diabetic patient the importance of seeing a podiatrist on a regular basis and having the nails trimmed only by the podiatrist or health care professionals.

Patient Problems, Goals, and Outcome Criteria: Nail Disorder

Patient Problems	Goals and Outcome Criteria
Potential for injury related to improper nail trimming, poor peripheral circulation	Decreased potential for injury: properly trimmed nails; absence of injury: no evidence of inflammation (e.g., redness, swelling, pain, excess warmth)

Patient Problems, Goals, and Outcome Criteria: Nail Disorder—cont'd

Patient Problems	Goals and Outcome Criteria
Inability to manage treatment program related to lack of understanding of proper nail care and treatment of nail disorders	Effective management of therapeutic measures: demonstrates correct nail care and prescribed treatments

Interventions

Teach patients how to trim their nails correctly and the importance of wearing properly fitting shoes. Toenails should be cut straight across and even with the end of the toe. Show patients with PVD or DM how to inspect their feet daily and advise them to seek medical attention for any abnormality. A seemingly minor foot infection can have drastic consequences, including amputation, for the patient with poor circulation. If the patient cannot care for the feet adequately, seek a referral to a podiatrist. Teach the patient with DM, PVD, or both the importance of bathing the feet daily; wearing clean, dry socks; and wearing shoes that fit properly. These patients should be discouraged from going barefoot.

PSORIASIS

Pathophysiology

Psoriasis is a chronic inflammatory skin condition characterized by defined areas of thickened, inflamed, erythematous skin, frequently covered with silvery scales (Fig. 57.3). *Chronic plaque psoriasis* is the most common form of psoriasis. The lesions usually are located on the scalp, elbow folds, knees and the gluteal cleft (space between the buttocks). Although the onset can occur at any age, psoriasis most often begins in adults. It is a multisystem disorder associated with multiple comorbidities (multiple illnesses at the same time), including *psoriatic arthritis*, obesity, metabolic syndrome, hypertension, diabetes, and atherosclerotic disease. About one-third of people with psoriasis have psoriatic arthritis, in which there is joint swelling and stiffness as well as severe nail problems.

Cause and Risk Factors

Psoriasis is caused by a combination of immune, genetic, and environmental factors. Particular stressors that can aggravate psoriasis are bacterial and viral infections; stress; overuse of alcohol; smoking; and drugs such as lithium, antimalarials, angiotensin-converting enzyme (ACE) inhibitors, and beta-blockers.

Medical Diagnosis

Psoriasis is diagnosed based on the health history and the physical examination.

Medical Treatment

No cure for psoriasis exists, but it can be treated topically or systemically. Over-the-counter emollients, especially petroleum jelly or thick creams, can help keep skin soft and moist. The emollients should be rubbed onto the skin after a bath or shower. Patients with mild psoriasis are usually treated with topical medications: corticosteroids, tazarotene, Estar, and vitamin D derivatives (calcipotriene [Dovonex]). Topical salicylic acid may be used with the corticosteroids. Tazarotene (Tazorac) is a topical retinoid agent that stays in the skin longer, leading to longer remissions. Anthralin (Anthra-Derm) may be used to remove heavy scales. With a gloved hand, it is applied only to the lesions. After a specified period, anthralin is removed with tissues, after which the patient removes the residue by showering or bathing. The medication must be handled carefully because it stains hair, skin, fingernails, furniture, and bathroom fixtures. Newer preparations that may not stain (e.g., Estar gel) are now available. Ultraviolet B (UVB) may be used to enhance topical therapy with tar and anthralin.

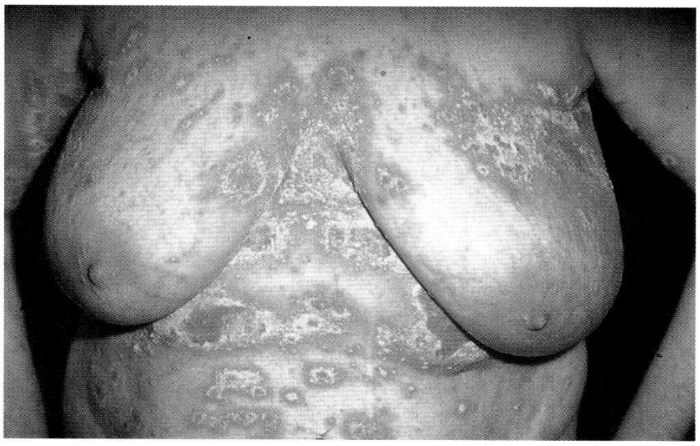

Fig. 57.3 Psoriasis. (Courtesy Columbia Presbyterian Dermatology Associates, New York, NY.)

Moderate to severe psoriasis may be treated with psoralen and ultraviolet A (PUVA), a combination of methotrexate and UVA. Methotrexate suppresses the immune response that triggers the disease and frequently is used to treat psoriatic arthritis. Other drugs include oral retinoids (acitretin [Soriatane]) and biologic agents (etanercept [Enbrel]). Patients receiving biologic agents should be monitored closely for infections because these agents tend to decrease the number of circulating T cells. Oral retinoids may reduce the risk of skin cancers associated with PUVA. Systemic corticosteroids may be used on a short-term basis. Patients on most forms of systemic therapy require periodic liver testing and blood studies because of the adverse effects. Methotrexate and oral retinoids are contraindicated during pregnancy because of the risk of fetal harm.

Pharmacology Capsule

If a woman of childbearing age is taking methotrexate or oral retinoids, ensure that she understands that these drugs are harmful to a fetus. If the patient suspects she is pregnant, she should inform her physician immediately if taking either of these drugs. Instruct women of childbearing age to use appropriate methods to prevent pregnancy while on these drugs.

Pharmacology Capsule

Because of risks to the fetus, women should use reliable contraception during and for 3 years after therapy with Soriatane.

◆ NURSING CARE OF THE PATIENT WITH PSORIASIS

Focused Assessment

Relevant data for the patient with psoriasis include a description of symptoms and identification of treatments being used (see Nursing Care Plan: Patient With Psoriasis). Inspect the affected areas for lesions and scales. Document joint pain or stiffness because the condition may cause arthritis. Explore the effect of psoriasis on the patient's everyday life and the coping strategies used.

Patient Problems, Goals, and Outcome Criteria: Psoriasis

Patient Problems	Goals and Outcome Criteria
Inability to manage treatment program related to lack of knowledge about the skin condition and treatment	Effective management of treatment regimen: patient correctly describes and demonstrates self-care
Altered self-concept related to lesions and scales on skin	Improved self-concept: patient makes effort to improve appearance and makes positive remarks about self
Decreased socialization related to embarrassment about skin lesions	Increased socialization: patient shows continued involvement in social activities

Interventions

Inability to manage treatment program. The focus of nursing care is education that helps the patient to manage the prescribed regimen. The patient and family need to know that the condition is chronic but not contagious and usually responds to treatment. Teach the patient about the prescribed medications and treatments. Tell the patient to report signs of secondary infection (i.e., fever, purulent discharge, increased redness) to the health care provider. In addition, encourage adequate rest, good nutrition, and stress management. If taking drugs that suppress the immune system, the patient should practice good hygiene, stay away from crowds, and avoid people with infections.

Altered self-concept. Give the patient the opportunity to express feelings about psoriasis and the effects on their life. Demonstrate acceptance of the patient's appearance and the feelings that are expressed. Learning to manage the condition can help the patient to feel more hopeful, realizing that remission will occur.

Decreased socialization. Encourage the patient to maintain social contacts and plan strategies to deal with exacerbations without undue stress.

INTERTRIGO

Pathophysiology

Intertrigo is inflammation of the skin where two skin surfaces touch: axillae, abdominal skinfolds, and the area under the breasts. The affected area is usually red and "weeping," with clear margins. The area may be surrounded by vesicles and pustules.

Cause and Risk Factors

The inflammation of intertrigo results from heat, friction, and moisture between two touching body surfaces. These factors create the perfect environment for infection by *Candida albicans* (yeast) or bacteria.

Nursing Care Plan **Patient With Psoriasis**

FOCUSED ASSESSMENT

Health History

A 45-year-old police officer came to the health care provider's office because of a "rash" on his trunk. He reports that he is in good health and has had no major injuries or illnesses except a left knee injury sustained in a fall as a teenager. He is taking no medications but is allergic to penicillin. He is alarmed by the rash and is afraid it might spread and be something serious. The health care provider diagnoses psoriasis. The patient is divorced and enjoys socializing, especially dancing. He is concerned about how people might react to his condition.

Physical Examination

Vital signs: blood pressure 144/88 mm Hg, pulse 84 beats per minute, respiration 16 breaths per minute, temperature 98.2°F (36.8°C) measured orally. Height 5′10″, weight 164 lb. He is alert and oriented but mildly anxious. The skin on the face, arms, and legs is normal. Bright-red lesions with silvery scales are distributed over the anterior and posterior chest, abdomen, buttocks, and hands. Heart and breath sounds are normal. The abdomen is soft, with bowel sounds present in all four quadrants. Full range of motion of all joints is possible, with crepitation in the left knee. Peripheral pulses are strong and symmetric. The extremities are warm and dry.

Nursing Care Plan Patient With Psoriasis—cont'd

Patient Problems	Goals and Outcome Criteria	Interventions
Inability to manage treatment program related to lack of knowledge of psoriasis and its treatment	Correctly describe psoriasis and prescribed treatment measures.	Explain that psoriasis typically has periods of exacerbation and remission, that it is not contagious, and that symptoms can be improved with treatment. Explain the prescribed treatment, including proper application of topical medications and side and adverse effects of drug therapy. For oral drugs, provide information about the schedule as well as adverse and side effects. Warn of signs of secondary infection (i.e., fever, purulent drainage, increased redness) that should be reported to the health care provider. Encourage the patient to plan for adequate rest and eat a balanced diet. Explore stress management strategies. Refer the patient to a mental health counselor if needed. Supplement verbal teaching with written material.
Altered self-concept related to lesions and scales on skin	Expresses positive statements about self.	Demonstrates acceptance of the patient through eye contact and touch. Be aware of personal reaction to lesions. Encourage the patient to share feelings about the condition. Help the patient to feel "in control" by providing information about the management of psoriasis.
Decreased socialization related to embarrassment about skin lesions	Continues social activities and identify strategies to deal with social situations.	Explore how the patient thinks others will react to his condition. Role-play strategies to use in social situations. Encourage continued activity. Emphasize expected improvement.

CRITICAL THINKING QUESTIONS

1. Why is stress management important in the treatment of psoriasis?
2. What are the psychosocial effects of a diagnosis of psoriasis?

Medical Diagnosis and Treatment

The medical diagnosis is based on the site and appearance of the inflamed skin and the presence of *C. albicans* as confirmed by potassium hydroxide (KOH) examination and culture of skin scrapings. If the skin is not broken, it can be washed with water twice daily. The area is then rinsed and patted dry. Soft gauze may be used to separate layers of body tissue and absorb moisture. Cornstarch is contraindicated because it supports the growth of *C. albicans*. For severe inflammation or fungal infection, treatment may include a topical corticosteroid or antifungal. Examples of topical antifungals are nystatin, ketoconazole, clotrimazole, and terbinafine. Vytone 1% is a combination corticosteroid, antibacterial, and antifungal preparation. Wet soaks with tap water or Burow solution are sometimes ordered to remove exudate if an infection is present.

NURSING CARE OF THE PATIENT WITH INTERTRIGO

Focused Assessment

Intertrigo is fairly common among patients in long-term care facilities. Investigate complaints of pain, irritation, or redness in body folds. Monitor body temperature to detect possible infection. Inspect susceptible areas (i.e., axillae, groin, beneath breasts, abdominal skinfolds) on a daily basis.

Patient Problems, Goals, and Outcome Criteria: Intertrigo

Patient Problems	Goals and Outcome Criteria
Disrupted skin tissue integrity related to inflammation	Improved skin tissue integrity: intact skin without redness
Potential for infection related to moist environment, broken skin, and medications	Absence of infection: no fever, pain, or redness

Interventions

Areas where skin surfaces are in close contact must be kept clean and dry. Apply topical medications (antifungals and corticosteroids) as ordered. Report increasing redness and tenderness, fever, and broken skin to the health care provider. Encourage women with pendulous breasts to wear a soft, supportive bra. If incontinence has contributed to perineal intertrigo, positioning the patient with the legs apart allows moisture to evaporate. Encourage clients to keep nails short and to report excessive scratching to the health care provider so that additional medication can be provided to decrease pruritus.

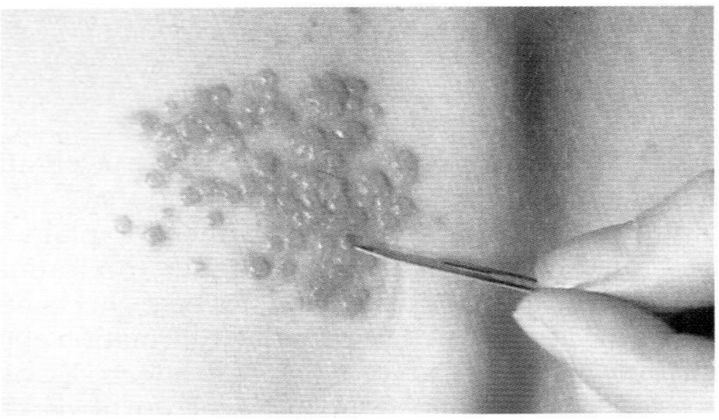

Fig. 57.4 Herpes simplex lesions. (From Lookingbill DP, Marks JG: *Principles of dermatology*, ed 2, Philadelphia, 1993, Saunders.)

HERPES SIMPLEX

Cause and Risk Factors

The herpes simplex virus (HSV) causes an infection that begins with itching and burning and progresses to the development of vesicles that rupture and form crusts (Fig. 57.4). Sites most often infected by the virus are the nose, lips, cheeks, ears, and genitalia. Two types of HSV are HSV-1 and HSV-2. Most infections on the face and upper body are caused by HSV-1; most genital infections are caused by HSV-2. However, either type may cause oral or genital infections. HSV-1 is transmitted through close contact via infected oral secretions. After initial infection, HSV-1 establishes a chronic infection in neural ganglia and reactivates on mucosa and skin. Clinical manifestations include recurrent oral lesions, commonly called *cold sores* or *fever blisters,* skin and mucous membrane lesions, and ocular infections (herpetic keratitis). Patients typically have repeated outbreaks and remissions. Because HSV can be transmitted by direct contact, genital infection is considered an STI and is discussed in detail in Chapter 55.

Medical Diagnosis

Diagnostic tests used to identify herpes infections include laboratory studies of exudate from a lesion and blood studies to detect specific antibodies.

Medical Treatment

Herpes simplex infections are treated with acyclovir (Zovirax) or, for cold sores, docosanol (Abreva). Antiviral drugs are not curative but may reduce the severity and frequency of outbreaks. Oral acyclovir is more effective than the topical preparation for initial and recurrent infections. Analgesics and topical anesthetics may be prescribed for pain.

◆ NURSING CARE OF THE PATIENT WITH HERPES SIMPLEX

Nursing care consists primarily of patient education about the nature of the herpes simplex infection and its treatment and prevention. Emphasize that the condition is contagious and tends to recur. Prevention of sexually transmitted herpes simplex is discussed in Chapter 5. This section focuses on HSV-1.

Focused Assessment

In the health history, describe how the patient developed the herpetic lesions. Document sexual contacts so that the patient can be advised of the need for medical evaluation. A complete medical history is taken with particular attention to disorders or medications that might suppress the immune response. The physical examination includes a careful inspection of the lesions. The examiner should wear gloves to avoid direct contact with lesions.

Patient Problems, Goals, and Outcome Criteria: Herpes Simplex

Patient Problems	Goals and Outcome Criteria
Pain related to herpetic lesions	Pain relief: states pain relief; rates pain below 4 on a 1–10 pain scale; relaxed expression
Inadequate coping related to anticipated recurrent lesions, embarrassment	Adequate coping: demonstrates ability to cope with condition with positive outlook
Inability to manage treatment program related to lack of knowledge of disease, treatment, and risk of transmission	Effective management: describes self-care, follows plan of care, takes precautions to protect partner

Interventions

Pain. Document patient reports of pain. Administer analgesics and topical anesthetics as ordered or instruct the patient in self-medication. Compresses saturated with astringent solutions such as Burow solution sometimes are ordered.

Inadequate coping. Explore the patient's knowledge and concerns about HSV-1. Lesions on the face may be especially distressing because they are so obvious. Demonstrate acceptance of the patient's feelings and provide factual information to enable the patient to cope with the condition.

Inability to manage treatment program. Topical and oral drugs may be ordered. Instruct the patient in use of the drugs. Stress that HSV remains in a dormant state in the body after the initial infection. Periodic recurrences are expected and may be triggered by stressors, including emotional distress, fever, trauma, sunburn, or fatigue. The patient may be able to identify personal triggers and should try to avoid or minimize them. Recurrent episodes are typically less severe than the initial one.

To prevent transmission of the infection to others, advise the patient to avoid oral contact while the lesions are present. The patient should exercise good hand washing and avoid touching the lesions.

Immunosuppressed patients are especially susceptible to herpes infections and must be protected from infected people. Patients who do not follow adequate self-management practices may experience secondary skin infections that may require additional treatment. Most of these infections occur secondary to scratching. Advise the patient to keep nails short, bathe daily, and use medications as prescribed. A health care provider may prescribe medication to decrease itching.

Pharmacology Capsule

Acyclovir (Zovirax) does not cure herpes simplex virus (HSV) infections. Patients can still transmit the infection to others despite antiviral therapy and the absence of lesions.

HERPES ZOSTER

Cause and Risk Factors

Herpes zoster infection, commonly called *shingles*, is caused by the varicella-zoster virus, the same organism that causes chickenpox. In some people who have had chickenpox, the virus remains latent (alive but inactive) in nerve tissue until the infection is activated in the form of shingles. People who have never had chicken pox or the vaccine may acquire chicken pox from direct skin to skin contact with a shingles blister. The virus occurs more frequently in people over age 50 years. Older adults are especially susceptible to complications, which include postherpetic neuralgia, trigeminal herpes zoster (affecting the facial and acoustic nerves), and ophthalmic involvement. With postherpetic neuralgia, pain and itching may persist for years. Immunosuppressed people are at increased risk for herpes zoster infections and may have serious systemic complications.

Clinical Manifestations

The shingles rash most commonly affects the chest, abdomen and back, but may show up on almost any part of the body. If a rash develops near the eye, it can permanently impair vision if left untreated. The first symptoms are pain, itching, burning and heightened sensitivity along a nerve pathway, followed by the formation of vesicles in the area. Crusts form on the lesions, which remain infectious for about 7 to 10 days (Fig. 57.5). The rash lasts approximately 3 to 4 weeks leaving residual scarring or changes in skin color. The pain is limited to the areas of the skin affected by the rash and can be mild or severe, sharp, stabbing, or burning. It often is worse in older adults, possibly severe enough to interfere with daily activities and sleep. When the mucous membranes are affected, ulcers develop. The infection is contagious to people who have not had previous exposure to the virus. Home health providers and nurses working in the clinic may be the first to recognize herpes zoster and should report their findings immediately to the client's health care provider.

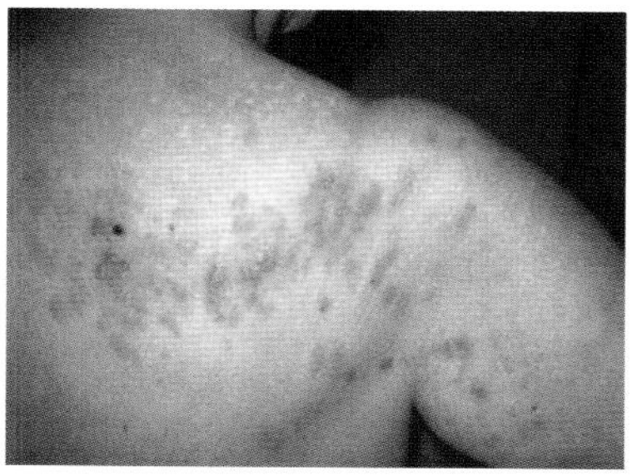

Fig. 57.5 Herpes zoster lesions (i.e., shingles). (From Lookingbill DP, Marks JG: *Principles of dermatology*, ed 2, Philadelphia, 1993, Saunders.)

Medical Diagnosis

A diagnosis of herpes zoster infection can be made on the basis of the health history and physical examination findings. The diagnosis can be confirmed by a Tzanck test or a viral culture of material from a lesion.

Medical Treatment

Herpes zoster infection is treated with antivirals. Topical agents are available but are used primarily to treat herpes simplex. The most commonly prescribed drugs include acyclovir, famciclovir, valacyclovir, and foscarnet. Oral administration of medications is effective for most patients. However, the intravenous route is used for persons who have impaired immune system function. Treatment is most effective if initiated within 72 hours of the onset of the rash. Wet dressings soaked in Burow solution may be ordered to loosen crusts, decrease oozing, and soothe the affected areas. Pain may be treated with analgesics and sedatives. After crusts form, a topical antibiotic ointment may be administered 2 or 3 times a day. Systemic corticosteroids seem to be helpful in reducing pain and may or may not decrease the risk of herpetic neuralgia.

Postherpetic neuralgia is treated with a variety of analgesics, anticonvulsants, and antidepressants. Topical antiinflammatory and anesthetic drugs may be applied. Other methods that may be tried to relieve pain are transcutaneous electrical nerve stimulation (TENS), nerve blocks, and acupuncture.

Individuals 60 years of age and older may receive a vaccine for herpes zoster. Anyone younger than 60 years of age who has herpes zoster also can be given the vaccine. The initial patient assessment should note whether the individual has been given this vaccine.

◆ NURSING CARE OF THE PATIENT WITH HERPES ZOSTER

Focused Assessment

Describe the patient's present illness. A complete medical history is needed to identify conditions or treatments that might cause the patient to have a reduced immune response. Explore the effect of the symptoms on the patient's life. If this is a recurrent infection, evaluate the patient's understanding of the condition. In the physical examination, document the distribution and appearance of the lesions.

Patient Problems, Goals, and Outcome Criteria: Herpes Zoster

Patient Problems	Goals and Outcome Criteria
Disrupted skin integrity related to lesions	Improved skin integrity: absence of vesicles and pruritus
Pain related to lesions, inflammation, or postherpetic neuralgia	Pain relief: states pain relief, less than 4 on the 1–10 pain scale; relaxed manner
Inadequate coping related to chronic pain associated with postherpetic neuralgia	Effective coping: patient uses strategies to cope with chronic pain

Interventions

Disrupted skin integrity. Inspect the lesions each day. Apply cool medicated compresses and administer antipruritics as ordered. Individuals who have not had chickenpox are susceptible to herpes zoster infection and should avoid contact with the lesions. To promote healing and prevent transmission, provide information about the cause, course, treatment, and communicability of herpes zoster.

Pain. Administer prescribed analgesics and antiviral medications or instruct the patient in self-medication. Follow up to determine the effectiveness of the drugs to relieve pain. Inform the health care provider if the patient's pain persists despite medication.

Inadequate coping. Emotional support is especially important for the patient who has chronic pain. Management of chronic pain is discussed in detail in Chapter 8.

NECROTIZING FASCIITIS

Necrotizing fasciitis, also known as flesh eating disease, is an infection of the deep fascial structures under the skin. Aerobic and anaerobic organisms may be present, including *Streptococcus*, *Staphylococcus*, *Peptostreptococcus*, *Bacteroides*, and *Clostridium* species. About one-third of the cases are as a result of methicillin resistant staphylococcus aureus (MRSA). The organisms excrete enzymes that destroy tissue, including blood vessels that supply the affected area. Deprived of blood flow, tissue necrosis occurs.

Risk factors include immunosuppression, diabetes, obesity, alcoholism, intravenous drug use and peripheral artery disease. The most common areas of the body affected are the extremities, perineum, and genitals. Necrotizing fasciitis should be suspected when a patient has a small external wound with evidence of larger underlying inflammation. The infection may progress rapidly with loss of large amounts of tissue and can result in death. Good handwashing and wound care can reduce infection from a wound. Treatment involves extensive debridement, intravenous and topical antibiotics, and eventual skin grafting. Amputations may occur depending on response to therapy. Patients and family need to be aware of the severity of the disease process, and nursing staff should collaborate with other members of the health care team in providing emotional, spiritual, and psychological support.

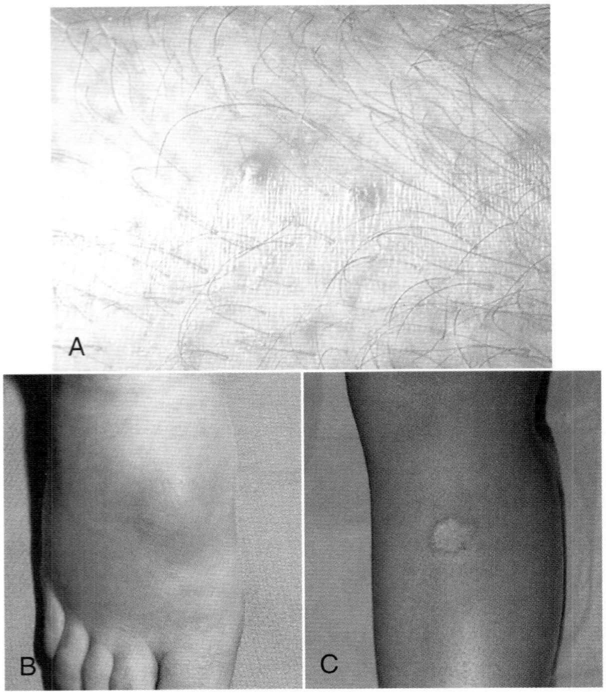

Fig. 57.6 (A) Folliculitis. (B) Furuncle and abscess. (C) Tinea corporis. (From Lookingbill DP, Marks JG: *Principles of dermatology*, ed 2, Philadelphia, 1993, Saunders.)

OTHER INFECTIONS

A number of skin infections can occur in addition to those discussed in this chapter. Some of the more common conditions (i.e., impetigo, folliculitis, furuncles, carbuncles, erysipelas, cellulitis, warts) are presented in Fig. 57.6 and Table 57.1.

INFESTATIONS

Lice and scabies infestations are described in Table 57.2. Pediculosis is illustrated in Fig. 57.7.

PEMPHIGUS

Pemphigus is a chronic autoimmune condition in which bullae (blisters) develop on the face, back, chest, groin, and umbilicus. The blisters rupture easily, releasing a foul-smelling drainage. Potassium permanganate baths, Domeboro solution, and oatmeal products with oil may be ordered to soothe the affected areas, reduce

Table 57.1 Additional Skin Infections

INFECTION	CAUSE	SIGNS AND SYMPTOMS	TREATMENT
Impetigo	Group A streptococci	Vesicle or pustule that ruptures, leaving a thick crust	Antibiotic therapy: erythromycin or dicloxacillin
Folliculitis	*Staphylococcus aureus*	Inflamed hair follicles with white pustules	Warm compresses, topical antibiotics
Furuncle (boil)	*Staphylococcus aureus*	Inflamed skin and subcutaneous tissue with deep, inflamed nodules	Warm compresses, topical antibiotics
Carbuncle	*Staphylococcus aureus*	Clustered, interconnected furuncles	Systemic antibiotics, incision and drainage
Erysipelas	Beta-hemolytic group A streptococci	Round or oval patches that enlarge and spread; redness, swelling, tenderness, warmth	Systemic antibiotics, usually penicillin
Cellulitis	Usually *Streptococcus pyogenes*	Local tenderness and redness at first, then malaise, chills, and fever; site becomes more erythematous; nodules and vesicles may form; vesicles may rupture, releasing purulent material identified by culture	For *S. pyogenes*: penicillin, a cephalosporin, or vancomycin; other antibiotics for other organisms
Verruca (wart)	Human papillomavirus	At first, small shiny lesions; they enlarge and become rough	Electrical current to destroy lesion followed by removal with curette, cryotherapy (freezing), topical medications

Table 57.2 Infestations of the Skin

INFECTION	CAUSE	SIGNS AND SYMPTOMS	TREATMENT
Scabies	*Sarcoptes scabiei*, sometimes called *itch mite*	Thin, red lines on skin; itching	Topical scabicide applied and repeated 1 week later; clothing and bed linens washed in hot water or dry-cleaned
Lice	*Pediculus humanus* or *Phthirus pubis*	Itching of hairy areas of body (head, pubis); nits (eggs) seen as tiny white particles attached to hair shafts	Head lice: pediculicide shampoo applied to dry hair, then hair combed with fine-toothed comb to remove nits and dead lice; also treat brushes and combs Body or pubic lice: apply pediculicide lotion as directed For both sites: wash clothing and bed linens in hot water or have dry-cleaned; usually need to treat all members of household Assure patient that infestations are common and not caused by unsanitary living

odor, and decrease the risk of infection. Treatments may include corticosteroids, other immunosuppressants, and oral or topical antibiotics. Patients with extensive skin loss require the same care as burn patients (see the section "Nursing Care of the Patient With Burn Injury").

CANCER

Skin lesions may be suspected as cancerous because of their appearance and location. The diagnosis is confirmed by microscopic examination of cells obtained from the excised lesion or a tissue sample obtained by biopsy. Skin cancers are classified as *nonmelanoma* or *melanoma.* Nonmelanoma skin cancers include basal cell carcinoma and squamous cell carcinoma. Risk factors for skin cancer are sun exposure, fair skin with freckling, light-colored hair and eyes, male gender, cigarette smoking, tanning beds, and a tendency to sunburn easily (see the Cultural Considerations box). Tanning beds have been specifically labeled *carcinogenic to humans* after years of controversy and study. The risk of melanoma increases by 75% among people who begin using them before age 30 years, as well as with the severity of sunburn. The risk of nonmelanoma skin cancers increases with the total amount of sun exposure. See Chapter 7 for detailed nursing care of the patient with cancer.

Cultural Considerations

What Does Culture Have to Do with Skin Cancer?

White Americans have an increased incidence of skin cancer compared with either Black Americans or Native Americans. Patients with light skin who live in sunny climates should protect themselves from excessive exposure and routinely assess for skin changes.

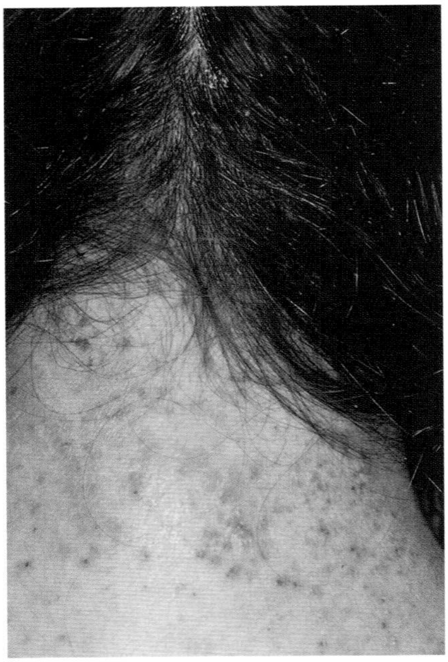

Fig. 57.7 Pediculosis. (From Lookingbill DP, Marks JG: *Principles of dermatology*, ed 2, Philadelphia, 1993, Saunders.)

ACTINIC KERATOSIS

Actinic keratoses are precancerous lesions most often found on the face, neck, forearms, and backs of the hands—all areas exposed to sunlight. They may become malignant if not treated. Actinic keratoses are most common among White older adults. They typically appear as papules or plaques of irregular shape. The hard scale on the lesion may shed and reappear (see Fig. 57.8A).

Treatments for actinic keratosis include drug therapy, cryotherapy, electrodessication, and surgical excision. Drugs used to treat actinic keratosis are topical 5-fluorouracil and diclofenac sodium. Another choice is topical aminolevulinic acid with blue light photoactivation after 14 to 18 hours. Because topical treatments may cause irritation and photosensitivity, caution patients to avoid direct sun exposure. Cryotherapy is the use of liquid nitrogen to freeze and destroy the lesion, causing a blister to form. With electrodessication, the patient is given a local anesthetic, and an electrical current destroys the lesion, which is then scraped off. Surgical excision may be done in several ways, and the patient may or may not have sutures.

NONMELANOMA SKIN CANCER

Basal Cell Carcinoma

Basal cell carcinomas usually begin as painless, nodular lesions that have a pearly appearance (see Fig. 57.8B). They are thought to be related to sun exposure. Basal cell carcinomas grow slowly and rarely metastasize. Nevertheless, they should be removed because they can cause local tissue destruction. Basal cell

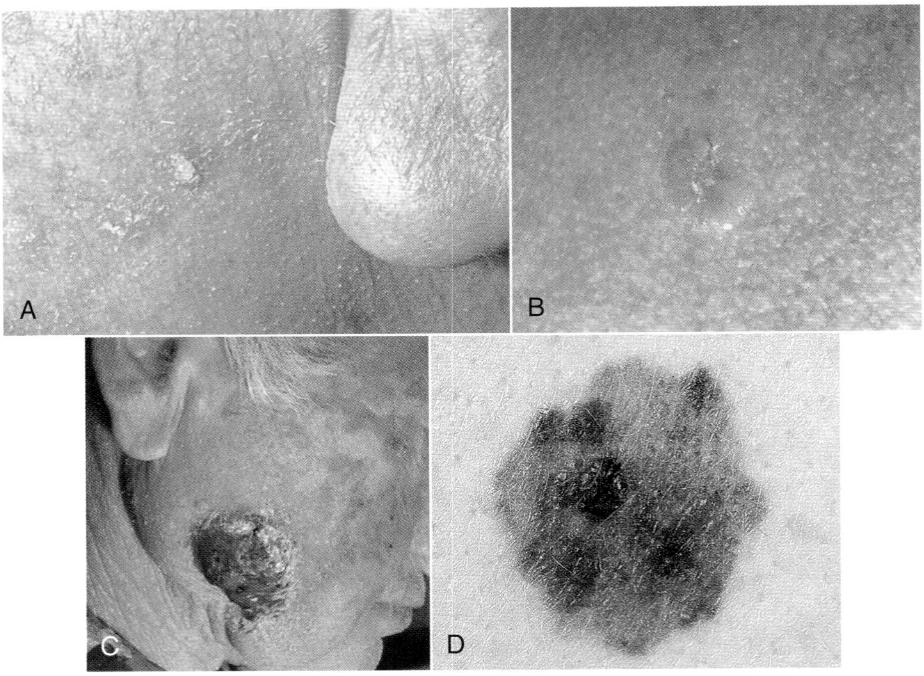

Fig. 57.8 Skin cancers. (A) Actinic keratosis (a premalignant lesion). (B) Basal cell carcinoma. (C) Squamous cell carcinoma. (D) Malignant melanoma. (A to C, From Lookingbill DP, Marks JG: *Principles of dermatology*, ed 2, Philadelphia, 1993, Saunders. D, From Habif TP, Campbell JL Jr., Chapman MS, et al.: *Skin disease: diagnosis and treatment*, ed 3, St. Louis, 2011, Saunders.)

carcinomas are treated with surgical excision, Mohs micrographic excision, electrodissection and curettage, cryotherapy, radiation, or drugs that are applied topically or injected into the lesion. Mohs surgery is a technique in which microscopic tissue samples are studied to determine the margins of the malignancy.

Squamous Cell Carcinoma

Squamous cell carcinomas may appear as scaly ulcers or raised lesions with no clear margins (see Fig. 57.8C). Like basal cell carcinomas, they most often develop on sun-exposed areas, including the lips and in the oral cavity. Squamous cell carcinomas frequently are associated with overuse of tobacco and alcohol. Unlike basal cell carcinomas, they grow rapidly and metastasize. Treatment may include surgical excision, cryotherapy, and radiation therapy.

MELANOMA

A malignant melanoma arises from the pigment-producing cells in the skin. It is the most serious form of skin cancer because it can be fatal if metastasis occurs. Melanomas can be found anywhere on the body, not just on sun-exposed areas. Typical melanomas have irregular borders and uneven coloration (see Fig. 57.8D). The lesions may begin as a tan macule that enlarges and becomes either very dark or light in color. Malignant melanomas are removed surgically, with Mohs technique to avoid leaving malignant tissue around the excised lesion. Thus, a wide area around a melanoma is excised. Chemotherapy and immunotherapy also may be used.

CUTANEOUS T-CELL LYMPHOMA

Cutaneous T-cell lymphoma is characterized by the migration of malignant T cells to the skin. Several manifestations of cutaneous T-cell lymphoma exist, including mycosis fungoides and Sézary syndrome. At first, cutaneous T-cell lymphoma may resemble eczema, with macular lesions appearing on areas that are protected from the sun. They form tumors, enlarge, and can spread to distant sites. When confined to the skin, this type of lymphoma can be cured with topical chemotherapy, systemic PUVA, or superficial radiotherapy (or a combination of these treatments).

KAPOSI SARCOMA

Kaposi sarcoma forms in the lining of the blood and lymph vessels. The lesions appear as painless purplish spots predominately on the legs, feet or face, but also can appear in the genitals, mouth or lymph nodes. (See Chapter 32, Fig. 32.1B). Kaposi sarcoma is caused by the human herpesvirus 8 (HHV-8) and is manifested in people with weakened immune systems. Patients with human immunodeficiency virus (HIV) infection are at the highest risk for Kaposi sarcoma. Recipients who are immuno-suppressed after organ transplants also are at risk. Local lesions may be excised or injected with intralesional chemotherapy; applied with a vitamin A-like drug (retinoid); burned (electrodessication) or frozen (cryotherapy); or given low dose radiation, especially in the mouth. For HIV/AIDS related Kaposi sarcoma, an antiviral drug reduces the amount of virus that causes AIDS and increases the number of immune cells in the body.

Systemic lesions are treated with chemotherapy, immune therapy, and radiotherapy.

PRESSURE INJURY

Pressure injuries are localized areas of tissue necrosis (tissue death) that develop when soft tissue is compressed between a bony prominence and an external surface.

Development of Pressure Injuries

An area of **erythema** (redness) is the beginning of a pressure injury and a sign that capillaries in the area have become congested because of impaired blood flow. Erythema can occur within 1 to 2 hours in a person with healthy skin and adequate circulation. Persons who are malnourished, obese, aged, or suffering from circulatory disease are even more likely to develop erythematous areas that progress rapidly to an ulcerated stage.

In addition to immobility, factors that contribute to the development of pressure injuries are shearing forces, friction, chemical irritants such as urine, sedation, and poor nutrition. **Shearing forces** exert a downward and forward pressure on tissues underlying the skin. Shearing action occurs when a patient slumps down while sitting in bed or in a chair; it can also occur when boosting a patient up in bed (Fig. 57.9). *Friction* occurs when surfaces rub the skin and injure epithelium, for example, when a patient is pulled across the bed linen. *Pressure points* are areas over bony prominences such as the elbows, hips, shoulders, and sacrum.

Pressure injuries are expensive to treat, result in longer hospital stays, increase the likelihood of placement in a long-term care facility, and increase mortality. Therefore, prevention is vital, and nursing care is a major factor in pressure injury prevention.

Preventing Pressure Injuries

The first step in the prevention of pressure injuries is to identify patients who are at risk for developing them. The Braden Scale is a tool used to assess the patient's risk factors for pressure injury. The risk factors include sensory perception, moisture, activity, mobility, nutrition, and friction and shear. Scores on each category range from 1 (highest risk) to 4 (lowest risk); a total score of 15 to 18 is mild risk, 13 to 14 is moderate risk, 10 to 12 is high risk, and 9 or less is very high risk (Fig. 57.10).

A pressure injury prevention protocol consists of proper skin care, pressure reduction, accessible support systems, improved mobility, adequate nourishment,

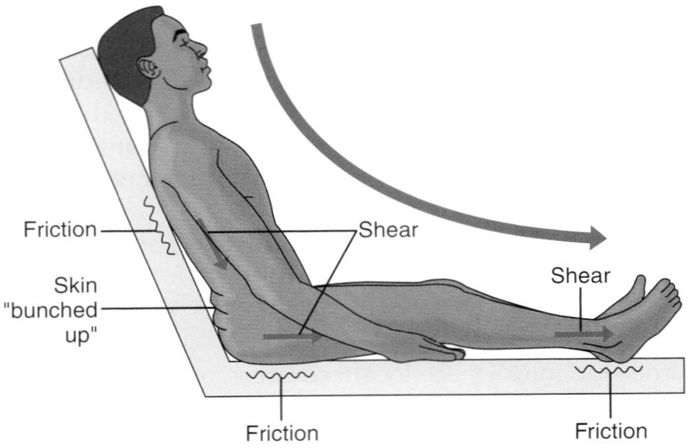

Fig. 57.9 Shearing forces pulling skin layers away from deeper tissue. The skin is "bunched up" against the back of the mattress while the rest of the bone and muscle in the area presses downward on the lower part of the mattress. Blood vessels become kinked, obstructing circulation and leading to tissue death. (From Ignatavicius DD, Workman, ML, Rebar CR, Heimgartner NM: *Medical-surgical nursing: concepts for interprofessional collaborative care*, ed 10, St. Louis, 2021, Elsevier.)

education, and effective communication (see Chapter 12). If pressure injuries develop despite all preventive measures, assess and precisely describe the stage of the injury. Proper documentation helps to evaluate the effectiveness of treatment and progress toward healing and repair. Documenting the skin condition and presence of pressure injuries on admission to a health care facility is especially important.

Stages of Pressure Injuries

Pressure injuries are classified into six stages (Fig. 57.11).

Stage I: nonblanchable erythema. The major characteristic of stage I pressure injuries is erythema (redness) that does not blanch (turn white at the point of pressure) when pressed. Before stage I begins, a finger pressed on a reddened area causes temporary blanching, followed by a return of the erythema when the finger is removed. In stage I, blanching does not occur. The area of redness reflects the shape of the object creating the pressure or the bony prominence underlying the skin. Pain and tenderness may be present with warmth, swelling, and hardening of the tissue, but the skin is intact. In individuals with dark skin, there may not be visible blanching, and the affected skin may appear a different color from surrounding tissue. At this stage, little destruction of tissue has occurred, and the condition is reversible.

Stage II: partial thickness. In stage II, some skin loss has occurred in the epidermis and dermis. A blister or shallow ulcer develops. The ulcer bed is pink without dead tissue or bruising. The ulcer is surrounded by a broad, irregular, and painful reddened area that is warmer than normal.

Stage III: full-thickness skin loss. Stage III is characterized by full-thickness skin loss involving damage or necrosis of the dermis and subcutaneous tissue. Subcutaneous fat may be visible but not bone, tendon, or muscle. A craterlike sore with a distinct outer margin has formed as the epidermis thickens and rolls over the edge toward the ulcer base. The wound may be infected and usually is open and draining with a loss of fluid and protein. The patient may have fever, dehydration, anemia, and leukocytosis (increased white blood cells in the blood).

Stage IV: full-thickness tissue loss. In stage IV, full-thickness skin loss has occurred with extensive destruction and exposure of bone, tendons, or muscles. The ulcer usually is extensively infected and may appear black with exudation, foul odor, and purulent drainage.

Additional stages. In the United States, two additional stages are used. The first is labeled *Unstageable/Unclassified: Full-thickness skin or tissue loss—depth unknown.* In this stage, slough (yellow, green, tan, gray, or brown) or eschar (tan, brown, or black) covers the base of a full-thickness ulcer. The true stage cannot be determined until at least part of the wound base can be examined. The second additional stage is *Deep Tissue Injury—depth unknown.* This stage is characterized by purple or maroon color to intact skin or blood-filled blisters. The actual depth of tissue injury cannot be determined at this point.

Treatment

The first step in treating pressure injuries is to continue all preventive measures. A pressure injury cannot heal unless measures are taken to relieve the pressure that initially caused it. Numerous treatments are used to promote wound healing. The National Pressure Ulcer Advisory Panel provides an excellent summary of research-based recommendations for prevention and treatment. These materials are available under Educational and Clinical Resources at www.npiap.org. In general, stage I and II pressure injuries should be cleaned with water or normal saline. Avoid pastes, creams, ointments, and powder because they may interfere with healing. In addition, alcohol, antiseptics, and disinfectants are not used because their effectiveness has not been proven; they may actually cause harm. Stage I and II ulcers generally are not infected, therefore topical and oral antibiotics are not appropriate. Heat is not used because a rise in temperature increases the metabolic demands of the tissue and places additional stress on the affected area.

The most effective dressing for a stage I or II pressure injury is one that provides a moist environment and maintains a temperature close to body temperature. All wound covers should allow oxygen to pass through. Wound healing is enhanced when the ulcer

Patient's name ______	Evaluator's name ______			Date of assessment		
Sensory perception Ability to respond meaningfully to pressure-related discomfort	**1. Completely limited** Unresponsive to painful stimuli (does not moan, flinch, or grasp) because of diminished level of consciousness or sedation OR limited ability to feel pain over most of body surface	**2. Very limited** Responds only to painful stimuli; cannot communicate discomfort except by moaning or restlessness OR has a sensory impairment that limits the ability to feel pain or discomfort over half of the body	**3. Slightly limited** Responds to verbal commands but cannot always communicate discomfort or need to be turned OR has some sensory impairment that limits ability to feel pain or discomfort in one or two extremities	**4. No impairment** Responds to verbal commands; has no sensory deficit that would limit ability to feel or voice pain or discomfort		
Moisture Degree to which skin is exposed to moisture	**1. Constantly moist** Skin is kept moist almost constantly by perspiration, urine; dampness is detected every time the client is moved or turned	**2. Very Moist** Skin is often but not always moist; linen must be changed at least once a shift	**3. Occasionally moist** Skin is occasionally moist, requiring an extra linen change approximately once a day	**4. Rarely moist** Skin is usually dry; linen requires changing only at routine intervals		
Activity Degree of physical activity	**1. Bedfast** Confined to bed	**2. Chairfast** Ability to walk severely limited or nonexistent; cannot bear own weight and must be assisted into chair or wheelchair	**3. Walks occasionally** Walks occasionally during the day but for very short distances, with or without assistance; spends the majority of each shift in bed or chair	**4. Walks frequently** Walks outside the room at least twice a day and inside the room at least once every 2 hours during waking hours		
Mobility Ability to change or control body position	**1. Completely immobile** Does not make even slight changes in body or extremity position without assistance	**2. Very limited** Makes occasional slight changes in body or extremity position but unable to make frequent or significant changes independently	**3. Slightly limited** Makes frequent though slight changes in body or extremity position independently	**4. No limitations** Makes major and frequent changes in position without assistance		
Nutrition Usual food intake pattern	**1. Very poor** Never eats a complete meal; rarely eats more than a third of any food offered; eats two servings or less of protein (meat or dairy products) per day; takes fluids poorly; does not take a liquid dietary supplement OR is NPO or maintained on clear liquids or IV for more than 5 days	**2. Probably inadequate** Rarely eats a complete meal and generally eats only about half of any food offered; protein intake includes only three servings of meat or dairy products per day; occasionally will take a dietary supplement OR receives less than optimal amount of liquid diet or tube feeding	**3. Adequate** Eats over half of most meals; eats a total of four servings of protein (meat, dairy products) each day; occasionally will refuse a meal, but will usually take a supplement if offered OR is receiving tube feeding or total parenteral nutrition, which probably meets most nutritional needs	**4. Excellent** Eats most of every meal; never refuses a meal; usually eats a total of four or more servings of meat and dairy products; occasionally eats between meals; does not require supplementation		
Friction and shear	**1. Problem** Requires moderate to maximum assistance in moving; complete lifting without sliding against sheets is impossible; frequently slides down in bed or chair, requiring frequent repositioning with maximum assistance; spasticity, contractures, or agitation leads to almost constant friction	**2. Potential problem** Moves feebly or requires minimum assistance during a move; skin probably slides to some extent against sheets, chair, restraints, or other devices; maintains relatively good position in chair or bed most of the time but occasionally slides down	**3. No apparent problem** Moves in bed and in chair independently and has sufficient muscle strength to lift up completely during move; maintains good position in bed or chair at all times			
Scoring system: 15–16 = mild risk, 12–14 = moderate risk, <11 = severe risk				Total score		

Fig. 57.10 The Braden Scale for predicting pressure sore risk. (From Barbara Braden and Nancy Bergstrom. ©1988. Reprinted with permission. From Ignatavicius DD, Workman, ML, Rebar CR, Heimgartner NM: *Medical-surgical nursing: concepts for interprofessional collaborative care*, ed 10, St. Louis, 2021, Elsevier.)

Stage I

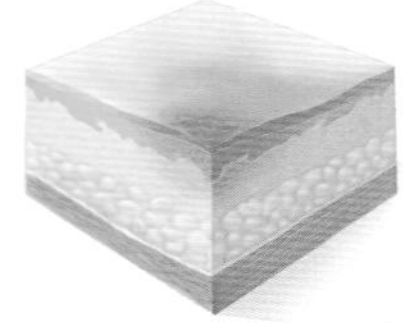

Intact skin with non-blanchable redness of a localized area usually over a bony prominence. Darkly pigmented skin may not have visible blanching; its color may differ from the surrounding area

The area may be painful, firm, soft, warmer, or cooler as compared to adjacent tissue. Stage I may be difficult to detect in individuals with dark skin. May indicate "at risk" persons (a heralding sign of risk)

Stage II

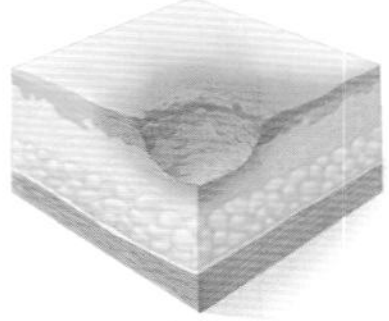

Partial-thickness loss of dermis presenting as a shallow open ulcer with a red pink wound bed, without slough. May also present as an intact or open/ruptured serum-filled blister

Presents as a shiny or dry shallow ulcer without slough or bruising.* This stage should not be used to describe skin tears, tape burns, perineal dermatitis, maceration, or excoriation

*Bruising indicates suspected deep-tissue injury

Stage III

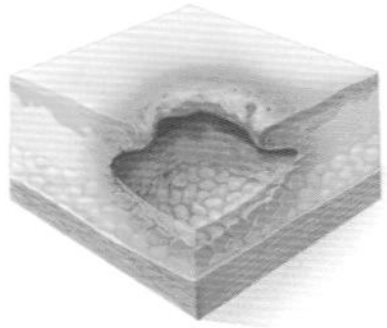

Full-thickness tissue loss. Subcutaneous fat may be visible, but bone, tendon, or muscle are not exposed. Slough may be present but does not obscure the depth of tissue loss. May include undermining and tunneling

The depth of a stage III pressure ulcer varies by anatomical location. The bridge of the nose, ear, occiput, and malleolus do not have subcutaneous tissue, and stage III ulcers can be shallow. In contrast, areas of significant adiposity can develop extremely deep stage III pressure ulcers. Bone/tendon is not visible or directly palpable

Stage IV

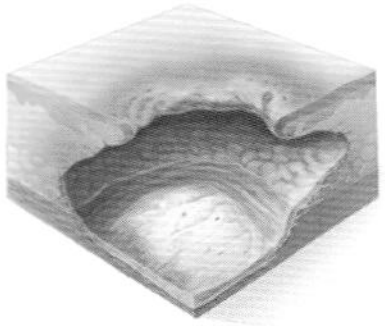

Full-thickness tissue loss with exposed bone, tendon, or muscle. Slough or eschar may be present on some parts of the wound bed. Often includes undermining and tunneling

The depth of a stage IV pressure ulcer varies by anatomical location. The bridge of the nose, ear, occiput, and malleolus do not have subcutaneous tissue and these ulcers can be shallow. Stage IV ulcers can extend into muscle and/or supporting structures (e.g., fascia, tendon, or joint capsule), making osteomyelitis possible. Exposed bone/tendon is visible or directly palpable

Unstageable

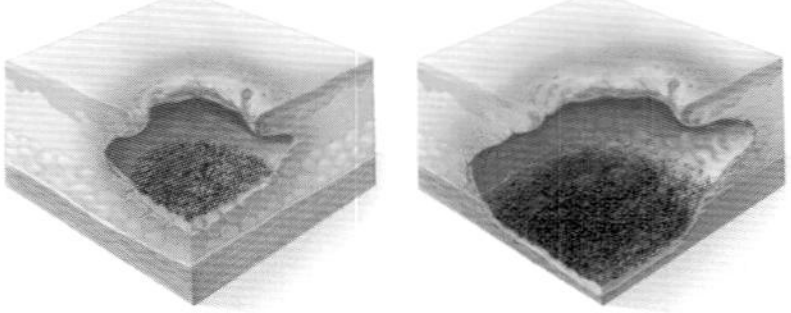

Full-thickness tissue loss in which the base of the ulcer is covered by slough (yellow, tan, gray, green, or brown) and/or eschar (tan, brown, or black) in the wound bed

Until enough slough and/or eschar is removed to expose the base of the wound, the true depth, and therefore stage, cannot be determined. Stable (dry, adherent, intact without erythema or fluctuance) eschar on the heels serves as the body's natural (biological) cover and should not be removed

Deep tissue injury

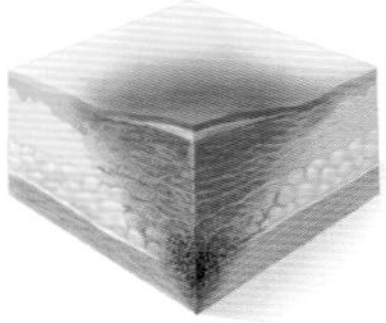

Purple or maroon localized area of discolored intact skin or blood-filled blister due to damage of underlying soft tissue from pressure and/or shear. The area may be preceded by tissue that is painful, firm, mushy, boggy, warmer, or cooler as compared to adjacent tissue

Deep-tissue injury may be difficult to detect in individuals with dark skin. Evolution may include a thin blister over a dark wound bed. The wound may further evolve and become covered by thin eschar. Evolution may be rapid, exposing additional layers of tissue even with optimal treatment

Fig. 57.11 Classification of pressure injuries. (From Black JM, Hawks JH: *Medical-surgical nursing: clinical management for positive outcomes*, ed 8, St. Louis, 2009, Saunders.)

and surrounding tissues can take up oxygen and eliminate carbon dioxide freely.

Stage III and IV pressure injuries require more extensive treatment and supportive care. Mechanical devices used for irrigation include spray bottles, bulb and piston syringes, and other specialized irrigating devices such as a Waterpik. Excess pressure can cause trauma and may force bacteria into the wound; therefore, the Waterpik should be used only on the lowest setting. Cleansing solutions and antimicrobials may be needed if the wound is infected or has debris. Debridement of necrotic tissue is necessary to promote granulation of new, healthy tissue. Common methods of debridement are surgery; autolysis; and enzymatic, mechanical, and biosurgical (maggot therapy) techniques. Debridement is sufficiently done when the ulcer bed appears pink, indicating healthy granulation tissue. Negative-pressure wound care, described in Chapter 12, can significantly decrease the healing time for pressure injuries. Supportive care consists of measures to treat anemia, dehydration, and protein depletion. Nutritional intervention consists of oral supplements high in protein and vitamins, nasogastric feedings, or parenteral nutrition to provide the additional nutrients necessary for healing.

Stage II, III, and IV pressure injuries are normally colonized with bacteria. Good wound care usually prevents the bacteria from causing a clinical infection. Topical broad-spectrum antibiotics may be ordered if the wound fails to heal despite good care. If evidence of widespread infection exists, systemic antibiotics are indicated.

Patients may have pain associated with pressure injuries. Administer an analgesic before dressing changes and debridement procedures. Topical opioids are sometimes applied to the ulcer surface. Allow time for the drug to take effect before the procedure. Patients with chronic ulcer pain may be treated with a local anesthetic and an antidepressant or antiepileptic agent. Transcutaneous electrical nerve stimulation (TENS) may be helpful.

Pressure injuries are difficult to resolve. About 70% of stage II ulcers heal in 6 months with appropriate treatment, but only about 50% of stage III and IV ulcers heal within this period. Surgical consultation should be obtained if ulcers do not respond to optimal care. Surgical approaches include direct closure and skin grafts. Adaptive touch nonadhering silicon dressing also is used. Newer therapies involve electrical stimulation (ES) to create an electrical flow throughout the tissues. ES is said to increase blood flow and stimulate healing.

Rates of surgical complications and recurrence rates are high. Osteomyelitis is the major cause of injury after surgery, and bone biopsy is recommended to make a diagnosis. Bacteremia may occur causing fever, tachycardia, hypotension, or altered mental status. Overall mortality is high, and antibiotics pending culture results should cover methicillin-resistant organisms.

NURSING CARE OF THE PATIENT WITH A PRESSURE INJURY

Focused Assessment

A complete health history is important to identify conditions that may contribute to the development of a pressure injury. Patients who are older, with previous illnesses that can contribute to immobility, inadequate nutrition, impaired cognition, or incontinence are more likely to develop a pressure injury.

Describe the patient's present illness. Document vital signs; skin color, turgor, and presence or absence of pressure injuries; mobility; level of consciousness; orientation, and elimination habits. If a pressure injury is present, record the location, appearance and stage of development.

Patient Problems, Goals and Outcome Criteria: Pressure Injury

Patient Problems	Goals and Outcome Criteria
Potential for disrupted skin tissue integrity related to decreased mobility, incontinence, inadequate nutrition, impaired cognition, older age	Absence of disrupted skin tissue integrity: no appearance of pressure injury, especially over pressure points; skin warm, dry, no discoloration
Disrupted skin tissue integrity related to pressure injury	Increased skin tissue integrity: healing evident in pressure injury; no deterioration of the wound
Potential for infection related to pressure injury	Absence of infection in pressure injury: no increase in temperature, redness, drainage

Interventions

Ensure that preventive measures are carried out. Inspect skin regularly for reddened or darkened areas. Keep skin clean and dry. Remove pressure from patient's bony areas. Take steps to reduce immobility, friction and shearing forces. Turn and position patients as needed (some patients may require turning as often as every hour; others may only require turning every three hours). Provide adequate nutrition and hydration for healthy skin. Do not massage pressure points or reddened areas.

Clean stage I and II pressure injuries with water or normal saline and apply a warm, moist dressing. Stage III and IV pressure injuries require more extensive treatment than stage I and II. The wounds are deeper and may be infected. Good wound care is essential, and if infection occurs, a topical antibiotic may be applied. The injury needs to be irrigated and debrided to promote granulation of new, healthy tissue.

BURNS

Burns are tissue injuries that are described as *thermal* (i.e., flame, flash, scalding liquids, hot objects), *chemical*, *electrical*, *radiation*, or *inhalation*. Burns are a leading cause of accidental death despite improved survival rates attributed to advances in the care of burn patients. Sadly, 75% of all burn injuries could have been prevented. Educating the public about ways to prevent burns is essential.

Emergency treatment of the burn patient is discussed in Chapter 63. Acute care of seriously burned patients is an advanced specialty that is beyond the scope of this book; therefore, this section provides a limited discussion of nursing care of the patient after they reach a medical facility.

CLASSIFICATION OF BURNS

Burns are classified by the size and depth of the tissue injury. It is important to reevaluate the burn periodically because evidence of the extent of the injury can change over time. Size is often defined as the percentage of body surface area affected. To describe depth, a burn is classified as *partial thickness* or *full thickness*, depending on the layers of tissue injured.

Burn Size

Burn size may be estimated using the Wallace rule of nines or the Lund and Browder method. The rule of nines estimates the percentage of body surface area burned. Areas of the body are assigned percentage values of nine or multiples of nine (Fig. 57.12). The percentages are totaled to estimate burn size. For example, in an adult, if one arm and hand are burned, the burn size is estimated as 9.5%.

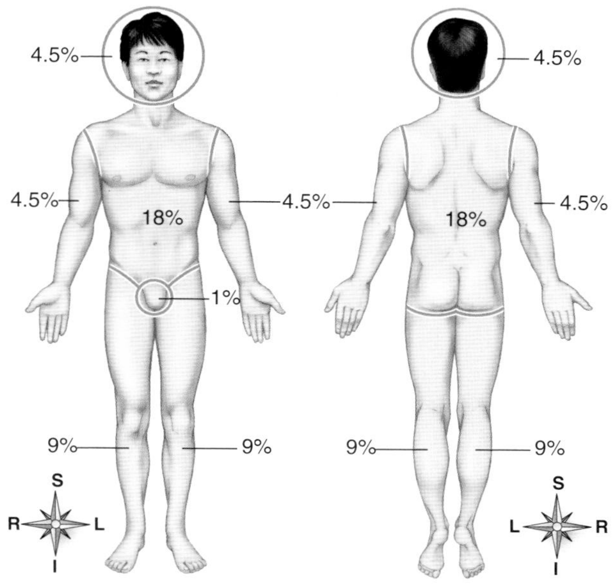

Fig. 57.12 Rule of nines. (From Patton KT, Thibodeau GA: *The human body in health & disease*, ed 7, St. Louis, 2018, Elsevier.)

Body area	0-1 Years	1-4 Years	5-9 Years	10-14 Years	15 Years	Adult
Head	19	17	13	11	9	7
Neck	2	2	2	2	2	2
Ant. trunk	13	13	13	13	13	13
Post. trunk	13	13	13	13	13	13
R. buttock	2.5	2.5	2.5	2.5	2.5	2.5
L. buttock	2.5	2.5	2.5	2.5	2.5	2.5
Genitalia	1	1	1	1	1	1
R. u. arm	4	4	4	4	4	4
L. u. arm	4	4	4	4	4	4
R. l. arm	3	3	3	3	3	3
L. l. arm	3	3	3	3	3	3
R. hand	2.5	2.5	2.5	2.5	2.5	2.5
L. hand	2.5	2.5	2.5	2.5	2.5	2.5
R. thigh	5.5	6.5	8	8.5	9	9.5
L. thigh	5.5	6.5	8	8.5	9	9.5
R. l. leg	5	5	5.5	6	6.5	7
L. l. leg	5	5	5.5	6	6.5	7
R. foot	3.5	3.5	3.5	3.5	3.5	3.5
L. foot	3.5	3.5	3.5	3.5	3.5	3.5

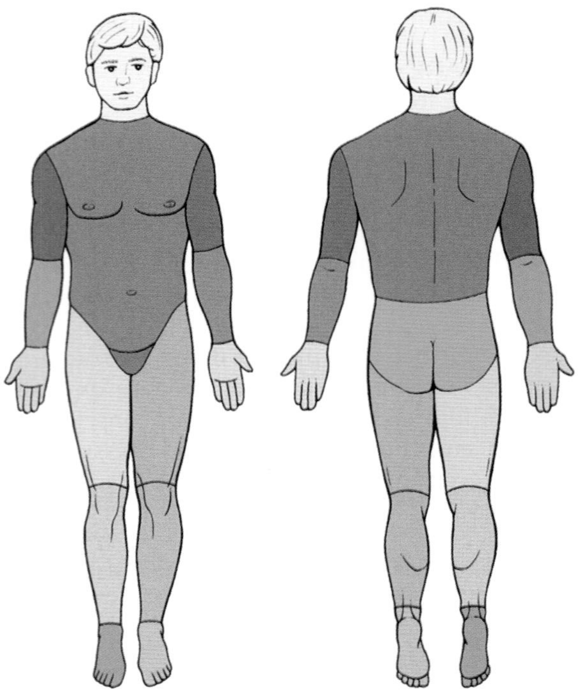

Fig. 57.13 Berkow's adaptation of the Lund and Browder method of estimating body surface area burned. (From Monahan FD, Drake DT, Neighbors M, editors: *Medical-surgical nursing: foundations for clinical practice*, ed 2, Philadelphia, 1998, Saunders.)

The Lund and Browder method also estimates the percentage of body surface burned, but the body is divided into smaller segments. Various percentages are assigned to body parts depending on the patient's age. This is more accurate than the rule of nines because it accounts for differences in body proportions. For example, the head of an infant is 19% of the total body surface area, whereas the head of an adult is only 7% of the total body surface area. Fig. 57.13 is an example of the Lund and Browder chart as modified by Berkow. A quick method of estimating the percentage of body surface burned is to use the patient's palm. The size of the palm represents 1%.

Burn Depth

Partial-thickness burns are sometimes called *first-degree* or *second-degree* burns. A burn affecting only the epidermis is called a *superficial* (or *first-degree*) burn. A burn that affects the epidermis and the dermis is a *superficial* or *deep partial-thickness* (or *second-degree*) burn, depending on the tissues affected. Burns that extend into even deeper tissue layers are called *full-thickness* (or *third degree, fourth degree burns*) (Figs. 57.14 and 57.15). In some cases, the full-thickness burns are categorized more specifically into *fourth degree* (extends into fat), *fifth degree* (extends into muscle), and *sixth degree* (extends into bone).

Superficial burns. A superficial burn, like a sunburn, is pink to red and painful.

Superficial partial-thickness burns. Superficial partial-thickness burns are painful and usually appear blistered or weepy and pale to red or pink. A severe sunburn can be a superficial partial-thickness burn.

Deep partial-thickness burns. A deep partial-thickness burn is characterized by large, thick-walled blisters or by edema and weeping, cherry-red, exposed dermis. It is painful and sensitive to cold air.

Full-thickness burns. Full-thickness burns involve the epidermis, dermis, and underlying tissues, including fat, muscle, and bone. Full-thickness burns typically appear dry, feel leathery, and may be red, white, brown, or black. The burned tissue usually lacks sensation.

Burn Severity

Burn severity is based on size, depth, location, age, general health status, and mechanism of injury. Various criteria are used to define major burns. The American Burn Association criteria for a major burn in an adult are the following:

1. Burn size: 25% or more body surface area for people younger than 40 years of age; 20% or more body surface area for people older than 40 years of age
2. Disfiguring or disabling injuries to the face, eyes, ears, hands, feet, or perineum
3. High-voltage electrical burn injury
4. Inhalation injury (any time you see black soot around the mouth and nose, an inhalation injury should be suspected)
5. Major trauma in addition to the burn

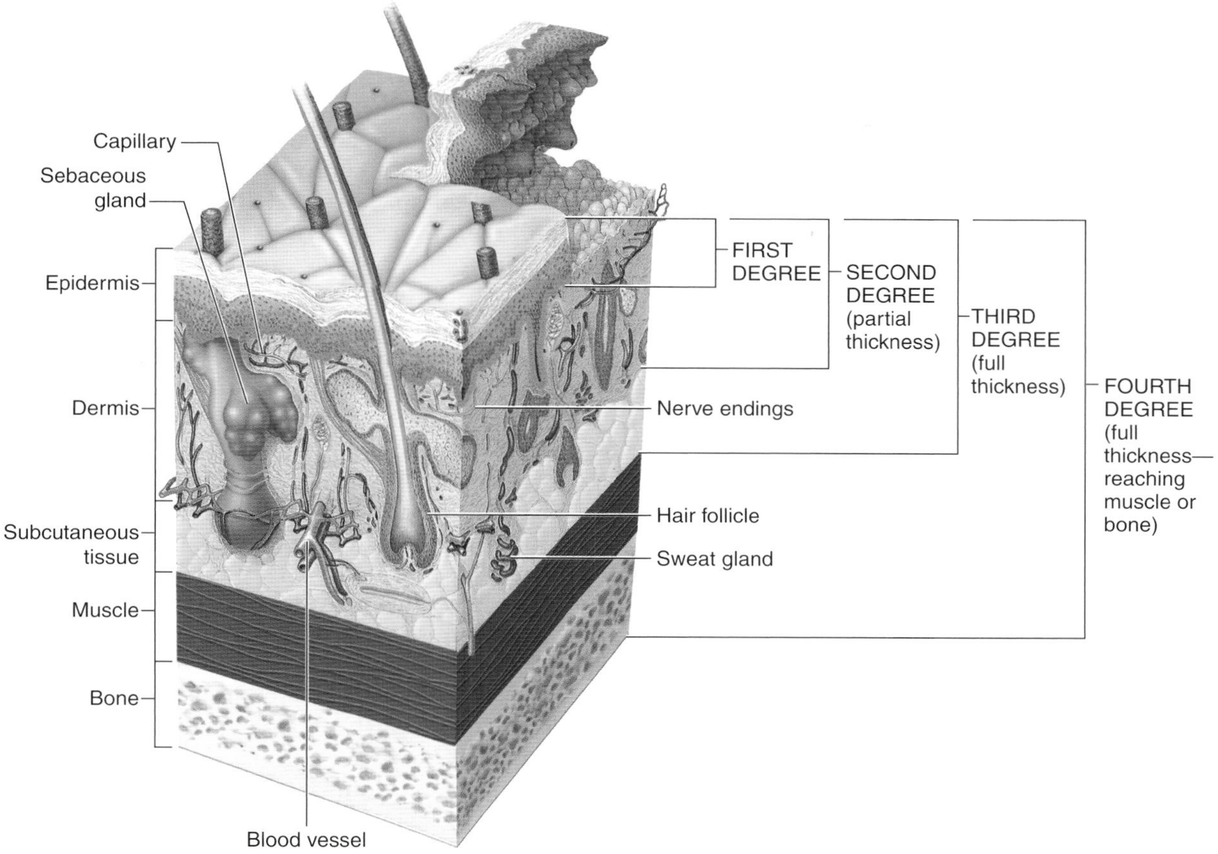

Fig. 57.14 Burn classification by depth. (From Patton KT, Thibodeau GA: *The human body in health & disease*, ed 7, St. Louis, 2018, Elsevier.)

Baux Score

The Baux score is a simple way to predict the probability of mortality because of burns. The original Baux score was based on the calculation of a patient's age plus the amount of total body surface affected by burning as determined by the Wallace rule of nines or the Lund and Browder chart. In recent years, the total score has been revised to include inhalation injury, which was determined to add 17 points to the total score. The revised Baux score is expressed as:

Baux score = (percent body surface burned) + (patient's age) + 17 (inhalation injury). A score over 140 is considered to be nonsurvivable, depending on available treatment resources.

PATHOPHYSIOLOGY OF BURN INJURY

Local Effects

Burn-injured tissue releases chemicals that cause increased capillary permeability, which permits plasma to leak into the tissues. Injury to cell membranes permits excess sodium to enter the cell and allows potassium to escape into the extracellular compartment. These shifts in fluids and electrolytes cause local edema and a decrease in cardiac output. Fluid evaporates through the wound surface, further contributing to the declining blood volume. Eighteen to 36 hours after a burn injury, capillary permeability begins to normalize, and reabsorption of edema fluid begins. Cardiac output returns to normal and then increases to meet increased metabolic demands.

Systemic Effects

Fluid balance. The shift of plasma proteins from the capillaries may result in hypoproteinemia, which causes fluid to shift from the bloodstream to the extracellular tissue. This shift decreases blood volume and causes generalized edema in the early postburn period. Blood is shunted from the kidneys to compensate for the fluid volume deficit and urine output falls. These fluid shifts, if not corrected, result in decreased tissue perfusion and decreased cardiac output that may lead to hypovolemic shock. Fluid resuscitation is critical during the first 24 to 48 hours. Intake and output should be strictly monitored to prevent shock.

As the capillaries recover and edema fluid is reabsorbed, the patient's blood volume increases. If kidney function is adequate, urine output increases to prevent hypervolemia.

Gastrointestinal function. Blood flow to the intestines decreases and an ileus may develop. Some patients

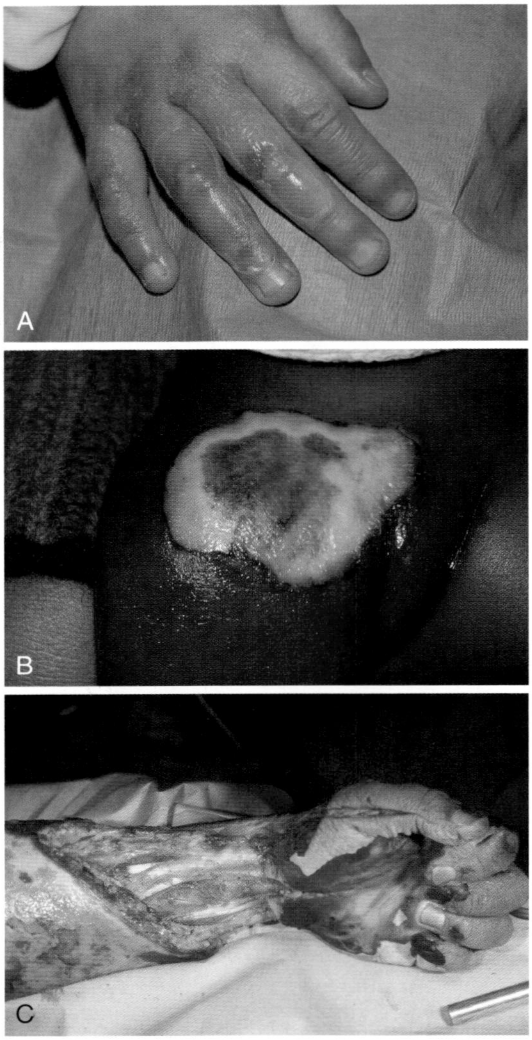

Fig. 57.15 Burn depth. (A) Partial-thickness (i.e., second-degree). (B) Full-thickness (i.e., third-degree). (C) Full-thickness (i.e., fourth-degree). (From Davis PJ, Cladis FP: *Smith's anesthesia for infants and children*, ed 9, Philadelphia, 2017, Elsevier.)

have stress ulcers, sometimes called *Curling ulcers*, after severe burns. Thus, they are routinely treated with antacids to neutralize gastric acid and H2 receptor blockers to reduce gastric acid secretion.

Immune system. Because immunity is depressed after a serious burn, the patient is less able to resist infection. The loss of the protective skin barrier also puts the patient at risk for life-threatening infection. Burn patients are monitored closely for signs of infection. The most common are methicillin-resistant *Staphylococcus aureus* (MRSA) and vancomycin-resistant *Enterococcus* (VRE). Because of military commitments, a threat also exists for infections related to organisms that are not routinely seen in the United States. The most common organism that may be seen in burn patients that come from overseas is *Acinetobacter*. Members of the military who return to the United States for burn treatment should be routinely cultured on admission to rule out any of the mentioned infections.

Respiratory system. The burn patient may suffer inhalation injuries, including carbon monoxide poisoning, smoke poisoning, and thermal damage. Inhalation injury occurs with flame burns or from being trapped in an enclosed space filled with smoke. Suspect inhalation injury if the patient has facial burns, redness and swelling of the pharynx, restlessness, cough, dyspnea, or sooty sputum. Carbon monoxide displaces oxygen (O_2) on hemoglobin (Hgb), so the blood is unable to transport O_2 to the tissues. The patient will show signs of hypoxia and die if the condition is not corrected (see Chapter 63 for additional discussion of carbon monoxide poisoning).

Smoke poisoning is the result of inhaling combustion by-products. Thermal damage to the lower airway is rare but can happen if the patient was unconscious or inhaled live steam. With inhalation injury, pulmonary edema develops and may progress to adult respiratory distress syndrome. Anyone suspected of having an inhalation injury needs to have the airway protected and should be evaluated immediately for any signs of respiratory distress. Before being discharged from the hospital, anyone with an inhalation injury should have pulmonary function studies completed to evaluate lung function.

Myocardial depression. Evidence exists of myocardial depression in the early postburn period. Laboratory studies usually are done to evaluate the effects of burns on the myocardium. Patients should be evaluated for the need for beta-blockers.

Psychologic effects. Psychologic responses to burn injuries are highly individual. A psychologist, psychiatric nurse practitioner, or psychiatric clinical nurse specialist should be involved with the care of the patient and the family from the beginning. Four stages of psychologic response have been identified: (1) impact, (2) retreat or withdrawal, (3) acknowledgment, and (4) reconstruction. Because of the effects that burns have on the patient and their return to home and community, the burn patient may need a psychologic evaluation to determine the need for further counseling and support. Psychosocial support may be needed for months and years after the burn because the patient may experience long-term effects such as posttraumatic stress disorder.

STAGES OF BURN INJURY

Care of the burn patient is often described in terms of three stages: (1) emergent, (2) acute, and (3) rehabilitation. The emergent stage begins with the injury and ends when fluid shifts have stabilized. The acute stage begins with fluid stabilization. Some sources mark the end of the acute stage when all but 10% of the burn wounds are closed, but others define the acute stage as extending until all wounds are closed. The rehabilitation stage follows the acute stage and lasts as long as efforts continue to promote improvement or adjustment. Some overlap exists between the acute and rehabilitation stages because nursing care in the acute stage can significantly affect the potential for rehabilitation. In reality, rehabilitation starts as soon as the patient stabilizes. Physical therapy and occupational therapy should be consulted immediately when the patient is admitted.

MEDICAL TREATMENT IN THE EMERGENT STAGE

In the emergency department, the staff first assess airway, breathing, and circulation and then determine whether the patient has injuries in addition to the burn. If inhalation injury is suspected, O_2 therapy is started. The patient may require intubation if the airway is compromised. Intravenous lines are established to begin fluid resuscitation and to provide emergency vascular access. An indwelling urinary catheter and a nasogastric tube usually are inserted. Blood is drawn for baseline laboratory studies (hematocrit, electrolytes, and blood gases, if indicated). Tetanus prophylaxis may be administered. Pain is assessed and analgesics are ordered. The wound is then cleaned, debrided, and inspected. Unless the patient is at a major burn center, the burns may not be debrided immediately. If the patient is to be transported, the burns are covered with clean sheets.

Once the initial care is completed, the patient with serious burns is transferred to a burn specialty care unit or a critical care unit. Intravenous fluid therapy is an essential aspect of care during the first few days of burn treatment. Several formulas are used to select the volumes and solutions to be administered. Volume is based on the patient's weight and extent of injury. For the first 24 hours, intravenous fluids may consist of various combinations of electrolyte, colloid, and dextrose solutions. However, specific formulas vary among specialty care units. For example, some formulas prescribe only electrolyte solutions in the first 24 hours.

For the second 24 hours, fluid volume is decreased based on urine output. Fluids then consist of different combinations of electrolyte, colloid, and dextrose solutions. Some formulas omit electrolyte solutions in the second 24 hours.

In addition to fluids, medical care may include antibiotic therapy and surgical procedures.

WOUND CARE

Wound care after a burn injury is intended to promote healing, prevent infection, control heat loss, retain function, and minimize disfigurement. Burn wounds may be treated by the open or closed method. The method of wound care is based in part on the state of the wound. The open method involves the use of topical antimicrobials but no dressings. Open care is less restrictive and simpler than closed care but provides increased opportunity for loss of fluid and heat through the wound surface. Closed care uses topical medications covered by dressings. Because some areas of the wound may be deeper than other areas, it is not unusual to see open care for some of the patient's wounds and closed care for others. Examples of topical medications that may be used are silver sulfadiazine (Silvadene) and mafenide acetate (Sulfamylon). To prevent tetanus, a tetanus toxoid booster may be given if the patient has not been immunized within the past 5 years. Patients who have never been immunized are given tetanus immune globulin and the first in a series of tetanus toxoid.

For clean partial-thickness wounds that will heal without grafting, temporary wound coverings generally are used. Temporary wound coverings include amniotic membranes, grafts from cadavers or pigs, and a number of synthetic materials that promote wound healing or protect donor or graft sites. Grafted areas in need of protection often are covered by temporary wound coverings that prevent grafts from shifting during the first 72 hours. Graft sites also are treated with negative pressure wound therapy. Donor sites are treated with a variety of products, including fine-mesh gauze and synthetic and biosynthetic products. Donor sites are more painful than graft sites because of the exposure of nerve endings.

Debridement

A partial-thickness burn may blister, peel, and heal with minimal long-term effects. A full-thickness burn, however, often is covered by a thick, leathery layer of burned tissue (eschar) that shelters microorganisms and inhibits healing. Eschar must be removed before healing can take place. Further, if eschar encircles a limb, it may need to be incised to permit tissue swelling without compromising circulation. **Debridement** is the removal of debris and necrotic (dead) tissue from a wound. In the case of a burn wound, debridement includes removal of eschar. Debridement may be accomplished by mechanical means (using scissors and forceps), surgical excision, or the use of enzymes. Enzymatic debridement is the use of topical medications containing enzymes capable of dissolving necrotic tissue. These substances are applied directly to the wound but should not be applied to wounds that communicate with major body cavities or to exposed nerves. Enzymatics may cause pain and bleeding.

Complementary and Alternative Therapies

Maggot debridement therapy (MDT) has been used since ancient times to remove necrotic tissue from wounds. MDT can help to reduce infection and promote faster tissue growth, as well as decrease the length of antibiotic therapy and hospitalization.

Skin Grafting

A burn wound may be covered using the patient's own skin, called an *autograft*. The graft is usually taken from the thigh or buttocks using a tool called a *dermatome*. The thickness of the graft determines whether it is a split-thickness or a full-thickness graft. If a thin layer of skin is used, it is considered a split-thickness graft. A split-thickness graft may be a sheet graft (an intact section of skin) or a meshed graft. A meshed graft has multiple tiny slits that allow the skin to be stretched to cover a larger area. The slits also allow for wound exudate to be absorbed by the cover dressing. Grafts vary in size, with the smallest being pinch and postage stamp grafts. Larger grafts may be needed to cover all or part of the burn.

For very deep burns and burns of the face, neck, or hands, a full-thickness graft may be preferred. A full-thickness graft includes skin and subcutaneous tissue and provides better cosmetic results. Another type of full-thickness graft is a pedicle or flap graft, in which one end of a section or tube of donor tissue is sutured to the recipient site while another section remains attached to the donor site. This type of graft continues to receive blood from the donor site. Once the graft "takes" or attaches to the recipient site, the pedicle or flap is cut free from the donor site.

After grafting, the recipient site is inspected for bleeding under the graft that could interfere with survival of the graft. The area is immobilized for 3 to 7 days to permit attachment of the graft to the wound base. Splints, traction, and restraints may be used for immobilization. In most burn centers, the grafts are inspected on day 3 to assess the degree of attachment. The graft is inspected again on day 5 and a determination is made about removal of staples. By day 7, all staples should be removed. After an autograft, the patient's donor site requires care as well. The donor site usually is covered with fine-mesh gauze or synthetic dressings and bandages. The dressings generally are removed 24 hours after surgery to allow the site to air dry. If the donor site is still wet, a heat lamp may be used to assist in the drying process. As the donor site dries, the fine-mesh gauze or Xeroform will begin to lift off the skin. The excess material is trimmed as it lifts off the treated area.

Scarring

The formation of burn scars can be minimized by the use of pressure dressings in the early stages of care, followed by the use of custom-fitted garments that apply continuous pressure. These garments are worn 23 hours a day and may be prescribed for as long as 2 years (Fig. 57.16). Explain to the patient that the garments need to be tight to be effective. Massage of the area either by hand or with a battery-operated device also helps to reduce the appearance of scars.

Patients with facial burns should be encouraged to do facial exercises that will decrease the appearance of scar tissue.

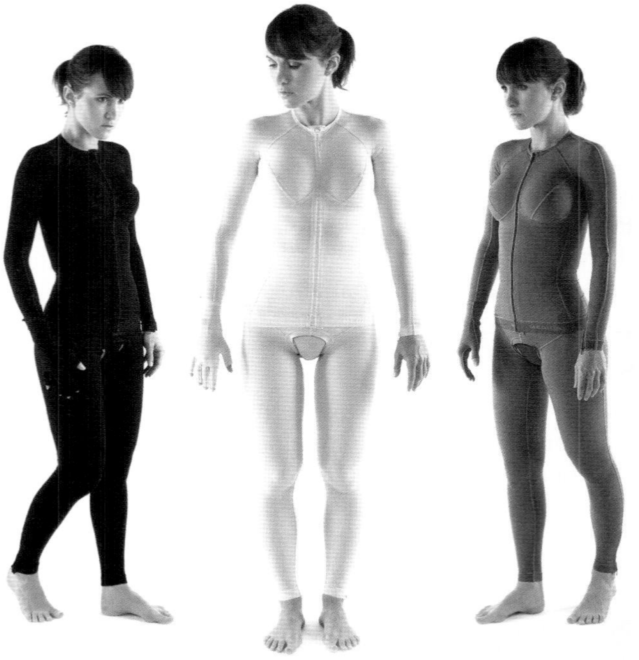

Fig. 57.16 A pressure garment minimizes the hypertrophic scarring that is common after burn injuries. (Courtesy Medical Z.)

◆ NURSING CARE OF THE PATIENT WITH BURN INJURY

Focused Assessment

When the patient is stabilized, a complete assessment should be done. As priorities change, additional relevant data will be needed.

Health History

In the history of the present illness, describe the circumstances surrounding the burn injury. In the past medical history, document any chronic diseases, surgeries, or hospitalizations. Identify medications and allergies. Take a family history even though it is not specific to burn injuries because it may alert the staff to other problems. The review of systems detects current problems with each body system. In the functional assessment, describe the patient's habits and lifestyle, roles and responsibilities, stressors, and coping strategies.

Physical Examination

The physical examination begins with vital signs. The examiner should be alert for abnormalities that suggest hypoxia (i.e., restlessness, tachypnea), excess fluid volume (i.e., bounding pulse, hypertension), deficient fluid volume (i.e., tachycardia, hypotension), hypovolemia (i.e., hypotension, tachycardia), or infection (i.e., fever, tachycardia). If the patient's condition is stable enough, measure their height and weight as soon as possible.

Throughout the examination, inspect the skin for burn wounds and other lesions. Note wound color and the presence of any eschar. Palpate intact skin for temperature and turgor. Observe chest expansion and auscultate the lungs for wheezing, stridor, or atelectasis. Auscultate the apical pulse for rate and rhythm. Assess the abdomen for active bowel sounds and distention. Inspect the extremities for injury and deformity. Delay range-of-motion assessment if an extremity is immobilized.

Patient Problems, Goals, and Outcome Criteria: Burn Injury

Depending on the severity and type of burn, patient problems with a burn injury may include those listed in this table. The first two problems are most likely to occur in the emergent stage; the remaining problems may be made in the emergent, acute, or rehabilitation stages.

Patient Problems	Goals and Outcome Criteria
Inadequate circulation related to hypovolemia secondary to shift of fluid from vascular to extracellular compartment	Adequate circulation: pulse and blood pressure (BP) consistent with patient norms
Fluid volume excess related to changes in capillary permeability and accumulation of fluid in body tissues	Normal fluid balance: edema decreasing or absent; increased urine output
Acute pain related to tissue trauma of burn injury	Pain relief: patient statement of pain relief, below 4 on a 1 to 10 pain scale; more relaxed manner
Potential for infection related to disrupted skin tissue integrity	Absence of infection: normal body temperature and white blood cell (WBC) count, negative wound cultures
Decreased body temperature related to impaired heat-regulating ability of injured skin	Normal body temperature: temperature within patient norms
Inadequate nutrition related to high metabolic demands	Adequate nutrition: stable body weight
Decreased mobility related to contractures, therapeutic immobilization, pain	Adaptation to physical limitations: minimal contractures, clear breath sounds, bowel movement at least every 2 to 3 days
Inadequate coping related to possible disfigurement, dysfunction, fear of death	Adequate patient coping: positive patient statements about future, participates in rehabilitation efforts
Inadequate family coping related to uncertain outcome, fear of patient death, and altered family function	Adequate family coping: positive family statements about the future, family interest in ways to help patient's recovery

Interventions

Inadequate circulation. The risk of inadequate circulation is greatest in the emergent stage when fluid has shifted from the blood to the extracellular compartment. If blood volume is not maintained, the patient's blood pressure (BP) falls, and tissue perfusion is impaired. To monitor cardiac output, record the patient's vital signs and fluid intake and output. Signs of inadequate circulation include hypotension, tachycardia, and decreased urine output. Inadequate tissue perfusion may be manifested by cool, pale, or cyanotic skin; restlessness; and confusion. Administer intravenous fluids as ordered with close, continuous monitoring of fluid status. Strict monitoring of intake and output is essential. The patient may also need invasive lines, such as a pulmonary artery catheter, to monitor cardiac output.

Fluid volume excess. Increased fluid volume may result from the retention of fluid in the extracellular compartment. As capillary permeability returns to normal and fluid is reabsorbed, the patient's blood volume increases. If the patient's kidneys can eliminate the excess fluid efficiently, the patient suffers no ill effects from the increasing blood volume. Because of the possibility that the patient's circulatory system may be unable to adapt to the increased volume, the patient is at risk for heart failure (HF).

Monitor the patient's vital signs for hypertension, dyspnea, and full, bounding pulse. Measure urine output and compare it with fluid intake. Administer intravenous fluids as ordered and monitor the patient closely. Document data collected for the assessments.

Acute pain. Partial-thickness wounds are typically very painful. Full-thickness burns lack sensation because of the destruction of the superficial nerves. However, burns are often uneven in depth, so patients with full-thickness burns often have pain as well. The burn patient is given opioid analgesics, such as morphine, as ordered. An opioid agonist such as fentanyl (Sublimaze) may be given intravenously or orally before performing painful wound care. If given orally, administer the medication 45 minutes before the procedure. If given intravenously, administer the drug 5 to 10 minutes ahead of time. The intramuscular route is not routinely used until fluid shifts have stabilized because absorption is less reliable. Nonsteroidal anti-inflammatory drugs (NSAIDs) also may be prescribed. Pain is aggravated by anxiety, so use measures to reduce fear and anxiety in the management of pain. Document the patient's response to interventions. Additional nursing measures for pain are described in Chapter 8.

Potential for infection. The burn patient, without protective skin, is at great risk for infection. Routinely monitor for signs of local infection (i.e., pus, foul odor, increased redness) and systemic infection (i.e., fever, increased white blood cell [WBC] count). Infection can come from the staff, visitors, the environment, and the patient's own body. Specific infection control measures vary with the agency. Strict hand washing should be practiced by the patient and all who enter the room. Body hair around wounds is usually shaved or cut to prevent wound contamination. However, do not shave the eyebrows—if shaved, they tend to grow back in a disorganized pattern. Carry out wound care as ordered or according to routines of the specialty care unit.

Decreased temperature. Loss of heat through the burn wound surface places the patient at risk for hypothermia (i.e., low body temperature). This is especially problematic for older adults whose ability to maintain body temperature is already compromised because of various age-related changes.

Monitor the patient's temperature to detect any changes. Keep the room warm and use external heat sources as needed. The room temperature should be above 76°F. In a burn intensive care unit, the temperature may be above 85°F. Attempt to limit body surface area exposure during wound care. Body heat loss may be increased if the patient is on an air-fluidized bed, so carefully monitor the temperature of the bed.

Inadequate nutrition. Healing of a large burn wound requires considerable energy. Therefore, it is critical that adequate nutrition be provided to meet the increased metabolic demands. Consult with the dietitian about the patient's nutritional needs and preferences. Calorie needs may be as much as twice the patient's baseline needs. Regular meals may need to be supplemented with between-meal feedings. Stress to the patient the need for increased intake during the recovery period. Try to create an environment conducive to eating and encourage the patient to eat all food served. Provide assistance with meals, if needed. Some patients require tube feedings or total parenteral nutrition (TPN) to meet their calorie needs. Encourage the patient to drink protein drinks rather than water. Calorie counts may be done at the bedside to ensure that the patient is consuming enough calories to meet the increased metabolic needs associated with burns.

Decreased mobility. Patients with burns may have mobility restrictions imposed by the injury or the treatment. The hazards of immobility, including pressure sores, joint contractures, pneumonia and atelectasis, constipation, and urinary infections, are discussed in Chapter 12. Monitor range of motion in affected joints and perform passive or active exercises unless contraindicated. Keep injured limbs in functional positions as much as possible (Fig. 57.17). In addition, exercise unaffected joints to maintain flexibility and strength. Impaired mobility may interfere with the patient's ability to participate in their own care. Evaluate patient's ability to manage self-care and provide assistance as needed. As the patient moves toward recovery, the rehabilitation team helps them to adapt self-care activities to permanent injuries.

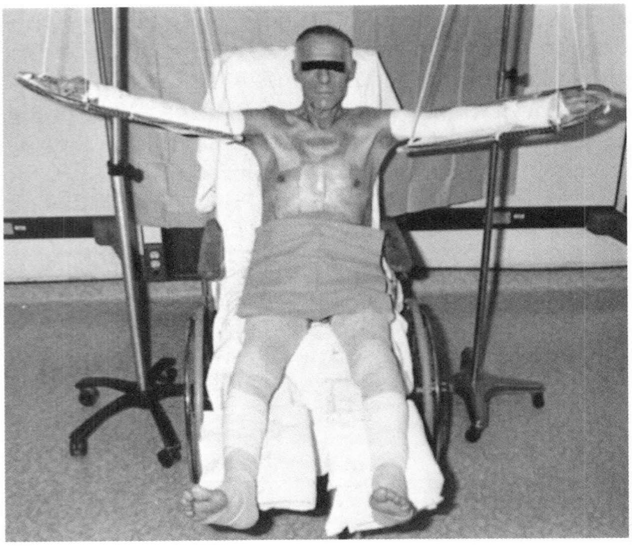

Fig. 57.17 Therapeutic positioning. This patient's arms are extended to prevent flexion contractures. Pressure dressings on legs prevent edema and minimize scarring. (From Black JM, Matassarin-Jacobs E: *Luckmann and Sorenson's medical-surgical nursing: clinical management for continuity of care*, ed 5, Philadelphia, 1997, Saunders.)

Inadequate coping. Severe burns can result in disfigurement and loss of function. The patient faces a long and difficult recovery period. The emotional responses of the burn patient are often like those of any grieving person: shock, disbelief, anger, withdrawal, denial, and depression. Demonstrate acceptance of the patient regardless of the emotional state. Provide opportunities for the patient to express their thoughts and feelings. The patient may find it helpful to talk to a nurse practitioner, counselor, or spiritual adviser. Some patients find support groups helpful in learning to live with their injuries. Encourage the patient to identify and use coping strategies that have been effective in the past. If effective coping strategies are used, the patient eventually incorporates the physical and functional changes into a new body image (see the Patient Teaching box).

Patient Teaching

Burns

When the patient is acutely ill, patient teaching consists of telling the patient what is being done, why, and what to expect. As the patient stabilizes, the teaching plan should include the following points:

- You can help to prevent wound infection by practicing good hygiene and avoiding others with infections.
- Because your nutritional needs are greatly increased as a result of the healing that needs to occur, you must eat all food provided, including meal supplements. You should try to eat six small meals plus supplements while you are healing.
- Positioning, exercise, and splints help to prevent stiffening of joints, skin breakdown, and blood clots in your legs.
- Pain management is possible, so tell the nurse or physician if your pain is not controlled.
- Protect grafts from pressure and shearing force so they can heal.
- Clothing, make-up, hairpieces, and prostheses can be used to conceal scars and improve appearance.
- Adaptive devices are available to compensate for disabilities.
- Rehabilitation resources will be provided once the acute phase has passed.

Inadequate family coping. A serious burn injury that may require months or years of therapy has a tremendous effect on the family. Significant others must be included in the patient's care. When the family arrives after the trauma, a health care provider advises them of the patient's injuries, what to expect when they see the patient, and what is being done for the patient. The family should be offered an opportunity to talk with a social worker, nurse practitioner, counselor, or spiritual adviser. A social worker or case manager should be assigned to the patient soon after admission.

CONDITIONS TREATED WITH PLASTIC SURGERY

Plastic surgery includes aesthetic (cosmetic) and reconstructive procedures. Aesthetic surgical procedures are performed to improve appearance, whereas reconstructive procedures are done to correct abnormalities. In addition to usual surgical approaches, plastic surgery may include use of flaps and grafts, skin expansion, implants, liposuction, and microvascular surgery.

Aesthetic Surgery

In general, aesthetic surgery alters a body feature that is structurally normal but perceived by the patient as unattractive. Examples of aesthetic surgery are rhytidectomy, blepharoplasty, chin implants, rhinoplasty, abdominoplasty, breast augmentation, and breast reduction. A rhytidectomy, commonly called *a facelift*, is done to remove facial wrinkles and tighten sagging tissue (see the Complementary and Alternative Therapies box). A blepharoplasty is the removal of excess tissue around the eyes. It is usually an aesthetic procedure but may be done to improve function if droopy eyelids impair vision. Chin implants are done by placing a prosthesis to correct a receding chin. A rhinoplasty alters the shape or size, or both, of the nose. In an abdominoplasty, excess skin and adipose tissue are removed and the abdominal muscles are tightened.

Breast augmentation is breast enlargement, which may be performed to increase the size of both breasts or to improve breast symmetry. A variety of techniques have been used for breast augmentation. The most common procedure has been to implant a silicone rubber implant filled with saline. Silicone implants have been used since 2006 after a 14-year ban because of concerns about possible adverse effects of silicone leakage. Breast reduction decreases breast size and may be requested to improve appearance or body proportion or to eliminate discomfort associated with excessively large breasts. Liposuction is the removal of excess adipose tissue with a suction device, most commonly used on the thighs, abdomen, arms, and buttocks.

Reconstructive Surgery

A number of procedures may be classified as *reconstructive.* Reconstructive surgery may be done to repair disfiguring scars, to restore body contours after radical surgery such as mastectomy, to eliminate benign lesions such as birthmarks, to restore features damaged by trauma or disease, and to correct developmental defects.

◆ NURSING CARE OF THE PATIENT HAVING PLASTIC SURGERY

When working with people who are having plastic surgery, you must be aware of your own biases and feelings. If you view cosmetic procedures as vain or frivolous, you may have difficulty being supportive of patients who choose to have these procedures done. Many factors may motivate people to have aesthetic surgery. Physical appearance is a component of body image and may affect self-esteem. Some people believe that a change in appearance will benefit their personal or professional lives. A person who is very self-conscious about a physical feature can benefit immensely from aesthetic surgery. It is important not to judge the patient's motivation for seeking surgery. It is also important to be alert to the patient's unrealistic expectations for the surgical outcome.

Although each procedure may require some specific nursing interventions, this section addresses general nursing care for the patient having plastic surgery. Some specific procedures are presented in Table 57.3.

Table 57.3 Complications of Common Plastic Surgery Procedures

PROCEDURE	DESCRIPTION	COMPLICATIONS
Rhytidectomy (facelift)	Removal of excess skin and tissue from face	Hematoma, hemorrhage, temporary or permanent facial nerve damage, wound infection, bruising, edema, skin necrosis, hair loss
Blepharoplasty	Removal of bulging fat and excess skin around eye	Hematoma, ectropion, corneal injury, visual loss (rare), wound infection (rare)
Rhinoplasty	Removal of excess cartilage and tissue from nose with correction of septal defects if indicated	Hematoma, hemorrhage, temporary bruising and edema, wound infection, septal perforation, minor skin irritation
Augmentation mammoplasty	Insertion of breast-shaped synthetic implants	Hematoma, hemorrhage, wound infection, phlebitis, capsule formation and contraction
Reduction mammoplasty	Excision of excessive breast tissue and skin	Hematoma; hemorrhage; infection; fat necrosis; wound dehiscence; necrosis of nipple, areola, and skin flap

Modified from Ignatavicius DD, Workman MS, Mishler MA, editors: *Medical-surgical nursing across the health care continuum*, ed 3, Philadelphia, 1999, Saunders.

◆ PREOPERATIVE NURSING CARE

Many of these procedures may be done in day surgery or short-stay surgical units. Thus, patient preparation emphasizes teaching for self-care. Initial teaching may be done by a health care provider.

Focused Assessment

Health history. Document the patient's description of the problem being treated with plastic surgery and what the patient expects the procedure to accomplish. The past medical history may elicit conditions that might affect wound healing, such as DM, circulatory disorders, and impaired blood coagulation. In the review of systems, the surgical area should receive special attention. For example, if a blepharoplasty is being done, visual acuity should be tested and documented. The functional assessment describes the patient's lifestyle and usual activities, which may require some temporary modification after plastic surgery.

Physical examination. The routine preoperative physical examination is performed as described in Chapter 17. Describe the condition that is being treated. Most plastic surgeons have preoperative photographs made to document the condition. If the nurse takes the photograph, they should be sensitive to the patient's discomfort or embarrassment.

Patient Problems, Goals, and Outcome Criteria: Plastic Surgery, Preoperative

Patient Problems	Goals and Outcome Criteria
Anxiety related to uncertain outcome, anticipated change in appearance, surgical procedure	Reduced anxiety: patient's statement of less anxiety, absence of trembling or tachycardia, relaxed expression
Lack of knowledge related to unfamiliarity with surgical routines	Understanding of surgical routines: patient correctly describes routines, identifies any actions to be carried out before admission and postoperatively

Interventions

Anxiety. Note whether the patient seems anxious by observing for nervousness, trembling, increased pulse, and difficulty concentrating. Share such observations and ask how the patient feels about the planned surgery. Anxiety may be reduced by encouraging the patient to express concerns, acknowledging that these feelings are normal, and providing information about what to expect.

Lack of knowledge. Determine the patient's perception of the procedure and its outcome. Discuss surgical preoperative and postoperative procedures and self-care. Advise the patient if swelling, bruising, and scars are expected in the immediate postoperative period. Patients usually are told not to take drugs that prolong bleeding time, including aspirin and herbal products, before surgery. Smoking is discouraged because nicotine causes vasoconstriction, which can interfere with healing. The patient may be instructed to scrub the surgical area at intervals before the procedure. Specific teaching depends on the exact procedure and the surgeon's orders or agency's protocol.

◆ POSTOPERATIVE NURSING CARE

Routine postoperative nursing care is detailed in Chapter 17. This section emphasizes special considerations when a patient has plastic surgery.

Focused Assessment

The patient may have had general, regional, or local anesthesia. Monitor vital signs and level of consciousness. Inspect dressings for drainage or bleeding but do not remove them without specific orders. Some dressings, such as those used after rhinoplasty, may serve as splints, so they must not be disturbed. Observe flaps and grafts for color and evidence of fluid accumulation; palpate for warmth. If drains are present, inspect and measure the contents each shift. The fluid should gradually lighten from sanguineous (red) to serosanguinous (pink) to serous (pale yellow). Remember that it is important to monitor the patient's comfort level.

Patient Problems, Goals, and Outcome Criteria: Plastic Surgery, Postoperative

Patient Problems	Goals and Outcome Criteria
Acute pain related to tissue trauma	Reduced pain: patient states pain is relieved and under 4 on a 1 to 10 pain scale; relaxed manner
Potential for infection related to surgical incision	Absence of infection: no fever or foul drainage, decreasing redness and edema
Potential for inadequate tissue perfusion related to decreased circulation to grafted tissue, pressure created by edema or implants, nerve damage	Adequate tissue perfusion: normal tissue warmth and color, normal neuromuscular function (i.e., sensation, movement, reflexes)
Potential for fluid volume deficit related to effects of liposuction	Normal fluid balance: vital signs consistent with patient norms, fluid intake equal to output
Altered self-concept related to change in appearance	Healthy body image: patient expresses understanding of temporary appearance, expresses satisfaction with outcome
Inability to manage self-care related to lack of information about postoperative care	Appropriate postoperative self-care: patient describes and demonstrates self-care correctly

Interventions

Acute pain. Minor procedures such as blepharoplasty usually cause minimal pain, but major procedures such as grafting or abdominoplasty can be very painful. Pain is treated with analgesics as ordered. Aspirin usually is not ordered because it prolongs bleeding time. After surgery on the face or head, the head of the bed is elevated, and cold compresses are ordered to decrease swelling. Document the effects of interventions. Notify the health care provider if the patient reports increasing pain or if pain is not responsive to treatment.

> **Complementary and Alternative Therapies**
>
> In addition to analgesics, recommend comfort measures, such as positioning, relaxation, and imagery, to decrease pain.

Potential for infection. Monitor for signs and symptoms of infection (although these are unlikely to be seen during a brief hospitalization). Instruct the patient to report increasing redness, swelling, drainage, or fever. The nurse should use gloves and, along with the patient, exercise good hand washing before any contact with the incisions, flaps, or grafts. Give antimicrobial drugs as ordered. Some plastic surgeons order topical antimicrobials applied to the incisions. After rhytidectomy, the patient usually is not permitted to shampoo the hair for several days to avoid contamination of the incisions.

Potential for inadequate tissue perfusion. After plastic surgery, inspect the affected tissues for evidence of adequate circulation. Grafts rely on blood flow in underlying tissue to supply nutrients and O_2 and to remove wastes. Thus, grafts must be protected from trauma and pressure. Pallor, cyanosis, and coolness in a graft suggest inadequate circulation and must be reported to the surgeon immediately. If fluid accumulates under the graft, it separates the graft from the underlying tissue, depriving it of O_2 and nutrients. Swelling or blisters must be reported to the surgeon, who may remove the accumulated fluid with a small-gauge needle and syringe.

Rhytidectomy poses a risk of injury to the facial nerve, which is manifested by facial asymmetry. If asymmetry is observed, notify the surgeon immediately. The patient may be returned to surgery to relieve the pressure on the nerve and prevent permanent damage.

After blepharoplasty, monitor the patient's visual status. Although the risk is slight, the eye could be injured during the procedure.

After abdominoplasty, the patient may be required to protect the operative site by remaining in a flexed position for a specified period of time. Familiarize yourself with specific postoperative orders of your patient's surgeon. Position the bed so that the patient's head and knees are elevated to reduce stress on the suture line. When out of bed, the patient may be required to continue the flexed position. The patient is gradually permitted to straighten up; however, such directions vary with different surgeons.

After breast augmentation, monitor the patient for bleeding, infection, and altered sensation. The patient also is at risk for capsule formation, in which scar tissue gradually encloses the implant, causing the breast to become hard and misshaped. The surgeon may advise the patient to massage the breast to reduce the risk of capsule formation. This procedure involves pushing each breast up, to the side, and toward the center of the chest, holding each position to the count of 10. For a period specified by the surgeon, the patient should avoid raising the arms above the head.

Potential for fluid volume deficit. Patients who have liposuction are at risk for hypovolemia because of excessive fluid loss. Intravenous fluids may be ordered after surgery, and oral fluids are usually encouraged when the patient is fully alert. Monitor vital signs for tachycardia and hypotension associated with fluid volume deficit. Use caution when assisting patients out of bed. If the blood volume is low, the patient may feel dizzy or faint.

Altered self-concept. In the immediate postoperative period, the patient often has edema and bruising as well as visible incisions. Assure the patient that these effects will gradually resolve. You can explore measures to conceal the evidence of trauma, but no makeup should be applied to surgical incisions until they are well healed.

Inability to manage self-care. In preparing for discharge, provide verbal and written instructions for self-care. The following topics must be included: drug therapy (names of drugs ordered, schedule), wound care, signs and symptoms of infection, activity restrictions, and measures to prevent complications.

Put On Your Thinking Cap!

A patient who has just returned from surgery complains of being cold. Your assessment reveals pale hands and feet, weak pedal pulses, and slight shivering. Both feet and ankles are cold to the touch. Her vital signs are normal, and her wound dressing is dry. Explain the basis of each of the assessment findings.

You obtain a warmed blanket and cover the patient snugly, increase the temperature in the room, and ask her to call you if she does not feel better soon. When you return in 15 minutes, her hands and feet are warm and pedal pulses are palpable. She is resting quietly with no shivering. Explain the physiology behind her condition changes.

Get Ready for the NCLEX® Examination!

Key Points

- Pruritus (itching) is a symptom rather than a disease. It is treated by correction or removal of the underlying cause, by skin moisturizers, and by drugs such as antihistamines, corticosteroids, and local anesthetics.
- Atopic dermatitis, one type of eczema, is abnormally dry, itchy skin that is treated with moisturizers, antihistamines, antibiotics, and corticosteroids.
- Seborrheic dermatitis is a chronic inflammatory disease of the skin caused by increased sebum production. It is treated with medicated shampoos for the scalp and topical corticosteroids and antibiotics for other body sites.
- Acne, which is characterized by comedones, pustules, and cysts primarily on the face, neck, and upper trunk, may be treated with topical medications, oral antibiotics, estrogen, spironolactone, and retinoids.
- Psoriasis, characterized by bright-red lesions with silvery scales, may require treatment with topical corticosteroids, keratolytics, vitamin A derivatives, antipsoriatics, oral retinoids, biologic agents, ultraviolet light, and vitamin D derivatives (calcipotriene [Dovonex]).
- Fungal infections, including tinea pedis, tinea manus, tinea cruris, tinea corporis, tinea barbae, and candidiasis, are usually treated with antifungal drugs.
- The two major conditions affecting the nails are (1) infections and (2) inflammation caused by ingrown nails.
- Necrotizing fasciitis, a serious infection that affects the fascia under the skin, is treated with antibiotics, debridement, and skin grafting.
- HSV-1 and HSV-2, which cause outbreaks of vesicles that rupture and form crusts, is treated with antiviral drugs that reduce the frequency and severity of outbreaks but are not curative.
- Herpes zoster infection (shingles) causes pain and itching along a nerve pathway and may respond to antiviral drugs such as acyclovir.
- Common patient problems for the patient with an infectious or inflammatory skin disorder include disrupted skin integrity, pain, potential for (secondary) infection, altered self-concept, decreased socialization, and inability to manage treatment program.
- Lice and scabies are tiny parasites that may infest the hair and skin, causing intense itching.
- Pemphigus is a chronic autoimmune condition in which fragile bullae develop and rupture, spilling a foul drainage.
- Skin cancers include basal cell carcinoma, squamous cell carcinoma, melanoma, cutaneous T-cell lymphoma, and Kaposi sarcoma; actinic keratosis is a premalignant lesion.
- Pressure injuries are most likely to occur in patients with sensory and perceptual loss; excess moisture on the skin; decreased level of activity; decreased mobility; and inadequate nutrition and in the presence of friction and sheer.
- Stages of pressure injuries are (I) nonblanchable erythema, (II) partial thickness, (III) full- thickness skin loss, and (IV) full-thickness tissue loss.
- Burns are classified by size and depth of the tissue injury.
- Serious burns affect not only the skin but also fluid balance, GI function, respiratory function, and the immune system.
- The three stages of burn injury are (1) emergent, (2) acute, and (3) rehabilitation.
- Wound care after burn injury is intended to promote healing, prevent infection, control heat loss, retain function, and minimize disfigurement.
- Nursing care of the burn patient may address inadequate circulation; increased fluid volume; pain; potential for

infection; decreased body temperature; inadequate nutrition; decreased mobility; inadequate individual coping; inadequate family coping; and inability to manage treatment regimen.

Additional Learning Resources

SG Go to your Study Guide for additional learning activities to help you master this chapter content.

Go to your Evolve website (http://evolve.elsevier.com/Linton/medsurg) for the following learning resources and much more:

- Fluid & Electrolyte Tutorial
- Review Questions for the NCLEX® Examination

Review Questions for the NCLEX® Examination

1. You are caring for a client who is experiencing severe itching secondary to atopic dermatitis. Which of the following measures should be recommended to help prevent scratching and skin injury? (Select all that apply.)

1. Maintain the room temperature around 70°F
2. Apply keratolytic agents liberally to affected areas
3. Wash new clothing before wearing it
4. Take daily hot baths
5. Wear loose clothing

NCLEX Client Need: Health Promotion and Maintenance

2. You are caring for a client who asks you about the causes of contact dermatitis. You understand that contact dermatitis is caused by which of the following?

1. Infestations of parasites
2. Reactions to drugs
3. Excessive skin dryness
4. An allergic response

NCLEX Client Need: Physiological Integrity: Reduction of Risk Potential

3. You are giving a lecture to a group of clients who have psoriasis. Your discussion should include which of the following? (Select all that apply.)

1. Psoriasis can usually be cured with drug therapy.
2. Direct contact with others can transmit psoriasis.
3. Anthralin must be kept on the skin continuously.
4. Psoriasis can be aggravated by stress.
5. Treatment may include methotrexate and ultraviolet light (UVA).

NCLEX Client Need: Physiological Integrity: Physiological Adaptation

4. While assessing an obese older patient in a long-term care facility, you notice that the patient has intertrigo in body folds (axilla, beneath the breasts). Which measure is *most* appropriate to reduce the risk of a recurrence?

1. Keep body folds clean and dry
2. Reduce bathing to 3 times each week
3. Liberally sprinkle cornstarch on body creases
4. Scrub affected areas with topical antiseptics

NCLEX Client Need: Physiological Integrity: Physiological Adaptation

5. You are caring for a female patient who is being treated with isotretinoin (Accutane) at the clinic for severe acne after other treatments have failed. All of the following statements should be included in the teaching plan. Which of the following statements is *most* important?

1. "Your skin may become very dry and peel."
2. "It may take several months to see improvement."
3. "You will sunburn very easily while on this drug."
4. "If sexually active, you must use reliable contraception."

NCLEX Client Need: Health Promotion and Maintenance

6. Which of the following is a drug used to treat HSV-1?

1. Hydrocortisone (Cortizone)
2. Isotretinoin (Accutane)
3. Acyclovir (Zovirax)
4. Methoxsalen (Oxsoralen)

NCLEX Client Need: Physiological Integrity: Reduction of Risk Potential

7. What is the *best* way to prevent skin cancer?

____

NCLEX Client Need: Physiological Integrity: Pharmacological Therapies

8. Characteristics of typical melanomas include which of the following?

1. Nodular lesion with a pearly appearance
2. Irregular lesion with uneven coloration
3. Scaly ulcer with no clear margins
4. Painful red, blue, or purple macules

NCLEX Client Need: Health Promotion and Maintenance

SLO/Objective: Apply knowledge of anatomy and physiology and pathophysiology to determine which assessment data require follow-up from the nurse.

NGN Item Type: Enhanced Hot Spot

Cognitive Skill: Recognize Cues

A 45-year-old patient is hospitalized in the acute stage of recovery from second-and third-degree burns over 40% of her body, which she sustained from a house fire. All but 10% of the burn wounds are closed, and she is beginning the rehabilitation stage of recovery.

- Blood pressure 120/68 mm Hg
- Pulse 100 beats per minute
- Respirations 18 breaths per minute
- Temperature 102°F
- Rates pain as 6 on the 1 to 10 pain scale
- Facial scarring
- Anxiety
- Fatigue and weakness
- Strong peripheral pulses
- Enteral feedings

Highlight or place a check mark next to the assessment findings that require follow up by the nurse.

58 Special Senses: Vision and Hearing Introduction

http://evolve.elsevier.com/Linton/medsurg

Objectives

1. Identify the anatomy and physiology of the eye and ear.
2. List the data to be collected in the nursing assessment of vision and hearing.
3. Identify the nursing responsibilities for patients having diagnostic tests or procedures to diagnose vision and hearing disorders.
4. Explain the administration, actions, and side effects of common drugs used to treat vision and hearing disorders.
5. Describe the nursing care of patients who require surgery for vision and hearing disorders.

Key Terms

cataract (KĂT-ă-răkt)
cerumen (sĕ-ROO-mĕn)
equilibrium (ē-kwĭ-LĬB-rē-ŭm)
hyperopia (hī-pĕr-Ō-pē-ă)
miotic (mī-ŎT-ĭk)
mydriatic (mĭd-rē-ĂT-ĭk)
otalgia (ō-TĂL-jē-ă)
otic (Ō-tĭk)
ototoxic (ō-tō-TŎK-sĭk)
presbycusis (prĕz-bē-KŪ-sĭs)
presbyopia (prĕz-bē-Ō-pē-ă)
refraction (rē-FRĂK-shŭn)
scotomata (skō-TŌ-mă-tă)
tinnitus (tĭ-NĪ-tĭs)
tonometry (tō-NŎM-ĕ-trē)
tympanic membrane (tĭm-PĂN-ĭk MĔM-brān)
vertigo (VĔR-tĭ-gō)

VISION AND HEARING

Vision and hearing play an important part in overall health and wellness. The two senses work together to help people perceive and participate in the world around them. The eyes and ears send signals to the brain to promote vision and hearing, and along with the muscles and joints also maintain balance and coordination. Eye movement sparks vibrations in the eardrum, even in the absence of sounds, indicating that motion in the ears and eyes is controlled by the same sensory pathways and motor commands deep within the brain. For example, hearing the direction of a movement, like a car driving down the road, enhances the ability to see the direction that the car is moving.

Visually impaired older people are more likely to experience hearing loss, which has a cumulative effect on function and well-being. Vision and hearing loss in older adults also is related to gradually reduced brain functioning and cognitive decline. In addition, loss of sight and hearing have been linked to lower social interaction, higher rates of depression, cognitive decline and dementia. Factors that contribute to vision and hearing loss include genetic conditions, premature birth, illness (chicken pox, measles, meningitis, brain tumors, diabetes, and certain cancers), medications (antibiotics, pain relievers, cholesterol medications), injuries, and older age.

To preserve vision and hearing, people are advised to maintain a healthy lifestyle, including a diet of fish—especially salmon and tuna, and dark, colorful fruits and vegetables—exercise, and smoking cessation.

EYE AND VISION

In the United States, an estimated 21 million people have some vision impairment even when wearing glasses or contact lenses. American adults aged 40 years and older are at the greatest risk for eye diseases. Nurses can play an important role in the prevention of vision loss, treatment of disorders of the eye, and rehabilitation of people with vision disturbances.

ANATOMY AND PHYSIOLOGY OF THE EYE

The eyeball is the primary structure involved in seeing. Several structures, in addition to the eyeball, make up the visual system. The external structures of the visual system include the eyelids, eyelashes, conjunctiva, cornea, sclera, and extraocular muscles.

EXTERNAL STRUCTURES

The external structures of the visual system protect and move the eyeball. The eyelids and eyelashes protect the eye by keeping it moist and shielding it from foreign substances. The lids are lined with a mucous membrane called the *palpebral conjunctiva.* The membrane continues from the inner eyelid margins to form a pocket around the eye and then covers the sclera up to the margin of the iris. The portion of the membrane that covers the anterior sclera is the *bulbar conjunctiva.*

Lacrimal glands located above the eyes secrete tears into the eyes through lacrimal ducts in the upper eyelids. Spontaneous blinking (approximately 15 times a minute) bathes the eyeballs in tear fluid. Tear fluid provides oxygen (O_2) and some nutrients to the cornea. Tear fluid flows through the lacrimal sac and is the route through which the eye can absorb eye drops. The fluid then goes to the rest of the body; thus, eye drops can have systemic effects. With excessive fluid production, tears flow from the eyes. Increased tear production occurs with trauma, irritation, or emotional distress. Decreased tear production occurs to some extent with aging. Severe deficiencies in tear fluid cause dry eyes, making the cornea susceptible to injury (Fig. 58.1).

Normal vision requires both eyes to move simultaneously in the same direction, called *conjugate movement.* Eye movements are coordinated by three cranial nerves and six extraocular muscles.

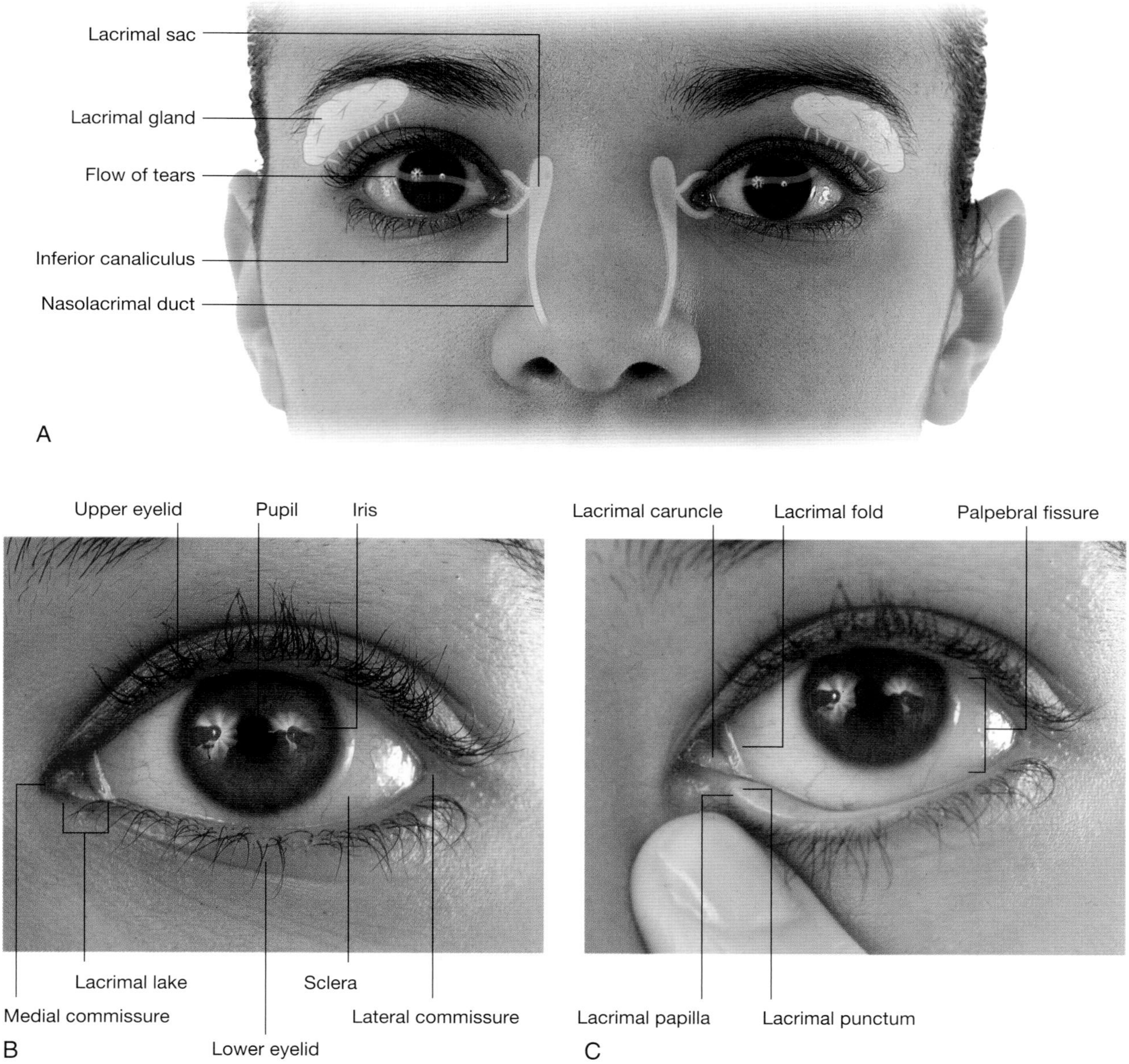

Fig. 58.1 A, B, C Lacrimal structures. (From Drake RL, Vogl AW, Mitchell AWM: *Gray's anatomy for students*, ed 3, Philadelphia, 2015, Churchill Livingstone.)

EYEBALL

The eyeball consists of three layers of tissue: (1) the sclera, (2) the choroid, and (3) the retina (Fig. 58.2).

Sclera

The sclera, the tough outer layer of the eyeball, is a white, opaque membrane except for the clear covering over the cornea. The cornea allows light to enter the eye for vision and provides approximately 65% to 75% of the focusing power of the eye. A protective membrane called the *conjunctiva* covers the cornea.

Choroid

The choroid or middle layer, located between the sclera and the retina, contains connective tissue and is rich in blood vessels that deliver nourishment to the retina in the back of the eye. The colored part of the eye, called the *iris*, is in front of the choroid and behind the cornea. The hole in the center of the iris is the *pupil*. The iris contracts and relaxes to control the amount of light entering the eye through the pupil. Dim light or severe stress causes the iris to contract, triggering the pupil to dilate, or enlarge. Bright light causes the iris to relax, leaving the pupil constricted, or smaller.

Retina

The retina, the inner lining of the eyeball, is composed of two layers: (1) the sensory retina, which contains nerve cells that process visual information sent to the brain, and (2) the retinal pigment epithelium (RPE), which lies between the sensory retina and the wall of the eye.

The RPE receives nutrients and O_2 from the choroid and supplies the sensory layer.

The area at the back of the eyeball contains light-sensitive receptors called *rods* and *cones*. Rods are most important for vision in dim light and is perceived only in black and white. Cones are used for daylight vision and color perception. The area of sharpest vision on the retina is the *macula*. Because the macula has no blood vessels, it depends on the choroid for nourishment.

Optic Nerve

The optic nerve enters the back of the eyeball and sends visual messages to the brain for interpretation. When the eye is examined with an ophthalmoscope, the part of the optic nerve that can be seen is referred to as the *optic disc*.

Fluid Chambers

Anterior chamber. Within the eyeball are two chambers separated by the lens. The anterior chamber,

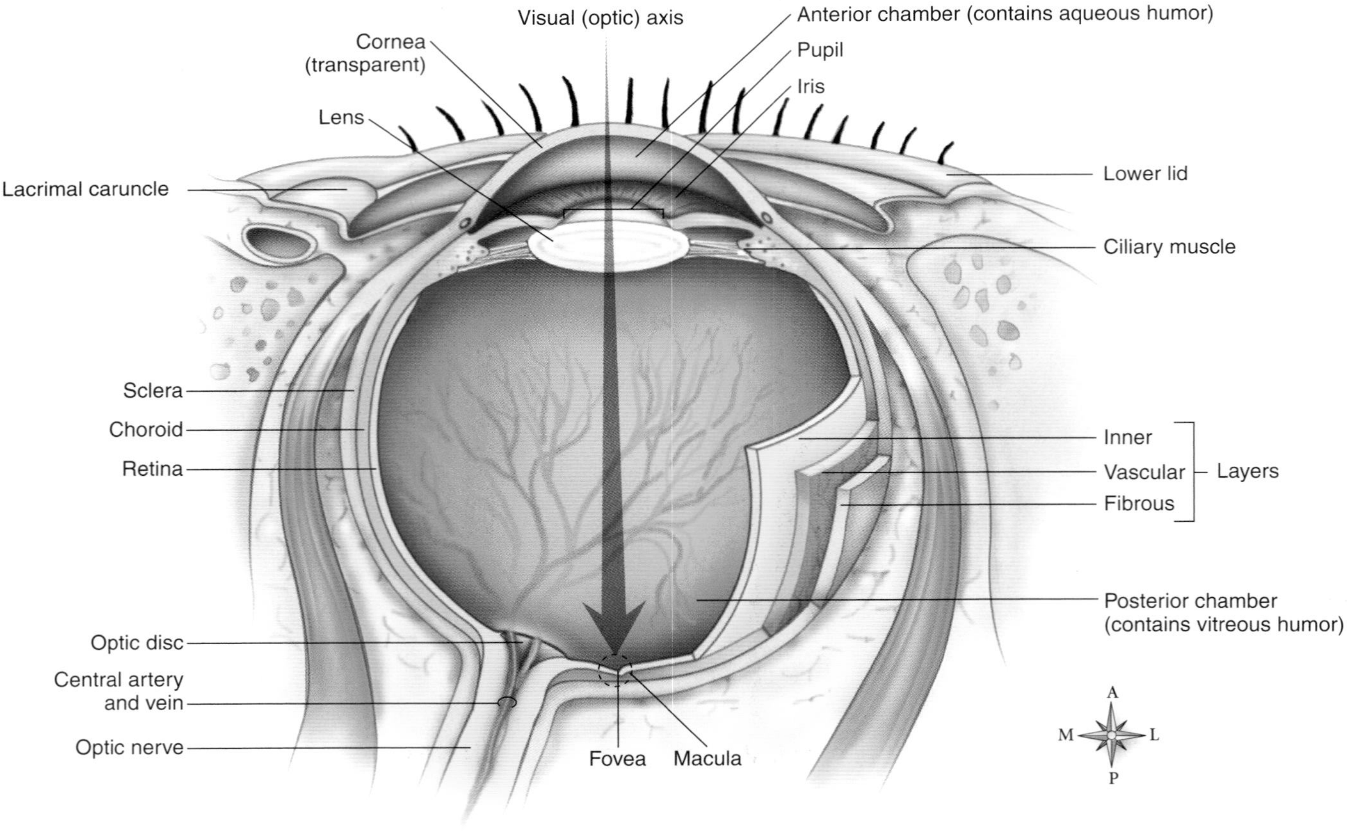

Fig. 58.2 Internal structures of the eye. (From Patton KT, Thibodeau GA: *Human body in health & disease*, ed 7, St. Louis, 2018, Elsevier.)

located between the iris and the cornea, is filled with aqueous humor, a clear, watery fluid. Aqueous humor is produced in the ciliary body. It flows over the lens, through the pupil, and out through the trabecular meshwork into the canal of Schlemm. The *trabecular meshwork* is a spongy tissue that lies in the drainage angle located between the iris and the cornea. The majority of aqueous humor flows through the trabecular meshwork. The *canal of Schlemm* returns the fluid to the venous circulation. The function of aqueous humor is to provide nutrition to the eye and to maintain intraocular pressure (IOP). The production and drainage of the fluid from the eye must be balanced to maintain normal pressure within the eye. The flow of aqueous humor is illustrated in Fig. 58.3.

Posterior chamber. The larger posterior chamber behind the lens is filled with vitreous humor, a clear, gelatinous material that helps to hold the retina in place.

Lens

The lens is a transparent structure behind the iris. It is attached to the ciliary muscle. The ciliary muscle relaxes and contracts to change the shape of the lens. This process, called *accommodation*, permits the eye to focus on objects at different distances. To focus on a near object, the ciliary muscle contracts, making the lens curve. For distance, the muscle relaxes, making the lens flatten.

VISUAL PATHWAY

As light enters the eye, it passes through the transparent cornea, aqueous humor, lens, and vitreous humor. These structures are called *refractive media*. They refract (bend) horizontal and vertical light rays so that the light rays focus on the retina.

On the retina, the light rays reflected from the image are reversed and upside down. Images are carried as impulses through the optic nerve. At the optic chiasm, fibers from the left field from each eye join to form the left optic tract. Fibers from the right field of each eye join to form the right optic tract. Images are transmitted to the brain by way of the optic tracts (Fig. 58.4).

AGE-RELATED CHANGES IN THE EYE

As people age, typical changes occur in the structures and function of the eye. The skin around the eye becomes wrinkled and looser. The eyelids usually have some excess tissue, which is not important clinically unless it interferes with vision. The amount of fat around the eye decreases, permitting the eyeball to sink deeper into the orbit. Tear secretion diminishes, and the cornea becomes less sensitive. The pupil usually is smaller in an older person and responds somewhat more slowly to light.

A ring of gray, white, or yellow in the outer edge of the cornea, which is made up of fat and cholesterol deposits, is called the *arcus senilis*. Some disagreement exists about the significance of the arcus senilis. It does not affect vision but may be related to elevated serum lipid levels (see Fig. 58.4).

Vision changes associated with age are related to changes in the lens and the ciliary muscle. The lens becomes less elastic and more dense, opaque, and yellow. These changes have several significant effects. First, light passing through the lens scatters, causing the patient to be sensitive to glare. The second, more important effect is that the ability to focus on near objects is impaired. This farsightedness (**hyperopia**) in older people is called **presbyopia**, causing most older people to wear glasses for reading or other close work. Older people may report seeing specks moving across the field of vision. These dark spots, called *floaters*, are actually bits of debris in the vitreous. Despite the age-related changes in the eye, older people generally retain adequate vision for daily activities.

NURSING ASSESSMENT OF THE EYE

HEALTH HISTORY

Present Health

When collecting data for assessment of the eye, record changes in vision, including blurring, diplopia (double vision), spots, floaters, flashes of light, tunnel vision, altered color perception, halos around lights, blind spots (**scotomata**), and diminished visual fields. If the patient reports pain, inquire about its location and nature (e.g., sharp, stabbing, aching, burning). Document sensitivity to light, called *photophobia*. Describe any drainage from the eyes such as tears, purulent discharge, or crusting of the eyelids or eyelashes. Note whether the eyes feel dry or irritated and if there is redness or swelling of the lids or periorbital area (around the eyes).

Past Health

Because visual disturbances can be associated with conditions other than problems with the eye or related structures, obtain a good history of past medical problems. Be alert for the following conditions:

- Diabetes. Elevated blood glucose can cause temporary blurring of vision. Permanent changes in the retina associated with diabetes can cause blindness.
- Neurologic disorders. Brain tumors, head injuries, and strokes are examples of conditions that may impair vision. Effects may be blurred vision, diplopia (double vision), inability to move eyes, or loss of part of the visual fields.
- Thyroid disease. Hyperthyroidism may cause exophthalmos (i.e., bulging eyes).
- Hypertension. Elevated blood pressure can cause changes in the blood vessels of the eye, eventually leading to vision loss.

Note any eye injury or previously diagnosed eye disease, including date of last examination and treatment.

A current medication history also is important in assessing vision problems. Some drugs can cause

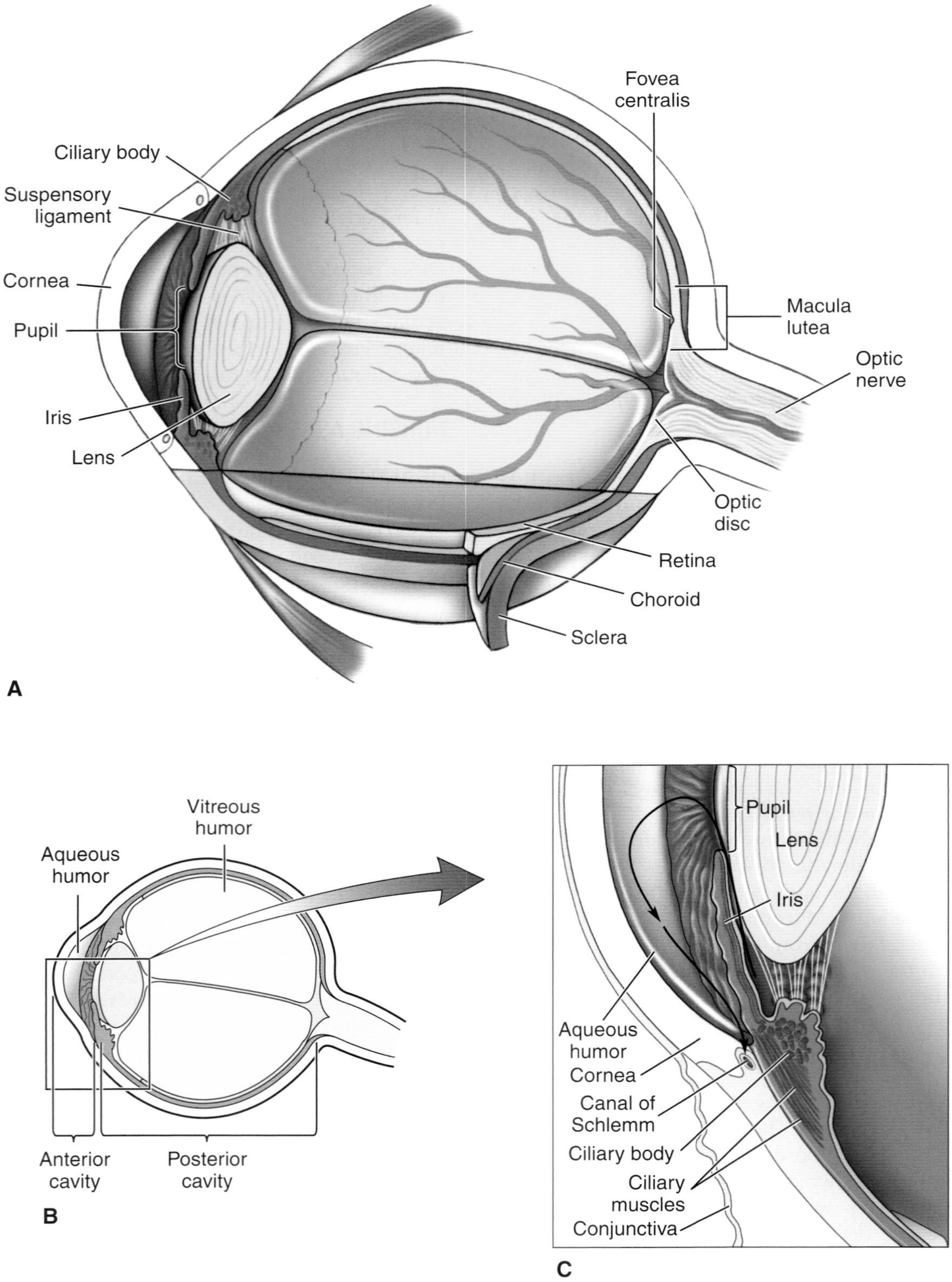

Fig. 58.3 The flow of aqueous humor through the eye. **A** Fluid is produced by the ciliary body. **B** It flows through the pupil **C** into the anterior chamber and out through the trabecular meshwork and the canal of Schlemm. (From Herlihy B: *The human body in health and illness*, ed 5, St. Louis, 2014, Saunders.)

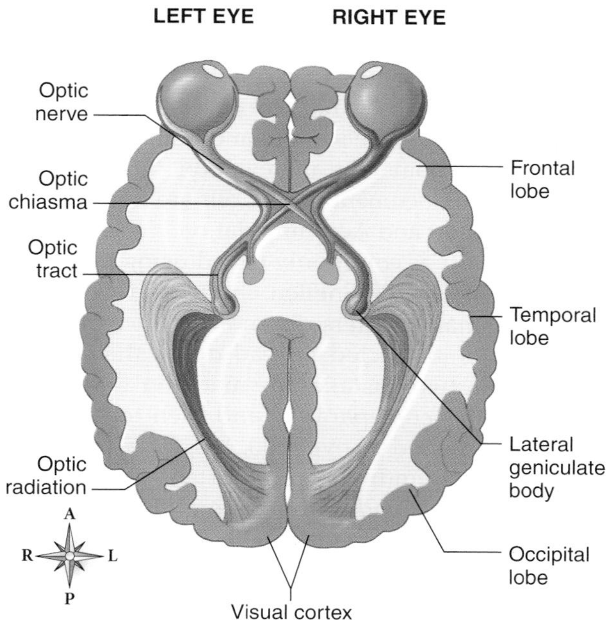

Fig. 58.4 The visual pathway. (From Patton KT, Thibodeau GA: *Human body in health & disease*, ed 7, St. Louis, 2018, Elsevier.)

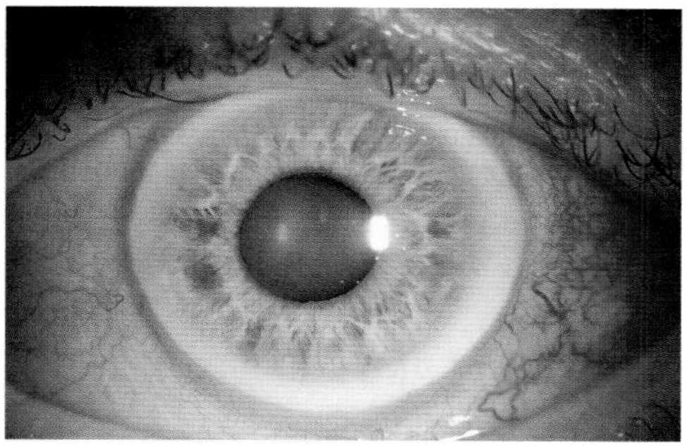

Fig. 58.5 Arcus senilis or age-related degeneration of the cornea. (From Kanski JJ: *Clinical ophthalmology: a synopsis*, ed 2, New York, 2009, Butterworth-Heinemann, in Harding MM, Kwong J, Roberts D, Hagler D, Reinisch C: *Medical-surgical nursing: assessment and management of clinical problems*, ed 11, St. Louis, 2020, Elsevier.)

temporary or permanent changes in visual acuity and color vision. Others may contribute to the development of **cataracts** or glaucoma.

Pharmacology Capsule

Drugs that are especially likely to be related to visual disturbances are digitalis, corticosteroids, indomethacin, and sulfisoxazole. Patients taking thioridazine, chlorpromazine, or ethambutol also should be monitored for ocular toxicity.

Family History

The family history includes any known eye diseases as well as a history of arteriosclerosis, diabetes, and thyroid disease.

Functional Assessment

In the functional assessment, document the patient's occupation, roles, and usual activities. Ascertain the effect of visual impairment on the ability to carry out activities of daily living. Be alert for activities that might pose a risk to the eyes.

When assessing the eyes, be alert for the signs of trouble listed in Box 58.1. If any of these are present, refer the patient to a health care provider for evaluation. The nursing assessment of the patient with an eye disorder is summarized in Box 58.2.

Box 58.1 Signs of Eye Problems in Adults

If you notice any of these signs of possible eye problems, see an eye doctor for a complete eye examination:

- Unusual trouble adjusting to dark rooms
- Difficulty focusing on near or distant objects
- Squinting or blinking because of unusual sensitivity to light or glare
- Change in color of iris
- Red-rimmed, encrusted, or swollen lids
- Recurrent pain in or around eyes
- Double vision
- Dark spots in the center of viewing
- Lines and edges appear distorted or wavy
- Excess tearing or "watery eyes"
- Dry eyes with itching or burning
- See spots, ghost-like images

The following may be indications of potentially serious problems that might require emergency medical attention:

- Sudden loss of vision in one eye
- Sudden hazy or blurred vision Flashes of light or black spots Halos or rainbows around light Curtain-like blotting out of vision Loss of peripheral (side vision)

From Prevent Prevent Blindness: Signs of eye disease and vision problems. https://preventblindness.org, 2021.

Put On Your Thinking Cap!

What are some ways you could assess gross visual acuity when diagnostic charts are not available or not practical?

PHYSICAL EXAMINATION

A health care provider performs a complete examination, including inspection of the inner eye. However, the nurse can inspect the external eye, assess the response of the pupil to light, and evaluate gross visual acuity. If abnormalities are suspected, inform a health care provider or advise the patient to seek medical evaluation.

In the eye examination, first inspect the eyelids for redness, drainage, and position. The lids should cover the eyeball completely when closed. When the eyes are open, the lower lid should be at the level of the iris. The upper lid should barely cover the upper margin of the iris. The lids should fit closely to the eyeball and the eyelashes should not turn toward the eye. Describe any crusting or drainage on the lids or the lashes.

Inspect the eyeball for color and moisture. The sclera should be clear white. Excessive redness

Box 58.2 Assessment of the Patient With an Eye or Ear Disorder

HEALTH HISTORY
Present Health
Eye: Changes in vision; symptoms of eye disorders: pain, photophobia, drainage, dryness, irritation, redness, swelling
Ear: Changes in the external ear, hearing acuity, or balance; pain in ear or throat, tinnitus (ringing in the ear), dizziness, vertigo, nausea, vomiting
Past Health History
Eye: Diabetes, neurologic disorders, thyroid disease, hypertension, previously diagnosed eye disease or injury, date of last eye examination, current medications (specifically, digitalis, corticosteroids, indomethacin, sulfonamides)
Ear: Sinus infections, dental problems, allergies, upper respiratory infections, hypertension, diabetes mellitus (DM), hypothyroidism, surgery on ear or throat, recent head injury, rubella and rubella immunization, recent and current medications

FAMILY HISTORY
Known eye diseases, hearing impairments, arteriosclerosis, diabetes, thyroid disease, arthritis

FUNCTIONAL ASSESSMENT
Occupation, roles, usual activities, changes required by eye problems
Exposure to excessively loud noise, use of hearing aid

PHYSICAL EXAMINATION
Eye
Eyelids: Redness, drainage, position, closure, crusting, inversion, or eversion
Eyeball: Color, moisture
Sclera: Color, redness, jaundice
Pupils: Size, equality, reaction to light, accommodation
Visual Acuity: Measured with Snellen chart, gross acuity
Visual fields
Extraocular movements
Corneal reflex
Inner Eye: Ophthalmoscopic examination of anterior chamber, lens, vitreous, and fundus (inner surface of retina)
Ear
General Survey: Response to normal voice; gait, posture, and balance
External Ear: Position of auricles; lesions, tenderness, or nodules
Lymph Nodes: Enlargement of lymph nodes in front of or behind ear
Mastoid: Tenderness
External Auditory Canal: Obstruction, lesions, drainage
Tympanic Membrane: Redness, bulging

may be caused by irritation or inflammation. A yellow color, called *icterus*, is associated with liver dysfunction.

Observe the pupils for size, equality, and reaction to light. Pupils that are unequal or dilated or do not respond to light suggest neurologic problems. Some medications also can affect pupil characteristics. Test accommodation by having the patient focus on the examiner's finger held at a distance and then having the patient watch the finger as it slowly moves toward the patient's nose. The pupils should constrict and the eyes converge, meaning that the pupils become smaller and both eyes move to fix on the same point. The abbreviation PERRLA is commonly used to document that Pupils are Equal, Round, Reactive to Light and Accommodation.

Visual acuity is commonly tested using the Snellen chart (Fig. 58.6). The Snellen chart has rows of progressively smaller letters. From a distance of 20 feet, the patient is instructed to read down the chart until more than two mistakes are made on a single line. Each eye is tested separately and then together. The lines are numbered 20 over 200, 100, 70, 50, 40, 30, 25, 20, and 15. The findings are reported as the last line the person could read with no more than two errors. That is, if the person reads the 20/30 line with one error but made three errors on the 20/25 line, the vision would be recorded as 20/30 in the eye tested. This means that the person could read at 20 feet what a person with normal vision could read at 30 feet. The Snellen chart may be used for vision screening in clinic and office settings. In the hospital, it may be more practical to test acuity by simply asking the patient to read available print.

Advance practice nurses learn to assess visual fields, extraocular movements, and the corneal reflex. In addition, several tests are used to detect strabismus (crossed eyes).

DIAGNOSTIC TESTS AND PROCEDURES

Various health professionals are trained to assess and treat conditions of the eye. An ophthalmologist is a physician with specialized training in diagnosing and treating eye conditions. The ophthalmologist prescribes corrective lenses for refractive errors and treats other eye conditions with medications and surgery. An optometrist is trained to diagnose errors of refraction and to prescribe corrective lenses. An optician fills prescriptions written by an ophthalmologist or optometrist and fits the prescribed lenses.

Nursing care related to diagnostic tests and procedures for disorders of the eye is described in Table 58.1.

OPHTHALMOSCOPIC EXAMINATION

The ophthalmoscopic examination involves using an ophthalmoscope (Fig. 58.7) to examine the lens, vitreous humor, retina, and optic disc. A solution such as phenylephrine ophthalmic preparation may be instilled in the eye first to dilate the pupil. This permits a better view of the inner eye. A darkened room also causes the pupil to dilate.

The examiner studies the cornea, lens, and vitreous for opacities. The blood vessels at the back of the eyeball (fundus) are inspected for evidence of disease. Degenerative changes of the retina may be observed.

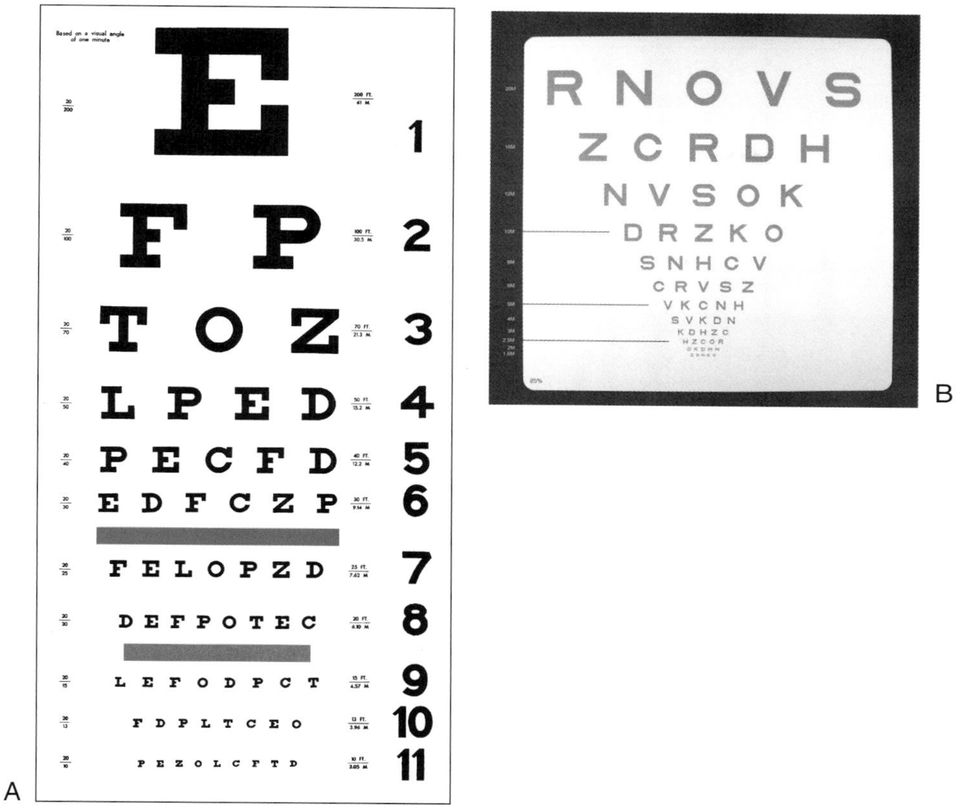

Fig. 58.6 A, B The Snellen chart is used to measure visual acuity. (From Ball JW, Dains JE, Flynn JA, et al: *Seidel's guide to physical examination: an interprofessional approach*, ed 9, St. Louis, 2019, Elsevier.)

REFRACTOMETRY

As light enters the eye, it passes through the aqueous humor, lens, and vitreous humor. The light rays bend so that they focus on the retina, a process called **refraction.** Refractive errors occur when the light does not bend properly, causing alterations in vision (discussed in the section titled "Errors of Refraction"). To assess refraction, the pupil is dilated, and the patient reads a chart through a series of lenses. The patient identifies which lens permits the clearest image. This procedure, called *refractometry*, enables the examiner to detect refractive errors. The procedure requires no special preparation or aftercare. In patients who cannot cooperate, retinoscopy may be done to measure refractive error.

VISUAL FIELDS

Visual fields include the area a person can see while looking straight ahead without moving the head. Some conditions, such as glaucoma, retinal detachment, and certain neurologic abnormalities, cause loss of parts of the visual fields. To assess visual fields the patient's field of vision is compared with that of a normal examiner (Fig. 58.8). The patient and examiner sit facing each other. The examiner moves their hand out of the line of vision and then brings it into the expected line of vision in a specific pattern. The patient states when the examiner's fingers are seen. No special preparation, equipment, or postprocedure care is needed.

TONOMETRY

Tonometry is the measurement of intraocular pressure in the anterior chamber of the eye. Normal intraocular pressure (IOP) is 10 to 20 mm Hg. Routine measurement of IOP is important to detect high pressures that damage the retina if untreated.

Several procedures are used to measure IOP. The most accurate procedure is called *applanation*, which is performed with a slit lamp microscope. The Tono-Pen is a handheld instrument that is touched to the surface of the eye several times; the resulting pressure measurements are averaged (Fig. 58.9). Procedures in which the instrument touches the eye require that the cornea be anesthetized with eye drops such as proparacaine 0.5% (Ophthaine). The Diaton tonometer measures pressure through the closed eyelid. The pneumatonometer is an instrument that directs a puff of air to the surface of the eye. It measures IOP by measuring resistance to the air.

MEASUREMENT OF ELECTRICAL POTENTIAL

Because the retina is composed of nerve tissue, it has an electrical potential that can be measured. This is useful in detecting retinal disorders, including retinitis pigmentosa, massive ischemia, widespread infection, and some chemical toxicities. One procedure used to measure electrical potential is electroretinography. For electroretinography, anesthetic drops are instilled. Then a contact lens electrode is placed on the eye and exposed

Table 58.1 **Diagnostic Tests and Procedures: The Eye**

TEST AND PURPOSE	PATIENT PREPARATION	POSTPROCEDURE NURSING CARE
Ophthalmologic examination: Examines the inner eye through the pupil to diagnose abnormalities of retina, optic disc, and blood vessels.	Administer mydriatic medication if ordered to dilate pupil. Room is darkened during examination. Visual acuity may be reduced because of pupil dilation.	If pupils are dilated, eyes will be sensitive to light. Clinics usually have inexpensive disposable "sunglasses" that can be given to the patient. If visual acuity is poor, patient will need someone else to drive home.
Refractometry: Identifies refractive errors and corrective lens needed.	No special preparation. If pupils are dilated, eyes will be sensitive to light.	If pupils are dilated, patient will need sunglasses until pupils return to normal.
Tonometry: One of several instruments used to measure intraocular pressure (IOP).	For procedures in which an instrument touches cornea, anesthetic drops are ordered. Inform patient of need to remain still during procedure.	Advise patient not to rub eyes for 15 minutes after the procedure because injury could occur when eye is anesthetized.
Fluorescein angiography: Pictures of blood vessels in the eye are taken after a dye is injected into a vein in the hand or arm. Permits diagnosis of abnormalities of vessels and retina.	Signed consent required. Administer mydriatic or cycloplegic medication as ordered to dilate the pupil. Assess allergies to iodine and seafood. Notify physician if patient is allergic. Diphenhydramine (Benadryl) may be ordered to reduce risk of allergic reaction to dye; have emergency supplies available in case of severe allergic reaction. Tell patient a dye will be given intravenously, then photographs taken through the pupil. A blue light that will flash when photos are taken may cause temporary vision disturbance. Flashing light can trigger seizure activity in patients with epilepsy.	Dye may cause a yellowish skin color for 6 to 24 hours. Urine may be greenish as dye is eliminated. Visual acuity may be reduced because of pupil dilation. Advise patient to wear sunglasses. May need someone to drive patient home.
Visual fields: Identifies the area a person can see while looking straight ahead. Assessed by comparing the fields the patient can see with those of an examiner with normal visual fields. Patient and examiner sit facing each other. They cover opposite eyes. Examiner moves their hand out of line of vision, then brings it into expected line of vision in a specific pattern. Patient states when examiner's fingers are seen.	No preparation needed.	No postprocedure care needed.
Electroretinography: Used to detect some retinal disorders. A contact lens electrode is placed, and the eye is exposed to flashes of light. The retinal response is recorded.	Anesthetic eye drops will be administered. The patient will need to remain still and focus on a target.	Advise patient not to rub eye because of risk for injury while anesthetized.

to flashes of light at varying intensities and speeds. The response of the retina is recorded. The patient must fix their gaze on a target and remain very still.

FLUORESCEIN ANGIOGRAPHY AND CORNEAL STAINING

To detect abnormal blood vessels or blood flow, fluorescein is injected intravenously and the retina is observed and photographed as the dye circulates (Fig. 58.10). Preparation for fluorescein angiography includes (1) the use of mydriatic drops to dilate the pupil and (2) initiation of intravenous access. The patient should be asked about allergies to dyes. A signed consent form is required. The dye causes the patient's skin to appear yellow for several hours after the test. Encourage the patient to drink fluids to promote elimination of the

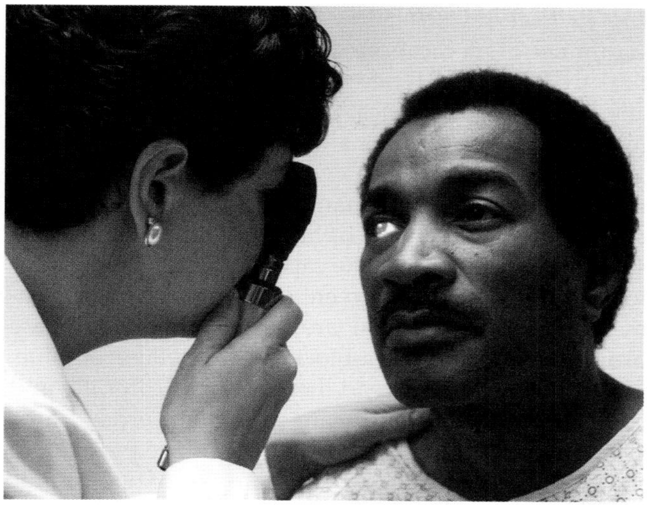

Fig. 58.7 An ophthalmoscope is used to examine the inner structure of the eye. (From Ignatavicius DD, Workman ML: *Medical-surgical nursing: patient-centered collaborative care*, ed 8, St. Louis, 2016, Saunders.)

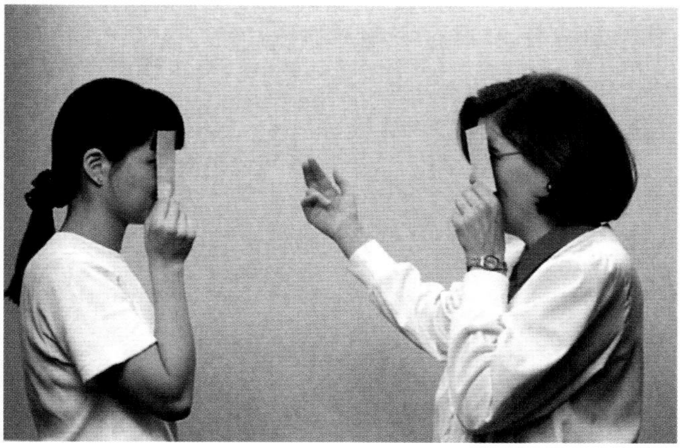

Fig. 58.8 Assessment of visual fields. (From Wilson SF, Giddens JF: *Health assessment for nursing practice*, ed 5, St. Louis, 2013, Mosby.)

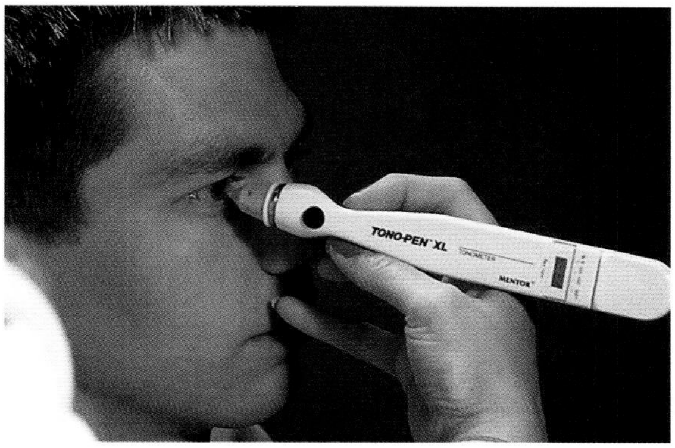

Fig. 58.9 Tono-Pen tonometry. (From Monahan F, Sands J, Neighbors M, et al: *Phipps' medical-surgical nursing: health and illness perspectives*, ed 8, St. Louis, 2006, Mosby.)

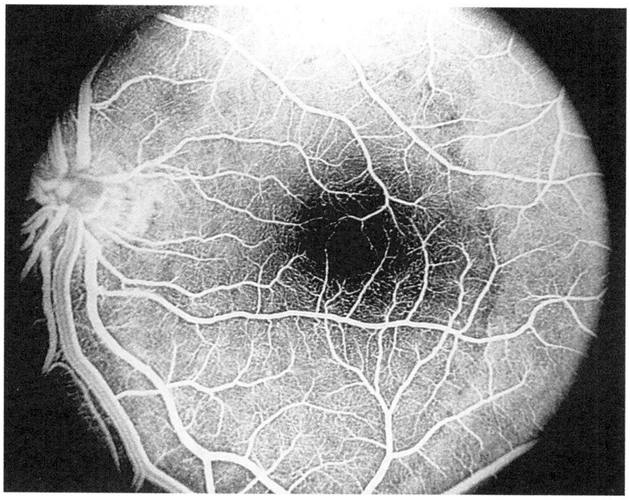

Fig. 58.10 Fluorescein angiography permits visualization of the blood vessels of the eye to examine the inner structure of the eye. (From Black JM, Hawks JH, Keene AM: *Medical-surgical nursing: clinical management for continuity of care*, ed 6, Philadelphia, 2001, Saunders.)

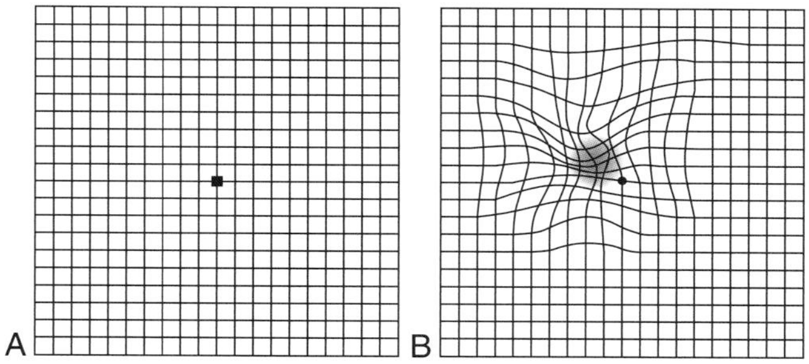

Fig. 58.11 Amsler grid. (A) Normal grid. (B) Abnormal grid as seen by a person with macular degeneration. (From Harding MM, Kwong J, Roberts D, Hagler D, Reinisch C: *Medical-surgical nursing: assessment and management of clinical problems*, ed 11, St. Louis, 2020, Elsevier.)

dye. As the dye is excreted, the urine appears bright green. Patients frequently feel nauseated after the procedure.

Fluorescein also can be used to detect abrasions of the cornea. Fluorescein is applied to the surface of the eye, followed by a saline rinse. The cornea is then examined through a blue filter. Dye permits scratches to be seen more readily.

IMAGING PROCEDURES

Ultrasonography may be used to obtain images of the eye for diagnostic purposes.

AMSLER GRID TEST

The Amsler grid test is used to monitor for changes in vision with macular disease. A card with grid lines that has a dot in the center is provided to the patient. The patient is asked to fixate on the dot and identify anything abnormal in the shape, clarity, or completeness of the grid (see Fig. 58.11).

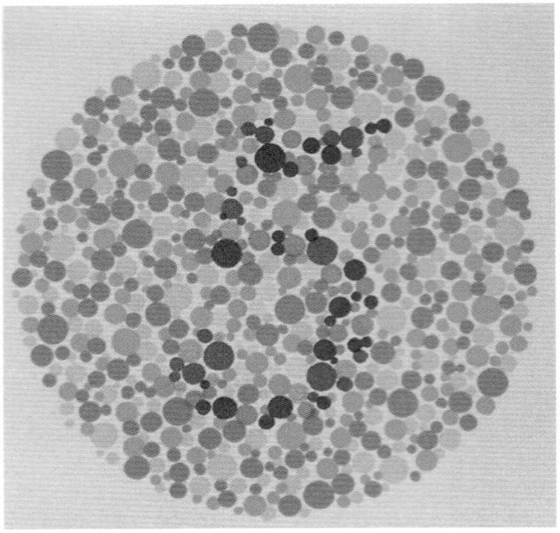

Fig. 58.12 An Ishihara color plate for testing color vision. (From Ignatavicius DD, Workman LM, Rebar CR, Heimgartner NM: *Medical-surgical nursing: concepts for interprofessional Collaborative Care*, ed 10, St. Louis, 2021, Elsevier, 2020.)

COLOR BLINDNESS

Color blindness, or color deficiency, occurs when one or all three cones (red, green and blue) in the retina do not detect color. This typically happens between greens and reds, and occasionally blues. People may have trouble seeing colors and the brightness of colors or may have an inability to tell the difference between the shades of the same or similar colors. Color blindness is an inherited trait, usually passed down from a color blind father, through a daughter who carries the gene but has normal color vision, to her son. Thus, color blindness is most common in men and rarely occurs in women. The test for color blindness is simple and can be done by looking at images that have numbers embedded in dots of color. The numbers are a different color from the background (see Fig. 58.12).

COMMON THERAPEUTIC MEASURES

EYE IRRIGATION

Irrigations are performed to remove irritating chemicals from the eye. Sterile normal saline is the best solution to use. Plain water also is acceptable, especially in emergencies. In the hospital or clinic setting, a health care provider sometimes orders irrigations with ophthalmic medications. Key points in irrigating the eye include the following:

1. While wearing gloves, cleanse the eyelids and eyelashes.
2. Position the patient with the affected eye down so that contaminated fluid does not run into the unaffected eye.
3. Place a basin and waterproof pad to collect the fluid.
4. Gently direct the fluid into the lower conjunctival sac from the inner canthus (corner of the eye) to the outer canthus.
5. Do not touch the eye with the tip of the irrigating syringe.
6. Have the patient blink occasionally to move particles toward the lower conjunctival sac.
7. If extended irrigation is needed, special irrigation systems may be used.

TOPICAL MEDICATIONS

A number of medications are available for application directly to the eye. These include miotics, mydriatics, anesthetics, cycloplegics, antibiotics, and antiinflammatory drugs. **Mydriatics** dilate the pupils, **miotics** constrict the pupils, and cycloplegics prevent accommodation. Some drug manufacturers color code the caps and labels of topical ophthalmic drugs to help you select the correct drug. The caps and labels of mydriatics are red; miotics are green; nonsteroidal antiinflammatory drugs (NSAIDs) are gray; antiinfectives are brown or tan; and beta-blockers are yellow or blue. Nevertheless, always read the drug label carefully and compare it to the health care provider's order. Some systemic drugs, such as diuretics to reduce pressure in the eye, also may be ordered. Examples of ophthalmic drugs are included in Table 58.2.

The following are key points to remember when administering topical eye medications:

1. Be careful that medications labeled for ophthalmic use are put only in the eye!
2. Drops should be room temperature when administered. Rolling the bottle between the palms is a good way to warm the medication.
3. Tell the patient to tilt their head back and look at the ceiling. The head can be turned slightly so that excess medication runs out the outer canthus of the eye and does not contaminate the opposite eye.
4. Place your finger below the lower lid and gently pull the eyelid down to expose the conjunctival sac and create a pouch.
5. Brace the hand holding the medication and then drop the medication into the conjunctival sac without touching the eyelid with the container to avoid contaminating the medication container.
6. Tell the patient to close their eyes and move them as if looking around. This distributes the medication over the eye.
7. You or the patient should apply gentle pressure to the lacrimal sac at the inner canthus of the eye for approximately 1 minute. This reduces the amount of the medication entering body fluids, thereby reducing systemic effects (Fig. 58.13).
8. If more than one medication is being given, wait 5 minutes between each medication administration.

PROTECTION OF THE EYES AND VISION

Maintaining adequate vision involves the prevention of injuries and the treatment of abnormalities. Nurses must be knowledgeable about the protection and care of the eyes.

PATIENT TEACHING

Nurses can teach people how to care for their eyes to protect vision. Adults younger than 40 years of age should have their eyes examined every 3 to 5 years. After the age of 40 years, eye examinations should be performed every 2 years and should include

Table 58.2 **Drug Therapy: Disorders of the Eye**

General Nursing Considerations

1. Advise the patient to follow directions exactly.
2. If the condition worsens or does not improve, notify the physician.
3. If multiple ophthalmic drugs are ordered, wait 5 min between them.
4. After administering ophthalmic solutions, apply gentle pressure to inner canthus for approximately 1 min to decrease absorption and systemic effects.
5. Teach the patient or family member the correct technique for drug administration.
6. Emphasize that patients should never share eye medication.

DRUG	USE AND ACTION	SIDE EFFECTS	NURSING INTERVENTIONS
Adrenergics			
epinephrine bitartrate (Epitrate) dipivefrin HCl (Propine) phenylephrine (Neo-Synephrine), oxymetazoline (Visine L.R., OcuClear)	Dilate pupil. Used in open-angle (chronic) glaucoma. Decrease corneal congestion. Control hemorrhage.	Cardiac stimulation, headache, brow pain, insomnia, nervousness, allergy, worsening of acute (narrow-angle) glaucoma. Rebound redness.	Sunglasses needed for 6 h. Tell patient to report eye pain immediately; may be caused by increased intraocular pressure (IOP).
alpha-2 adrenergic agonists: apraclonidine, brimonidine	Alpha-2 agonists decrease aqueous formation to lower IOP in open-angle glaucoma.	Headache, dry mouth, dry nose, altered taste, conjunctivitis, lid reactions, pruritus.	
Anticholinergics (Antimuscarinics)			
atropine (Isopto Atropine) homatropine (Isopto Homatropine) scopolamine (Isopto Hyoscine) cyclopentolate (Cyclogyl) tropicamide (Mydriacyl)	Dilate pupil. Used before eye examinations and for uveitis. Decrease lacrimal gland secretion. Cyclopentolate and tropicamide have shorter duration of action.	Photophobia, inability to accommodate, corneal dryness and irritation.	Apply at ordered time before eye examination. If eye pain occurs, may indicate undetected glaucoma. Safety measures while pupils dilated because vision is blurred. Artificial tears may be needed.
Antibacterials			
gentamicin sulfate (Garamycin Ophthalmic) erythromycin (Ilotycin) polymyxin B sulfate (neomycin sulfate, bacitracin) sulfonamides (Sulamyd Ophthalmic) ciprofloxacin (Ciloxan)	Treatment or prevention of eye infections.	Allergic reaction, conjunctivitis.	Screen for previous allergic reactions; withhold drug and notify physician if allergic. Inspect eyes and lids for increasing redness.
Antifungals			
natamycin (Natacyn)	Effective against some fungal infections of eye.	Rarely: allergic reaction, conjunctival edema.	Advise patient to continue treatment as prescribed (usually 14–21 days). Notify physician if symptoms continue or if edema develops.
Antivirals			
vidarabine (Vira-A)	Treatment of herpes simplex, keratitis.	Irritation, redness, edema, pain, itching, photophobia. Rarely: allergic reactions.	Advise sunglasses for sensitivity. Refrigerate.
Topical Anesthetics			
proparacaine HCl (Ophthaine, Ophthetic) tetracaine HCl (Pontocaine)	Block sensation in external eye for tonometry, removal of sutures or foreign bodies, some surgical procedures.	Stinging, irritation. Allergic reactions rare.	Do not use discolored solution. Caution patient not to touch or rub eye or insert contact lens until sensation returns.

Continued

Table 58.2 **Drug Therapy: Disorders of the Eye—cont'd**

Antiinflammatories			
Corticosteroids: prednisolone acetate prednisolone sodium phosphate dexamethasone fluorometholone	Prevent redness and swelling caused by inflammation from causes other than bacterial infection. For short-term use only.	Systemic effects possible if sufficient drug is absorbed. Adverse effects with long-term use include cataracts, eye infection, increased IOP, fluid retention, nausea, mood swings, hypokalemia, and many others.	Apply pressure to lacrimal sac for 1–2 min after application to reduce absorption. Monitor blood studies. Remove contact lenses before using. Reinsert in 10 min if no redness.
Nonsteroidal antiinflammatory drugs (NSAIDs) ketorolac tromethamine (Acular) Mast cell stabilizers cromolyn sodium (Cromolyn, Opticrom) lodoxamide tromethamine (Alomide) H1-receptor blocker emedastine difumarate (Emadine) Decongestant: phenylephrine (Neo-Synephrine)	Treats allergic conjunctivitis; relieves inflammation. Mast cell stabilizers take several weeks for full effect. H1-receptor blocker provides immediate relief of symptoms.	Eye irritation, allergic reactions.	Tell patient on mast cell stabilizers it will be several days before full effect is evident. Ask about allergies to NSAIDs; if allergic, withhold ophthalmic NSAIDs and notify supervisor or physician. Risk of bleeding if taken with oral NSAIDS or anticoagulants.
Angiotensin Inhibitors			
ranibizumab (Lucentis) aflibercept (Eylea) bevacizumab (Avastin)	Injected into the vitreous humor to slow progression of wet macular degeneration. May improve vision. Repeated every 1 to 2 months.	Inflammation in the eye, blurred vision, corneal edema, conjunctival hemorrhage, increased IOP, "floaters," eye discomfort.	Advise patient to notify physician immediately if pain, light sensitivity, or redness occur (may have inflammation). Reinforce need for follow-up and repeat treatments.

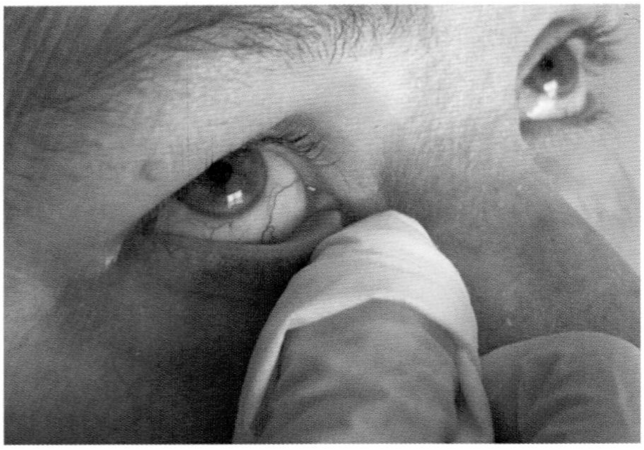

Fig. 58.13 Applying punctal occlusion to prevent systemic absorption of eye drops. (From Workman ML, LaCharity L: *Understanding pharmacology*, ed 2, St. Louis, 2016, Saunders, in Ignatavicius DD, Workman LM, Rebar CR, Heimgartner NM. *Medical-surgical nursing: concepts for interprofessional collaborative care*, ed 10, St. Louis, 2021, Elsevier.)

testing for glaucoma. After age 60 years, eye exams should be performed every 1 to 2 years. Regular eye exams aid in early detection and treatment of eye disorders.

Tell patients to report sharp, stabbing eye pain or deep, throbbing eye pain. Other symptoms that should be reported to a health care provider are photophobia (sensitivity to light), blurred or double vision, loss of part of the visual fields, halos around lights, and floaters. Floaters are spots that appear to move across the field of vision. Some patients describe floaters as being like birds or bugs swooping past one's face. Other symptoms that require medical evaluation are burning sensations, itching, excessive tearing, and the presence of drainage from the eyes.

When symptoms of eye problems exist, patients should seek medical advice rather than try home remedies. First aid for eye injuries is explained in Chapter 63.

Nutrition Considerations

1. Vitamin A is essential for normal vision.
2. An early symptom of vitamin A deficiency is night blindness.
3. Severe vitamin A deficiency causes clinical eye disease that leads to blindness.

Prevention of Injuries

Injuries caused by foreign objects are a major cause of vision loss. Teach young children the danger of throwing or poking objects at the faces of playmates. Assess toys for safety. Adult activities that produce sparks or cause fragments to be dispersed also cause injuries. Advise protective eyewear for such potentially dangerous activities.

Basic Eye Care

Gently cleanse the eyelids each time the face is washed. Use a clean cloth without soap. Wash the eye from the inner canthus (near the nose) toward the outer canthus. Dry crusts on the eyelids and eyelashes usually can be wiped off. If necessary, place a warm, damp cloth on the lids for several minutes to soften the crusts.

Routine eye rinses and drops are unnecessary for most people. Exceptions are people with inadequate tear production and those whose eyes do not close completely. Lubricating drops called *artificial tears* are available over the counter. Sometimes eye patches are applied, or the lids are taped shut to prevent drying of the cornea.

EFFECT OF VISUAL IMPAIRMENT

Vision loss has significant effects on all areas of an individual's life. Mild losses may require only some adaptations. More serious losses affect independence, mobility, employment, and interpersonal relationships. In addition, pleasure in seeing the people and things an individual treasures is lost.

The loss of vision triggers a grief response. People grieve for the lost function just as they might grieve after the loss of a loved one. Factors that affect a person's response to this loss include personality, usual coping style, effect of vision loss on the person's life, and the circumstances of the loss. If grief is resolved in a healthy manner, adaptation and acceptance eventually occur. People who have progressive loss of vision may experience anticipatory grief. Nursing care to help the person who is grieving is discussed in Chapter 19.

NURSING CARE OF THE VISUALLY IMPAIRED PATIENT

When people hear the word *blind*, they think of someone who is unable to see. However, degrees of visual impairment exist. Although some visually impaired people are unable to see at all, many others have partial vision. Therefore, medical literature is more likely to use terms such as *visual impairment* or *visually handicapped* rather than *blind*. In addition, a stigma may be attached to the word *blind*, as some people automatically associate blindness with helplessness.

Trauma, disease, and some congenital defects account for visual handicaps throughout the life span. Some types of visual disturbances are more common in older people.

To work with the visually impaired, be aware of their thoughts and feelings about visual handicaps. Assume that people with visual impairments could be independent and productive. Pity has no place in this situation because it encourages hopelessness and helplessness. The person needs help with some tasks but should still be treated as an adult.

The extent of vision loss determines the types of assistance that might be needed. Many people have visual problems that can be corrected with eyeglasses, drug therapy, or surgical treatment. Many products are available to enable visually impaired people to function more independently. When planning care, consider whether the patient's condition is temporary, permanent, correctable, treatable, or progressive.

◆ FOCUSED ASSESSMENT

The nursing assessment of the patient with an eye disorder is summarized in Chapter 58, Box 58.2.

Patient Problems, Goals, and Outcome Criteria: Visual Impairment

Patient Problem	Goals and Outcome Criteria
Lack of knowledge related to strategies to adapt to altered reception, transmission, and interpretation of visual stimuli	Adaptation to vision impairment: patient has no falls or other traumatic injuries, uses assistive devices and techniques to maintain as much independence as possible
Inadequate coping related to decreased independence, threat to body image, denial	Effective coping: patient makes efforts to adapt, participates in self-care to maximum degree possible
Potential for injury related to inability to walk safely because of impaired vision, anxiety	Absence of injury: patient walks safely; uses strategies to move about safely
Inability to manage treatment regimen related to lack of knowledge of treatment of vision impairment	Effective management of treatment regimen: prescribed plan of care is managed appropriately; patient carries out plan of care and participates in rehabilitation programs if indicated

◆ INTERVENTIONS

Lack of Knowledge

When a visually impaired person is admitted to a health care facility, provide an orientation to the environment. The fact that the patient has visual impairment should be reflected in the nursing care plan. In addition, a sign may be posted to alert other caregivers and employees.

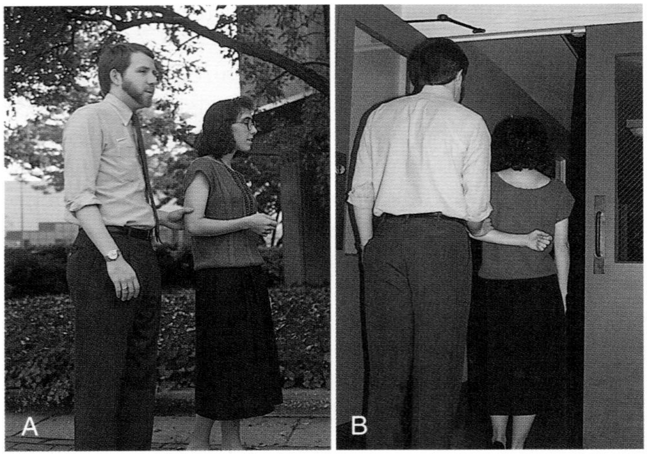

Fig. 58.14 (A) To escort a visually impaired person, allow the person to grasp your upper arm. (B) To enter a narrow passage or doorway, bring your arm behind your back to alert the person. (Courtesy Cleveland Sight Center, Cleveland, OH. www.clevelandsightcenter.org.)

Safety is a primary consideration for these patients. Measures to support the patient with impaired vision and to prevent injury include the following:

1. When you enter the room, announce your presence and introduce yourself to avoid startling or embarrassing the patient.
2. Speak before touching the patient to avoid startling them.
3. Speak in a normal tone of voice. People tend to act as if those who cannot see cannot hear, so a tendency exists to raise one's voice when talking to the visually impaired.
4. Address the patient in the appropriate manner for their age and intellectual ability. Visual impairment is not associated with mental impairment.
5. Advise the patient about what to expect during procedures.
6. Tell the patient when you leave the room.
7. Leave the bed in low position.
8. Place the call bell within reach and ensure that the patient knows how to use it.
9. Keep doors either open or closed so that the ambulatory patient does not run into a partially closed door.
10. Do not rearrange the room after orienting the patient.
11. Eliminate meaningless noise from the environment as much as possible.
12. To lead a blind person, have them take your arm (Fig. 58.14).

The environment significantly influences the visually impaired patient's ability to function. It should be safe and promote maximal independence. As mentioned, orientation to the setting is especially important. Ensure that the patient can use the call system, locate personal items, and use the bathroom. Tell the patient if any new equipment or furniture is brought into the room. Keep pathways in the room free of clutter.

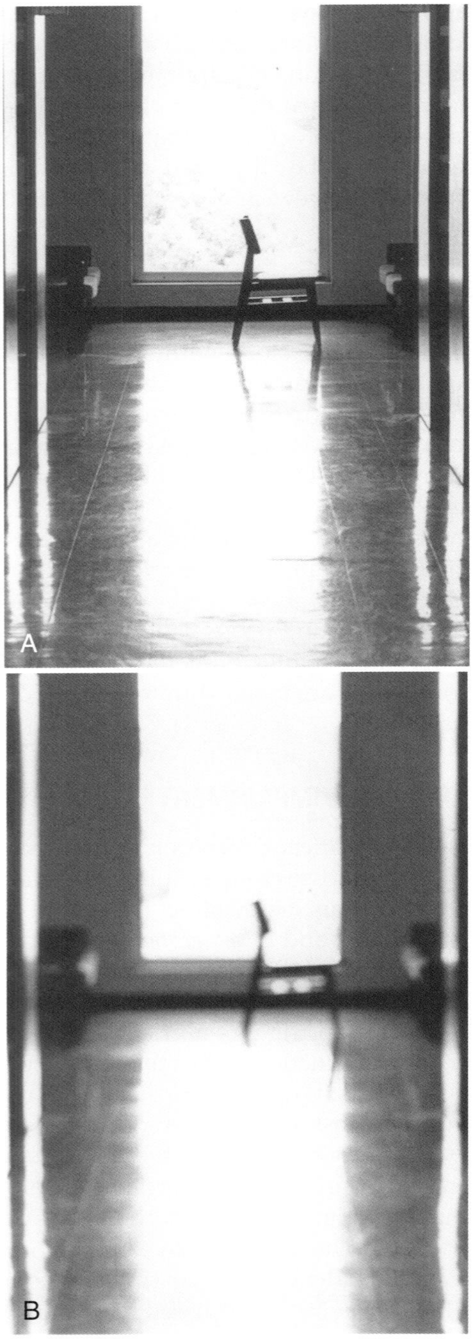

Fig. 58.15 Glare perceived by (A) a person with normal vision and (B) an older person who has undergone age-related changes. (From Linton AD, Lach H: *Matteson and McConnell's gerontological nursing*, ed 3, Philadelphia, 2007, Saunders.)

For patients who are partially sighted, lighting is very important. Glare must be reduced because it interferes with vision. Windows should have adjustable shades, blinds, or sheers. Floors should not be highly polished (Fig. 58.15). Color can provide important cues to enable the partially sighted person to function. This is especially true of the older person whose color perception may have changed. Older people perceive warm colors (e.g., red, orange, yellow) more accurately than cool colors (e.g., blue, green). Furniture color should be distinctly different from the color of floors and walls. Light switches, handrails, and steps marked with contrasting colors are easier to locate. Dishes and cups with colored rims facilitate self-feeding and reduce spills.

Inadequate Coping

People who have lived with visual impairment usually have developed routines and strategies to cope with the situation. Ask about such routines and maintain them as much as possible. If the patient uses assistive devices such as eyeglasses or magnifying glasses, make sure they are available and encourage their use. The older person who becomes confused during hospitalization may show dramatic improvement when eyeglasses are provided.

Encourage diversional activities when appropriate. The patient with some vision may be able to enjoy reading with magnifiers or large-print reading material. Talking books are available without charge through the American Foundation for the Blind. Many bookstores stock audio books (i.e., books recorded on compact disks [CDs]), and eBooks are available online or through libraries. Those who have been trained can use Braille for reading material and computers. Braille uses arrangements of raised dots to represent letters. The reader reads the material by moving the fingertips over the characters. Not everyone is able to master reading Braille because of the sensitive touch needed. Special telescopic lenses and magnifiers can enable some patients to read, write, and use a computer. Canes and guide dogs permit independent ambulation. Voice recognition programs permit computer use without typing.

Ask the patient about what assistance is required instead of assuming that help is needed. Many patients are quite independent despite impaired vision. Do not encourage dependence during hospitalization. To orient the patient to the location of foods, fluids, or other objects on the tray or table, think of their arrangement as a clock face (e.g., "your meat is at 3 o'clock").

Potential for Injury

A consistent environment enables the patient to be more independent with less risk of injury. Do not move furniture, personal effects, and equipment without patient consent. Rehabilitation experts teach patients techniques and adaptive equipment to facilitate physical mobility.

Some visually impaired people have guide dogs that enable them to move about more independently. These dogs are trained to guide their owners inside and outside the home. They can usually go anywhere their owners go. Laws that restrict pets in public places usually do not apply to guide dogs. When the dogs are wearing their harnesses, they are working and should not be distracted by friendly strangers.

Inability to Manage Treatment Regimen

Teach patients with diseases of the eye to perform prescribed measures to promote healing. Ensure that the patient is able to use eye drops properly and be sure that oral medications are kept in a place that is easily accessible and labeled in large letters so that they are taken correctly.

EAR AND HEARING

Approximately 15% of American adults (37.5 million) report some degree of hearing loss, and 50% of those older than 75 years of age have disabling hearing loss. Loss of hearing can have significant impact on most aspects of an individual's life.

Hearing loss is the third most common chronic physical condition after high blood pressure and arthritis. In addition, hearing loss is among the most common work-related conditions and is almost always permanent. Impaired hearing is associated with depression; cognitive decline; isolation; loss of enjoyment when sounds are muted and lack quality; and decreased safety at home or at work.

Health care providers can reduce disability by teaching people how to prevent hearing loss, identifying and addressing treatable causes of hearing loss, and by helping to rehabilitate those who are impaired.

ANATOMY AND PHYSIOLOGY OF THE EAR

The ears are essential organs for hearing, position sense, and equilibrium. **Position sense** enables a person to know the position of body parts without looking. **Equilibrium** is the state of balance needed for walking, standing, and sitting. As noted earlier, the sensory and motor neuronal pathways to and from the ear are significantly intertwined with the pathways of the eye for hearing and vision functioning.

ANATOMY

The ear has three major sections: (1) the external ear, (2) the middle ear, and (3) the inner ear (Fig. 58.16).

External Ear

Auricle. The external ear includes the auricle and the external auditory canal. The auricle, also called the *pinna*, is the visible part of the ear.

Innervation. Because many nerves innervate the ear, ear pain can sometimes be traced to disorders of the nose, mouth, or neck. Of special importance is the facial nerve (the seventh cranial nerve), which lies alongside the auditory canal. The facial nerve is protected in the canal by a thin bony covering. It exits from the skull just in front of the ear and branches across the face to control muscle movement.

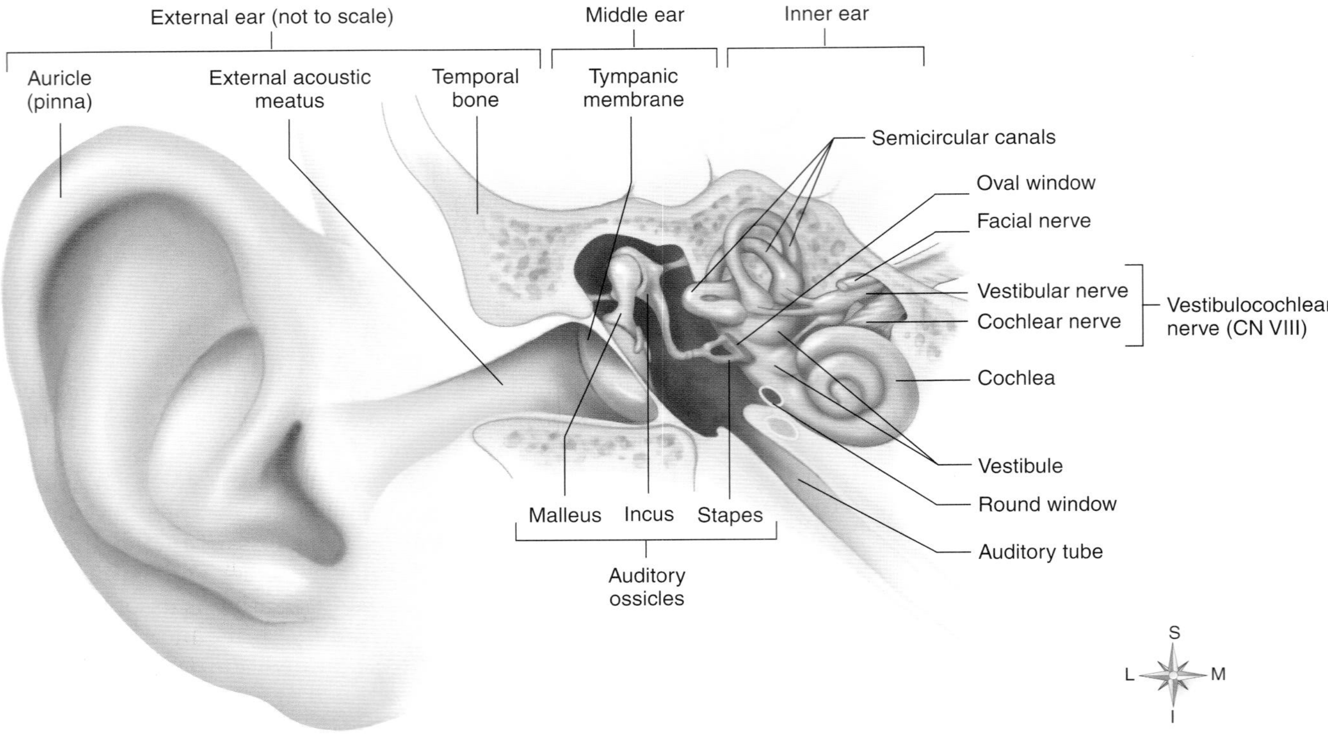

Fig. 58.16 Anatomic structure of the ear illustrating the three major sections: (1) the external ear, (2) the middle ear, and (3) the inner ear. *CN*, Cranial nerve. (From Patton KT, Thibodeau GA: *Anatomy and physiology*, ed 8, St. Louis, 2013, Mosby.)

Lymph drainage. Lymph nodes located in front of, behind, and below the auricle drain the ear. In the presence of ear infections, they may become enlarged.

External auditory canal. The external auditory canal extends from the external opening of the ear to the tympanic membrane. The **tympanic membrane** commonly is called the *eardrum*. The canal is lined with cells that secrete **cerumen** (earwax). The waxy secretion coats and protects the canal.

Tympanic membrane. The tympanic membrane at the end of the external auditory canal is shiny and pearl gray. Sound waves entering the external auditory canal cause the membrane to vibrate.

Middle Ear

Bones. The middle ear is an air-filled space in the temporal bone. It contains three ossicles (small bones): (1) malleus (hammer), (2) incus (anvil), and (3) stapes (stirrup). The function of these bones is to conduct the sound waves transmitted by the tympanic membrane to the inner ear.

The malleus lies directly under the tympanic membrane. One portion of the malleus is attached to the membrane and another portion is connected to the incus. The incus is connected to the stapes. The stapes has a footplate that fits into the oval window. The oval window, which opens into the vestibule, separates the middle ear from the inner ear. Sound waves are transmitted from the tympanic membrane to the malleus, the incus, the stapes, and then the oval window.

Eustachian tube. An important structure in the middle ear is the eustachian tube. The eustachian tube extends from the middle ear to the nasopharynx, as illustrated in Fig. 58.17. It creates an air passage to the middle ear so that air pressure remains the same on both sides of the tympanic membrane.

Mastoid process. The mastoid process is the bony structure behind the auricle. The interior is made up of air cells that are directly connected to the middle ear. The mastoid process is very close to the brain.

Inner Ear

The inner ear consists of the membranous labyrinth and the bony labyrinth. The membranous labyrinth contains fluid called *endolymph*. Endolymph moves with changes in body position and is important to both hearing and balance.

The parts of the bony labyrinth are the vestibule, semicircular canals, and cochlea. The oval window opens into the vestibule. Receptors in the vestibule monitor the position of the head to maintain posture balance. Receptors in the semicircular canals monitor changes in rate or direction of movement to maintain balance during movement. The cochlea is a coiled tube that looks like a snail. It contains the organ of Corti, which is the receptor end-organ

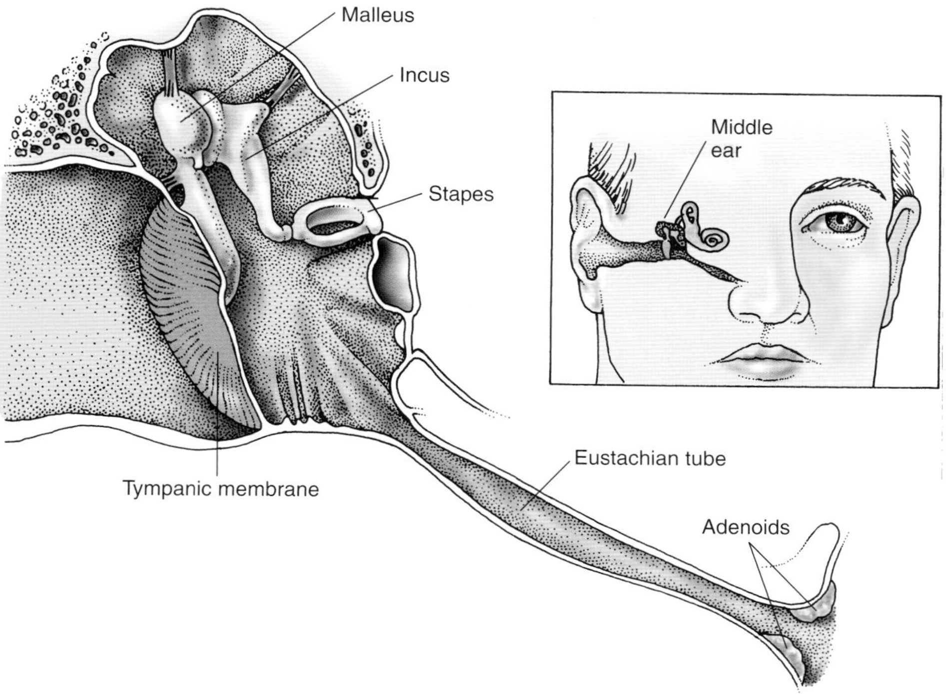

Fig. 58.17 The eustachian tube extends from the middle ear to the nasopharynx. (From Ignatavicius DD, Workman ML: *Medical-surgical nursing: patient-centered collaborative care*, ed 6, St. Louis, 2010, Saunders.)

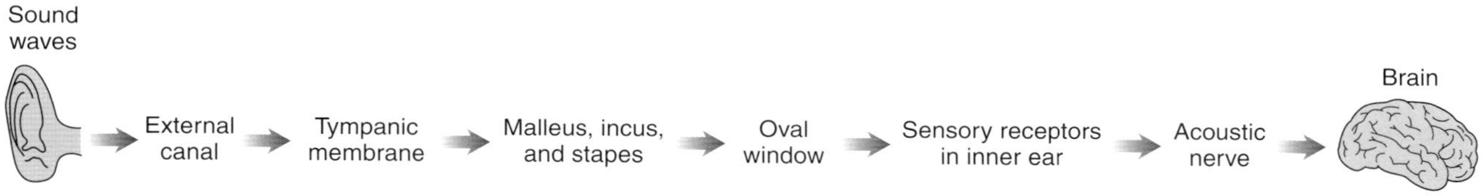

Fig. 58.18 Physiology of hearing.

of hearing. The organ of Corti transmits stimuli from the oval window to the acoustic (auditory) nerve.

PHYSIOLOGY OF HEARING

The perception and interpretation of sound depend on a complex series of steps. A malfunction at any step can result in some type of hearing impairment. Fig. 58.18 illustrates the steps involved in the hearing process.

Loudness and intensity are two different types of sounds. Loudness refers to how one perceives audible sounds; intensity is the amount of sound energy in a confined space as measured in decibels (dB). The risk of hearing damage increases with the intensity of a sound rather than loudness. A whisper is about 30dB, normal conversation is about 60dB, motorcycle engine running is about 95dB, and loud entertainment venues such as concerts, bars, restaurants and loud listening devices are about 105 to 110dB. Noise above 70 dB over a long period of time can slowly damage hearing; loud noise above 120 dB can cause immediate damage (Fig. 58.19).

Damage to any part of the ear can cause hearing loss, which can be temporary or permanent. Loud noise is particularly harmful to the cochlea or inner ear. Most people are born with about 16,000 hair cells in the cochlea. Around 30% to 50% of hair cells can be damaged before changes in hearing are detected. By the time there is noticeable hearing loss, many hair cells have been destroyed and cannot be repaired. After attending a loud event, short term hearing loss may occur because high decibel sounds cause the hair cells to bend; then, in many cases, they will become straight again after a recovery period. However, if loud noise has damaged too many of the hair cells, some of them will die. In addition to damaging hair cells, high decibel noise can damage the auditory nerve, which can make it difficult to hear in noisy places. The effect of noise over time can influence the degree of hearing loss in later life.

TINNITUS

Approximately 50 million Americans suffer from chronic **tinnitus** lasting more than 6 months, and about 25% of those have symptoms severe enough to interfere with daily activities. It occurs more frequently in men than in women and becomes more common with aging.

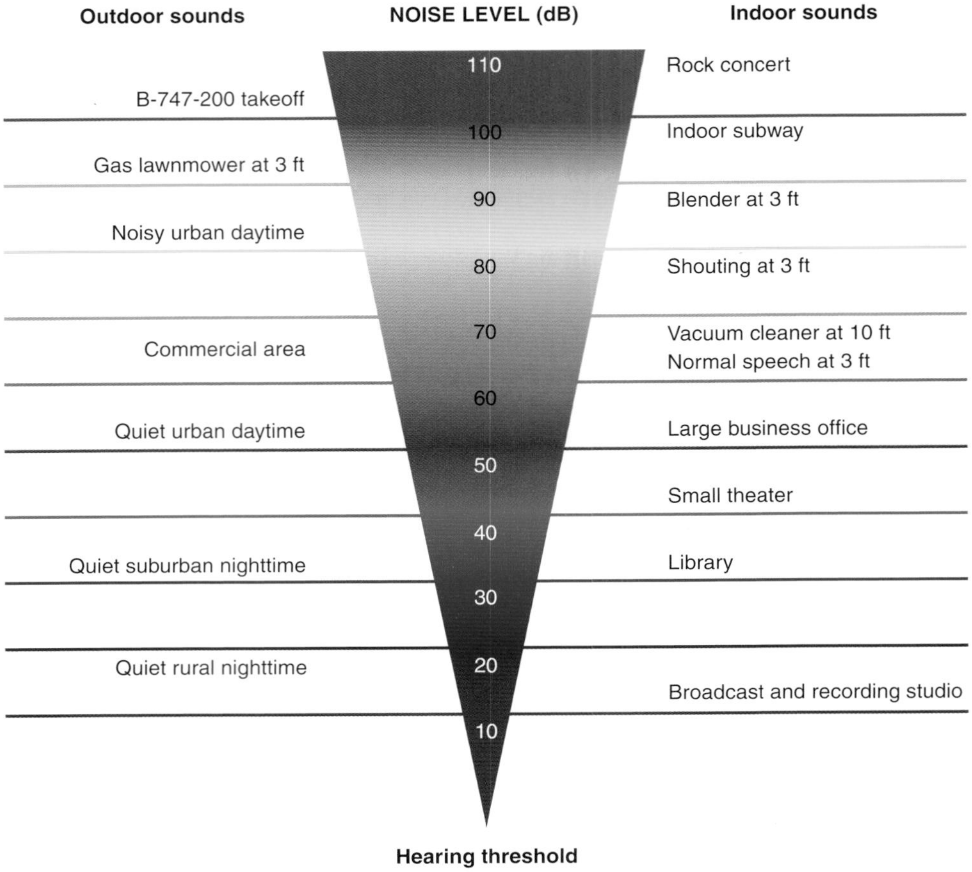

Fig. 58.19 Range of common environmental sounds. (From Harding MM, Kwong J, Roberts D, Hagler D, Reinisch C: *Medical-surgical nursing: assessment and management of clinical problems*, ed 11, St. Louis, 2020, Elsevier.)

Tinnitus, often called ringing in the ears, is the perception of a ringing, buzzing, hissing, or roaring sound in one or both ears heard only by the patient. It may be continuous or intermittent, pulsing, or steady, and range in severity from a soft buzz to a loud ring. Tinnitus is caused by damage to the tiny hairs in the cochlea that results from very loud noises, certain medications, injury, disease, or normal aging. The damage may be temporary, but the noise may be permanent. Other causes not related to the auditory system include disorders of the temporomandibular joint, severe anxiety, and neck injuries. Hearing aids that increase clarity of sound to mask the tinnitus may help to alleviate the condition. People who have difficulty sleeping because of the tinnitus may be treated with medication and/or behavior changes to improve sleep.

AGE-RELATED CHANGES IN THE EAR

Changes occur in the external, middle, and inner ear with aging. Some changes have no functional significance, but others can lead to serious problems with hearing or balance.

The skin of the auricle may become dry and wrinkled. Dryness of the external canal causes itching. Cerumen production declines and the protective wax dries. Hairs in the canal become coarser and longer, especially in men. The combination of dry cerumen and coarse hairs may lead to obstruction of the canal.

The eardrum thickens and the bony joints in the middle ear degenerate somewhat, but these changes are not thought to impair hearing significantly.

Degenerative changes in the inner ear include atrophy of the cochlea, the cochlear nerve cells, and the organ of Corti, which can affect sensitivity to sound, understanding of speech, and balance. The result is that many older people have some degree of hearing loss and some have problems with balance. Older adults with hearing loss also are more likely to develop dementia than adults with normal hearing.

Older people have difficulty hearing high pitched sounds such as various consonants (d, b, c, etc.), birds chirping, high-pitched voices, etc. This type of hearing loss most often associated with age is called **presbycusis**. Presbycusis is discussed further in Chapter 60.

NURSING ASSESSMENT OF THE EXTERNAL EAR, HEARING, AND BALANCE

The nursing assessment of the ear includes inspection of the external ear and evaluation of hearing and balance. In addition to collecting data about the patient's hearing and balance, the licensed vocational nurse/licensed practical nurse (LVN/LPN) may be trained to perform some specific diagnostic procedures to evaluate hearing. To collect data from the patient, the health care provider must first determine if the patient has a hearing impairment that interferes with verbal communication. If the patient's hearing impairment is severe, determine the usual means of communication. It may be necessary to call on a family member or a sign language interpreter or to use written communication during the assessment.

HEALTH HISTORY

Present Health

Determine the problem that has led the patient to seek medical care. Provide a full description of any symptoms that may reflect problems with the ear, including changes in hearing acuity, pain, tinnitus, dizziness, **vertigo**, nausea, vomiting, and problems with balance. Describe changes in hearing acuity including the kind of change that occurred and whether it was sudden or gradual. Ask the patient to describe the nature of the pain (e.g., sharp, throbbing, dull) and when it occurs. Pain in the ear is called **otalgia**. If tinnitus is present, ask if the sound heard is continuous or intermittent. Document dizziness, vertigo, nausea, vomiting, or problems with balance and the circumstances under which they occur.

Past Health

Ask about any previous acute or chronic ear problems. Acute conditions that may affect hearing or balance include sinus infections, dental problems, allergies, and upper respiratory infections. Chronic conditions that may be significant are hypertension, diabetes mellitus, and hypothyroidism. Note recent surgical procedures on the ear or throat or a recent head injury.

Hearing impairments often are congenital (present at birth). One cause of hearing loss in an infant is rubella (measles) during the mother's pregnancy. Therefore, it is significant to note whether female patients have had rubella or have been immunized for the infection. Document any family history of hearing loss for all patients.

Identify any drugs in the medication history that might be ototoxic. A drug that can damage the eighth cranial nerve or the organs of hearing and balance is termed **ototoxic**. Examples of drugs that can have ototoxic effects are aspirin and aminoglycoside antibiotics. Ototoxicity is discussed more fully in Chapter 60 in the section titled "Nursing Care of the Patient with Ototoxicity."

> **Pharmacology Capsule**
>
> Some drugs, including aspirin, are ototoxic. Signs and symptoms of ototoxicity are tinnitus, hearing loss, dizziness, and ataxia.

Functional Assessment

In the functional assessment, describe exposure to excessively loud noise such as amplified music, firearm use, or noisy machinery. Note the use of any assistive hearing devices.

The nursing assessment is outlined in Box 58.2.

PHYSICAL EXAMINATION

Some general observations of the patient give important clues about hearing and balance. Observe how the patient responds to a normal voice. Patients who do not hear well use many adaptive behaviors. They may turn a good ear toward the speaker, ask people to repeat things, ask "what?" frequently, or watch the speaker's mouth closely. Note the presence of a visible hearing aid. The patient's posture and balance while walking and sitting alert the examiner to possible inner ear problems.

External Ear

The position of the auricles is significant. Normally, the top of the auricle is at approximately the level of the eye. The ears should be positioned symmetrically. The auricles should be examined for shape, lesions, and nodules. The auricles and the mastoid process are palpated for tenderness. Palpation in front of, below, and behind the ear may locate enlarged lymph nodes.

External Auditory Canal

Use a penlight to inspect the outer portion of the external auditory canal for any obvious obstructions or drainage. The only normal secretion in the canal is *cerumen*. It should be golden to brown in color and should not block the opening to the canal. If any drainage is seen, record the color, amount, and odor.

Some nurses are taught to use an otoscope to inspect the external canal and the tympanic membrane. The tympanic membrane should be shiny and pearl gray.

DIAGNOSTIC TESTS AND PROCEDURES

Several specialists handle different aspects of the diagnosis and treatment of hearing disorders. An otologist is a physician who specializes in the medical and surgical treatment of ear related disorders. An otolaryngologist is a physician who specializes in diseases of the ears and throat. An audiologist is not a medical doctor but has specialized training to identify and treat hearing and balance disorders that are not treatable with medicine or surgery. An audiologist or hearing instrument specialist performs tests to determine whether a hearing aid will help a particular patient. If it is thought that a patient would benefit from a hearing aid, the audiologist or certified hearing instrument specialist also identifies the best kind of hearing aid.

The otoscopic examination and tuning fork tests for gross hearing acuity are usually part of the general physical examination. Various procedures and tests may be used to assess auditory and vestibular function. Auditory function tests include pure tone audiometry, speech audiometry, auditory evoked potential (AEP), electrocochleography, auditory brainstem response (ABR), and tympanometry. Tests of vestibular function are the caloric test stimulus, electronystagmography (ENG), posturography, and rotary chair testing.

Diagnostic tests and procedures for patients with disorders of the ear, hearing, and balance are described in Table 58.3.

OTOSCOPIC EXAMINATION

The otoscope is the instrument used to examine the external auditory canal and tympanic membrane. The examination permits diagnosis of inflammatory and infectious processes as well as obstructions of the external canal. When using an otoscope, you should do the following:

Table 58.3 Diagnostic Tests and Procedures: Disorders of the Ear, Hearing, and Balance

TEST AND PURPOSE	PATIENT PREPARATION	POSTPROCEDURE NURSING CARE
Audiometry		
Pure tone audiometry tests: detect hearing impairment by assessing the patient's ability to hear a range of sounds.	Tell the patient the test will be conducted in a sound-isolated room. The examiner will place earphones on the patient and introduce tones. The patient will be asked to identify when sounds are heard and when they disappear. A tuning fork will be placed near the patient's ear and the patient will be asked when vibrating sound is heard and when it ceases. No other preparation is needed.	No special postprocedure care.
Speech audiometry: measures the ability to hear spoken words.	The patient will listen to simple words through earphones and repeat the words that are understood. No special preparation is needed.	No special postprocedure care.
Auditory brainstem evoked potentials (ADEPs): used to estimate magnitude of hearing loss and determine whether a lesion is in the cochlea, eighth cranial nerve, or brainstem. Useful in assessing infants or others who cannot communicate.	Electrodes are placed on the scalp and earlobes. The patient is exposed to a series of clicks via earphones.	The scalp should be clean before electrodes are placed. After the test, remove electrode gel.
Electrocochleography: used to measure electrical activity in cochlea and auditory nerve in patients who cannot cooperate.	The nurse is not usually directly involved in the test but can inform the patient that electrodes will be placed on the head and a tiny microphone and earphone will be placed in the outer ear canal. The patient will be instructed to relax while a series of clicking sounds are made. No patient response is required.	No specific nursing interventions.
Auditory brainstem response (ABR): measures electrical activity along auditory pathway to detect certain tumors, brainstem problems, and stroke.	Although the nurse does not usually participate in this test, tell the patient electrodes will be applied to the head (like those applied to the chest for an ECG) and brain wave activity recorded in response to sound. The patient is encouraged to rest or sleep during the test because no response is required.	No specific nursing interventions.
Tympanometry: assesses response of middle ear to pressure changes.	Although the nurse is not likely to participate in the test, tell the patient that a device that creates pressure will be placed in the external ear canal. Loud noises may be heard. The patient needs to remain still and quiet and not swallow during the test.	No specific nursing interventions.
Vestibular Tests		
Caloric test: the ears are irrigated with warm or cool water to assess for dizziness. Dizziness is consistent with a diagnosis of Menière disease.	Tell the patient that the ears will be irrigated to assess for dizziness. Tell the examiner if the patient has had central nervous system depressants, alcohol, or barbiturates because they alter test response. The examiner will then observe the patient for nystagmus, nausea, vomiting, or dizziness.	Assess for nausea. Offer small amounts of clear liquids at first. Safety measures if dizzy.

Table 58.3 Diagnostic Tests and Procedures: Disorders of the Ear, Hearing, and Balance—cont'd

TEST AND PURPOSE	PATIENT PREPARATION	POSTPROCEDURE NURSING CARE
Electronystagmography: used to detect lesions in the vestibule.	Nothing by mouth for 3 h before the test. No alcohol or caffeine for 24–48 h before the test. Take eyeglasses to the test. Withhold medications as ordered. Tell the patient electrodes will be placed around the eyes and they will be asked to focus on specific targets. The ears are irrigated, and the patient is turned in various positions in a special chair.	Assess for nausea. Offer small amounts of clear fluids at first. Safety precautions if dizzy.
Posturography assesses for lesions affecting balance.	Inform the patient that they will be placed in a box with a floor that moves to assess balance. Inform patient that test is uncomfortable and can be stopped at any time if patient requests.	Assess for nausea. Offer small amounts of clear fluids at first. Safety precautions if dizzy.
Rotary chair testing: assesses balance.	Tell patient the room will be darkened. A light meal before the test is advised. Patient will sit in a chair that is rotated by a motor. Sedatives are best withheld for 24 h before test.	Assess for nausea. Offer small amounts of clear fluids at first. Safety precautions if dizzy.

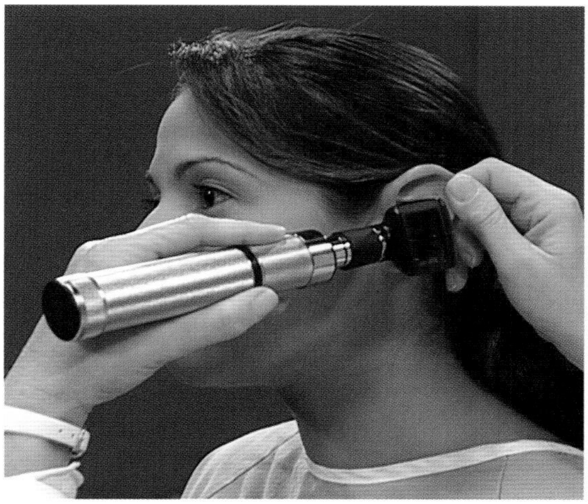

Fig. 58.20 Correct technique for using an otoscope to examine the external auditory canal and the tympanic membrane. The adult auricle is pulled up and back; the examiner's hand is stabilized against the patient's face. (From Seidel HM, Ball JW, Dains JE, et al.: *Mosby's guide to physical examination*, ed 7, St. Louis, 2010, Mosby.)

1. Use the largest speculum that fits the ear canal easily.
2. For adult patients, pull the auricle up and back to straighten the canal; then guide the speculum gently into the canal.
3. Steady the otoscope by resting the little finger against the patient's cheek, as illustrated in Fig. 58.20.
4. Never force the speculum into the ear.
5. If the patient is unable to cooperate, have someone hold the head still during the examination.
6. Clean or replace the speculum between patients and between ears on each patient.

The appearance of the normal tympanic membrane is illustrated in Fig. 58.21.

TUNING FORK TESTS

Rinne and Weber tests use a tuning fork to assess the conduction of sound by air and by bone. These are useful in determining the nature of the hearing loss and in selecting the best treatment. Some nurses are taught to perform these tests. The procedures are described here in the event that you are required to implement them.

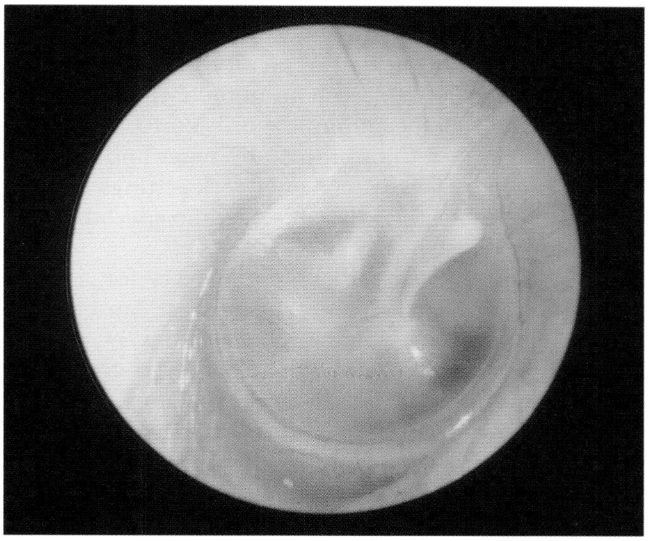

Fig. 58.21 Normal appearance of the tympanic membrane through the otoscope. (From Ignatavicius DD, Workman ML, Mishler MA: *Medical-surgical nursing across the health care continuum*, ed 3, Philadelphia, 1999, Saunders.)

Rinne Test

For the Rinne test, tap the tuning fork on the hand to activate it. Then place the base of the tuning fork on the patient's mastoid bone. If the vibration is conducted through the bone, the patient hears a humming sound. When the sound no longer is heard, move the fork so that the tines of the tuning fork are near but not touching the ear canal. Ask the patient if they can hear the sound and, if so, to report when the sound disappears. This assesses the patient's ability to hear sound waves conducted through the air.

Normally, air conduction is better than bone conduction. Therefore, the patient should be able to hear the sound transmitted through air even after it can no longer be heard through bone. This normal finding is recorded as "AC > BC" (air conduction is greater than bone conduction). If bone conduction is greater than air conduction, the patient may have a conductive hearing loss.

Weber Test

For the Weber test, place the base of an activated tuning fork on the midline of the skull. Ask the patient to identify the side in which the sound is loudest. With normal hearing in both ears, the sound is heard equally on each side. The sound is louder in an ear with conductive hearing loss and softer in an ear with sensorineural hearing loss.

AUDIOMETRY

Pure tone audiometry is the assessment of the ability to hear simple sound waves. Audiometry gives a precise measurement of hearing acuity using a machine called an *audiometer*. Speech audiometry evaluates the patient's ability to hear simple words correctly. Special training is needed to use the audiometer and to interpret test results. Nurses in some work settings learn to do audiometry testing. Patients need no special preparation for the tests.

The nurse can do other simple tests for a gross assessment of hearing. The whisper test can be done easily in any setting. Stand 1 to 2 feet from the patient, facing away from them. Have the patient cover the ear on the opposite side. Exhale and then speak in a low whisper. Ask the patient to tell you what was whispered. The words can be repeated louder until the patient is able to hear them. After assessing one ear, change sides and assess the other ear. This simple test gives you an idea about the patient's general hearing ability.

CALORIC TEST

The caloric test is used to diagnose disorders in the vestibular system or its central nervous system (CNS) connections. The ear is irrigated with warm or cold water and the patient is observed for reactions that suggest vestibular problems. A person with a labyrinth disorder responds with nystagmus (involuntary rapid eye movements), vertigo, and nausea and vomiting. A person with vestibular disease has a decreased or absent response to the test. Test results are altered by CNS depressants, barbiturates, and alcohol. Inform the examiner if the patient has had any of these drugs before the examination.

ELECTRONYSTAGMOGRAPHY

Electronystagmography is used to detect lesions in the vestibule. Electrodes are placed around the eyes and eye movements are measured as the patient focuses on specific targets as the ears are irrigated with water, as air is blown into the ears, and as the head position is changed. Nystagmus is a normal response.

The patient usually is allowed nothing by mouth (NPO) for 3 hours before the test. No caffeine or alcoholic beverages should be consumed for 24 to 48 hours before the test. Medications may be withheld on the physician's directions. Patients who normally wear eyeglasses are instructed to bring them to the test. After the test, the patient may report nausea and may vomit. If the patient is dizzy, take appropriate safety precautions.

OTHER AUDITORY AND VESTIBULAR TESTS

Electrocochleography, tympanometry, posturography, and rotary chair testing are described in Table 58.3. Computed tomography (CT) and magnetic resonance imaging (MRI) scans may be used to locate lesions that affect hearing and balance.

HEARING LOSS

Hearing loss is a frequent cause of disability and is most common among older adults. About 25% of Americans aged 65 to 74 and about 50% cent over age 75 years have hearing loss.

TYPES OF HEARING LOSS

The term *hard of hearing* can describe any level of impairment, including the total inability to hear (deafness). Millions of Americans have some degree of hearing impairment. Hearing losses are classified into categories. The categories of hearing loss discussed here are *conductive*, *sensorineural*, *mixed*, and *central*.

Conductive Hearing Loss

Conductive hearing loss results from interference with the transmission of sound waves from the external or middle ear to the inner ear. Conductive hearing loss may be caused by obstruction of the external canal or eustachian tube, and otosclerosis. Otosclerosis is a condition in which the stapes in the middle ear does not vibrate. Patients with conductive hearing loss hear better in noisy settings than in quiet settings. They do not speak loudly because bone conduction allows them to hear their own voices.

Most conditions that cause conductive hearing loss are treatable. Obstructions can usually be removed. Otosclerosis can be treated surgically with a procedure called a *stapedectomy*. This condition is discussed in more detail in Chapter 60 in the section titled "Nursing Care of the Patient Having Stapedectomy." Hearing aids usually are helpful for patients with conductive hearing loss.

Sensorineural Hearing Loss

Sensorineural hearing loss is sometimes called *nerve deafness*. It is a disturbance of the neural structures in the inner ear or the nerve pathways to the brain. Sensorineural hearing loss may be congenital, but it can also be caused by noise, trauma, aging, Menière disease, ototoxicity, diabetes, and syphilis.

Patients with sensorineural hearing loss can hear sounds but have difficulty understanding speech. They often complain that speech sounds are muffled. This type of hearing loss is not as easily corrected. Hearing aids may help by amplifying the sound, but it will still be muffled.

Mixed Hearing Loss

Mixed hearing loss is a combination of conductive and sensorineural losses. Treatment of any reversible problems often results in improvement of mixed hearing loss.

Central Hearing Loss

Central hearing loss is caused by some problem in the CNS. The patient either cannot perceive or cannot interpret sounds that are heard.

CLINICAL MANIFESTATIONS

Most hearing loss progresses over time so that patients may not recognize the loss until it becomes severe. They may complain that their hearing is fine but that others are mumbling. Many behaviors should lead the nurse to suspect hearing loss. The patient may lean in or turn one ear toward the speaker. The patient with a hearing loss may fail to follow directions, speak while others are speaking, or turn the radio or television up very loudly. Irritability and even hostility are not uncommon. Some people become very suspicious of others because they cannot hear what others are saying. Hearing loss may have no other symptoms; however, otalgia (ear pain), dizziness, and tinnitus (ringing in the ears) may be present with certain types of disorders.

EFFECT OF HEARING IMPAIRMENT

People with obvious physical disabilities usually receive some consideration and understanding from strangers. People who have hearing impairments may not be treated as well.

Those who had impairments in early childhood usually have speech difficulties. If speech is not clear, others may assume that the person is intellectually impaired. Sadly, the phrase *deaf and dumb* has been used to refer to people who neither hear nor speak. These terms are understandably offensive to the hearing-impaired person. The term *deaf* is not offensive but suggests a total inability to hear. Hearing impairment, on the other hand, implies a range of abilities.

Most adults seem to accept the use of eyeglasses fairly easily but are often resistant to using a hearing aid. A tendency exists to deny one's hearing loss. When a person refuses to admit to a hearing loss, family members and others may stop trying to communicate. The hearing-impaired person may alienate those who would like to be close and supportive.

People with severe hearing impairment probably suffer the most severe social isolation of those with any sensory disorders. A decrease in hearing and social isolation leads to greater incidence of cognitive impairment (memory problems, difficulty learning and making decisions) in older populations. Nurses can help by educating the public about hearing loss.

ADAPTATIONS TO HEARING LOSS

Some hearing impairments can be corrected. If not, the patient and family need to learn to cope with the loss. For many people, hearing aids produce at least some improvement in hearing. Many patients read lips and observe body language closely to enhance understanding of spoken messages.

Sign language uses hand signals to communicate. There is not a universal sign language shared by all hearing-impaired people; various countries can have different hand signals. Sign language provides a very effective means of communicating as long as others know how to use it. Unfortunately, most nurses are not trained in this skill.

Several electronic devices are available to serve people with hearing impairments. Telephones can be adapted to send and receive written messages. Earphones are readily available for use with radios, stereos, and televisions so that the volume can be adjusted as needed, in addition to reducing environmental noises. Some television channels provide closed-captioned programming, in which a written script is shown on the bottom of the screen. A portable telecommunication device for the deaf makes telephone communication possible. In the home, flashing lights can be used to alert the person to doorbells, telephone rings, and alarm clocks. For the person who does not speak, small handheld computers called *personal communicators* print out messages typed by the user.

For many years, guide dogs have been used to help people with visual impairments. A similar intervention is being used with dogs trained to assist the hard of hearing. These dogs are taught to recognize common sounds (e.g., doorbell, telephone, smoke alarm, crying baby) and to get the attention of the owner.

COMMON THERAPEUTIC MEASURES

Problems of the ear and related structures sometimes require medications or surgery. Other therapeutic measures for problems of the ear include irrigations and the use of hearing aids. You may encounter patients who are being treated by any of these measures.

EAR DROPS

Medications placed directly into the external ear canal are called **otic** drops or simply *eardrops*. Eardrops may be ordered to treat infection or inflammation, to reduce pain, or to soften earwax. Determine if a perforation (hole) in tympanic membrane is present before administering eardrops. Some eardrops can damage the ossicles and are not safe to administer in the presence of a perforation. When administering eardrops, keep the following points in mind:

1. Be sure to use an otic solution.
2. Warm the drops to body temperature by rolling the bottle between the palms.
3. Have the patient tilt the head so that the ear to be treated is positioned toward you.
4. Straighten the external auditory canal of an adult by pulling the auricle up and back. For a child, pull the auricle down and back.
5. Hold the dropper at the opening of the canal but do not contaminate the tip by touching the skin.
6. Instruct the patient to keep the treated ear up for several minutes to keep the medication from leaking out of the ear. The health care provider may order a cotton ball to be placed loosely in the canal to keep the medicine in place.

Examples of commonly used otic medications are listed in Table 58.4.

Pharmacology Capsule

Medications administered into the external ear are called *otic drugs*.

IRRIGATION

Irrigation is the use of a solution to cleanse the external ear canal or to remove something from the canal. A common indication for irrigation is impacted cerumen. Impacted cerumen is dried earwax that blocks the canal. The nurse may perform the irrigation, if agency policy permits, or may assist with the procedure. If the tympanic membrane (eardrum) is perforated, the canal should *not* be irrigated because fluid could be forced into the middle ear causing pain and injury.

The following key points should be remembered when irrigating an ear:

1. Select the correct solution as ordered by the health care provider.
2. Warm the solution to body temperature (95°F to 105°F).
3. Have the patient sit up and hold an emesis basin under the ear to be irrigated.

Table 58.4 Drug Therapy: The Ear, Hearing, and Balance

DRUG	USE AND ACTION	SIDE EFFECTS	NURSING INTERVENTIONS
Antibiotics			
chloramphenicol (Chloromycetin otic)	Broad-spectrum antibiotic used to treat infections of lining of external auditory canal.	Hypersensitivity: redness, rash, swelling, burning, pain.	If patient shows signs of hypersensitivity, withhold drug and notify physician.
Topical Corticosteroids			
Cipro HC (ciprofloxacin and hydrocortisone) Ciprodex (ciprofloxacin and dexamethasone) Floxin otic (ofloxacin alone)	Treat inflammation, pruritus, and allergic response. Usually combined with antibacterial or antifungal.	Can encourage microbial resistance to fluoroquinolones.	May be used in the presence of a tympanic membrane perforation. Caution to avoid eye contact.
Antibacterials and Softening Agents			
carbamide peroxide with glycerin (Debrox, Murine ear drops)	Soften earwax. Treat aphthous ulcers.	Redness, irritation, superinfection.	Contraindications: ear surgery, perforated tympanic membrane; ear drainage, redness, pain, or tenderness. Teach patient not to clean ear with cotton swabs, which force wax deeper into ear.
Drying Agents			
Boric acid in isopropyl alcohol (Ear-Dry, Swim-Ear)	Dry external canal after swimming or bathing. Decrease risk of infection.	Local irritation.	Instilled in external canal immediately after swimming or bathing. Contraindicated with perforated tympanic membrane.
Antiemetics			
scopolamine (Transderm Scop) dimenhydrinate (Dramamine) meclizine (Antivert) chlorpromazine (Thorazine)	Prevent or treat nausea, vomiting, motion sickness.	Sedation, drowsiness, tremor, fever, tachycardia, hypotension, constipation, dry mouth.	Safety precautions for drowsiness. Monitor pulse and blood pressure. Monitor stools and urinary output. Mouth care.

4. Drape the shoulder under the basin.
5. Straighten the external canal of an adult by pulling the auricle up and back. For a child, pull the auricle down and back.
6. Select an irrigating syringe or bulb syringe with a tip that is smaller than the canal.
7. Do not allow the syringe tip to completely block the canal.
8. Direct the solution toward the top of the canal in a steady stream, not toward the eardrum.
9. The procedure can be repeated several times if needed.
10. Eardrops may be ordered to soften impacted cerumen before irrigating.
11. Describe any substances flushed out of the ear.
12. If the impacted cerumen or foreign body does not wash out, inform the health care provider.

HEARING AIDS

Following an evaluation, the audiologist or hearing instrument specialist can inform the patient what, if any, technology is most likely to be beneficial. Technologic options include assisted listening devices, hearing aids, and cochlear implants. Assisted listening devices include such options as an amplified telephone receiver or a personal television listening device.

A hearing aid is a device that amplifies sound; that is, it makes sound louder. All hearing aids have four components: (1) a microphone to receive sound waves and convert them to electrical signals, (2) an amplifier to strengthen the signals, (3) a receiver to convert signals to sound waves, and (4) a battery to power the device. Various aids are worn in the ear, behind the ear, or in the middle of the chest. The device worn in the middle of the chest (i.e., "body hearing aid") is the most powerful. It consists of a wire that connects the ear speaker to an amplifier and battery worn on the body (Fig. 58.22).

Technology is advancing so that modern hearing aids have overcome many limitations of older models. Improvements include features such as noise cancellation, wind noise reduction, wireless capabilities, and the ability to assess the environment and automatically determine the best hearing condition for the patient. The hearing aid requires some care. Daily cleaning and proper nighttime storage are important to maintain the function of the hearing aid. Proper cleaning of hearing aids varies with different models, so consult with the audiologist or hearing instrument specialist for instructions. When it is not being worn, turn the aid off and store it in a protective case with the battery compartment open. Ensure that the case is labeled with the patient's name. Keep extra batteries on hand.

If the hearing aid is not working, first check to ensure that it is turned to the on position. If it is on, check the ear mold to see if it needs cleaning. The next step is to check battery placement. If the battery is not inserted correctly, the hearing aid will not work. If the hearing aid has a cord, check it to see if it is broken or unplugged. If these checks fail to locate the problem, change the battery. If a new battery does not correct the problem, the cord, if present, can be changed. Should the hearing aid still not work, return it to the dealer for service.

Nurses and other health care providers need to be familiar with hearing aids and how they work. The patient's nursing care plan should indicate that the patient usually wears a hearing aid. Confusion and auditory deprivation (increased hearing loss related to decreased auditory stimulus) in some older patients might be avoided if the hearing aid were kept in place. The cost of hearing aids can range from several hundred to several thousand dollars if both ears are involved. When patients are hospitalized, take care to prevent loss of these devices.

Many people deny their hearing loss and may be resistant to using hearing aids. It may take considerable encouragement from family members and

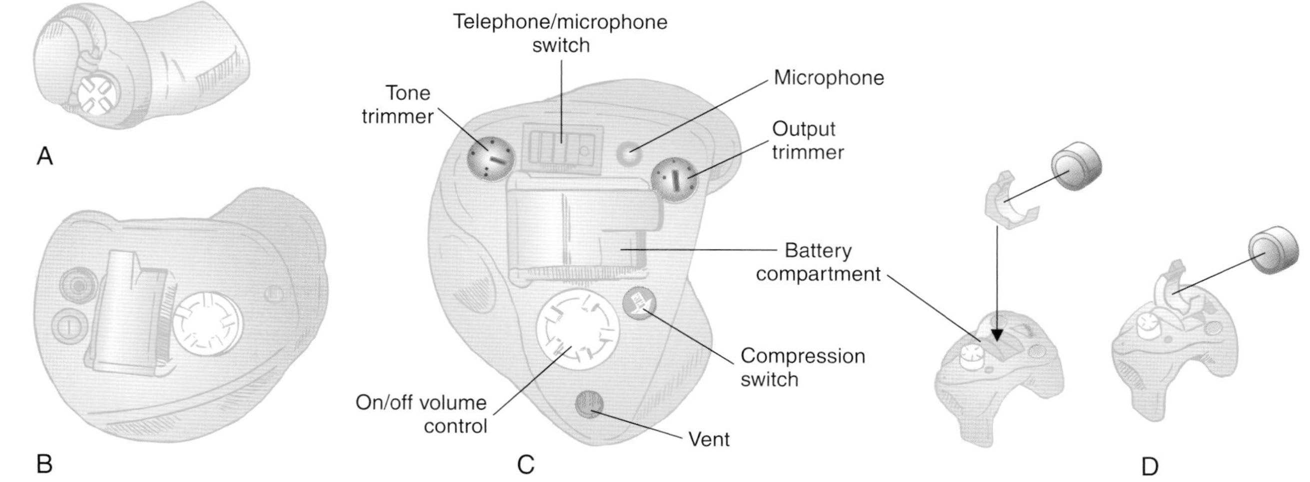

Fig. 58.22 Types of hearing aids and components. (A) In-the-canal aid. (B) In-the-ear aid. (C) Hearing aid components. (D) Battery compartment. (Courtesy Arnold G. Schuring, MD.)

health care providers to get a hearing-impaired person to try a hearing aid. It may be helpful to point out the benefits of improved hearing in the patient's everyday life.

Hearing aids amplify all sounds, including background noise. This is especially annoying when a person first tries to use an aid. Multiple visits to a hearing specialist usually are required to gradually increase the volume of the hearing aids. Patients are advised to wear the aid first in quiet settings. Once they learn to adjust the volume and tone comfortably, they can try it in noisy settings. It may take several months before a hearing aid feels comfortable.

Pharmacology Capsule

Among the drugs that can cause hearing impairment are salicylates, furosemide, ethacrynic acid, aminoglycoside antibiotics, and some chemotherapeutic drugs.

COCHLEAR IMPLANTS

A cochlear implant may be recommended for people with moderate to severe sensorineural hearing loss and those who cannot benefit from regular hearing aids. It is a surgically implanted prosthetic device that uses electrical stimulation to provide hearing. Patients need not be totally deaf, and most patients have some hearing with some sentence recognition. People with bilateral hearing loss benefit from bilateral implants, which improve speech perception, allow better hearing in conditions with significant background noise, enhance sound localization, and allow the patient to hear sound coming from either side without turning one's head. Cochlear implants provide significant benefit and increased quality of life even for adults aged 70 years and older.

The cochlear implant consists of a microphone, a processor, a transmitter, and a receiver. The microphone, at ear level, picks up sounds that are then amplified by the processor (Fig. 58.23). The sound, in the form of magnetic signals, is transmitted electronically to the receiver. The receiver is surgically implanted behind the ear. Electrodes attached to the receiver stimulate nerve fibers in the cochlea to produce sound. Several months of training are needed to learn to tell sounds apart. Thus, candidates for the cochlear implant must be highly motivated and carefully screened. Current efforts to improve cochlear

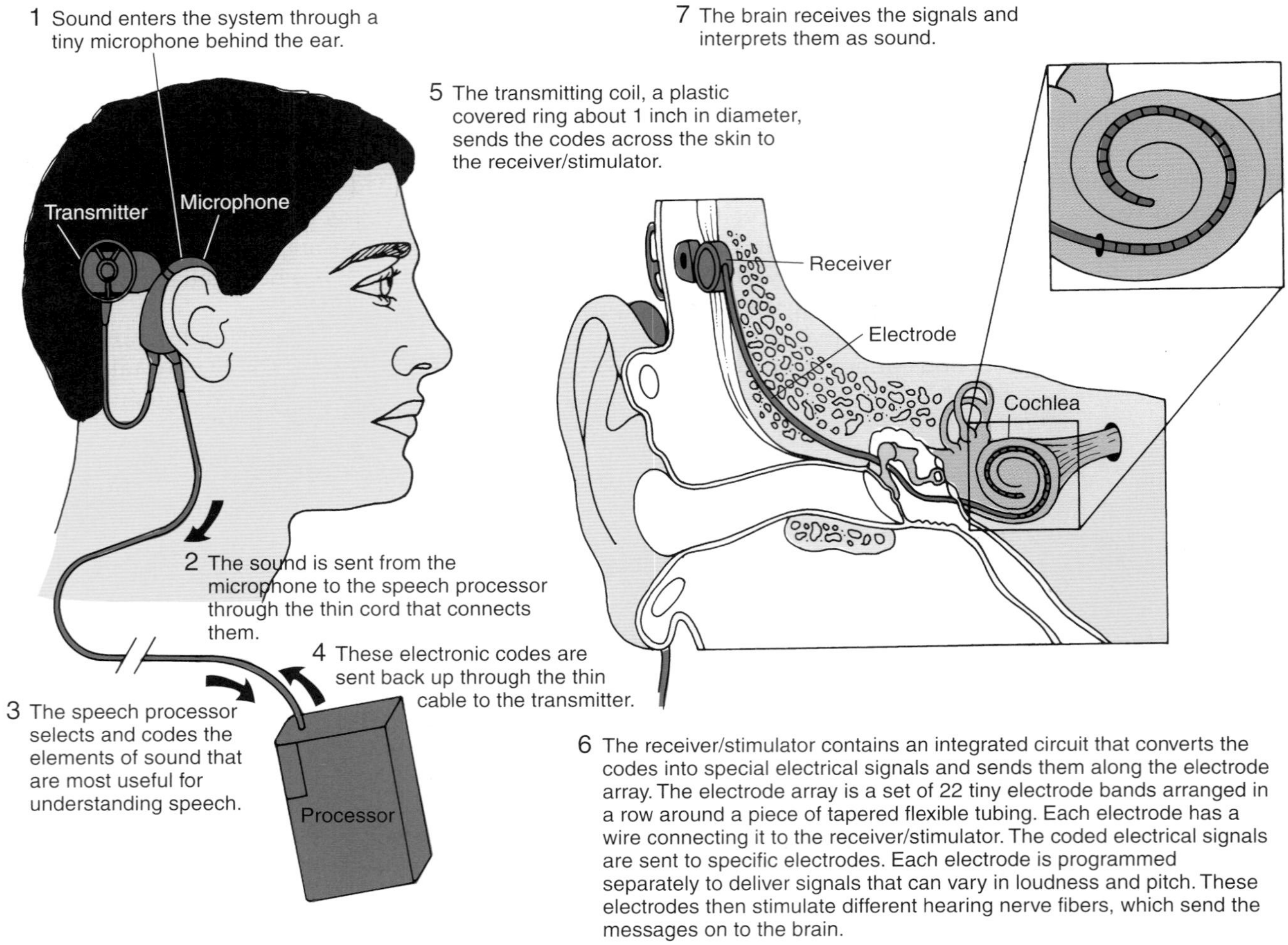

Fig. 58.23 Cochlear implant to restore hearing. (Modified from Black JM, Hawks JH: *Medical-surgical nursing: clinical management for positive outcomes*, ed 8, St. Louis, 2009, Saunders.)

implants include greater use of bilateral implants and development of a totally implantable device.

NURSING CARE OF THE PATIENT WITH A HEARING IMPAIRMENT

Focused Assessment

Assessment of the patient with a hearing impairment is summarized in Box 58.2.

Patient Problems, Goals, and Outcome Criteria: Hearing Impairments

Patient Problem	Goals and Outcome Criteria
Inability to communicate effectively related to impaired hearing	Effective communication: patient and others use alternative means of communication
Decreased socialization related to inability to communicate verbally	Reduced social isolation: participation in social activities
Inadequate coping related to change in social interaction, threat to body image, or denial	Effective coping with permanent hearing impairment: patient has satisfying social interactions, makes positive statements about self, plans realistically
Lack of knowledge regarding prevention, diagnosis, and treatment of hearing impairment	Patient knowledge of prevention and treatment: patient correctly practices preventive measures and describes treatments and resources for adaptation

INTERVENTIONS

Inability to Communicate Effectively

Many techniques are available to improve communication for people with hearing impairments. You can use these approaches and teach others to use them. When working with a hearing-impaired patient, follow these guidelines:

1. Ensure that the patient knows you are present. Try to move into the patient's line of vision before touching them.
2. Find out the patient's usual means of communication and ensure that they have access to any assistive devices.
3. Speak slowly and distinctly.
4. Ensure that the patient can see your face clearly. Do not turn away while speaking.
5. Do not eat, smoke, or chew gum if the patient reads lips.
6. Provide adequate lighting directed toward your face. A strong light behind you creates a glare and makes it hard to see your features.
7. Lower your voice tone. High-frequency hearing loss typically occurs first, then progresses to low-frequency hearing loss.
8. Assess the patient's ability to hear a normal voice tone. The volume can be increased a little if needed but shouting simply distorts the message. People who wear hearing aids often complain that everyone shouts at them.
9. If the patient has a good ear, speak toward that side.
10. Amplify your voice, if necessary, by using a rolled-up sheet of paper or a stethoscope. To use the stethoscope, put the earpieces in the patient's ears and speak into the bell.
11. Help patients to follow spoken messages by informing them of the topic to be addressed.
12. Use short sentences or phrases.
13. Use body language to support the verbal message.
14. Have a writing pad, picture board, or another similar device available. Use it if the patient cannot understand you or if you do not understand the patient.
15. Try to validate patient understanding by encouraging feedback and assessing whether directions are followed.
16. When a hearing-impaired patient is hospitalized, ensure that a call bell is provided but remind staff that the patient cannot use the intercom.

Decreased Socialization

The preceding guidelines may improve communication with the hearing-impaired person. However, the most important thing you can do is to have a positive attitude toward trying to communicate with the patient. Genuine interest and attention encourage the patient to express themselves in whatever way is possible.

When other people seem hurried or annoyed, they discourage the patient's attempts to communicate. Some patients withdraw from social interactions. They may become isolated and depressed. Encourage the patient to learn new communication methods. Teach the patient how to use assistive devices. Provide information about community resources for the hard of hearing. Explore the type of activities that are satisfying to the patient and encourage continued involvement. Advise the health care professional if the patient becomes increasingly sad or withdrawn. Counseling with a mental health professional may be suggested.

Inadequate Coping

The way people cope with hearing loss varies with the individual. Some deny the problem for as long as possible; others deliberately learn everything they can about treatments and adaptive strategies. Recognize that both of these behaviors are responses to a stressful situation. It is important to explore the patient's feelings about hearing loss. If the patient is anxious, you may use stress reduction techniques (e.g., relaxation exercises, massage, meditation). The patient who denies hearing loss is often resistant to teaching, so they may not take advantage of opportunities to deal with the problem effectively.

Lack of Knowledge

Most people with hearing impairment have some hearing ability. Emphasize measures to reduce the risk of additional impairment. Advise the patient to seek prompt treatment of any symptoms of infection such as fever, pain in the ear, or drainage. Hearing protection is recommended in excessively noisy settings. Patients who are taking ototoxic drugs are told to contact the health care provider if hearing acuity worsens or tinnitus develops (see the Patient Teaching box). If eardrops or irrigations are ordered, demonstrate the procedure and reinforce the prescriber's orders. Patients also need instruction in the use of hearing aids, as described in the section titled "Hearing Aids."

Patient Teaching

Hearing Impairments

- Many types of hearing loss are correctable or at least capable of being improved.
- Hearing is not related to intelligence.
- No one should be ashamed of a hearing impairment.
- Measures can be taken to reduce the risk of certain types of hearing loss.
- All women of childbearing age should be immunized for rubella to prevent one form of congenital hearing impairment.

SURGICAL INTERVENTION FOR THE EYE AND EAR

A number of visual and hearing conditions are treated or corrected with surgery. Nursing care of patients having specific surgical procedures is discussed with the appropriate pathophysiologic processes in Chapters 59 and 60. However, some general measures apply to most patients before and after surgery on the eye and ear.

PREOPERATIVE NURSING CARE

FOCUSED ASSESSMENT

Preoperative assessment and care are discussed in detail in Chapter 17. Before surgery, determine what the patient understands about the procedure and supply needed information about the preoperative and postoperative routines. Ask whether the patient is feeling nervous, anxious, or fearful that the procedure may not be successful or that some complication will lead to further loss of vision or hearing. If the patient is anxious, explore the specific concerns. Sometimes patient teaching and reassurance are sufficient to reduce anxiety. Notify the surgeon if the patient is very anxious.

Determine whether any current or future activity limitations exist. If the patient has poor vision or hearing, document the type of help needed. In addition, note the physician's orders for intravenous fluids and/or preoperative medications. Food and fluid intake is usually restricted from the evening before surgery to reduce the risk of nausea, vomiting, and aspiration after surgery. Because many procedures on the eye and ear are done in day surgery facilities, ensure that the patient understands the preoperative routine. Document who will take the patient home after the procedure because the patient will not be able to drive until cleared to do so by the surgeon.

Immediate preoperative care usually includes having the patient remove any articles such as eyeglasses or hearing aids. The hearing-impaired person going to surgery may feel very helpless without the hearing aid. Notify the operating room staff and ask if the patient can wear the hearing aid to the surgical suite. Place a note on the front of the chart to alert caregivers to the patient's hearing impairment and the presence of a hearing aid. Carefully track the location of the hearing aid to avoid losing it in the perioperative period.

Patient Problems, Goals, and Outcome Criteria: Preoperative

Patient Problems	Goals and Outcome Criteria
Anxiety related to uncertain outcome, lack of knowledge about surgery and surgical routines	Reduced anxiety: patient states anxiety is reduced, relaxed manner
Inability to manage self-care related to visual and hearing impairments	Ability to manage self-care: self-care performed successfully

INTERVENTIONS

Anxiety

Explore the patient's feelings about the surgery and provide information. Refer specific questions about the surgical procedure, risks, complications, or outcomes to the surgeon. Explain general surgical and postoperative routines.

Inability to Manage Self-Care

On admission, orient the visually or hearing-impaired patient to the room. Keep objects in one place and advise the patient of any new equipment or articles in the environment. Follow agency policy for obtaining consent for surgery. Offer to read any written material to the visually impaired patient or provide written materials to the hearing-impaired patient.

POSTOPERATIVE NURSING CARE

FOCUSED ASSESSMENT

After surgery, check the patient's vital signs and level of consciousness during recovery from anesthesia. Inspect the dressing on the operative eye or ear for bleeding or drainage; document drainage color, odor, and amount. In addition, ask about pain and nausea. If vision is impaired, inspect the environment for safety hazards. Monitor the patient for pain, nausea, dizziness, and fever. Before discharge, determine the patient's understanding of and ability to administer prescribed medications by having the patient or caregiver demonstrate self-medication.

Patient Problems, Goals, and Outcome Criteria: Postoperative

Patient Problems	Goals and Outcome Criteria
Potential for injury related to pressure or trauma on the eye; dizziness or vertigo, fluid accumulation, pressure in the ear	Decreased potential for injury: patient avoids potentially harmful activities (e.g., rubbing eye, bending forward); maintains prescribed position, avoids behavior that increases pressure Absence of injury: patient does not fall
Acute pain related to tissue trauma or edema	Pain relief: patient states pain is reduced or absent; reports less than 4 on a 1–10 pain rating scale; relaxed manner
Anxiety related to temporary visual or hearing impairment	Decreased anxiety: patient states is less anxious; calm demeanor
Potential for infection related to surgical procedure	Healing without infection: normal body temperature and white blood cell (WBC) count
Inability to communicate effectively related to packing and edema in affected ear	Effective communication: patient and nurse use effective strategies to facilitate verbal communication
Inability to manage treatment regimen related to lack of understanding of self-care measures and usual postoperative course	Adequate management of treatment regimen: patient adheres to plan of care, demonstrates appropriate self-care

INTERVENTIONS

Potential for Injury

Straining is contraindicated because it increases pressure in both the eye and the ear. The patient should avoid nose blowing, coughing, and sneezing; however, if these are unavoidable, the mouth should be kept open to relieve pressure. Stool softeners may be ordered to prevent constipation and straining with bowel movements.

An important aspect of the postoperative care of patients having eye surgery is to prevent increased IOP. Caution the patient against activities that increase pressure, including straining, leaning forward, lifting, and lying on the affected side. The physician will specify how long restrictions are necessary. Because vomiting and retching raise IOP, treat nausea promptly.

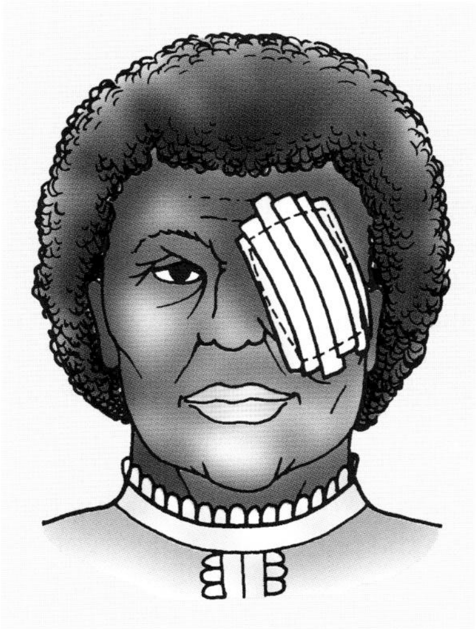

Fig. 58.24 The shield protects the operative eye from pressure or rubbing. (From Ignatavicius DD, Workman ML, Mishler MA: *Medical-surgical nursing across the health care continuum*, ed 3, Philadelphia, 1999, Saunders.)

After eye surgery, the physician may prescribe limitations on activity, position, or both. The head of the bed is usually elevated. The patient may be wearing a bulky dressing or a small eye patch. Either may be covered with a lightweight metal or plastic shield (Fig. 58.24). The dressing absorbs any drainage and the shield protects the eye from rubbing. Instruct the patient not to rub the eye. Check the surgeon's orders to determine whether the dressing can be changed. Eye drops or ointments may be ordered and may be different from those used before surgery. When an eye is patched, take safety precautions to prevent injury.

After ear surgery, dizziness and vertigo are common. Dizziness is a feeling of unsteadiness, whereas **vertigo** is the sensation that one's body or the room is spinning.

Sudden movements often trigger vertigo, so advise the patient to move slowly and carefully. Instruct the patient to call for help when getting up and assist the patient for as long as dizziness or vertigo is a problem. Nursing interventions such as the use of side rails as assistive devices and leaving the bed in a low position will help prevent injuries.

The ear is commonly packed and covered with a dressing after surgery. A drain may be in place; only the surgeon may remove the packing. A specific position may be ordered after surgery. If drainage is being encouraged, the patient is most likely positioned on the affected side. However, if the procedure includes a graft on the tympanic membrane, the patient is usually positioned on the unaffected side.

Put On Your Thinking Cap!

After eye surgery, patients typically go home on the same day. Considering the usual restrictions imposed to prevent increased intraocular pressure (IOP), what are some obstacles the patient might encounter? What strategies might you suggest to the patient?

Acute Pain

Although one might expect eye surgery to be painful, postoperative pain usually is mild to moderate, whereas pain after ear surgery may be more severe. Determine the nature of the patient's pain and have the patient rate the pain on a scale from 1 to 10, with 10 being the worst pain imaginable. If a patient reports severe pain of the eye, notify the physician. Pain usually requires analgesics for several days after ear surgery. Give analgesics as ordered. In addition, use measures such as positioning and massage to promote relaxation.

Anxiety

To reduce anxiety, explain what is being done and why, and encourage the patient to express concerns and ask questions.

Potential for Infection

Take measures to reduce the risk of postoperative infection. Advise the patient to avoid crowds and people with colds for several weeks. The ear canal should be kept dry for 2 to 4 weeks as instructed by the surgeon. Shampooing and other activities that expose the surgical site to moisture usually are disallowed for 2 weeks, although it is restricted longer in some cases.

Inability to Manage Treatment Regimen

Patients typically are discharged with some medications. Provide careful directions and a written schedule for the medications. To determine the ability to self-administer eye or ear medications, ask the patient to demonstrate the procedure before discharge. If necessary, instruct a family member in administering the medications.

Put on Your Thinking Cap!

An 80-year-old male patient is being discharged after ocular surgery. He has several topical ophthalmic drugs that must be applied twice daily. One eye is to remain patched until he sees the surgeon in 1 week. What information would you want to gather to determine whether he will be able to manage at home?

Get Ready for the NCLEX® Examination!

Key Points: Vision

- An estimated 21 million people in the United States have some vision impairment.
- Increased IOP must be controlled to prevent permanent vision loss.
- Vision loss affects all aspects of a person's life: independence, mobility, employment, communication, and interpersonal relationships.
- After eye surgery, nursing care addresses potential for injury, inadequate coping, pain, anxiety, and inadequate self-care.
- Common patient problems with impaired vision include inadequate knowledge, anxiety, inadequate coping, inadequate adherence, inability to perform self-care, and impaired mobility

Key Points: Hearing

- Approximately half of all adults older than 75 years of age have some hearing loss.
- Hearing losses are classified as *conductive*, *sensorineural*, *mixed*, or *central.*
- Adaptations for the hard of hearing include sign language, electronic devices, television closed captioning, personal communicators, telephones for the deaf, and trained dogs.
- Nursing care of the patient with hearing impairment addresses inability to communicate effectively, decreased socialization, inadequate coping, and lack of knowledge.
- Cerumen (earwax) can become impacted and obstruct the external ear canal, causing pain and hearing impairment.
- Hearing aids are useful in the patient with conduction hearing loss.
- Cochlear implants are beneficial in patients with moderate to severe sensorineural hearing loss.
- Common patient problems after ear surgery include pain, potential for injury, potential for infection, and inability to communicate effectively.

Additional Learning Resources

SG Go to your Study Guide for additional learning activities to help you master this chapter content.

Go to your Evolve website (http://evolve.elsevier.com/Linton/medsurg) for the following learning resources and much more:
- Fluid & Electrolyte Tutorial
- Review Questions for the NCLEX® Examination

Clinical Judgment and Next-Generation NCLEX® Examination-Style Questions

1. Which of the following is the fluid that fills the anterior chamber of the eye?

1. Aqueous humor
2. Ciliary fluid
3. Vitreous humor
4. Refractive fluid

NCLEX Client Need: Physiological Integrity: Physiological Adaptation

2. Your examination of the eyes of an older adult reveals eyeballs slightly sunken in the orbits, small pupils that do not respond to light, a grayish ring around the iris, and a complaint that the eyes feel dry sometimes. Which of these would you consider *normal* in an older adult? (Select all that apply.)

1. Eyeballs slightly sunken
2. Small pupils
3. Pupils not responsive to light
4. Grayish ring around iris
5. Eyes that feel dry sometimes

NCLEX Client Need: Physiological Integrity: Physiological Adaptation

3. **You are assisting with a community vision screening project. A participant says, "The nurse says my vision is 20/40 in both eyes. What does that mean?" Your response should be:**
   1. "You see best at 20 to 40 feet from objects."
   2. "You cannot see more than 40 feet in the distance."
   3. "At 40 feet, you can read what most people can read at 20 feet."
   4. "At 20 feet, you can read what a person with normal vision could read at 40 feet."

   NCLEX Client Need: Health Promotion and Maintenance

4. **When a patient comes to the office for an eye examination, the ophthalmologist administers phenylephrine 2.5% eye drops for which of the following reasons?**
   1. To reveal any scratches on the cornea
   2. To dilate the pupil
   3. To anesthetize the cornea
   4. To dilate retinal blood vessels

   NCLEX Client Need: Health Promotion and Maintenance

5. **For an otoscopic examination of the external auditory canal of an adult, the examiner should do which of the following?**
   1. Pull the auricle straight up
   2. Pull the earlobe down
   3. Pull the auricle up and back
   4. Pull the auricle straight back

   NCLEX Client Need: Physiological Integrity: Physiological Adaptation

6. **During the Rinne test, a patient reports hearing the tuning fork when it is placed on the mastoid bone and when the tines are then positioned near the ear canal. How should this information be interpreted?**
   1. The patient probably has an obstruction in the ear canal.
   2. The patient probably has a conductive hearing loss.
   3. The patient's response to this test is normal.
   4. The patient probably has a sensorineural hearing loss.

   NCLEX Client Need: Physiological Integrity: Reduction of Risk Potential

7. **Normal age-related changes in the ears of the older adult include which of the following?**
   1. Increased cerumen secretion
   2. Coarser hair in the ear canal
   3. Progressive hearing loss
   4. Thinning of the eardrum

   NCLEX Client Need: Physiological Integrity: Reduction of Risk Potential

8. **A resident in a long-term care facility points to her ear and loudly says, "I can't hear!" The patient's hearing aid appears to be positioned correctly in her ear canal. What is the first thing you should do?**
   1. Remove the aid and clean it
   2. Replace the battery
   3. Turn up the volume
   4. See if it is set to the on position

   NCLEX Client Need: Health Promotion and Maintenance

9. **During shift change, it is noted that a new patient is severely hard of hearing. What is the most important question for you to ask about this patient initially?**
   1. What means of communication does the patient use?
   2. Is the patient aware of the latest technology to assist the hard of hearing?
   3. Has the patient ever been hospitalized before?
   4. Can a family member stay with the patient to interpret?

   NCLEX Client Need: Health Promotion and Maintenance

10. **You are preparing to administer otic drops when you notice that the patient has gauze in the affected ear with a piece of narrow gauze extending from the ear. What should you do?**
    1. Gently remove the packing, instill the drops, and replace the packing.
    2. Apply the drops to the narrow piece of gauze for transport into the ear.
    3. Trim the gauze so that the packing is not accidentally pulled out of the ear.
    4. Inform the registered nurse (RN) that the drops cannot be given at this time.

    NCLEX Client Need: Health Promotion and Maintenance

10. **SLO/Objective: Apply knowledge of anatomy and physiology and pathophysiology to determine which assessment data require follow-up by the nurse.**

    NGN Item Type: Enhanced Hot Spot

    Cognitive Skill: Recognize Cues

    A 76-year-old man lives alone at home and receives weekly visits from a home health nurse to monitor his medications and functional and cognitive abilities. His vision and hearing are impaired significantly, and his recent memory is somewhat impaired. He is an insulin-dependent diabetic, hypertensive and has osteoarthritis in both knees, right hand, and left hip. The nursing assessment on a recent visit includes the following:
    - Blood pressure 150/68 mm Hg
    - Pulse 72 beats per minute and regular
    - Respirations 22 breaths per minute
    - Temperature 99.6°F
    - NPH insulin 20 units and Regular insulin 10 units q am self-administered injection
    - Metoprolol 50 mg HS
    - HCTZ 25 mg q am
    - Presbycusis, no hearing aid
    - Presbyopia, bifocal lens glasses
    - Blurred vision
    - Walks with aid of walker or cane.

    Highlight or place a check mark next to the assessment findings that require follow-up by the nurse.

59 Eye and Vision Disorders

http://evolve.elsevier.com/Linton/medsurg

Objectives

1. List measures to reduce the risk of eye injuries.
2. Describe the pathophysiology, signs and symptoms, diagnosis, and treatment of selected eye conditions.
3. Assist in developing a nursing care plan for the patient with an eye disorder.

Key Terms

astigmatism (ă-STĬG-mă-tĭzm)
blepharitis (BLĔF-ă-RĪ-tĭs)
cataract (KĂT-ă-răkt)
chalazion (kă-LĀ-zē-ŭn)
conjunctivitis (kŏn-jŭnk-tĭ-VĪ-tĭs)
cycloplegic (sī-klō-PLĒ-jĭk)
ectropion (ĕk-TRŌ-pē-ŏn)
entropion (ĕn-TRŌ-pē-ŏn)
enucleation (ē-nū-klē-Ā-shŭn)
hordeolum (hŏr-DĒ-ŭh-lūm)
hyperopia (hī-pĕr-Ō-pē-ă)
keratitis (kĕr-ă-TĪ-tĭs)
miotic (mī-ŎT-ĭk)
mydriatic (mĭd-rē-ĂT-ĭk)
myopia (mī-Ō-pē-ă)
presbyopia (prĕz-bē-Ō-pē-ă)
refraction (rē-FRĂK-shŭn)

EXTERNAL EYE DISORDERS

INFLAMMATION AND INFECTION

The eye is a potential site for infectious and inflammatory conditions. Because of the sensitivity of the eye, such disorders can cause considerable discomfort. Some may even threaten vision if not treated. They typically are treated on an outpatient basis, but the clinic nurse or long-term care nurse may interact with patients affected by these disorders.

Eyelid Infection and Inflammation

Blepharitis is an inflammation of the hair follicles along the eyelid margin most often caused by staphylococci bacteria. Seborrheic blepharitis frequently is found with seborrhea of the scalp and eyebrows. Symptoms include itching, burning, and photophobia. Scales or crusts may be seen on the lid margins. The patient may report that dried crusts seal the eyelids shut on awakening.

Untreated blepharitis could lead to inflammation of the cornea or formation of a stye. The health care provider may prescribe an antibiotic ointment for the condition. Be certain that any medication applied to the eye is an ophthalmic preparation. The eyelids also can be gently cleansed with baby shampoo solution.

Hordeolum (stye) is a common acute staphylococcal infection of the eyelid margin that originates in a lash follicle. The affected area of the lid is red, swollen, and tender. If a person has repeated infections, these may be related to staphylococcal infections at some other location on the body. The primary treatment is the application of warm, moist compresses several times a day. The health care provider may order ophthalmic antibiotics or may incise and drain the stye.

Chalazion is an inflammation of the glands in the eyelids. Swelling prevents fluid from leaving the glands, causing them to become enlarged and tender. Warm compresses may bring some relief. Treatment may include a corticosteroid injection into the chalazion to reduce inflammation or incision and drainage of the lesion.

Conjunctivitis

Conjunctivitis is an inflammation of the conjunctiva caused by bacteria, viruses, allergy, or chemical irritants. Warm or cool compresses, antiinflammatory eye drops, and topical vasoconstrictors may be ordered. Mast cell stabilizers with or without antihistamines may be ordered for long-term management of allergic conjunctivitis.

Bacterial conjunctivitis, commonly called *pinkeye*, is characterized by redness of the conjunctiva, mild irritation, and purulent drainage. The condition usually clears up spontaneously, but topical antibiotics may be prescribed.

Viral conjunctivitis can be caused by adenoviruses, herpes simplex virus type 1 (HSV-1), and herpes zoster virus. Viral infections are characterized by redness and drainage. The drainage in viral infections is watery rather than purulent. White or gray round, raised areas called *follicles* may be seen on the conjunctiva.

Viral infections tend to persist longer than bacterial infections and are more likely to produce severe eye damage. The medical management varies with the causative organism. Infections caused by HSV-1 are treated with idoxuridine (HerpEX) ointment or other topical medications. Corticosteroids are contraindicated with viral conjunctivitis because they may contribute to deep corneal ulcers and other complications.

Other organisms that can cause conjunctivitis include chlamydia and fungi that are more common in developing countries but are seen occasionally in the United States. They are treated with topical or systemic antimicrobial medications. Conjunctivitis that is caused by an infectious agent can be passed from one person to another. Thus, infected people should practice good hand washing and should avoid sharing washcloths.

ENTROPION AND ECTROPION

Proper closure of the eyelids is important to protect the eye and keep the cornea moist. **Entropion** is a condition in which the lower lid turns inward. Eyelashes rub against the eye, causing pain and possibly scratching the cornea. Surgical correction usually is recommended.

Ectropion is a condition in which the lower lid droops and turns outward. The eye does not close completely, causing it to become dry and irritated. The dry cornea is easily injured. Ectropion may be treated symptomatically or surgically.

FOREIGN BODY

Everyone has experienced the discomfort of having a foreign body in the eye. Blinking and tearing usually will wash small irritants from the eye. If the foreign body remains in the eye, evert the upper and lower lids as illustrated in Fig. 59.1. If the object is clearly visible and does not appear to be embedded in the eye, you may attempt to remove it. Use a sterile cotton swab to touch the object gently. If the object is not embedded, it usually clings to the swab and can be removed. A health care provider should remove foreign bodies that are embedded in the eye.

CHEMICAL SPILLS AND SPLASHES

Chemical spills and splashes are discussed in Chapter 63.

KERATITIS

Keratitis is inflammation, infection, or both of the cornea. The portion of the cornea in front of the pupil has no blood vessels because it must remain transparent. This means that it has no direct blood supply, making it especially vulnerable to infections.

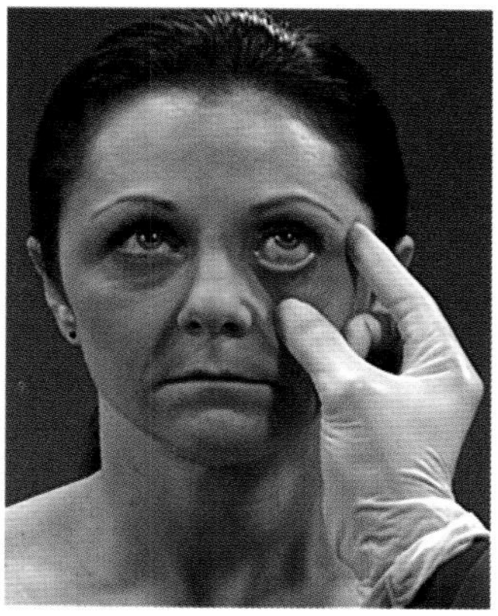

Fig. 59.1 Eversion of the eyelids for inspection of the sclera and conjunctiva. (From Ball JW, Dains JE, Flynn JA, et al.: *Seidel's guide to physical examination: an interprofessional approach*, ed 9, St. Louis, 2019, Elsevier.)

Sources of infection include bacteria, viruses, and fungi. In addition, chemical or mechanical injuries cause inflammation that may be followed by infection. If scar tissue forms, that portion of the cornea becomes cloudy, and vision is impaired. In addition, the infection can extend to the inner structures of the eye. Serious lesions can rupture if the eye is rubbed. Therefore, prompt treatment of keratitis is important to preserve vision.

Keratitis does not produce noticeable drainage, but it does cause considerable pain. Medical treatment includes topical antibacterials or antivirals and topical corticosteroids. Systemic antibiotics also may be ordered after culture and sensitivity results are obtained. Sometimes the health care provider injects antibiotics directly into the conjunctiva. Topical anesthetics are not used because the patient might accidentally cause additional injury to the anesthetized cornea. Eye pads are not used with keratitis because they provide a dark, damp environment for microorganisms to grow.

CORNEAL OPACITY

A healthy cornea is clear, allowing light to enter the pupil. When the cornea is injured by infection or trauma, scar tissue may form. In some cases, a rigid contact lens can correct the uneven corneal surface. If scar tissue prevents light from entering the eye, varying degrees of vision impairment occur. *Phototherapeutic keratectomy* (PTK) uses an excimer laser to destroy corneal abnormalities. The procedure has a high rate of success and a recovery period of only a few days. If PTK fails or is not an option, the only other treatment for corneal opacity is removal of the scarred cornea and replacement with a healthy cornea. The surgical procedure is called a *keratoplasty.*

Healthy corneas are obtained from donors shortly after death. The donor may authorize the transplant before death or by the family. The donated tissue is removed and preserved, preferably within 4 hours of death. Eye tissue is easier to preserve than other

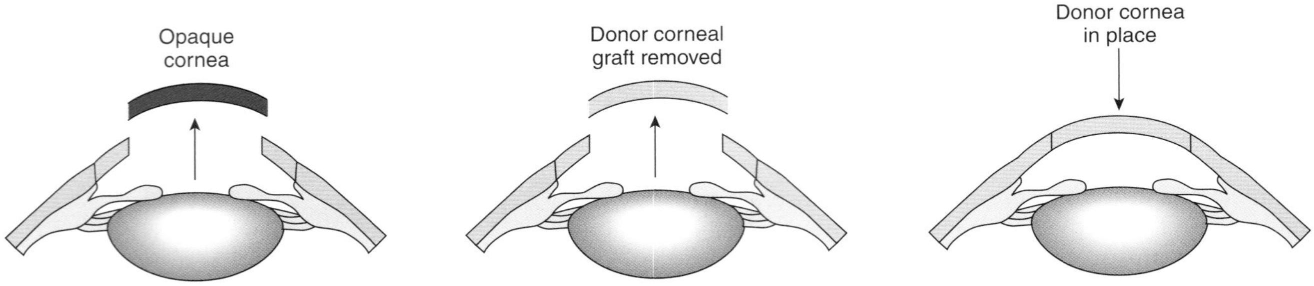

Fig. 59.2 Keratoplasty. The damaged cornea is removed and then replaced with a corneal graft from a donor eye.

body tissues permitting the keratoplasty to be done as a scheduled procedure rather than as an emergency on-call procedure. Before surgery, which is performed under local anesthesia, eye drops may be ordered to either dilate or constrict the pupil. Drops that constrict the pupil (**miotics**) pull the iris over the lens like a curtain and protect the lens during surgery. Sometimes, however, it is necessary to remove the lens as well as the cornea. Lens extraction is necessary if the lens is cloudy because of injury or age-related changes. In this case, preoperative *mydriatic* drops that dilate the pupil are ordered to allow access to the lens.

The types of grafts used in keratoplasty vary in depth. A *penetrating keratoplasty* is used for a corneal transplant where the central two-thirds of the damaged cornea is removed and replaced with a healthy cornea from a human donor. An *endothelial keratoplasty involves the removal of the abnormal inner lining of the cornea, known as the endothelium.* In a *deep anterior lamellar keratoplasty*, only the outermost layers of the cornea are removed. The type of graft used depends on the extent of injury to the recipient's cornea.

During a keratoplasty, the surgeon first removes the patient's damaged cornea. An identically sized graft is then taken from the donor eye and secured to the recipient's eye with very fine sutures, as shown in Figs. 59.2 and 59.3A. When a penetrating keratoplasty is done, the aqueous humor is lost from the anterior chamber of the eye. The surgeon replaces the fluid with a saline solution.

❖ NURSING CARE OF THE PATIENT HAVING KERATOPLASTY

Nursing care of the patient having eye surgery is discussed in Chapter 58 in the section titled "Surgical Intervention: Eye and Ear." In addition to routine postoperative care after eye surgery, the following specific care may apply after keratoplasty.

After surgery, the keratoplasty patient has an eye pad and a metal shield over the operative eye. Sometimes the other eye is temporarily patched as well because the eyes normally track together. This reduces eye movement until the operative eye heals. Corticosteroid eye drops may be ordered to reduce inflammation. Unlike other tissue transplants, corneal transplants do not require immunosuppressant therapy to prevent tissue rejection.

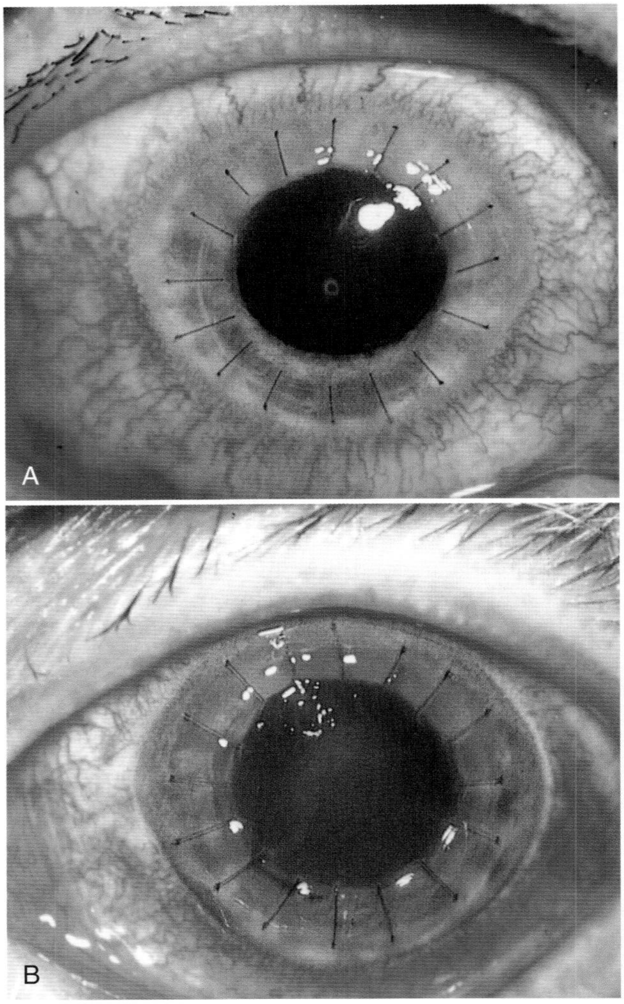

Fig. 59.3 Keratoplasty. (A) Appearance of the eye soon after keratoplasty. (B) Acute corneal rejection. (Courtesy Ophthalmic Photography at the University of Michigan, W.K. Kellogg Eye Center, Ann Arbor, Mich.)

Focused Assessment

Inspect the dressing for drainage and ask if the patient is having any pain or nausea. After the dressing is removed, inspect the eye for corneal opacity. In addition, evaluate the patient's visual acuity. Vision is usually blurry for the first few weeks followed by gradual improvement. Complete recovery may take as long as 6 to 12 months.

The normal appearance of the eye soon after keratoplasty is shown in Fig. 59.3A.

Patient Problems, Goals, and Outcome Criteria: Keratoplasty, Postoperative

Patient Problems	Goals and Outcome Criteria
Potential for injury related to activities that increase intraocular pressure (IOP)	Decreased potential for injury: patient avoids activities that increase IOP (e.g., bending forward, lifting, straining)
Acute pain related to tissue trauma	Pain relief: patient states pain is relieved, under 4 on a 1–10 pain scale, relaxed manner
Decreased visual acuity related to inflammation or rejection of transplanted tissue	Adaptation to temporary decrease in vision: patient performs usual activities with minimal assistance Gradual improvement in visual acuity: patient reports improved visual acuity scores
Inability to manage treatment regimen related to lack of understanding of usual postoperative course	Effective management of prescribed plan of care: patient correctly describes and demonstrates self-care measures

Interventions

Potential for injury. Caution the patient to avoid any activities that increase pressure in the eye, including rubbing the eye, bending forward, lifting, straining at stool, and coughing. Report and promptly treat nausea because vomiting raises intraocular pressure (IOP). Administer stool softeners as ordered to prevent constipation. The patient will probably be instructed to wear the shield for several weeks while sleeping to prevent accidental trauma.

Acute pain. Only mild to moderate pain is expected after keratoplasty. The health care provider usually orders analgesics such as acetaminophen to be given as needed. Notify the health care provider of severe or increasing pain because it suggests increased IOP or infection.

Decreased visual acuity. Rejection of corneal grafts is not common, but it can happen. When rejection occurs, blood vessels appear in the cornea and the cornea becomes cloudy (see Fig. 59.3B). Corticosteroid drops are ordered to reduce inflammation and the risk of rejection. Patients should know that symptoms of rejection include redness, swelling, decreased vision, and pain. Other topical medications that are usually ordered are antibiotics to prevent infection and **mydriatics** to dilate the pupil.

Inability to manage treatment program. Nurses and patients should realize that the grafted eye must heal just like any other body part that has undergone surgery. In the movies, the health care provider removes the dressing dramatically. The patient blinks a few times, and the world comes into focus. In reality, it takes a while before the patient's vision clears. Reassure the patient that this is normal.

Before discharge, determine what medications the patient will be taking at home. Review the medications with the patient, demonstrate proper self-administration, and have the patient return the demonstration. Instruct the patient to promptly report symptoms of graft rejection, which include unusual redness in the eye, eye pain, sudden change in visual acuity, and increased light sensitivity.

ERRORS OF REFRACTION

Light must pass through the cornea, aqueous humor, lens, and vitreous humor to reach the retina. These structures through which light passes are called *refractive media.* In the eye, the term **refraction** refers to the bending of light rays so that they focus on the retina. Abnormalities, called *errors of refraction*, occur when refractive media do not bend light rays correctly. Myopia, hyperopia, and astigmatism are common problems caused by variations in the structure of the eyeball. Fig. 59.4 illustrates these variations and the type of correction required.

TYPES OF ERRORS OF REFRACTION

Myopia and Hyperopia

Myopia is the medical term for *nearsightedness.* In myopia, the lens is situated too far from the retina, and light rays come together to focus in front of the retina. People with myopia have difficulty seeing distant images clearly. Often recognized in the early school years, the condition typically progresses slowly until adolescence. Biconcave lenses are used for correction, and new eyeglasses usually are needed approximately every 2 years.

When the lens is too close to the retina, light rays come together behind the retina. This condition creates **hyperopia**, commonly known as *farsightedness.* The hyperopic person sees clearly in the distance but has difficulty focusing on close objects. Biconvex lenses are needed for correction.

Astigmatism

When irregularities in the cornea or lens exist, **astigmatism** results. Most people have some degree of astigmatism. If the condition is mild, the natural lens can correct for the abnormality. If it is severe, however, then vision is distorted, and corrective lenses are needed. A person can have astigmatism with myopia or hyperopia.

Presbyopia

Presbyopia is another disorder that is classified with errors of refraction. Presbyopia is poor accommodation that is caused by loss of elasticity of the ciliary muscles.

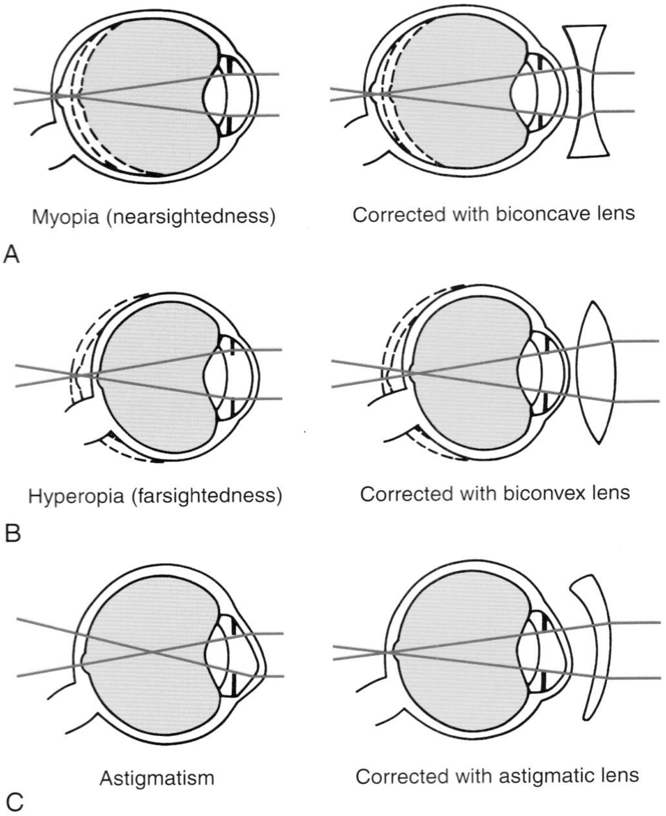

Fig. 59.4 Refraction. (A) Myopia: light rays converge before they reach the retina because the lens is too far from the retina. (B) Hyperopia: light rays converge beyond the retina because the lens is too close to the retina. (C) Astigmatism: uneven surfaces of the cornea bend light rays in a way that causes distortion of the image. (From Black JM, Hawks JH, Keene AM: *Medical-surgical nursing: clinical management for positive outcomes*, ed 8, Philadelphia, 2009, Saunders.)

Accommodation is the adjustment of the lens for near and distant vision. It is accomplished by contraction or relaxation of the ciliary muscles, which causes the lens to change shape.

Presbyopia is considered a normal age-related change that most often develops after 40 years of age. As it progresses, people may be observed holding reading material at arm's length. People who are already hyperopic tend to have presbyopia at an earlier age than other people. Myopic people usually are able to read small print by holding it close.

Corrective lenses are needed when the visual changes become bothersome. Bifocal lenses often are prescribed. Bifocals have two different lenses. The upper part of the lens is used for distant vision and the lower part is used for near vision. Trifocals have three lenses, for distant, closer, and near vision. Progressive lenses gradually blend the lens needed for seeing various distances. The wearer scans the lens to find the area needed for a particular task. Reading lenses usually must be changed every 2 to 3 years.

MEDICAL TREATMENT

Corrective lenses are the primary treatment for refractive errors, and eyeglasses are most commonly used. The major advantage of eyeglasses is that they require no special skills to use. Disadvantages are heavy frames and dirty lenses.

Contact lenses are tiny plastic and silicone disks made to fit over the patient's cornea. The lenses float on the tear film over the cornea. The primary advantages of contact lenses are convenience and appearance. Disadvantages include cost, the need for training and dexterity to insert and remove the lenses, and the risk of corneal injury.

Contact lenses are either rigid or soft. Rigid lenses are standard or gas permeable. Gas-permeable lenses are made of materials that allow oxygen (O_2) and carbon dioxide (CO_2) to pass through them. This is important because the cornea exchanges gasses through the tear film beneath the contact lens. Hard lenses must be removed from the eye at the end of the day to prevent damage to the cornea.

Soft lenses include several variations: standard, high water content, toric, disposable, and daily disposable. Standard and daily disposable lenses must be removed at night. The other varieties may be used for daily or extended wear. Disposable extended-wear contact lenses can be worn for as long as 2 weeks. For this reason, they may be prescribed for older patients who have cataract surgery. The patient is cautioned to follow the prescribed cleaning routine for the type of lenses worn.

SURGICAL TREATMENT

Surgical correction of refractive errors has advanced dramatically in recent years. Photorefractive keratectomy (PRK) uses an excimer laser to reshape the cornea for treatment of myopia, hyperopia, and astigmatism. An alternative procedure to correct those problems is the laser-assisted in situ keratomileusis (LASIK) procedure. LASIK involves peeling back a thin layer of the cornea and using a laser to reshape the middle layer of the cornea. Intracorneal ring segments (ICRS) are implanted between layers of the cornea to treat mild myopia. Intraocular lenses (IOLs) can correct both myopia and hyperopia. Phakic IOLs are implanted in front of the natural lenses. Refractive IOLs actually replace the patient's natural lens, making it a more invasive procedure with a higher risk of complications.

The surgical procedures are performed under local anesthesia in outpatient facilities. To be selected for surgery, the patient must have a healthy eye and be free of active autoimmune or vascular disease, severe dry eyes, keratitis, or other eye conditions. Postoperatively, patients may complain of dry eyes and difficulty with night driving and glare. The outcomes cannot be evaluated immediately because refraction stabilizes slowly after surgery; however, 10-year follow-up studies for PRK and LASIK surgery found that after 2 years, visual correction remained stable with high patient satisfaction.

NURSING CARE OF THE PATIENT WITH ERRORS OF REFRACTION

Nursing responsibilities for the patient with errors of refraction are limited to encouraging periodic examinations and knowing if the patient uses corrective lenses. In emergency situations, the nurse may have to remove contact lenses for the patient. When caring for patients who have laser surgery, it may be your responsibility to teach postoperative care to the patient. You should include proper use of any prescribed eye drops, measures to protect the eye, and symptoms to be reported to the surgeon.

INTERNAL EYE DISORDERS

CATARACT

A **cataract** is an opacity of the lens in the eye that may cause blurred or distorted vision, problems with glare; or in advanced cases, blindness. Most cataracts are age-related, and by age 80, more than half of the people in the United States have cataracts or have had cataract surgery. Cataracts are the leading cause of blindness worldwide, and the leading cause of vision loss in the United States. They may be congenital, traumatic, or degenerative. Congenital cataracts are those that are present at birth. Traumatic cataracts are caused by chemical, mechanical, heat, or radiation injury. Degenerative cataracts are more common with aging but they occur earlier in people with diabetes or Down syndrome.

Risk factors for developing cataracts include age, smoking, alcohol consumption, sunlight exposure, family history of cataracts, diabetes mellitus, HIV/AIDS, and steroid use. Preventive measures to protect eyes and delay the formation of cataracts include wearing sunglasses and a hat with a brim to block the sun; quitting smoking; eating plenty of fruits and vegetables, especially leafy greens like spinach, kale and collard greens; and, if over 60 years of age, getting a dilated eye examination every 2 years.

Pathophysiology

The lens is composed of cells that contain a high content of cytoplasmic protein that provides transparency in the lens. Unlike other epithelial cells, the lens cannot shed the cells that die. Over time, these cells are compressed into the center of the lens so that they begin to lose their transparency and become more opaque or cloudy. As opacity increases, light rays become less able to penetrate the lens, so that vision becomes blurry. Blindness eventually results if a cataract is untreated. With age, both eyes generally are affected, although they may not change at the same rate. Injuries tend to cause opacity rapidly, whereas age-related opacity progresses slowly.

Clinical Manifestation

Cataracts can cause cloudy or blurry vision; faded looking colors; poor night vision; halos around lights; double vision; spots or ghost images, and floaters. The pattern of visual changes depends on the location of the developing cataract. A central cataract is located in the center of the lens. Patients with central cataracts may have fairly good peripheral vision. They may see better in dim light because the pupil dilates, allowing them to see around the cloudy center of the lens. Conversely, patients who have peripheral cataracts can see straight ahead but not to the side. As cataracts develop, people who initially were hyperopic may have temporary improvements in near vision. This is called *second sight.*

Cataracts also are described as either immature or mature. With an immature cataract, there is still enough transparency in the lens for the light rays to reach the retina, resulting in limited vision. With a mature cataract, the opaque lens prohibits the light rays from reaching the retina, resulting in severely impaired vision.

Medical Treatment

The only curative treatment for cataract is removal of the lens, although mydriatics may be helpful in the early stages. Cataract extraction is the most frequently performed eye operation in the United States. Several

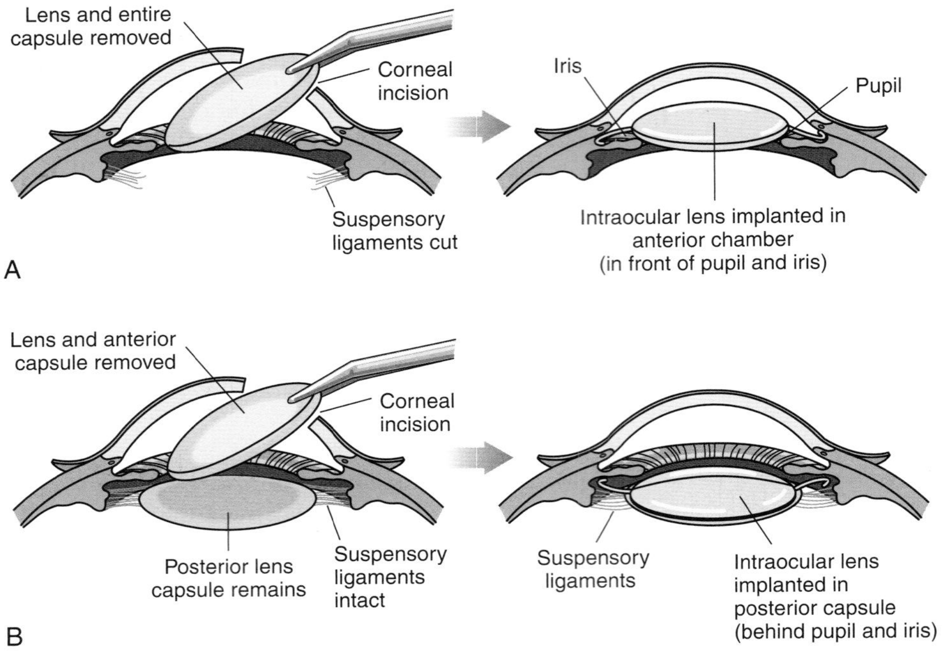

Fig. 59.5 Methods of cataract extraction. (A) Intracapsular cataract extraction with removal of entire lens and capsule. (B) Extracapsular cataract extraction leaving the posterior lens capsule intact. (From Monahan F, Sands J, Neighbors M, et al.: *Phipps' medical-surgical nursing: health and illness perspectives*, ed 8, St. Louis, 2006, Mosby.)

types of cataract extraction exist, as illustrated in Fig. 59.5. If the lens and capsule are removed, it is called an *intracapsular cataract extraction.* The preferred procedure is the *extracapsular cataract extraction* in which the lens is removed, leaving the capsule in place. A small incision is made in the eye. Then the surgeon extracts the lens or uses sound waves to break up the lens (phacoemulsification) followed by aspiration of the fragments out of the eye. Cataract extraction typically is accompanied by placement of an artificial lens behind the iris. Sometimes the remaining capsule becomes cloudy, causing vision to become blurred again. This usually can be corrected easily with laser treatment.

Cataract extraction commonly is performed on an outpatient basis. Most patients tolerate the procedure well with just a mild sedative and local anesthesia. In some cases, general anesthesia may be preferred. Cataract surgery generally is considered safe, even for those who are very old.

Complications

Complications that sometimes occur include leakage of vitreous humor, hemorrhage into the eye, and opening of the incision.

Lens Replacement

Once the lens has been removed, the eye is said to be *aphakic.* The patient is extra farsighted and unable to accommodate for changes in object size. Some type of artificial lens is needed for correction.

Contact lenses. Whereas contact lenses have many advantages over eyeglasses, they have drawbacks as well. Considerable dexterity is required to insert, remove, and care for contact lenses. This makes them impractical for some older patients. The main complication of contact lens use is corneal injury.

Intraocular lenses. A plastic lens that can be implanted in the eye is called an *intraocular lens.* The intraocular lens typically is implanted immediately after removal of the natural lens. Complications of insertion include corneal edema, secondary glaucoma, lens displacement, and retinal detachment. Although some new intraocular lenses accommodate for near and far vision, the patient still may require reading glasses for close work.

❖ NURSING CARE OF THE PATIENT WITH CATARACTS

Because cataract extractions typically are performed on an outpatient basis with monitored intravenous sedation and local anesthesia, you may have limited opportunity for patient and family teaching. Care of the patient having eye surgery is presented in Chapter 58 under "Surgical Intervention: Eye and Ear." This section emphasizes additional care specific to cataract surgery.

PREOPERATIVE NURSING CARE

Eye drops often are ordered at frequent intervals before cataract surgery. The orders must be followed exactly. Common drops used before cataract surgery are mydriatics, **cycloplegics**, antibiotics, and nonsteroidal antiinflammatory drugs (NSAIDs). Mydriatics dilate the pupil, making it easier for the surgeon to access the lens. Cycloplegics temporarily paralyze the muscles of accommodation, keeping the eye still during the procedure. Antibiotics reduce the risk of infection and NSAIDs reduce inflammation. A sedative may be given to decrease anxiety.

POSTOPERATIVE NURSING CARE

Focused Assessment

After cataract surgery, ask about pain and nausea. The patient is likely to return from surgery wearing a patch and shield over the operative eye. Note the presence of the patch and any apparent drainage. In addition, note the patient's level of consciousness and orientation (see Nursing Care Plan: Patient Having Cataract Surgery, Postoperative).

Nursing Care Plan — Patient Having Cataract Surgery, Postoperative

FOCUSED ASSESSMENT

Health History

A 72-year-old retired welder is seeking medical care because of cloudy vision that has become increasingly worse. He reports spots moving across his field of vision. Cataracts were diagnosed, with the right lens affected more severely than the left. He had a right extracapsular cataract extraction under local anesthesia this morning in the outpatient surgery department. He says that he has mild pain in the eye area at this time. His record reveals a history of myocardial infarction 5 years ago and surgery for prostate enlargement 6 months ago. Although he is retired, he works every day on his small farm. He lives with his wife and an adult daughter.

Physical Examination Vital signs: blood pressure 142/68 mm Hg, pulse 88 beats per minute, respiration 18 breaths per minute, temperature 98°F (36.7°C) measured orally. Height 5′7″, weight 155 lb. Alert, oriented, and in semi-Fowler or sitting position. An eye pad is in place over the right eye, protected with a metal shield. A small amount of clear drainage is noted seeping below the dressing.

Patient Problems	Goals and Outcome Criteria	Interventions
Potential for injury related to increased intraocular pressure (IOP), trauma	Decreased potential for injury: patient avoids activities that increase IOP. IOP remains 12 to 21 mm Hg.	Administer antiemetics immediately as ordered for nausea and vomiting. Change damp pad as allowed. Administer eye drops (antimicrobials and corticosteroids) as ordered. Instruct the patient to avoid stress on operative eye, rubbing the operative eye, straining, leaning forward, or lying on the affected side. Encourage patient to take stool softeners as ordered to prevent constipation.
Lack of knowledge about postoperative care	The patient will adapt to visual impairment and function in environment without injury.	The patient will probably go home after outpatient surgery. Until then, keep in a sitting position. When the patient returns home, some assistance with activities of daily living (ADL) may be needed for a day or two.
Acute pain related to tissue trauma	Pain level below 4 on a 0 to 10 pain scale, relaxed appearance.	Assess pain. Notify the surgeon if severe (may indicate increased IOP). Administer analgesics as ordered and evaluate effects.
Anxiety related to temporary vision impairment, activity restrictions	Decreased anxiety and calm appearance.	Explain what is being done and why. Be sensitive to concerns about surgery. Answer questions. Respond promptly to needs.
Inability to manage treatment program related to lack of understanding of condition, self-care, and limitations	Effective management of treatment program: the patient (and family member) will demonstrate instillation of medications and state activity limitations.	Explain postoperative limitations. Someone must drive patient home from surgery. No lifting over 5 lb, bending forward, or straining until cleared by health care provider. Review procedure for eye drops and have patient or family member demonstrate instillation. Supplement verbal instructions with written information.

CRITICAL THINKING QUESTIONS

1. Why is it important to prevent constipation in a patient who has had cataract surgery?
2. Explain why activities that increase IOP must be avoided postoperatively.

Patient Problems, Goals, and Outcome Criteria: Cataract Surgery: Postoperative

Patient Problems	Goals and Outcome Criteria
Inability to manage self-care related to lack of knowledge of postoperative care	Patient is aware of procedures for postoperative care of cataract surgery to prevent strain on the eye
Potential for injury related to increased intraocular pressure (IOP), vision impairment	Reduced potential for injury: patient avoids activities that increase IOP, IOP remains 12 to 20 mm Hg. Patient demonstrates self-care, maneuvers in environment without injury, administers medications properly

Interventions

Inability to manage self-care. After cataract surgery, it is most important to prevent strain on the operative eye. Examples of restrictions intended to decrease strain are sleeping on the unaffected side, not lifting more than 5 lb, and avoiding bending forward. Administer stool softeners as ordered to prevent straining with defecation or instruct the patient in self-medication. If nausea occurs, promptly administer an antiemetic as ordered. Reinforce postoperative limitations specified by the surgeon. Caution the patient to avoid rubbing the eye. You may see less restrictive postoperative care in some settings because researchers are questioning some of the traditional practices. However, you should follow the orders of the individual surgeon or agency protocols until newer guidelines are issued.

Potential for injury. Always be aware of safety precautions after cataract surgery. When one eye is patched, the patient has limited peripheral vision. The unoperated eye often has some degree of impairment as well. Medications may be ordered that cause blurred vision. Outpatient surgery allows the patient to return to a familiar setting on the same day. If the patient resides in a long-term care facility, ensure that the environment is uncluttered, and personal items are conveniently placed.

Confusion sometimes occurs in the postoperative period, especially in those who are very old. The confused person may fail to follow safety precautions or may place strain on the operative eye. Therefore, monitor mental status until the person returns to their preoperative mental state.

Medications prescribed after cataract surgery usually include antibiotics and corticosteroids or NSAIDs. You may need to teach a family member or friend how to give the medications until the patient is able to administer them.

A mild analgesic generally is ordered as needed. Postoperative patients with cataract surgery should not have severe pain. If a patient complains of severe pain, notify the health care provider. Severe pain may indicate hemorrhage or rising intraocular pressure.

GLAUCOMA

After cataracts, glaucoma is the second leading cause of blindness worldwide. Glaucoma occurs in infants, children, and adults, which often goes undiagnosed. Blindness from glaucoma is 6 to 8 times more common among Black Americans than among White Americans. Risk factors for developing glaucoma include age over 60 years, Black American or Hispanic/Latino over age 40 years, and family history of glaucoma.

Pathophysiology

Glaucoma is a condition that results from damage to the optic nerve, often associated with increased intraocular pressure (IOP). Normally, aqueous humor enters and leaves the anterior chamber of the eye so that IOP is maintained between 8 and 22 mm Hg. Glaucoma is a condition in which IOP is increased above normal. It can be caused by a number of changes that affect the outflow of aqueous humor from the anterior chamber.

Types of Glaucoma

The two most common types of glaucoma are (1) open-angle glaucoma and (2) angle-closure glaucoma. They are similar in that increased IOP may be present, but in some cases, increased intraocular pressure can be absent. The main adverse effect of increased IOP is damage to the optic nerve with subsequent vision loss. Both chronic open-angle and acute angle-closure glaucoma are considered *primary glaucomas.* Increased IOP because of other conditions is called *secondary glaucoma.*

Open-angle glaucoma. Open-angle glaucoma is more common than angle-closure glaucoma. Open-angle glaucoma results from either increased aqueous production and/or decreased outflow in the eye causing IOP. Excess pressure damages the back portion of the eye. It impairs blood flow to the optic nerve and retina, resulting in vision impairment. Peripheral vision is lost first. The field of vision gradually narrows until the patient has tunnel vision. The patient who has tunnel vision can see only a small circle, as if looking through a tube or a tunnel. Complete blindness eventually occurs as the disease progresses. Vision may be restored if glaucoma is treated early; otherwise, vision loss is permanent.

People with open-angle glaucoma rarely experience symptoms, and the condition is detected primarily during a comprehensive eye examination. High elevations of IOP (up to 40 mm Hg) generally do not cause pain, redness, or visual symptoms. As long as the central vision is preserved, there is no loss of visual acuity.

Open-angle glaucoma is treated by lowering IOC. Options for treatment may include prescription eyedrops, oral medications, laser treatment, surgery, or a combination of any of these. Prescription eyedrop medications include prostaglandins, beta-blockers, alpha-adrenergic agonists, carbonic anhydrase inhibitors, rho kinase inhibitors, and miotic or cholinergic agents. If eyedrops do not bring the IOP down to desired levels, oral medicine such as carbonic anhydrase inhibitors generally are used. Drugs work either by decreasing the production of aqueous humor or by improving the outflow of aqueous humor.

Beta-blockers frequently are the first drugs used in the treatment of glaucoma. These drugs probably lower IOP by decreasing the production of aqueous humor. Adrenergics decrease IOP by decreasing the formation of aqueous humor. Cholinergic miotics facilitate the outflow of aqueous humor. These drugs constrict the pupil, which permits fluid to flow more easily through the angle where the iris meets the cornea and into the trabecular meshwork. A disadvantage of many currently used miotic agents is that they must be administered frequently. Some new preparations, including ocular inserts, are effective for a longer period of time. Carbonic anhydrase inhibitors reduce IOP by decreasing the production of aqueous humor. Various forms are available for oral, topical, and parenteral use. Hyperosmotic agents, including oral glycerin and intravenous mannitol, promote movement of fluid from the intraocular structures.

Examples of each classification of drugs used to treat glaucoma as well as additional details are provided in Table 59.1.

Surgical intervention may be recommended when drugs do not reduce pressure adequately; the patient does not use prescribed drugs properly; or adverse reactions interfere with drug therapy. Surgical procedures for glaucoma include laser trabeculoplasty, trabeculectomy, and cyclocryotherapy. Laser trabeculoplasty may be tried first because it can be performed under local anesthesia in an outpatient setting. A laser is used to create multiple holes in the trabecular meshwork, which improves drainage of aqueous humor from the anterior chamber. If the procedure is successful, IOP falls over a period of time. Meanwhile, the health care provider usually has the patient continue using glaucoma medications.

A trabeculectomy is one of several surgical procedures that create a channel to allow aqueous humor to drain under the conjunctiva. If this procedure is not effective, cyclocryotherapy may be performed. A cold probe, called a *cryoprobe*, is used to freeze part of the ciliary body. Freezing destroys some of the tissue, resulting in decreased production of aqueous humor. Minimally invasive glaucoma surgery (MIGS) can be used to lower eye pressure and has less risk than trabeculectomy.

Angle-closure glaucoma. Angle-closure glaucoma also is called *acute glaucoma*. It accounts for approximately 10% of all glaucomas. With angle-closure glaucoma, the flow of aqueous humor through the pupil is blocked. Pressure forces the iris forward, causing it to block the trabecular meshwork. A rapid rise in IOP occurs, increasing to greater than 50 mm Hg. If the pressure is not lowered promptly, permanent blindness can result. Therefore, angle-closure glaucoma is considered a medical emergency. Unlike open-angle glaucoma, angle-closure glaucoma causes sudden, acute pain. Other signs and symptoms are blurred vision, halos around lights, nausea and vomiting, and headache on the affected side.

The goal of medical treatment is to reduce the intraocular pressure quickly. Drugs initially used to treat angle-closure glaucoma include miotics and oral or intravenous carbonic anhydrase inhibitors (see Table 59.1). After the pressure has been lowered, iridotomy or iridectomy usually is recommended to prevent recurrence. Laser peripheral *iridotomy* (LPI) is a procedure used to treat angle-closure glaucoma caused by blockage of the pupil. LPI eliminates pupillary block by allowing the aqueous to pass directly from the posterior chamber into the anterior chamber bypassing the pupil. The procedure may be performed on both eyes because the healthy eye is likely to experience similar problems in the future. Laser peripheral *iridectomy* is a procedure in which the surgeon makes an incision into the anterior chamber and surgically excises a small amount of iris tissue to create a passage for aqueous humor to reach the angle.

Cultural Considerations

Glaucoma is the leading cause of blindness in Black Americans. Open-angle glaucoma is most common in people of European or African descent; angle-closure glaucoma is more common among populations of Asian descent.

NURSING CARE OF THE PATIENT WITH GLAUCOMA

Nurses who work in acute care settings are most concerned with preserving vision with drug therapy and patient teaching for self-care. Patients with chronic glaucoma who are hospitalized for other reasons still require management of their glaucoma.

Focused Assessment

General assessment of the patient with an eye disorder is outlined in Chapter 58, Box 58.2. Nurses who work in specialty clinics or units also may be trained to measure IOP. When a patient has glaucoma, collect data about the patient's knowledge of the disease and treatment as well as about the patient's ability to carry out self-care.

If the patient has impaired vision, additional assessment may be appropriate. These are discussed in detail in Chapter 58 in the section titled "Nursing Care of the Visually Impaired Patient."

Table 59.1 Drug Therapy: Glaucoma

General Nursing Considerations

1. Teach patient or caregivers, or both, the proper way to administer eye drops.
2. Recognize that failure to control IOP can result in permanent blindness.
3. Avoid corticosteroids, succinylcholine, and anticholinergics in glaucoma patients.
4. Ophthalmic solutions should be tightly capped and protected from light.
5. Ophthalmic solutions should not be used if they change color or other characteristics.
6. Be alert for systemic effects of ophthalmic drugs.

DRUG	USE AND ACTION	SIDE EFFECTS	NURSING INTERVENTIONS
Beta-Adrenergic Blockers			
timolol (Timoptic) metipranolol (OptiPranolol) carteolol (Ocupress) levobunolol (Betagan Liquifilm) betaxolol (Betoptic)	Treatment of chronic open-angle glaucoma. Decreases aqueous formation. Often used in combination with other drugs.	Eye irritation. Possible systemic effects of beta-blockers: bronchospasm, heart failure. All contraindicated with asthma except betaxolol, which is beta-1 selective. See drug handbook for individual beta-blocker adverse effects.	Monitor pulse, BP, and respiration. Assess for wheezing, bronchospasm, bradycardia, hypotension, dysrhythmias. Question order for nonselective beta-blocker in patient with asthma.
Cholinergic Agonists			
pilocarpine (Pilopine HS) carbachol (Isopto Carbachol)	All cholinergics increase aqueous outflow. Constrict pupil.	Myopia. Poor vision in dim light. Lacrimation (tearing). Systemic effects (i.e., change in pulse rate or rhythm, bronchospasm, decreased BP, nausea, diarrhea, headache).	Advise patient to use caution for tasks requiring distant vision or vision in dim light. Antidote: atropine. Minimize side effects by applying pressure over lacrimal duct after administering drug.
pilocarpine (Ocusert ocular system)		Few side effects.	Ocusert therapeutic system lasts 1 week. More costly.
echothiophate iodide (Phospholine Iodide)		Blurred vision, brow ache, eyelid twitching, watering eyes, nausea, diarrhea, tachycardia.	Assess pulse.
Alpha-2 Adrenergic Agonists			
apraclonidine (Iopidine)	Short-term use only.	Headache, dry mouth, conjunctivitis, ocular itching.	Oral hygiene. Assess conjunctiva for redness, itching.
brimonidine (Alphagan)	Long-term use with open-angle glaucoma or ocular hypertension.	Hypertension with Alphagan, but not with Iopidine. Headache, dry mouth and nose, altered taste, conjunctivitis.	Monitor BP. Oral hygiene. Assess conjunctiva for redness, itching.
Prostaglandin Analogs			
latanoprost (Xalatan) travoprost, bimatoprost tafluprost	Increases aqueous outflow in open-angle glaucoma and ocular hypertension.	Permanent darkening of green-brown, yellow-brown, and blue/gray/brown irises of the eyes. Also blurred vision, burning, headache, sensation of having foreign body in eye.	Inform patient of possible sensation of having foreign body in eye.
Oral Carbonic Anhydrase Inhibitors			
acetazolamide (Diamox) dichlorphenamide methazolamide (Neptazane)	Treatment of acute and chronic glaucoma. Decreases aqueous formation. Used less now than in past.	Increased urinary output, potential hypokalemia. Possible allergic response in people who are allergic to sulfonamides. Tingling of fingers and toes (paresthesia). Itching. Sore throat, skin rash, and fever may suggest serious blood disorders.	Monitor intake and output. Withhold and notify physician if patient is allergic. Assess for hypokalemia (pulse changes, mental status changes, muscle weakness, abdominal distention). Expect increased urine output. Provide access and assistance to toilet. Do not give at bedtime.
Topical Carbonic Anhydrase Eye Drops			
brinzolamide (Azopt) dorzolamide (Trusopt)	Open-angle glaucoma.	Irritation, bitter taste.	Monitor for local and systemic allergic reactions.

Table 59.1 Drug Therapy: Glaucoma—cont'd

DRUG	USE AND ACTION	SIDE EFFECTS	NURSING INTERVENTIONS
Rho Kinase Inhibitors			
Netarsudil Rhopressa	Increases aqueous outflow	Red eye and ocular irritation	Assess pain levels and amount of irritation in eyes. Monitor for local and systemic allergic reactions.
Combined Medications			
Dorzolamide HCL & timolol maleate (Cosopt) (Cosopt PF)	Combined action of beta-blocker and carbonic anhydrase inhibitor.	See each type.	See each type. Contraindicated with asthma.
netarsudil & latanoprost ophthalmic solution 0.02%/0.005% (Rocklatan)	Combined rho kinase inhibitor and prostaglandins analog.	See each type. Eye redness and stinging.	See each type.
brimonidine tartrate & timolol maleate ophthalmic solution 0.2%/0.5% (Combigan)	Combined beta blocker and alpha agonist.	See each type.	See each type.
brinzolamide & brimonidine tartrate 1%/0.2%	Combined carbonic anhydrase inhibitor and alpha agonist.	Blurred vision, eye irritation, bad taste, dry mouth, and eye allergy.	See each type.

BP, Blood pressure; *IOP*, intraocular pressure; *IV*, intravenous.

Patient Problems, Goals, and Outcome Criteria: Glaucoma

Problems	Goals and Outcome Criteria
Potential for injury related to increased intraocular pressure (IOP)	Decreased risk for injury: adherence to prescribed measures to reduce IOP, normal IOP readings
Anxiety related to fear of actual or potential loss of vision	Decreased anxiety: patient states feeling less fearful
Inability to manage treatment program related to lack of understanding of disease, treatment, and complications	Effective management of condition: patient correctly describes and adheres to prescribed drug therapy
Acute pain related to sudden increase in IOP, inflammation caused by corrective procedures	Pain relief: patient states pain is reduced or relieved, relaxed manner

Interventions

Potential for injury. One of the most important things you can do to prevent damage to the optic nerve is to keep IOP within normal limits by administering prescribed medications. Be extremely cautious in selecting and administering ophthalmic medications. Different medications are often ordered for the affected and the unaffected eye. The procedure for applying eye drops and ointments is described in Chapter 58 in the section titled "Topical Medications."

Anxiety and inability to manage treatment program. You must be sensitive to the patient's fears about glaucoma leading to blindness (see the Patient Teaching box). Emphasize that adherence to prescribed drug therapy usually can control IOP and reduce the risk of complications. Because open-angle glaucoma is painless, the patient may not appreciate the need for ongoing treatment. Stress the importance of keeping regular appointments for evaluation of IOP. Unfortunately, noncompliance with drug therapy is a frequent patient problem with glaucoma. Remember (and teach the patient) that any drugs that dilate the pupil are contraindicated. Patients may not be aware that many nonprescription cold and allergy remedies contain drugs that dilate the pupil. The health care provider should be consulted before taking any additional drugs.

Patient Teaching

Glaucoma

- Glaucoma usually responds to treatment, but it can lead to blindness if untreated.
- Regular checkups are essential to monitor intraocular pressure (IOP) because glaucoma is usually painless.
- Consult with a health care provider before taking any new medication.
- Wear a medical alert tag.
- Take along spare medication when traveling.
- Notify your health care provider if visual acuity or peripheral vision decreases.

Patients who have glaucoma should wear a bracelet to alert health care providers to the condition. They should keep their medications on hand at all times. When traveling, the patient with glaucoma should keep spare medications in separate locations in case one is lost. It is helpful to have a wallet card stating the exact medication schedule in case the patient becomes ill and is unable to give this information.

Acute pain. Pain in acute glaucoma attacks is treated with drugs that reduce IOP. Analgesics may be given as ordered. If the patient has surgery for glaucoma, postoperative care is similar to the general care after eye surgery, described in Chapter 58 in the section titled "Postoperative Nursing Care." Monitoring IOP is especially important after glaucoma surgery. Postoperative pain can usually be treated with nonopioid analgesics. Report increasing or unrelieved pain to the surgeon.

Many drugs are contraindicated with glaucoma (see the Complementary and Alternative Therapies box).

Complementary and Alternative Therapies

Caution patients to avoid taking over the counter (OTC) drug products without consulting the health care provider. Many OTC drugs, including herbal medications, can raise intraocular pressure (IOP).

RETINAL DETACHMENT

Pathophysiology

Retinal detachment is a separation of the sensory (light-sensitive) layer of the eyeball from the pigmented layer. The detachment begins when a tear in the retina allows fluid to collect between the sensory and pigmented layers causing the two layers to separate. Separation deprives the sensory layers of nutrients and O_2 that normally are supplied by the blood vessels in the choroid. This leads to damage to the nerve tissue in the sensory layer, resulting in partial or complete loss of vision. Retinal tears may occur spontaneously or as a result of trauma. They are more common in older people; and in people with myopia, diabetic retinopathy, and other eye diseases.

Clinical Manifestations

Signs and symptoms of retinal detachment depend on the location and extent of the detachment. Patients may report seeing flashes of light or floaters, cloudy vision, or a dark shadow on the sides or in the middle of the field of vision. If the area of detachment is large, vision may be lost completely. Some patients say that it seems as if a curtain has come down or across the line of vision, which can be very frightening (Fig. 59.6).

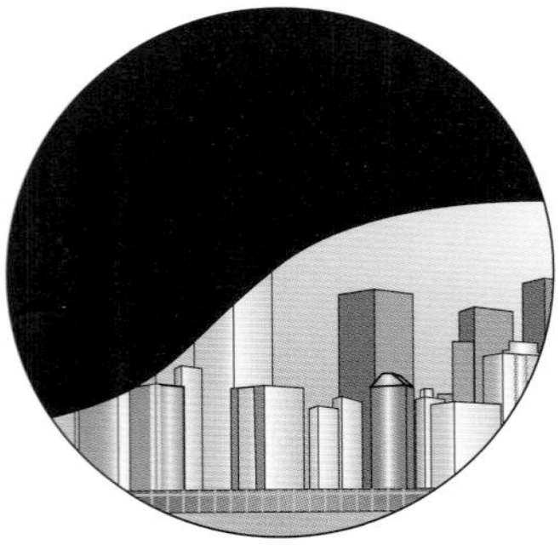

Detached retina

Fig. 59.6 Loss of partial field of vision because of retinal detachment. (Courtesy National Industries for the Blind, Alexandria, VA.)

Medical and Surgical Treatment

Retinal detachment is considered a medical emergency. The symptoms come on quickly, so people are advised to go to an eye doctor or emergency department immediately to avoid further detachment and the risk of permanent vision loss. Special procedures are required to repair retinal detachments. Most holes or tears must be sealed promptly. Laser photocoagulation, a procedure in which intense light burns the detached portion of the retina, commonly is used. As the area heals, scar tissue forms and seals the tear. Cryotherapy also causes scar tissue to form, but it uses a cold probe applied to the eyeball behind the tear. The cold radiates through the layers of tissue, freezing the torn tissue. Another procedure that may be used is retinopexy, in which gas is injected into the eye to apply pressure to the tear. Laser, cryotherapy, and retinopexy procedures may be performed on an outpatient basis.

Scleral buckling frequently is performed along with laser treatment or cryotherapy. The patient may have local or general anesthesia, and usually is discharged the same day. The scleral buckle is a silastic band that is secured around the eyeball under the sclera. Small silicone implants are sutured under the band opposite the area of detachment. The layers of tissue are brought back together by pressing from the outside. The band is left in place permanently (Fig. 59.7). The health care provider may inject an air bubble or normal saline into the vitreous humor after the surgical procedure to apply internal pressure to the detached portion of the retina.

Sometimes tears cause bleeding into the vitreous. Significant amounts of blood in the vitreous interfere with vision. When this occurs, the ophthalmologist may perform a vitrectomy to remove the bloody tissue. Vitrectomy also is indicated when the vitreous is creating traction on the retina.

NURSING CARE OF THE PATIENT WITH RETINAL DETACHMENT

Before corrective measures are taken, the patient usually is placed on strict bed rest with the head elevated. In the preoperative period, many patients are very anxious. Encourage them to talk about their fears and to ask questions. Even though the procedure is performed under local anesthesia, oral intake may be

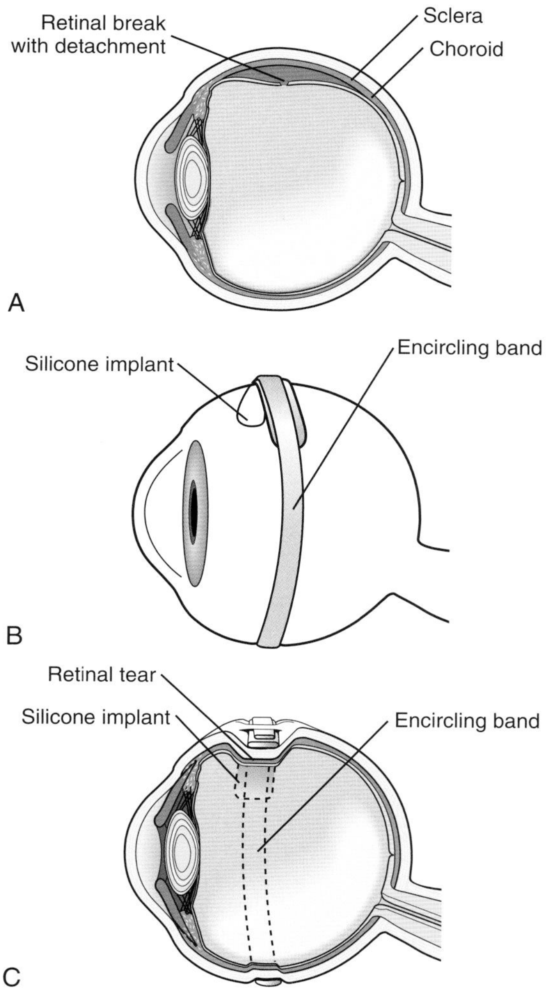

Fig. 59.7 (A) Retinal detachment. (B and C) Scleral buckle and silicone implant in place to treat retinal detachment. (From Lewis SM, Heitkemper MM, Dirksen SR, et al.: *Medical-surgical nursing: assessment and management of clinical problems*, ed 9, St. Louis, 2015, Mosby.)

restricted to reduce the risk of postoperative vomiting. Intravenous fluids may be ordered.

Postoperative care is essentially the same as for other patients undergoing eye surgery, as described in Chapter 58 in the section titled "Postoperative Nursing Care." Positioning orders may be very specific for these patients. If an air bubble has been injected, it will rise to the top of the eye. If the patient's detachment is in the back of the eye, a face-down position is necessary to keep the bubble in the right place. Saline travels down rather than up, so the same patient would need to stay face up if saline had been injected. The surgeon prescribes any activity limitations. The length of hospitalization varies depending on the location and severity of the tear, the type of repair, and the surgeon's routines.

SENILE MACULAR DEGENERATION

The macula is the part of the retina that is responsible for central vision. As people age, changes in the eye cause the macula to degenerate. The two forms of

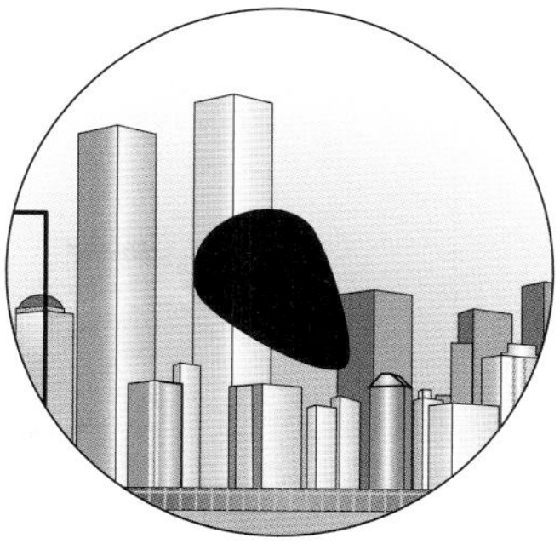

Fig. 59.8 Vision of the patient with macular degeneration. (Courtesy of the National Industries for the Blind, Alexandria, VA.)

macular degeneration are dry (strophic) and wet (exudative). The dry form is most common and is characterized by the appearance of drusen (yellow deposits) in the macula. As the yellow deposits grow and become more numerous, vision may dim or be distorted, and central vision gradually gets worse. The dry form tends to worsen slowly, so patients keep most of their vision. They often report difficulty reading or doing close work (Fig. 59.8).

The dry form usually occurs first and can progress to the wet form; however, only 10 per cent of people with macular degeneration have the wet form. In the wet form, blood vessels grow underneath the macula and leak blood and fluid into the retina. Vision becomes blurry and distorted, with blind spots and loss of central vision. The wet form is the leading cause of permanent vision loss. Both the wet and dry types are progressive. Peripheral vision remains intact.

Regular eyeglasses do not improve vision with macular degeneration. Special telescopic lenses may be helpful. Laser treatments or vitrectomy may offer hope to some patients with macular degeneration. The most promising treatment is a series of intraocular injections of an angiogenesis inhibitor (a drug that inhibits the growth of new blood vessels) such as ranibizumab (Lucentis). This procedure is performed in a clinic setting and is relatively painless. At best, the patient actually has some improvement in vision. For others, the progression of the condition is slowed. The nurse should help the patient and family members to learn to cope with the level of vision impairment the patient experiences. The nursing care is like that described in Chapter 58 in the section titled "Nursing Care of the Visually Impaired Patient" (see the Complementary and Alternative Therapies box).

Complementary and Alternative Therapies

Some practitioners believe that high doses of vitamins C and E, beta-carotene, and zinc may slow the progression of age-related dry macular degeneration. Note that smokers should not take large doses of beta-carotene.

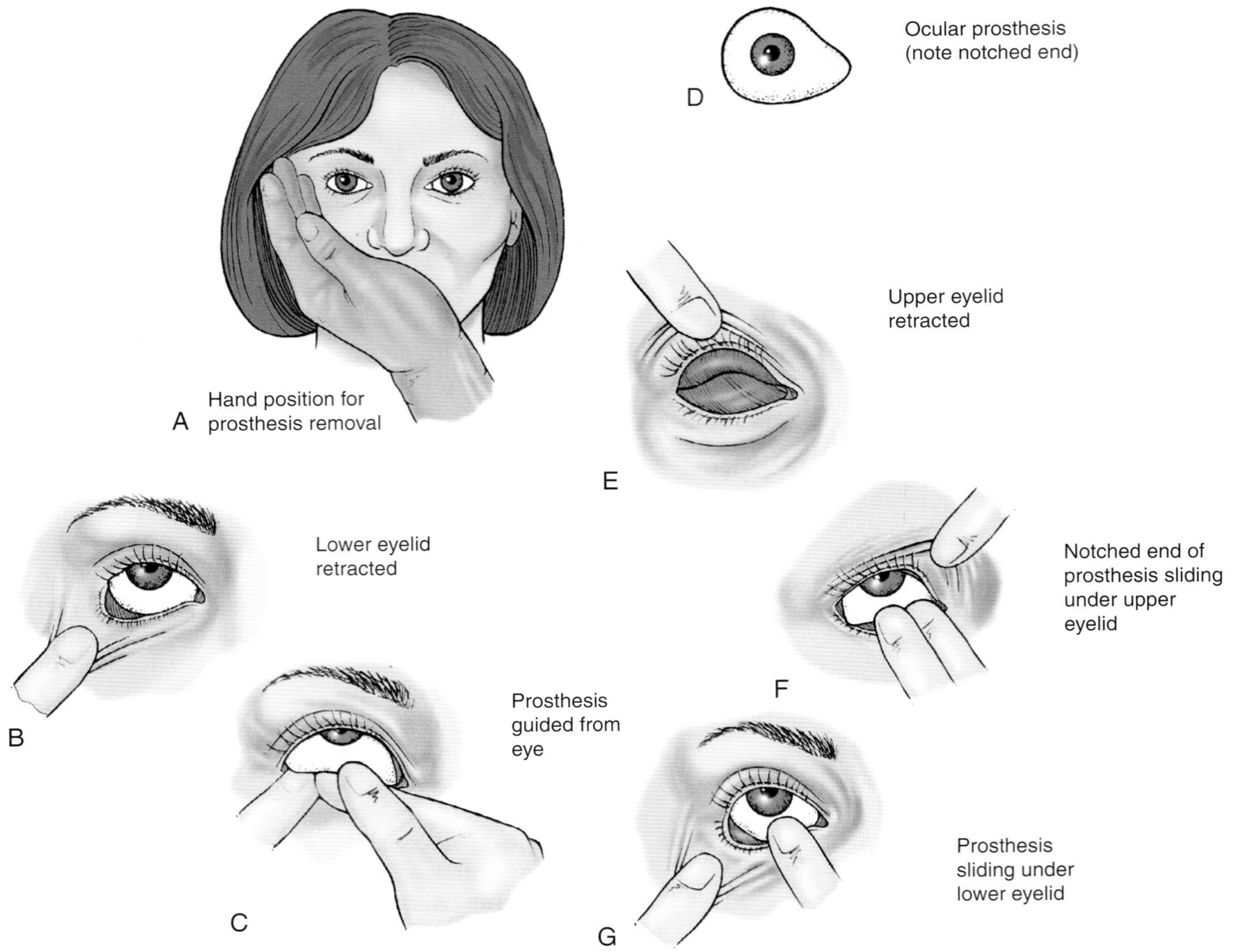

Fig. 59.9 Removal (A to C) and insertion (D to G) of an eye prosthesis. (From Monahan FD, Drake DT, Neighbors M, editors: *Medical-surgical nursing: foundations for clinical practice*, ed 2, Philadelphia, 1998, Saunders.)

ENUCLEATION

Some eye conditions are so serious that removal of the eyeball is the only treatment. **Enucleation** is the term used for removal of the eyeball. Conditions that may result in enucleation include injury, infection, sympathetic ophthalmia, and some glaucomas and malignancies.

During the surgical procedure, the eyeball is removed. A round device is placed in the cavity, and muscles are sutured over it. The conjunctiva is then sutured over the muscle. This procedure creates a foundation for the future placement of an eye prosthesis. The patient returns from surgery with a temporary shell called a *conformer* in the prosthesis base, which is covered with a pressure dressing. Observe for excessive bleeding or increasing pain. Report any temperature elevation. After the pressure dressing is removed, the surgeon may order wound care and topical medications.

Approximately 1 month after the enucleation, an optician can fit a prosthesis. The prosthesis is carefully made to look like the patient's natural eye. The patient must learn to insert, remove, and clean the prosthesis. Nurses should also know how to care for an eye prosthesis as illustrated in Fig. 59.9. The steps to remove and clean a prosthesis are as follows:

1. Wash hands thoroughly and apply gloves.
2. Gently depress and pull the lower lid down.
3. Allow the prosthesis to slip out over the lower lid.
4. Wash the prosthesis under running water, using the fingers to remove any debris.

If the prosthesis is to be stored, it should be placed in a container with normal saline or water.

To reinsert the prosthesis, do the following:

1. Raise the upper lid by pressing it up against the orbit.
2. Slip the top of the prosthesis under the orbit.
3. Pull the lower lid down so that the prosthesis can slip into place.

The patient's nursing care plan should always inform staff that the patient has an eye prosthesis.

Get Ready for the NCLEX® Examination!

Key Points

- Infectious and inflammatory conditions of the eye include blepharitis, hordeolum, chalazion, conjunctivitis, and keratitis.
- Entropion is inversion of the lower lid; ectropion is eversion of the lower lid.
- Only a health care provider should remove a foreign body embedded in the eye.
- Corneal opacity is treated with removal of the scarred cornea and replacement with a healthy donor cornea in a procedure called *keratoplasty.*
- Errors of refraction include myopia, hyperopia, and astigmatism and are often correctable with corrective lenses.
- An opaque lens, called a *cataract*, can be removed and vision restored with a lens replacement in the form of eyeglasses, contact lenses, or intraocular lenses.
- Glaucoma, increased IOP, is a leading cause of blindness and is treated with drug therapy, surgery, or both.
- Nursing care of the patient with glaucoma focuses on potential for injury, fear, inability to manage treatment program, and pain.
- Retinal detachment is separation of the sensory layer of the eyeball from the pigmented layer and can result in partial or complete loss of vision.
- Treatments for retinal detachment include laser therapy, cryotherapy, retinopexy, scleral buckling, and vitrectomy.
- Senile macular degeneration causes progressive loss of central vision but may be slowed or improved by intraocular injections of an angiogenesis inhibitor.
- Enucleation is removal of the eyeball necessitated by injury, infection, sympathetic ophthalmia, and some glaucomas and malignancies.
- After enucleation, a prosthesis can be used to restore the patient's normal appearance.

Additional Learning Resources

SG Go to your Study Guide for additional learning activities to help you master this chapter content.

Go to your Evolve website (http://evolve.elsevier.com/Linton/medsurg) for the following learning resources and much more:

- Fluid & Electrolyte Tutorial
- Review Questions for the NCLEX® Examination

Clinical Judgment and Next-Generation NCLEX® Examination-Style Questions

1. **A patient is being discharged after cataract surgery. Discharge instructions should include which of the following statements? (Select all that apply.)**
   1. "Always lie on the unaffected side."
   2. "Avoid pressure on the operative eye."
   3. "Moderate to severe pain is expected."
   4. "Resume usual activities immediately."
   5. "Expect a small amount of bleeding."

   NCLEX Client Need: Physiological Integrity: Reduction of Risk Potential

2. **After keratoplasty, you observe that the patient's cornea is cloudy. What should you do?**
   1. Reassure the patient that cloudiness is normal for several weeks after surgery.
   2. Elevate the patient's head and encourage increased fluid intake.
   3. Report signs of corneal rejection to the health care provider.
   4. Prepare the patient for emergency surgery.

   NCLEX Client Need: Physiological Integrity: Reduction of Risk Potential

3. **Drugs used to treat open-angle glaucoma act by which of the following mechanisms? (Select all that apply.)**
   1. Increasing aqueous outflow
   2. Dilating the canal of Schlemm
   3. Relaxing the trabecular meshwork
   4. Decreasing aqueous formation
   5. Reducing systemic blood pressure

   NCLEX Client Need: Physiological Integrity: Pharmacological Therapies

4. **A patient came to the clinic complaining of severe eye pain. The physician diagnosed acute angle-closure glaucoma. The nurse understands that the most serious complication of angle-closure glaucoma is:**
   1. Rupture of the eyeball
   2. Permanent blindness
   3. Nausea and vomiting
   4. Increased intracranial pressure

   NCLEX Client Need: Physiological Integrity: Reduction of Risk Potential

5. **Two patients had surgery for retinal detachments this morning. Postoperatively, one is positioned on the left side with the head of the bed flat. The other is in Fowler position. What factors determined the best postoperative position for these patients? (Select all that apply.)**
   1. Patient preference
   2. Intraocular pressure
   3. Location of the repaired tear
   4. Use of air or saline to support the repair
   5. Whether or not a scleral buckle was applied

   NCLEX Client Need: Physiological Integrity: Physiological Adaptation

6. **(Take Action Using Matrix Test Item)**

   A 72-year-old woman had cataract surgery on her left eye with a lens replacement. The nurse assesses the patient and plans health teaching for the patient in preparation for her discharge.

   Use an X for the health teaching below that is *Indicated* (appropriate or necessary), *Contraindicated* (could be harmful), or *Nonessential* (makes no difference or not necessary) before the patient's discharge at this time.

HEALTH TEACHING	INDICATED	CONTRAINDICATED	NONESSENTIAL
"Arrange for someone to drive you home."			
"Avoid bending forward."			
"Take a stool softener to avoid straining on defecation."			
"Eat a high protein diet."			
"Always sleep on your left side."			
"Do not lift more than 5 lb."			
"Report severe pain in the affected eye to your health care provider."			

Ear and Hearing Disorders

60

http://evolve.elsevier.com/Linton/medsurg

Objectives

1. Describe the pathophysiology, signs and symptoms, complications, and medical or surgical treatment for selected ear and hearing disorders.
2. Assist in the development of a nursing care plan for a patient with a disorder of the ear, hearing, or balance.

Key Terms

ototoxicity
presbycusis (prĕz-bē-KŪ-sĭs)
tinnitus (tĭ-NĬ-tĭs)
tympanic membrane (tĭm-PĂN-ĭk MĔM-brān)
vertigo (VĔR-tĭ-gō)

HEARING DISORDERS

Hearing disorders may occur in the external ear and canal, and the middle and inner ears. Disorders causing hearing loss in each section of the ear are shown in Fig. 60.1.

DISORDERS OF EXTERNAL EAR AND CANAL

FOREIGN BODIES AND CERUMEN

Occasionally, foreign bodies get into the external ear canal. Most small objects can be flushed from the ear by gentle irrigation, but only if the **tympanic membrane** (eardrum) is intact. If the eardrum is ruptured, the fluid may be forced into the inner ear and cause an infection. Insects can be killed by instilling a small amount of mineral oil, which is then flushed from the canal. An alternative method is to hold a flashlight near the auricle. The insects are attracted to the light and may move toward the light beam out of the canal.

One of the most common causes of obstruction of the external ear canal is impacted cerumen. The dry cerumen may be gold to dark brown and may fill the entire canal in one or both ears. The patient is not always aware of the obstruction but may complain of hearing loss, ear pain, or **tinnitus**. When a large amount of hardened cerumen is present, the health care provider may order eardrops to soften the cerumen before irrigation. The procedure may have to be repeated several times before all cerumen is removed. If the foreign body or cerumen is not removed by irrigation, ear forceps or a cerumen spoon can be used.

INFECTION AND INFLAMMATION

Infection or inflammation of the lining of the external ear canal is called *external otitis* or *swimmer's ear*. Swimming can lead to external otitis by washing out protective cerumen, which leaves the lining of the external canal susceptible to infectious agents. Infection and inflammation also may be caused by scratching or cleaning the ear with sharp objects. Allergic external otitis may result from contact with cosmetics, hair sprays, earphones, earrings, or hearing aids. Infection results from staphylococcal or streptococcal bacteria but also may be fungal in origin (Fig. 60.2).

The most characteristic symptom of external otitis is pain that increases when the auricle is pulled. Infected skin becomes red, swollen, and tender to touch or movement, which can lead to hearing loss. Other symptoms include dizziness, fever, and drainage. Drainage may be purulent or blood tinged.

Medical Treatment

Topical antibacterial or antifungal drugs are used to treat external otitis. Corticosteroid drops may be ordered to reduce inflammation unless the infection is caused by a fungus. In that case, corticosteroids are contraindicated. If the external canal is obstructed by edema, the health care provider may insert an ear wick through the blocked canal. An ear wick is a long piece of gauze that extends out of the ear canal. Medication placed on the external portion of the ear wick soaks the gauze and distributes the medication in the canal. Moist heat, topical anesthetic drops, and mild analgesics may be ordered for pain. Any drainage from the ear should be treated as infected material and handled carefully. External otitis is typically treated on an outpatient basis.

❖ NURSING CARE OF THE PATIENT WITH A DISORDER OF THE EXTERNAL EAR

Focused Assessment

Nurses, especially in long-term care facilities, need to inspect the ear canal routinely for impacted cerumen

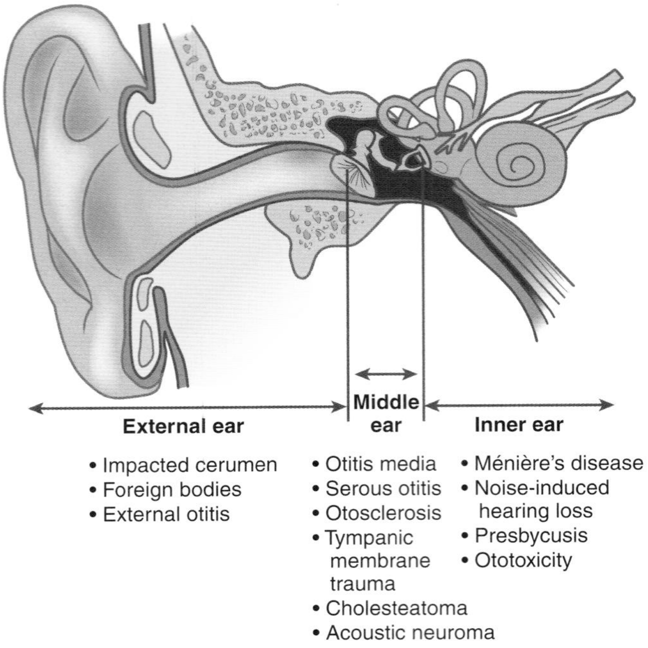

Fig. 60.1 Causes of hearing loss.

or drainage. Note any presenting symptoms of pain or irritation.

Patient Problems, Goals and Outcome Criteria: External Ear Disorder

Patient Problems	Goals and Outcome Criteria
Inability to communicate effectively related to obstruction of the external auditory canal	Effective communication: patient able to hear adequately after removal of obstruction
Lack of knowledge related to cause and treatment of decreased hearing	Patient seeks care for external ear obstruction, inflammation or infection
Acute pain related to obstruction or inflammation of external ear canal	Pain relief after irrigation or medical treatment of external ear

Interventions

Inability to communicate effectively. The goal is removal of the obstruction to improve hearing. Report findings to the health care provider and carry out orders for eardrops. Ensure that drops are at room temperature; cold could trigger dizziness. Remember, ear irrigations and most eardrops are contraindicated in the presence of a perforation in the tympanic membrane.

Lack of knowledge. Educate patients to avoid trying to remove cerumen with cotton-tipped applicators or other tools. These efforts can harm the ear canal or the tympanic membrane, in addition to forcing cerumen or foreign bodies further into the canal. Because it is awkward to put drops into one's own ear, you may also need to teach a family member how to do it.

Teach patients to prevent external otitis by refraining from the use of sharp instruments to clean the auditory canal and by avoiding suspected irritants such as hair spray and earphones. Advise the use of earplugs while swimming. The health care provider may instruct the patient to use a drying agent (e.g., Ear-Dry) after swimming or bathing.

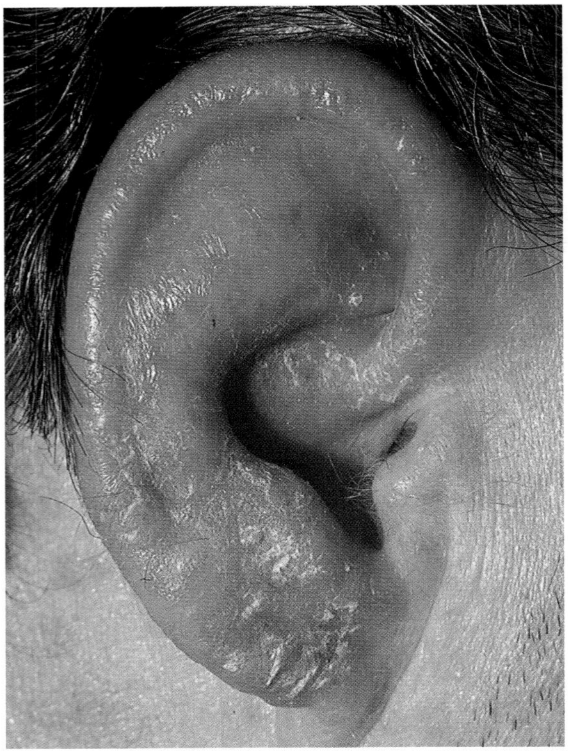

Fig. 60.2 External otitis. (From Habif TP: *Clinical dermatology*, ed 6, Philadelphia, 2016, Elsevier.)

Acute pain. Oral analgesics, topical corticosteroids, and antibiotics are given as ordered to treat pain and to reduce inflammation and infection. Administer the prescribed drops or teach the patient or caregiver the procedure. Apply heat to the affected ear for 20 minutes three times a day using a heated towel or heating pad. Soak the towel in warm water, wring, and put in a plastic bag. Pain may be reduced by minimizing head movements.

MIDDLE EAR

Conditions of the middle ear are serious because of the risk for complications, including permanent hearing loss and involvement of the inner ear.

OTITIS MEDIA

Otitis media also is known as a *middle ear infection*. The middle ear connects to the throat by way of the eustachian tube, through which fluid drains. This helps to even out the pressure between the outer and inner ear. A cold, allergy, sore throat, or respiratory infection can irritate the eustachian tube or cause it to swell, preventing fluid from draining from the middle ear. The fluid builds up against the tympanic membrane where bacteria and viruses can grow, resulting in infection. The most common symptoms of otitis media are ear pain, feeling of fullness in the ear, fluid draining from the ear, fever, and hearing loss. Untreated ear infections can lead to infections in other parts of the head, permanent hearing loss, or speech and language problems. Cigarette smoke as well as smoke from vaping devices, such as e-cigarettes and electronic nicotine, can increase the chances of infection. Thus, to help prevent ear infections, homes should be free of these devices.

The types of otitis media include *acute otitis media*, *otitis media with effusion (serous otitis media)*, and *chronic otitis media*.

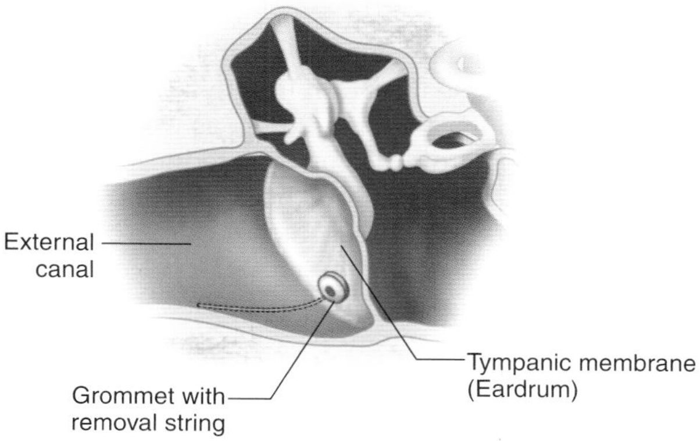

Fig. 60.3 Grommet through the tympanic membrane. A small grommet is placed through the tympanic membrane away from the margins, which allows prolonged drainage of fluids from the middle ear.

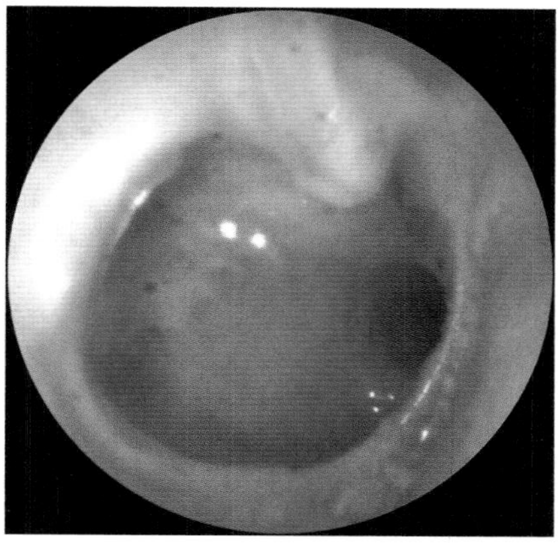

Fig. 60.4 Perforation of the tympanic membrane. (From Flint P, Haughey B, Lund V, Niparko JK, editors: *Cummings otolaryngology. Head and neck surgery*, ed 5, St. Louis, 2010, Mosby.)

Acute Otitis Media

Acute otitis media develops suddenly, usually after an upper respiratory infection. Edema leads to blockage of the eustachian tubes, and fluid and pus accumulate, causing painful pressure on the eardrum. Clinical manifestations include fever, pain, malaise, drainage, and reduced hearing in the ear. The eardrum may rupture, resulting in scarring and subsequent hearing loss. Acute otitis media is more common in children than in adults.

Medical treatment. Although acute otitis media occurs suddenly with redness and swelling, fever and ear pain, it often resolves without intervention; oral antibiotics may be prescribed in some circumstances. Another option is topical ear drops, usually combinations of antibacterials and corticosteroids, that are given for 1 week. Before the drops are administered, the canal should be cleared of debris. Instruct the patient to lie on the unaffected side for a few minutes after instilling the drops to promote flow of the medication into the canal. If a wick has been placed in the canal because of swelling, apply the ear drops directly to the wick. Antihistamines may be ordered if allergies are thought to be contributing to the problem. Sometimes a *myringotomy* is performed. Myringotomy is the creation of a small opening in the tympanic membrane to reduce pressure and allow fluid to drain. If infection is eliminated, the tympanic membrane should heal without permanent damage. A tympanostomy tube or grommet may be placed to allow for continuous drainage for a patient with chronic otitis media (Fig. 60.3). The health care provider may suggest *autoinsufflation*, which helps adjust the air pressure in the ear. The patient is told to pinch the nose and gently exhale, forcing the air back into the eustachian tube.

Otitis Media With Effusion (Serous Otitis Media)

Otitis media with effusion (OME) is an inflammation of the middle ear in which fluid or mucus builds up next to the eardrum caused by swelling or blockage of the eustachian tube. Common causes are allergies, irritants (particularly cigarette smoke), and respiratory infections. Drinking while lying on the back, or a sudden increase in air pressure such as a descending in an airplane, also my cause swelling or blockage. The middle ear feels full, which can last for months and affect hearing.

Chronic Otitis Media

Chronic otitis media may follow repeated attacks of otitis media and is characterized by inflammation and purulent drainage that may involve the ossicles, auditory canal, and mastoid bone. The condition usually is not painful; however, nausea and dizziness may occur. On examination, the eardrum may be perforated or shows signs of a healed perforation (Fig. 60.4). An audiogram may detect some conductive hearing loss if the bones in the middle ear have been damaged by the chronic infection.

Possible complications of chronic otitis media include mastoiditis, meningitis, labyrinthitis, cholesteatoma, and hearing impairment.

Mastoiditis. Because the middle ear is directly connected to the air cells in the mastoid bone, infection in the middle ear can extend into the mastoid bone. In addition, because the brain lies next to the mastoid bone, the infection can spread there as well. Signs and symptoms of mastoiditis include redness, swelling, tenderness and pain behind the ear; thick, purulent discharge from the ear; headache, malaise and irritability; fever and elevated white blood cell (WBC) count; and hearing loss. The symptoms often appear after a recurring or severe ear infection. Mastoiditis is very serious because it can lead to a brain abscess, meningitis (i.e., inflammation of the covering of the brain), a blood clot, or paralysis of the facial muscles. Treatment consists of antibiotics, surgery to drain the middle ear (*myringotomy*), or removal of part of the mastoid bone.

Cholesteatoma. A **cholesteatoma** is a growth in the middle ear. It can be congenital (present at birth) or acquired (usually caused by multiple ear infections). Cholesteatomas are formed when excess cells accumulate in a cyst or sac near the tympanic membrane. The cells form a ball of tissue that grows and may damage the facial nerve, the ossicles, and the labyrinth. A cholesteatoma must be removed surgically.

Medical treatment. Chronic otitis media is treated with systemic antibiotics and, if the eardrum is intact, irrigations to remove debris. If the tympanic membrane does not heal, tympanoplasty may be performed to repair it. The procedure may be carried out through the ear canal or through an incision behind the auricle. Sometimes grafts of the patient's tissue are used to repair the tear. If the ossicles in the middle ear are diseased, they may be replaced with prostheses.

If the infection has extended to the mastoid bone, a mastoidectomy typically is performed at the same time. A mastoidectomy can be modified (simple) or radical. In a modified procedure, infected mastoid tissue is removed but the middle ear is left intact. In a radical mastoidectomy, all structures in the middle ear are removed. Although used frequently in the past, the radical procedure is rarely performed today.

❖ NURSING CARE OF THE PATIENT HAVING A MASTOIDECTOMY

General care of the patient having surgery on the ear is discussed in Chapter 58 in the section titled "Surgical Intervention for the Eye and Ear." Before mastoid surgery, the emphasis is on patient teaching and reduction of anxiety. Primary considerations after surgery on the middle ear include comfort, safety, prevention of infection, and prevention of pressure on the tympanic membrane. Nausea is another common problem after middle ear surgery. Keep an emesis receptacle nearby. The health care provider usually orders antiemetics to be given as needed for nausea. If the patient vomits frequently, a risk of dehydration exists. Monitor intake and output and give intravenous fluids if ordered.

The type of dressing varies. It may be small and placed over the auricle. However, if the surgeon entered through the mastoid bone, expect a large head dressing with a drain. Inspect the dressing and describe any drainage but do not disturb or remove the dressing. Assist the patient the first time out of bed in case dizziness is a problem. The patient should avoid any activity that creates pressure on the tympanic membrane (e.g., blowing the nose, coughing, sneezing, straining). If unavoidable, encourage the patient to cough or sneeze with the mouth open.

OTOSCLEROSIS

Otosclerosis is a condition in which an abnormal growth causes the footplate of the stapes to become fixed. The fixed stapes cannot vibrate, so sound waves cannot be transmitted to the inner ear. The effect of this abnormality is a conductive hearing loss. If the disease also involves the inner ear, the patient has sensorineural hearing loss as well. The condition affects both ears but may progress faster in one ear than in the other.

Otosclerosis is most common among middle-aged Caucasian women and is thought to be hereditary. The primary symptom of otosclerosis is slowly progressive hearing loss in the absence of infection. In the early stages, the patient may report tinnitus or the inability to hear low-pitched sounds or whispers. Some people experience dizziness or balance problems. The Rinne test reveals bone conduction to be greater than air conduction.

Medical Treatment

Although mild otosclerosis can be treated with a hearing aid, the most common treatment is a surgical procedure called a *stapedectomy*. The surgeon advises the patient of the surgical risks, including complete hearing loss, infection, prolonged vertigo, and damage to the facial nerve. Stapedectomy is done in an outpatient setting under local anesthesia. The stapes is removed and replaced with a prosthesis made of plastic or metal. Some fatty tissue is taken from a small incision behind the ear and placed over the oval window. The surgeon puts packing in the ear canal at the completion of the stapedectomy. A small dressing is then placed over the ear. Hearing starts to return about one week after surgery, then continues to improve. When the graft heals, hearing is restored permanently in most patients (Fig. 60.5).

Patients return home the same day of surgery and are encouraged to rest and avoid strenuous work for one week. Drugs are prescribed to control nausea and vertigo. The patient may be allowed to lie on the back or the unaffected side, but specific position restrictions may be ordered.

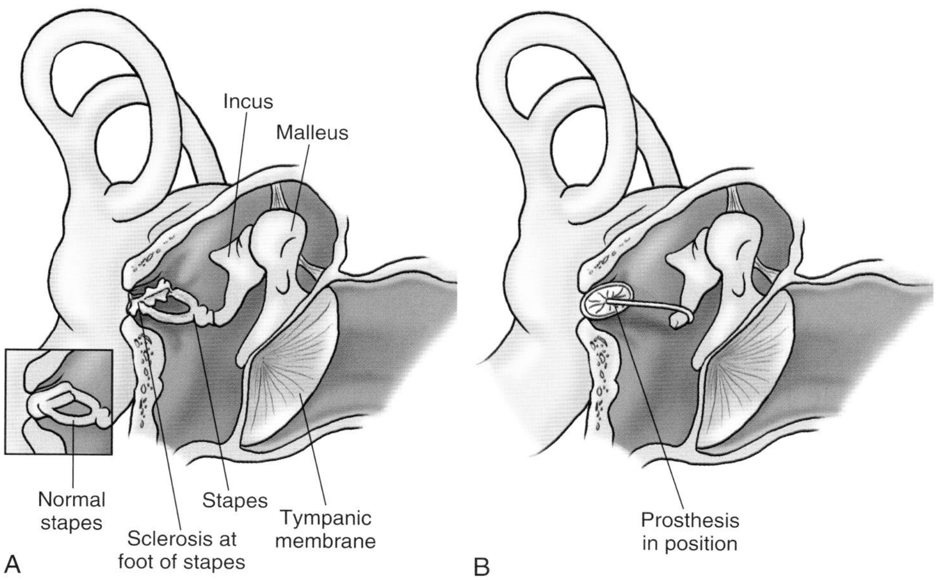

Fig. 60.5 Otosclerosis: (A) before and (B) after stapedectomy. (From Monahan FD, Drake DT, Neighbors M, editors: *Medical-surgical nursing: foundations for clinical practice*, ed 2, Philadelphia, 1998, Saunders.)

NURSING CARE OF THE PATIENT HAVING STAPEDECTOMY

Care of the patient having ear surgery is detailed in Chapter 58 in the section titled "Surgical Intervention of the Eye or Ear." In addition to the usual preoperative teaching, tell the patient having stapedectomy that hearing usually is worse immediately after surgery but improves gradually over approximately 6 weeks.

After surgery, focus on pain relief, safety, prevention of infection, and avoidance of pressure in the ear. Because pressure can cause the graft to separate, it is especially important for the patient to avoid anything that increases pressure in the ear. After stapedectomy, nausea, vomiting, and vertigo are common.

The packing in the ear should not be disturbed. The surgeon removes it approximately 1 week after the surgery. After the dressing and packing are removed, the patient usually is advised to keep the ear dry for at least 2 weeks. Swimming and showering typically are not permitted for approximately 6 weeks; however, in many cases, showering may be done with a protective covering on the affected ear.

The patient should avoid contact with people who have colds, flu, or other infectious respiratory illnesses. A balanced diet and adequate rest are needed for tissue healing and resistance to infection. Vertigo may persist after discharge, so the patient must plan for assistance with activities of daily living (ADLs). Emphasize that hearing improvement is gradual.

INNER EAR

LABYRINTHITIS

Labyrinthitis, or inflammation of the labyrinth, may be acute or chronic, caused by a virus, or occasionally, bacteria. Acute labyrinthitis may follow an acute upper respiratory infection, acute otitis media, pneumonia, or influenza. It also can be an adverse effect of some drugs (see the Complementary and Alternative Therapies box). *Suppurative labyrinthitis* is an inner ear infection that usually follows an upper respiratory infection, ear infection, or ear surgery. The effects can destroy the labyrinth and cochlea, causing permanent deafness. Increased risks for labyrinthitis include drinking large amounts of alcohol; fatigue; recent viral illness, respiratory or ear infection; smoking; stress; and using certain prescription or nonprescription medications, particularly aspirin.

Complementary and Alternative Therapies

Caution patients who have inner ear disorders that many herbal products can cause dizziness, nausea, and vomiting. Drowsiness is another side effect of many herbals, which may enhance the sedative effects of drugs used to manage vertigo.

Clinical Manifestations

Signs and symptoms of labyrinthitis include dizziness, vertigo, loss of balance, nausea, vomiting, headache, anorexia, nystagmus (rapid eye movement), and sensorineural hearing loss on the affected side. **Vertigo** is a sensation of movement that causes dizziness and nausea. Patients may say that the room seems to be spinning or that they feel as though they are spinning. A feeling of fullness and pressure in the ear often precedes a vertigo attack. Attacks may last several minutes to several hours. Sudden movement during an attack of vertigo can cause vomiting.

Severe symptoms last about one week; most people are completely better within 2 to 3 months. Older people are more likely to have dizziness that lasts longer. Additional symptoms of suppurative labyrinthitis are tinnitus and hearing loss. Symptoms can start suddenly and usually ease after a few days. Balance typically returns in two to six weeks or longer. In very rare cases, hearing loss is permanent.

Medical Treatment

Labyrinthitis is treated with antiemetics such as prochlorperazine; antihistamines; medications to relieve dizziness such as meclizine or scopolamine; sedatives such as diazepam (Valium); corticosteroids, and antiviral medications until it resolves.

❖ NURSING CARE OF THE PATIENT WITH LABYRINTHITIS

Focused Assessment

During an acute episode of labyrinthitis, describe the patient's symptoms. Monitor intake and output, daily weights if possible, and food intake if persistent vomiting occurs.

Patient Problems, Goals, and Outcome Criteria: Labyrinthitis

Patient Problems	Goals and Outcome Criteria
Potential for injury related to vertigo	Safety: absence of injury or falls
Inadequate nutrition related to anorexia and nausea	Adequate nutrition: stable body weight
Potential for fluid volume deficit related to vomiting	Adequate hydration: equal fluid intake and output, moist mucous membranes, vital signs consistent with patient norms
Anxiety related to acute illness	Reduced anxiety: patient states anxiety is reduced, calm manner

Interventions

Safety is a major concern for the patient with vertigo. Assist and supervise the patient when they are out of bed. Give antiemetics as prescribed for nausea and vomiting. If vomiting persists, the patient is at risk for development of fluid and electrolyte imbalances (i.e., hypokalemia, dehydration) and intravenous fluids may be needed. The patient needs reassurance that the condition resolves in time.

MÉNIÈRE DISEASE

Ménière disease (endolymphatic hydrops) is a disorder of the labyrinth. The onset usually occurs in people between 40 and 60 years of age. The cause is unknown, but the symptoms are related to an accumulation of fluid in the inner ear. Some things that have been found to trigger attacks include alcohol, nicotine, stress, and certain stimuli such as bright lights and sudden movements of the head.

Clinical Manifestations

The seriousness of symptoms of Ménière disease varies among patients. Acute attacks occur at intervals and last for hours to days, and the frequency of attacks can be reduced with medical treatment. During an acute attack, the classic symptoms are hearing loss, vertigo, and a feeling of fullness in the ear (*aural fullness*), accompanied by pallor, sweating, nausea, and vomiting. The hearing loss is unilateral, meaning that only one ear is affected. Tinnitus may accompany acute attacks and is heard as a high pitched buzzing sound that sometimes becomes a roar. Hearing usually improves between attacks, but some loss of low-frequency sounds may remain. Patients who have had many attacks may eventually have permanent sensorineural hearing loss.

Medical Diagnosis

Diagnosis of Ménière disease is based on the history and physical findings. The patient describes hearing and balance disturbances as noted earlier. An audiogram often reveals a loss of the ability to hear low-frequency sounds. If the caloric test or electronystagmography is performed, the patient with Ménière disease has a severe attack of vertigo. A glycerol test involves audiometry testing before and after giving the patient oral glycerol (a diuretic that draws fluid from the inner ear). Improved hearing after glycerol is given suggests Ménière disease.

Ménière disease is diagnosed by ruling out other conditions that can cause similar symptoms. Therefore, the health care provider may order a number of radiographs and other tests to detect any neurologic, allergic, or endocrine disorders.

Medical Treatment

Ménière disease may be treated medically or surgically (see the Complementary and Alternative Therapies box). Drugs prescribed during an acute attack include atropine, epinephrine, benzodiazepines such as diazepam (Valium), antihistamines, antiemetics, anticholinergics, vasodilators, and diuretics. To lessen the severity of an attack of vertigo, motion sickness medications such as meclizine or diazepam (Valium) may reduce the spinning sensation and help control nausea and vomiting. In addition, antinausea medications such as promethazine may control nausea and vomiting during an episode of vertigo. Gentamicin and steroids, injected into the middle ear and absorbed into the inner ear, also are drugs used to improve vertigo symptoms. Drugs that may be prescribed between attacks to reduce their frequency and severity are diuretics and drugs that help to control vertigo. Meclizine and transdermal scopolamine are less sedating than many other agents and may allow the patient to maintain a more normal life.

Complementary and Alternative Therapies

Biofeedback, self-hypnosis, and relaxation techniques may be recommended to help the patient learn to live with Ménière disease.

A low-sodium diet and diuretics seem to increase the length of time between attacks by reducing edema in the inner ear. If moderate sodium restriction is not effective, the patient may be put on a strict sodium-free diet (see the Nutritional Considerations box). Caffeine, nicotine, and alcohol are discouraged. Vestibular rehabilitation is a series of exercises performed to help the patient develop a tolerance for vertigo. It begins with moving the eyes and head up and down and side to side and progresses to more vigorous activity. The physical therapist usually teaches vestibular rehabilitation. Most patients respond positively to conservative medical treatment. Positive pressure therapy employs a device called a Meniett pulse generator to reduce fluid buildup in the middle ear. The device fits into the external ear and delivers pressure to the middle ear intermittently. Patients use it at home 3 times a day for 5 minutes each time. Positive pressure therapy has shown improvement in symptoms of vertigo, tinnitus, and aural pressure in some patients.

Nutrition Considerations

A low-salt diet is sometimes prescribed for people with Ménière disease. Caffeine, alcohol, chocolate, and nicotine may aggravate or trigger an attack.

See the Patient Teaching box for managing vertigo.

Patient Teaching

Dos and Don'ts for Managing Vertigo

DO

- Stay still and rest
- Lie in a dark room if you feel very dizzy
- Avoid noise and bright lights during attacks
- Avoid sudden movements or position changes
- Get enough sleep—tiredness can make symptoms worse
- Rest during severe episodes. Slowly resume activity. You may need help walking when you lose your balance during attacks
- Drink plenty of water. If you're sick, it's best to drink little and often
- Start to go for walks outside as soon as possible—it may help to have someone with you to steady you until you become confident
- When you're out and about, keep your eyes focused on a fixed object, rather than looking around all the time
- Ask your health care provider about balance therapy. This may help once nausea and vomiting have passed

DON'T

For 1 week after symptoms disappear:

- Drive, cycle or use tools or machinery if you feel dizzy
- Operate heavy machinery
- Climb
- Drink alcohol—it can make symptoms worse

Surgical Treatment

Surgery is advised only when all other measures have failed. Surgical procedures drain excess fluid from the inner ear (endolymphatic shunt) or cut the part of the acoustic nerve that controls balance (vestibular nerve section). The incision may be inside or behind the ear. In general, these surgical procedures pose some risk for permanent hearing loss. A more destructive surgical procedure is a labyrinthectomy, which is a surgical excision of the labyrinth. This procedure is reserved for conditions that have not responded to other measures. It is only performed if the affected ear already has profound hearing loss.

Potential complications of surgery for Ménière disease include infection, hearing loss, loss of cerebrospinal fluid (CSF), and damage to the seventh cranial nerve. The leakage of CSF may occur with procedures that require opening the skull. The seventh cranial nerve is the facial nerve that is located very close to the ear canal. It controls the movement of certain muscles of the face. Surgical procedures in and around the ear can result in trauma to the facial nerve.

NURSING CARE OF THE PATIENT WITH MÉNIÈRE DISEASE

Focused Assessment

The pattern of acute attacks should be documented (see Nursing Care Plan: Patient With Ménière Disease). Note substances or stimuli that trigger the episodes. Document specific symptoms, including nausea, vomiting, vertigo, and tinnitus. Determine how the condition affects the patient's life, what the patient knows about the disease, and what coping mechanisms are used.

Patient Problems, Goals, and Outcome Criteria: Ménière Disease

Patient Problems	Goals and Outcome Criteria
Potential for injury related to vertigo	Safety: absence of falls and injuries
Potential for fluid volume deficit related to vomiting	Normal hydration: equal fluid intake and output, normal vital signs, moist mucous membranes
Anxiety related to acute illness or disruption of usual lifestyle	Reduced anxiety: patient states anxiety is reduced, calm manner
Inability to manage self-care related to lack of knowledge about management of Ménière disease	Effective self-management: appropriate self-care, patient correctly describes and demonstrates self-care measures

Interventions

Potential for injury. Safety is a major concern. Attacks come on suddenly and can be dangerous in many

Nursing Care Plan — Patient With Ménière Disease

FOCUSED ASSESSMENT

Health History

A 62-year-old man has had repeated episodes of nausea, hearing loss, and vertigo over the past year. His attacks last 2 to 3 hours, during which he is completely incapacitated. His wife brought him to the emergency department after he vomited repeatedly and seemed very weak. His health history reveals repeated urinary tract infections but no other serious illness or injuries. He is an accountant who owns his own business.

Physical Examination

Vital signs: blood pressure 136/82 mm Hg, pulse 88 beats per minute, respiration 16 breaths per minute, temperature 98°F (36.7°C) measured orally. Height 5′4″, weight 200 lb. Patient appears acutely ill and unable to sit or stand. Physical findings are normal except for mild hearing loss. The health care provider's diagnosis is probable Ménière disease.

Patient Problems	Goals and Outcome Criteria	Interventions
Potential for injury related to vertigo	A safe environment is provided: The patient will have no injuries during acute episodes.	Assist the patient to bed and allow him to remain still. Raise the side rails and put the bed in low position. Place the call bell within reach and caution him to refrain from getting up unassisted. Darken the room and keep it quiet. Postpone nonessential care. Provide a urinal for voiding. When the attack subsides, assist the patient out of bed until he is no longer dizzy.
Potential for fluid volume deficit related to vomiting	The patient is adequately hydrated, as evidenced by vital signs consistent with patient's norms, moist mucous membranes, and fluid intake equal to output.	Give antiemetics and antihistamines as ordered. Provide an emesis receptacle. If the patient vomits, promptly empty, clean, and return the emesis receptacle or provide a new one. Administer intravenous fluids as ordered.
Anxiety related to acute illness, disruption of usual lifestyle	The patient states that anxiety is reduced and will appear more relaxed.	Be available but let patient lie quietly. When the patient is able to talk, explore how the condition affects his life and how he can deal with it. Tell him that the condition usually can be improved with treatment.
Inability to manage treatment program related to lack of knowledge of condition and treatment	The patient describes measures to manage acute attacks and to reduce frequency of attacks.	Explain drugs to patient, including dosage, schedule, side effects, and information that should be reported to the health care provider. If sodium restriction is prescribed, explain that some patients benefit from the restriction. Request dietary consult if special diet is ordered.

CRITICAL THINKING QUESTIONS

1. Why is it important to let the patient lie still and remain undisturbed as much as possible?
2. Why do some patients with Ménière disease benefit from sodium restriction?

circumstances. Fortunately, many people can recognize an aura, or peculiar feeling, that precedes an attack. They should know to seek safety promptly when an aura occurs. If driving, the patient should pull over and stop the car as soon as possible.

Potential for fluid volume deficit. During an acute attack while in the hospital, have the patient remain still because movement may trigger vomiting. Keep the room dark and quiet. Postpone nonessential care such as bathing. Promptly give medications for nausea and vomiting and keep an emesis receptacle close to the patient. An intravenous infusion usually is ordered to provide fluids, medications, or both. After the symptoms subside, assist the patient when getting up until dizziness goes away.

Anxiety. Patients with Ménière disease may be anxious about the condition and the limitations it imposes. Encourage the patient to share concerns and help the patient to learn how to manage the condition (see the Patient Teaching box).

Patient Teaching

Ménière Disease

- You need to know about prescribed medications and how to manage their side effects (provide specifics).
- Alcohol, caffeine, and tobacco may make your symptoms worse.

Inability to perform self-care. Interventions involve patient teaching as presented in the Patient Teaching box.

Put On Your Thinking Cap!

Think about a routine day. Consider how a person's life might be affected by frequent attacks of Ménière disease.

Postoperative Nursing Care

If the patient has surgery for Ménière disease, postoperative care depends on the type of procedure. Carefully check the surgeon's orders for position and activity limitations. General nursing care is concerned with safety, comfort, and detection of complications. On the first few days after surgery, the patient's symptoms may be severe. Antiemetics are ordered to control nausea and vomiting. Delay nonessential care until the patient tolerates movement. Assist patients when getting up and walking until they are able to walk steadily. The call bell always should be within reach. Patients can be dizzy for several days and unsteady for several weeks.

Observe for facial nerve damage by having the patient smile and show their teeth. If the facial nerve is damaged, the muscles on the affected side do not respond and the patient's face is not symmetric. Immediately notify the surgeon of any evidence of facial nerve damage. Nerve damage may be reversible if treated promptly.

Put On Your Thinking Cap!

Explain why patients with inner ear disorders may have problems with balance as well as with hearing.

Box 60.1 Ototoxic Drugs

ANTIBIOTICS
Aminoglycosides
amikacin sulfate (Amikin)
gentamicin sulfate (Garamycin)
kanamycin sulfate (Kantrex)
neomycin sulfate
streptomycin sulfate
tobramycin sulfate (Nebcin)
Erythromycins
erythromycin estolate (Ilosone)
erythromycin ethylsuccinate (Pediamycin)
erythromycin stearate (Erythrocin)
erythromycin lactobionate (Erythrocin)

TETRACYCLINE
minocycline (Minocin)

MISCELLANEOUS AGENT
vancomycin

DIURETICS
furosemide (Lasix)
ethacrynic acid (Edecrin)

ANTIDYSRHYTHMIC AGENTS
quinidine

ANTIINFLAMMATORIES/ANALGESICS
aspirin
ibuprofen (Motrin)
indomethacin (Indocin)

ANTINEOPLASTIC AGENTS
bleomycin (Blenoxane)
cisplatin (Platinol, CDDP)
dactinomycin (Cosmegen)
mechlorethamine (nitrogen mustard, Mustargen)

PRESBYCUSIS

Although many older people hear very well, approximately half of those older than 75 years of age have some difficulty hearing. **Presbycusis** is the term used to describe hearing loss associated with aging. It is the result of changes in one or more parts of the cochlea. The extent of the disability depends on the location of the changes in the cochlea.

People with presbycusis may hear well in quiet surroundings but hear poorly in noisy places. They have diminished hearing for high frequency sounds, such as consonants (b, d, c, etc.), birdsong, and higher pitched voices. Some patients deny that they don't hear well and may blame others for mumbling or not speaking clearly.

Medical Diagnosis and Treatment

A thorough hearing evaluation is indicated for the older person whose hearing seems to be declining. Many people have the mistaken idea that hearing loss in older adults is inevitable and not treatable. In fact, many patients with presbycusis benefit from hearing aids. If a hearing aid is recommended, the patient needs to learn how to use and care for it, as described in Chapter 58 in the section titled "Hearing Aids." Hearing aids are helpful but are not the only way to improve communication. The patient must be willing to tell others how they can be understood more easily. The patient also can practice and improve listening skills. A speech-language pathologist (specialist in communication) can teach patients various skills to improve communication in the presence of a hearing loss.

In addition to hearing aids, other electronic devices are available to improve hearing. These are described in Chapter 58 in the section titled "Adaptations to Hearing Loss" and include phone amplifiers and personal earphones for radios and televisions.

NURSING CARE OF THE PATIENT WITH PRESBYCUSIS

Nursing assessment, patient problems, goals, and interventions for the patient with impaired hearing are described in Chapter 58 under "Nursing Care of the Patient with Impaired Hearing." In addition, nurses should educate people about hearing loss and aging. They also can work to overcome the resistance that many people have to admitting hearing loss. Once the problem has been diagnosed, nurses can help the patient to adapt and learn to use supportive devices.

OTOTOXICITY

Ototoxicity is damage to the ear or eighth cranial nerve caused by specific chemicals, including some drugs. Common ototoxic drugs are salicylates (i.e., aspirin) and aminoglycoside antibiotics. These and other ototoxic drugs that pose a threat to hearing are listed in Box 60.1. Ototoxicity can range from reversible tinnitus to permanent hearing loss. Hearing, balance, or both may be affected. Tinnitus is frequently the first sign of ototoxicity, and when the offending drug is discontinued, the condition disappears. Sometimes the effects of ototoxic drugs (hearing and balance problems) are permanent. The extent of impairment depends on the drug dosage and how long it was given. Patients who have poor renal or liver function are at special risk for ototoxicity because drugs are excreted more slowly, increasing the likelihood of toxicity.

NURSING CARE OF THE PATIENT WITH OTOTOXICITY

The primary nursing responsibilities are early detection and prevention of progressive hearing loss caused by ototoxic drugs. To reduce the risk of ototoxicity, be familiar with these drugs. Instruct patients to report hearing loss, tinnitus, or problems with balance. Promptly report such symptoms to the health care provider. In addition, teach patients that aspirin is not a harmless drug. Monitor the urine output of patients on ototoxic drugs because low urine output may mean that the potentially toxic drug is excreted slowly, increasing the risk of toxicity. Report low urine output to the health care provider. The nursing care plan should alert all staff to the potential for ototoxicity.

Disorders that impair hearing or balance can have a profound effect on a person's life and well-being. The nurse plays an important role in the prevention, early detection, and treatment of hearing and balance disturbances.

Get Ready for the NCLEX® Examination!

Key Points

- Cerumen (earwax) can become impacted and lead to obstruction of the external ear canal, resulting in pain and hearing impairment.
- External otitis, infection and inflammation of the external ear canal, is treated with topical antibiotics and corticosteroids.
- Otitis media, infection of the middle ear, can generate permanent hearing loss and inner ear problems.
- Otosclerosis is a condition in which the stapes becomes fixed, producing a conductive and sometimes sensorineural hearing loss.
- Labyrinthitis, which is inflammation of the labyrinth, induces vertigo and nausea and may be treated with antiemetics and antibiotics.
- Ménière disease, characterized by attacks of hearing loss and vertigo, may be treated with drug therapy, low-sodium diet, surgical intervention, or a combination of these.
- Nursing care of the patient with Ménière disease may address potential for injury, potential for fluid volume deficit, anxiety, and inability to manage treatment program.
- Presbycusis is hearing loss associated with aging that may be improved with a hearing aid.
- Ototoxicity is damage to the eighth cranial nerve producing effects that may range from tinnitus to permanent hearing loss.

Additional Learning Resources

SG Go to your Study Guide for additional learning activities to help you master this chapter content.

Go to your Evolve website (http://evolve.elsevier.com/Linton/medsurg) for the following learning resources and much more:

- Fluid & Electrolyte Tutorial
- Review Questions for the NCLEX® Examination

Clinical Judgment and Next-Generation NCLEX® Examination-Style Questions

1. You are preparing to administer otic drops when you notice that the patient has gauze in the affected ear with a piece of narrow gauze extending from the ear. What should you do?

1. Gently remove the packing, instill the drops, and replace the packing.
2. Apply the drops to the narrow piece of gauze for transport into the ear.
3. Trim the gauze so that the packing is not accidentally pulled out of the ear.
4. Inform the registered nurse (RN) that the drops cannot be given at this time.

NCLEX Client Need: Health Promotion and Maintenance

2. Which nursing measures are appropriate for the patient who is having an acute attack of Ménière disease? (Select all that apply.)

1. Keep the room quiet and dark
2. Advise the patient to drink additional fluids
3. Delay routine care until the patient is no longer dizzy
4. Monitor vitals every hour until stable and then every 4 hours
5. Assist the patient to sit up in the bedside chair for 1 hour twice a day

NCLEX Client Need: Physiological Integrity: Reduction of Risk Potential

3. When a patient is taking an aminoglycoside antibiotic, instructions should include which of the following?

1. "Let me know if you have any 'ringing' in your ears."
2. "Check the white part of your eyes for a color change."
3. "Restrict your fluid intake to 1 L each day."
4. "Change position slowly in case your blood pressure (BP) drops."

NCLEX Client Need: Physiological Integrity: Reduction of Risk Potential

4. Stapedectomy is used to correct which of the following?

1. Sensorineural hearing loss
2. Ménière disease
3. Otosclerosis
4. Otitis media

NCLEX Client Need: Physiological Integrity: Pharmacological Therapies

5. **Patients who are considering having a cochlear implant should be told which of the following?**
   1. "This procedure restores perfect hearing in 99% of patients."
   2. "Complications of cochlear implant are often disabling."
   3. "Results vary from minimal to excellent improvement in hearing."
   4. "Cochlear implants cannot enable you to discriminate speech."

   NCLEX Client Need: Physiological Integrity: Reduction of Risk Potential

6. **SLO/Objective: Determine appropriate nursing actions for patients experiencing Meniere disease.**

   NGN item Type: Extended Drag and Drop

   Cognitive Skill: Take Action

   (Take Action Using Matrix Test Item)

   A 78-year-old woman, with a history of hypertension, osteoarthritis, bilateral knee replacements, back pain, and Ménière disease, resides in a long-term care facility. Recently she has been diagnosed with an acute attack of Ménière disease in her left ear. She complains of hearing loss and tinnitus in her left ear and shows signs of vertigo, nausea, and vomiting. The nurse assesses the patient and plans health teaching for the patient so that she can return to her normal way of living.

   Use an X for the health teaching below that is *Indicated* (appropriate or necessary), *Contraindicated* (could be harmful), or *Nonessential* (makes no difference or not necessary) before the patient's discharge at this time.

HEALTH TEACHING	INDICATED	CONTRAINDICATED	NONESSENTIAL
"You can keep the TV on to distract you from your symptoms."			
"Lie still in bed while the symptoms last."			
"Take a stool softener to avoid straining on defecation."			
"Eat a high protein diet."			
"We will give you medications to ease your symptoms."			
"Do not get out of bed without help from your nurse."			
"Keep the emesis receptacle handy and report if you have vomited."			

61 Psychobiologic Disorders

http://evolve.elsevier.com/Linton/medsurg

Objectives

1. Describe the differences between social relationships and therapeutic relationships.
2. Describe key strategies in communicating therapeutically.
3. Describe the components of the mental status examination.
4. Identify target symptoms, behaviors, and potential side effects for the following types of medications: antianxiety (anxiolytic), antipsychotic, and antidepressant drugs.
5. Summarize current thinking about the causes of schizophrenia and major depressive and bipolar disorders.
6. Identify key features of the mental status examination and their relevance in anxiety disorders, obsessive-compulsive and related disorders, schizophrenia, major depressive and bipolar disorders, cognitive disorders, and personality disorders.
7. Identify common patient problems, goals, and interventions for persons with anxiety disorders, obsessive-compulsive and related disorders, schizophrenia and schizoaffective disorders, major depressive and bipolar disorders, cognitive disorders, and personality disorders.

Key Terms

biologic approach (bī-ō-LŎ-jĭk)
cognitive-behavioral approach
denial (dē-NĪ-ăl)
depersonalization (dē-PĔR-sŭn-ŭl-ĭ-ZĀ-shŭn)
extrapyramidal side effects (EPS) (ĕks-tră-pĭ-RĂM-ĭ-dăl)
interpersonal approach
milieu therapy
parkinsonian syndrome
projection
psychosis (sī-KŌ-sĭs)
repression
schizoaffective disorder
schizophrenia (skĭ-zō-FRĔN-ē-ŭh)
sensorium (sĕn-SŌ-rē-ŭm)
tardive dyskinesia (TĂR-dĭv dĭs-kĭ-NĒ-zē-ă)

The goal of this chapter is to introduce the reader to essential aspects of nursing care when working with individuals who have a comorbid psychiatric illness in addition to their medical and/or surgical problems.

How individuals, families, and populations think about and explain mental health and mental illness varies from one geographic location to another, and from culture to culture, as well as from one period of time to another. It is now understood that many factors contribute to the development of a mental illness and many strategies are available for helping people with psychiatric disorders.

Traditional treatment settings that focused on providing care for people with psychiatric disorders include outpatient, intensive outpatient, partial hospitalization, and inpatient hospitalization as well as treatment in residential settings. Within these settings, treatment methods include milieu therapy, individual psychotherapy, group or family psychotherapy, educational groups, and treatment with medications. New and safer medications allow treatment primarily on an outpatient basis. Nursing interventions are diverse and geared toward helping patients and families to cope with the mental illness, manage their lives, and enhance quality of life. Mental illness and mental health exist along a continuum. Some people who are experiencing a psychiatric disorder may experience acute symptoms and require hospitalization. Others may have chronic and persistent mental illness. Therefore, nursing interventions are delivered in many settings including the hospital and the community.

Nurses who work with patients in other health care settings such as medical clinics, medical and surgical inpatient units, or intensive care units also see patients who have psychiatric difficulties along with their other health problems. The ability to provide a high quality of nursing care to patients with mental illness in any work setting is important.

Nursing interventions are based on several theoretical approaches, which are described according to biological, psychodynamic, interpersonal, cognitive-behavioral, and other theories. **Milieu therapy** or **therapeutic community** is defined as "a scientific structuring of the environment to effect behavioral changes and to improve the psychological health and functioning of the individual" (American Nurses Association Standards of Psychiatric Mental Health Nursing Practice, mccc.edu). In this setting, patients learn adaptive coping, interaction, and relationship skills that can be generalized to other aspects of their lives. Examples of therapeutic community settings include alcohol and drug rehabilitation facilities, weight loss groups, and behavioral disorder treatment clinics. Patients feel safe and trust that they are able to try out new coping skills without feeling self-conscious.

The **biologic approach** assumes that mental disorders are related to physiologic changes within the central nervous system (CNS). With this perspective, mental illness is managed with medications, much as any other acute or chronic illness—such as diabetes—is managed. The biologic approach dominates much of the current thinking about psychiatric disorders, but it is only one aspect of treatment.

The **psychodynamic approach** is based on the theory that (1) humans function at different levels of awareness, ranging from conscious to unconscious, and (2) people use ego defense mechanisms such as **repression**, **denial**, and **projection** to prevent or minimize anxiety.

The **interpersonal approach** has three components: (1) anxiety is often communicated interpersonally, (2) the patient learns new ways of coping or maturing in a therapeutic relationship, and (3) the establishment of trust is an important first step in working with patients. The interpersonal approach is of particular concern to nurses because, as Hildegard Peplau (often considered the mother of psychiatric nursing) stated in her seminal work, "Nursing is a significant, therapeutic, interpersonal process." Dr. Peplau (1992) pointed out that "The central feature of nursing practice is the nurse–patient relationship."

Key ideas from the **cognitive-behavioral approach** are that (1) behavior is learned, (2) behavior increases because of a response to that behavior from the environment (i.e., reinforcement), and (3) the way a person thinks about things (their thoughts) influences emotional states and behavior.

Put On Your Thinking Cap!

Four patients are receiving different treatments for mental illness. An aspect of each type of treatment is listed. Can you identify the theoretic approach behind each treatment?

- A patient is helped to develop new coping skills through a therapeutic relationship.
- A patient is guided to recall events that could be related to her present illness.
- A patient is helped to understand the consequences of his behavioral patterns.
- A patient is prescribed an antianxiety (anxiolytic) drug.

ESTABLISHING THERAPEUTIC RELATIONSHIPS

In caring for a patient with a psychiatric disorder, you must first establish a therapeutic (rather than a social) relationship (Table 61.1). A range of interpersonal strategies has been found to be particularly helpful in promoting the patient's level of comfort with the nurse. They include being available, listening, clarifying, sharing observations, and accepting silence. Therapeutic use of self is key to providing good care to patients with psychiatric illness, avoiding advice giving, and assisting patients at their level of comprehension.

BEING AVAILABLE

When you are working with a patient, direct all your attention completely toward that person. Avoid involvement in any other activity that might be interpreted by the patient as lack of availability, such as focusing on entering information in their chart or computer while they are talking with you. Avoid interruptions in your conversation with the patient as much as possible.

LISTENING

Use empathy when you are listening to the patient. Concentrate on what the patient is saying and remember that you are trying to hear how they experience and describe their life. When listening therapeutically, make every effort to avoid cutting the patient off or

Table 61.1 Therapeutic Relationships Versus Social Relationships

THERAPEUTIC	SOCIAL
Purpose is to benefit the patient.	Purpose is to benefit both participants in the relationship.
Relationship develops purposefully.	Relationship develops spontaneously.
Focus is on personal and emotional needs of patient.	Focus is on personal and emotional needs of both participants.
Helper has responsibility for evaluating the interaction and the changing behavior.	Participants are not formally responsible for evaluating their interaction.
Relationship has some boundaries (i.e., purpose, place, time) and a clear ending.	Relationship may or may not have clear boundaries and a clear ending.

jumping to conclusions. You are trying to get the essence of how the patient perceives their situation, experiences certain symptoms, and describes their circumstances.

To listen well, you must be aware of your own thoughts and feelings. These feelings are an important source of data for you because you may experience a wide range of feelings while interacting with patients. If you are aware of your own feelings, you will be able to manage your physical (body language) and verbal responses. Listening is done by concentrating on the patient and by refraining from thinking of responses while the patient is speaking.

CLARIFYING

Clarifying is one way of validating that you understand what the patient is saying. For example, you might ask, "So what you are saying is that you are feeling very sad right now?" Asking questions may also help patients to clarify their thoughts. For example, if a patient says, "I have problems at home," you might ask, "What is happening at home that is troubling you?" If a patient states, "My world is falling apart," you might say, "Tell me more about what you mean when you say, 'My world is falling apart.'" It is helpful to avoid the word *why* when asking questions. For example, instead of asking, "Why do you feel that way?" try asking "How did you come to feel that way?"

SHARING OBSERVATIONS

Patients benefit from knowing what you see and hear while listening. For example, you might say, "You are saying that your life is falling apart, and I notice that you are fidgeting and tapping your foot. It looks like this is really difficult for you." This statement provides the patient with input that they are heard and that you are really listening.

ACCEPTING SILENCE

Sometimes it is therapeutic to allow moments of silence between you and the patient. This is called *therapeutic silence.* It is important that you feel comfortable with silence because silence enables patients to consider their own thoughts as well as what you are communicating to them. Although they may feel strange at first, silences allow patients to sort through their feelings and organize their thinking.

◆ NURSING ASSESSMENT OF THE PSYCHIATRIC PATIENT

Health History

The nursing assessment of the patient with mental illness provides the foundation for patient problems and development of the plan of care. The observations of the licensed vocational nurse/licensed practical nurse (LVN/LPN) contribute important data to the assessment. In addition to the usual data for the physical assessment, you will want to understand what brings the patient to the care setting where you are practicing. Ask the patient to tell you what has been happening recently that has caused them to seek treatment, to describe the symptoms and acuity, onset, duration, and length of time each symptom has been present. Inquire about the person's past psychiatric history by asking they have ever felt like this before or have been treated in the past for anxiety, depression, or other mental health problems. Included in the past psychiatric history are past hospitalizations and outpatient treatment as well as any past medications used and the patient's response to them.

List all medications the patient has been taking, including both medications taken to treat psychiatric problems and all other medications and over-the-counter (OTC) medications, herbal remedies, and vitamin supplements. A family and social history is collected to document family history of mental illness, substance abuse, current family configuration, employment or school activities, and resources available to the patient. Collecting information on current and recent use of tobacco, alcohol, prescription drugs, cannabinoids, and other psychoactive substances is also essential to determine if the patient is at risk for substance related problems such as withdrawal (see the Complementary and Alternative Therapies box). This also provides information on how the patient may attempt to cope with stressors.

> **Complementary and Alternative Therapies**
>
> Be aware of any herbal supplements the patient is taking. Some can interact with drugs used for mental illness.

Mental Status Examination

Another major feature of a complete health assessment of the patient with psychiatric problems is the mental status examination. This examination is usually conducted as part of the admission process and is an ongoing assessment tool throughout the course of treatment. The mental status examination is based on observations made by the nurse and patient responses to questions used to evaluate several domains of mental functioning including psychomotor activity, speech, behavior, mood, emotional expressions (affect), sensorium, cognitive processing, and perceptions and thinking. The mental status examination is an organized assessment providing additional data to round out the assessment (Table 61.2).

Appearance/activity. The first step in a mental status examination is to observe how a person looks. Specific data include the following:

- Appearance in relation to stated age (Does the patient look their stated age?)
- Appropriateness of clothing in relation to the patient's particular peer group or subculture, temperature in the room, or the weather

Table 61.2 Components of the Mental Status Examination

COMPONENT	RELEVANT DATA
Appearance	Age, clothing, personal hygiene, unusual physical characteristics
Activity	Recent change in activity level, hyperactivity, agitation, psychomotor retardation, repetitive mannerisms, stereotypes
Mood and affect	Happiness, sadness, worry; constricted or expanded feelings; intensity; lability; appropriateness
Speech and language	Mutism, paucity, pressured speech, tangential speech, blocking, loose associations, word salad
Thought content	Obsessions, compulsions, phobias, delusions
Perceptual disturbances	Illusions, hallucinations
Insight and judgment	Potential for suicide
Sensorium	Orientation to time, place, person; level of consciousness
Memory and attention	Remote and recent memory, attention, calculation
General intellectual level	Vocabulary, knowledge of current events, abstract thinking

- Personal grooming and hygiene
- Unusual physical characteristics (tattoos, etc.)
- Motor activity

Note any recent change in the patient's activity level (increased or decreased). Other types of activity that are observed include the following:

- Hyperactivity or activity at a level considerably above average purposeful activity
- Agitation or purposeless activity, such as wringing of hands, pacing, picking a clothing, foot tapping
- Psychomotor retardation or a decrease in movement; slowness; delayed actions, thoughts, and speech
- Repetitive movements that are part of a purposeful activity (mannerisms)
- Repetitive movements that are not part of purposeful activity (stereotypy)

Also note the patient's cooperativeness with you as the examiner. Describe the patient's behavior toward you. Was your patient friendly and engaging with you, or did they seem indifferent and reluctant to answer questions?

Speech and language. Assessment includes characteristics of speech and language. Normally, speech is of appropriate rate, rhythm, and volume. Unusual findings in the assessment of speech include mutism (i.e., not speaking), long pauses before responding, minimal or very little speech (i.e., paucity), and pressured speech (i.e., loud, and insistent, rapid).

Mood and affect. *Mood* is a sustained feeling state or emotion that a person experiences in several aspects of life. Mood is assessed in terms of its intensity, depth, duration, and fluctuation. Words that may be used to describe mood include irritable, anxious, depressed, euphoric, labile (up-and-down), and despairing. In the assessment, in addition to observing the patient's mood, the nurse asks the patient to describe how they feel.

Affect describes a person's external presentation of a feeling state or emotional responsiveness—your impression of their emotional state. Affect ranges from blunted, flat, and constricted to euphoric, expansive, and intense. A normal affect exists when the person's body language, mannerisms, and verbal responses are consistent with the person's mood and within an average range of emotional intensity. Affect is also described according to its appropriateness and congruence. Appropriate affect exists when the person's outward emotional expression matches what they are saying or doing. For example, a patient who is discussing sadness and despair might be tearful and look sad. An example of an inappropriate affect is when someone tells you that they are sad and feeling guilty about something that happened but at the same time smiling, laughing, and very animated. In the latter example, the affect is considered incongruent with mood. The intensity of feelings may be increased or decreased (diminished). Feelings also may be stable or consistent rather than labile or rapidly changing.

Consciousness and cognition. **Sensorium** focuses intellectual and cognitive functions—the patient's ability to take in, process, and communicate information.

Orientation. Assess orientation in terms of time, date, place, person, and self as well as the situation or circumstance in which the patients find themselves. These data are obtained by asking the patient direct questions (e.g., "What time is it now?" "What day is today?" "Where are we now?" "Can you tell me your name?"). The patient's level of consciousness also is noted. The four levels of consciousness are (1) comatose, (2) stuporous, (3) drowsy (somnolent, lethargic), and (4) alert. Also note if the patient is confused and/or disoriented.

Memory. Assess remote memory (i.e., memory of the distant past) by comparing the patient's memory of personal and past events with what is recalled by other reliable historians including family or friends. If you are collecting data related to memory or the ability to recall new information, ask the patient to learn three unrelated words and to recall these words 5 minutes later. A quick way to determine recent memory is to ask what was eaten at the previous meal.

General intellectual functioning. General intellectual functioning is estimated by determining the patient's vocabulary and knowledge of current events. For example, ask the patient to name the current president of the United States and the name of the previous president. Asking the patient to subtract 7s from 100 or 3s from 20 or to spell a word like "world" backward challenges the patient's attention as well as their ability to calculate (an aspect of general intellectual level). Abstract thinking is another area of general intellectual level (concrete versus formal operational thought). Data that provide evidence of the abstract reasoning can be collected by asking the patient to identify common elements of two objects such as a banana and an apple (e.g., "What do a banana and apple have in common?") or asking the patient to interpret a proverb (e.g., "What does the phrase 'a rolling stone gathers no moss' mean?"). A word of caution about asking a patient to interpret a proverb; consider the patient's language and cultural background and if they are familiar with the proverb. People from cultures different from that of the nurse or whose first language is not English may not be familiar with common proverbs and may not be able to interpret them, which does not necessarily reflect a deficit in abstract reasoning.

Perceptual disturbances. Perceptual disturbances may involve any one of the senses such as vision, hearing, taste, touch, and smell. One type of perceptual disturbance is an illusion, in which a specific stimulus, such as a spot on the wall, is misinterpreted (e.g., a spot is perceived as a bug). Another perceptual disturbance is a hallucination, which is a sensory experience that occurs without an external stimulus (e.g., a person sees nonexistent bugs crawling on the floor [visual hallucination], hears voices when no one is around [auditory hallucination], or feels nonexistent bugs crawling on the skin [tactile hallucination]). Sometimes this is referred to as *internal stimuli*. Evidence of this may include a person sitting alone but talking as if someone were present, or looking around as if someone were talking to them.

Thought process. The evaluation of a person's thinking includes two parts: the thought process and the thought content. An individual's thought process refers to the individual's ability to think clearly, logically, and in a goal-directed fashion that is coherent. A normal thought process is then described as logical, linear, goal-directed, and coherent. Abnormal or unusual findings related to thought process include tangential, circumstantial, impoverished, or illogical thought processes. Additional abnormal findings relative to thought process include thought blocking, such as when a person stops speaking before reaching the point. Loose associations include continual shifting from one topic to another and shifting between topics to the point of incoherence, which also is described as *word salad*.

Thought content. Thought content refers to thoughts that patients describe throughout the interview related to descriptions of symptoms or circumstances of their illness as well as the presence of self-injurious thoughts, suicidal ideations, or homicidal thoughts. Thought content also refers to any delusions (false beliefs) that the patient may have (e.g., "I know the FBI is following me and my house is bugged"). The presence or absence of obsessions, compulsions, phobias, and perseverations are also noted in the description of thought content.

This area must be assessed with clear and direct questions such as "Do you have any thoughts of harming yourself or killing yourself?" Further assessment includes determining whether the patient has constructed any plans to hurt themselves. If the patient endorses suicidal thoughts, you must ask whether the patient has made any plans to commit suicide. If yes, ask them to describe the plans. This information is useful in assessing the lethality of the plans. Another part of the assessment includes determining whether the patient has any means available to carry out a suicide plan. For example, if the patient has planned to shoot themselves, is a gun available at home? If the patient has thoughts of overdosing on medication, does the patient have available supplies of medications at home?

Insight and judgment. Insight is the ability of the person to understand the correct cause or meaning of the situation, and judgment is the ability to assess the situation accurately and determine the appropriate course of action. Insight and judgment are often considered in relation to suicide potential. One way of assessing insight is to consider if the patient has a basic understanding of their situation, such as their illness and what the appropriate course of treatment or action should be. Regarding judgment, some people ask a social judgment question such as "If you were walking down the street and you found an envelope lying on the ground which was stamped and had an address on the front, what would you do?" An example of good judgment would be that the patient would drop the envelope in a nearby mailbox. Another way of evaluating judgment is if patients express a desire to recover from their illness and engage in treatment to achieve that outcome.

Suicide risk assessment. As described in evaluating the thought content, you can assess suicide risk by asking the patient if they have had or are currently having any thoughts or ideas about suicide (suicidal ideation). Ask the patient if they have ever attempted suicide (past suicide attempts). Asking the patient if they have ever had or currently have any ideas about how to commit suicide provides information about suicide plans (plans). Finally, ask the patient if they have ever had or currently have any intention to carry out a plan to commit suicide (intention). The three main elements of suicide risk assessment in the mental status examination are (1) suicidal ideations (thoughts), (2) suicide plans (plans or means of committing suicide), and (3) intent to follow through with a suicide plan (intention). The patient who is considered suicidal may not be left alone for any reason, and a sitter is placed with the patient continuously.

TYPES OF PSYCHIATRIC DISORDERS

Psychiatric disorders are classified in the *Diagnostic and Statistical Manual of Mental Disorders* published by the American Psychiatric Association. This publication is updated periodically and is authored in part by a task force of various workgroups consisting of more than 1000 experts in different fields of psychiatric and mental health science. The DSM-5 is the current edition and is organized by major categories (e.g., Depressive and Related Disorders) and by subcategories of diagnoses.

ANXIETY DISORDERS

Generalized Anxiety Disorder

Individuals with generalized anxiety disorder (GAD) have a difficult time controlling their worry and anxiety. To meet the diagnostic criteria for these diagnoses, the individual must have had anxiety occurring more days than not for at least 6 months with worries and anxieties about multiple situations and events. The intensity, frequency, and duration of their worry is out of proportion to the things they worry about. Their thoughts and worries interfere with their ability to function in their day-to-day activities. These individuals worry about everyday routine life situations such as work responsibilities, health, finances, family members, and minor matters. What distinguishes GAD from day-to-day anxiety that is not pathologic is that the worries are excessive and typically interfere significantly with the individual's ability to function in their world, and these individuals perceive their concerns as difficult to manage. Their worries are more pervasive, pronounced, and distressing and are often accompanied by physical symptoms such as feeling restless and tense. These individuals are distressed by their worry and have difficulty functioning. Although generalized anxiety disorder (GAD) can occur in childhood and adolescence, it is estimated that at some time in their lives approximately 5.7% of adults will experience this type of anxiety (Generalized Anxiety Disorders, National Institutes of Mental Health, 2020. nimh.NIH.gov). The prevalence peaks in middle age and declines across the later years of life (Kessler et al., 2012; Gum et al., 2009).

Treatment of GAD includes individual psychotherapy such as cognitive behavioral therapy (CBT) and pharmacotherapy with first-line agents including the selective serotonin reuptake inhibitors (SSRIs). Judicious use of a benzodiazepine may be helpful at the beginning of treatment until the SSRI becomes effective; however, long-term use of benzodiazepines should be avoided because of the potential for addiction.

Panic Disorder

In panic disorder, the person experiences recurrent panic attacks, which are episodes of intense fear or discomfort that reach a peak within minutes. Panic attacks vary in length but generally do not exceed 10 to 15 minutes, may progress to the point of terror, and are often accompanied by feelings of impending doom. The panic attacks are usually unexpected in which there is no obvious trigger and seem to occur out of the blue regardless of whether the person is in a calm or anxious state. Physical symptoms of severe anxiety include increased pulse, elevated blood pressure, trembling, diaphoresis, shortness of breath, chest pain, nausea, dizziness, and paresthesia (numbness or tingling sensations). Psychologic symptoms include feelings of unreality or feeling of being detached from oneself and fear of dying, or fear of losing control or "going crazy." Those with panic disorder also experience persistent concern or worry about having additional panic attacks or their consequences, and they often develop significant maladaptive changes in behavior related to these attacks designed to avoid having future attacks.

Treatment of panic disorder includes individual psychotherapy such as cognitive behavioral therapy (CBT) and pharmacotherapy with first-line agents including the SSRIs. Initially short-term use of a benzodiazepine may be helpful, but it should be noted that panic attacks are self-limiting in their duration, and by the time an oral medication is absorbed and becomes active, the panic attack has usually subsided. Panic disorder may be present with or without agoraphobia.

Specific Phobia

A phobia is a disorder in which the patient experiences a marked and persistent fear that is excessive, unreasonable, or both. The fear is precipitated by the presence or anticipation of a particular object or situation (e.g., the presence of a spider, as is the case with arachnophobia). The phobia is specific in that it pertains to a specific object or situation (e.g., animals, flying, heights, other people). Any object or situation can precipitate a phobia. The four major categories of specific phobias are: (1) natural environment, (2) animals, (3) mutilation/medical treatment, and (4) situations. (Table 61.3).

Patients with specific phobias typically recognize the fear as disproportionate to the object or situation, but they may have anxiety or panic when encountering or anticipating the object or situation, resulting in significant distress. These patients work hard at avoiding the object or situation that precipitates these symptoms.

Table 61.3 The Four Major Specific Phobias Categories

Natural Environment	Animals
• Astraphobia: Thunderstorms • Hydrophobia: Water • Dendrophobia: Trees	• Batrachophobia: Amphibians • Cynophobia: Dogs • Equinophobia: Horses
Mutilation/Medical Treatment	**Situations**
• Trypanophobia: Needles/ injections • Dentophobia: Dentists • Hemophobia: Blood	• Claustrophobia: Confined spaces • Aerophobia: Flying • Glossophobia: Speaking in public

OBSESSIVE-COMPULSIVE AND RELATED DISORDERS

Formerly considered under the broad category of anxiety disorders, obsessive-compulsive and related disorders are now found in their own category in the DSM-5. Included in this broad category are obsessive-compulsive disorder (OCD), body dysmorphic disorder, hoarding disorder, trichotillomania, excoriation (skin picking) disorder, and related disorders.

Obsessive-Compulsive Disorder

OCD consists of recurrent obsessions (i.e., thoughts), compulsions (i.e., behaviors), or both that produce distress, are time-consuming, and interfere with functioning. Obsessions frequently involve intrusive thoughts about unpleasant or even violent acts that a person cannot stop. For example, a person may be obsessed with the idea of being dirty and needing to wash. Compulsive behaviors typically evolve to reduce the internal sense of distress experienced because of obsessive thoughts. Examples of compulsions are hand washing, counting, and checking (e.g., repeated checking to see whether the door is locked). The person experiencing obsessions and compulsions knows that these thoughts and behaviors are not "normal" and may be embarrassed by them. However, if the compulsion is resisted, the internal sense of distress may become too overwhelming to handle.

Research has found that neurophysiology plays a role in the origin of this disorder. Some studies have shown that changes in electroencephalography findings are seen in people with OCD.

Recently, advanced neuroimaging has also shed some light on these disorders. The current thinking is that the biological basis of these disorders is related to communication with the frontal cortex and deeper areas in the brain (subcortical structures) with dysfunction in the serotonin transport system. Many people with OCD have considerably reduced their symptoms with a tricyclic antidepressant (TCA) or an SSRI. Cognitive-behavioral psychotherapy in combination with medication management is a standard of treatment.

Body Dysmorphic Disorder

Persons with body dysmorphic disorder become preoccupied with one or more perceived flaws in their physical appearance. These individuals believe they look unattractive, abnormal, deformed, or ugly. The flaws they perceive are not generally observable to others or only appear slight to others. Their distorted perceptions can range from believing they are mildly "unattractive" to severe such as believing they look hideous or monster-like. Individuals with body dysmorphic disorder may have good or fair insight that their perceptions are probably not true, or they may have poor insight or even absent insight in that they believe their body is genuinely significantly flawed. These individuals are often drawn to repetitive behaviors or mental acts such as comparing themselves to what they believe is normal. These activities become time-consuming and difficult to resist or control. Individuals with body dysmorphic disorder can become preoccupied with checking their perceived deficits, examining them directly, grooming excessively, and attempting to camouflage their deficits, and it can sometimes lead to compulsive behaviors like skin picking, which can result in skin damage, infections, and even damaged blood vessels. Rates of suicidal ideation and suicide attempts are higher in people with this disorder than in the general population.

Hoarding Disorder

Persons with hoarding disorder demonstrate persistent problems discarding or parting with possessions regardless of their actual value. These individuals cannot part with belongings because of the perceived need for these items in the future or some aesthetic value or strong sentimental attachment to their possessions. They commonly fear losing important information as well. Commonly saved items can include newspapers, magazines, old clothing, and other items, but virtually any item can or should be saved. Persons with hoarding disorder experience distress when facing the prospect of discarding their belongings. Their saving these items is intentional, and their living space can become unmanageable. Although some individuals with hoarding disorder have some degree of insight that they have a problem, others lack insight despite psychosocial consequences. They may be resistant to others such as family members attempting to point out that they have a problem. Hoarding behavior tends to run in families, with about 50% of persons reporting they have a relative who also hoards.

Trichotillomania

Persons with trichotillomania demonstrate the behavior of recurrent pulling out of their hairs, resulting in hair loss. Typically, they have repeated attempts to decrease or stop pulling their hair out. This pulling out of hair causes significant distress and/or impairment in social, occupational, or other important areas of functioning. True trichotillomania is not caused by the result of body dysmorphic disorder. Although the hair pulling may occur in any region of the person's body, the most common sites are the scalp, eyebrows, and eyelids. The hair pulling can be preceded by emotional distress or accompanied by some type of psychosocial stress. Although the hair pulling does not usually occur in the presence of others, it does sometimes occur in the presence of family members. Research demonstrates that there is evidence of a genetic vulnerability to trichotillomania. The disorder is more common in people who have a first-degree relative with obsessive-compulsive disorder.

Excoriation (Skin-Picking) Disorder

Individuals with excoriation disorder demonstrate the behavior of recurrent picking at their own skin. The most common areas where the skin is picked are the face, arms, and hands, although some individuals pick for multiple body sites. Persons with this disorder either pick at healthy skin or at some minor skin irregularities such as pimples, calluses, or scabs. They spend an inordinate amount of time involved in the picking behavior, and the behavior may last for months or even years. The behavior causes significant distress or impairment in the individual's social or occupational functioning and can lead to embarrassment, shame, and infections of the skin. Some persons with skin picking disorder attempt to hide their behavior and, as with trichotillomania, may have a desire to stop picking but find they are unable to do so.

TRAUMA- AND STRESSOR-RELATED DISORDERS

Although formerly under the broad category of anxiety disorders, trauma- and stressor-related disorders are now in a separate category. Within this category, and for the purposes of this chapter, we will examine posttraumatic stress disorder (PTSD) and acute stress disorder.

Posttraumatic Stress Disorder

PTSD is a cluster of symptoms experienced after a distressing event that is outside the range of normal events (e.g., watching one's family being murdered) and in which the person experienced intense fear, helplessness, horror, or a combination of these feelings. Examples of symptoms include reexperiencing the trauma through repeated and intrusive recall of the event (at times as a flashback); avoiding situations that in some way remind the person of the event; feeling detached from other people; and having a heightened sense of arousal, which is experienced as difficulty falling asleep, hypervigilance, an exaggerated startle response, or a combination of these. Recommended treatment uses psychotherapy and pharmacotherapy. Evidence-based pharmacotherapy includes SSRIs such as sertraline.

Patrick's admission provides a clinical example of PTSD with nursing interventions.

Patrick was admitted to the psychiatric inpatient unit with the diagnosis of PTSD. Two months before admission, he and his coworker friend were in a truck accident on an overpass. Patrick watched in horror as his friend fell out of the truck, which was hanging over the edge. The fall killed his friend instantly. Patrick was able to climb out of the passenger side and sustained injuries to his back and legs. He received physical therapy for his injuries. For the past 2 weeks, he has been continually preoccupied by the event, has had persistent insomnia and nightmares, repeatedly says that he should have been the one to die, becomes easily irritable, does not show feelings when with others, and jumps whenever he hears a loud noise, or someone touches him unexpectedly. The nurse assigned to work with Patrick found him pacing. She remained with him as he paced. The following patient problems were immediately relevant: anxiety, disturbed sleep pattern, post trauma syndrome, and complicated grieving. Patrick and the nurse decided together that the priorities were to decrease his anxiety and to improve his sleep. Patrick was willing to learn a progressive relaxation exercise (which involves relaxing one group of muscles at a time until the body is relaxed). After learning the exercise, Patrick worked on deep abdominal breathing and agreed to use this strategy when he found himself preoccupied with the accident. The nurse did not purposefully probe the details of the event, but if Patrick had brought it up, she would have listened attentively and offered support and empathy.

Acute Stress Disorder

As in PTSD, the person with acute stress disorder has been exposed to a distressing event that is outside the range of normal events. The event or events have happened recently. The symptoms last from 3 days to 1 month. This disorder is characterized by the following:

- Intrusion symptoms: recurrent distressing dreams, recurrent memories of the traumatic event, or flashbacks of the event that in serious cases may occur with complete loss of awareness of present surroundings
- Negative mood: persistent inability to experience feelings of happiness, satisfaction, or love
- Dissociative symptoms: feeling a sense of detachment; having a reduced awareness of one's surroundings; inability to remember aspects of the traumatic event
- Avoidance symptoms: avoiding distressing memories or external reminders of the traumatic event
- Arousal symptoms: sleep disturbances, irritability, angry outbursts, problems with concentration, or exaggerated startle response

SOMATIC SYMPTOM AND RELATED DISORDERS

Individuals with somatic symptom and related disorders experience multiple, current physical symptoms that are distressing or result in significant disruption of daily life. Symptoms in this category are usually persistent and may involve pain or other physical symptoms. Individuals tend to worry excessively about illness and often think the worst about their health.

Somatic Symptom Disorder

Persons with somatic symptom disorder experience one or more physical symptoms that they experience as distressing and/or result in significant disruption in their daily life. In addition, these individuals experience excessive thoughts, feelings, or behaviors related to the symptoms or associated health concerns they feel. Their thoughts, feelings, and behaviors are disproportionate to the seriousness of the symptom and are persistent. These individuals spend excessive time and energy devoted to their symptoms and their health concerns. The course of this illness can be persistent, with symptoms lasting 6 months or more, and the severity can be mild, moderate, or severe. Persons with somatic symptom disorder are not intentionally trying to pretend they are sick. This is true whether or not there is a medical explanation for their symptoms. These individuals have high levels of worry about illness.

Illness Anxiety Disorder

In illness anxiety disorder, formerly known as *hypochondriasis*, individuals are preoccupied with having or acquiring a serious underlying illness. They are convinced that they have a serious medical problem despite the absence of any concrete medical findings. They will seek other opinions if one health care provider does not validate their concerns, and they often take multiple prescription medications from various other health care providers. Concern about the feared illness often becomes a central part of people's lives and may impair social, occupational, or other important areas of functioning. In some cases of illness anxiety disorder, the person does not recognize that the concerns about having a serious illness are excessive or unreasonable.

Conversion Disorder (Functional Neurologic Symptom Disorder)

In conversion disorder, symptoms may include blindness, deafness, or paralysis of the legs without a physiologic cause. Usually, the symptoms are neurologic and can occur in response to some threatening or traumatic event. The symptoms are real and not created; they can cause significant distress or impairment in social, occupational, or other important areas of functioning. In some cases, a true physiologic cause for the symptoms has been discovered years later; therefore, a diagnosis of conversion disorder is usually tentative and provisional.

DISSOCIATIVE DISORDERS

Dissociative disorders involve a change in identity, memory, consciousness, motor control, and behavior. The change may be sudden or gradual, may be transient or occur over a long period, and is thought to be an escape from anxiety. In a sense, persons unconsciously dissociate or remove themselves psychologically from anxiety-provoking situations because the situations are too much to bear. Even normal persons may experience **depersonalization** under severe stress. In this case, individuals feel that they are outside of themselves or floating overhead watching what is happening, as if it were happening to someone else. Examples of dissociative disorders are amnesia or dissociative identity disorder (formerly multiple personality disorder).

Dissociative amnesia is characterized by a gap in memory, usually of a traumatic or stressful nature, that is too extensive to be explained by normal forgetfulness. Five major types of amnesia exist: (1) localized amnesia, or difficulty remembering anything about the first few hours after a profoundly disturbing event; (2) selective amnesia, or the ability to remember some but not all of the events surrounding a traumatic experience; (3) generalized amnesia, or failure to remember one's entire life; (4) continuous amnesia, or inability to recall events after a specific time up to and including the present; and (5) systematized amnesia, or loss of memory for certain categories of information, such as all memories related to one's family or to a particular person.

Dissociative identity disorder is a relatively rare dissociative disorder with two major components: (1) presence of two or more distinct personality states and (2) possession. In the first, two or more distinct personalities exist within the person and at least two personalities repeatedly take control of the person's behavior. Legal identity is retained by the "host personality." Other personalities within the body are called *alter personalities*. Individuals with this disorder experience frequent gaps in memory for personal history, both remote and recent. Most patients with dissociative identity disorders report severe childhood abuse, including physical, sexual, or ritual cult abuse; however, these experiences are difficult to verify. In the second, possession form, identities appear as though a spirit, supernatural being, or outside person has taken control so that the individual begins speaking or acting in a distinctly different manner. For example, a person who appears to be possessed by the devil may take on the characteristics of a satanic entity. The identities that are present are recurrent, unwanted, and involuntary; cause significant distress or impairment; and are not a normal part of cultural or religious practice.

MEDICAL TREATMENT

The category of medications used to treat the acute symptoms of anxiety is the anxiolytic category. The first-line anxiolytic (antianxiety) medications are the serotonin reuptake inhibitors (e.g., SSRI's—paroxetine

Table 61.4 Drug Therapy: Common Anxiolytics (Antianxiety Medications) in the Benzodiazepine Class

DRUG NAME	NURSING IMPLICATIONS	PATIENT TEACHING
alprazolam (Xanax) chlordiazepoxide (Librium) clonazepam (Klonopin) clorazepate (Tranxene) diazepam (Valium) halazepam (Paxipam) lorazepam (Ativan)	The drugs may vary in the length of their half-life (short, intermediate and long). Effective in the treatment of anxiety and panic disorders. However, a short half-life may lead to rebound anxiety. Sometimes used to treat acute alcohol withdrawal. Depresses the central nervous system (CNS). A long half-life allows for once- or twice-a-day dosing. May potentiate other CNS depressants; therefore, administer these drugs with caution with other CNS depressants. Administer with extreme caution in older adults and those who are frail because these patients may be more sensitive to the effects of these medications and more prone to confusion or falls. Abrupt cessation after prolonged or excessive use may result in withdrawal, including seizures and death. An intermediate half-life allows dosing at 3 or 4 times per day.	Avoid alcohol when taking medications in this class because alcohol will intensify their effects and potentially cause respiratory depression. Rebound anxiety may result when medication wears off, especially when taking those with short half-lives. If this happens, report it to your practitioner. Do not take more medication at one time than prescribed or use medication more frequently in a day than prescribed. May impair driving, decrease attention and concentration, and cause drowsiness. Avoid driving or operating dangerous machinery until the effects of the medicine on coordination, reaction time, motor control, and judgment are known. Do not abruptly stop taking this medication without consulting with your practitioner.

[Paxil], sertraline [Zoloft], and fluoxetine [Prozac]) and benzodiazepines (e.g., diazepam [Valium], chlordiazepoxide hydrochloride [Librium], lorazepam [Ativan], alprazolam [Xanax], and clonazepam [Klonopin]). The nursing implications and patient teaching needs related to anxiolytic drug therapy are described in Table 61.4.

Antidepressants are used much more commonly to treat anxiety disorders, acute and posttraumatic stress disorder, and obsessive-compulsive and related disorders either alone or in combination with anxiolytics. Antidepressants, such as the SSRIs and some newer antidepressants such as venlafaxine (Effexor), nefazodone (Dutonin, Nefadar [formerly Serzone]), and duloxetine (Cymbalta), often are useful in reducing anxiety, decreasing distress, and improving overall functioning. This is especially true when the patient suffers from depression as well as anxiety.

SSRI's may be prescribed for months to years; however, benzodiazepines are usually prescribed for brief periods. Side effects associated with benzodiazepines include sedation, such as drowsiness, fatigue, dizziness, and confusion. Because physical and psychologic dependence occur, withdrawal from these medications must be medically supervised. Abrupt cessation of benzodiazepines may result in withdrawal symptoms, including seizures and even death. Thus, these medications are typically used at the initial phase of treatment to reduce symptoms until other medications can take effect.

Pharmacology Capsule

Benzodiazepines, which are given for anxiety disorders or as an adjunct medication for treating schizophrenia, may have side effects such as drowsiness, loss of coordination, fatigue, confusion, blurred vision, and psychologic dependence.

◆ NURSING CARE OF THE PATIENT WITH AN ANXIETY DISORDER, ACUTE AND POSTTRAUMATIC STRESS DISORDER, SOMATIC SYMPTOM DISORDER, OR DISSOCIATIVE DISORDER

Focused Assessment

The patient's self-report of symptoms and their objective observations help to determine the presence and level of anxiety (i.e., mild, moderate, severe, or panic). Particularly relevant mental status examination categories include motor activity, speech and language, and thought content.

Patient Problems, Goals, and Outcome Criteria: Anxiety, Acute and Posttraumatic Stress Disorder, Somatic Symptom Disorder, and Dissociative Disorders

Patient Problems	Goals and Outcome Criteria
Anxiety related to inadequate opportunity to prepare for stressor as evidenced by alteration in concentration, sleeping pattern, or communication pattern, or difficulty organizing information	Reduced anxiety: patient will express understanding of the relationship between emotional state and behavior, (or) patient will become actively involved in planning own care, (or) patient will identify effective and ineffective coping techniques and implement effective coping techniques

Interventions

Strategies to help patients reduce anxiety from a panic state center on remaining calm; speaking firmly with short, simple instructions (e.g., "Sit down with me here"); and moving to a less stimulating area. Once the anxiety is reduced to a manageable level, assist patients in exploring what happened, clarifying their usual ways of relieving anxiety (e.g., by expressing anger or experiencing somatic symptoms instead of more typical anxiety symptoms), and identifying what triggered the anxiety (e.g., feelings of self-doubt regarding finding employment after discharge). You can assist clients in problem-solving decisions and can teach ways to prevent and manage heightened anxiety in the future (see the Complementary and Alternative Therapies box).

Complementary and Alternative Therapies

Useful techniques to manage anxiety include relaxation techniques such as diaphragmatic deep breathing exercises, warm baths, positive self-talk, and physical exercise. Cognitive-behavioral psychotherapy is also used as an evidence-based treatment for individuals with anxiety disorders.

SCHIZOPHRENIA AND SCHIZOAFFECTIVE DISORDERS

Schizophrenia is a term used to refer to a group of usually chronic thought disorders in which psychotic symptoms primarily impair the affected person's ability to interpret the world accurately. Schizophrenia is characterized by disturbances in thinking, mood, and behavior. **Psychosis** is a state in which a person has distorted perceptions of reality. Psychotic symptoms include delusions, hallucinations, disorganized thinking (speech), grossly disorganized or abnormal motor behavior, and negative symptoms. The symptoms are characterized as either *positive* or *negative.* Positive symptoms appear to reflect an excess or distortion of normal functions and include delusions, hallucinations, problems with communication, and bizarre behavior. Negative symptoms appear to reflect a decrease or loss of normal functions and include diminished emotional expression (i.e., flattened affect), slowed thinking and speech, and difficulty initiating goal-directed behavior.

Typically, patients with schizophrenia have functioned normally in early life. The symptoms usually begin in adolescence or early adulthood with a first diagnosis made in late teens to early thirties; however, some types of schizophrenic disorders are more often diagnosed in later life. The person with schizophrenia has trouble functioning in the areas of work, interpersonal relationships, and/or self-care. These abilities deteriorate significantly during acute episodes and may not return to baseline after the first psychotic episode. With each subsequent episode, the ability to function independently continues to deteriorate, intelligence quotient (IQ) levels drop, and thinking becomes very concrete. These patients struggle to tolerate even the typical stressors of daily living. However, newer medications have been highly successful in helping people to return to their previous activities.

Cause and Risk Factors

The cause of schizophrenia disorder is not certain. The model that integrates diverse potential causes states that patients who are most vulnerable to acquiring the disorder encounter factors (stress) that precipitate the disorder. The model is called the *stress-diathesis model.* Researchers have established that people with schizophrenia probably were genetically vulnerable to the disorder. The range of biologic factors being investigated includes (1) neurotransmitters (e.g., dopamine, norepinephrine, and gamma-aminobutyric acid) and their receptors; (2) structural abnormalities such as degeneration of the limbic system, enlargement of the lateral and third ventricles, and loss of neurons in the temporal lobe; (3) infectious agents; and (4) hormonal deregulation.

In males, the disorder first occurs in the early to mid-20s whereas in females the age of onset is generally in late 20s. The incidence is between 0.3% and 0.8%, although there is variation by race/ethnicity and country of origin and in various countries. Psychotic symptoms tend to decrease as people age, possibly caused by age-related declines in dopamine activity. Some 20% of people with schizophrenia attempt suicide on one or more occasions; 5% to 6% die by suicide. About half of those with schizophrenia also have another co-occurring mental or behavioral health disorder.

Medical Treatment

The most commonly prescribed medications for people with schizophrenia are antipsychotic (neuroleptic) medications and antiparkinsonism medications, which are at times administered to prevent or relieve some of the side effects of the antipsychotics. (The nursing implications and patient teaching needs related to drug therapy are described in Table 61.5.) Anxiolytic medications may also be administered in conjunction with the antipsychotics to decrease agitation and akathisia (a potential side effect of antipsychotics in which the patient is restless and unable to sit still). Two broad categories of antipsychotics exist: (1) first-generation agents (FGAs) and (2) second-generation agents (SGAs). FGAs are also referred to as *conventional* or *typical agents.* They are the older agents that were very useful in treating the positive symptoms of schizophrenia such as auditory and visual hallucinations; however, they were not particularly useful in treating the negative symptoms such as poverty of thought, delayed thinking, and decreased function. Many of the SGAs are known to help with both positive and negative symptoms and have a reduced incidence of side effects compared with the older FGAs.

When working with patients who are receiving antipsychotics, you are responsible for observing and recording accurately all data relevant to the target behaviors and symptoms of the medications as well as the

Table 61.5 Drug Therapy: Selected Antipsychotics (Neuroleptics)

DRUG NAME	NURSING IMPLICATIONS	PATIENT TEACHING
First-Generation (Conventional) Antipsychotics		
chlorpromazine (Thorazine) fluphenazine (Prolixin) haloperidol (Haldol) loxapine (Loxitane) mesoridazine (Serentil) perphenazine (Trilafon) thioridazine (Mellaril) thiothixene (Navane) trifluoperazine (Stelazine)	These agents are helpful in the treatment of positive symptoms of schizophrenia and other psychotic processes. They may cause drowsiness and sedation, postural hypotension, dry mouth, and blurred vision (especially in frail and older people). Watch for extrapyramidal side effects (EPS), such as Parkinson syndrome–like involuntary movements, muscle rigidity, dystonia, akathisia, and oculogyric crisis. Long-term administration may result in tardive dyskinesia.	Caution the patient to rise slowly from a lying position to a sitting position and from sitting to standing to avoid a sudden drop in blood pressure (BP). Caution patients to avoid driving or operating dangerous machinery until the effects of the medicine on coordination, reaction time, motor control, and judgment are known. Assess the patient for abnormal, involuntary movements and report these to the prescribing practitioner. Administer medications to treat motor movement side effects as ordered. Provide the patient with hard candy or sugarless chewing gum to help with dry mouth. Provide dietary teaching to help the patient avoid or manage weight gain and diabetes associated with these and other neuroleptics.
Second-Generation (Atypical) Antipsychotics		
aripiprazole (Abilify) asenapine (Saphris) brexpiprazole (Rexulti) cariprazine (Vraylar) clozapine (Clozaril) iloperidone (Fanapt) lurasidone (Latuda) olanzapine (Zyprexa) paliperidone (Invega) quetiapine (Seroquel) risperidone (Risperdal) ziprasidone (Geodon)	Many of these agents treat both the positive and the negative symptoms of schizophrenia and other psychotic disorders. They may cause drowsiness and sedation, postural hypotension, dry mouth, and blurred vision (especially in frail and older people). Watch for EPS, such as Parkinson syndrome–like movements, muscle rigidity, dystonia, akathisia, and oculogyric crisis. Although these side effects are less common with second-generation agents, they are still seen in patients taking these drugs. Long-term administration also may result in tardive dyskinesia, although this may be less likely.	Caution the patient to rise slowly from a lying position to a sitting position and from sitting to standing to avoid a sudden drop in BP. Caution patients to avoid driving or operating dangerous machinery until the effects of the medicine on coordination, reaction time, motor control, and judgment are known. Assess the patient for abnormal, involuntary movements and report these to the prescribing practitioner. Administer medications to treat motor movement side effects as ordered. Provide the patient with hard candy or sugarless chewing gum to help with dry mouth. Provide dietary teaching to help the patient avoid or manage weight gain and diabetes associated with these and other antipsychotics.
	In addition to the implications mentioned earlier, the patient taking clozapine may experience a significant drop in white blood cell (WBC) count. Routine blood count monitoring must be done to identify any drop in WBC count. If this happens, the medication is withheld (and usually discontinued).	In addition to the other side effects associated with taking clozapine, teach the patient taking atypical neuroleptics to watch for and report immediately to the prescribing practitioner a sore throat, fever, chills, and any other signs of infection.

potential side effects. A variety of potential side effects exists, some of which have rapid onset and require immediate treatment.

One side effect that can be managed with nursing interventions and patient teaching is orthostatic hypotension (or postural hypotension), which is a drop in blood pressure (BP) when a person changes position from lying down to sitting or from sitting to standing. This problem, which creates a risk for falls, occurs most frequently in the early weeks of treatment and is more common in the morning, after the patient has been in bed during the night, as well as after a large meal. Older adults and those in poor physical health are at particular risk for this side effect. See Chapter 34 for details on the assessment and management of orthostatic hypotension.

Another group of side effects are referred to as **extrapyramidal side effects (EPS)** and stem from the effect of the antipsychotic agents on the extrapyramidal tracts of the CNS. These tracts play a role in the control of involuntary movements. Different EPS may occur at different periods during medication therapy and are described as follows.

Acute dystonic reactions may occur after one dose of medication or during the first few days of treatment. The reactions consist of severe muscle contractions involving the tongue, face, neck (i.e., torticollis), and back (i.e., opisthotonos). The larynx also may be constricted (i.e., laryngospasm), which compromises the patient's airway. The reaction is reversed with benztropine mesylate (Cogentin), given intramuscularly or intravenously as ordered, or with diphenhydramine hydrochloride (Benadryl), administered intravenously as ordered. Acute dystonia is a medical emergency and must be treated immediately. It is important to note that certain antiemetics such as promethazine (Phenergan) and prochlorperazine (Compazine) may also cause dystonic reactions.

After 1 to 2 weeks of treatment with antipsychotic medications, the **parkinsonian syndrome**—consisting of masklike face, rigid posture, shuffling gait, and resting tremor—may occur. Other extrapyramidal syndromes that may occur in treatment are akathisia, a reversible restlessness manifested as an urge to pace and difficulty sitting still. Some references state that akathisia is the most common side effect of neuroleptic medications.

Tardive dyskinesia is usually an irreversible syndrome that may occur after prolonged use of antipsychotic drug therapy. It consists of persistent involuntary movements of the face, jaw, and tongue that lead to grimacing, jerky movements of the upper extremities, and tonic contractions of the neck and back. Treatment includes discontinuing the causative agent; however, the symptoms may continue. First line medications to decrease involuntary movements include valbenazine (Ingrezza), deutetrabenazine (Austedo), and tetrabenazine (Xenazine). *Gingko biloba* extract and vitamin E also may be used for treatment.

Neuroleptic malignant syndrome occurs in 1% of people receiving antipsychotic (neuroleptic) agents and certain antiemetics such as prochlorperazine (Compazine). Mortality rates reported for people with this condition range from 14% to 30%. The first symptom is usually muscular rigidity accompanied by akinesia (i.e., emotional unresponsiveness and blunted affect) and respiratory distress and may include involuntary muscle movements, but the cardinal sign is hyperthermia (a temperature of ≥101°–103°F). Neuroleptic malignant syndrome is a medical emergency that requires immediate intervention and intensive care because it may result in permanent impairment or even death.

One antipsychotic drug, clozapine (Clozaril), presents a risk for the blood disorder known as *agranulocytosis*, an extreme decrease in granulated white blood cells (WBCs), which frequently manifests as a sore throat and fever. Patients receiving this medication require close supervision and frequent WBC counts. If the WBC drops significantly or if the patient experiences sore throat, fever, and flulike symptoms (or a combination of these symptoms), the medication must be withheld, and the physician must be notified at once. Severe infection may result when the WBC counts drop below acceptable levels.

In monitoring a patient for drug side effects, a wide range of data is relevant (from vital signs to facial expression). Pay close attention to all patient descriptions of symptoms.

After a period of time, patients taking FGAs almost always experience EPS such as akathisia and pseudoparkinsonism. Tardive dyskinesia also is a significant risk when patients are taking FGAs; thus, SGAs are now considered first-line agents, although tardive dyskinesia has been reported in patients taking second-generation antipsychotics (SGAs) as well.

Weight gain, hyperglycemia, and onset of type 2 diabetes have all been associated with the use of SGAs. Therefore, it is important that you teach patients taking these medications about proper diet, exercise, and the need for regular checkups. A few of the SGAs may cause an abnormal increase in serum progesterone (i.e., hyperprolactinemia), which can lead to an enlargement of the breasts (i.e., gynecomastia) and production of milk (i.e., galactorrhea) in both men and women.

◆ NURSING CARE OF THE PATIENT WITH SCHIZOPHRENIA

Focused Assessment

The following data contribute to the mental status examination of the person with schizophrenia:

- Appearance: may have poor grooming and failure to bathe
- Activity: may exhibit agitation, bizarre postures, catatonic excitement or stupor, mannerisms or stereotypes, or stiff body movements
- Mood and affect: may have flat affect or inappropriate rage or happiness
- Speech and language: mutism, tangential speech, blocking, or loose associations
- Thought content: delusions that may be persecutory, grandiose, religious, or somatic
- Perceptual disturbances: auditory hallucinations (most common) and visual hallucinations (next most common)
- Insight and judgment: usually little insight into illness
- Sensorium: oriented to person, place, and time
- Memory: usually intact (but difficulties with attention make assessment difficult)

Patient Problems, Goals, and Outcome Criteria: Schizophrenia

Patient Problems	Goals and Outcome Criteria
Impaired cognition related to delusions (i.e., false beliefs), loose associations, concrete thinking, and symbolism, as evidenced by patient statements such as that the president is out to get them	Orientation: patient differentiates illusions from reality, fewer loose associations, more logical thinking

Patient Problems, Goals, and Outcome Criteria: Schizophrenia—cont'd

Patient Problems	Goals and Outcome Criteria
Altered personal identity related to hallucinations, illusions, and heightened response to irrelevant stimuli, as evidenced by patient's inability to tolerate group therapy, talking to themselves, and looking for something when nothing is there	Improved sensory perceptual function: reduced frequency of hallucinations, less response to irrelevant environmental and other stimuli
Inability to communicate effectively related to delayed thinking as evidenced by very slow and delayed speech	Improved verbal communication: patient expresses thoughts clearly
Inability to manage self-care related to withdrawal and loss of motivation and judgment, as evidenced by poor hygiene, poor grooming, and avoiding others	Improved self-care: patient manages activities of daily living (ADL) with maximum independence in relation to level of ability

Interventions

Impaired cognition. Nursing interventions include speaking in a gentle and nonconfrontational manner, decreasing unwanted environmental stimuli, focusing on reality (i.e., real events, real people), letting the patient know that you do not share the delusion without directly confronting the delusion (do not argue or try to disprove the delusion), encouraging the patient to express feelings and anxiety, and connecting delusions with anxiety-provoking situations (see interventions for anxiety, discussed earlier under "Nursing Care of the Patient With an Anxiety Disorder, Somatic Symptom Disorder, or Dissociative Disorder").

Altered personal identity. Interventions include making brief, frequent contacts with the patient (to interrupt hallucinatory experiences); encouraging the patient to pay attention to what is occurring in the environment (instead of internal stimuli); encouraging involvement in quiet activities; and informing patients that hallucinations are part of the disease process.

Inability to communicate effectively. Interventions may include seeking clarification and verbalizing the implied, which may be useful if the patient is not speaking (e.g., "It must have been difficult for you when your father didn't come after he told you he would"). You will also want to provide regular contact with the patient and use gentle encouragement, understanding that the patient's thinking may be slowed.

Inability to perform self-care. Possible interventions include providing recognition for all constructive self-care actions (e.g., "I see you've bathed and washed your hair"), demonstrating how to perform an activity if necessary, intervening to assist when necessary, offering finger foods or cans of food for the patient to open, or serving meals family style if the patient believes that food has been poisoned.

Schizoaffective Disorder

Schizoaffective disorder has similar features to schizophrenia with the additional symptoms of a major mood disorder throughout the illness. An individual may have impaired occupational functioning, restricted social contact, and difficulties with self-care, but negative symptoms are usually less severe and persistent than in schizophrenia. The disorder is about one-third as common as schizophrenia, and the age of onset is usually in young adulthood. Treatment and nursing care are similar for patients with schizophrenia and those with mood disorders.

MOOD DISORDERS

Major Depressive Disorder

Major depressive disorder is one of the most common psychiatric disorders, with a 12-month prevalence of 7.1%. An estimated 17.3 million adults in the United States had at least one major depressive episode in 2017. Unfortunately, approximately 35% of adults with major depression and 60% of adolescents did not receive treatment in 2017, the last year measured. The occurrence is 3 times higher in people aged 18 to 29 years than in people over 60 years of age. Beginning in adolescence, 1.5 to 3 times as many women as men are diagnosed with major depression. There is a greater risk for family members with major depressive disorder and people with depressive personality traits. Stress is also related to the onset of major depressive disorder. The diagnosis is made by the presence of a depressed mood most of the day, most days of the week, which persists for more than two weeks and is accompanied by such symptoms as appetite disturbance, weight loss, or weight gain; problems with initiating sleep, remaining asleep, or waking too early in the morning; loss of interest in activities that used to bring pleasure or joy; loss of energy; fatigue; impairment in attention and concentration; and sometimes suicidal ideation. In its most severe form, major depression can also include psychotic symptoms.

Bipolar Disorders

People with bipolar disorders experience significantly elevated (or very irritable) or depressed moods. There are three primary types of bipolar disorder—bipolar I, bipolar II, and cyclothymic disorder. Bipolar I disorder is marked by experiencing episodes of elevated (mania) or irritable mood that lasts a week or longer or are so severe that a person becomes hospitalized. Some episodes of depression may occur as well. A person can also experience what is known as a mixed episode with both mania and depressive symptoms occurring at the same time. In severe episodes of mania or depression, psychotic symptoms may also occur.

In bipolar disorder type II, there are intermittent episodes of major depressive disorder alternating with episodes of hypomania for at least four days, including an elevated mood or very irritable mood, but not to the level of full mania.

Cyclothymic disorder is experienced as fluctuating periods of alternating episodes of hypomania or depression for two years in adults and one year in children.

The lifetime prevalence of bipolar disorder is 4.4%, with the mean age of onset at 25 years. Rates are similar for men and women and are higher among single and divorced people than among married people. People in higher socioeconomic groups and those with lower levels of education have higher rates of bipolar disorder.

Cause and Risk Factors

Causes of major depressive and bipolar disorders have not been definitively established. The most recent research suggests that mood disorders are caused by a combination of genetic, biological, environmental, and psychologic factors. Probable causes include neurotransmitter dysregulation, neuroreceptor deficits, neuroendocrine dysfunctions, genetic factors, loss of significant others, learned helplessness, and negative thoughts about life experiences.

Medical Treatment

For major depressive disorder, several types of antidepressant medications are available: SSRIs; SNRIs; TCAs; and less commonly used monoamine oxidase inhibitors (MAOIs), and others. (Important considerations related to drug therapy are listed in Table 61.6). As the patient responds to antidepressant medication and the energy level increases, the risk of suicide also increases.

For bipolar disorder types I and II, the use of antidepressants is controversial. Second generation (atypical) antipsychotics and/or mood-stabilizing agents are the most effective treatments. The manic phase of bipolar disease typically is treated with lithium or divalproex (Depakote) alone or with an atypical antipsychotic. (Nursing implications and patient teaching needs are described in Table 61.7.) When administering medications, you are responsible for ensuring that medication has been swallowed and not held in the mouth and later discarded or saved for an overdose (see the Complementary and Alternative Therapies box).

Complementary and Alternative Therapies

Many people use the herbal preparation St. John's wort to relieve depression. However, additional study is needed before it can be recommended as a replacement for conventional drugs used to treat major mental illnesses. Patients should be educated to avoid using St. John's wort if they are taking prescribed medications such as an antidepressant that increases serotonin, because St. John's wort also increases serotonin, and taking the two together can result in a life-threatening syndrome, the serotonin syndrome.

Pharmacology Capsule

Although newer medications such as the SSRIs are safer to use in treating depression, occasionally a patient may require the use of a tricyclic antidepressant. The side effects of tricyclic antidepressants (TCAs) are drowsiness, fatigue, orthostatic hypotension, dry mouth, blurred vision, urinary retention, and constipation. TCAs often are difficult to tolerate in older adults.

MAOIs sometimes are prescribed for patients with a depression that is resistant to the SSRIs, TCAs, and other antidepressants. A 2-week period should elapse between ending most antidepressants and beginning an MAOI. The very serious side effect of a hypertensive crisis occurs if the patient taking an MAOI ingests tyramine-containing food or drink, such as avocados, bananas, beer, bologna, canned figs, chocolate, cheese (except cottage cheese), liver, papaya products, pâté, herring, fava beans, raisins, salami, sausage, sour cream, soy sauce, some wines, and yogurt. These foods also must be avoided for 3 weeks after stopping treatment with an MAOI. Symptoms of a hypertensive crisis, which requires immediate treatment, include headache, palpitations, visual changes, neck stiffness, nausea, vomiting, sweating, sensitivity to light, pupil changes, and bradycardia or tachycardia. A "washout" period of about 4 weeks must elapse when discontinuing an MAOI before starting most other antidepressants.

Sexual dysfunction (i.e., anorgasmia, delayed or absent ejaculation, decreased libido) may occur with any antidepressant but seems to be more common when a patient is taking an SSRI. Some antidepressants such as nefazodone and bupropion (Wellbutrin) are much less likely to cause this troublesome side effect.

Put On Your Thinking Cap!

A patient with bipolar disorder is being treated for severe depression in an inpatient facility with bupropion (Wellbutrin) and divalproex sodium (Depakote). Identify the nursing implications related to these medications.

◆ NURSING CARE OF THE PATIENT WITH MAJOR DEPRESSION

Focused Assessment

Data that are relevant to the mental status assessment of a patient who has depression include the following:

- Activity: the patient is likely to exhibit psychomotor retardation and possibly no spontaneous movements, with a downcast gaze; however, a patient may exhibit agitation (e.g., hand wringing and hair pulling), especially if an older adult.
- Mood and affect: the patient may or may not have depressed feelings and may not appear depressed.
- Speech and language: the patient's speech volume and rate may be decreased. In addition, responses to questions may be delayed and mutism may be present.

Table 61.6 Drug Therapy: Antidepressant Drugs

DRUG	CONSIDERATIONS
SSRIs	
citalopram (Celexa) escitalopram (Lexapro) fluoxetine (Prozac) fluvoxamine (Luvox) paroxetine (Paxil) sertraline (Zoloft)	SSRIs can be taken once a day, making adherence to a prescribed treatment easier for the patient. SSRIs are not considered cardiotoxic; thus an overdose is unlikely to cause life-threatening dysrhythmias. Besides depression, SSRIs may be useful in generalized anxiety disorder, panic disorder, and OCD. Most patients tolerate the medications in the morning, whereas others may feel tired and thus should take the SSRIs in the evening. Some may cause weight gain. All of these can cause sexual dysfunction.
SNRIs	
desvenlafaxine (Pristiq) duloxetine (Cymbalta) levomilnacipran (Fetzima) venlafaxine (Effexor)	SNRI's may additionally have some efficacy in treatment of multiple pain syndromes. Duloxetine also used for diabetic peripheral neuropathy, generalized anxiety disorder, chronic musculoskeletal pain, and fibromyalgia. Avoid abrupt withdrawal.
Tricyclics	
amitriptyline (Elavil) clomipramine (Anafranil) desipramine (Norpramin) doxepin (Sinequan) imipramine (Tofranil) nortriptyline (Pamelor)	TCAs affect not only serotonin but also epinephrine and norepinephrine. As such, they may cause cardiac complications. Severe and life-threatening dysrhythmias may result from an overdose. Side effects may be more problematic in this group of medications than with SSRIs. Many of these medicines cannot be taken once a day; bid or tid dosing must be used to reach the total daily dose.
Tetracyclics	
maprotiline (Ludiomil) mirtazapine (Remeron)	These agents are at least as potentially dangerous as TCAs; significant sedation may occur. May be given in single or divided doses. Note Remeron is contraindicated in patients with glaucoma.
Other Agents	
bupropion (Wellbutrin) nefazodone (Serzone) trazodone (Desyrel)	Dosing schedules vary. Bupropion can cause seizures; does not cause weight gain or sexual dysfunction—unlike SSRIs. Although not common, nefazodone can cause severe liver injury. Trazodone is sedating; often used to relieve antidepressant-induced insomnia.
MAOIs	
phenelzine (Nardil) tranylcypromine (Parnate)	Phenelzine (Nardil) is not a first-line (i.e., first choice) drug. Strict diet restrictions are necessary for patients taking these medications. Interactions with foods containing tyramine, other antidepressants, and many other drugs can lead to life-threatening hypertensive crisis. Must be given in divided doses. Warn patients to avoid OTC medications until approved by prescriber of MAOI.

bid, twice a day; *MAOI*, monoamine oxidase inhibitor; *OCD*, obsessive-compulsive disorder; *OTC*, over-the-counter; *SNRI*, serotonin norepinephrine reuptake inhibitors; *SSRI*, selective serotonin reuptake inhibitor; *TCA*, tricyclic antidepressant; *tid*, three times a day.

- Thought content: the patient expresses a generally negative view of self and world, and may ruminate about loss, guilt, suicide, and depression. A psychotic patient may have delusions of guilt, failure, worthlessness, or terminal illnesses.
- Insight and judgment: suicidal ideation can occur during major depressive episodes. Risk factors include history of past suicide attempts or threats, males over 65, substance use, chronic illness, family violence, traumatic experiences, having firearms in the home, being single or living alone, social isolation, and feeling hopeless. Insight into illness may be impaired because of negative perceptions of reality.
- Sensorium: the patient is oriented but may not have energy to answer questions.
- Memory and attention: the patient often complains of impaired focus, concentration, and forgetfulness.

Patient Problems, Goals, and Outcome Criteria: Major Depression

Patient Problems	Goals and Outcome Criteria
Potential for self-harm related to hopelessness and increased energy level associated with treatment, as evidenced by patient endorsing suicidal ideations	Reduced potential for self-harm: patient seeks out staff member if an urge to harm self is experienced; develops coping skills to replace self-destructive behavior and displays acceptable ways of expressing anger, rage, and hostility; mobilizes social support systems; if suicidal, never left alone
Impaired self-concept related to negative feelings about self	Improved self-concept: patient accepts own body, has positive feelings about self, identifies aspects of self they like; identifies thoughts about self

Continued

Table 61.7 Drug Therapy: Mood Stabilizers

DRUG NAME	NURSING IMPLICATIONS	PATIENT TEACHING
carbamazepine (Tegretol)	Used in the treatment of bipolar mood disorder as well as in seizure disorders. Requires careful monitoring of liver enzymes and drug levels. May cause anemia. May cause life-threatening allergic skin reactions (Stevens-Johnson syndrome); watch for development of rash, hold medication if rash develops and notify prescriber immediately. May cause dizziness, drowsiness, unsteady gait. May result in fetal abnormalities if used during pregnancy.	Take exactly as prescribed, notify prescriber at once if rash develops, and hold medication until further advice from a health care provider. Keep all medical appointments and have blood work done as ordered. Notify your prescriber immediately if you suspect you are pregnant. Do not breastfeed while taking this medication.
lamotrigine (Lamictal)	Used in the treatment of bipolar disorders as well as seizure disorders. May cause life-threatening allergic skin reactions (Stevens-Johnson syndrome); watch for development of rash, hold medication if rash develops and notify prescriber immediately. May cause dizziness, drowsiness, unsteady gait. Must be started at a low dose and titrated up slowly, not more than once every 1 to 2 weeks. May result in fetal abnormalities if used during pregnancy.	Take exactly as prescribed. Do not double up for missed dosages. Swallow the regular tablets whole; do not split, chew, or crush them. Tell your doctor if you are pregnant, plan to become pregnant, or are breast-feeding. If you become pregnant while taking lamotrigine, call your doctor.
lithium (lithium carbonate, Lithobid, lithium SR)	Used in the treatment of bipolar disorders; occasionally used as adjunct treatment for depression. Narrow therapeutic range of 0.5 to 1.5 mEq/L (check your local laboratory reference range). Watch for signs of lithium toxicity (tremulousness, nausea, vomiting, diarrhea, changes in level of consciousness). Maintain adequate hydration. Monitor renal function (serum creatinine and BUN) and report abnormal findings. Monitor serum level of lithium. Do not change from immediate release to sustained release or vice versa unless directed by prescriber because this may alter serum levels unexpectedly.	Take exactly as prescribed. Drug must be taken regularly to achieve and maintain adequate blood level. Do not alter salt intake. Do not double up on doses if one is missed. Maintain adequate fluid intake, especially in hot weather. Avoid excessive use of caffeinated beverages. Keep follow-up appointments and have blood levels drawn as directed. Report signs of toxicity at once.
valproic acid, divalproex sodium (Depakote, Depakene)	Used in the treatment of bipolar disorders. Serum levels must be monitored for therapeutic range (50–100 μg/mL). Metabolized by the liver, so periodic monitoring of liver enzymes is necessary. May cause some sedation. May cause hair loss; if moderate to severe, notify prescribing practitioner. Report moderate to severe abdominal pain immediately to prescriber (may cause pancreatitis).	Take medication exactly as prescribed. Drug must be taken regularly to achieve and maintain adequate blood level. Do not double up on medication if a dose is missed. Avoid driving or operating dangerous machinery until exact effects of medication are known. Keep follow-up appointments and have blood levels drawn as directed. Report moderate to severe abdominal pain immediately to prescriber (may cause pancreatitis).

BUN, Blood urea nitrogen.

Patient Problems, Goals, and Outcome Criteria: Major Depression—cont'd

Patient Problems	Goals and Outcome Criteria
Inadequate nutrition related to anorexia	Adequate nutrition: achieves and maintains ideal weight and has more energy
Sleep disturbance related to anxiety	Improved sleep: patient sleeps within 30 minutes of retiring and remains asleep for 6 to 8 uninterrupted hours

Interventions

Potential for self-harm. Interventions may include establishing a no-harm contract; frequently assessing a patient's suicidal potential (see the section titled "Nursing Assessment of the Psychiatric Patient"); taking necessary suicide precautions; removing dangerous objects such as pantyhose, belts, and any sharp objects; maintaining continuous one-to-one contact if indicated; encouraging honest expression of feelings; assisting in identifying symbols of hope in the patient's life; identifying community resources for times of crisis; and communicating the message that the patient is worthwhile.

Impaired self-concept. Interventions may include helping the patient to identify positive aspects and limitations regarding his or her body; to like the body despite its imperfections; to improve hygiene, grooming, and posture, which makes positive affirmations about self; to limit self-criticism; to be aware of negative self-statements; to learn to give and receive compliments; and to develop social skills.

Inadequate nutrition. Possible interventions include involving a dietitian in planning an adequate diet for the patient; directly assisting patients to make healthy choices regarding their menu and eating choices; documenting intake; determining food preferences and attempting to satisfy those preferences; and offering small, frequent meals.

Sleep disturbance. For patients with a sleep disturbance, discourage sleep during the day; provide sleep-producing measures such as a light, small snack, and warm bath; and teach relaxation movements that can be used before retiring. The patient should avoid exercising before bedtime, watching television or electronic devices in bed, and ingesting caffeine after 2 PM. The patient may be asked to keep a sleep diary (see Nursing Care Plan: Patient with Major Depression).

Nursing Care Plan **Patient With Major Depression**

FOCUSED ASSESSMENT

Health History

A 53-year-old woman is admitted to a psychiatric hospital with a diagnosis of major depression. During the past few weeks, she has become increasingly listless, apathetic, and disinterested in anyone or anything. She cries frequently and says that her life has not seemed to be worth living. She complains that she cannot sleep and has no appetite. She frequently talks about wanting to commit suicide. She was referred to a psychiatrist, who recommended that she be admitted to the hospital for treatment.

Physical Examination

Vital signs: blood pressure 110/70 mm Hg, pulse 78 beats per minute, respirations 22 breaths per minute, temperature 98.8°F (37.1°C) measured orally. Height 5′4″, weight 120 lb. Appears apathetic, sad, and cries frequently. Somewhat disheveled. Gaunt and tired looking.

Patient Problems	Goals and Outcome Criteria	Interventions
Potential for self-harm related to suicidal feelings	The patient will not harm herself, as evidenced by seeking out nursing staff if she experiences the urge to harm herself; developing coping skills to replace self-destructive behavior; and developing acceptable ways to express anger, rage, and hostility.	Frequently assess her suicidal potential and take necessary suicide precautions—create a safe environment—remove dangerous objects; maintain continuous one-to-one contact; encourage honest expression of feelings; and assist in identifying symbols of hope in the patient's life, such as recognizing personal strengths or setting small, realistic goals. Encourage the patient to reach out to staff if suicidal thoughts arise or worsen. Never leave the patient alone; provide a sitter for her.
Impaired self-concept related to depression	The patient will maintain or enhance self-concept, as evidenced by acceptance of her own body and sense of self, identification of negative thoughts about herself, and identification of aspects of herself she likes.	Help the patient to identify positive aspects and limitations regarding her body and to accept her body regardless of limitations. Encourage the patient to improve her hygiene. Assist the patient to accept compliments and to limit self-criticism.
Inadequate nutrition related to anorexia or lack of interest in food	The patient will gain weight and experience a higher energy level, as evidenced by more participation and interaction in activities with others.	Involve the dietitian in planning an adequate diet. Determine food preferences and attempt to satisfy those preferences. Offer small, frequent meals.
Sleep disturbance related to depression relapse	The patient will sleep within 30 minutes of retiring and remain asleep for 6 to 8 uninterrupted hours.	Provide sleep-producing measures such as small snacks, warm baths, and relaxation exercises before the patient retires.

CRITICAL THINKING QUESTIONS

1. Explain why the patient requires close monitoring when she begins to feel more energetic.
2. What are some examples of symbols of hope in a person's life?

◆ NURSING CARE OF THE PATIENT WITH BIPOLAR DISORDER WITH MANIC EPISODES

Focused Assessment

The nurse may observe the following:

- Appearance: the patient's form of dress is often inappropriate (e.g., bright, nonmatching colors; excessive make-up and jewelry).
- Activity: the patient is hyperactive and has a decreased need for sleep.
- Mood, affect, and feelings: although frequently euphoric, the patient may also be very irritable, angry, and hostile (based on low frustration tolerance) as well as emotionally labile.
- Speech and language: the patient is talkative and uses pressured speech that is difficult to interrupt. In addition, they have a flight of ideas (i.e., continuous, rapid shift from one topic to another), and the rate and volume of speech is increased.
- Thought content: themes of self-confidence, self-aggrandizement, and possibly delusions of grandeur (e.g., a false belief that one has great wealth or power) or delusions of persecution are noted.
- Sensory perception: the patient may experience hallucinations.
- Judgment and insight: the patient often has little insight regarding their illness. In addition, the patient's judgment is impaired, as evidenced by actions such as large spending sprees, substance use, sexual activities incongruent with usual behavior, suicide attempts, and homicide attempts.

Patient Problems, Goals, and Outcome Criteria: Bipolar Disorder With Manic Episodes

Patient Problems	Goals and Outcome Criteria
Potential for injury related to impaired judgment	Reduced potential for injury: patient does not exhibit potentially injurious activities
Potential for violence toward others related to impaired judgment, low frustration tolerance, and emotional lability	Reduced potential for violence toward others: patient does not harm others, verbalizes anger appropriately
Inadequate nutrition related to hyperactivity	Balanced nutrition: patient consumes necessary daily nutrients in appropriate form for manic state, maintains body weight
Sleep disturbance related to hyperactivity	Improved sleep: patient sleeps at least 6 uninterrupted hours
Mood disturbance related to disinhibition	The patient will verbalize a realistic understanding of the meaning of their own symptoms The patient will not engage in risky behavior

Interventions

Potential for injury. Interventions include decreasing environmental stimuli (e.g., providing a quiet, simply decorated room), discouraging group activities, encouraging a few one-to-one contacts, removing hazardous objects and substances from the environment, and providing a structure that includes physical activities such as brisk walks.

Potential for violence toward others. Interventions include decreasing environmental stimuli, observing the patient frequently, removing harmful objects, finding physical outlets, demonstrating a show of strength if necessary, administering prescribed medications, and restraining the patient if other measures have failed. The goal is to provide the least restrictive environment possible; however, there may arise a need to protect patients from harming themselves or others. Restraints should be applied following an established protocol by staff who have been educated to restrain patients in a safe and humane manner. The patient in restraints should be checked at least every 15 minutes to make certain that circulation to extremities is satisfactory and to assess needs regarding nutrition and elimination.

Inadequate nutrition. Interventions include providing foods that can be consumed on the run, attempting to have the patient's favorite foods and easy-to-eat and finger foods available, and educating the patient on the importance of satisfactory nutrition (see the Nutrition Considerations box).

Nutrition Considerations

- During manic episodes, patients may not meet nutritional needs because of increased physical activity and difficulty sitting down to complete a meal.
- Anorexia may be a problem for depressed patients.

Sleep disturbance. Interventions may include ensuring that the environment is free from excessive stimuli; observing closely for signs of fatigue, such as fine tremor and puffy, dark circles below the eyes; and encouraging warm baths and soft music at bedtime.

Mood disturbance. Initiate precautions to reduce risks related to disinhibition (temporary loss of inhibition). Disinhibited patients may require increased observation and frequent redirection to avoid risky behaviors. Assist the patient to evaluate effectiveness of their strategies to meet new goals emphasizing recovery.

The key medications for people with manic episodes are divalproex sodium (Depakote) or lithium carbonate. Because relief from symptoms may take up to 3 weeks, the patient may also receive an antipsychotic (neuroleptic) medication.

The therapeutic level of divalproex sodium in the blood is 50 to 100 μg/mL (depending on the laboratory). The patient may develop toxicity if the blood level exceeds the therapeutic range. Therefore, a valproic acid level is done at intervals to assess blood levels. Because divalproex is metabolized by the liver, patients with liver disorders may receive lower dosages.

Lithium is excreted by the kidneys and has a narrow therapeutic range. The therapeutic blood level for acute mania is 0.5 to 1.5 mEq/L (depending on the laboratory). If the level is greater than 1.5 mEq/L (or lower in the elderly), symptoms of toxicity occur. It is critical for the patient taking lithium to stay well hydrated. If a patient taking lithium becomes dehydrated, they can easily become lithium toxic. Signs and symptoms of lithium toxicity include tremor, nausea, vomiting, diarrhea, and changes in level of consciousness.

Pharmacology Capsule

Older adults and medically compromised patients are exceptionally vulnerable to experiencing the side effects of all psychotropic medications, especially postural hypotension, falls, and confusion.

NEUROCOGNITIVE DISORDERS

The key problems for people with cognitive disorders stem from impairments in cognition (thinking) and/or memory. These deficits are acquired rather than developmental (such as an intellectual disability), meaning they represent a change from the individual's baseline functioning. The neurocognitive disorders include delirium and major and mild neurocognitive disorders. Delirium and dementia are two very different disorders that involve deficits in orientation, memory, language comprehension, and judgment.

Delirium

Delirium is almost always reversible whereas dementia usually is not. Dementia is slow in its onset. Delirium is rapid in onset, with changes occurring within hours or a couple of days. Delirium can be evidenced in a hospitalized patient and must be identified and addressed urgently to prevent serious and potentially fatal outcomes.

Common causes of delirium are meningitis, neoplasms, drugs ranging from alcohol to steroids, prescribed medications—especially anticholinergics—medication interactions, electrolyte imbalance, endocrine dysfunction, liver abnormalities, renal failure, thiamine deficiency, acute infections, and postoperative states. Delirium represents a life-threatening emergency. The nurse must be able to identify changes in levels of consciousness; orientation to person, place, time, and circumstance; confusion; and other changes from the patient's baseline mental status. Immediate intervention is necessary to determine the cause and correct the underlying medical condition.

Major and Minor Neurocognitive Disorders

Major and minor (mild) neurocognitive disorders are disorders of cognition that progress gradually and can be caused by many underlying etiologies. The distinction between a major and minor disorder is the level of impairment evidenced by the patient in their thinking, memory, and ability to problem solve. As the name implies, major neurocognitive disorders are evidenced by more severe impairments in multiple areas of functioning, whereas minor neurocognitive disorders are less severe on presentation. Major and minor neurocognitive disorders, formerly referred to as *dementias*, are categorized by the type of presentation, the underlying disease, and the areas of the brain involved. Common types of major and minor neurocognitive disorders can be caused by Alzheimer disease, Parkinson disease, Huntington disease, vascular disease, frontotemporal lobar degeneration, Lewy body disease, chronic substance/alcohol use, traumatic brain injury, human immunodeficiency virus infection, prion disease related, or multifactorial. Delirium and dementia are discussed in greater detail in Chapter 13.

PERSONALITY DISORDERS

Every individual exhibits particular personality traits. A person may be shy, aggressive, dependent, or manipulative. When personality traits become inflexible and dysfunctional, a person may have a personality disorder. The essential features of a personality disorder are that it is pervasive (it concerns all aspects of one's life), chronic, and maladaptive. Examples of personality disorders are as follows:

- Antisocial personality disorder: a pattern of disregard for and violation of the rights of others. (The individual repeatedly breaks the law; lies; fails to plan ahead; shows a reckless disregard for the safety of self and others; is irresponsible; and lacks remorse for having hurt, mistreated, or stolen from another.)
- Avoidant personality disorder: a pattern of social inhibition accompanied by feelings of inadequacy and hypersensitivity to negative evaluation. (Individuals avoid occupational activities that involve interpersonal activities because of fear of criticism, disapproval, or rejection. In addition, the individuals are unwilling to get involved with people unless certain of being liked, are preoccupied with being criticized or rejected in social situations, view self as inferior to others, and are unusually reluctant to take personal risks.)
- Borderline personality disorder: a pattern of instability in interpersonal relationships, self-image, and affect as well as marked impulsivity. (The individual makes frantic efforts to avoid real or imagined abandonment; has chronic feelings of emptiness; shows inappropriate, intense anger or has difficulty controlling anger; has an unstable self-image or sense of self; and exhibits recurrent suicidal behavior, gestures, or threats.)

- Narcissistic personality disorder: a pattern of grandiosity, need for admiration, and lack of empathy. (The individual has an exaggerated sense of self-importance; requires excessive admiration; takes advantage of others to achieve their own ends; is often envious of others; and exhibits arrogant, haughty behaviors or attitudes. Note: People with antisocial, borderline, histrionic, or narcissistic personality disorder often appear dramatic, highly emotional, or erratic.)
- Obsessive-compulsive personality disorder: difficulty establishing and sustaining close relationships associated with a pattern of preoccupation with orderliness, perfectionism, and control. (The individuals are preoccupied with details, rules, lists, order, organization, or schedules to the extent that a major part of the activity is lost. In addition, they show perfectionism, rigidity, stubbornness, and restricted emotional expression.)
- Schizotypal personality disorder: a pattern of difficulties in social and interpersonal relationships in which the person suffers from acute discomfort with close relationships and therefore has a decreased capacity for such relationships. (The individual also has cognitive and perceptual distortions as well as eccentricities of behavior that make close relationships difficult.)

Borderline Personality Disorder

The person with borderline personality disorder has patterns involving unstable relationships, unstable self-image, and unstable mood. Two theories offer explanations for the cause of this disorder. First, a genetic influence is thought to exist—there may be another family member with this personality disorder. The second explanation is related to developmental experiences. Early childhood abandonment, neglect, and trauma may have an impact. Some theorists view an essential component of psychosocial development as separation-individuation. Some feel that problems with attachment exist. It is thought that between 2 and 3 years of age, the child separates from the parents as a unique self. If the parents are nonaccepting or ambivalent about the child's increasing autonomy, and if the parents reinforce dependent behavior, the child does not fully experience self as separate. This problem with separation-individuation is thought to form the basis of *splitting*, a frequently used mechanism in borderline personality disorder. Persons who are splitting view others as all good or all bad and may shift their views of a particular other from all good to all bad. A person who has a clearly developed sense of self and who does not split, views others as having a mix of good qualities and negative qualities. The case of a patient called Bonnie and her recent hospitalization provides a clinical example of borderline personality disorder:

Nora, an LVN, worked part-time on a psychiatric unit. She reported to work at 11 PM one night after 5 days of not working to discover that Bonnie had been readmitted after opening the suture line on her wrists with a steak knife. One year ago, Bonnie had cut this wrist, saying that she was trying to feel something. Bonnie told Nora that she had missed her terribly and she hoped Nora would work with her that night. Nora said that Susan (the full-time registered nurse [RN]) would work with her that night. Bonnie swore and returned to her room. When Nora made rounds, Bonnie said that she was sure something was wrong and began walking around the room with a staggering gait. Bonnie said that she had not taken anything to create this problem. Her vital signs were stable, and her pupils were normal in size and reaction to light. Nora reported the situation to Susan and reflected on her responses to Bonnie. Initially she felt anger, telling herself that Bonnie was manipulative when she did not have her way. She thought about how Bonnie manipulates others when she feels helpless (she has no idea of how to meet her own needs). She also thought about Bonnie's splitting (seeing Nora as good nurse and Susan as a bad nurse). Nora felt less angry as she considered the reasons for Bonnie's behavior. When Susan entered Bonnie's bedroom, Bonnie's gait was normal. Susan conversed with Bonnie for two 10-minute periods (at the beginning and end of her shift), during which time Bonnie could share whatever was on her mind and discuss her goals and plans for the following day.

◆ NURSING CARE OF THE PATIENT WITH BORDERLINE PERSONALITY DISORDER

Focused Assessment

The most relevant aspects of the mental status examination are the following:

- Mood, affect, feeling: the patient may experience mood swings or chronic feelings of emptiness and boredom or intense anger.
- Insight and judgment: the patient makes repeated suicidal threats and gestures and exhibits self-mutilating behavior.

Patient Problems, Goals, and Outcome Criteria: Borderline Personality Disorder

Patient Problems	Goals and Outcome Criteria
Potential for self-harm related to episodes of anger and impaired judgment	Absence of self-harm: patient does not harm or mutilate self
Decreased socialization related to unstable relationships	Improved social interaction: patient maintains relationships
Impaired self-concept related to splitting	Improved sense of self: patient clarifies own unique characteristics; differentiates thoughts and feelings of self and others; less splitting, clinging, and disturbing behaviors

Interventions

Potential for self-harm. In addition to the interventions identified in the sections titled "Major Depressive Disorder" and "Bipolar Disorders," various interventions are more specific to the issues of borderline personality disorder. It is important to be aware of your own feelings to refrain from any automatic responses that are not helpful (e.g., avoiding the patient who has cut themselves). If patients mutilate themselves, it is important to care for wounds without acting in a way that might reinforce the self-mutilation (e.g., offering sympathy). Conversely, it is not appropriate to express disgust or in any way denigrate the patient. Ask patients to talk about feelings that occurred just before the self-mutilation. You can act as a role model for constructive expression of angry feelings and acknowledge the patient's positive expressions of negative feelings.

Decreased socialization. Interventions include assisting patients in examining their own behaviors in relationships, communicating availability, acknowledging (reinforcing) independent behavior, and setting limits as appropriate.

Impaired self-concept. Interventions include helping the patient to discuss and take ownership of their own thoughts and feelings, clarifying values while being cautious not to impose one's own values, and avoiding empathetic responses that may be viewed as mind reading (e.g., "I know how you feel").

SUMMARY

Nurses work with patients with psychiatric disorders in a variety of settings, including psychiatric inpatient units. Treatment for psychiatric disorders is influenced by the culture, place, and acuity of the present illness. You can use various strategies in communicating therapeutically with patients. The mental status examination is one aspect of the assessment of patients and is particularly relevant on a psychiatric unit. Systematically use the mental status examination with patients on admission and on an ongoing basis. For each of the major psychiatric disorders, possible observations for the relevant mental status examination categories are presented. Possible patient problems, goals, and interventions have been suggested for each disorder.

Get Ready for the NCLEX® Examination!

Key Points

- According to current thinking, mental illnesses are related to specific physiologic changes in the CNS.
- Milieu therapy or therapeutic community is providing a structured environment to effect behavioral changes and to improve the psychological health and functioning of the individual. Patients learn adaptive coping, interaction, and relationship skills that can be generalized to other aspects of their lives.
- The psychoanalytic approach to mental illness is based on the theory that humans function at different levels of awareness, ranging from conscious to unconscious, and that people use ego defense mechanisms to prevent anxiety.
- The interpersonal approach to mental illness has three components: (1) anxiety is often communicated interpersonally, (2) the patient learns new ways of coping or maturing in a therapeutic relationship, and (3) establishing trust is an important first step in the nurse's work with patients.
- Key ideas from the cognitive behavioral approach to mental illness are that behavior is learned, that behavior changes in response to positive consequences (positive reinforcement) or in response to the removal of negative stimuli (negative reinforcement), and that thoughts influence emotional states.
- In caring for a patient with a psychiatric disorder, nurses establish therapeutic (as opposed to social) relationships.
- The mental status examination consists of observations regarding appearance, activity, mood and affect, speech and language, thought content, perceptual disturbances, insight and judgment, sensorium, and memory and attention.
- A patient with an anxiety disorder experiences either the highly uncomfortable feeling of fear directly or a symptom such as compulsive hand washing that prevents or reduces the occurrence of anxiety.
- In panic disorder a patient experiences recurrent panic attacks, which are intense episodes of apprehension, at times to the point of terror; often these attacks are accompanied by the feeling of impending doom.
- A person with a specific phobia is fearful of a particular entity or situation. The four categories of phobias are fears of the natural environment, fears related to animals, fear related to medical treatments or issues, and fears related to specific situations.
- OCD involves recurrent obsessions (thoughts), compulsions (behaviors), or both that produce distress and interfere with functioning.
- PTSD and acute stress disorder are clusters of symptoms experienced after a distressing event that is outside the range of normal events.
- Individuals with a somatic symptom disorder, such as conversion disorder or illness anxiety disorder, are convinced that they have serious medical problems despite the absence of concrete medical findings.
- Dissociative disorders involve a change in identity, memory, or consciousness, usually to escape from anxiety.
- Goals for the nursing care of patients with anxiety, somatic symptom disorders, and dissociative disorders are to decrease anxiety to a point at which problem solving can occur and to teach methods such as relaxation techniques to interrupt anxiety as it escalates.

- The term *schizophrenia* refers to a highly problematic group of biologic disorders in which symptoms of psychosis exist, including delusions, hallucinations, marked loosening of associations, catatonia, and flat or inappropriate affect.
- People with major depressive disorder experience a significantly depressed mood for more than 2 weeks accompanied by other physical symptoms.
- People with bipolar disorders experience a significantly elevated (or severely irritable) mood, alternating with significantly depressed mood, or both.
- Neurocognitive disorders include major and mild neurocognitive disorders (dementia) or delirium. These disorders are characterized by cognitive deficits sufficiently severe enough to impair social or occupational functioning. Delirium is rapid in its onset. The dementias are gradual in onset.
- Personality disorders occur when personality traits become inflexible and dysfunctional and are pervasive, chronic, and maladaptive.
- Drug therapy for people with psychiatric disorders uses anxiolytics, antidepressants, antipsychotics, and mood stabilizers.

Additional Learning Resources

SG Go to your Study Guide for additional learning activities to help you master this chapter content.

Go to your Evolve website (http://evolve.elsevier.com/Linton/medsurg) for the following learning resources and much more:
- Fluid & Electrolyte Tutorial
- Review Questions for the NCLEX® Examination

Clinical Judgment and Next-Generation NCLEX® Examination-Style Questions

1. **Which of the following is the primary focus of nursing care for patients with mental illness and their families?**
   1. Helping them to cope with and manage mental illness
   2. Administering medications
   3. Protecting other people from the patient
   4. Controlling the patient's behavior

   NCLEX Client Need: Psychosocial Integrity

2. **Which of the following are important characteristics of a therapeutic relationship? (Select all that apply.)**
   1. The purpose is to benefit both the patient and the nurse.
   2. The relationship has a clear purpose and ending.
   3. The relationship has no clear boundaries.
   4. The relationship develops purposefully.
   5. The nurse's emotional needs are met.

   NCLEX Client Need: Psychosocial Integrity

3. **Which statement best illustrates the strategy of *clarifying* in a nurse-patient interaction?**
   1. "When you mention your son, you look very sad."
   2. "What were you saying while I was on the telephone?"
   3. "Why do you get quiet when I ask about your husband?"
   4. "Are you saying that you are afraid of him?"

   NCLEX Client Need: Psychosocial Integrity

4. **In the mental status examination, the nurse collects data on multiple areas, including which of the following? (Select all that apply.)**
   1. Thought content
   2. Mood and affect
   3. Appearance
   4. Reaction time
   5. Memory and attention

   NCLEX Client Need: Psychosocial Integrity

5. **Mr. Brooks was hospitalized after a major automobile accident in which another person died. Mr. Brooks reports having no sensation in his legs and is unable to move them. Diagnostic studies reveal no physical basis for his symptoms. The patient's symptoms are typical of which of the following?**
   1. Illness anxiety disorder
   2. PTSD
   3. Conversion disorder
   4. Panic disorder

   NCLEX Client Need: Psychosocial Integrity

6. **John is a young college student who has just been diagnosed with schizophrenia. His concerned parents ask for information about his diagnosis. Which reply would be correct and appropriate?**
   1. "Schizophrenia is a mental illness that affects a person's thinking and distorts their view of reality."
   2. "Most people with schizophrenia eventually require permanent care in a psychiatric facility."
   3. "At this time, no medications or treatments are available for schizophrenia."
   4. "Most episodes of schizophrenia resolve within 1 or 2 weeks."

   NCLEX Client Need: Psychosocial Integrity

7. **Nursing interventions to promote communication with the person who has schizophrenia include which of the following? (Select all that apply.)**
   1. Let the patient know that you do not share their delusions
   2. Encourage the patient to attend to activities in the environment
   3. Point out the flaws in the patient's illogical statements
   4. Inform the patient that hallucinations are part of the disease
   5. Ask the patient to explain why they behave as they do

   NCLEX Client Need: Psychosocial Integrity

8. **Several residents in a long-term care facility have been taking a first-generation antipsychotic for a prolonged period of time. Which data should the LVN/LPN collect related to this drug therapy? (Select all that apply.)**
   1. Dry mouth
   2. Shuffling gait
   3. Muscle rigidity
   4. Abnormal movements
   5. Faintness upon changing from a sitting to a standing position

   NCLEX Client Need: Physiological Integrity: Pharmacological Therapies

9. **People who are arrogant, need excessive admiration, and take advantage of others for their own gain may have which type of personality disorder?**

   NCLEX Client Need: Psychosocial Integrity

10. **A patient with bipolar disorder who is taking divalproex (Depakote) is advised that blood samples will be taken periodically to monitor for which adverse effect?**

    1. Liver damage
    2. Dystonic reactions
    3. Kidney damage
    4. Extrapyramidal syndromes

    NCLEX Client Need: Physiological Integrity: Pharmacological Therapies

11. **SLO Objective:** Apply knowledge of anatomy and physiology and pathophysiology to determine which assessment data require follow-up by the nurse.

    NGN Item Type: Enhanced Hot Spot

    Cognitive Skill: Recognize Cues

    A 49-year-old woman comes to the clinic because she is experiencing days when she is so tired that she can't get out of bed. She cries all the time and says that life is not worth living. During the past year she unsuccessfully attempted suicide using medications that she stored up. The patient has been diagnosed with major depression and has not been taking the SSRIs that her psychiatrist has ordered. She doesn't like her psychiatrist, which is why she has come to the general medical clinic. The nurse documents these findings as part of the assessment.

    - Temperature 97° F
    - Pulse 76 beats per minute and regular
    - Respirations 20 breaths per minute
    - Blood pressure 135/80 mm Hg
    - Cries softly with a downcast gaze
    - Appears disheveled, pale
    - Feelings of hopelessness
    - Says life is not worth living
    - Can't remember the names of her medications and is not taking them

    Highlight or place a check mark next to the assessment findings that require follow up by the nurse.

62 Substance-Related and Addictive Disorders

http://evolve.elsevier.com/Linton/medsurg

Objectives

1. Apply the biologic, environmental, and behavioral theories to the risks of substance-related and addictive disorders.
2. Discuss prevention and treatment for substance-related and addictive disorders.
3. Describe the development, course, and outcomes of substance-related disorders.
4. Describe the development, course, and outcomes of gambling addiction.
5. Describe the data to be collected for the nursing assessment of a patient with substance-related and addictive disorders.
6. Describe the patient problems and interventions associated with substance-related and addictive disorders.
7. Discuss populations that present special problems in relation to substance use and gambling addiction.

Key Terms

12-step program
addiction
codependent
comorbidity and dual diagnosis
delirium tremens
tolerance
withdrawal

THE SCIENCE OF ADDICTION

Addiction has become a problem of such worldwide significance since the 1960s that a large amount of energy and financial resources has been targeted toward a better understanding of the disorder. The consequences of addiction affect people of all ages, and the cost in the United States is upward of half a trillion dollars a year, when calculated considering their combined medical, economic, criminal, and social impact. In the United States, drug-involved overdose contributes to the death of more than 70,000 Americans per year (NIDA, 2021). Alcohol related deaths per year in this country are estimated at 95,000 lives lost (68,000 males, 27,000 females) (NIAAA, 2021). Lastly, tobacco is associated with an estimated 480,000 U.S. deaths per year (CDC, 2021). Researchers are attempting to discover the specific causes of substance-related disorders and addiction to prevent and treat them more effectively.

According to the National Institute on Drug Abuse (NIDA), addiction is a "chronic, relapsing brain disease that is characterized by compulsive drug seeking and use, despite harmful consequences." A person with a substance use disorder continues to use a substance despite significant cognitive, behavioral, and physiologic symptoms associated with its use. Research has shown that drugs change the structure of the brain and how it works, and the effects may be long lasting and sometimes irreversible. Addiction also affects behavior to the degree that judgment, decision-making, learning, memory, and self-control are impaired.

The fifth edition of the *Diagnostic and Statistical Manual of Mental Disorders* (DSM-5) describes drug use and addictive disorders as mental illnesses because drugs can cause an intense activation of the brain's reward system leading to neglect of normal activities and behaviors. In addition, the use of some drugs can also cause negative psychologic changes such as anxiety, mood disorders, and psychosis. The diagnosis of the disorder is grouped into four different categories: (1) impaired control, (2) social impairment, (3) risky use, and (4) pharmacologic criteria. Impaired control features the need to increase the amount of substance over a period of time; multiple unsuccessful attempts to decrease or discontinue use; an inordinate amount of time spent obtaining, using, or recovering from the effects of the substance; and an intense craving for the substance. Social impairment consists of a failure to fulfill major role obligations at work, school, or home; continued use of the substance despite social or interpersonal problems; reduced social or recreational activities; and withdrawal from family activities and hobbies to use the substance. Risky use is characterized by continued use despite physically hazardous conditions and despite physical or psychologic problems associated with use. Pharmacologic criteria include increased **tolerance** to the degree that more of the substance is needed to gain the same effect, and **withdrawal** that occurs when blood and tissue levels of the drug decline after prolonged use.

The DSM-5 no longer uses the terms *dependence* and *abuse* in association with substance-related disorders. Rather, the conditions are described in terms of severity based on the number of symptom criteria an individual demonstrates. For example, a mild disorder is indicated by the presence of two to three symptoms, a moderate disorder by four to five symptoms, and a severe disorder by six or more symptoms. It takes time for new terminology to be widely accepted. Therefore many practitioners may still use the more familiar terms *drug abuse* and *addiction* when diagnosing and treating substance-related and addictive disorders.

CAUSE AND RISK FACTORS

In recent years, scientists have studied the effects that drugs have on the brain and behavior and have found that many factors combine to influence whether a person becomes addicted. The biologic makeup of an individual, which can be influenced by gender, ethnicity, developmental stage, and the surrounding environment, may be a major risk factor (Fig. 62.1). Predisposition to addiction differs among individuals, and the more risk factors a person has, the greater the chance for the disease of addiction.

Initially, people may take drugs to feel good or achieve a sense of euphoria, to relieve stress or anxiety, to enhance performance, or—especially among adolescents—in response to peer pressure. Most addictions begin with casual or social use of a drug, leading to habitual and more frequent use. Gradually, there may be a need for larger doses to get high, followed by the need for the drug just to feel good. Finally, it may be increasingly difficult to go without the drug, and individuals may reach the point where they seek and take the drugs despite the problems caused to themselves and loved ones. Stopping may cause intense cravings and withdrawal symptoms.

Biology and Genes

Research completed through family and twin studies support that addictions are heritable (Bevilacqua & Goldman, 2009). Genetic factors account for 40% to 60% of an individual's vulnerability to addiction; in addition, people with mental disorders are at greater risk for substance use disorder and addiction than the general population. Substance use disorders and mental disorders often coexist; mental illnesses may precede addiction or addiction may worsen the mental illness.

Scientists have identified specific areas of the brain where every major drug that is associated with substance use disorders, including opiates, methamphetamine, cocaine, tobacco, alcohol, and marijuana, has its initial effects. With repeated drug exposure, significant disruptions in these brain circuits cause the circuits to "reset," leading to compulsive behavior to seek and use drugs. Thus, the medical community considers addiction to be a chronic medical illness, like those that have the following characteristics: (1) incurability, (2) a genetic predisposition to develop under the right conditions, and (3) a potential to be treated effectively only by total abstinence from the substance that the body cannot handle.

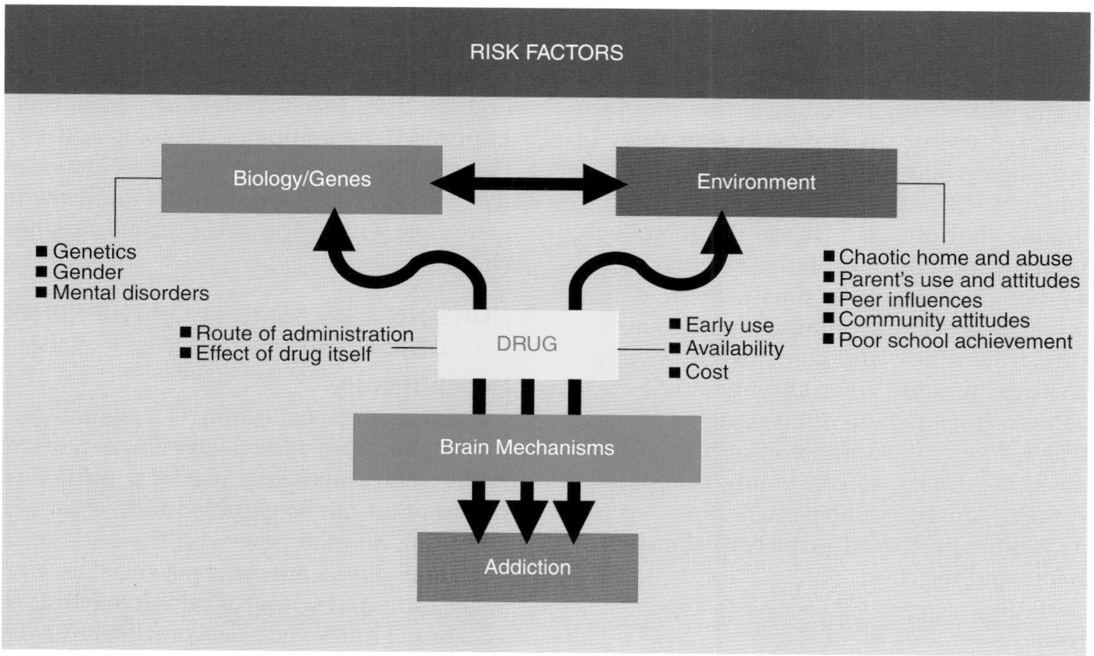

Fig. 62.1 The overall risk for addiction is affected by the biologic makeup of the individual and their surrounding social environment. (Modified from National Institute on Drug Abuse, National Institutes of Health: *Drugs, brain and behavior: the science of addiction*. Washington, DC, 2010, U.S. Department of Health & Human Services.)

Environmental Factors

Major environmental factors that may play a role in the process of becoming addicted are the home environment, and peer and school influences. Children who live in a home where older adults have substance or alcohol use disorders or who engage in criminal behavior may be at increased risk for addiction; in addition, at-risk children may have been subjects of verbal or physical abuse. In adolescence, friends and schoolmates can influence even teens without risk factors to try drugs for the first time. Academic failure and poor social skills can also put a teen at risk for developing an addiction.

The coronavirus disease (SARS-CoV-2 [COVID-19]) pandemic starting in 2019 also affected substance use in this country. Approximately 13% of young adults aged 18 to 24 years reported starting or increasing substance use because of perceived stress, and difficulties with coping (Czeisler et al., 2020). This also disproportionally affected racial/ethnic minorities, essential workers, and unpaid adult caregivers.

The ways in which biologic sex and gender interact with each other and with substance use are complex. Drugs, reasons for use, and consequences frequently vary by sex and gender. Gender is influenced by sociocultural factors, such as expected social roles and behaviors that often differ according to race and class and that can change over time. In general, the overall rate of substance use is greater in males than in females; however, some studies have shown that females demonstrate different reactions to drugs than males in brain responses, risk factors, reasons for abusing prescription drugs, benefits of treatment, and reasons for relapsing.

Many people who live in poverty and in crime-ridden areas use drugs to relieve the stress inherent in these environments. In contrast, it can be observed that individuals with strong religious values that prohibit the excessive use of drugs have lower rates of addiction. Among certain subcultures, the use of certain drugs can be a rite of entry into a gang or a badge of honor proving that one has "made it." In college, students may be exposed to alcohol and other drugs in ways they have not been previously. Binge drinking, for example, is not an uncommon phenomenon in college dorms, fraternities, and sororities, sometimes starting as a rite of initiation. Even among middle-class Americans, the average person often parties to excess on New Year's Eve, for example. Certain cultural groups, such as the Irish, are commonly stereotyped as heavy drinkers. Among country music fans, "crying in your beer" is often portrayed as the typical means of coping with loss and rejection.

Other Factors

Other factors that increase the risk of addiction are early use, availability, cost, and method of administration. Research has shown that the earlier individuals begin to use substances, the more likely they are to develop more serious use disorders. This may be explained by the harmful effect on the developing brain, genetic susceptibility, mental illness, unstable family relationships, and exposure to physical or sexual abuse.

Smoking or injecting a substance into a vein increases its addictive potential. The drug enters the brain within seconds, producing a powerful rush of pleasure or "high" that lasts only a few minutes, followed by a "low" after the drug has worn off. It is thought that addiction results from the need to continually achieve the high associated with the substance used.

Cost and availability of substances also affect predisposition to addiction. The lower the cost and the easier it is to obtain drugs, the more likely a person will become addicted.

COMORBIDITY

Comorbidity, sometimes called **dual diagnosis**, is a term used to describe a situation in which two disorders or illnesses occur in the same person at the same time or when one follows the other. This may result in interactions between the illnesses that affect the course and prognosis of both.

Many people who are addicted to drugs are also diagnosed with mental illnesses and vice versa. Surveys have found that individuals diagnosed with mood or anxiety disorders are almost twice as likely to suffer from a drug use disorder and that individuals diagnosed with drug use disorders are twice as likely to suffer from mood and anxiety disorders. In addition, there is a higher prevalence of smoking among patients with mental disorders. Three possibilities for comorbidity exist: (1) drug use can cause abusers to experience one or more symptoms of another mental illness; (2) mental illness can lead to drug use, particularly as a form of self-medication to relieve symptoms; and (3) both drug use disorders and other mental illnesses are caused by combined biologic and environmental factors. Because there is a high incidence of comorbidity between drug use disorders and mental illness, a comprehensive approach to diagnosis and treatment should be used.

◆ NURSING ASSESSMENT OF THE PERSON WITH AN ADDICTION

Health History

Thorough data collection is essential to initiate the nursing process effectively when working with patients with substance use and addictive disorders. Information can be gathered from a variety of sources, including an interview with the patient, family members, and significant others; a social assessment; medical records; and school or military records. The licensed vocational nurse/licensed practical nurse (LVN/LPN) may participate in the collection of data from these sources. Many people with substance use and addictive disorders have sustained major losses—of jobs, relationships, property, self-esteem, and health. They may face legal charges. Often, they will not seek professional help until they have "hit bottom." Even then, they may seek help only when given an ultimatum of some type, typically from their family, employer, or a court of law.

Questioning the patient produces the most reliable data when the questioning is nonjudgmental, direct, and specific and the answers are verified by more than one source when possible. For example, if the patient reports drinking a couple of beers after work each night, you should ask exactly how many were ingested, how many ounces each contained, or how big the bottle or glass used was. It is also important to know when the patient ingested the drug last and how much was taken to predict the possibility and timing of physical withdrawal symptoms. A nonjudgmental and matter-of-fact manner is the least likely to alienate an already defensive patient. Finding the most appropriate balance of support and reality-based confrontation is a highly developed skill that increases the likelihood that patients will continue in the treatment process. Some team members who work in substance use disorder treatment centers are recovering from addiction themselves, which often helps the client to be more honest and less defensive, and feel less hopeless and alone.

Patterns and consequences of substance use and addictive disorders. The patient who has been abusing one or more substances will describe typical patterns of behavior and a combination of physical or psychologic withdrawal symptoms characteristic of the substances used. A few patients may not experience any physical withdrawal symptoms despite a history of prolonged, frequent, and heavy use, even of some substances that usually are physically addicting. Much depends on the stage of addiction, the habitual patterns of use, the patient's baseline physical status, and the combinations and interactions of the drugs used.

Many people with substance use and addictive disorders experience erratic and unprovoked mood swings. They may describe a lifestyle revolving almost totally around obtaining and using the substance of choice, starting early in the day, often alone, and requiring more of the substance over time to get the desired effects. Many with substance abuse disorders make efforts to hide the extent of their habit from others and, despite their best efforts, have been unsuccessful in limiting use of the substance. Blackouts may have occurred when under the influence of a particular substance (especially alcohol). Blackouts are episodes of amnesia in which the individual does not remember what happened during a period of time. Patients often have significant work problems or damaged relationships as a result of being unable to meet the expectations placed on them.

Defense mechanisms. Typical defense mechanisms used by individuals with substance use and addictive disorders include denial, rationalization, intellectualization, and projection. Denial is readily apparent when patients state that they do not have a problem with drug use despite evidence to the contrary. Individuals also may initially minimize the problems they have had with using drugs. Some deny that they need help in staying clean and sober. Some insist that they do not need to change friends or attend a **12-step program** meeting such as Alcoholics Anonymous (AA) regularly.

Rationalization is a defense mechanism in which addicts attempt to justify the reasons for substance use. This is an "excuse" for addiction. An example is the individual who insists that they had to use heroin because no other way to cope with the pain of a physical injury was available: "The drugs my doctor gave me weren't working."

Intellectualization is closely related to rationalization but differs in that the person focuses only on objective facts as a way of avoiding dealing with unconscious conflicts and the emotions they evoke. For example, an alcoholic who killed someone while driving under the influence of alcohol would be intellectualizing if they stated that it was better that the victim die suddenly rather than live as a paraplegic.

Projection in persons with substance use and addictive disorders involves shifting the blame for their behavior onto someone or something else. Drug users using projection might insist that they became addicted to alcohol as a result of the pressure to drink at work-related social functions to keep colleagues from thinking they were prudes. They also may blame a spouse or loved one.

PHYSICAL EXAMINATION

On physical examination, many people with substance abuse disorders appear malnourished and poorly cared for. Evidence of physical trauma from falls, abrasions, or fights may be present. Jaundice or discolored sclera of the eyes may suggest cirrhosis or other liver problems. Hypertension is a critical sign of withdrawal and is often accompanied by the physical signs of fluid retention in the legs or a protuberant abdomen swollen by liver ascites. Tooth decay and severe gum disease may arise from drug-induced physical changes to the mouth that arise with methamphetamine use. Changes in mental status such as anxiety, confusion, irritability, memory loss, tremors, lack of coordination, and other neurologic signs are significant and may be associated with several causes, including nutritional deficits (see the Nutrition Considerations box). It is important to recognize and report these findings because they may indicate that the patient is entering physical withdrawal and may be at risk for **delirium tremens** (DTs) and seizures if the drug being used is alcohol, a benzodiazepine, or both. Be alert for needle tracks in unexpected parts of the body (e.g., between the toes, in tattoos) in an individual who is believed to have been using substances intravenously. The atypical client may not have any obvious signs of physical problems, but abnormalities may be found on laboratory tests done when the client enters a treatment program.

Nutrition Considerations

1. Heavy drug or alcohol intake has a negative effect on nutrition because it displaces foods in the diet that are more nutritious and impairs absorption and metabolism of nutrients in the body.
2. The nutritional goals for persons with alcoholism are to support them in avoiding alcohol and to correct nutritional deficits.
3. Individuals with chronic alcoholism may need supplements of folate and vitamin B_6.
4. Stimulants may induce anorexia; however, as the effects of the stimulants subside, hunger develops.

DIAGNOSTIC TESTS

To assess the patient's physical status, a thorough physical examination is done on initiation of treatment, along with a basic laboratory screen chosen to identify problems in any of the major organ systems. Abnormalities often are seen on liver function tests, in electrolyte values, and on tests reflecting nutritional status and gastric function. Diseases such as hepatitis B and hepatitis C that can be spread through blood and body fluids may be identified, especially among intravenous drug users. Syphilis rates are increasing, and the escalating rate of HIV infection in this population is of national concern. Infections of various kinds are common. Special neurologic, neuropsychologic, and imaging studies may disclose brain damage from chronic drug use.

BLOOD ALCOHOL STUDY

A blood alcohol study is the most accurate type of test available to measure the degree of intoxication on initiation of treatment for alcohol use. A blood alcohol level greater than 0.3% requires treatment for overdose; at concentrations greater than 0.4%, risk for coma or death markedly rises from suppression of vital life functions. Legal intoxication definitions vary from state to state but are commonly determined when a person's blood alcohol level is greater than 0.05%.

URINE DRUG SCREENING

Urine drug screening is the preferred way to screen for the recent use of an unknown drug and is commonly done along with the initial laboratory work. Drugs that are most likely to be identified in this way on a routine 10-panel drug test can include amphetamines, barbiturates, benzodiazepines, cannabis (marijuana), cocaine ("crack, coke"), opiates, phencyclidine (PCP), lysergic acid diethylamide (LSD), opioid analgesics, sedatives, and stimulants. With this test, drug metabolites can be identified for days or weeks after use, depending on the drug used. A special screen may be necessary when looking for inhalants or anabolic steroids.

Typically, to ensure that tampering with the specimens or substitution of another person's urine has not occurred, a staff member of the same sex witnesses the collection of a urine specimen. After collection, the sample is kept under chain of custody (i.e., each person handling the sample signs a special document that accompanies the sample until it can be analyzed). Any temporary storage of the sample is maintained under secure conditions.

Sometimes a false positive test can occur in which a urine drug screen indicates that an illicit substance was used; however, the results may be attributed to a cross-reactivity of a commonly used medication, food, or substance (such as nonsteroidal antiinflammatory drugs, hemp-containing food, poppy seeds, dextromethorphan). Positive samples may then be sent to a reference laboratory for confirmatory testing.

HAIR ANALYSIS

Hair analysis is a recent addition to the methods for detection of substance use. It requires sensitive technology but may be very helpful in monitoring patients for relapse. Typically, hair samples detect drug use for up to 90 days after only 2 or 3 days of use. However, the presence of addiction or whether the person is currently under the influence of the substance cannot be inferred from a positive finding.

GAMBLING DISORDER

Gambling disorder was added to the DSM-5 list of mental illnesses related to addiction. A gambling disorder is a persistent and recurrent problematic gambling behavior leading to a clinically significant impairment or distress. Gambling involves risking something of value in the hopes of gaining something of greater value, causing disruptions in personal, family, and/or vocational pursuits. An individual needs to gamble with increasing amounts of money to achieve the desired excitement but, after losing the money, often returns on another day to get even ("chasing" one's losses). The person lies to conceal the extent of involvement with gambling and may rely on others to provide money to relieve desperate financial situations caused by the gambling.

The prevalence of gambling disorder is higher in males, lower education and socio-economic status, and youth (Abbott, 2020). Those who have experienced adverse childhood events (trauma and abuse), have feelings of marginalization, and experience psychological distress may also be at greater risk to engage in problematic gambling. The addiction usually develops over a course of years, gradually increasing in frequency and amount. Only about 10% of those with a gambling addiction seek treatment.

PRESCRIPTION DRUG ADDICTION

The nonmedical use of prescription drugs, particularly opioid pain relievers (fentanyl, hydrocodone, oxycodone, methadone, morphine), attention deficit hyperactivity disorder (ADHD) stimulants, and antianxiety drugs, is highest among young adults (18–25 years of age). More males than females use prescription drugs nonmedically. They may use these substances to get high or because the stimulants may help them to study better. Since 1999, 841,000 people have died from a drug overdose and in 2019, 70% of those deaths involved an opioid (CDC, 2021, March 25).

PREVENTION

Because early use of drugs increases a person's risk for addiction, prevention is the best strategy to reduce the possibility of developing a substance-use disorder. National drug use surveys indicate that some children are already addicted to drugs by age 12 or 13 years. Therefore, adolescence is a critical time for preventing drug addiction. Teenagers are still developing judgment and decision-making skills, which limits their ability to assess risks accurately and make sound decisions about drugs. Although alcohol use has decreased among teens, marijuana use has increased, especially among boys. Several principles of prevention can be applied to most substances (see the Health Promotion box).

Health Promotion

Preventing Alcohol Use Among Children

- Alcohol use often begins at an early age, and the proportion of young people who drink frequently or heavily is alarming. The Leadership to Keep Children Alcohol Free initiative is a coalition of federal government agencies and private foundations dedicated to mobilizing resources to combat this public health problem.
- Research has shown that adolescents who abuse alcohol recall 10% less of what they have learned than those who do not drink. Alcohol use also may lead to increased sexual activity, unplanned pregnancy, sexually transmitted infections, criminal activity (including drunk driving), suicide attempts, and other destructive or violent behavior.
- The age at which a person first uses alcohol is a powerful predictor of lifetime alcohol abuse and dependence. An epidemiologic study published in the *Journal of Substance Abuse* found that more than 40% of those who begin drinking before 15 years of age will develop alcohol abuse or alcohol dependence at some time in their lives.

As a health professional, talking to people about this issue will help to keep it high on the public agenda. Here are some suggestions:

- Talk to children about the dangers of early alcohol use. As appropriate, encourage your patients, friends, and neighbors to talk to their children. Some organizations, such as Mothers Against Drunk Driving (MADD) and Students Against Drunk Driving (SADD), provide speakers free of charge.
- Ask other health care professionals, such as pediatric nurses, to discuss alcohol use during children's annual physicals.
- Share literature about preventing alcohol abuse with members of your community.
- Support recreational alternatives to drinking in your community.
- Encourage parents to learn about their responsibilities regarding alcohol access and serving alcohol to minors in their homes.
- Talk to teachers, counselors, school administrators, and school board members to ensure that school prevention programs put equal emphasis on alcohol and illicit drug use.
- Place the issue of alcohol use by children on agendas for meetings of the parent-teacher association, the city council, faith groups, the Rotary Club, the local chamber of commerce, and other community groups and organizations.
- Involve young people in peer support roles in your community's prevention efforts.
- Write letters to the editors of your local newspapers asking them to print articles about the dangers of early alcohol use.
- Contact elected and appointed officials at local and state levels to inform them about the problem and what can be done to solve it.
- Enlist support for immediate and consistent enforcement of underage alcohol-related drinking laws in your community.

Modified from National Institute on Alcohol Abuse and Alcoholism, National Institutes of Health: Leadership to keep children alcohol free. In Keep kids alcohol free: *strategies for action.* Available at https://files.eric.ed.gov/fulltext/ED496019.pdf

TREATMENT

Addiction is a treatable disease that can be managed successfully like other chronic illnesses. According to NIDA, key principles have emerged based on scientific research since the 1970s, as follows:

- Addiction is a complex but treatable disease that affects brain function and behavior.
- No single treatment is appropriate for everyone.
- Treatment needs to be readily available.
- Effective treatment attends to multiple needs of the individual, not just to their drug abuse.
- Remaining in treatment for an adequate period of time is critical.
- Counseling—individual and/or group—and other behavioral therapies are the most commonly used forms of addiction therapy.

- Medications are an important element of treatment for many patients, especially when combined with counseling and other behavioral therapies.
- An individual's treatment and service plan must be assessed continually and modified as necessary to ensure that it meets their changing needs.
- Many drug-addicted individuals also have other mental disorders.
- Medically assisted detoxification is only the first stage of addiction treatment and by itself does little to change long-term drug abuse.
- Treatment does not need to be voluntary to be effective.
- Drug use during treatment must be monitored continuously, as lapses during treatment do occur.
- Treatment programs should assess patients for the presence of human immunodeficiency virus/acquired immunodeficiency syndrome (HIV/AIDS), hepatitis B and C, tuberculosis, and other infectious diseases as well as provide targeted risk-reduction counseling to help patients modify or change behaviors that place them at risk of contracting or spreading infection.

SUBSTANCE-RELATED DISORDERS

In DSM-5, 10 separate classes of drugs associated with substance-related disorders are identified: (1) alcohol, (2) caffeine, (3) cannabis (marijuana), (4) hallucinogens, (5) inhalants, (6) opioids, (7) sedatives, hypnotics, and anxiolytics, (8) stimulants, (9) tobacco, and (10) other or unknown substances (Table 62.1).

ALCOHOL AND ALCOHOLISM

Alcoholism is the most common drug-related disorder in the United States. According to the American Society of Addiction Medicine, alcoholism is:

> *A primary, chronic disease with psychosocial and environmental factors influencing its development and manifestations. The disease is often progressive and fatal. It is characterized by continuous or periodic impaired control over drinking, preoccupation with the drug alcohol, use of alcohol despite adverse consequences, and distortions in thinking, most notably denial.*

Environmental risks for the disease are cultural attitudes toward drinking, availability, peer pressure, and ineffective coping with stress. Genetic predisposition accounts for 40% to 60% of the risk for alcoholism, and males have higher rates of alcohol-related disorders than do females. However, females may develop higher blood alcohol levels per drink than males because they have more fat and less water in their bodies and metabolize less alcohol in their esophagus and stomach.

Pharmacology Capsule

The American Society of Addiction Medicine defines alcohol as a *drug* because it has addictive qualities like those associated with other drug-related disorders. Simple intoxication from alcohol usually lasts less than 12 hours and is followed by the unpleasant experience of a hangover beginning about 4 to 6 hours after the last drink. Typical symptoms include headache, upset stomach, vomiting, sweating, thirst, fatigue, and blurred vision or "seeing stars." The cause of these symptoms has not been pinpointed; however, it is believed to be a result of hypoglycemia, dehydration, and the buildup of acetaldehyde and lactic acid in the blood.

Chronic use involves the regular daily ingestion of large quantities of alcohol, regular heavy drinking only on weekends, or binges of heavy drinking followed by long periods of abstinence. Physical addiction occurs when alcohol becomes integrated into physiologic processes at the cellular level. The cell becomes dependent on the alcohol to carry on certain metabolic processes; if alcohol is no longer available, the cell goes into "shock" and is unable to compensate for the loss quickly. Thus, alcohol withdrawal syndrome begins after the individual stops or decreases the amount ingested. Heavy chronic drinkers may experience the onset of withdrawal without stopping drinking because they are no longer able to ingest enough alcohol to meet the body's demands for the substance to function.

Alcohol withdrawal syndrome involves physiologic and behavioral symptoms that begin when the individual's blood alcohol level drops. It is divided into two stages, depending on the onset and severity of symptoms. The first stage usually occurs within 6 to 12 hours after the last drink and is called *early withdrawal.* Symptoms begin with anxiety, agitation, and irritability. If the patient does not drink, tremors may be observed. Blood pressure (BP), pulse, and temperature all begin to rise. Sweating, nausea, vomiting, and diarrhea are typical.

The second stage, *major withdrawal,* begins with the onset of seizures and hallucinations and can advance to life-threatening delirium tremens. This stage usually occurs after approximately 3 days (sometimes less) without alcohol or treatment and can be predicted from extreme elevations in temperature, pulse, and BP. The patient typically becomes disoriented and confused. Hallucinations are often visual and "animal" in nature. Bugs, snakes, and rats are commonly described, sometimes perceived to be crawling on the person. Familiar jokes about seeing "pink elephants" probably evolved out of this type of withdrawal experience.

Alcohol withdrawal is the most life-threatening withdrawal syndrome compared with those associated with other types of drugs, even heroin. (Withdrawal from barbiturates and benzodiazepines can also result in delirium tremens; both types of drugs have similar central nervous system [CNS] depressant effects.)

Table 62.1 Common Mood-Altering Chemicals

DRUG NAME	EFFECTS	SITE OF ACTION	LENGTH OF EFFECT
Alcohol			
Alcohol, beer, wine (as beverages)	Relaxation, sedation, release of inhibitions, objective signs (i.e., incoordination, nausea, vomiting, slurred speech)	Central nervous system (CNS), respiratory system	Onset: 20 minutes to 1 hour Duration: dose-related
Caffeine			
Coffee, tea, chocolate, caffeinated drinks	Stimulation, restlessness, anxiety, objective signs (i.e., increased heart and respiratory rates, diarrhea, gastric disorder, insomnia, tremors)	CNS	Onset: 10 to 30 minutes Duration: 3 to 7 hours
Cannabis			
Marijuana, hashish	Failure in judgment and memory, euphoria, mild intoxication, relaxation, sexual arousal, panic states, visual hallucinations, objective signs (i.e., reddened eyes, dry mouth, incoordination, heart rate to 140 beats per minute)	CNS, cardiovascular system, respiratory system	Onset: 20 to 30 minutes Duration: 3 to 7 hours (Administration- and dose-dependent)
Hallucinogens			
Psilocybin ("magic" mushrooms), lysergic acid diethylamide (LSD), mescaline (from peyote cactus), dimethoxymethamphetamine (DOM), STP (no chemical name), 3,4-methylenedioxyamphetamine (MDMA, ecstasy)	Altered body image, euphoria, sharpened perceptions, somatic effects (i.e., dizziness, tremors, weakness, nausea), psychosis-like symptoms, emotional swings, suspiciousness, bizarre behavior, increased blood pressure (BP), increased temperature, objective signs (i.e., dilated pupils, flushing, tremors)	CNS	Onset: 40 to 60 minutes Duration: 6 to 12 hours
Hallucinogens			
Phencyclidine (PCP, "angel dust")	Detachment from surroundings, decreased sensory awareness, illusions of superhuman strength, acute intoxication, objective signs (i.e., flushing, fever, sweating, coma, agitation, confusion, hallucinations, paranoia, violence)	CNS	Onset: 2 to 3 minutes, up to 45 minutes (rapid onset) Duration: drug- and dose-related
Inhalants			
Benzene (paint thinner, cleaning fluid, glue), nitrites, nitrous oxide	Euphoria, giddiness, headache, fatigue, drowsiness, objective signs (i.e., dysrhythmias, damage to kidneys, liver abnormalities)	CNS, cardiac effect	Onset: immediate Duration: 20 to 45 minutes

Continued

Table 62.1 Common Mood-Altering Chemicals—cont'd

DRUG NAME	EFFECTS	SITE OF ACTION	LENGTH OF EFFECT
Opioids, Semisynthetics, and Synthetic Analgesics			
Codeine, morphine, heroin, hydromorphone (Dilaudid), methadone, meperidine (Demerol), propoxyphene (Darvon), designer drugs	Analgesia, euphoria, escape, reduced sexual and aggressive drives, respiratory depression, sedation, sleepiness, objective signs (i.e., hypertension, pupillary constriction, constipation)	CNS (opioid receptors), respiratory system	Onset: 20 to 30 minutes Duration: 4 to 8 hours
Sedatives, Hypnotics, and Anxiolytics			
Barbiturates (secobarbital [Seconal], phenobarbital [Nembutal], amobarbital [Amytal], amobarbital/secobarbital [Tuinal]) Barbiturate-like agents (methaqualone [Quaalude]) Benzodiazepines (alprazolam [Xanax], chlordiazepoxide [Librium], diazepam [Valium], lorazepam [Ativan])	Drowsiness, sedation, euphoria, escape, loss of aggressive and sexual drives, emotional lability, poor judgment	CNS, cardiovascular system, respiratory system	Onset: 30 to 40 minutes Duration: varies with each drug (barbiturates may have longer half-life than benzodiazepines, depending on the drug.)
Stimulants			
Amphetamine (methamphetamine, Dexedrine, Benzedrine), methylphenidate (Ritalin), cocaine, crack	Euphoria, grandiosity, wakefulness, relief of fatigue, stimulation, energy, anxiety, depression, suppression of appetite, aggressive feelings, paranoia, objective signs (i.e., sweating, dilated pupils, increased BP, rapid heart and respiratory rates, tremors, seizures)	CNS, peripheral nervous system, cardiovascular system	Onset: 10 to 30 minutes (route-related) Duration: drug-related
Nicotine			
Cigarettes, smokeless tobacco	Stimulation, enhanced performance	CNS, respiratory system, cardiovascular system, endocrine system	Onset: immediate Duration: 5 to 15 minutes

From Naegle MA: Substance-related disorders. In Haber J, Krainovich B, McMahon AL, et al., editors: *Comprehensive psychiatric nursing*, ed 5, St. Louis, 1997, Mosby.

Thus, it is critical to counsel alcoholics never to attempt to withdraw on their own or "go cold turkey." They always should seek medical treatment. Most require inpatient hospitalization and administration of medications such as lorazepam (Ativan) or chlordiazepoxide (Librium) to prevent the severe consequences of withdrawal and to ensure early detection and treatment of symptoms. When any patient is hospitalized for non–substance-related causes, be sure to directly discuss prior alcohol use. If a heavy drinker suddenly stops ingesting alcohol during their stay, they can experience seizures as well.

Medical Complications

Common medical complications of chronic alcoholism include cirrhosis of the liver, pancreatitis, gastrointestinal (GI) bleeding (often from esophageal varices), Wernicke encephalopathy, Korsakoff psychosis, and fetal alcohol syndrome.

Wernicke encephalopathy. Wernicke encephalopathy is caused by vitamin B_1 (thiamine) deficiency. Its symptoms include delirium, confabulation because of memory loss, unsteady gait, a sense of apprehension, and altered levels of consciousness that can proceed to coma. If it is not properly treated with vitamin supplementation, Korsakoff psychosis may develop.

Korsakoff psychosis. In this disorder, both thiamine and niacin deficiencies contribute to the degeneration of the cerebrum and the peripheral nervous system. Symptoms include amnesia, confabulation, disorientation, and peripheral neuropathies. Despite treatment, some residual problems persist in both Wernicke encephalopathy and Korsakoff psychosis. However, dementia is permanent if the patient progresses to Korsakoff psychosis. Both disorders are classified as *alcohol amnesic disorders*.

Fetal alcohol syndrome. Fetal alcohol syndrome is a medical complication that is of great concern in many countries. If a woman drinks alcohol during pregnancy, the unborn child is at risk for symptoms such as low birth weight, mental retardation, growth deficiencies, heart defects, facial malformations, learning disabilities, and hyperactivity. Recent controversy has arisen over whether maternal alcoholism constitutes child abuse and is thus reportable under child protection statutes.

Treatment for Alcohol Addiction

Because alcoholism affects everyone in the family system, active family involvement in the treatment of an alcohol-related disorder has come to be seen as a critical factor in the success of treatment outcomes. Alcoholism often produces predictable patterns of individual behavior or changes in roles that may significantly handicap various family members in getting their needs met. Examples of some of the labels given to these atypical roles are the hero, the mascot, the lost child, and the scapegoat. Adult children of alcoholics may struggle with issues throughout their lives as a result of dysfunctional patterns of thoughts and behaviors learned in childhood through the enactment of these types of roles. Spouses of alcoholics frequently struggle with "enabling" behaviors. These are described as any behavior that "covers up" or protects alcoholics from the consequences of their drinking behaviors. For example, a woman might lie to her husband's boss about why he will not be at work, when the husband is too "hung over" to perform adequately. Those who enable are sometimes considered **codependent**, in that their behavior is highly structured around managing and adapting to the alcoholic's dysfunctional behavior.

Family, peer pressure, and confrontation can be critical factors in inducing the alcoholic to seek treatment. Through participation in a 12-step self-help support group for the significant others of persons with a substance use disorder, called *Al-Anon* and *Alateen*, spouses, children, friends, and coworkers can learn new ways of coping with issues and how to avoid enabling the alcoholic so that it becomes harder for them to continue the destructive pattern of drinking.

Intervention. An intervention is a planned, structured meeting by family and friends to confront the alcoholic with the effect that the person's alcohol use has on each member of the group. Often the alcoholic or substance user is brought into the meeting without prior notification about the intervention. The intervention is led by a specially trained interventionist who helps those involved in the process to prepare by writing down the ways in which the person's alcohol use affects them personally. The interventionist offers suggestions on how to word ideas in ways less likely to evoke defensiveness and how to focus on the issues to reject the problem drinking but not the person. During the intervention, all the participants have an opportunity to read their letters aloud to the alcohol user. At the end of each letter, the reader requests that the alcoholic go into treatment to get help. Usually, after experiencing a confrontation from a roomful of significant people, users will go unhappily, but voluntarily, directly from the intervention into a treatment program that has been arranged for in advance.

The use of this strategy has come under criticism because the user confronted in this way often feels coerced into treatment. After the intervention, the user may harbor angry feelings directed at members of the family for being critical, pushy, and having "tricked" them. Ideally, for treatment to be most effective, individuals should choose to go voluntarily. Proponents of the use of intervention respond that the user may die or suffer terrible consequences of the disease before seeking help on a totally voluntary basis, and thus the end justifies the means.

Detoxification. Detoxification is usually done in an inpatient hospital or rehabilitation center. During detoxification, the patient's vital signs are monitored frequently. The Clinical Institute Withdrawal Assessment for Alcohol–Revised (CIWA-Ar) is a ten-item scale of common symptoms that may be completed by nurses to assess alcohol withdrawal. The CIWA-Ar can be completed in about 5 minutes and assesses symptoms such as nausea and vomiting, anxiety, tremor, sweating, auditory disturbances, visual disturbances, tactile disturbances, headache, agitation, and clouding of sensorium. Drugs from the anxiolytic (benzodiazepine) group are most often used in detoxification of the alcohol-dependent patient. The two most common benzodiazepines used to treat acute alcohol withdrawal are lorazepam (Ativan) and diazepam (Valium). Intravenous magnesium sulfate may be used to prevent seizures in rare cases. Scheduled anticonvulsant agents are prescribed if seizures occur. Fluids are encouraged to combat dehydration, and vitamin replacement therapy is instituted. Rest and nutrition are emphasized. Initially, patients do not participate in group therapy because of their physical status but once stabilized may benefit from supportive services and counseling.

Rehabilitation. Once patients are medically stable, they are referred to either an inpatient or an outpatient treatment program, depending on individual needs and resources. The traditional inpatient programs typically can last from 30, 60, or 90 days and can include highly structured scheduling of drug education films and presentations; increasingly confrontational individual, group, and family therapy; recreational and occupational therapy; milieu therapy; motivational interviewing approach, and introduction to AA or other self-help support group. New tools are currently being developed for diagnosis and treatment of addiction including deoxyribonucleic acid (DNA) testing and treatments focused on specific areas of the brain. The availability of third-party reimbursement for an inpatient rehabilitation stay varies among facilities. Patients may also be referred to partial hospitalization programs (day treatment programs) and outpatient therapy as well as to other community resources. Less common is an extended residential program in therapeutic communities that may last 180 days or longer.

Alcoholics Anonymous. AA is a nonprofit, worldwide organization of alcoholics who meet anonymously in small groups at various times during the day throughout the year to assist one another in staying sober. The organization uses a strong spiritual base, which is controversial, and a 12-step program (Box 62.1) involving discussions and written exercises designed around each of the 12 steps as a means of keeping the alcoholic from relapsing. Members identify another participant of the same sex who is seasoned in the recovery process, and to whom they can relate, to act as their sponsor. The sponsor agrees to be available to the person for support and advice in staying sober. Service work in the community is also seen as integral to focusing outside oneself.

Members use regular readings from *Alcoholics Anonymous*, known as 'The Big Book', written by founding members to keep them on track (Box 62.2 lists the 12 traditions of AA). No dues are required from AA members; instead, the organization relies on donations. In addition, AA has no political affiliations and makes no endorsements of candidates or products. Everyone involved participates on a voluntary basis. Even group leaders are volunteers and are not professional counselors. Meetings may be advertised in the community using the title "Friends of Bill W." as a means of maintaining the anonymity of participants (Bill W. was one of two originators of the organization). Before discharge from an inpatient treatment program, alcoholics can attend various community AA meetings to increase the odds of continued outpatient participation and to begin the process of finding a "home group" to which they can connect.

Recently, research has begun to question what works in alcohol rehabilitation. Actual outcomes of the traditional types of treatment approaches have not been documented clearly. As a result, many insurance companies no longer fund 30-day inpatient treatment. Many 30-day inpatient treatment programs have been forced to close because of a lack of clients able to afford the cost of this intensive treatment. Treatment facilities have been forced to provide brief and creative

Box 62.1 Twelve Steps of Alcoholics Anonymous

1. We admit we were powerless over alcohol—our lives had become unmanageable.
2. Came to believe that a Power greater than ourselves could restore us to sanity.
3. Made a decision to turn our will and lives over to the care of God, as we understood Him.
4. Made a searching and fearless moral inventory of ourselves.
5. Admitted to God, to ourselves, and to another human being the exact nature of our wrongs.
6. Were entirely ready to have God remove all these defects of character.
7. Humbly asked Him to remove our shortcomings.
8. Listed all persons we had harmed and became willing to make amends to them all.
9. Made direct amends whenever possible, except when to do so would injure them or others.
10. Continued to make personal inventory and when we were wrong promptly admitted it.
11. Sought through prayer and meditation to improve our conscious contact with God, as we understood Him, praying only for knowledge of His will for us and the power to carry it out.
12. Having had a spiritual awakening as the result of these steps, we tried to carry this message to alcoholics and to practice these principles in all our affairs.

inpatient rehabilitation with rapid referral to an outpatient program and aftercare.

One trend is toward using more nontraditional treatment approaches that have produced successful outcomes. Some components of alcohol rehabilitation that have been shown to be very useful in maintaining continued sobriety are the teaching of stress management, social skills training, behavioral approaches, marital therapy, and matching clients with a therapist who uses a style most likely to benefit their personality type. A move is also underway in which treatment programs are attempting to group patients with similar lifestyles and characteristics together rather than to group everyone together. Other factors being considered in developing more homogeneous small groups are styles of thinking (abstract versus concrete thinkers), sex role–related issues, ethnicity, and age. The current trend is away from a "cookie cutter" approach to treatment that is expected to work for anyone who

Box 62.2 Twelve Traditions of Alcoholics Anonymous

1. Our common welfare should come first; personal recovery depends on Alcoholics Anonymous (AA) unity.
2. For our group purpose, there is but one ultimate authority—a loving God as He may express Himself in our group conscience. Our leaders are but trusted servants; they do not govern.
3. The only requirement for AA membership is a desire to stop drinking.
4. Each group should be autonomous except in matters affecting other groups or AA as a whole.
5. Each group has but one primary purpose—to carry its message to the alcoholic who still suffers.
6. An AA group ought never endorse, finance, or lend the AA name to any related facility or outside enterprise, lest problems of money, property, and prestige divert us from our primary purpose.
7. Every AA group ought to be fully self-supporting, declining outside contributions.
8. AA should remain forever nonprofessional, but our service centers may employ special workers.
9. AA, as such, ought never be organized; but we may create service boards or committees directly responsible to those they serve.
10. AA has no opinion on outside issues; hence the AA name ought never be drawn into public controversy.
11. Our public relations policy is based on attraction rather than promotion; we need always maintain personal anonymity at the level of press, radio, and films.
12. Anonymity is the spiritual foundation of all our traditions, ever reminding us to place principles before personalities.

is an alcoholic (see Nursing Care Plan: Patient Who Is Abusing Alcohol).

Cost containment has stimulated the development of many new types of outpatient programs for the treatment of alcoholism. Most day treatment or partial hospitalization programs are very similar to the traditional inpatient milieu and offer similar types of therapies, but they allow patients to return to their own homes at night. In this case, the risk of relapse often requires the use of medication such as disulfiram (Antabuse) or metronidazole (Flagyl), which makes the user ill if mixed with alcohol. Usually, involvement in the program is intensive but does not last for the traditional 30 days.

Other individuals use active involvement in AA as the primary means for recovery by attending at least 90 meetings in 90 days. Other community programs also are available to assist the alcoholic in the recovery process and should not be overlooked. Some are church related; some are focused on getting the recovering user back to work by providing job placement or an opportunity to return to school. One example of a community recovery program that exists in various parts of the country is the Patrician Movement. In addition, halfway houses may be available in the local area as a service of community mental health organizations.

Relapse prevention. Relapse prevention is a key component in the treatment of persons with substance use disorder. Relapse prevention involves assisting patients to identify triggers to their substance use. For example, a person may identify friends who consistently use the abused substance or may identify places where drinking or using occurs. The person then recognizes that being with those friends or in those places sets them up to drink or use. As part of the relapse prevention strategy, the person then actively avoids those people and places. Other coping strategies are developed that can be used if the person encounters a trigger.

Aftercare and recovery. One of the newer aspects of the recovery process involves various types of aftercare services to assist alcoholics who have completed a treatment program successfully to make a gradual transition back into the community with the support necessary to prevent relapses. Many inpatient substance disorder use programs now provide aftercare groups to discharged patients as a supplement to continued involvement in AA and other 12-step support groups such as Adult Children of Alcoholics and Co-Dependents Anonymous.

Medications. The treatment team may recommend the use of disulfiram (Antabuse) to assist a patient who is highly motivated to remain sober but who recognizes that poor impulse control may increase the odds of relapse. Disulfiram inhibits the metabolism of alcohol in the body, producing an uncomfortable, potentially life-threatening reaction to exposure to alcohol. This medication is taken daily and lasts in the body for up to 2 weeks. If there is an urge to drink, the presence of the drug in the system usually provides the necessary negative reinforcement to resist that impulse. Signs and symptoms of a disulfiram-alcohol reaction include flushing, headache, nausea, vomiting, dizziness, rapid heart rate, difficulty breathing, sweating, confusion, and hypotension that may lead to coma, convulsions, and death. The severity of the symptoms varies from person to person and symptoms can last for 30 to 60 minutes or more.

Naltrexone (Revia) is a newer medication used to treat cravings or desires for alcohol once the individual

Nursing Care Plan Patient Who Is Abusing Alcohol

FOCUSED ASSESSMENT

Health History

A 37-year-old man was admitted for alcohol detoxification. He was found lying on the floor at home, unconscious, and appeared to have vomited and been incontinent of urine and feces. He has a long history of alcohol use but claims that he does not have a problem because he drinks only beer. He recently lost his job because he was not reporting for work on time, and his wife has threatened to leave him if he does not stop drinking. His two children, 8 and 10 years of age, are afraid of him when he drinks. His usual intake of alcohol is two six-packs of beer a day. He has been detoxified in the hospital and is now ready for the rehabilitation phase of his treatment.

Physical Examination Vital signs: blood pressure 128/72 mm Hg; pulse 80 beats per minute; respiration 20 breaths per minute; temperature 97.6°F (36.4°C), measured orally. Height 5′10″, weight 160 lb. The patient's skin and eyes have a slightly yellowish tinge. There is a cast on his left arm from below the elbow to the fingers. He appears thin and wasted.

Patient Problems	Goals and Outcome Criteria	Interventions
Denial related to continued alcohol use	The patient will acknowledge that he has a problem, stop ingesting alcohol, and attend Alcoholics Anonymous (AA) meetings on a regular basis.	Use confrontational techniques to help the patient accept the diagnosis of alcoholism and support his 12-step program of rehabilitation.
Inadequate coping related to alcohol ingestion as a means of coping with stressors	The patient will overcome his impulse to drink alcohol until intoxicated and to use alcohol as a coping mechanism, as evidenced by stopping ingestion of alcohol and substituting other coping mechanisms.	Help the patient to overcome cravings by introducing new coping mechanisms such as exercise and stress management skills. Encourage him to attend his treatment program and AA meetings on a regular basis.
Chronic altered self-concept related to loss of control, guilty feelings	The patient will maintain a satisfactory self-concept, as evidenced by lessened self-criticism, good hygiene, and positive interactions with others. The patient will develop a realistic sense of self, verbalize positive aspects of self and begin to forgive himself, and express his true feelings.	Help the patient to maintain a satisfactory self-concept after confrontational therapy sessions by allowing him to vent his feelings and acting as a role model for dealing with others. Allow the patient to vent his feelings about his illness and to explore his feelings about his past behaviors. Support the patient in his 12-step program of rehabilitation.
Potential for injury related to excessive use of alcohol and high risk for relapse	The patient will not injure himself or others as a result of excessive ingestion of alcohol.	Encourage the patient to abstain from drinking by supporting his participation in rehabilitation activities. Intervene at the first signs of impending relapse.

CRITICAL THINKING QUESTIONS

1. Describe two techniques you might use to help the patient vent his feelings.
2. Describe in detail two coping mechanisms that may help the patient to overcome cravings for alcohol.

has quit drinking. It is believed that this medication helps to reduce the desire to drink by blocking receptors in the brain responsible for taking up opiates and resulting in euphoria. Naltrexone is an opioid antagonist that acts at opiate receptors to competitively inhibit the effects of opiate agonists. It has no analgesic activity of its own. This medication is not a cure for alcoholism; however, clinical trials have demonstrated an increase in the number of days sober after quitting alcohol compared with those who attempted to abstain from alcohol without this medication. Studies have demonstrated the effectiveness of treatment with this medication combined with psychosocial treatments such as individual psychotherapy. Side effects may include nausea, headache, constipation, dizziness, nervousness, insomnia, drowsiness, or anxiety. Patients should be warned to avoid opioid analgesics such as codeine, hydrocodone, oxycodone, morphine, hydromorphone, and heroin. Patients must wait 7 to 10 days after taking opioids before taking naltrexone or risk acute withdrawal symptoms.

Pharmacology Capsule

Disulfiram (Antabuse) is sometimes used to assist a recovering alcoholic who is highly motivated to remain sober but who recognizes that poor impulse control may increase the odds of relapse.

Pharmacology Capsule

Naltrexone (Revia) does not cure alcoholism but may help to decrease the desire to drink, thereby extending the length of time an individual maintains sobriety. Patients must wait 7 to 10 days after discontinuing opioids before starting this medication and may not use opioids of any kind while on naltrexone.

Pharmacology Capsule

To avoid a disulfiram-alcohol reaction, patients who are taking disulfiram (Antabuse) must be instructed to avoid alcohol in foods (e.g., sauces, candies), topical preparations (e.g., cologne, aftershave), mouthwashes, and medications (e.g., over-the-counter [OTC] cold preparations, cough syrup).

The danger of giving disulfiram to a person who is poorly motivated to stop drinking is that they might either stop taking the medication or drink despite taking the medication and become seriously ill. As a result, careful patient teaching is essential. The patient must be taught to avoid alcohol in foods (e.g., salad dressings, sauces, candies, chocolate prepared with liqueurs), topical preparations (e.g., cologne, aftershave, liniments), medications (e.g., over-the-counter [OTC] cold preparations or cough syrups), and mouthwashes containing alcohol. Alcohol wipes cannot be used by the nurse to cleanse the skin in preparation for an injection without a topical reaction. Because of the risks of accidental exposure to a substance containing alcohol, patients are encouraged to wear a medical alert bracelet or carry a card in their wallets to alert emergency care personnel to a possible disulfiram-alcohol reaction if they are found unconscious. Patients also are asked to sign a consent form for the use of the drug before it is prescribed to document those proper instructions about diet, risks, precautions, and type of emergency care needed in the event of exposure to alcohol have been offered and are understood. It is important for the nurse to be alert for patient attempts to bypass the prohibitive effects of disulfiram by ingesting large doses of vitamin C to have a drink on occasion. Patients who are addicted are often very knowledgeable about drug treatment and can easily find out that massive doses of vitamin C are given intravenously for the treatment of overdose or disulfiram-alcohol reaction.

Pharmacology Capsule

Do not use alcohol to cleanse injection sites if the patient is taking disulfiram (Antabuse).

The use of disulfiram is contraindicated in individuals with impaired liver function, heart problems, or significant debilitation. Obviously, safe use of the drug also requires that the person have no memory impairments, self-destructive intentions, or poor judgment.

Sometimes, metronidazole (Flagyl) is used for similar purposes because it also produces an uncomfortable reaction when combined with alcohol but does not produce the severe life-threatening reactions described for disulfiram. In addition, it does not remain in the system for an extended period and can be given in the event of many medical problems for which disulfiram is contraindicated.

Research efforts continue to attempt to identify other types of drugs that could assist alcoholics to go through withdrawal more comfortably and avoid relapse. Medications currently under scrutiny for this purpose include naltrexone hydrochloride (Trexan); antidepressants such as amitriptyline hydrochloride (Elavil), gabapentin (Neurontin), desipramine hydrochloride (Norpramin), and fluoxetine hydrochloride (Prozac); and angiotensin-converting enzyme (ACE) inhibitors such as enalapril maleate (Vasotec).

CAFFEINE

Caffeine is derived from coffee, tea leaves, kola nuts, and cocoa beans, and the content varies among varieties of food. OTC pain relievers, cold medications, and diet pills and even decaffeinated coffee may contain caffeine. Because caffeine is a central nervous system stimulant, regular use may cause mild physical dependence, altering mood and behavior; however, there are few health and adverse social consequences compared with other addictive substances. Withdrawal occurs within 12 to 24 hours after stopping caffeine intake and may lead to mild to moderate withdrawal symptoms, including headache, fatigue, anxiety, irritability, depressed mood, and difficulty concentrating.

CANNABIS (MARIJUANA)

Marijuana, "pot," "weed," "grass," or "hemp" is a mixture of dried leaves, stems, seeds, and flowers of the *Cannabis* or hemp plant. The drug is smoked or taken orally in capsules or food. Individuals experience heightened awareness; euphoria, followed by drowsiness or relaxation; impaired short-term memory, attention, judgment, coordination, and balance; increased heart rate; and increased appetite. Marijuana is psychologically addicting in about 9% of its users. Controversy persists about the negative effects of chronic use of this drug. Long-term use in vulnerable individuals is associated with mental disorders such as schizophrenia, depression, and anxiety as well as memory loss. In the medical community, derivatives of marijuana show promise as medication for the treatment of glaucoma, asthma, nausea and vomiting as a result of chemotherapy, and as an appetite stimulant.

HALLUCINOGENS

Hallucinogens include lysergic acid diethylamide (LSD or "acid"), phencyclidine (PCP or "angel dust"), and 3,4-methylenedioxymethamphetamine (MDMA or "ecstasy" and "Adam").

Lysergic Acid Diethylamide

LSD is not physically addicting but can produce physical symptoms of altered perceptions that are dreamlike, often with an altered sense of time and feelings that one has attained special insight. Emotions are intensified and labile. Individuals often experience depersonalization, in which they feel as if they are floating outside of themselves or in unreal surroundings. The drugs are typically used to enhance self-awareness and are usually taken episodically (approximately twice a week). Acute adverse reactions are most often described as a "bad trip" involving paranoia, depression, frightening hallucinations, and confusion. The person experiencing a bad trip is responsive to verbal support and reassurance. The primary danger of the use of these drugs is accidental death as a result of perceptual distortions (e.g., attempting to fly off a building) or seizures related to the cutting agent used. Cutting agents are chemicals that may be quite toxic, which are used in the manufacturing or dilution of the final drug product. Chronic long-term adverse reactions include psychosis, depression, paranoia, and flashbacks. LSD use is regaining popularity.

Phencyclidine

PCP differs from other hallucinogens in that users experience a psychotic state like that observed in schizophrenics. Brain reward areas are stimulated so that users can stimulate themselves mentally in a pleasurable way. Studies also suggest that this drug is strongly physically addictive, with a severe withdrawal reaction occurring after binge use. Unexpected sensory stimuli that interrupt the individual's internal experience may provoke unpredictable violence. The person may possess enormous strength and may feel no pain. The risks of use thus involve serious injury to oneself or others, in addition to severely elevated temperature, hypertensive crisis, and renal failure. Under acute intoxication, patients are best managed by reducing stimuli as much as possible, often by seclusion, even to the point of avoiding talking or performing routine treatments until the patient is stabilized. If violent, mechanical restraint is necessary.

INHALANTS

A very dangerous type of substance use involves misuse of four general categories of inhalants: volatile solvents, aerosols, gases, and nitrites. Examples of chemicals often inhaled for the mind-altering response include paint, glue, aerosol sprays, Wite-Out correction fluid, and gasoline. These products usually are inhaled after being placed in a plastic bag or other container that is placed over the nose and mouth, a process also known as *huffing*. Symptoms appearing in the individual under the influence of the drug depend on the substance inhaled and include nosebleeds, bloodshot eyes, infected lesions around the nose and mouth, and severe disorientation or unconsciousness. The risks include progressive brain damage, asphyxiation, seizures, depressed bone marrow leading to aplastic anemia, liver or kidney damage, or cardiac dysrhythmias. No physical withdrawal syndrome is seen.

This group of drugs often is misused among teenagers because of its easy availability and low cost. The cumulative brain damage from chronic use is a very serious problem among poor and minority adolescents.

OPIOIDS

Opioids are either made directly from the opium poppy plant or manufactured using the same chemical structure. Prescription opioids are used for pain management and work by blocking pain signals between the brain and the body. However, this medication can be misused—either by taking higher than recommended doses or using the drug to get high. Regular use of prescribed opioids can increase tolerance and dependence, and for many, long term opioid use can lead to addiction The opioids most often misused are heroin, morphine, oxycodone (Oxycontin), hydrocodone, pentazocine (Talwin), methadone, and meperidine (Demerol). In the United States, deaths involving synthetic opioids, especially fentanyl and its analogues are continuing to rise.

Heroin

Heroin is a highly addictive opioid that produces euphoria on intravenous use. The person experiences a "rush" and then gradually nods off to sleep. On awakening, the person feels immune to stressors until the withdrawal symptoms begin to trigger the need to "cop a fix" again. This usually occurs 8 to 12 hours after the last use. Risks of chronic use of heroin include overdose, malnutrition, and respiratory arrest as well as hepatitis B, hepatitis C, and HIV infections from shared needle use. To support their ever-increasing habit, many people addicted to heroin resort to crime, such as stealing. Sometimes they seek detoxification only to reduce the level of the dose needed to experience the pleasurable response to the drug, because a lower dose is less expensive to obtain.

Symptoms of withdrawal include tearing of the eyes, runny nose, gooseflesh, sweating, alternating fever and chills, muscle and joint pain, upset stomach, diarrhea, loss of appetite, restlessness, and irritability. Individuals usually are in such subjective distress that they inappropriately seek medications from the staff while in treatment. It is particularly challenging to work with patients experiencing this type of withdrawal and care must be taken to remain nonjudgmental.

SEDATIVES, HYPNOTICS, AND ANXIOLYTICS

Sedatives, hypnotics, and anxiolytics are drugs that generally are obtained by prescription for anxiety or insomnia or are purchased illegally. They are typically taken orally and can become addictive. Symptoms of overdose include oversedation, respiratory depression, impaired coordination, and brain damage. Intoxication with barbiturates is even more dangerous than with benzodiazepines. Although benzodiazepines and barbiturates are like alcohol in terms of dangerous physical withdrawal reactions (e.g., delirium tremens, seizures), barbiturate overdose induces an anesthesia-like state. Symptoms of barbiturate withdrawal usually occur somewhat later, sometimes days after the last use, depending on the half-life of the drug. Once a person is addicted, abruptly stopping any of these drugs may trigger psychosis.

STIMULANTS

Stimulants include amphetamines ("speed"), methamphetamine ("meth" and "crystal meth") and similar drugs, and cocaine or "crack."

Amphetamines

Amphetamines typically are used orally or intravenously, daily or on binges. They are very psychologically addictive; the dose is gradually increased over time to produce the euphoria (or "high") that is extremely pleasurable. Symptoms often include hyperactivity, irritability, combativeness, and paranoia after extended use. A person intoxicated by amphetamines may be very dangerous and experience paranoia and agitation. No physical withdrawal symptoms are noted, but the user typically experiences a profound depression and sense of exhaustion called *crashing*. Selective serotonin reuptake inhibitors (SSRIs) and other types of antidepressants such as bupropion (Wellbutrin) commonly are used to treat the depression, which may persist in chronic users for up to 2 years after the last amphetamine use. Toxic psychosis may occur in approximately 90% of chronic users up to 1 year past the last use. Unfortunately, 5% to 15% of these individuals never fully recover. Neuroleptics may be used to treat toxic psychosis.

Methamphetamine

Methamphetamine is an illegal drug sold on the streets that may also be known as meth, crank, speed, crystal meth, and ice. The substance is a white, odorless, bitter-tasting crystalline powder that easily dissolves in water or alcohol. This drug is taken orally, intranasally (snorting the drug powder into the nose), by injecting the drug through a needle, or by smoking. Methamphetamine causes rapid release of the neurotransmitter dopamine while also blocking dopamine's natural reuptake into the neuron. This rapid release of dopamine occurs in reward regions of the brain, causing intense euphoria or a "rush" in the user. Over time, chronic methamphetamine use causes several alterations in brain function, with actual changes in structure and neuronal function. Effects last up to 14 hours; the user often will do anything to obtain the drug and is considered at risk for being very dangerous while under the influence. Long-term use may lead to symptoms such as insomnia, major mood swings, delusional behavior, and extreme paranoia. In addition, users may display repeated infections, missing and rotted teeth (called "*meth mouth*"), severe weight loss, skin sores, and heart attack or stroke. Large doses can result in agitation, chest pain, heart attack, difficulty breathing, kidney damage or failure, paranoia, seizures, and (in extreme cases) cardiac arrest or coma.

Cocaine

Cocaine is a highly addictive alkaloid of the plant *Erythroxylum coca*, which grows mainly in Peru and Bolivia. Cocaine produces an intense feeling of euphoria that usually lasts only 30 to 60 minutes; however, the substance remains in the brain for about 10 days after use. Pure forms of cocaine are quite expensive. The drug typically is inhaled nasally or mixed with other drugs, such as heroin, and injected intravenously ("speedballs"). Symptoms of chronic inhalation include runny nose, sniffles, frequent colds, weight loss, hyperactivity, and damage to the nasal mucosa or septum that may be severe enough to require surgical repair. In instances when the drug is injected, severe allergic reactions may result, and there is increased risk for HIV, hepatitis C, and other bloodborne diseases from contaminated needles.

Cocaine is very psychologically addicting, which is thought to be the result of overstimulation of the pleasure centers of the brain. Users may lose interest in their usual activities and demonstrate abrupt mood swings, poor judgment, impatience, and ultimately suspiciousness and hallucinations. Cocaine constricts blood vessels; dilates pupils; increases body temperature, heart rate, and blood pressure; and causes headaches, abdominal pain and nausea, and decreased appetite. Cocaine is a very dangerous drug in that strokes, seizures, and heart attacks that are sometimes fatal can occur even in first-time users.

Withdrawal occurs when heavy cocaine users decrease or stop use of the drug and experience a "crash." Treatment often consists of diazepam (Valium) or phenobarbital for their sedative effects. Neuroleptics may be used in the event of psychosis. Many clients are severely depressed for up to 2 years after quitting. Studies have shown that damage to the brain may impair the patient's ability to experience pleasure. Antidepressants such as bupropion (Wellbutrin), beta-blockers such as propranolol hydrochloride (Inderal), or calcium-channel blockers may be helpful in this event.

Crack

Crack is a hardened form of cocaine that is smoked. It presents major problems in many urban areas of the United States because it is readily available and inexpensive compared with other drugs. It produces a tremendously addicting, short-acting euphoria that is quickly followed by "crashing," which stimulates continued cravings and use. The cravings are so intense that, as with "ice," the user will do almost anything to obtain more of the drug and often resorts to violence if thwarted. Overdose of this drug is life threatening because no drug is available to counteract the overstimulation, which results in respiratory failure.

TOBACCO

Nicotine, the addictive substance in tobacco, increases the level of dopamine, a neurotransmitter that acts on the reward centers of the brain. Within 10 seconds of inhaling a cigarette, the drug level peaks in the brain. However, the effects decrease rapidly so that the smoker must continue dosing to maintain the drug's pleasurable effects and prevent withdrawal. Pharmacologic effects of withdrawal produce symptoms including irritability, craving, depression, anxiety, cognitive and attention deficits, sleep disturbances, and increased appetite. These symptoms may occur within the first few days after smoking cessation and usually subside within a few weeks; however, symptoms can last for months. Behavioral factors related to the actual activity associated with smoking such as handling, lighting, and smoking the cigarette can also influence the severity of symptoms and difficulty in stopping tobacco use.

Nearly half of all smokers try to quit each year. Success is greatest when behavioral counseling is used along with smoking cessation aids. First-line pharmacologic aids are nicotine-based products that deliver nicotine via a patch, chewing gum, lozenge, nasal spray, or inhaler and the nicotine-free products varenicline (Chantix) and bupropion (Wellbutrin, Zyban).

Some have tried to use electronic cigarettes ("e-cigarettes") in their attempts to reduce tobacco consumption. E-cigarettes are battery-operated products that deliver nicotine, flavor, and other chemicals. The nicotine levels can be adjusted according to user need. The chemicals are converted into an aerosol that the user inhales. To date, research on the use of e-cigarettes to assist with smoking cessation is uncertain regarding efficacy.

OTHER OR UNKNOWN SUBSTANCES

A new group of used drugs on the illegal market includes synthetic drugs especially designed to sidestep categorization with any of the drugs identified as illegal in the United States. Although use of these drugs may not be technically illegal, their misuse presents unique hazards. Ecstasy, also called *Adam,* is an example of a synthetic drug generally grouped with the hallucinogens. A very similar second-generation designer drug is called *Eve*. China White is an example of a synthetic type of heroin that acts in much the same way as heroin. "Synthetic marijuana" (known commonly as *Spice, K2, Kronic, Blue Lotus*) is an ever-changing mixture of herbs, spices, and laboratory-created cannabinoid-like chemicals that can cause users to experience catatonia, hypertension, seizures, anxiety, paranoia, and hallucinations. Major risks are present when the user mixes these drugs with those from the other groups because the results are unpredictable.

CONDITIONS ASSOCIATED WITH SUBSTANCE USE DISORDERS

The risk of human immunodeficiency virus (HIV) disease, the illness that precedes AIDS, continues to present the greatest danger for patients with substance use disorders who are using intravenous drugs because of the common practice of sharing needles. The Centers for Disease Control and Prevention (CDC) indicate an alarming number of new cases of HIV-positive diagnoses among intravenous drug users and their sexual partners. Nursing care for these patients now includes teaching them how to clean their "works" with bleach and how to use condoms correctly.

Individuals who have or are predisposed to a serious psychiatric illness may have an active case of the mental disorder. By altering levels of brain chemicals that control emotions, thought processes, and behavior, misuse of these chemicals can trigger an exacerbation of an existing illness.

Another major area of concern is the effect of intrauterine exposure to these chemicals on the fetus. Fetuses carried by mothers who are physically addicted to an opioid are born addicted and may also experience developmental delays and a prolonged lack of the capacity to feel pleasure even after they have been successfully weaned from the substance used. "Cocaine babies" are currently being studied for clues to the consequences of prenatal exposure to the drug. Findings suggest that attention deficit disorder (with or without hyperactivity) occurs more often in this population, along with dyslexia, other neurologic problems, and learning disabilities.

Clients with chronic pain disorders are also very vulnerable to the substance use disorders, especially those of the opioid and depressant groups, because of their frequent frustration over an inability to manage their pain effectively. In addition, many lack knowledge of the risks of regular use of pain medication. They often feel betrayed by their physician and other caregivers because they were not informed about prescribed analgesics and pain management (e.g., the importance of temperate use along with the use of exercise and other types of supportive techniques to manage pain and avoid addiction).

TREATMENT FOR SUBSTANCE USE DISORDERS

Treatment of substance use disorders is very similar to alcohol detoxification and rehabilitation. Narcotics Anonymous (NA) is structured much like AA but focuses on drugs other than alcohol. Often inpatient treatment programs place recovering addicts with persons with alcohol use disorder for educational and therapy groups. However, the rate of relapse is much higher for most drug abuse patients, especially those who use highly addicting intravenous drugs. A booming area of research is the identification of alternative treatments and medications that will help drug users to detoxify more comfortably from the chemicals that they are addicted to and reduce the risks of relapse. Currently, some support exists for treating drug use disorders separately from alcohol use disorder.

As with treatment for alcohol use disorder, family involvement in the process is very important. Al-Anon is the support group for family members or significant others of a substance-abusing person. It is recommended that members of the family begin attending meetings as soon as they realize that the person is using some type of drug. The intervention process described earlier under "Treatment for Alcohol Abuse" may be used to get the person into treatment.

Many patients who use drugs have legal problems, which may provide the catalyst for seeking help. Sometimes they are mandated by the courts to go into treatment; at other times their attorney recommends treatment before the case goes to court to influence the judge favorably before sentencing. In the past, many individuals were involuntarily committed to state hospital drug treatment programs for 30 days. However, many state hospital systems across the country are closing their drug and alcohol treatment units because of the program expense and the need to provide additional services to the seriously mentally ill, which is often judged more of a priority.

DETOXIFICATION

Detoxification from physically addicting drugs is very complex because of the likelihood of polysubstance use and the uncertainty of what to expect when two or more drugs are mixed. Usually, inpatient hospitalization is recommended for safety. However, some individuals who have been using drugs that are primarily psychologically addicting may not demonstrate many physical symptoms but rather experience intense psychologic cravings. For example, if a conversation about past drug use occurs within the recovering addict's hearing or if something in the environment triggers memories of the "high" sensation that they experienced while using, the person may experience cravings that stimulate feelings of restlessness, itching, hives, flushing, and elevated BP and pulse, which are believed to be psychogenic in origin. These patients need a great deal of support to help them overcome the profound urge to use. This experience puts the patient at very high risk for relapse.

MEDICATIONS

Methadone

Methadone is one drug used in the treatment of heroin addiction. However, some controversy exists about using this medication because the drug is a synthetic opioid analgesic (full opioid agonist) that may also be prescribed appropriately for chronic severe pain. Given orally (in diskette or liquid form), it is absorbed slowly and does not produce the "rush" normally experienced with the intravenous use of heroin. It also alleviates the cravings for more opioids for a short period of time, depending on the dose given. In detoxification, the dose of the drug is gradually reduced without telling patients exactly what dose they are getting. Although this process is one of substituting another addictive drug for the one misused by the client, some believe it to be justified in that withdrawal from methadone is less uncomfortable for the patient. The patient also risks severe respiratory depression if heroin is injected while methadone is in the system. The most typical problematic side effects of methadone include severe constipation and profound sweating. Some states require daily visits to a methadone clinic and in other states, limited medications are allowed for take-home treatment.

Pharmacology Capsule

Methadone is a synthetic opioid analgesic that may be used in the detoxification of heroin-related opioid addiction.

Buprenorphine and Buprenorphine/Naloxone

Buprenorphine binds partially to opioid receptors in the brain, reducing cravings and thus illicit opioid use. Buprenorphine can be given sublingually. It is also available as four implants that last for six months (Probuphine) or subcutaneous injections given every month (Sublocade). Suboxone is a combination sublingual medication of buprenorphine plus naloxone. Naloxone is a mu opioid receptor antagonist that reverses, and thus blocks, the rewarding (high) effects of buprenorphine if snorted or injected, lessening misuse potential. Unlike methadone use in recovery, specialty clinic visits are not a requirement and patients may feel less stigmatized in treatment.

Clonidine

Clonidine hydrochloride (Catapres) has become a more popular means of assisting the substance user through detoxification. It is a nonopiate antihypertensive drug that partially blocks withdrawal symptoms. Clonidine does not completely remove the unpleasant feelings that accompany heroin withdrawal (see the Complementary and Alternative Therapies box). Unfortunately, some may leave treatment because of the inherent discomfort and unrealistic expectations that they should not feel sick at all while using the drug to withdraw.

Complementary and Alternative Therapies

Some herbal remedies are being studied for use as agents to reduce withdrawal symptoms.

Naloxone

Naloxone hydrochloride (Narcan) and nalmefene (Selincro) are opioid antagonists that counteract the dangerous respiratory depressant effects of heroin or another opiate overdose. When Narcan is given to a person who is addicted and under the influence of an opiate, the person may experience acute withdrawal symptoms.

Many other drugs are currently under investigation to determine whether they could assist the person with a substance use disorder by reducing the cravings for the drug abused or by counteracting the long-term psychologic consequences of use of certain drugs. Examples of these include some of the antidepressants, anticonvulsants, and various herbal agents.

Still other medications may be used in the supportive treatment of those undergoing opiate withdrawal to control symptoms such as diarrhea, abdominal cramping, and generalized, diffuse pain.

Put On Your Thinking Cap!

Can you explain why Narcan would cause a person who is addicted to an opioid to experience acute withdrawal symptoms?

REHABILITATION

In most cases, the process of rehabilitation for substance use disorder is very similar to that for alcohol use disorder. Instead of attendance at AA meetings, the client often participates in NA at least some of the time. This support group is based on the 12 steps of AA, except that the word *drugs* replaces the word *alcohol* in all the literature. In addition, the case histories used for reading assignments are about other addicts in recovery related specifically to the use of drugs other than alcohol; this is to help the client identify with people with similar struggles. Relapse rates for individuals abusing drugs other than alcohol alone are much higher and present unique issues. Trends suggest that future treatment programs will be more likely to separate clients into small groups of people facing similar issues and having similar characteristics; this is to individualize the recovery process much more than is done in most settings today. Most current settings may advertise more than one "track" for substance abuse treatment. However, clients share the same facilities and participate in most of the traditional programming despite different learning styles and other issues. It has been suggested that this practice may place clients who do not fit the traditional mold at higher risk for relapse.

On an outpatient basis, clients are encouraged to participate in NA on a regular basis (90 meetings in the first 90 days), just as those recovering from alcoholism. Attempts usually are made to allow the client to experience different group locations and times before discharge from the inpatient setting to increase the likelihood that the client will participate as recommended. Various other community programs may be available, such as the Patrician Movement, which provides outpatient treatment on an ongoing basis for those who cannot afford more costly inpatient rehabilitation. Many private health care systems are opening day treatment programs for people with substance use disorders as insurance reimbursement for long-term inpatient programs become less available.

AFTERCARE AND RECOVERY

Individuals recovering from substance use disorders may be offered an opportunity to participate in a support group provided by the hospital at which they received treatment. Many of the same people who went through treatment at the same time participate together. Because the relationships built during this time of crisis are often intense, the groups can be very helpful in preventing relapse. It is hoped that clients also will continue regular participation in NA groups on an ongoing basis. Some individuals do well in halfway houses, which allow for a new living environment surrounded by other recovering addicts during the difficult transition back into the community. Sometimes it is recommended that patients do not return to work until their ability to cope with stress is more developed.

METHADONE MAINTENANCE

Some patients who have experienced multiple relapses into heroin use after treatment may have sustained permanent damage to chemical receptor sites in the brain, which decreases their ability to resist relapse. As a result, methadone maintenance is not uncommon. In this process, the person goes to a methadone clinic on a daily or 3-times-a-week basis to receive a dose or doses of the medication to cover the next 24 to 72 hours. A single dose may be administered in liquid form or in a diskette dissolved in juice, and the person is carefully observed by clinic staff members to ensure that the medication is taken and not hoarded in any way. The patient may continue this process indefinitely, often for many years. Sometimes the dose of the methadone is maintained at the same level without attempts to reduce it while at other times gradual titration is attempted.

Methadone maintenance programs have been criticized across the United States because the process is often viewed as exchanging one addiction for another without attempts to detoxify the patient. In addition, clinic records and security have been lax in many instances, resulting in clinic methadone thefts and illegal sales on the street. Supporters of the programs counter these arguments by pointing out that criteria for involvement in these programs require that patients have been unsuccessful in remaining "clean" after detoxification on more than one occasion and that patients are no longer "forced" into crime to support their habits. In addition, methadone is administered in such a way that no rush is experienced, allowing the person to return to school or work and reintegrate into society without the risk of losing everything to relapse. Methadone maintenance programs also are more cost effective than residential treatment or incarceration.

The controversy over methadone maintenance has resulted in the frequent use of naltrexone (Trexan) as an alternative. This drug is related to naloxone (Narcan) and is a pure opioid antagonist. This means that the drug reduces or completely blocks the effects of any intravenous opioids in the patient's system. The detoxified patient is placed on this drug to help prevent use of heroin. If the patient takes small doses of heroin while on naltrexone, no effect is experienced; however, if the patient injects large doses, they will become very physically ill and may die or sustain serious injury such as coma. An addicted person taking naltrexone soon after regular use of heroin will experience withdrawal symptoms because of the antagonist actions of the drug.

Pharmacology Capsule

Methadone maintenance is used for patients who have experienced multiple relapses into heroin use after standard treatment and rehabilitation efforts.

Research is underway to evaluate the use of various types of other psychotropic medications to stabilize neurochemical and neurophysiologic alterations in the brains of addicted persons. This may eventually provide an answer to the high rates of relapse in individuals with substance use disorder involving opioids.

NURSING CARE OF THE PERSON WITH A SUBSTANCE USE DISORDER

Focused Assessment

The initial step in developing a nursing plan of care for the patient with a substance use disorder is always a thorough assessment. The data you collect on first contact with the patient can help to identify and prioritize problems that must be addressed to maximize the likelihood that the patient will remain sober. Examples of the types of problems often seen in substance use disorders of any kind are denial, poor impulse control, high risk for injury, high risk for relapse, guilt, and low self-esteem. Detailed assessment of the person with a substance disorder is detailed earlier in the section titled "Nursing Assessment of the Person With Addiction."

Patient Problems, Goals, and Outcome Criteria: Substance Use Disorder

Patient Problems	Goals and Outcome Criteria
Inadequate coping related to substance use, as evidenced by using substances to deal with anxiety, emotional discomfort, and stress	Improved coping: identifies and uses healthy alternative coping strategies to deal with anxiety, emotional discomfort, and stress; patient verbalizes strategies to prevent relapse
Denial related to substance use and refusal to acknowledge actual consequences of substance use	Verbalizes an internalized sense that the substance use is unhealthy and out of control and that the treatment is required
Potential for injury related to excessive use of the drug and high risk for relapse, manifested by a history of falls, driving while under the influence, combining the substance used with other substances, being aggressive while under the influence, reduced attendance at Alcoholics Anonymous (AA) or Narcotics Anonymous (NA) meetings, frequent dreams of drug use, returning to places where one used drugs, and not seeking relief for high stress	Decreased potential for injury to self and others: patient does not engage in dangerous activities when under drug's influence

Interventions

Nursing interventions for persons with substance use disorders in detoxification involve regular physical assessment (with the frequency determined by the severity of symptoms), administration of appropriate medications, and teaching the patients about their actions and consequences. Providing adequate nutrition is critical because the patient may have been eating irregularly and maybe become dehydrated. High levels of anxiety during detoxification also require a great deal of reassurance and support, providing the opportunity to help the patient begin to process the impending decision to continue in rehabilitation.

Once the patient has agreed to participate in rehabilitation, the focus of nursing care changes from one of primarily attending to the physical concerns of the patient to assisting the client in processing the meaning of their substance use disorder and planning for a future without continued use of that substance. The biggest issue to be addressed at first is the heavily entrenched denial that most substance users possess. Often, they minimize the severity of the use, perhaps lying outright about how much they were using. You must work toward penetrating this denial without further damaging the individual's self-esteem. This has traditionally demanded more confrontational techniques than appropriate in other types of psychiatric treatment. In many "substance use only" treatment programs, the style of confrontation used was often overly hostile and critical. This approach is no longer seen as the most helpful to the patient. Studies now show that patients who were treated in this way were far more likely to leave treatment early to return to their "drugging and drinking." This is of great concern because the person may never return to treatment and may die or be seriously injured as a result of the continued substance abuse.

You can also be extremely helpful in assisting the patient to work through the 12-step process. After intense educational AA or NA meetings and group therapy sessions during most of the day, patients often want to vent feelings and process thoughts about what they are learning. Conflicts with family members, bosses, friends, or parents often may be overwhelming. Patients usually lack the skills to handle these types of interpersonal stressors because of habitual avoidance of issues through past substance use. You can act as an ally in helping patients to cope and begin to practice new ways of reacting. Teaching stress management and practicing these new skills with patients can greatly increase the odds that they will not relapse after discharge.

Relapse prevention is a critical area to attend to in dealing with each patient. The patient must be taught to recognize symptoms that often lead to relapse. Examples of these include overtiredness or poor health, being unnecessarily dishonest with others, impatience, argumentativeness, depression, self-pity, cockiness, forgetting or minimizing the risk of relapse, unreasonable expectations of self and others, decreased or irregular participation in AA or NA meetings or daily meditation and self-inventory, use of a chemical other than those previously abused, forgetting to be thankful that their lives are better, and feeling all-powerful.

Another effective means of intervention is to act as a good role model in handling feelings, participating appropriately in meetings, and communicating to the patient in a way that supports the program. For example, telling patients that participation in AA meetings is not necessary for recovery could undermine their struggle to initiate the profound changes in lifestyle necessary to stay drug free.

SPECIAL PROBLEMS FOR POPULATIONS OF PEOPLE WITH SUBSTANCE USE DISORDERS

The unique characteristics of many groups of individuals influence the process of recovery and contribute to a high risk for relapse into chronic use of whatever substance the person has used. Recent research in addressing these problems has proved very promising. As mentioned earlier, the trend is to provide specially designed treatment approaches for groups of individuals who have common traits and problems that may contribute to their dependency on alcohol or other drugs.

OLDER ADULTS

Although older adults use approximately 25% of the medications used in the United States, only about 2% to 5% of men and less than 1% of women older than 65 years of age have alcohol use disorder. Substance use disorder among older adults is more likely to involve use of OTC and prescription sleeping pills, pain medications, or tranquilizers than the use of illegal drugs such as cocaine. Misuse is seldom for recreational purposes among this age group.

Because of a decreased ability to metabolize and eliminate alcohol or drugs from the body, older adults with substance use disorders over extended periods of time may experience significant medical problems as a result. The most typical physical consequences of alcohol use disorder among older adults include malnutrition, cirrhosis of the liver, bone thinning, gastritis, poor memory, and decreased cognitive ability to process new information. If the person combines alcohol with any other medication that has CNS depressant effects, the danger of oversedation, impaired responses, or respiratory depression is very great.

Many older adults with alcohol use disorder have maintained a regular pattern of use over many years without obvious problems. As their bodies age, their ability to tolerate the same quantities decreases, putting them at risk for falls or other injuries as a result of intoxication. Others turn to first-time or heavier patterns of use to cope with anxiety produced by the typical stressors of aging such as retirement, losses of significant others, family conflict, health problems, social isolation, and loss of self-worth. Among older adults who move to more affluent retirement communities, a rise in alcoholism has been noted. This may be because of involvement in cocktail parties, regular drinking with meals, and peer pressure to participate to be accepted.

Problems of substance use disorder in the older population are usually diagnosed by the health care provider as a result of complaints related to the psychologic or physical effects of alcohol use disorder, such as memory impairment or insomnia. Older adults often deny that they have a substance use problem and may resist treatment without the support and pressure of their family.

Treatment of alcoholism in older adults is like that of younger individuals, except that the period of withdrawal must be monitored more closely and must occur more slowly because of the older person's physical frailty. Rehabilitation groups and educational programs ideally should be structured to permit processing information more slowly to allow for the cognitive

Get Ready for the NCLEX® Examination!

Key Points

- Many experts in substance-related disorders subscribe to the biologic theory that proposes that faulty physiologic processes contribute to addiction to a specific substance and that addiction is a physical illness.
- Some theorists contend that sociocultural factors contribute to the development of substance-related disorders.
- According to behavioral and learning theories, a substance-related disorder is a learned maladaptive way of coping with stress and anxiety.
- Although the specific causes of addiction have not been established, it is most likely that the true cause involves a combination of biologic, cultural, and behavioral factors.
- To obtain reliable data when questioning a person about a substance-related disorder, the nurse must be nonjudgmental, direct, and specific. More than one person should verify the information obtained when possible.
- The lifestyle of an addicted person may focus entirely on obtaining and using the substance of choice, with an increasing need for more and more to get the desired effects.
- Individuals with substance-related disorders often have erratic and unprovoked mood swings, blackouts, significant work problems, and damaged relationships.
- Typical defense mechanisms used by addicts include denial, rationalization, intellectualization, and projection.
- Many people abusing alcohol appear malnourished and poorly cared for, have evidence of physical trauma from falls or violence, appear jaundiced, and when in withdrawal may be hypertensive with signs of fluid retention.
- Tests for detecting substance use include a blood alcohol study, a urine drug screen, and hair analysis.
- Chronic alcoholism involves the regular daily ingestion of large amounts of alcohol, regular heavy drinking only on weekends, or binges of heavy drinking followed by long periods of abstinence.
- Physical addiction occurs when the cells of the body are dependent on alcohol to carry out certain metabolic processes; without the alcohol, the cells go into shock.
- Alcohol withdrawal syndrome begins after an individual stops or decreases the amount of alcohol ingested and involves physiologic and behavioral symptoms that begin when the individual's blood alcohol level drops.
- Alcoholism influences the entire family. Family and peer pressure can be critical factors in inducing an alcoholic to seek treatment.
- Strategies that have been successful in alcohol rehabilitation are 12-step programs, stress management, social skills training, behavioral approaches to marital therapy, and matching clients with therapists who use a style most likely to benefit their personality type.
- Substance-related disorders encompass the following classes of drugs: (1) alcohol; (2) caffeine; (3) cannabis; (4) hallucinogens; (5) inhalants; (6) opioids; (7) sedatives, hypnotics, and anxiolytics; (8) stimulants; (9) tobacco; and (10) other or unknown substances.
- Treatment for drug addiction is like alcohol detoxification and rehabilitation; however, relapse rates are higher, and treatment may need to be more individualized.
- Methadone maintenance may be used for long-term heroin users who have sustained permanent damage to chemical receptor sites in the brain and therefore have a decreased ability to resist relapses or who have failed multiple attempts at rehabilitation.

Additional Learning Resources

SG Go to your Study Guide for additional learning activities to help you master this chapter content.

Go to your Evolve website (http://evolve.elsevier.com/Linton/medsurg) for the following learning resources and much more:

- Fluid & Electrolyte Tutorial
- Review Questions for the NCLEX® Examination

Clinical Judgment and Next-Generation NCLEX® Examination-Style Questions

1. **The theory that substance dependence is caused by faulty physiologic processes is the ____________ theory.**

   NCLEX Client Need: Psychosocial Integrity

2. **Mr. White was arrested for public intoxication and was advised by his attorney to enroll in an alcohol treatment program. A nurse interviews him when he comes to a mental health center. He tells the nurse that he really does not have a problem with alcohol and that he just had a few too many drinks while celebrating with a friend. This is an example of which defense mechanism?**

   NCLEX Client Need: Psychosocial Integrity

3. **What is the chief advantage of using hair analysis to detect drug use?**
   1. Hair samples can be taken without patient permission.
   2. Hair samples will reveal drug use as long as 90 days later.
   3. It is not possible for a patient to substitute someone else's hair.
   4. The chain of custody is unnecessary with hair samples.

   NCLEX Client Need: Physiological Integrity: Reduction of Risk Potential

4. **An alcoholic patient was injured in an automobile accident. She said that she had her last drink 2 hours before the accident. About 8 hours after admission, she developed symptoms of early alcohol withdrawal. You should anticipate delirium tremens by ______ hours after her last drink.**

   NCLEX Client Need: Psychosocial Integrity

5. **Mr. Jones calls the hospital to report that his wife, a dietitian, cannot come to work because she has the "flu." She consumed a large amount of alcohol the previous evening and has a hangover. This has happened several times in the past. Mr. Jones' behavior is an example of which of the following?**
   1. Support
   2. Enabling
   3. Rationalization
   4. Compensation

   NCLEX Client Need: Psychosocial Integrity

6. **When a patient who is taking disulfiram (Antabuse) consumes alcohol, expected outcomes include which of the following? (Select all that apply.)**
   1. Hypotension
   2. Tachycardia
   3. Confusion
   4. Nausea and vomiting
   5. Pallor

   NCLEX Client Need: Physiological Integrity: Pharmacological Therapies

7. **Young people should be warned that inhalants can cause which of the following?**
   1. Progressive brain damage
   2. Sexual dysfunction
   3. Schizophrenia
   4. Aggressive behavior

   NCLEX Client Need: Psychosocial Integrity

8. **A patient being treated for an overdose of opioids is given Narcan. Narcan is given for which of the following reasons?**
   1. To stimulate the heart
   2. To raise BP
   3. To treat respiratory depression
   4. To sedate the patient and prevent seizures

   NCLEX Client Need: Physiological Integrity: Pharmacological Therapies

9. **Which of the following are among the drugs most used by older adults with substance use disorder? (Select all that apply.)**
   1. Cocaine
   2. Pain medications
   3. Sleeping aids
   4. Alcohol
   5. Marijuana

   NCLEX Client Need: Physiological Integrity: Pharmacological Therapies

10. **Which statement most accurately describes drug use among adolescents?**
    1. Only 1 in 10 adolescents have problems with substance use.
    2. Adolescents tend to deny any possible negative outcomes of drug use.
    3. Most adolescents seek treatment for substance use on their own.
    4. Adolescents should be treated with adults who can model mature behavior.

    NCLEX Client Need: Psychosocial Integrity

11. **SLO/Objective:** **Prioritize nursing care for patients with substance abuse.**

    NGN Item Type: Cloze

    Cognitive Skill: Prioritize Hypotheses

    A 42-year-old male has been admitted to a rehabilitation center for detoxification. He has a long history of alcoholism and has been in treatment several times over the past 15 years. He appears malnourished and disheveled. He has abrasions on his arms and hands, and his legs are edematous. The patient is disoriented and uncoordinated. His blood alcohol level is 4.0.

    - Blood pressure 180/100 mm Hg
    - Pulse 98 beats per minute
    - Respirations 24 breaths per minute
    - Blood alcohol 4.0%
    - Disoriented
    - Uncoordinated
    - Edema in ankles and feet
    - Disheveled
    - Malnourished

    Choose the *most likely* options for the information missing from the statements below by selecting from the list of options provided.

    The patient is experiencing confusion, disorientation, hypertension, and edema. His appearance and symptoms are most likely the result of ______ and _______, and need to be closely monitored. Failure to recognize these conditions can lead to _______.

OPTIONS
Pain
Dehydration
Blood alcohol level
Malnutrition
Nausea and vomiting
Coma
Alcohol withdrawal effects
Death

First Aid, Emergency Care, and Disaster Management

63

http://evolve.elsevier.com/Linton/medsurg

Objectives

1. List the principles of emergency and first-aid care.
2. List the steps of the initial assessment and interventions for the person requiring emergency care.
3. Describe the components of the nursing assessment of the person requiring emergency care.
4. Outline the steps of the nursing process for emergency or first-aid treatment of victims of cardiopulmonary arrest, choking, shock, head injury, hemorrhage, traumatic injury, burns, heat or cold exposure, poisoning, bites, and stings.
5. Discuss the roles of nurses and nursing students in relation to bioterrorism, natural disasters, and epidemics and pandemics.
6. Explain the legal implications of administering first aid in emergency situations.
7. Explain the implications of the Good Samaritan doctrine.

Key Terms

avulsion (ă-VŬL-zhŭn)
cardiac tamponade (KĂR-dē-ăk tăm-pōn-ĀD)
epidemic hemorrhage (HĔM-ŏr-ĭj)
hemothorax (hē-mō-THŌ-răks)
hyperthermia (hī-pĕr-THĔR-mē-ă)
hypothermia (hī-pō-THĔR-mē-ă)
pandemic
poison
sprain
strain

In the inpatient setting, the nurse is often the first person on the scene when accidents or emergencies occur. Nurses also need to be prepared to act in emergency situations in homes and other community settings. Prompt intervention can make a dramatic difference in patient outcomes. Knowledge of first aid can mean the difference between life and death in many situations. This chapter addresses first-aid interventions for common emergencies seen in homes and community settings. Some emergency conditions that require further medical attention are covered in greater detail elsewhere in this book.

GENERAL PRINCIPLES OF EMERGENCY CARE

When accidents or emergencies occur, the victim and any observers are often anxious and frightened. Knowing that a nurse is present can be very reassuring to them, but you must remember the cardinal rule: Remain calm! Victims react to emergencies in various ways, from stunned silence to hysteria. Your priority is to preserve life and minimize the effects of injuries, but the manner in which you conduct yourself can also soothe and reassure the victim.

The nursing process is used in emergencies just as it is in other nursing situations. The important difference is that assessment and intervention must be accomplished very quickly and efficiently to identify and treat priority needs immediately.

SURVEY THE SCENE

The first step in initiating first aid is to survey the scene. You must determine if the area is safe for you, the victim(s), and any bystander(s) before you proceed. Once you have determined safety, the next steps are to determine how many are injured, how are they injured, and who is around that can help. Identify yourself as a nurse and obtain the victim's consent to provide them with care; then activate, or have a bystander activate, the emergency response system (i.e., call 911). If the victim is unable to provide consent, the emergency doctrine allows treatment to be provided under the assumption that the person would consent if able.

PRIMARY AND SECONDARY SURVEYS

The focused assessment begins when approaching the victim so that they do not have to move their head to see you. Ask the victim's name to determine whether they can speak, which would reveal airway or neurologic problems. Determine the nature of the emergency; for instance, was the injury caused by a motor vehicle accident, a fall, a diving accident, or an electrocution? In addition, look for any hazards to the victim and the rescuer. For example, is the victim in a burning vehicle or lying in the middle of the highway? Failure to recognize such dangers may result in injuries to the rescuer and additional injuries to the victim.

A primary survey is performed to detect life-threatening injuries. A primary survey consists of checking airway-breathing-circulation, disability, exposure, and facilitation of family. The nurse should intervene immediately if indicated in the following sequence:

1. Evaluate the airway for breathing and immobilize the cervical spine.
2. Initiate cardiopulmonary resuscitation or rescue breathing as needed. Use the jaw thrust maneuver to open the airway on an unconscious patient.
3. Look for uncontrolled bleeding, identify the source, and apply pressure to the source.
4. Assess for disability, which includes the level of consciousness.
5. Assess for exposure by removing clothing and observing for injury.
6. Facilitate the family by allowing them to be close to the patient.
7. Look for a medical alert tag, usually a necklace or a bracelet.

After the primary survey, once again conduct a systematic head-to-toe inspection (called the *secondary survey*) to detect significant changes and other findings that might have been missed initially.

GUIDELINES FOR FIRST AID TREATMENT

General guidelines for first-aid treatment of emergency patients are as follows:

1. Protect the airway.
2. Splint injured parts in the position they are found.
3. Prevent chilling but do not add excessive heat.
4. Do not remove penetrating objects.
5. Do not give anything by mouth to an unconscious person or to one with potentially serious injuries.
6. Stay with the injured person until medical care or transportation arrives.

NURSING ASSESSMENT IN EMERGENCIES

Patient emergencies can occur in every setting. In some situations, nurses observe the events and know what has happened, but at other times evidence at the scene is needed to determine the circumstances. Intervening appropriately in emergencies whose cause cannot be immediately determined can be difficult. Be prepared to make a quick appraisal and then act promptly to provide appropriate care that may save a life. The health history and physical examination are presented separately here but, in fact, may be conducted almost simultaneously in emergencies. Depending on the nature of the injury outside the health care setting, the assessment focuses on the specific injury. The more complete assessment described next would be conducted in the health care setting where the licensed vocational nurse/licensed practical nurse (LVN/LPN) may assist with data collection.

HEALTH HISTORY

If the victim is able to speak or a witness is available, obtain a brief health history of the victim. Data collection is limited in emergency situations and should include the chief complaint, any treatment given, and the relevant medical history. The acronym SAMPLE may help you to remember to inquire about Symptoms, Allergies, current Medications, Past illness/Pregnancy, Last oral intake, and Events related to injury.

Reason for Seeking Care

Determine the nature of the problem, the signs and symptoms, and the circumstances under which the injury or illness occurred. If the victim is or has been unconscious, note the length of time that the person has been unconscious if possible.

Medical Treatment

Determine whether any treatment has been given and, if so, the effect of the treatment. In the presence of an injury, note whether the victim has been moved.

Past Health History

If possible, determine known health problems, including diabetes and cardiac or pulmonary disease, which may provide important clues to the immediate problem or influence the care provided. Check for a medical alert tag, which may provide essential information if the patient cannot. If possible, identify current medications and known allergies. Note any evidence of alcohol or other drugs.

Pharmacology Capsule

The medical alert tag can provide clues about medical emergencies and alert rescuers to known allergies and chronic conditions.

PHYSICAL EXAMINATION

Determine if the patient is responsive, then begin collecting objective data. The first assessment priorities must be the ABCs: Airway, Breathing, and Circulation—followed by D (Disability) and E (Exposure). Watch the victim's chest for rhythmic breathing and listen near the patient's mouth and nose for air movement. Palpate the carotid and peripheral pulses. Once the adequacy of respiration and circulation has been established, assess for uncontrolled bleeding and shock. Note the level of consciousness, pupil response, and gross sensory and motor function to determine disability. Exposure refers to the removal of clothing to permit a more complete inspection for injuries. If no evidence of uncontrolled bleeding or shock is noted, the next step is a systematic head-to-toe examination. At each step, look for obvious injury, bleeding, swelling, bruising, and drainage. Note circulation, mobility, sensation, symmetry, and alignment of the entire body. Also note skin color, warmth, and temperature at each step of the head-to-toe assessment.

The systematic assessment, or secondary survey, will be a more thorough assessment of the injured person. It begins with a head-to-toe assessment. Speak to the victim and evaluate the response to determine level of consciousness (alert, disoriented, unresponsive). Evaluate comprehension by asking the patient to follow simple commands such as opening and closing the eyes. Inspect the eyes for pupil size, equality, and reaction to light. Ask the alert victim about neck pain or stiffness and the ability to swallow. Inspect the chest for symmetry of the chest wall movement. Next, assess respiratory effort, dyspnea, and abnormal sounds associated with respirations. Examine the contour of the abdomen to detect distention. Use light palpation to detect areas of pain or tenderness. Inspect the extremities for deformity or injury and evaluate movement. Then assess peripheral pulses and warmth and sensation in the extremities. Box 63.1 summarizes the focused assessment of the patient who requires first aid or emergency care.

SPECIFIC EMERGENCIES

CARDIOPULMONARY ARREST

When the heart stops beating, a person is in cardiac arrest. When respirations cease, the person is in respiratory, or pulmonary, arrest. Cardiopulmonary arrest is the absence of a heartbeat and respirations. The cardiac and respiratory systems are so dependent on each other that when one fails, the other quickly fails as well.

Nerve tissue is susceptible to hypoxia (low levels of oxygen), and brain cells begin to die after 4 minutes without oxygen. Unless circulation and oxygenation are restored very quickly after cardiopulmonary arrest, permanent brain damage or death results. Prompt recognition and treatment of cardiopulmonary arrest can maintain the oxygen supply to the brain until circulation and respiration are restored.

Cardiopulmonary resuscitation (CPR) can be part of basic life support or advanced life support. Basic life support is the immediate care given to maintain oxygenation of the brain until advanced life support is available. To obtain the latest recommended interventions, see materials published by the American Heart Association (AHA) and the American Red Cross. All nurses should be familiar with the automated external defibrillator (AED), which is available in many public places.

Box 63.1 Assessment of the Patient Who Requires First Aid or Emergency Care

HEALTH HISTORY

Reason for Seeking Care

Nature of illness or injury, signs and symptoms, circumstances of illness or injury, how long unconscious

Treatment: Efforts that have been made, effects, whether moved after injury

Past Health History

Current health problems, current medications, allergies

PHYSICAL EXAMINATION

ABCs: Airway, breathing, circulation
Skin: Color, temperature, obvious injury
Head: Level of consciousness
Eyes: Opening, pupil size, equality, response to light
Neck: Stiffness, pain, ability to swallow
Chest: Symmetry of movement, dyspnea, respiratory rate and effort
Abdomen: Contour, rigidity, distention, pain, tenderness
Extremities: Deformity, movement, sensation, peripheral pulses

Causes

Among the causes of cardiopulmonary arrest are myocardial infarction, heart failure, electrocution, drowning, drug overdose, anaphylaxis, and asphyxiation.

Signs and Symptoms

Victims of cardiopulmonary arrest collapse and quickly lose consciousness. They have no pulse or respiration.

Focused Assessment

In cardiopulmonary arrest, assessment and interventions are quickly interwoven. Only patient problems and goals are provided here.

Patient Problems	Goals and Outcome Criteria
Inadequate circulation related to cessation of heartbeat Decreased cardiac output related to cessation of heartbeat	Adequate circulation until heartbeat and respirations are restored: improving skin color, palpable pulse, spontaneous respirations
Inadequate ventilation related to inadequate or absent respirations	Effective ventilation: spontaneous respirations, improving skin color

Interventions

Refer to the latest AHA guidelines for CPR because the guidelines are revised at intervals.

CHOKING OR AIRWAY OBSTRUCTION

Choking is airway obstruction caused by a foreign body that enters the airway.

Focused Assessment

The initial response when a person appears to be choking depends on the severity of the airway obstruction.

Mild airway obstruction. If the victim has good air exchange, is responsive, and can cough forcefully, do not interfere.

1. Encourage the victim's efforts to breathe and cough.
2. If symptoms persist, activate the emergency response system.

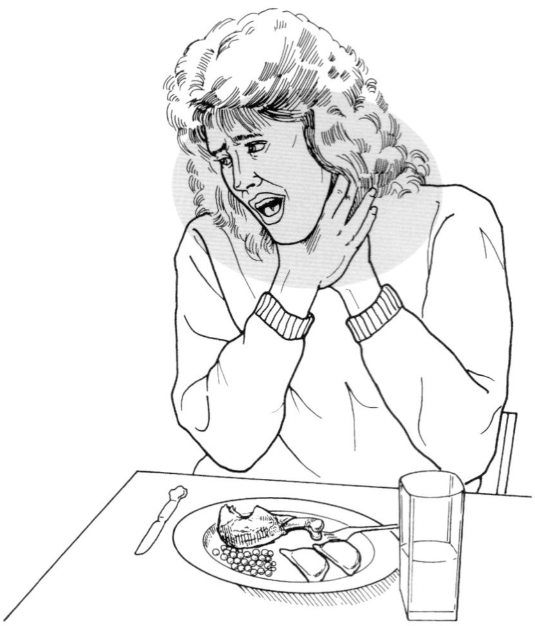

Fig. 63.1 The universal choking sign.

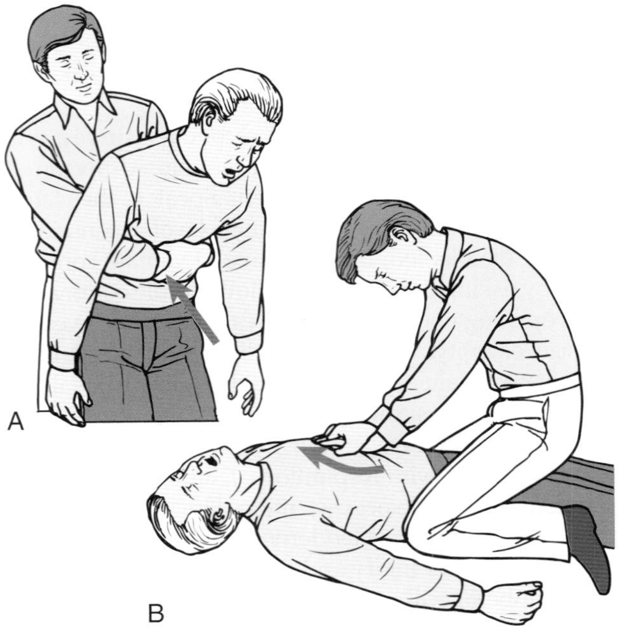

Fig. 63.2 (A) Abdominal thrusts for the conscious choking victim. (B) Abdominal thrusts for the unconscious choking victim. (A, From Lewis SM, Heitkemper MM, Dirksen SR, et al.: *Medical-surgical nursing: assessment and management of clinical problems*, ed 7, St. Louis, 2007, Mosby. B, From Lewis SM, Heitkemper MM, Dirksen SR. *Medical-surgical nursing: assessment and management of clinical problems*, ed 5, St. Louis, 2000, Mosby.)

Severe airway obstruction. Signs of severe airway obstruction are poor or no air exchange, poor or no cough, high-pitched noise known as stridor on inhalation, respiratory distress, cyanosis, inability to speak, inability to move air, and clutching the neck (the universal choking sign, depicted in Fig. 63.1).

Patient Problems, Goals, and Outcome Criteria: Choking

Patient Problems	Goals and Outcome Criteria
Airway obstruction related to inability to expel an aspirated foreign object	Patent airway with normal respirations: expulsion of foreign object, audible respirations, improving skin color, decreased coughing, reduced anxiety, normal pulse

Interventions

Perform abdominal thrusts for the conscious or unconscious choking victim per the latest AHA guidelines for choking (Fig. 63.2). Adaptive measures should be taken for obese or pregnant individuals.

Complications from abdominal thrusts. Because of the risk for damage to internal organs, a person who has received abdominal thrusts should subsequently be examined by a health care provider.

Prevention

Most choking deaths could be prevented if people would do the following:

1. Cut food into small pieces, eat slowly, and chew food thoroughly before swallowing.
2. Avoid laughing and talking while chewing and swallowing.
3. Perform abdominal thrusts promptly when a person is in distress because of an obstructed airway.

SHOCK

Shock results from acute circulatory failure caused by inadequate blood volume, heart failure, overwhelming infection, severe allergic reactions, or extreme pain or fright. Because of the complexity of the topic, shock is covered in detail in Chapter 9.

HEMORRHAGE

Hemorrhage is the loss of a large amount of blood. The loss of more than 1 liter of blood in an adult may lead to hypovolemic shock. Continued uncontrolled bleeding results in death. Bleeding may be external or internal. Internal bleeding is suspected if a trauma victim shows signs of shock but no external bleeding is evident.

Focused Assessment

Assess for signs and symptoms of hemorrhage, which may include obvious bleeding; cool, sweaty, pale skin; weak, thready pulse; rapid respirations; and decreasing alertness. The victim who is bleeding internally may also have abdominal distention, pain, hematemesis, or dyspnea, depending on the site of the bleeding. Ask if the patient has a bleeding disorder or takes any drugs that affect blood coagulation.

Patient Problems, Goals, and Outcome Criteria: Hemorrhage

Patient Problems	Goals and Outcome Criteria
Decreased cardiac output related to hypovolemia	Increased cardiac output: pulse and blood pressure within normal range, skin warm and dry, no visible bleeding
Fear related to possible impending death	Decreased fear: patient appears more relaxed, states is less fearful

Interventions

The immediate treatment for external bleeding is direct, continuous pressure with or without gauze. Ideally, a sterile dressing is placed over the wound. If sterile supplies are unavailable, use a clean cloth. Place the patient in a supine position. To provide stabilization, immobilize an injured part. Elevation of the feet 6 to 12 inches is permitted unless it causes pain. Elevation decreases blood flow to the area. After the bleeding stops, secure a large dressing, if available, over the wound. Reinforce the dressing but do not change it.

If direct wound pressure and elevation fail to control bleeding, apply indirect pressure, that is, pressure to the main artery that supplies the area (Fig. 63.3).

The use of a tourniquet to control severe bleeding in an extremity is an option. However, tourniquets that are inappropriately placed or left in place too long may result in complications such as amputations. Therefore, tourniquets should be applied only by people with advanced training in first aid. Some sources do not recommend a tourniquet under any circumstances; others indicate that it should be used only as a last resort when a limb is mangled, crushed, or amputated. The least dangerous tourniquet is a pneumatic one, such as a blood pressure cuff, which allows control of pressure. If a blood pressure cuff is used, inflate the cuff above the victim's systolic blood pressure. If the victim's blood pressure cannot be measured, the cuff should be inflated until the bleeding stops. Once the cuff is inflated, only a physician should remove it. When a victim with a tourniquet is transferred, the receiving caregiver must be informed that a tourniquet is in place.

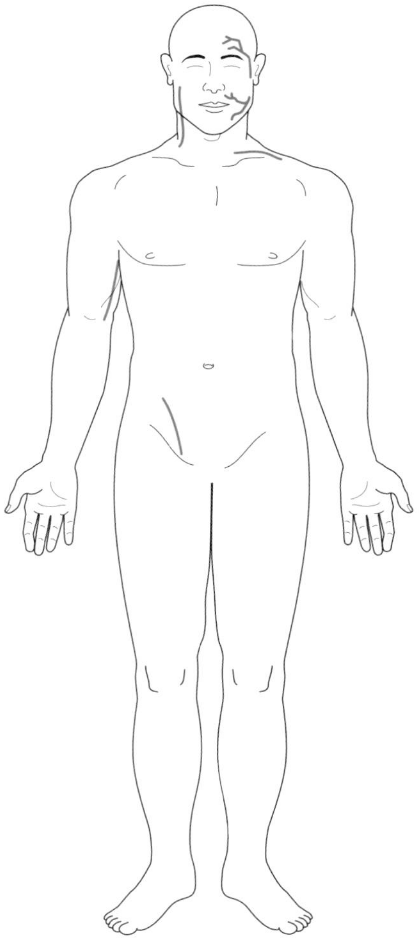

Fig. 63.3 Major arterial pressure points.

Epistaxis

One type of bleeding that requires special intervention is epistaxis (nosebleed). Blood may come from the anterior or the posterior portion of the nose. Most anterior nosebleeds respond to pressure. Instruct the patient to sit down and lean the head forward to prevent aspiration of blood. Pinch the nostrils of the patient shut for at least 10 minutes (Fig. 63.4). Pinching the nostrils provides pressure that decreases bleeding. In most cases, this action stops the bleeding. Afterward, advise the patient not to blow or pick at the nose for several hours. Continued bleeding or bleeding from the posterior area of the nose requires medical treatment (see Chapter 26).

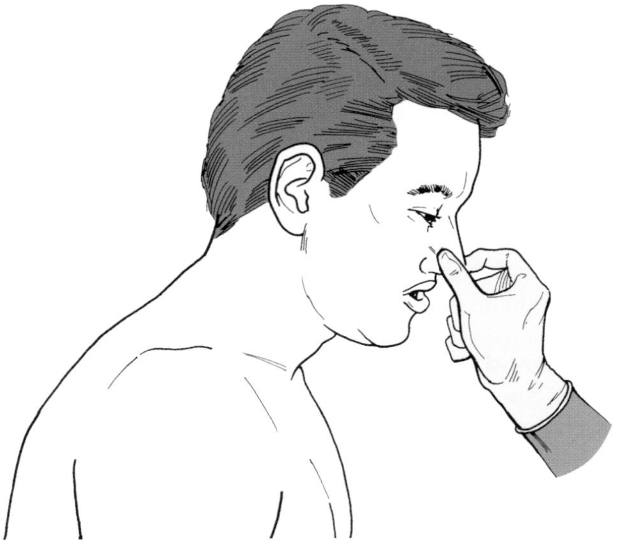

Fig. 63.4 Epistaxis may be controlled by having the patient sit up and lean forward slightly. Then pinch the patient's nostrils closed.

TRAUMATIC INJURY

Traumatic injuries result from a variety of events. Sports injuries, motor vehicle accidents, falls, and acts of violence often require emergency treatment at the scene of the injury.

Fractures

A fracture is a break in a bone that may be described as simple or compound, open or closed, complete or incomplete. A simple (closed) fracture does not break the skin. A compound (open) fracture is one in which the ends of the broken bone protrude through the skin. In a complete fracture, the broken ends are separated. The bone ends in an incomplete fracture are not separated. (See Chapter 45 for a discussion of other types of fractures.)

Focused Assessment. Check the victim of traumatic injury for signs and symptoms of fractures. The primary symptom is pain, although some people, especially older adults, do not always have severe pain with fractures. Numbness and tingling may be present because of injury to nerves and blood vessels. Objective signs of fracture include deformity, swelling, discoloration, decreased function, and bone fragments protruding through the skin. Suspected fractures should be treated as such until they are ruled out by the physician.

Patient problem, goal, and outcome criterion: fractures. The primary patient problem for the emergency treatment of the person with a suspected fracture is risk for injury related to movement of unstable fractures. The goal is reduced risk for injury, and the outcome criterion is stabilization of the fractured bone with minimal tissue damage.

Interventions. The key to emergency management of fractures is immobilization. Immobilize the injured part, including the joints above and below the injury, to prevent further trauma to the bone and surrounding soft tissue. Do not attempt to straighten a broken bone. Instead, splint the bone in the position in which it was found, with as little movement as possible. Boards, sticks, magazines, and strips of cloth can all be used to immobilize an injured limb. A cool pack may be applied to reduce swelling.

Severe bleeding may be present with compound fractures. In such cases, apply direct pressure to the artery above the injury. Give the victim nothing by mouth and seek transportation to a medical care facility as soon as possible.

Strains and Sprains

Strains are injuries to muscles or to the tendons that attach muscles to bones, or to both. **Sprains** are injuries to ligaments. Ligaments are bands of tissue that hold bones in position in the joints. These injuries are painful, and swelling may be present. Emergency treatment for both injuries is immobilization, elevation, and application of a cool pack. The victim should see a physician for further evaluation.

Head Injury

Head injury is not always apparent immediately after an accident. It should be suspected with any type of blow to the head or any unexplained loss of consciousness. A critical complication of head injury is increased intracranial pressure caused by bleeding or swelling associated with trauma. Increased intracranial pressure progressively impairs brain function and may lead to cessation of breathing.

Older adults are at special risk for head injuries because they are more likely than younger people to have sensory deficits, unstable gait, or circulatory disorders. Head injury in an older person may be overlooked if a state of confusion is attributed to age without determining the person's usual level of mental function.

Focused Assessment. When head injury is suspected, the focused assessment includes inspection and palpation of the head and evaluation for signs and symptoms of increased intracranial pressure. Signs of increased intracranial pressure are as follows:

- Change in behavior, agitation, confusion
- Decreasing level of consciousness
- Pupil dilation or constriction, pupillary inequality, slow or no pupillary response to light
- Impaired sensory or motor function
- Increasing blood pressure with widening pulse pressure
- Decreasing pulse and respiratory rates
- Projectile vomiting

Be alert for the leakage of cerebrospinal fluid (CSF) that occurs with basilar skull fractures. CSF leakage is usually seen as clear, colorless fluid draining from the nose or ear. If the fluid drains onto a white cloth, it appears as a yellowish stain. If blood is in the fluid, a yellow "halo" is produced around the pink (bloody) center. Although other fluids can also produce the "halo" sign, it is one piece of data in assessing for CSF leakage.

Patient Problems, Goals, and Outcome Criteria: Head Injury

Patient Problems	Goals and Outcome Criteria
Inadequate oxygenation related to neurologic trauma	Adequate oxygenation: normal respiratory rate and depth, normal pulse, oxygen saturation of at least 95%
Potential for injury to brain or spinal column related to increasing intracranial pressure, improper movement after spinal fracture	Decreased potential for injury: prompt recognition of rising intracranial pressure (altered mental function, unequal pupils, abnormal response of pupils to light), secure immobilization of spine

Interventions. The victim of a head injury must be assessed by a physician as soon as possible. Because head injuries often accompany spinal injuries, always treat the victim as if a spinal injury has occurred until it is ruled out. This precaution is especially important when the victim is unconscious or when no history can be obtained. Immobilize the neck and keep the victim flat with proper alignment of the neck and head. A backboard should be used to transport the victim.

Even if the head injury seems to be minor, the physician may admit the victim to the hospital for observation as a precaution. This safety measure is initiated because bleeding and swelling are sometimes so slow that signs and symptoms of increased intracranial pressure may not appear until hours or even weeks after the initial injury. (See Chapters 21 and 22 for detailed neurologic assessment and care of the hospitalized patient with a head injury.)

Neck and Spinal Injuries

Suspect neck and spinal injuries in any patient with a head injury, especially if the victim has had a diving or motor vehicle accident. Do not move the victim during the initial assessment unless absolutely necessary. Improper movement of the patient with a spinal injury may increase the damage to the spinal cord, causing permanent paralysis. After a diving injury, the neck and back should be immobilized while removing the victim from the water.

Focused Assessment. When a victim has a neck or spinal injury, first evaluate the victim's breathing and circulation and then begin resuscitation if needed. Use the jaw thrust method to open the airway. DO NOT use the head tilt–chin lift technique until the spine has been cleared by a physician! Then determine the victim's movement and sensation in all extremities.

Patient problem, goal, and outcome criteria: neck and spinal injuries. The priority patient problem for the person with a neck or spinal injury is potential for injury related to improper movement of the fractured spine. The goal is decreased potential for additional injury. Outcome criteria include continuous immobilization of the spine and transport for medical care.

Interventions. Immediately summon an expert emergency team when neck or spinal injury is suspected. A professional team has the equipment and the expertise to immobilize and transport the victim properly. In remote or life-threatening settings, the victim may have to be moved. If so, a rolled towel or article of clothing can be used as a collar to support the neck. The victim can then be moved by logrolling to one side and then rolling back onto a board, keeping the spine as straight as possible. Throughout the movement, one rescuer supports the head while two others support the shoulders, hips, and legs.

Eye Injury

Eye conditions that warrant immediate attention include presence of foreign bodies, chemical contact, perforation of the globe, and eyelid trauma.

Focused Assessment. After an injury of the eye, inspect the patient's eyelid for trauma and the eye itself for redness, foreign bodies, or penetrating objects. If the eye has been exposed to a chemical irritant, attempt to determine what the substance is.

Patient problem, goal, and outcome criteria: eye injury. The primary patient problem is potential for injury related to foreign body, direct trauma, or exposure to harmful substances. The goal is to minimize the risk of injury to the eye. Outcome criteria, depending on the nature of the injury, may be removal of a foreign body or chemical or protection of the eye from further damage while medical attention is being obtained.

Interventions. Interventions are summarized in Table 63.1.

Ear Trauma

The position and structure of the external ear make it vulnerable to traumatic injury. The most serious injury to the external ear is avulsion. **Avulsion** means that all or part of the auricle is torn loose.

Focused Assessment. Determine the extent of the injury; note whether any tissue is fully separated and the severity of bleeding. If necessary, apply direct pressure to the site of the injury to control bleeding.

Patient problem, goal, and outcome criteria: ear trauma. If bleeding is under control, the priority patient problem for a traumatic injury to the auricle is disrupted tissue integrity related to trauma. The goal is to preserve the tissue to maximize successful repair. Outcome criteria for successful interventions are recovery and protection of avulsed tissue.

Interventions. If the injured part is actually separated, reattachment may be possible. Retrieve the tissue, wrap it in plastic, keep it cool, and transport it with the victim.

Chest Injury

Injuries to the chest can result in serious impairment of respiratory function. Chest injuries are described as open or closed. The most critical injuries are open pneumothorax, flail chest, massive **hemothorax**, and **cardiac tamponade**. Any injury at or below the nipple line may cause both chest and abdominal injuries.

Table 63.1 Interventions for Specific Eye Injuries

TYPE OF INJURY	EMERGENCY INTERVENTION
Foreign bodies	If not embedded: remove by irrigation or by gently touching the object with the corner of a clean cloth or gauze pad or a moistened cotton-tipped applicator. Embedded foreign bodies should be removed only by a physician.
Chemical contact	Immediately flush the eye for at least 20 min. Sterile normal saline or water is ideal, but tap water may be used. Direct the irrigating fluid to flow from the inner canthus to the outer canthus of the eye. Even if the flushing seems to relieve all symptoms, the patient should be examined by a physician to assess the eye for injury.
Perforation of the globe	Do not attempt to remove an object that has perforated the eye! You could cause additional harm. Instead, limit movement of the object and the eye, and transport the victim for immediate medical care. Protect the injured eye by covering it with a shield that does not touch the object. An inverted paper cup can be taped over the eye. Patch the unaffected eye as well because the eyes move together. This precaution limits movement in both eyes. Tell the patient why both eyes need to be covered.
Eyelid trauma	Seek medical evaluation because injury of the globe, as well as the lid, is always possible. Do not apply direct pressure to a bleeding eyelid. If the globe has been injured, pressure could cause additional harm. Apply a loose dressing and transport the victim for medical care.

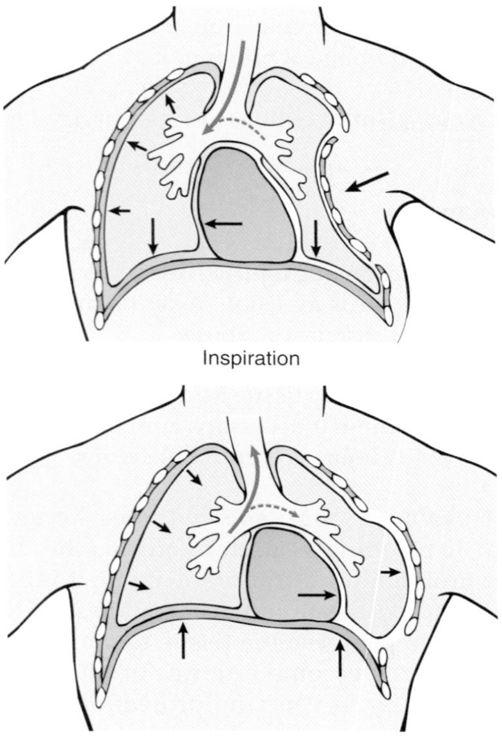

Fig. 63.5 Paradoxical motion caused by loss of chest wall support. (From Lewis SM, Dirksen SR, et al.: *Medical-surgical nursing: assessment and management of clinical problems*, ed 9, St. Louis, 2015, Mosby.)

Focused Assessment. Assessment of respiratory status always takes first priority when the victim has sustained a chest injury. Note the rate and character of the victim's respirations, skin color, pulse rate and rhythm, symmetry of the chest wall movement, and the presence of any apparent injuries to the chest. Signs and symptoms of chest injuries that impair respirations are dyspnea, tachycardia, restlessness, cyanosis, asymmetric or other abnormal chest wall movement, and abnormal sounds associated with breathing (Fig. 63.5). Note the patient's mental state and level of consciousness.

Patient problem, goal, and outcome criteria: chest injury. For the patient with a chest injury, the priority patient problem is inadequate oxygenation related to altered anatomic structure. The goal is adequate oxygenation, and the outcome criteria are absence of dyspnea, normal pulse and respiratory rates, and normal skin color.

Interventions. Interventions for emergency management of specific chest injuries are briefly described in Table 63.2. (See "Nursing Care of the Patient With Pneumothorax in Chapter 27 for a more detailed discussion.)

Abdominal Injury

Focused Assessment. Assess the abdomen for evidence of injury. In addition to asking the patient about abdominal symptoms, inspect the abdomen for abnormalities. Suspect internal abdominal injuries when the patient complains of abdominal pain or the abdomen shows evidence of trauma or distention. The protrusion of internal organs through a wound is called *evisceration*. Eviscerated organs are subject to trauma and drying.

Patient Problems, Goals, and Outcome Criteria: Abdominal Injury

Patient Problems	Goals and Outcome Criteria
Disrupted tissue integrity related to traumatic injury or exposed internal organs	Protection of eviscerated tissue: proper covering of wound to maintain moisture and warmth
Potential for infection related to break in skin, possible injury to intestinal tract	Decreased potential for infection: wound protected from contamination

Table 63.2 Emergency Interventions for Chest Injuries

TYPE OF INJURY	EMERGENCY INTERVENTION
Pneumothorax: an open chest wound penetrates the pleural cavity, allowing air to enter, which collapses lung on affected side. *Signs and symptoms:* Dyspnea, asymmetric chest wall movement, "sucking" sound as air moves in and out of wound with respirations.	Apply vented dressing: sealed on three sides so air can escape but not enter the wound.
Flail chest: several adjacent ribs are broken in more than one place, causing a loss of support in the affected section of the chest wall. *Signs and symptoms:* The affected section moves inward on inspiration and outward on expiration. This abnormal chest wall movement, called *paradoxical motion*, impairs gas exchange (see Fig. 63.5).	Provide support for the injured area. Hold or tape a small pad or pillow over the injury to splint the ribs.
Hemothorax: accumulation of blood in the pleural cavity; causes the lung or lungs to collapse. *Signs and symptoms:* Increasing respiratory or circulatory failure.	Cannot be diagnosed directly or treated by the first-aid care provider. The victim requires prompt treatment in a medical facility.
Cardiac tamponade: presence of blood in the pericardial sac. *Signs and symptoms:* Increasing respiratory or circulatory failure.	Cannot be diagnosed directly or treated by first-aid care. Causes decreased cardiac output. The victim requires prompt treatment in a medical facility.

Interventions. Possible internal injuries require medical evaluation. Do not give the patient anything by mouth while preparing for transport. Do not attempt to replace eviscerated organs in the abdomen because additional harm may result. Cover eviscerated organs with some material such as plastic wrap or foil to conserve moisture and warmth. A saline-soaked sterile dressing is ideal but is not likely to be available at the scene of an accident. Cover the wound with a clean cloth and seek transportation to a hospital.

Traumatic Amputation

If body tissue has been partially or completely detached, reattachment may be possible. If supplies are available, clean the wound surfaces with sterile water or saline and place the tissue in its normal position. Ideally, a body part that is completely detached should be wrapped in sterile gauze moistened with sterile saline, placed in a watertight container such as a resealable plastic bag, and placed in an iced saline bath. The tissue should not be frozen or placed in contact with ice. Amputated extremities may be healthy enough for reattachment for 4 to 6 hours whereas digits (fingers and toes) may be viable for as long as 8 hours.

BURNS

Care of the burn patient is discussed in detail in Chapter 57. This chapter addresses only emergency measures for burn care. When a burn accident occurs, the immediate concern is to stop the burning process. A victim whose clothing is burning should be told to drop to the ground and roll to extinguish the flames. Smother the flames with coats or blankets or extinguish the flames with water if no chemicals or flammable liquids are present on the clothing. Remove burning or smoldering materials from the victim. Protection of the airway is of primary importance in a burn patient.

Focused Assessment

First determine the type of burn that has occurred. If the victim has had a flame burn or has been in a closed, smoke-filled area, begin with assessment of respirations. Assess airway patency. The patient who has singed areas around the mouth or nose, or any areas of blackness around the mouth and nose or the eyes, must be treated as having an inhalation injury. Then determine the extent and depth of the burns. Inspect the skin for color, blisters, and tissue destruction. Superficial burns are typically pink or red and painful. Deeper burns may be red, white, or black and may destroy not only the skin but also the underlying tissues. The deepest burns are not painful because nerves have been destroyed. However, because the depth of a burn is often not uniform, patients with deep burns can still have pain. Determining the extent of the body surface area injured is very important. (See guidelines for assessing the extent of burn injury in Chapter 57.)

Electrical burns are difficult to assess initially because the full extent of tissue damage may not be apparent for several days. In the event of chemical burns, note and immediately remove any remaining chemical.

Interventions

Ensuring a patent airway and respirations for burn victims is critical. If the burns have been caused by flames, fumes, or chemicals, the victim may have inhaled substances that cause respiratory impairment. Immediately apply oxygen and anticipate an order for arterial blood gas analysis. Rescue breathing, if needed, is described in AHA publications under Cardiopulmonary Arrest. Other interventions are addressed in Table 63.3 for each of the major types of burns.

Patient Problems, Goals, and Outcome Criteria: Burns

Depending on the severity and type of the burn patient, problems and goals for the burn victim immediately after the injury may include the following.

Patient Problems	Goals and Outcome Criteria
Inadequate oxygenation related to inhalation or thermal injury, edema of airway tissues	Improved oxygenation: normal pulse and respiratory rates; no dyspnea, confusion, or cyanosis; normal arterial blood gases
Potential for complications (continued tissue damage) related to thermal destruction, chemical injury	Absence of complications: no additional damage after initial burn, skin surfaces protected and free of burning materials
Pain related to thermal injury	Reduced pain: victim calmer, states pain is lessened

Table 63.3 Emergency Interventions for Burns

TYPE OF BURN	EMERGENCY INTERVENTION
Minor or superficial	Immerse the injured body part in cool water for 2 to 5 minutes. Applying butter to the burn is contraindicated. Medical care is usually not required.
Sunburn	Topical preparations with benzocaine may be soothing. Many people believe that *Aloe vera* is very effective in treating minor burns, but this treatment is still being studied. Children and older adults with extensive sunburn may require hospitalization for dehydration.
Extensive burns	Apply cool water only until the burned area is cool. Do not apply butter, lotions, ice, medications, or absorbent materials. Call the nearest burn center for instructions before applying any dressing. You may be advised to cover burns with a clean, dry dressing or cloth. Wrap burned fingers and toes separately to prevent sticking together. Have the victim transported for medical care immediately.
Chemical burns	Remove contaminated clothing. Thoroughly dust powdered chemicals from the skin and then flush with water for 30 minutes. If the dry chemical is not removed before flushing, the water may cause the chemical to become caustic, resulting in additional injury. Flush liquid chemicals from the skin with running water for at least 30 min. Apply a dressing or covering and have the victim transported for medical care.

HEAT AND COLD EXPOSURE

Extreme heat or cold may have local or systemic effects. Several mechanisms work to maintain body temperature within a fairly narrow range. If the body temperature rises or falls excessively, vital functions begin to fail. Infants and older adults are less able to adapt to temperature extremes than other people. This tendency places them at increased risk for excessive alterations in body temperature.

Hyperthermia

Excessive heat exposure may cause **hyperthermia**, a condition in which body temperature rises above 37.2°C (99°F). Heat edema and heat cramps are mild degrees of hyperthermia. These mild forms of hyperthermia usually can be treated by moving the individual into a cool place and providing fluids with electrolytes such as sports drinks. Salt tablets are not generally recommended. Heat exhaustion and heat stroke are more serious. Treatment details are presented in Table 63.4. (See also the Patient Teaching box.)

Patient Teaching

Prevention of Heat Exhaustion

- Avoid strenuous activities outdoors when the temperature or humidity is very high.
- Increase fluid intake to replace excessive fluid loss.
- Take frequent rest breaks when working in hot, humid weather.

Pharmacology Capsule

Diuretics and anticholinergics increase the risk of heat stroke by affecting the body's heat-reducing defenses.

Hypothermia

Hypothermia is a decrease in body core temperature below 35°C (95°F). It may be caused by prolonged exposure to cold, extremely cold temperatures, or immersion in cold water. Hypothermia causes depression of vital functions and, if it is not corrected, death results from cardiac dysrhythmias. Hypothermia is classified based on core body temperature as mild (32°C–35°C), moderate (28°C–32°C), or severe (<28°C). In the mild stage, the patient shivers to generate body heat. Blood vessels in the extremities are constricted and performance of complex motor tasks is impaired. Persons in moderate hypothermia appear dazed and have poor motor coordination, slurred speech, and violent shivering; they also may behave irrationally. Severe hypothermia is characterized by waves of shivering, rigid

Table 63.4 Emergency Interventions for Heat and Cold Exposure

TYPE OF EXPOSURE OR INJURY	EMERGENCY INTERVENTION
Heat Exhaustion	
Caused by excessive fluid loss when exposed to high environmental temperature and humidity. Rising body temperature and metabolic rate increase oxygen demand. Cardiac output and heart rate first increase then fall. Loss of fluids causes hypovolemia (low blood volume) and electrolyte imbalances. *Signs and symptoms:* Dizziness, headache, muscle cramps, nausea and vomiting, and collapse. Skin is usually pale and damp. Elevated rectal temperature; may be as high as 41.1°C (106°F).	Move the person to cooler environment, preferably one that is air-conditioned, and loosen clothing. Splash cool water on the skin. If the victim is alert, offer fluids such as commercially prepared electrolyte drinks, if available.
Heat Stroke	
Body core temperature of 41.1°C (106°F) or greater. Temperature-regulating mechanisms in the brain fail. Heart, kidneys, and central nervous system functions are depressed. The victim is unable to sweat and will die if the temperature is not lowered. Usually associated with strenuous activity in hot, humid weather. *Signs and symptoms:* Similar to heat exhaustion at first: dizziness, weakness, nausea. As the condition worsens, the skin becomes red, hot, and dry. *Perspiration is noticeably absent*. If the condition is not reversed, the victim may collapse and have seizures. The body temperature may reach as high as 43.3°C (110°F).	Cooling the person quickly is critical. Immediate transport for medical care is recommended. Anyone who cannot be transported immediately should be moved into the shade or to an air-conditioned area if possible. Apply wet, cool towels to the trunk and the extremities and place ice packs on the forehead and axillae. If a tub is available, the victim can be placed in a cool bath. Continue cooling measures until the body temperature falls below 38.3°C (101°F).
Frostbite	
Serious cold injury. Blood vessels in the skin and the extremities constrict when exposed to extreme cold. Blood clots form and circulation to the affected areas decreases. Cells die because of lack of oxygen and nutrients and because of formation of crystals that cause them to swell and rupture. Nose, cheeks, fingers, and toes are affected most often. *Signs and symptoms:* Pain is noted at first, then tingling followed by numbness.	Patient should be transported for medical treatment as soon as possible. If transport is delayed, seek a setting where warm water is available. *Do not attempt to thaw the tissue unless warmth can be maintained*. Frostbitten extremities are best rewarmed by immersion in a warm water bath of 37.7°C–40.5°C (100°F–105°F). Handle affected areas very gently to prevent additional tissue trauma. Do not rub, massage, or apply cold to the tissue. As tissue warms, the skin turns bright pink and blisters. Rewarming is very painful. If the procedure is performed in a medical facility, analgesics will be ordered before rewarming. After warming the extremities, pat dry and wrap in sterile dressings. Wrap each finger or toe separately to prevent injured tissues from sticking together. Immobilize and elevate affected parts. With severe or deep frostbite, thawed tissue dies and eventually has to be surgically debrided (removed).
Hypothermia	
Rectal temperature lower than 35°C (95°F). *Signs and symptoms:* Mild hypothermia: shivering and impaired performance. Progressive chilling: decreasing heart and respiratory rates and blood pressure. Irregular heart and breathing patterns; cardiopulmonary arrest if not treated.	Mild hypothermia: wrap victim in warm, dry clothing and blankets. Severe hypothermia: transport immediately for treatment. Victim must be rewarmed aggressively but gradually because excessive rewarming sends lactic acid and cold blood from the extremities to the heart, possibly triggering cardiac dysrhythmias. Warm the torso first. It may be wrapped in blankets or immersed in tepid water. Once the rectal temperature reaches 35°C (95°F), turn attention to warming the extremities also. Internal rewarming (warmed oxygen and intravenous fluids, peritoneal lavage, and extracorporeal blood warming) may be ordered in a medical facility.

muscles, and pale skin. The pulse rate is slow, and the pupils are dilated.

Older adults are susceptible to hypothermia because of loss of subcutaneous fat, diminished circulation, and reduced neural control over circulation; they are also unable to conserve heat effectively. Research shows that confusion in some older people is the result of hypothermia. (See Table 63.4 for treatment of systemic responses to heat and cold exposure and local cold injuries. Local thermal injuries were discussed earlier under "Burns.")

POISONING

A **poison** is any substance that, in small quantities, is capable of causing illness or harm after ingestion, inhalation, injection, or contact with the skin. Large quantities of most chemicals, including all medications, can act as poisons. Even common drugs such as aspirin, acetaminophen, and vitamins can be poisonous if taken in excessive amounts.

Carbon Monoxide Poisoning

Carbon monoxide is an odorless, invisible gas emitted by internal combustion engines, gas stoves and furnaces, and burning charcoal and other combustible materials. When carbon monoxide is inhaled, it enters the bloodstream and promptly binds with hemoglobin. Carbon monoxide binds to hemoglobin much more readily than oxygen. Therefore it soon occupies many of the sites on the hemoglobin needed to transport oxygen to the cells. The victim becomes hypoxemic and can die.

Focused Assessment. Evaluate for early signs and symptoms of carbon monoxide poisoning, which include headache and shortness of breath with mild exertion. Dizziness, nausea, vomiting, and mental changes appear next. As the amount of carbon monoxide in the bloodstream rises, the victim loses consciousness and develops cardiac and respiratory irregularities. A victim usually dies when the carbon monoxide bound with hemoglobin exceeds 70%. Although a cherry-red skin color is a clear indicator of carbon monoxide poisoning, skin color is often found to be pale or bluish with reddish mucous membranes.

Patient problem, goal, and outcome criteria: carbon monoxide poisoning. The primary patient problem for the victim of carbon monoxide poisoning is inadequate oxygenation related to carbon monoxide poisoning. The goal of nursing care for the emergency treatment of the victim of carbon monoxide poisoning is normal oxygenation. Criteria for evaluating the effects of nursing interventions are regular pulse with a rate of 60 to 100 beats per minute, oxygen saturation of 95% or higher, regular respirations with a rate of 12 to 20 breaths per minute, and alert mental state.

Interventions. Immediately move the victim of carbon monoxide poisoning to fresh air. If the person is not breathing, start rescue breathing. Seek emergency medical assistance immediately. Give the victim oxygen as soon as it is available. At the hospital, the patient may be placed in a hyperbaric oxygen chamber. A hyperbaric chamber uses pressure to force oxygen into the blood and tissues. See the Patient Teaching box for ways to prevent carbon monoxide poisoning.

Patient Teaching

Prevention of Carbon Monoxide Poisoning

- Keep gas furnaces and stoves in proper repair.
- Burners that use gas must be vented to the outside.
- Do not use charcoal or wood-burning devices in a closed area without ventilation.
- Never let an engine run in a closed garage.
- Use a carbon monoxide detection alarm device.

Pharmacology Capsule

Common drugs such as aspirin, acetaminophen, and vitamins can be poisonous if taken in excessive amounts.

Drug or Chemical Poisoning

Poisoning by drugs or chemicals can result from accumulation, excessive dose level, drug interactions, or ingestion of inappropriate substances.

Focused Assessment. In situations that suggest poisoning, collect data about relevant signs and symptoms. The signs and symptoms vary with the type of poison. The history is an important part of the assessment of a poisoning victim and should include the following:

1. Name of the drug or chemical involved (If the victim cannot provide the information, look for clues and save the container.)
2. Amount of substance consumed
3. Length of time since the substance was taken
4. Last food consumed: amount, time
5. Signs and symptoms that may be caused by poisons
6. Victim's age and approximate weight
7. Other medications, drugs, or alcohol ingested

Patient problem, goal, and outcome criterion: drug or chemical poisoning. The primary patient problem for the victim of drug or chemical poisoning is potential for injury related to poison. The general goal of nursing intervention for a poisoning victim is decreased or minimized risk for injury caused by the poisoning agent. The criterion for evaluating successful intervention for drug or chemical poisoning is the absence of ill effects from the substance.

Interventions. In the event of poisoning, immediately call the American Association of Poison Control Centers at 1-800-222-1222 to be put in contact with your local poison control center. Having the product container with you is helpful because specific interventions depend on knowing exactly what poison was consumed. The poison control center staff person will ask about the condition, age, and weight of the individual; exactly when the poisoning occurred; and your name and telephone number. Although some poisonings can be treated at home, the patient should see a health care provider if the following are present: Temperature over 100.4°F (38°C), severe abdominal pain, inability to eat or drink, or bloody stool or emesis.

Several options are available for treatment of poisoning in an emergency facility. Fortunately, most cases of poisoning respond well to only supportive measures. For example, if the poison has caused hypotension, the hypotension will be treated medically. The choice of treatment depends on the potential severity of the poisoning, the time from ingestion, the risks associated with a specific intervention, and the availability of a specific antidote for the ingested poison. Activated charcoal (AC) may be administered if the poison had been consumed within the past two hours. AC binds to many poisons, thus preventing their absorption. However, not all poisons are adsorbed by AC. Efforts to decontaminate (i.e., remove the poison) from the digestive tract may employ gastric lavage, whole bowel irrigation (WBI), and/or cathartics. Gastric lavage is rarely used because the poison usually remains in the stomach for less than an hour after ingestion. Bowel lavage causes rapid transit of the poison through the intestinal tract for elimination. It may be used when the poison does not bind with AC, sustained release or enteric-coated drugs were ingested, or packets of illicit drugs were swallowed for concealment. Cathartics are not used alone, but may be given with the initial dose of AC (Hendrickson, 2021).

Food Poisoning

Food poisoning is caused by ingesting contaminated food. Contaminants can be bacteria, chemicals, or natural toxins. Bacteria most often associated with food poisoning in the United States are norovirus, *Salmonella*, *Clostridium perfringens*, and *Campylobacter* (Table 63.5).

Focused Assessment. Victims of food poisoning often recognize the relationship between their symptoms and the ingestion of food. The most common symptoms of food poisoning are nausea, vomiting, abdominal cramps, and diarrhea. Botulism caused by *C. botulinum* is rare but very serious because it produces neurotoxic effects, including difficulty breathing, seeing, and swallowing. An important clue that food poisoning is causing the victim's symptoms is that all who consumed a certain food become ill. To assist in identifying poisons, samples of stool or vomited materials may be collected for possible laboratory analysis.

Patient problem, goal, and outcome criterion: food poisoning. The primary patient problem for the victim of food poisoning is potential for injury related to poisoning. The specific type of injury depends on the action of the contaminant. In general, the treatment of food poisoning involves identifying the poison and decreasing the symptoms. The goal of nursing care

Table 63.5 Common Agents Implicated in Food Poisoning in the United States

ORGANISM	SOURCE	SIGNS AND SYMPTOMS	TREATMENT	PREVENTION
Norovirus	Fecal–oral route. Contaminated surfaces, food, water. Airborne vomitus droplets	Nausea and vomiting, watery diarrhea (not bloody), abdominal pain. Can be asymptomatic	No specific drug therapy. Fluid replacement: oral rehydration fluids Intravenous fluids if dehydrated	Avoid contact with infected people. Rinse fruits and vegetables before eating. Thoroughly cook shellfish. Wash hands often. Disinfect surfaces that could be contaminated.
Clostridium perfringens	Improper canning; inadequately cooked meat or poultry	Onset 6–12 h after ingestion: abdominal cramps, diarrhea	Antidiarrheals	Thorough cooking
Salmonella	Contaminated food; undercooked meat, eggs	Abdominal cramps, diarrhea, nausea and vomiting	Antidiarrheals, antiemetics, intravenous fluids	Thorough washing and cooking
Campylobacter	Usually foodborne most often chicken. Also waterborne or via direct contact with animal or animal products	Cramping pain around umbilicus, diarrhea (sometimes bloody). Complications: reactive arthritis, Guillain-Barré syndrome	Hydration and electrolytes as needed. Severe disease: azithromycin	Cook chicken thoroughly. Wash cutting boards, utensils, etc. used in preparation

for the victim of food poisoning is the absence or reduction of ill effects from the poison. The criterion for evaluating the effects of intervention for food poisoning is diminished symptoms (e.g., decreased pain, respiratory rate of 12–20 breaths per minute, depending on the poison).

Interventions. Medical care is necessary if symptoms are severe or persistent, especially in children and older adults. Treatment is largely symptomatic with emphasis on fluid and electrolyte balance. Intravenous fluids may be prescribed with severe vomiting and diarrhea. Patients with botulism may require ventilatory support.

Prevention. Most cases of food poisoning can be attributed to improper cooling, storage, or preparation of perishable foods. People need to be taught the importance of cleanliness when handling and cooking food and the correct way to cool and prepare food for storage.

Pharmacology Capsule

Many drugs and chemicals have antidotes. Antidotes are substances that block or reverse the effects of other substances. If the poisonous substance is known, an antidote may be ordered.

BITES AND STINGS

Snakes, ticks, bees, wasps, household pets, and even humans are capable of causing serious harm with their bites or stings. The most serious effects of bites are anaphylactic shock, infection, and tissue destruction.

Focused Assessment

Try to determine the type of bite the patient has received. Inspect the bite wound to identify the characteristics of the actual bite site and any changes in surrounding tissue. Ask the patient about any symptoms that developed after the bite, such as pain, edema, numbness, tingling, nausea, fever, dizziness, and dyspnea.

Patient Problems, Goals, and Outcome Criteria: Bites and Stings

Patient Problems	Goals and Outcome Criteria
Potential for infection related to break in skin by bite of human, animal, or insect	Reduced potential for infection: clean wound
Potential for injury related to exposure to allergens or toxins	Reduced potential for injury: antihistamine, epinephrine, or antitoxin drugs prevent dyspnea or other specific toxic effects

◆ Interventions

See Table 63.6 for interventions related to bites. The Patient Teaching boxes discuss insect bite allergy and Lyme disease.

Patient Teaching

Insect Bite Allergy

People who are very sensitive to venom should be taught how to avoid and treat bites. The teaching plan should include the following:

- Always wear a medical alert tag stating: "Allergic to insect bites."
- Obtain an emergency allergy treatment kit. Learn to use it. Teach a family member to use it. Carry it with you at all times.
- Avoid perfumes, hair spray, and bright colors when working outside. Insects are drawn to strong scents and bright colors.
- Wear long pants and sleeves, shoes and socks, and gloves when gardening.
- Keep the car windows closed when driving.
- Consider desensitizing injections if recommended by a physician. These injections gradually reduce sensitivity to venom.
- Use an insect repellant containing DEET.

Patient Teaching

Lyme Disease

Untreated Lyme disease, transmitted by the deer tick, can have serious chronic effects on the brain, eyes, joints, muscles, heart, blood vessels, lungs, skin, liver, spleen, stomach, and intestines. Adherence to the following guidelines can reduce the risk of contracting Lyme disease:

- After engaging in outdoor activities, inspect body folds and hairy areas for ticks. If ticks are removed within 36 hours, the odds of getting Lyme disease are greatly reduced.
- If you have a tick bite and develop influenza-like symptoms within 7 to 10 days, seek medical care. Antibiotic therapy can arrest Lyme disease at this early stage.

EPIDEMICS AND PANDEMICS

When a disease affects a significant proportion of a given demographic such as a college campus or a military installation at the same time, it is called an **epidemic**. When it sweeps across borders affecting many populations, it is called a **pandemic**. Most Americans have heard of Ebola, SARS, and Zika, but relatively few have been touched by these personally or professionally. The distance we felt between ourselves and potentially deadly infections was suddenly very small when COVID-19 swept across the globe. As of mid-2021, 175 million people around the world have been infected resulting in 3.78 million deaths. At the time of writing, in the United States, 33.4 million cases have been confirmed and 599,000 have died (Johns Hopkins, June 11, 2021).

Table 63.6 Interventions for Specific Bites

TYPE OF BITE	EFFECTS	INTERVENTIONS
Snake bite	Venom that is injected through the fangs into the victim may affect the nervous system or the blood and blood vessels. Venom that affects the nervous system is *neurotoxic* and can cause nausea, vomiting, dizziness, tachycardia, muscle twitching, and respiratory distress. *Local effects:* Discoloration, pain, mild to severe edema. Bites of poisonous snakes usually leave two distinct fang marks, although a finger or a toe may be pierced by only one fang.	Seek medical care immediately. A description of the snake (shape of head, color) assists in identification, which may affect treatment. To limit absorption of venom, immobilize the part where the bite is located and keep it at or below the level of the heart. Try to keep the patient still. Wipe the wound. If available, a suction cup can be applied to aspirate the wound. Antivenin, which may be given to counteract the effects of the venom, is most effective if given within 6 hours of the bite. Some tissue around the bite often becomes necrotic and must be removed surgically. *No longer recommended* (risks outweigh benefits): Tourniquet, ice, incision, and suction.
Insect bite or sting	*Common reactions:* Local itching, edema, and erythema. People who have serious allergies react with systemic symptoms of urticaria (hives), edema, and possibly fatal anaphylaxis. Characteristics of anaphylaxis are difficulty breathing and a drop in blood volume and blood pressure. If the process is not reversed, the victim quickly loses consciousness and dies (see Chapter 5).	Especially anticipate anaphylaxis in victims who develop systemic symptoms rapidly. *Mild reactions:* Calamine lotion or a paste of baking soda or meat tenderizer is soothing. *Severe allergic responses:* the patient with severe allergies should be taken to a medical facility. Epinephrine (intramuscular), diphenhydramine chloride (Benadryl), and corticosteroids (dexamethasone) may be administered after a bite or sting to prevent anaphylaxis. *Prevention:* people who are severely allergic to insect venom should carry emergency epinephrine that can be given intramuscularly after a bite or sting to prevent anaphylaxis. Only the honeybee leaves its stinger, which continues to inject venom into the victim. Immediately remove the stinger with a scraping motion rather than by grasping and pulling on it. Pinching the stinger to grasp it injects additional venom.
Animal bite	All animal bites should be taken seriously because of the risk of wound infections and rabies. Rabies is an infection of the central nervous system that is almost always fatal.	Clean the wound thoroughly; apply a bulky dressing. Advise the patient to have a tetanus booster if immunizations are not current. Patient should see a physician for antibiotic therapy. Follow local protocol to assess whether the animal has rabies. If the animal shows signs of rabies or cannot be located, *previously unvaccinated people* should receive four injections of human diploid cell vaccine (HDCV) intramuscularly at 0, 3, 7, and 14 days. In addition, the patient should receive rabies immune globulin (HRIG) at the same time as the first dose of the HDCV vaccine to provide rapid protection that persists until the vaccine works. If the victim was bitten on the face or head, the virus may reach the central nervous system more quickly. Therefore treatment may be started before the disease is confirmed in the animal.
Human bite	Human bites are potentially very dangerous because of the risk of infection. The most common site is the hand or fingers, caused by hitting a person in the mouth.	Clean thoroughly and apply a dressing. Advise the victim to seek medical attention for antibiotic therapy.

Continued

Table 63.6 Interventions for Specific Bites—cont'd

TYPE OF BITE	EFFECTS	INTERVENTIONS
Tick bite	Tick bites require attention because ticks carry organisms that cause Lyme disease and Rocky Mountain spotted fever. *Lyme disease:* *Early localized stage:* Influenza-like symptoms with or without a ring-shaped reddened area around the bite ("bull's-eye lesion"). *Early disseminated stage:* Fatigue, anorexia, vomiting, neurologic symptoms. *Late disseminated stage:* Joint (Lyme "arthritis") and muscle involvement, progressive neurologic symptoms ("arthritis"). *Rocky Mountain spotted fever:* *Symptoms*: Appear 3 to 10 days after the bite: chills, fever, headache, pain behind the eyes, joint and muscle pain, and a rash that begins on the wrists and ankles and spreads to the extremities, the trunk, and sometimes the face. Can be fatal if not treated.	When a tick is discovered, remove it promptly. *CDC recommendation*: Grasp the tick near the skin with tweezers and use a firm, steady motion to remove the tick. After tick removal, inspect to see if it is intact (no part remaining in the victim's skin). Wash the site with soap and water; apply antiseptic. *Lyme disease:* Tell the patient to notify the physician if influenza-like symptoms or a "bull's-eye lesion" develops in next 7 to 10 days. *Diagnosis:* Skin biopsy to detect the causative organism, *Borrelia burgdorferi*. A blood test can detect antibodies about 2 months after onset of the infection. *Treatment:* Early localized or disseminated stages: doxycycline or amoxicillin. *Lyme "arthritis" and neurologic symptoms:* Penicillin, cephalosporin, or chloramphenicol. *Rocky Mountain spotted fever treatment:* Tetracycline and chloramphenicol.
Spider bite	Most spider bites cause only local irritation.	For any bite, wash the site and apply a cool compress. Transport the victim for medical care if bite was by black widow or brown recluse.
	Black widow: Venom is neurotoxic; causes pain, nausea and vomiting, fever, weakness, muscle cramps, headache. *More serious effects:* Respiratory distress, hypertension, seizures, and shock.	*Black widow* is shiny black with red hourglass on abdomen. *Treatment:* Antivenin is available for black widow spider bites.
	Brown recluse: Bite not especially painful; area usually swells within a few hours. Initially, a bluish ring appears around the bite. Later it is surrounded by a white ring with a red "halo." Some people experience nausea and vomiting, fever, and joint pain. Severe cardiac, renal, and neurologic reactions are uncommon. In 3–4 days after a bite, the affected tissue becomes necrotic.	*Brown recluse* is light brown with a fiddle-shaped mark on the thorax. Medical attention should be sought for these bites. *Treatment:* No specific antivenin is available to counteract the venom of the brown recluse. Eventually the tissue sloughs off or needs to be debrided. The injury can be so extensive that reconstructive surgery is needed.

CDC, Centers for Disease Control and Prevention.

As it became apparent that this was not "just another flu," all levels of government took notice and implemented policies and guidelines to stem the rising tide of infections. Scientists raced to develop vaccines and deliver them to the public. The pharmaceutical industry sought drugs that would slow or stop the deadly coronavirus SARS-CoV-2 that causes COVID-19. In many cities, hospitals were suddenly overwhelmed with critically ill patients and the health care system was stretched to the limit. At the level of the bedside, it has been nurses on the frontline nurses on the frontline putting themselves at risk to care for patients with a disease that was not fully understood. It became clear that the nation, the health care system, and the health care professions were not adequately prepared to respond to a pandemic.

Just as cases appeared to be waning, new variants emerged resulting in new surges. The effectiveness of existing vaccines against the variants is being evaluated. Nurse organizations and leaders have banded together to find ways to improve our readiness for future pandemics that are bound to occur. Efforts have focused on: (1) Meeting the need for increased bedside nurses to care for the surge of patients, (2) Preparing the current and future nursing workforce for such events, and (3) Providing a safe work environment for those nurses who put themselves at risk.

INCREASE THE ACTIVE NURSING WORKFORCE

As the need for additional nurses became clear, state boards of nursing, with recommendations by the National Council of State Boards of Nursing (NCSBN), implemented policies to address the workforce deficit. Because each state board could make its own policies, there was no consistency across the nation. Examples of policies that have been implemented are:

- The process for retired and inactive nurses to obtain active licenses and return to practice were streamlined.
- Rules on the temporary practice of nurses in states other than the ones where they were licensed were relaxed.
- Nurses with suspended licenses not related to patient safety issues were reviewed and their licenses restored if appropriate.

PREPARE CURRENT AND FUTURE NURSES FOR PANDEMIC RESPONSE

- The NCSBN in collaboration with 10 national nursing organizations encouraged nursing programs and health care facilities to work together. For example, facilities could hire students and faculty to provide care that would meet the students course requirements and support facility staff.
- Schools of nursing and professional organizations need to provide training for current and future nurses in relation to pandemic responses.
- Nursing school curricula need to include required content related to nursing in a pandemic.
- Nursing faculty need the opportunity to enhance their knowledge and skills for a pandemic response.
- Discussions of ethical issues that nurses and nursing students caring for pandemic patients face must take place: dealing with person risk, possibility of putting significant others at risk, caring for one's family versus continuing clinical work

PROVIDE A SAFE WORK ENVIRONMENT FOR HEALTH CARE PROVIDERS

For frontline nurses, COVID-19 was at first an unknown. It was not clear how it was transmitted and how nurses could best protect themselves from infection. Among the tasks for health care facilities were to:

- Design different staffing patterns to maximize use of employees
- Assure adequate personal protective equipment (PPE) and train personnel in its use
- Cross train nurses to cover areas (e.g., ICUs) where the need is greatest
- If not already in place, set up plans, procedures, and human resources to deal with the surge of new employees
- Provide resources for emotional support of nurses working in a high-stress environment.

We all hope that COVID-19 will be the last pandemic we see for a long time, but we have to assume the next one is on the horizon and that nurses will again be on the frontline.

ROLES OF THE LICENSED VOCATIONAL NURSE/ LICENSED PRACTICAL NURSE DURING A PANDEMIC

Because each state board of nursing specifies the scope of practice for LVNs/LPNs, it is vital that you go to your board with questions about practice during a pandemic. The Texas Board of Nursing, for example, states "The RN and LVN scope of practice remains unchanged in a disaster" (Texas Board of Nursing, 2018). Therefore, nurses are not permitted to perform acts of medical diagnosis or to prescribe therapeutic measures under normal circumstances, or in disaster/pandemic situations. To provide medications, a valid order by a physician, podiatrist, or dentist is required. An exception is vaccine administration which is considered preventative and does not require a medical diagnosis or order. Student nurses can also administer vaccines under the direct supervision of an RN faculty member or preceptor as long as the student has the training, skills, knowledge, and abilities to provide the vaccine safely.

In Texas, disasters constitute exceptions to the rules that prohibit mandatory overtime. If a nurse is given an assignment that they think is unsafe, the nurse can invoke "safe harbor" which provides immunity from board action against the nurse's license. Policies and procedures regarding safe harbor should be clearly spelled out in each board of nursing rules and regulations. The priority consideration is patient safety. Keep in mind that this information is obtained from the Texas Board of Nursing and may differ from other state policies.

Put On Your Thinking Cap!

Go to the Board of Nursing website in your state and access information about LVN/LPN and student roles during disasters including pandemics.

ACTS OF BIOTERRORISM

In recent decades, numerous events, including the terrorist attacks on the World Trade Center and Pentagon, have made us aware that we are vulnerable to attacks using various means. Bioterrorism is the deliberate release of pathogens to kill and injure people. The biologic agents most likely to be used in terrorism attacks are anthrax, botulism, plague, smallpox, and tularemia. Because these agents are easily spread, they have the potential to cause many deaths. Imagine the public panic that might follow an outbreak of smallpox! A major problem in the United States is lack of experience in recognizing and treating these infections. Basic information about the biologic agents most likely to be used as bioterrorism weapons is provided in Table 63.7.

Table 63.7 Biologic Agents Most Likely to Be Used as Bioterrorism Weapons

BIOLOGIC AGENT	CHARACTERISTICS	TREATMENTS AND OUTCOMES
Anthrax	After exposure, symptoms may appear in 7 to 42 days. Three types: 1. Skin (cutaneous): painless lesion begins as small sore and then blisters, ulcerates, and blackens. 2. Lungs (inhalation): sore throat, mild fever, muscle aches, cough, shortness of breath. 3. Digestive tract (gastrointestinal): nausea, anorexia, bloody diarrhea, severe stomach pain.	Antibiotic treatment with fluoroquinolones used for prevention following exposure (along with vaccine); antibiotics alone for infection Cutaneous: usually responds to antibiotics Gastrointestinal: fatal in 25% to 50% of cases Inhalation: fatal in about one-half of all cases
Botulism	Toxins are ingested in foods. Onset of symptoms 6 hours to 2 weeks after ingestion. Causes progressive paralysis with double vision, drooping eyelids, slurred speech, and dry mouth. Progresses downward to arms, chest, and legs. Can paralyze muscles of respiration.	Centers for Disease Control and Prevention stocks antitoxin, which can reduce severity of symptoms if given early. Most people recover after weeks to months of supportive care.
Pneumonic plague	Normally spread by infected rodent fleas but can be spread in an aerosol form and then transmitted from one person to another. Causes fever, weakness, rapidly developing pneumonia, shortness of breath, and cough.	Prompt antibiotic therapy (within 24 h after onset of symptoms) may be effective in prevention after exposure. Antibiotics include streptomycin, gentamicin, and tetracyclines.
Smallpox	Caused by a virus transmitted from person to person. Onset of symptoms 10 to 12 days after exposure includes high fever and pain. Rash with small papules progresses to pustules and then to scabs.	Can be prevented with vaccine, but this is not routinely given now in the United States. No specific treatment is available. Among infected persons who have not been vaccinated, 25% to 30% die.
Tularemia	In nature, is carried by rodents and rabbits. As a weapon, can be made into an aerosol or dispersed in food or water. Onset of symptoms usually 3 to 5 days after exposure. Manifestations: sudden fever, chills, headache, diarrhea, muscle aches, joint pain, dry cough, progressive weakness.	Antibiotics are usually effective. Efforts to have a vaccine approved are underway.

From Centers for Disease Control and Prevention Bioterrorism https://www.cdc.gov/anthrax/bioterrorism/index.html; Disease Control and Prevention: *Emergency preparedness and response, 2012*. https://emergency.cdc.gov/bioterrorism/prep.asp; Pneumonic Plague: https://wwwnc.cdc.gov/travel/yellowbook/2018/infectious-diseases-related-to-travel/plague-bubonic-pneumonic-septicemic.

In the event of an outbreak of disease related to bioterrorism, health care providers must know how to protect themselves and others. Health care facilities should have readily available information on resources, including from the local health department and the Centers for Disease Control and Prevention (CDC). Staff should know where to obtain personal protective equipment and what types of precautions (e.g., patient isolation) should be taken. Staff members who are exposed should obtain prophylactic therapy if appropriate. Persons with weakened immune systems should not provide direct care for affected individuals.

DISASTER PLANNING

A challenge for the health care system is to be ready for natural disasters that often occur with short warning. Organizations such as the American Red Cross and the Salvation Army, which are experienced in handling these situations, quickly move in to help. However, a call for nurse volunteers usually follows. Regardless of the area of clinical expertise, each nurse can certainly contribute. The American Red Cross offers courses in disaster training for nurses and nursing students. With appropriate supervision, nursing students can assist with many services in disaster situations. When Hurricanes Katrina, Harvey, and Sandy struck the United States, local nurses, nursing faculty, and nursing students were indispensable in providing care to persons affected and displaced by the storm. See the Health Promotion box for a review of how the Health Insurance Portability and Accountability Act (HIPAA) applies during disaster response situations.

Internet resources for emergency preparedness information include the following:

- US Department of Health and Human Services, Office of the Assistant Secretary for Preparedness and Response: https://www.phe.gov/emergency/events/COVID-19/Pages/default.aspx.
- Federal Emergency Management Agency (FEMA): www.fema.gov
- Centers for Disease Control and Prevention: www.cdc.gov

Health Promotion

HIPAA Privacy and Disclosures in Emergency Situations

The HIPAA Privacy Rule allows patient information to be shared to assist in disaster relief efforts, such as those that occurred after Hurricane Katrina. Providers and health plans covered by the HIPAA Privacy Rule can share patient information in all of the following ways.

TREATMENT

Health care providers can share patient information as necessary to provide treatment. Treatment includes:

- Sharing information with other providers (including hospitals and clinics)
- Referring patients for treatment (including linking patients with available providers in areas where the patients have relocated)
- Coordinating patient care with others (e.g., emergency relief workers or others who can help in finding patients appropriate health services)

NOTIFICATION

Health care providers can share patient information as necessary to identify, locate, and notify family members, guardians, or other persons responsible for the individual's care or the individual's location, general condition, or death. Thus when necessary, the hospital may notify the police, the media, or the public at large to the extent necessary to help locate, identify, or otherwise notify family members and others as to the location and general condition of their loved ones.

IMMINENT DANGER

Providers can share patient information with anyone as necessary to prevent or lessen a serious and imminent threat to the health and safety of a person or the public, consistent with applicable law and the provider's standards of ethical conduct.

FACILITY DIRECTORY

Health care facilities that maintain a directory of patients can tell people who call or ask about individuals whether the individual is at the facility, the individual's location in the facility, and the individual's general condition.

Of course, the HIPAA Privacy Rule does not apply to disclosures if they are not made by entities covered by the Privacy Rule. Thus for instance, the HIPAA Privacy Rule does not restrict the American Red Cross from sharing patient information.

HIPAA, Health Insurance Portability and Accountability Act.
From www.hhs.gov/ocr/hipaa.

LEGAL ASPECTS OF EMERGENCY CARE

Although we do not ordinarily treat people without their permission, in emergencies patients may be unable to consent to care. In such cases, treatment can be provided under the assumption (called the *emergency doctrine*) that the patient would have consented if able.

In the first-aid treatment of emergencies outside the hospital, the nurse is expected to demonstrate the same skill, knowledge, and care that would be provided by other nurses in the same community with the same credentials. The Good Samaritan doctrine in most states is intended to limit liability and provide protection against malpractice claims when health care providers render first aid at the scene of an emergency. Although many Good Samaritan laws cover nurses, not all do. An important point to remember is that these laws do not protect the nurse in the event of gross negligence or willful misconduct. In addition, recent court cases have challenged the Good Samaritan doctrine.

Be aware that situations involving legal matters may depend on evidence at the scene of the injury. Remember that clothing and other materials may provide important information and should not be discarded. Victims who require first aid have the same rights to privacy and confidentiality as those treated in health care facilities. Do not disclose to the public any information about the victim's condition or treatment. In cases involving possible criminal activity, preserving all evidence, such as soiled or damaged clothing and body fluids, may be critical.

Put On Your Thinking Cap!

You are traveling with your spouse when a van in front of you swerves, runs off the road, and rolls over. You summon assistance on your cellphone and then stop to help. You find the following: Mr. A., in the driver's seat, complains of severe chest pain from striking the steering wheel; Mrs. B., lying on the ground, has an open compound fracture that is bleeding heavily; Teenager C., in the back seat, complains of severe neck pain; Teenager D., beside the van, has blood streaming from her nose and a cut on her forehead; and Grandmother E. is wandering around in a dazed state with her hands to her head. Fill in the table below to show the type of injury you think each person may have sustained, the priority of each injury, the assessment (relevant data), and interventions for each injury, and the sequence of your interventions. Compare your completed table with that of your classmates and reach agreement on the best answers.

VICTIM	TYPE OF INJURY	PRIORITY	ASSESSMENT	INTERVENTIONS
Mr. A.				
Mrs. B.				
Teen C.				
Teen D.				
Grandmother E.				

Get Ready for the NCLEX® Examination!

Key Points

- Knowledge of first aid can make the difference between life and death in many situations.
- The cardinal rule in emergency situations: Remain calm!
- The primary survey includes evaluation of airway, breathing, and circulation.
- Look for medical alert tags, which may give some clues about the patient's health status.
- Critical interventions that may be needed are CPR or rescue breathing, application of pressure to control bleeding, head-to-toe inspection, and immobilization of injured spine or limbs.
- Because brain cells begin to die after 4 minutes without oxygen, treatment of cardiopulmonary arrest must begin immediately.
- The universal sign of choking is grabbing the throat with one or both hands.
- Abdominal thrusts use pressure on the diaphragm to force air and obstructions out of the airway.
- Shock results from acute circulatory failure caused by inadequate blood volume, heart failure, overwhelming infection, severe allergic reactions, and extreme pain or fright.
- The immediate treatment for external bleeding is direct, continuous pressure.
- Tourniquets are controversial but may be used to control bleeding as a last resort.
- For epistaxis, the patient should be told to sit down and lean forward; then pinch the nostrils shut for at least 10 minutes.
- The key to emergency management of fractures is immobilization.
- Sprains and strains are treated initially with immobilization, elevation, and cool packs.
- Monitor for signs and symptoms of increased intracranial pressure with any head injury.
- Improper movement of the patient with a spinal injury may damage the spinal cord, causing permanent paralysis.
- Only a physician removes foreign bodies embedded in the eye.
- When tissue is actually torn from the body, it should be retrieved, wrapped in saline-moistened gauze, placed in a plastic bag, kept cool, and transported with the patient for possible reattachment.
- When a chest injury occurs, assessment of respiratory status always takes first priority.
- Open chest wounds that penetrate the pleural cavity allow air to enter (pneumothorax), causing the lung on the affected side to collapse.
- Cover eviscerated organs with some material such as plastic or foil to conserve moisture and warmth; do not attempt to replace the organs in the abdomen.
- The first concern with burns is to stop the burning process and then to ensure a patent airway and respirations.
- Cover large burns with clean, dry dressings and transport the victim to a care facility immediately.
- Extreme heat or cold can have serious local or potentially fatal systemic effects.
- People with heat stroke will die if the body temperature is not lowered quickly.
- Perspiration is noticeably absent with heat stroke.
- Victims of severe hypothermia must be rewarmed gradually to prevent triggering cardiac dysrhythmias.
- A hyperbaric oxygen chamber may be used to treat carbon monoxide poisoning.
- Instructions about treatment of poisoning should be obtained from the poison control center; instructions may also be found on product labels.
- In the event of poisoning, the first action is to call the local poison control center for expert guidance
- The most serious effects of bites and stings are anaphylactic shock, infection, and tissue destruction.
- Lyme disease, transmitted by tick bites, can lead to chronic cardiac, neuromuscular, and musculoskeletal disorders.
- Among the agents used as bioterrorism weapons are anthrax, botulism, pneumonic plague, smallpox, and tularemia.
- HIPAA privacy rules allow patient information to be shared to assist in disaster relief efforts.
- The emergency doctrine assumes that people would give consent for treatment of life-threatening conditions if they were able.
- Good Samaritan laws do not protect nurses against gross negligence or willful misconduct.

Additional Learning Resources

SG Go to your Study Guide for additional learning activities to help you master this chapter content.

Go to your Evolve website (http://evolve.elsevier.com/Linton/medosurg) for the following learning resources and much more:

- Fluid & Electrolyte Tutorial
- Review Questions for the NCLEX® Examination

Clinical Judgment and Next-Generation NCLEX® Examination-Style Questions

1. **After determining that an accident victim is breathing and has a pulse, the nurse should next assess for:**
   1. Loss of sensation in extremities
   2. Bleeding
   3. Level of consciousness
   4. Ability to speak

   NCLEX Client Need: Physiological Integrity: Physiological Adaptation

2. **Circulation must be restored within 4 minutes of cardiopulmonary arrest because:**
   1. Irreversible kidney failure develops
   2. The blood begins to coagulate
   3. The lungs fill with fluid
   4. Brain cells begin to die

   NCLEX Client Need: Physiological Integrity: Physiological Adaptation

3. **A person with dementia living at home is found with an empty bottle of aspirin. The caregiver suspects that the patient has consumed an unknown quantity of the drug. What should the caregiver's *first* action be?**
   1. Have the victim drink a large glass of water
   2. Administer syrup of ipecac
   3. Call the poison control center for guidance
   4. Drive the victim to the emergency department

   NCLEX Client Need: Physiological Integrity: Physiological Adaptation

4. **Which of the following is the primary maneuver used to dislodge a foreign body from the airway?**
   1. Blow to the upper back
   2. Mouth-to-mouth ventilation
   3. Abdominal thrusts
   4. Chest compressions

   NCLEX Client Need: Physiological Integrity: Physiological Adaptation

5. **During a hike, a participant falls and injures his leg. Suspecting a fracture, the first-aid care provider should take what action?**
   1. Immobilize the leg in the position in which it was found
   2. Gently straighten the leg and immobilize it
   3. Apply a tourniquet above the fracture if bleeding is present
   4. Elevate the injured part above the level of the victim's heart

6. **SLO Objective: Outline the steps of the nursing process for emergency or first-aid treatment of victims of head injury.**

   NGN Item Type: Cloze

   Cognitive Skill: Prioritize Hypotheses

A middle-aged man has just been in an auto accident. The nurse who arrives on the scene calls EMS and collects the following data:
- large wound on forehead
- moderate bleeding from scalp wound
- conscious but confused about the accident
- headache
- respiration 14 breaths per minute
- heart rate 54 beats per minute, bounding
- unequal pupils
- moves all four extremities on command
- pain in left shoulder with movement.

Choose the *most* likely options for the information missing from the statements below by selecting from the list of options provided.

The immediate priority is to (1)_________. The nurse recognizes that (2)________ heart rate and respiratory rate and (2)________ in the presence of a head injury suggest possible (2)__________. Failure to obtain prompt medical care could result in (2)___________ and (2)___________.

OPTIONS FOR 1	OPTIONS FOR 2
Immobilize the spine	Slow
Provide some form of sugar	Rapid
Orient the patient	Heart rate
Apply pressure to the wound	Respiratory rate
Initiate rescue breathing	Confusion
Tilt his head back to open the airway	Hypoglycemia
Ask if any bystanders have an EpiPen	Increased intracranial pressure
Initiate cardiopulmonary resuscitation	Anaphylaxis
Assist the patient to call a family member	Respiratory arrest
Take photos of the accident scene	Death
	Ketoacidosis

NCLEX Client Need: Physiological Integrity: Physiological Adaptation

7. **While at a picnic at the lake, a person catches his clothing on fire while trying to start a charcoal fire. What should bystanders do *first*?**
   1. Tell him to run and jump in the lake
   2. Try to extinguish the flames with their hands
   3. Tell him to drop to the ground and roll
   4. Run to a telephone to call for help

   NCLEX Client Need: Physiological Integrity: Reduction of Risk Potential

8. **A high school football player collapses during practice on a hot, humid day. He is breathing but not responding verbally. His skin is hot, red, and dry. Which of the following actions should be taken? (Select all that apply.)**
   1. Move him to a cool location
   2. Activate the emergency medical services system
   3. Notify his parents to take him to the hospital
   4. Encourage him to take sips of ice cold liquids
   5. Apply cool, wet towels

   NCLEX Client Need: Physiological Integrity: Physiological Adaptation

9. **The patient with hypothermia must be *gradually* rewarmed to prevent ________________________.**

   NCLEX Client Need: Physiological Integrity: Reduction of Risk Potential

10. **The nurse in an immunization clinic notices a peculiar ring-shaped, reddened area on the leg of a child. When asked about it, the mother states that she removed a tick from that area last week. What should the nurse do?**
    1. Suspect early Lyme disease and refer the child for medical treatment
    2. Advise the mother to apply antibiotic ointment to the lesion daily
    3. Recognize the bite of a black widow spider and apply a constrictive band
    4. Contact the physician for an order for brown recluse spider antivenin

    NCLEX Client Need: Physiological Integrity: Physiological Adaptation

Bibliography and Reader References

CHAPTER 1: ASPECTS OF MEDICAL-SURGICAL NURSING

Academy of Medical-Surgical Nurses. (2012). *Scope and standards of medical-surgical nursing practice* (5th ed.). https://amsn.org.

Dupler, A. E. (2017). Legal implications in nursing practice. In P. A. Potter, A. G. Perry, P. A. Stockert, et al. (Eds.), *Fundamentals of nursing* (9th ed.). St. Louis: Elsevier.

National Association For Practical Nurse Education and Service. (2007). *Standards of practice*. https://napnes.org/drupal-7.4/sites/default/files/pdf/standards/standards_2009.pdf.

NCSBN. (April 29, 2019). *National guidelines for nursing delegation*. Retrieved from https://www.ncsbn.org/NGND-PosPaper_06.pdf.

Park, L. J. (Jul 22, 2020). Using the SBAR handover tool. *British Journal of Nursing*, *29*(14).

Texas Board of Nursing. (2007). Texas administrative code chapter 217: Licensure, peer assistance and practice. Retrieved Oct 12, 2020 from https://www.bon.texas.gov/rr_current/217-11.asp.

CHAPTER 2: MEDICAL-SURGICAL PRACTICE SETTINGS

Center for Medicare Services. *What medicare covers, N.d.* Medicare.gov.

Taylor, M. G., Lynch, S. M., & Urena, S. (Feb, 2018). Race differences in ADL disability decline 1984-2004. *Aging Health*, *30*(2), 167–189.

Texas Board of Nursing. (2016). *Currently employed Texas LVNs by county and primary place of employment*. https://www.bon.texas.gov/pdfs/2016TexasStatistics/Sept2016/LVNs%20BY%20county%20and%20clinical%20practice%20area2.pdf.

Texas Board of Nursing. (2016). *Currently employed Texas LVNs by county and primary place of employment*. https://www.bon.texas.gov/pdfs/2016TexasStatistics/Sept2016/LVNs%20BY%20county%20and%20employment%20field2.pdf.

US Department of Health and Human Services Centers for Medicare and Medicaid Services. (November 5, 2018). *MLN Matters Number: SE1436*.

US Department of Health and Human Services, Centers for Medicare and Medicaid. (Jan 1, 2019). *MLN Matters #SE 1436. Eligibilityfor home health services*.

US Department of Health and Human Services NIH office of Extramural Research. (1990). *Individuals with disabilities*. https://extramural-diversity.nih.gov/diversity-matters/individuals with disabilities. Retrieved Sep 15, 2020.

US Equal Employment Opportunity Commission. (January 1, 1992). *Your employment rights as an individual with a disability*. Retrieved Sep 15, 2020 from https://www.eeoc.gov/laws/guidance/your-employment -rights-individual with a disability.

CHAPTER 3: MEDICAL-SURGICAL PATIENTS: INDIVIDUALS, FAMILIES, AND COMMUNITIES

American Cancer Society Guidelines for the Early Detection of Cancer. https://www.cancer.org/healthy/find-cancer-early-screening-guidelines/screening-recommendations-by-age.html#30-39.

American Dental Association. (2013). *American dental association statement of regular dental visits*. ADA.org.

Bureau of Labor Statistics, U.S. Department of Labor. (2020). Licensed practical and licensed vocational nurses. *Occupational Outlook Handbook*. Retrieved November 11, 2020 from https://www.bls.gov/ooh/healthcare/licensed-practical-and-licensed-vocational-nurses.htm#tab-3.

Centers for Disease Control and Prevention. (October 30, 2019). Vaccine information statement PCV13. *Patient Pamphlet*.

Centers for Disease Control and Prevention. (October 30, 2019). Vaccine information statement Recombinant zoster (shingles). *Patient Pamphlet*.

Centers for Disease Control and Prevention. (2017). *Are you getting enough sleep?*. https://www.cdc.gov/features/sleep/index.html.

Centers for Disease Control and Prevention. (2016). *Pneumococcal vaccination*. http://www.vaccines.gov/disease/pneumonia/index.html.

Department of Health and Human Services – Office of Disease Prevention and Health Promotion. (2017). *Healthy people 2020*. https://www.healthypeople.gov/2020/topics-objectives.

National Center for Health Statistics. (2018). *Ten leading causes of death by age group, United States*.

National Institute on Aging. (April 10, 2020). *Shots for safety*. Retrieved November 12, 2020 from https://www.nia.nih.gov/health/shots-safety.

National Institutes for Health-National Heart, Lung, and blood Institute. (2008). Recommendations for physical activity. https://www.nhlbi.nih.gov/health/health-topics/topics/phys/recommend.

Internet Resources

Centers for Disease Control and Prevention: cdc.gov/vaccines.

National Sleep Foundation. (2015). *National sleep foundation recommends new sleep times*. https://sleepfoundation.org/press-release/national-sleep-foundation-recommends-new-sleep-times.

CHAPTER 4: HEALTH, ILLNESS, STRESS, AND COPING

Agency for Healthcare Research and Quality. (2018). *Next steps after your diagnosis*. Retrieved October 18, 2020 from https://www.ahrq.gov/health-literacy/patient-education/diagnosis/support.html.

American Dental Association. (2013). *American dental Association statement of regular dental visits*. ADA.org.

Centers for Disease Control and Prevention. (2017). *Are you getting enough sleep?*. https://www.cdc.gov/features/sleep/index.html.

Centers for Disease Control and Prevention. (2016). *Pneumococcal vaccination*. http://www.vaccines.gov/disease/pneumonia/index.html.

Department of Health and Human Services – Office of Disease Prevention and Health Promotion. (2017). *Healthy people 2020*. https://www.healthypeople.gov/2020/topics-objectives.

National Institutes for Health-National Heart, Lung, and Blood Institute. (2008). Recommendations for physical activity. https://www.nhlbi.nih.gov/health/health-topics/topics/phys/recommend. www.MouthHealthy.org.

National Sleep Foundation. (2015). *National sleep foundation recommends new sleep times*. https://sleepfoundation.org/press-release/national-sleep-foundation-recommends-new-sleep-times.

Piercy, K. L., Trolano, R. P., Ballard, R. M., Carlson, S. A., Fulton, J. E., Galucka, D. A., et al. (2018). *The physical activity guidelines for Americans*. Retrieved October 18, 2020 from https://pubmed.ncbi.nlm.nih.gov/30418471/#:~text=The Physical Activity Guidelines for Americans.

US Department of Health and Human Services. (2019). *Healthy people 2030*. Retrieved October 15, 2020 from https://health.gov/healthypeople.

CHAPTER 5: IMMUNITY, INFLAMMATION, AND INFECTION

Anderson, D. J., & Harris, A. (last updated March 11, 2020). Infection prevention: Precautions for preventing transmission of infection. *UpToDate*. Retrieved October 20, 2020 from https://www.uptodate.com/contents/infection-prevention-precautions-for-preventing-transmission-of-infection?source=history_widget.

Black, J. M., & Hawks, J. H. (2009). *Medical-surgical nursing: Clinical management for positive outcomes* (8th ed.). St. Louis: Saunders.

Centers for Disease Control and Prevention. (2017). *2017 National notifiable condition*. https://wwwn.cdc.gov/nndss/conditions/notifiable/2017/.

Centers for Disease Control and Prevention. (2016). *Antibiotic prescribing and use in hospitals and long-term care*. https://www.cdc.gov/antibiotic-use/healthcare/index.html.

Centers for Disease Control and Prevention. (2017). *Healthcare Infection Control Practices Advisory Committee (HICPAC)*. https://www.cdc.gov/hicpac/index.html.

Centers for Disease Control and Prevention. (2017). *Immunization schedules*. https://www.cdc.gov/vaccines/schedules/.

Centers for Disease Control and Prevention. (2017). *Infection control: Isolation precautions*. https://www.cdc.gov/infectioncontrol/guidelines/isolation/index.html.

Centers for Disease Control and Prevention. (2017). *Infection control: Multidrug-Resistant Organisms (MDRO) management*. https://www.cdc.gov/infectioncontrol/guidelines/MDRO/index.html. Last updated February 15, 2017.

Centers for Disease Control and Prevention. (2016). *Injection safety*. https://www.cdc.gov/injectionsafety/index.html.

Centers for Disease Control and Prevention. (2016). *Public health image library: Bioterrorism diseases/agents*. https://phil.cdc.gov/bt.aspx.

Kim, A. Y., & Gandhi, R. T. (Oct 23, 2020). Coronavirus disease 2019: Management in hospitalized adults. *UpToDate*. Retrieved October 27, 2020 from uptodate.com/.

McCance, K. L., & Huether, S. E. (2009). *Pathophysiology: The biologic basis for disease in adults and children* (9th ed.). St. Louis: Mosby-Elsevier.

Monahan, F. D., Drake, D. T., & Neighbors, M. (Eds.). (1998). *Medical-surgical nursing: Foundations for clinical practice* (2nd ed.). Philadelphia: Saunders.

Patton, K. T., & Thibodeau, G. A. (2018). *Human body in health & disease* (7th ed.). St. Louis: Mosby Elsevier.

US Department of Health and Human Services. Centers for Disease Control and Prevention. (n.d.). *Protect your patients, combat antibiotic resistance*. Retrieved October 25, 2020 from https://www.cdc.gov/drugresistance/pdf/threats-report/Actions-For-Healthcare-508.pdf.

US Department of Health and Human Services. Centers for Disease Control and Prevention Healthcare Infection Control Advisory Committee. (2006; last reviewed November 5, 2015). Management of MDROs in healthcare settings. Retrieved October 20, 2020 from http://www.cdc.gov/infection control/guidelines/MDRO/index.html.

World Health Organization. (2018). *Clean care is safer care: Clean hands protect against infection*. http://www.who.int/gpsc/clean_hands_protection/en/.

CHAPTER 6: FLUID, ELECTROLYTE, AND ACID-BASE BALANCE

Burchum, J. R., & Rosenthal, L. D. (2016). *Lehne's pharmacology for nursing care* (9th ed.). St. Louis: Elsevier-Saunders.

Faller-Kopman, D. J. (April 1, 2020). The evaluation, diagnosis, and treatment of the adult patient with acute hypercapnic respiratory failure. *UpToDate*. Retrieved October 27, 2020 from www. uptodate.com.

Hyzy, R. C., & McSparron, J. I. (June 26, 2020). Non-Invasive ventilation in adults with acute respiratory failure: Benefits and contraindications. *UpToDate*. Retrieved October 27, 2020 from www. uptodate.com.

Johnson, C. S., & Sacks, G. (2017). Nutrition and aging. In H. M. Fillit, K. Rockwood, & J. Young (Eds.), *Brocklehurst's textbook of geriatric medicine and gerontology* (8th ed.) (pp. 660–666). Philadelphia: Elsevier.

Mahan, L. K., & Raymond, J. L. (2017). *Krause's food and the nutrition care process* (14th ed.). St. Louis, MO: Elsevier.

Mayo Clinic Staff. (2014). *Nutrition and healthy eating*. http://www.mayoclinic.org/healthy-lifestyle/nutrition-and-healthy-eating/in-depth/water/art-20044256.

Mount, D. B. (August 20, 2019). Treatment and prevention of hyperkalemia in adults. *UpToDate*. Retrieved October 27, 2020 from https://www.uptodate.com/contents/treatment-and-prevention-of-hyperkalemia-in-adults?search=hyperkalemia%20treatment&source=search_result&selectedTitle=1~150&usage_type=default&display_rank=1.

Mount, D. B. (December 2, 2019). Clinical manifestations and treatment of hypokalemia in adults. *UpToDate*. Retrieved October 27, 2020 from www. uptodate.com.

Seifter, J. L. (2016). Acid-base disorders. (pp. 762-774). In L. Goldman, & A. I. Schafer (Eds.), *Goldman-Cecil medicine* (2nd ed 5.) (pp. 755–762). St. Louis: Elsevier-Saunders.

Seifter, J. L. (2016). Potassium disorders. In L. Goldman, & A. I. Schafer (Eds.), *Goldman-Cecil medicine* (2nd ed 5.) (pp. 755–762). St. Louis: Elsevier-Saunders.

Slotki, I. S., & Skorecki, K. (2016). Disorders of sodium and water homeostasis. In H. M. Fillit, K. Rockwood, & J. Young (Eds.), *Brocklehurst's textbook of geriatric medicine and gerontology* (8th ed.) (pp. 741–755). Philadelphia: Elsevier.

Sterns, R. H., & Hoorn, E. I. (July 23, 2020). Treatment of hypernatremia in adults. *UpToDate*. Retrieved October 27, 2020 from www. uptodate.com.

Sterns, R. H. (2020). Treatment of hyponatremia: SIADH and reset osmostat. *UpToDate*. Retrieved October 27, 2020 from www. uptodate.com.

CHAPTER 7: THE PATIENT WITH CANCER

Abebe, W. (2002). Herbal medication: Potential for adverse interactions with analgesic drugs. *Journal of Clinical Pharmacy and Therapeutics*, 27(6), 391–401.

Abrams, A. C. (2013). *Clinical drug therapy* (10th ed.). Philadelphia: Lippincott–Williams & Wilkins.

American Cancer Society. https://www.cancer.org/content/dam/cancer-org/online-documents/en/pdf/infographics/diet-physical-activity-guidelines-infographic.pdf.

American Cancer Society. (last rev 7-30-2020). *Guidelines for the early detection of cancer*. Retrieved October 27, 2020 from https://www.cancer.org/healthy/find-cancer-early/cancer-screening-guidelines/american-cancer-society-guidelines-for-the-early-detection-of-cancer.html.

American Cancer Society. *Cancer facts & figures for African Americans: 2016-2018*. (website). https://www.cancer.org/content/dam/cancer-org/research/cancer-facts-and-statistics/cancer-facts-and-figures-for-african-americans/cancer-facts-and-figures-for-african-americans-2016-2018.pdf.

American Cancer Society. (2016). *Cancer facts and figures*. (website). https://www.cancer.org/research/cancer-facts-statistics/all-cancer-facts-figures/cancer-facts-figures-2016.html.

American Cancer Society. (2017). *Complementary and alternative medicine*. (website). http://www.cancer.org/treatment/treatmentsandsideeffects/complementaryandalternativemedicine/index.

Barnes, P. M., Bloom, B., & Nahin, R. L. (*CDC National Health Statistics report #12, 2007*. Complementary and alternative medicine use among adults and children: United States, (serial online). https://nccih.nih.gov/research/statistics/2007/camsurvey_fs1.htm.

Block, A. S., Grant, B., Hamilton, K. K., et al. (2013). *Complete guide to nutrition for cancer survivors: Eating well, staying well during and after*. Bethesda, Md: ACS.

Burchum, J. R., & Rosenthal, L. D. (2019). *Lehne's pharmacology for nursing care* (10th ed.). St Louis MO: Elsevier.

Burke, C. C. (Ed.). (2012). *Psychosocial dimensions of oncology nursing care* (2nd ed.). Pittsburgh: Oncology Nursing Society.

Cancer treatment tables (2020). Retrieved November 10, 2020 from https://www.cancerquest.org/patients/treatments/cancer-treatment-tables.

Centers for Disease Control and Prevention (last updated September 22, 2020). Cancer screening. Retrieved October 25, 202 from https://www.cdc.gov/cancer/dcpc/prevention/screening.html.

Concus, A. P., & Singer, M. I. (2011). Head and neck cancer. In L. Goldman, & J. C. Bennett (Eds.), *Goldman's Cecil textbook of medicine* (24th ed.). Philadelphia: Saunders.

Doenges, M., Moorhouse, M., & Murr, A. (2009). *Nursing care plans: Guidelines for individualizing client care across the life span*. Philadelphia: F. A. Davis Co.

Franks, H. M., & Roesch, S. C. (2007). Appraisals and coping in people living with cancer: A meta-analysis. *Psycho-Oncology*, *15*(12), 1027–1037.

Harris, D. J. (2010). Transplantation. In J. Eggert (Ed.), *Cancer basics*. Pittsburgh: Oncology Nursing Society.

Levine, A. (2010). Chemotherapy. In J. Eggert (Ed.), *Cancer basics*. Pittsburgh: Oncology Nursing Society.

Lewis, M. A., Hendrickson, A. W., & Moynihan, T. J. (2011). Oncologic emergencies: Pathophysiology, presentation, diagnosis, and treatment. *CA Cancer Journal of Clinics*, *61*(5), 287–314.

Lewis, S. M., Heitkemper, M. M., Dirksen, S. R., et al. (Eds.). (2010). *Medical-surgical nursing: Assessment and management of clinical problems* (8th ed.). St. Louis: Mosby.

McMullen, L. (2013). Patient navigation in the oncology care setting. *Seminars in Oncology Nursing*, *29*(2), 105–117.

National Center for Complementary and Integrative Health. (2017). *10 things to know about dietary supplements for children and teens*. (website). https://nccih.nih.gov/health/tips/children.

National Comprehensive Cancer Network. (2017). *NCCN clinical practice guidelines in oncology™, hepatobiliary cancers*. (website). www.nccn.org/professionals/physician_gls/pdf/hepatobiliary.pdf.

National Institutes of Health. (2015). *Cancer vaccines*. (website). https://www.cancer.gov/about-cancer/causes-prevention/vaccines-fact-sheet.

Nipp, R. D., Greer, J. A., El-Jawahri, A., et al. (2017). Coping and prognostic awareness in patients with advanced cancer. *Journal of Clinical Oncology*, *35*(22), 2551–2557.

Pagana, K. D., & Pagana, T. J. (2012). *Mosby's diagnostic and laboratory test reference* (11th ed.). St. Louis: Mosby.

Polovich, M., Olsen, M., & LeFebvre, K. (Eds.). (2014). *Chemotherapy and biotherapy guidelines and recommendations for practice* (4th ed.). Pittsburgh: Oncology Nursing Society.

Rigotti, N. A., & Kalkhoran, S. (updated: Oct 06, 2020). *Vaping and e-cigarettes*. Retrieved October 3, 2020 from uptodate.com/.

Sigal, J. J., Claude, O. M., Margolese, R., et al. (2008). How patients with less-advanced and more-advanced cancer deal with three death-related fears: An exploratory study. *Journal of Psychosocial Oncology*, *26*(1), 53–68.

Wu, K., Ghantous, H., & Birnkrant, D. (2008). Current regulatory toxicology perspectives on the development of herbal medicines to prescription drug products in the United States. *Food and Chemical Toxicology*, *46*(8), 2606–2610.

Internet Resources

American Cancer Society. http://www.cancer.gov.

Centers for Disease Control and Prevention. cdc.gov/vaccines.

National Cancer Institute. http://www.cancer.gov.

Oncology Nursing Society. http://www.ons.org.

Additional Resources

The following resources are available on the Internet and are free to download and save electronically or print. There are many practical tips for the patient:

American Cancer Society. (2004). *A cancer source book for nurses* (8th ed.). Atlanta: ACS.

National Cancer Institute. (2007). *Chemotherapy and you (NIH Publication No. 88–7156)*. Bethesda, Md: National Cancer Institute.

National Cancer Institute. (2011). *Eating hints: Recipes and tips for better nutrition during cancer treatment (NIH Publication No. 11–2079)*. Bethesda, Md: National Cancer Institute.

National Cancer Institute. (2007). *Radiation therapy and you (NIH Publication No. 11–7157)*. Bethesda, Md: National Cancer Institute.

The University of Kansas. (2009). *Guide to extravasation management in adult and pediatric patients (Adapted from Saint Francis Hospital Department of Pharmacy services Protocol)*. Lawrence: University of Kansas.

CHAPTER 8: PAIN

American Pain Society. (2016). *Principles of analgesic use* (6th ed.). Glenview, IL: American Pain Society.

Benzon, H. T. (2014). *Practical management of pain. [electronic resource]*. Philadelphia: Elsevier/Saunders.

Brant, J. M., Mohr, C., Coombs, N. C., et al. (2017). Original article: Nurses' knowledge and attitudes about pain: Personal and professional characteristics and patient reported pain satisfaction. *Pain Management Nursing*, *18*, 214–223. https://doi.org/10.1016/j.pmn.2017.04.003.

D'Arcy, Y. M. (2011). *Compact clinical guide to chronic pain management: An evidence-based approach for nurses*. New York: Springer Publishing Company.

Ddeveza, L. A., Hunter, D., & Curtis, M. R. (July 14, 2020). Management of knee osteoarthritis. *UpToDate*. Retrieved October 7, 2020 from uptodate.com.

Goldman, L., & Schafer, A. I. (2016). *Goldman-Cecil medicine. [electronic resource]*. Philadelphia, Pa: Elsevier/Saunders.

Herdman, T. H., & Kamitsuru, S. (2014). *Nursing diagnoses 2015-17. [electronic resource]: Definitions and classification*. Chichester, England: Wiley Blackwell.

McCaffery, M., & Beebe, A. (1989). *Pain: Clinical manual for nursing practice*. St. Louis: Mosby.

McCaffrey, M., & Beebe, A. (1989). *Pain: Clinical manual for nursing practice*. St. Louis MO: C.V Mosby.

McMahon, S. B. (2013). *Wall and Melzack's textbook of pain. [electronic resource]*. Philadelphia, Pa: Elsevier/Saunders.

National Comprehensive Cancer Network. (2014). NCCN clinical practice guidelines in oncology, version 1. *Adult cancer pain*. (website) http://www.nccn.org/professionals/physician_gls/pdf/pain.pdf.

Oliver, J., Coggins, C., Compton, P., et al. (2012). American society for pain management nursing position statement: Pain management in patients with substance use disorders. *Pain Management Nursing, 13*(3), 169–183. https://doi.org/10.1016/j.pmn.2012.07.001.

Parsons, G., & Preece, W. (2010). *Principles and practice of managing pain. [electronic resource]: A guide for nurses and allied health professionals*. Berkshire, England: McGraw-Hill: Open University Press, 2010.

Pasero, C., & McCaffery, M. (2011). *Pain assessment and pharmacologic management*. St. Louis: Mosby.

Pasero, C., Quinlan-Colwell, A., Rae, D., et al. (2016). Position statement: American society for pain management nursing position statement: Prescribing and administering opioid doses based solely on pain intensity. *Pain Management Nursing, 17*, 170–180. https://doi.org/10.1016/j.pmn.2016.03.001.

Tauben, D., Fishman, S., & Crowley, M. (May 6, 2020). Pharmacologic management of chronic non-cancer pain in adults. *UpToDate*. Retrieved October 7, 2020 from uptodate.com.

Waldman, S. D. (2015). *Atlas of interventional pain management. [electronic resource]*. Philadelphia: Elsevier/Saunders.

Waldman, S. D. (2017). *Atlas of pain management injection techniques. [electronic resource]*. St. Louis: Elsevier.

Waldman, S. D. (2014). *Atlas of uncommon pain syndromes. [electronic resource]*. Philadelphia: Saunders/Elsevier.

Waldman, S. D. (2011). *Pain management. [electronic resource]*. Philadelphia: Elsevier/Saunders.

Waldman, S. D. (2016). *Physical diagnosis of pain. [electronic resource]: An atlas of signs and symptoms*. St. Louis: Elsevier.

Wynn, H. R. (2017). *Youmans and Wynn neurological surgery[electronic resource]* (7th ed.). Philadelphia: Elsevier.

Internet Resources

Agency for Healthcare Research and Quality. www.ahrq.gov.

American Academy of Pain Management. http://www.aapainmanage.org/.

American Cancer Society. www.cancer.org.

American Pain Society. www.ampainsoc.org.

American Society for Pain Management Nursing. www.aspmn.org.

Arthritis Foundation. www.arthritis.org.

City of Hope Pain & Palliative Care Resource Center. http://prc.coh.org.

Hospice Foundation of America. www.hospicefoundation.org.

Institute for Safe Medication Practices. http://www.ismp.org.

International Association for the Study of Pain. https://www.iasp-pain.org/.

National Center for Complementary and Integrative Health. https://nccih.nih.gov/.

The Joint Commission. http://www.jointcommission.org/topics/pain_management.aspx.

U.S. Food and Drug Administration. www.fda.gov.

World Health Organization. http://www.who.int/cancer/palliative/painladder/en/.

CHAPTER 9: SHOCK

Anderson, M. W., & Watson, G. A. (2013). Traumatic shock: The fifth shock. *Journal of Trauma Nursing, 20*(1), 37–43.

Balk, R. A. (2014). Systemic inflammatory response syndrome (SIRS). *Virulence, 5*(1), 20–26.

Ballentine JR: *Severe allergic reaction, Emedicinehealth*. (website): www.emedicinehealth.com/severe_allergic_reaction_anaphylactic_shock/article_em.htm.

Brooks, M. (2014). Oral health in the ICU: Something to smile about, medscape medical news from the American Association of Critical-Care Nurses (AACN) 2014 National teaching institute and critical care exposition. *Medscape*. (website) http://www.medscape.com/viewarticle/825553.

Burchum, J. R., & Rosenthal, L. D. (2019). *Lehne's Pharmacology for nursing care* (10th ed.). St. Louis: Elsevier.

Chinn, L. (2013). Spinal cord injuries. *Medscape*. (website). http://emedicine.medscape.com/article/793582.

Colwell C: *Initial evaluation and management of shock in adult trauma, UpToDate*. (website): https://www.uptodate.com/contents/initial-evaluation-and-management-of-shock-in-adult-trauma. Updated Dec 11, 2015.

Dellinger, R., Schorr, C., & Levy, M. (2017). A users' guide to the 2016 surviving sepsis guidelines,. *Critical Care Medicine, 45*(3), 381–385.

deMoya, M. (*Shock, merck manual, professional version (website)*. http://www.merckmanuals.com/professional/critical-care-medicine/shock-and-fluid-resuscitation/shock Updated Oct 2013.

Gaieski D, Mikkelsen M: *Definition, classification, etiology, and pathophysiology of shock in adults, UpToDate*. (website): https://www.uptodate.com/contents/definition-classification-etiology-and-pathophysiology-of-shock-in adults?source=search_result&search=types%20of%20shock&selectedTitle=1~150. Updated: May 25, 2016.

Gaieski, D. F., & Mikkelsen, M. E. (last updated Jan 10, 2020). *Definition, classification, etiology, and pathophysiology of shock in adults*. Retrieved November 1, 2020 from uptodate.com.

Gaieski, D. F., & Mikkelsen, M. E. (last updated April 1, 2020). *Evaluation of and initial approach to the adult patient with undifferentiated hypotension and shock*. Retrieved November 1, 2020 from uptodate.com.

Hochman, J. S., & Reyentovich, A. (last updated April 27, 2020). *Prognosis and treatment of cardiogenic shock complicating acute myocardial infarction*. Retrieved November 1, 2020 from uptodate.com.

Kalil, A. *Septic shock treatment & management, Medscape*. (website): http://emedicine.medscape.com/article/168402-treatment. Updated: Sep 07, 2017.

Kaplan, L. *Systemic inflammatory response syndrome, Medscape*. (website): http://emedicine.medscape.com/article/168943-overview. Updated: Sep 13, 2017.

Kleinpell, R., Aitken, L., & Schorr, C. (2013). Implications of the new sepsis guidelines for nursing care. *American Journal of Critical Care, 22*(3), 211–222.

Kolecki, P. *Hypovolemic shock*, Medscape. (website): http://emedicine.medscape.com/article/760145-overview. Updated Oct 13, 2016.

Lessnau, K. *Distributive shock*, Medscape. (website): http://emedicine.medscape.com/article/168689-overview. Updated: Oct 08, 2015.

Levi, M. *Disseminated intravascular coagulation*, Medscape. (website): http://emedicine.medscape.com/article/199627-overview. Updated: Sep 29, 2016.

Mandel, J., & Palevsky, P. M. (last updated Aug 29, 2019). *Treatment of severe hypovolemia or hypovolemic shock in adults*. Retrieved November 2, 2020 from uptodate.com.

Miranda, M., Balarini, M., Caixeta, D., et al. (2016). Microcirculatory dysfunction in sepsis: Pathophysiology, clinical monitoring, and potential therapies. *American Journal of Physiology - Heart and Circulatory Physiology, 311*(1), H24–H35.

Moya, M. *Shock, Merck Manual, Professional Version (Website)*: http://www.merckmanuals.com/professional/critical-care-medicine/shock-and-fluid-resuscitation/shock Updated Oct 2013.

Neviere, R. (last updated Feb 03, 2020). *Sepsis syndromes in adults: Epidemiology, definitions, clinical presentation, diagnosis, and prognosis*. Retrieved November 3, 2020 from uptodate.com.

Nickson, C. Shock, 2017. LifeInTheFastLane. (website): https://lifeinthefastlane.com/ccc/shock-ddx/Shock.

Perel, P., Robers, I., & Kerr, K. (2013). Colloids versus crystalloids for fluid resuscitation in critically ill patients. *Cochrane Database of Systematic Reviews* (2), CD000567.

Ren, X., Lenneman, A. *Cardiogenic Shock*, Medscape. (website): misc.medscape.com/pi/android/medscapeapp/html/A152191-business.html. Updated Jan 11, 2017.

Rhodes, A., Evans, L., Alhazzani, W., et al. (2017). Surviving sepsis campaign: International guidelines for the management of sepsis and septic shock: 2016. *Critical Care Medicine, 45*, 486–552.

Richards, J., & Wilcox, S. (2014). Diagnosis and management of shock in the emergency department. *Emergency Medicine Practice, 16*(3), 1–24.

Rittenberger, J. C., & Callaway, C. W. (last updated June 9, 2020). *Post cardiac arrest management in adults*. Retrieved November 1, 2020 from uptodate.com.

Schmidt, G. A., & Mandel, J. (last updated April 17, 2020). *Evaluation and management of suspected sepsis and septic shock in adults*. Retrieved November 1, 2020 from uptodate.com.

Singer, M., Deutschman, C., Seymour, C., et al. (2016). The third international consensus definitions for sepsis and septic shock (Sepsis-3),. *Journal of the American Medical Association, 315*(8), 801–810.

Skidmore-Roth, L. (2021). *Mosby's 2021 nursing drug reference* (34th ed.). St. Louis MO: Elsevier.

Strickler, J. (2013). Halting the downward spiral of traumatic hypovolemic shock, *Nursing 2012. Critical Care, 7*(2), 42–47.

U.S. Department of Health and Human Services. (2000). *Healthy people 2020*. Rockville, Md: U.S. Department of Health and Human Services.

CHAPTER 10: THE OLDER ADULT PATIENT

Administration on Aging. (2013). *A profile of older Americans: 2012*. (website). www.aoa.gov/Aging_Statistics/Profile/2012/14.aspx.

Alzheimer's Association. (2013). *Alzheimer's disease facts and figures*. (website). http://www.alz.org/alzheimers_disease_facts_and_figures.asp#prevalence.

American Academy of Dermatology. (2011). *How do I prevent skin cancer?*. (website). www.aad.org/spot-skin-cancer/understanding-skin-cancer/how-do-i-prevent-skin-cancer.

American Association of Suicidology. (2009). *Elderly suicide fact sheet*. (website). www.suicidology.org.

American Cancer Society. (2013). *American Cancer Society recommendations for early breast cancer detection in women without breast symptoms*. (website). www.cancer.org/cancer/breastcancer/moreinformation/breastcancerearlydetection/breast-cancer-early-detection-acs-recs.

American Geriatrics Society 2012. Beers criteria update expert panel. (2012). American Geriatrics Society updated beers criteria for potentially inappropriate medication use in older adults. *Journal of the American Geriatrics Society*. (serial online). www.americangeriatrics.org/files/documents/beers/2012BeersCriteria_JAGS.pdf.

Burchum, J. R., & Rosenthal, L. D. (2016). *Lehne's pharmacology for nursing care* (9th ed.). St. Louis: Elsevier.

Centers for Disease Control and Prevention. (2012). *Cervical cancer screening guidelines for average-risk women*. (website). www.cdc.gov/cancer/cervical/basic_info/screening.htm.

Centers for Disease Control and Prevention. (2012). *Depression is not a normal part of growing older*. (website). www.cdc.gov/aging/mentalhealth/depression.htm.

Centers for Disease Control and Prevention, Injury Prevention and Control. *Data and statistics. Ten leading causes of injury deaths by age group highlighting unintentional injury deaths, United States – 2010*. (website): www.cdc.gov/injury/wisqars/pdf/10LCID_All_Deaths_By_Age_Group_2010-a.pdf.

Centers for Disease Control and Prevention, National Center for health statistics. *2011 life expectancy in the U. S.*, 2012. (website): http://www.cdc.gov/nchs.hus/contents2012.htm#018.

Cooper, T. K., & Smith, O. M. (2017). Gynecologic disorders in older women. In H. M. Fillit, K. Rockwood, & J. Young (Eds.), *Brocklehurst's textbook of geriatric medicine and gerontology* (8th ed.). St. Louis: Saunders.

Eliopoulos, C. (2014). *Gerontological nursing* (8th ed.). Philadelphia: Wolters Kluwer Health/Lippincott Williams & Wilkins.

Erikson, E. (1963). *Childhood and society*. New York: Norton.

Federal Trade Commission Consumer Information. (2008). *Lasik and other vision-correcting surgeries: Health information for older people*. (website). www.consumer.ftc.gov/articles/0322-lasik-and-other-vision-correcting-surgeries-health-information-older-people.

Fillit, H. M., Rockwood, K., & Young, J. (Eds.). (2017). *Brocklehurst's textbook of geriatric medicine and gerontology* (8th ed.). St. Louis: Saunders.

Gunter, L., & Estes, C. (1979). *Education for gerontologic nursing*. New York: Springer.

Kirkwood, T. B. L. (2017). Evolution theory and the mechanisms of aging. In H. M. Fillit, K. Rockwood, & J. Young (Eds.), *Brocklehurst's textbook of geriatric medicine and gerontology* (8th ed.). St. Louis: Elsevier.

Maddox, M. A., & Madison, H. E. (2015). Theories of aging. In S. E. Meiner (Ed.), *Gerontologic nursing* (5th ed.). St. Louis: Elsevier.

Martin, J., & Li, C. (2017). Normal cognitive aging. In H. M. Fillit, K. Rockwood, & J. Young (Eds.), *Brocklehurst's textbook of geriatric medicine and gerontology* (8th ed.). St. Louis: Saunders.

National Center for Biotechnology Information. *Inpatient hospital stays by diagnosis*. (website). www.ncbi.nlm.nih.gov/books/NBK52720#sec2.s4.

Rolland, Y., Matteo, C., & Vellas, B. (2017). Sarcopenia. In H. M. Fillit, K. Rockwood, & J. Young (Eds.), *Brocklehurst's textbook of geriatric medicine and gerontology* (8th ed.). St. Louis: Elsevier.

Thomas, J. M., Cooney, M., Jr., & Fried, T. R. (2013). Systematic review: Health-related characteristics of elderly hospitalized adults and nursing home residents associated with short-term mortality. *Journal of the American Geriatrics Society, 61*, 902–911.

Woodruff, K. (2010). Preventing polypharmacy in older adults. *American Nurse Today, 5*(10). (serial online) www.americannursetoday.com/article.aspx?id=7132&fid=6852#.

CHAPTER 11: FALLS

American Nurses Association. (2009). *Patient falls*.

Capezuti, E., Talerico, K. A., Cochran, I., et al. (1999). Individualized interventions to prevent bed-related falls and reduce siderail use. *Journal of Gerontological Nursing, 25*(11), 26–33.

Cauley, J. A., Lacroix, A. Z., Wu, L., et al. (2008). Serum 25-hydroxyvitamin D concentrations and risk for hip fractures. *Annals of Internal Medicine, 149*(4), 242–250.

Centers for Disease Control. (2012). *Falls in nursing homes*. www.cdc.gov/HomeandRecreationalSafety/Falls/nursing.html#restraints.

Centers for Disease Control. (2016). *Falls are leading cause of injury and death in older Americans*.

DeMoss, M. (2013). Patient safety. In P. A. Potter, A. G. Perry, P. A. Stockert, et al. (Eds.), *Fundamentals of nursing* (8th ed.). St. Louis: Mosby.

Gillespie, W. J., Gillespie, L. D., & Parker, M. J. (2010). Hip protectors for preventing hip fractures in older people. *Cochrane Database of Systematic Reviews* (10), CD001255.

Gillespie, L. D., Robertson, M. C., Gillespie, L. D., et al. (2013). Interventions for preventing falls in older people living in the community. *Cochrane Database of Systematic Reviews* (7).

Healey, F., Oliver, D., Milne, A., et al. (2008). The effect of bedrails on falls and injury: A systematic review of clinical studies *Age and Ageing, 37*(4), 368–378.

Howe, T. E., Rochester, L., Jackson, A., et al. (2007). Exercise for improving balance in older people. *Cochrane Database of Systematic Reviews* (4), CD004963.

Lyons, R. A., John, A., Brophy, S., et al. (2008). Modification of the home environment for the reduction of injuries. *Cochrane Database of Systematic Reviews* (3), CD003600.

McClure, R., Turner, C., Peel, N., et al. (2005). Population-based interventions for the prevention of fall-related injuries in older people. *Cochrane Database of Systematic Reviews* (3), CD001220.

Meiner, S. E., & Miceli, D. G. (2000). Safety. In A. G. Lueckenotte (Ed.), *Gerontologic nursing* (2nd ed.). St. Louis: Mosby.

Neyens, J. C., van Haastregt, J. C., Dijcks, B. P., et al. (2011). Effectiveness and implementation aspects of interventions for preventing falls in elderly people in long-term care facilities: A systematic review of RCTs. *Journal of the American Medical Directors Association*, *12*(6), 410–425.

Parker, M. J., Gillespie, W. J., & Gillespie, L. D. (2005). Hip protectors for preventing hip fractures in older people. *Cochrane Database of Systematic Reviews* (2), CD001255.

The Joint Commission (TJC). (2008). *2008 national patient safety goals*. Oakbrook Terrace, IL: The Commission. http://www.jointcommission.org/standards_information/npsgs.aspx.

Tzeng, H., & Yin, C. (2008). The extrinsic risk factors for inpatient falls in hospital patient rooms. *Journal of Nursing Care Quality*, *23*(3), 233–241.

World Health Organization. (2016). *Falls, Media centre*.

Internet Resources

Matter of Balance. www.aoa.gov/AoARoot/AoA_Programs/HCLTX/Evidence_Based/.

Evidence-based health programs. http://www.healthyagingprograms.org.

National Council on Aging. www.ncoa.org.

Legal Eagle Eye Newsletter for the Nursing Profession. www.nursinglaw.com.

Prevent Falls. www.fallprevention.org.

CHAPTER 12: IMMOBILITY

Burchum, J. R., & Rosenthal, L. D. (2016). *Lehne's pharmacology for nursing care* (9th ed.). St. Louis: Elsevier.

Colwell, J. (2013). Skin integrity and wound care. In P. A. Potter, A. G. Perry, P. A. Stockert, et al. (Eds.), *Fundamentals of nursing* (8th ed.). St. Louis: Mosby.

European Pressure Ulcer Advisory Panel and National Pressure Ulcer Advisory Panel. (2009). *Prevention of pressure ulcers: Quick reference guide*. (website). www.npuap.org.

European Pressure Ulcer Advisory Panel and National Pressure Ulcer Advisory Panel. (2009). *Treatment of pressure ulcers: Quick reference guide*. (website). www.npuap.org.

Guimaraes, M. M. F., El Dib, R. P., Smith, A. F., et al. (2009). Incentive spirometry for prevention of postoperative pulmonary complications in upper abdominal surgery. *Cochrane Database of Systematic Reviews* (0), CD006058.

McInnes, E., Jammali-Blas, A., Bell-Syer, S. E. M., et al. (2011). Support surfaces for pressure ulcer prevention. *Cochrane Database of Systematic Reviews* (0), CD001735.

National Pressure Ulcer Advisory Panel. *NPUAP pressure ulcer prevention points*. (website). www.npauap.org/resources/educational-and-clinical-resources/pressure-ulcer-prevention-points/.

National Pressure Ulcer Advisory Panel. *NPUAP pressure ulcer stages/categories*. (website). www.npauap.org/resources/educational-and-clinical-resources/npuap-pressure-ulcer-stagescategories/.

Pieper, B., & Ratliff, C. (2010). *Registered nurse competency-based curriculum: Pressure ulcer prevention*. (website). www.npuap.org.

Tritak, A. B. (2013). Mobility and immobility. In P. A. Potter, A. G. Perry, P. A. Stockert, et al. (Eds.), *Fundamentals of nursing* (8th ed.). St. Louis: Mosby.

Young, T., & Clark, M. (2008). Re-positioning for pressure ulcer prevention (protocol). *The Cochrane Collaboration*, *4*. (serial online). http://www.thecochranelibrary.com.

CHAPTER 13: DELIRIUM AND DEMENTIA

American Psychiatric Association. (2016). *APA releases new practice guidelines on the use of antipsychotics in patients with dementia*.

Cerejeira, J. *Mukaetova-Ladinska: Nursing research and practice: A clinical update on delirium: From early recognition to effective management*. Volume 2011. ArticleID 875196.

Deichendes, C. L., & McCurry, S. M. (2009). Current treatments for sleep disturbances in individuals with dementia. *Current Psychiatry Reports*, *11*(1), 20–26.

DSM-5, American Psychiatric Association. (2013). *Diagnostic and statistical manual of mental disorders* (5th ed.). Washington, DC: APA. (DSM-V).

Eeles, E., Davis, D., & Bhat, R. (2017). Delirium. In H. M. Fillit, K. Rockwood, & J. Young (Eds.), *Brocklehurst's textbook of geriatric medicine and gerontology* (8th ed.). Elsevier.

Khachiyants, N., Trinkle, D., et al. (2011). Sundown syndrome in persons with dementia: An update. *Psychiatry Investigation*, *8*(4), 275–287.

Lewis, S. L. (2017). Nursing management: Dementia, and delirium. In SM Lewis, L Bucher, MM Heitkemper, et al. (Eds.), *Medical-surgical nursing: Assessment and management of clinical problems* (10th ed.). St. Louis: Elsevier.

Lyons, D. L., Grimley, S. M., & Sydnor, L. (2008). Double trouble: When delirium complicates dementia. *Nursing*, *38*(9), 48–54.

Matteson, M. A., Linton, A. D., & Barnes, S. J. (1996). Cognitive development psychiatry investing: Approach to dementia. *Journal of Nursing Scholarship*, *28*(3), 233–240.

Matteson, M. A., Linton, A. D., Barnes, S. J., et al. (1996). The relationship between Piaget and cognitive levels in persons with Alzheimer's disease and related disorders,. *Aging (Milano)*, *8*(1), 61–69.

Sewell, M., Li, C., & Sano, M. (2017). Neuropsychology in the diagnosis and treatment of dementia. In H. M. Fillit, K. Rockwood, & J. Young (Eds.), *Brocklehurst's textbook of geriatric medicine and gerontology* (8th ed.). Elsevier.

Weiser, M. L. (2008). Antipsychotics: Restraints for the elderly. *American Journal of Nursing*, *108*(12), 11.

Internet Resources

Alzheimer's.org. *Alzheimers association research roundtable*. http://emedicine.com/article 288890-medication.

CHAPTER 14: INCONTINENCE

American Society of Colon and Rectal Surgeons. (2012). *Bowel incontinence*. (website). http://www.fascrs.org/patients/conditions/bowel_incontinence/.

American Urological Association. *Guidelines for the surgical management of stress urinary incontinence, 2012 update*. (website). www.auanet.org/common/pdf/education/clinical-guidance/Incontinence/pdf.

American Urological Association Foundation. (2009). *Loss of bladder control*. (website). http://www.urologyhealth.org/_media/_pdf/Urinary%20Incontinence%20Brochure%202009.pdf.

Baumgartner, U. (2012). The artificial sphincter: Therapy for faecal incontinence [abstract]. *Zentralblatt Fur Chirurgie*, *137*(4), 340–344.

Brown, S. R., Wadhawan, H., & Nelson, R. L. (2013). Surgery for faecal incontinence in adults. *Cochrane Database of Systematic Reviews* (7), CD001757.

Campbell, S. E., Glazener, C. M., Hunter, K. E., et al. (2012). Conservative management for postprostatectomy urinary incontinence. *Cochrane Database of Systematic Reviews* (0), CD001843.

Harari, D. (2017). Constipation and fecal incontinence in old age. In H. M. Fillit, K. Rockwood, & J. Young (Eds.), *Brocklehurst's textbook of geriatric medicine and gerontology* (8th ed.). Elsevier.

Madjar, S., Raz, S., & Gousse, A. E. (2001). Fixed and dynamic urethral compression for the treatment of post-prostatectomy urinary incontinence: Is history repeating itself? *Journal of Urology*, *166*(2), 411–415.

Mantoo, S., Meurette, G., Podevin, J., et al. (2012). The magnetic anal sphincter: A new device in the management of severe fecal incontinence. *Expert Review of Medical Devices*, *9*(5), 483–490.

Medtronic. *About sacral neuromodulation*. (website). http://professional.medtronic.com/pt/uro/snm/.

Moore, K. N., Schieman, S., Ackerman, T., et al. (2004). Assessing comfort, safety, and patient satisfaction with three commonly used penile compression devices. *Urology*, *63*, 150–154.

National Association for Continence. (2012). *Management products for men*. (website). www.nafc.org/find-a-product/male-products/.

National Association for Continence. (2012). *Management products for women*. (website). www.nafc.org/find-a-product/female-products/.

Resnick, N. M. (2016). Incontinence. In L. Goldman, & A. I. Schafer (Eds.), *Goldman-Cecil medicine* (25th ed.). St. Louis: Elsevier.

Robert, M., Schulz, J. A., Harvey, M. A., et al. (2013). Technical update on pessary use. *Journal of Obstetrics and Gynaecology Canada*, *35*(7), 664–674.

Unscheid, C., Gould, C., & Pegues, D. A. (November 13, 2008). *Guidelines for preventing catheter-associated urinary tract infections*. Washington DC: Presented at HICPAC Meeting.

Van Wunnik, B. P., Visschers, R. G., van Asselt, A. D., et al. (2012). Cost-effectiveness analysis of sacral neuromodulation for faecal incontinence in The Netherlands. *Colorectal Disease*, *14*(12), e807–e814.

Wagg, A. (2016). Urinary incontinence. In L. Goldman, & A. I. Schafer (Eds.), *Goldman-Cecil medicine* (25th ed.). St. Louis: Elsevier.

CHAPTER 15: NUTRITION

Burchum, J. R., & Rosenthal, L. D. (2016). *Lehne's pharmacology for nursing care* (9th ed.). St. Louis: Elsevier.

FDA. (2013). *How to understand and use the nutrition facts label*. https://www.fda.gov/Food/Ingredients/PackagingLabeling/LabelingNutrition/ucm274593.htm.

Mahan, L. K., & Raymond, J. L. (2017). *Krause's food and the nutrition care process* (14th ed.). St. Louis: Elsevier.

News and Media/Healthgov. (2016). *Top things you need to know about the 2015-2020 dietary guidelines for Americans*. https://health.gov/news/dietary-guidelines-digital-press-kit/2016/01/top-10-things-you-need-to-know/.

Perreault, L. (Aug 24, 2020). Obesity in adults: Drug therapy. *UpToDate*. Retrieved December 20, 2020 from http://www.uptodate.com.

Seres, D. (Oct 14, 2020). Nutritional support in critically ill patients: An overview. *UpToDate*. Retrieved December 20, 2020 from http://www.uptodate.com.

U.S. Departments of Health and Human Services (HHS) and of Agriculture (USDA). (2015). *2015-2020 Dietary guidelines for Americans*. https://health.gov/dietaryguidelines/2015/guidelines.

US Department of Health and Human Services. (2018). *Physical activity guidelines for Americans* (2nd ed.). Washington DC: US DHHS.

US Departments of Health and Human Services and of Agriculture. (2020). *2020–2025 Dietary guidelines for Americans*. Washington DC: US DHHS.

USDA. (2016). *Find your healthy eating style and maintain it for a lifetime*. https://choosemyplate-prod.azureedge.net/sites/default/files/misc/dietaryguidelines/MyPlateMyWins.pdf.

CHAPTER 16: INTRAVENOUS THERAPY

Alexander, M., Corrigan, A., Gorski, L., & for the Infusion Nurses Society., et al. (2010). *Infusion nursing: An evidence-based approach* (3rd ed.). St. Louis: Saunders.

Extending short peripheral catheter dwell time. (2017). A best practice discussion: Erratum. *Journal of Infusion Nursing*, *40*(4), 252.

Infusion Nurses Society. Infusion therapy standards of practice crosswalk: 2011/2016.

Krenik, K. M., Smith, G. E., & Bernatchex, S. F. (2016). Catheter securement systems for peripherally inserted and nontunneled central vascular access devices: Clinical evaluation of a novel sutureless device. *Journal of Infusion Nursing*, *39*(4), 210–217.

Kumar, A., & Lyon, C. (2011). How often do you need to change a PICC line. *Evidence-Based Practice*, *14*(1), 8–9.

Lewis, S. M., Heitkemper, M. M., Dirksen, S. R., et al. (Eds.). (2015). *Medical–surgical nursing: Assessment and management of clinical problems*, (9th ed.). St. Louis: Mosby.

Mattox, E. A. (2017). Complications of peripheral venous access devices: Prevention, detection, and recovery strategies. *Critical Care Nurse*, *37*(2), e1–e15.

Potter, P. A., & Perry, A. G. (Eds.). (2017). *Fundamentals of nursing* (9th ed.). St. Louis: Mosby.

Walker, M. D. (2016). Fluid and electrolyte imbalances: Interpretation and assessment. *Journal of Infusion Nursing*, *39*(6), 382–386.

Internet Resources

Intravenous Nurses Society. http://www.ins1.org.

Lippincott's Nursing Center. http://nursingcenter.com/.

CHAPTER 17: SURGERY

Askari, R., & Romanowski, K. S. (October 12, 2020). Overview of perioperative nutritional support. *UpToDate*. Retrieved November 10, 2020 from uptodate.com.

Barnett, S. (Feb 22, 2019). Anesthesia for the older adult. *UpToDate*. Retrieved November 12, 2020 from uptodate.com.

Bateman, B. T., Cole, N., Sun-Edelstein, C., & Lay, C. L. (August 26, 2020). Post dural puncture headache. *UpToDate*. Retrieved November 13, 2020 from https://www.update.com.

Burchum, J. R., & Rosenthal, L. D. (2019). *Lehne's pharmacology for nursing care* (10th ed.). St. Louis MO: Elsevier.

Glick, D. B., Holt, N. F., & Nussmeier (March 21, 2019). Overview of post-anesthesia care for adult patients. *UpToDate*. Retrieved November 12, 2020 from uptodate.com.

King, A. (May 4, 2020). General anesthesia: Intravenous induction agents. *UpToDate*. Retrieved November 14, 2020 from uptodate.com.

Mizell, J. S. (June 29, 2020). Principles of abdominal wound closure. *UpToDate*. Retrieved November 5, 2020 from uptodate.com.

Muluk V., Cohn SL, & Whinney C. Perioperative medication management. *UpToDate*. Retrieved November 13, 2020 from uptodate.com.

Renew, J. R. (November 13, 2020). Clinical use of neuromuscular blocking agents in anesthesia. *UpToDate*. Retrieved Nov14, 2020 from uptodate.com.

Wahr, J. A. (Appril 7, 2020). Safety in the operating room. *UpToDate*. Retrieved November 13 from uptodate.com.

CHAPTER 18: THE PATIENT WITH AN OSTOMY

Fichera, A. (October 13, 2020). Restorative proctocolectomy with ileal pouch-anal anastomosis: Laparoscopic approach. *UpToDate*. Retrieved November 22, 2020 from uptodate.com.

Fleischer, I., & Wise, P. (2009). *Continent urostomy guide*. United Ostomy Associations of America, Inc.
Fleshner, P. R. (February 24, 2020). Surgical management of ulcerative colitis. *UpToDate*. Retrieved November 22, 2020 from uptodate.com.
Francone, T. D. (March 24, 2020). Overview of surgical ostomy for fecal diversion. *UpToDate*. Retrieved November 22, 2020 from uptodate.com.
Landmann, R. G., & Cashman, A. L. (June 9, 2020). Ileostomy or colostomy care and complications. *UpToDate*. Retrieved November 22, 2020 from uptodate.com.
Shariat, S. F., Bochner, B. H., Donahue, T. F., & Pietzak, E. J. (January 8, 2020). Urinary diversion and reconstruction following cysectomy. *UpToDate*. Retrieved November 22, 2020 from uptodate.com.

CHAPTER 19: PALLIATIVE AND HOSPICE CARE

Center to Advance Palliative Care. *About palliative care, n.d.* https://www.capc.org/about/palliative-care/.
DHHS Centers for Medicare and Medicaid services. (2020). *Medicare and you 2021*. Baltimore MD.
Hospice Foundation of America. *What is hospice? n.d.* http://hospicefoundation.org/End-of-Life-Support-and-Resources/Coping-with-Terminal-Illness/Hospice-Services.
National Hospice and Palliative Care Organization. (August 2020). *2020 Edition: Hospice facts and figures*. Alexandria, VA: National Hospice and Palliative Care Organization. Retrieved November 21, 2020 from www.nhpco.org/factsfigures.nhpco.org.
National Hospice and Palliative Care Organization. (2015). *NHPCO's Facts and figures: Hospice care in America*. Alexandria VA: NHPCO. (updated 2017).
NIH National Cancer Center. (2010). *Palliative care in cancer*. https://www.cancer.gov/about-cancer/advanced-cancer/care-choices/palliative-care-fact-sheet.
Upchurch, L. A. L. (2017). Palliative care at end of life. In SL Lewis, L Bucher, MM Heitkemper, et al. (Eds.), *Medical-surgical nursing* (10th ed.) (pp. 129–143). St. Louis: Elsevier.

CHAPTER 20: COMPLEMENTARY AND ALTERNATIVE THERAPIES AND INTEGRATIVE HEALTH CARE

Ahn, A. C. (Last updated October 27, 2020). Acupuncture. *UpToDate*. Retrieved November 29, 2020 from uptodate.com.
Antioxidant vitamin and mineral supplements to slow down the progression of age-related macular degeneration (AMD). (2017). *Cochrane Review*. http://www.cochrane.org/CD000253/EYES_antioxidant-vitamin-and-mineral-supplements-prevent-development-age-related-macular-degenation-amd.
Burchum, J. R., & Rosenthal, L. D. (2016). *Lehne's pharmacology for nursing care* (9th ed.). St. Louis: Elsevier.
Fujita, T., Feng, C., & Takano, T. (2017). Presence of caffeine reversible interferes with efficacy of acupuncture-induced analgesia. *Scientific Reports*, *7*, 3397.
Herman, P. M., Anderson, M. L., Sherman, K. J., et al. (2017). Cost effectiveness of mindfulness-based stress reduction vs cognitive behavioral therapy or usual care among adults with chronic low-back pain. *Spring*.
Kemper, K. J. (last updated November 11, 2019). *UpToDate*. Retrieved November 29, 2020 from uptodate.com.
Koithan, M. (2017). Complementary and alternative therapies. In P. A. Potter, A. G. Perry, P. A. Stockert, et al. (Eds.), *Fundamentals of nursing* (9th ed.). St. Louis: Elsevier.
NCCIH. (last updated May 2019). *What is yoga and how does it work?*. Retrieved November 28, 2020 from ncchi.nih.gov.
NCCIH: 2015. https://www.nih.gov/health/homeopathy.
NCCIH. (2016). *Complementary, alternative, or integrative health: What's in a Name?*. https://nccih.nih.gov/health/integrative-health#types.
Saper, R. B. (last updated December 16, 2019). Overview of herbal medications and dietary supplements. *UpToDate*. Retrieved November 29, 2020 from uptodate.com.
Saper, R. B. (last updated July 22, 2019). Clinical use of echinacea. *UpToDate*. Retieved November 29, 2020 from uptodate.com.
Wang. (January 1, 2020). Chinese herbal medicine for treatment of allergic disorders. *UpToDate*. Retrieved November 29, 2020 from uptodate.com.

CHAPTER 21: NEUROLOGIC SYSTEM INTRODUCTION

Carroll, V. S. (2011). AANN core curriculum for neuroscience nursing (5th ed.). *Journal of Neuroscience Nursing*, *43*(2), 118.
Jepson, R., Despain, K., & Keller, D. C. (2008). Unilateral neglect: Assessment in nursing practice. *Journal of Neuroscience Nursing*, *40*(3), 142–149.
Lassiter, T. F., & Henkel, A. I. (2013). Pharmacologic management of neuroscience patients. In J. V. Hickey (Ed.), *The clinical practice of neurological and neurosurgical nursing* (7th ed.). Philadelphia: Wolters Kluwer/Lippincott–Williams & Wilkins .
Lorimer, M. S., Tucker-Lipscomb, B., & Sanders, D. B. (2018). Neuromuscular junction and muscle disease. In E. Barker (Ed.), *Neuroscience nursing: A spectrum of care* (3rd ed.). St. Louis: Elsevier.
Thompson, T. (2007). Neurologic assessment of the older adult: A guide for nurses. In *AANN clinical practice guideline series*. Chicago: American Association of Neuroscience Nurses.

CHAPTER 22: NEUROLOGIC DISORDERS

Ben-Zacharia, A. B., & Del Bene, M. L. (2018). Inflammatory demyelinating diseases. In E. Barker (Ed.), *Neuroscience nursing: A spectrum of care* (3rd ed.). St. Louis: Elsevier.
Blank-Reid, C., McClelland, R. N., & Santora, T. A. (2018). Neurotrauma: Traumatic brain injury. In E. Barker (Ed.), *Neuroscience nursing: A spectrum of care* (3rd ed.). St. Louis: Elsevier.
Cellar, J. S., Khan, J., Lah, J. J., et al. (2018). Management of dementia and motor neuron disease. In E. Barker (Ed.), *Neuroscience nursing: A spectrum of care* (3rd ed.). St. Louis: Elsevier.
Clinical pharmacology, Tampa, Fla: *Gold Standard, Inc*, 2006. (website): http://clinicalpharmacology.com/?epm=2_1. Updated February 2006.
Cox, D., & Stone, J. (2006). Managing self-injection difficulties in patients with relapsing-remitting multiple sclerosis. *Journal of Neuroscience Nursing*, *38*(3), 167–171.
Foster, R. E., & Long, L. (2007). *Care of the patient with seizures* (2nd ed.). Chicago: American Association of Neuroscience Nurses.
Fowler, S., & Newton, L. (2006). Complementary and alternative therapies: The nurse's role. *Journal of Neuroscience Nursing*, *38*(4), 261–264.
Johnson, K., Mowrey, K., & Bergman, M. J. (2018). Neurotrauma: Spinal injury. In E. Barker (Ed.), *Neuroscience nursing: A spectrum of care* (3rd ed.). St. Louis: Elsevier.
Kraemer, D. A., & Barker, E. (2018). Management of seizures and epilepsy. In E. Barker (Ed.), *Neuroscience nursing: A spectrum of care* (3rd ed.). St. Louis: Elsevier.
McIlvoy, L., & Meyer, K. (2008). Nursing management of adults with severe traumatic brain injury. In H. J. Thompson (Ed.), *AANN clinical practice guideline series*. Chicago: American Association of Neuroscience Nurses.
Paolino, A., Baker, K., Featherstone, K., et al. (2006). Guide to the care of the patient with craniotomy post-brain tumor resection. In *AANN reference series for clinical practice*. Chicago: American Association of Neuroscience Nurses.
Ross, A. P., Hackbarth, N., Rhol, C., et al. (2008). Effective multiple sclerosis management through improved patient assessment. *Journal of Neuroscience Nursing*, *40*(3), 150–157.
Shen-Yeng, L., & Fox, S. H. (2008). An update on the management of Parkinson's disease. *Geriatrics of Aging*, *11*(4), 215–222.

Whitney, C. M., Maddux, B. N., & Riley, D. E. (2018). Management of Parkinson's disease and movement disorders. In E. Barker (Ed.), *Neuroscience nursing: A spectrum of care* (3rd ed.). St. Louis: Elsevier.

CHAPTER 23: CEREBROVASCULAR ACCIDENT

Adams RJ, Albers G, Alberts MJ, et al: *Update to the AHA/ASA recommendations for the prevention of stroke in patients with stroke and transient ischemic attack, Stroke*. (serial online): http://stroke.ahajournals.org/cgi/content/full/39/5/1647.

Alberts, M. J., Hademenos, G., Latchaw, R. E., et al. (2000). Recommendations for the establishment of primary stroke centers: Brain attack coalition. *Journal of the American Medical Association*, *283*, 3102–3109.

Alexander, S., Gallek, M., Presciutti, M., et al. (2012). Care of the patient with aneurysmal subarachnoid hemorrhage. In H. J. Thompson (Ed.), *AANN clinical practice guideline series*. Chicago: American Association of Neuroscience Nurses.

Benjamin, E. J, Blaha, M. J, & On behalf of the American Heart Association Statistics Committee and Stroke Statistics Subcommittee, et al. (2017). Heart disease and stroke statistics – 2017 update: A report from the American heart association. Benjamin (Ed.). (2017). *Circulation*. (serial online). http://circ.ahajournals.org/content/135/10/e146.

Centers for Disease Control and Prevention.*FastStats on cerebrovascular disease or stroke*. (website). https://www.cdc.gov/nchs/fastats/stroke.htm.

del Zoppo, G. J., Saver, J. L., Jauch, E. C., et al. (2009). Expansion of the time window for treatment of acute ischemic stroke with intravenous tissue plasminogen activator: A science advisory from the American Heart Association. *Stroke*. (serial online). http://stroke.ahajournals.org/cgi/content/full/40/8/2945.

Easton, J. D., Saver, J. L., Albers, G. W., & Definition and evaluation of transient ischemic attack, et al. (2009). A scientific statement for healthcare professionals from the American Heart Association/American Stroke Association Stroke Council; Council on Cardiovascular Surgery and Anesthesia; Council on cardiovascular Radiology and intervention; Council on Cardiovascular Nursing; and the Interdisciplinary Council on Peripheral Vascular Disease. *Stroke*. (serial online) http://stroke.ahajournals.org/cgi/content/full/40/6/2276.

Frizzell, J. P., Argour, R., & March, K. (2005). Acute stroke: Pathophysiology, diagnosis, and treatment. *AACN Clinical Issues*, *4*(16), 421–440.

Kernan, W. N., Ovbiagele, B., et al. (2014). Guidelines for the prevention of stroke in patients with stroke and transient ischemic attack: A guideline for healthcare professionals from the American Heart Association/American Stroke Association. *Stroke*. (serial online). http://stroke.ahajournals.org/content/45/7/2160.

Kumar, B., Kumar, G., & Misra, U. K. (2009). Central poststroke pain: A review of pathophysiology and treatment. *Anesthesia & Analgesia*, *108*(5), 1645–1657.

Powers, W. J., Derdeyn, C. P., et al. (2015). AHA/ASA focused update of the 2013 guidelines for the early management of patients with acute ischemic stroke regarding endovascular treatment: A guideline for healthcare professional from the American Heart Association/American Stroke Association. *Stroke*. (serial online). http://stroke.ahajournals.org/content/46/10/3020.

Pugh, S., Mathiesen, C., Meighan, M., et al. (2012). Guide to the care of the hospitalized patient with ischemic stroke. In H. J. Thompson (Ed.), *AANN clinical practice guideline series*. Chicago: American Association of Neuroscience Nurses.

Solenski, M. J. (2004). Transient ischemic attacks: Part I. Diagnosis and evaluation. *American Family Physician*, *69*(7), 1665–1674.

Summers, D., Leonard, A., Wentworth, D., et al. (2009). Ischemic stroke patient: A scientific statement from the American heart association. *Stroke*. (serial online). http://stroke.ahajournals.org/cgi/content/full/40/8/2911.

Weber, R., Weimar, C., & Diener, H. C. (2009). Medical prevention of stroke and stroke recurrence in patients with TIA and minor stroke. *Expert Opinion on Pharmacotherapy*, *10*(12), 1883–1894.

Wolff, T., Miller, T., & Ko, S. (2009). Aspirin for the primary prevention of cardiovascular events: An update of the evidence for the U.S. Preventive services task force. *Annals of Internal Medicine*, *150*(6), 405–410.

Internet Resources

ABCD2. http://www.mdcalc.com/abcd2-score-for-tia.

Centers for Disease Control. www.cdc.gov/stroke/facts_statistics.htm.

Council on Cardiovascular and Stroke Nursing. http://my.americanheart.org/professional/Councils/CVN/Council-on-Cardiovascular-and-Stroke-Nursing_UCM_320474_SubHomePage.jsp.

National Institutes of Health. http://stroke.nih.gov.

National Stroke Association. http://www.stroke.org.

CHAPTER 24: SPINAL CORD INJURY

Boling, J., Fields-Ryan, S., & Georgievski-Resser, T. S. (2007). Cervical spine surgery: A guide to preoperative and postoperative patient care. In A. L. Strayer, & J. Haymore (Eds.), *AANN reference series for clinical practice*. Chicago: American Association of Neuroscience Nurses.

Clinical pharmacology, Tampa, Fla: *Gold Standard, Inc*, 2006. (website): http://clinicalpharmacology.com/?epm=2_1. Updated February 2006.

Hickey, J. V. (2013). Infections of the central nervous system. In J. V. Hickey (Ed.), *The clinical practice of neurological and neurosurgical nursing* (7th ed.). Philadelphia: Wolters Kluwer/Lippincott–Williams & Wilkins.

Hickey, J. V. (2013). Neurodegenerative diseases. In J. V. Hickey (Ed.), *The clinical practice of neurological and neurosurgical nursing* (7th ed.). Philadelphia: Wolters Kluwer/Lippincott–Williams & Wilkins.

Hickey, J. V. (2013). Seizures and epilepsy. In J. V. Hickey (Ed.), *The clinical practice of neurological and neurosurgical nursing* (7th ed.). Philadelphia: Wolters Kluwer/Lippincott–Williams & Wilkins.

Hickey, J. V. (2013). Vertebral and spinal cord injuries. In J. V. Hickey (Ed.), *The clinical practice of neurological and neurosurgical nursing* (7th ed.). Philadelphia: Wolters Kluwer/Lippincott–Williams & Wilkins.

Starkweather, A. (2006). Posterior lumbar interbody fusion: An old concept with new techniques. *Journal of Neuroscience Nursing*, *38*(1), 13–20 30.

Starkweather, A., Pagnotta, P., Emmons, D., et al. (2006). Lumbar spine surgery: A guide to preoperative and postoperative patient care. In A. L. Strayer, & J. Haymore (Eds.), *AANN reference series for clinical practice*. Chicago: American Association of Neuroscience Nurses.

CHAPTER 25: RESPIRATORY SYSTEM INTRODUCTION

Boruchoff, S. E., & Weinstein, M. P. (September 23, 2019). Microbiological specimen collection and transport. *UpTo Date*. Retrieved December 5, 2020 from uptodate.com.

Burchum, J. R., & Rosenthal, L. D. (2019). *Lehne's pharmacology for nursing care*. St. Louis MO: Elsevier.

Centers for Disease Control and Prevention. (September 1, 2016). *Fact Sheets | Testing & Diagnosis | Testing for Tuberculosis (TB)*. Retrieved December 4, 2020 from https://cdc.gov.

Chow, A. W. (September 21, 2020). Evaluation of acute pharyngitis in adults. *UpToDate*. Retrieved December 3, 2020 from https://www.uptodate.com.

Cystic Fibrosis Foundation (n.d.). *Airway clearance*. Retrieved December 2, 2020 from https://www.cff.org.

Huggins, J. T., Carr, S. R., & Woodward, G. A. (October 30, 2020). Thoracostomy tubes and catheter management and removal. *UpToDate*. Retrieved December 2, 2020 from https://www.uptodate.com.

Islam, S. (September 29, 2020). Flexible bronchoscopy in adults: Overview. *UpToDate*. Retrieved December 2, 2020 from https://www.uptodate.com.

Pagana, K. D., & Pagana, T. J. (2014). *Mosby's manual of diagnostic and laboratory tests* (5th ed.). St. Louis MO: Elsevier.

Sheski, F. D. (August 12, 2020). Flexible bronchoscopy. *UpToDate*. Retrieved December 2, 2020 from https://www.uptodate.com.

Simon, R. H. (October 14, 2020). Cystic fibrosis: Overview of treatment of lung disease. *UpToDate*. Retrieved December 2, 2020 from https://www.uptodate.com.

Skidmore, L. (2021). *Mosby's 2021 nursing drug reference* (34th ed.). St. Louis MO: Elsevier.

Smetana, G. W. (June 12, 2020). Strategies to decrease postoperative complications in adults. *UpToDate*. Retrieved December 2, 2020 from https://www.uptodate.com.

CHAPTER 26: UPPER RESPIRATORY DISORDERS

Acerra, J. R., & Pritchard, J. P. (2017). *Pharyngitis clinical presentation*. emedicine.medscape.com/article/764304-clinical.

Acerra, J. R., & Pritchard, J. P. (2017). *Pharyngitis treatment and management*. emedicine.medscape.com/article/764304-clinical.

American Cancer Society. *Surgery for laryngeal and hypopharyngeal cancers*. www.cancer.org/cancer/laryngeal-and-hypopharyngeal-cancer/treating/surgery.html.

American Cancer Society. *What are the key statistics about laryngeal and hypopharyngeal cancers?* www.cancer.org/cancer/laryngeal-and-hypopharyngeal-cancer/about/key-statistics.html.

American Cancer Society. *What are the key statistics about nasal cavity and paranasal sinus cancers?* www.cancer.org/cancer/nasal-cavity-and-paranasal-sinus-cancer/about/key-statistics.html.

American Cancer Society. (*What happens after treatment for laryngeal or hypopharyngeal cancer?* www.cancer.org/cancer/laryngeal-and-hypopharyngeal-cancer/after-treatment/follow-up.html.

Brockstein, B. E., Stenson, K. M., & Sher, D. J. (January 21, 2020). *Treatment of locoregionally advanced (stage III and IV) head and neck cancer: The larynx and hypopharynx*. *UpToDate*. Retrieved December 9, 2020 from http://www.uptodate.com.

Lewin, J. S., Hoffman, H. T., & Sperry, S. M. (Feb 10, 2020). Alaryngeal speech rehabilitation. *UpToDate*. Retrieved December 9, 2020 from http://www.uptodate.com.

Lewis, S. M., Bucher, L., Heitkemper, M. M., et al. (Eds.). (2017). *Medical-surgical nursing: Assessment and management of clinical problems* (10th ed.) Elsevier.

Mayo Clinic. *Recurring strep throat: When is tonsillectomy useful?* www.mayoclinic.org/diseases-conditions/strep-throat/expert-answers/recurring-strep-throat/FAQ-20058360?p=1.

Medline Plus. *Tonsillitis*. medlineplus.gov/tonsillitis.html.

National Cancer Institute. *Paranasal sinus and nasal cavity cancer treatment*. www.cancer.gov/types/head-and-neck/patient/paranasal-sinus-treatment.

Patel, Z. M., & Hwang, P. H. (September 25, 2020). Uncomplicated acute rhinosinusitis in adults: Treatment. *UpToDate*. Retrieved December 9, 2020 from http://www.uptodate.com.

Quoc, A. N., Meyers, A. D., et al. (2017). *Epistaxis treatment and management*. http://emedicine.medscape.com/article/863220-treatment.

Skidmore-Roth, L. (2017). *Mosby's drug guide for nursing students*. St. Louis: Mosby.

CHAPTER 27: ACUTE LOWER RESPIRATORY TRACT DISORDERS

Caliendo, A. M., & Hanson, K. E. (December 3, 2020). Coronavirus disease 2019 (COVID-19): Diagnosis. *UpToDate*. Retrieved December 11, 2020 from http://www.uptodate.com.

Cohen, P., & Blau, J. (November 30, 2020). Coronavirus disease 2019 (COVID-19): Outpatient evaluation and management in adults. *UpToDate*. Retrieved December 11, 2020 from http://www.uptodate.com.

Dolin, R. (May 31, 2019). Treatment of seasonal influenza in adults. *UpToDate*. Retrieved December 11, 2020 from http://www.uptodate.com.

Dolin, R. (November 18, 2020). Epidemiology of influenza. Transmission, clinical manifestations, and complications. *UpToDate*. Retrieved December 11, 2020 from http://www.uptodate.com.

Dolin, R. (September 7, 2020). Seasonal influenza in adults: Transmission, clinical manifestations, and complications. *UpToDate*. Retrieved December 11, 2020 from http://www.uptodate.com.

Drabkin Alan. (2015). Clinical dvisor, *18*(9), 112-114. 3p. (Journal Article pictorial) ISSN: 1524-7317.

Karlson, K. A., & French, A. (November 25, 2019). Initial evaluation and management of rib fractures. *UpToDate*. Retrieved December 11, 2020 from http://www.uptodate.com.

Kim, A. Y., & Gandhi, R. T. (December 7, 2020). Coronavirus disease 2019 (COVID-19): Management in hospitalized adults. *UpToDate*. Retrieved December 11, 2020 from http://www.uptodate.com.

Lewis, S. L., et al. (2017). *Medical-surgical nursing: Assessment and management of clinical problems* (10th ed.). St. Louis: Elsevier.

Light, R. W., & Lee, Y. C. G. (April 10, 2020). Pneumothorax: Definitive management and prevention of recurrence. *UpToDate*. Retrieved December 17, 2020 from http://www.uptodate.com.

Light, R. W., & Lee, Y. C. G. (September 28, 2020). Pneumothorax in adults: Epidemiology and Etiology. *UpToDate*. Retrieved December 17, 2020 from http://www.uptodate.com.

Lip, G. Y. H., & Hull, R. D. (March 6, 2020). Venous thromboembolism: Initiation of anticoagulant (first 10 days). *UpToDate*. Retrieved December 17, 2020 from http://www.uptodate.com.

Lip, G. Y. H., & Hull, R. D. (Mary 7, 2020). Overview of pulmonary embolism. *UpToDate*. Retrieved December 17, 2020 from http://www.uptodate.com.

Lip, G. Y. H., & Hull, R. D. (September 19, 2019). Rationale and indications for indefinite anticoagulation in patients with venous thromboembolism. *UpToDate*. Retrieved December 17, 2020 from http://www.uptodate.com.

McIntosh, K. (November 20, 2020). Coronavirus disease 2019 (COVID-19): Clinical features. *UpToDate*. Retrieved December 11, 2020 from http://www.uptodate.com.

Sarani, B. (May 12, 2020). Surgical management of severe rib fractures. *UpToDate*. Retrieved December 17, 2020 from http://www.uptodate.com.

Sarani, B. (October 25, 2019). Inpatient management of traumatic rib fractures. *UpToDate*. Retrieved December 17, 2020 from http://www.uptodate.com.

Siegel MD. Acute respiratory distress syndrome: Clinical features, diagnosis, and complications in adults. . Retrieved December 17, 2020 from http://www.uptodate.com.

Thompson, B. T., Kabrhel, C., & Pena, C. (January 30, 2020). Clinical presentation, evaluation, and diagnosis of the non-pregnant adult with suspected pulmonary embolism. *UpToDate*. Retrieved December 17, 2020 from http://www.uptodate.com.

Winkle, J. M., & Legome, E. (May 5, 2020). Initial evaluation and management of penetrating thoracic trauma in adults. *UpToDate*. Retrieved December 17, 2020 from http://www.uptodate.com.

Zachary, K. C. (Jan 9, 2020). Treatment of seasonal influenza in adults. *UpToDate*. Retrieved December 17, 2020 from http://www.uptodate.com.

https://www.cdc.gov/features/rhinoviruses/index.html.

https://www.uptodate.com/contents/the-common-cold-in-adults-treatment-and-prevention?source=search_result&search=treatment+for+the+common+cold&selectedTitle=1~149.

https://www.cdc.gov/flu/about/viruses/types.htm.

https://www.cdc.gov/flu/professionals/vaccination/index.htm.

https://www.cdc.gov/flu/pdf/professionals/antivirals/antiviral-summary-clinician.pdf.

https://www.cdc.gov/pneumonia/index.html.

https://www.cdc.gov/Features/Pneumonia/.

https://www.uptodate.com/contents/pneumococcal-vaccination-in-adults?source=search_result&search=which%20medical%20conditions%20that%20patients%20have%20require%20a%20pneumonia%20vaccine&selectedTitle=1~150.

https://www.uptodate.com/contents/pneumococcal-pneumonia-in-adults?source=see_link.

https://www.uptodate.com/contents/pneumococcal-pneumonia-in-adults?source=machineLearning&search=symptoms%20of%20pneumonia&selectedTitle=1~150&sectionRank=1&anchor=H1267666844#H1267666844.

https://www.uptodate.com/contents/nutritional-support-in-advanced-lung-disease?source=search_result&search=nurtional%20support%20for%20patients%20with%20respiratory%20failure&selectedTitle=8~150.

https://www.uptodate.com/contents/nutritional-support-in-advanced-lung-disease?source=search_result&search=nurtional%20support%20for%20patients%20with%20respiratory%20failure&selectedTitle=8~150#H19.

https://www.uptodate.com/contents/initial-evaluation-and-management-of-chest-wall-trauma-in-adults?source=search_result&search=chest%20trauma&selectedTitle=1~150.

https://www.uptodate.com/contents/initial-evaluation-and-management-of-rib-fractures?source=search_result&search=rib%20fracture%20adult&selectedTitle=1~103.

https://www.uptodate.com/contents/clinical-presentation-evaluation-and-diagnosis-of-the-nonpregnant-adult-with-suspected-acute-pulmonary-embolism?source=search_result&search=signs%20of%20pulmonary%20emboli&selectedTitle=1~150.

https://www.uptodate.com/contents/treatment-prognosis-and-follow-up-of-acute-pulmonary-embolism-in-adults?source=search_result&search=treatment%20of%20pulmonary%20embolism&selectedTitle=1~150.

https://www.uptodate.com/contents/acute-respiratory-distress-syndrome-supportive-care-and-oxygenation-in-adults?source=search_result&search=treatment%20of%20ards&selectedTitle=2~150.

CHAPTER 28: CHRONIC LOWER RESPIRATORY TRACT DISORDERS

Accurso, F. J. (2016). Cystic fibrosis. In L. Goldman, & A. I. Schafer (Eds.), *Goldman-Cecil medicine* (Vol. 1) (2nd ed 5.). Philadelphia: Elsevier/Saunders.

Barker, A. F. (October 30, 2020). Bronchiectasis in adults: Maintaining lung health. *UpToDate*. Retrieved December 30, 2020 from https://www.uptodate.com.

Barker, A. F. (October 30, 2020). Bronchiectasis in adults: Treatment of acute exacerbations and advanced disease. *UpToDate*. Retrieved December 30, 2020 from https://www.uptodate.com.

Berg, K., & Wright, J. L. (2016). The pathology of chronic obstructive pulmonary disease. *Archives of Pathology & Laboratory Medicine*, *2016*(140), 1423–1428.

Blair, M. (2016). Care of patients with infectious respiratory problems. In D. D. Ignatavicius, & M. L. Workman (Eds.), *Medical-surgical nursing: Patient centered collaborative care* (8th ed.). St. Louis: Elsevier.

Burchum, J. R., & Rosenthal, L. D. (2019). *Lehne's pharmacology for nursing care* (10th ed.). St. Louis: Elsevier.

Collazo, S. (2017). Obstructive pulmonary diseases. In SL Lewis, L Bucher, MM Heitkemper, et al. (Eds.), *Medical-surgical nursing: Assessment and management of clinical problems*. St. Louis: Elsevier.

Condren, M. E., & Bradshaw, M. D. (2013). Ivacaftor: A novel gene-based therapeutic approach for cystic fibrosis. *Journal of Pediatrics Pharmacology Therapics*, *18*(1), 8–13.

Drazen, J. M. (2016). Asthma. In L. Goldman, & A. I. Schafer (Eds.), *Goldman-Cecil medicine* (Vol. 1) (2nd ed 5.). Philadelphia: Elsevier/Saunders.

Ellner, J. J. (2016). Tuberculosis. In L. Goldman, & A. I. Schafer (Eds.), *Goldman-Cecil medicine* (Vol. 1) (2nd ed 5.). Philadelphia: Elsevier/Saunders.

Ferguson, G. T., & Make, B. (December 17, 2019). Stable COPD: Initial pharmacologic management. *UpToDate*. Retrieved December 30, 2020 from https://www.uptodate.com.

Iannuzzi MC: Sarcoidosis. In Goldman L, Schafer AI, editors: *Goldman-Cecil medicine*, (Vol. 1) (2nd ed 5.). Philadelphia, Elsevier/Saunders.

Khouri FR: Lung cancer and other pulmonary neoplasms. In Goldman L, Schafer AI, editors: *Goldman-Cecil medicine*, (Vol. 1) (2nd ed 5.). Philadelphia, Elsevier/Saunders.

Kim, V., Davey, A., Comellas, A. P., et al. (2014). Clinical and computed tomographic predictors of chronic bronchitis in COPD: A cross sectional analysis of the COPDGene study. *Respiratory Research*, *2014*(415), 52.

Lange, P., & Vestbo, J. (2016). Chronic mucus hypersecretion and the natural history of chronic obstructive pulmonary disease. *American Journal of Respiratory and Critical Care Medicine*, *193*(6). https://doi-org.libproxy.uthscsa.edu/10.1164/rccm.201601-0001ED.

National Heart, Lung, and Blood Institute. (2012). *Asthma care quick reference: Diagnosing and managing asthma*. https://www.nhlbi.nih.gov/files/docs/guidelines/asthma_qrg.pdf.

NHLBI. (2020). *2020 Focused updates to the asthma management guidelines*. Retrieved 12-20-2020 from https://www.nhlbi.nih.gov/health-topics/asthma-management-guidelines for the diagnosis, management, and treatment of asthma.

Niewoehner, D. E. (2016). Chronic obstructive pulmonary disease. In L. Goldman, & A. I. Schafer (Eds.), *Goldman-Cecil medicine* (Vol. 1) (2nd ed 5.). Philadelphia: Elsevier/Saunders.

O'Donnell, A. E. (2016). Bronchiectasis, atelectasis, cysts, and localized lung disorders. In L. Goldman, & A. I. Schafer (Eds.), *Goldman-Cecil medicine* (Vol. 1) (2nd ed 5.). Philadelphia: Elsevier/Saunders.

Politis, A., Ioannidis, V., Gourgoulianis, K. I., et al. (2017). Effects of varenicline therapy in combination with advanced behavioral support on smoking cessation and quality of life in inpatients with acute exacerbation of COPD, bronchial asthma, or community-acquired pneumonia: A prospective, open-label, preference-based, 52 week, follow-up trial. *Chronic Respiratory Disease*. https://doi.org/10.1177/1479972317740128. From: https://www.ncbi,nlm.nih.gov/pubmed/29117796 Downloaded December 2, 2017.

Raghu G: Interstitial lung disease. In Goldman L, Schafer AI, editors: *Goldman-Cecil medicine*, (Vol. 1) (2nd ed 5.). Philadelphia: Elsevier/Saunders.

Rossi, A., Butorac-Petanjek, B., Casio, B. G., et al. (2017). *International Journal of Chronic Obstructive Pulmonary Disease*, *12*, 2593–2610. Downloaded from: https://www.dovepress.com/.

Schmit, K. M., Wansaula, Z., Pratt, R., et al. (2017). *Tuberculosis – United States 2016*.

Tarlo SM: Occupational lung disease. In Goldman L, Schafer AI, editors: *Goldman-Cecil medicine*, (Vol. 1) (2nd ed 5.). Philadelphia: Elsevier/Saunders.

Workman, M. L. (2016). Care of patients with noninfectious lower respiratory problems. In D. D. Ignatavicius, & M. L. Workman (Eds.), *Medical-surgical nursing: Patient centered collaborative care* (8th ed.). St. Louis: Elsevier.

Zieger, R. S., Tran, T. N., Butlet, R. K., et al. (2017). Relationship of blood eosinophil count to exacerbations in chronic obstructive pulmonary disease. *Journal of Allergy Clinical Immunology Practice*. From: https://wwwl.ncbi.nlm.nih.gov/pubmed/29153881 Downloaded December 1, 2017.

CHAPTER 29: HEMATOLOGIC SYSTEM INTRODUCTION

Burchum, J. R., & Rosenthal, L. D. (2019). *Lehne's Pharmacology for nursing care* (10th ed.). St. Louis: Elsevier.

Burchum, J. R., & Rosenthal, L. D. (2016). *Lehne's pharmacology for nursing care* (9th ed.). St. Louis: Elsevier.

Pagana, K. D., & Pagana, T. J. (2014). *Mosby's manual of diagnostic and laboratory tests* (5th ed.). St. Louis: Elsevier/Mosby.

Potter, P. A., Perry, A. G., Stockert, P. A., et al. (2017). *Fundamentals of nursing* (9th ed.). St. Louis: Elsevier.

Zehnder, J. L. (Jan 31, 2020). Bone marrow aspiration and biopsy: Indications and techniques. *UpToDate*. Retrieved Jan 8, 2021 from www.uptodate.com.

CHAPTER 30: HEMATOLOGIC DISORDERS

Brugnara, C., & Brodsky, R. A. (August 7, 2020). Warm autoimmune hemolytic anemia (AIHA) in adults. *UpToDate*. Retrieved January 11, 2021 from http://www.uptodate.com.

Burchum, J. R., & Rosenthat, L. D. (2019). *Lehne's pharmacology for nursing care* (10th ed.). St. Louis MO: Elsevier.

Field JJ, & Vichinsky EP. (12-9-20)l. Overview of management and prognosis of sickle cell disease. *UpToDate*. Retrieved January 11, 2021 from http://www.uptodate.com.

Hoots, W. K., & Shapiro, A. D. (September 23, 2020). Hemophilia A and B: Routine management including prophylaxis. *UpToDate*. Retrieved January 15, 2021 from http://www.uptodate.com.

Hoots, W. K., & Shapiro, A. D. (September 27, 2019). Clinical manifestations and diagnosis of hemophilia. *UpToDate*. Retrieved January 15, 2021 from http://www.uptodate.com.

Leung, L. L. K. (January 4, 2021). Disseminated intravascular coagulation (DIC) in adults: Evaluation and management. *UpToDate*. Retrieved January 10, 2021 from www.uptodate.com.

Means RT, & Fairfield KM. (4-28-20). Clinical manifestations and diagnosis of vitamin B^{12} and folate deficiency. *UpToDate*. Retrieved January 11, 2021 from http://www.uptodate.com.

Means RT, & Fairfield KM. (6-23-20). Treatment of vitamin B_{12} and folate deficiency. *UpToDate*. Retrieved January 11, 2021 from http://www.uptodate.com.

Olson, T. S. (July 18, 2019). Aplastic anemia: Pathogenesis, clinical manifestations, and diagnosis. *UpToDate*. Retrieved January 11, 2021 from http://www.uptodate.com.

Olson, T. S., & Dunbar, C. E. (July 8, 2020). Treatment of aplastic anemia. *UpToDate*. Retrieved January 11, 2021 from http://www.uptodate.com.

Tefferi, A. (March 11, 2020). Clinical manifestations and diagnosis of polycythemia vera. *UpToDate*. Retrieved January 11, 2021 from http://www.uptodate.com.

Tefferi, A. (November 22, 2019). Prognosis and treatment of polycythemia vera. *UpToDate*. Retrieved January 11, 2021 from http://www.uptodate.com.

Vichinsky EP. (10-27-20). Disease-modifying therapies for prevention of vaso-occlusive pain and management of chronic pain in sickle cell disease. *UpToDate*. Retrieved January 11, 2021 from http://www.uptodate.com.

CHAPTER 31: IMMUNOLOGIC SYSTEM INTRODUCTION

Burchum, J. R., & Rosenthal, L. D. (2019). *Lehne's pharmacology for nursing care* (10th ed.). St. Louis MO: Elsevier.

Burchum, J. R., & Rosenthal, L. D. (2016). *Lehne's pharmacology for nursing care* (9th ed.). St. Louis: Elsevier.

Centers for Disease Control and Prevention. (2014). *HIV PrEP guidelines*. https://wwwn.cdc.gov/hivrisk/decreased_risk/medicines/prep.html.

Centers for Disease Control and Prevention. (2017). *HIV testing*. https://www.cdc.gov/hiv/testing/laboratorytests.html.

Centers for Disease Control and Prevention. (2017). *Post-exposure prophylaxis (PEP) for preventing HIV after exposure*. https://wwwn.cdc.gov/hivrisk/decreased_risk/medicines/pep.html.

Centers for Disease Control and Prevention. (2017). *Pre-Exposure prophylaxis*. www.cdc.gov/pdf/guidelines/PrEPguidelines2014.pdf.

Ignatavicius, D. D., & Workman, M. L. (2016). *Medical-surgical nursing* (8th ed.). St. Louis: Elsevier.

Lewis, S. L., Bucher, L., Heitkemper, M. M., et al. (2017). *Medical-surgical nursing*. St. Louis: Elsevier.

Pagana, K. D., & Pagana, T. J. (2014). *Mosby's manual of diagnostic and laboratory tests* (5th ed.). St. Louis: Elsevier.

Sax, P. E. (January 21, 2020). Acute and early HIV infection: Treatment. *UpToDate*. Retrieved January 20, 2021 from http://www.uptodate.com.

Sax, P. E. (November 11, 2020). Acute and early HIV infection: Clinical manifestations. *UpToDate*. Retrieved January 20, 2021 from www.uptodate.com.

Skidmore-Roth, L. (2021). *2021 Mosby's nursing drug reference* (X ed.). St. Louis MO: Elsevier.

Skidmore-Roth, L. (2017). *Mosby's 2017 nursing drug reference* (30th ed.). St. Louis: Elsevier.

UCSF HIV Insite. (2012). *Adverse effects of antiretroviral drugs*. http://hivinsite.ucsf.edu/InSite?page=ar-05-01#S2.5X.

CHAPTER 32: IMMUNOLOGIC DISORDERS

Abrams, C. S. (2016). Thrombocytopenia. In L. Goldman, & A. I. Schafer (Eds.), *Goldman-Cecil medicine* (Vol. 1) (2nd ed 5.). Philadelphia: Elsevier/Saunders.

American Cancer Society. (2021). *Cancer facts and figures 2021*. Atlanta GA: American Cancer Society.

American Cancer Society. (2017). *Treating acute lymphocytic leukemia*. https://www.cancer.org/cancer/acute-lymphocytic-leukemia/treating.html.

Applebaum, F. R. (2016). The acute leukemias. In L. Goldman, & A. I. Schafer (Eds.), *Goldman-Cecil medicine* (Vol. 1) (2nd ed 5.). Philadelphia: Elsevier/Saunders.

Bierman, P. J., & Armitage, J. O. (2016). Non-Hodgkin lymphomas. In L. Goldman, & A. I. Schafer (Eds.), *Goldman-Cecil medicine* (Vol. 1) (2nd ed 5.). Philadelphia: Elsevier/Saunders.

Breman, D. C., Alhamad, T., & Mallone, A. (Dec 8, 2020). Kidney transplantation in adults: Clinical features and diagnosis of acute renal allograft rejection. *UpToDate*. Retrieved Jan 28, 2021 from uptodate.com.

Burchum, J. R., & Rosenthal, L. D. (2019). *Lehne's pharmacology for nursing care* (10th ed.). St Louis MO: Elsevier.

Centers for Disease Control and Prevention Division of HIV/AIDS Prevention, National Center for HIV/AIDS, Viral Hepatitis, STDs, and TB Prevention. (Nov 24, 2020). *HIV* surveillance report Vol. 2020; 31.

Centers for Disease Control and Prevention. (2014). *HIV PrEP guidelines*. https://wwwn.cdc.gov/hivrisk/decreased_risk/medicines/prep.html.

Centers for Disease Control and Prevention. (2016). *HIV surveillance report: Diagnosis of HIV Infection in the United States and Dependent areas 20916* (Vol. 28). https://www.cdc.gov/hiv/statistics/overview/index.html.

Centers for Disease Control and Prevention. (2017). *Opportunistic infections*. www.cdc.gov.

Clarke, J. (Feb 24, 2020). Initial management of discoid lupus and subacute cutaneous lupus. *UpToDate*. Retrieved Jan 28, 2021 from uptodate.com.

Connors, J. M. (2016). Hodgkin lymphoma. In L. Goldman, & A. I. Schafer (Eds.), *Goldman-Cecil medicine* (Vol. 1) (2nd ed 5.). Philadelphia: Elsevier/Saunders.

Crow, M. K. (2016). Systemic lupus erythematosus. In L. Goldman, & A. I. Schafer (Eds.), *Goldman-Cecil medicine* (vol II) (2nd ed 5.). Philadelphia: Elsevier/Saunders.

del Rio, C., & Cohen, M. S. (2016). Prevention of human immunodeficiency virus infection. In (2nd ed 5.). L. Goldman, & A. I. Schafer (Eds.), *Goldman-Cecil medicine* (vol II). Philadelphia: Elsevier/Saunders.

DiNenno, E. A., Prejean, J., Irwin, K., et al. (2017). Recommendations for HIV screening of gay, bisexual, and other men who have sex with men — United States. *MMWR. Morbidity and Mortality Weekly Report*, *2017*(66), 830–832.

Drew, W. L. (2016). Cytomegalovirus. In L. Goldman, & A. I. Schafer (Eds.), *Goldman-Cecil medicine* (vol II) (2nd ed 5.) (p. 2016). Philadelphia: Elsevier/Saunders.

Feldweg, A. M., & TePas, E. (Jan 8, 2021). What's new in allergy and immunology. *UpToDate*. Retrieved Jan 28, 2021 from uptodate.com.

Galgiani, J. N. (2016). Coccidioidomycosis. In L. Goldman, & A. I. Schafer (Eds.), *Goldman-Cecil medicine* (vol II) (2nd ed 5.). Philadelphia: Elsevier/Saunders.

George, J. N., & Cuker, A. (9-30-2019). Acquired thrombocytopenic purpura: Initial treatment. *UpToDate*. Retrieved February 3, 2021 from www.uptodate.com.

George, J. N., & Cuker, A. (9-30-2019). Acquired thrombocytopenic purpura: Clinical manifestations and diagnosis. *UpToDate*. Retrieved February 3, 2021 from www.uptodate.com.

Gulick, R. M. (2016). Antiretroviral therapy of human immunodeficiency virus and acquired immunodeficiency syndrome. In L. Goldman, & A. I. Schafer (Eds.), *Goldman-Cecil medicine* (vol II) (2nd ed 5.). Philadelphia: Elsevier/Saunders.

Kauffman, C. A. (2016). Candidiasis. In L. Goldman, & A. I. Schafer (Eds.), *Goldman-Cecil medicine* (vol II) (2nd ed 5.). Philadelphia: Elsevier/Saunders.

Kauffman, C. A. (2016). Cryptococcosis. In L. Goldman, & A. I. Schafer (Eds.), *Goldman-Cecil medicine* (vol II) (2nd ed 5.). Philadelphia: Elsevier/Saunders.

Kauffman, C. A. (2016). Histoplasmosis. In L. Goldman, & A. I. Schafer (Eds.), *Goldman-Cecil medicine* (vol II) (2nd ed 5.). Philadelphia: Elsevier/Saunders.

Kovacs, J. A. (2016). Pneumocystis pneumonia. In L. Goldman, & A. I. Schafer (Eds.), *Goldman-Cecil medicine* (vol II) (2nd ed 5.). Philadelphia: Elsevier/Saunders.

Leukemia and Lymphoma Society. (2017). *Facts and statistics*. https://www.lls.org/http%3A/LLsorg.prod.acquia-sites.com/facts-and-statistics-overview/facts-and-statistics#Leukemia.

Lewis, S. L. (2016). Altered immune responses and transplantation. In SL Lewis, L Bucher, MM Heitkemper, et al. (Eds.), *Medical-surgical nursing* (10th ed.). St. Louis: Elsevier.

Lima, A. A. M., & Guerrant, R. L. (2016). Cryptosporidiosis. In L. Goldman, & A. I. Schafer (Eds.), *Goldman-Cecil medicine* (vol II) (2nd ed 5.). Philadelphia: Elsevier/Saunders.

Masur, H., Healey, L. M., & Hadigan, C. (2016). Infectious and metabolic complications of human immunodeficiency virus and acquired immunodeficiency syndrome. In L. Goldman, & A. I. Schafer (Eds.), *Goldman-Cecil medicine* (vol II) (2nd ed 5.). Philadelphia: Elsevier/Saunders.

Mayo Clinic. (2017). *Idiopathic thrombocytopenic purpura (ITP)*. https://www.mayoclinic.org/diseases-conditions/idiopathic-thrombocytopenic-purpura/diagnosis-treatment/drc-20352330?p=1.

Mitta, A., Curtis, B. R., Reese, J. A., & George, J. N. (2019). Drug-induced thrombocytopenia: 2019 update of clinical and laboratory data. *American Journal of Hematology*, *2019*(94), E76.

National Cancer Institute. (2017). *Adult lymphoma treatment (PDQr) - health professional version*. https://www.cancer.gov/types/lymphoma/hp/adult-hodgkin-treatment-pdq.

National Cancer Institute. (2017). *Adult non-Hodgkin lymphoma treatment (PDQr) - health professional version*. https://www.cancer.gov/types/lymp;homa/hp/adult-nhl-pdq.

National Heart, Lung, and Blood Institute. (2014). *What is thrombotic thrombocytopenic purpura?* https://www.nhlbi.nih.gov/health/health-topics/topics/ttp.

National Resource Center on Lupus. (Last updated Jan 23, 2021). *Medications used to treat lupus*. Retrieved Jan 31, 2021 from https://www.lupus.org/resources.

O/Brien, S., & Jabour, E. (2016). The chronic leukemias. In L. Goldman, & A. I. Schafer (Eds.), *Goldman-Cecil medicine* (Vol. 1) (2nd ed 5.). Philadelphia: Elsevier/Saunders.

Pichler, W. J. (Feb 18, 2019). Drug hypersensitivity: Classification and clinical features. *UpToDate*. Retrieved Jan 28, 2021 from uptodate.com.

Roberts, D. (2016). Arthritis and connective tissue diseases. In SL Lewis, L Bucher, MM Heitkemper, et al. (Eds.), *Medical-surgical nursing* (10th ed.). St. Louis: Elsevier.

Skidmore-Roth, L. (2021). *Mosby's 2021 nursing drug reference* (34th ed.). St. Louis MO: Elsevier.

Wallace, D. J., & Gladman, D. D. (Dec 10, 2019). Clinical manifestations and diagnosis of systemic lupus erythematosus in adults. *UpToDate*. Retrieved Jan 28, 2021 from uptodate.com.

Walsh, T. J. (2016). Aspergillosis. In L. Goldman, & A. I. Schafer (Eds.), *Goldman-Cecil medicine* (vol II) (2nd ed 5.). Philadelphia: Elsevier/Saunders.

CHAPTER 33: CARDIOVASCULAR SYSTEM INTRODUCTION

Aldea, G. (2016). Minimally invasive coronary artery bypass graft surgery: Definitions and techniques. *UpToDate*. https://www.uptodate.com/contents/minimally-invasive-coronary-artery-bypass-graft-surgery-definitions-and-technical-issues?source=search_result&search=totally%20endoscopic%20coronary%20artery%20bypass&selectedTitle=1~150.

American Heart Association. *Heart disease and stroke statistics 2009 update: a report from the American Heart Association Statistics Committee and Stroke Statistics Subcommittee, Circulation* (serial online): http://circ.ahajournals.org/cgi/content/full/119/2/e21.

American Heart Association. (2006). *Know the facts, get the stats 2007 (AHA Publication No. 55–1041)*. Dallas: American Heart Association.

American Heart Association. (2016). *Myocardial perfusion imaging*. http://www.heart.org/HEARTORG/Conditions/HeartAttack/DiagnosingaHeartAttack/Myocardial-Perfusion-Imaging-MPI-Test_UCM_446352_Article.jsp#.WbqTJjOZNBw.

American Heart Association. (2017). *The skinny on fats*. http://www.heart.org/HEARTORG/Conditions/Cholesterol/PreventionTreatmentofHighCholesterol/The-Skinny-on-Fats_UCM_305628_Article.jsp#.Wbq4EzOZNBw.

Benjamin, E., et al. (2017). Heart disease and stroke statistics-2017 Update. *A Report from the American Heart Association*. http://circ.ahajournals.org/content/135/10/e146.

Birks, E. (2017). Immediate and long-term mechanical circulatory support. *UpToDate*. https://www.uptodate.com/contents/intermediate-and-long-term-mechanical-circulatory-support?source=search_result&search=ventricular%20assist%20device&selectedTitle=2~97.

Burchum, J. R., & Rosenthal, L. D. (2016). *Lehne's pharmacology for nursing care* (9th ed.). St. Louis: Elsevier.

Cleveland Clinic. (2019). *Multigated Acquisition Scan (MUGA)*. www.myclevelandclinic.org.

Danias, P. G., & Chang, J. D. (Nov 2020). *Approach to evaluation of the right ventricle in adults*. Retrieved from http://www.uptodate.com.

Fogoros, R. N. (2018). *Cardiac biomarkers, cardiac enzymes, and heart disease*. Very Well Health.

Healthy People 2020. (2013). *Heart disease and stroke*. https://www.healthypeople.gov/2020/topics-objectives/topic/heart-disease-and-stroke/objectives.

Jaffe, A., & Morrow, D. (2016). Troponin testing. Clinical use. *UpToDate*. https://www.uptodate.com/contents/troponin-testing-clinical-use?source=see_link.

Jarvis, C. (2016). *Physical examination and health assessment* (7th ed.). St. Louis: Elsevier.

Lewis, S. M., Bucher, L., Heitkemper, M. M., et al. (Eds.). (2017). *Medical-surgical nursing: Assessment and management of clinical problems* (10th ed.). St. Louis: Elsevier.

Mayoclinic.com: *High blood pressure (hypertension): Risk factors*. (website): http://www.mayoclinic.org/diseases-conditions/high-blood-pressure/basics/risk-factors/con-20019580.

McCance, K., Huether, S., Brashers, V., et al. (2014). *Pathophysiology: The biologic basis for disease in adults and children* (7th ed.). St. Louis: Mosby.

Mozaffarian, D., Benjamin, E., Go, A., et al. (2016). Heart disease and stroke statistics—2016 update. *Circulation*. https://doi.org/10.1161/CIR0000000000000350.

Mukhurjee, D. (2016). Direct oral anticoagulants: Practical management approaches. *American College of Cardiology*. http://www.acc.org/latest-in-cardiology/ten-points-to-remember/2016/07/27/02/50/direct-oral-anticoagulants.

Pagana, K., Pagana, T., & Pagana, T. (2017). *Mosby's diagnostic and laboratory test reference* (13th ed.). St. Louis, MO: Elsevier.

Porter, R. S. (2017). *The Merck manual of diagnosis and therapy* (20th ed.). Whitehouse Station, NJ: Merck & Co., Inc.

Potter, P. A., Perry, A. G., Stockert, P. A., et al. (Eds.). (2017). *Fundamentals of nursing* (9th ed.). St. Louis: Elsevier.

Rubenfire, M. (2016). Aspirin for primary prevention of CVD and colorectal cancer. *American College of Cardiology*. http://www.acc.org/latest-in-cardiology/ten-points-to-remember/2016/04/21/14/54/aspirin-use-for-the-primary-prevention-of-cardiovascular-disease.

Sexton, D. (2017). Patient education: Antibiotics before procedures. (beyond the basics). *UpToDate*. Texasheartinstitute.org: Coronary artery disease. (website) http://www.texasheartinstitute.org/HIC/Topics/Cond/Coronaryarterydisease.cfm.

Wu, A. H. B. (Ed.). (2006). *Tietz clinical guide to laboratory tests* (4th ed.) (pp. 306–307). St. Louis: Saunders Elsevier.

CHAPTER 34: HYPERTENSION

(2019). *ACA/ACC clinical performance and quality measures for adults with high BP*. American College of Cardiology.

Alexander. (2019, February 22). *Hypertension Guidelines*. (E. H. Yang, Ed.) Retrieved Nov 24, 2020, from Medscape: https://emedicine.com/article/241381-guidelines.

American Heart Association. (2018, October 30). *Is vaping better than smoking?*: Retrieved November 23, 2020, from www.cdc.gov/tobacco/basic_information/e-cigarettes.

Arnett, D. K., & B., R. (2019, March 17). 2019 ACC/AHA guideline on the primary prevention of cardiovascular disease. *Journal American College of Cardiology*.

Bohm, M. (2020, May 2). Efficacy of catheter based renal denervation in the absence of antihypertensive medications. *Lancet*, *395*(10234), 1444–1451.

Chen. (2019, February 19). Inflammation and apparent treatment-resistent hypertension in patients with CKD. *Hypertension*.

Elliott, W. J. (2019, Dec 3). Drugs used for hypertensive emergencies. *UpToDate*.

Ford. (1997, September). Ambulatory blood pressure monitoring: A 24 hour tool. *ADVANCE for Nurse Practitioners*.

JNC 8 Guidelines for the Management of Hypertension in Adults. (2014, October 1). *American Family Physician*, *90*(7), 503–504.

Kumbhani. (2017, August 08). Systolic blood pressure intervention trial - SPRINT. *American College of Cardiology*.

Mayo Clinic staff. (2019, January 9). *10 ways to control high blood pressure without medication*.

MD, & Townsend, R. R. (2020, November 24). *Director hypertension program, professor of medicine*. Philadelphia, PA, USA: University of Pennsylvania. (V. Ford, Interviewer).

Merelli. (2019, October 17). *High Blood Pressure (Hypertension) Medications*. (O. Ogbru, Ed.) Retrieved November 24, 2020, from Rxlist: https://rxlist.com/high_blood_pressure_hypertension_medications/drug-class htm.

R, A. (2019, February 2019). *Hypertension Guidelines: Guideline Summary*. (E. Yang, Ed.) Retrieved November 24, 2020, from Medscape: https://emedicine.medscape.com/article 241381-guidelines.

Unger, T., & B., C. (2020, May 6). 2020 International society of hypertension global hypertension guidelines. *Hypertension*, *75*, 1334–1357.

Weber. (2019, June 24). Renal devervation for treating hypertension: Current scientific and clinical evidence. *JACC Cardiovascular Intervention*, *12*(12), 1095–1105.

CHAPTER 35: CARDIAC DISORDERS

Aldea, G. (2016). Minimally invasive coronary artery bypass graft surgery: Definitions and techniques. *UpToDate*. https://www.uptodate.com/contents/minimally-invasive-coronary-artery-bypass-graft-surgery-definitions-and-technical-issues?source=search_result&search=totally%20endoscopic%20coronary%20artery%20bypass&selectedTitle=1~150.

American Heart Association. (2006). *Know the facts, get the stats 2007 (AHA Publication No. 55–1041)*. Dallas: American Heart Association.

American Heart Association. (2016). *What is Pericarditis?* http://www.heart.org/HEARTORG/Conditions/More/What-is-Pericarditis_UCM_444931_Article.jsp#.WcEsMzOZNBw.

Amsterdam, E. A., Wenger, N. K., Brindis, R. G., et al. (2014). AHA/ACCC guideline for the management of patients with non-ST-elevation acute coronary syndrome: A report of the American College of Cardiology/American Heart Association task force on practice guidelines. *Journal of the American College of Cardiology*, *64*, e139–e228.

Benjamin, E. J., Blaha, M. J., & On behalf of the American Heart Association Statistics Committee and Stroke Statistics Subcommittee., et al. (2017). Heart disease and stroke statistics – 2017 update: A report from the American heart association. *Circulation*. (serial online): http://circ.ahajournals.org/content/135/10/e146.

Birks, E. (2017). Immediate and long-term mechanical circulatory support. *UpToDate*. https://www.uptodate.com/contents/intermediate-and-long-term-mechanical-circulatory-support?source=search_result&search=ventricular%20assist%20device&selectedTitle=2~97.

Colucci, W. (2017). Treatment of acute decompensated heart failure. *UpToDate*. https://www.uptodate.com/contents/treatment-of-acute-decompensated-heart-failure-components-of-therapy?source=search_result&search=oxygen%20and%20Heart%20failure&selectedTitle=1~150.

Cooper, L. T. (Nov 2020). Etiology and pathogenesis of myocarditis. Retrieved from http://www.uptodate.com.

Cooper, L. T. (Nov 2020). Treatment and prognosis of myocarditis in adults. Retrieved from http://www.uptodate.com.

Healthy People 2020. (2013). *Heart disease and stroke*. https://www.healthypeople.gov/2020/topics-objectives/topic/heart-disease-and-stroke/objectives.

Heart Disease Facts, & Centers for disease control and prevention. (2020). *CDC 24/7: Saving lives, protecting people.*

Holger, T., & Abbott, J. D. (Nov 2020). Acute myocardial infarction: Mechanical complications. Retrieved from http://www.uptodate.com.

Jaffe, A., & Morrow, D. (2016). Troponin testing. Clinical use. *UpToDate.* https://www.uptodate.com/contents/troponin-testing-clinical-use?source=see_link.

Kannam, J., Aroesty, J., & Gersch, B. (2016). Stable ischemic heart disease. Overview of care. *UpToDate.* https://www.uptodate.com/contents/stable-ischemic-heart-disease-overview-of-care?source=search_result&search=angina%20management&selectedTitle=1~150.

Kondur, A., Powan, H., & Afonso, L. (2014). *Complications of MI.* http://emedicine.medscape.com/article/164924-overview#a2.

Mancini, D. (2020). Heart transplantation in adults: Indications and contraindications. Retrieved from www.uptodate.com.

Mancini, D. (2017). Indications and contraindications for cardiac transplantation in adults. *UpToDate.* https://www.uptodate.com/contents/indications-and-contraindications-for-cardiac-transplantation-in-adults?source=search_result&search=cardiac%20transplantation&selectedTitle=1~150https://www.uptodate.com/contents/antibiotics-before-procedures-beyond-the-basics.

Mozaffarian, D., Benjamin, E., Go, A., et al. (2016). Heart disease and stroke statistics—2016 update. *Circulation.* https://doi.org/10.1161/CIR0000000000000350.

O'Gara, P., et al. (2012). *2013 ACCF/AHA guideline for the management of ST-elevation myocardial infarction: A report of the American College of Cardiology Foundation/American Heart Association task force on practice guidelines.* https://www.heart.org/idc/groups/heart-public/@wcm/@mwa/documents/downloadable/ucm_453635.pdf.

Reeder, G., & Kennedy, H. (2016). Overview of the acute management of ST elevation myocardial infarction. *UpToDate.* https://www.uptodate.com/contents/overview-of-the-acute-management-of-st-elevation-myocardial-infarction?source=search_result&search=STEMI%20management&selectedTitle=1~150.

Reilly, C., Anderson, K., Baas, L., et al. (2015). American association of heart failure nurses best practice paper: Literature synthesis and guideline review for dietary sodium restriction. *Heart & Lung, 44*, 289–298.

Sexton, D. (2017). Patient education: Antibiotics before procedures. (beyond the basics). *UpToDate.* Texasheartinstitute.org: Coronary artery disease. (website). http://www.texasheartinstitute.org/HIC/Topics/Cond/Coronaryarterydisease.cfm.

Simons, M., & Lahara, R. S. (Nov 2020). *New therapies for angina pectoris.* Retrieved from http://www.uptodate.com.

Svensson L. Heart Valve Replacement: Which Type is Best for You? How mechanical and biological valves differ. Cleveland Clinic, June 14, 2018/Heart Health.

Virani, S. S., Alonso, A., Benjamin, E. J., Bittencourt, M. S., Calloway, C. W., Carson, A. P., et al. (2020). *Circulation, 141*(9) e139–e5.

Wilson, W., Taubert, K. A., Gewitz, M., et al. (2007). Prevention of infective endocarditis: Guidelines from the American Heart Association: A guideline from the American Heart Association rheumatic fever, endocarditis, and Kawasaki disease committee, council on cardiovascular disease in the young, and the council on clinical cardiology, council on cardiovascular surgery and anesthesia, and the quality of care and outcomes research interdisciplinary working group. *Circulation, 116*, 1736.

Yancy, C. W., et al. (2013). ACCF/AHA guideline for the management of heart failure: A report of the American College of Cardiology Foundation/American Heart Association task force on practice guidelines. *Circulation.* (serial online) http://circ.ahajournals.org/content/early/2013/06/03/CIR.0b013e31829e8776.

Zafari, A. M. (2019). Myocardial infarction. *Medscape.*

CHAPTER 36: VASCULAR DISORDERS

Akar, A. R., & I.B. (2019). *Thromboangiitis obliterans (buerger disease)* (9th ed.). Philadelphia, PA, USA: Elsevier.

American Heart Association. (2018, Oct 30). *Is vaping better than smoking?* Retrieved from www.cdc.gov/tobacco/basic_information/e-cigarettes.

American Society of Hematology. (2020, February 7). *Venous thromboembolism (blood clots)* (C. f. Prevention, Editor). Retrieved from https://www.cdc.gov/ncbddd/dvt/facts.html.

Blood Clot Recovery. (2020, June 12). *Stop your anxiety.* Retrieved November 6, 2020, from Anxiety Archives: https://bloodclotrecovery.net/tag/anxiety.

Chen, M. (2020, October 08). *MedlinePlus medical encyclopedia* (U. N. Medicine, Editor). Retrieved from medlineplus.gov/ency/article/00102.htm.

Firnhaber, J. M., & P. C (2019, Mar 15). Lower extremity peripheral artery disease: Diagnosis and treatment. *America Family Physician, 99*(6), 362–369.

Ginsberg, J. (2016). Peripheral venous disease. In L. Goldman, & A. I. Schafer (Eds.), *Goldman-Cecil medicine* (25th ed.). Philadelphia: Elsevier Saunders.

Jaff, M. R., & Bartholomer, J. R. (2016). Other peripheral arterial diseases. In L. Goldman, & A. I. Schafer (Eds.), *Goldman-Cecil medicine* (25th ed.). St. Louis: Elsevier.

John Hopkins Medicine. (2020). *Chronic venous insufficiency.* Retrieved October 29, 2020, from Heart and Vascular: https://www.hopkinsmedicine.org/health/heart-and-vascular.

Mayo Clinic. (2019, July 17). *Varicose veins.* Retrieved November 13, 2020, from https://www.mayoclinic.org/diseases-conditions/varicose-veins/diagnosis-treatment.

Medical News Today. (2019, April 29). *Lymphangitis: Causes, symptoms, and pictures.* Retrieved November 13, 2020, from https://medicalnewstoday.com/articles/325069.

Nature Reviews Cardiology. (2018, November 15). Abdominal aortic aneurysm: Update on pathogenesis and medical treatments. *Nature, 16*, 225–242.

NHLBI, NIH. (2019, December 17). *Aortic aneurysm.* Retrieved November 9, 2020, from Health Topics: https://www.nhlbi.nih.gov/health-topics/aneurysm.

P, M. (2019, April 12). *5 Deep vein thrombosis nursing care plans* (Nurseslabs, Editor). Retrieved from Nurseslabs: https://nurseslab.com/deep-vein-thrombosis-nursing-care-plans/2/.

Pascarella, L., & S.C. (2019). *Rutherford's vascular surgery and endovascular therapy* (P. B. Sidawy AN, Ed.) (9th ed.). Philadelphia, PA, USA: Elsevier.

Penn Medicine Updates. (2017). *The cold truth about raynaud's.* Retrieved from www.pennmedicine.org/updates/blogs/health-and-wellness/2017/december/raynauds.

Penn Medicine. (2020). *Aortic dissection.* Retrieved November 10, 2020, from Penn Medicine.org. https://www.pennmedicine.org/conditions-treated-a-toz/aortic-dissection.

Upchurch, G. R., & E.G. (2020, July 3). Guidelines for thoracic endovascular aneurysm repair (Tevar). *Journal of Vascular Surgery.*

White, C. J. (2016). Atherosclerotic peripheral arterial disease. In L. Goldman, & A. I. Schafer (Eds.), *Goldman-Cecil medicine* (25th ed.). St. Louis: Elsevier.

Wipke-Tevis, D., & Rich, K. (2017). Vascular disorders. In SM Lewis, L Bucher, MM Heitkemper, et al. (Eds.), *Medical-surgical nursing: Assessment and management of clinical problems* (10th ed.). St. Louis: Elsevier.

CHAPTER 37: DIGESTIVE SYSTEM INTRODUCTION

Burchum, J. R., & Rosenthal, L. D. (2019). *Lehne's pharmacology for nursing care* (10th ed.). St Louis MO: Elsevier.

Burchum, J. R., & Rosenthal, L. D. (2016). *Lehne's pharmacology for nursing care* (9th ed.). St. Louis: Elsevier.

Cave D. (2-25-21). Wireless video capsule endocscopy. *UpToDate*. Retrieved Feb 27, 2021 from uptodate.com. UpToDate. Retrieved Feb 27, 2021 from uptodate.com.

Collares, F. B., & Anderson, S. (1-10-2020). Transjugular liver biopsy. *UpToDate*. Retrieved Feb 27, 2021 from uptodate.com.

Douberi, C. (March 18, 2020). Tests for screening for colorectal cancer. *UpToDate*. Retrieved Feb 27, 2021 from uptodate.com.

FDA. (2017). *FDA approved Mavyret for hepatitis C*. https://www.fda/gov/newsevents/newsroom/pressannouncements/ucm570038.htm.

Fillit, H. M., Rockwood, K., & Young, J. (2017). *Brocklehurst's textbook of geriatric medicine and gerontology* (8th ed.). Philadelphia: Elsevier.

Gaglio, P. J., & Cotler, S. J. (Nov 6, 2019). Liver transplantation in adults: Long term management of transplant recipients. *UpToDate*. Retrieved Mar 4, 2021 from uptodate.com.

Hodin, R. A., & Bordeianou, L. (March 17, 2020). Inpatient placement and management of nasogastric and nasoenteric tubes in adult. *UpToDate*. Retrieved Feb 27, 2021 from uptodate.com.

Lamont, J. T. (April 2, 2020). Indications and diagnostic tests for *H. pylori* infection. *UpToDate*. Retrieved Mar 4, 2021 from uptodate.com.

Pagana, K. D., & Pagana, T. J. (2014). *Mosby's manual of diagnostic and laboratory tests* (5th ed.). St. Louis: Elsevier.

Potter, P. A., Perry, A. G., Stockert, P. A., et al. (2017). *Fundamentals of nursing* (9th ed.). St. Louis: Elsevier.

Seres, D. (February 4, 2019). Nutrition support in critically ill patients. *UpToDate*. Retrieved Mar 4, 2021 from uptodate.com.

Skidmore-Roth, L. (2021). *Mosby's 2021 nursing drug reference*. St. Louis MO: Elsevier.

Vollmer, C. M., Zakko, S. F., & Afdahl, N. H. (Dec 12, 2020). *UpToDate*. Retrieved Mar 4, 2021 from uptodate.com.

CHAPTER 38: UPPER DIGESTIVE TRACT DISORDERS

Amarasinghe, G., & Sifrim, D. (2014). Functional esophageal disorders: Pharmacological option. *Drugs*, *74*, 1335–1344.

American Cancer Society. (2017). *Cancer facts and figures*. (website). www.cancer.org/research/cancerfactsfigures/cancerfactsfigures/cancer-facts-figures-2017.

Castle, K. (2012). Novel methods of imaging the GI tract in endoscopy. *Gastrointestinal Nursing*, *10*(5), 38–43.

Gupta, N., Bansal, A., Wani, S. B., et al. (2011). Endoscopy for upper GI cancer screening in the general population: A cost-utility analysis. *Gastrointestinal Endoscopy*, *74*(3), 610–624e2.

Jarvis, C. (2016). *Physical examination and health assessment* (7th ed.). Philadelphia: Saunders.

Kim, M. (2018). *Toupet fundoplication*. Retrieved Feb 27, 2020 from https://drminkim.com/procedure/esophageal/toupet-fundoplication/.

Lewis, S. L., Dirksen, S. R., & Heitkemper, M. M. (2014). Nursing management: Upper gastrointestinal problems. In SM Lewis, MM Heitkemper, SR Dirksen, et al. (Eds.), *Medical-surgical nursing: Assessment and management of clinical problems* (9th ed.). St. Louis: Mosby.

National Cancer Institute at the National Institutes of Health website. https://www.cancer.gov/types/head-and-neck/patient/lip-mouth-treatment-pdq#section/_48.

Reedy, S. (2009). An evidence-based review of obesity and bariatric surgery. *The Journal for Nurse Practitioners*, *5*(1), 22–29.

Scott, R., & Enns, R. (2015). Advances in capsule endoscopy. *Gastroenterology and Hepatology*, *11*(9), 612–617.

Shephard, R. J. (2017). Cancers of the esophagus and stomach: Potential mechanisms behind the beneficial influence of physical activity. *Clinical Journal of Sport Medicine*, *27*(4), 415–421.

Sobieraj, D. M., Coleman, S. M., & Coleman, C. I. (2011). US prevalence of upper gastrointestinal symptoms: A systematic literature review. *American Journal of Managed Care*, *17*(11), e449–e458.

Patel, D. A., Lappas, B. M., & Vaezi, M. F. (2017). An overview of achalasia and its subtypes. *Gastroenterology and Hepatology*, *13*(7), 411–420.

Wu JH, Guo Z, Kumar S, et al: Incidence of serious upper and lower gastrointestinal events in older adults with.

CHAPTER 39: LOWER DIGESTIVE TRACT DISORDERS

American Cancer Society. (2017). *Cancer facts and figures*. (website). www.cancer.org.

American Gastroenterological Association. (2014). *Guidelines for management of Crohn's disease*. (website). www.gastro.org/guidelines/drug-therapy-for-crohn-s.

Apovian, C. M. (2016). The obesity epidemic-understanding the disease and the treatment. *New England Journal of Medicine*, *374*, 177–179.

Bakshi, A., Stephen, S., Borum, M. L., et al. (2012). Emerging therapeutic options for celiac disease: Potential alternatives to a gluten-free diet. *Gastroenterology and Hepatology*, *8*(4), 582–588.

Bibbins-Domingo., et al. (2017). Screening for celiac disease: US preventive services task force recommendation statement. *Journal of the American Medical Association*, *317*(12), 1252–1257.

Cawley, J. (2015). An economy of scales: A selective review of obesity's economic causes, consequences, and solutions. *Journal of Health Economics*, *43*, 244–268.

Cobbols, A., & Lord, S. (2012). Treatment and management of obesity: Is surgical intervention the answer? *Journal of Perioperative Practice*, *22*(4), 114–121.

Croghan, A. (2014). Nursing assessment: Gastrointestinal system. In SM Lewis, MM Heitkemper, SR Dirksen, et al. (Eds.), *edical-surgical nursing: assessment and management of clinical problems* (9th ed.). St. Louis: Mosby.

DuBois, R. N. (2008). Neoplasms of the large and small intestine. In L. Goldman, & D. Ausiello (Eds.), *Cecil textbook of medicine* (23th ed.). Philadelphia: Saunders.

Fleming, V., & Wade, W. E. (2010). A review of laxative therapies for treatment of chronic constipation in older adults,. *The American Journal of Geriatric Pharmacotherapy*, *8*(10), 51.

Grodner, M., Roth, S. L., & Walkingshaw, B. C. (2012). *Nutritional foundations and clinical applications* (5th ed.). St. Louis: Mosby.

Jarvis, C. (2016). *Physical examination and health assessment* (7th ed.). Philadelphia: Saunders.

Kushner, R. F., & Ryan, D. H. (2014). Assessment and lifestyle management of patients with obesity: Clinical recommendations from systematic reviews. *Journal of the American Medical Association*, *312*(9), 943–952.

Lafon, C., & Lawson, L. (2012). Postoperative ileus in GI surgical patients: Pathogenesis and interventions. *Gastrointestinal Nursing*, *10*(2), 45–49.

Lewis, S. L., Dirksen, S. R., & Heitkemper, M. M. (2015). Nursing management: Lower gastrointestinal problems. In SM Lewis, MM Heitkemper, SR Dirksen, et al. (Eds.), *Medical-surgical nursing: Assessment and management of clinical problems* (9th ed.). St. Louis: Mosby.

MedlinePlus. *Hernia*. website. http://www.nlm.nih.gov/medlineplus/hernia.html.

Merck Manuals. *Hernias of the abdominal wall*. (website). http://www.merckmanuals.com/professional/gastrointestinal_disorders/acute_abdomen_and_surgical_gastroenterology/hernias_of_the_abdominal_wall.html.

National Institute of Diabetes and Digestive and Kidney Diseases. (2013). *Crohn's disease* (website). www.digestive.niddk.nih.gov.

National Institute of Diabetes and Digestive and Kidney Diseases. (2013). *Ulcerative colitis* (website). www.digestive.niddk.nih.gov.

Ogden, J. (2016). Improving recognition and management of coeliac disease, Prescriber. *The Journal of Prescribing and Medicines Management March*, 44–47.

Parian, A. (2017). Disease management strategies for moderate to severe IBD in adults. *Journal Management Care Medicine*, *20*(2), 15–20.

Scott, R., & Enns, R. (2015). Advances in capsule endoscopy. *Gastroenterology and Hepatology*, *11*(9), 612–617.

Skidmore-Roth, L. (2017). *Mosby's nursing drug reference*. St. Louis: Mosby.

Werutsky, G., Ducreux, M., Lutz, M., et al. (2012). The EORTC gastrointestinal tract cancer group: 50 years of research contributing to improved gastrointestinal cancer management,. *EJC Supplements*, *10*(1), 51–57.

Wu, J. H., Guo, Z., Kumar, S., et al. (2011). Incidence of serious upper and lower gastrointestinal events in older adults with and without Alzheimer's disease. *Journal of the American Geriatrics Society*, *59*(11), 2053–2061.

CHAPTER 40: LIVER, GALLBLADDER, AND PANCREATIC DISORDERS

American Cancer Society. (2021). *Gallbladder cancer*. Retrieved March 15, 2021 from cancer.org.

Bajaj, J. S., & Sanyal, A. J. (Oct 28, 2020). Methods to achieve hemostasis in patients with acute variceal hemorrhage. *UpToDate*. Retrieved March 17, 2021 from uptodate.com.

Burchum, J. R., & Rosenthal, L. D. (2019). *Lehne's pharmacology for nursing care* (10th ed.). St. Louis MO: Elsevier.

Centers for Disease Control and Prevention. (2021). *Recommended child and adolescent immunization schedule for ages eighteen years or younger, United States 2021*. Retrieved March 1, 2021 from https://www.cdc.gov/vaccines/schedules/hcp/imz/adults.html.

Collares FB, & Anderson S. (Jan 10, 2020). Transjugular liver biopsy. Retrieved March 1, 2021 from *UpToDate*. Retrieved March 17, 2021 from uptodate.com.

Freedman, S. D. (Jan 27, 2021). Treatment of chronic pancreatitis. *UpToDate*. Retrieved March 17, 2021 from uptodate.com.

Gaglio, P. J., & Cotler, S. J. (Nov 6, 2019). *Liver transplantation in adults: Long-term management of transplant recipients*.

Goldberg, E., & Chopra, S. (Nov 6, 2019). Cirrhosis in adults: Overview of complication, general management, and prognosis. *UpToDate*. Retrieved March 17, 2021 from uptodate.com.

Goldberg, E., Chopra, S., & Rubin, J. N. (Sep 21, 2020). Acute liver failure in adults: Management and prognosis. *UpToDate*. Retrieved March 17, 2021 from uptodate.com.

Kim, A. Y. (June 12, 2019). Epidemiology and transmission of hepatitis C virus infection. *UpToDate*. Retrieved March 17, 2021 from uptodate.com.

Lewis, S. L., Bucher, L., Heitkemper, M. M., et al. (2017). *Medical-surgical nursing* (10th ed.). St. Louis: Elsevier.

Negro, F., & Lok, A. S. I. (Jul 31, 2020). Pathogenesis, epidemiology, natural history, and clinical manifestation of hepatitis D virus infection. *UpToDate*. Retrieved March 17, 2021 from uptodate.com.

Olson, M. C. (2020). Liver, biliary tract, and pancreas problems. In M. M. Harding (Ed.), *Lewis's medical surgical nursing* (11th ed.). St. Louis MO: Elsevier.

Pawlotsky, J.-M. (2016). Acute viral hepatitis. In L. Goldman, & A. I. Schafer (Eds.), *Goldman-Cecil medicine* (2nd ed 5.).

Raijman, I. (Dec 30, 2019). Endoscopic management of bile duct stones: Standard technique and mechanical lithotripsy. *UpToDate*. Retrieved March 17, 2021 from uptodate.com.

Runyon, B. A. (Jan 11, 2021). Ascites in adults with cirrhosis: Initial treatment. *UpToDate*. Retrieved March 17, 2021 from uptodate.com.

Ryan, D. P., & Mamon, H. (Dec 15, 2020). Initial chemotherapy and radiotherapy for nonmetastatic, locally advanced, unresectable and borderline resectable exocrine pancreatic cancer. *UpToDate*. Retrieved March 17, 2021 from uptodate.com.

Vege, S. S. (Mar 8, 2021). Management of acute pancreatitis. *UpToDate*. Retrieved March 17, 2021 from uptodate.com.

Vollmer, C. M., Zakko, S. F., & Afdahl, N. H. (Dec 20, 2020). Treatment of acute calculous cholecystitis. *UpToDate*. Retrieved March 17, 2021 from uptodate.com.

Zakko, S. F., & Afdahl, N. H. (Nov 10, 2020). Acute calculous cholecystitis: Clinical features and diagnosis. *UpToDate*. Retrieved March 17, 2021 from uptodate.com.

CHAPTER 41: UROLOGIC SYSTEM INTRODUCTION

Brennon, D. C., & Malone, A. (Feb 27, 2020). Kidney transplantation in adults: Treatment of acute T-cell mediated (cellular) rejection of the renal allograft. *UpToDate*. Retrieved Mar 14, 2021 from uptodate.com.

Clemens, J. Q. (Jan 4, 2021). Management of interstitial cystitis/bladder pain syndrome. *UpToDate*. Retrieved Mar 14, 2021 from uptodate.com.

Curhan, G. C., Aronson, M. D., & Preminger, G. M. (Jul 2, 2019). Diagnosis and acute management of suspected nephrolithiasis in adults. *UpToDate*. Retrieved Mar 14, 2021 from uptodate.com.

Hardinger, K., & Brennon, D. C. (Aug 7, 2020). Kidney transplantation in adults: Maintenance immunosuppressive therapy. *UpToDate*. Retrieved Mar 14, 2021 from uptodate.com.

Hooton, T. M., & Gupta, K. (Mar 15, 2021). Acute simple cystitis in women. *UpToDate*. Retrieved Mar 20, 2021 from uptodate.com.

Hooton, T. M., & Gupta, K. (Mar 19, 2021). Acute complicated urinary tract infection (including pyelonephritis in adults. *UpToDate*. Retrieved Mar 20, 2021 from uptodate.com.

Niaudet, P. (May 20, 2020). Poststreptoccal glomerulonephritis. *UpToDate*. Retrieved Mar 14, 2021 from uptodate.com.

Pagana, K., Pagana, T., & Pagana, T. (2017). *Mosby's diagnostic & laboratory test reference* (13th ed.). St. Louis: Elsevier.

Schaeffer, A. J. (Jul 2, 2019). Placement and management of urinary bladder catheters in adults. *UpToDate*. Retrieved Mar 14, 2021 from uptodate.com.

CHAPTER 42: UROLOGIC DISORDERS

Altok, M., et al. (2017). Ureteral orifice involvement by urothelial carcinoma: Long term oncologic and functional outcomes. *International Braz Journal of Urology*, *43*(6), 1052–1059.

American Cancer Society. (2021). *Facts and figures 2021*.

Appel, G. B., & Kaplan, A. A. (Sep 16, 2020). Overview of the classification and treatment of rapidly progressive (crescentic) glomerulonephritis. *UpToDate*. Retrieved Mar 23, 2021 from uptodate.com.

Atkins, M. B. (Feb 25, 2021). Overview of the treatment of renal cell carcinoma. *UpToDate*. Retrieved Mar 23, 2021 from uptodate.com.

Atkins, M. B. (Jul 16, 2020). Clinical manifestations, evaluation, and staging of renal cell carcinoma. *UpToDate*. Retrieved Mar 23, 2021 from uptodate.com.

Atkins, M. B., & Choueiri, T. K. (Jan 26, 2021). Epidemiology, pathology, and pathogenesis of renal cell carcinoma. *UpToDate*. Retrieved Mar 23, 2021 from uptodate.com.

Brennon, D. C., & Malone, A. (Feb 27, 2020). Kidney transplantation in adults: Treatment of acute T-cell mediated (cellular) rejection of the renal allograft. *UpToDate*. Retrieved Mar 14, 2021 from uptodate.com.

Burchum, J. R., & Rosenthal, L. D. (2019). *Lehne's pharmacology for nursing care* (10th ed.). St. Louis MO: Elsevier.

Chapman, A. B., Rahbari-Oskoui, F. F., & Bennett, W. M. (Oct 19 2020). Autosomal dominant polycystic kidney disease in adults: Treatment. *UpToDate*. Retrieved Mar 23, 2021 from uptodate.com.

Clemens, J. Q. (Jan 4, 2021). Management of interstitial cystitis/bladder pain syndrome. *UpToDate*. Retrieved Mar 23, 2021 from uptodate.com.
Curhan, G. C. (Feb 26, 2021). Prevention of recurrent calcium stones in adults. *UpToDate*. Retrieved Mar 23, 2021 from uptodate.com.
Curhan, G. C. (Nov 2, 2020). Kidney stones in adults: Epidemiology and risk factors. *UpToDate*. Retrieved Mar 25, 2021 from uptodate.com.
Curhan, G. C., Aronson, M. D., & Preminger, G. M. (Jul 2, 2021). Diagnosis and acute management of suspected nephrolithiasis in adults. *UpToDate*. Retrieved Mar 25, 2021 from uptodate.com.
Curhan, G. C., Preminger, G. M., & Taylor, E. N. (Dec 11, 2019). Renal complications of extracorporal shock wave lithotripsy. *UpToDate*. Retrieved Mar 25, 2021 from uptodate.com.
Dirkes, S. (2015). Acute kidney injury: Causes, phases, and early detection. *American Nurse Today*, *10*(7). https://www.americannursetoday.com/acute-kidney-injury/.
Doyle, J., & Forni, L. (2016). Acute kidney injury: Short-term and long-term effects. *Critical Care*, *20*(188). https://ccforum.biomedcentral.com/articles/10.1186/s13054-016-1353-y.
Edvardsson, V., et al. (2013). Hereditary causes of kidney stones and chronic kidney disease. *Pediatric Nephrology*, *28*(10), 1923–1942.
George, D., & Jonasch, E. (Feb 15, 2021). Systemic treatment of advanced clear cell renal carcinoma. *UpToDate*. Retrieved Mar 23, 2021 from uptodate.com.
Hardinger, K., & Brennon, D. C. (Aug 7, 2020). Kidney transplantation in adults: Maintenance immunosuppressive therapy. *UpToDate*. Retrieved Mar 14, 2021 from uptodate.com.
Hooton, T. M., & Gupta, K. (Mar 15, 2021). Acute simple cystitis in women. *UpToDate*. Retrieved Mar 23, 2021 from uptodate.com.
Hooton, T. M., & Gupta, K. (Mar 19, 2021). Acute complications of urinary tract infection (including pyelonephrosis) in adults. *UpToDate*. Retrieved Mar 23, 2021 from uptodate.com.
Hooton, T. M. (Jul 20, 2020). Acute simple cystitis in men. *UpToDate*. Retrieved Mar 23, 2021 from uptodate.com.
Huether, S., & McCance, K. (2017). *Understanding pathophysiology* (6th ed.). St. Louis: Elsevier.
Jarvis, C. (2016). *Physical examination and health assessment* (7th ed.). St. Louis: Elsevier.
Lianglos, O., & Jaber, B. L. (Feb 26, 2020). Kidney and patient outcomes after acute kidney injury in adults. *UpToDate*. Retrieved Mar 23, 2021 from uptodate.com.
Mailloux, L., & Heinrich, W. (2017). *Patient survival and maintenance dialysis*. www.uptodate.com.
McCance, K., & Huether, S. (2014). *Pathophysiology: The biologic basis for disease in adults and children* (7th ed.). St. Louis: Elsevier.
National Cancer Institute. (2017a). *Cancer stat facts: Bladder cancer*. https://seer.cancer.gov/statfacts/html/urinb.html.
National Cancer Institute. (2017b). *Renal cell cancer treatment*. https://www.cancer.gov/types/kidney/patient/kidney-treatment-pdq#section/all.
National Cancer Institute. (2017c). *SEER cancer stat facts: Kidney and renal pelvis cancer*. http://seer.cancer.gov/statfacts/html/kidrp.html.
National Kidney Foundation. (2016). *Kidney stones*. https://www.kidney.org/atoz/content/kidneystones.
Niaudet, P. (May 20, 2020). Poststreptococcal glomerulonephritis. *UpToDate*. Retrieved Mar 23, 2021 from uptodate.com.
Okusa, M., & Rosner, M. (2017). *Overview of the management of acute kidney injury in adults*. www.uptodate.com.
Okusa, M. D., & Rosner, M. H. (Oct 22, 2019). Overview of the management of Acute Kidney Injury (AKI) in adults. *UpToDate*. Retrieved Mar 23, 2021 from uptodate.com.
Pagana, K., Pagana, T., & Pagana, T. (2017). *Mosby's diagnostic & laboratory test reference* (13th ed.). St. Louis: Elsevier.
Prezioso, D., et al. (2015). Dietary treatment of urinary risk factors for renal stone formation. A review of CLU Working Group. *Archivio Italiano di Urologia, Andrologia*, *87*(2), 105–120. https://air.unimi.it/retrieve/handle/2434/369628/557185/5413-19480-3-PB.pdf.
Radhakrishman, J. (April 16, 2020). Glomerular disease: Evaluation and differential diagnosis in adults. *UpToDate*. Retrieved Mar 23, 2021 from uptodate.com.
Richie, J. P. (Sep 17, 2019). Definitive surgical management of renal cell carcinoma. *UpToDate*. Retrieved Mar 23, 2021 from uptodate.com.
Rosenberg, M. (2017). *Overview of the management of chronic kidney disease in adults*. www.uptodate.com.
Shariat, S. F., Bocher, B. H., & Pietzak, E. J. (Jan 8, 2020). Urinary diversion and reconstruction following cystectomy. *UpToDate*. Retrieved Mar 23, 2021 from uptodate.com.
Torres, V. E., & Bennett, W. M. (Jan 11, 2021). Autosomal dominant polycystic kidney disease in adults: Epidemiology, clinical presentation, and diagnosis. *UpToDate*. Retrieved Mar 23, 2021 from uptodate.com.
United Network for Organ Sharing. (2017). *Qualifications*. https://transplantliving.org/living-donation/being-a-living-donor/qualifications/.
U.S. Department of Health & Human Services. (2016). *Organ donation statistics*. https://www.organdonor.gov/statistics-stories/statistics.html.

CHAPTER 43: MUSCULOSKELETAL SYSTEM INTRODUCTION

Burchum, J. R., & Rosenthal, L. D. (2016). *Lehne's pharmacology for nursing care* (9th ed.). St. Louis: Elsevier.
Cantu, R. V. (2017). Orthopedic geriatrics. In H. M. Fillit, K. Rockwood, & J. Young (Eds.), *Brocklehurst's textbook of geriatric medicine and gerontology* (9th ed.). St. Louis: Elsevier.
Huether, S. E., & McCance, K. L. (2016). *Understanding pathophysiology* (6th ed.). St. Louis: Elsevier.
Jarvis, C. (2016). *Physical examination and health assessment* (7th ed.). St. Louis: Elsevier.
Kizior, R. J., & Hodgson, B. B. (2016). *Saunders nursing drug handbook*. Elsevier.
Lewis, S. M., Bucher, L., Heitkemper, M. M., et al. (Eds.). (2017). *Medical-surgical nursing: Assessment and management of clinical problems* (10th ed.). St. Louis: Elsevier.

CHAPTER 44: CONNECTIVE TISSUE DISORDERS

Block, J. A., & Scanzello, C. (2016). Osteoarthritis. In L. Goldman, & A. I. Schafer (Eds.), *Goldman-Cecil medicine* (25th ed.). St. Louis: Elsevier.
Centers for Disease Control and Prevention. (2020). *Arthritis*. CDC 24/7: Saving lives, protecting people.
Centers for Disease Control and Prevention. (July 27, 2020). What is osteoarthritis (OA)? Centers for disease control and prevention, National center for chronic disease prevention and health promotion. *Division of Population Health*.
Centers for Disease Control and Prevention. (2017). *Arthritis*. https://www.cdc.gov/arthritis/index.htm.
Cleveland Clinic. (2020). *Osteoporosis: Management and treatment*.
Cohen, S., & Canella, A. (2020). *Patient education: Disease-Modifying Antirheumatic Drugs (DMARDs) in rheumatoid arthritis*. Retrieved from http://www.uptodate.com.
Edwards, N. L. (2016). Crystal deposition diseases. In L. Goldman, & A. I. Schafer (Eds.), *Goldman-Cecil medicine* (25th ed.). St. Louis: Elsevier.
Erens, G. A., Walter, B., & Crowley, M. (2020). *Total hip arthroplasty*. Retrieved from http://www.uptodate.com.
Gaffo, A. L. (2020). *Treatment of gout flares*. Retrieved from http://www.uptodate.com.

Hopkins medicine. (2020). *Minimally invasive spine surgery*. Retrieved from http://www.hopkinsmedicine.org/health.

Inman, R. D. (2016). The spondyloarthropathies. In L. Goldman, & A. I. Schafer (Eds.), *Goldman-Cecil medicine* (25th ed.). St. Louis: Elsevier.

Institute of Medicine. (2010). *Dietary reference intakes for calcium and vitamin D*. (website). www.iom.edu.

Mackenzie, C. R., & Edwin, P. S. (2016). Surgical treatment of joint diseases. In L. Goldman, & A. I. Schafer (Eds.), *Goldman-Cecil medicine* (25th ed.). St. Louis: Elsevier.

Mahan, L. K., Escott-Stump, S., & Raymond, J. L. (Eds.). (2017). *Krause's food and the nutrition care process* (14th ed.). St. Louis: Elsevier.

Mariette, X. (2016). Sjögren's syndrome. In L. Goldman, & A. I. Schafer (Eds.), *Goldman-Cecil medicine* (25th ed.). St. Louis: Elsevier.

Martin, G. M., & Harris, I. (2021). *Total knee arthroplasty*. Retrieved from http://www.uptodate.com.

Mayo, Clinic. (2019). *Osteoporosis*.

Nair, P., Ting, J., Keen, H. I., et al. (2017). Arthritis in older adults. In H. M. Fillit, K. Rockwood, & J. Young (Eds.), *Brocklehurst's textbook of geriatric medicine and gerontology* (8th ed.). St. Louis: Elsevier.

National Health Service. (2019). *United Kingdom*. NSAIDs. http://www.nhs.uk.

NIH. (2019). National center for complementary and integrative health. *Rheumatoid arthritis: In depth*. U.S. Department of Health and Human Services National Institutes of Health.

O'Dell, J. R. (2016). Rheumatoid arthritis. In L. Goldman, & A. I. Schafer (Eds.), *Goldman-Cecil medicine* (25th ed.). St. Louis: Elsevier.

Office of Dietary Supplements. (2013). *NIH: Dietary supplement fact sheet*, (website): ods.od.nih.gov/factsheets/Calcium-HealthProfessional#h2.

Patient care & health information. (2021). *Rheumatoid arthritis*. Mayo clinic.

Pietrangelo, A., & Klein, E. (2020). 20 remedies for rheumatoid arthritis flare-ups. *Healthline*.

Price, M. C. (2017). Musculoskeletal problems. In SM Lewis, SR Dirksen, MM Heitkemper, et al. (Eds.), *Medical-surgical nursing: Assessment and management of clinical problems* (10th ed.). St. Louis: Elsevier.

Roberts, D. (2017). Arthritis and connective tissue diseases. In SM Lewis, L Bucher, MM Heitkemper, et al. (Eds.), *Medical-surgical nursing: Assessment and management of clinical problems* (10th ed.). St. Louis: Elsevier.

Schur, P. H., & Gibofsky, A. (2020). *Nonpharmacologic therapies for patients with rheumatoid arthritis*. Retrieved from http://www.uptodate.com.

Spiera, R. F. (2016). Polymyalgia rheumatica and temporal arteritis. In L. Goldman, & A. I. Schafer (Eds.), *Goldman-Cecil medicine* (25th ed.). St. Louis: Elsevier.

Stone, J. H. (2016). The systemic vasculitides. In L. Goldman, & A. I. Schafer (Eds.), *Goldman-Cecil medicine* (25th ed.). St. Louis: Elsevier.

Vaishnay, A. S., Othman, Y. A., Virk, S. S., Gang, C. H., & Qureshi, S. A. (2019 Jun; 5). Current state of minimally invasive spine surgery. *Journal of Spine Surgery* (Suppl. 1), S2–S10.

Varga, J. (2016). Systemic sclerosis (scleroderma). In L. Goldman, & A. I. Schafer (Eds.), *Goldman-Cecil medicine* (25th ed.). St. Louis: Elsevier.

Weber, T. J. (2016). Osteoporosis. In L. Goldman, & A. I. Schafer (Eds.), *Goldman-Cecil medicine* (25th ed.). St. Louis: Saunders.

CHAPTER 45: FRACTURES

Centers for Disease Control and Prevention. (2010). *Hip fractures among older adults*. (website). www.cdc.gov/HomeandRecreationalsSafety/Falls/adulthipfx.html.

Cheshire, W. P. (2016). Jr: Autonomic disorders and their management. In L. Goldman, & A. I. Schafer (Eds.), *Goldman-Cecil medicine* (25th ed.). St. Louis: Elsevier.

Matteson, E. L., & Osmon, D. R. (2016). Infections of the bursae, joints, and bones. In L. Goldman, & A. I. Schafer (Eds.), *Goldman-Cecil medicine* (25th ed.). St. Louis: Elsevier.

Petron, D. J. (2021). *Distal radius fractures in adults*. Retrieved from http://www.uptodate.com.

WebM D. (2021). *Colles' fracture*. Retrieved from www.webmd.com.

Weitz, J. I. (2016). Pulmonary embolism. In L. Goldman, & A. I. Schafer (Eds.), *Goldman-Cecil medicine* (25th ed.). St. Louis: Elsevier.

Wollan, M. K. (2017). Musculoskeletal trauma and orthopedic surgery. In Lewis SM, Bucher L, Heitkemper MM, et al., Eds.), *Medical-surgical nursing: Assessment and management of clinical problems* (10th ed.). St. Louis: Elsevier.

CHAPTER 46: AMPUTATIONS

Amputee Coalitions. (2017). *Limb loss statistics*. (website). www.amputee-coalition.org.

Assiotis, A., Sachinis, N. N. P., & Chalidis, B. E. (2012). Pulsed electromagnetic fields for the treatment of tibial delayed unions and nonunions: A prospective clinical study and review of the literature. *Journal of Orthopaedic Surgery and Research*, *7*(24). (serial online) http://www.josr-online.com/content/7/1/24.

Kosharskyy, B., Almonte, W., Shaparin, N., et al. (2013). Intravenous infusions in chronic pain management. *Pain Physician*, *16*(3), 231–249.

Mulvey, M. R., Bagnall, A., Johnson, M. I., et al. (2013). Transcutaneous electrical nerve stimulation (TENS) for phantom pain and stump pain following amputation in adults. *Cochrane Database of Systematic Reviews*, CD007264.

Mayo Clinic. (2018). *Phantom pain*. (website). www.mayoclinic.org.

Porshinsky, B. S., Grossman, S. S., Beery, P. R., et al. (2011). Clinical uses of the medicinal leech: A practical review. *Journal of Postgraduate Medicine*, *57*(1), 65–71.

Scott, L. T., Tintle, M., Baechler, M. F., et al. (2010). Traumatic and trauma-related amputations: Part II: Upper extremity and future directions. *The Journal of Bone and Joint Surgery*, *92*(18), 2934–2945.

Shi, H., Xiong, J., Chen, Y., et al. (2013). Early application of pulsed electromagnetic field in the treatment of postoperative delayed union of long-bone fractures: A prospective randomized controlled study. *BMC Musculoskeletal Disorders*, *14*(35).

Wollan, M. K. (2017). Musculoskeletal trauma and orthopedic surgery. Lewis SM, Bucher L, Heitkemper MM, et al., (Eds.), *Medical-surgical nursing: Assessment and management of clinical problems* (10th ed.). St. Louis: Elsevier.

CHAPTER 47: ENDOCRINE SYSTEM INTRODUCTION

Burchum, J. R., & Rosenthal, J. R. (2016). *Lehne's pharmacology for nursing care* (9th ed.). St. Louis: Elsevier.

Burchum, J. R., & Rosenthal, L. D. (2019). *Lehne's pharmacology for nursing care* (10th ed.). St Louis MO: Elsevier.

Cushing Syndrome. (n.d.). Retrieved May 1, 2021 from niddk.nih.gov/health-information/endocrine-diseases/Cushings-syndrome.

Kelly, K. A. (2017). Assessment of endocrine system. Table 47–6. In Lewis SM, Bucher L, Heitkemper MM, et al., (Eds.), *Medical-surgical nursing: Assessment and management of clinical problems*. St. Louis: Elsevier.

Melmed, S., & Katznelson, L. (Aug 26, 2019). Diagnosis of acromegaly. *UpToDate*. Retrieved April 15, 2021 from uptodate.com.

Nieman, L. K. (May 29, 2020). Establishing a diagnosis of Cushing's syndrome. *UpToDate*. Retrieved April 5, 2021 from uptodate.com.

Nieman, L. K. (Oct 16, 2019). Diagnosis of adrenal insufficiency in adults. *UpToDate*. Retrieved April 5, 2021 from uptodate.com.

Pagana, K. D., & Pagana, T. J. (2014). *Mosby's manual of diagnostic and laboratory tests* (5th ed.). St. Louis: Elsevier.

Perrone, R. D., & Inker, L. A. (Oct 29, 2020). *Patient education: Collection of a 24 hour urine specimen.*

Ross, D. S. (Dec 11, 2019). Laboratory assessment of thyroid function. *UpToDate*. Retrieved April 5, 2021 from uptodate.com.

Skidmore-Roth, L. (2021). *Mosby's 2021 nursing drug reference* (34th ed.). St Louis MO: Elsevier.

Skidmore-Roth, L. (2017). *Nursing drug reference* (30th ed.). St. Louis: Elsevier, 2017.

Sterns, R. H. (Sep 15, 2020). Diagnostic evaluation of adults with hyponatremia. *UpToDate*. Retrieved April 5, 2021 from uptodate.com.

CHAPTER 48: PITUITARY AND ADRENAL DISORDERS

Burchum, J. R., & Rosenthal, L. D. (2019). *Lehne's pharmacology for nursing care* (10th ed.). St Louis MO: Elsevier.

Bichet, D. G. (Nov 5, 2020). Treatment of central diabetes insipidus. *UpToDate*. Retrieved April 15, 2021 from uptodate.com.

Cushing Syndrome. (n.d.). Retrieved May 1, 2021 from niddk.nih.gov/health-information/endocrine-diseases/Cushings-syndrome.

Eugster, E. A. (Mar 1, 2021). Pituitary gigantism. *UpToDate*. Retrieved April 15, 2021 from uptodate.com.

Kahn, A. (Aug 28, 2020). *Everything you need to know about Cushing's syndrome*. Retrieved April 15, 2021 from healthline.com/health/cushings-syndrome.

Melmed, S., & Katznelson, L. (Dec 3, 2020). Treatment of acromegaly. *UpToDate*. Retrieved April 15, 2021 from uptodate.com.

Melmed, S., & Katznelson, L. (Aug 26, 2019). Diagnosis of acromegaly. *UpToDate*. Retrieved April 15, 2021 from uptodate.com.

Nieman, L. K. (Feb 25, 2021). Causes of secondary and tertiary adrenal insufficiency in adults. *UpToDate*. Retrieved April 15, 2021 from uptodate.com.

Nieman, L. K. (Jul 31, 2020). Treatment of adrenal insufficiency in adults. *UpToDate*. Retrieved April 15, 2021 from uptodate.com.

Nieman, L. K. (May 29, 2020). Establishing a diagnosis of Cushing's syndrome. *UpToDate*. Retrieved April 5, 2021 from uptodate.com.

Nieman, L. K. (Feb 28, 2020). Causes of primary adrenal insufficiency. *UpToDate*. Retrieved April 15, 2021 from uptodate.com.

Nieman, L. K. (Dec 6, 2019). Primary therapy of Cushing's disease: Transsphenoidal surgery and pituitary irradiation. *UpToDate*. Retrieved April 15, 2021 from uptodate.com.

Nieman, L. K. (Oct 30, 2019). Overview of the treatment of Cushing's syndrome. *UpToDate*. Retrieved April 5, 2021 from uptodate.com.

Nieman, L. K. (Oct 16, 2019). Diagnosis of adrenal insufficiency in adults. *UpToDate*. Retrieved April 5, 2021 from uptodate.com.

Nieman, L. K. (Oct 16, 2019). Diagnosis of adrenal insufficiency in adults. *UpToDate*. Retrieved April 5, 2021 from uptodate.com.

Nieman, L. K. (Oct 26, 2018). Diagnosis of adrenal insufficiency in adults. *UpToDate*. Retrieved April 15, 2021 from uptodate.com.

Perrone, R. D., & Inker, L. A. (Oct 29, 2020). Patient education: Collection of a 24 hour urine specimen. *UpToDate*. Retrieved April 15, 2021 from uptodate.com.

Skidmore-Roth, L. (2021). *Mosby's 2021 nursing drug reference* (34th ed.). St Louis MO: Elsevier.

Snyder, P. J. (Mar 19, 2019). Treatment of hypopituitarism. *UpToDate*. Retrieved April 15, 2021 from uptodate.com.

Sterns, R. H. (Apr 16, 2021). Overview of the treatment of hyponatremia in adults. *UpToDate*. Retrieved April 16, 2021 from uptodate.com.

Young, W. F., & Kebebew, E. (Feb 12, 2021). *Treatment of pheochromocytoma.*

CHAPTER 49: THYROID AND PARATHYROID DISORDERS

Burchum, J. R., & Rosenthal, L. D. (2016). *Lehne's pharmacology for nursing care* (9th ed.). St. Louis MO: Elsevier.

Davies, T. F. (Jan 3, 2020). Pathogenesis of Hashimoto's thyroiditis. *UpToDate*. Retrieved May 8, 2021 from uptodate.com.

Goltzman, D. (Mar 12, 2021). Treatment of hypocalcemia. *UpToDate*. Retrieved May 8, 2021 from uptodate.com.

Kim, M., & Ladensorn, P. W. (2016). Thyroid. In L. Goldman, & A. I. Schafer (Eds.), *Goldman-Cecil medicine* (Vol. 11) (2nd ed 5.). Philadelphia: Elsevier.

Milas, M. (Jan 7, 2020). Parathyroidectomy in end-stage kidney disease. *UpToDate*. Retrieved May 5, 2021 from uptodate.com.

Pagana, K. D., & Pagana, T. J. (2014). *Mosby's manual of diagnostic and laboratory tests* (5th ed.). St. Louis: Elsevier.

Ross, D. S. (Apr 3, 2020). Diagnostic approach to treatmentof thyroid nodules. *UpToDate*. Retrieved April 15, 2021 from uptodate.com.

Ross, D. S. (Dec 11, 2019). Laboratory assessment of thyroid function. *UpToDate*. Retrieved May 8, 2021 from uptodate.com.

Ross, D. S. (Jul 20, 2019). Disorders that cause hyperthyroidism. *UpToDate*. Retrieved May 3, 2021 from uptodate.com.

Ross, D. S. (Oct 12, 2020). Clinical presentation and evaluation of goiter in adults. *UpToDate*. Retrieved May 8, 2021 from uptodate.com.

Silverberg, S. J., & Fuleihan, G. E. (May 22, 2019). Primary hypoparathyroidism: Management. *UpToDate*. Retrieved May 8, 2021 from uptodate.com.

Skidmore-Roth, L. (2017). *Mosby's 2017 nursing drug reference* (30th ed.). St. Louis: Elsevier.

Thacker, R. V. (2016). The parathyroid glands, hypercalcemia, and hypocalcemia. In L. Goldman, & A. I. Schafer (Eds.), *Goldman-Cecil medicine* (Vol. 11) (2nd ed 5.). Philadelphia: Elsevier.

CHAPTER 50: DIABETES AND HYPOGLYCEMIA

American Diabetes Association. (1990). Diabetes Control and Complications Trial (DCCT). *Diabetes Care*, *13*(4), 427–433.

American Diabetes Association. (2017). *Diabetes forecast consumer guide.* http://www.diabetesforecast.org/2017/mar-apr/diabetes-medications.html.

American Diabetes Association. (2017). Standards of medical care in diabetes. *Diabetes Care*, *40*(Suppl. 1).

American Diabetes Association. (2021). Standards of medical care in diabetes. *Diabetes Care*, *44*(Suppl. 1).

American Diabetes Association. *The cost of diabetes.* (website). www.diabetes.org/advocacy/news-events/cost-of-diabetes.html.

Centers for Disease Control and Prevention. (2017). *National diabetes statistics report, 2017*. Atlanta: Centers for Disease Control and Prevention.

Chamberlain, J., Herman, W., Leal, S., et al. (2017). Pharmacologic therapy for type 2 diabetes. *Annals of Internal Medicine*, *166*(8), 572–579.

Desimone, M. E., & Weinstock, R. S. (2017). Non-diabetic hypoglycemia [updated Sept 2017]. In L. S. DeGroot, G. Chrousos, & K. Dungan (Eds.), *Endotext*. MD: South Dartmouth (MA). Text.com.

Desimone, M. E., & Weinstock, R. S. (2017). Non-diabetic hypoglycemia [updated Sept 2017]. In L. S. DeGroot, G. Chrousos, & K. Dungan (Eds.), *Endotext*. MD: South Dartmouth (MA). Text.com.

Diabetes and Your Feet. *Centers for disease control and prevention.* Retrieved 5/24/21 https://www.cdc.gov/diabetes/library/features/healthy-feet.

Dickinson, J. K. (2020). Diabetes mellitus. In M. M. Harding, J. Kwong, D. Hagler, D. Roberts, & C Reinisch (Eds.), *Lewis's medical-surgical nursing: Assessment and management of clinical problems* (11th ed.). St. Louis MO: Elsevier.

Disease State. *Diabetes, U.S. Pharmacist.* Retrieved 5/28/21 https://www.uspharmacist.com/topic/diabetes.

Freeland, B. (2017). Hypoglycemia in diabetes mellitus. *Home Healthcare Now, 35*(8), 415–419.

Funnell, M., & Piatt, G. (2017). Incorporating diabetes self-management education into your practice. *The Journal for Nurse Practitioners, 13*(7), 468–474.

Gerard, S., & Ritchie, J. (2017). Challenges of inpatient glycemic control. *Journal of Nursing Care Quality, 32*(3), 267–271.

National Center for Chronic Disease Prevention and Health Promotion (NCCDPHP): Power of Prevention, Atlanta, Centers for Disease Control and Prevention. Retrieved 6/4/21 https://www.cdc.gov/chronicdisease/programs-impact/pop/diabetes.htm.

National Diabetes Statistics Report, 2020, Atlanta, Centers for Disease Control and Prevention. Retrieved 6/4/21 https://www.cdc.gov/diabetes/library/features/diabetes-stat-report.html.

Reusch, J., & Manson, J. (2017). Management of type 2 diabetes in 2017: Getting to goal. *Journal of the American Medical Association, 317*(10), 1015–1016.

Umpierrez, G. E., Smiley, D., Jacobs, S., et al. (2011). Randomized study of basal-bolus insulin therapy in the inpatient management of patients with type 2 diabetes undergoing general surgery (RABBIT 2 surgery). *Diabetes Care, 34*(2), 256–261.

Umpierrez, G. E., Smiley, D., Jacobs, S., et al. (2011). Randomized study of basal-bolus insulin therapy in the inpatient management of patients with type 2 diabetes undergoing general surgery (RABBIT 2 surgery). *Diabetes Care, 34*(2), 256–261.

Zhou, X., Siegel, K. R., Ng, B. P., Jawanda, S., Proia, K. K., Zhang, X., et al. (2020). Cost-effectiveness of diabetes prevention interventions targeting high-risk individuals and whole populations: A systematic review. *Diabetes Care, 43*, 1593–1616.

CHAPTER 51: FEMALE REPRODUCTIVE SYSTEM INTRODUCTION

American Cancer Society. (2015). *Cancer facts for women.* (website). http://www.cancer.org.

American Cancer Society. (Apr 22, 2021). *Breast cancer early detection and treatment.* Retrieved May 10, 2021 from cancer.org/cancer/breast-cancer/screening-tests-and-early-detection.html.

Burchum, J. R., & Rosenthal, L. D. (2019). *Lehne's pharmacology for nursing care* (10th ed.). St Louis MO: Elsevier.

Burchum, J. R., & Rosenthal, L. D. (2016). *Lehne's pharmacology for nursing care* (9th ed.). St. Louis: Elsevier.

Elmore, J. G., & Lee, C. I. (Dec 8, 2020). Screening for breast cancer: Evidence for effectiveness and harm. *UpToDate.* Retrieved May 10, 2020 from uptodate.com.

Skidmore-Roth, L. (2021). *Mosby's 2021 nursing drug reference* (34th ed.). St. Louis MO: Elsevier.

CHAPTER 52: FEMALE REPRODUCTIVE DISORDERS

American Cancer Society. (2021). *ACS Breast cancer early detection recommendations.* Retrieved May 12, 2021 from https://www.cancer.org/cancer/breast-cancer/screening-tests-and-early-detection/.

Burchum, J. R., & Rosenthal, L. D. (2019). *Lehne's pharmacology for nursing care* (10th ed.). St. Louis MO: Elsevier.

Chen, K. T. (Jan 12, 2021). Bartholin gland masses: Diagnosis and management. *UpToDate.* Retrieved May 10, 2021 from uptodate.com.

Chiebowski, R. T. (May 13, 2021). Factors that modify breast cancer risk in women. *UpToDate.* Retrieved May 20, 2021 from uptodate.com.

Clemons, J. L. (Feb 25, 2021). Vaginal pessaries: Indications, devices, and approach to selection. *UpToDate.* Retrieved May 16, 2021 from uptodate.com.

Dixon, J. M. (Jan 15, 2020). Lactational mastitis. *UpToDate.* Retrieved May 10, 2021 from uptodate.com.

Esserman, L. J., & Joe, B. N. (May 30, 2019). Diagnostic evaluation of women with suspected breast cancer. *UpToDate.* Retrieved May 17, 2021 from uptodate.com.

Frumovitz, M. (Apr 14, 2021). Invasive cervical cancer: Epidemiology, risk factors, clinical manifestations, and diagnosis. *UpToDate.* Retrieved May 17, 2021 from uptodate.com.

Kaunitz, A. M. (Feb 2, 2021). Approach to abnormal uterine bleeding in nonpregnant reproductive age patients. *UpToDate.* Retrieved May 10, 2021 from uptodate.com.

Kushung, W., & Hornstein, M. D. (Mar 8, 2021). Evaluation of female infertility. *UpToDate.* Retrieved May 10, 2021 from uptodate.com.

Mehrara, B. (Feb 5, 2021). Breast cancer associated lymphedema. *UpToDate.* Retrieved May 10, 2021 from uptodate.com.

NIH Office of Dietary Supplements. (updated Jun 3, 2020). *Black cohosh: Fact sheet for health professionals.* Retrieved May 9, 2021 from ods.od.nih.gov/factsheets/BlackCohosh-HealthProfessionals/.

Powell, A. M. (Jan 27, 2020). Acute cervicitis. *UpToDate.* Retrieved May 10, 2021 from uptodate.com.

Roe, A., Bartz, B. A., & Douglas, P. S. (Feb 8, 2021). *Combined estrogen-progestin contraception: Side effects and health concerns.*

Schenken, R. S. (Apr 27, 2021). Endometriosis: Pathogenesis, clinical features, and diagnosis. *UpToDate.* Retrieved May 10, 2021 from uptodate.com.

Schenken, R. S. (Dec 1, 2020). Endometriosis: Treatment of pelvic pain. *UpToDate.* Retrieved May 10, 2021 from uptodate.com.

Sobel, J. D. (Feb 26, 2021). Candidal vulvovaginitis: Treatment. *UpToDate.* Retrieved May 11, 2021 from uptodate.com.

Sobel, J. D. (Mar 26, 2021). Bacterial vaginosis: Treatment. *UpToDate.* Retrieved May 10, 2021 from uptodate.com.

Sobel, J. D. (Mar 3, 2021). Approach to females with symptoms of vaginitis. *UpToDate.* Retrieved May 11, 2021 from uptodate.com.

Sobel, J. D., & Mitchell, C. (Sep 4, 2020). Bacterial vaginosis: Clinical manifestations and diagnosis. *UpToDate.* Retrieved May 10, 2021 from uptodate.com.

Stewart, E. A. (May 13, 2021). Uterine fibroids (Leiomyomas): Treatment overview. *UpToDate.* Retrieved May 16, 2021 from uptodate.com.

Welt, C. K., & Barbieri, R. L. (Nov 10, 2020). Evaluation and management of primary amenorrhea. *UpToDate.* Retrieved May 10, 2021 from uptodate.com.

Wiesenfeld, H. C. (Feb 10, 2021). Pelvic inflammatory disease: Treatment in adults and adolescents. *UpToDate.* Retrieved May 12, 2021 from uptodate.com.

CHAPTER 53: MALE REPRODUCTIVE SYSTEM INTRODUCTION

Burchum, J. R., & Rosenthal, L. D. (2019). *Lehne's pharmacology for nursing care* (10th ed.). St. Louis: Elsevier.

Burchum, J. R., & Rosenthal, L. D. (2016). *Lehne's pharmacology for nursing care* (9th ed.). St. Louis: Elsevier.

Freedland, S. (Apr. 29, 2021). Measurement of prostate-specific antigen. *UpToDate.* Retrieved May 30, 2021 from uptodate.com.

Kelly, K. A. (2017). Endocrine problems. In Lewis SL, Bucher L, Heitkemper MM, & et al (Eds.), *Medical-surgical nursing: Assessment and management of clinical problems* (10th ed.). St. Louis: Elsevier.

McVary, K. T. (Jan. 25, 2021). Medical treatment of benign prostatic hypertrophy. *UpToDate*. Retrieved May 30, 2021 from uptodate.com.

Pagana, K. D., & Pagana, T. J. (2014). *Mosby's manual of diagnostic and laboratory tests* (5th ed.). St. Louis: Elsevier.

Pagana, K. D., & Pagana, T. J. (2014). *Mosby's manual of diagnostic and laboratory tests* (5th ed.). St. Louis: Elsevier.

Skidmore-Roth, L. (2017). *Mosby's 2017 nursing drug reference* (30th ed.). St. Louis: Elsevier.

CHAPTER 54: MALE REPRODUCTIVE DISORDERS

American Cancer Society. (Apr 23, 2021). *Recommendations for prostate cancer early detection*. Retrieved 5-25-2021 from cancer.org/cancer/prostate-cancer/detection-diagnosis-staging/ACS-recommendations.html.

American Cancer Society. (2017). *Cancer facts and figures, 2017*. Atlanta GA.

Barrisford, G. W. (Sep 23, 2019). Balanitis in adults. *UpToDate*. Retrieved 5/29/2021 from uptodate.com.

Brandt, W. O., Bello, A. J., & Lue, T. F. (May 5, 2021). Surgical management of Peyronie disease. *UpToDate*. Retrieved 5/25/2021 from uptodate.com.

Brandt, W. O., Bello, A. J., & Lue, T. F. (Jan 29, 2021). Peyronie disease: Diagnosis and medical management. *UpToDate*. Retrieved 5/25/2021 from uptodate.com.

Burchum, J. R., & Rosenthal, L. D. (2017). *Lehne's pharmacology for nursing care* (9th ed.). St. Louis: Elsevier.

Cross, W., & Prescott, S. (2016). The prostate. In H. M. Fillit, K. Rockwood, & J. Young (Eds.), *Brockelhurst's textbook of geriatric medicine and gerontology* (8th ed.). Philadelphia: Elsevier.

Dawson, N. A. (Jan 29, 2021). Overview of the treatment of disseminated castration-sensitive prostate cancer. *UpToDate*. Retrieved 5/29/2021 from uptodate.com.

Dawson, N. A., & Leger, P. (May 27, 2021). Overview of the treatment of castration and resistant prostate cancer (CRPC). *UpToDate*. Retrieved 5/29/2021 from uptodate.com.

Diveci, S. (Oct 16, 2019). Priapism. *UpToDate*. Retrieved 5/25/2021 from uptodate.com.

Einhorn, L. H. (2016). Testicular cancer. In L. Goldman, & A. I. Schafer (Eds.), *Goldman-Cecil medicine* (Vol. 1) (2nd ed 5.). Philadelphia: Elsevier.

Hoffman, R. M. (May 3, 2021). Screening for prostate cancer. *UpToDate*. Retrieved 5/25/2021 from uptodate.com.

Kaplan, S. A. (2016). Benign prostatic hyperplasia and prostatitis. In L. Goldman, & A. I. Schafer (Eds.), *Goldman-Cecil medicine* (Vol. 1) (2nd ed 5.). Philadelphia: Elsevier.

Khera, M. (Jun 23, 2020). Nonoral drugs for sexual dysfunction. *UpToDate*. Retrieved 5/25/2021 from uptodate.com.

Klein, E. A. (1-21-2021). Prostate cancer: Risk stratification and choice of initial treatment. *UpToDate*. Retrieved 5/29/2021 from uptodate.com.

Klein, E. A. (Nov 16, 2020). Patient education: Prostate cancer treatment: Stage I to III cancer (Beyond the Basics). *UpToDate*. Retrieved 5/29/2021 from uptodate.com.

McVary, K. T. (Jul 9, 2020). Surgical treatment of benign prostatic hyperplasia. *UpToDate*. Retrieved 5/26/2021 from uptodate.com.

Meyrier, A., & Fekete, T. (Oct 16, 2020). Chronic bacterial prostitis. *UpToDate*. Retrieved 5/25/2021 from uptodate.com.

Oh, W. K. (Apr 13, 2020). Overivew of the treatment of testicular germ cell tumors. *UpToDate*. Retrieved 5/25/2021 from uptodate.com.

Pettaway, C. A. (Jan 25, 2021). Cancer of the penis: Epidemiology, risk factors, and pathology. *UpToDate*. Retrieved 5/25/2021 from uptodate.com.

Quallich, S. A. (2017). Male reproductive and genital problems. In Lewis SL, Bucher L, Heitkemper MM, et al., (Eds.), *Medical-surgical nursing* (10th ed.). St. Louis: Elsevier.

Small, E. J. (2016). *Prostate cancer*.

Steele, G. S., Richie, J. P., & Michaelson, M. D. (Jan 25, 2021). Clinical manifestations, diagnosis, and staging of testicular gern cell tumors. *UpToDate*. Retrieved 5/25/2021 from uptodate.com.

Swerdloff, R. S., & Wand, C. (2016). The testis and male hypogonadism, infertility, and sexual dysfunction. In L. Goldman, & A. I. Schafer (Eds.), *Goldman-Cecil medicine* (Vol. 1) (2nd ed 5.). Philadelphia: Elsevier.

CHAPTER 55: SEXUALLY TRANSMITTED INFECTIONS

Albrecht, M. A. (Jun 4, 2019). Treatment of genital herpes simplex virus infection. *UpToDate*. Retrieved Jun 1, 2021 from uptodate.com.

American Nurses Association. (2015). *Nursing Informatics: Scope and standards for practice* (2nd ed.). Silver Spring, MD: American Nurses Association.

Anderson, C., & Sensmeier, J. (2015). *Nursing*. Hagerstown, MD: Lippincott Williams & Wilkins, *8* (45).

Bartlett, J. G., & Weber, D. J. (2015). Management of healthcare personnel exposed to HIV. *UpToDate*. Waltham, MA: UpToDate Inc www.uptodate.com.

Burchum, J. R., & Rosenthal, L. D. (2019). *Lehne's pharmacology for nursing care* (10th ed.). St. Louis MO: Elsevier.

CDC. (2016). Use of a 2-dose schedule for human papillomavirus vaccination — updated recommendations of the advisory committee on immunization practices. *MMWR. Morbidity and Mortality Weekly Report*, *65*(49), 1405–1408. https://www.cdc.gov/mmwr/index.html.

Centers for Disease Control and Prevention. (Jan 25, 2021). *CDC estimates 1 in 5 people in the U.S. have a sexually transmitted infection*. Retrieved May 28, 2021 from cdc.gov/media/releases/2021/p.0125-sexually-transmitted-infection.html.

Centers for Disease Control and Prevention. (last rev Feb 12, 2021). *Recommended adult immunization schedule for ages 19 or older*. Retrieved Jun 1, 2021 from https://www.cdc.gov/vaccines/schedules/hcp/imz/adult.html#.

Centers for Disease Control and Prevention: Condom Effectiveness. (2016). *National Center for HIV/AAIDS, Viral hepatitis, STD, and TB prevention Centers for disease control and prevention*. https://www.cdc.gov/condomeffectiveness/index.html.

Centers for Disease Control and Prevention. (2015). Sexually transmitted diseases treatment guidelines, 2015. *Morbidity and Mortality Weekly Report Recommendations and Reports*, *64*(RR3), 1–137. https://www.cdc.gov/mmwr/.

Centers for Disease Control and Prevention. (2017). *Sexually transmitted disease Surveillance*. Atlanta, GA: Department of Health and Human Services.

Cox, J. T., & Palefsky, J. M. (Oct 30, 2020). Human papillomavirus vaccination. *UpToDate*. Retrieved Jun 1, 2021 from uptodate.com.

Food and Drug Administration. (Aug 21, 2020). *Gardasil*, 9. Retrieved Jun 1, 2021 from https://www.fda.gov/vaccines-blood-biologics/vaccines/gardasil-9.

Glassman KS, Rosenfeld P: *Data makes the difference: The smart nurse's handbook for using data to improve care*. Silver Spring, MD: American Nurses Association.

Haddad, R. J. (Sep 10, 2020). Epidemiology, staging, and clinical presentation of HPV associated head and neck cancer. *UpToDate*. Retrieved May 30, 2021 from uptodate.com.

Healthcare Information and Management Systems Society. (2015). *Impact of informatics nurse survey*. http://www.himss.org/ni-impact-survey.

Jarrell, K. (2016). Nursing management: Sexually transmitted infections. *Nurse Key*. https://nursekey.com/nursing-management-sexually-transmitted-infections/.

Johnston, C., & Wald, A. (Dec 9, 2019). Epidemiology, clinical manifestations, and diagnosis of herpes simplex virus type 1 infection. *UpToDate*. Retrieved Jun 1, 2021 from uptodate.com.

Linnen, D. (2016). The promise of big data: Improving patient safety and nursing practice. *Nursing, 46*(5). Hagerstown, MD: Lippincott Williams & Wilkins.

Mayo Foundation for Medical Education and Research. (2017). *Patient care and health information guide: Diseases and conditions-Sexually Transmitted Diseases (STDs)*. http://www.MayoClinic.Org/diseases.

McCormick, K., Sensmeier, J., Dykes, P., et al. (2015). Exemplars for advancing standardized terminology in nursing to achieve sharable, comparable quality data based upon evidence. *Online Journal Nursing Information, 19*(2).

Mmeje, O., Wallett, S., Kolenic, G., et al. (2017). Impact of Expedited Partner Therapy (EPT) implementation on chlamydia incidence in the USA. *Sexually Transmitted Infections*. https://doi.org/10.1136/sextrans-2016-052887.

National Center for HIV/AIDS, & Viral Hepatitis, and Tuberculosis Prevention, Division of Sexually Transmitted Disease Prevention. (revised Dec, 2020). *Sexually transmitted diseases: Summary of CDC treatment*. Retrieved May 29 from cdc.gov/std/tg2015/2015-wall-chartpdf.

Palefsky, J. M. (Nov 21, 2019). Virology of human papilloma virus infections and the link to cancer. *UpToDate*. Retrieved May 30, 2021 from uptodate.com.

Rebelo, A. (2017). Austin Regional Clinic implements Wolters Kluwer's UpToDate anywhere for streamlined access to clinical decision support within EMR. *UpToDate*. Waltham, MA: UpToDate Inc www.uptodate.com.

Sobel, J. D. (Mar 31, 2021). Patient education: Bacterial vaginosis (beyond the basics). *UpToDate*. Retrieved May 30, 2021 from uptodate.com.

Sobel, J. D., & Mitchell, C. (Apr 20, 2021). Trichomoniasis. *UpToDate*. Retrieved May 30, 2021 from uptodate.com St. Louis MO: Elsevier.

Workowski, K. A. (2015). Centers for disease control and prevention sexually transmitted diseases treatment guidelines. *Clinical Infectious Diseases, 8*. https://doi.org/10.1093/cid/civ771.

Wyner, L. M. (2015). NP to the rescue. *Nursing, 2015*(45), 8 Hagerstown, MD: Lippincott Williams & Wilkins.

CHAPTER 56: INTEGUMENTARY SYSTEM INTRODUCTION

Burchum, J. R., & Rosenthal, L. D. (2016). *Lehne's pharmacology for nursing care* (9th ed.). St. Louis: Elsevier.

Gallagher, D. L. (2017). Assessment of integumentary system. In Lewis SM, Bucher L, Heitkemper MM, et al., (Eds.), *Medical-surgical nursing: Assessment and management of clinical problems* (10th ed.). St. Louis: Elsevier.

Gallagher, D. L. (2017). Integumentary problems. In Lewis SM, Bucher L, Heitkemper MM, et al., (Eds.), *Medical-surgical nursing: Assessment and management of clinical problems* (10th ed.). St. Louis: Elsevier.

Tobin, D. J., Veysey, E. C., & Finlay, A. Y. (2017). Aging of the skin. In H. M. Fillit, K. Rockwood, & J. Young (Eds.), *Brocklehurst's textbook of geriatric medicine and gerontology* (8th ed.). St. Louis: Elsevier.

Werth, V. P. (2016). Principles of therapy of skin diseases. In L. Goldman, & A. I. Schafer (Eds.), *Goldman-Cecil medicine* (25th ed.). St. Louis: Elsevier.

CHAPTER 57: SKIN DISORDERS

Albrecht, M. A., Hirsch, M. S., & Mitty, J. (2021). *Patient education: Shingles (beyond the basics)*. Retrieved from http://www.uptodate.com.

Albrecht, M. A., & Levin, M. J. (2021). *Epidemiology, clinical manifestations, and diagnosis of herpes zoster*. Retrieved from http://www.uptodate.com.

Albrecht, M. A. (2021). *Patient education: Genital herpes (beyond the basics)*. Retrieved from http://www.uptodate.com.

Bazalinski, D., Kozka, M., Karnas, M., & Wiech, P. (2019). Effectiveness of chronic wound debridement with the use of larvae of *Lucilia Sericata*. *Journal of Clinical Medicine, 8*(11), 1845.

Bierman PJ, Armitage JO: Non-Hodgkin's lymphomas. In Goldman L, Schafer AI, (Eds.), *Goldman-Cecil medicine* (25th ed.). St. Louis, Elsevier.

Burchum, J. R., & Rosenthal, L. D. (2016). *Lehne's pharmacology for nursing care* (9th ed.). St. Louis: Elsevier.

Burn evaluation. (2020). *National Institutes of Health/U.S. Library of medicine*. Retrieved from https://medlineplus.gov/lab-tests/burn-evaluation.

Burns. (2020). *National Institute of general medical sciences*.

Evans, E. C., & Gray, M. (2003). What interventions are effective for the prevention and treatment of cutaneous candidiasis? *Journal of Wound Ostomy and Continence Nursing, 30*, 11–16.

Feldman, S. R. (2020). *Patient education: Psoriasis (beyond the basics)*. Retrieved from http://www.uptodate.com.

Feldman, S. R. (2020). *Psoriasis: Epidemiology, clinical manifestations, and diagnosis*. Retrieved from http://www.uptodate.com.

Geilen, C. C., & Orfanos, C. E. (2002). Standard and innovative therapy of psoriasis. *Clinical & Experimental Rheumatology, 20*(6 Suppl. 28), S81–S87.

Hornung, R. L., Magee, K. H., Lee, W. J., et al. (2003). Tanning facility use: Are we exceeding food and drug administration limits? *Journal of the American Academy of Dermatology, 49*(4), 655–661.

Itchy skin. (2021). *American Academy of Dermatology Association*. www.aad.org.

Johnston, C., & Wald, A. (2021). *Epidemiology, clinical manifestations, and diagnosis of herpes simplex virus type 1 infection*. Retrieved from http://www.uptodate.com.

Kaposi's sarcoma. (2020). *Mayo clinic*. http://mayoclinic.org.

Leone, G., Rolston, K., & Spaulding, G. (2003). Alefacept for chronic plaque psoriasis: A selective therapy with long-lasting disease remissions and encouraging safety profile. *Dermatology Nursing, 15*(3), 216–220.

Montefour, K., Frieden, J., Hurst, S., et al. (2008). *Acinetobacter baumannii*: An emerging multidrug resistant pathogen in critical care. *Critical Care Nurse, 28*(1), 15–25.

Nikkels, A. F., & Piérard, G. E. (2002). Oral antivirals revisited in the treatment of herpes zoster: What do they accomplish? *American Journal of Clinical Dermatology, 3*(9), 591–598.

Osler, T., Glance, L. G., & Hosmer, D. W. (2010). Simplified estimates of the probability of death after burn injuries. Extending and updating the baux score. *The Journal of Trauma, 68*(3), 690–697.

Sasseville, D. (2020). *Seborrheic dermatitis in adolescents and adults*. Retrieved from http://www.uptodate.com.

Snowden, R. V. (2009). Tanning beds pose serious cancer risk, agency says. *ACS News Center*. (website) http://www.cancer.org/Cancer/news/tanning-beds-pose-serious-cancer-risk-agency-says.

Weston, W. L. (2020). *Patient education: Eczema (atopic dermatitis) (beyond the basics)*. Retrieved from http://www.uptodate.com.

CHAPTER 58: SPECIAL SENSES: VISION AND HEARING

American Foundation for the Blind. *Statistical snapshots from the American Foundation for the Blind*. (website). http://www.afb.org/info/blindness-statistics/2.

Baloh, R. W., & Jen, J. C. (2016). Hearing and equilibrium. In L. Goldman, & A. I. Schafer (Eds.), *Goldman-Cecil medicine* (25th ed.). St. Louis: Saunders.

Braverman, B. (2020). Will my sight be affected by my hearing loss? *Vision*. allaboutvision.com.

Brodie, S. E., & Francis, J. H. (2017). Aging and disorders of the eye. In H. M. Fillit, K. Rockwood, & J. Young (Eds.), *Brocklehurst's textbook of geriatric medicine and gerontology* (8th ed.). St. Louis: Elsevier.

Burchum, J., & Rosenthal, L. (2015). *Pharmacology for nursing care* (9th ed.). St. Louis: Elsevier.

Duke University. (2018). When the eyes move, the eardrums move too. *Science Daily*. www.sciencedaily.com.

Eyes and ears: More in common than you think. (2021). *The hearing and tinnitus center of dallas fort worth, Irving, TX.*

Fast facts of common eye disorders. (2020). *Centers for disease control and prevention*. cdc.gov.

How does loud noise cause hearing loss?. (2018). *Centers for disease control and prevention*. cdc.gov.

Huether, S. E., & McCance, K. L. (2016). *Understanding pathophysiology* (6th ed.). St. Louis: Elsevier.

Jarvis, C. (2016). *Physical examination and health assessment* (7th ed.). St. Louis: Elsevier.

Kizior, R. J., & Hodgson, B. B. (2016). *Saunders nursing drug handbook*. Elsevier.

Lehne, R. A. (2013). *Pharmacology for nursing care* (8th ed.). St. Louis: Saunders.

Lewis, S. M., Bucher, L., Heitkemper, M. M., et al. (Eds.). (2016). *Medical-surgical nursing: Assessment and management of clinical problems* (10th ed.). St. Louis: Elsevier.

Noise and hearing loss prevention: Preventing hearing loss. (2018). *Centers for disease control and prevention*. cdc.gov.

Quick statistics about hearing. (2021). *U.S. Department of health & Human services, NIH, National Institute on Deafness and other Communication disorders. Hearing amplification in adults. (2021).* Retrieved from UpToDate http://www.uptodate.com.

Rishiq, D. (2016). *Cognitive decline and the role of hearing aids*. (website). https://starkeypro.com/pdfs/technicalpapers/Cognitive_Decline_and_the_Role_of_Hearing_Aids.pdf.

Rodemerk, K. S. (2016). *Auditory deprivation: Use it or lose it*. (website). https://starkeypro.com/pdfs/technical-papers/Auditory_Deprivation-Use_it_or_Lose_it.pdf.

Smith, S. C., & Neely, S. (2016). Nursing assessment: Visual and auditory systems. In Lewis SM, Bucher L, Heitkemper MM, et al., (Eds.), *Medical-surgical nursing: Assessment and management of clinical problems* (10th ed.). St. Louis: Elsevier.

Tips to prevent vision loss. (2019). *Centers for disease control and prevention*. cdc.gov.

Turbert, D. (2021). *What is color blindness?* Eye Health A-Z.

Vision impairment and chronic health conditions. (2021). *Centers for disease control and prevention*. cdc.gov.

Vision loss and age. (2020). *Centers for disease control and prevention*. cdc.gov.

What noises cause hearing loss? (2019). *Centers for disease control and prevention*. cdc.gov.

Internet Resources

American Foundation for the Blind. http://www.igc.apc.org/afb/index.html.

Guide Dogs for the Blind. http://www.guidedogs.com.

Talking Books. *National library service for the blind and visually handicapped*. http://www.loc.gov/nls/.

National Institute on Deafness and Other Communication Disorders. (2016). *Quick statistics*. (website). www.nidcd.nih.gov/health/statistics/Pages/quick.aspx.

Page, T. S. (2017). *Application of Evidence-based practices to global interprofessional collaborations aimed at reducing hearing-related health disparities*. (website). http://www.nursinglibrary.org/vhl/bitstream/10755/621815/1/Page_85772_presentation.pdf.

CHAPTER 59: EYE AND VISION DISORDERS

Bower, K. S. (2020). Laser refractive surgery. *UpToDate*. Retrieved from http://www.uptodate.com.

Cataracts. (2020). *National eye Institute*. Retrieved from https://nei.nih.gov.

Centers for Disease Control and Prevention. (2015). *Common eye disorders*. https://www.cdc.gov/visionhealth/basics/ced/index.html.

Centers for Disease Control and Prevention. (2017). *Don't let glaucoma steal your sight!* (website). https://www.cdc.gov/features/glaucoma-awareness/index.html.

Endothelial keratoplasty. (2020). *Cincinnati eye Institute*. Retrieved from http://www.cincinnatieye.com.

Glaucoma Research Foundation. (2013). *Glaucoma facts and stats*. (website). www.glaucoma.org/glaucoma/glaucoma-facts-and-stats.php.

Glaucoma. (2020). *National eye Institute*. Retrieved from https://nei.nih.gov.

Glaucoma. (2021). *Mayo clinic*. Retrieved from www.mayoclinic.org.

Jacobs, D. S. (2021). Open-angle glaucoma: Epidemiology, clinical presentation, and diagnosis. *UpToDate*. Retrieved from http://www.uptodate.com.

Jacobs, D. S. (2021). Open-angle glaucoma: Treatment. *UpToDate*. Retrieved from www.uptodate.com.

Jacobs, D. S. (2021). Cataract in adults. *UpToDate*. Retrieved from http://www.uptodate.com.

Kozarsky, A. (2019). Age-related macular degeneration. *WebMD*. Retrieved from http://www.webmd.com.

Medication Guide: Glaucoma. (2020). *Glaucoma research foundation*. Retrieved from http://www.glaucoma.org.

MedlinePlus. (2012). *Corneal transplant*. (website). http://www.nlm.nih.gov/medlineplus/ency/article/003008.htm.

National Institutes of Health. *NEI Health information: Facts about the cornea and corneal disease. (website)*. www.nei.nih.gov/health/cornealdisease#19.

Ou, Y. (2018). *Side effects of laser iridotomy Bright Focus foundation*. Retrieved from www.brightfocus.org.

Retinal detachment. (2020). *National eye Institute*. Retrieved from https://nei.nih.gov.

Shahbazi, S., Studnicki, J., & Warner-Hillard, C. W. (2015). A cross-sectional retrospective analysis of the racial and geographic variations in cataract surgery. *PLoS One*. https://doi.org/10.1371/journal.pone.0142459.

Shoss, B. L., & Tsai, L. M. (2013). Postoperative care in cataract surgery [abstract]. *Current Opinion in Ophthalmology, 24*(1), 66–73.

Weizer, J. S. (2021). Angle-closure glaucoma. *UpToDate*. Retrieved from http://www.uptodate.com.

Yi, C., Lee, D., Chung, E., et al. (2010). A comparison of posterior lamellar keratoplasty modalities: DLEK vs. DSEK. *Korean Journal of Ophthalmology, 24*(4).

CHAPTER 60: EAR AND HEARING DISORDERS

Kacker, A., Pierce-Smith, D., & Fraser, M. (2021). *Middle ear infection (otitis media) in adults*. Rochester, NY: University of Rochester Medical Center.

Labyrinthitis and vestibular neuritis. (2020). *National health Service*. http://www.nhs.uk.

Labyrinthitis Penn Medicine, Baloh, R. W., & Jen, J. C. (2020). Hearing and equilibrium. In L. Goldman, & A. Schafer (Eds.), *Goldman-cecil medicine* (26th ed.). Philadelphia, PA: Elsevier. chap. 400.

Mastoiditis. (2019). *National Health Service (NHS), United Kingdom*. www.nhs.uk.

Mayo Clinic. (2015). *Meniere's disease*. (website). http://www.mayoclinic.org/diseases-conditions/menieres-disease/basics/definition/con-20028251.

Medscape reference. (2015). *Overview (labyrinthectomy)*. (website). emedicine.medscape.com/article/2051423-overview.
Meniere's disease. (2017). *National Institute on Deafness and other Communication disorders. (NIC). USDHHS, National Institutes of health*. https://www.nidcd.nih.gov/health/clearinghouse.
Meniere's disease. (2020). *Diagnosis and treatment. Mayo clinic staff*. Rochester, MN: Mayo Clinic. http://www.mayoclinic.org.
Meniere's disease. (2020). *Symptoms and causes. Mayo clinic staff*. Rochester, MN: Mayo Clinic. http://www.mayoclinic.org.
National Institute on Deafness and Other Communication Disorders. (2017). *Meniere's disease*. (website). http://www.nidcd.nih.gov/health/balance/pages/meniere.aspx.
Otitis media (middle ear infection) in adults. (2021). *Columbia University Irving medical Center*. http://entcolumbia.org.
Otitis media with effusion. (2020). *Medline Plus. National Institutes of health/U.S. National library of medicine*. https://medlineplus.gov/ency/article/007010.
Otosclerosis and stapedectomy. (2021). *Center for hearing and Balance*. NY: Icahn School of Medicine at Mount Sinai.
Otosclerosis. (2018). *National Institute on Deafness and other Communication disorders (NID). USDHHS*. National Institutes of Health, NIH Pub. No. 13, 4234.
Vestibular Disorders Association. *Dietary considerations*. (website). vestibular.org/understanding-vestibular-disorders/treatment/vestibular-diet.
Weinstein, B. E. (2017). Disorders of hearing. In H. M. Fillit, K. Rockwood, & J. Young (Eds.), *Brocklehurst's textbook of geriatric medicine and gerontology* (8th ed.). St. Louis: Saunders.

CHAPTER 61: PSYCHOBIOLOGIC DISORDERS

American Psychiatric Association. (2013). *Diagnostic and statistical manual of mental disorders, (5th ed.). (DSM-5)*. Washington, DC: APA. drug tables.
Gum, A. M., King-Kallimanis, B., & Kohn, R. (2009). Prevalence of mood, anxiety, and substance-abuse disorders for older Americans in the national comorbidity survey-replication. *The American Journal of Geriatric Psychiatry, 17*(9), 769–781.
Kessler, R. C., Petukhova, M., Sampson, N., et al. (2012). Twelve-month and lifetime prevalence and lifetime morbid risk of anxiety and mood disorders in the United States. *International Journal of Methods in Psychiatric Research, 21*(3), 169–184.
Linton, A. D. (2014). *Pharmacology companion for introductory nursing care of adults*. Philadelphia: Saunders.
National Institute of Mental Health. (2021, May). *Anxiety disorders*. https://www.nimh.nih.gov/health/topics/anxiety-disorders/.
National Institute of Mental Health. (2021, May). *Bipolar disorder*. https://www.nimh.nih.gov/health/statistics/bipolar-disorder.
National Institute of Mental Health. (2021, May). *Major depression*. https://www.nimh.nih.gov/health/statistics/major-depression.
National Institute of Mental Health. (2021,May). *Schizophrenia*. https://www.nimh.nih.gov/health/statistics/schizophrenia.
National Institute of Mental Health. (2014). *Turning discovery into health. website*. http://www.nimh.nih.gov/health/publications.
Peplau, H. E. (1992). Interpersonal relations: A theoretical framework for application in nursing practice. *Nursing Science Quarterly, 5*(1), 13–18.
Pertusa, A., Frost, R. O., Fullana, M., et al. (2010). Refining the diagnostic boundaries of compulsive hoarding: A critical review. *Clinical Psychology Review, 30*(4), 371–386.
Phelps, L. L. (Ed.). (2017). *Sparks and Taylor's nursing diagnosis reference manual* (10th ed.). Printed in the Wolters Kluwer.
Puzantian, T., & Carlat, D. J. (2020). *Medication fact book for psychiatric practice* (5th ed.). Carlat Publishing.
Sachs, G., & Erfurth, A. (2018). Obsessive compulsive and related disorders: From the biological basis to a rational pharmacological treatment. *International Journal of Neuropharmacology, 21*(1), 59–62.
Sadock, B. J., & Sadock, V. A. (2015). *Kaplan & Sadock's synopsis of psychiatry: Behavioral sciences/clinical psychiatry* (11th ed.). Philadelphia: Lippincott Williams & Wilkins.
Stahl, S. M. (2021). *Stahl's essential psychopharmacology: Prescriber's guide* (7th ed.). Cambridge University Press.

Internet Resources

American Psychiatric Association. apa@psych.org.
Mayo Foundation for Medical Education and Research. www.mayoclinic.org.
Plus, M., & U.S. National Library of Medicine, National Institutes of Health. www.nlm.nih.gov/medlineplus.
National Alliance of Mental Illness. http://www.nami.org.
National Institute of Mental Health: Prevalence of major depressive episode among adults. (2017). https://www.nimh.nih.gov/health/statistics/major-depression.shtml.

CHAPTER 62: SUBSTANCE-RELATED AND ADDICTIVE DISORDERS

Abbott, M. (2020). Gambling and gambling-related harm: Recent World Health Organization initiatives. *Public Health, 184*, 56–59.
Adams, Z. M., Ginapp, C. M., Price, C. R., Qin, Y., Madden, L. M., Yonkers, K., et al. (2021). "A good mother": Impact of motherhood identity on women's substance use and engagement in treatment across the lifespan. *Journal of Substance Abuse Treatment, 130*, 108474.
American Psychiatric Association. (2013). *Diagnostic and statistical manual of mental disorders* (5th ed.). Washington, DC: APA.
Bevilacqua, L., & Goldman, D. (2009). Genes and addictions. *Clinical Pharmacology and Therapeutics, 85*(4), 359–361.
Center for Disease Control. (2017). *CDC–Alcohol and drug use*. https://www.cdc.gov/stltpublichealth/didyouknow/topic/alcohol.html.
Center for Disease Control. (2017). *FastStats: Illegal drug use-CDC*. https://www.cdc.gov/nchs/fastats/drug-use-illegal.htm.
Centers for Disease Control and Prevention. (2021, March 25). *The drug overdose epidemic: Behind the numbers*. https://www.cdc.gov/drugoverdose/data/index.html.
Centers for Disease Control and Prevention. (2021, May 15). *Smoking and tobacco use*. https://www.cdc.gov/tobacco/data_statistics/fact_sheets/fast_facts/index.htm.
MÉ, C., Lane, R. I., Petrosky, E., et al. (2020). Mental health, substance use, and suicidal ideation during the COVID-19 pandemic — United States, June 24–30, 2020. *MMWR. Morbidity and Mortality Weekly Report 69*, 1049–1057.
Mayo Clinic Staff. (2014). *Drug addiction*. (website). http://www.mayoclinic.com/health/drug-addiction/DS00183.
McCrady, B. S., Epstein, E. E., & Fokas, K. F. (2020). Treatment interventions for women with alcohol use disorder. *Alcohol Research: Current Reviews, 40*(2), 08.
National Drug Intelligence Center. (2011). *The economic impact of illicit drug use in American society*. Washington, DC: U.S. Department of Justice.
National Institute on Alcohol Abuse and Alcoholism. (2021, May). *Alcohol use in the United States*. https://www.niaaa.nih.gov/publications/brochures-and-fact-sheets/alcohol-facts-and-statistics.
National Institute on Drug Abuse. (2021, May 15). *Overdose death rates*. https://www.drugabuse.gov/drug-topics/trends-statistics/overdose-death-rates.
National Institute on Drug Abuse. (2003). *Preventing drug use among children and adolescents, a research-based guide for parents, educators, and community leaders* (2nd ed.). Washington, DC: U.S. Department of Health and Human Services.

National Institute on Drug Abuse. (2014). *The science of drug abuse and addiction (NIDA Drug Publications)*. Washington, DC: U.S. Department of Health and Human Services.

University of Michigan Center for Advancing Research and Solutions for Society. (2014). *Sex, gender & alcohol/other drug use*. (website). www.carss.umich.edu/evolving-projects/sex-gender-alcoholother-drug-use/.

CHAPTER 63: FIRST AID, EMERGENCY CARE, AND DISASTER MANAGEMENT

2020 American Heart Association, Inc, and The American National Red Cross. AHA/RED CROSS GUIDELINE FOCUSED UPDATE 2020 American Heart Association and American Red Cross Focused Update for First Aid Circulation https://www.ahajournals.org/journal/circ.

2020 American Heart Association and American Red Cross Focused Update for First Aid. (27 October 2020). *Circulation, 142*(17), e287–e303.

Allos BM. Clinical manifestations, diagnosis, and treatment of Campylobacter infection. *UpToDate*. Retrieved Jun 8, 2021 from uptodate.com.

American Nurses Association. (2020). *Nurses, ethics and the response to COVID-19 pandemic*. Retrieved Jun 8, 2021 from nursingworld.org/.495c6c/globalassets/practiceandpolicy/work-environment/halth-safety/coronavirus/nurses-ethics-and-the-response-to-the-covid-19-pandemic.pdf.

Amesh, A. A. (Apr 24, 2020). Identifying and managing casualties of biological terrorism. *UpToDate*. Retrieved Jun 4, 2021 from uptodate.com.

Benton, D. (2018). Disasters, regulation, and proactive response. Is nursing ready for the next disaster? *American Nurse Today, 1*(13), 32–33.

Bucher, L. (2017). Emergency and disaster nursing. In *Medical surgical nursing assessment and management of clinical problems* (10th ed.) (pp. 1628–1650). United States: Elsevier.

Centers for Disease Control and Prevention. (2021). National Center for emerging and Zoonotic infections diseases. *Division of Foodborne Waterborne, and Environmental Disease*.

Centers for Disease Control and Prevention. https://www.cdc.gov.

Circulation. (2020). *142*(16 suppl 2), S336, originally published October 21, 2020, https://doi.org/10.1161/CIR.0000000000000929.

Circulation. 2020;142:e287–e303.

Estimated annual number of episodes of illnesses caused by 31 pathogens transmitted commonly by food, United States. Retrieved Jun 4, 2021 from cdc.gov.

Hendrickson, R. G. (May 6, 2021). Gastrointestinal decontamination of the poisoned patient. *UpToDate*. Retrieved Jun 8, 2021 from uptodate.com.

Johns Hopkins University Bloomberg School of Public Health Center for Health Security. (Jun 10, 2020). *Recommendations for improving national nurse preparedness for pandemic response: Early lessons from COVID-19*. Retrieved Jun 11, 2021 from centerfor healthsecutiry.org/oour-work/publications/recommendations-for-improving-national-nurse-preparation-for-pandemic-response-early-lessons-from-covid-19.

LaRocque, R., & Harris, J. B. (Jun 26, 2020). Approach to the patient with acute diarrhea in resource-rich settings. *UpToDate*. Retrieved Jun 4, 2021 from uptodate.com.

LaRocque, R., & Harris, J. B. (May 17, 2019). Patient education: Foodborne illness beyond the basics. *UpToDate*. Retrieved Jun 4, 2021 from uptodate.com.

Linda bucher chapter 68, Medical surgical nursing assessment and management of clinical problems 10th edition.

National Council of State Boards of Nursing. (March 27, 2020). *Policy Brief: U.S. Nursing leadership supports practice/academic partnerships to assist the nursing workforce during the COVID-19 crisis*. Retrieved Jun 8, 2021 from ncsbn.org/practice-academic-partnership.htm.

National Council of State Boards of Nursing (n.d.). (*Policy Brief: Evaluating board of nursing discipline during the COVID-19 pandemic*. Retrieved Jun 8, 2021 from ncsbn.org/Policy-Brief-US-Nursing-Discipline-COVID19.pdf.

O'Ryan, N. G. (Feb 21, 2020). Norovirus. *UpToDate*. Retrieved Jun 8, 2021 from uptodate.com.

Pegram, P. S., & Stone, S. M. (Dec 7, 2020). Botulism. *UpToDate*. Retrieved Jun 4, 2021 from uptodate.com.

Pellegrino, J., L, Charlton, N., P, Flores, G., E., Goolsby, C., A., Hoover, A., V, Kule, A., et al. (2020). 2020 American Heart Association, Inc, and The American National Red Cross. AHA/RED CROSS GUIDELINE FOCUSED UPDATE 2020 American Heart Association, Inc, and The American National Red Cross. AHA/RED CROSS GUIDELINE FOCUSED UPDATE 2020 American Heart Association and American Red Cross Focused Update for First Aid. *Circulation*. 142, (17):e287–e303.

Singletary, E. M., Charlton, N. P., Epstein, J. L., et al. (2015). 2015 American Heart Association and American red cross guidelines update for first aid. *Circulation, 132*(Suppl. 2), S574–S589. https://doi.org/10.1161/CIR.0000000000000269.

Texas Board of Nursing. (2020). Regulatory cooperation: Working with the Board of Nursing to quickly respond to a crisis. *Texas Nursing Magazine Issue, 2*(2020), 10.

Texas Board of Nursing. (2018). FAQS relating to nursing practice in disaster areas. Retrieved Jun 8, 2021 from https://www.bon.texas.gov/covid-19practicefaq.asp.

Index

b indicates boxes, *f* indicates illustrations, and *t* indicates tables.

C

H

M

P